A Practical Approach to Infectious Diseases

W9-AMC-429

A Practical Approach to
Infectious Diseases

Fourth Edition

A Practical Approach to Infectious Diseases

Edited by

Richard E. Reese, M.D.
Clinical Professor of Medicine, Columbia
University College of Physicians and
Surgeons, New York; Attending Physician,
Infectious Disease Unit, Bassett Healthcare,
Cooperstown, New York

Robert F. Betts, M.D.
Professor of Medicine, University of Rochester
School of Medicine and Dentistry; Associate
Physician in Medicine, Strong Memorial
Hospital, Rochester, New York

Little, Brown and Company
Boston New York Toronto London

Copyright © 1996 by Richard E. Reese and Robert F. Betts
Fourth Edition

Previous editions copyright © 1983 and 1986 by Richard E. Reese and R. Gordon Douglas, Jr.; 1991 by Richard E. Reese and Robert F. Betts

All rights reserved. No part of this book may be reproduced in any form or by any electronic or mechanical means, including information storage and retrieval systems, without permission in writing from the publisher, except by a reviewer who may quote brief passages in a review.

Library of Congress Cataloging-in-Publication Data
A practical approach to infectious diseases / [edited by] Richard E.
    Reese, Robert F. Betts. — 4th ed.
        p.   cm.
    Includes bibliographical references and index.
    ISBN 0-316-73721-6
    1. Communicable diseases—Handbooks, manuals, etc. I. Reese,
Richard E. II. Betts, Robert F.
    [DNLM: 1. Communicable Diseases—handbooks. WC 39 P895 1996]
RC112.P79 1996
616.9—dc20
DNLM/DLC
for Library of Congress   96-11889
                                                                      CIP

Printed in the United States of America

KP

Editorial: Nancy E. Chorpenning
Production Editor: Marie A. Salter
Copyeditor: Lois Hall
Indexer: Nancy Newman
Production Supervisor/Designer: Louis C. Bruno, Jr.
Cover Designer: Sally Bergman-Costello
Cover image courtesy of Lynn Margulis and Ricardo Guerrero

To our students, house officers, and patients, who stimulated the writing of this book

Editor's Note

A portion of the proceeds of this book will be given annually to The College of Wooster (Wooster, OH) in honor of the life of Elizabeth Hope Weaver, who left us too soon while on a mission project serving others

(R.E.R.)

Contents

Preface

This book is intended for medical students, house officers, practicing physicians, nurses, infection control practitioners, and other health care providers who treat inpatients or outpatients for infections. It also should be useful to the microbiology laboratory supervisor or technician who wants to correlate microbiology laboratory results with potential clinical implications.

The book attempts to be a practical, day-to-day guide to the diagnosis and treatment of common infectious diseases and their attendant problems; it includes specific recommendations on antimicrobial dosage, route of administration, and duration of therapy.

During the mid-1970s, we realized that there was no readily available, concise, and well-referenced book or manual discussing the approach to and treatment of clinical infectious diseases and related problems. The standard textbooks contain excellent discussions of basic pathophysiology and specific diseases of single microbial etiology, but the texts usually do not emphasize, as we do here, how to approach common problems such as pneumonias, bacteremias, wound infections, or pharyngitis. In addition, for the busy clinician who may not be able to find answers quickly in the comprehensive textbook, the outline format in this book facilitates information retrieval.

The topics discussed in the first edition were selected after a careful review, over a period of several years, of the questions posed most often to the infectious disease consultation service at The Strong Memorial Hospital, Rochester, New York, and after assessment of the infections commonly seen in the emergency room, outpatient clinic, and office settings. New material added to the second, third, and fourth editions stems in part from the questions and problems raised by medical students, house staff, attending physicians, and referring physicians at the teaching institutions represented by the contributing authors, as well as the rapidly expanding and changing developments in infectious diseases.

Based on very positive feedback about the earlier editions, we were encouraged to revise the book because of the rapid advances in antibiotic therapy and in infectious disease treatments in general. The fourth edition contains new information on emerging infectious diseases including *Escherichia coli* 0157:H7, *Helicobacter pylori,* human ehrlichiosis, and vancomycin-resistant enterococci. The increasing problems of antibiotic-resistant bacteria, including penicillin-resistant *Streptococcus pneumoniae,* are reviewed. New 1995 USPHS/IDSA recommendations to prevent opportunistic infections in patients positive for human immunodeficiency virus are summarized. Other new discussions include deep neck soft-tissue infections, multidrug resistant tuberculosis, acute pancreatitis, new antibiotics (e.g., piperacillin-tazobactam), and new criteria to diagnose endocarditis.

In general, the length of the chapters has been dictated by the frequency or importance of the clinical problems, or both. Four exceptions to this are Eye Infections (Chap. 6), Infections Due to Fungi, *Actinomyces,* and *Nocardia* (Chap. 18), Infections in Transplantation (Chap. 20), and Antiviral Agents (Chap. 26). Eye and transplant infections are presented in some detail because this information is very difficult to glean from the literature and because the primary care physician may be the one who deals initially with these infections. Fungal infections are seen frequently in the compromised host (especially with underlying HIV infection) and at times in the traveler, and, therefore, the clinical aspects of these infections are discussed in some detail. Chapter 26, Antiviral Agents, is a detailed discussion intended for the practitioner, which delineates when and why certain antiviral agents are currently useful or are anticipated to be useful; it provides important background information and practical clinical advice, including dosages. The last chapter, Antibiotic Use, was carefully revised so that it is as up-to-date as possible. A carefully selected list of references follows each section of the chapter.

There are many controversial areas in the diagnosis and management of infectious disease problems. In these cases, we try to point out several different approaches and outline our preferred approach. Each author has stressed a practical clinical approach. One of the editors (R.E.R.), who does 25 percent general internal medicine and 75 percent infectious disease consultation, has tried carefully to ensure that a useful and realistic approach is presented.

The text material was originally presented in outline format to help the reader find information as quickly as possible. We have retained this format in the fourth edition because of its popularity and usefulness. The references at the end of each chapter have been carefully selected and are often annotated to guide the reader.

We have included color photographs of a limited number of important clinical findings (e.g., rashes) that may aid in diagnosing an important infection.

We thank Marilyn Dunckel, Meg Preston, and the Word Processing Unit personnel at Office Services, Bassett Healthcare, for their help in typing and preparing portions of the manuscript. We especially thank Linda Muehl (Librarian, Bassett Healthcare), who has assisted us in numerous literature searches. In addition, we thank Robin L. Phillips (librarian assistant), Joseph S. Bertino, Jr., Pharm. D., Edward G. Timm, Pharm. D., Michael A. Foltzer, M.D., James Bordley IV, M.D., and Alan J. Kozak, M.D., at Bassett Healthcare for their useful advice. One of the editors (R.E.R.) thanks Walter A. Franck, M.D. (Physician-in-Chief, Department of Medicine, Bassett Healthcare), for his continued encouragement and support of this writing project, and Henry F.C. Weil, M.D. (Bassett Healthcare), for his continued encouragement. We also thank Nancy Chorpenning, Priscilla Hurdle, and Marie Salter of Little, Brown and Company, for their guidance throughout the publication process for this edition.

Finally, we thank our wives, Shirley and Sherrill, for their encouragement, patience, and support during the preparation of this text.

R.E.R.
R.F.B.

Contributing Authors

David V. Alcid, M.D.	Associate Professor of Clinical Medicine, UMDNJ-Robert Wood Johnson Medical School; Chief of Infectious Disease Unit and Microbiology Laboratory, Department of Medicine, St. Peter's Medical Center, New Brunswick, New Jersey
Paula W. Annunziato, M.D.	Assistant Professor and Attending Physician, Department of Pediatrics, Columbia University College of Physicians and Surgeons, New York
Ann Sullivan Baker, M.D.	Associate Professor of Medicine (Ophthalmology), Harvard Medical School; Director, Infectious Disease Service, Massachusetts Eye and Ear Infirmary, Boston
Robert F. Betts, M.D.	Professor of Medicine, University of Rochester School of Medicine and Dentistry; Associate Physician in Medicine, Strong Memorial Hospital, Rochester, New York
Stanley W. Chapman, M.D.	Professor of Medicine, University of Mississippi School of Medicine; Director, Infectious Diseases Unit, University of Mississippi Medical Center, Jackson, Mississippi
Susan E. Cohn, M.D., M.P.H.	Assistant Professor of Medicine, University of Rochester School of Medicine and Dentistry; Associate Director, AIDS Clinical Trials Unit, Division of Infectious Diseases, Strong Memorial Hospital, Rochester, New York
John J. Condemi, M.D.	Clinical Professor of Medicine, University of Rochester School of Medicine and Dentistry, Rochester, New York
Raphael Dolin, M.D.	Charles A. Dewey Professor of Medicine, University of Rochester School of Medicine and Dentistry; Physician-in-Chief, Department of Medicine, Strong Memorial Hospital, Rochester, New York
Marlene L. Durand, M.D.	Instructor in Medicine, Harvard Medical School; Clinical Assistant in Medicine, Infectious Disease Unit, Massachusetts General Hospital, Boston

Paul J. Edelson, M.D. — Associate Professor of Pediatrics, Cornell University Medical College, New York; Chairman, Department of Pediatrics, New York Methodist Hospital, Brooklyn, New York

Walter A. Franck, M.D. — Professor of Clinical Medicine, Columbia College of Physicians and Surgeons, New York; Physician-in-Chief, Department of Medicine, Bassett Healthcare, Cooperstown, New York

Alice C. Furman, M.D. — Clinical Fellow, Department of Medicine, Cornell University Medical College; Fellow, Division of Infectious Disease, The New York Hospital, New York

Paul S. Graman, M.D. — Associate Professor of Medicine and Clinical Director, Infectious Diseases Unit, University of Rochester School of Medicine and Dentistry; Hospital Epidemiologist and Attending Physician, Department of Medicine, Strong Memorial Hospital, Rochester, New York

Mala R. Gupta, M.D. — Senior Instructor in Infectious Diseases, University of Rochester School of Medicine and Dentistry; Associate Hospital Epidemiologist, Department of Infectious Diseases, Strong Memorial Hospital, Rochester, New York

Caroline Breese Hall, M.D. — Professor of Pediatrics and Medicine, Division of Infectious Diseases, University of Rochester Medical Center, Rochester, New York

Harold M. Henderson, M.D. — Assistant Professor of Medicine, Department of Internal Medicine, University of Mississippi, and Division of Infectious Diseases, University of Mississippi Medical Center, Jackson, Mississippi

David R. Hill, M.D. — Associate Professor of Medicine, University of Connecticut School of Medicine; Director, International Traveler's Medical Service, University of Connecticut Health Center, Farmington, Connecticut

Sally H. Houston, M.D. — Assistant Professor of Medicine, Division of Infectious Diseases, University of South Florida; Assistant Epidemiologist, Department of Infectious Diseases, Tampa General Hospital, Tampa, Florida

Jerome F. Hruska, M.D., Ph.D. — Associate Professor of Medicine and Consultant in Infectious Diseases, Department of Internal Medicine, University of Nevada School of Medicine, Las Vegas

Nancy Epifano Hughes, M.D.	Assistant Physician, Department of Medicine, Bassett Healthcare, Cooperstown, New York
John A. Jernigan, M.D.	Assistant Professor of Medicine, Emory University School of Medicine; Hospital Epidemiologist, Emory University Hospital, Atlanta
Stephen R. Jones, M.D.	Associate Professor of Medicine, Oregon Health Sciences University; Chief, Department of Medicine, Good Samaritan Hospital and Medical Center, Portland, Oregon
Adolf W. Karchmer, M.D.	Professor of Medicine, Harvard Medical School; Chief, Division of Infectious Diseases, New England Deaconess Hospital, Boston
Gerald A. Landry, M.D.	Chief Medical Resident, Department of Medicine, Bassett Healthcare, Cooperstown, New York
C. Richard Magnussen, M.D.	Associate Professor of Medicine, University of Rochester School of Medicine and Dentistry; Head, Infectious Diseases Unit, St. Mary's Hospital, Rochester, New York
Marilyn A. Menegus, Ph.D.	Professor of Microbiology and Immunology, University of Rochester School of Medicine and Dentistry; Associate Director, Microbiology Laboratories, Strong Memorial Hospital, Rochester, New York
David J. Mock, M.D.	Clinical Assistant Professor of Medicine, University of Rochester School of Medicine and Dentistry and Parkridge Hospital, Rochester, New York
Taimor Nawaz, M.D., M.R.C.P.	Fellow and Instructor, Division of Infectious Diseases, University of Rochester School of Medicine and Dentistry, Rochester, New York
Rathel L. Nolan, M.D.	Associate Professor of Medicine, Department of Infectious Diseases, University of Mississippi Medical Center, Jackson, Mississippi
Katherine L. O'Brien, M.D.	Instructor, Department of Pediatric Infectious Disease, Johns Hopkins Medical Institutions, Baltimore
Richard D. Pearson, M.D.	Professor of Internal Medicine and Pathology, University of Virginia School of Medicine; Attending Physician, Department of Internal Medicine, University of Virginia Health Sciences Center, Charlottesville, Virginia
Robert L. Penn, M.D.	Professor of Medicine, Louisiana State University School of Medicine in Shreveport; Chief, Section of Infectious Diseases, Louisiana State University Medical Center, Shreveport, Louisiana

Keith R. Powell, M.D.

Professor and Associate Chair, Department of Pediatrics, University of Rochester School of Medicine and Dentistry; Attending Physician, Department of Pediatrics, Strong Memorial Hospital, Rochester, New York

Daniel W. Rahn, M.D.

Professor and Vice Chairman, Department of Medicine, Medical College of Georgia; Program Director, Internal Medicine Residency Training Program, Medical College of Georgia, Augusta, Georgia

Richard E. Reese, M.D.

Clinical Professor of Medicine, Columbia University College of Physicians and Surgeons, New York; Attending Physician, Infectious Disease Unit, Bassett Healthcare, Cooperstown, New York

Michael F. Rein, M.D.

Professor of Medicine, University of Virginia School of Medicine; Attending Physician, Department of Medicine, University of Virginia Medical Center, Charlottesville, Virginia

Gregory J. Riley, M.D.

Clinical Assistant Professor of Medicine, University of Rochester School of Medicine and Dentistry; Senior Attending Physician, Department of Medicine, The Genesee Hospital, Rochester, New York

Norbert J. Roberts, Jr., M.D.

The Paul R. Stalnaker, M.D., Distinguished Professor of Internal Medicine, and Professor of Microbiology and Immunology; Director, Division of Infectious Diseases, The University of Texas Medical Branch, University of Texas Medical School at Galveston, Galveston, Texas

Robert H. Rubin, M.D.

Director, Center for Experimental Pharmacology and Therapeutics, Harvard–MIT Division of Health Sciences and Technology, Cambridge, Massachusetts; Chief of Transplantation Infectious Disease, Massachusetts General Hospital, Boston

W. Michael Scheld, M.D.

Professor of Medicine and Neurosurgery, Division of Infectious Diseases, University of Virginia School of Medicine, Charlottesville, Virginia

Deborah E. Sentochnik, M.D.

Staff Physician, Department of Infectious Diseases, Lahey Clinic, Burlington, Massachusetts

Kent A. Sepkowitz, M.D.

Assistant Professor of Medicine, Cornell University Medical College; Assistant Attending Physician, Division of Infectious Diseases, New York Hospital, and Assistant Physician, Infectious Disease Service, Memorial Sloan-Kettering Cancer Center, New York

JoAnn Palumbo Shea, A.R.N.P., M.S.N.

Clinical Instructor in Internal Medicine, University of South Florida College of Medicine; Manager, Employee Health and Wellness, Tampa General Healthcare, Tampa, Florida

Michael G. Sheehan, M.D.

Attending Physician, St. Joseph's Hospital, Syracuse, New York

John T. Sinnott, M.D.

Professor and Director, Division of Infectious Disease, University of South Florida College of Medicine; Chief of Staff, Tampa General Hospital, Tampa, Florida

Rosemary Soave, M.D.

Associate Professor of Medicine and Public Health, Cornell University Medical College; Associate Attending Physician, Department of Medicine, The New York Hospital–Cornell Medical Center, New York

Eugene L. Speck, M.D., Ph.D.

Associate Professor of Medicine, University of Nevada School of Medicine; Co-Director, Infectious Disease Unit, University Medical Center, Las Vegas

Mark C. Steinhoff, M.D.

Associate Professor of Infectious Diseases, Johns Hopkins School of Medicine; Medical Staff, Department of Pediatrics, Johns Hopkins Hospital, Baltimore

Richard L. Sweet, M.D.

Professor of Obstetrics, Gynecology, and Reproductive Sciences, University of Pittsburgh School of Medicine; Chair, Department of Obstetrics, Gynecology, and Reproductive Sciences, Magee-Women's Hospital, Pittsburgh

Anne M. Traynor, M.D.

Fellow, Division of Hematology/Oncology, University of Iowa Hospitals and Clinics, Iowa City, Iowa; Former Chief Resident in Medicine, Bassett Healthcare, Cooperstown, New York

John J. Treanor, M.D.

Associate Professor of Medicine, University of Rochester School of Medicine and Dentistry, Rochester, New York

Allan R. Tunkel, M.D., Ph.D.

Associate Professor of Medicine, Medical College of Pennsylvania and Hahnemann University School of Medicine, Philadelphia

David H. Walker, M.D.

Director, Center for Tropical Diseases, University of Texas Medical Branch; Professor and Chairman, Department of Pathology, University of Texas Medical Branch, University of Texas Medical School at Galveston, Galveston, Texas

Thomas T. Ward, M.D.

Associate Professor of Medicine, Oregon Health Sciences University School of Medicine; Chief of Infectious Diseases Section, Veterans Administration Medical Center, Portland, Oregon

Henry F.C. Weil, M.D.

Assistant Clinical Professor of Medicine, Columbia University College of Physicians and Surgeons, New York; Attending Physician, Department of Internal Medicine, Bassett Healthcare, Cooperstown, New York

Harold C. Wiesenfeld, M.D.

Assistant Professor of Obstetrics, Gynecology, and Reproductive Sciences, University of Pittsburgh School of Medicine; Co-Director, Sexually Transmitted Diseases Clinic, Allegheny County Health Department, Pittsburgh

A Practical Approach to
Infectious Diseases

Drug Notice. The authors of this book have made a special effort to ensure that the dosage recommendations are accurate and in agreement with the standards accepted by the general medical community at the time of publication. The medications described do not necessarily have specific approval by the Food and Drug Administration for use in the diseases and dosages for which they are recommended. Since dosage regimens may be modified as new research and laboratory studies accumulate, readers are advised to check the package insert data to see whether changes approved by the FDA have been made in the recommended dosages and/or contraindications for use. This is particularly important with new or infrequently used agents.

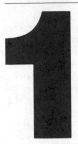

Fever and Fever of Unknown Etiology

Eugene L. Speck and
Norbert J. Roberts, Jr.

For centuries, fever has been recognized as a characteristic sign of infection. However, fever may also be due to such noninfectious causes as tumor, collagen vascular diseases, and drugs. Close to a third of patients admitted to the hospital will have an episode of fever, particularly on medical and surgical services [1]. The clinician must remain aware, however, that very young and very old individuals may present with serious infections without showing a febrile response, as can individuals with significant malnutrition [2] or with preceding stress to their thermoregulatory systems. An example of the latter circumstance would be an individual admitted with hypothermia due to exposure [3]: As many as 41% of such patients had serious infections in one study, and more than a third of the infections were not diagnosed at the time of admission.

The **pathophysiology** of fever has been elucidated only relatively recently, and the thermometer remains an essential diagnostic tool even in this era of sophisticated technology. Fever had been viewed as a beneficial response to disease until the last century, when the concept that fever itself required treatment gained acceptance. This transition may have occurred because the antipyretic agents that came into widespread use had additional antiinflammatory and analgesic activities, and the treated patients improved in regard to several parameters of illness.

Fever phobia (undue parental fear of fever in their children) was clearly documented in 1980 [4] and, despite recent efforts to inform medical practitioners and the public, persists even today, at least in part because of mixed messages to the public [5]. The role and impact of fever in host responses to challenge continue to be reassessed [6–10]. **The data and the analyses suggest that routine suppression of a febrile response is not warranted.** Judgment should be applied regarding therapeutic intervention (antipyresis) in any individual case, with consideration of both the potential benefits and the deleterious effects of temperature elevation for the individual. See the text by Mackowiak [9] for in-depth discussions of thermoregulation, fever, fever of unknown etiology, and other relevant aspects of this host response.

Fever

I. **Definitions**
  A. **Normal basal body temperature** often is thought to be 37°C (98.6°F), determined orally, but should more accurately be considered as a temperature that falls within specified ranges for different times of the day, with variation among individuals. The normal oral temperature range ($\geq$ 99% of healthy young adults) over an entire day is 36–37.7°C (96.8–99.9°F) with diurnal variation as discussed in sec. **C** [11]. **Rectal temperatures are higher by approximately 0.6°C (1°F).** The usual temperature range of an individual can rarely be determined beforehand in clinical practice. Therefore, an oral temperature exceeding 37.2°C (98.9°F) in the early morning and 37.7°C (99.9°F) in the late afternoon or evening may ordinarily be considered higher than the usual normal range for healthy adults 40 years of age or younger, as judged by recent studies [11].
  B. The **method used to determine the body temperature** is important with regard to both the expected range and the accuracy of the reading (related to confounding factors). Routine temperature measurements in most clinical settings have generally relied on oral and rectal sites, now often measured using digital electronic thermometers, which have become widely available (including for home use). **Ear thermometry** has been developed and applied more recently [12]. This form of

infrared thermometry measures the flow of heat from the surfaces of the tympanic membrane and the ear canal. The method is quick and more acceptable to some adults and to children, but the methodology is relatively new, and its reliability has yet to be fully established. More patients with high temperatures need to be studied. The patient factors (e.g., very young age, presence of ear pathology) and environmental factors (e.g., warm ambient temperature) that can affect measurements and conversion to equivalent oral or rectal temperatures are still being characterized [12].

C. **Diurnal variation.** Diurnal variation may normally be as much as 1°C (1.8°F) or more in any given individual, but the mean diurnal temperature oscillation is approximately 0.5°C (0.9°F) [11], with women having slightly higher normal temperatures than men overall. **Temperature is lowest in the early morning and highest in the late afternoon or early evening** (4–8 PM).

The diurnal rhythm is consistent in each person and usually is preserved with a fever [13], with the absolute temperature range elevated for that individual. Its absence may suggest the possibility of factitious fever if other etiologies for the fever cannot be identified (assuming no hypothalamic disorder exists).

D. **Fever and hyperthermia** are two distinct processes physiologically [14, 15].

1. **Fever** is said to exist whenever the body temperature rises above the maximum of the normal range, in a physiologically regulated manner, in response to a new temperature set point that has been established (see sec. II).

2. **Hyperthermia** does not involve the resetting of the normal temperature set point. Hyperthermia most commonly results from thermoregulatory responses that are inadequate for the body's needs or from adverse reactions to anesthetics or other pharmacologic agents. Hyperthermia is more likely to develop in those individuals with less effective thermoregulation (the very young and the very old) but may occur even in healthy young adults (e.g., as a result of prolonged intense exercise in warm, humid weather, such as with participation in a marathon). Heat production exceeds heat loss, and the temperature exceeds the individual's set point. Heat stroke and malignant hyperthermia are extreme and highly dangerous examples of hyperthermia [15–17].

3. A **practical clinical concept** that results from this distinction is that antipyretics (drugs that lower the set point) are effective in treating fever but are unlikely to affect hyperthermia. Therefore, physical measures to lower the body temperature usually must be applied in hyperthermia cases.

E. **Lethal temperature ranges.** Body temperature is very actively and effectively controlled, both in the basal state and in response to the higher set point that is induced by an exogenous pyrogenic challenge. In the latter case, temperatures exceeding 41°C are very uncommon, even with infections that are characteristically associated with high fevers [18].

1. **The lower lethal temperature** is approximately 26°C (78.8°F) (excluding therapeutic hypothermia).

2. **The average upper lethal limit** is approximately 43°C (109.4°F), although morbidity and mortality of such supraphysiologic temperatures are related to both the degree and the duration of the temperature elevation. Thus, temperatures in excess of 42.5°C commonly are required and used to produce hyperthermic treatment of tumors. Such temperatures do affect the immune system [19] but, with appropriate control of the intensity and duration of the hyperthermia (especially if applied locally to the tumor), are well tolerated by patients.

II. **Physiology of fever and associated responses**

A. **Proinflammatory cytokines, fever, and associated responses.** Fever results when exogenous pyrogens (bacteria, viruses, fungi, other microorganisms, allergens, etc.) or pyrogenic factors (immune complexes, lymphokines from sensitized lymphocytes, etc.) encounter circulating monocytes or monocyte-derived tissue macrophages, the major sources of biologically defined endogenous pyrogen (EP), which eventually was molecularly defined and termed *interleukin 1* (IL-1) [20]. IL-1 also proved to be a cytokine responsible for the biologically defined activity known as *leukocyte endogenous mediator* (LEM), responsible for induction of the acute-phase response and other metabolic aspects of an infectious challenge, and the biologic activity known as *lymphocyte-activating factor* (LAF), responsible for initiating the activation and proliferation of lymphocytes specific to the challenging microorganism or other exogenous pyrogen [20].

Although many cells are capable of producing IL-1, it appears that the prime source of this EP is the monocyte-macrophage. Extensive studies determined that

IL-1 is only one of several proinflammatory cytokines produced primarily by monocytes-macrophages that can act as EPs and produce fever [21, 22]. Thus, it is probably wise at this time to consider the major EPs to be the proinflammatory cytokines IL-1, tumor necrosis factor–alpha (TNF), and IL-6. IL-1 and TNF have pleiotropic activities that overlap remarkably and include the previously noted biologic activities associated with infection and fever. The precise roles of these different cytokines are still under investigation because IL-1 can induce its own production as well as that of TNF, TNF can induce its own production as well as that of IL-1, and both can induce the production of IL-6. Animal models of experimental bacteremia have suggested that TNF is induced first after endotoxin challenge, followed rapidly by IL-1 and then (to a lesser extent) by IL-6 induction [22]. Overall, the extensive available data link IL-1 most closely with a febrile response to challenge. In some models, however, the production of IL-6 appears to be under the control of IL-1, and the best correlations for the severity of an infectious disease with any cytokine are with the level of IL-6, not IL-1 or TNF [21]. IL-6 does not induce production of IL-1 or TNF and, therefore, may provide an eventual, quantitative "readout" for the proinflammatory cytokine response. Furthermore, mice with a disrupted IL-6 gene show impaired immune and acute-phase responses [23].

A relatively recent (yet active) field of investigation has arisen from the recognition that exogenous pyrogens such as viruses induce the concomitant production of both IL-1 and inhibitors of IL-1, or IL-1 receptor antagonists (IL-1ra), by monocytes-macrophages [21, 24]. In fact, in studies involving challenge of healthy human volunteers with experimental endotoxemia, the IL-1ra was induced as quickly as, and in greater amounts (quantitative plasma levels by radioimmunoassay) than, IL-1 [25]. TNF inhibitors have also been identified. The full breadth of biologic activity of these inhibitors of IL-1 and TNF are currently being determined, and it is likely that the febrile and other acute responses to infection or similar pyrogenic challenges will be regulated in an integrated fashion by the several mediators that are produced [10].

In addition, potential biologic negative feedback loops are also activated by IL-1. IL-1 induces the release of several hypothalamic and pituitary peptides, including endorphins and adrenocorticotropic hormone (ACTH), and can also act directly on the adrenal gland to augment steroid synthesis [10, 21]. Corticosteroids can, in turn, block IL-1 production and release [10, 21].

B. **The sepsis syndrome and septic shock.** Sepsis is discussed in detail in Chap. 2. It is important to note here that many of the features of the sepsis syndrome and septic shock have been related to production of the proinflammatory cytokines associated with fever, particularly TNF [26, 27]. These cytokine mediators or their receptors (combined with several other identified factors) are being targeted in efforts to reduce the morbidity and mortality of sepsis and septic shock [22, 26]. Such non-etiology-specific intervention would be likely to affect the outcome by providing support until specific medical intervention (administration of antimicrobial or other appropriate agents) or specific immune responses become effective. Such an approach would also be more broadly applicable than agents such as antilipopolysaccharide (anti-LPS) antibodies, which would not affect sepsis or septic shock due to infection by gram-positive bacteria or many other microbes.

C. **Central nervous system events in the production of fever.** IL-1 is a potent pyrogen that appears rapidly to affect structures in the CNS, leading to the febrile response. The preoptic area (POA) of the anterior hypothalamus is the region that evokes the most rapidly developing and most intense febrile response to locally injected IL-1, although ablation of the area does not abolish the febrile response to pyrogens [28]. IL-1 may thus also act at extra-POA sites, and these have been described [28]. There is thus far no direct evidence that circulating IL-1 crosses the blood-brain barrier and localizes in the IL-1-sensitive sites [21, 28], but entry pathways have been postulated [28]. There have been extensive studies regarding which neurotransmitters within the CNS are involved in the IL-1-induced febrile response. Among the various factors that have been assessed for a possible role in induction or control of fever, adequate (if controversial) evidence exists only for prostaglandins of the E series [28].

The field of neuroimmunoendocrinology is only now beginning to map precisely the cascade of responses to exogenous pyrogens and, in particular, the neurochemical identities as well as the organization of factors responding to a pyrogenic challenge. The regulation and integration of responses to a pyrogen will likely be shown to be bidirectional, as suggested by extensive recent mapping of neuro-endocrine-immune interactions [29]. Such observations already extend our knowledge well beyond the long-recognized activation of the pituitary-adrenal axis during an infection, and the cortisol-mediated or other glucocorticoid-mediated suppression of the immune response, including production of the proinflammatory cytokines IL-1, TNF, and IL-6.

III. **Metabolic and physiologic responses, and the acute-phase reaction.** A variety of physiologic and metabolic alterations begin at the onset of an infection or shortly thereafter [2, 20, 30–32]. Many of these changes formerly were considered to be the results of the accompanying fever, but they might also ensue from the direct action of the proinflammatory cytokine mediators induced by the invading microorganisms or their products (see sec. **II.A**). The extent to which physiologic responses are due to, or aggravated by, temperature elevation of a fever as opposed to resulting from direct coordinated effects of proinflammatory cytokines is still being delineated.

A. Prominent **metabolic changes** associated with pyrogenic infections and other etiologies of fever include:

1. **Metabolic rate increases** of approximately 10–12% with each 1°C elevation in body temperature. If the need for calories and amino acids is not met, body wasting can eventually ensue.

2. **Increased insensible water loss,** which is influenced by the degree of fever, hyperpnea, humidity, and ambient temperature. Generally, there will be an increase of 300–500 ml/m^2/°C/day.

3. **Heart rate increases** of up to 15 bpm per degree Celsius increase in temperature, which could induce heart failure or angina in individuals with significant cardiovascular disease.

4. **Electrolyte depletion** through loss via sweating and, if associated with the infection, via diarrhea or vomiting.

B. **Secondary nutritional consequences** (the "costs") of an acute infection or recurrent mild infections are unlikely to be significant for the well-nourished child or adult but may be substantial for those who are marginally nourished and are severely or frequently challenged by infection [2]. The latter individuals are susceptible to a vicious cycle: malnutrition leading to increased susceptibility to infection leading to increasing malnutrition [2]. Infection with the human immunodeficiency virus (HIV), combined with associated opportunistic infections, vividly illustrates this course.

C. **Altered hepatocyte functions** in acute generalized infection include [31, 33]: increased uptake of free amino acids from plasma, increased gluconeogenesis with glycogenolysis, increased ureagenesis, increased liponeogenesis, impaired ketogenesis, increased uptake and sequestration of iron (in transferrin and hemosiderin) and zinc (with metallothionein), and synthesis of acute-phase proteins (see sec. **D**).

Some metabolic changes vary during the course of an infection. For example, hyperglycemia may be a prominent feature early in the infection, whereas hypoglycemia secondary to depletion of carbohydrate stores may be troublesome later in the course of an uncontrolled infection.

D. In the **acute-phase response**, certain proteins synthesized by the liver, referred to collectively as **acute-phase reactants,** are synthesized in response to the proinflammatory cytokines IL-1, TNF, and IL-6 [30, 32, 34], with responses enhanced by glucocorticoids. Changes in these proteins (C-reactive protein, alpha$_1$-antitrypsin, haptoglobin, serum amyloid P component, serum amyloid A protein, and others) commonly are associated with the temperature elevation of a fever, but their precise roles in host defense are not entirely clear [34]. Furthermore, additional changes in other body constituents such as circulating iron or zinc, which decrease in this setting [31, 33], are commonly associated with infection and the febrile response and may play integrated roles in host defense [33] (see sec. **V.A.3.b**).

IV. **Fever patterns**

A. **Background.** Before the advent of modern diagnostic techniques, the pattern of the febrile response was stressed as an important diagnostic clue. **Generally, a fever pattern (temperature course) cannot be considered pathognomonic for a particular infectious agent in a given patient** [13]. (See **B.6** and the next major section of this chapter regarding drug fever, which illustrate this important point.) Despite this general concept, in certain circumstances (and especially when combined with other information) the fever curve may provide a clue to the etiology of the fever.

B. **Types of fever** (temperature over time). Because fever patterns often are discussed in the literature and at times provide some clinical clues, they are briefly summarized here. As noted earlier, diurnal variation often is preserved during a febrile episode, with more than 90% of patients with remittent or intermittent fever due to infection showing diurnal variation in one study [13].

  1. **Intermittent fevers** are characterized by wide swings in temperature (> 0.3°C [0.5°F] and < 1.4°C [2.5°F]), with the temperature returning to normal at least once during any 24-hour period. This is the second most common type of fever encountered by an infectious diseases consulting service [13].

     a. Pyogenic abscesses and irregular use of antipyretics are the most common causes of the intermittent pattern. This pattern can also be seen in disseminated tuberculosis, acute pyelonephritis with bacteremia, and malaria.

     b. **A double fever spike** occurring daily is said to be suggestive of gonococcal endocarditis and has been noted with miliary tuberculosis. It is also much more commonly associated with sporadic use of antipyretics in a febrile patient.

     c. **Variants of intermittent fevers**
        (1) Alternate-day fever may be seen in *Plasmodium vivax* infections and steroid withdrawal fevers (patients on alternate-day dosage schedules).
        (2) Fever spikes every third day occur in *Plasmodium malariae* infections.
        (3) Any form of malaria in the early stages of infection may present with intermittent or remittent fevers without periodicity.

  2. **Remittent fever** is similar to intermittent fever except the fluctuations in temperature are less dramatic and the temperature does not return to normal. This is the most common type of fever encountered by an infectious diseases consulting service [13]. Examples include acute respiratory viral infections, mycoplasmal pneumonia, and *Plasmodium falciparum* malaria.

  3. **Hectic ("septic") fever** can be either an intermittent or a remittent fever with a difference of 1.4°C (2.5°F) or more between peak and trough temperatures.

  4. **Sustained (continuous) fever** is a moderately persistent elevation in temperature with only minimal fluctuations. Examples include gram-negative bacterial pneumonia, brucellosis, typhoid fever, tularemia, psittacosis, pneumococcal pneumonia, rickettsial infections, and fever in a comatose patient with CNS damage.

  5. **Relapsing (recurrent) fever** is characterized by periods of fever and periods of normal temperature alternating cyclically. During the febrile episodes, the fever may follow any of the previously listed patterns. Examples include lymphomas, rat-bite fever, borreliosis, and dengue.

  6. **Temperature-pulse disparity** (i.e., high temperature with a relatively slow pulse) may be seen in factitious fever, brucellosis, typhoid fever, psittacosis, and Legionnaires' disease. A clue to factitious fever may be the absence of diurnal variation when there is no hypothalamic disease.

  7. **Drug fever** may present with any of the patterns described in secs. **1–5** [13, 35]. Hectic fever spikes may simulate sepsis at times. Drug fever is discussed in more detail later in this chapter.

C. **Hyperpyrexia** (extreme temperature elevation) often generates concern in both parents and physicians. However, as noted earlier, temperatures exceeding 41°C (105.8°F) are rare even with infections commonly associated with high fevers [18]. On the basis of one retrospective study of patients (with a relatively small number of children) selected from an infectious disease consultation service [36], it appears that infections are the single most common cause (39%) of extreme temperature elevation. Thermoregulatory failure alone may account for 18% of cases, and 32% of cases of extremely high temperatures are caused by the simultaneous occurrence of thermoregulatory failure and infection [36]. Even in these selected, often very ill patients, there was little evidence of direct tissue damage caused by fever per se, with two patients dying at the time of extreme pyrexia (one with heat stroke, and one with gram-negative bacteremia and fulminant hepatitis following renal transplantation). A case-control study of hyperpyrexia in children [37] showed that such a presentation led to a significantly larger number of diagnostic procedures but was not associated with an increased rate of serious infection, such as bacteremia or meningitis, relative to children with more moderate fevers. **Hyperpyrexic individuals need to be evaluated as carefully and thoroughly as other febrile individuals but probably do not require additional diagnostic tests.**

1. **Infections more likely to be associated with extreme fever** are gram-negative bacteremia, Legionnaires' disease, abacteremic pyelonephritis, bacterial meningitis, viral encephalitis, typhoid fever, and malaria, but very high temperatures also commonly occur in children with respiratory virus infections such as influenza [38].

2. **Noninfectious causes of extreme pyrexia** are likely to be heat stroke, intracerebral hemorrhage, hemorrhagic pancreatitis, and the malignant hyperthermia associated with general anesthesia or with neuroleptic drugs, e.g., neuroleptic malignant syndrome (NMS) [16, 17, 39, 40]. See related discussion in sec. **III.D.** under Drug Fever.

D. **Attenuated fever responses.** Although significant infection may exist, fever sometimes may be absent.

1. **Seriously ill newborns** with infection may lack a fever or may even have subnormal temperatures. (In contrast, young children may have exaggerated febrile responses to relatively insignificant infections.)

2. **Elderly patients** occasionally do not exhibit a febrile response [41] or, when febrile, have a limited response as compared to a younger patient.

3. Patients with **uremia** may not have a fever or may have a fever with temperatures normally not considered febrile. (Such patients may have a basal temperature somewhat lower than normal, and a temperature in the usual high-normal range might therefore represent a fever for them.)

4. **Significantly malnourished individuals** may show reduced production of the proinflammatory cytokines and a diminished febrile response [2].

5. Patients receiving **corticosteroids** or **continuous treatment with antiinflammatory** or **antipyretic agents** may not have a febrile response.

V. **Potential reasons for not treating fever.** There seems to be a tendency—almost a reflex—among physicians as well as parents to attempt to lower body temperature in a patient with fever. Fever per se has not been shown to be harmful or even uncomfortable in humans [42, 43]. Temperatures in excess of 41°C (106°F) due to infection are uncommon [18], and temperatures in the high physiologic range (39–41°C; 102–105°F) in the adult do not appear to be harmful unless they persist for long periods or produce associated adverse effects (see sec. **VI**) [42, 44]. Conservation of the febrile response over time and across species argues for a beneficial role of fever for the species if not for the individual host in the setting of an infection or other pyrogenic challenge [8, 10]. Such a concept, in turn, argues for **judgment in each case regarding suppression of fever.** There are certainly data from both in vivo (largely animal models) and in vitro (including human leukocytes) studies that support a generally beneficial role for fever in the setting of infection [8, 10]. It remains controversial, however, whether fever affords the human any survival advantage, although it is reasonable to suspect that it does and there have been hints that this is so [45].

A. There are three **general ways in which fever could enhance resistance to or recovery from an infection or other challenge.** These potential mechanisms are indicated only briefly here but are discussed in detail elsewhere [8, 10].

1. **Direct temperature effects on the offending microorganism.** There are a number of published reports showing that temperature elevations that are within the physiologically febrile range of an animal may have direct adverse effects on the growth of some microorganisms [8]. Overall, however, this is not a common or likely major mechanism for postulated beneficial effects of fever, especially considering the narrow range from basal to physiologically febrile temperatures for most hosts.

2. **Effects on activities of antimicrobial agents or biologic factors against offending microorganisms.** This mechanism overlaps with the preceding one, and there are data to suggest that, for some microorganisms (e.g., *T. pallidum* and some gram-positive and gram-negative bacteria), **antibiotics may show greater antimicrobial effects at temperatures in the human febrile range compared to normal basal temperatures** [8, 46, 47].

This mechanism may play a role in the current era of antimicrobial therapy, but it is unlikely to have selected for the febrile response through evolution. Data exist, however, that suggest the existence of such mechanisms related to the host's own natural immunologic and nonspecific soluble mediators potentially involved in the evolution of fever for defense. For example, antibodies have been described that bind to and inactivate poliovirus at 39°C but not at 37°C [48]. In addition, the adverse effects of low plasma iron levels on

bacterial growth during infection are particularly manifest at febrile temperatures [33, 49]. Thus, **the susceptibility of a microorganism to a host factor or response may be altered by the physiologic rise in temperature of the host.**
3. Most data supporting a beneficial effect for fever support the concept that **host immunologic defenses are enhanced at febrile temperatures** [8, 10].
   a. **Effects of fever** and associated responses from **animal models of infection.** Numerous studies, using many species of animals, have shown a survival benefit (reduced morbidity or mortality) of fever or hyperthermia in the setting of challenge by bacteria, viruses, fungi, and other pathogens [8]. An elegant series of integrated investigations by Kluger and colleagues [7, 50] used the poikilothermic lizard as an animal model to control and examine the role of temperature in defense against an infectious challenge. The mortality of the animals challenged with bacteria was inversely related to temperature, with the greatest survival evident at temperatures in the febrile range for the animals [7, 50]. The range of temperatures studied had no direct effects on the bacteria, but the febrile response was clearly associated with enhanced survival [7, 50]. This suggested that fever affected host defense mechanisms. The febrile animals had lower titers of bacteria in body tissues than did animals with normal temperatures, and they had sterile blood cultures (with less dissemination of bacteria after inoculation) [51]. Such findings were associated with a greater accumulation of leukocytes at the site of bacterial inoculation. Thus, local containment of a bacterial infection by prompt leukocyte responses appeared to occur to a greater extent in the context of fever. The fever did not have to be continuous to benefit the host, and effective antipyretic administration was associated with decreased survival relative to the animals that were allowed to maintain a fever [52]. Furthermore, the benefit of an associated acute-phase (metabolic) response was demonstrated. A defensive role could be attributed to the depressed level of plasma iron during the animal's fever [49].
   Elevated temperatures have also been associated with enhanced immunologic defenses against in vivo viral challenge [8, 10]. **Overall, in vivo observations regarding fever and survival from infectious challenge suggest beneficial effects of the temperature elevation on immunologic functions and host defense** [8, 10].
   b. **Fever, immunologic responses, and host defense.** Temperature elevation, either as a result of the febrile response or occurring by exogenous application of hyperthermia, has been associated with effects on recognition, recruitment, and effector phases of the immune response, including responses of human leukocytes assayed in vitro [10].
   Immunologic pathogen-specific responses are generally enhanced in the setting of temperature elevation within the physiologic range [8, 10]. Temperature elevation appears to affect primarily the phase of recognition and sensitization or activation of mononuclear leukocytes. T-lymphocyte responses (or their interactions with monocytes-macrophages) are enhanced for generation of effector cells, such as antibody-producing B lymphocytes or cytotoxic T lymphocytes (CTL). The activities of the effector cells, once generated, usually either are not enhanced (e.g., CTL) or are depressed (B lymphocytes) by the temperature elevation. In the latter case, the adverse effect is more than offset by the increased T helper function. **Overall, the data suggest that temperature elevations that occur as a result of the febrile response constitute a beneficial component of effective host defense** [8, 10].
   Note: Although fever appears to be associated with enhanced function of the immune system, a direct connection between such phenomena and the beneficial effect of fever on outcome from infectious challenge is not yet established.
B. **Reasons not to treat fever**
   1. Fever may be a generally beneficial host defense–related response (see **A**).
   2. Other events and responses (e.g., metabolic, such as restriction of iron availability) that accompany fever may interact with fever and thereby contribute to host defense (see secs. **III** and **V.A.3.a**).
   3. Fever is an indicator of disease, and its resolution rather than its persistence may aid in the evaluation of a chosen therapeutic regimen. Pharmacologic suppression of the fever may create a false sense of improvement and may

delay needed alterations in the antimicrobial regimen or other targeted intervention [44].

Because fever may have many causes (e.g., infections, autoimmune diseases, or tumors), suppressing a fever of uncertain origin may mislead the clinician and should be avoided unless deemed appropriate for the particular patient (see sec. **VI**). Only uncommonly does the pattern of the fever curve offer a clue to the etiologic diagnosis (see sec. **IV**).

4. There are well-recognized potential harmful effects of antipyretic agents that might be encountered unnecessarily, such as gastrointestinal bleeding or Reye's syndrome associated with the use of aspirin.

   In addition, studies have shown adverse effects of aspirin or acetaminophen therapy on parameters associated with recovery from infection (e.g., prolonged shedding of rhinovirus or varicella virus [during chickenpox] by antipyretic-treated subjects [53]).

5. Iatrogenic stress could ensue for the patient if PRN administration of antipyretics is used in the setting of persistent infection. The patient will expend energy alternately to decrease and increase body temperature (to match the varying set point) if the exogenous pyrogen has not yet been eradicated and the antipyretic effect wanes (see sec. **VII**).

6. "Social benefits" of fever may help the population at large—that is, the febrile individual often feels sick (probably not related to the elevated temperature per se) and remains home or even in bed. Antipyresis or analgesia would lead to early exposure of others (see also **4**).

VI. Potential reasons to treat fever. The preceding section discusses reasons why most individuals and the human species overall may benefit from the existence of the febrile response. Nonetheless, individual subjects may be anticipated to have morbidity—derived from the fever—that is unacceptable in the context of current therapeutic capabilities and sound medical judgment regarding relative risks. Risks considered in the analysis should also include nonmedical factors such as interference with required daily activities due to illness (that might be alleviated by analgesia or antipyresis). It is thus reemphasized that **the decision regarding whether to suppress a fever should be specific for the individual patient.** Several examples can be cited to illustrate judicious antipyresis.

A. **To avoid potentially harmful secondary effects** in episodes such as the following:

   1. The **elderly individual with pulmonary or cardiovascular disease,** for whom the additional metabolic and cardiovascular effects of a fever-related temperature elevation could lead to greater morbidity or even increased risk of mortality. Congestive heart failure could be precipitated by fever-related tachycardia in such patients. Thus, while an increased temperature after a myocardial infarction might select for the strongest of the species and may enhance wound repair for those individuals, medical responsibility for the care of the individual patient (as well as current concerns for preservation of the species) may recommend judicious use of antipyretics.

   2. **The patient at additional risk from the hypercatabolic state** with hyperventilation, sweating, and loss of fluids, exacerbating poor nutrition or dehydration, particularly if the fever is prolonged.

   3. The young (< 3 or 4 years of age) **child with a history of febrile convulsions** during previous febrile episodes. **Note:** Recurrent febrile convulsions were observed to be more frequent at lower (38–38.9°C) than higher (≥ 40°C) temperatures in one study [54].

   4. The **individual exhibiting toxic encephalopathy or delirium** or known to be mentally disturbed, whose condition may be exacerbated by a fever, and the elderly when the fever appears to precipitate an encephalopathy.

   5. It is controversial whether high fevers could be teratogenic during certain periods of pregnancy. When effects have been shown in animal models, they have depended on the degree and the duration of the temperature elevation.

B. **For the patient's comfort.** Although patients may be unaware of their fevers, some are very uncomfortable. As noted earlier, it is not clear that discomfort is due to fever per se, but the combination of fever and associated (e.g., neuroendocrine or metabolic) responses may lead to discomfort. Once the diagnosis is clearly established or the workup is judiciously initiated, suppression of temperature may be reasonable to make the patient more comfortable (see sec. **VII**).

VII. Methods of lowering temperature. Antipyretic orders commonly are written imprecisely and as a routine for hospitalized patients; acknowledgment of the intervention appears in the progress notes for only a small percentage of patients, with a rationale appearing even less frequently [55].

The most common antipyretic order may be for PRN administration, often not even prompted by detection of a fever. **If aspirin or another antipyretic agent is given intermittently in response to fever spikes, its use may cause precipitous drops in temperature and produce a temperature chart with a hectic appearance.** Both the fall in temperature in response to antipyretic medication (with resetting of the thermoregulatory set point) and the subsequent rise in temperature again (if the exogenous pyrogen—microorganism or other—has not yet been controlled or eliminated) are physiologic, energy-consuming processes that produce more stress for the host than would continued maintenance of the febrile temperature. The alternating episodes of fever spikes, antipyretic administration, and drenching sweats are also very unpleasant for the patient.

If the decision is made to suppress a patient's fever, it is usually more appropriate to do so by continuous administration of the antipyretic for a period of time (24–48 hours) after the fever's characteristics have been noted, followed by withholding of the antipyretic agent to determine whether the fever persists. The withholding of antipyretic therapy allows one to observe the temperature curve for evidence of therapeutic efficacy if antimicrobial or other agents have been administered (i.e., absence of fever with appropriate specific therapy for the infection or illness responsible for inducing the fever) and, in the absence of such evidence, indicates the potential need for further evaluation.

A. **Antipyretics**
   1. **Aspirin** is the most common and often the most effective way to reduce body temperature. However, aspirin occasionally will reduce temperatures to hypothermic levels.
      a. **Dosages.** Adults: 325–650 mg PO or PR q4–6h. Children: 10–15 mg/kg/dose PO q4–6h, not to exceed a total daily dose of 3.6 g.
      b. **Duration.** In patients with infectious causes of fever, specific antibiotic therapy alone usually will control infection and fever within 24–72 hours (or, in a viral syndrome, the acute febrile phase may be over in 1–3 days). At this point if not before, it is advantageous to withhold antipyretic therapy as noted previously and to monitor the temperature to determine whether it would be appropriate to discontinue the aspirin (or alternate antipyretic agent).
      c. **Viral infections in children.** It is currently **advisable to avoid salicylates to treat fever in children with viral illnesses, particularly chickenpox and influenzalike illnesses, because salicylate use has been associated with Reye's syndrome** (see Chap. 8).
   2. **Alternatives to salicylates** are necessary in allergic or anticoagulated patients, or in patients who have hemostatic or platelet abnormalities or GI tract ulcers, or who are otherwise intolerant of these agents. **Acetaminophen** often is used as an aspirin substitute and is approximately as effective as aspirin in reducing fever in either adults or children [56]. The usual dosages are as follows—adults: 325–650 mg PO or PR q4–6h (maximum 4 g/day for short-term use); children: 10–15 mg/kg/dose q4–6h (not to exceed 5 doses per 24 hours).
B. **Sponging the body** with isopropyl alcohol or water may be done. As water has the highest heat of vaporization, it is the preferred liquid. Tepid (rather than cold) water may decrease the tendency toward peripheral vasoconstriction, a counterproductive reflex.
C. The **Turkish massage of Weinstein** [42] is a method of reducing fever by rubbing the patient's skin with a Turkish towel and tepid water. This method takes advantage of the heat of vaporization while encouraging cutaneous vasodilation. The increased cutaneous blood flow will function as a heat exchanger, and core temperature will be lowered.
D. **Cooling blankets** also are popular and may have an appropriate role in temperature reduction. These blankets enhance conductive heat loss and are effective. However, the clinician should not attempt to reduce the temperature to normal as this may result in hypothermia by "overshooting." The body will respond with peripheral vasoconstriction and shivering, making the patient feel miserable. **The cooling blanket should be turned off when body temperature reaches approximately 37.7–38.3°C (100–101°F), to minimize overshooting.** When possible, an antipyretic drug should be used in association with the cooling blanket in an attempt to blunt wide swings in temperature.

E. **Extreme hyperpyrexia (body temperature equal to or exceeding 41°C [106°F]).**
For those very uncommon instances in which an infectious process results in very high body temperature elevations, and especially for malignant hyperthermia and heat stroke, extreme measures may be required. A rapid decrease in temperature is essential. Perhaps the most effective measure is to immerse the patient in an ice-water bath until the temperature is reduced to 39.5°C (103°F). At this point, more moderate measures (see secs. **A, B, D**) should be continued to control the fever. **Dantrolene sodium is considered the drug of choice to treat malignant hyperthermia** (2.5 mg/kg IV initially, with total doses up to 10.0 mg/kg IV to control the event) [16].

VIII. **The decision regarding whether to treat a fever per se (and if so, how) should be a considered decision every time,** not merely a routine, predetermined response to detection of a fever.

Drug Fever

Drugs are a fairly common cause of fever [35, 57, 58]. Because fever is a hallmark of infections, drug fever, especially if associated with chills or rigors, may initially be interpreted as the presence of infection. Drug fever may complicate the evaluation of a patient who is already being treated with appropriate antibiotics for a given infection. In fact, as a group, **antimicrobial agents have been linked to the greatest proportion of cases** [35] (Table 1-1). In addition, a drug fever may occur in patients undergoing long-term therapy (e.g., with methyldopa or allopurinol). Relatively few individuals will have a history of atopic disease (2%) or a history of a previous drug allergy (11%) [35].

I. **Pathogenesis of drug fever.** Fever caused by drugs can be due to contamination of the drug with a pyrogen or microorganism, can be related to the pharmacologic action of the drug itself (e.g., amphotericin B), or can be due to an allergic (hypersensitivity) reaction to the drug.

II. **Clinical presentation**
A. **Fever pattern.** The fever may be sustained (10%), remittent (28%), intermittent (21%), or hectic (41%) [35]. It is often out of proportion to the clinical picture (e.g., the patient may feel and look well but still have fevers). Hectic fever patterns, rigors, and leukocytosis can mimic a bacterial or other septic process.
  1. **With associated findings.** Rigors (43% [corrected calculation]), myalgias (25%), rashes (18%; less than half pruritic), headache (18%), leukocytosis (22%), eosinophilia (22%), serum sickness, abnormal liver function tests, and proteinuria may occur [35]. In this series, relative bradycardia (pulse rate ≤ 100/min during fever) was uncommon. Associated organ dysfunction may be seen in more than a third of episodes but is most often mild [35].
  2. **Fevers with no associated systemic manifestations.** Antibiotic-induced fevers commonly occur without systemic manifestations, but this can also be the case with agents such as antihistamines, barbiturates, procainamide, quinidine, and others.
B. **Onset and duration**
  1. **Onset** occurs typically within 10 days after a patient begins taking a drug [59], although drug fevers, even those that are immunologically mediated, can develop with the first dose or any time thereafter. The median time of onset has recently been reported to be 8 days [35].
  2. The **duration** is variable. Once the offending drug has been discontinued, the fever usually subsides in 24–48 hours, although rarely it may take 4–5 days to subside, especially with drugs that have a long half-life, such as trimethoprim-sulfamethoxazole.
III. **Diagnosis and treatment**
A. **Drug fever should be suspected** whenever a fever occurs (with or without associated findings) in a patient who is taking a drug known to produce fever (see Table 1-1). The diagnosis should always be considered, but **especially when the patient either looks and feels well** on the current therapy and has no obvious uncontrolled or superimposed infections or is at least hemodynamically stable with no localized infection.
B. **Discontinuation of the suspect drug** with a decrease in the temperature within 1 or 2 days will lend support to the diagnosis and help avoid such potentially

Table 1-1. Agents responsible for episodes of drug fever[a]

Cardiovascular (38)
  Alpha methyldopa (16)
  Quinidine (13)
  Procainamide (6)
  Hydralazine
  Nifedipine
  Oxprenolol
Antimicrobial (46)
  Penicillin G (9)
  Ampicillin (2)
  Methicillin (6)
  Cloxacillin (2)
  Cephalothin (7)
  Cephapirin
  Cephamandole
  Tetracycline (2)
  Lincomycin
  Sulfonamide (2)
  Sulfamethoxazole-trimethoprim
  Streptomycin[b]
  Vancomycin
  Colistin
  Isoniazid (5)
  Paraaminosalicylic acid
  Nitrofurantoin (2)
  Mebendazole
Antineoplastic (12)
  Bleomycin (3)
  Daunorubicin
  Procarbazine
  Cytarabine
  Streptozocin (2)
  6-Mercaptopurine
  L-Asparaginase
  Chlorambucil
  Hydroxyurea

Central nervous system (30)
  Diphenylhydantoin (11)
  Carbamazepine (3)
  Chlorpromazine
  Nomifensine (2)
  Haloperidol
  Triamterene
  Benztropine[b]
  Thioridazine (2)
  Trifluoperazine[b]
  Amphetamine (2)
  Lysergic acid (5)[b]
Antiinflammatory (3)
  Ibuprofen
  Tolmetin
  Aspirin
Other (19)
  Iodide (6)
  Cimetidine (2)
  Levamisole
  Metoclopramide
  Clofibrate
  Allopurinol
  Folate
  Prostaglandin E_2 (2)
  Ritodrine
  Interferon (2)
  Propylthiouracil

[a]Numbers in parentheses indicate number of episodes induced by drugs responsible for several episodes.
[b]Fever seen during drug overdose.
Source: P. A. Mackowiak and C. F. LeMaistre, Drug fever: A critical appraisal of conventional concepts. An analysis of 51 episodes in two Dallas hospitals and 97 episodes reported in the English literature. *Ann. Intern. Med.* 106:728, 1987.

dangerous complications as thrombocytopenia, pancytopenia, exfoliative dermatitis, or a vasculitis. **Rechallenge with the offending agent is not generally recommended** unless done carefully in a controlled setting (i.e., in a hospital). However, a recent study suggested that rechallenge with agents responsible for drug fever (> 45% of cases reported) was associated with a low risk of serious sequelae, although it was not altogether free from risk [35].

C. In most clinical circumstances, the offending drug should be discontinued and an alternative drug provided [59]. **Under special circumstances**—for example, where a particular antibiotic is indispensable and no effective alternative is available—drug fever and a macular rash may not be absolute contraindications to continuing the drug. In these circumstances, consultation with an infectious disease or allergy specialist should be sought and careful attention must be directed to the potential development of sequelae such as renal, hepatic, vascular, or dermatologic complications (see Chap. 27).

D. **Neuroleptic malignant syndrome** (NMS) [39, 40] is precipitated by the effects of neuroleptic drugs (e.g., butyrophenones, loxapine, phenothiazines, thioxanthenes, antidepressants, and antiemetics), although other unknown factors may be involved as well. **The cardinal signs of NMS are hyperthermia** (temperatures to 41°C and higher), **hypertonicity, fluctuating consciousness, and autonomic nervous system lability** with diaphoresis, tachycardia, blood pressure instability, and/or cardiac arrhythmias. Laboratory findings are nonspecific although elevated CPK levels (secondary to myonecrosis) can occur. Symptoms may last over several days, even after discontinuation of the offending agent.

As is true with malignant hyperthermia, sodium dantrolene appears to be effective therapy for NMS [39, 40] (see sec. **VII.E** under Fever). Other potentially useful therapeutic drugs are bromocriptine mesylate, amantadine, and levodopa combined with dopadecarboxylase inhibitor (carbidopa); no controlled or comparative studies have been reported for any of these drugs.

Fever of Unknown Etiology

I. Definitions. Fever of unknown origin (FUO) was defined by Petersdorf and Beeson [60] in 1961 as a febrile illness of more than 3 weeks' duration. To qualify as FUO, temperatures must exceed 38.3°C (101°F) on several determinations with no diagnosis reached after 1 week of study in the hospital. These criteria are chosen because they tend to eliminate acute, self-limited infectious illnesses such as common viral diseases, postoperative fevers, and febrile illnesses of obvious cause; the criteria exclude patients who defervesce spontaneously, and they also allow time for the completion of the usual initial laboratory studies. Because of the expense of hospitalization and the frequent ability to investigate an FUO as an outpatient, **Petersdorf** [61] **has modified this definition** by proposing that, in lieu of 1 week in hospital, 1 week of intelligent and intensive investigation be undertaken, which in most patients is possible on an outpatient basis.

Durack and Street [62] **have recommended further modifications. They have proposed subdividing FUO into four groups:**

A. Classic FUO
1. Fever of 38.3°C (101°F) or higher on several occasions.
2. Fever of more than 3 weeks' duration.
3. Diagnosis uncertain, despite appropriate investigations, after at least three outpatient visits or at least 3 days in hospital.

B. Nosocomial FUO
1. Fever of 38.3°C (101°F) or higher on several occasions in a hospitalized patient receiving acute care.
2. Infection not present or incubating on admission.
3. Diagnosis uncertain after 3 days despite appropriate investigation, including at least 2 days' incubation of microbiologic cultures.

C. Neutropenic FUO
1. Fever of 38.3°C (101°F) or higher on several occasions.
2. Fewer than 500 neutrophils/mm^3 within 1–2 days.
3. Diagnosis uncertain after 3 days despite appropriate investigation, including at least 2 days' incubation of microbiologic cultures.

D. HIV-associated FUO [62a]
1. Fever of 38.3°C (101°F) or higher on several occasions.
2. Confirmed positive serology for HIV infection.
3. Fever of more than 4 weeks' duration for outpatients or more than 3 days' duration in hospital.
4. Diagnosis uncertain after 3 days despite appropriate investigation, including at least 2 days' incubation of microbiologic cultures.

II. Causes of FUO [60, 63, 64]
A. Table 1-2 compares the results of three major studies of **the causes of FUO** in patients. These studies were carried out in university-based referral centers. Although infections are still the most common cause of FUOs, the incidence of multisystem or collagen vascular diseases remains significant, and there has been a decrease in the number of tumors presenting as FUOs. However, Barbado and colleagues [65] find that collagen vascular diseases, especially vasculitides, are more frequent (29%) than infections (11%). Endocarditis, abdominal abscesses, and hepatobiliary diseases have become less important causes of FUOs in recent years. Tuberculosis remains an important cause of FUOs, and cytomegalovirus has become an increasingly frequent cause of FUO.

Table 1-2. Causes of fever of unknown origin: Comparison of three reports

	Petersdorf and Beeson [60] (100 cases)	Patients (%)	Larson et al. [63] (105 cases)	Patients (%)	Knockaert et al. [64] (199 cases)	Patients (%)
Infections	Tuberculosis Intraabdominal abscess Hepatobiliary disease Endocarditis Cirrhosis and bacteremia Pyelonephritis Psittacosis Brucellosis Malaria Gonococcal urethritis	36	Tuberculosis Intraabdominal abscess Wound infection Catheter infections Cytomegalovirus Urinary tract infections Sinusitis Candidiasis Amebic hepatitis Osteomyelitis	31	Tuberculosis Intraabdominal abscess Hepatobiliary disease Endocarditis Cytomegalovirus	23
Neoplasms	Leukemia and lymphoma Carcinomatosis Solid tumor No histologic diagnosis	19	Leukemia and lymphoma Hodgkin's disease Solid tumor	31	Leukemia and lymphoma Myeloma Solid tumor	7
Collagen vascular disease	Lupus erythematosus Rheumatic fever Cranial arteritis Unclassified	15	Polyarteritis Rheumatic fever Giant cell arteritis Panaortitis and arteritis Still's disease	9	Lupus erythematosus Polymyalgia Temporal arteritis Still's disease	20

Table 1-2 (continued)

	Petersdorf and Beeson [60] (100 cases)	Patients (%)	Larson et al. [63] (105 cases)	Patients (%)	Knockaert et al. [64] (199 cases)	Patients (%)
Miscellaneous	Pulmonary sarcoidosis Factitious fever Familial Mediterranean fever (periodic disease) Pericarditis Granulomatous hepatitis Ruptured spleen and pancreatitis Myelofibrosis Erythema multiforme Drug fever Thyroiditis Weber-Christian disease	23	Pulmonary sarcoidosis Factitious fever Familial Mediterranean fever (periodic disease) Pericarditis Granulomatous hepatitis Crohn's disease Myxoma Hematomas	17	Pulmonary sarcoidosis Factitious fever Familial Mediterranean fever (periodic disease) Allergic alveolitis Lymph node pseudotumor Crohn's disease Drug fever Thyroiditis Hyperthyroidism Hyperthermia Silicone embolization Femoral aneurysm Castleman disease Vogt-Koyanagi-Harada syndrome	24
Undiagnosed		7		12		26

1. **Infections (23–36%).** Tuberculosis; bacterial endocarditis due to slow-growing organisms; culture-negative endocarditis; localized suppurative process within the biliary tract, liver, or kidney; intraabdominal abscesses; septic pelvic vein thrombophlebitis; and certain viral infections such as cytomegalovirus (CMV), Epstein-Barr virus (EBV), or primary infection with HIV type 1 should be considered. (See Chaps. 17 and 19.)

2. **Neoplasms (7–31%).** Lymphoma, leukemia, renal cell carcinoma, gastrointestinal tumor, and metastatic ovarian carcinoma are the most common neoplasms. In the most recent studies of FUOs [64], there was a marked decrease in the incidence of neoplasms. This is believed to be due to the widespread use of ultrasonography and CT scanning.

3. **Collagen vascular diseases (9–20%).** Systemic lupus erythematosus, rheumatoid arthritis, mixed connective tissue diseases, temporal arteritis, juvenile rheumatoid arthritis of the adult (adult Still's disease), and vasculitis can present as an FUO.

4. **Miscellaneous causes (17–24%)** are drug fever, recurrent pulmonary emboli, inflammatory bowel disease (especially regional enteritis), sarcoidosis, and factitious or fraudulent fever. However, there are numerous unusual causes of FUOs [66, 67].

5. **In adults, 10% of FUOs will remain undiagnosed.** In Knockaert's study [64], there was a noticeably higher incidence of undiagnosed cases (26%). This is because, in contrast to other reports, Knockaert and coworkers [64] categorized as FUOs fever in patients with diseases of unknown origin, such as granulomatous hepatitis or pericarditis; these were labeled *nondiagnosis* rather than being relegated to the miscellaneous category [61]. It is reassuring, though, that the vast majority of patients that remain undiagnosed do well in follow-up [68, 69, 70].

6. **The spectrum of causes** of FUOs among community hospital patients and the elderly ($\geq$ 65 years old) is similar to the general population, with a few noticeable differences [71–73].

    In the community hospital group, infections (abscesses, tuberculosis, endocarditis, acute HIV infection, and CMV) represented approximately 33% of the FUO population; neoplasms, primarily lymphomas, were present in 24% of the population; and 16% had collagen vascular diseases. Alcoholic hepatitis and recurrent pulmonary emboli are relatively common in this group. The most common causes of FUOs in the elderly are leukemias, lymphomas, abscesses, tuberculosis, and temporal arteritis.

B. **Factitious fever** refers to fever produced artificially by the patient.

1. **A diagnosis of factitious fever** [74] should be considered in any FUO, especially in young women or persons with medical training or if the patient looks clinically well and there is a disparity between temperature and pulse. The advent of digital thermometers has reduced the frequency of this diagnosis.

2. **Absence of the normal diurnal pattern** should alert the physician to this diagnostic possibility.

3. Some practitioners recommend several temperature determinations in the presence of a nurse or physician. Others have suggested the use of a thermocoupling device (electric thermometer) to allow immediate recording of results. Urine temperatures have also been suggested as a means to uncover factitious fever due to manipulation of the glass thermometer [75].

4. The diagnosis should be considered especially in paramedical personnel.

C. **Fraudulent fever** is akin to factitious fever. In this case, the fever is authentic but is induced by the patient's self-inoculation or ingestion of foreign material.

III. **Approach to the FUO.** Although the clinical investigation of a patient with FUO should be individualized, Knockaert [76] has developed a detailed diagnostic strategy for the patient with an FUO. This report also presents an algorithmic approach to the diagnosis of FUOs.

A. **Rule out common infections or other causes of fever.** Although it may seem obvious, initial assessment of the nonseptic febrile patient must rule out the common infections causing fever, including respiratory and urinary tract infections, wound and pelvic infections, gastrointestinal infections, and superficial and deep phlebitis, including intravenous-related phlebitis in hospitalized patients.

1. **A careful history** and **physical examination** and **basic laboratory screens** such as blood count, urinalysis and urine culture, chest x-ray, stool examination, and two or three blood cultures are indicated.

      2. The patient's current medications should be carefully evaluated to help exclude a drug fever.

  B. Determine whether the patient has a true FUO. Before launching what may be an intensive workup for FUO, the fever should be present, at least by history, for 3 weeks and the routine evaluation should be unremarkable. Only then may a case be defined as an FUO.

  C. Workup of the patient with a true FUO. Although fever is a common manifestation of infection, the causes of FUO often are noninfectious in origin. The differential diagnosis (see Table 1-2) must be kept in mind. **Most of these patients have a treatable or curable disease that is presenting in an uncommon manner.**

    1. Careful history taking is essential to discover clues from the patient's travel background, exposure to tuberculosis, animal exposure, drug use, work environment, hobbies, geographic origins, HIV risk factors, and other habits. With the differential diagnosis of FUO in mind, the physician explores each of the diagnostic categories. If the workup is unrewarding initially, **serial follow-up histories** may provide additional clues to a specific diagnosis. Interviews with the immediate family or close relatives may be helpful.

    2. A complete and careful physical examination should be repeated if the patient is believed to have a true FUO. Again, the differential diagnosis is kept in mind and particular attention is paid to the following points:

      a. Skin. Look for peripheral stigmata of **bacterial endocarditis** (BE), which may be present in only 20–30% of patients with BE, a subtle rash of vasculitis, skin lesions that may be biopsied, rash of juvenile rheumatoid arthritis, and so on.

      b. Lymph nodes may provide the diagnosis when biopsied.

      c. Hepatomegaly may provide the diagnosis when the liver is biopsied.

      d. Abdominal masses or areas of tenderness may reflect an intraabdominal abscess.

      e. Rectal and pelvic examinations may provide evidence of an abscess or another septic process.

      f. Cardiac examination may provide evidence of underlying valvular disease, which may predispose the patient to endocarditis. It must be recalled that the absence of murmur does not exclude the diagnosis of BE, especially in the patient older than 60 years; in one study, approximately 33% of elderly patients with subacute BE did not have a murmur at presentation [77].

      g. Serial physical examinations are crucial! While the patient is hospitalized, his or her clinical status might change, and a new lymph node, murmur, or rash could appear and provide an important clue to the diagnosis.

    3. Laboratory examinations and biopsies. By definition, the routine CBC, urine and sputum cultures, chest x-ray, and other determinations have already been unrewarding in the early evaluation of the FUO. Studies of antibodies to EBV and CMV, especially IgM antibodies, may be helpful (see Chap. 17). **Further testing must be individualized,** as a variety of tests are available.

IV. Laboratory and diagnostic aids in the FUO evaluation

  A. Initial blood culture reports

    1. In continuous bacteremia (such as endocarditis), three sets of blood cultures will usually be adequate to recover the organism in more than 95% of cases [78]. However, any oral or parenteral antibiotic therapy given before the initial blood cultures are drawn may inhibit the growth of the organisms (e.g., in partially treated BE). In addition, some fastidious organisms may take several days or weeks (e.g., *Brucella*) to grow or may have special growth requirements. Additional blood cultures may have to be ordered, and the microbiology laboratory may need to be notified that a fastidious organism might be involved (e.g., *Haemophilus* spp.). See related discussions in Chaps. 2 and 10.

    2. Culture-negative endocarditis. Culture-negative endocarditis is a recognized entity that accounts for 5–15% of cases of endocarditis (see Chap. 10) [79]. It can occur even in patients who have had no prior exposure to antibiotics and is well described in the literature of the preantibiotic era. **This diagnosis should be considered in the patient with FUO, negative initial blood cultures, and underlying cardiac disease** (such as rheumatic or congenital heart disease). When possible, infectious disease consultation should be sought for such patients before one commits a patient to a prolonged course of antibiotics.

  B. Tissue biopsies

    1. Lymph nodes that are pathologically enlarged should be biopsied early in the workup, as underlying malignancy or granulomatous disease might be uncovered.

  2. **Liver.** In patients with hepatomegaly, abnormal liver function tests, or possible miliary tuberculosis or disseminated fungal disease, a liver biopsy may provide the diagnosis either by histologic examination or by culturing.
      a. **Granulomatous hepatitis** may have multiple origins but, in 20–26% of cases, a cause cannot be found [80].
      b. **The biopsy should be cultured aerobically and anaerobically and for acid-fast organisms and fungi.** Rarely, the organism involved in infective endocarditis may be cultured from the liver biopsy.
  3. **Skin nodules and rashes** may provide a clue to metastatic disease or an underlying vasculitis.
  4. **Temporal artery biopsy** (bilateral) may be diagnostic in the elderly patient with an unexplained elevated erythrocyte sedimentation rate.
C. **Skin tests**
  1. **The intermediate purified protein derivative (PPD) test** should be done routinely unless the patient is known to be a reactor. A negative test should be repeated in approximately 1 week to test for a "booster effect," and anergy should be ruled out (see Chap. 9) [81].
  2. **Rule out anergy.** Other antigens should be tested, such as *Candida*, trichophyton, streptokinase-streptodornase, and mumps. The patient must be examined within 4 hours of the mumps antigen test to be certain the result is negative at that time.
  3. **Fungal skin tests** generally are not helpful diagnostically (see Chap. 18). For example, skin tests with histoplasmin and blastomycin are not useful diagnostically, especially in an endemic area. In addition, these tests may induce an antibody response that would either lead to a false diagnosis or preclude future serologic studies.
D. **Serology.** As a general rule, serologic tests assume importance when a fourfold or greater rise in titer can be demonstrated (see Chap. 25). However, a *Histoplasma* complement fixation test result of 32 or greater is strongly suggestive of acute infection, whereas a negative test does not rule out the diagnosis.
  1. **An acute-phase blood sample** should be drawn; serum should then be frozen and set aside in an FUO evaluation. This will assure an early specimen if careful serologic studies are indicated as the workup proceeds.
  2. **Blood for convalescent titer** usually is drawn 2–4 weeks after the acute titer.
  3. Occasionally, only a single serum specimen is available for study. Characteristic titer elevations may be very suggestive, or even diagnostic, in certain clinical settings. For example, an indirect fluorescent antibody titer of 1:1,024 or greater to *Toxoplasma gondii* is suggestive of toxoplasmosis. A specific IgM antibody response is highly suggestive of a recent primary infection, more so than is the presence of IgG antibody (see Chaps. 17 and 25).
  4. The term **febrile agglutinins** refers to a group of agglutination tests that include *Salmonella* spp., *Brucella* spp., *Francisella tularensis,* and *Proteus* OXK, OX2, OX19 (see sec. **5.c**). *Salmonella* infections, including typhoid fever, can easily and more reliably be diagnosed by appropriate cultures. Because brucellosis can cause FUOs and have an atypical presentation, serologic testing is probably cost-effective. Tularemia usually is diagnosed on clinical and cultural data; serologic tests generally are not used.
      Febrile agglutinins are not useful as a screening test. These tests have low specificity and cross-reactions. One should order individual tests with a particular disease entity in mind.
  5. **Examples of cases in which serologic studies may aid in FUO evaluations**
      a. **Viral disease.** If an FUO has lasted more than 3 weeks, most viral infections can be excluded. However, CMV and EBV mononucleosis in young children and, most importantly, CMV in adults (especially middle-aged adults) are viral illnesses that can cause prolonged fevers. HIV serology is discussed in Chap. 19.
      b. **Toxoplasmosis.** The diagnosis of toxoplasmosis can be difficult, and serologic tests such as the IgM immunofluorescent antibody assay (IFA) have been helpful in confirming a clinical suspicion (see Chap. 17 for further discussion).
      c. **Rickettsial disease.** The diagnosis of rickettsial disease is supported by

positive agglutination tests with one or more of the *Proteus vulgaris* antigens (OXK, OX2, OX19), which cross-react with certain *Rickettsiae*. With the exception of Q fever, serologic tests have only a minor confirmatory role in the diagnosis of *Rickettsiae*. Enzyme-linked immunosorbent assay, (ELISA), complement fixation, and IFA are all useful in diagnosing Q fever, although ELISA is considered the most sensitive of the three.

   d. **Legionnaires' disease** can be detected by culture and direct fluorescent staining of sputum, bronchial washings, pleural fluid, or tissue. Indirect fluorescent antibody testing is also available (see Chap. 9). Serologic confirmation is established when a single convalescent serum sample has a titer of 1:256 or greater or when there is at least a fourfold rise in titer to a minimum titer of 1:128. A direct fluorescent antibody technique also is available for testing tissue (see Chap. 9).

   e. **Psittacosis** is most readily diagnosed by demonstrating a fourfold or greater rise in complement-fixing antibody.

E. **Sedimentation rate.** The usefulness of the erythrocyte sedimentation rate (ESR) in FUO is under debate. The ESR often is elevated in endocarditis, but it can be normal. Noninfectious causes of elevated ESR are common, as, for example, in uremia. For the most part, a normal ESR is comforting in the FUO workup, although very uncommonly serious disease can be present while the ESR is normal. In the older patient ($\geq$ 55 years) with FUO and an ESR in excess of 100, the diagnosis of **temporal arteritis** should be considered. The patient's history should be reviewed carefully with respect to headaches, visual problems, and myalgias. One should carefully palpate the temporal arteries, looking for tenderness. However, the diagnosis may exist in the absence of physical findings or typical history [82]. **When temporal arteritis is suspected, the patient should undergo bilateral temporal artery biopsies** for definitive diagnosis. Initiation of high-dose steroid therapy (e.g., prednisone, 60–80 mg/day PO) may help to prevent blindness, a major complication of temporal arteritis.

F. **Collagen vascular disease screening.** Because up to 15% of adult patients with FUO have a collagen vascular disease, histories must be elicited carefully.

   1. **ESR** and **antinuclear antibody** studies generally are used for screening.

   2. **Muscle or skin biopsies** (or both) of suspicious rashes may uncover a vasculitis.

G. **Radiographic contrast studies**

   1. **An intravenous pyelogram (IVP) with nephrotomograms** may help in diagnosing a hypernephroma that presents as an FUO [83] or a perinephric abscess. Computerized axial tomography and ultrasonography have replaced the IVP to a great extent. However, the IVP will be abnormal in 93% of cases with renal tuberculosis [84].

   2. **Gastrointestinal studies.** Gastrointestinal tumors are an uncommon cause of FUO [66]. However, inflammatory bowel disease may, at times, present with a rather benign history, and an upper GI series with small-bowel follow-through may help establish the diagnosis. In addition, contrast x-rays, such as barium enema, may help identify and localize a space-occupying intraintestinal process. Colonoscopy and barium studies are complementary. Nonetheless, GI contrast studies **should not be viewed as routine;** the yield is low unless there are symptoms or other clues pointing to the GI system [76].

H. **Radionuclide scans** [76, 85–90]. Sulfur colloid labeled with technetium 99M has fallen into disuse with the advent of gallium 67 and indium 111 scanning. Total-body gallium scanning has occasionally been useful in detecting occult abscesses and lymphoma as well as thyroiditis and unusual tumors, such as leiomyosarcoma and pheochromocytoma. Indium is less likely to accumulate in noninfected foci. Bone scans and indium 111 scans appear to be useful in distinguishing osteomyelitis from a cellulitis that is in close proximity to the bone. Three-phase bone scanning frequently is not specific enough to delineate clearly cellulitis from osteomyelitis (see Chap. 16).

Gallium 67 scanning has been helpful in defining pneumonia in patients with AIDS who are hypoxic and have a normal or near-normal chest x-ray. Indium 111 probably is equally as useful. Gallium 67 and indium 111 scanning should be considered complementary and as second- or third-line diagnostic procedures.

Gallium 67– and indium 111–labeled leukocytes are being attached to nonspecific immunoglobulins in an effort to achieve greater sensitivity. Further studies are required to determine the usefulness of this technique.

Overall, we seldom use radionuclide scanning in the FUO workup. CT scanning is preferred (see **J**).

I. Ultrasonography

1. Particularly in culture-negative or suspected endocarditis, the noninvasive imaging procedure of ultrasonography may be useful to detect **vegetations**. Transesophageal echocardiography (see Chap. 10) has added a new dimension to the sensitivity of detecting valvular vegetations, especially those on prosthetic valves. It is also a sensitive tool for detecting **atrial myxomas**.

2. **Abdominal or pelvic studies** may help localize an abscess or differentiate a solid from a cystic mass. Ultrasonography is useful in visualizing hepatobiliary and renal abnormalities. This technique is also effective in detecting dissecting abdominal aortic aneurysms, which rarely can present as an FUO.

J. Computed tomography [76, 91, 92] is a useful and sensitive tool for identifying and localizing intracranial, intraabdominal, and intrathoracic abscesses. **CT scanning appears to be more sensitive than gallium scanning and is the cause of the decreased number of normal biopsies.** Most patients with an FUO should have an abdominal CT scan to help rule out an occult abscess.

Magnetic resonance imaging (MRI) is a promising new radiologic development. At present, its usefulness in infectious diseases is for identifying cerebral toxoplasmosis and epidural abscesses of the spine and to help resolve questionable cases of osteomyelitis. The role of MRI in assessing an FUO has not been defined.

V. Miscellaneous diseases that cause FUOs

A. Granulomatous hepatitis may be documented by a liver biopsy performed as part of the FUO evaluation [80]. This represents a histologic reaction pattern with many etiologies, among which are tuberculosis, histoplasmosis, brucellosis, Q fever, syphilis, sarcoidosis, Hodgkin's disease, berylliosis, Wegener's granulomatosis, and drug reactions. In approximately 20–25% of patients with a diagnosis of granulomatous hepatitis, a cause cannot be determined. In such patients, a trial of antituberculous therapy may be appropriate. If this is unsuccessful, alternate-day corticosteroids might be tried. It is advisable to consult with an infectious disease specialist, if possible, for this problem.

B. Juvenile rheumatoid arthritis is characterized in children by fever; polyarticular or monoarticular arthritis; salmon-colored, nonpruritic, evanescent macular or maculopapular rash; generalized lymphadenopathy; hepatosplenomegaly; and, occasionally, pericarditis (rarely, myocarditis). Iridocyclitis occurs frequently and should be sought by an ophthalmologist, even if ocular symptoms are minimal. Rheumatoid factor is absent. A similar clinical picture may be seen in young adults.

C. Familial Mediterranean fever (periodic disease) is an autosomal recessive disease characterized by periodic fevers contracted predominantly by men, particularly those of Italian, Sephardic Jewish, or Irish descent. Peritonitis, pleuritis, arthritis, and skin lesions may accompany the fever.

D. Whipple's disease is seen in middle-aged to older men and is characterized by low-grade fever, progressive weight loss, diarrhea, malabsorption, arthralgias, abdominal pain, increased skin pigmentation, and lymphadenopathy. Jejunal biopsy can establish the diagnosis.

E. Bacterial hepatitis is comprised of chronic nonsuppurative bacterial infections of the liver (e.g., *Staphylococcus aureus*) other than those causing a granulomatous reaction [93]. Fever and minimally elevated alkaline phosphatase may be the only evidence of liver involvement. A liver biopsy will be helpful and, as usual, the biopsy should be cultured aerobically and anaerobically.

F. Hyperimmunoglobulinemia D and periodic fever is a syndrome described in six patients of Dutch ancestry in 1984 [94]. The clinical picture was similar to familial Mediterranean fever.

G. Ehrlichiosis. The majority of symptomatic patients with ehrlichiosis present with an abrupt onset of fever, chills, and headache often accompanied by nausea, myalgias, arthralgias, and malaise. A recent report discusses six patients in whom the principal finding was protracted fever ranging from 17–51 days' duration. The diagnosis was delayed due to the lack of consideration of the diagnosis, patient's delay in seeking medical care, or both [94a]. See Appendix A.

H. Other unusual etiologies of FUO have been described [66, 67].

VI. Indications for exploratory laparotomies in patients with FUO. Exploratory laparotomy seldom is indicated if scanning procedures, ultrasound studies, and percutaneous biopsies are used appropriately. Laparotomy is not considered a routine procedure but is reserved as a concluding step in the workup of selected patients [92, 95, 96] and when abnormalities apparent on scanning need clarification, biopsy, or possible drainage. However, laparoscopy should be considered first if it is technically feasible [97].

VII. **Therapeutic drug trials in patients with FUO.** In general, the use of medication in the absence of a definitive diagnosis is discouraged. However, a therapeutic trial may be justified if, after one has done a careful investigation and culturing, the clinical and laboratory data support certain etiologies but a definitive diagnosis cannot be reached. **Infectious disease consultation should be sought in these situations.**

　　A. **Granulomatous hepatitis** may warrant a trial of antituberculous drugs for 2–3 weeks [80]. If the signs and symptoms of an inflammatory process persist, a trial of corticosteroids may be rewarding.

　　B. If untreated, **blood culture–negative endocarditis** has a high mortality [79]. If clinical data indicate that this entity is the most likely possibility, a trial of antibiotics may be lifesaving. The combination of penicillin and an aminoglycoside often is recommended. Patients with prosthetic valves that were inserted recently should receive antibiotics active against *Staphylococcus epidermidis* (see Chap. 10).

　　C. **Tuberculosis** may be suspected in a patient with a history of that illness. A 2- to 3-week trial of antituberculous therapy is likely to cause a defervescence in fever if active tuberculosis is the cause.

　　D. In the **cancer patient** with FUO, the fever may respond to naproxen or indomethacin if the fever is due to the neoplasm. Infections, of course, should be ruled out by an appropriate workup.

VIII. **Recurrent or episodic FUO.** In some patients with a classic FUO, the fever spontaneously resolves for at least 2 weeks and then recurs. On further workup, only 20% or so of these patients will have underlying infection, tumor, or connective tissue diseases [70]. Miscellaneous causes (e.g., Crohn's disease, factitious fever) are common. Overall, these patients generally do well [70] and often can simply be followed carefully and assessed serially as outpatients.

References

1. McGowen, J.E., et al. Fever in hospitalized patients: With special reference to the medical service. *Am. J. Med.* 82:580, 1987.
2. Santos, J.I. Nutrition, infection, and immunocompetence. *Infect. Dis. Clin. North Am.* 8:243, 1994.
   Reviews the impact of nutrition on susceptibility to infection as well as the impact of infection on nutrition.
3. Lewin, S., Brettman, L.R., and Holzman, R.S. Infections in hypothermic patients. *Arch. Intern. Med.* 141:920, 1981.
4. Schmitt, B.D. Fever phobia: Misconceptions of parents about fever. *Am. J. Dis. Child.* 134:176, 1980.
5. May, A., and Bauchner, H. Fever phobia: The pediatrician's contribution. *Pediatrics* 90:851, 1992.
6. Bennett, I.L., Jr., and Nicastri, A. Fever as a mechanism of resistance. *Bacteriol. Rev.* 24:16, 1960.
   A review that precipitated the modern reassessment of the role of fever.
7. Kluger, M.J., Ringler, D.H., and Anver, M.R. Fever and survival. *Science* 188:166, 1975.
   An elegant study that was definitive for its field as well as catalytic for the many recent studies by other investigators that have reassessed the role of fever.
8. Roberts, N.J., Jr. Temperature and host defense. *Microbiol. Rev.* 43:241, 1979.
   A concise but extensive review of the data, both pro and con, involving the role of temperature as a host defense mechanism.
9. Mackowiak, P.A. *Fever: Basic Mechanisms and Management.* New York: Raven, 1991.
   The entire text addresses relevant data and concepts. For a related discussion see C.A. Dinarello and S.M. Wolff, Pathogenesis of Fever and the Acute Phase Response. In G.L. Mandell, J.E. Bennett, and R. Dolin (eds.), Principles and Practice of Infectious Diseases (4th ed.). New York: Churchill Livingstone, 1995.
10. Roberts, N.J., Jr. The impact of temperature elevation on immunological defenses. *Rev. Infect. Dis.* 13:462, 1991.

An update of [8], with attention limited to temperature elevation and extensive recent immunologic studies.

11. Mackowiak, P.A., Wasserman, S.S., and Levine, M.M. A critical appraisal of 98.6°F, the upper limit of the normal body temperature, and other legacies of Carl Reinhold August Wünderlich. *J.A.M.A.* 268:1578, 1992.

12. Beach, P., and McCormick, D. Fever and tympanic thermometry. In Proceedings of a symposium, January 18, 1991, San Diego, Calif. *Clin. Pediatr.* 30(Suppl.):1, 1991. *A supplement dedicated to analyses of ear thermometry.*

13. Musher, D.M., et al. Fever patterns. Their lack of clinical significance. *Arch. Intern. Med.* 139:1225, 1979.

14. Stitt, J.S. Fever versus hyperthermia. *Fed. Proc.* 38:39, 1979. *Discusses and compares the differing physiologic characteristics.*

15. Simon, H.B. Hyperthermia. *N. Engl. J. Med.* 329:483, 1993. *A clear review of causes and consequences of hyperthermia (as opposed to fever).*

16. Heiman-Patterson, T.D. Malignant hyperthermia. *Semin. Neurol.* 11:220, 1991.

17. Iaizzo, P.A., and Palahniuk, R.J. Malignant hyperthermia: Diagnosis, treatment, genetics, and pathophysiology. *Invest. Radiol.* 26:1013, 1991.

18. DuBois, E.F. Why are fever temperatures over 106°F rare? *Am. J. Med. Sci.* 217:361, 1949. *For a recent review, see P.A. Mackowiak and J.A. Boulant, Fever's glass ceiling. Clin. Infect. Dis. 22:525, 1996.*

19. Roberts, N.J., Jr., Lu, S.-T., and Michaelson, S.M. Hyperthermia and human leukocyte functions: DNA, RNA, and total protein synthesis after exposure to < 41° or > 42.5° hyperthermia. *Cancer Res.* 45:3076, 1985.

20. Dinarello, C.A. Interleukin-1. *Rev. Infect. Dis.* 6:51, 1984. *Reviews the experimental data equating EP, LEM, and LAF biologic activities (many references).*

21. Dinarello, C.A. Role of interleukin-1 in infectious diseases. *Immunol. Rev.* 127:119, 1992. *An update of [20], reviewing intervening observations.*

22. Cerami, A. Inflammatory cytokines. *Clin. Immunol. Immunopathol.* 62:S3, 1992. *A concise review of the proinflammatory cytokines.*

23. Kopf, M., et al. Impaired immune and acute-phase responses in interleukin-6-deficient mice. *Nature* 368:339, 1994.

24. Roberts, N.J., Jr., Prill, A.H., and Mann, T.N. Interleukin 1 and interleukin 1 inhibitor production by human macrophages exposed to influenza virus or respiratory syncytial virus: Respiratory syncytial virus is a potent inducer of inhibitory activity. *J. Exp. Med.* 163:511, 1986.

25. Granowitz, E.V., et al. Production of interleukin-1-receptor antagonist during experimental endotoxaemia. *Lancet* 2:1423, 1991.

26. Glauser, M.P., et al. Pathogenesis and potential strategies for prevention and treatment of septic shock: An update. *Clin. Infect. Dis.* 18(Suppl. 2):S205, 1994.

27. Bone, R.C. The pathogenesis of sepsis. *Ann. Intern. Med.* 115:457, 1991.

28. Blatteis, C.M. Neural mechanisms in the pyrogenic and acute-phase responses to interleukin-1. *Int. J. Neurosci.* 38:223, 1988. *Recent review of IL-1 and the nervous system: entry of IL-1, neuronal responses and neurotransmitters.*

29. Reichlin, S. Neuroendocrine-immune interactions. *N. Engl. J. Med.* 329:1246, 1993.

30. Beisel, W.R. Effects of infection on nutritional status and immunity. *Fed. Proc.* 39:3105, 1980.

31. Beisel, W.R. Magnitude of the host nutritional responses to infection. *Am. J. Clin. Nutr.* 30:1236, 1977. *A classic and still very pertinent review.*

32. Baumann, H., and Gauldie, J. The acute phase response. *Immunol. Today* 15:74, 1994. *Current review of the acute-phase response cascade and its regulation.*

33. Weinberg, E.D. Iron and infection. *Microbiol. Rev.* 42:45, 1978. *A classic review, comprehensive.*

34. Steel, D.M., and Whitehead, A.S. The major acute phase reactants: C-reactive protein, serum amyloid P component and serum amyloid A protein. *Immunol. Today* 15:81, 1994.

35. Mackowiak, P.A., and LeMaistre, C.F. Drug fever: A critical appraisal of conventional concepts. An analysis of 51 episodes in two Dallas hospitals and 97 episodes reported in the English literature. *Ann. Intern. Med.* 106:728, 1987. *A recent evaluation and review that challenges earlier concepts.*

36. Simon, H.B. Extreme pyrexia. *J.A.M.A.* 236:2419, 1976.
37. Alpert, G., Hibbert, E., and Fleisher, G.R. Case-control study of hyperpyrexia in children. *Pediatr. Infect. Dis. J.* 9:161, 1990.
38. Putto, A., Ruuskanen, O., and Meurman, O. Fever in respiratory virus infections. *Am. J. Dis. Child.* 140:1159, 1986.
39. Caroff, S.N., and Mann, S.C. Neuroleptic malignant syndrome. *Med. Clin. North Am.* 77:185, 1993.
40. Heiman-Patterson, T.D. Neuroleptic malignant syndrome and malignant hyperthermia: Important issues for the medical consultant. *Med. Clin. North Am.* 77:477, 1993. *See related report by B.H. Guze and L.R. Baxter, Neuroleptic malignant syndrome.* N. Engl. J. Med. *313:163, 1985.*
41. Collins, K.J., and Exton-Smith, A.N. Thermal homeostasis in old age. *J. Am. Geriatr. Soc.* 31:519, 1983.
42. Keusch, G.T. Fever: To be or not to be. *N. Y. State J. Med.* 76:1998, 1976.
43. Kluger, M.J. Fever revisited. *Pediatrics* 90:846, 1992.
44. Done, A.K. Treatment of fever in 1982: A review. *Am. J. Med.* 74:27, 1983.
45. Weinstein, M.P., et al. Spontaneous bacterial peritonitis: A review of 28 cases with emphasis on improved survival and factors influencing prognosis. *Am. J. Med.* 64:592, 1978.
46. Manzella, J.P., Roberts, N.J., Jr., Robertson, R.G., et al. Temperature elevation, bacterial growth and antibiotic activity. *J. Antimicrob. Chemother.* 6:795, 1980.
47. Mackowiak, P.A. Direct effects of hyperthermia on pathogenic microorganisms: Teleologic implications with regard to fever. *Rev. Infect. Dis.* 3:508, 1981.
48. Delaet, I., and Boeye, A. Monoclonal antibodies that disrupt poliovirus only at fever temperatures. *J. Virol.* 67:5299, 1993.
49. Grieger, T.A., and Kluger, M.J. Fever and survival: The role of serum iron. *J. Physiol.* 279:187, 1978.
50. Vaughn, L.K., Bernheim, H.A., and Kluger, M.J. Fever in the lizard *Dipsosaurus dorsalis*. *Nature* 252:473, 1974.
51. Bernheim, H.A., et al. Effects of fever on host defence mechanisms after infection in the lizard *Dipsosaurus dorsalis*. *Br. J. Exp. Pathol.* 59:76, 1978.
52. Bernheim, H.A., and Kluger, M.J. Fever: Effect of drug-induced antipyresis on survival. *Science* 193:237, 1976.
53. Stanley, E.D., et al. Increased virus shedding with aspirin treatment of rhinovirus infection. *J.A.M.A.* 231:1248, 1975.
54. El-Radhi, A.S., and Banajeh, S. Effect of fever on recurrence rate of febrile convulsions. *Arch. Dis. Child.* 64:869, 1989.
55. Issacs, S.N., Axelrod, P.I., and Lorber, B. Antipyretic orders in a university hospital. *Am. J. Med.* 88:31, 1990.
56. Koch-Weser, J. Acetaminophen. *N. Engl. J. Med.* 295:1297, 1976.
57. Lipsky, B.A., and Hirschmann, J.V. Drug fever. *J.A.M.A.* 245:851, 1981.
58. Mackowiak, P.A. Drug fever: Mechanisms, maxims and misconceptions. *Am. J. Med. Sci.* 294:275, 1987.
59. Anderson, J.A. Allergic reactions to drugs and biological agents. *J.A.M.A.* 268:2845, 1992.
60. Petersdorf, R.G., and Beeson, P.B. Fever of unexplained origin. Report on 100 cases. *Medicine* (Baltimore) 40:1, 1961. *Classic study. See update [63].*
61. Petersdorf, R.G. Fever of unknown origin. An old friend revisited [editorial]. *Arch. Intern. Med.* 152:21, 1992.
62. Durack, D.T., and Street, A.C. Fever of unknown origin—reexamined and redefined. *Curr. Clin. Top. Infect. Dis.* 11:35, 1991. *For a related review, see J.A. Gelfand and S.M. Wolff, Fever of Unknown Origin. In G.L. Mandell, J.E. Bennett, and R. Dolin (eds.), Principles and Practice of Infectious Disease (4th ed.). New York: Churchill Livingstone, 1995. Also see M.J. Arbo et al., Fever of nosocomial origin: Etiology, risk factors, and outcomes.* Am. J. Med. *95:505, 1993.*
62a. Mirales, P., et al. Fever of unknown origin in patients infected with the human immunodeficiency virus. *Clin. Infect. Dis.* 20:872, 1995. *Recent review of this topic. Report from Spain in which a cause of FUO in patients (with median CD4+ cell count, 71/mm³) was found in 44 of 50 patients. Tuberculosis,* Mycobacterium avium *complex infection, and visceral leishmaniasis were the most frequent diagnoses. Examination of lymph node aspirates, bone marrow biopsy, and*

culture of clinical specimens for mycobacteria were the procedures with the highest diagnostic yield. Study also points out that visceral leishmaniasis has been a frequent cause of FUO where such infection is prevalent.

63. Larson, E.B., Featherstone, H.J., and Petersdorf, R.G. Fever of undetermined origin: Diagnosis and follow-up of 105 cases, 1970–1980. *Medicine* (Baltimore) 61:269, 1982.
    Follow-up study of FUO by the author who standardized the concept. Compares these results with original study 30 years ago.

64. Knockaert, D.C., Vanneste, L.J., Vanneste, S.B., and Bobbaers, H.J. Fever of unknown origin in the 1980's. *Arch. Intern. Med.* 152:51, 1992.
    Most recent update of the diagnostic spectrum of FUOs.

65. Barbado, F.J., et al. Pyrexia of unknown origin: Changing spectrum of diseases in two consecutive series. *Postgrad. Med. J.* 68:884, 1992.

66. Wolff, S.M., Fauci, A.S., and Dale, D.C. Unusual etiologies of fever and their evaluation. *Annu. Rev. Med.* 26:277, 1975.
    A discussion of less obvious, or infrequent, causes of FUOs. A few rare causes not included in Chap. 1 of this text are discussed.

67. Mackowiak, P.A., et al. Dissecting aortic aneurysm manifested as fever of unknown origin. *J.A.M.A.* 236:1725, 1976.

68. Kerttula, Y., Hirvonen, P., and Petterson, I. Fever of unknown origin: A follow-up investigation of 34 patients. *Scand. J. Infect. Dis.* 15:185, 1983.

69. Weinstein, L. Clinically benign fever of unknown origin: A personal retrospective. *Rev. Infect. Dis.* 7:692, 1985.
    An expert's expert highlights benign causes of FUO and offers clues in identifying these individuals.

70. Knockaert, D.C., Vanneste, L.J., and Bobbaers, H.J. Recurrent or episodic fever of unknown origin. *Medicine* 72:184, 1993.
    Details of 45 cases with a literature survey. A slightly different slant on the classic FUO description, but the vast majority of patients did well.

71. Kazanjian, P.H. Fever of unknown origin: Review of patients treated in community hospitals. *Clin. Infect. Dis.* 15:968, 1992.
    This study, which was carried out from 1984 through 1990, updates our understanding of FUOs in the community hospital setting.

72. Goetz, M.B. Fever of unknown origin in the elderly. *Infect. Dis. Clin. Pract.* 2:377, 1993.

73. Cunha, B.A. Commentary: FUO in the elderly. *Infect. Dis. Clin. Pract.* 2:380, 1993.

74. Aduan, R.P., et al. Factitious fever and self-induced infection. A report of 32 cases and review of the literature. *Ann. Intern. Med.* 90:230, 1979.
    Discusses nature of underlying psychiatric illnesses.

75. Murray, H.W., et al. Urinary temperature: A clue to early diagnosis of factitious fever. *N. Engl. J. Med.* 296:23, 1977.
    An easy and reliable method of diagnosing factitious fever.

76. Knockaert, D.C. Diagnostic strategy for fever of unknown origin in the ultrasonography and computed tomography era. *Acta Clin. Belg.* 47:100, 1992.
    A detailed and logical approach to the diagnosis of FUOs.

77. Thell, R., Martin, F.H., and Edwards, J.E. Bacterial endocarditis in subjects 60 years of age and older. *Circulation* 51:174, 1975.
    Almost 33% of these patients had no obvious murmurs.

78. Aronson, M.D., and Bor, D.H. Blood cultures. *Ann. Intern. Med.* 106:246, 1987.

79. Pesanti, E.L., and Smith, I.M. Infective endocarditis with negative blood cultures. An analysis of 52 cases. *Am. J. Med.* 66:43, 1979.
    Although this is a retrospective study, there were autopsy data for approximately half the cases.

80. Simon, H.B., and Wolff, S.M. Granulomatous hepatitis and prolonged fever of unknown origin: A study of 13 patients. *Medicine* (Baltimore) 52:1, 1973.
    A detailed report with a comprehensive discussion. See related discussion by W.C. Maddrey, Granulomatous Liver Disease: Clinical Aspects. In L.B. Schiff and J.H. Lewis (eds.). Current Perspectives in Hepatology. New York: Plenum, 1989. Pp. 309–326; and by J.S. Sartin and R.C. Walker. Granulomatous hepatitis: A retrospective review of 88 cases at the Mayo Clinic. Mayo Clin. Proc. 66:914, 1991.

81. Thompson, N.J., et al. The booster phenomenon in serial tuberculin testing. *Am. Rev. Respir. Dis.* 119:587, 1979.

82. Ghose, M.K., Shensa, S., and Lerner, P.I. Arteritis of the aged (giant cell arteritis) and fever of unexplained origin. *Am. J. Med.* 60:429, 1976.
    Emphasizes that temporal arteritis may occur without classic signs and symptoms.

83. Cronin, R.E., et al. Renal cell carcinoma: Unusual systemic manifestations. *Medicine* (Baltimore) 55:291, 1976.
    Fever occurs in 16–68% of patients with these tumors.
84. Simon, H.B., Weinstein, A.J., Pasternack, M.S., et al. Genitourinary tuberculosis. Clinical features in a general hospital population. *Am. J. Med.* 63:410, 1977.
85. Wegener, W.A., and Alavi, A. Diagnostic imaging of musculoskeletal infection. *Orthoped. Clin. North Am.* 22:401, 1991.
86. Fineman, D.S., et al. Detection of abnormalities in febrile AIDS patients with In-111-labeled leukocytes and Ga-67 scintigraphy. *Radiology* 170:677, 1989.
87. Knockaert, D.C., Mortelmans, L.A., Deroo, M.C., and Bobbaers, H.J. Clinical value of Gallium-67 scintigraphy in the investigation of fever or inflammation of unknown origin in the ultrasound and computed tomography era. *Acta Clin. Belg.* 44:91, 1989.
88. Jacobsen, A.F., Harley, J.D., Lipsky, B.A., and Pecoraro, R.E. Diagnosis of osteomyelitis in the presence of soft-tissue infection and radiologic evidence of osseous abnormalities: Value of leukocyte scintigraphy. *Am. J. Radiol.* 157:807, 1991.
89. Davies, S.G., and Garvie, M.W. The role of Indium-labelled leukocyte imaging in pyrexia of unknown origin. *Br. J. Radiol.* 63:850, 1990.
90. McAfee, J.G., Gagne, G., Subramanian, G., and Schneider, R.F. The localization of Indium-111-leukocytes, Gallium-67-polyclonal IgG and other radioactive agents in acute focal inflammatory lesions. *J. Nucl. Med.* 32:2126, 1991.
91. Rowland, M.D., and Del Bene, V. Use of body computed tomography to evaluate fever of unknown origin. *J. Infect. Dis.* 156:408, 1987.
92. McNeil, B.J., et al. A prospective study of computed tomography, ultrasound, and gallium imaging in patients with fever. *Radiology* 139:647, 1981.
93. Weinstein, L. Bacterial hepatitis: A case report on an unrecognized cause of fever of unknown origin. *N. Engl. J. Med.* 299:1052, 1978.
94. Van Der Meer, J.W.M., et al. Hyperimmunoglobulinaemia D and periodic fever: A new syndrome. *Lancet* 1:1087, 1984.
94a. Roland, W.E., et al. Ehrlichiosis: A cause of prolonged fever. *Clin. Infect. Dis.* 20:821, 1995.
    Authors conclude that ehrlichiosis should be considered for patients with FUO and in particular for those with a history of tick exposure in an endemic area. Polymerase chain reaction (PCR) of blood and / or serologic titers were used to make the diagnosis. Patients responded to doxycycline therapy. See also Appendix A.
95. Rothman, D.L., Schwarts, S.I., and Adams, J.T. Diagnostic laparotomy for fever or abdominal pain of unknown origin. *Am. J. Surg.* 133:273, 1977.
    Positive findings on laparotomy of 21 of 24 FUO patients who were thoroughly investigated preoperatively.
96. Greenall, M.J., Gough, M.H., and Kettlewell, M.G. Laparotomy in the investigation of patients with pyrexia of unknown origin. *Br. J. Surg.* 70:356, 1983.
    Supports the study of Rothman et al. [95]. Laparoscopy may be a useful prelude to laparotomy and, in some instances, may obviate laparotomy.
97. Henning, H. Value of laparoscopy in investigating fever of unexplained origin. *Endoscopy* 24:687, 1992.

2

Bacteremia and Sepsis

Nancy Epifano Hughes
and David V. Alcid

A positive blood culture is a common problem in hospitalized patients. In a large series reported in 1987, of 29,542 inpatient blood cultures, 9.7% were positive [1]. It is estimated that 30% of patients with true bacteremia will die because of the bacteremia or associated complications [2].

This chapter reviews the pathogenesis and pathophysiology of bacteremia as well as the epidemiology of both nosocomial and community-acquired bacteremia, plans a rational approach to the patient with sepsis of unknown etiology or septic shock and the leukopenic patient with fever, and briefly considers selected gram-positive and gram-negative bacteremias and bacteremias in specific clinical situations.

General Concepts

I. **Definitions**
   A. **Bacteremia** means the presence of viable bacteria in the blood as demonstrated by a positive blood culture. (False positive blood cultures are discussed later [see sec. I under Positive Blood Cultures]). A patient with bacteremia may or may not have symptoms and may have only a low-grade temperature. The duration of bacteremia has direct clinical implications in terms of identifying both the source of bacteremia and the duration of antibiotic therapy.
      1. **Transient bacteremias** are common. The precise duration of a transient bacteremia is poorly defined. Most bacteremias following dental extraction and endoscopy last only 5–15 minutes. Thus, it is reasonable to think of a transient bacteremia as **lasting for several minutes**, not several hours or days. Transient bacteremias occur in diseases such as bacterial pneumonia, meningitis, and pyelonephritis, and in nondisease states such as chewing, toothbrushing, instrumentation, or manipulation of various infected mucosal sites (see Chap. 28B under Prevention of Bacterial Endocarditis).
      2. **Sustained or continuous bacteremias** are defined by multiple positive blood cultures obtained over several hours to several days. These are suggestive of an intravascular source (infected artery, vein, arteriovenous shunt, or heart valve). In the setting of poor host defense, occasional extravascular infections (e.g., abdominal abscess) may cause continuous bacteremia.
      3. **Intermittent bacteremias** are defined as those in which blood cultures are intermittently positive (without therapy); they are recurrent transient bacteremias. This suggests intermittent obstruction of an infected site (e.g., biliary or genitourinary) or intermittent manipulation of an extravascular source.
   B. **Sepsis—new definitions.** A recent consensus conference of the American College of Chest Physicians and the Society of Critical Care Medicine resulted in a useful framework of definitions and criteria for the disease states and physiologic alterations formerly and variously termed *septicemia, sepsis syndrome, septic shock,* and *organ failure* [3].
      1. **Systemic inflammatory response syndrome (SIRS).** This syndrome is a set of acute physiologic responses to any of various insults, infectious or noninfectious. SIRS may occur as the result of burns, trauma, pancreatitis, or other noninfectious severe insults (Fig. 2-1). SIRS is defined by the presence of two or more of the following clinical manifestations:

Revised from M.A. Foltzer and R.E. Reese, Bacteremia and Sepsis. In R.E. Reese and R.F. Betts (eds). *A Practical Approach to Infectious Diseases* (3rd ed.). Boston: Little, Brown, 1991.

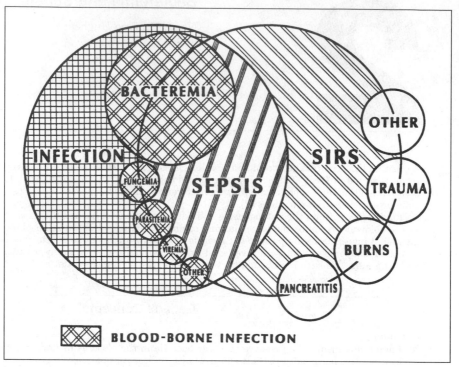

Fig. 2-1. The interrelationship between systemic inflammatory response syndrome (*SIRS*), sepsis, and infection. (From R. C. Bone et al., Definitions for sepsis organ failure and guidelines for the use of innovative therapies in sepsis. *Chest* 101:1644, 1992.)

  a. Temperature less than 36°C or greater than 38°C.
  b. Pulse rate greater than 90 bpm.
  c. Respiratory rate greater than 20 per minute or hyperventilation as shown by a $PaCO_2$ of less than 32 mm Hg.
  d. A white blood cell count less than 4,000/mm³ or greater than 12,000/mm³, or greater than 10% immature polymorphonuclear leukocytes.
 2. Sepsis. If SIRS is caused by infection, then the syndrome is called *sepsis.* Thus, the clinical manifestations just listed apply for the definitions of sepsis.
 3. Septic shock is sepsis with hypotension (systolic blood pressure of < 90 mm Hg or a reduction of > 40 mm Hg from baseline) despite adequate fluid resuscitation. Perfusion abnormalities are present and may result in lactic acidosis, oliguria, or acute alteration of mental status. Perfusion abnormalities may persist after a patient has been rendered normotensive by the administration of inotropes or pressor agents.
 4. Severe sepsis is sepsis with organ dysfunction, hypotension, or hypoperfusion abnormalities included but not limited to those listed in **3.** This represents a definable phase in the disease continuum from sepsis to septic shock.
 5. Multiple organ dysfunction syndrome (MODS) is altered organ function requiring intervention for the preservation of homeostasis. Although MODS may develop as a primary process following, for example, trauma with lung injury or rhabdomyolysis with acute renal failure, with regard to sepsis, MODS occurs in response to the systemic inflammatory response to infection. (See Septic Shock.)
 II. Pathogenesis of bacteremia. Intravascular sources—endocarditis, infection of arteriovenous shunt, vein, or artery, and intravascular catheters—inoculate the bloodstream directly. **Extravascular sources**—wound, abscess, pneumonia, and manipulation—seed the blood via lymphatic drainage [4]. In the latter, bacteremia occurs when regional lymph node function is overwhelmed by excessive bacteria reaching the node, increased perfusion pressure of the lymphatics (pressure of edema or manipulation

of the area), or involvement by unusually virulent organisms. Focal extravascular containment of infection requires circulating neutrophil influx. Ingestion and killing often are augmented by immunoglobulin or complement, or both. If bacteremia occurs, macrophages in the liver and spleen phagocytize the bacteria. Bacteria opsonized by IgG are cleared primarily by the spleen, whereas bacteria to which C3b is bound are cleared primarily by the liver. Circulating granulocytes are not effective scavengers of intravascular bacteria. Thus, successful containment of infection requires local defenses based primarily in the activation of granulocyte phagocytosis backed by the local lymphatic macrophage. Clearing of bacteremia is enhanced by functional immunoglobulin and complement, which act largely as opsonins in the efficient phagocytosis by splenic and hepatic macrophages.

III. **Pathophysiology of bacteremias.** The **manifestations of bacteremia** are varied; all organ systems may be involved (Table 2-1). Although gram-negative organisms more commonly produce septic shock, **it is not possible, on the basis of clinical presentation, to differentiate between gram-positive and gram-negative bacteremias** (see under Sepsis of Unknown Etiology and Septic Shock for more discussion).

After bacteria or endotoxin is introduced, a period of active cytokine (tumor necrosis factor [TNF], interleukin-1 [IL-1]) synthesis precedes the appearance of fever (30–90 minutes). Therefore, a blood culture drawn at the time of fever spike may be clear (transient bacteremia), whereas one drawn an hour earlier might have contained bacteria. **Blood cultures drawn before the temperature spike and rigor may have the highest yield.**

IV. **Epidemiology of bacteremias.** Gram-negative bacteria continue to be the leading cause of nosocomial bacteremia. More recently, studies show an increased incidence of gram-positive nosocomial bacteremia [5, 6].

   A. **Organisms involved.** Table 2-2 summarizes the current trend of nosocomial bacteremia in the United States [6]. A rise in the incidence of all gram-positive infections is apparent. Several points are noteworthy:

   1. Except as reported for small nonteaching hospitals, **coagulase-negative staphylococci** were responsible for the greatest increase in bloodstream infections. This may be related to the more common use of intravascular devices or to greater surveillance for bacteremia with more frequent blood culture collection and reporting of the organism as a pathogen rather than a contaminant [6].

Table 2-1. Manifestations of sepsis

Common	Less common or seen only in severe sepsis
Fever, rigors, myalgias	Hypothermia
Tachycardia	Shock
Tachypnea (respiratory alkalosis)	Lactic acidosis
Hypoxemia	Adult respiratory distress syndrome
Proteinuria	
Leukocytosis (left shift, toxic granules, Döhle bodies)	Azotemia, oliguria
	Leukopenia, leukemoid reaction
Eosinopenia	Thrombocytopenia
Hypoferremia	Disseminated intravascular coagulation
Irritability, lethargy	
Mild liver function abnormalities	Anemia
Hyperglycemia in diabetics	Stupor, coma*
	Overt upper gastrointestinal tract bleeding
	Cutaneous lesions
	Funduscopic lesions
	Hypoglycemia

*See L. A. Eidelman et al., The spectrum of septic encephalopathy. *J.A.M.A.* 275:470, 1996.
Source: R. L. Harris et al. Manifestations of sepsis. *Arch. Intern. Med.* 147:1895, 1987. Copyright 1987, American Medical Association.

Table 2-2. Percentage increase in primary bloodstream infection rates, 1980–1989, in the United States as reported to the Centers for Disease Control[a]

	Small teaching hospital[b] (%)	Large teaching hospital[b] (%)
Coagulase-negative staphylococci	424	754
Candida species	219	487
Enterococci	197	120
S. aureus	122	176
Aerobic gram-negative organisms	19	−1

[a]From data reported by National Nosocomial Infectious Surveillance (NNIS) System hospitals.
[b]All the increases during 1980–1989 were highly significant ($p < .0001$) except for the nonsignificant changes in rates due to gram-negative bacilli.
Source: Adapted from S. N. Bannerjee et al., Secular trends in nosocomial primary bloodstream infections in the United States, 1980–1989. *Am. J. Med.* 91(Suppl. 3B):885, 1991.

2. **Gram-negative bacteremias** remain the major nosocomial infectious problem. The most common isolates are the Enterobacteriaceae (*Escherichia coli* and *Klebsiella, Serratia, Enterobacter,* and *Proteus* spp.).
3. **Fungemias** also are occurring more frequently, with increased reporting of blood cultures positive for *Candida* spp.
B. **Community-acquired bacteremias** are most commonly attributable to *E. coli* (22%), *Streptococcus pneumoniae* (16%), and *Staphylococcus aureus* (12%) [7].
C. Multivariate analysis of **factors associated with the highest mortality** include a respiratory tract source, nosocomial infection, hypotension, isolation of enterococci or fungi, gram-negative bacteremia, body temperature lower than 38°C, age greater than 40 years, and underlying illness such as cirrhosis or malignancy [2]. A possible explanation for poor prognosis with enterococcal bacteremia is that only the most compromised hosts or those previously treated with multiple antibiotics develop enterococcemia.

Sepsis of Unknown Etiology

In the emergency room or hospital, the physician often is confronted with a patient with the initial diagnosis of sepsis [7a]. Because the mortality of known cases of bacteremia is high, especially with gram-negative and staphylococcal infections, a rapid yet meticulous approach is needed.

I. **Ruling out a primary site of infection.** The initial history, physical examination, and screening laboratory tests (blood count, urinalysis, chest x-ray, sputum Gram stain, and Gram stains of any exudates) are performed in hopes of establishing a primary site of infection. Some patients will have an obvious focus (e.g., pneumonia, pyelonephritis, cellulitis, wound infection, or postpartum infection). **If such a primary source can be identified, therapy can be directed to the likely organisms.** Even after a careful initial evaluation, the source of infection may be unclear. **The patient is said to have sepsis of unclear etiology only if the initial evaluation does not yield an obvious focus.**
   A. **Leukopenic patients may not have the usual manifestations of a primary focus of infection.** These patients are discussed separately under Fever in the Leukopenic Patient.
   B. **A second look.** Special additional steps will need to be taken to evaluate further those patients in whom there is no obvious focus. Physical findings change, and so **repeated examination is very important.**
II. **Further evaluation.** A careful approach to sepsis of unclear etiology is important so that the physician can provide optimal treatment rather than just routinely obtaining a culture from the patient and beginning a combination of antibiotics—for example, an aminoglycoside and a cephalosporin. Although this combination may cover many organisms, it may not be optimal for some organisms such as *Pseudomonas,* staphylococci, enterococci, *Bacteroides fragilis,* or meningococci. If such organisms are highly

suspected, different antibiotics or combinations may provide better therapy and improve the prognosis for the patient.

Gram-negative, gram-positive, and fungal bloodstream infections may all have a similar clinical presentation, so the presentation itself cannot distinguish the general type of organism. Nevertheless, certain aspects of the workup may provide clues as to the potential pathogens.

A. **History**
   1. **Community- versus hospital-acquired infections.** In the hospitalized or recently hospitalized patient, the organisms causing the bacteremia may be more resistant. This affects the choice of antibiotics, particularly aminoglycosides, depending on the resistance patterns at one's local hospital.
   2. **Prior or current medications.** If the patient has been using antipyretics, the temperature curve may be suppressed or otherwise affected. Recent intake of oral or parenteral antibiotics may preclude positive cultures as well as select out more resistant bacteria. Medications may cause a sepsislike picture (e.g., drug fever with quinidine use). Corticosteroids and nonsteroidal antiinflammatory drugs may mask the signs and symptoms of infection. Beta-blockers may give the impression of temperature-pulse disproportion (fever with relative bradycardia).
   3. **Recent manipulations or surgery.** A history of recent cystoscopy, dental extraction, wound manipulation, intravenous or hyperalimentation line placement, or attempted abortion may be important in determining the pathogenesis of the sepsis.
   4. **Underlying diseases** may predispose the patient to particular problems or organisms.
      a. **Underlying heart disease,** such as rheumatic heart disease and congenital valvular lesions, should raise concern about endocarditis.
      b. **Splenectomized patients** are particularly prone to fulminant infections due to *Haemophilus influenzae, Neisseria meningitidis,* or *S. pneumoniae* (see sec. III.F under Positive Blood Cultures).
      c. **Intraabdominal sepsis** may be of particular concern in patients with inflammatory or other known bowel or biliary tract disease. The potential role of anaerobes, particularly *B. fragilis,* may affect selection of specific antibiotic therapy.
      d. **The potential of a septic abortion or pelvic infection** should be considered as mixed aerobic and anaerobic infections are common.
      e. **Intravenous drug abuse** predisposes to infection with staphylococci and gram-negative bacilli.
      f. **Immunocompromised patients** are at particular risk for nosocomial pathogens and fungi (see Fever in the Leukopenic Patient).
   5. **Travel history** may be important to alert the physician to unusual diseases that may have a septic presentation such as Rocky Mountain spotted fever [8] (endemic areas include North Carolina, Virginia, and the mid-Southeastern states), babesiosis (acquired in Nantucket, Martha's Vineyard, Shelter Island, Long Island), malaria, or infection with *Vibrio* spp. (e.g., exposure to raw oysters or salt water), typhoid fever, or the like [9].
B. **Physical examination: further clues.** If the initial examination did not reveal an obvious primary focus of infection, further information must be sought.
   1. **Skin.** Meticulous serial inspections may provide some clues initially missed.
      a. **Furuncles** or intravenous drug abuse marks should be sought.
      b. **Intravenous sites** should be carefully inspected. Approximately one-half of patients with intravenous-related sepsis will have clinically evident phlebitis. Any peripheral plastic catheter in place for more than 48–72 hours is suspect in the septic patient.
      c. **Rash.** A characteristic rash may provide a clue to the underlying bacteremia [10]. The rash of an acutely ill, febrile patient can provide a clue to the underlying diagnosis. Table 2-3 summarizes some of the diagnoses associated with certain types of rashes. The reader is referred to an excellent series of color photographs and clinical descriptions of these entities in references [11, 11a] and, for further reading on rashes and bacterial infections in children, the book *Infectious Diseases of Children* by Krugman and colleagues [12].

Table 2-3. Rash and fever in the acutely ill febrile patient: Diagnosis according to lesion type

Purpuric macules, purpuric papules, or purpuric vesicles	Vesicles, bullae, or pustules	Macules or papules
Bacteremias	Varicella (chickenpox)	Drug hypersensitivities
Meningococcemia	Generalized herpes zoster	Scarlet fever
Gonococcemia	Disseminated herpes simplex	Kawasaki disease
Staphylococcemia	Enterovirus infections	Viral exanthems (measles, infectious mononucleosis,
Pseudomonas	Toxic epidermal necrolysis	ECHO virus, coxsackievirus, and varicella)
Bacterial endocarditis	Erythema multiforme	Secondary syphilis
Drug hypersensitivities	Drug hypersensitivities	Erythema multiforme
Enterovirus infections (ECHO virus, and coxsackievirus)	Bacteremias	Erythema marginatum
Rickettsial diseases	Meningococcemia	SLE
Rocky Mountain spotted fever	*Pseudomonas* bacteremia	Serum sickness
Typhus (louse-borne)	Staphylococcal bacteremia	Allergic vasculitis with urticaria
Allergic vasculitis	Bacterial endocarditis	TSS and SSSS
Acquired immunodeficiency syndrome (AIDS)	Erysipelas	AIDS
Systemic lupus erythematosus (SLE)	SLE	Rickettsial disease (e.g., Rocky Mountain spotted fever)
	Staphylococcal scalded skin syndrome (SSSS)	Typhoid fever
	Staphylococcal toxic shock syndrome (TSS)	Lyme disease (erythema chronicum migrans)
		Bacteremias
		Meningococcemia
		Bacterial endocarditis
		Toxic epidermal necrolysis

Source: Adapted from T. B. Fitzpatrick and R. A. Johnson, Differential Diagnosis of Rashes in the Acutely Ill Febrile Patient and in Life-Threatening Diseases. In T. B. Fitzpatrick et al. (eds.), *Dermatology in General Medicine* (3rd ed.). New York: McGraw-Hill, 1987. Atlas 3, pp. A21–A30. (See also related discussion in reference [11a].)

(1) **Meningococcemia** can present with a fulminant course over several hours. Initially, the rash may be macular or petechial, but it may appear ecchymotic or purpuric, and this implies a worse prognosis. Scrapings of these skin lesions may demonstrate gram-negative diplococci on Gram stain (see Plate I A–D).

(2) **Disseminated gonococcal infections** may present with distal extremity (fingers and fingertips), petechial, pustular, papular, or hemorrhagic lesions (see Plate I F and G and Chap. 13).

(3) *Pseudomonas* **bacteremias** occasionally can present with what were previously believed to be characteristic lesions, **ecthyma gangrenosum** (see Plate III B). These oval or round lesions have a rim of erythema and induration, and the center may go on to ulcerate. Other bacteremias, such as *Aeromonas hydrophila,* can present with similar lesions.

(4) *S. aureus* **bacteremia** may mimic the skin lesion of meningococcemia.

(5) **Candidemias** can present with raised, discrete, pink-red skin nodules (see Plate III A). A punch biopsy of these lesions will demonstrate the pathogen. (See under Candidiasis in Chap. 18.)

d. **Peripheral stigmata of bacterial endocarditis** (e.g., splinter hemorrhages, Osler nodes) are present only in a minority of patients (fewer than 30%), so their absence in a given patient does not rule out this diagnosis. However, subconjunctival hemorrhages are more common.

e. **Jaundice** of abrupt onset, particularly in the compromised host or patient with a wound infection, may be seen in clostridial sepsis with hemolysis. Acute biliary tract obstruction must also be considered. Jaundice is, however, a nonspecific finding in sepsis of any etiology [13].

2. **Head examination.** A head, eyes, ear, nose, and throat (HEENT) examination may reveal local infection that may provide a focus for an unsuspected meningitis (i.e., chronic ear infections or sinus infection), although initial physical examination should have raised the possibility of a localized CNS infection. Funduscopy may reveal the retinal changes seen in systemic candidemia, as discussed in Chap. 18.

3. **Heart.** A careful baseline cardiac examination is important for purposes of comparison, in case a murmur develops or changes. The absence of a murmur does not exclude the diagnosis of bacterial endocarditis, particularly in the patient older than 60 years. A murmur of underlying rheumatic heart disease will make one more suspicious of possible endocarditis in the septic patient.

4. **Lungs.** The lungs initially may sound clear in the elderly, dehydrated patient with an early pneumonia. With hydration and time, rales may become audible, and an infiltrate may become obvious on chest roentgenography. The compromised host may show minimal findings on lung examination but may have an abnormal chest x-ray.

5. **Abdomen and rectal and pelvic examination.** In the septic patient who is an unreliable informant or who is unable to give a history, **the abdominal scar of a splenectomy** should be sought. Localized abdominal findings may be subtle in the elderly or in patients on steroids.

   In addition to a routine abdominal examination, rectal and pelvic examinations are very important. A rectal abscess may be a primary source of infection in patients with inflammatory bowel disease or in leukopenic patients. Both the rectal and pelvic examinations should have been done earlier in the workup when one was trying to exclude a primary focus but, on occasion, these examinations may have been deferred initially in the septic patient.

6. **Extremities.** The physician should look for any evidence of a phlebitis with associated pulmonary emboli that could explain the patient's hypotension, elevated respiratory rate, or fever. A full skeletal evaluation should include **examination for point tenderness over the spine for the possibility of osteomyelitis** (see Chap. 16).

7. **CNS.** Obtundation may be seen in the septic patient without CNS infection, **especially the elderly.** In the febrile, toxic patient seen because of a cerebrovascular accident, the possibility of bacterial endocarditis presenting primarily with neurologic findings must be considered (see Chap. 10 under Infective Endocarditis). A lumbar puncture should be performed if there is any suspicion of CNS infection.

8. **Wounds.** Foul-smelling wounds or exudates may suggest anaerobic infections. Although gas in the subcutaneous tissue or muscle can suggest a clostridial

infection, this is usually a relatively late finding in true *Clostridium perfringens* myonecrosis. Other organisms can also cause soft-tissue gas, among them *Klebsiella* spp., *E. coli,* anaerobic streptococci, and *Bacteroides* spp. (see Chap. 4 under Anaerobic Soft-Tissue Infections).

C. **Special laboratory tests.** Much of the preliminary laboratory work is undertaken during the search for a focal infection. The blood count may show signs of a bacterial infection (e.g., a left shift, toxic granulation, Döhle bodies, or fragmented red blood cells suggestive of disseminated intravascular coagulation [DIC]). Thrombocytopenia is commonly seen in sepsis, especially involving gram-negative organisms, in the absence of DIC.

1. **Blood cultures are essential** for making a specific etiologic diagnosis and for helping to determine the duration of a given bacteremia. **Multiple blood cultures** should be obtained. In the critically ill patient, **two to three blood cultures should be drawn 15–20 minutes apart,** before any medications are given. Multiple separate blood cultures will help determine the type of the bacteremia (transient versus continuous), which may, in turn, determine the duration of antibiotic therapy. At least 20–30 ml of blood per venipuncture in the adult patient is the optimal volume of blood for increased yield [14].

   If fungi are highly likely (compromised host or hyperalimentation-related sepsis), special media may be available from the microbiology laboratory that will increase the yield of fungal blood cultures, although *Candida* spp. often will grow in routine blood culture media (see Chaps. 18 and 25).

2. **Skin lesion aspirates or biopsy.** Skin lesions should be aspirated, Gram-stained, and cultured. This approach may be especially helpful in identifying disseminated gonorrhea and meningococcal or staphylococcal infections. A punch biopsy of the maculopapular lesion of disseminated candidemia can be diagnostic (see Chap. 18).

3. **Review of recent culture data.** For the hospitalized, or recently hospitalized, patient, there may be available recent culture data suggesting a potential pathogen, or antibiotic resistance may be apparent on susceptibility data.

4. **Liver and renal function testing** will be important because the results may affect antibiotic choices and doses.

D. **Initial therapy.** If an obvious focus cannot be identified in the septic- or bacteremic-appearing patient, empiric antibiotics are initiated after cultures have been obtained. Regimens should include activity against common isolates [7a, 15].

1. Table 2-4 summarizes common initial regimens [15a].
   a. **Bactericidal agents and synergistic combinations** are used whenever possible.
   b. The **intravenous** route should be used to ensure adequate serum antibiotic levels.
   c. In **renal failure,** the standard initial dose of antibiotics can be given. Subsequent doses may need modification, depending on the antibiotic used (see Chap. 28).
   d. **New antibiotics. Imipenem-cilastatin** has the potential for monotherapy because of its broad spectrum of activity. **Aztreonam** may be an alternative to the aminoglycoside in combination therapy (see Chap. 28 for a discussion).

2. **Monitor** the patient for signs of septic shock.

3. Antibiotic regimens can be altered appropriately when susceptibility data become available for the blood isolate.

Septic Shock

Despite ongoing advances in our understanding of the pathogenetic mechanisms that produce sepsis and septic shock, septic shock ranks first as a cause of death in intensive care units, with a mortality from 30 to 70%. Some trends that have contributed to the rise in the incidence of sepsis are the increasingly common use of invasive devices and immunosuppressive agents and the increased life span of chronically ill populations [16].

I. **Pathogenesis.** The first step is invasion of the bloodstream by the organism from the infectious source. The response to this invasion is the production of a vast array of endogenous mediators resulting in circulatory dysregulation with attendant organ

Table 2-4. Empiric regimens in suspected bacteremias or sepsis syndrome in various settings

Setting	Organisms highly suspected	Therapy (adult doses, normal renal function)[a]
Leukopenia without an obvious focal infection	Enteric gram-negative bacilli, Pseudomonas species	Antipseudomonas penicillin (e.g., piperacillin 3 g q4h or 4 g q6h) or similar agent and an aminoglycoside[b-d]
	Gram-positive cocci (if a Hickman line-related infection is present or highly suspicious)	Vancomycin can be added[d,e]
Rheumatic or congenital heart disease with possible endocarditis	S. aureus, viridans streptococci, and enterococci	Penicillin (2–3 million units q4h) or ampicillin 1.5 g q4h, low-dose gentamicin, and cefazolin 1 g q6h[f]
Prosthetic cardiac valve endocarditis	S. epidermidis, streptococci, S. aureus	Vancomycin[e,g] and gentamicin[h]
Splenectomized patient, without an obvious focus	S. pneumoniae, H. influenzae	Ceftriaxone (2 g q24h) or ampicillin-sulbactam (3 g q6h)
Intra-arterial or intravenous or deep-line catheter (e.g., Hickman or Broviac catheter)	S. aureus, S. epidermidis, nosocomial gram-negatives, enterococci (fungi)	Vancomycin[e] ± nafcillin, and an aminoglycoside[b,i] until cultures are available
Underlying bowel disease (e.g., peritonitis)	Mixture of aerobic and anaerobic flora	Ceftriaxone[j,k] (2 g q24h) and metronidazole (15 mg/kg loading dose and then 7.5 mg/kg q6h IV)
		or
		cefotaxime[j,k], 2 g q8h, and metronidazole
		or[k]
		piperacillin-tazobactam or ampicillin-sulbactam with or without an aminoglycoside[b]
		or
		imipenem 500 mg–1 g q6–8h (see Chap. 28G)
Possible meningococcemia[l]	N. meningitidis	Aqueous penicillin (2 million units IV q2h); in the patient with a delayed penicillin allergy, ceftriaxone (2 g q12h); in the patient with an immediate severe reaction to penicillin, chloramphenicol (1g q6h)
No underlying focal infection Community-acquired 1. Mild to moderately ill patient	Community-acquired gram-negatives, occult S. aureus infection	Cefazolin[m] (1 g q6h)

Table 2-4 (continued)

No underlying infection		
Community-acquired (cont'd)		
2. Severely ill	Gram-positive cocci, gram-negative bacilli	A third-generation cephalosporin (e.g., ceftriaxone, 2 g q24h, or cefotaxime, 2 g q8h); a first-generation cephalosporin (e.g., cefazolin, 1 g q6h) and an aminoglycoside[b]; a semisynthetic penicillin (e.g., oxacillin, 1.5–2 g q4h) and an aminoglycoside[b]
	If enterococci are a concern, special considerations apply[j,k]	Imipenem (1 g q6–8h); ampicillin-sulbactam (3 g q6h) with or without gentamicin, or piperacillin-tazobactam, especially if enterococci are a concern[j]
Hospital-acquired	Gram-negative bacilli with *P. aeruginosa* a potential concern, gram-positive cocci, including methicillin-susceptible staphylococci	Piperacillin (3 g q4h or 4 g q6h), plus cefazolin (1 g q6–8h) plus an aminoglycoside[b,d,n], a third-generation cephalosporin[o] and an aminoglycoside[b]; ampicillin-sulbactam[o], ticarcillin-clavulanate[o] or piperacillin-tazobactam[o], and an aminoglycoside[b]; imipenem and an aminoglycoside
	Nosocomial gram-negative bacilli and methicillin-resistant staphylococci (e.g., line-related sepsis)	Vancomycin[e,p] and an aminoglycoside +/− piperacillin
Neonatal sepsis	See Chap. 3	

[a]For pediatric dosages and doses in renal failure, see individual discussions in Chap. 28.

[b]Usually tobramycin or gentamicin is used at 2.0 mg/kg/dose for 12–24 hr, and then 1.5 mg/kg/dose (see Chap. 28H for details). If gentamicin or tobramycin resistance is known or highly likely, amikacin is indicated, 15 mg/kg/day, with divided doses q8h. Ideally, aminoglycoside serum levels should be monitored (see Chap. 28H). Aztreonam (see Chap. 28G) can be substituted if it is desirable to avoid an aminoglycoside.

[c]Although ceftazidime is useful in the therapy of the stable febrile leukopenic patient without a focus of infection (see Chap. 28F), as is imipenem (see Chap. 28G), we do not favor the use of it as monotherapy in the septic- or bacteremic-appearing patient.

[d]Although gram-positive bacteria are increasing in frequency in this setting, they are less life-threatening than gram-negative bacteremias, and antibiotic therapy can be modified after culture and susceptibility data are available. Therefore, empiric vancomycin therapy is not routinely indicated (see Chap. 28O). If the patient with a central line has, on clinical evaluation, a probable or possible line-related infection, vancomycin should be added pending cultures.

[e]In patients with normal renal function, the usual starting dose of vancomycin is 1 g IV (slow infusion over 2 hr) q12h. See Chap. 28O for the details of dosing vancomycin. See also discussion of antistaphylococcal activity of vancomycin in Chap. 28O.

[f]This is a vigorous regimen: The penicillin-aminoglycoside or ampicillin-aminoglycoside combination is aimed at streptococci, including enterococci. The cefazolin provides activity against *S. aureus* and avoids using two penicillin agents (e.g., penicillin and oxacillin). Low-dose gentamicin is 1 mg/kg/dose. In the penicillin-allergic patient, vancomycin can be used with low-dose gentamicin to provide activity against streptococci, including enterococci and *S. aureus*. The role of monotherapy with ampicillin-sulbactam is unclear in this setting.

[g]Vancomycin is used empirically to ensure good activity against coagulase-negative staphylococci. In known or cases highly suspicious for early prosthetic valve endocarditis due to *S. epidermidis*, rifampin (300 mg PO q8h) is often added. See Chap. 10.

[h]In this setting, low-dose gentamicin, 1.0 mg/kg/dose, is used to help achieve synergy.

[i] If *Pseudomonas* species is a major concern in a Hickman- or deep-line catheter infection (e.g., tunnel infection), piperacillin (3 g q4h, or 4 g q6h) should be added to the aminoglycoside to provide synergy. The vancomycin can also be used while awaiting culture data.

[j] Although enterococci may be cultured from peritoneal fluid, in recent reviews of intra-abdominal infection, authors conclude enterococci are not usually pathogens. Therefore, therapy aimed at enterococci is usually not necessary. This topic is discussed and referenced in detail in Chap. 11 under Intra-abdominal Infection.

[k] In urosepsis (especially if the urine Gram stain shows gram-positive cocci suggesting enterococci) or in the critically ill patient with intra-abdominal sepsis in whom one wants to cover enterococci while awaiting cultures (see [j]), only certain antibiotics will be active against enterococci; e.g., ampicillin-aminoglycoside combinations, ampicillin-sulbactam, piperacillin, or piperacillin-sulbactam are active against most enterococci. (See Chap. 28H for a discussion of gentamicin-resistant enterococci and Chap. 28O for a discussion of vancomycin-resistant enterococci [VRE].) Imipenem is active against a majority of enterococci. Cephalosporins are not active in vivo against enterococci. In the penicillin-allergic patient, vancomycin can be used for enterococci (see Chap. 28O).

[l] The presentation and rash of toxic shock syndrome (TSS) may appear similar to meningococcemia. Since TSS initially needs supportive therapy primarily, while awaiting culture data it is critical to treat patients for life-threatening meningococcemia if this is in the differential diagnosis (see text).

[m] Cefazolin alone will cover *S. aureus*, most *S. pneumoniae*, and many community-acquired gram-negatives and may often be a reasonable agent in the patient who is not very ill.

[n] Piperacillin (ticarcillin)-aminoglycoside combinations provide synergistic activity against gram-negative bacteria, including *P. aeruginosa*. Cefazolin provides activity against methicillin-susceptible staphylococci and allows one to use a cephalosporin rather than an antistaphylococcal penicillin. Furthermore, which aminoglycoside is chosen may depend on hospital susceptibility data (see Chap. 28H and footnote [b]). Aztreonam can be substituted for an aminoglycoside. Since imipenem alone may not be adequate for pseudomonal bacteremia, we would not use it as monotherapy.

[o] Because many hospital-acquired gram-negative pathogens (e.g., *Enterobacter* species, *P. aeruginosa*, *Citrobacter* species) may be resistant to the third-generation cephalosporins or ampicillin-sulbactam, ticarcillin-clavulanate, or piperacillin-tazobactam, monotherapy with these agents for hospital-acquired sepsis is not advised. Ceftazidime has inadequate activity against staphylococci; ceftriaxone or cefotaxime has acceptable activity against methicillin-susceptible staphylococci while awaiting culture data. Ceftazidime can be used as an alternative to piperacillin in the patient with a delayed penicillin allergy.

[p] If methicillin-resistant staphylococci are a significant pathogen in your hospital, vancomycin is the agent of choice.

Source: Adapted from R. E. Reese and R. F. Betts (eds.), *Handbook of Antibiotics* (2nd ed.). Boston: Little, Brown, 1993. Pp. 600–603; and from Medical Letter. The choice of antibiotic drugs. *Med. Lett. Drugs Ther.* 36:53, 1994 with update 38:25, 1996.

dysfunction. These dysfunctions may include myocardial depression, renal or hepatic failure, adult respiratory distress syndrome (ARDS), DIC, and CNS depression [17] (Fig. 2-2).

A. **Inflammatory cascade.** A detailed discussion of this very active area of research is beyond the scope of this chapter.

B. The **proinflammatory cytokines TNF-α and IL-1** are produced in response to a bacterial (whole organism, component, or toxin) insult. TNF and IL-1 share many of the same biologic properties, including those that are beneficial to the host such as induction of fever and increased production as well as enhancement of phagocytic activity. Cytokines also induce hemodynamic compromise and stimulate release of other inflammatory mediators such as platelet-activating factor (PAF), leukotrienes, prostaglandins, and other interleukins. Cytokines together produce a given case of **SIRS** in a dynamic regulatory and counterregulatory fashion. The precise interplay of these various proteins has not been elucidated and is complicated by the differences in host susceptibility to these agents; host susceptibility probably determine what syndrome a particular patient will develop (sepsis, septic shock, SIRS, MODS) [18, 19].

II. **Continuum of sepsis.** Formerly, septic shock was divided into two phases, early (characterized by low systemic vascular resistance and normal or elevated cardiac output) and late (characterized by falling cardiac output and cellular metabolic failure, acidosis, and hypotension, which will not be volume-responsive as it may be earlier in the course of the disease). Current conventional wisdom, however, is to **view the septic states as occurring or progressing over continuum of severity.**

III. **Differential diagnosis of fever and shock. Patients presenting with fever and hypotension may not always have septic shock.** The initial evaluation usually will help exclude the following other possibilities.

A. **Purulent bacterial pericardial effusion.** This is likely to occur after open heart surgery, spreading from an adjacent pneumonia or empyema or seeding of a sterile effusion during bacteremia.

B. **Peritonitis.**

C. **Pneumonia with severe hypoxia.**

D. **Mediastinitis.** This may occur following esophageal manipulation (esophagoscopy, variceal sclerotherapy) or gunshot or stab wound.

E. **Anaphylaxis** induced by antibiotics prescribed for a known infection.

F. **Staphylococcal toxic shock syndrome** (TSS), a clinical syndrome first described in 1978 and initially seen **primarily** in menstruating women who use tampons. However, there has been a significant decrease in the number of cases of menstruation-related TSS over the last decade [20].

The syndrome is designated as either *menstrual* (MTSS) or *nonmenstrual* (NMTSS), depending on the clinical setting. Clinically, NMTSS occurs in a heterogeneous group of individuals with various clinical presentations other than those of the MTSS group. NMTSS frequently is associated with renal and CNS effects and fewer musculoskeletal complaints than is MTSS [21, 22].

1. **Pathogenesis. TSS is due to an exotoxin, TSST-1, usually produced by S. aureus,** that colonizes the vagina and cervix as well as other foci such as furuncles and surgical wounds. Bacteremia is not a necessary condition and rarely occurs.

2. **Clinical manifestations. TSS may complicate any focal staphylococcal infection.** The diagnosis is clinical, based on the criteria of the Centers for Disease Control (Table 2-5). Although isolation of *S. aureus* is not required, culture of blood, vagina, cervix, nares, urine, wound, and cerebrospinal fluid (CSF) should be obtained where indicated. The differential diagnosis includes meningococcemia, leptospirosis, Rocky Mountain spotted fever, scarlet fever, severe viral exanthem (measles), septic shock, and streptococcal TSS. Meningococcemia should be excluded initially, as none of the agents listed in sec. **3.b** is a drug of choice for *N. meningitidis.*

3. **Treatment**

a. **Initial therapy is supportive.** Antistaphylococcal therapy does not modify the initial course because the course usually is toxin-mediated, although bacteremia has occasionally been reported [23].

b. **Penicillinase-resistant antistaphylococcal therapy is useful in the prevention of relapse,** and the authors recommend oxacillin or nafcillin (e.g., in adults, 1.0–1.5 g IV q4h). A first-generation cephalosporin or vancomycin is used in the penicillin-allergic patient. Intravenous therapy for 1 week,

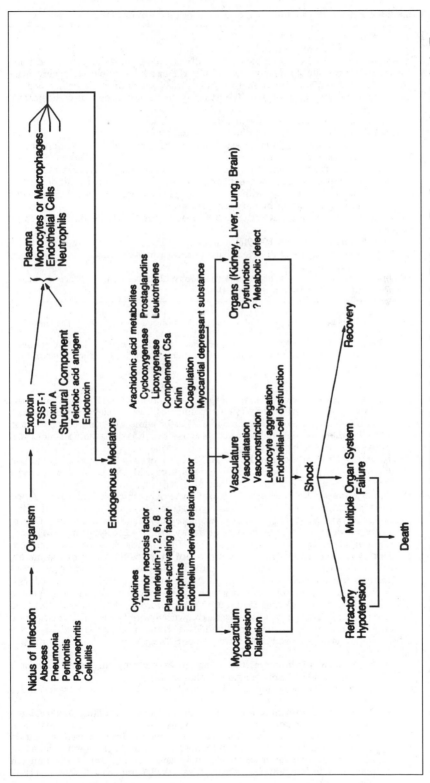

Fig. 2-2. Pathogenetic sequence of the events in septic shock. TSST-1 = toxic shock syndrome toxin; Toxin A = *Pseudomonas aeruginosa* toxin A. (From J. E. Parillo, Pathogenetic mechanisms of septic shock syndrome. Reprinted by permission of the *New England Journal of Medicine*, 328:1471, 1993.)

Table 2-5. Criteria for the diagnosis of toxic shock syndrome (TSS)

1. Fever: temperature $\geq$ 38.9°C (102°F)
2. Rash: diffuse macular erythroderma
3. Desquamation 1 to 2 weeks after onset of illness, particularly of palms and soles
4. Hypotension: systolic blood pressure $\leq$ 90 mm Hg for adults or below fifth percentile by age for children younger than 16 years; orthostatic drop in diastolic blood pressure $\geq$ 15 mm Hg from lying to sitting, orthostatic syncope, or orthostatic dizziness
5. Multisystem involvement—three or more of the following:
    Gastrointestinal: vomiting or diarrhea at onset of illness
    Muscular: severe myalgia or creatine phosphokinase level fivefold the upper limit of normal for laboratory
    Mucous membrane: vaginal, oropharyngeal, or conjunctival hyperemia
    Renal: blood urea nitrogen or creatinine at least twice the upper limit of normal for laboratory or urinary sediment with pyuria ($\geq$ 5 leukocytes per high-power field) in the absence of urinary tract infection
    Hepatic: total bilirubin, SGOT, SGPT at least twice the upper limit of normal for laboratory
    Hematologic: platelets $\leq$ 100,000/mm^3
    Central nervous system: disorientation or alterations in consciousness without focal neurologic signs
6. Negative results of the serologic tests for Rocky Mountain spotted fever, leptospirosis, and measles (when indicated)

SGOT = serum aspartate transaminase; SGPT = serum alanine transaminase.
Source: Adapted from A. L. Reingold et al., Toxic shock syndrome surveillance in the United States, 1980–1981. *Ann. Intern. Med.* 96 (pt. 2):875, 1982; and from F. A. Waldvogel, *Staphylococcus aureus* (including toxic shock syndrome). In G. L. Mandell, J. E. Bennett, and R. Dolin (eds.), *Principles and Practice of Infectious Diseases* (4th ed.). New York: Churchill Livingstone, 1995. P. 1766.

followed by 1 week of oral therapy, is recommended. Eradication of the carrier state, assessed by follow-up cultures, is of uncertain significance.

If meningococcemia cannot be excluded, while awaiting cultures, it is reasonable to treat for this also because this life-threatening illness will respond to antibiotic therapy.

G. **Streptococcal toxic shock syndrome** (STSS) is an invasive streptococcal infection that affects young, otherwise healthy adults, aged 20–50 years, in a sporadic fashion. See related discussions in Chap. 4.

1. **Pathogenesis.** The syndrome is caused by a pyrogenic exotoxin produced by certain strains of group A beta-hemolytic streptococci, especially the M-1 and M-3 serotypes. Most often, there is a recent history of soft-tissue injury. Streptococcal infection of other body sites also may produce the syndrome [24].

2. **Clinical manifestations.** Pain at the site of trauma is the most common presenting complaint. **Hypotension is present in more than half of the cases, and early organ dysfunction is a striking feature in this syndrome.** Myonecrosis and necrotizing fasciitis may develop during the course of illness. Bacteremia occurs in 60% of cases, and culture of the infected soft-tissue site will yield positive cultures for group A streptococci in 95% of cases [25]. The course of the illness is rapidly progressive, with a fatality rate of approximately 30%, despite its occurrence in a young, nonimmunocompromised host. See Table 2-6 for a proposed case definition of STSS.

3. **Therapy**
    a. **Early surgical drainage, debridement, fasciotomy, or amputation** of a clearly defined site of infection is indicated.
    b. **Supportive therapy** should be instituted for hypotension and organ failure (see sec. **IV**).
    c. **Antibiotic options include penicillin, erythromycin, or clindamycin. Ceftriaxone is an alternative.** In some cases of accelerated soft-tissue destruction, indicating accompanying rapid toxin production, direct protein synthesis inhibitors (erythromycin and clindamycin) may prove more efficacious [24, 26]. Overall, **we favor clindamycin** in this setting, unless clindamycin resistance is common. (See Chap. 4, sec. **IV.B.1** under Cellulitis, p. 112.)

Table 2-6. Proposed case definition for the streptococcal toxic shock syndrome*

I. Isolation of group A streptococci (*Streptococcus pyogenes*)
   A. From a normally sterile site (e.g., blood, cerebrospinal, pleural, or peritoneal fluid, tissue biopsy, surgical wound)
   B. From a nonsterile site (e.g., throat, sputum, vagina, superficial skin lesion)
II. Clinical signs of severity
   A. Hypotension: systolic blood pressure ≤ 90 mm Hg in adults or less than the fifth percentile for age in children
   and
   B. At least two of the following signs
      1. Renal impairment: creatinine ≥ 177 μmol/L (≥ 2 mg/dL) for adults or greater than or equal to twice the upper limit of normal for age. In patients with preexisting renal disease, a twofold or greater elevation over the baseline level
      2. Coagulopathy: platelets ≤ 100 × 10^9/L (≤ 100,000/mm^3) or disseminated intravascular coagulation defined by prolonged clotting times, low fibrinogen level, and the presence of fibrin degradation products
      3. Liver involvement: alanine aminotransferase (SGOT), aspartate aminotransferase (SGPT), or total bilirubin levels greater than or equal to twice the upper limit of normal for age. In patients with preexisting liver disease, a twofold or greater elevation over the baseline level
      4. Adult respiratory distress syndrome defined by acute onset of diffuse pulmonary infiltrates and hypoxemia in the absence of cardiac failure, or evidence of diffuse capillary leak manifested by acute onset of generalized edema, or pleural or peritoneal effusions with hypoalbuminemia
      5. A generalized erythematous macular rash that may desquamate
      6. Soft-tissue necrosis, including necrotizing fasciitis or myositis, or gangrene

*An illness fulfilling criteria I.A and II.A and B can be defined as a *definite* case. An illness fulfilling criteria I.B and II.A and B can be defined as a *probable* case if no other etiology for the illness is identified.
Source: The Working Group on Severe Streptococcal Infections, Defining the group A streptococcal toxic shock syndrome: Rationale and consensus definition. *J.A.M.A.* 269:390, 1993.

   H. **Other causes of hypotension and fever** include acute myocardial infarction, pulmonary embolism, myocarditis, volume depletion, or GI bleeding with focal infection (i.e., pneumonia), pancreatitis, and adrenal insufficiency.
IV. **Therapy for sepsis of unclear etiology.** A favorable outcome is related to early aggressive intervention.
   A. **Patient monitoring** is critical; vital signs, urine output, and mentation are helpful clinical parameters. Swan-Ganz catheterization may be useful [13]. Optimal pulmonary capillary wedge pressure (PCWP) for patients with septic shock is considered to be 10–14 mm Hg, although individual assessment of cardiac output response to frequent fluid challenges has been recommended [27]. (For example, a 250-ml bolus of crystalloid solution can be given every 15 minutes until cardiac output plateau is reached.)
   B. **Volume replacement is essential.** Both crystalloid and colloid solutions have been used in fluid resuscitation, and no consensus has been reached regarding the most efficacious solution type. However, some authors suggest that a lower incidence of pulmonary edema occurs with colloid solutions.
   C. **Correction of hypoxia and acidosis.** Supplemental oxygen or assisted ventilation (when required) should be liberally utilized to maximize tissue oxygenation. Although acidosis should be reversed by improved tissue oxygenation, bicarbonate administration may at times be needed, especially if the pH is below 7.0–7.1. Nonetheless, the current role of bicarbonate in modifying the course and outcome of septic shock is unknown, and correction of the underlying pathophysiologic process remains the basis of therapy [28].
   D. **Antibiotics** administered early in the course of therapy have been shown to decrease mortality. Optimal selection of initial antibiotic therapy should be based on individual settings, as summarized in Table 2-4.
      1. **Intravenous bactericidal drugs** are preferred.

2. **Adequate doses** must be used and serum levels monitored where indicated (i.e., aminoglycosides). (See Chap. 28 for proper loading dose and doses in renal failure.)

3. **Antibiotic combinations** have been advocated for possible synergy, to provide broad coverage while one awaits culture data [29]. Synergy may be especially important in the leukopenic host and particularly in patients in whom *P. aeruginosa* and enterococcal bacteremia are either suspected or documented. The necessity of combination therapy in the future may be lessened by the introduction of single antibiotics with broad-spectrum activity (e.g., imipenem) to which organisms are sensitive (see sec. **IV.B.2.d** under Fever in the Leukopenic Patient).

E. **Pressor therapy** should be used as a **supplement** to volume expansion. Therapy is empiric and the optimal agent uncertain. Dopamine alone has been recommended, as has norepinephrine in combination with low-dose dopamine. A recent double-blind, randomized therapeutic trial comparing dopamine and norepinephrine found norepinephrine at 1.5 ± 1.2 µg/kg/min to be more efficacious in restoring adequate tissue perfusion in those with hyperdynamic septic shock [30]. The therapy must be guided by the clinical characteristics of the patient, with the knowledge that higher-than-usual doses of pressors may be required owing to down-regulation of adrenergic receptors in the septic patient. Potentially antagonistic drugs such as calcium channel blockers and angiotensin-converting enzyme (ACE) inhibitors should be discontinued.

F. **Septic sources** must be removed, including abscess drainage and removal of infarcted bowel or viscera. An intravascular catheter that is suspected of being the septic source should be removed or replaced.

G. **High-dose corticosteroids. There currently is no proven benefit of administering pharmacologic doses of corticosteroids to the septic patient** [31].

H. **Other agents. Immunotherapies are experimental** and are aimed at stemming the tide of inflammatory response.

1. **Antiendotoxin monoclonal antibodies.** Early clinical trials show some improvement in survival in different patient subsets for the two agents **E-5,** a murine IgM, and **HA-1A,** a human IgM. E-5 appears to be effective in patients without shock, whereas HA-1A appears to be effective in treating gram-negative bacteremia with shock as compared to placebo. Results of subsequent clinical trials are inconclusive. These agents had not been approved for clinical use as of early 1996. The reader is referred to three excellent current reviews [7a, 32, 32a].

2. **Anti-TNF antibodies.** Early clinical studies show disappointing results using anti-TNF antibodies, with increased mortality in a subgroup of patients [33].

3. **IL-1 receptor antagonists (IL-1ra) are endogenous inhibitors of IL-1.** In animal models of sepsis, recombinant IL-1ra administration attenuates cardiovascular depression and enhances survival. Results of early human clinical trials are inconclusive [34].

Fever in the
Leukopenic Patient

Infection secondary to the leukopenia that occurs in the course of disease or as a consequence of chemotherapy is the leading cause of death in leukemia and other malignancies. Early institution of empiric antibiotic therapy has decreased infection-related morbidity and mortality.

I. **Urgent problems.** Although fever may be due to the underlying malignancy, **until proved otherwise fever in a leukopenic patient is assumed to be due to infection, and therapy must be instituted before culture results are available.** It is estimated that 60% of febrile neutropenic patients have infection, with bacteremia present in 20% [35]. Culture-negative causes for fever may include the underlying disease, drug fever, viral hepatitis, adrenal insufficiency, graft-versus-host disease, leukocyte transfusion reactions, and pulmonary emboli.

A. **Granulocytopenia** ($<$ 500/mm^3 or falling counts near this level) **and fever** (oral temperature $>$ 38°C on more than one or two occasions or $>$ 38.5°C once) have been recommended as the threshold for initiation of empiric therapy.

B. The **risk of bacteremia is greater if the granulocyte count is lower than 100/mm^3** [36]. Likewise, prolonged granulocytopenia predisposes to infection. Thus, prolonged profound granulocytopenia may define a high-risk group (see sec. **IV.B**) [37]. A lower-risk group is defined by granulocyte counts in the 100–500/mm³ range, an average duration of leukopenia of approximately 7–10 days, and clinical stability (i.e., not hypotensive, no ARDS and, ideally, younger patients).

C. **Initial approach. Leukopenic patients with fever require immediate evaluation and therapy.** Major considerations are discussed later.

1. A careful history must be obtained, with specific attention directed toward prior surgery (e.g., splenectomy); recent therapy including cytotoxic agents, radiation, and current medications (especially corticosteroids); and prior infectious episodes (and organisms). These data may influence decisions concerning empiric antibiotic therapy (see later discussion in sec. **IV**).

2. An **obvious focus** of infection that can be treated specifically should be sought.

3. If there is no obvious focus, determine an initial and rational antibiotic regimen (i.e., empiric antibiotic therapy).

4. **Baseline laboratory workup.** For the reasons discussed in sec. **II**, these patients routinely need at least the following:
   a. **A chest x-ray,** even if pulmonary symptoms are absent.
   b. **A urine culture,** even if the urinalysis appears benign.
   c. **Blood cultures.** Two cultures, at least 15–20 minutes apart, are suggested.
   d. **Examination and culture of any exudates** (sputum, wound, or drainage).

5. **Early antibiotic therapy** is essential. One cannot await the results of cultures before initiating therapy.

II. **An obvious site of infection.** Remember that the patient with leukopenia may not manifest the usual signs of infection (pus, inflammation, infiltrates, etc.) [38].

A. **Pneumonia.** Cough, sputum production, and **purulent sputum** on Gram stain become **less reliable** as the absolute granulocyte count decreases. The chest x-ray usually will reveal an infiltrate if a pneumonia is present; therefore, x-ray must be performed routinely. Rarely, a patient may present with an early gram-negative pneumonia with normal chest x-ray, but these patients usually have symptoms indicating that the infection is localized in the lung.

B. **Urinary tract infection (UTI)** may occur without pyuria or dysuria. Cultures should be obtained routinely.

C. **Skin infections** lack the classic signs of inflammation, although erythema and local pain or tenderness may be present. Therefore, a high index of suspicion must be maintained in these patients.

D. **Pharyngitis.** Leukopenic patients often will have no exudate but will complain of a sore throat and have erythema of the pharynx.

E. **Anorectal infection** [39] may be remarkable only for slight perirectal discomfort with stool passage. One gentle rectal examination may disclose slight induration and associated discomfort. A hemorrhoid with an uninfected fissure will not cause fever [37]. This may be the source of anaerobic infection and has specific implications for therapy (see sec. **IV**). **Abscess aspiration** can be performed to help confirm the diagnosis and to assist therapeutically. These patients do not form normal amounts of pus, and only a minimal amount of watery fluid may be obtained. On Gram stain, few polymorphonuclear leukocytes may be seen, but many gram-negative organisms often are present. The aspirated fluid should be cultured both aerobically and anaerobically.

F. **Central venous catheters** may be the source of bacteremia and require careful evaluation of the tract and exit site (see later discussion under Catheter-Related Sepsis).

G. **Miscellaneous.** In Sickles' series [38], meningitis, peritonitis, sinusitis, and esophagitis were seen infrequently. Occasionally, these patients may have a primary **dental focus** of infection, and a careful inspection of the oral cavity, including percussion of the teeth to assess local tenderness, is indicated.

III. **No obvious primary site.** Often after a careful history, physical examination, and laboratory screens have been performed to look for a primary site of infection, no focus of infection is identified.

A. **Assume occult bacteremia.** Leukopenic patients frequently will have a bacteremia, presumably from an endogenous source. It generally is assumed that many of the infections originate in the GI tract. Organisms, particularly gram-negative aerobes (*Pseudomonas* spp., *Klebsiella* spp., and *E. coli*), presumably enter the bloodstream by way of small ulcerations or bleeding sites in the bowel wall.

B. **Approach.** After full cultures are obtained, empiric therapy is started, directed primarily against gram-negative bacilli.

IV. Therapy is started as soon as the clinical assessment and baseline cultures have been completed.

A. For localized infection, antibiotics are directed against the commonly isolated organisms, as is discussed in Chap. 28 and in individual chapters on specific infections.

    1. Whenever possible, **bactericidal antibiotics are selected.**

    2. Synergistic combinations and optimal drug doses are used, with serum level monitoring of aminoglycosides. Simultaneous use of two drugs active against infecting organisms may be associated with improved clinical outcome [29, 36]. However, monotherapy to reduce toxicity may be a consideration (see sec. **B.2.d**).

    3. Abscesses should be drained. However, conservative management of perirectal infection with the addition of either clindamycin or metronidazole is recommended [39].

    4. Antibiotic therapy usually is continued for at least 10–14 days and sometimes longer (i.e., until the granulocyte count is > 500/mm^3).

B. Occult infection must be presumed in the febrile leukopenic patient if there is no obvious source. This situation also requires immediate empiric antibiotic therapy [40].

    1. Goal. Empiric antibiotic therapy is directed against the most commonly isolated organisms, which historically have been *Pseudomonas* spp., *E. coli*, and *Klebsiella* spp. *Pseudomonas* spp. have become a less frequent cause of infection in neutropenic cancer patients in the last decade, allowing for broader selection of empiric antimicrobial therapy. *Enterobacter* and *Citrobacter* spp. are isolated more frequently than in the past and often elicit beta-lactamases. Alpha-hemolytic streptococci may cause life-threatening infection. Streptococcal and enterococcal infections may develop in those on oral quinolone prophylaxis (see Chap. 28S). In the past decade, coagulase-negative staphylococcal infections have become more common [41–43]. *Corynebacterium jeikeium* has been more frequently isolated in venous catheter–associated infections as well. Although anaerobic bacteria are uncommon causes of primary infection in granulocytopenia, they may be present in polymicrobial bacteremias [41] (see sec. **4**).

    2. An aminoglycoside and a broad-spectrum penicillin (e.g., piperacillin) are a common combination used in this setting and are the standard regimen to which other regimens are compared [44]. Unless organisms are resistant to gentamicin, newer aminoglycosides do not lower mortality.

        a. Dosage

            (1) Aminoglycoside. Either **gentamicin** or **tobramycin** (a 2-mg/kg dose initially, followed by a 1.7-mg/kg dose q8h if the patient has normal renal function) is used in adults. Serum levels ideally should be monitored in these patients to ensure adequate levels and to minimize toxicity (see Chap. 28H).

                Amikacin is useful when dealing with suspected resistant gram-negative bacteremia, usually in a patient previously treated with aminoglycosides or in the hospital setting where more resistant organisms are found. (For dosing, see Chap. 28 under Aminoglycosides.)

            (2) Antipseudomonal penicillins (ticarcillin, mezlocillin, and piperacillin) are used. Piperacillin, 3 g q4h or 4g q6h, is suggested. Doses are adjusted in renal failure. **Empirically,** all agents have similar success rates (see Chap. 28E).

            (3) Penicillin allergy. Ceftazidime in combination with an aminoglycoside is often recommended in the patient with a delayed reaction to penicillin.

        b. Triple antibiotic combinations (e.g., cephalosporin, antipseudomonal penicillin, and aminoglycoside) have not shown clear advantage over double-drug regimens and are **not advised.**

        c. Vancomycin has been advocated by some for empiric use, in view of the increased incidence of gram-positive bacteremia in neutropenic patients. However, there is no proved reduction in patient morbidity or mortality from empiric use of this agent. Clinical response is observed when vancomycin is added at the time that gram-positive organisms are isolated [45]. One study reported a reduction in the eventual need for the use of amphotericin B in regimens containing empiric vancomycin [46]. Because gram-positive bacteremias appear to be more readily tolerated than gram-negative infections, **vancomycin is not routinely recommended empirically unless a central venous catheter is suspected as a source of fever. Vancomycin is added when culture data indicate a need for it.**

   d. Monotherapy

      (1) Imipenem. Studies support the use of imipenem alone [47, 48]. The precise role for monotherapy remains undefined [49] but, based on recent data on imipenem use and its favorable resistance patterns (see Chap. 28G), it is reasonable to recommend its use, especially in institutions where *P. aeruginosa* bacteremia is declining. Some experts believe that patients with known or highly suspected gram-negative bacteremia deserve double-drug therapy to provide synergy. (See further discussion in Chap. 28G.)

      (2) Ceftazidime has been used successfully as monotherapy [50]. The possible emergence of resistance in monotherapeutic treatment of *P. aeruginosa* bacteremia is a concern, especially for patients recently treated with other third-generation cephalosporins. In a patient who has recently received one or more courses of ceftazidime for similar bouts of leukopenic fever and who is very ill, we would avoid monotherapy with ceftazidime in case a resistant gram-negative bacilli were involved. Also, if species of *Enterobacter, Citrobacter,* or *Serratia* are found with notable frequency in a particular hospital, Pizzo [51] suggests that monotherapy with a third-generation cephalosporin be avoided because of the ease with which beta-lactamase is induced in these organisms, which increases the likelihood that resistant organisms will emerge.

   e. Alternative combinations. In the setting where aminoglycoside usage is discouraged (e.g., an elderly patient with renal insufficiency for whom aminoglycoside monitoring is not available, or a patient receiving concurrent nephrotoxic drugs), ceftazidime combined with piperacillin has been recommended [52], although an increased incidence of rash has been noted with this double-beta-lactam combination [53] and marrow toxicity has been suggested in other double-beta-lactam regimens (e.g., moxalactam plus piperacillin). **We do not advocate these alternative regimens.**

   f. Outpatient oral antibiotic therapy for carefully selected febrile leukopenic patients is undergoing clinical study. Accepted guidelines are not available as of early 1996 [53a].

3. Duration of therapy

   a. Positive blood cultures. Specific therapy usually is continued for 10–14 days; it may be extended if granulocytopenia persists. Although narrow (organism-specific) therapy is encouraged in normal hosts, in the patient with severe prolonged neutropenia broad coverage has been suggested to reduce the incidence of superinfection [54]. Enterococcal superinfections, however, do occur more frequently with third-generation cephalosporin use in the neutropenic patient.

   b. Negative blood cultures. In a patient who defervesces, antibiotic therapy usually is continued until the granulocyte count rises to more than 500/mm^3 [55] or for 14 days, whichever is shorter, because prolonged antibiotic therapy has been associated with invasive fungal disease. Several authors have suggested that relatively few adverse consequences occur if empiric antibiotics are discontinued in the persistently neutropenic patient when infection is either controlled or doubtful; their reports included patients who remained persistently febrile as well as those who defervesced and apparently responded to initial antibiotic therapy [56, 57]. **Nonetheless, this remains a controversial area, especially in the persistently febrile patient, and infectious disease consultation is recommended when discontinuation of therapy is contemplated.**

4. Some patients remain febrile despite empiric or specific antibacterial therapy. Approximately 75% of patients will defervesce within the first week of therapy [56].

   a. Review optimal therapy. In the setting of documented gram-negative bacteremia, peak bactericidal levels may be a useful parameter to monitor. Granulocytopenic patients with peak bactericidal levels of 1:16 or greater had a better outcome than those with levels of 1:8 in one study [58].

   b. Rather than random substitution for an initial antibiotic combination, **systematic addition of agents may be reasonable.** Mucositis or perirectal or abdominal tenderness would favor anaerobic coverage with either clindamycin or metronidazole [41].

   c. **Serial thorough physical examinations should be performed.** The use of imaging studies to localize a site of infection in the absence of symptoms has been disappointing. Some experts have suggested that chest CT scans may at times be helpful [51] in selected patients who may have subtle or questionable underlying changes on chest radiographs. For example, if the question of pulmonary nodules is raised by routine chest radiographs, a chest CT scan will help clarify whether there is more extensive pulmonary disease (e.g., suggesting early invasive pulmonary aspergillosis). Nevertheless, the cause of fever often cannot be identified [51].

   d. **Empiric antifungal therapy (amphotericin B)** has been advocated on the seventh febrile day for presumed treatment of occult fungal infections while patients continue broad-spectrum antibiotics [41]. In practice, many **authorities will initiate antifungal therapy after 3–5 days in the persistently febrile patient despite broad-spectrum antibiotics** or will immediately institute amphotericin therapy in the patient with prolonged neutropenia, multiple antibiotics, and clinical deterioration suggesting occult infection. Addition of amphotericin B for the patient with either persistent unexplained fever or unexplained clinical deterioration appears to be the most reasonable empiric therapy. (See also discussion in **e** and in Chap. 18.)

   e. **Hepatic candidiasis** has recently been described as a cause of persistent fever in cancer patients who recover from an episode of neutropenia [59]. The suggestive symptoms include fever and right upper quadrant pain accompanied by elevated alkaline phosphatase. Confirmation should be made by CT scan or ultrasonography followed by liver biopsy. Amphotericin B and fluconazole have been used in this setting. See Chap. 18 for additional discussion.

   f. **Recurrent fever** in a neutropenic patient who initially defervesced should suggest possible fungemia, or bacteremia with a resistant pathogen. In this situation, patients must be carefully reassessed, and usually amphotericin B must be added and a change to broader gram-negative antimicrobial activity (e.g., amikacin) may be necessary [60].

   g. **Granulocyte transfusions.** The precise role of white blood cell transfusions in the infected granulocytopenic patient remains controversial. Currently, it is suggested that granulocyte transfusions may be reasonable in the setting of documented bacterial infection with failure to improve after 48 hours of adequate therapy. The potential toxicity and narrow therapeutic margin of granulocyte transfusions limit their use to large institutions with sophisticated patient support mechanisms [61].

   h. **Granulocyte-stimulating factors** are discussed in sec. **V.A.4.**

 V. **Prevention of infection in leukopenic patients.** Infection often delays the initiation or continuation of antineoplastic therapy. Methods have been devised to decrease the incidence of infection in leukopenic patients.

   A. **Methods to decrease exposure**

   1. Avoid unnecessary hospitalization and invasive procedures.

   2. **Isolation procedures.** Infection is often due to endogenous bacteria from the patient's GI tract. Special forms of protective isolation have not been shown to be superior to routine care with hand-washing [62]. Modified protective isolation for both patient care personnel and visitors is a reasonable compromise. This includes the following:

   a. A private room is desirable to reduce opportunity for patient cross-contamination.

   b. **Good hand-washing is the most effective way** to decrease spread of nosocomial organisms to the leukopenic patient.

   c. Masks should be worn by caregivers and visitors with an upper respiratory infection.

   3. **Prophylactic oral antibiotics** to prevent endogenous infection from the GI tract have been studied, with conflicting results. Although trimethoprim-sulfamethoxazole (TMP-SMZ) has been advocated for selective suppression of aerobic gram-negative GI flora without suppressing the anaerobic population, its use lengthens the duration of neutropenia, leads to allergic reactions, and selects for resistant gram-negative bacteremia. The fluoroquinolones norfloxacin and ciprofloxacin have been shown to reduce aerobic gram-negative bacteremia

when compared with placebo and TMP-SMZ, respectively [63]. However, no improvement in mortality was seen, so the criteria for their use for selective GI decontamination remains undefined. **At this point, we would not advise routine use of the fluoroquinolones or other oral agents to prevent infectious complications** unless the patient is part of a controlled clinical study that seeks to assess the role of these regimens. (See related discussions in Chaps. 28K and 28S.)

4. **The use of cytokines with hematopoietic growth-stimulating effect** [63, 64, 64a]. Granulocyte-macrophage colony-stimulating factors (GM-CSF) and granulocyte colony-stimulating factor (G-CSF) have been shown to reduce the number of days of leukopenia and neutropenia after aggressive chemotherapy in patients with advanced cancer. Most important is the reduction in the number of days of neutropenia with a neutrophil count of less than 0.1×10^9/L [64a]. The precise role of these agents is being better defined as further experience is accumulating. Pizzo [51] concludes that the use of a colony-stimulating factor, although safe and well tolerated, adds to the cost of care. For patients with prolonged neutropenia, the use of such an agent may be beneficial and can be justified. For patients with neutropenia of short duration (< 1 week), in whom the risk of infection is low, these agents are unnecessary [51].

   In a recent editorial comment on this topic, addressing whether growth factors should be administered concomitantly with empiric antibiotic therapy in the febrile leukopenic patient, Schimpff suggests that G-CSF and GM-CSF may benefit patients with febrile neutropenia just beginning to receive empiric antibiotics and in whom the granulocyte count is expected to remain at less than 0.1×10^9/L [64a]. A related editorial emphasizes the need for more studies [64b].

B. **Improve host defenses**
   1. Respect normal skin boundaries where possible. Minimize invasive procedures and intravenous lines.
   2. Administer polyvalent pneumococcal vaccine once (if the patient has not received this previously).
   3. Administer yearly influenza vaccine.
   4. Avoid live vaccines (BCG, yellow fever, and oral polio).
   5. Avoid corticosteroid administration when possible.

Positive Blood Cultures

When a blood culture is reported to be positive, the clinician must decide whether the results represents true bacteremia or a contaminant. In addition, certain pathogens isolated from blood cultures may be associated with special characteristics, including typical sources that need to be investigated, special implications for therapy, and prognosis. The technique of obtaining and timing blood cultures is discussed in Chap. 25, sec. I, under Culture Techniques. During an acute episode, it is helpful to draw two to three separate blood cultures. Multiple cultures will help the clinician interpret the implications of blood cultures as they become available.

I. **True bacteremia versus contaminated blood cultures.** Prior studies have shown that between 5 and 30% of positive blood cultures represent contamination (i.e., they are **false positive** blood cultures). Some of the characteristics of true bacteremia, as opposed to contaminated, cultures have been established [65, 66]. **The final decision as to whether the organism isolated is real or a contaminant is** *still* clinical.
   A. **Type of organism isolated**
      1. Bacteria that are usually **true pathogens are virulent organisms** such as group A streptococci, *S. pneumoniae, E. coli,* meningococci, *Proteus mirabilis, H. influenzae, Haemophilus parainfluenzae,* and *S. aureus.* If a single blood culture yields one of these organisms, it almost always indicates a true positive.
      2. **Common contaminants**
         a. **Staphylococcal coagulase-negative** organisms (*S. epidermidis* or *S. saprophyticus*) are commonly isolated and, in some series, represent 15–30% of positive blood culture isolates. Approximately 90% of these are contaminants, although **they can be pathogenic,** as is discussed in sec. **II.B.**
         b. **Streptococci** (i.e., alpha-streptococci) and enterococci do not always mean true bacteremia.

      c. **Diphtheroids,** or corynebacteria, are normal colonizers of the skin and pharynx. They frequently contaminate blood cultures and usually have no clinical significance. When isolated on multiple occasions—for example, in a patient with a prosthetic heart valve—these organisms may represent the pathogen causing endocarditis [67]. They might also represent a bloodstream infection related to an indwelling catheter.

      d. *Bacillus subtilis* is a gram-positive rod that usually is not a pathogen.

   B. **Number of positive cultures.** As a general rule, multiple blood cultures yielding the same organism usually indicate true bacteremia. In the special settings where organisms such as coagulase-negative staphylococci or diphtheroids are causing disease, most blood cultures will be positive.

II. **Implications of specific bacteremias**

   A. *S. aureus* **(coagulase-positive) bacteremia.** Although gram-negative bacteremias have increased in recent years, studies reveal that 10–15% of positive blood cultures yield *S. aureus*. *S. aureus* rivals *E. coli* in causing nosocomial bacteremia. *S. aureus* bacteremias are associated with a high mortality (30–40%), even with appropriate therapy. Penicillin-sensitive and penicillin-resistant *S. aureus* seem equally virulent. **Some individuals are prone to *S. aureus* bloodstream infections because of high carriage rates of the organism. Among these groups are** (1) those with atopic dermatosis, (2) diabetics, (3) intravenous drug users, (4) chronic renal dialysis patients, and (5) patients with chronic indwelling catheters. Other risk factors include recent high-dose glucocorticosteroid therapy and prior hospitalization within 30 days of the onset of illness. *S. aureus* infections have recently been reviewed [68–71].

      1. **Source.** There is often a definable source of staphylococcal infection such as a cutaneous wound, abscess, or intravenous catheter. **In 20–30% of cases, no primary site of infection is found, which is a marker for a high probability of endocarditis.** Secondary foci of infection (multiple lung, renal, splenic, or bone abscesses) are also common markers for underlying endocarditis. Patients with bacteremia without an identifiable source carried a higher mortality, which is attributed to delay in instituting the proper antistaphylococcal therapy [71].

      2. **Clinical evaluation.** Multiple blood cultures drawn before the initiation of therapy are extremely important in patients with suspected staphylococcal bacteremia. Duration of therapy is contingent on differentiation between transient bacteremia (usually requiring only short-term therapy) and prolonged bacteremia (requiring long-term therapy). Daily evaluation of the patient must include a search for secondary (metastatic) foci of infection. The latter imply a complicated infection that requires prolonged therapy.

        a. **Sustained bacteremia.** Multiple positive blood cultures over several hours to days confirms prolonged bacteremia with presumed high risk for bacterial endocarditis, often in the absence of peripheral stigmata. An extended course of antibiotics (4–6 weeks) is recommended in this situation.

        b. **Bacteremia with a removable focus.** If a patient has a transient bacteremia, presumably due to an indwelling catheter, generally 2 weeks of parenteral antibiotic therapy is recommended. The risk of endocarditis and metastatic infection is believed to be acceptably low in this situation [72]. A recent retrospective study of catheter-related *S. aureus* bacteremia showed a significant relapse rate in those with initially complicated courses (fever and or bacteremia for 3 days after catheter removal) who were treated with parenteral antibiotics for fewer than 10 days [73]. (See related discussion in sec. **V.D.2** under Catheter-Related Sepsis.) If any question exists concerning the duration or etiology of the *S. aureus* bacteremia, extended parenteral antibiotics should be given (see Chap. 10), and infectious disease consultation is advised. Any patient with prolonged bacteremia before removal of the catheter and onset of therapy probably deserves long-term therapy (i.e., 4 weeks). Some experts also suggest that prolonged therapy is indicated in the following conditions: (1) a suppurative catheter site; (2) severe underlying disease such as poorly controlled diabetes, cirrhosis, immunodeficiency, malnutrition, or malignancy; (3) a hemodynamically significant murmur; (4) appearance of a new murmur; (5) persistence of fever and bacteremia even after several days of therapy [74]; or (6) development of clinical evidence for a metastatic focus while the patient is receiving the 14-day course.

   c. A febrile patient may have only **one blood culture drawn before antibiotics**
      are started. If this is positive for *S. aureus,* the significance of the culture
      may be difficult to determine owing to the problem of differentiating be-
      tween transient and prolonged bacteremia. To avoid this dilemma, two or
      three blood cultures (drawn 20–25 minutes apart) should be obtained before
      therapy is started.
   d. **Only one of several blood cultures is positive.** At times in a febrile patient,
      only one of several blood cultures may prove positive for *S. aureus.* This
      may occur in the setting of an occult focus of infection (e.g., liver abscess,
      osteomyelitis).
3. **Therapy.** The majority of community- and hospital-acquired staphylococci are
   penicillin-resistant. Therefore, initial therapy is a semisynthetic penicillin (oxacillin or nafcillin, 9–12 g/day IV in adults). The incidence of methicillin-resistant
   staphylococci (MRSA) is high in some institutions. If MRSA is a concern, initial
   therapy would be vancomycin. (If renal function is normal, the usual dose is
   500 mg q6h or 1 g q12h. See Chap. 28O.) If the organism is penicillin-susceptible
   (minimum inhibitory concentration [MIC] < 0.1 µg/ml), penicillin is the drug
   of choice and 16–20 million units daily is suggested in adults with normal
   renal function.
   a. **Combination therapy.** The combination of a beta-lactam or vancomycin
      with an aminoglycoside has experimentally demonstrated more rapid steril-
      ization of cardiac valve vegetations but no improvement in clinical morbid-
      ity or mortality [68]. Rifampin has been advocated recently in lieu of the
      aminoglycoside component; however, in vitro synergism, antagonism, or
      indifference may occur and can be dose-dependent. In general, combination
      therapy is not recommended.
   b. **Penicillin-allergic patients.** In the patient with a delayed reaction to peni-
      cillin, cephalosporins are not contraindicated (see Chap. 27). Cephalothin,
      1.5–2.0 g IV q4h, or cefazolin, 1 g IV q6h in adults, has been used. The
      second-generation (e.g., cefoxitin) and third-generation cephalosporins are
      less active against *S. aureus* (see Chap. 28F). Vancomycin can be used in
      the patient with a history of severe immediate penicillin allergy. If renal
      function is normal, the usual dose is 500 mg q6h or 1 g q12h. This bacteri-
      cidal drug has good antistaphylococcal activity and is the favored agent of
      many experts, although failures of therapy can occur [75]. (See Chap. 28O
      for further discussion of vancomycin, including dosing in renal failure.)
   c. **Methicillin resistance.** Vancomycin is the drug of choice in the case of
      methicillin resistance. Those with proven or suspected endocarditis tend
      to have a delayed clinical response to the drug but are generally without
      serious complications. The addition of rifampin has not been shown to
      enhance clinical response [76]. Despite in vitro susceptibility by standard
      disc method, there are many reports of failure of cephalosporins alone or
      in combination with an aminoglycoside in treating MRSA.
   d. **Duration of therapy** is discussed previously and in Chap. 10. Because
      at times optimal duration is a matter of controversy, infectious disease
      consultation may be helpful.
B. *S. epidermidis* **(coagulase-negative) bacteremia** has long been recognized as a
   common cause of contaminated blood cultures. *S. epidermidis* now is recognized
   as a frequent hospital-acquired pathogen [77]. It accounts for approximately 9%
   of primary nosocomial bacteremias and is a complication of insertion of orthopedic
   devices, prosthetic heart valves, and intravenous catheters. It can cause bacteremia in granulocytopenic patients. Mortality from *S. epidermidis* bacteremia has
   been reported to be in the 30–34% range [5, 77], similar to that reported for
   S. aureus.
   1. **Source.** These organisms are found in the normal skin flora and usually are
      of low virulence; cutaneous breaks in host defense allow invasion. They produce
      mucoid adherence factors and cause erosive changes on smooth catheter sur-
      faces and therefore are well adapted for indolent infection [78].
   2. **Clinical evaluation.** A single positive blood culture may be difficult to interpret.
      However, in some reports, more than 90% of patients with *S. epidermidis*
      bacteremias had previously had central or arterial lines. **The following clinical
      guidelines should suggest true bacteremia with coagulase-negative staphy-
      lococci:** multiple positive blood cultures obtained over a brief period of time

(hours to days), detection of growth in less than 48 hours, growth in both aerobic and anaerobic bottles [65], and an in situ foreign body such as an intravascular catheter or prosthetic cardiac valve (see Chap. 10). Quantification with lysis centrifugation technique can be very helpful in drawing conclusions.

3. **Therapy.** Because of antibiotic pressure, many S. *epidermidis* organisms are methicillin-resistant.
   a. **Single-drug therapy.** Vancomycin is the drug of choice, although methicillin or oxacillin can be used if susceptibility data are available [78]. (Vancomycin resistance is very unusual. See Chap. 28O.)
   b. **Combination therapy.** In the presence of deep-seated infections or endocarditis [79], vancomycin plus rifampin is recommended (see Chap. 10).
   c. **Surgery.** The combined medical-surgical approach would appear to offer the best chance of cure for prosthetic valve endocarditis, prosthetic hips, vascular grafts, and CNS shunts. Central venous catheter infections (septicemia), however, have been successfully treated without line removal (see sec. V under Catheter-Related Sepsis).

C. **Beta-hemolytic group A streptococci** can occasionally cause a fulminant bacteremia [80–82].
   1. **Setting and source.** Underlying diseases such as solid tumors, lymphoproliferative and collagen vascular disease, diabetes mellitus, and alcohol and intravenous drug abuse predispose patients, but normals are also at risk. The skin and the respiratory tract are the usual foci of infection. However, **in a recent review, 33% of bacteremia cases due to group A streptococci did not have an obvious source,** more than half of the patients had a malignant disease and, in this study, the mortality was 20% [82]. The upper respiratory tract is a source of bacteremia primarily in children with leukemia; group A streptococci are not found in the normal flora of any body site in adults [81]. Nosocomial epidemics have been reported.
   2. **Therapy**
      a. **Penicillin** typically is the drug of choice. In adults with normal renal function, 2 million units q4h is suggested. In children, 200,000–300,000 units/kg/day is suggested. The intravenous route should be used. If a bacteremia occurred in the setting of invasive streptococcal infection, we would favor clindamycin 600 mg IV q8h in adults (see sec. **III.G** under Septic Shock).
      b. **Penicillin-allergic patients.** In many patients, a first-generation cephalosporin can be used (see Chap. 28F). In adults, cefazolin, 1 g IV q6h (or its equivalent), provides more than adequate levels. In children, 75–100 mg/kg/day is suggested. If a cephalosporin is contraindicated, vancomycin can be used, as it is bactericidal against the streptococci.
   3. **Duration of therapy.** The duration of therapy of group A streptococcal bacteremia is **poorly defined in the literature.** Endocarditis rarely is caused by this organism. If endocarditis is documented, these patients would require at least 4 weeks of therapy. Because of the potential virulence of the organism, for sustained bacteremias the authors treat patients with 3 weeks of parenteral antibiotics **even in the absence of overt endocarditis.** For a well-documented transient bacteremia, 10–14 days of therapy probably are adequate.

D. **Group B streptococci** (*Streptococcus agalactiae*) are a common cause of bacteremia in neonates. Group B streptococcal peripartum infections carry significant morbidity and mortality in women. It is apparent that the organism is detected with an increased frequency in nonpregnant adults as well [83, 84].
   1. **Neonatal bacteremias** are discussed in Chap. 3.
   2. **Adult bacteremias**
      a. **Setting.** Group B streptococcal infections, including bacteremias, are most frequently traceable to female genitourinary or postpartum infections. However, infections can be seen in both men and women with underlying diabetes, liver disease, HIV infection, and malignancy (especially after chemotherapy or radiation therapy). Other chronic diseases of the renal, cardiac, and respiratory systems also predispose to infection. The most common sources include skin, bone, urinary tract, and lung; primary bacteremia is not uncommon.
      b. **Spectrum of bacteremias.** Transient benign bacteremias as well as acute and subacute endocarditis and fulminant sepsis can occur. Polymicrobial bacteremias have been reported.

c. **Therapy.** Currently, 10–14 days of high-dose penicillin (12–18 million units/day) or ampicillin (8–12 g/day) are recommended, if renal function is normal, for transient bacteremia. The MIC for group B streptococci, which are penicillin-susceptible, may be fourfold to eightfold higher than the MIC for group A streptococci. Combination therapy with penicillin and an aminoglycoside (see sec. **E.3**) has been suggested for bacteremia caused by **tolerant** group B streptococci. A first-generation cephalosporin and vancomycin are alternatives in the patient with a delayed penicillin allergy. Some strains of group B streptococci are resistant to clindamycin and erythromycin. (In neonates and infants, ampicillin and an aminoglycoside are commonly used [see Chap. 3].) Group B streptococcal vaccines and passive immunotherapy are presently undergoing clinical trials.

E. **Enterococcal (streptococcal group D) bacteremias**
   1. **Source.** The enterococcus is a common isolate from the colon and the female genital tract. A primary focus of infection can usually be identified and includes the **genitourinary tract** of men and women (Chap. 12), **pelvic** infections in women (Chaps. 13, 14), **intraabdominal abscess and cholangitis** (Chap. 11), mixed **wound infections** (Chap. 4), and intravascular catheter-related infections (see sec. **VII.B** under Catheter-Related Sepsis).
   2. **Special considerations.** Enterococcal bacteremia is not synonymous with endocarditis. **A number of clinical points should suggest endocarditis** [85]: isolated (nonpolymicrobial) enterococcemia, community-acquired bacteremia, known valvular heart disease, and absence of known extracardiac focus.
      The frequency of nosocomial enterococcal bacteremia is increasing, usually among patients given broad-spectrum antibiotics, including third-generation cephalosporins, imipenem, and aztreonam [86]. The incidence of enterococcal bacteremia also is rising in patients with solid and hematologic malignancies and is attributed to increasing use of prophylactic antibiotics against gram-negative bacteremia [87].
      The enterococcus is resistant to many antibiotics. Bactericidal activity is seen with high doses of ampicillin alone; however, **the synergistic combination of penicillin or ampicillin and gentamicin or streptomycin is more reliably bactericidal** and so is recommended for endocarditis. We favor a penicillin and gentamicin combination because, with prolonged use, penicillin may be better tolerated than ampicillin. Recently, high-level gentamicin resistance has been reported (see Chap. 28H), and routine testing of gentamicin sensitivity in endocarditis and persistent bacteremia has been suggested. (See Chap. 10 for further discussion.) Enterococcal isolates resistant to multiple agents (beta-lactams, glycopeptides, aminoglycosides) have been reported in nosocomial outbreaks and are associated with higher mortality. (See related discussions in Chaps. 28H and 28O, which cover vancomycin-resistant enterococci.)
   3. **Therapy.** For prolonged bacteremias, endocarditis, and gentamicin-resistant enterococci see the discussion of therapy in Chaps. 10 and 28H. For documented transient bacteremias with gentamicin-susceptible strains, the authors would treat an adult patient with normal renal function with aqueous penicillin (2–3 million units IV q4h) or ampicillin (1.5–2.0 g IV q4h) and gentamicin (1 mg/kg/dose) for 10–14 days. Alternatives for the penicillin-allergic patient are discussed in Chap. 10.

F. *S. pneumoniae* **bacteremia.** Transient bacteremias are said to occur in 20–30% of pneumonias caused by *S. pneumoniae*. The pneumococcus remains an important pathogen, still with the potential for significant mortality. In one report, the mortality rate for bacteremic patients was 34% [88]. The majority of deaths occur within the first 48 hours despite initiation of effective antibiotic therapy, probably because of poor host defenses [88].
   1. **Source.** An obvious pneumonia is the most common source. However, meningitis, otitis, and peritonitis must also be considered. Endocarditis is unusual but, in one review, comprised 2.2% of cases of pneumococcal bacteremia [88]. An occult bacteremia (without defined focus) can occur, possibly from an undetectable pulmonary nidus, and is more common in patients younger than 30 years.
   2. **Special considerations.** Bacteremia is more prevalent in patients with preexisting diseases, especially in those older than 20 years. Diseases compromising normal respiratory function predominate. Previous splenectomy and sickle cell disease are well-recognized risks for pneumococcal sepsis. **An increasingly**

important risk factor is human immunodeficiency virus (HIV) infection. Young patients (e.g., < 40–45 years of age) with pneumococcal bacteremia should be tested for HIV [89]. A review found that 77% of bacteremia strains were represented in the 23-valent vaccine and that patients at high risk for bacteremia were identified by previous hospitalization and multiple underlying risk factors [90]. Therefore, specific target groups (immunocompromised) for vaccination have been identified, often with disappointing antibody response (see Chap. 9).

3. **Therapy.** Treatment of pneumococcal pneumonia (with bacteremia) is discussed in Chap. 9 and endocarditis in Chap. 10. Therapy of prolonged bacteremia without overt endocarditis is controversial; for penicillin-susceptible isolates, the authors suggest 2–3 weeks of intravenous penicillin G, 12–18 million units daily or cefazolin 1 g q8h in adults.

   Penicillin-resistant pneumococci are increasingly prevalent. Pneumococcal resistance to penicillin has become a worldwide problem, especially in South Africa, Spain, Hungary, and France, where up to 50% of isolates are resistant to penicillin. In the United States, the frequency of resistance is 1–25% or more, with higher rates seen in certain geographic areas [91]. **See detailed discussion of this topic in Chap. 28C.** Bacteremia with pneumococci moderately resistant to penicillin (MIC < 0.1–1.0 μg/ml) may still be treated effectively with high-dose penicillin [91]. However, endocarditis and meningitis with resistant organisms (i.e., MIC > 2 μg/ml) are not effectively treated with high-dose penicillin, and vancomycin is suggested instead. (See Chaps. 28C and 28O.) **Laboratories should test for penicillin resistance in all isolates from blood, CSF,** or other normally sterile sites. (See Chap. 28C for further discussion of penicillin resistance.)

G. *Streptococcus bovis* **bacteremias.** *S. bovis* is a group D nonenterococcal streptococcus that can cause endocarditis. Unlike group D enterococcal streptococci, *S. bovis* is penicillin-susceptible.

   1. **Implications.** Studies have shown that patients with carcinoma of the colon have a significantly increased fecal carriage rate of *S. bovis*. In addition, underlying carcinoma and polyps of the colon have been noted commonly in patients with bacteremias due to *S. bovis*. Presumably, these GI lesions are the portals of entry of this organism. These observations have led Klein and colleagues [92] to **recommend careful evaluation of the GI tract** (e.g., barium contrast studies, colonoscopy) **of all patients with *S. bovis* bacteremias or endocarditis.**

   2. **Therapy** is discussed in Chap. 10. Intravenous penicillin is the drug of choice. Cefazolin can be used in patients with delayed penicillin allergies.

H. **Viridans streptococci.** Although viridans streptococci commonly cause subacute bacterial endocarditis (30–40% of cases in many series) [93], the isolation of viridans streptococci from a blood culture does not automatically mean the patient has endocarditis.

   1. **Setting and source.** Viridans streptococci are normal inhabitants of the upper respiratory and intestinal tract and are sometimes present on the skin. Therefore, oral and dental manipulations can be associated with transient bacteremias. Positive blood cultures can also result from skin contamination [93].

      Isolates are likely to be significant when (1) two or more separate cultures are positive, (2) cultures are not polymicrobial, and (3) positive cultures are seen in association with a clinical picture of endocarditis or septicemia [93]. The identification of certain species may also be significant.

      Streptococcus milleri frequently produces suppurative infections, such as deep abscesses; **therefore, the isolation of *S. milleri* from the blood should prompt one to look for deep abscesses** [94]. Because it is important not to undertreat endocarditis, infectious disease consultation is advised if the significance of culture data is unclear. (See also Chap. 10.)

   2. **Therapy.** Intravenous penicillin G (9–12 million units/day in adults) is the drug of choice for viridans streptococcal bacteremia. Although relative resistance to penicillin (MIC > 0.1 μg/ml) has been reported, the clinical significance is unknown. In the absence of endocarditis, 10–14 days of intravenous therapy is recommended. A first-generation cephalosporin or erythromycin is recommended for the penicillin-allergic patient. (See Chap. 10 for a discussion of therapy of endocarditis due to viridans streptococci.)

I. **Group G streptococci** are included in the normal flora of skin, pharynx, vagina, and GI tract. Bacteremia with these organisms may cause life-threatening disease such as endocarditis or septic arthritis [95, 96]. Meningitis occurs less frequently.

1. **Therapy.** Despite in vitro susceptibility to penicillin, the clinical response often is suboptimal, even with the use of high-dose parenteral penicillin. Most cephalosporins, including cefotaxime, are active as is vancomycin. Combinations of gentamicin with either penicillin, cefotaxime, or vancomycin are synergistic against 80–90% of isolates [95].
2. In the penicillin-allergic patient, a cephalosporin (first-generation) or vancomycin is recommended [96]. If CNS penetration is required, a third-generation cephalosporin (ceftriaxone or cefotaxime) is suggested. Clindamycin and erythromycin are not effective bactericidal agents. Note that vancomycin tolerance has been reported (see Chap. 28O). Vancomycin treatment of tolerant strains should include an aminoglycoside (as in **1**).

J. **Gram-negative bacteremias.** The **low risk of endocarditis** due to gram-negative organisms is discussed in Chap. 10. Infections that warrant additional emphasis are the following:

1. **Meningococcal sepsis or bacteremia.** The meningococci can cause a transient bacteremia or septicemia, with or without an associated meningitis. Rarely, chronic meningococcemia can occur in a relatively healthy-appearing host [97]. Mortality with meningitis is estimated at 2–10%, whereas septicemia (without meningitis) has a mortality estimated at 20–30% and perhaps higher [98]. Poor prognostic signs include (1) the absence of meningitis, (2) hypotension, (3) prompt appearance of petechiae, (4) hyperpyrexia, (5) the absence of leukocytosis, and (6) thrombocytopenia.

   a. **Implications.** Meningococcemia can be a rapid, fulminant infection requiring immediate intervention and should be considered in the differential diagnosis of the febrile patient with a rash that may be macular, purpuric, petechial, or ecchymotic. Gram stain of the buffy coat or skin-lesion scraping may reveal the pathogen. *S. aureus* and pneumococci can produce a similar rash.

      Studies have suggested that patients with recurrent *N. meningitidis* and *N. gonorrhoeae* bacteremia should be evaluated for terminal complement deficiencies as a predisposing factor [99]. Close contacts of index cases (those who share eating and sleeping quarters) are at high risk of contracting invasive meningococcal disease (clinically apparent within 5 days in 50% of cases), and they should be considered for prophylaxis and careful serial clinical evaluations for the development of invasive disease (see Chap. 5 for discussion of prophylaxis after exposure to meningococcal meningitis). Medical personnel treating infected patients run little added risk unless there is intimate contact (e.g., mouth-to-mouth resuscitation) [98].

      b. **Therapy.** Penicillin is the drug of choice. Adult dosage if renal function is normal is 2 million units IV q2h; in children, 300,000 units/kg/day often is recommended. (See the dose adjustments for patients with renal failure in Chap. 28C.)

      The duration of therapy for meningococcemia with or without meningitis is controversial, though short regimens (4 days of IV therapy) have been effective. We recommend 7–10 days of IV antibiotics. We do not advise oral therapy.

      In the penicillin-allergic patient, a third-generation cephalosporin such as ceftriaxone or cefotaxime is very effective. Chloramphenicol and TMP-SMZ are alternatives when beta-lactam use is absolutely contraindicated.

2. **Disseminated gonococcal infections** are discussed in Chap. 13.
3. ***Salmonella.*** Nontyphoid *Salmonella* bacteremia has been reviewed [100, 101]. The following points deserve emphasis. (See related discussion in Chap. 11.)

   a. **Metastatic sites** of infection should be carefully excluded. The bacteremia may seed the meninges, joints, bones, endocardium, and vascular system.
   b. **Endothelial infection** (endocarditis or arteritis) recently has been shown to occur most frequently in patients older than 50 years as well as those with prior vascular surgery. *Salmonella choleraesuis* is particularly likely to cause vascular infection; its isolation should prompt a vigorous search for arteritis. Surgical resection and prolonged antibiotics will be necessary [102].
   c. **Therapy.** Bacteremia usually requires parenteral therapy. Currently, resistance to chloramphenicol, TMP-SMZ, and ampicillin has been recognized (this is a regional phenomenon), most commonly in nontyphoid species. Third-generation cephalosporins and ciprofloxacin are highly active against

Salmonella spp. No standard recommendations exist for treatment of bacteremia; however, several generalizations can be made (see Chap. 11 for further discussion):

(1) Chloramphenicol will not eradicate the organisms or prevent development of a carrier state. It should also not be used where an intravascular infection (arteritis) is suspected; a bactericidal agent is needed.

(2) Drugs of choice for intravascular infection are third-generation cephalosporins or ciprofloxacin, pending susceptibility data.

(3) Initially, intravenous therapy is advised (e.g., 3–5 days of an IV third-generation cephalosporin). If the patient does well, is afebrile for 48 hours, and is compliant, the initial IV therapy might be followed by oral therapy (e.g., ciprofloxacin if not contraindicated) to complete 14 days of antibiotics. Metastatic or intravascular infection requires prolonged (4-week) intravenous therapy. We would also consider prolonged therapy in an immunocompromised bacteremic patient.

4. **_E. coli_ bacteremia** is the most frequently seen gram-negative bacteremia. Primary foci include localized infections in the genitourinary tract, pelvis, biliary system, and GI tract. Nosocomial bacteremias are common and include catheter-related infections. In uncomplicated cases (without abscess or prolonged bacteremia), we would administer parenteral antibiotics at least until the patient is afebrile for 24–48 hours. This may then be followed with oral antibiotics to complete a 14-day course (total) of antibiotics in a compliant patient.

5. **_Klebsiella_** spp. bacteremias occur in settings similar to those described in **4.** Third-generation cephalosporins are active against community-acquired *Klebsiella* spp. (see Chap. 28F). A cephalosporin and aminoglycoside combination may be used to achieve synergy. Recent studies show that seriously ill patients fared better when given combination therapy [103, 104]. Nosocomial *Klebsiella* spp. can be resistant to third-generation cephalosporins; imipenem is active against these [104a].

6. **_P. aeruginosa_** bacteremias can occur [105]. They usually are hospital-acquired and often are polymicrobial. Patients frequently have underlying debilitating diseases, particularly malignancies. Severe pseudomonal infections and sepsis have been reported in patients with HIV infection with AIDS, especially those patients who are leukopenic [106]. Initial sites of infection are the genitourinary tract, respiratory tract, intravascular devices, and skin. Studies reveal that, even with antibiotic therapy, the mortality is high.

   Combination therapy with a full-dose aminoglycoside and an antipseudomonal penicillin remains the treatment of choice. Tobramycin (2 mg/kg/dose for the first 24 hours of therapy, followed by 1.7 mg/kg/dose ideally with pharmacokinetic dosing) and ticarcillin or piperacillin often are recommended. If tobramycin resistance is suspected, amikacin should be used. Ceftazidime (combined with an aminoglycoside) is recommended in the patient with a delayed penicillin allergy. A minimum of 14 days of IV therapy is suggested. The potential roles in this setting of aztreonam, imipenem, and ticarcillin-clavulanate or piperacillin-tazobactam are reviewed in Chap. 28, but monotherapy with these agents is not recommended. In the unusual circumstance where an aminoglycoside cannot be used, a combination of piperacillin and aztreonam is a consideration, and infectious disease consultation is suggested.

7. **_Vibrio_ spp. may cause bacteremias in patients with a history of ingestion of raw shellfish or saltwater exposure or immersion.** Patients with underlying hepatic disease may be at an increased risk for infections due to these pathogens, which can cause sepsis, gastroenteritis, cellulitis, septic thrombophlebitis, and conjunctivitis [9].

8. **_Campylobacter jejuni_** is an unusual cause of bacteremia but may especially be seen in the extremes of life or in patients with underlying disease. In a recent review, enteritis was present in approximately 70% of cases, and the GI tract was presumed to be the source of sepsis. In the other 30% of patients, diarrhea was not present and the source of the infection is speculative. Antibiotics of choice include erythromycin and aminoglycosides; fluoroquinolones are also active against this organism and may prove to be the agent of choice. The mortality is approximately 25%; death occurs mostly in compromised patients with protracted bacteremia [107].

In a recent review [107a] bacteremia was noted in < 1% of patients with *C. jejuni* infection. This low frequency may, in part, reflect that physicians rarely culture the blood of patients with diarrheal illness, even when fever is present. Three patterns of bacteremia have been described. First, transient bacteremia in a normal host with *Campylobacter* enteritis may occur. The bacteremia may be discovered several days after blood cultures are obtained and, in the interim, the patient may recover completely without antibiotic therapy. The course is benign and no antibiotics are indicated in these patients [107a]. Second, there may be a sustained bacteremia in a normal host, usually with enteritis, and these patients do well with antibiotic therapy. Third, sustained bacteremia may occur in a compromised host, even without enteritis. Prolonged antimicrobial therapy is usually required for control of these infections [107a].

Therefore, *C. jejuni* **bacteremia should be considered in the differential diagnosis of febrile patients with diarrhea.** Because blood cultures are processed in a special manner in the microbiology laboratory (proper media and incubation at 42°C), it is wise to alert the microbiology laboratory that you are concerned about *C. jejuni* in the blood (and stool) cultures.

III. **Special types of bacteremia**
   A. **Breakthrough bacteremia.** Persistently positive blood cultures, despite initiation of adequate therapy, indicate what are called **breakthrough bacteremias,** which are classified as either early (occurring within the first 72 hours of therapy) or late [108]. Aerobic gram-negative rods are most commonly isolated, and patients frequently have chronic medical problems [108, 109]. Early bacteremias have been attributed to inadequate antibiotic dosing, and late bacteremias to undrained foci of infection or resistant organisms.
      1. **Clinical evaluation**
         a. Reconfirm antibiotic susceptibility and perform an MIC on the isolate.
         b. Reconsider doses and route of administration. Oral agents usually are unacceptable. Drugs with narrow toxic-therapeutic ratios (i.e., aminoglycosides) often will necessitate determination of serum levels.
      2. **Prolonged gram-negative bacteremias** [110] are fairly common, and organisms involved include *Klebsiella* spp., *Enterobacter* spp., *E. coli,* and *B. fragilis.* Common portals of entry include intraabdominal abscesses (especially liver and genitourinary) and intravascular infections. An abdominal CT scan is generally warranted in these patients.
   B. **Polymicrobial bacteremias** are defined by multiple organisms from the same blood culture and account for 6–18% of bacteremias. There are no pathognomonic features of these bacteremias, although mortality may be high (35–63%) [7, 111]. Improvement in mortality clearly depends on correct antibiotic therapy for all involved bacteria or fungi [111].

      Sources of polymicrobial sepsis include abscesses in the abdomen, gallbladder, decubitus ulcers and, much less commonly, the respiratory tract. As expected, multiple predisposing factors are seen, including leukopenia. Polymicrobial bacteremia is frequently a nosocomial infection. Occasionally, it may be a clue that a patient is injecting himself or herself with feces or sputum. Microorganisms isolated in a recent series showed (in order of frequency) Enterobacteriaceae (*E. coli, Klebsiella* spp., etc.), anaerobes and streptococci including enterococci (excluding pneumococci and group A streptococci), *Staphylococcus* spp., *Pseudomonas* spp., and fungi. The combination of Enterobacteriaceae and streptococci or anaerobic gram-negative bacilli was highly suggestive of a primary focus of infection from a GI source [111].
   C. **Decubitus ulcer sepsis.** Bacteremias secondary to decubitus ulcers are **often polymicrobial** [112]. Common pathogens include *S. aureus,* enterococci, enteric gram-negative organisms, and anaerobes. In a recent series of bacteremic patients with spinal cord injury, 19% of the bacteremias were secondary to pressure sores (decubitus ulcers). The most common isolates were anaerobes, followed by *S. aureus* [113].
      1. **Special considerations.** These bacteremias may be persistent if adequate **surgical debridement** is not carried out. Patients commonly develop a contiguous **osteomyelitis.**
      2. **Therapy. Adequate surgical debridement is essential.** Pending cultures, antibiotic regimens are similar to those for intraabdominal-related infections (see Chap. 11); for example, clindamycin and ceftriaxone or clindamycin and an

aminoglycoside might be used. Such regimens will not cover enterococci, but these organisms uncommonly invade the bloodstream in this setting.

If monotherapy is desirable, cefoxitin, ticarcillin-clavulanate, ampicillin-sulbactam, piperacillin-tazobactam and imipenem-cilastatin are possible options, as discussed in Chap. 28. For severe infections if monotherapy is desired, imipenem-cilastatin is suggested while awaiting culture data.

D. Occult bacteremia in children [114–119]. When febrile children, who have no localizing signs and in whom the fever remains unexplained after a routine history and physical examination, have been studied in outpatient settings, approximately 5–10% have positive blood cultures. This topic has been reviewed in detail elsewhere [118].

Studies have shown that if these children are not treated with antibiotics at the time of the initial encounter, 5–10% will return with bacterial meningitis, 10% with localized infection, and another 30% with continued fever and persistent bacteremia [118]. Prior studies have shown the risk of meningitis is highest with *H. influenzae* type b infection [117]. However, with the availability and use of conjugated *H. influenzae* b vaccines and subsequent decline in invasive *H. influenzae* b infections [120], this organism is believed to be less important in vaccinated patients in this setting.

   1. **Types of bacteremia.** The most common pathogens are *S. pneumoniae* (approximately 90% of cases), *H. influenzae* type b and, infrequently, *N. meningitidis* and *S. aureus* [118].
   2. **Risk factors** associated with a higher probability that children will be bacteremic in this setting include the following [114–116]:
      a. Younger than 24 months.
      b. Temperature higher than 40°C.
      c. Peripheral WBC 15,000/mm^3 or greater.
      d. Peripheral blood smear with toxic granulations or vacuolation of polymorphonuclear leukocytes, thrombocytopenia.
      e. Underlying diseases including immunodeficiency, malnutrition, and sickle cell disease.
      f. Clinical appearance of being ill (toxic) or unhappy, inconsolable, irritable or lethargic; not eating or drinking well.
   3. **Therapy.** In prior studies, patients initially treated with antibiotics fared better than those not treated initially. Whether to treat a patient must be individualized after an assessment of the preceding risk factors. If the physician decides to start antibiotics while awaiting blood culture results, such antibiotic therapy should provide adequate coverage for *S. pneumoniae*. A recent prospective multicenter study of children at increased risk for occult bacteremia (see **2**) randomized subjects to receive a single IM injection of ceftriaxone (75 mg/kg up to 1 g maximum) or oral amoxicillin-clavulanate (40 mg/kg/day) in three divided 8-hourly doses. **Both regimens were equally effective,** but the group that received amoxicillin-clavulanate had a higher incidence of antibiotic-associated diarrhea and remained febrile longer [119]. **Careful follow-up with additional antibiotics** [19] **is essential, and patients whose blood cultures are positive warrant reevaluation.**

E. Anaerobic bacteremias. Although studies in the 1970s showed that up to 10% of bacteremias involve anaerobes, recent studies have shown a declining rate of anaerobic bacteremias accounting for 1.5–3% of positive blood cultures [121]. These may be polymicrobial in nature, and *B. fragilis* is the most common single isolate.

   1. ***B. fragilis*** bacteremias commonly originate from intraabdominal or pelvic infections. Mortality is particularly high in patients with underlying malignancies, although a recent study suggests significant mortality and morbidity with just the presence of *B. fragilis* group bacteremia [121a]. Metronidazole, a bactericidal agent, is very effective against *B. fragilis* and is the drug of choice for bacteremia. Imipenem-cilastatin, ticarcillin-clavulanate, and ampicillin-sulbactam are also very active against *B. fragilis*.
   2. **Clostridial bacteremias** (*C. perfringens* and other *Clostridium* spp.) can be present as incidental findings [122] (i.e., a positive blood culture in a febrile but otherwise asymptomatic patient) or, in contrast, may be associated with evidence of severe systemic sepsis in the setting of peripartum or abortion-related infection, mixed wound infection, or true myonecrosis, GI disease such

as ischemic colitis, and biliary disease. In addition, patients with solid tumors appear particularly prone to clostridial bacteremia, especially that caused by *Clostridium septicum.*

There is no typical clinical presentation. However, **shock, intravascular hemolysis, and jaundice should suggest clostridial bacteremia.** The highest mortality is seen with polymicrobial infection, multiple blood cultures positive for *Clostridium* spp. alone, and bacteremia associated with clinical sepsis [123].

The **drug of choice is high-dose aqueous penicillin** (18–24 million units/day in adults with normal renal function). Metronidazole, clindamycin, and chloramphenicol are alternatives in the penicillin-allergic patient.

F. **Splenectomy-related sepsis.** See Table 2-4 for empiric antibiotic therapy.

1. **Splenectomized children** are believed to be at increased risk for infection [124]. Overwhelming sepsis, most often due to pneumococci, can occur, particularly within 2 years after splenectomy [125]. This has led many authorities to recommend chronic oral penicillin prophylaxis as well as pneumococcal vaccine in splenectomized children.

2. **Splenectomized adults** with Hodgkin's disease who have undergone radiation therapy or chemotherapy are also at risk for overwhelming sepsis with *S. pneumoniae* and *H. influenzae.* These patients may be in complete remission and therefore not leukopenic when they present with sepsis [124, 126]. A healthy adult who has undergone splenectomy for trauma is at risk for overwhelming pneumococcal sepsis, but the incidence is much lower than in young children. (See the related discussion in Chap. 28B, sec. **IV.B.**)

3. *Capnocytophagia canimorsus* [formerly called **dysgonic fermenter 2** (DF-2)] bacteremia occurring after a dog bite is particularly virulent in the splenectomized patient [128]. This is a gram-negative, slow-growing, fastidious bacillus that often is seen on buffy coat Gram stain. Penicillin is effective, as are ampicillin-sulbactam and amoxicillin-clavulanate, which are agents of choice for dog-bite wounds, as discussed in detail in Chap. 4.

4. **Babesiosis** may be particularly virulent in the asplenic patient [127].

5. **Prevention.** Pneumococcal, *H. influenzae* b, and meningococcal vaccines may provide partial protection for these patients and are suggested. The role of penicillin prophylaxis is discussed in Chap. 28B, sec. **IV.B.**

G. **Bacteremias in AIDS.** See Chap. 19.

H. **Bacteremia and intravenous drug use.** In a review of intravenous drug use in Detroit [129], the organisms most frequently seen (in order of decreasing frequency) were *S. aureus,* streptococci, polymicrobial infection, and *P. aeruginosa.* Nearly half of the *S. aureus* cases were methicillin-resistant. Predictive variables of methicillin resistance included regular antibiotic use or recent hospitalization for any reason. Enterococci, often seen in earlier studies, were absent. Occasionally, *H. parainfluenzae* is seen. The sources of bacteremia were (in order of decreasing frequency) endocarditis (41%), soft-tissue or skin infection (34%), mycotic aneurysm (9%), and thrombophlebitis (4%). Endocarditis was not seen in those with a clearly defined focus of infection [130]. Extension of this experience to other urban areas may not be valid, however. Empiric antibiotic use in intravenous drug users (prior to culture data) must be based on local drug abuse practices and local epidemiology.

Catheter-Related Sepsis

Intravascular catheters and devices have become indispensable in the management of severely ill patients. Infections that carry significant morbidity and mortality are the most frequent complications related to these devices [131, 132]. It is estimated that more than 60% of nosocomial bacteremias and endocarditides are derived from intravascular devices [131]. **Ninety percent of catheter-related infections occur in the setting of a central venous catheter** [132], **so the focus here will be on this type of device.** The following is an overview of definitions, pathogenesis, diagnosis, prevention, and management of catheter-related sepsis. (For a detailed review see [132a].)

I. **Definitions** [131, 133]

A. **Exit- or insertion-site infection** indicates the presence of purulent drainage and erythema at the point where the device penetrates the skin, without evidence of bloodstream infection.

B. **Tunnel infection** is a complication of long-term catheters, such as Hickman and Broviac devices. There is usually cellulitis over the intradermal segment of the catheter (i.e., erythema and tenderness over the tunnel segment). This often occurs at the time of insertion but can occur later and present as fever of unexplained origin with local pain.

C. **Catheter-related septicemia** (CRS) denotes a bloodstream infection that is:
   1. **Related** to a vascular catheter, as evidenced by quantitative blood or catheter cultures that **microbiologically match** peripheral blood culture results.
   2. **Probably related** to a vascular device based on any of the following findings:
      a. There is evidence of local catheter infection.
      b. Sepsis resolves within 48 hours of catheter removal.
      c. Sepsis persists despite 72 hours of appropriate antimicrobial therapy.

II. **Pathogenesis.** Microorganisms are introduced into the bloodstream by the following routes [131, 134, 135].
   A. **Skin insertion site,** the most frequent source of infections related to short-term catheters (i.e., indwelling ≤ 10 days).
   B. **Hub contamination,** the most frequent source of infection with long-term catheters (i.e., indwelling > 3 weeks). Contaminating organisms are introduced by personnel manipulating the catheter hub, thereby producing colonization of the intraluminal surface of the catheter and possibly bloodstream invasion. The most commonly involved organism is coagulase-negative staphylococcus [134].
   C. **Hematogenous seeding** of the catheter from a remote infectious source. This is rare.
   D. **Contaminated infusate.** This too is relatively uncommon. It may go unrecognized until an epidemic occurs. Responsible organisms are often *Klebsiella* or *Enterobacter* spp.

III. **Laboratory diagnosis.** No laboratory diagnostic method is considered a "gold standard" [131]. **Methods described here require a simultaneous blood culture obtained from a separate venipuncture site.**
   A. **The roll-plate, semiquantitative method of catheter culture**
      1. This technique is limited in that it demonstrates external catheter surface colonization.
      2. Culture of the catheter tip is indicated in fever of undetermined source or in the presence of exit-site or tunnel infection. Routine catheter tip culture is not indicated.
   B. **Sonication** of the intravascular catheter segment (and culture of the sonicate) may help to identify intraluminal contaminants.
   C. **Quantitative blood cultures** are those simultaneously obtained through a catheter and through a peripheral vein. A differential colony count of 10:1, respectively, has been proposed to indicate CRS [132].

IV. **Prevention of CRS is the most effective form of management** [132, 136]. Measures include:
   A. **Use of maximal sterile conditions during device insertion,** including gown, gloves, mask, and large drape.
   B. **Reduction of flora at the skin insertion site with use of uncontaminated topical disinfectants,** such as betadine or chlorhexidine gluconate. There is evidence that the latter preparation is the better one for this purpose [136].
   C. **Antibiotic ointments** applied at the insertion site, though these have not conclusively proven effective.
   D. **Dressings.** Some experts prefer simple dressings of a high-quality sterile gauze, whereas others still use a transparent, breathable dressing. Both can be changed every 24–48 hours with close monitoring.
   E. **Employment of an expert team** for the insertion and maintenance of intravenous devices. This practice has been shown to lower the incidence of CRS significantly in several studies [132].
   F. Scheduled guidewire exchange of short-term catheters has not proved useful in preventing CRS.
   G. Peripherally inserted central venous catheters may prove to be a lower-risk form of venous access for extended periods in certain patient subgroups [137].
   H. Newer technologies may include antibiotic-bonded catheters and attachable silver-impregnated cuffs. It is hoped that these new materials will be associated with lower infection rates [136].

V. Management of CRS requires careful consideration of several factors together.
(Refer to the excellent reviews by Raad and Body [132] and Maki [132a].

   A. Exit-site infection is treated with intravenous antibiotics without catheter removal, unless the offending organism is a *Pseudomonas* species (see **D**). Failure of a persistently septic patient to respond to appropriate antibiotics necessitates catheter removal.

   B. Tunnel infections are more serious and most often require catheter removal along with intravenous antibiotics.

   C. Bacteremia related to a catheter will, most commonly, be **uncomplicated** [73, 132], which is defined in the literature as a bloodstream infection that responds to antibiotic therapy within approximately 48 hours. By contrast, **complicated CRS** is a bloodstream infection associated with bacterial endocarditis, prolonged bacteremia, septic thrombosis, septic emboli, osteomyelitis, or abscess. These complicated CRS (deeper infections) require prolonged courses of intravenous antibiotics, generally 4–6 weeks [132].

   D. The etiologic organism is an important determinant of the course of therapy.

      1. **Coagulase-negative staphylococcal infections** are usually successfully treated with 5–7 days of intravenous antimicrobial therapy without catheter removal. However, a recent analysis demonstrated a nearly sevenfold rate of recurrence of bacteremia in those whose catheters remained in place [132]. Therefore, the best course of action is not clear, pending further clinical studies. Infectious disease consultation is advised.

      2. *S. aureus* **CRS** has been associated with a variable frequency of complications, up to 45% in compromised individuals [132].

         a. **Uncomplicated** bacteremia responds to 10–14 days of intravenous therapy [132, 132a].

         b. **Complicated CRS**, indicated by persistent fever, sepsis, or positive blood cultures despite 48 hours of appropriate antibiotics and catheter removal, requires 4 weeks of intravenous therapy.

      3. **Catheter-related candidemia** also may be either complicated or uncomplicated. A 10- to 14-day course of intravenous amphotericin is recommended for uncomplicated catheter-related candidemia. Removal of the catheter is recommended if candidemia persists for more than 48 hours after amphotericin B institution.

      4. **Gram-negative rods infrequently** cause CRS. Hospital-acquired species, such as *Pseudomonas, Acinetobacter,* and *Xanthomonas* spp., can be involved. One week of intravenous antimicrobial therapy generally suffices. In the case of pseudomonal CRS, the catheter should be removed to eradicate the infection [132].

      5. *Corynebacterium jeikeium* may produce CRS, especially in the neutropenic population. Catheter removal is advised, and vancomycin is the drug of choice.

      6. **Atypical mycobacterium** (*M. fortuitum* or *M. chelonei*) tunnel infections require catheter removal, sometimes along with tunnel excision. Cefoxitin and amikacin together have been effective therapy [132].

VI. Peripheral inserted central venous catheters (PICC) have a low rate of complications and are being employed more frequently [132a, 137].

VII. Peripheral catheters

   A. Intravenous catheter-related infections. Peripheral plastic catheters left in place for more than 48–72 hours are associated with an increasing risk of phlebitis or bacteremia. A secondary bacteremia is seen in 2–8% of patients with prolonged catheter use.

      1. **Common pathogens** include *S. aureus, Klebsiella* spp., and other gram-negative bacilli.

      2. On physical examination, **obvious phlebitis** is present in only a **minority** of patients with intravenous-related sepsis. Therefore, in a bacteremic patient without an obvious source of infection, the plastic catheter must be suspect. In this setting:

         a. Remove the suspect catheter, infusion lines, and solution container.

         b. Culture the catheter tip as described by Maki and colleagues [133] by rolling the amputated catheter tip across a blood agar plate rather than just placing the tip into broth medium.

         c. Milk the involved vein and Gram stain any exudate.

         d. Save or culture the intravenous fluid, because the fluid itself may be contaminated.

   e. Draw two or three separate **blood cultures** in an attempt to determine
   whether there is a prolonged bacteremia.
   3. Therapy. Once the catheter has been removed, antibiotics are directed against
   common pathogens (see Table 2-4).
   4. Prevention. The date of insertion of plastic (or Teflon) catheters should be
   clearly marked so they can be routinely removed in 48–72 hours. **To minimize
   the risk of intravenous-related phlebitis,** it is important to **rotate the catheter
   (or needle) site every 48–72 hours.**
**B. Arterial catheters. Catheters left in place for more than 4 days have an increased
   likelihood of developing localized infections or bacteremias** [138]. The risk of
   bacteremia increases if the catheter was inserted by cutdown, if there is local
   inflammation, or both.
   1. Organisms. Common organisms isolated from the bloodstream are enterococci,
   Klebsiella spp., *S. aureus,* and *E. coli.* Candidemia can occur.
   2. Approach. The approach to this problem is similar to that outlined for intravenous catheter-related infections in sec. **1.** Bacteremias can occur in the absence
   of local inflammation. Bacteremia from another site may seed these catheters.
   In a bacteremia from any source, these lines should ideally be removed as soon
   as possible.
   3. Therapy. Because of the possibility of enterococcal infections, vancomycin and
   an aminoglycoside can be used while awaiting cultures (see Table 2-4).
   4. Prevention. The catheters should be inserted percutaneously with sterile technique, and sites ideally should be rotated every 4 days.

References

1. Stillman, R.I., Wenzel, R.P., and Donowitz, L.C. Emergence of coagulase negative
   staphylococci as major nosocomial bloodstream pathogens. *Infect. Control* 8:108, 1987.
2. Weinstein, M.P., et al. The clinical significance of positive blood cultures. A comprehensive analysis of 500 episodes of bacteremia and fungemia in adults. Clinical observations with special reference to factors influencing prognosis. *Rev. Infect. Dis.* 5:54,
   1983.
3. Bone, R.C., et al. American College of Chest Physicians/Society of Critical Care Medicine Consensus Conference: Definitions for sepsis organ failure and guidelines for
   the use of innovative therapies in sepsis. *Crit. Care Med.* 20:864, 1992.
   An attempt to standardize definitions of commonly used terms, such as sepsis *and*
   septic shock.
4. Bennett, I.V., Jr., and Beeson, P.B. Bacteremia: A consideration of some experimental
   and clinical aspects. *Yale J. Biol. Med.* 26:241, 1954.
5. Ponce DeLeon, S., and Wenzel, R.P. Hospital-acquired bloodstream infections with
   Staphylococcus epidermidis. Am. J. Med. 77:639, 1984.
6. Banerjee, S.N., et al. Secular trend in nosocomial primary blood stream infection in
   the United States, 1980–1989. *Am. J. Med.* 91(Suppl. 3b):86S, 1991.
7. Weinstein, M.P., et al. The clinical significance of positive blood cultures: A comprehensive analysis of 500 episodes of bacteremia and fungemia in adults: I. Laboratory
   and epidemiology observations. *Rev. Infect. Dis.* 5:35, 1983.
7a. Cunha, B.A. Antibiotic treatment of sepsis. *Med. Clin. North Am.* 79:551, 1995.
   *A recent review of this topic with an emphasis on the clinical approach and antimicro-
   bial therapy.*
8. Helmick, C.J., Bernard, K.W., and D'Angelo, L.J. Rocky Mountain spotted fever:
   Clinical, laboratory and epidemiologic features of 262 cases. *J. Infect. Dis.* 150:480,
   1984.
9. Klontz, K.C., et al. Syndromes of *Vibrio vulnificus* infections: Clinical and epidemiologic features in Florida cases, 1981–1987. *Ann. Intern. Med.* 109:318, 1988.
   For additional information on systemic and other infections related to Vibrio *spp., see*
   *D.L. Dworzack, R.B. Clark, and P.J. Padgitt, New causes of pneumonia, meningitis,
   and disseminated infections associated with immersion.* Infect. Dis. Clin. North Am.
   *1:615, 1987; and M.K. Hill and C.V. Sanders, Localized and systemic infection due
   to* Vibrio *species.* Infect. Dis. Clin. North Am. *1:687, 1987.*
10. Kingston, M.E., and Mackey, D. Skin clues in the diagnosis of life-threatening infections. *Rev. Infect. Dis.* 8:1, 1986.

11. Fitzpatrick, T.B., and Johnson, R.A. Differential Diagnosis of Rashes in the Acutely Ill Febrile Patient and in Life-Threatening Diseases. In T.B. Fitzpatrick et al. (eds.), *Dermatology in General Medicine* (3rd ed.). New York: McGraw-Hill, 1987. Atlas 3, pp. A21–A30.

11a. Levin, S., and Goodman, L.J. An approach to acute fever and rash in the adult. *Curr. Clin. Top. Infect. Dis.* 15:19, 1995.

12. Krugman, S., et al. (eds.). *Infectious Diseases of Children* (9th ed.). St. Louis: Mosby, 1992.
This book has excellent photographs and descriptions of childhood diseases presenting as exanthemas.

13. Harris, R.L., et al. Manifestations of sepsis. *Arch. Intern. Med.* 147:1895, 1987.
A complete review of potential organ system dysfunction seen in sepsis. See also J.M. Quale, Clinical significance and pathogenesis of hyperbilirubinemia associated with Staphylococcus aureus *septicemia.* Am. J. Med. *85:615, 1988.*

14. Smith, S.E., and Weinstein, M.P. Blood cultures. *Infect. Dis. Clin. North Am.* 7:221, 1993.

15. Liebovici, L., et al. Bacteremia and fungemia of unknown origin in adults. *Clin. Infect. Dis.* 14:436, 1992.
A prospective survey of bacteremia of unknown etiology that demonstrated the following: 62% of isolates were gram-negative; (2) 10% were polymicrobial; (3) staphylococci were isolated from cultures of 67% of hemodialysis patients and 37% of diabetic patients; and (4) Pseudomonas spp. were responsible for 15% of hospital-acquired bacteremias.

15a. Gross, P.A., et al. Quality standard for the treatment of bacteremia. *Clin. Infect. Dis.* 18:428, 1994.
Includes literature review emphasizing that when a proper antibiotic is used for bacteremias (with and without sepsis) mortality is improved. Part of the quality standard series.

16. Parillo, J.E. Management of septic shock: Present and future. *Ann. Intern. Med.* 115:491, 1991.
An excellent review on the topic.

17. Parillo, J.E. Pathogenetic mechanisms of septic shock syndrome. *N. Engl. J. Med.* 328:1471, 1993.
See related review by R.P. Wenzel et al., Current understanding of sepsis. Clin. Infect. Dis. *22:407, 1996.*

18. Pennington, J.A. Therapy with antibody to tumor necrosis factor in sepsis. *Clin. Infect. Dis.* 17(Suppl. 2):S515, 1993.

19. Bone, R.C. The pathogenesis of sepsis. *Ann. Intern. Med.* 115:457, 1991.
A very good discussion of the pathogenesis of septic shock syndrome.

20. Tofte, R.W., and Williams, D.N. Clinical and laboratory manifestations of toxic shock syndrome. *Ann. Intern. Med.* 96(Pt. II):843, 1982.
An extensive review of the syndrome is contained within this issue. For an exhaustive review of TSS, see the International Symposium on Toxic Shock Syndrome. Rev. Infect. Dis. *11:(Suppl. 1), 1989.*

21. Manjouri, L., et al. Reporting of toxic shock syndrome Staphylococcus aureus, 1980–1990. *J. Infect. Dis.* 164:1245, 1991.

22. Kain, K.C., Schulzer, M., and Chow, A.W. Clinical spectrum of nonmenstrual toxic shock syndrome (NMTSS): Comparison with menstrual TSS by multivariate analysis. *Clin. Infect. Dis.* 16:100, 1993.

23. Crowther, M.A., et al. Menstrual toxic shock syndrome complicated by persistent bacteremia: A case report and review. *Clin. Infect. Dis.* 16:288, 1993.

24. Stevens, D.L. Invasive group A streptococcal infections. *Clin. Infect. Dis.* 14:2, 1992.
A state-of-the-art article, with a complete discussion of the pathogenesis of streptococcal TSS.

25. Hoge, C.W., Schwartz, B., Talkington, D.F., et al. The changing epidemiology of invasive group A streptococcal infections and the emergence of streptococcal toxic shock–like syndrome. *J.A.M.A.* 269:384, 1993.
A good clinical description of streptococcal TSS.

26. Stevens, D.L., et al. The Eagle effect revisited: The efficacy of clindamycin, erythromycin, and penicillin in the treatment of streptococcal myositis. *J. Infect. Dis.* 158:23, 1988.

27. Rackow, E.C., Astiz, M.E., and Weil, M.H. Cellular oxygen metabolism during sepsis and shock. The relationship of oxygen consumption to oxygen delivery. *J.A.M.A.* 259:1989, 1988.

28. Narins, R.G., and Cohen, J.J. Bicarbonate therapy for organic acidosis: The case for its continued use. *Ann. Intern. Med.* 106:615, 1987.
    Not all authors agree. See P.W. Stacpoole, Lactic acidosis: The case against bicarbonate therapy [editorial]. Ann. Intern. Med. *105:276, 1986.*

29. Allan, J.D., Jr. Antibiotic combinations. *Med. Clin. North Am.* 71:1079, 1987.

30. Martin, C., et al. Norepinephrine or dopamine for the treatment of hyperdynamic septic shock? *Chest* 103:1826, 1993.

31. McGowan, J.E., et al. Infectious Diseases Society of America. Guidelines for the use of systemic glucocorticosteroids in the management of selected infections. *J. Infect. Dis.* 165:1, 1992.

32. Glauser, M.P., et al. Pathogenesis and potential strategies for prevention and treatment of septic shock: An update. *Clin. Infect. Dis.* 18(Suppl.):S205, 1994.

32a. Natanson, C., et al. Selected treatment strategies for septic shock based on proposed mechanisms of pathogenesis. *Ann. Intern. Med.* 120:771, 1994.
    This Clinical Staff Conference held at the National Institutes of Health, Bethesda, Md., concludes that no new therapy (e.g., core-directed antiendotoxin and anticytokine therapy for sepsis) has shown clinical efficiency.

33. Cross, A.S. Biotech strategies for treatment of sepsis. *Endotoxin Newsletter* 3:2, 1993.

34. Fisher, C.J., et al. Human recombinant interleukin-1 receptor antagonist (IL-1ra) in the treatment of patients with sepsis syndrome. *Circ. Shock* Suppl. 1:42, 1993.

35. Klastersky, J. Concept of empiric therapy with antibiotic combinations: Indications and limits. *Am. J. Med.* 80(Suppl. 5C):2, 1986.

36. Love, L.J., et al. Improved prognosis for granulocytopenic patients with gram-negative bacteremia. *Am. J. Med.* 68:643, 1980.

37. Brown, A.E. Neutropenia, fever and infection. *Am. J. Med.* 76:421, 1984.
    A good overview of infectious complications in the neutropenic host. There is a brief reference to the emerging problem of enterococcal superinfection in patients treated with third-generation cephalosporins. This problem continues to increase.

38. Sickles, E.A., Greene, W.A., and Wiernick, P.H. Clinical presentation of infection in granulocytopenic patients. *Arch. Intern. Med.* 135:715, 1975.
    Still a useful discussion about the limited signs of infection.

39. Rolston, K.V., and Bodey, G.P. Diagnosis and management of perianal and perirectal infection in the granulocytopenic patient. *Curr. Clin. Top. Infect. Dis.* 13:164, 1993.

40. Hughes, W.T., et al. Guidelines for the use of antimicrobial agents in neutropenic patients with unexplained fever. *J. Infect. Dis.* 161:381, 1990.
    Report from the Infectious Disease Society of America.

41. Pizzo, P.A., et al. Approaching the controversies in antibacterial management of cancer patients. *Am. J. Med.* 76:436, 1984.
    Excellent discussion of multiple clinical problems. Several articles covering many aspects of infection in the leukopenic patient are included in this issue. See related article by Pizzo [51].

42. Press, O.W., et al. Hickman catheter infections in patients with malignancies. *Medicine* (Baltimore) 63:189, 1984.
    A good review. See also D.K. Henderson, Bacteremia Due to Percutaneous Intravascular Devices. In G.L. Mandell, J.E. Bennett, and R. Dolin (eds.), Principles and Practice of Infectious Diseases (4th ed.). New York: Churchill Livingstone, 1995.

43. Wade, J.C., et al. *Staphylococcus epidermidis:* An increasing cause of infection in patients with granulocytopenia. *Ann. Intern. Med.* 97:503, 1982.
    The respiratory and alimentary tracts were the sites of origin of infection. Increased use of the central venous catheter was not found to be a cause.

44. Young, L.S. Empirical antibiotic therapy in the neutropenic host [editorial]. *N. Engl. J. Med.* 315:580, 1986.
    Editorial response to Pizzo et al. [50]. Dr. Young emphasizes the importance of avoiding monotherapy in the bacteremic patient. Additional support for using ceftazidime in combination with an aminoglycoside for bacteremias in cancer patients with granulocytopenia is shown in the EORTC International Antimicrobial Group Report. N. Engl. J. Med. 317:1692, 1987.

45. Rubin, M., et al. Gram-positive infections and the use of vancomycin in 550 episodes of fever and neutropenia. *Ann. Intern. Med.* 108:30, 1988.

46. Karp, J.E., et al. Empiric use of vancomycin during prolonged treatment-induced granulocytopenia. *Am. J. Med.* 81:237, 1986.

47. Liang, R., et al. Ceftazidime versus imipenem-cilastatin as initial monotherapy for

febrile neutropenic patients. *Antimicrob. Agents Chemother.* 34:1336, 1990.
Study from Hong Kong in which 89 neutropenic patients were randomized to be treated with either agent as monotherapy. The in vitro susceptibilities and the clinical response suggested that with the exception of P. aeruginosa, imipenem was more effective than ceftazidime. The majority of failures, relapses, and superinfections were related to resistant organisms such as methicillin-resistant staphylococci, Pseudomonas species, or fungi.

48. Bodey, G.P., et al. Imipenem-cilastatin as initial therapy for febrile cancer patients. *Antimicrob. Agents Chemother.* 30:211, 1986.

49. Wade, J.C., Johnson, D.E., and Bustamante, C.I. Monotherapy for empiric treatment of fever in granulocytopenic cancer patients. *Am. J. Med.* 80(Suppl. 5C):85, 1986.

50. Pizzo, P.A., et al. A randomized trial comparing ceftazidime alone with combination antibiotic therapy in cancer patients with fever and neutropenia. *N. Engl. J. Med.* 315:552, 1986.
Initial study that has been expanded by the report of B.E. DePauw et al. for the Intercontinental Antimicrobial Study Group, ceftazidime compared with piperacillin and tobramycin for the empiric treatment of fever in neutropenic patients with cancer: A multicenter randomized trial. Ann. Intern. Med. 120:834, 1994. Study involved 696 patients (83% acute leukemia or bone marrow transplants) receiving either IV ceftazidime, 2 g q8h, or piperacillin (12–18 g/day in four to six divided doses) plus tobramycin (1.7–2.0 mg/kg/dose q8h). Conclusion was that ceftazidime alone was as effective but safer than combination therapy, even in those with profound and prolonged granulocytopenia.
Some experts may still prefer double drug regimens for known or highly suspect bacteremic cases, with the hopes of achieving synergy if a gram-negative organism is involved.

51. Pizzo, P.A. Management of fever in patients with cancer and treatment-induced neutropenia. *N. Engl. J. Med.* 328:1323, 1993.
Recent summary by national expert. Reviews basis for empiric theory, changes in prominent organisms, and antimicrobial options.

52. Young, L.S. Fever and Septicemia. In R.H. Rubin and L.S. Young (eds.), *Clinical Approach to Infection in the Compromised Host* (3rd ed.). New York: Plenum, 1994. Pp. 67–104.

53. Anaissie, E.J., et al. Randomized trial of beta-lactam regimens in febrile neutropenic cancer patients. *Am. J. Med.* 84:581, 1988.

53a. Freifeld, A.G., and Pizzo, P.A. The outpatient management of febrile neutropenia in cancer patients. *Oncology* 10:599, 1996.

44. Pizzo, P.A., Landisch, S., and Robichaud, K.J. Treatment of gram-positive septicemia in cancer patients. *Cancer* 45:206, 1980.

55. Pizzo, P.A., et al. Duration of empiric therapy in granulocytopenic patients with cancer. *Am. J. Med.* 67:194, 1979.

56. Joshi, J.H., et al. Can antibacterial therapy be discontinued in persistently febrile granulocytopenic cancer patients? *Am. J. Med.* 76:450, 1984.

57. DiNubile, M.J. Stopping antibiotic therapy in neutropenic patients. *Ann. Intern. Med.* 108:289, 1988.
A potential approach to a complex clinical situation given the proper circumstances and close observation; many neutropenic patients are stable when broad-spectrum antibiotics are discontinued. This remains a controversial topic.

58. Sculier, J.P., and Klastersky, J. Significance of serum bactericidal activity in gram-negative bacillary bacteremia in patients with and without granulocytopenia. *Am. J. Med.* 76:429, 1984.

59. Thaler, M., et al. Hepatic candidiasis in cancer patients: The evolving picture. *Ann. Intern. Med.* 108:88, 1988.
The mode of infection may be via portal seeding; therefore, hepatic candidiasis often occurs in the absence of documented candidemia.

60. Wingard, J.R., Santos, G.W., and Saral, R. Differences between first and subsequent fevers during prolonged neutropenia. *Cancer* 59:844, 1987.

61. Wright, D.G. Leukocyte transfusions: Thinking twice. *Am. J. Med.* 76:637, 1984.

62. Nauseef, W.M., and Maki, D.G. A study of the value of simple protective isolation in patients with granulocytopenia. *N. Engl. J. Med.* 304:448, 1981.
See related discussion by P.J. van den Broek, Infection control during neutropenia. J. Hosp. Infect. 11(Suppl. A):7–14, 1988.

63. Verhoef, J. Prevention of infections in the neutropenic patient. *Clin. Infect. Dis.* 17(Suppl. 2):S359, 1993.
An excellent up-to-date review.

64. Dale, D.C. Potential role of colony stimulating factors in the prevention and treatment of infectious diseases. *Clin. Infect. Dis.* 18(Suppl.):S180, 1993.

64a. Schimpff, S.C. Growth factors and empiric therapy with antibiotics: Should they be used concurrently? *Ann. Intern. Med.* 121:538, 1994.
Editorial comment by national expert. See related article in same issue.

64b. Hussein, A.M., et al. The use of growth factors with antibiotics in the setting of neutropenic fever. *Am. J. Med.* 100:15, 1996.

65. Kirchoff, L.V., and Sheagren, J.N. Epidemiology and clinical significance of blood cultures positive for coagulase-negative *Staphylococcus*. *Infect. Control* 6:479, 1985.

66. Strand, C.L., and Shulman, J.A. *Bloodstream Infections: Laboratory Detection and Clinical Considerations.* Chicago: American Society Clinical Pathology Press, 1988. P. 18.

67. Van Scoy, R.E., et al. Coryneform bacterial endocarditis. *Mayo Clin. Proc.* 52:216, 1977.
For a related discussion, see B.A. Lipsley et al., Infections caused by nondiphtheria corynebacteria. Rev. Infect. Dis. 4:1220, 1982.

68. Sheagren, J.N. *Staphylococcus aureus:* The persistent pathogen (Pt. 1). *N. Engl. J. Med.* 310:1368, 1984.

69. Sheagren, J.N. *Staphylococcus aureus:* The persistent pathogen (Pt. 2). *N. Engl. J. Med.* 310:1437, 1984.

70. Mylotte, J.M., McDermott, C., and Spooner, J.A. Prospective study of 114 consecutive episodes of *Staphylococcus aureus* bacteremia. *Rev. Infect. Dis.* 9:891, 1987.

71. Lautenschlager, S., Herzog, C., and Zimmerli, W. Course and outcome of bacteremia due to *Staphylococcus aureus:* Evaluation of different clinical definitions. *Clin. Infect. Dis.* 16:567, 1993.

72. Ehni, W.F., and Reller, L.B. Short-course therapy for *S. aureus* catheter infections. *Arch. Intern. Med.* 149:533, 1989.

73. Raad, I.I., and Sabbagh, M.F. Optimal duration of therapy for catheter *Staphylococcus aureus* bacteremia: A study of 55 cases and review. *Clin. Infect. Dis.* 14:75, 1992.

74. Galpin, J.E., et al. Short-course therapy for *S. aureus* catheter infections. *Infect. Dis. Alert* 8:53, 1989.
An editorial comment on and summary of [72].

75. Small, P.M., and Chambers, H.F. Vancomycin for *Staphylococcus aureus* endocarditis in intravenous drug users. *Antimicrob. Agents Chemother.* 34:1227, 1990.
In this review, 5 of 13 patients failed therapy with vancomycin. This study raises the question of the equivalence of efficacy of vancomycin and penicillinase-resistant beta-lactam agents.

76. Levine, D.P., et al. Slow response to vancomycin or vancomycin plus rifampin in methicillin-resistant *Staphylococcus aureus* endocarditis. *Ann. Intern. Med.* 115:674, 1991.

77. Martin, M.A., et al. Coagulase-negative staphylococcal bacteremia. Mortality and hospital stay. *Ann. Intern. Med.* 110:9, 1989.
In this series, coagulase-negative staphylococci (primarily S. epidermidis) were the leading cause of hospital-acquired bacteremias, which often prolonged hospital stays.

78. Lowy, F.D., and Hammer, S.M. *Staphylococcus epidermidis* infections. *Ann. Intern. Med.* 99:834, 1983.

79. Karchmer, A.W., Archer, G.L., and Dismukes, W.E. *Staphylococcus epidermidis* causing prosthetic valve endocarditis: Microbiologic and clinical observations as guides to therapy. *Ann. Intern. Med.* 98:447, 1983.

80. Duma, R.J., et al. Streptococcal infections: A bacteriologic and clinical study of streptococcal bacteremia. *Medicine* (Baltimore) 48:87, 1969.
Detailed study of groups A, B, and D and other streptococcal bacteremias. Still useful.

81. Bibler, M.R., and Rouan, G.W. Cryptogenic group A streptococcal bacteremia at an urban general hospital and review of the literature. *Rev. Infect. Dis.* 8:941, 1986.

82. Burkert, T., and Watanakunakorn, C. Group A streptococcal bacteremia in a community teaching hospital. *Clin. Infect. Dis.* 14:29, 1992.

83. Farley, M., et al. A population based assessment of invasive disease due to group B streptococcus in non-pregnant adults. *N. Engl. J. Med.* 328:1807, 1993.
See related paper by L.A. Jackson et al., Risk factors for group B streptococcal disease in adults. Ann. Intern. Med. 123:415, 1995.

84. Schwartz, B., et al. Invasive group B streptococcal disease in adults. *J.A.M.A.* 266:1112, 1991.
85. Maki, D.G., and Agger, W.A. Enterococcal bacteremia: Clinical features, the risk of endocarditis, and management. *Medicine* (Baltimore) 67:248, 1988.
86. Granninger, W., and Ragette, R. Nosocomial bacteremia due to *Enterococcus faecalis* without endocarditis. *Clin. Infect. Dis.* 15:49, 1992.
87. Awada, A., et al. Streptococcal and enterococcal bacteremia in patients with cancer. *Clin. Infect. Dis.* 15:33, 1992.
88. Gransden, W.R., Eyckyn, S.J., and Phillips, I. Pneumococcal bacteremia: 325 episodes diagnosed at St. Thomas's Hospital. *Br. Med. J.* 290:505, 1985.
    For a recent update, see J.F. Plouffe et al., Bacteremia with Streptococcus pneumoniae: *Implications for therapy and prevention.* J.A.M.A. *275:194, 1996.*
89. Redd, S.C., et al. The role of human immunodeficiency virus in pneumococcal bacteremia in San Francisco residents. *J. Infect. Dis.* 162:1012, 1990.
90. Fanciullo, G.J., et al. Serotyping of 1,458 pneumococcal isolates with analysis of bacteremia in 84 patients. *South. Med. J.* 79:1370, 1986.
91. Applebaum, P.C. Antimicrobial resistance in *Streptococcus pneumoniae:* An overview. *Clin. Infect. Dis.* 15:77, 1992.
92. Klein, R.S., et al. *Streptococcus bovis* septicemia and carcinoma of the colon. *Ann. Intern. Med.* 91:560, 1979.
93. Swenson, F.J., and Rubin, S.J. Clinical significance of viridans streptococci isolated from blood cultures. *J. Clin. Microbiol.* 15:725, 1982.
94. Gossling, J. Occurrence and pathogenicity of the *Streptococcus milleri* group. *Clin. Infect. Dis.* 14:120, 1988.
95. Johnson, C.C., and Tunkel, A.R. Viridans and Groups C and G Streptococci. In G.L. Mandell, J.E. Bennett, and R. Dolin (eds.), *Principles and Practice of Infectious Diseases* (4th ed.). New York: Churchill Livingstone, 1995.
96. Lam, K., and Bayer, A.S. Serious infections due to group G streptococci: Report of 15 cases with in vitro–in vivo correlations. *Am. J. Med.* 75:561, 1983.
97. Benoit, F.L. Chronic meningococcemia: Case report and review of the literature. *Am. J. Med.* 35:103, 1963.
    Meningococcemia can present as an indolent infection in a previously healthy host.
98. Peltola, H. Meningococcal disease: Still with us. *Rev. Infect. Dis.* 5:71, 1983.
99. Peterson, B.H., et al. *N. meningitidis* and *N. gonorrhoeae* bacteremia associated with C(sub 6), C(sub 7), or C(sub 8) deficiency. *Ann. Intern. Med.* 90:917, 1979.
100. Goldberg, M.B., and Rubin, R.H. The spectrum of *Salmonella* infection. *Infect. Dis. Clin. North Am.* 2:571, 1988.
     Includes summary of bacteremias.
101. Cherubin, C.E., Neu, H.C., and Imperato, P.J. Septicemia with non-typhoid *Salmonella. Medicine* (Baltimore) 53:365, 1974.
102. Cohen, P.S., et al. The risk of endothelial infection in adults with *Salmonella* bacteremia. *Ann. Intern. Med.* 89:931, 1978.
103. Watanakunakorn, C., and Jura, J. *Klebsiella* bacteremia: A review of 196 episodes during a decade (1980–1989). *Scand. J. Infect. Dis.* 23:399, 1991.
104. Kovick, J.A., et al. Prospective observational study of *Klebsiella* bacteremia in 230 patients: Outcome of antibiotic combinations versus monotherapy. *Antimicrob. Agents Chemother.* 36:2639, 1992.
104a. Meyer, K.S., et al. Nosocomial outbreak of *Klebsiella* infection resistant to late-generation cephalosporins. *Ann. Intern. Med.* 119:353, 1993.
105. Gallagher, P.G., and Watanakunakorn, C. *Pseudomonas* bacteremia in a community teaching hospital, 1980–1984. *Rev. Infect. Dis.* 11:846, 1989.
106. Kielhofner, M., et al. Life-threatening *Pseudomonas aeruginosa* infections in patients with human immunodeficiency virus infection. *Clin. Infect. Dis.* 14:403, 1992.
107. Dhawan, V.K., et al. *Campylobacter jejuni* septicemia—epidemiology, clinical features and outcome. *West. J. Med.* 144:324, 1986.
107a. Blaser, M.J. Campylobacter and related species. In G.L. Mandell, J.E. Bennett, and R. Dolin (eds.), *Principles and Practice of Infectious Diseases* (4th ed.). New York: Churchill Livingstone, 1995. Pp. 1948–1956.
108. Anderson, E.T., Young, L.S., and Hewitt, W.L. Simultaneous antibiotic levels in "breakthrough" gram-negative rod bacteremia. *Am. J. Med.* 61:493, 1976.
109. Weinstein, M.P., and Reller, L.B. Clinical importance of "breakthrough" bacteremia. *Am. J. Med.* 76:175, 1984.

110. Harris, J.A., and Cobbs, C.G. Persistent gram-negative bacteremia. *Am. J. Surg.* 125:705, 1973.
111. Weinstein, M.P., et al. Clinical importance of polymicrobial bacteremia. *Diagn. Microbiol. Infect. Dis.* 5:185, 1986.
     For another review, see A.G. Reuben et al., Polymicrobial bacteremia: Clinical and microbiologic patterns. Rev. Infect. Dis. 11:161, 1989.
112. Galpin, J.E., Chow, A.W., and Bayer, A.S. Sepsis associated with decubitus ulcers. *Am. J. Med.* 61:346, 1976.
113. Montgomerie, J.Z., et al. Low mortality among patients with spinal cord injury and bacteremia. *Rev. Infect. Dis.* 13:867, 1991.
     A significant percentage of these patients had underlying decubitus ulcers.
114. Teele, D.W., et al. Bacteremia in febrile children under two years of age: Results of cultures of blood of 600 consecutive febrile children seen in a "walk-in" clinic. *J. Pediatr.* 87:227, 1975.
115. McLellan, D., and Giebink, G.S. Perspectives on occult bacteremia in children. *J. Pediatr.* 109:1, 1986.
116. Rubin, L.G., and Carmody, L. Pneumococcal and *Haemophilus influenzae* type B antigen detection in children at risk for occult bacteremia. *Pediatrics* 80:92, 1987.
117. Shapiro, E.D., et al. Risk factors for development of bacterial meningitis among children with occult bacteremia. *J. Pediatr.* 109:15, 1986.
118. Lorin, M.I., and Feigin, R.D. Fever Without Localizing Signs and Fever of Unknown Origin. In R.D. Feigin and J.D. Cherry (eds.), *Textbook of Pediatric Infectious Diseases* (3rd ed.). Philadelphia: Saunders, 1992. Pp. 1012–1022.
119. Bass, J.W., et al. Antimicrobial treatment of occult bacteremia: A multicenter cooperative study. *Pediatr. Infect. Dis.* 12:466, 1993.
120. Centers for Disease Control. Progress toward elimination of *Haemophilus influenzae* type b disease among infants and children—United States, 1987–1993. *M.M.W.R.* 43:144, 1994.
121. Lombardi, D.P., and Engelberg, N.C. Anaerobic bacteremia: Incidence, patient characteristics, and clinical significance. *Am. J. Med.* 92:53, 1992.
     See related paper from Mayo Clinic by C.W. Dorsher et al., Anaerobic bacteremias: Decreasing rate over a 15-year period. Rev. Infect. Dis. 33:633, 1991. Authors speculate the decline may be related to earlier recognition and treatment of localized anaerobic infection, widespread preoperative use of agents before bowel surgery, and use of broad-spectrum antimicrobial regimens that include agents with activity against anaerobes. See also V.A. Peralno et al., Incidence and significance of anaerobic bacteremia in a community hospital. Clin. Infect. Dis. 16(Suppl. 4):S288, 1993, in which anaerobic bacteremia was uncommon but when present was often associated with a change in antimicrobial therapy.
121a. Redondo, M.C., et al. Attributable mortality of bacteremia associated with the *Bacteroides fragilis* group. *Clin. Infect. Dis.* 20:1492, 1995.
     Study suggests an excess mortality of 19% attributable to B. fragilis group bacteremia. Authors still favor the routine use of anaerobic media for blood cultures.
     For a recent related paper on the importance of anaerobic bacteremia, see A. Arzese et al., Anaerobe-induced bacteremia in Italy: A nationwide survey. Clin. Infect. Dis. 20(Suppl. 2):S230, 1995. Of strains isolated, B. fragilis group species accounted for 34.5% of isolates.
122. Gorbach, S.L., and Thadepelli, H. Isolation of clostridium in human infections: Evaluation of 114 cases. *J. Infect. Dis.* 131(Suppl. 5):81, 1975.
123. Pietraritta, J.J., and Deckers, P.J. Significance of clostridial bacteremia. *Am. J. Surg.* 143:519, 1982.
     See related article by G.P. Bodey et al., Clostridial bacteremia in cancer patients: A 12-year experience. Cancer 87:1928, 1991.
124. Styrt, B. Infection associated with asplenia: Risks, mechanisms, and prevention. *Am. J. Med.* 88(Suppl. 5N):33N, 1990.
125. Ein, S.H., et al. The morbidity and mortality of splenectomy in childhood. *Ann. Surg.* 185:307, 1977.
     Overwhelming sepsis is usually due to pneumococci and is seen within 2 years after splenectomy. For an update, see [124].
126. Weitzman, S., and Aisenberg, A.C. Fulminant sepsis after the successful treatment of Hodgkin's disease. *Am. J. Med.* 62:47, 1977.
127. Rosner, R., et al. Babesiosis in splenectomized adults: Review of 22 reported cases. *Am. J. Med.* 76:696, 1984.

128. Hicklin, H., Verghese, A., and Alvarez, S. Dysgonic fermenter 2 septicemia. *Rev. Infect. Dis.* 9:884, 1987.
    Acquired through dog bites, the predisposed patient either is asplenic or has alcoholic liver disease. In the asplenic patient, fulminant sepsis with accompanying peripheral gangrene and disseminated intravascular coagulation is seen. See related discussion in Chap. 4 under Animal Bites.

129. Crane, L.R., et al. Bacteremia in narcotic addicts at the Detroit Medical Center: I. Microbiology, epidemiology, risk factors and empiric therapy. *Rev. Infect. Dis.* 8:364, 1986.

130. Levine, D.P., et al. Bacteremia in narcotic addicts at the Detroit Medical Center: II. Infectious endocarditis: A prospective comparative study. *Rev. Infect. Dis.* 8:374, 1986.

131. Mermel, L.A. Prevention and management of infections from intravascular devices: Magnitude of the problem and definitions. Symposium presented at the International Conference on Antimicrobial Agents and Chemotherapy, New Orleans, October 1993.

132. Raad, I.I., and Bodey, G.P. Infectious complications of indwelling vascular catheters. *Clin. Infect. Dis.* 15:197, 1992.
    For related reviews, see R.N. Garrison and M.A. Wilson, Intravenous and central catheter infections. Surg. Clin. North Am. 74:557, 1994 and G.L. Malanoski et al., Staphylococcus aureus catheter-associated bacteremia: Minimal effective therapy and unusual infectious complications associated with arterial sheath catheters. Arch. Intern. Med. 155:1161, 1995. Data support 10–15-day course of IV antibiotics in patients without early complications.

132a. Maki, D.G. Infections caused by intravascular devices used for infusion therapy: Pathogenesis, prevention, and management. In A.L. Bisno and F.A. Waldvogel (eds.), *Infections Associated with Indwelling Medical Devices* (2nd ed.). Washington, D.C.: ASM Press, 1994. Pp. 155–212.
    For other related discussions, see D.K. Henderson. Bacteremia due to percutaneous intravascular devices. In G.L. Mandell, J.E. Bennett, and R. Dolin (eds.), Principles and Practice of Infectious Diseases. New York: Churchill Livingstone, 1995. Pp. 2587–2599; and I.I. Rand et al., The relationship between the thrombotic and infectious complications of central venous catheters. J.A.M.A. 271:1014, 1994.

133. Maki, D.G., Weise, C.E., and Sarafin, H.W. Semi-quantitative culture method for identifying intravenous catheter-related infection. *N. Engl. J. Med.* 296:1305, 1977.
    The semiquantitative culture method described in this article remains the standard for identifying catheter-related septicemia. Distinguishes contamination from true infection. Study looked at peripheral catheters as well as subclavian and internal jugular central venous pressure monitor catheters.

134. Maki, D.G. Infections due to Infusion Therapy. In J.V. Bennett and P.S. Brachman (eds.), *Hospital Infections.* Boston: Little, Brown, 1992.

135. Daschner, F.D., and Frank, U. Intravenous catheter and device-related infection. *Curr. Opin. Infect. Dis.* 2:663, 1989.

136. Maki, D.G. Prevention and management of infections from intravascular devices: Pathophysiology and strategies for prevention. Symposium presented at 33rd Interscience Conference on Antimicrobial Agents and Chemotherapy, New Orleans, October 1993.

137. Merrell, S.W., et al. Peripherally inserted central venous catheters. Low risk alternatives for ongoing venous access. *West. J. Med.* 160:25, 1994.

138. Band, J.D., and Maki, D.G. Infections caused by arterial catheters used for hemodynamic monitoring. *Am. J. Med.* 67:735, 1979.

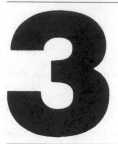

Neonatal Sepsis and Infections

Katherine L. O'Brien
and Mark C. Steinhoff

The frequency and severity of bacterial infections are greater in the newborn period than at any time thereafter. The newborn often does not manifest the classic clinical signs of infection usually observed in children and adults. Moreover, the maturing physiology of the newborn requires that drug therapy be carefully individualized. This chapter is designed to help practitioners manage infectious diseases in these especially vulnerable patients.

I. **Background.** Infection and disease caused by bacteria and viruses are not uncommon events in newborn infants (Table 3-1). Systemic bacterial infection occurs in fewer than 1% of newborns, and viral disease may occur in 6–8% of all neonates. The rate of septicemia is 2.7/1,000 full-term infants [1]. Nosocomial bacterial infection has been reported in 2–25% of newborns in intensive care nurseries [2]. **The mortality of neonates from infections varies among nurseries but has been reported as 15–50% for early-onset sepsis and 10–20% for late-onset sepsis. Mortality is higher still for prematures.** These percentages show that, even in this antibiotic era, the morbidity and mortality from neonatal infections are extraordinarily high. We shall examine some of the reasons for higher incidence and increased severity of neonatal infections in the following sections.

A. **Definitions**
1. **Fetus:** from eighth week of gestation to birth.
2. **Neonate:** birth to 28 days of age.
3. **Infant:** 1 month to 1 year.
4. **Early-onset neonatal infection:** occurs within the first 7 days of life and usually is caused by organisms acquired during the intrauterine or intrapartum stages.
5. **Late-onset neonatal infection:** occurs after 7 days and frequently results from postpartum (often nosocomial) colonization.

B. **Perinatal environments.** Infections may be caused by pathogenic organisms acquired before, during, or after birth. In passing from intrauterine to independent existence, the newborn is exposed to and becomes colonized with many microorganisms.
1. **Intrauterine.** The fetus develops in a sterile ecosphere, protected from maternal microorganisms by the placenta and the amniotic membranes. Intrauterine infection can result from:
   a. **Transplacental passage of pathogens** with placentitis, as seen in **viral infection** (e.g., rubella, cytomegalovirus [CMV], herpes simplex, hepatitis, human immunodeficiency virus [HIV], mumps), **bacterial infections** (syphilis, tuberculosis, *Listeria,* and *Salmonella* infections), and **protozoal infections** (toxoplasmosis and malaria).
   b. **Infection that ascends** through the cervix, causing amnionitis.
2. **Intrapartum.** During normal delivery, the sterility of the amniotic space is lost when the membranes rupture. As the neonate passes through the birth canal, he or she is newly colonized with the wide variety of organisms resident in the maternal cervicovaginal canal. Common organisms include streptococci, *Escherichia coli,* and other aerobic and anaerobic enteric pathogens. The neonate may also be exposed to *Chlamydia, Neisseria gonorrhoeae,* herpes simplex viruses, and CMV if the mother is infected.
3. **Postpartum.** In the postpartum period, the neonate is in contact first with the hospital nursery and then with the household. If ill, the newborn will be exposed to a large number of nursery staff as well as the devices used for respiratory and metabolic support, all of which increase the likelihood of infection. Organisms that may spread in the nursery include enteroviruses, herpes simplex, respiratory syncytial virus, and parainfluenza viruses.

Table 3-1. Frequency of perinatal infections due to selected microorganisms

Microorganism	Mother (per 1,000 pregnancies)	Fetus (intrauterine per 1,000 live births)	Neonate (intrapartum per 1,000 live births)
Cytomegalovirus			
During pregnancy	16–130	5–15	—
At delivery	110–280	—	50–100
Hepatitis B[a]	1–2 acute	Rare	0.1–0.3
	5–15 chronic		
Chlamydia	40–50	—	10–60 (conjunctivitis)
			3–10 (pneumonia)
Rubella			
Epidemic	20–40	4–30	0
Interepidemic	0.1–1.0	—	0.2
Toxoplasma gondii	1.5–6.4	1.3–7.0	0
Herpes simplex	1–10	Rare	0.1–0.5
Hepatitis C[b]	0–43	Unknown	Unknown
(incomplete data)			
Treponema pallidum	0.2	0.1	0
Group B streptococcus	50–250	—	1–2
Escherichia coli	Common	—	1–2

[a]International Federation of Gynecology and Obstetrics. Hepatitis in pregnancy. ACOG Tech. Bull. No. 174, November 1992. *Int. J. Gynecol. Obstet.* 42:189, 1993.
[b]N. S. Silverman et al. Hepatitis C virus in pregnancy: Seroprevalence and risk factors for infection. *Am. J. Obstet. Gynecol.* 169:583, 1993.
Source: Modified and updated from J. S. Remington and J. O. Klein, *Infectious Diseases of the Fetus and Newborn Infant.* Philadelphia: Saunders, 1976.

II. **Ontogeny of the immune system.** In addition to movement from one environment to another, the newborn also progresses from one level of immune function to another. The fetus may be viewed as a compromised host in a protected, sterile environment. Similarly, the newborn is a less compromised host whose immune function matures rapidly while in contact with the normal environment [3]. Because of the unique environment and the maturing immunocompetence of the neonate, the microorganisms that cause disease are different from those seen later in childhood or in adults.
   A. **B lymphocytes** are present by the tenth week of gestation. **Antibody production** is noted by the twentieth week (Fig. 3-1). Virtually all the IgG present at birth has been passively transferred from the maternal circulation. This transfer occurs predominantly between 32 weeks' gestation and birth; consequently, premature newborns have lower levels of IgG than do full-term infants. The half-life of this maternally derived IgG is approximately 25 days; the nadir is reached at 2–4 months, before the child's own production increases (see Fig. 3-1). Infants have a diminished antibody response to the polysaccharide antigens of the encapsulated bacteria (*Streptococcus pneumoniae, Haemophilus influenzae,* and *Neisseria meningitidis*). These are not common causes of neonatal disease, probably because of specific antibody acquired from the mother.
   B. **T lymphocytes.** There is little information about the early development of T lymphocytes. Homograft rejection is present by the fifth month of gestation. T-cell function probably is intact at birth but may not be fully effective because the nonspecific inflammatory response is deficient in newborns.
   C. **Leukocytes** are present early in gestation: granulocytes at 2 months, lymphocytes at 3 months, and monocytes at 4–5 months. Leukocytes probably are normal in their bactericidal function at birth, but they have abnormal chemotaxis and probably deficient phagocytosis.
   D. **Humoral factors. Complement** is synthesized and present early in gestation but, at birth, serum **C1q, C2, C3, C4, C5, factor B,** and total hemolytic levels are **low.** The **opsonic activity** of the sera of premature and term neonates is decreased, as is the **chemotactic activity** when compared with adult sera.

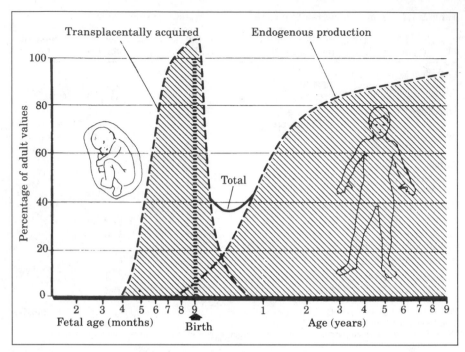

Fig. 3-1. Plasma IgG concentration at difference ages. (From A. S. Goldman and R. M. Goldblum, Primary deficiencies in humoral immunity. *Pediatr. Clin. North Am.* 24:280, 1977.)

   E. **Passive immunity**
     1. **Transplacental transport of maternal IgG** provides some transient protection against the following microorganisms (if the mother has antibodies): *S. pneumoniae,* other *Streptococcus* spp., *Staphylococcus* spp., *H. influenzae,* and the common viral agents (measles, rubella, chickenpox). Usually, little protection is transferred against the enteric gram-negative organisms.
     2. **Breast milk** is rich in **secretory IgA** directed against respiratory and enteric microorganisms. It also contains active T and B lymphocytes, leukocytes, macrophages, and nonspecific inhibitors of bacterial and viral replication.

Pharmacology and Use of Antibiotics in Neonates

In addition to the changes in immune function mentioned earlier, the newborn also experiences rapid physiologic changes that are important in terms of drug dosage. **In the practice of pediatrics, all drugs are administered on the basis of surface area or weight until the child reaches adult size.**

I. **Pharmacology**
   A. **Route of administration.** Absorption of an oral drug may be affected by the initial decreased gastric acidity of newborns and by the decreased intestinal motility of prematures. The vasomotor instability of neonates may make the subcutaneous and intramuscular routes uncertain. For these and other reasons, **antibiotics for severe neonatal infections should be administered intravenously.**
   B. **Antibiotic distribution** in infants is unique because of the rapid changes in body composition and compartments that occur after birth.
     1. **The extracellular fluid** (ECF) compartment comprises up to 50% of total body weight in neonates and drops to 25% by 1 year and to 20% in adulthood. **Because the ECF compartment comprises such a high percentage of the neonate's total body weight, the volume of distribution of some drugs, such**

as the aminoglycosides, is increased, requiring larger doses relative to weight.

   2. **Serum albumin** is quantitatively and qualitatively different in neonates relative to adults, being lower in concentration and showing less affinity for the penicillins. In neonates, albumin is important as a binder of bilirubin. Drugs that displace bilirubin from albumin (sulfonamides and selected cephalosporins) must be used with care to avoid kernicterus [4, 5].

C. **Antibiotic metabolism** in the newborn is different from that in adults and children and changes rapidly in the first week of life.

   1. **Hepatic.** Some **hepatic enzyme systems** are not fully developed at birth, and drugs rendered inactive by those systems must be administered in lower doses. Because of the decreased glucuronidation of chloramphenicol, newborns require less frequent and lower doses to avoid the gray-baby syndrome.

   2. **Renal.** Renal blood flow, glomerular filtration, and tubular function are all diminished at birth.

      a. **The glomerular filtration rate** is only 30% of adult levels, and this increases the half-life of the aminoglycosides and chloramphenicol.

      b. **Tubular secretion** is decreased to 20% of adult levels. Thus, the half-life of the penicillin family is lengthened.

II. **Some principles of antibiotic use**

A. **Dosages. Table 3-2** gives recommended dosages for selected antibiotics. This table is necessarily complex, to allow consideration of body mass and physiologic maturity in determining the optimal dosage. **Note that drug amounts are listed per dose, not per day.**

   1. **Aminoglycosides.** Because of the wide individual variation among infants in the excretion of the aminoglycosides, their prolonged use (> 5 days) should be guided by serum levels to avoid toxic or ineffectual levels (see Chap. 28H).

   2. **Chloramphenicol** doses should likewise be guided by monitoring of **serum levels** (see sec. **B.3**).

B. **Adverse reactions**

   1. **Penicillins.** The penicillin group of drugs is safe in neonates and infants. IgE-mediated immediate reactions are very rare, even in children born to allergic mothers. Methicillin-induced renal toxicity has been reported but is rare in neonates.

   2. **Aminoglycosides.** The older agents (kanamycin and gentamicin) appear to be safe when used as recommended. Experience with amikacin and tobramycin reveals no acute toxicity in newborns when used in recommended doses and when serum levels are monitored.

   3. **Chloramphenicol** is well documented as the cause of the **gray-baby syndrome** in neonates. It should be used only when less toxic drugs will not suffice, and serum levels should be monitored. Careful observation for early signs of the gray-baby syndrome (vomiting, abdominal distention, diarrhea, poor sucking, and respiratory distress) should be undertaken with complete blood counts and platelet counts at least twice weekly to detect hematologic abnormalities. (See Chap. 28J for additional discussion of chloramphenicol and the role of monitoring serum drug levels.)

C. **Special limitations of use of antibiotics in neonates**

   1. **Sulfonamides** have only bacteriostatic effects on bacteria. They can cause kernicterus by their competition with unconjugated bilirubin for albumin-binding sites. Because of this toxic effect and because of the availability of other drugs for previous indications, there is **no current indication for sulfonamides in neonates** except in the treatment of toxoplasmosis and *Pneumocystis carinii* pneumonia.

   2. **Tetracyclines** are bacteriostatic and have considerable toxicity. They bind to bone and teeth by chelation with calcium, causing decreased bone growth and permanent discoloration of teeth. **The use of this group of drugs should be avoided from the second trimester of gestation to the eighth year of life.**

   3. **Cephalosporins.** The first-generation agents (e.g., cephalothin and cefazolin) as well as most second-generation agents (e.g., cefuroxime and cefoxitin) do not adequately penetrate the cerebrospinal fluid (CSF). The third-generation cephalosporins (cefotaxime and ceftriaxone) are able to penetrate the CSF well and are active against many gram-negative bacilli. These agents are discussed in detail in Chap. 28F. **Ceftriaxone should be avoided in the first 4 weeks of life as it affects bilirubin-albumin binding and may increase the risk of bilirubin**

Table 3-2. Recommended dosages of selected antibiotics for neonates by age and birth weight

Antibiotic	Route of administration	Dose (mg/kg) at age 0–7 days		Dose (mg/kg) at age 8–30 days	
		Wt < 2,000 g	Wt > 2,000 g	Wt < 2,000 g	Wt > 2,000 g
Acyclovir	IV	10 q8h	10 q8h	10 q8h	10 q8h
Amikacin[a]	IV, IM	7.5 q12h	7.5–10 q12h	7.5–10 q8h	10 q8h
Ampicillin[b]	IV, IM	25–50 q12h	50–100 q8h	50–100 q8h	25–50 q6h
Amphotericin B	IV	0.25–1.0 q24h	0.25–1.0 q24h	0.25–1.0 q24h	0.25–1.0 q24h
Cefotaxime[c]	IV, IM	50 q12h	50 q8–12h	50 q8h	50 q6–8h
Ceftazidime	IV, IM	50 q12h	50 q12h	50 q8h	50 q8h
Chloramphenicol[a,d]	IV, PO	25 q24h	25 q24h	25 q24h	25 q12h
Clindamycin	IV, IM, PO	5 q8h	5–10 q6h	5–10 q6h	5–10 q6h
Erythromycin	PO	10 q12h	10 q12h	10 q12h	10 q8h
Gentamicin[a]	IV, IM	2.5 q12h	2.5 q12h	2.5 q8h	2.5 q8h
Methicillin	IV, IM	25–50 q12h	25–50 q8h	25–50 q8h	25–50 q6h
Nafcillin[e]	IV	25 q12h	25 q8h	25 q8h	25 q6h
Oxacillin	IV, IM	25 q12h	25 q8h	25 q8h	25 q6h
Penicillin G[f]	IV, IM	25,000–50,000 units q12h	25,000–50,000 units q8h	25,000–75,000 units q8h	25,000–50,000 units q6h
Penicillin, benzathine[f]	IM	50,000 units once (max. 2.4 million)	50,000 units once	50,000 units once	50,000 units once
Penicillin procaine[f]	IM	50,000 units q24h (max. 4.8 million)	50,000 units q24h	50,000 units q24h	50,000 units q24h
Ticarcillin	IV, IM	75 q12h	75 q8h	75 q8h	100 q8h
Tobramycin[a]	IV, IM	2.5 q12h	2.5 q12h	2.5 q8h	2.5 q8h
Vancomycin[a]	IV	10–15 q12–18h	10–15 q8–12h	10–15 q8h	10–15 q8h

[a] Serum antibiotic levels must be monitored. Listed doses are for initiation of therapy.
[b] Group B streptococcal meningitis requires 300–400 mg/kg/day of ampicillin.
[c] Cefotaxime and other third-generation cephalosporins are described in detail in Chap. 28F.
[d] Loading dose of 20 mg/kg IV or PO.
[e] Excretion predominantly hepatic; use with caution in young and premature infants.
[f] Penicillin doses are expressed in units per kilogram. Group B streptococcal sepsis requires 200,000 units/kg/day of penicillin G. Group B streptococcal meningitis requires 500,000 units/kg/day of penicillin G.

encephalopathy in jaundiced neonates [4, 6]; therefore cefotaxime is preferred in the neonate [7–9].

4. **Nafcillin should not be used in premature or very young infants.** Its excretion is predominantly by hepatic mechanisms, which may be deficient in these young infants.

III. **Antibiotic use in the pregnant or lactating woman** (see Chap. 28A)

A. **Placental transfer of antibiotics.** As a general rule, pregnant women should avoid **all** drugs because of the risk of fetal toxicity. Table 3-3 shows the infant-maternal serum concentration of selected antibiotics.

Sulfonamides given to mothers late in pregnancy have caused kernicterus or hemolytic anemia in infants deficient in glucose-6-phosphate dehydrogenase (G6PD). Similarly, **tetracycline** has caused dental deformities and discoloration. Of the aminoglycosides, **streptomycin** used during pregnancy has been associated with eighth nerve dysfunction in neonates. The documented fetal toxicity of these antibiotics warrants careful evaluation of their use in pregnancy [10, 11].

B. **Antibiotics in breast milk.** There are limited data on nursing neonates regarding adverse effects associated with antibiotics administered to their mothers [11, 12]. Nevertheless, nursing mothers should avoid all drugs if possible. Table 3-4 shows the concentrations of selected antibiotics in breast milk and their milk-plasma ratios. An important consideration is the total daily "dose" a nursing baby would receive; in many cases, this dose is not toxicologically significant.

1. **Nalidixic acid and sulfonamides,** when administered to the lactating mother, have been reported to cause hemolytic anemias in G6PD-deficient infants; consequently, nitrofurantoin may also do so. If a nursing mother must receive these drugs, breast-feeding should be stopped. (See related discussions in Chaps. 28K and 28T.)

2. The use of certain antibiotics by the nursing mother entails **theoretic risks** to her infant. **Metronidazole** is carcinogenic in rodents; **penicillins** may sensitize the infant; **tetracyclines** may cause dental staining; **chloramphenicol** may suppress hematopoiesis; and any antimicrobial may alter enteric flora. None

Table 3-3. Placental transfer of antibiotics

Infant/maternal serum concentrations	Antibiotic
50–100%	Ampicillin Carbenicillin Chloramphenicol* Methicillin Nitrofurantoin* Penicillin G Sulfonamides* Tetracyclines*
30–50%	Amphotericin B Cefamandole Cephalothin Clindamycin Gentamicin* Kanamycin* Streptomycin*
0–30%	Amikacin* Cefazolin Ceftriaxone Dicloxacillin Erythromycin Nafcillin Oxacillin Tobramycin*

*Potential for adverse effect on the fetus.
Source: Modified from G. H. McCracken and J. D. Nelson, *Antimicrobial Therapy for Newborns.* New York: Grune & Stratton, 1977; and from J. S. Remington and J. O. Klein, *Infectious Diseases of the Fetus and Newborn Infant* (3rd ed.). Philadelphia: Saunders, 1990.

Table 3-4. Antibiotics in breast milk

Maternal milk-plasma concentration	Antibiotic	Milk concentration (μg/ml)
50–100%	Ampicillin	0.07
	Chloramphenicol*	16–25
	Clindamycin	0.5–3.1
	Erythromycin	0.4–1.6
	Isoniazid	6–12
	Metronidazole*	NA
	Sulfapyridine*	30–130
	Tetracycline*	0.5–2.6
	Trimethoprim-sulfamethoxazole	2
< 30%	Amoxicillin	0.014–0.10
	Cefotaxime	0.26
	Cephazolin	1.5
	Kanamycin*	18.4
	Nalidixic acid*	4
	Oxacillin	0.2
	Penicillin G	0.01–0.04
	Streptomycin*	0.3–1.3

NA = not available.
*Potential toxicity for nursing infant.
Source: Modified from G. H. McCracken and J. D. Nelson, *Antimicrobial Therapy for Newborns.* New York: Grune & Stratton, 1977; and from J. S. Remington and J. O. Klein, *Infectious Diseases of the Fetus and Newborn Infant* (3rd ed.). Philadelphia: Saunders, 1990.

of these effects has been reported in infants, but it would be prudent to stop breast-feeding if metronidazole or chloramphenicol must be given to the mother. (These agents are detailed in Chaps. 28J and 28P.)

Neonatal Sepsis
(Sepsis Neonatorum)

I. **Bacteriology.** The organisms that most commonly cause sepsis and meningitis in the United States have changed over the decades. In the 1940s, the group A streptococci and, in the 1950s, the staphylococci (especially phage group I) were prominent. Since the early 1960s, *E. coli* and, currently, the group B streptococci have been the major causative bacteria [1]. The prevalent pathogenic organisms in a single nursery change with time and may not be similar to organisms found on other wards. It is valuable to be aware of the most common pathogens in one's own nursery as well as of their antibiotic susceptibilities.

A. **E. coli** is one of the maternal enteric organisms that colonizes the gastrointestinal tract of the newborn, from which it can invade the blood and meninges. (This organism is discussed further under Neonatal Meningitis.)

B. **Group B streptococci have become the most common cause of bacteremia and sepsis in many nurseries** [13].

1. **Acquisition of group B streptococci.** The organisms can be acquired **intrapartum** from the maternal cervix or vagina and colonize the skin and upper respiratory and GI tracts of the neonate. Colonization rates among pregnant women range from 5 to 40% depending on the population and culture technique. **Of infants born to colonized mothers, 40–75% are themselves colonized and 1–2% will develop early-onset disease.** The infants are colonized with the strains borne by their mothers. The presence of specific maternal antibody appears to protect the infant from early-onset sepsis. Determining the most efficacious and cost-effective time to screen for group B streptococcal colonization has been hampered by lack of sensitive and specific rapid diagnostic techniques, poor adherence to prenatal care, and the intermittent nature of maternal group B streptococcal colonization. **New prevention guidelines** from

the Centers for Disease Control, American Academy of Pediatrics, and American College of Obstetrics and Gynecology **recommend** either screening by culture for group B streptococci carriage at 35 to 37 weeks' gestation followed by intrapartum prophylaxis with intravenous penicillin for all carriers, or no screening but prophylaxis based on defined risk factors [14]. No economic analysis of this strategy is available, but analyses of similar prevention strategies have demonstrated cost savings [15].

2. **Syndromes caused by group B streptococci**
   a. **Early-onset disease** occurs in the first 5–7 days of life, often as an overwhelming sepsis with apnea and shock [16, 17]. This devastating presentation frequently is associated with obstetric complications and prematurity. The pulmonary manifestations may be difficult to differentiate clinically or radiologically from the respiratory distress syndrome. Meningitis will occur in 15–30% of cases. Mortality rates of 50% in the 1960s and 1970s have declined to 10–20% with early aggressive management. Recurrences of disease occur in approximately 3% of cases.
   b. **Late-onset disease** occurs after 7 days of age (to 4 months of age) and usually presents as sepsis, meningitis, or another localized infection in moderately ill infants.

C. *Listeria monocytogenes* is a gram-positive rod that may cause congenital disease resulting in abortion or stillbirth. It is likely that peripartum colonization leads, in some neonates, to early- or late-onset disease [18].
   1. **Early-onset disease** appears in the first week of life, often in premature infants, with pneumonia, shock, and salmon-colored dermal papules. Assisted ventilation often is required, and mortality may reach 50%.
   2. **Late-onset disease** often presents as meningitis in full-term infants. In some cases, the CSF will be characterized by a lymphocytosis rather than polymorphonuclear leukocytes; however, this is unusual [19]. Therapy with ampicillin alone or in combination with gentamicin results in a lower mortality than that of early-onset disease.

D. **Anaerobes** may cause sepsis. Approximately 10–25% of all neonatal bacteremias are due to anaerobes [20]. Although only a portion of affected neonates will be septic, the clinical manifestations of neonatal anaerobic bacteremia are indistinguishable from other causes of neonatal sepsis. Therefore, **anaerobic cultures** using special media **should be performed routinely in neonates with suspected sepsis,** especially when aerobic cultures have been negative.

E. **Miscellaneous.** Many other bacteria are rare causative agents of neonatal sepsis and meningitis. Most frequent among these are group D streptococci, *H. influenzae* (commonly nontypeable), and enteric gram-negative organisms [21, 22]. In the high-risk newborn population, *Staphylococcus epidermidis* is a common cause of vascular catheter-associated bacteremia [23].

F. **Nonbacterial causes of sepsis syndrome.** Herpes simplex virus and enteroviruses can present with a clinical picture similar to bacterial sepsis in the newborn (see sec. **X** under Selected Specific Infections in the Newborn and under Disseminated Intrauterine Infections). Noninfectious diseases such as inborn errors of metabolism and congenital heart disease must also be included in the differential diagnosis of these infants.

II. **Clinical features.** The signs and symptoms of neonatal sepsis are **often subtle** and may be noted only by close observers such as the mother or nurse. **A high level of suspicion must be maintained** for the possibility of neonatal sepsis. Neonatal meningitis is a common complication of neonatal sepsis.

A. **Factors associated with neonatal sepsis** are listed in Table 3-5. When any of these factors is present, at least a CBC and blood culture should be performed. Most neonates with suspected sepsis are started empirically on antibiotics after appropriate laboratory studies have been obtained. In some cases, the infant may simply be observed for further signs of illness before antibiotics are started.

B. **Symptoms and signs** in neonatal sepsis are shown in Table 3-6.

III. **Diagnosis. The clinician must suspect sepsis with the report of any of the signs in Table 3-6.** A history and physical examination will provide further information [24, 25].

A. **Samples of blood, urine, and CSF** [25a] must be obtained, examined, and cultured. Body surface cultures (ear canal, nasopharynx, axilla, umbilicus, groin, and gastric aspirate) are of limited value in predicting the etiology of sepsis except with herpes simplex virus disease [26].

Table 3-5. Factors associated with neonatal sepsis

Source or cause	Remarks
Early-onset sepsis	
Maternal perinatal infection	Fever, pyuria, and foul amniotic fluid are signs of maternal infection.
Prolonged rupture of the membranes	Variably defined as > 12, 18, or 24 hr.
Prolonged labor, difficult delivery	Meconium staining may reflect stress and hypoxia of infant.
Prematurity and low birth weight	Rate of septicemia is inversely correlated with birth weight and gestational age.*
Low Apgar score, resuscitation	Hypoxia, hypoperfusion, aspiration, and intubation are all associated with septicemia.
Late-onset sepsis	
Congenital anomalies	Meningomyelocele, sinus tracts, and the like provide routes for infection.
Prolonged intensive care nursery admission	Increased risk of nosocomial infection.
Procedures or manipulations	Fetal monitoring electrodes, umbilical vein or artery catheters, chest tubes, arterial cannulas, and such provide routes and sites for infection.
Gender	Male infants are more likely to become septic than are female infants.

*Data from K. C. Buetow, S. W. Klein, and R. B. Lane, Septicemia in premature infants. *Am. J. Dis. Child.* 110:20, 1965.

B. **Laboratory tests** may be useful in making the diagnosis.
   1. **Peripheral WBC** count is a useful test (Table 3-7). Many infected infants, particularly premature infants, will exhibit leukopenia rather than leukocytosis. Leukopenia should heighten concern about possible infection, although it is not a specific finding. Other conditions including birth asphyxia, pregnancy-induced hypertension, prematurity, and low birth weight also may cause a low WBC count [27]. Various hematologic scoring systems have been studied, including the ratio of immature to total neutrophils, but these scoring systems are not commonly used [28].
   2. **Counterimmunoelectrophoresis (CIE) or latex agglutination (LA)** will detect the majority of culture-proved group B streptococcal infections. (See Chap. 25 for the details of CIE testing.)
   3. **Other tests,** when used individually, are unreliable indicators of neonatal sepsis. These include the erythrocyte sedimentation rate, nitroblue tetrazolium test, C-reactive protein, leukocyte alkaline phosphatase, and endotoxin detection by the limulus lysate test. A combination of a complete leukocyte count, microerythrocyte sedimentation rate, and C-reactive protein may be more accurate than any single test [28–30].
C. **Presumptive therapy.** Ultimately, the clinical condition of the baby should determine whether the next step of presumptive therapy is taken. **Because neonatal sepsis often progresses rapidly and has a very high mortality, early presumptive therapy must be instituted when this diagnosis is suspected, as soon as cultures are obtained.** Many infants are treated for minimal indications, and only a few will prove to have sepsis.
   In one report [31], 6.5% of 1,551 infants in two nurseries were treated with antibiotics for presumed sepsis, but only 6% of those treated had positive blood cultures. Rapid early treatment is essential, even though it is recognized that many patients may be treated unnecessarily.
IV. **Therapy** (Table 3-8)
   A. **Antibiotics**
      1. **Early-onset disease.** Therapy for early-onset disease must be directed against group B streptococci, other gram-positive cocci including enterococcus, gram-

Table 3-6. Symptoms and signs in neonatal sepsis

Signs and symptoms	Approximate percentage of cases
Temperature	
Hyperthermia	50
Hypothermia	15
Pulmonary	
Dyspnea	20
Periodic breathing or apnea	20
Cyanosis	25
Cardiovascular (tachycardia, bradycardia, hypotension, shock)	25
Gastrointestinal	
Anorexia	30
Vomiting	20
Abdominal distention	20
Diarrhea	10
Hepatic	
Hepatomegaly	30–50
Jaundice	30
Hematologic (bleeding diathesis)	2–10
CNS	
Lethargy	35
Irritability or jitteriness (or both)	15
Seizure	15
Asymptomatic	6–9

Source: Data from K. C. Buetow, S. W. Klein, and R. B. Lane, Septicemia in premature infants. *Am. J. Dis. Child.* 110:29, 1965; L. Gluck, H. F. Wood, and M. D. Fousek, Septicemia of the newborn. *Pediatr. Clin. North Am.* 13:1131, 1966; G. H. McCracken Jr. and H. R. Shinefield, Changes in the pattern of neonatal septicemia and meningitis. *Am. J. Dis. Child.* 112:33, 1966; and W. L. Nyhan and M. D. Fousek, Septicemia of the newborn. *Pediatrics* 22:268, 1958.

Table 3-7. Range of WBC ($\times$ 1,000/mm^3) and ratios for normal infants of all weights and gestational ages

Age	Total neutrophils	Immature (band) neutrophils
Birth	1.8–6.0	0–1.1
12 hr	7.8–14.5	0–1.4
1 d	7.2–12.6	0–1.3
2 d	3.6–8.1	0–0.8
5 d	1.8–5.4	0–0.5
28 d	1.8–5.4	0–0.5

Source: Adapted from B. L. Manroe et al., The neonatal blood count in health and disease: I. Reference values for neutrophilic cells. *J. Pediatr.* 95:89, 1979.

negative enteric organisms, and *Listeria.* **Intravenous ampicillin** and either an **aminoglycoside** (the aminoglycoside choice will depend on local susceptibility patterns) or **cefotaxime** intramuscularly or intravenously should be used initially. Culture results will allow more specific therapy [9, 32, 33].

2. **Late-onset disease** is caused by the same organisms listed for early-onset disease, with the addition of hospital-acquired staphylococci and gram-negative organisms. **Ampicillin and either an aminoglycoside or cefotaxime** are most often used parenterally for initial therapy. If methicillin-resistant *S. aureus* or *S. epidermidis* is an epidemiologically important cause of sepsis in the neonatal intensive care population, **vancomycin and a third-generation cephalosporin** should be used until culture and sensitivity results are available.

Table 3-8. Suggested initial empiric antibiotic therapy of neonatal infections

Clinical syndrome	Suggested therapy
Early-onset sepsis, meningitis	Ampicillin *and* either gentamicin or cefotaxime
Late-onset sepsis, meningitis	Ampicillin *and* cefotaxime
Early-onset pneumonia	Ampicillin *and* either gentamicin or cefotaxime
Catheter sepsis	Vancomycin *and* cefotaxime
Necrotizing enterocolitis	Ampicillin, gentamicin, *and* clindamycin

3. **Duration of therapy.** Specific management must be tailored to each infant, taking into consideration maternal antibiotic therapy prepartum and intrapartum, quality of culture specimens, culture results, and the infant's overall clinical course. In some instances, infants are treated empirically in the face of negative cultures. General guidelines are as follows.
   a. **If initial cultures are negative** and the infant is asymptomatic, most clinicians would stop antibiotic therapy after 3–5 days and observe closely.
   b. **If initial blood cultures are positive** and meningitis is not present, most authorities recommend a 7- to 10-day course of treatment with the appropriate antibiotic, based on susceptibility data.
4. Anaerobic infection should be suspected in any infant not doing well on the recommended initial therapy.
B. **Ancillary care** is as important as antibiotic therapy and usually requires an intensive care nursery.
   1. **Vital signs,** including blood pressure and blood gases, should be monitored.
   2. **Ventilatory support** often is required because of hypoxia and hypercapnia.
   3. **Fluid and electrolytes** must be monitored closely, as acidosis, hypoglycemia, and electrolyte imbalances are common in the ill neonate.
   4. **Red blood cell transfusions** may be necessary to improve intravascular volume and oxygen-carrying capacity.
   5. **Other blood products** such as white cells, intravenous immunoglobulin (Ig), and fresh frozen plasma have all been used as adjuncts to antibiotic therapy [34]. Use of prophylactic intravenous Ig for premature neonates has been advocated [35], but a recent trial showed no benefit, thereby contributing to the conflicting evidence regarding benefit [36]. Preliminary data for the use of intravenous Ig as adjuvant therapy in septic neonates suggest a benefit, but the data are inconclusive and intravenous Ig is not used routinely [37]. Group B streptococcal hyperimmunoglobulin has been compared with standard intravenous Ig and does not appear to improve outcome [38]. Fresh frozen plasma should be used for infants with disseminated intravascular coagulation and has been advocated to improve the diminished serum complement and opsonic activity of neonates. The data on the efficacy of granulocyte transfusions in neonates is mixed and incomplete. Use of granulocytes varies by center.

Neonatal Meningitis

I. **Clinical features.** The presenting features of meningitis in the neonate may not be different from those listed for sepsis (see Table 3-6). In some series, convulsions, irritability, or lethargy were more prominent. Only rarely will an infant with meningitis exhibit a bulging fontanelle or nuchal rigidity.
II. **Diagnosis.** Samples of blood, CSF, and urine should be obtained, examined, and cultured. The tests listed in sec. **III** under Neonatal Sepsis may be useful for diagnosis, especially detection of antigen by CIE and the LA test. Table 3-9 lists the mean and ranges for normal values for CSF analysis in newborns.
III. **Bacteriology.** In a large series, *E.coli* and group B streptococci cause up to 70% of neonatal meningitis, with *L. monocytogenes* accounting for another 5%. Of the many types of *E. coli,* those with the polysaccharide capsular antigen K1 are associated with neonatal meningitis. Eighty percent of all *E. coli* meningitides are due to organisms

Table 3-9. Composition of normal cerebrospinal fluid in newborns

Age	Total WBC/mm³		ANC		Glucose (mg/dl)		Protein (mg/dl)	
	Mean	Range	Mean	Range	Mean	Range	Mean	Range
Premature newborn	9.0	0–29	NR	NR	50	24–63	115	65–150
Term newborn	8.2	0–22	NR	NR	52	34–119	90	20–170
0–4 wk	11.0	0–50	0.40	0–7.5	46	36–61	84	35–189
4–8 wk	7.1	0–50	0.18	0–2.1	46	29–62	59	19–121

ANC = absolute neutrophil count; NR = no data.
Source: Adapted from W. A. Bonadio. The cerebrospinal fluid: Physiologic aspects and alterations associated with bacterial meningitis. *Pediatr. Infect. Dis. J.* 11:423, 1992.

carrying the K1 antigen. Approximately 30% of all newborn babies are colonized with K1 strains, and the rate of meningitis is estimated to be 1 of every 100 colonized infants. Carriage of K1 strains has been demonstrated in a high percentage of nursery personnel, so infants may be colonized postnatally as well. The severity of disease and the presence of sequelae have been correlated positively with the presence and concentration of the K1 antigen in the CSF. Other pathogens known to cause meningitis, particularly in the low-birth-weight infant, are *S. aureus, S. epidermidis, Citrobacter diversus* [39], and *Candida* spp.

IV. **Therapy**
   A. **Antibiotics**
      1. **Initial therapy. Parenteral ampicillin and either an aminoglycoside or cefotaxime should be used. The highest of the doses indicated in Table 3-2 should be administered** because of the limited penetration of some of these antibiotics into the CSF. If gram-negative bacilli are seen on the Gram stain of the CSF, some experts would combine ampicillin with both an aminoglycoside and cefotaxime while awaiting cultures [40–42].
      2. **Group B streptococci (suspected or proved).** Because of the relative resistance of group B streptococci to penicillin and reports of relapse after therapy, the recommended doses of penicillin have been raised. Aqueous penicillin should be given at 500,000 units/kg/day (see Table 3-2). Some authors recommend treating this organism with both penicillin and an aminoglycoside until results of tolerance assays are known (minimum inhibitory [MIC] and minimum bactericidal [MBC] concentrations) and until CSF cultures are negative. Therapy should be continued for at least 14 days after negative CSF cultures have been documented by repeat lumbar puncture. If there is no clinical improvement despite therapy, consultation with an infectious disease specialist is recommended.
      3. **L. monocytogenes** should be treated with parenteral ampicillin or penicillin. The duration of therapy is as recommended for group B streptococci (see sec. 2). Some experts add a parenteral aminoglycoside (e.g., gentamicin) for synergy.
      4. **Enteric gram-negative bacteria** are more difficult to eradicate from the CSF than gram-positive bacteria, in part because of the low levels of aminoglycosides achieved therein. Several routes of antibiotic administration have been studied, including the intralumbar and intraventricular routes. Controlled trials have shown either no additional benefit over the intravenous route or detrimental effects [43]. Parenteral antibiotics of appropriate type, combination, dose, and interval remain the standard of care.
         a. **Third-generation cephalosporins.** Among the third-generation cephalosporins, cefotaxime appears useful and safe in infants [8, 9, 33]. It has activity against gram-negative enteric bacteria—in some cases, better than aminoglycosides, ampicillin, and the second-generation cephalosporins. However, this third-generation agent is not active against *Pseudomonas* spp., group D enterococci, or *L. monocytogenes* and does not have optimum activity against most staphylococci. Ceftriaxone, although similar to cefotaxime in spectrum of activity, affects bilirubin-albumin binding and may increase

the risk of bilirubin encephalopathy in jaundiced neonates; therefore, it should be avoided if possible [4, 6]. Ceftazidime has a spectrum of activity similar to cefotaxime, with the added benefit of antipseudomonal activity. It may be used in the setting where *Pseudomonas* is a suspected pathogen.

b. **Aminoglycosides** remain important agents in the management of meningitis, particularly with penicillin-tolerant strains of group B streptococci and enteric gram-negative organisms. This class of antibiotic is almost always used in combination with another antibiotic, usually of the beta-lactam class.

c. **Chloramphenicol** has been used in patients with susceptible bacteria, but this is not an ideal agent. Serum levels must be carefully monitored in neonates to avoid toxicity. Furthermore, chloramphenicol is usually bacteriostatic rather than bactericidal against gram-negative bacilli.

d. **Recommendation.** Because of the difficulties and controversies involved in treating enteric gram-negative bacilli meningitis, the authors **suggest an infectious disease consultation** and careful consideration of the use of a third-generation cephalosporin if susceptibility studies show that the agent is active. If a *Pseudomonas* species is causing the meningitis and it is not susceptible to ceftazidime, an aminoglycoside may still be necessary in conjunction with another antipseudomonal drug (synthetic penicillins, ceftazidime, imipenem). (See the discussion of these agents in Chap. 28.)

In general, repeat lumbar punctures are done to document sterilization of the CSF, and therapy is continued for 14 days after sterilization or for a total of 21 days.

B. **Ancillary care** (see sec. **IV.B** under Neonatal Sepsis). It is particularly important to monitor free water intake to avoid the hyponatremia due to inappropriate secretion of antidiuretic hormone associated with meningitis. However, above all, support of blood pressure and perfusion must be optimized. The role of corticosteroids has not been studied in the neonate, and we do not advocate their use. (See the related discussion in Chap. 5.)

Selected Specific Infections in the Newborn

I. **Ophthalmia neonatorum,** or **conjunctivitis** in the infant less than 4 weeks of age, usually is caused by organisms acquired in the birth canal [44]. *Chlamydia trachomatis,* staphylococci, gonococci, streptococci, and viruses including herpes simplex virus are all documented as etiologic agents of this disease. Prophylaxis is mandated in most of the United States. Silver nitrate drops, 1% (Crede's solution), tetracycline, or erythromycin ointment have efficacy against gonococcal conjunctivitis. One of these three products should be applied to the neonate's eyes within an hour of birth. The silver nitrate solution may cause an early, nonpurulent discharge that should resolve within 24–48 hours. Conjunctivitis due to *N. gonorrhoeae* and other gram-negative organisms requires appropriate parenteral antibiotics. Ophthalmia caused by staphylococci and gonococci often is of earlier onset than conjunctivitis caused by *C. trachomatis* or adenovirus.

The approach to and therapy for this problem are discussed further in Chap. 6 (sec. **IV** under Conjunctivitis). **The conjunctival discharge is infectious, so handwashing control measures are important to prevent spread** to attendants and other patients in the nursery.

II. **Upper respiratory tract infections. Otitis media** is common in infants with cleft palate and not uncommon in normal newborns. This infection may present in isolated fashion or as part of a generalized septicemia. A full review of this topic is available [45]. (See additional discussion of otitis media in Chap. 7.)

A. **Bacteriology.** Published reports implicate gram-negative organisms such as *E. coli* and *Klebsiella* spp., as well as the expected respiratory tract pathogens such as *S. aureus, Haemophilus* spp., and streptococci.

B. **Diagnosis** is based on the finding of a gray or red tympanic membrane with decreased mobility. Tympanocentesis should be attempted to confirm the diagnosis and to direct therapy, because sepsis or meningitis may be a consequence of inappropriate therapy. A full sepsis workup should be performed for all ill-appearing infants. If a tympanocentesis is not done, close follow-up must be assured to evaluate for possible treatment failures.

C. Therapy. Initial therapy is controversial. We would advocate tympanocentesis followed by parenteral ampicillin and either an aminoglycoside or a third-generation cephalosporin for all neonates with otitis media, until culture results are available. Others would suggest that outpatient amoxicillin therapy in a well-appearing infant is safe and sufficient initial therapy. Treatment should continue for 7–10 days or longer if purulent tympanic abnormalities persist (see Table 3-2 for doses).

III. **Lower respiratory tract infections** in neonates can be classified as congenital, intrapartum, or postnatal, depending on when the pathogen was acquired. The physical findings of rales, decreased breath sounds, and percussion dullness may be difficult to detect in the neonate. **The finding of respiratory distress should lead to chest x-ray, which is the most useful tool in confirming or ruling out a pneumonia.** A CBC and blood culture should also be done.

   A. Congenital pneumonia usually is part of a transplacental infection. Rubella, CMV, herpes simplex virus, congenital syphilis, and *Toxoplasma gondii* can all cause this type of pneumonia.

      1. **Clinical features.** Infants with transplacental congenital pneumonia are often small for gestational age and bear the other stigmata of their infection. (See the discussion under Disseminated Intrauterine Infections.)

      2. **Therapy.** There is no therapy for rubella and CMV infections. The pneumonias associated with toxoplasmosis, congenital syphilis, and herpes virus should be treated as discussed under Disseminated Intrauterine Infections, later in this chapter.

   B. Intrapartum pneumonia is due to the aspiration of maternal cervicovaginal organisms or of infected amniotic fluid and is manifested at birth or shortly thereafter.

      1. **Clinical presentation.** Babies with bacterial pneumonia may present as asphyxiated newborns with fulminant disease. Group B streptococci may cause devastating early-onset sepsis with pneumonia and respiratory distress.

      2. **Cultures.** Cultures of blood and respiratory secretions should be obtained. The best approach to the latter is to obtain a tracheal aspirate under direct vision with a laryngoscope. If a pleural effusion is present, a needle aspiration should be performed for diagnostic studies.

      3. **Therapy.** Intrapartum pneumonia should be treated by administration of parenteral ampicillin and either an aminoglycoside or cefotaxime for 10 days. If group B streptococci are suspected, the higher dose of ampicillin in Table 3-2 should be doubled.

   C. Postpartum pneumonia often is nosocomial in origin, the infant acquiring an organism from the nursery attendants or equipment.

      1. **Etiology.** Of particular concern are hospital-acquired staphylococcal and gram-negative bacterial pneumonias. Respiratory syncytial virus, parainfluenza type 3 virus, influenza virus, and enteroviruses are all fairly common causes of postnatally acquired pneumonia. Unfortunately, these agents often cause respiratory tract disease that cannot, with certainty, be clinically distinguished from bacterial disease. Therefore, initial antibiotic therapy is mandatory in all lower respiratory tract disease of acute onset.

      2. **Clinical features.** These neonates present with the development of respiratory distress: tachypnea, cough, apnea, expiratory grunting, nasal flaring, and subcostal and sternal retractions.

      3. **Cultures** should be performed as discussed under sec. **B.2.** Viral cultures also should be obtained from skin, rectum, conjunctiva, throat, and nasopharynx.

      4. **Therapy.** Postpartum pneumonia should be treated initially with broad-spectrum parenteral antibiotics (e.g., cefotaxime and an aminoglycoside) (see Table 3-8). If the organism is either staphylococcus or a gram-negative, therapy with the appropriate antibiotic should continue for 3 weeks.

   D. Chlamydial pneumonitis is a clinically distinct syndrome in infants who are infected intrapartum. Of those neonates who are exposed, 10–20% develop pneumonitis (see Table 3-1).

      1. **Clinical features.** Symptoms usually become apparent at 4 to 12 weeks of age. Half of the infants have a history of conjunctivitis. There is a gradual worsening of cough, which may occur in staccato paroxysms that result in cyanosis. There is no whoop, and fever is very rare. Inspiratory crepitations and abnormal tympanic membranes are common features found on physical examination. X-rays show patchy alveolar infiltrates and hyperinflation. Many affected in-

fants have eosinophilia of more than 400/mm^3 [46, 47]. Infants may excrete *C. trachomatis* for up to 2 years [48].

2. **Diagnosis** is made by the history and clinical features. Culture of *C. trachomatis* is not widely available. A recently introduced commercial immunofluorescent technique may be useful for diagnosis.

3. **Therapy** consists of 2 weeks of erythromycin, 40 mg/kg/day, or sulfisoxazole, 150 mg/kg/day [49].

E. *Ureaplasma urealyticum* **and** *Mycoplasma hominis* have been associated with pneumonia in the newborn. Colonization rates of up to 80% have been estimated among pregnant women; 15–30% of their newborns are surface-colonized at birth. The presence of these organisms in the placenta has been associated with chorioamnionitis, spontaneous abortion, prematurity, and congenital pneumonia. High antibody levels to *U. urealyticum* have been found in infants with respiratory disease and chronic lung disease [50].

1. **Clinical features.** There are no unique clinical findings in pneumonia caused by these organisms.

2. **Diagnosis.** Because of high colonization rates among pregnant women, these pathogens should be considered when pneumonia is diagnosed. Isolation of these organisms requires special media.

3. **Therapy.** Erythromycin has been recommended for treatment of *U. urealyticum* cases [51], but no efficacy data for this agent are available.

IV. **Gastrointestinal infections**

A. **Diarrheal disease** is more prevalent in infancy and childhood than at any later period; this may be due to the diminished immunocompetence previously mentioned. Local antimicrobial factors such as gastric pH, peristalsis, and secretory IgA are also altered in the neonate's GI tract and may contribute to increased susceptibility. Breast milk probably compensates for some of the deficiencies of local immunity, but only a fraction of neonates receive it. Enteric pathogens may be acquired orally, either intrapartum or postpartum.

1. **Etiology.** It is possible that a proportion of neonatal diarrheal disease is not infectious in origin, being due instead to changes in the composition and volume of the diet or to changes in bowel function. Of the infectious diarrheas, rotavirus is the most frequent cause; *Salmonella* and *Shigella* spp. and *E. coli* account for some of the remainder [52]. *Campylobacter* enteritis has occurred in neonates (these infections are discussed in Chap. 11 under Gastroenteritis and Food Poisoning). It is likely that other agents exist that are not yet identified.

2. **Evaluation.** In an infant with diarrhea, a fresh stool smear should be examined for leukocytes by methylene blue staining to determine whether an invasive organism is responsible. Fecal leukocytes are often present in diarrhea caused by *Salmonella* and *Shigella* spp. or invasive *E. coli,* whereas they are usually absent in toxicogenic bacterial or viral disease. (For further discussion of the implications of fecal leukocytes, see Chap. 11 under Gastroenteritis and Food Poisoning.) **Fresh stools should be cultured** for enteric pathogens, and blood cultures should be obtained.

3. **Therapy**

a. **Replacement of fluid losses** is the most important aspect of treatment. Monitoring of the infant's output, weight, and vital signs must be meticulous to accomplish this.

b. **Antibiotic therapy** for bacterial diarrhea is somewhat controversial. The following are suggested guidelines.

(1) *Salmonella* **and** *Shigella* **spp.** A neonate ill with the invasive organisms *Salmonella* and *Shigella* should be treated initially with parenteral cefotaxime (pending susceptibility data) because of the risk of systemic involvement and metastatic infection. Antibiotic sensitivities should be determined on all bacterial isolates to guide further therapy, which should be administered for at least 5–7 days. Treatment of *Salmonella* gastroenteritis may cause the infant to become a carrier. These asymptomatic carriers should be followed with stool cultures [53].

(2) *E. coli.* Diarrhea in neonates and infants has been associated with certain enteropathogenic serotypes of *E. coli* (mechanism unknown), invasive *E. coli,* or strains of *E. coli* that produce an enterotoxin. Unfortunately, the tests for identification of the latter two groups of *E. coli* are not widely available. An infant with prolonged diarrhea who has

an enteropathogenic serotype of *E. coli* in the stools might benefit from a course of oral neomycin (100 mg/kg/day) or colistin (15 mg/kg/day).

   (3) *Campylobacter.* Erythromycin has been suggested to treat such infection (see Chap. 11).

c. **Isolation. The affected infant should be isolated immediately to prevent nosocomial spread.** Infection control methods such as isolation, the placing of infants in cohorts, and enforced gowning and hand-washing for all care-givers are paramount in the management of enteric infections in the nursery.

B. **Necrotizing enterocolitis** is an illness of unknown primary etiology, but it is often associated with sepsis and peritonitis [54]. It occurs both sporadically and as a nursery epidemic. It has an incidence of up to 5% of all prematures, and the mortality is 20–40%. Blood cultures are positive in up to 50% of cases. The organisms found in the blood are similar to the enteric flora seen in peritoneal fluid, with *E. coli, Klebsiella,* and *Enterobacter* spp. predominating [54].

   1. **Diagnosis**
      a. **Presenting signs** are often nonspecific and include temperature instability, apnea, lethargy, and gastric residuals. Many of these infants have abdominal distention, vomiting, and blood in the stools. Physical signs in advanced disease will include peritonitis and crepitance or cellulitis of the abdominal wall.
      b. **Roentgenographic evaluation** may show ileus, bowel distention, pneumatosis intestinalis, portal vein gas, or free peritoneal gas.
      c. **Laboratory tests** are nonspecific. Thrombocytopenia and neutropenia often occur in this illness. The stool may exhibit reducing substances, occult blood, or gross blood. Blood cultures may be positive up to 50% of the time.

   2. **Medical therapy** should be instituted as soon as this diagnosis is suspected.
      a. **Fluid and nutritional maintenance.** Oral feedings are stopped and naso-gastric suction begun. Because oral feedings must be discontinued for 2 or 3 weeks, intravenous alimentation should be started by the central or peripheral route as soon as the baby is stable.
      b. **Antibiotics.** Parenteral ampicillin and an aminoglycoside should be started. Some neonatologists advocate the use of parenteral clindamycin for anaerobes; there is no evidence that these antibiotics improve outcome [54, 55].
      c. **Transfusion** may be necessary for volume repletion, and some authors advocate the use of fresh frozen plasma.
      d. **Serial x-rays.** Repeat lateral and supine x-ray views of the abdomen should be obtained every 8 hours to detect advancement or perforation.
      e. **Surgical intervention** is indicated for clinical or x-ray evidence of perforation, cellulitis of the anterior abdominal wall, or clinical deterioration of the medical regimen.

V. **Genitourinary (GU) infections.** Urinary tract infections are not uncommon in the newborn; in this period, they are more common in boys than in girls. Reported rates for bacteriuria range from 1% in full-term infants to 3% for prematures. The most common causative organisms are *E. coli, Klebsiella* spp., and enterococci [56, 57].

A. **Clinical presentation.** Failure to gain weight, vomiting, fever, and jaundice are the most common symptoms. Local symptoms are very rare; occasionally, a poor urinary stream in boys may draw attention to the GU tract. Bacteriuria may be the first sign of sepsis.

B. **Diagnosis.** Examination of clean-catch urines can be confused by the presence of WBCs from circumcision or vaginal discharge. Most authors accept that a clean-catch urine with 20–25 WBC/mm^3 or more in the first week and 10–25 WBC/mm^3 or more in the second week is abnormal. A suprapubic bladder tap or bladder catheterization provides uncontaminated urine for urinalysis, Gram staining, and culture. The presence of any bacterial growth in a bladder tap or catheterized specimen is significant and is an indication for blood cultures and the initiation of therapy.

C. **Initial treatment** should be guided by findings on Gram stain and usually consists of ampicillin and an aminoglycoside. Urine should be sterile in 48 hours after initiation of therapy, and specific treatment should be continued for 10–14 days.

D. **Further investigation.** After control of the infection, **renal ultrasonography** and **voiding cystourethrography** are mandatory, as GU malformations are found in 5–10% of these patients. **Follow-up urine cultures** after completion of therapy are also important because reinfection is a frequent occurrence. (See related discussions in Chap. 12.)

VI. **Musculoskeletal infections**

   A. **Neonatal osteomyelitis** is rare but important because of its morbidity [58]. This entity is discussed further in Chap. 16 under Hematogenous Osteomyelitis.

   1. **Pathogenesis.** Pathogens gain access to the bone through bacteremia, direct inoculation (e.g., monitoring electrodes or venipuncture), or spread from adjacent infection. Because the fetal vascular connections extend from the metaphysis through the epiphyseal plate into the epiphysis and persist until 18 months of age, epiphysitis (with permanent damage of the growth plate) and secondary arthritis can result (see Chap. 16, sec. **I.B** under Hematogenous Osteomyelitis). The femur, humerus, tibia, and radius are the most commonly affected bones. Ninety percent of neonatal osteomyelitis is due to *S. aureus,* streptococci, *H. influenzae,* and pneumococci. Coliforms are rare causative agents.

   2. **Clinical presentation.** Affected infants often appear well, are afebrile, and may manifest only guarding of the affected area with decreased spontaneous movement, local swelling, and tenderness. Other babies may exhibit septicemic symptoms that overshadow the local findings.

   3. **Diagnosis**

      a. **X-ray findings** are very useful. Because of the rapid remodeling of bone in infants, changes may be evident within 7 days. **Bone scans** may be positive within days of onset of symptoms.

      b. **Needle aspiration** of the involved bone and secondarily infected joint space will provide material for Gram staining and culture.

   4. **Therapy.** If organisms are gram-positive on stain, a penicillinase-resistant penicillin should be given, parenterally at first. If gram-negative organisms are seen, ampicillin and an aminoglycoside should be adequate. If no organisms are seen, a penicillinase-resistant penicillin and an aminoglycoside should be employed. Drainage may be required if there is localization of pus. Specific parenteral therapy should continue for at least 3 weeks. If available, infectious disease and orthopedic consultations should be obtained.

   B. **Septic arthritis.** A primary infectious arthritis without involvement of nearby bone may be secondary to a bacteremia or to direct inoculation (as by femoral venipuncture). *S. aureus,* gram-negative organisms (*E. coli, Pseudomonas* spp., *Haemophilus* spp., gonococci), and *Streptococcus* spp. account for most cases [59]. This presents in a manner identical to osteomyelitis in the newborn. The affected joint should be aspirated. The initial therapy and duration of therapy are similar to that suggested for osteomyelitis. Drainage and immobilization of the joint are important elements of treatment.

VII. **Skin infections.** The neonate is particularly susceptible to local skin infections because of the presence of one or two wounds (umbilical cord and circumcision), the immaturity of the stratum corneum, and the initial absence of the normal dermal bacterial flora. Only some local infections will be discussed here.

   A. **Superficial pustular rashes** are usually due to streptococci or staphylococci and can be treated locally with hexachlorophene or an antibiotic ointment. Widespread or invasive lesions should be Gram-stained and cultured and treatment started with parenteral antibiotics to prevent septicemia. Cellulitis, erysipelas, folliculitis, and impetigo should all be treated presumptively with a parenteral penicillinase-resistant penicillin while one is awaiting cultures.

   B. **Staphylococcal scalded skin syndrome** may appear in any one of its manifestations, either sporadically or as a nursery outbreak (see Plate III E) [60]. Staphylococci in phage group II that produce an exotoxin (exfoliatin) may cause (1) bullous impetigo, (2) Ritter's disease in infants, (3) Lyell's disease or toxic epidermal necrolysis in older children, or (4) a scarlatiniform rash (staphylococcal scarlet fever).

   1. **Clinical presentation.** Initially, the rash is erythematous, and at times tender, and it often has a sandpaper texture. Skin creases may have increased erythema (Pastia's lines). Within 2 days, the epidermis peels off at sites of minor trauma (Nikolsky's sign), and large, flaccid bullae appear, which may also exfoliate. The areas of exfoliation dry out, and seborrhealike flakes appear. These flakes often are found around the mouth. The flakes desquamate over 3–5 days, leaving normal skin underneath. During the exfoliative stage of the disease, infants are febrile, irritable, and uncomfortable, but usually not severely ill. Children with the scarlatiniform rash syndrome do not develop a strawberry tongue and do not exfoliate.

2. **Diagnosis** is by the clinical findings, because the toxicogenic staphylococci may not be recovered from the local lesion.
3. **Therapy.** All forms of this disease should be treated with a parenteral penicillinase-resistant penicillin. Fluid therapy may be necessary because of the increased insensible fluid loss through the damaged skin.

C. **Omphalitis** occurs when pathogenic bacteria predominate in the normally necrotic **umbilical stump.** It is manifested by oozing and purulent discharge from the stump and by local periumbilical inflammation and erythema. The most common causative organisms are staphylococci, *Streptococcus* spp., and coliforms. Gram staining and culture should be done. Because omphalitis can serve as the source of an ascending phlebitis (funisitis) leading to peritonitis or septicemia, it should be vigorously treated with local care and parenteral antibiotics—initially a penicillinase-resistant penicillin and either an aminoglycoside or cefotaxime.

D. **Circumcision wound infections** are caused by the same organisms that cause omphalitis and should be treated similarly.

E. **Neonatal breast abscess** is common in full-term infants. It is usually unilateral and occurs more often in girls. *S. aureus* is the most common pathogen, although streptococci and coliforms have also been described. Early in the course of infection, fluid should be expressed from the iodine-cleansed nipple for Gram staining and culture. In early infection, parenteral antibiotics probably will suffice for cure. Incision and drainage may be required in advanced cases. In either situation, treatment should begin with penicillinase-resistant penicillin and an aminoglycoside and should continue for 10 days with the appropriate drug (see Table 3-2).

VIII. **Hepatitis B virus** (HBV) has a unique natural history in newborns, who have difficulty clearing the infection; these infants have a high probability of becoming chronic carriers of the virus. Chronic carriers of HBV have an estimated 25% risk of developing cirrhosis or hepatocellular carcinoma. (See Chap. 11 for a discussion of HBV epidemiology.) **Since 1991, universal immunization of infants with HBV vaccine has been recommended as the best approach to eliminating transmission of HBV** [61]. We will discuss the specific recommendations for prevention of perinatal transmission. (See further discussion of HBV vaccine in Chap. 22.)

A. **Infants acquire HBV from their mothers.** The probability of infection of the infant is increased if the maternal HBV infection is symptomatic or occurs late in pregnancy. Mothers who are positive for hepatitis surface or e antigen (HBsAg or HBeAg) will transmit the virus to 80% of their infants. Most of these infants will not have symptomatic disease, but **90% will become chronic HBV carriers, and up to 25% will die of chronic liver disease in adulthood** [61].

B. **Passive protection with either HBV immunoglobulin (HBIG) or immunization with HBV vaccine** is approximately 70% effective in reducing the probability of chronic infection in the newborn. Both passive and active immunization used together are 90% effective. **Current recommendations** [62] are that all infants born to HBsAg-positive mothers, regardless of the mother's HBeAg or anti-HBe status, should receive both **HBIG** (0.5 ml IM) within 12 hours of birth and **HBV vaccine** (0.5 ml IM in the anterolateral thigh) within 12 hours of birth, and additional doses as outlined in Chap. 22. Immunized infants should be tested for HBsAg and anti-HBs at 12–15 months.

C. **All pregnant women,** particularly those at increased risk, **should be routinely tested for HBsAg during an early prenatal visit in each pregnancy.** If screening has not been done during pregnancy or the results are not available, an HBsAg test should be done at the time of admission or soon afterward. **Infants of mothers with pending tests or of mothers who did not receive prenatal care should receive HBIG and HBV vaccine** within 12 hours of birth in the dosage appropriate for infants born to HBsAg-positive mothers (5 µg Recombivax HB or 10 µg Engerix-B).

D. **Infants should be managed with hepatitis precautions in the nursery.** There is no contraindication to breast-feeding.

IX. **Hepatitis C virus** (HCV) is the major cause of non-A non-B hepatitis. Mothers with HCV can transmit the virus to their infants, although there are conflicting and insufficient data to evaluate this risk firmly in an individual case. It appears from small preliminary studies that the risk of transmission is very low (< 5%) but that maternal coinfection with HIV likely increases the risk. The natural history of perinatal HCV infection is unknown. Treatment with recombinant interferon-alpha is under evaluation for adults and children; however, no data exist for its use in the neonatal period [63]. (See further discussion of HCV in Chap. 11.)

X. **Enteroviruses,** specifically **coxsackievirus,** have been implicated in neonatal disease [64, 64a]. They probably infect the neonate in the peripartum or postpartum period. Echoviruses and coxsackie B serotypes have caused nursery outbreaks during community epidemics. Most enteroviruses are capable of causing meningoencephalitis or GI disease. They can be the cause of an undifferentiated febrile illness that leads to the consideration of sepsis in neonates. Coxsackie B serotypes have caused a serious disease consisting of encephalitis, myocarditis, and hepatitis, whereas echoviruses are associated with a hepatitis-sepsis syndrome.

   Diagnosis is by culture (stool, urine, throat, nasopharynx) or serologic evaluation and treatment is supportive. Intravenous Ig has been used by some authors. **Infants with suspected coxsackievirus disease should be isolated** to prevent spread of this devastating infection.

XI. **Varicella** is a rare infection in the neonate but is discussed here because of the availability of therapy [65]. Infection of the fetus early in pregnancy is associated with a congenital syndrome in 2.3% of neonates, consisting of cutaneous scars, limb hypoplasia and paralysis, encephalitis, and chorioretinitis [66]. **The outcome of perinatal varicella depends on the time of exposure of the infant.** If maternal disease occurs more than 5 days before delivery, there is little or no risk of dissemination or sequelae. If maternal disease occurs within 5 days before or 2 days after delivery, approximately half the newborns will develop varicella with a risk of severe disseminated varicella and a 30% mortality.

   Infants in the high-risk group should receive zoster immune globulin (125 units, 1.25 ml IM) as soon as possible after delivery [62]. If clinical varicella develops, **acyclovir** should be used. There is little clinical experience with acyclovir in neonates, and an infectious disease consultation is advised (see also Chap. 26). Infants born to mothers with varicella should be isolated in the nursery.

XII. *Candida* **spp.** are the most common cause of fungal infection seen in newborns. True congenital candidiasis may be either local cutaneous or systemic disease and differs from neonatal systemic candidiasis by age at onset and organ involvement. Neonatal systemic candidiasis usually involves multiple organs (rarely is skin involved) and can be divided into two forms: catheter-associated sepsis and disseminated candidiasis. Premature infants and infants with hyperalimentation catheters or with prolonged exposure to broad-spectrum antibiotics are at highest risk of disease [67, 68].

   A. **Diagnosis** is made by recovery of *Candida* organisms from blood, CSF, or joint, pleural, or other normally sterile fluid. Antigen and antibody detection techniques have not been useful in diagnosis.

   B. **Therapy.** Most authorities recommend removal of vascular catheters and administration of amphotericin B, in graduated doses up to 1.0 mg/kg/day, commencing at 0.1–0.25 mg/kg/day IV over a period of 4–6 hours. Flucytosine (5-FC) may provide additional therapeutic benefit in selected fungal infections (100–150 mg/kg/day in three to five divided doses orally). Conclusive clinical data are available only for the use of 5-FC in *Cryptococcus neoformans* meningitis. The duration of antifungal therapy remains controversial. In disseminated infection, a total dose of 25–30 mg/kg of amphotericin B has been recommended. Some authorities suggest limiting the maximum maintenance dose of amphotericin B to 0.5 mg/kg/day in the very low-birth-weight ($< 1,500$ g) infant [68, 69]. Both drugs are nephrotoxic and hepatotoxic; appropriate monitoring of organ function and antifungal blood levels are recommended, as is an infectious disease consultation. (See Chap. 2 for further discussion of vascular catheter-related infections and Chap. 18 for further discussion of antifungal agents.)

   For a recent review of antifungal agents in neonatal systemic candidiasis, see [69a].

Disseminated Intrauterine Infections

The syndrome of disseminated intrauterine infection is caused by diverse organisms that generally result in distinguishable clinical conditions with overlapping features. These infections have been lumped under the acronym *TORCH* (toxoplasmosis, other, rubella, cytomegalovirus, herpes), which has led to the false perception that these infections are clinically identical and uniformly diagnosed by serology, commonly referred to as *TORCH titers*. These titers usually refer to measurement of organism-specific IgG; however, an infant's IgG is maternal in origin. IgM assays for these congenital infections do not have a high enough sensitivity or specificity to make them useful single diagnostic tests. Therefore, **a single TORCH titer is not a complete laboratory evaluation.** A comprehensive diagnostic evaluation for suspected perinatal infection includes consideration of epidemiologic factors, maternal history, physical examination, and ancillary laboratory and radiographic findings [70]. The laboratory investigation of a child with a suspected intrauterine infection must be undertaken in a logical, reasoned, timely manner. Every attempt should be made to arrive at a definitive diagnosis as prognosis and treatment vary by disease; however, a firm diagnosis cannot always be made immediately. Careful clinical and serologic follow-up for 6–15 months may be necessary before an infection can be definitively excluded or implicated.

Intrauterine infections may present with a variety of clinical manifestations or no clinical findings at all. **Some signs that should lead to consideration of an intrauterine infection are listed in Table 3-10.** These signs are not unique to congenital infections; therefore, other diagnostic possibilities must also be explored (e.g., cardiac disease, inherited metabolic defects, immunologic disease). **In many situations, infants with congenital infections share the following characteristics:** (1) inapparent or mild disease in the mother, (2) a wide range of severity of infection in the fetus, (3) overlapping clinical features, and (4) variability of long-term sequelae.

Infectious agents that may cause congenital infections (disseminated or localized, intrauterine or peripartum) **include but are not limited to** toxoplasmosis, syphilis, rubella, CMV, enterovirus, parvovirus B19, HIV, herpes simplex virus, varicella-zoster virus, HBV, and HCV. A brief summary of the common causes of disseminated intrauterine infections follows. For an in-depth discussion, refer to the textbook of Remington and Klein [2].

I. *Toxoplasma gondii* is a protozoa that may infect the fetus by transplacental passage during maternal parasitemia. Approximately 50% of the infants born to mothers who seroconvert during pregnancy are infected, although only 10% of these infants have clinical manifestations. The estimated frequency of clinically evident infection in the United States is 1–4 per 1,000 live births [2].

A. **Clinical presentation.** The affected newborn exhibits chorioretinitis, CSF pleocytosis and elevated protein, microcephaly, and cerebral calcifications. Petechiae, hepatosplenomegaly, jaundice, a maculopapular rash, and interstitial pneumonitis have been described in these infants.

B. **Diagnosis** is by the following methods:
1. Documentation of rising *Toxoplasma*-specific IgG titers over the first 4–6 months of life
2. IgM assays (double-sandwich technique, state or reference laboratory)
3. Direct demonstration of tachyzoites in placenta or infant tissue
4. Culture of *Toxoplasma* from infant blood, cord blood, placenta, CSF, amniotic fluid

C. **Therapy** should include a combination of pyrimethamine (1 mg/kg or 15 mg/m²/day or every 2 days, maximum 25 mg/day) and sulfadiazine or trisulfapyrimidine (75–100 mg/kg/day in two doses), with folinic acid (5 mg IM every 3 days) to prevent bone marrow toxicity. Alternating courses of pyrimethamine and sulfadiazine

Table 3-10. Common clinical features associated with intrauterine infection in neonates

Growth retardation	Cardiac abnormalities
Hepatosplenomegaly	Chorioretinitis
Jaundice	Keratoconjunctivitis
Hemolytic anemia	Cataracts
Petechiae, ecchymoses	Glaucoma
Microcephaly, hydrocephalus	Nonimmune hydrops
Intracranial calcification	Bone abnormalities
Pneumonitis	
Myocarditis	

with spiramycin for a year is the recommended practice. The schedule of alterna-
tion is determined by the severity of symptoms [2]. CBC and platelet counts should
be monitored twice weekly. Corticosteroids (prednisone, 1–2 mg/kg/day) may be
added for patients with active macular chorioretinitis. An infectious disease consultation is recommended.

II. **Rubella.** Congenital rubella is still a problem [71]. Fetal infection with rubella may
result in teratogenesis or abortion if it occurs in the first 2 months of gestation.
Infection after the first trimester is associated with disseminated disease.
   A. **Clinical presentation.** The majority (up to 68%) of neonatal infections are subclinical. The classic presentation is of a small, full-term, "blueberry-muffin" baby with
   thrombocytopenic purpura, cataracts, cardiac lesions, and hepatosplenomegaly.
   Pneumonitis, metaphyseal radiolucencies, and CNS involvement, with bulging
   fontanelles, are also seen. Hearing defects and mental retardation may become
   apparent only later in childhood.
   B. **Diagnosis** is made by any one of these tests:
      1. High or rising complement fixation or hemagglutination inhibition titers (IgG)
      2. Elevated specific IgM
      3. Viral culture from respiratory secretions or urine
   C. **Therapy is symptomatic. Infected neonates may excrete the virus for months,
   and they should be placed on strict isolation.**

III. **Cytomegalovirus** is the most common virus of neonates [72]. It may be acquired by
the infant transplacentally, peripartum, or postnatally. Of pregnant women, 4% have
cytomegaloviruria, and 10–15% have positive cervical cultures. It is likely that infants
infected early in utero are affected more than those who acquire the agent later.
Cytomegaloviruria has been demonstrated in 1% of neonates (range, 0.2–2.0%); most
of these acquired the organism transplacentally. Maternal antibody does not prevent
infection of the fetus, but it does appear to ameliorate severity. Infants of mothers
with primary CMV infection who presumably did not have passive antibody were
more likely to symptomatic infection and sequelae [73].
   A. **Clinical presentation.** It is estimated that 95% of all babies with intrauterine
   CMV infection are asymptomatic. Symptomatic disseminated intrauterine disease
   is characterized by: (1) intrauterine growth retardation, (2) hepatosplenomegaly,
   (3) jaundice, (4) petechiae, and (5) pulmonary involvement. In a recent report of
   106 symptomatic cases, 70% had hepatosplenomegaly, petechiae and jaundice,
   and 53% had microcephaly at birth [74].
   B. **Diagnosis** of CMV intrauterine disease is by any of these tests:
      1. Viral culture from urine or throat in the first 2 weeks of life
      2. Persistently high complement fixation titers (IgG)
      3. Persistently high IgM fluorescent antibody assay
   C. **Therapy** is symptomatic. Careful hand-washing and secretion precautions are
   advised.
   D. **Prognosis.** Mortality is 12% in those with disseminated disease, as there is no
   treatment other than supportive measures [74]. Survivors may develop chorioretinitis, periventricular cerebral calcifications, and deafness. **The cytomegaloviruria
   may continue intermittently for years.**

IV. **Herpes simplex virus** (HSV) usually is acquired peripartum but may be transmitted
transplacentally as well. Both HSV types 1 and 2 cause disease in neonates.
   A. **Clinical manifestations. One should suspect this diagnosis when caring for a
   septic neonate** [75]. Three syndromes are recognized: skin, eyes, and mouth
   (SEM), CNS, and disseminated disease. However, not all exposed infants will be
   infected. Rates of infection in newborns are 30–50% following exposure to primary
   maternal disease and 3–5% following recurrent maternal disease. Although there
   are many more women with recurrent disease than primary disease, the higher
   attack rate for the latter results in 50% of the neonatal cases. **Neonatal HSV
   disease cannot be ruled out on the basis of maternal history** [76, 77].
      1. **Disseminated infections.** These infants may have jaundice, hepatomegaly,
      pneumonitis, bleeding diathesis, and CNS manifestations. Only half of those
      with disseminated disease develop the typical vesicular rash. Mortality in this
      form is 80%, and most survivors have sequelae.
      2. **Local disease** implies involvement of only one organ system—CNS, or skin,
      eyes, or mouth.
   B. **Diagnosis** may be made by any one of the following tests:
      1. Viral culture of skin, rectum, throat, nasopharynx, conjunctiva, urine, stool,
      and CSF

2. Cytologic evaluation of skin lesion (multinucleate giant cells on Tzanck smear)
3. Rising complement fixation titers
4. Elevated specific IgM titers

C. **Treatment** of all forms of HSV infection or suspected HSV infection with **acyclovir** (10 mg/kg/dose IV q8h for 10–21 days) should be started as soon as viral cultures have been obtained [78, 79]. Vidarabine (30 mg/kg/day IV infused over 12 hours) may also be used, but the large fluid volume required makes it less practical. The use of suppressive oral acyclovir therapy following intravenous therapy for disease in a neonate is also controversial. Advice should be sought from a pediatric infectious disease consultant. The evaluation and management of a well infant born to a mother with active herpetic lesions is more controversial (see **D**). Chapter 26 provides further discussion of antiviral therapy.

D. **Prevention.** When the mother has documented active genital HSV infection, cesarean section has reduced neonatal acquisition rates from 50% to 6% in some studies. Evaluation and management of an exposed infant is controversial. Some experts recommend the use of routine serial weekly cultures for 6–8 weeks from birth, with initiation of intravenous acyclovir if any cultures obtained after 48 hours of life are positive [77]. Close follow-up by a physician and immediate evaluation of the infant for any signs of illness are the cornerstones of management. (See Chap. 13, sec. **III** under Genital Lesions, for further discussion.)

V. **Syphilis. The number of cases of congenital syphilis has increased steadily since the 1980s, in parallel with adult primary cases,** so clinicians must again be alert for this important intrauterine infection, which has devastating sequelae if untreated. The treponema usually is acquired transplacentally, although intrapartum acquisition is possible. A mother with untreated primary or secondary syphilis is unlikely to have any normal children; half will be premature or suffer perinatal death, and the remainder will have congenital syphilis [80]. The rates of these outcomes decrease with maternal infection in late gestation to 10% perinatal death and 10% congenital syphilis.

A. **Clinical presentation.** Approximately 50% of infected newborns are initially asymptomatic. Infants with congenital infection may demonstrate a vesicular or bullous rash that includes the palms and soles; they may have chronic rhinitis (snuffles), maculopapular rash, abnormal CSF, pneumonitis, myocarditis, nephrosis, pseudoparalysis, nonimmune hydrops, condylomata lata, hepatosplenomegaly, and generalized lymphadenopathy. These manifestations may not be apparent at birth but may develop during the first few weeks of life [81, 82].

   Bony lesions appear roentgenographically at 1–3 months and are characteristic: symmetric metaphyseal involvement with elevation of the periosteum, and osteomyelitic lesions, most often involving the humerus and tibia. These bone changes are said to occur in 90% of infants who manifest congenital syphilis [83]. The osteochondritis and periostitis may be painful and may be manifested by the pseudoparalysis of a limb due to pain (pseudoparalysis of Parrot).

B. **Diagnosis may be problematic.** Therefore, infection often is assumed and appropriate treatment administered without a definitive diagnosis. **Because the risks of therapy with penicillin are minimal and the sequelae of untreated syphilis can be permanent, treatment is advised in doubtful cases.** Infants born to mothers with no prenatal care should be tested by VDRL or a similar serologic screening test for syphilis.

1. **Diagnosis depends on the following:**
   a. Identification of the spirochete in any of the skin lesions or in the nasal discharge by **dark-field examination,** or
   b. **Serologic evaluation** (see Chap. 13 under Genital Lesions). Serum from the mother or infant is preferred over cord blood specimens for serology, because of false positives and false negatives in the latter [84]. Infected infants are often asymptomatic at birth and, if maternal or infant infection occurred late in pregnancy, infected infants may also be seronegative. The VDRL test usually is used for screening, and the fluorescent treponemal antibody absorption (FTA-ABS) test is used for confirmation. Maternal antibody is transmitted to the infant, and these tests measure both IgG and IgM.

2. **All newborns suspected of having congenital syphilis on the basis of maternal history or physical findings should be fully evaluated by** (1) careful examination for clinical signs of syphilis; (2) serology, including IgM if available; (3) radiologic survey of long bones; and (4) a lumbar puncture to collect CSF

for routine analysis, a dark-field examination, and a VDRL (not RPR) test. If
available, the placenta should be examined for focal villositis and the presence
of spirochetes.
C. **Therapy.** Recommendations for therapy were changed in 1988 because of reports
of **failure of benzathine penicillin** treatment. The initiation of therapy is based
on maternal and infant serology, clinical findings, and history of maternal treatment. The mother's data is assessed first. If the serologically positive mother did
not receive adequate therapy or received nonpenicillin therapy, or if adequate
follow-up is not assured, her infant should be treated with penicillin at birth [85].
    **Infants with proven or probable disease should receive 10–14 days of therapy
    with aqueous crystalline penicillin G.** Current Centers for Disease Control and
American Academy of Pediatrics recommendations are for 10–14 days of intravenous therapy with crystalline penicillin G 50,000 units/kg/dose q12h for the first
week and q8h after the seventh day [62, 85]. Some authorities suggest procaine
penicillin (50,000 units/kg/day IM in one dose) for 10–14 days. A few infants will
manifest a Herxheimer reaction to therapy, with a fever spike 6–8 hours after
the first penicillin dose. (See Chap. 13.)
    Management of **asymptomatic infants** with normal CSF and normal long-bone
radiographs is also determined by the adequacy of maternal therapy. Only if the
mother received documented adequate penicillin therapy more than 1 month
before delivery, and follow-up of the infant is ensured, can observation without
therapy be contemplated. For all other situations (which are likely to be the
majority of cases), **10–14 days of intravenous aqueous crystalline penicillin
is recommended.**
D. **Follow-up.** Treated infants should be seen in follow-up at 3 months and then at
6-month intervals for repeat serologic evaluation, CSF examinations, and clinical
reevaluation, until it is clear that VDRL titers are falling. Untreated or benzathine-
treated infants should be seen at 1, 2, 4, 6, and 12 months. The infant's VDRL
titers should decrease by 3 months of age, and FTA-ABS titers should decrease
by 6 months. If antibody titers remain stable or increase, reevaluation and therapy
are mandatory.
VI. **Human parvovirus B19,** the etiologic agent of erythema infectiosum, has been associated with adverse fetal outcome following maternal infection. Case reports describe
a spectrum including spontaneous abortions, hydrops fetalis, and stillbirths, as well
as normal infants. There are not yet adequate data to determine fully the risk of
fetal morbidity and death following acute maternal infection with parvovirus B19.
Available studies suggest that the risk of fetal death following acute maternal infection
in the first 20 weeks of gestation is 3–9%, whereas the risk following household
exposure of a woman with unknown serologic status is approximately 1–2% [86].
A. **Clinical presentation.** The principal adverse fetal outcome has been nonimmune
hydrops with severe ascites and pericardial and pleural effusions, which result
from severe anemia caused by direct infection and destruction of reticulocytes by
parvovirus B19 (aplastic crisis) [70, 87, 88].
B. **Diagnosis** may be made by any of the following tests:
    1. Specific IgM determination in cord or neonatal blood
    2. Polymerase chain reaction (PCR) for viral DNA
    3. Persistent infant B19 IgG at 12 months of age and IgM; although these are
    not readily available
    Until such tests and further data are available, the findings of elevated maternal
    alpha-fetoprotein levels, hydrops fetalis, and fetal aplastic crisis may be the best
    indicators of B19 infection.
C. **Therapy.** No specific therapy is available.
VII. **HIV** can be transmitted from mothers to infants in utero, intrapartum, or postpartum
through breast milk. The risk of **perinatal transmission** varies according to patient
population and geographic location but is in the range of 25% in most North American
settings. Issues of concern in the neonatal period center around early diagnosis of
HIV infection, evaluation for *Pneumocystis carinii* prophylaxis, and management of
associated conditions such as low birth weight, drug withdrawal, congenital syphilis,
or hepatitis. A recent placebo-controlled trial of zidovudine (ZDV; formerly azidothymidine [AZT]), in pregnant women and their newborn infants demonstrated a significantly reduced transmission rate compared with placebo (8% versus 25%) [89]. (See
related discussions in Chaps. 19 and 26.)
A. **Clinical presentation.** No recognizable dysmorphic syndrome has been associated

with HIV infection. **Most perinatally infected infants are asymptomatic at birth.** A small number of infants may develop symptoms within the first few days or weeks of life, including *P. carinii* pneumonia (PCP), active CMV disease, or acute bacterial infections. There appear to be two distinct patterns of natural history among perinatally infected children. One group of infants develops symptoms within the first year of life, whereas the other group remains asymptomatic for 3–5 years or more. Ongoing studies are attempting to delineate the factors responsible for this variation in disease progression. When symptoms do occur, they most commonly include oral candidiasis, failure to thrive, developmental delay, loss of developmental milestones, lymphadenopathy, recurrent or severe bacterial infections, pneumonia (PCP), lymphocytic interstitial pneumonitis, chronic or recurrent diarrhea, and hepatosplenomegaly [90].

B. **Diagnosis.** Because infants acquire maternal IgG transplacentally, routine HIV testing with IgG antibody–based assays [enzyme-linked immunosorbent assay (ELISA), Western blot] are not diagnostically useful. It is, however, **important to establish the diagnosis by other means as early as possible for preventive, therapeutic, and prognostic reasons.** Evaluation should include more specific assays such as PCR, p24 antigen, HIV-IgA, and culture, as well as an evaluation of the infant's immune status by measurement of T-cell subsets. **In most cases, a referral to a local or regional pediatric HIV specialist is advised** [91].

C. **Therapy.** Age-specific CD4 counts (infants younger than 12 months, T4 < 1,500 or < 20%) should be used to evaluate the need for **PCP prophylaxis** with trimethoprim-sulfamethoxazole [92]. (See further discussion in Chap. 24.) There are no well-defined CD4 counts for initiation of antiretroviral therapy; consequently, this therapy usually is initiated on the basis of symptomatology. Adjunctive therapy may include intravenous Ig or prophylactic penicillin in certain settings. Immunization schedules also vary slightly for these children. Oral polio vaccine should be replaced by inactivated polio vaccine. These decisions should be made in consultation with a pediatric HIV specialist [91, 93].

VIII. **Other infectious agents** should be considered when evaluating an infant with a suspected intrauterine infection. These include tuberculosis [94], *L. monocytogenes, Leptospirosis,* hepatitis B, enteroviruses, adenoviruses, varicella-zoster virus, and Epstein-Barr virus. Infants with these infections have demonstrated findings included in Table 3-10. As more is learned about the pathogenesis of old and new microbial agents, identification of other agents active in intrauterine infection will undoubtedly continue to expand.

Although much is known about neonatal infections, controlled trials of therapy are limited in number [95]. As a consequence, many recommendations are expert opinions based on limited data. Therefore, close individualized care should be afforded all ill neonates.

References

1. Gladstone, I.M., Ehrenkranz, R.A., Edberg, S.C., and Baltimore, R.S. A ten-year review of neonatal sepsis and comparison with the previous fifty-year experience. *Pediatr. Infect. Dis. J.* 9:819, 1990.
   A review of 280 cases of sepsis among neonates at a single medical center showed the changing patterns of etiology.
2. Remington, J.D., and Klein, J.O. *Infectious Disease of the Fetus and Newborn Infant* (4th ed.). Philadelphia: Saunders, 1995.
   Comprehensive reference textbook.
3. Wilson, C.B. Immunologic basis for increased susceptibility of the neonate to infection. *J. Pediatr.* 108:1, 1986.
4. Robertson, A., Fink, S., and Karp, W. Effect of cephalosporins on bilirubin-albumin binding. *J. Pediatr.* 112:291, 1988.
   Cephalosporins displace bilirubin from albumin, increasing free bilirubin.
5. Fink, S., Warren, K., and Robertson, A. Effect of penicillins on bilirubin-albumin binding. *J. Pediatr.* 113:566, 1988.
6. Martin, E., et al. Ceftriaxone-bilirubin-albumin interactions in the neonate: An vivo study. *Eur. J. Pediatr.* 152:530, 1993.
   In vivo evaluation of ceftriaxone in neonates demonstrating increases in fre

7. Jacobs, R.F., and Kearns, G.L. Cefotaxime pharmacokinetics and treatment of meningitis in neonates. *Infection* 17:72, 1989.
   A prospective clinical trial of 22 infants with gram-negative enteric meningitis successfully managed with cefotaxime.
8. Spritzer, R., Kamp, H.J.V.D., Dzoljic, G., and Sauer, P.J.J. Five years of cefotaxime use in a neonatal intensive care unit. *Pediatr. Infect. Dis.* 9:92, 1990.
   Susceptibility of gram-negatives to cefotaxime were unchanged in the face of increasing use of cefotaxime as empiric therapy.
9. Jacobs, R.F. Efficacy and safety of cefotaxime in the management of pediatric infections. *Infection* 19(Suppl. 6):S330, 1991.
10. Medical Letter. Safety of antimicrobial drugs in pregnancy. *Med. Lett. Drugs Ther.* 29:61, 1987.
11. Briggs, G.G., Freeman, R.K., and Yaffe, S.J. *Drugs in Pregnancy and Lactation* (4th ed.). Baltimore: Williams & Wilkins, 1994.
    Full review of all drugs, including antibiotics, and their transmission from mother to infant in breast milk and across the placenta.
12. American Academy of Pediatrics: Committee on Drugs. The transfer of drugs and other chemicals into human milk. *Pediatrics* 93:137, 1994.
    Recent policy regarding medications in breast milk.
13. Noya, F.J.D., and Baker, C.J. Prevention of group B streptococcal infection. *Infect. Dis. Clin. North Am.* 6:41, 1992.
    Review of approaches and recommendations.
14. Centers for Disease Control. Guidelines for prevention of perinatal group B streptococcal disease: A public health perspective. *M.M.W.R.* [in press, 1996].
    Detailed review and recommendations for maternal screening and management for group B streptococcal disease during pregnancy and labor.
15. Mohle-Boetani, J.C., et al. Comparison of prevention strategies for neonatal group B streptococcal infection. *J.A.M.A.* 270:1442, 1993.
    A population-based economic analysis supporting universal prenatal GBS screening and chemoprophylaxis of colonized women with labor complications.
16. Yagupsky, P., Menegus, M.A., and Powell, K.R. The changing spectrum of group B streptococcal disease in infants: An eleven-year experience in a tertiary care hospital. *Pediatr. Infect. Dis. J.* 10:801, 1991.
    Risk factors, clinical syndromes, and case fatality rates for early- and late-onset disease were documented.
17. Adams, W.G., et al. Outbreak of early onset group B streptococcal sepsis. *Pediatr. Infect. Dis. J.* 12:565, 1993.
18. Gellin, B.G., and Broome, C.F. Listeriosis. *J.A.M.A.* 261:1313, 1989.
    A complete review of microbiology, epidemiology, pathogenesis, and treatment of this microbial agent.
19. Schwarze, R., Bauermeister, C.D., Ortel, S., and Wichmann, G. Perinatal listeriosis in Dresden, 1981–1986: Clinical and microbiological findings in 18 cases. *Infection* 17:131, 1989.
    Study of bacteremia and meningitis caused by this organism.
20. Noel, G.J., et al. Anaerobic bacteria in a neonatal intensive care unit: An eighteen-year experience. *Pediatr. Infect. Dis. J.* 7:858, 1988.
    A recent review of the epidemiologic and clinical findings of anaerobic infections in the newborn.
21. Buchino, J.J., et al. Group D streptococcal infection in newborn infants. *Am. J. Dis. Child.* 133:270, 1979.
22. Kinney, J.S., et al. Early onset *Haemophilus influenzae* sepsis in the newborn infant. *Pediatr. Infect. Dis. J.* 12:739, 1993.
    Although rare, H. influenzae *can occur in the newborn.*
23. Baumgart, S., et al. Sepsis with coagulase-negative staphylococci in critically ill newborns. *Am. J. Dis. Child.* 137:461, 1983.
24. Gerdes, J.S. Clinicopathologic approach to the diagnosis of neonatal sepsis. *Clin. Perinatol.* 18:361, 1991.
    Presents data and suggested management algorithms for evaluation of ill neonates.
    Polin, R.A., and St. Geme III, J.W. Neonatal sepsis. *Adv. Pediatr. Infect. Dis.* 7:25, 1992.
    iew of epidemiology, etiology, risk factors, and approach to treatment of sepsis.
    ll, T.E., et al. No lumbar puncture in the evaluation for early neonatal sepsis: ingitis be missed? *Pediatrics* 95:803, 1995.

Some pediatricians advocate selective criteria to omit lumbar punctures in sepsis evaluations of newborn infants. This article shows that the use of these criteria will result in missed or delayed diagnosis of bacterial meningitis.

26. Evans, M.E., et al. Sensitivity, specificity, and predictive value of body surface cultures in a neonatal intensive care unit. *J.A.M.A.* 259:248, 1988.
Surface cultures are not useful in predicting the etiology of sepsis.

27. Baley, J.E., et al. Neonatal neutropenia: Clinical manifestations, cause, and outcome. *Am. J. Dis. Child.* 142:116, 1988.

28. Rodwell, R.L., Taylor, K.M.C.D., Tudehope, D.I., and Gray, P.H. Hematologic scoring system in early diagnosis of sepsis in neutropenic newborns. *Pediatr. Infect. Dis. J.* 12:372, 1993.
Hematologic profiles (neutropenia, immature: total neutrophils, total WBC, platelet count) of 1,000 neonates prospectively evaluated were found to identify sepsis early and predict prognosis.

29. Rozycki, H.J., Stahl, G.E., and Baumgart, S. Impaired sensitivity of a single early leukocyte count in screening for neonatal sepsis. *Pediatr. Infect. Dis. J.* 6:440, 1987.

30. Gerdes, J.S., and Polin, R.A. Sepsis screen in neonates with evaluation of plasma fibronectin. *Pediatr. Infect. Dis. J.* 6:443–446, 1987.
Positive total WBC, immature-total neutrophil ratio, C-reactive protein, and micro-erythrocyte sedimentation rate had a sensitivity of 100%, specificity of 85%. Fibronectin levels were not helpful, and this technique did not identify late-onset sepsis in preterm infants.

31. Hammerschlag, M.R., et al. Patterns of use of antibiotics in two newborn nurseries. *N. Engl. J. Med.* 296:1268, 1977.
Documents high rates of presumptive therapy with antibiotics in 1970s; rates may be higher now.

32. Bradley, J.S. Neonatal infections. *Pediatr. Infect. Dis. J.* 4:315, 1985.
Brief summary with good management suggestions.

33. Word, B.M., and Klein, J.O. Current therapy of bacterial sepsis and meningitis in infants and children: A poll of directors of programs in pediatric infectious diseases. *Pediatr. Infect. Dis. J.* 7:267, 1989.
Documents increasing use of cefotaxime with ampicillin for neonatal disease.

34. Cairo, M.S., et al. Randomized trial of granulocyte transfusion versus intravenous immune globulin therapy for neonatal neutropenia and sepsis. *J. Pediatr.* 120:281, 1992.
Pilot randomized study suggesting benefit of WBC transfusions in septic neonates with neutropenia.

35. Baker, C.J., et al. Intravenous immune globulin for the prevention of nosocomial infection in low birth-weight neonates. *N. Engl. J. Med.* 327:213, 1992.
A controlled trial of LBW infants concluded that intravenous immunoglobulin reduces nosocomial infections.

36. Fanaroff, A.A., et al. A controlled trial of intravenous immune globulin to reduce nosocomial infections in very-low-birth-weight infants. *N. Engl. J. Med.* 330:1107, 1994.
A controlled trial of intravenous immunoglobulin in 2,416 LBW neonates demonstrating no reduction in nosocomial infections.

37. Hill, H.R. Intravenous immunoglobulin use in the neonate: Role in prophylaxis and therapy of infection. *Pediatr. Infect. Dis. J.* 12:549, 1993.
A comprehensive, reasoned review of the topic.

38. Weisman, Col. L.E., et al. Comparison of group B streptococcal hyperimmune globulin and standard intravenously administered immune globulin in neonates. *J. Pediatr.* 122:929, 1993.

39. Kline, M.W. *Citrobacter* meningitis and brain abscess in infancy: Epidemiology, pathogenesis, and treatment. *J. Pediatr.* 113:430, 1988.
A complete review of this devastating disease.

40. McCracken, G.H., Jr., et al. Consensus report: Antimicrobial therapy for bacterial meningitis in infants and children. *Pediatr. Infect. Dis. J.* 6:501, 1987.

41. Klein, J.O., Feign, R.D., and McCracken, G.H. Report of the task force on diagnosis and management of meningitis. *Pediatrics* 78:959–979, 1986.

42. Plotkin, S.A., et al. Meningitis in infants and children. *Pediatrics* 81:904, 1988.
Update of [41], recommending cefotaxime or ceftazidime plus ampicillin for therapy of neonatal meningitis.

43. McCracken, G.H., Jr., Mize, S.G., and Threckeld, N. Neonatal meningitis cooperative study. Intraventricular gentamicin therapy in gram-negative bacillary meningitis of infancy: Report of the Second Neonatal Meningitis Cooperative Study Group. *Lancet* 1:787, 1980.
    This randomized trial demonstrated a deleterious effect of intraventricular amino-glycosides.
44. Hammerschlag, M.R. Neonatal conjunctivitis. *Pediatr. Ann.* 22(6):346, 1993.
    Review of etiologic agents, diagnosis, and management.
45. Burton, D.M., Seid, A.B., Kearns, D.B., and Pransky, S.M. Neonatal otitis media. *Arch. Otolaryngol. Head Neck Surg.* 119:672, 1993.
    A full update on diagnosis, etiologic agents, and management.
46. Beem, M.O., and Saxon, E.M. Respiratory tract colonization and a distinctive pneumonia syndrome in infants infected with *Chlamydia trachomatis*. *N. Engl. J. Med.* 296:306, 1977.
    Classic first report of this syndrome, with superlative clinical description.
47. Rettig, P.J. Perinatal infections with *Chlamydia trachomatis*. *Clin. Perinatol.* 15:321, 1988.
    Excellent complete recent review of maternal and neonatal disease. Prompt improvement with erythromycin or sulfonamide therapy is reported.
48. Bell, T.A., et al. Chronic *Chlamydia trachomatis* infections in infants. *J.A.M.A.* 267:400, 1992.
    Documents the chronic carriage of chlamydiae acquired perinatally.
49. Centers for Disease Control. Recommendations for the prevention and management of *Chlamydia trachomatis* infections, 1993. *M.M.W.R.* 42(RR-12):1, 1993.
50. Cassell, G.H., et al. *Ureaplasma urealyticum* intrauterine infection: Role in prematurity and disease in newborns. *Clin. Microbiol. Rev.* 6:69, 1993.
    Review of the data regarding this pathogen in newborns.
51. Waites, K.B., Crouse, D.T., and Cassell, G.H. Antibiotic susceptibilities and therapeutic options for *Ureaplasma urealyticum* infections in neonates. *Pediatr. Infect. Dis. J.* 11:23, 1992.
52. Steinhoff, M.C., and Smith, D.H. Diarrheagenic *E. coli*. In V.C. Vaughn, R.J. McKay, and R.E. Behrman (eds.), *Nelson Textbook of Pediatrics* (11th ed.). Philadelphia: Saunders, 1979. P. 769.
53. St. Geme, J.W., et al. Consensus: Management of *Salmonella* infection in the first year of life. *Pediatr. Infect. Dis. J.* 7:615, 1988.
    A consensus on management and therapy for Salmonella *infection. Each expert discusses his or her approach to a difficult problem. A good summary.*
54. Kliegman, R.M., and Walsh, M.C. Neonatal necrotizing enterocolitis: Pathogenesis, classification, and spectrum of illness. *Curr. Probl. Pediatr.* 17:219, 1987.
    An extensive review of this topic.
55. Faix, R.G., Polley, T.Z., and Grasela, T.H. A randomized, controlled trial of parenteral clindamycin in neonatal necrotizing enterocolitis. *J. Pediatr.* 112:271, 1988.
    Showed no effect of adding clindamycin to standard regimen of treatment.
56. Littlewood, J.M. Sixty-six infants with urinary tract infection in the first month of life. *Arch. Dis. Child.* 47:218, 1972.
57. Ginsburg, C.M., and McCracken, G.H. Urinary tract infections in young infants. *Pediatrics* 69:409, 1982.
58. Asmar, B.I. Osteomyelitis in the neonate. *Pediatr. Infect.* 6:117, 1992.
    Useful review of aspects unique to the neonate.
59. Dan, M. Septic arthritis in young infants: Clinical and microbiological correlations and therapeutic implications. *Rev. Infect. Dis.* 6:147, 1984.
60. Melish, M.E., and Glasgow, L.A. Staphylococcal scalded skin syndrome. The expanded clinical spectrum. *J. Pediatr.* 78:958, 1971.
    Classic review of the syndrome.
61. Centers for Disease Control. Hepatitis B virus: A comprehensive strategy for eliminating transmission in the United States through universal childhood vaccination. Recommendations of the Immunization Practices Advisory Committee (ACIP). *M.M.W.R.* 40(RR-13):1, 1991.
    Policy statement recommending universal immunization of infants.
62. Peter, G., et al. (eds.). *1994 Red Book: Report of the Committee on Infectious Diseases* (23rd ed.). Elk Grove Village, IL: American Academy of Pediatrics, 1994.
    Essential reference. Includes neonatal drug dose information; updated frequently.

63. A-Kader, H.H., and Balistreri, W.F. Hepatitis C virus: Implications to pediatric practice. *Pediatr. Infect. Dis. J.* 12:853, 1993.
See related paper by M.J. Koziel, Immunology of viral hepatitis. Am. J. Med. 100:98, 1996, with an update on hepatitis C virus.

64. Modlin, J.F., and Kinney, J.S. Perinatal Enterovirus Infections. In S.C. Aronoff et al. (eds.). *Advances in Pediatric Infectious Diseases,* Vol. 2. Chicago: Year Book, 1987. P. 57.

64a. Abzug, M.J., et al. Neonatal enterovirus infection: Virology, serology, and effects of intravenous immune globulin. *Clin. Infect. Dis.* 20:1201, 1995.
Report of 16 neonates including seven cases with echovirus and seven with coxsackievirus; data do not yet support widespread use of immunoglobulin for neonates with suspected or proven enterovirus infections.

65. Brunell, P.A. Varicella in pregnancy, the fetus, and the newborn: Problems in management. *J. Infect. Dis.* 166 (Suppl. 1):S42, 1992.
Summary of the issues of management of varicella occurring perinatally.

66. Pastuszak, A.L., et al. Outcome after maternal varicella infection in the first 20 weeks of pregnancy. *N. Engl. J. Med.* 330:901, 1994.
Documents 2.3% frequency of congenital syndrome in infants of infected mothers.

67. Butler, K.M., and Baker, C.J. Candida: An increasingly important pathogen in the nursery. *Pediatr. Clin. North Am.* 35:543, 1988.
An extensive review of an increasingly important pathogen in the intensive care nursery. Discussion of antifungal agents included.

68. Baley, J.E., Kliegman, R.M., and Fanaroff, A.A. Disseminated fungal infections in very low birth weight infants: Clinical manifestations and epidemiology. *Pediatrics* 73:144, 1984.

69. Koren, G., et al. Pharmacokinetics and adverse effects of amphotericin B in infants and children. *J. Pediatr.* 118:559, 1988.

69a. van den Anker, J.N., et al. Antifungal agents in neonatal systemic candidiasis. *Antimicrob. Agents Chemother.* 39:1391, 1995.
This "mini-review" presents an overview of the available pharmacokinetic data for amphotericin B, flucytosine, and azoles in the newborn. Dosages, dosage adjustments in the face of organ failure, and toxicity are reviewed.

70. Kinney, J.S., and Kumar, M.L. Should we expand the TORCH complex? A description of clinical and diagnostic aspects of selected old and new agents. *Clin. Perinatol.* 15:727, 1988.
This article provides a diagnostic approach to the laboratory diagnosis of suspected TORCH infection. New agents associated with perinatal infection are discussed.

71. Lee, S.H., Ewert, D.P., Frederick, P.D., and Mascola, L. Resurgence of congenital rubella syndrome in the 1990s. Report on missed opportunities and failed prevention policies among women of childbearing age. *J.A.M.A.* 267:2616, 1992.
Highlights issues of failure to vaccinate women of childbearing age and consequent morbidity of their infants.

72. Yow, M.D. Congenital cytomegalovirus disease: A new problem. *J. Infect. Dis.* 159:163, 1989.
Review of a common problem.

73. Fowler, K.B., et al. The outcome of congenital cytomegalovirus infection in relation to maternal antibody status. *N. Engl. J. Med.* 326:663, 1992.
Very helpful study for predicting outcomes and counseling parents.

74. Boppana, S.B., et al. Symptomatic congenital cytomegalovirus infection: Neonatal morbidity and mortality. *Pediatr. Infect. Dis. J.* 11:93, 1992.
Excellent review of 106 neonates with symptomatic congenital CMV.

75. Whitley, R.J. Neonatal herpes simplex virus infections. *Clin. Perinatol.* 15:903, 1988.
A complete review of a complex subject. See also R.J. Whitley et al., Changing presentation of herpes simplex virus in neonates. J. Infect. Dis. 158:109, 1988; and S. Kohl, The neonatal human's immune response to herpes simplex virus infection: A critical review. Pediatr. Infect. Dis. J. 8:67–74, 1989.

76. Brown, Z.A., et al. Neonatal herpes simplex virus infection in relation to asymptomatic maternal infection at the time of labor. *N. Engl. J. Med.* 324:1247, 1991.
An excellent study demonstrating the variability in risk of neonatal disease according to presence or absence of type-specific HSV maternal antibody. Neonatal HSV developed in 33% of infants born to mothers without type-specific antibodies compared with 3% of infants born to mothers with antibodies.

77. Prober, C.G., et al. The management of pregnancies complicated by genital infections with herpes simplex virus. *Clin. Infect. Dis.* 15:1031, 1992.
    A consensus paper from the Infectious Disease Society of America, with suggestions for management of this complex problem.
78. Whitley, R., et al. A controlled trial comparing vidarabine with acyclovir in neonatal herpes simplex virus infection. *N. Engl. J. Med.* 324:444, 1991.
    A landmark study demonstrating the clinical equivalence of vidarabine and acyclovir.
79. Whitley, R.J., and Gnann, J.W., Jr. Acyclovir: A decade later. *N. Engl. J. Med.* 326:782, 1992.
    A full review.
80. Reyes, M.P., Hunt, N., Ostrea, E.M., Jr., and George, D. Maternal congenital syphilis in a large tertiary-care urban hospital. *Clin. Infect. Dis.* 17:1041, 1993.
    A comprehensive update of congenital syphilis natural history. See also related paper by F.B. Coles et al., Congenital syphilis surveillance in upstate New York 1989–1992: Implications for prevention and management. J. Infect. Dis. 171:732, 1995.
81. Ikeda, M.K., and Jenson, H.B. Evaluation and treatment of congenital syphilis. *J. Pediatr.* 117:843, 1990.
    An excellent comprehensive review of the complex topic. See related paper by B.J. Stoll, Congenital syphilis: Evaluation and management of neonates born to mothers with reactive serologic tests for syphilis. Pediatr. Infect. Dis. J. 13:845, 1994.
82. Zenker, P.N., and Berman, S.A. Congenital syphilis: Trends and recommendations for evaluation and management. *Pediatr. Infect. Dis. J.* 10:516, 1991.
    Latest Centers for Disease Control recommendations for evaluation and management.
83. Hira, S.K., et al. Early congenital syphilis: Clinicoradiologic features in 202 patients. *Sex. Transm. Dis.* 12:177, 1985.
    Description of syphilis from the 1980s.
84. Chhabra, R.S., et al. Comparison of maternal sera, cord blood, and neonatal sera for detecting presumptive congenital syphilis: Relationship with maternal treatment. *Pediatrics* 91:88, 1993.
    Demonstrates difficulties using cord blood and advocates use of infant serum.
85. Centers for Disease Control. 1993 Sexually transmitted diseases treatment guidelines. *M.M.W.R.* 42(RR-14):1, 1993.
    Complete recommendations for management of infants, children, and adults.
86. American Academy of Pediatrics: Committee on Infectious Diseases. Parvovirus, erythema infectiosum, and pregnancy. *Pediatrics* 85:131, 1990.
    Policy statement describing minimal risk to the fetus.
87. Centers for Disease Control. Risks associated with human parvovirus B19 infection. *M.M.W.R.* 39:81, 1989.
    A thorough review of this topic.
88. Ware, R. Human parvovirus infection. *J. Pediatr.* 114:343, 1989.
    Another thorough review of this topic.
89. Centers for Disease Control. Zidovudine for the prevention of HIV transmission from mother to infant. *M.M.W.R.* 43(16):285, 1994.
    Controlled trial of zidovudine (ZDV) in mothers and infants showed reduction in transmission from 23% to 8%.
90. Falloon, J., et al. Human immunodeficiency virus infection in children. *J. Pediatr.* 114:1, 1989.
    A thorough review of pathogenesis, epidemiology, and clinical manifestations of pediatric AIDS. There is a complete discussion of management issues for human immunodeficiency virus infection.
91. Pizzo, P.A., and Wilfert, C.M. (eds.). Perspectives on pediatric human immunodeficiency virus infection. *Pediatr. Infect. Dis. J.* 12:513, 1993.
    Comprehensive recent review.
92. Centers for Disease Control. Guidelines for prophylaxis against *Pneumocystis carinii* pneumonia for children infected with human immunodeficiency virus. *J.A.M.A.* 265:1637, 1991.
    An important table for deciding when to start PCP prophylaxis in children.
93. Working Group on Antiretroviral Therapy. Antiretroviral therapy and medical management of the human immunodeficiency virus–infected child. *Pediatr. Infect. Dis. J.* 12:513, 1993.
    Recommendations for routine laboratory evaluation, medications, and management.

94. Cantwell, M.F., et al. Brief report: Congenital tuberculosis. *N. Engl. J. Med.* 330: 1051, 1994.
    A good description of the pathophysiology and management of this rare condition.
95. Sinclair, J.C., and Bracken, M.B. (eds.). *Effective Care of the Newborn Infant.* Oxford: Oxford University Press, 1992.
    A complete formal review with assessment of validity and meta-analysis of all randomized controlled trials done in newborns. The relative lack of controlled trials of therapy for infection is notable: Two trials of therapy for necrotizing enterocolitis and five trials of therapy for meningitis, 1980–1987.

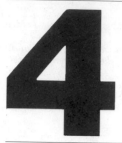

Skin and Soft-Tissue Infections

C. Richard Magnussen

Skin and soft-tissue infections are common problems. In organizing this chapter, more limited, superficial skin problems will be addressed first (e.g., impetigo, cutaneous abscess, puncture wounds); then more involved infections (e.g., cellulitis, necrotizing soft-tissue infections, neck infections); and finally principles of wound management and tetanus.

Impetigo

Simple superficial impetigo is the most common skin condition seen in children. It generally is diagnosed and treated on clinical grounds alone and is reviewed in detail elsewhere [1]. In the United States, so-called bullous impetigo occurs less commonly and is seen in fewer than 10% of cases of impetigo but may be more common in Britain [1].

I. **Clinical characteristics**
   A. **Simple superficial impetigo** [1] is an indolent, well-tolerated infection with lesions typically found on exposed areas of skin, especially the extremities. Typical lesions can begin at a traumatized area (e.g., insect bite or abrasion) with an erythematous papule, which then evolves to a crusted form ranging in size from several millimeters to 1–2 cm or more. The crust is amber or honey-colored and thick. When the crust is removed, amber serous fluid may exude from the base. An erythematous margin may surround the crust. Initial discrete lesions may enlarge and coalesce. Because the patient is nontoxic, lesions may be present for 2–3 weeks before the patient seeks medical attention.
   B. **Bullous impetigo** is less common in the United States. Superficial bullae (0.5–3.0 cm in diameter) arise from normal-appearing skin. The bullae are usually flaccid and contain fluid that varies from thin and translucent to cloudy or even purulent-appearing. A thin margin of erythema often surrounds the bullae. After they rupture, a flat, thin, varnishlike coating forms over the denuded area. In neonates, lesions are most often on the perineum, periumbilical area, or both; in older children, the extremities are more involved [1].

II. **Epidemiology**
   A. **Simple superficial impetigo** is primarily a disease of children and is more prevalent during **warm, humid weather.** It occurs both endemically and in epidemics and can spread within families and among those in close physical contact [1]. **Group A streptococci** have been considered to be the primary etiologic agent, although some cultures of lesions typically yield a mixed flora of group A streptococci and *S. aureus.* Cutaneous trauma is important in the development of skin lesions [1].
   B. **Bullous impetigo** is due exclusively to staphylococci (*S. aureus*), which can be isolated from culture of bullae fluid aspirates. Phage type 71 has been commonly reported. The bullae are caused by the epidermolytic toxin produced by the staphylococci [1].

   Nursery-associated epidemics have been reported in the United States among neonates exposed to high rates of staphylococcal colonization. The skin infection may not become apparent until 3–4 weeks after discharge [1]. In older children, sporadic cases may be seen.

III. **Diagnosis and therapy**
   A. **Simple superficial impetigo**

1. **Diagnosis** is based on **clinical appearance** of the lesions, their superficial nature, and the absence of systemic toxicity. Bacterial cultures are not routinely advised unless the presentation is atypical or the patient fails to respond to usual therapy [1].
2. **Therapy is directed at both staphylococci and streptococci,** as prior studies have shown therapy directed only at streptococci is less effective [1]. Pediatric oral antibiotic doses are given in Chap. 28. Lesions should be cleansed and covered, at least initially.
   a. **Oral therapy** with 10 days of erythromycin, cephalexin, dicloxacillin, or clindamycin is effective.
   b. **Topical mupirocin** therapy, applied tid for 10 days, is as effective as oral regimens [2, 3] and **often is preferred** by patients and their parents [3]. (See further discussions of mupirocin, Chap. 28U.)
   c. Some experts prefer oral systemic therapy in some settings, including multiple lesions or impetigo in multiple family members, childcare groups, or athletic teams [4].

B. **Bullous impetigo**
   1. **Diagnosis** can be confirmed by aspirating the bullae, demonstrating polymorphonuclear leukocytes and gram-positive cocci in the aspirate, and culturing staphylococci from the aspirate [1]. In extensive cases, skin biopsy sometimes is used.
   2. **Therapy.** Systemic oral **antistaphylococcal agents** are recommended; the role of mupirocin in this setting has not been investigated [1]. A 10-day course of dicloxacillin, a first-generation cephalosporin, erythromycin, or clindamycin usually is recommended. In patients with very extensive disease, initial therapy with an antistaphyloccal parenteral agent may be indicated.

IV. **Prophylaxis**
A. **Simple superficial impetigo**
   1. **Normal cleanliness** with regular bathing is useful.
   2. **Prompt attention to minor wounds** has been suggested. Some suggest applying antibiotic ointment to insect bites and early infected lesions to prevent the development of overt disease [1].
   3. Prophylactic administration of penicillin has been employed in some epidemic outbreaks, but its routine use is not advised [1]. This may be an important public health consideration if there is an epidemic with a nephritogenic group A streptococcal strain in a community.
   4. Children with impetigo should not return to school or daycare until at least 24 hours after beginning antibiotic therapy [4].
B. **Bullous impetigo** usually is not associated with recurrent disease requiring prophylaxis.

V. **Prognosis**
A. **Simple superficial impetigo** usually has a good outcome. Severe local and distant metastatic suppurative complications are rare [1].
   1. **Acute poststreptococcal glomerulonephritis** (AGN) can occur and is more likely when the skin infection has been caused by nephritogenic strains such as M-types 2, 49, 55, 56, and 31 [1]. Titers of anti-DNAse B are more reliable indicators of recent skin infection than is the antistreptolysin O (ASO) titer (see Chap. 25). Appropriate antibiotic therapy does not appear to prevent the development of AGN once the infection is established.
   2. Acute rheumatic fever apparently does not occur following streptococcal pyoderma.
B. **Bullous impetigo.** Because bullous impetigo is due to staphylococci, the nonsuppurative sequelae seen with streptococci are not a concern.

VI. **Role of antibiotic therapy in prevention of impetigo sequelae.** Antimicrobial therapy can definitely be justified to achieve the following objectives: (1) as a public health measure, to decrease the size and duration of a streptococcal reservoir; (2) to prevent very rare, but serious, complications such as endocarditis or meningitis; (3) to prevent local extension of the lesions; and (4) to improve the appearance of the afflicted individual.

VII. **Prophylaxis. Impetigo is contagious, and contact should be prevented until the crust disappears.** The lesions should be cleansed and covered with a clean dressing. Treatment of contacts with benzathine penicillin probably is not warranted unless a nephritogenic strain begins to propagate in a community.

Cutaneous Abscesses

Cutaneous abscesses are among the most common soft-tissue infections encountered in clinical practice. They are found on all areas of the body and involve a variety of aerobic and anaerobic bacteria. The most prevalent types of cutaneous abscesses are discussed here.

I. **Types of cutaneous abscesses**
   A. **Isolated furuncles.** Furuncles (common boils) are *S. aureus* infections of obstructed hair follicles or sebaceous glands. Fever and constitutional symptoms are infrequent. Spontaneous or surgical drainage usually affords prompt relief. However, **lesions on the lips and nose can spread through the facial and emissary veins, possibly resulting in cavernous sinus thrombosis or brain abscess.** Lesions on the lips and nose should not be physically manipulated in any manner, and surgical drainage is contraindicated. Treatment of lip and nose furuncles should consist of warm soaks to the area; antistaphylococcal antibiotics are not routinely indicated, unless the patient is febrile or has evidence of extension of the process to adjacent tissues.
   B. **Recurrent furuncles** or other staphylococcal skin infections occur in some otherwise healthy adults for no obvious reason. These are more common in patients who have diabetes mellitus, are on chronic hemodialysis, or abuse intravenous drugs. These patients are chronic nasal carriers of *S. aureus,* and the skin is repeatedly inoculated from the nasal reservoir. No treatment regimen has proven to be universally effective, but a topical agent to eradicate staphylococcal nasal carriage in combination with an oral antistaphylococcal antibiotic is currently the favored approach. Mupirocin (see Chap. 28U) applied to the anterior nares twice daily for 5 days often is effective in eradicating staphylococcal carriage [5]. Clindamycin given by the oral route, along with topical mupirocin, may be the most effective regimen. In one controlled trial, 150-mg clindamycin once daily for 3 months eliminated recurrent staphylococcal skin infections in a high percentage of patients [6]. Oral rifampin combined with an antistaphylococcal penicillin (such as dicloxacillin) or combined with a fluoroquinolone (such as ciprofloxacin) has also been advocated. These agents and doses are discussed in Chap. 28.
   C. **Carbuncles.** Carbuncles are large cutaneous abscesses initiated by *S. aureus* infections of an obstructed hair follicle. These large abscesses are erythematous, warm, painful, and often accompanied by fever and constitutional symptoms. Bacteremia, with spread of staphylococcal infection to bone, endocardium, brain, or other sites, can occur, and therefore blood cultures should be drawn in the febrile patient. Surgical drainage is usually necessary, and systemic antibiotic therapy is required if there is a surrounding cellulitis or if the patient is toxic. As is discussed in sec. **II.B.2,** patients with underlying heart lesions should be treated with antibiotics (antistaphylococcal) before the cutaneous lesions are incised.
   D. **Mixed cutaneous abscesses.** It is not widely appreciated that cutaneous abscesses can be caused by a variety of bacterial species other than *S. aureus.* Anaerobes, either in pure culture or mixed with coliforms, are characteristic of abscesses in the perineal region. Nonperineal abscesses are more likely to be secondary to aerobic bacteria, but anaerobic bacteria can be present. Incision and drainage is the most effective treatment, and antibiotics are used only in high-risk patients or when signs of systemic infection are present.
II. **Evaluation of cutaneous abscesses.** The following recommendations are suggested as guidelines for the initial evaluation of cutaneous abscesses:
   A. **Clinical evaluation**
      1. Assess degree of illness (i.e., fever, chills, sweats, or constitutional symptoms). If the patient is febrile, blood cultures should be obtained.
      2. Assess degree of risk (i.e., diabetes mellitus, valvular heart disease, immunologic disorder, or immunosuppressive chemotherapy).
      3. Assess location of abscess (i.e., lips or nose, perineum, or other site).
      4. **Obtain Gram stains** of drainage or aspirated material.
      5. **Culture** drainage or aspirated material for aerobes and anaerobes.
   B. **Incision and drainage**
      1. Abscesses on the lips and nose should not be drained.
      2. **Antibiotic prophylaxis** is indicated for patients with underlying **cardiac valve disease** (see Chap. 28B). Because drainage of subcutaneous abscesses may

result in staphylococcal or streptococcal bacteremia and drainage of perineal abscesses may result in gram-negative bacilli or enterococcal bacteremia, the prophylactic regimen will differ depending on the site of the abscess. Refer to Chap. 28B for a more detailed discussion of antibiotic prophylaxis during abscess drainage.

III. **Treatment.** Most cutaneous abscesses will require incision and drainage for successful eradication. Antibiotic therapy will be necessary in certain situations.
  A. **Incision and drainage** should be performed except for abscesses on the lips and nose.
  B. **Antibiotics** should be reserved for the following situations:
    1. **High-risk patients** with impaired host defenses (i.e., diabetes mellitus, immuno-suppressed patients).
    2. **Extension of infection** to adjacent tissues (i.e., cellulitis, osteomyelitis).
    3. **Bloodstream invasion.**
    4. **Underlying cardiac valve disease** in which prophylaxis is indicated.
  C. **Initial antibiotic regimens** can be chosen based on the Gram stain of the abscess drainage or aspirate. In adults, the following regimens are suggested:
    1. **Gram-positive cocci**
      a. **Oral therapy.** Dicloxacillin, 250–500 mg q6h, can be given. A first-generation oral cephalosporin can be used in the patient with a delayed penicillin allergy or in the patient for whom the potential GI side effects of dicloxacillin should be avoided. Cephalexin or cephradine, 750–1,000 mg q6h, can be used in the adult (see Chap. 28F for dosage discussion). In the penicillin-allergic patient in whom cephalosporins are contraindicated or in the cephalosporin-allergic patient, oral clindamycin (300–450 mg q8h) could be used.
      b. **Parenteral therapy.** Nafcillin or oxacillin, 1–2 g IV q4–6h, is recommended. In the patient with a delayed penicillin allergy, cefazolin, 750 mg q8h, could be used.
    2. **Gram-negative bacilli** (perineal area abscess)
      a. **Oral therapy.** Amoxicillin (250–500 mg tid) and clindamycin (300–450 mg tid) or amoxicillin (250 mg)–clavulanate (125 mg) (Augmentin) will cover the majority of pathogens while one is awaiting culture results.
      b. **Parenteral therapy.** Cefazolin and clindamycin or ampicillin-sulbactam (Unasyn) can be used. Cefoxitin (or cefotetan) alone is a reasonable alternative (see Chap. 28). If a more resistant organism is suspected or documented, an aminoglycoside or a second- or third-generation cephalosporin could be used, depending on susceptibility results.
      c. **In a penicillin-allergic patient,** a first-generation cephalosporin may be used if it is not contraindicated. Clindamycin also is suggested for anaerobic coverage. Cefoxitin (or cefotetan), each of which provides coverage in many cases of *B. fragilis,* may be a reasonable single agent (see Chap. 28).

Puncture Wounds (of Feet)

I. **Clinical characteristics.** Nail puncture wounds are a universal problem, occurring most commonly in the feet of children or young adults during warm weather [7]. This type of wound can have such serious complications as tetanus, cellulitis, local soft-tissue infection, or underlying osteomyelitis. It is estimated that 3–15% of these wounds become infected, resulting in cellulitis or localized deep-tissue abscess and that 0.6–1.8% are complicated by osteochondrosis with or without pyoarthrosis. In more than 90% of cases, the infecting organism is *Pseudomonas aeruginosa* [8].

II. **Treatment. Initial management** of the puncture wound should include the following procedures:
  A. Cleanse the wound with a detergent or iodophor.
  B. Surgically debride devitalized tissue.
  C. Probe the wound for the presence of residual foreign bodies.
  D. Institute proper tetanus prophylaxis.
  E. **Prophylactic antibiotics are not routinely indicated** unless the wound has gone unattended for more than 6 hours or unless adjacent soft-tissue infection has already occurred.

III. **Complications.** If cellulitis, local soft-tissue infection, or abscesses result from the puncture wound, these infections should be managed as outlined in other sections of this chapter. Osteomyelitis of the small bones of the foot may occur (*P. aeruginosa* is the most common pathogen) and will require proper antibiotic and surgical therapy, as discussed in Chap. 16.

In a recent report on the therapy of foot infections that occurred following a nail puncture wound, initial treatment of the wound was surgical and included extensive incision and debridement of the affected tissue and drainage of pus. Oral ciprofloxacin was then used for 7 days in patients with cellulitis or deep-tissue abscess, and for 14 days in patients with osteochondritis [8].

Animal Bites and
Rabies Prevention

Bite wounds account for approximately 1% of all hospital emergency room visits. Of the 1–2 million bite wounds that occur annually in the United States, the majority (approximately 80%) cause only minor injury, and the victims neither need nor seek medical care. Management of bite wounds has been extensively reviewed [9].

I. **Types of bite wounds**
  A. **Dog bites.** Dogs are responsible for nearly 80% of animal bite wounds, and approximately **15–20% of these dog-bite wounds become infected.** The risk of infection is greatest (approximately 40%) for crush injuries, puncture wounds, and wounds of the hand [9].
    1. **Bacteriology** [9]. All these organisms can be found in the oral flora of the dog.
      a. **Alpha-hemolytic streptococci** are isolated from the majority of wounds.
      b. *Pasteurella multocida* organisms are identified in 20–30%.
      c. *S. aureus* is detected in 20–30%.
      d. **Other aerobic pathogens** include streptococci (among them enterococci), *Eikenella corrodens, Capnocytophaga canimorsus* (formerly dysgonic fermenter 2 [DF-2]) and, infrequently, other gram-negative bacilli.
    2. **Antibiotic therapy.** A number of studies have attempted to address the pros and cons of prophylactic antibiotic therapy, but this issue remains unclear. In his excellent review, Goldstein [9] emphasizes that no large-scale randomized trial involving a group of injuries of similar severity and site has been done. Furthermore, whereas most clinicians would treat wounds that are severe and those that involve the hand or a joint, and a few would treat trivial wounds, optimal management of the moderate category of wounds remains uncertain [9].
        Pending definitive data, Goldstein [9] suggests that because more than 80% of dog-bite wounds harbor potential pathogens and because it cannot be predicted which 15–20% will become infected, it **seems prudent to administer antimicrobial treatment for 3–5 days** after most dog bites. Trivial wounds need not be treated.
      a. See Table 4-1 for options. **For the non-penicillin-allergic patient, amoxicillin-clavulanate is suggested for outpatient therapy.** For an infected wound requiring parenteral antibiotics, ampicillin-sulbactam is suggested.
      b. **In the penicillin-allergic patient,** the single optimal agent is not clear. Erythromycin is not an ideal choice. See Table 4-1 for options.
    3. **Irrigation** with normal saline, **debridement,** and **surgical repair** will depend on the severity of the injury. Infected wounds and those that are seen more than 24 hours after the bite occurs should be left open. Whether to close wounds seen less than 8 hours after the bite and not yet clinically infected remains controversial [9]. Elevation of the injured area is useful.
    4. **Tetanus prophylaxis** should be assessed.
    5. **Rabies** risk needs assessment. See the discussion in sec. **III.**
  B. **Cat bites.** Because the incidence of infection is greater than 50%, persons bitten by cats should usually receive antibiotics. Cat teeth are slender and extremely sharp, so they easily penetrate into bones and joints, with a proportionate increase in rates of septic arthritis and osteomyelitis [9].
    1. **Bacteriology.** The organisms isolated are those found in the oropharynx of the cat.
      a. *P. multocida* is the pathogen isolated the most frequently, in more than 50% of cases. Otherwise, the spectrum of bacteria is similar to that for a dog (see sec. **A.1**).
      b. Cat-scratch disease can follow a bite or scratch (see Chap. 17).
    2. **Antibiotic therapy.** Although trivial wounds probably do not merit therapy, because of the potential deep inoculation of bacteria and subsequent infection,

it seems **prudent to use antibiotics for 3–5 days for most cat bites,** following the same principles as for dog bites. Full therapeutic courses of antibiotics are used for infected wounds.

3. Tetanus, rabies, and surgical approach are as outlined in sec. **A.3–5.**

C. **Human bites** generally are **very serious and more prone to infection** and complications than animal bites. In the preantibiotic era, up to 20% of human-bite victims required amputation of the infected body part. Even now, amputation of an infectious complication is not uncommon [9].

   1. **Occlusional bites** (i.e., a wound sustained when human teeth bite part of the human anatomy)
      a. **Bacteriology.** *S. aureus, E. corrodens, H. influenzae,* and beta-lactamase producing oral anaerobes are potential pathogens.
      b. **Antibiotics.** Most clinicians administer 3–5 days of early-treatment (prophylactic) antibiotics in this setting.
         In the non-penicillin-allergic patient, amoxicillin-clavulanate is suggested. In the allergic patient (see sec. **A.2.b**), options can be based on flora and the data in Table 4-1.
   2. **Clenched-fist injuries** are the **most serious** and are sustained to the metacarpophalangeal joint (knuckle) of the dominant hand when the fist of one person strikes the teeth of another [9]. **Because these wounds often are complicated by deep-space infections, septic arthritis, and osteomyelitis, patients with these wound infections need hospitalization and attention by physicians experienced with hand surgery** [9]. Often the patient has an overt wound infection at the time of presentation, so prophylaxis is not the key issue.
      a. **Bacteriology. Anaerobic bacteria,** some of which produce beta-lactamase, occur in the majority of wounds. *E. corrodens* is detected in 25% of cultures.
      b. For parenteral therapy, ampicillin-sulbactam is an appealing single agent and, for oral therapy, amoxicillin-clavulanate can be used. See Table 4-1 for options to consider in the allergic patient. See also sec. **1.b.**
      c. If an injury is seen within hours of its occurrence, prophylactic antibiotics are advised for 3–5 days.

D. **Exotic animal bites.** Few data are available on the bacteriology of wounds from bites of exotic animals. Monkey bites seem more serious and prone to infection [9]. Infectious disease consultation is advised.

II. **Miscellaneous** [9]
   A. **Cultures** for aerobic and anaerobic bacteria should be obtained from any **infected bite wound** and initially from moderate to serious bite wounds inflicted by an animal other than a cat or dog.
   B. **Irrigation** of wounds with normal saline and **debridement** of devitalized tissue and any foreign material is recommended. Wound closure must be individualized. If a fracture is suspected, a roentgenogram is indicated. Elevation of the extremity that is wounded is useful.
   C. **Rabies** and **tetanus** immunization need assessment.
   D. **Patients with antibiotic allergies** may be difficult to treat with monotherapy. See possible options in Table 4-1. Tetracycline is contraindicated in pregnant women and in children younger than 8 years. If erythromycin is used, the clinical response of the patient needs to be carefully monitored [9].
   E. *C. canimorsus* (formerly DF-2) is an unusual gram-negative bacillus that has been identified as a cause of fulminant sepsis from infected dog-bite wounds [10]. Splenectomized individuals are at particularly high risk for septic shock and disseminated intravascular coagulopathy due to this pathogen. See Table 4-1 for susceptibility data.

III. **Rabies prophylaxis.** Rabies in humans has decreased from an average of 22 cases per year in 1946–1950 to 0–5 cases per year since 1960 [11–13]. However, an **enzootic rabies epidemic,** especially in raccoons, is currently occurring in the mid-Atlantic states, New York, and New England. As a result, more animal cases of rabies are being reported to the Centers for Disease Control (CDC) than at any time in the past 40 years. This development heightens the importance of an understanding of the epidemiology of rabies and correct postexposure treatment [11, 12].
   A. **Considerations prior to antirabies therapy.** Rabies prophylaxis cannot be instituted after every animal bite. The decision to begin prophylaxis must be based on the following considerations:
      1. **Species of biting animal.** Carnivorous animals (especially skunks, foxes, coyotes, raccoons, dogs, and cats) and bats are more likely to be rabid than rodents (which never have produced a case of human rabies in the United States).

Table 4-1. Antimicrobial susceptibilities of bacteria frequently isolated from animal-bite wounds

Agent	Percentages of isolates susceptible					
	S. aureus	E. corrodens	Anaerobes	P. multocida	C. canimorsus	S. intermedius
Penicillin	10	99	50/95*	95	95	70
Dicloxacillin	99	5	50	30	NS	100
Amoxicillin-clavulanate	100	100	100	100	95	100
Cephalexin	100	20	40	30	NS	95
Cefuroxime	100	70	40	90	NS	NS
Cefoxitin	100	95	100	95	95	NS
Erythromycin	100	20	40	20	95	95
Tetracycline	95	85	60	90	95	NS
TMP-SMZ	100	95	0	95	V	NS
Quinolones	100	100	40	95	NS	NS
Clindamycin	95	0	100	0	95	95

TMP-SMZ = trimethoprim-sulfamethoxazole; NS = not studied; V = variable.
*Percentage of human-bite isolates/percentage of animal-bite isolates.
Note: Data are compiled from various studies.
Source: E. J. C. Goldstein, Bite wounds and infection. *Clin. Infect. Dis.* 14:633, 1992. Published by University of Chicago Press.

2. **Circumstances of biting incident.** An unprovoked attack (not related to attempts to handle or feed an apparently healthy animal) increases the likelihood that the animal is rabid.
3. **Type of exposure.** The chance of inoculation with infectious saliva is greatest by bite; however, scratches, abrasions, open wounds, mucous membranes, or cornea contaminated by saliva should be considered potentially infected.
4. **Vaccination status of biting animal.** Properly immunized animals have only a minimal chance of acquiring rabies and transmitting the virus, and if the animal has a documented record of rabies immunization, prophylaxis is not warranted for a provoked attack. Therefore, this information should be obtained as soon as possible when domestic animal bites are involved.
5. **Presence of rabies in the region.** The species of animal most likely to be infected with rabies varies from region to region. Local and state health officials should be consulted for current interpretations of the risk of rabies in the various animal species of their region.

B. **Recommendations for management of potential rabies exposure.** Management of a potential rabies exposure necessitates immediate action. The following recommendations may be modified according to knowledge of the five factors involved in the biting incident. Recommendations for management of potential rabies exposure [11] are as follows:
1. **The suspected animal should be caught.** A healthy pet should be observed by a veterinarian for 10 days, and ill pets or wild animals should be sacrificed. (The healthy-appearing pet can be sacrificed for an immediate answer.) The skull should be left intact, and the head should be transported, on ice, to the nearest regional rabies laboratory for immediate immunofluorescent staining of the brain for rabies antigen, which will provide an answer within several hours.
2. **Cleansing of the wound.** See sec. I.
3. **Tetanus prophylaxis** and measures to control infection should be used as indicated as discussed at the end of this chapter.
4. **Postexposure prophylaxis.** A combination of passive and active immunization (vaccine and immunoglobulin) is recommended.
   a. **Passive immunity** is provided by **human rabies immunoglobulin (RIG)** which is administered only once, at the beginning of antirabies therapy. The recommended dose is 20 IU/kg, half of which should be infiltrated around the wound and the other half given intramuscularly in the buttocks. (The CDC does not provide RIG, which is manufactured by Bayer Corporation, which has a 24-hour emergency telephone through which RIG can be ordered: (800) 288-8370.
   b. **Active immunization.** Currently, two formulations of inactivated rabies vaccine are available for human use in the United States.
      (1) **Human diploid cell rabies vaccine (HDCV)** is an inactivated virus vaccine prepared from fixed rabies virus grown in human diploid embryo cell tissue culture. HDCV should be given in conjunction with RIG. Five 1-ml doses of HDCV should be given intramuscularly in the deltoid muscles. The first dose should be given as soon as possible after the exposure; an additional dose should be given on days 3, 7, 14, and 28 after the first dose. Routine serologic testing of normal hosts receiving recommended regimens is no longer believed to be necessary [11]. For known or highly suspect immunocompromised patients, follow-up serologic studies are important to assure protective antibody levels. Table 4-2 can be used as a postexposure antirabies treatment guide [11].
      Reactions to HDCV were initially considered to be uncommon, but systemic allergic reactions ranging from hives to anaphylaxis have been increasingly reported, especially following 2-year booster doses of HDCV given to individuals at risk for continued rabies exposure. Until this reaction problem can be resolved, **HDCV use for routine 2-year booster immunizations must be carefully assessed on an individual basis and should not be used indiscriminately.**
      (2) **Rabies vaccine adsorbed (RVA)** is a relatively new vaccine produced by the Michigan Department of Health (telephone 517-335-8119). The virus is grown in fetal rhesus monkey lung cells and adsorbed on aluminum phosphate. RVA should be given in conjunction with RIG. Five 1.0-ml doses are given intramuscularly in the deltoid muscle on days

Table 4-2. Guidelines for rabies prophylaxis[a]

Species of animal	Condition of animal at time of attack	Treatment of exposed person
Domestic: dog, cat	Healthy and available for 10 days of observation	None, unless animal develops rabies[b]
	Rabid or suspected rabid	RIG and HDCV or RVA
	Unknown (escaped)	Consult public health officials; if treatment is indicated, give RIG and HDCV or RVA
Wild: skunk, bat, fox, coyote, raccoon, bobcat, and other carnivores	Regard as rabid unless proved negative by laboratory tests[c]	RIG and HDCV or RVA
Other: livestock, rodents, rabbits, and hares	Consider individually; local and state public health officials should be consulted; bites of squirrels, hamsters, guinea pigs, gerbils, chipmunks, rats, mice, other rodents, rabbits, and hares almost never require antirabies prophylaxis	

RIG = rabies immunoglobulin; HDCV = human diploid cell rabies vaccine; RVA = rabies vaccine adsorbed.

[a]These recommendations are only a guide. They should be applied in conjunction with knowledge of the animal species involved, circumstances of the bite or other exposure, vaccination status of the animal, and the presence of rabies in the region. If antirabies treatment is indicated, both RIG and vaccine should be given as soon as possible, regardless of the interval since exposure.
[b]Begin treatment with RIG plus vaccine at first sign of rabies in biting dog or cat during 10-day holding period. The symptomatic animal should be killed and tested immediately.
[c]The animal should be killed and tested as soon as possible. Holding for observation is not recommended. Discontinue vaccine if fluorescent antibody tests of the killed animal are negative.
Source: From Centers for Disease Control, Rabies prevention: United States, 1991. *M.M.W.R.* 40 (RR-3):1–19, 1991.

0, 3, 7, 14, and 28. Serum sickness–like reactions may be less common with RVA, but direct comparisons with HDCV are lacking.

   (3) Additional information on postexposure prophylaxis can be obtained from state health departments.

  5. Preexposure prophylaxis is indicated for the following high-risk groups: veterinarians, animal control officers, wildlife workers, spelunkers, workers in a rabies virus laboratory, and travelers to foreign countries (for $\geq$ 1 month) where canine rabies is endemic [11]. Either HDCV or RVA can be used for preexposure prophylaxis, as follows:

   a. HDCV or RVA, 1.0 ml IM (deltoid area), can be administered in three doses on days 0, 7, and 21 or 28.

   b. HDCV, 0.1 ml, can be administered *intradermally* (skin over deltoid area) in three doses on days 0, 7, and 21 or 28. RVA should not be given by the intradermal route.

   c. Chloroquine phosphate (for malaria chemoprophylaxis) interferes with the antibody response to HDCV, and so HDCV should not be administered by the intradermal route to persons receiving chloroquine.

   d. A postvaccination rabies antibody titer should be checked every 2 years in high-risk groups, and an intramuscular or intradermal booster dose of vaccine should be administered if the titer is less than complete neutralization at a 1:5 serum dilution. Alternatively, a booster can be administered every 2 years without checking the antibody titer.

   e. Preexposure prophylaxis does not eliminate the need for prophylaxis after a rabies exposure. RIG is not necessary, but two intramuscular doses (1.0 ml each) of either HDCV or RVA should be administered, one immediately and one 3 days later.

Mucocutaneous Vesicles

The patient who presents with an acute eruption of mucosal or cutaneous vesicles often poses a difficult differential diagnostic problem for the physician. Several viral diseases are manifested by a mucosal or cutaneous vesicle eruption. The differential clinical characteristics can be subtle, and the laboratory evaluation often does not yield an immediate diagnosis. A description of the common mucocutaneous vesicular diseases is presented here and is followed by a logical scheme for the initial evaluation of mucocutaneous vesicles.

I. **Herpes simplex.** Herpes simplex virus (HSV) is a DNA virus that causes several types of clinical syndromes. HSV genital infections are discussed in Chap. 13 under Genital Lesions.

   A. **HSV acute gingivostomatitis.** The majority of initial HSV infections are subclinical, but acute gingivostomatitis can occur.

      1. **Clinical presentation.** This syndrome is characterized by a vesicular eruption of the buccal mucosa, pharynx, and tongue, accompanied by pain, fever, and malaise.

      2. **Differential diagnosis.** Differentiation from hand-foot-and-mouth disease, herpangina, and the pharyngeal vesicles caused by other enteroviruses (coxsackieviruses B1–B5, A7, and A9, and echoviruses 9 and 16) can be made by noting that **only HSV produces vesicles on the buccal mucosa, lips, gums, and tongue. Vesicular eruptions due to the enteroviruses are usually confined to the posterior mouth.** Also, the vesicles of HSV contain large syncytial cells, with many nuclei containing intranuclear inclusion bodies visible with Giemsa staining. Enterovirus vesicles do not contain multinucleate giant cells. HSV can be isolated from the mouth vesicles in the earlier stages, and a rise in HSV-specific antibody titer will occur in response to primary gingivostomatitis.

      3. **Therapy** (see related discussion in Chap. 26)

         a. **In the normal host,** topical acyclovir is of no clinical benefit. Oral (or parenteral) acyclovir reduces the duration of symptoms and viral shedding in primary herpetic gingivostomatitis and is a reasonable treatment option. In adults, acyclovir, 200 mg PO five times daily, can be given.

         b. The **immunocompromised host** is at risk for developing potentially severe disseminated HSV infection. In the compromised host with acute (or recurrent) necrotizing mucocutaneous HSV infection, intravenous [14] and oral acyclovir [15] have been used effectively to decrease viral shedding, accelerate lesion healing, and decrease pain. Parenteral acyclovir should not be given to every immunocompromised patient with mucocutaneous HSV but should be reserved for those at highest risk whose lesions do not heal rapidly. Topical acyclovir is never indicated. Therapy with acyclovir is discussed in detail in Chap. 26 and has recently been reviewed [16].

   B. **Recurrent herpes simplex.** The manifestation, commonly known as **cold sores** or fever blisters, occurs in those who have previously been infected and who possess circulating antibody to HSV. Small crops of thin-walled vesicles on an erythematous base occur most often on the mucocutaneous junction of the lips, but they may occur elsewhere on the face. In contrast to primary gingivoglossitis, recurrent lesions rarely occur inside the mouth unless the patient is immunocompromised. Eruptions also may occur elsewhere on the skin and may follow a zosteriform distribution. The virus can be isolated from these lesions. Multinucleate giant cells with acidophilic intranuclear inclusion bodies can be detected on Giemsa staining or with Tzanck preparation. However, in contrast to primary infection, a diagnostic rise in HSV-specific antibody titer may not occur.

   Oral acyclovir at a dose of 200–400 mg five times daily provides a slight clinical benefit if initiated early enough [15, 16], but this is not recommended routinely. Local application of acyclovir is not recommended either, for it is not effective in this setting and it may serve to select out resistant strains.

   For immunocompetent adults with frequent recurrences of herpes labialis (i.e., six or more episodes annually), one recent study suggests that oral acyclovir (400 mg bid) is effective in suppressing recurrences [17].

C. Other skin manifestations. HSV infection occasionally can manifest itself as a local or generalized cutaneous eruption with a close resemblance to varicella, variola, coxsackieviruses A9, A16, and B3, and herpes zoster.

II. **Varicella (chickenpox) and herpes zoster (shingles).** Varicella and herpes zoster are caused by the **same virus, varicella-zoster virus (VZV).** Varicella is a manifestation of disease in a nonimmune individual, and zoster represents recrudescence of latent infection in a partially immune host.

A. Varicella begins as discrete, erythematous, maculopapular lesions that rapidly become vesicular and then pustular, followed by a crusting stage. The rash is typically of a centripetal distribution, primarily involving the thorax and proximal extremities. Mucous membrane involvement closely resembling herpes simplex may occur.

1. **Transmission.** Patients with an uncomplicated clinical course may transmit varicella to susceptible individuals from 1 day before onset of skin lesions until 5 days after onset of the lesions. Patients with a prolonged clinical course and recurring skin lesions can shed virus for an indeterminate period of time.

2. **Immunity.** Individuals usually are considered immune to varicella infection if one or more of the following is present:
   a. History of chickenpox or shingles at some time in the past.
   b. Positive serum titer for varicella antibody.
   c. Cared for a child with chickenpox or resided in the same house with a case sometime in the past.

3. **Differential diagnosis.** Varicella may resemble variola (smallpox), impetigo, coxsackievirus and echovirus eruptions, and cutaneous herpes simplex. The latter can usually be differentiated on the basis of setting and other clinical characteristics. The remainder can be ruled out by the absence of multinucleate giant cells in vesicle scrapings (Tzanck preparation; see Chap. 25) and viral isolation studies.

4. **Therapy with acyclovir**
   a. **Therapy for any adult** with varicella should be considered because the disease often is more severe in adults than in children. Oral acyclovir at a dose of 800 mg five times daily for 7 days reduces the duration of the illness if started within 24 hours of onset of the eruption [18]. Longer duration or addition of steroids is of no obvious value.
   b. **For normal children,** oral acyclovir at a dose of 20 mg/kg of body weight (not to exceed 800 mg) given four times daily for 5 days reduces the duration and severity of varicella, but routine use in children is not recommended [19]. Parenteral acyclovir at a dose of 500 mg/m^2 IV q8h for 7 days has proved beneficial for varicella infection in immunocompromised children [20]. Infectious disease consultation is advised (see also Chap. 26).
   c. **For a detailed discussion of the use of acyclovir, see Chap. 26.**

5. **Vaccine.** The new varicella vaccine [21] is discussed in Chap. 22.

B. Herpes zoster. Herpes zoster results from reactivation of latent VZV in dorsal root ganglia. The characteristic dermatomic distribution of vesicles usually should prevent diagnostic confusion. However, HSV rarely can cause a similar segmental distribution, and herpes zoster can disseminate beyond the initial dermatome to resemble varicella closely. The vesicle of HSV, varicella, and zoster are histologically identical, and all possess multinucleate giant cells with intranuclear inclusions. Differentiation will depend primarily on clinical characteristics, testing of vesicular fluid for virus, or detection of viral antigen.

1. **Transmission.** Herpes zoster is less communicable than varicella, but contact with a patient with herpes zoster can result in varicella in approximately 15% of susceptible individuals.

2. **Treatment**
   a. **Segmental herpes zoster**
      (1) **Analgesia.** Prescription analgesics such as oxycodone or other codeine derivatives may be necessary to control the pain of acute herpes zoster.
      (2) **Corticosteroids are not recommended.** A recently completed study in immunocompetent adults with segmental herpes zoster showed that the addition of prednisolone to oral acyclovir therapy did not diminish postherpetic neuralgia [22]. Although steroids reduced the intensity of acute pain, the authors conclude that use of oral corticosteroids is not recommended in this setting [22].

(3) Acyclovir is discussed in detail in Chap. 26.

(a) Normal hosts. Both parenteral and oral acyclovir have been effective in reducing pain and enhancing the healing of localized herpes zoster in normal hosts, **but most healthy patients should not be treated, especially if lesions have been present for more than 72 hours and are limited to one dermatome** [23]. **Acyclovir should be considered for healthy patients if** cutaneous dissemination is present (i.e., more than 15 lesions outside the primary and adjacent dermatomes) or if the patient is older than 60 years and has underlying disease or if pain is very severe at onset. Some experts would treat those patients with ophthalmic VZV.

Oral acyclovir at a dose of 600–800 mg PO five times daily for 7–10 days enhances healing if started within 72 hours of the appearance of lesions [24]. **Intravenous acyclovir** at a dose of 5 mg/kg q8h for 5 days enhances relief of pain and accelerates healing [25]. None of the acyclovir regimens has been shown to reduce the severity of postherpetic neuralgia. The management of shingles has recently been reviewed [27].

The new antiviral agents famciclovir and valacyclovir are discussed in Chap. 26 (pp. 977–980). These agents may offer modest advantages in the immunocompetent host.

(b) Immunocompromised host. At present, most authorities recommend use of **intravenous acyclovir as soon as possible** for localized herpes zoster in the immunocompromised patient.

b. Disseminated herpes zoster. Herpes zoster may disseminate, particularly in the immunocompromised patient. Acyclovir at a dose of 500 mg/m² IV q8h for 7 days can halt the progression of disease, reduce the period of viral shedding, and prevent visceral dissemination, especially if started within 72 hours of onset of disease [28]. Infectious disease consultation is advisable.

3. Prophylaxis is discussed in sec. **V.**

III. Other viruses commonly causing vesicles

A. Hand-foot-and-mouth disease is caused by coxsackieviruses A16, A10, A5, B2, and B5. Anywhere from a few lesions to 100 lesions distribute characteristically on the margins of the palms and soles, on the dorsa of the hands and feet, and on the **posterior oropharynx.** The lesions begin as erythematous macules or papules, in the center of which arises an oval vesicle that rapidly ulcerates. The entire disease usually lasts only 7–10 days. Differential diagnosis includes herpes simplex and cutaneous eruptions of other enteroviruses. Herpes simplex vesicle scrapings contain multinucleate giant cells. Differentiation of hand-foot-and-mouth disease from other enteroviral diseases will depend on virus isolation from vesicle fluid and throat and stool cultures or diagnostic rises in antibody titers.

B. Herpangina can be caused by any one of six different group A coxsackievirus types (A2, A4, A5, A6, A8, or A10). The gray-white papulovesicular lesions are indistinguishable from those of herpes simplex but usually are confined to the **anterior pillars of the tonsillar fauces, soft palate, uvula, and tonsils.** Gingivitis, however, is a common manifestation of herpes simplex and not of the group A coxsackieviruses. There is rapid ulceration, and the entire course lasts only 4–6 days. The differential diagnosis includes herpes simplex gingivostomatitis and oropharyngeal lesions due to other enteroviruses. In contrast to herpangina, HSV causes lesions on the buccal mucosa, tongue, lips, and gums, with cervical adenopathy and hemorrhage of gums. Culture of the lesions, throat, and stool, along with acute and convalescent antibody titers, is the only way to distinguish herpangina from other enteroviral pharyngeal eruptions. There is no specific treatment.

C. Several **other enteroviruses** have a propensity to cause cutaneous or oropharyngeal vesicular eruptions. These include coxsackieviruses A7, A9, and B1–B5, and echoviruses 9, 16, and 19. The nature of the eruption cannot be used to determine the specific viral etiology. The rash resembles that caused by rubella; the lesions usually are maculopapular, discrete, and nonpruritic. The rash may be associated with aseptic meningitis and is more prevalent in the summer and fall. Differentiation may be based on culture of vesicular fluid, throat, stool, and cerebrospinal fluid (if meningitis is present), and on serologic studies.

D. **Other causes of oral ulcerations and vesicles** include aphthous ulcers which, if very severe, should suggest Behçet's syndrome. Stevens-Johnson syndrome occurs in association with an allergic reaction. Squamous cell carcinoma and lichen planus are to be considered. Hyperplastic or pseudomembranous candidiasis and pemphigoid are other lesions for which biopsy or fungal or viral culture may be required for differentiation.

E. **Ecthyma contagiosum (Orf)** is an uncommon condition resulting from cutaneous inoculation of a poxvirus harbored in sheep and goats. The characteristic lesion resembles the lesion following vaccination with vaccinia, presenting first as a small bulla with depressed central area, which evolves into a pustular lesion that then crusts. It occurs on the hands and arms and usually is benign and self-limited. Diagnosis can be made by skin biopsy. Once the lesion is recognized, unwarranted surgery can be avoided [29].

IV. **Evaluation of mucocutaneous vesicles.** A logical scheme for the initial evaluation of mucocutaneous vesicular eruptions can be summarized as follows:

A. **Clinical characteristics.** The distribution of the lesions is often an important clue to viral etiology, and the following characteristics should be noted (see preceding discussion):

1. Centripetal or segmental, or generalized cutaneous involvement.
2. Mucosal involvement (limited to posterior mouth) or the buccal mucosa, tongue, gums, and lips.

B. **Laboratory evaluation** can be a valuable adjunct to diagnosis. The proper virologic facilities may not always be available, however, and the following laboratory studies apply to the ideal situation or unusual case.

1. Collect vesicle fluid (if available) for viral isolation using sterile technique. Place the fluid in a viral holding or transport medium containing serum, and refrigerate unfrozen until tissue culture inoculation can be performed. If more than 24 hours is to elapse before it can be cultured, the specimen should be refrigerated and placed on ice during transportation to the laboratory.
2. Culture throat and stool for virus (see Chap. 25) if an enterovirus is suspected.
3. Obtain a serum sample as soon as possible (acute-phase). Separate RBCs from the serum, and store the serum at $-20°C$ until used.
4. Examine the vesicle for multinucleate giant cells. Rupture the vesicle, gently blot the fluid away, and scrape its base with a sterile knife to remove cells. Then smear cells on a slide, fix in methanol, and stain with Giemsa. The vesicular fluid may contain infectious viral particles and should be handled carefully.

V. **Prophylaxis**

A. **Varicella-zoster immunoglobulin (VZIG)** is currently licensed for passive immunization of susceptible immunodeficient patients exposed to VZV. VZIG is prepared from plasma obtained from healthy volunteer blood donors. It replaces an earlier product, ZIG, which had usually been in short supply because of the limited availability of the source material, zoster convalescent plasma. ZIG has been demonstrated to be effective for immunosuppressed patients exposed to varicella (chickenpox) or zoster and had previously been available for prophylaxis of varicella in immunosuppressed children. VZIG has now been shown to be as effective as ZIG in reducing the severity of varicella in immunodeficient children.

B. **Current recommendations for use of VZIG.** VZIG passive immunization is intended primarily to prevent the development of disseminated varicella in susceptible immunodeficient hosts exposed to VZV and to prevent postnatal chickenpox following intrauterine exposure. However, supplies of VZIG have now become plentiful enough to broaden the potential indications for VZIG to include individuals of any age, normal adults, pregnant women, and premature and full-term infants. Criteria for administration of VZIG are summarized as follows:

1. Negative or unknown prior varicella-zoster disease history.
2. One of the following **types of exposure** to varicella or zoster:
   a. Continuous household contact.
   b. Playmate contact (more than 1 hour of play indoors).
   c. Hospital contact (in same bedroom or adjacent beds in a large ward or prolonged face-to-face contact with an infectious staff member or patient).
   d. Newborn contact (newborn whose mother contracted chickenpox fewer than 5 days before delivery or within 48 hours after delivery).
3. **Age** of less than 15 years, with administration to immunocompromised adolescents and adults and to other older patients on an individual basis.

4. One of the following **underlying illnesses or conditions:**
   a. Leukemia or lymphoma.
   b. Congenital or acquired immunodeficiency.
   c. Immunosuppressive treatment.
   d. Newborn of mother who had onset of chickenpox within 5 days before delivery or within 48 hours after delivery.
   e. Premature infant (≥28 weeks' gestation) whose mother lacks a prior history of chickenpox.
   f. Premature infant (<28 weeks' gestation or ≤1,000 g of weight) regardless of maternal history.
   g. Pregnant women.
5. Time elapsed after exposure is such that **VZIG can be administered within 96 hours of exposure** but preferably sooner. VZIG should not be used if clinical infection has already become established, as evidenced by the onset of maculopapular or vesicular skin lesions.

C. **VZIG administration and cost.** VZIG is given by deep intramuscular injection. **It should never be administered intravenously.** Doses are based on body weight. Children weighing up to 10 kg are given 125 units (one vial). For children who weigh more than 10 kg, some experts recommend 125 units per 10 kg of body weight, to a maximum of 625 units (five vials) for children weighing more than 40 kg. The dose for adults is unknown, but five vials (625 units) is often recommended. Higher doses may be needed in immunocompromised adults.

VZIG is distributed in the United States by the American Red Cross Blood Services, Northeast Region (ARCBS-NE) through various regional blood centers. All requests for VZIG should be addressed to the nearest American Red Cross Blood Services Center.

D. **Varicella vaccine.** This live attenuated vaccine was licensed by the Food and Drug Administration in March 1995 [21] and is reviewed in Chap. 22.

Cellulitis and Related Skin Infections

Cellulitis is a superficial, spreading, warm, erythematous inflammation of the skin. There are several different types of cellulitis caused by a variety of pathogenic bacteria [30]. In the clinical approach to a given patient, it is important to try to separate out cellulitis (superficial infection) from those deeper infections (of subcutaneous fat and fascia and/or muscle) which are discussed in the next section under Necrotizing Soft-Tissue Infections. Furthermore, **sometimes a superficial cellulitis may be complicated by an extension of the infection into the contiguous soft tissue** (e.g., an invasive streptococcal A infection) so that early in the clinical presentation, it may be hard to separate these entities (superficial vs. deep); serial clinical assessment is therefore very important.

I. **Nonperineal cellulitis and related skin infections**
   A. **Diabetic foot infections** are discussed separately in Chap. 16.
   B. **Erysipelas.** This is manifested as a warm, shiny, red, edematous, and indurated lesion that begins as a small area of redness and spreads in the direction of the lymphatic flow. Classically, the advancing **elevated margin is sharply demarcated** from the surrounding skin and is easily palpable. **Group A beta-hemolytic streptococcus (occasionally group G) is almost always the cause of this syndrome.** It gains access via a small break in the skin and spreads rapidly. It is most common on the face but occurs on the extremities. When on the face, it can spread across the bridge of the nose and form a butterfly rash. Bullae may form, and serous fluid may be seen oozing from the raw surface. *S. aureus* rarely produces this appearance.
   C. **Cellulitis due to *S. aureus* with or without beta-hemolytic streptococcus.** When *S. aureus* and beta-hemolytic streptococci occur in conjunction, cellulitis can spread rapidly, be warm and tender, and be associated with significant systemic toxicity. **Because the clinical distinction** between erysipelas (see sec. **B**) due to group A streptococci and *S. aureus* cellulitis or mixed streptococcal and *S. aureus* cellulitis **is difficult, antibiotic treatment needs to be directed at both *S. aureus* and group A streptococcus.**

D. **Invasive group A streptococcal infections** have been reported with increased frequency since the mid-1980s [31–34]. Because some of these patients may initially start with what appears to be a severe but uncomplicated cellulitis (which then evolves into a more serious soft-tissue infection), we are including the discussion of this entity under cellulitis. For additional discussion, see under Necrotizing Soft-Tissue Infections.

1. **Streptococcal toxic shock syndrome (STSS)** is reviewed in detail in Chap. 2.
2. **Soft-tissue infections** are often the primary focus of infection in STSS [33]. In addition, severe soft-tissue infection, including myositis or fasciitis, can occur without the complete syndrome of STSS. **Clinical clues to severe invasive streptococcal infections include** the following:
   a. **Pain** at the site of soft-tissue infection, sometimes in severity out of proportion with the minor objective physical findings, sometimes abrupt in onset, and frequently necessitating the use of parenteral narcotic analgesics has been reported [33].
   b. Erythema, edema, and bullae can occur.
   c. **Immature granulocytes** (i.e., shift to the left), **lymphopenia,** hypoalbuminemia, and hypocalcemia may be clues to the diagnosis [33]. Bacteremia is not uncommon.
3. Therapy of soft-tissue infections includes surgical debridement of infected tissues and antibiotics. (See sec. **IV.B.1.**)
4. **Group A streptococcal necrotizing fasciitis** has been **reported in children following varicella infection** [35]. (See related discussion under Necrotizing Soft-Tissue Infections.)

E. **Group B streptococci** (*S. agalactiae*) can cause cellulitis and/or soft-tissue infections, especially in the elderly, those with diabetes and underlying malignancy, and those infected with human immunodeficiency virus (HIV) [36].

F. **Erysipeloid** cellulitis is caused by a slender, gram-positive rod, *Erysipelothrix rhusiopathiae,* and is to be distinguished from erysipelas. The infection usually occurs on the finger or hand, is violet or purple-red in color, and is warm and tender, with well-defined margins. It is limited almost exclusively to fishermen, butchers, and those handling raw fish or poultry.

G. *H. influenzae* **cellulitis** usually occurs in children.

1. **In children,** this bacterium can produce typical **blue-red to purple-red cellulitis.** Most of these children will have high fever and septicemia. The condition occurs most commonly on the face, less on the arms, and rarely elsewhere. The margins are indistinct, and this differentiates it from erysipelas; the blue-red or purple-red color distinguishes it from streptococcal and staphylococcal cellulitis. *H. influenzae* cellulitis is not exclusively a disease of children.
2. **In adults,** *H. influenzae* **type b rarely has caused** cellulitis of the neck and upper chest associated with *H. influenzae* type b respiratory tract infection and sepsis [37]. The characteristic purple-blue skin color may not be present. In any adult with cellulitis of the neck or upper chest associated with upper airway disease, *H. influenzae* should be considered in the differential diagnosis.

H. *P. aeruginosa* **cellulitis.** Various dermatologic manifestations of *P. aeruginosa* sepsis have been reported, including ecthyma gangrenosum (see Plate III B and Chap. 2, sec. **II.B** under Sepsis of Unknown Etiology), nodules, abscesses, vesicles, and cellulitis. In the immunocompromised host, *P. aeruginosa* sepsis has been associated with an erysipelaslike lesion on the extremities of the patient [38]. Therefore, systemic infection with *P. aeruginosa* should be considered in the differential diagnosis of any cellulitis or erysipelaslike lesion in the immunocompromised host. Until definitive culture results are available, empiric antibiotic therapy should probably include a broad-spectrum penicillin (ticarcillin, piperacillin, or mezlocillin) and tobramycin.

I. **Stasis dermatitis (stasis eczema, varicose eczema) of the calves may be confused with bacterial cellulitis** but should be suspected if the onset of distal lower-extremity erythema is **associated with** chronic peripheral **edema and** especially if the process **is bilateral.** Stasis dermatitis is a noninfectious eczemoid eruption of the lower legs secondary to venous hypertension [39]; a superimposed bacterial infection (e.g., with *S. aureus*) may occur. Dermatologic consultation may be useful.

1. **Differentiation** of stasis dermatitis from cellulitis may be assisted by the following features [39]:
   a. **Eczematous lesions** of the lower leg may be present without foot involve-

ment. Over time (days), weeping of skin areas may occur. Pruritus may be present.
   b. A "woody" sensation of the skin may result from recurrent and chronic disease.
   c. Ulcers, especially of the malleolus, may be present.
2. **Treatment** consists of the following:
   a. Elevation of the legs while sitting.
   b. Support stockings and compressive bandages.
   c. Diuretics if congestive heart failure with edema is present.
   d. Topical steroids of intermediate potency.
   e. Plain petrolatum for chronic maintenance.
   f. Antibiotics for any secondary cellulitis or infection.
3. If the process is acute and unilateral, the possibility of a deep venous thrombosis may need to be considered and excluded.
J. Saltwater-related wounds. Patients with underlying lacerations, puncture wounds, bites, fishing injuries, and the like who have contact with seawater may develop a wound infection due to *Vibrio vulnificus.* This has been reviewed [40] and can cause a **wide spectrum of wound infections,** including mild to severe cellulitis, vesicles and bullae, and myositis (i.e., a necrotizing soft-tissue infection). (Infections can mimic gas gangrene in their rapid progression and destructiveness.) Septicemia may occur, and infections may be fatal in immunocompromised hosts. (See Chap. 2 for further discussion.) Optimal antibiotic therapy is still under investigation, although in vitro organisms are susceptible to tetracycline and gentamicin. See related discussion under Necrotizing Soft-Tissue Infections.
K. Pyomyositis (bacterial myositis) is actually an infection of muscle but, at the time of presentation, the clinician may confuse this entity with an atypical cellulitis. Therefore, this topic is briefly discussed here and is reviewed elsewhere [41].
   1. The **usual pathogen** is *S. aureus.* This is a common problem in tropical countries (tropical pyomyositis). **Although previously considered rare in the United States and other temperate climates, pyomyositis is being reported with increasing frequency. Poorly controlled diabetes** mellitus appears to be an important **risk factor** [41].
   2. Presumably this problem is secondary to a transient bacteremia. Approximately 5–25% of patients will have positive blood cultures [41].
   3. **Clinical presentation.** The characteristic clinical scenario is a young person who first develops muscle pain followed by fever and a muscle that becomes swollen and indurated ("woody"). Fluctuance develops later, but obvious signs of inflammation may not be evident owing to the deep location of the infection. Multiple sites can be involved. Muscle enzyme studies (creatine phosphokinase [CPK] levels) are normal. In difficult cases, needle aspiration (with culture and Gram stain) and MRI scanning will help confirm the diagnosis. See related discussion under Necrotizing Soft-Tissue Infections.
   4. **Treatment** consists of drainage of the abscess and an antistaphylococcal antibiotic administered intravenously.
L. Familial Mediterranean fever (FMF) skin lesions. Erysipelas-like lesions can be seen in 10–45% of patients who have attacks of FMF, and these lesions may be the only manifestations, other than fever, of an FMF attack. The periodicity of the attacks and the lack of clinical response to antibiotics should raise consideration of this diagnosis [42].
II. Perineal cellulitis (i.e., perirectal or perivulvar area). When the perineal area is involved with a cellulitis and/or deep-tissue infection, the possibility that mixed aerobic-anaerobic bacteria are causing the problem increases.
   Enterobacteriaceae, accompanied by anaerobes, plays the paramount role in perineal cellulitis. Diabetes and obesity are very important predisposing factors. Whenever cellulitis occurs in this anatomic area, a mixed anaerobic and gram-negative (*E. coli, P. mirabilis, Klebsiella* spp.) infection is likely, spread is rapid and aggressive, and antibiotic and surgical therapy in combination often is essential.
III. Diagnosis. Evaluation of a clinically diagnosed cellulitis may include the following:
   A. Culture for aerobes and anaerobes may be attempted by either needle aspiration or punch biopsy. The yield of leading-edge cultures is low as changes at the leading edge of the cellulitis are often toxin-induced. Therefore, no bacteria are isolated. A swab culture (for aerobes) of the primary lesion or wound (if present) is of greater value and advised [43].

Needle aspirate or punch biopsy has been advocated for the following four limited clinical situations [44–46], but positive cultures are obtained only in a small minority of samples:

1. Identification of infecting organisms is essential.
2. Unusual organisms are suspected.
3. Antibiotic treatment is failing.
4. Diabetes mellitus or malignancy are underlying illnesses.

B. **Gram staining of the aspirated material** can lead to a tentative diagnosis.
C. **Blood cultures** frequently are positive and are advised in the febrile patient.
D. Antistreptolysin O (ASO) titers, if elevated, may help support the diagnosis of streptococcal disease (see Chap. 25).
E. Counterimmunoelectrophoresis (CIE) of blood and urine may be helpful if the diagnosis of *H. influenzae* cellulitis is suspected (see Chap. 25).

IV. **Treatment**

A. **General principles.** Initial antibiotic therapy should be based on the clinical impression and Gram stain of aspirated material, if available.
B. **Specific guidelines** for antibiotic therapy (using adult dosages) of the various cellulitides are as follows. (See Chap. 28 for equivalent pediatric dosages.)

1. **Streptococcal or staphylococcal cellulitis.** Because it is difficult to differentiate between these two possibilities, **empiric therapy is directed against both organisms.**

   a. **Severe infection.** Although in the past the antistaphylococcal penicillin agents have been considered drugs of choice for this type of infection, with clinical experience and with results from animal models, **clindamycin is now preferred.** Not only are the organisms more effectively killed, but also toxin production is ablated by clindamycin [30].

      (1) **Clindamycin.** In adults, 600 mg IV q8h is advised. In children, 30–40 mg/kg/day, divided into q8h doses, is suggested. See details of clindamycin in Chap. 28I. The one uncertainty with this regimen is that a small number of staphylococci or group A streptococci are resistant to clindamycin.

      (2) **Other options** include nafcillin-oxacillin, 1½ g q4h IV in adults and, for those with delayed penicillin allergy, cefazolin, 1 g q8h. For adult patients with a history of anaphylaxis to penicillin (or cephalosporins), vancomycin 1 g q12h can be used if renal function is normal.

   b. **Mild infection** in adults. If infection is mild, oral therapy can be selected. Dicloxacillin, 500 mg q6h, or high doses of a first-generation cephalosporin (cephradine or cephalexin, 750 mg–1.0 g qid) or clindamycin, 450–600 mg q8h, are all reasonable choices. Because dicloxacillin may cause GI side effects, a first-generation cephalosporin is a practical approach. (The rationale for a large oral cephalosporin dose is given in Chap. 28F.)
   Pediatric doses are reviewed in Chaps. 28D and 28F.

   c. **Culture-proven pure group A streptococcal disease.** If the process has become well controlled, then narrowing to penicillin in the nonallergic patient is a reasonable choice. If the disease remains severe and the organism is sensitive to clindamycin, the latter is the drug of choice (*vida supra*).

2. ***H. influenzae* cellulitis**

   a. **Mild infections.** Amoxicillin-clavulanate (Augmentin) is suggested. In the ampicillin- or penicillin-allergic patient, cefaclor, cefuroxime axetil, and trimethoprim-sulfamethoxazole are alternative oral agents.

   b. **Severe infections** often are associated with bacteremias. Because of this and the possibility of an ampicillin-resistant *H. influenzae* bacteremia, the author prefers to use intravenous cefuroxime or ceftriaxone until susceptibility data are available. (For doses, see Chap. 28F.) If the *H. influenzae* is susceptible to ampicillin, this agent can then be used.

3. **For documented group B streptococci** (*S. agalactiae*), ampicillin, a first-generation cephalosporin (e.g., cefazolin), ceftriaxone, and vancomycin are all considered active agents. (See Chap. 28A.) The optimal choice will depend on the clinical situation and whether other pathogens are known or highly suspected of being involved.

4. **Perineal or other suspected mixed cellulitis.** Unless there is strong reason to believe that resistant organisms are present, a cephalosporin, with either metronidazole or clindamycin, is suggested. Piperacillin-tazobactam is an op-

tion for monotherapy. The aminoglycosides are not sufficiently active in the anaerobic milieu to be relied on. It is reasonable, in a severely ill patient or where cephalosporin resistance is strongly suspected, to supplement the previously cited antibiotic regimen with an aminoglycoside until culture or sensitivity results become available. Some experts will use imipenem-cilastatin in this setting, but others, recognizing the need for an additional specific anaerobic agent and desiring to save imipenem, will opt not to use this agent in this setting. (See related discussion of mixed aerobic and anaerobic wound infections in sec. **IV.A** under Necrotizing Soft-Tissue Infections.)

   5. Erysipeloid. Procaine penicillin, 1.2 million units IM q12h, is reasonable.

C. **Follow-up.** Therapy may need to be adjusted in view of later blood and skin culture results. Surgical consultation should be obtained for evaluation of any rapidly advancing, fulminant, synergistic infection. Seven to ten days of therapy will usually be required. If there is rapid clinical improvement in severe infections, the course of therapy may often be completed with oral agents.

V. **Miscellaneous skin infections**

A. *Pseudomonas* **folliculitis** ("hot-tub folliculitis") is an infection associated with recreational use of contaminated whirlpools, hot tubs and, rarely, swimming pools [47]. Although not a true cellulitis, it is discussed here for it is not an uncommon condition.

   1. Clinical aspects. The typical rash occurs 2–4 days after exposure. Affected patients develop superficial papules, pruritic pustules, or violaceous red nodules that have a characteristic distribution in areas of moisture or friction or body areas covered by the patient's bathing suit (buttocks, hips, axillae, and lateral aspects of the trunk). The palms, soles, and mucous membranes are spared. The typical distribution allows the clinician to distinguish it from scabies, insect bites, contact dermatitis, staphylococcal folliculitis, or a viral eruption. Patients may have low-grade fever and malaise.

   2. Course and treatment. Although *P. aeruginosa* can be isolated from larger pustules, in the immunologically competent patient the rash is self-limited (resolving in 1 or 2 weeks) and no therapy is indicated. Corticosteroids are contraindicated, and their use may result in spread of the folliculitis.

B. **Pyoderma gangrenosum** is classically described as a characteristic progressive superficial skin lesion that begins as a tender erythematous nodule, then forms a pustule that rapidly ulcerates with edematous, dusky, overhanging borders and a surrounding margin of erythema. It has been described in patients with underlying inflammatory bowel disease, rheumatoid arthritis, and leukemia. Optimal therapy is not well defined, but medical control of the underlying disease, systemic corticosteroids, and also cytotoxic agents have been advocated. Because the condition mimics a poorly controlled cellulitis, concomitant antibiotics often are employed. Dermatologic and infectious disease consultations are advised.

C. **Kerions of the scalp** may appear as an impetigolike or soft-tissue infection that does not respond to antibiotic therapy [48]. This is a fungal infection of the scalp (tinea capitis) due to a variety of dermatophytes. The inflammatory form of this infection can start as a small furuncle and then progress to a boggy and indurated mass that may be tender and painful. Purulent material may be aspirated or may drain from the lesion. Bacterial cultures are usually negative, although secondary bacterial infections can occur. The lesion gradually evolves over several weeks to months. The diagnosis can be made by examining infected hairs under the microscope with a potassium hydroxide wet prep smear (see Chap. 25), although several samples may be required, or by culturing the infected hair or skin scrapings. Prolonged griseofulvin therapy (e.g., 3–6 weeks) has been successfully used and, at times, dermatologists will add systemic corticosteroids (e.g., for 3 weeks) to reduce the inflammatory response that can be associated with alopecia. Dermatologic consultation is advised as optimal therapy is debated.

D. **Ecthyma contagiosum** (or **Orf**) is an unusual viral infection [29], discussed in sec. **III.E** under Mucocutaneous Vesicles.

E. **Diphtheria.** The bacterium *Corynebacterium diphtheriae* can cause cutaneous and wound disease as well as upper respiratory infection. It occurs most commonly in humid, tropical areas with poor hygiene, although sporadic cases occur in temperate areas of the United States. The infection often begins as a tender, pustular lesion that breaks down and enlarges to form an oval, punched-out ulcer with a gray membrane at the base.

Diphtheria cellulitis is uncommon in developed countries. Oral erythromycin (2.0 g/day in adults) and procaine penicillin G, 600,000 units IM q6h in the adult, can be used; diphtheria antitoxin (if the patient is not allergic to horse serum), 10,000 units/day for no longer than 8–12 days, is also given.

Necrotizing Soft-Tissue Infections

Necrotizing soft-tissue infections (NSTI) include a variety of infections which have been reviewed elsewhere [30, 49]. These infections are characterized by rapidly progressing inflammation and necrosis of skin, subcutaneous fat and fascia, and sometimes muscle. Therefore, **they are deeper and more serious than an uncomplicated more superficial cellulitis.** In the **past,** several **terms** have been used to describe these problems, including **necrotizing fasciitis, synergistic gangrene,** nonclostridial crepitant cellulitis, and gram-negative **synergistic cellulitis** [49]. When muscle is involved with clostridial infection, it has been referred to as ***clostridial myonecrosis.*** Although a single pathogen may be isolated on culture (e.g., streptococcal group A), frequently these are mixed aerobic-anaerobic infections.

I. **Clinical setting.** The key to successful treatment of necrotizing soft-tissue infections is early diagnosis and treatment [49].

  A. **A high index of suspicion** is important, because early in the course of NSTI, the findings may be similar to a severe nonoperative cellulitis.

  1. **Impaired host defenses** are associated with NSTI, including advanced age, diabetes, peripheral vascular disease, malignancy, chronic alcoholism, chronic renal failure, and immunosuppressive therapy. Other risk factors include infections contaminated by soil or manure and infections secondary to trauma or ischemia.

  2. The initiating factor may, at times, be minor.

  3. **Clinical clues** to early recognition are **edema** beyond the area of erythema, **skin vesicles, crepitus** (or air in subcutaneous tissues on plain film) and the **absence of lymphangitis and lymphadenitis** [49]. These infections may spread rapidly along natural tissue planes.

   a. **Local spread** may lead to skin anesthesia, focal ecchymosis, or skin necrosis.

   b. **Systemic progression** may occur with hypotension, high fever, and septic appearance of the patient.

  4. It should be emphasized that the **presence of subcutaneous gas** discovered by palpation or x-ray **does not necessarily mean clostridial infection.** Enterobacteriaceae, anaerobic streptococci, and *Bacteroides* spp. can produce gas under appropriate metabolic conditions. **The distinction is important, because most of these organisms are not susceptible to the drug of choice for clostridial infections** (aqueous penicillin G), and infections caused by the nonclostridial organisms may not require the radical excision necessary in clostridial myonecrosis.

  B. **Diagnostic aids.** If NSTI is suspected, the following diagnostic maneuvers are indicated:

  1. **Gram staining** of tissue exudate.

  2. **Blood cultures,** aerobic and anaerobic.

  3. **Aerobic and anaerobic cultures** of a tissue section obtained at surgery or needle aspiration of a soft-tissue abscess; the material for anaerobic culture obtained at surgery should be transported rapidly to the microbiology laboratory in an oxygen-free environment.

  4. **Serial clinical assessments are important.** Usually the erythema will progress over the first 24 hours of therapy. Outlining the involved skin area with a pen may be beneficial. If there is very rapid progression of findings (e.g., erythema, crepitus) over hours, clostridial myonecrosis must be considered.

II. **Pathogenesis.** Four factors appear to be important [49]:

  A. **Anaerobic wound environment.** Infections in the perirectal or perivulvar area or those associated with soil or manure contamination or ischemia **are often due to a mixture of anaerobes and aerobes.**

B. **Toxic lytic enzymes** may be important in streptococcal group A infections and some progressive *Pseudomonas* spp. infections. Invasive streptococcal group A infections are discussed in sec. **I.D** under Cellulitis and Related Skin Infections.
C. **Bacterial synergy** appears important in animal models (e.g., together group A streptococcal infections and *S. aureus* cause a more severe infection than either alone). Invasive streptococcal group A infections are discussed in sec. **I.D** under Cellulitis and Related Skin Infections.
D. **Thrombosis of nutrient blood vessels.** With subcutaneous injury, skin necrosis may develop as a result of thrombosis of the nutrient vascular supply [49].

III. **Approach to therapy.** Once a NSTI has been recognized, **prompt and aggressive therapy** is essential. **Surgical consultation** and evaluation **is imperative.** Four aspects of therapy have been emphasized [49]:
A. **Resuscitation** includes fluid and electrolyte therapy and hemodynamic stabilization.
B. **Antibiotic therapy should be initiated immediately and is determined by the origin of the infection.** Suggested initial antibiotic regimens are necessarily broad spectrum, because the severity and rapid progression of anaerobic soft-tissue infections require aggressive therapy. All antibiotics should be given intravenously initially. Modifications can be made later, based on culture results and response to treatment (see sec. **IV**).
C. **Early aggressive surgical debridement** is essential [49, 50]. At exploration, gray necrotic fascia without frank pus is common [49]. Typically repeat debridement is required in 24–48 hours.
D. **Supportive treatment** is important (e.g., nutritional therapy). Heparin has been advocated by some [49].

IV. **Additional comments on antibiotic therapy**
A. **Antibiotic combinations** are commonly used, especially when perineal infections or serious infections are involved.
1. **Severe infection.** When the patient is very ill, there are **two** important **requirements:** first, that an antibiotic be used that has predictable **activity against the aerobic** organisms in the anaerobic milieu and, second, that an antibiotic specifically **active against the anaerobic** species must be included.
a. **For community-acquired infection, a broad-spectrum cephalosporin and either clindamycin or metronidazole** satisfy this requirement. Ampicillin and gentamicin are considered insufficient, the former because it lacks a broad enough spectrum and the latter because, in the anaerobic milieu, gentamicin is not adequately active.
Therefore, **clindamycin or metronidazole** could be used **in combination with** a third-generation cephalosporin (e.g., **ceftriaxone**). If culture data reveal a gram-negative organism susceptible to an earlier-generation and more cost-effective cephalosporin, the cephalosporin can be changed.
Although some authors suggest that monotherapy with imipenem or tazobactam-piperacillin is sufficient, if the infection is very severe we would generally avoid monotherapy in the very ill patient. (See the related discussion in Chap. 11, sec. **II** under Intra-abdominal Infections.)
b. **For hospital-acquired infection,** broader gram-negative antibiotic coverage seems appropriate while awaiting cultures. In this setting, an aminoglycoside, piperacillin, and metronidazole or clindamycin can be used.
2. **Mild or moderate infection.** In the case of moderate or mild infection, an antibiotic that has activity against both the aerobic gram-negatives and the anaerobes, which explains why drugs such as cefoxitin (or cefotetan) are successful. Although ampicillin-sulbactam is potentially useful in this setting, piperacillin-tazobactam is a better initial choice as the latter is more active against gram-negative aerobes. See Chap. 28E.
If oral therapy is appropriate, ampicillin-clavulanate or an oral quinolone or trimethoprim-sulfamethoxazole plus metronidazole or clindamycin are reasonable choices.
3. **Miscellaneous**
a. **Enterococci.** Often a major point of debate is whether to include enterococci in empiric coverage when treating mixed anaerobic-aerobic infection. Many experts believe that it is far more important to ascertain that gram-negative coverage is sufficiently broad than to include enterococcal coverage. In general, we do not consider it necessary to cover enterococci routinely.

(See the related discussion in Chap. 11, sec. **II,** under Intra-abdominal Infections.)

b. **Triple therapy** (ampicillin, gentamicin, and clindamycin). This combination of antibiotics has been used for suspected anaerobic infection in part because it possesses activity against enterococci. Nonetheless, it is far from ideal. Ampicillin's spectrum is inadequate against gram-negatives and, in the anaerobic milieu, gentamicin is insufficiently active at the tissue level. This is an example of sacrificing good aerobic activity to provide enterococcal coverage. **We do not advocate this combination.** (See the related discussion in Chap. 11, sec. **II,** under Intra-abdominal Infections.)

c. **In the patient with penicillin anaphylaxis.** In this setting, neither the penicillins nor the cephalosporins can be used with certain safety. **Aztreonam or an aminoglycoside** (despite its less than optimal activity) **or a quinolone** *plus* **an antianaerobic drug** (e.g., clindamycin or metronidazole) are used in combination.

d. **Clostridial infection.** When *Clostridium perfringens* infection is known or highly suspected (e.g., Gram stain of wound exudate reveals gram-positive rods in a very ill patient), aqueous penicillin G (e.g., 18 million units/d if renal function is normal) has been the drug of choice with or without hyperbaric oxygen.

The exact **role of hyperbaric oxygen therapy** in the therapy of clostridial myonecrosis **is unclear. In a recent murine model** of *C. perfringens* myositis [51], **clindamycin was the most effective antibiotic,** and its effect was not enhanced by hyperbaric oxygen therapy. With penicillin and metronidazole, there may be some additive benefit of hyperbaric oxygen therapy, but these combinations were less effective than clindamycin without hyperbaric oxygen therapy in this model [51]. In patients with delayed onset of therapy, hyperbaric oxygen may play a role, and infectious disease consultation is advised.

V. **Miscellaneous specific conditions**
A. **Fournier's gangrene of the scrotum** is one localized form of NSTI that deserves emphasis. Unfamiliarity with this syndrome frequently results in delayed diagnosis and inadequate treatment. Fournier's gangrene is a serious infection of the scrotum caused by anaerobic streptococci in association with other bacteria such as *Proteus* spp., *E. coli, S. aureus,* beta-hemolytic streptococci, various anaerobes and, occasionally, *Pseudomonas* spp.

1. **Clinical characteristics and diagnosis.** The condition may begin insidiously in an elderly debilitated patient or rapidly in a younger, healthier person. Scrotal swelling and pain are the first local symptoms; these are followed by progressive necrosis of scrotal skin and subcutaneous tissues. The patient may appear severely toxic and experience considerable pain. An initial diagnosis of systemic illness or acute abdomen may be made unless the genitalia are examined. Gangrene may involve the perineum and sometimes the penis, along with progressive necrosis of the scrotal skin and subcutaneous tissue. A putrid discharge may emanate from the necrotic scrotum.

2. **Treatment.** Aerobic and anaerobic cultures should be obtained along with the Gram stain of the purulent discharge. Initially, very broad-spectrum antibiotics are empirically started. A third-generation cephalosporin (e.g., ceftriaxone, 2 g/d), an aminoglycoside (see Chap. 28H for dosages), and clindamycin, 600 mg q8h IV, are suggested while awaiting cultures. However, **it should be stressed that a surgical approach with wide incision and drainage is mandatory,** along with replacement of fluids and electrolytes. **Immediate surgical consultation** should be requested. Because imipenem-cilastatin is active against the causative organisms previously cited, it is a candidate for monotherapy in this setting (see Chap. 28G). Piperacillin-tazobactam is another possible choice.

B. **Invasive group A streptococcal infections** are discussed in sec. **I.D,** under Cellulitis and Related Skin Infections.

C. NSTI in **diabetic foot infections** are discussed in Chap. 16.

D. *Vibrio vulnificus* **salt water wound infections** are discussed in sec. **I.H,** under Cellulitis and Related Skin Infections.

E. **Pyomyositis** is discussed in sec. **I.I,** under Cellulitis and Related Skin Infections.

Infections of Deep Spaces of the Neck

A variety of infections arising from the floor of the mouth and posterior pharynx involve the fascial planes of the neck and are remarkable for their potential for **rapid progression and potentially serious consequences** [52–54]. Although these infections usually are distinguished from one another by the different anatomic sites involved in the jaw and neck, several features are shared in common. **These infections usually are due to a polymicrobial mixture of normal mouth bacteria, spread rapidly to contiguous fascial spaces, and must be diagnosed and treated promptly to prevent serious complications** such as spread to the mediastinum, airway obstruction, and hematogenous dissemination.

I. **Anatomic considerations.** A detailed discussion of this topic is beyond the scope of this chapter and is well discussed elsewhere [54, 55]. However, several points warrant emphasis. Suppurative processes of the neck involve **three cervical spaces** that can be life-threatening. Complex fascial planes both separate and connect areas, thereby both limiting (at times) and facilitating (at other times) spread of infection.

   A. **Submandibular space** is shown in Fig. 4-1 and can be compromised by spreading infection involving the floor of the mouth and tongue tissue. **Ludwig's angina,** a bilateral, brawny cellulitis of the soft tissue (as shown in Fig. 4-1) is the major type of infection in the submandibular space. Patients will develop submandibular swelling and enlargement of the tongue and will have the potential for upper airway obstruction. Odontogenic infection is implicated in 70–90% of Ludwig's angina cases [54] (see sec. **IV.A**).

   B. **Lateral pharyngeal space** is divided into two functional units by the styloid process: the anterior (muscular) and the posterior (neurovascular) component. Each is vulnerable to infection with different clinical results. Both compartments abut the retropharyngeal space (Fig. 4-2).

   1. **Anterior compartment infection** is associated with soft-tissue swelling, which results in the following:

      a. **Unilateral trismus** due to irritation of the internal pterygoid muscle.

      b. **Induration and swelling along the angle of the jaw** (Fig. 4-3).

      c. **Bulging of the palantine tonsil** into the posterior pharynx (see Fig. 4-3).

      d. **Systemic toxicity** with fevers and rigors due to the uncontrolled abscess.

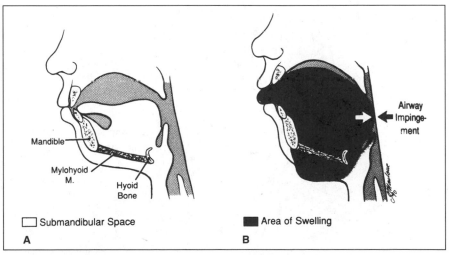

Fig. 4-1. Schematic representation of submandibular space. (A) Normal; (B) Ludwig's angina. (From T. E. Jacobs, R. S. Irwin, and V. Raptopoulos, Severe Upper Airway Infections. In J. M. Rippe, R. S. Irwin, J. S. Alpert, and M. P. Fink (eds.), *Intensive Care Medicine* (2nd ed.). Boston: Little, Brown, 1991. P. 702.)

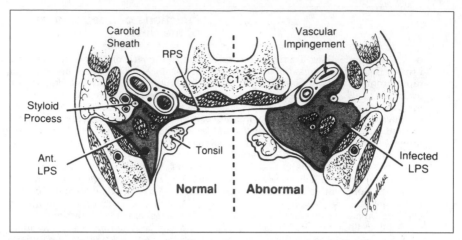

Fig. 4-2. Cross-sectional view of lateral pharyngeal space (*LPS*) showing normal anatomic landmarks and effects of space infection on them. *RPS* = retropharyngeal space. (From T. E. Jacobs, R. S. Irwin, and V. Raptopoulos, Severe Upper Airway Infections. In J. M. Rippe, R. S. Irwin, J. S. Alpert, and M. P. Fink (eds.), *Intensive Care Medicine* (2nd ed.). Boston: Little, Brown, 1991. P. 702.)

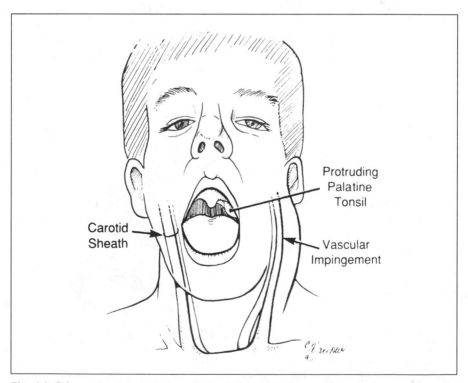

Fig. 4-3. Schematic representation of salient clinical findings of lateral pharyngeal space abscess. (From T. E. Jacobs, R. S. Irwin, and V. Raptopoulos, Severe Upper Airway Infections. In J. M. Rippe, R. S. Irwin, J. S. Alpert, and M. P. Fink (eds.), *Intensive Care Medicine* (2nd ed.). Boston: Little, Brown, 1991. P. 703.)

e. **Miscellaneous findings,** including dysphagia and ipsilateral neck or jaw pain or ipsilateral ear pain. Discomfort may worsen with turning of the head, which compresses infected tissue.

f. **Predisposing conditions include** a recent upper respiratory infection, pharyngitis, dental infection, or possibly otitis media with mastoiditis.

2. **Posterior compartment** infection can put the **carotid sheath** and its contents (e.g., internal carotid artery, internal jugular vein, vagus nerve, lymph nodes, cranial nerves IX through XII, and cervical trunks) at risk for compression or direct infection [54].

   a. **Signs of sepsis** (fever, leukocytosis, possibly hypotension) are not uncommon.

   b. **Absence of localizing signs** (e.g., trismus, tonsillar protrusion) is typical.

   c. **Signs and symptoms** relate to complications of involvement of the neurovascular structures.

      (1) **Suppurative jugular venous thrombosis** is the most common complication. It can cause bacteremia and septic emboli (see sec. **IV.B.4**).

      (2) **Carotid artery rupture** can occur. Arteritis develops from contiguous inflammation, which can result in false aneurysm formation. Because the carotid sheath is dense and not easily invaded, protracted infection of 1–2 weeks usually precedes arterial erosion. Cranial nerve palsies or Horner's syndrome can occur. Intermittent bleeding from the mouth or nose can occur and may suggest impending rupture [54].

      (3) **Enhanced CT** has been **very useful** to define lateral pharyngeal space neck infection [54]. (See sec. **IV.B.2**.)

C. **Retropharyngeal space** is shown in Fig. 4-4, which also **shows the location of the "danger space,"** so named because it is the pathway into the chest for all neck infections [54]. The danger space extends from the base of the skull to the diaphragm. Involvement of this space by infection is a result of extension from the

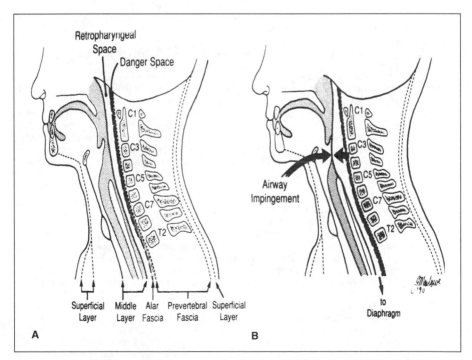

Fig. 4-4. Schematic representation of cervical fascial planes and spaces. (A) Normal; (B) retropharyngeal space abscess. (From T. E. Jacobs, R. S. Irwin, and V. Raptopoulos, Severe Upper Airway Infections. In J. M. Rippe, R. S. Irwin, J. S. Alpert, and M. P. Fink (eds.), *Intensive Care Medicine* (2nd ed.). Boston: Little, Brown, 1991. P. 699.)

retropharyngeal space or prevertebral space and may give rise to life-threatening complications from neck infection.

Retropharyngeal space abscesses are uncommon and most often seen in children younger than 6 years. The two chains of lymph nodes in this space are the source of most such abscesses. Therefore, **young children are at greater risk** because these nodes, which drain the nose, pharynx, middle ear, and paranasal sinuses, regress by about the age of 4 years [54].

D. **Descending infection**
   1. **Any deep neck infection can have access to the posterior mediastinum and diaphragm by the common pathway of the retropharyngeal space and the danger space.**
   2. **Aspiration pneumonia** and **lung abscess** are potential complications as there is pus in the oral cavity [54].

II. **Pathogenesis.** Many of these infections originate from an odontogenic source—infection of either the dental pulp or periodontal tissues. Diseased molar teeth of the mandible are an especially frequent source. A complex mix of normal oral bacterial flora initiates the infection and may involve *Bacteroides* spp., microaerophilic streptococci, aerobic streptococci, peptostreptococci, *Veillonella* spp., *Actinomyces* spp., and fusobacteria. Less commonly, enteric gram-negative bacilli, *S. aureus*, or *P. aeruginosa* may play a role. The infectious process rapidly takes the path of least resistance and burrows from the tooth structures into contiguous fascial spaces and planes, as discussed in sec. **I.**

Inadequately treated pharyngitis and tonsillitis can progress and extend to deep neck infections.

III. **Complications.** Direct extension of the infection can result in serious consequences. The anatomic basis of these complications was reviewed in sec. **I.** Because of these potential complications, deep neck infections often constitute urgent medical and surgical problems. The major complications are as follows:
   A. **Mediastinal suppuration** and mediastinitis can result in erosion of a great vessel with exsanguination.
   B. **Osteomyelitis** of the maxilla or mandible can occur.
   C. **Intracranial extension** can result in infection of the carotid sheath and life-threatening cavernous sinus thrombosis.
   D. **Airway obstruction** may ensue.
   E. Pleuropulmonary infection may eventuate in a necrotizing pneumonia or empyema.
   F. **Hematogenous dissemination** with a sepsis syndrome is possible.

IV. **Diagnosis and clinical syndromes.** Whenever possible, it is important to identify the space or spaces involved in deep neck infections so that appropriate treatment can be initiated, with the goal of preventing or minimizing complications noted in sec. **III.** The clinical picture may be confusing because of the involvement of multiple spaces and interference with the examination by trismus [54]. A **lateral neck radiograph, early consideration of a CT scan,** and **consultation with an otolaryngologist** are suggested. Leukocytosis and fever are common, nonspecific findings. The role of MRI scanning is undergoing evaluation; CT scans are less expensive and require less patient cooperation.

Several different clinical syndromes can be identified.
   A. **Ludwig's angina** is an infection of the **submandibular space.**
      1. **Anatomic considerations** are reviewed in sec. **I.A.**
      2. **Diagnosis** is based on **clinical findings.**
         a. These patients are febrile and toxic-appearing with brawny, tender, **bilateral** woody **swelling** of the **submandibular tissue** (see Fig. 4-1).
         b. Swelling of the floor of the mouth pushes the tongue upward and toward the roof of the mouth. The **tongue** may appear **enlarged** and protruding (see Fig. 4-1).
         c. **Trismus** is seen in approximately 50% of cases [54].
         d. **Airway compromise** may be imminent (see Fig. 4-1).
      3. Therapy is discussed in sec. **V.**
   B. **Lateral pharyngeal space abscess** must be promptly identified to prevent the life-threatening complication of spread to the carotid sheath, mediastinum, or bloodstream. This infection most commonly arises from submandibular space infection, pharyngitis, or peritonsillar abscess.
      1. **Anatomic considerations** are reviewed in sec. **I.B.**

2. **Diagnosis.** In addition to the clinical findings noted in sec. **I.B, CT scanning of the neck** (contrast-enhanced) is important to help define the anatomy and potential need for drainage. Ultrasonography probably is not as useful as CT [54]. In special circumstances, carotid artery angiography is done to locate a possible aneurysm before surgical repair (see sec. **I.B.2**).

3. **Therapy** typically involves surgical drainage and antibiotics (see sec. **V**).

4. **Postanginal sepsis** or **Lemierre syndrome** is a fulminant infection affecting healthy young adults or adolescents and is caused by acute oropharyngeal infection with secondary septic thrombophlebitis of the internal jugular vein [56]. Serious complications include septicemia (usually due to *Fusobacterium* spp.), metastatic infection of the lungs and pleural spaces, meningitis, brain abscess, and vocal cord paralysis. The cornerstone of therapy is prompt recognition and aggressive antibiotic therapy. Interestingly, this devastating infection can complicate a rather ordinary case of infectious mononucleosis [57].

C. **Retropharyngeal abscess**
   1. **Anatomic considerations** are reviewed in sec. **I.C.**
   2. **Pathogenesis.** These abscesses usually result from odontogenic infection, penetrating trauma (fish bone), or peritonsillar abscess. They are more common in children younger than 4 years, as emphasized in sec. **I.C.**
   3. **Clinical presentation**
      a. **In pediatric patients,** initial symptoms may be vague, including fever, irritability, and refusal to eat. The neck may be held stiffly and tilted away from the involved site. Interference with breathing and swallowing may occur depending on the degree of swelling (see Fig. 4-4). Spontaneous rupture of the abscess with aspiration is a potential complication [54].
      b. **Adults** usually will have signs and symptoms referable to the pharynx. There may be a history of trauma to the posterior pharynx (e.g., intubation or foreign bodies such as chicken bones). The most common symptoms are fever, sore throat, dysphagia, noisy breathing, stiff neck, and dyspnea.
   4. **Diagnosis** is aided by a **lateral neck radiograph** to identify prevertebral soft-tissue swelling.
   5. **Therapy** is discussed in sec. **V.** Rapid initiation of therapy is important in the hope of avoiding respiratory compromise or spread of infections via the danger space (see Fig. 4-4).

D. **Miscellaneous**
   1. **Peritonsillar abscess,** or **quinsy,** is an infrequent complication of acute tonsillitis in adolescents and young adults. The patient will present with fever, sore throat, difficulty swallowing, trismus, drooling, and a muffled ("potato") voice. Examination of the oropharynx usually reveals swelling of the anterior tonsillar pillar and soft palate. Incision and drainage will often be necessary to prevent spontaneous rupture, aspiration pneumonia, airway obstruction, and dissection to the lateral retropharyngeal space.
   2. **Epiglottitis** is discussed separately in Chap. 8.

V. **Therapy.** Patients with known or highly suspected deep neck infections deserve hospitalization with careful observation and otolaryngologic evaluation.
   A. **Airway management.** Establishment of an artificial airway is not universally required but should be done when evidence of airway obstruction, such as dyspnea and stridor, exists or there is inability to handle secretions [54].
      1. Upper airway obstruction is most likely to occur in infections of the submandibular space (see Fig. 4-1).
      2. Otolaryngologic consultation is advised as the options for optimal artificial airway management are still debated.
   B. **Intravenous antibiotics.** Culture specimens of abscess contents usually are not available unless a surgical drainage procedure is done (e.g., aspiration, incision). Any deep, surgically obtained specimen should be cultured aerobically and anaerobically.
      1. The mainstay of antibiotic therapy has been intravenous aqueous penicillin (e.g., 2 million units q4h in adults with normal renal function). For patients with peritonsillar abscess, this therapy still seems appropriate.
         Some oral *Bacteroides* spp. (e.g., *B. melaninogenicus*) may be relatively penicillin-resistant. Because of this, in the very ill patient, the use of clindamycin 600 mg q8h in adults or 40 mg/kg/day in children in q8h divided doses is preferred. Ampicillin-sulbactam is another option.

In children, it may sometimes be desirable to provide coverage for *H. influenzae,* and a combination of ceftriaxone and clindamycin is a consideration as ceftriaxone is not an optimal agent against anaerobes. However, if a child has received Hib vaccine, it probably is not necessary to use antibiotics directed against this pathogen due to the reduced incidence of invasive *H. influenzae* B infection in vaccine recipients [58]. In such a case, clindamycin alone may be used.

It seldom is necessary to treat for gram-negative bacilli, unless the patient is immunocompromised or has recently been hospitalized.

   2. **In the penicillin-allergic patient,** intravenous clindamycin is preferred in the dosages given in sec. **1.** If *H. influenzae* or community-acquired gram-negative bacilli are a concern and the patient has had a delayed penicillin-allergic reaction, ceftriaxone can be used in combination with clindamycin.

C. **Surgical drainage**
   1. Drainage is especially important for infections involving the retropharyngeal and lateral pharyngeal space. Up to 50% of cases of Ludwig's angina in the submandibular space can be cured without surgery [54].
   2. Otolaryngologic consultation is important. At times, intravenous antibiotics are used until the abscess has "matured," at which time it is drained surgically.

D. **Hyperbaric oxygen** therapy has been advocated as an adjunctive measure because involvement by anaerobic bacteria is so common and the consequences of progressive infection are so dire (see earlier discussion). Usually, however, this approach is unavailable to the clinician.

General Principles of Wound Infection Management

Wound infections can occur perioperatively or after accidental trauma to the skin. It is estimated that from 2 to 40% of surgical wounds become infected, depending on such factors as the type of operation (clean or contaminated), length of operation, and susceptibility of the host. Virtually all wounds, whether accidental or surgically induced, become contaminated with varying numbers and types of microbial pathogens. Even the cleanest, most technically correct surgical incision is subject to some microbial exposure owing to inability to sterilize the skin completely and to fallout from reservoirs of microbial growth in the operating room.

I. **Factors in development of wound infection.** The type of wound infection and the outcome of infection depend on a number of factors, the most important of which are the following:
   A. **Infecting organism.** Group A streptococcus produces rapid breakdown of the infected wound. *Staphylococcus aureus,* either methicillin-sensitive or methicillin-resistant (MRSA), is destructive also, though less so than group A streptococcus. (Actually, some infectious disease physicians believe that the preferred terminology for MRSA is *oxacillin-resistant S. aureus,* or ORSA, because oxacillin, not methicillin, is used for laboratory testing. We retain the use of the more commonly known acronym, MRSA, here.) Because MRSA resists standard antibiotics, wound infections can develop in the face of prophylaxis. Among the gram-negatives, *Proteus mirabilis* is quite destructive, but it is an infrequent cause of wound infection.
   B. **Inoculum size.** The numbers of infecting organisms introduced into a wound will affect the outcome (i.e., the larger the inoculum size, the greater the risk of wound infection).
   C. **Local and systemic host resistance factors.** The presence of foreign bodies, devitalized tissue, or hematomas, or poor surgical technique will hinder the normal host defense mechanisms; corticosteroid and immunosuppressive therapy will also hinder the normal host response.
   D. **Debilitation,** chronic illness, diabetes mellitus, cirrhosis, alcoholism, malignancy, and administration of steroids or cytotoxic drugs all predispose to development of wound infection.

II. **Epidemiology**
   A. **Nonsurgical wound contamination.** Wounds resulting from accidental trauma are contaminated at the time of injury by bacteria either in the immediate vicinity or introduced by the penetrating object. *S. aureus* remains the most common cause of community-acquired wound infection. In rural areas, soil and manure

contamination predispose to infections with Enterobacteriaceae, *Clostridium* spp., and *Bacteroides fragilis*.

B. **Surgical wound contamination.** Contamination of surgical wounds occurs during the operative procedure. The patient's endogenous bacterial flora is a common source of surgical wound infection. Other sources in the operating room are non-scrubbed personnel (circulating nurse, anesthesiologist, and other personnel not directly involved in the operation) and fallout from air contamination. Occasionally, certain scrubbed personnel are particularly prone to disseminate their bacteria into the area of the surgical wound. Holes in the surgeon's gloves and blood-soaked surgical gowns also predispose to transfer of bacteria from scrubbed personnel to the operative site.

C. The three most significant **risk factors for postoperative wound infection** are the probability that bacteria will contaminate the wound, the length of the operation, and the general health status of the patient. Surgical wounds can be **classified** into four categories based on risk of bacterial contamination of the wound at the time of surgery.

   1. **Clean wound.** A product of elective operations on uninfected tissue with no mucous membrane contact such as a herniorrhaphy. There is a risk of infection ranging from 0.5 to 1.5%.
   2. **Clean contaminated wound.** Results from elective operations in which mucous membranes are cut across. If no prophylaxis is provided, there is a 10–30% risk of wound infection depending on the type of surgery.
   3. **Contaminated wound.** Occurs in operations on fresh traumatic wounds or emergency entrance into the gastrointestinal tract (e.g., repair of a colonic perforation). In the absence of antibiotics, infection is almost certain; antibiotics are treatment rather than prophylaxis.
   4. **Dirty and infected wound.** Result of wound dehiscence, trauma incurred several hours or days earlier, or operations on frank abscesses. As for contaminated wounds, antibiotics are treatment rather than prophylaxis.

III. **Clinical characteristics.** Diagnosis of a wound infection is not difficult when the patient is febrile with an elevated WBC count and has a wound that is warm, erythematous, swollen, tender, and discharging purulent material. However, in many cases a patient will have a more benign-appearing wound with minimal discharge. **Unfortunately, wound cultures often are not diagnostic and can be misleading, because noninfected wounds frequently have bacterial colonization.** Therefore, microbial growth may represent merely wound colonization and not true wound infection. **Differentiation of colonization from infection may not be easy.** The type of bacteria isolated may be helpful in that organisms such as *Staphylococcus epidermidis*, *Neisseria* spp., and diphtheroids are infrequent tissue pathogens. However, organisms such as Enterobacteriaceae, *Pseudomonas* spp., *Clostridium* spp., and *S. aureus* can be serious pathogens of wounds or mere innocuous colonizers.

IV. **Clinical evaluation.** Because of the problems inherent in differentiating colonization from wound infection, the patient should undergo a thorough evaluation that includes the following points:

   A. **Consider the overall clinical state of the patient.** Evaluate for common indices of infection such as fever, diaphoresis, rigors, and elevated WBC count.
   B. **Evaluate the clinical status of the wound**
      1. **Visual inspection.** Copious discharge and large areas of **erythema** suggest that infection is present and may be severe, but these findings are usually not diagnostic of a specific organism.
      2. **Smell.** A putrid odor implicates anaerobes, although enterococci can be very malodorous. A grapelike smell suggests *Pseudomonas*.
      3. **Crepitance.** Anaerobes usually produce gas, but aerobes such as *Escherichia coli* also produce gas. This can be palpated as crepitance.
      4. **Gram staining** of any wound drainage is a potentially useful tool. For example, numerous polymorphonuclear cells and gram-positive cocci in clusters suggest *S. aureus*.
      5. **Miscellaneous.** In the neutropenic patient, typical clues (e.g., erythema) for inflammatory response are usually absent. The only clue may be the presence of pain at the site of infection. In patients with tetanus, often there is absolutely no evidence of inflammation at the wound site.
   C. **Obtain cultures of the discharge.** Using aseptic technique, aerobic cultures of the fresh wound exudate should be obtained. Not all wounds need anaerobic cultures. However, anaerobic cultures should be obtained when the wound has a

foul odor, evidence of crepitance, actual or potential contamination with fecal flora, or necrotic tissue (see Chap. 25).

D. Obtain blood cultures. Because wound infections sometimes result in bacterial invasion of the bloodstream, blood cultures should be obtained in the febrile patient. The presence of the same organism in wound and blood supports a diagnosis of wound infection.

E. The type of surgery may provide a clue to the causative organisms in postoperative wounds.

1. **Clean surgery:** *S. aureus,* group A beta-hemolytic streptococcus
2. **Clean surgery plus foreign body:** *S. aureus* or coagulase-negative staphylococci
3. **Bowel surgery:** *E. coli, P. mirabilis,* enterococci, and anaerobes
4. **Head and neck surgery:** mouth flora including anaerobes
5. **Vaginal hysterectomy:** group B beta-hemolytic streptococci, *E. coli,* enterococci, and anaerobes

V. Treatment. A combination of antibiotics and surgery (debridement, incision, and drainage) is often needed in the treatment of the wound infection. Antibiotics usually will need to be started before culture results are available. Clinical clues often must be used initially to decide which bacteria might be involved. Topical antibiotics have no role in an established wound infection, although mupirocin has been used effectively for impetigo (see earlier discussion). Selection of the administration route of the antibiotic (oral versus parenteral) is based on severity and the availability of active drugs. See Chap. 28 for pediatric doses; adult doses discussed below.

A. Antibiotic therapy based on presumed organisms

1. **Group A beta-hemolytic streptococcal infection.** Although penicillin G has been the standard of therapy for this infection, recent studies of deep-thigh group A infection in the rabbit model have suggested that clindamycin is preferable [59]. The latter not only is active when the organism is not replicating but also blocks toxin production. Therefore, in moderate to severe infection, clindamycin (600 mg IV q8h in adults) is suggested. If there is mixed infection with gram-negatives, a cephalosporin (e.g., cefazolin or ceftriaxone) may be useful depending on susceptibility data of the gram-negatives.

   For mild early infection, penicillin V, 1–2 g/day PO) is effective. If clindamycin is selected, 300–450 mg PO q8h is suggested. Cephalexin or cephradine, 500–750 mg q6h, is another option.

2. **Oxacillin-susceptible *S. aureus* infection.** Either nafcillin or oxacillin, 1.5 g q4h, is the drug of choice for moderate to severe infection, with the latter being less prone to cause phlebitis. Cefazolin, 1 g q8h, can be substituted in the patient with a delayed penicillin allergy (see Chap. 27). Intravenous vancomycin can be used in the patient with a history of immediate penicillin allergy. See Chap. 28 for dosing. Clindamycin or cephalosporins other than cefazolin are also effective, but there is no obvious advantage of the latter and the cost is higher.

   If the infection is mild, oral therapy such as dicloxacillin (500 mg qid), cephalexin (1 g qid), or clindamycin (300–450 mg q8h) is sufficient.

3. **Oxacillin-resistant *S. aureus* (ORSA or MRSA).** For the patient currently or recently hospitalized in a setting where this organism is frequently found, staphylococci must be considered resistant to oxacillin until proven otherwise. Furthermore, MRSA are, or will become, resistant to all other antibiotics except vancomycin, which is the treatment of choice. If renal function is normal, 1 g (over 2 hours) IV q12h is suggested.

4. **Gram-negative bacilli.** Until sensitivities become available, the third-generation cephalosporins are often well-suited. The exception is in the individual who has received a prolonged course of cephalosporins or who has received broad-spectrum antibiotics while hospitalized and in whom resistant bacteria may reside. For such a patient, an aminoglycoside is necessary until sensitivities are available.

   For milder infections, oral fluoroquinolones may be appropriate. If sensitivities are known, trimethoprim-sulfamethoxazole also may be useful.

5. **Anaerobes.** If the bowel is the site of infection, anaerobic organisms are accompanied by gram-negative organisms whereas, if the site is the oropharynx, gram-positive aerobes are present. Anaerobes often will be eradicated by the cephalosporin or penicillin being used to treat the aerobic infection, especially if of oral origin. However, if many features of serious anaerobic infection are present or if the GI tract is the origin of infection, supplementation with metronidazole or clindamycin is required. If antibiotics that have little anaero-

bic activity (e.g., a quinolone) are selected for the gram-negatives, antianaerobic treatment will need to be added, regardless of the severity.

6. **Enterococci.** Many experts believe that treatment for enterococci should be initiated only for unequivocal enterococcal wound infection. When that is present, ampicillin or vancomycin is the drug of choice. Piperacillin has sufficient activity if that is being used for other reasons.

In a mixed infection with only a small inoculum of enterococci, specific therapy aimed at enterococci often is unnecessary (see Chaps. 11 and 16).

B. **Surgical treatment. Debridement of devitalized tissue, drainage of associated abscesses, and removal of clots and foreign bodies are essential.** If these measures are performed inadequately, antibiotic therapy alone is unlikely to achieve clinical cure. More radical surgical procedures may be indicated for certain rapidly advancing necrotizing infections, which are discussed in more detail in the section on Anaerobic Soft-Tissue Infections.

VI. **Prophylaxis**

A. **Community-acquired wounds.** The role of prophylactic antibiotics in wound management remains a controversial, inadequately studied subject. Community-acquired wounds are contaminated at the time of trauma, and subsequent use of antibiotics is not truly prophylactic but is more correctly termed **early treatment.** No controlled double-blind prospective studies have been done to assess the relative efficacy of starting antibiotics immediately after community-acquired wounds have occurred, as compared to waiting until definite wound infection has developed.

B. **Surgical wounds.** The surgically induced wound has been studied in more detail than the community-acquired, and it is clear that antibiotics present in the tissue before, or at the time, wound contamination occurs can be highly effective in preventing infection. On the other hand, antibiotics instituted several hours after the occurrence of wound contamination have little or no ability to prevent subsequent infection. **See Chap. 28B for a detailed discussion of surgical antibiotic prophylaxis.** The usefulness of **topical antibiotics** and of **local antibiotic irrigation** of surgical wounds remains **controversial.** In general, the author does not advocate the use of either.

Tetanus

Tetanus is an infectious disease manifested by tonic muscle spasms and hyperreflexia caused by an exotoxin elaborated by the sporulated form of the causative bacterium. The causative agent of tetanus is an anaerobic, gram-positive rod, *Clostridium tetani* [60–62], which is in soil and can contaminate wounds. The clinical manifestations of the disease are not the result of invasive tissue injury but are secondary to the production of a potent toxin at the site of injury, usually a minor wound (such as from splinters of wood, a piece of metal, or a thorn). Chronic skin ulcers account for about 5% of such disease [63]. Disease is initiated by introduction of the sporulated form of the organism into the area of injury. Under the proper anaerobic conditions, the spores vegetate and begin to produce toxin. The incubation period is usually 3–21 days, and 88% of all human cases occur within 14 days. The incubation period is inversely proportional to the distance between the site of injury and the CNS.

I. **Prevention**

A. **Primary vaccination series and routine tetanus prophylaxis.** Everyone should receive routinely a complete primary vaccination series beginning at 2–3 months of age (see Chap. 22). A routine tetanus toxoid booster should be given every 10 years. For schoolchildren and adults, a complete primary vaccination series consists of three doses of tetanus and diphtheria toxoids, with 4–8 weeks separating the first and second doses and 6 months–1 year separating the second and third doses. It is each physician's responsibility to identify those patients who have not received a primary series of three tetanus injections and to ensure that such vaccinations are given promptly. **A routine toxoid booster should be given every 10 years.** For international travelers, a toxoid booster may be given every 5 years (see Chap. 21).

Serologic surveys have shown that men older than 60 years and women older than 40 often are not protected against tetanus because they have never been fully immunized or have not received necessary booster doses of tetanus toxoid. In the United States between 1989–1990, the risk of tetanus for adults older than 80 years was more than 10-fold greater than the risk for those aged 20–29 years

Table 4-3. Summary guide to tetanus prophylaxis in routine wound management

History of adsorbed tetanus toxoid (doses)	Clean minor wounds		All other wounds[b]	
	Td[a]	TIG[a]	Td[c]	TIG
Unknown or <3	Yes	No	Yes	Yes
≥3[d]	No[e]	No	No[f]	No

[a]Td = tetanus and diphtheria (adult type; see Chap. 22) adsorbed toxoids; TIG = human tetanus immunoglobulin: 250 units IM. (TIG is preferred over equine antitoxin.) When tetanus toxoid and TIG are given concurrently, the adsorbed toxoid is recommended. (Separate syringes and separate sites should be used.)
[b]Such as, but not limited to, wounds contaminated with dirt, feces, soil, saliva, and so on; puncture wounds; avulsions; and wounds resulting from missiles, crushing, burns, and frostbite.
[c]For children younger than 7 years; DTP (DT, if pertussis vaccine is contraindicated) is preferred to tetanus toxoid alone. For persons 7 years and older, Td is preferred to tetanus toxoid alone.
[d]If only three doses of fluid toxoid have been received, a fourth dose of toxoid, preferably an adsorbed toxoid, should be given.
[e]Yes, if more than 10 years since last dose.
[f]Yes, if more than 5 years since last dose. (More frequent boosters are not needed and can accentuate side effects.)
Source: Centers for Disease Control, Diphtheria, tetanus, and pertussis. Recommendations for vaccine use and other preventive measures. *M.M.W.R.* 40(RR-10):21–22, 1991.

[64]. **Protective antibodies decline over time.** In a recent survey of immunity to tetanus in the United States, 20% of children 10–16 years of age and 70% of adults older than 70 years did not have protective antibody levels and therefore were at risk for tetanus [65].

Physicians are cautioned against administering tetanus toxoid boosters at more frequent intervals: The boosters have been associated with urticaria, angioneurotic edema, and Arthus-like reactions.

B. **Tetanus prophylaxis in wound management.** Use of tetanus immunoglobulin (TIG) or tetanus toxoid must be considered when one is evaluating a patient with a wound. The current U.S. Public Health Service recommendations are given in Table 4-3 and are based on the prior history of tetanus immunizations and on classification of the wound as clean or not clean. **A clean, minor wound** is any wound less than 6 hours old that is clean and nonpenetrating and involves negligible tissue damage. **All other wounds** are those that are not clean. These are subject to a different set of guidelines for tetanus prophylaxis, as outlined in Table 4-3.

II. **Clinical characteristics of tetanus** [60, 61, 65]. Approximately one-third of patients who contract tetanus in the United States have no obvious wound or a wound considered by the patient to be trivial [62]. **Trismus** is the presenting symptom in more than 50% of cases, and sustained trismus produces a characteristic sardonic smile (*risus sardonicus*). Persistent contractions of the chest and back muscles result in **opisthotonos. Restlessness and irritability** may be followed by **tetanic seizures** manifested by a sudden burst of tonic contraction of muscle groups. Glottal or laryngeal spasm can impair air exchange, and dysphagia accompanied by hydrophobia may occur.

III. **Diagnosis.** Routine laboratory studies are of little use in the diagnosis of tetanus. The CSF of a patient with tetanus is normal, and Gram staining and anaerobic culture of the wound may not reveal the typical organisms. The diagnosis is based on clinical observations including a history of tissue injury followed by the development of the characteristic neurologic signs and symptoms described in sec. II.

Tetanus may be confused with more common conditions such as dystonic reactions to neuroleptic drugs (which typically involve lateral turning of the head, often with protrusion of the tongue—symptoms that are rarely, if ever, seen in tetanus), hysteria, local infection (dental or in the masseter muscle) with trismus, and, on rare occasions, dislocation of the mandible leading to "lockjaw" [63].

IV. **Treatment.** All the following treatment modalities should be instituted [60–62].
A. **Human tetanus immunoglobulin** (TIG) should be administered intramuscularly as soon as possible, although its efficacy is controversial [63]. A dose of 500 units may be as effective as the larger doses (≥ 3,000 units). No advantage has been

shown for injection of TIG into the area of the wound [61]. (In the event that TIG is not available, horse serum antitoxin may be used if intradermal tests have been done to rule out sensitivity to horse serum.)

B. **Surgical excision of the injured tissue** (site at which organisms are continuing to produce toxin) should be done if it would not be excessively mutilating.

C. **Intensive medical care** should be given in a quiet environment (the slightest disturbance may produce spasms, generalized seizures, or both). Benzodiazepines are the mainstay of treatment. To prevent spasms that last more than 5–10 seconds, diazepam is administered IV [63].

D. **Antibiotic therapy.** Often, procaine penicillin, 1.2 million units, has been given once daily, or 1.0 million units of aqueous penicillin G has been given IV q6h for 10 days in adults. Penicillin is no longer the drug of choice [63]. A prospective, open, nonrandomized clinical trial was carried out to compare the efficacy of procaine penicillin (1.5 million units IM q8h) versus metronidazole (e.g., 500 mg q6h) for 7–10 days. The patients who received metronidazole had a lower mortality, a shorter hospital stay, and an improved response to therapy [66].

V. **Prognosis.** The case-fatality ratio in 1989–1990 was 17% in persons 40–49 years old and was 50% in those 80 years or older [64]. Two forms of generalized tetanus have an especially poor outlook: (1) tetanus neonatorum, resulting from use of feces or articles soiled with feces to cover the severed umbilical cord after delivery, and (2) tetanus in heroin addicts.

Decubitus Ulcers

Decubitus ulcers are cutaneous ulcerations caused by prolonged pressure that results in ischemic necrosis of the skin surface and underlying soft tissue. They are most common in patients who are allowed to lie in bed without moving and in patients with sensory defects [67]. Malnutrition, fecal and urinary incontinence, fractures, and a low serum albumin are other potential risk factors [68].

I. **Clinical characteristics.** Decubitus skin ulcers are a common, and often vexing, problem occurring in patients with vascular insufficiency, neuropathy, or immobility. If these patients are allowed to progress unattended, the following **serious complications** can ensue: (1) cellulitis and deep-tissue necrosis, (2) osteomyelitis in adjacent bone, (3) septic thrombophlebitis, and (4) bacteremia.

II. **Evaluation of the decubitus ulcer as a source of fever.** A decubitus ulcer always should be considered as a possible source of fever. Cultures of the ulcer almost invariably will yield a mixed bacterial flora of aerobes and anaerobes, but the culture will not distinguish between bacterial colonization and tissue infection. The most common organisms are staphylococci, streptococci, coliforms, and a variety of anaerobes.

There is no definable difference between the bacteriology of uncomplicated ulcers and that of ulcers associated with serious infection. Extension of the process is related to such noninfectious features as local care, severity of ischemia, trauma, and diabetes control.

The origin of a fever can often be ascribed to a decubitus ulcer if there is no other obvious site and if there is a purulent exudate containing many neutrophils and bacteria on Gram staining, along with necrotic debris. Usually, there is a surrounding cellulitis, and there may be adjacent osteomyelitis.

III. **Treatment.** The decision to use antibiotics in the treatment of a decubitus ulcer depends on the associated clinical findings. Some guidelines for prevention and treatment follow.

A. **Mattresses and beds** that improve comfort and lessen skin pressure may have a role in preventing decubitus ulcers. Many types exist, ranging from the simple and inexpensive "egg-crate" foam mattress to complex and expensive air-fluidized beds.

B. **Nutritional supplementation** with oral high-calorie preparations and parenteral mixtures of amino acids may counteract the protein loss from tissue necrosis and promote wound healing.

C. **Chronic lesions** with minimal surrounding tissue inflammation **are unlikely to benefit from systemic antibiotics,** and treatment should be directed toward local care, with particular attention to debridement of necrotic tissue.

D. **Adjacent infection** such as cellulitis, osteomyelitis, or septic episodes will require antibiotic therapy. The diagnosis of contiguous osteomyelitis is often very difficult and may require bone biopsy, because both radionuclide scans and plain roentgenograms can give false positive results [69].

E. **Colonization of the decubitus ulcer** with pathogenic bacteria, detected on culture, is not an indication for use of antibiotics unless signs of tissue infection are present.

F. **Decubitus ulcer with sepsis** is a particularly serious complication [70, 71], and the high incidence of associated anaerobic bacteremia has been recognized (see Chap. 2, under Positive Blood Cultures). Initial therapy in adults should include either clindamycin, 600 mg IV q8h, or intravenous metronidazole to cover anaerobic bacteria, particularly *B. fragilis*. **Clindamycin** also will be effective against most *S. aureus* and non–group D streptococci. A **third-generation cephalosporin** will often cover the frequently involved coliform organisms. In the patient with a protracted hospital admission and, therefore, the possibility of more resistant gram-negative organisms, an aminoglycoside can be used while awaiting cultures. We do not believe it is necessary to use antibiotics routinely to provide activity against enterococci. Imipenem-cilastatin is a consideration for monotherapy in this setting as this agent alone is active against the mixed bacteria isolated. See Chap. 28 for a discussion of these agents.

   Surgical debridement in the septic patient may be just as important as antibiotic treatment. Prophylactic antibiotics may be administered just prior to surgical debridement to prevent bloodstream invasion during the procedure.

References

1. Melish, M.E. Bacterial Skin Infections. In R.D. Feigin and J.D. Cherry (eds.), *Textbook of Pediatric Infectious Diseases* (3rd ed.). Philadelphia: Saunders, 1992. Pp. 820–824.
2. Medical Letter. Mupirocin—a new topical antibiotic. *Med. Lett. Drugs Ther.* 30:55–56, 1988.
   Mupirocin is a safe and effective topical agent for impetigo.
3. Rice, T.D., Duggan, A.K., and DeAngelis, C. Cost-effectiveness of erythromycin versus mupirocin for the treatment of impetigo in children. *Pediatrics* 89:210–214, 1992.
   Erythromycin has commonly been a preferred agent for impetigo. In this study from Johns Hopkins, children were randomly assigned to receive oral erythromycin qid (46 patients) or topical mupirocin tid (47 patients) for 10 days. **Both regimens were equally effective.** *Although the overall costs (medication plus office visits) were more for the mupirocin recipients (because of a couple of extra clinic visits to assess slow resolution of lesions in the mupirocin recipients), those receiving erythromycin were more likely to have side effects or interference with a usual daily schedule. Therefore, mupirocin may be preferred by parents. See related article by J.J. Leyden,* Clin. Pediatr. 31:549, 1992.
4. Peter, G., et al. (eds.). *1994 Red Book: Report of the Committee on Infectious Diseases* (23rd ed.). Elk Grove Village, IL: American Academy of Pediatrics, 1994. P. 436.
5. Scully, B.E., et al. Mupirocin treatment of nasal staphylococcal colonization. *Arch. Intern. Med.* 152:353–356, 1992.
   This calcium in a paraffin-based preparation, used intranasal bid for 5 days, was effective in eliminating S. aureus *nasal carriage in medical staff at Columbia University College of Physicians and Surgeons. All 34 recipients of mupirocin tolerated this agent well.*
6. Klempner, M.S., and Styrt, B. Prevention of recurrent staphylococcal skin infections with low-dose oral clindamycin therapy. *J.A.M.A.* 260:2682–2685, 1988.
   A 3-month course of low-dose oral clindamycin prevented recurrent staphylococcal skin abscesses in 82% of patients during the treatment period.
7. Fitzgerald, R.H., and Cowan, J.D.E. Puncture wounds of the foot. *Orthop. Clin. North Am.* 6:965, 1975.
   Review of proper evaluation and treatment of puncture wounds.
8. Raz, R., and Miron, D. Oral ciprofloxacin for treatment of infection following nail puncture wounds of the foot. *Clin. Infect. Dis.* 21:194, 1995.
   In this report from Israel, 23 adult patients did well with a combination of surgical debridement and oral ciprofloxacin (750 mg PO bid). Culture data revealed P. aeruginosa *in only 18 patients and* S. aureus *in only 1 patient. Two patients had* S. aureus *alone and were susceptible to ciprofloxacin. Two cases had no isolated pathogens.*
9. Goldstein, E.J.C. Bite wounds and infection. *Clin. Infect. Dis.* 14:633, 1992.

Excellent state-of-the-art clinical review. For a related update, see E.J.C. Goldstein, Bites. In G.L. Mandell, J.E. Bennett, and R. Dolin (eds.), Principles and Practice of Infectious Diseases (4th ed.). New York: Churchill Livingstone, 1995. Pp. 2765–2769.

10. Hicklin, H., Verghese, A., and Alvarez, S. Dysgonic fermenter 2 septicemia. *Rev. Infect. Dis.* 9:884–890, 1987.
    DF-2 infection must be in the differential diagnosis of any splenectomized patient who develops life-threatening sepsis in combination with disseminated intravascular coagulation and peripheral gangrene.

11. Centers for Disease Control. Rabies prevention—United States, 1991. *M.M.W.R.* 40(RR-3):1–19, 1991.
    Updated recommendations from the Immunization Practices Advisory Committee for rabies prevention reflect the availability of the new rabies vaccine adsorbed (RVA). See also the related report from the Centers for Disease Control, Compendium of animal rabies control, 1994: National Association of State Public Health Veterinarians, Inc. M.M.W.R. 43(RR-10):1–9, 1994.

12. Fishbein, D.B., and Robinson, L.E. Rabies. *N. Engl. J. Med.* 329:1632–1638, 1993.
    Recent review of this topic.

13. Rosenthal, K.E., and Thornton, G.F. The 10 most common questions about rabies. *Infect. Dis. Clin. Pract.* 3:44–48, 1994.
    Up-to-date practical guidelines for both preexposure and postexposure rabies prophylaxis.

14. Meyers, J.D., et al. Multicenter collaborative trial of intravenous acyclovir for treatment of mucocutaneous herpes simplex virus infection in the immunocompromised host. *Am. J. Med.* 73(1A):229–235, 1982.
    Intravenous acyclovir decreased the time to cessation of pain, termination of viral shedding, and lesion healing.

15. Shepp, D.H., et al. Oral acyclovir therapy for mucocutaneous herpes simplex virus infection in immunocompromised recipients. *Ann. Intern. Med.* 102:783–785, 1985.

16. Whitley, R.J., and Gnann, J.W., Jr. Acyclovir: A decade later. *N. Engl. J. Med.* 327:782–789, 1992.
    An excellent review.

17. Rooney, J.F., et al. Oral acyclovir to suppress frequently recurrent herpes labialis: A double-blind placebo-controlled trial. *Ann. Intern. Med.* 118:268, 1993.

18. Wallace, M.R., et al. Treatment of adult varicella with oral acyclovir. A randomized placebo-controlled trial. *Ann. Intern. Med.* 117:358–363, 1992.

19. Brunell, P.A. Chickenpox: Examining our options. *N. Engl. J. Med.* 325:1577–1579, 1991.

20. Balfour, H.H., Jr. Intravenous acyclovir therapy for varicella in immunocompromised children. *J. Pediatr.* 104:134–136, 1984.
    A study of eight immunocompromised patients with varicella, which suggests that there is benefit of early administration of acyclovir. In four children who were treated with acyclovir within 2 days of onset of rash, the disease resolved quickly, whereas the other four who were treated after 5 days of onset of rash had progressive disease.

21. Committee on Infectious Diseases. Recommendations for the use of live attenuated varicella vaccine. *Pediatrics* 95:791, 1995.
    See also Medical Letter. Varicella vaccine. Med. Lett. Drugs Ther. 37:55, 1995.

22. Wood, M.J., et al. A randomized trial of acyclovir for 7 days or 21 days with and without prednisolone for treatment of acute herpes zoster. *N. Engl. J. Med.* 330:896–900, 1994.
    For acute herpes zoster in nonimmunocompromised adults, initiation of a 21-day course of oral acyclovir therapy within 72 hours of onset of rash along with prednisolone conferred no major advantage over the standard 7-day regimen of acyclovir. Neither additional acyclovir nor prednisolone reduced the frequency of postherpetic neuralgia.

23. Whitley, R., and Straus, S. Therapy for varicella-zoster virus infections: Where do we stand? *Infect. Dis. Clin. Pract.* 2:100–108, 1993.

24. McKendrick, W.M., et al. Oral acyclovir in acute herpes zoster. *Br. Med. J.* 293:1529–1534, 1986.

25. Bean, B., Braun, C., and Balfour, H.H., Jr. Acyclovir therapy for acute herpes zoster. *Lancet* 2:118–121, 1982.
    There was some benefit of intravenous acyclovir for herpes zoster in otherwise healthy adults.

26. Gilden, D.H. Herpes zoster with postherpetic neuralgia—persisting pain and frustration [editorial]. *N. Engl. J. Med.* 330:932–933, 1994.

Emphasizes that higher doses of acyclovir may reduce postherpetic neuralgia in the elderly, but the necessity of using the intravenous route is a disadvantage. New oral agents with enhanced bioavailability may surmount this problem.

27. Straus, S.E. Shingles. Sorrows, salves and solutions. *J.A.M.A.* 269:1836, 1993.
    Recent review of this topic.
28. Balfour, H.H., Jr., et al. Acyclovir halts progression of herpes zoster in immunocompromised patients. *N. Engl. J. Med.* 308:1448–1453, 1983.
    A prospective, double-blind, randomized, placebo-controlled trial demonstrating that acyclovir was able to halt progression of herpes zoster virus in immunosuppressed patients.
29. Huerter, C.J., Alvarez, L., and Stinson, R. Orf: Case report and literature review. *Cleve. Clin. J. Med.* 58:531–534, 1991.
    Case report of an infected sheep farmer with review of literature. Emphasizes clinical clues to assist in diagnosis and avoid unnecessary surgery or extensive diagnostic evaluation.
30. Swartz, M.N. Cellulitis and subcutaneous infections. In G.L. Mandell, J.E. Bennett, and R. Dolin (eds.), *Principles and Practice of Infectious Diseases* (4th ed.). New York: Churchill Livingstone, 1995. Pp. 909–929.
    Topics include streptococcal, staphylococcal, coliform, and Corynebacterium diphtheriae *skin infections.*
31. Stevens, D.L., et al. Severe group A streptococcal infections associated with a toxic shock–like syndrome and scarlet fever toxin A. *N. Engl. J. Med.* 321:1–7, 1989.
    Reports a cluster of 20 patients in the Rocky Mountain region who had severe streptococcal infections with local tissue destruction and life-threatening systemic toxicity.
32. Stevens, D.L. Invasive group A streptococcus infections. *Clin. Infect. Dis.* 14:2–13, 1992.
    State-of-the-art review of the reemergence of severe group A streptococcus infections including bacteremia, myositis, necrotizing fasciitis, and toxic shock syndrome.
33. Demers, B., et al. Severe invasion group A streptococcal infections in Ontario, Canada: 1987–1991. Clin. Infect. Dis. *16:792, 1993.*
    Summary of 50 cases. See also the editorial response. For a related discussion, see A.L. Forni et al., Clinical and microbiological characteristics of severe group A streptococcus infections and streptococcal toxic shock syndrome. Clin. Infect. Dis. *21:333, 1995.*
34. Working Group on Severe Streptococcal Infections. Defining group A streptococcal toxic shock syndrome. Rationale and consensus definition. *J.A.M.A. 269:390, 1993.*
    See companion article which indicates that in a study from Arizona, an underlying fasciitis was not a common finding in STSS.
35. Wilson, G.J., et al. Group A streptococcal necrotizing fasciitis following varicella in children: Case reports and review. *Clin. Infect. Dis.* 20:1933, 1995.
    See related paper by C.L. Peterson et al., Risk factors for invasive group A streptococcal infections in children with varicella: A case-control study. Pediatr. Infect. Dis. 15: 151, 1996, *and preceding article.*
36. Farley, M.M., et al. A population based assessment of invasive disease due to group B streptococci in nonpregnant adults. *N. Engl. J. Med.* 328:1807, 1995.
    See related editorial comment in same issue. Cellulitis, foot ulcers, and decubitus ulcers accounted for 36% of the infections reported in this series. Remember that penicillin/ampicillin, cephalosporins (see Chap. 28F), and vancomycin are active against group B streptococci.
37. Drapkin, M.S., et al. Bacteremic *Haemophilus influenzae* type b cellulitis in the adult. *Am. J. Med.* 63:449–452, 1977.
    Haemophilus influenzae type b should be considered in the differential diagnosis of any adult with cellulitis of the neck or upper chest and upper respiratory tract infection.
38. Roberts, R., et al. Erysipelaslike lesions and hyperesthesia as manifestations of *Pseudomonas aeruginosa* sepsis. *J.A.M.A.* 248:2156–2157, 1982.
    Physicians should be aware of the variety of cutaneous manifestations of Pseudomonas aeruginosa *sepsis, including cellulitis and erysipelaslike lesions with hyperesthesia.*
39. Clark, R.A.F., and Hopkins, T.T. The Other Eczemas. In S.L. Moschella and H.J. Hurley (eds.), *Dermatology* (3rd ed.). Philadelphia: Saunders, 1992. Pp. 473–476.
40. Klontz, K.C., et al. Syndrome of *Vibrio vulnificus* infections: Clinical and epidemiologic features in Florida cases, 1981–1987. *Ann. Intern. Med.* 109:318–323, 1988.
    See editorial response. For additional discussion and references on Vibrio spp. *infections, see Chap. 2 in this text.*
41. Walling, D.M., and Kaelin, W.G., Jr. Pyomyositis in patients with diabetes mellitus. *Rev. Infect. Dis.* 13:797–802, 1991.

Report of two cases of pyomyositis in patients with diabetes mellitus in the United States. Includes good review of the spectrum of this condition.

42. Jones, S.R. Diagnosis: Familial Mediterranean Fever [FMF]. *Clin. Infect. Dis.* 20:1547, 1995.
    One of the "photo-quiz" series. Contains nice color photo. Skin lesion may appear to be a "routine" cellulitis.

43. Hook, E.W., III, et al. Microbiologic evaluation of cutaneous cellulitis in adults. *Arch. Intern. Med.* 146:295–297, 1986.
    Aspiration cultures and skin biopsy cultures of the advancing edge of a cellulitis have a low yield.

44. Kielhofner, M.A., Brown, B., and Dall, L. Influence of underlying disease process on the utility of cellulitis needle aspirates. *Arch. Intern. Med.* 148:2451–2452, 1988.
    Needle aspirate of the leading edge of cellulitis was more likely to be positive in patients with either diabetes mellitus or malignancy.

45. Dunavel, T., et al. Quantitative cultures of biopsy specimens from cutaneous cellulitis. *Arch. Intern. Med.* 149:293–296, 1989.
    Central and peripheral biopsy cultures of cellulitis had a combined positive rate of only 18%.

46. Sachs, M.K. The optimum use of needle aspiration in the bacteriologic diagnosis of cellulitis in adults. *Arch. Intern. Med.* 150:1907–1912, 1990.
    Needle aspirate of the leading edge of cellulitis yielded pathogenic organisms in only 15% of patients. Although the yield is low, needle aspirate should be considered if knowledge of the organism is essential, initial antibiotic therapy has failed, or unusual pathogens are suspected.

47. Gregory, D.W., and Schaffner, W. *Pseudomonas* infections associated with hot tubs and other environments. *Infect. Dis. Clin. North Am.* 1:635–648, 1987.

48. Hay, R.J., Roberts, S.O.B., and Mackenzie, D.W.R. Mycology. In R.H. Champion, J.L. Burton, and F.J.G. Ebling (eds.), *Textbook of Dermatology* (5th ed.). London: Blackwell Scientific, 1992. P. 1151.

49. Lewis, R.T. Necrotizing soft-tissue infections. *Infect. Dis. Clin. North Am.* 6:693, 1992.

50. McHenry, C.R., et al. Determinants of mortality for necrotizing soft-tissue infections. *Ann. Surg.* 221:558, 1995.
    Emphasizes that early debridement was associated with a significant decrease in mortality. S. pyogenes infection was the most common cause of monomicrobial infection but was not associated with an excess mortality rate.

51. Stevens, D.L., et al. Evaluation of therapy with hyperbaric oxygen for experimental infection with *Clostridium perfringens. Clin. Infect. Dis.* 17:231, 1993.
    Interesting mouse model in which the efficacies of therapy with penicillin, metronidazole, or clindamycin, alone and in combination with hyperbaric oxygen, were compared. See two editorial responses in the same issue. The role of hyperbaric oxygen awaits further study.

52. Chow, A.W., Roser, S.M., and Brady, F.A. Orofacial odontogenic infections. *Ann. Intern. Med.* 88:392–402, 1978.
    Excellent review with discussion of pathogenesis, anatomic sites of infection, and variable clinical syndromes.

53. Chow, A.W., and Whiting, J.L. Life-threatening infections of the mouth and throat. *J. Crit. Illness* 2:36–58, 1987.
    Another excellent review with contemporary recommendations for antimicrobial regimens.

54. Jacobs, T.E., Irwin, R.S., and Raptopoulos, V. Severe Upper Airway Infections. In J.M. Rippe, R.S. Irwin, J.S. Alpert, and M.P. Fink (eds.), *Intensive Care Medicine* (2nd ed.). Boston: Little, Brown, 1991. Pp. 698–706.
    Contains an excellent discussion of the pathophysiology and anatomic considerations of deep cervical neck infections. Clear diagrams.

55. Chow, A.W. Life-threatening infections of the head and neck. *Clin. Infect. Dis.* 14: 991, 1992.
    "State-of-the-art" clinical article. Contains excellent figures of the anatomical issues.

56. Sinave, C.P., Hardy, G.J., and Fardy, P.W. The Lemierre syndrome: Suppurative thrombophlebitis of the internal jugular vein secondary to oropharyngeal infection. *Medicine* 68:85–94, 1989.
    Comprehensive review.

57. Dagan, R., and Powell, K.R. Postanginal sepsis following infectious mononucleosis. *Arch. Intern. Med.* 147:1581–1583, 1987.
    Routine cases of infectious mononucleosis can be followed by this serious complication.

58. Centers for Disease Control. Progress towards elimination of *Haemophilus influenzae* b disease among infants and children—United States, 1987–1993. *M.M.W.R.* 43: 144, 1994.
    Report documents marked decline in the incidence of invasive disease in children younger than 5 years in the United States since the introduction of Hib conjugate vaccines in 1988.
59. Stevens, D.L., Gibbons, A.E., Bergstrom, R., and Winn, V. The Eagle effect revisited: Efficacy of clindamycin, erythromycin and penicillin in the treatment of streptococcal myositis. *J. Infect. Dis.* 158:23–28, 1988.
60. Weinstein, L. Tetanus. *N. Engl. J. Med.* 289:1293–1296, 1974.
    A classic paper.
61. Bleck, T. *Clostridium tetani.* In G.L. Mandell, J.E. Bennett, and R. Dolin (eds.), *Principles and Practice of Infectious Diseases* (4th ed.). New York: Churchill Livingstone, 1995. Pp. 2173–2179.
    An excellent clinical discussion with detailed guidelines for therapy.
62. Bleck, T.P. Tetanus: Pathophysiology, management and prophylaxis. *Dis. Mon.* 37(9):545, 1991.
    Monograph devoted to this topic.
63. Sanford, J. Tetanus—Forgotten but not gone. *N. Engl. J. Med.* 332:812, 1995.
    Editorial comment on reference [65]. Nice concise discussion of tetanus.
64. Centers for Disease Control. Tetanus surveillance—United States, 1989–1990. *M.M.W.R.* [CDC Surveillance Summary] 41(8):1, 1992.
    Emphasizes the risk of tetanus in the elderly, especially those older than 80.
65. Gergen, P.J., et al. A population-based serologic survey of immunity to tetanus in the United States. *N. Engl. J. Med.* 332:761, 1995.
    Many Americans—especially the elderly—do not have immunity to tetanus.
66. Ahmadsyah, I., and Salim, A. Treatment of tetanus: An open study to compare the efficacy of procaine penicillin and metronidazole. *Br. Med. J.* 291:648–650, 1985.
    In this study from Indonesia, 76 patients received procaine penicillin and 97 patients received metronidazole. The authors concluded that metronidazole was more efficacious than penicillin in the treatment of tetanus.
67. Reuler, J.B., and Cooney, T.G. The pressure sore: Pathophysiology and principles of management. *Ann. Intern. Med.* 94:661–666, 1981.
    Excellent review.
68. Medical Letter. Treatment of pressure ulcers. *Med. Lett. Drugs Ther.* 32:17–18, 1990.
69. Sugarman, B. Pressure sores and underlying bone infection. *Arch. Intern. Med.* 147:553–555, 1987.
    Bone biopsy often is required for this diagnosis because radionuclide scans and plain roentgenograms may be falsely positive.
70. Bryan, C.S., Dew, C.E., and Reynolds, K.L. Bacteremia associated with decubitus ulcers. *Arch. Intern. Med.* 143:2093–2095, 1983.
    In-depth 5-year study of decubitus ulcer sepsis at four hospitals in one metropolitan area.
71. Montgomerie, J.Z., et al. Low mortality among patients with spinal cord injury and bacteremia. *Rev. Infect. Dis.* 13:867, 1991.
    In 103 episodes of bacteremia from 93 patients with spinal cord injury, infected pressure sores were the primary source in 19% of patients, second to urinary tract infections (47%).

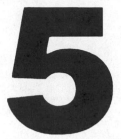

Central Nervous System Infections

Allan R. Tunkel
and W. Michael Scheld

Meningitis

Meningitis is defined as inflammation of the meninges that is identified by an abnormal number of white blood cells in the cerebrospinal fluid (CSF). The meningitis syndrome may be caused by a wide variety of infectious agents and may also be a manifestation of noninfectious diseases (Table 5-1). Here, we review the common infectious causes of meningitis, with particular emphasis on epidemiology and etiology, clinical presentation, diagnosis, treatment, and prevention.

I. **Epidemiology and etiology**

A. **Viruses.** Viruses are the major cause of the **acute aseptic meningitis syndrome,** a term used to define any meningitis (infectious or noninfectious), particularly one with a lymphocytic pleocytosis, for which a cause is not apparent after initial evaluation and routine stains and cultures of CSF [1, 2]. From 1982 through 1988, 8,300–12,700 cases of aseptic meningitis were reported to the Centers for Disease Control (CDC) annually, although these figures likely underestimate the importance of this syndrome as not all cases are reported and cases with a nonviral etiology are not reported as aseptic meningitis. The common viral etiologic agents that cause the acute aseptic meningitis syndrome are as follows:

1. **Enteroviruses.** Enteroviruses are currently the leading recognizable cause of the aseptic meningitis syndrome, accounting for 80–85% of all cases in which a pathogen is identified [2, 2a]. Enteroviruses are worldwide in distribution and are spread by the fecal-oral route; periods of warm weather and sparse clothing may facilitate spread of these organisms. Enteroviruses may also be recovered from houseflies, wastewater, and sewage [2, 3]. The predominant enteroviruses isolated from patients with meningitis during the years 1970–1983 in the United States were (in decreasing order) echovirus 11; echovirus 9; coxsackievirus B5; echoviruses 30, 4, and 6; coxsackieviruses B2, B4, B3, and A9; echoviruses 3, 7, 5, and 21; and coxsackievirus B1 [4].

   Infants and young children are the host populations most susceptible to enteroviral meningitis because there is absence of previous exposure and immunity. In one large cohort study from Finland, children younger than 1 year had an annual incidence of viral meningitis of 219 cases per 100,000 population versus an incidence of 19 cases per 100,000 population in children between the ages of 1 and 4 years [5]. Immunodeficiency and possibly physical exercise also predispose to enteroviral meningitis [2].

2. **Arboviruses.** The most common vector-transmitted cause of aseptic meningitis is St. Louis encephalitis virus, a flavivirus [2, 6]. Aseptic meningitis accounts for approximately 15% of all symptomatic cases of St. Louis encephalitis and may be as high as 35–60% in children. These infections are more common in warmer months when contact with the insect vector is more likely. Other arboviruses reported to cause aseptic meningitis include the California encephalitis group of viruses (e.g., La Crosse, Jamestown Canyon, and Snowshoe hare viruses, which are bunyaviruses) and the agent of Colorado tick fever, an orbivirus, which is seen in mountain and western regions of the United States and Canada [7].

3. **Mumps virus.** Infection with mumps virus commonly occurs in the winter and spring months, although the incidence of mumps has decreased markedly with widespread use of the attenuated live virus vaccine (from 76.3 cases per 100,000 population in 1968 to 2.1 cases per 100,000 population in 1988) [2, 8, 9]. CNS disease caused by mumps virus can occur in patients without evidence of

Table 5-1. Differential diagnosis of the meningitis syndrome

Infectious etiologies
Bacteria

Haemophilus influenzae
Neisseria meningitidis
Streptococcus pneumoniae
Listeria monocytogenes[a]
Streptococcus agalactiae
Aerobic gram-negative bacilli
Staphylococci
Other streptococci
Anaerobes
Pasteurella multocida
Leuconostoc spp.
Stomatococcus mucilaginosus
Brucella spp.[a]
Chlamydia psittaci
Chlamydia trachomatis
Mycoplasma pneumoniae[a]
Mycoplasma hominis[a]
Ureaplasma urealyticum
Nocardia spp.[a]
Actinomyces spp.[a]
Mycobacterium tuberculosis[a]

Viruses

Nonpolio enteroviruses[a,b]
Mumps virus[a]
Arboviruses[a,c]
Herpesviruses[a,d]
Lymphocytic choriomeningitis virus[a]
Human immunodeficiency virus[a]
Adenovirus[a]
Influenza A and B viruses[a]
Parainfluenza viruses
Measles virus (rubeola)[a]
Rubella virus (German measles)[a]
Poliovirus[a]
Rotavirus
Encephalomyocarditis virus
Vaccinia virus (cowpox)[a]

Fungi

Cryptococcus neoformans[a]
Candida spp.[e]
Coccidioides immitis[e]
Histoplasma capsulatum[a,e]
Aspergillus spp.[e]
Blastomyces dermatitidis[e]
Sporothrix schenckii[e]
Paracoccidioides brasiliensis[e]
Pseudallescheria boydii[e]
Cladosporium spp.[e]
Zygomycetes spp.[e]

Spirochetes

Treponema pallidum (syphilis)[a]
Borrelia burgdorferi (Lyme disease)[a]
Leptospira spp.[a]
Borrelia recurrentis (relapsing fever)[a]
Spirillum minor (rat-bite fever)

Rickettsiae

Rickettsia rickettsii (Rocky Mountain spotted fever)[a]
Coxiella burnetii (Q fever)
Rickettsia prowazekii (epidemic or louse-borne typhus)[a]
Rickettsia typhi (endemic or murine typhus)[a]
Rickettsia tsutsugamushi (scrub typhus)[a]
Ehrlichia spp.[a]

Protozoa and helminths

Naegleria fowleri[a]
Acanthamoeba spp.[a,e]
Angiostrongylus cantonensis
Toxoplasma gondii[a,e]
Taenia solium (cysticercosis)[e]
Trichinella spiralis[e]
Trypanosoma spp[a,e]
Paragonimus spp[e]
Echinococcus granulosus[e]
Strongyloides stercoralis (hyperinfection syndrome)[e]
Schistosoma spp.[e]
Entamoeba histolytica[e]
Gnathostoma spinigerum[e]
Multiceps multiceps[e]

Algae

Prototheca wickerhamii

Other infectious syndromes

Parameningeal foci of infection[f]
Infective endocarditis[a]
Bacterial toxins[g]
Viral postinfectious syndromes
Postvaccination[h]

Noninfectious etiologies and diseases of unknown etiology
Systemic illnesses

Systemic lupus erythematosus
Sarcoidosis
Behçet's disease[a]
Sjögren's syndrome
Mixed connective tissue disease
Rheumatoid arthritis
Polymyositis
Wegener's granulomatosis
Lymphomatoid granulomatosis
Polyarteritis nodosa
Granulomatous angiitis
Other cerebral vasculitides
Familial Mediterranean fever
Kawasaki's syndrome
Vogt-Koyanagi-Harada syndrome

Table 5-1 (continued)

Noninfectious etiologies and diseases of unknown etiology (cont.)

Medications
  Antimicrobial agents[i]
  Nonsteroidal antiinflammatory agents[j]
  Muromonab-CD3 (OKT3)
  Azathioprine
  Cytosine arabinoside (high-dose)
  Carbamazepine[k]
  Immunoglobulin[l]
  Phenazopyridine

Procedure-related
  Postneurosurgery
  Spinal anesthesia
  Intrathecal injections[m]
  Chymopapain injection

Miscellaneous
  Seizures
  Migraine or migrainelike syndromes
  Mollaret's meningitis
  Serum sickness
  Heavy metal poisoning

Malignancies
  Lymphomatous meningitis
  Carcinomatous meningitis
  Leukemia

Intracranial tumors and cysts
  Craniopharyngioma
  Dermoid or epidermoid cyst
  Pituitary adenoma
  Astrocytoma
  Glioblastoma multiforme
  Medulloblastoma
  Pinealoma
  Ependymoma
  Teratoma

---

[a]May also present as encephalitis.
[b]Primarily echoviruses and coxsackieviruses.
[c]In the United States, the major etiologic agents are the mosquito-borne California, St. Louis, Eastern equine, Western equine, and Venezuelan equine encephalitis viruses; and the tick-borne Colorado tick fever.
[d]Primarily herpes simplex virus type 2, but also herpes simplex virus type 1, varicella-zoster virus, cytomegalovirus, Epstein-Barr virus, and human herpesvirus-6.
[e]More commonly presents as chronic meningitis or focal CNS lesions.
[f]Brain abscess, sinusitis, otitis, mastoiditis, subdural abscess, epidural abscess, venous sinus thrombophlebitis, pituitary abscess, cranial osteomyelitis.
[g]Scarlet fever, streptococcal pharyngitis, toxic shock syndrome, pertussis, diphtheria.
[h]Mumps, measles, polio, pertussis, rabies, vaccinia.
[i]Trimethoprim, sulfamethoxazole, trimethoprim-sulfamethoxazole, ciprofloxacin, penicillin, isoniazid.
[j]Ibuprofen, sulindac, naproxen, tolmetin.
[k]In patients with connective tissue diseases.
[l]**Aseptic meningitis can occur after high-dose intravenous immunoglobulin.** For a review of this topic, see E. A. Sekul et al. Aseptic meningitis associated with high-dose intravenous immune globulin therapy: Frequency and risk factors. *Ann. Intern. Med.* 121:259, 1994. See also the editorial comment in same issue of *Ann. Intern. Med.,* and F. C. DeVlieghere et al. Aseptic granulocytopenic meningitis following treatment with intravenous gammaglobulin. *Clin. Inject. Dis.* 18:1008, 1994.
[m]Air, dyes, isotopes, antimicrobial agents, antineoplastic agents, steroids, dyes.

---

parotitis; 40–50% of patients with mumps meningitis have no evidence of salivary gland enlargement at presentation. **In an unimmunized population, mumps is one of the most common causes of aseptic meningitis and encephalitis,** with symptomatic meningitis estimated to occur in 10–30% of patients [9]. Males are affected 2–5 times more often than females, and the peak incidence is in children ages 5–9 years.

4. **Lymphocytic choriomeningitis virus.** Lymphocytic choriomeningitis virus was one of the earliest and seemingly most significant viruses to be associated with human aseptic meningitis, although it now is reported rarely as an etiologic agent [1, 2]. Lymphocytic choriomeningitis virus is transmitted to humans by contact with rodents (e.g., hamsters, rats, mice) or their excreta; the greatest risk of infection is in pet owners, persons living in impoverished and nonhygienic situations, and in laboratory workers [10]. Presumed routes of transmission are ingestion of food contaminated with animal urine and exposure of open wounds to dirt; there is no evidence of human-to-human transmission.

5. **Herpesviruses.** The herpesviruses are DNA viruses that include herpes simplex viruses (HSVs) types 1 and 2, varicella-zoster virus, cytomegalovirus (CMV), Epstein-Barr virus, human herpesvirus 6, and human herpesvirus 7.

The neurologic complications associated with the HSVs are the most significant [11]. HSVs account for nearly 0.5–3.0% of all cases of aseptic meningitis overall. The syndrome of HSV aseptic meningitis is **most commonly associated with primary genital infection with HSV type 2 [12]; meningitis is less likely with recurrences of genital herpes [13].** Primary genital infection with HSV type 1 and nonprimary genital infection with HSV of either type rarely result in meningitis [12].

Acute aseptic meningitis has also been associated with herpes zoster in patients with or without typical skin lesions [14, 15]. Single cases of Mollaret's recurrent meningitis have been associated with HSV type 1 [16] and Epstein-Barr virus [17]. Human herpesvirus 6 has also been associated with meningitis, in association with roseola infantum [18]. Cytomegalovirus and Epstein-Barr virus may cause aseptic meningitis in association with a mononucleosis syndrome, particularly in immunocompromised hosts. CMV infections of the nervous system in patients with acquired immunodeficiency syndrome (AIDS) have recently been reviewed [18a]. See related discussions in Chap. 19.

6. **Human immunodeficiency virus.** The human immunodeficiency virus (HIV) can infect the meninges early and persist in the CNS after initial infection [19]. Meningitis associated with HIV may occur as part of the primary infection or in an already infected patient; HIV has been isolated from the CSF in some of these cases [20]. However, acute meningitis does not occur in every individual who becomes infected, and it can be clinically silent. Retrospective studies have noted that 5–10% of HIV-infected patients develop an acute meningoencephalitis during or after the mononucleosislike syndrome that heralds initial infection [19, 21].

B. **Bacteria.** Bacterial meningitis remains an important problem worldwide; this topic has recently been reviewed [21a]. The overall annual attack rate for bacterial meningitis in the United States, as defined by a surveillance study of 27 states from 1978 through 1981, was approximately 3.0 cases per 100,000 population [22], although there was variability based on age, race, and gender. Furthermore, attack rates were 45.8 cases per 100,000 population in a study of 4,100 cases of bacterial meningitis at the Hospital Couta Maia in Salvador, Brazil, from 1973 through 1982 [23], indicating the importance of bacterial meningitis in this setting. Bacterial meningitis is also a significant problem in hospitalized patients. In a recent review of 493 episodes of bacterial meningitis in adults aged 16 years or older at the Massachusetts General Hospital from 1962 through 1988, 40% of episodes were nosocomial in origin, and these episodes carried a high mortality (35% for single episodes of nosocomial meningitis) [24].

The following sections review the epidemiology and etiology of specific bacterial meningeal pathogens.

1. *Haemophilus influenzae.* In the early 1980s, *H. influenzae* was isolated in 45–48% of all cases of bacterial meningitis in the United States; the overall mortality is 3–6% [22, 25]. Most cases were observed in infants and children younger than 6 years, with more than 90% caused by capsular type b strains. Isolation of this organism in older children and adults should suggest the presence of certain underlying conditions including sinusitis, otitis media, epiglottitis, pneumonia, diabetes mellitus, alcoholism, splenectomy or asplenic states, head trauma with CSF leak, and immunodeficiency (e.g., hypogammaglobulinemia) [26, 27]. **Recently, the incidence of invasive infections, specifically in young children, caused by *H. influenzae* type b in the United States has been profoundly reduced due, in part, to the recent widespread use of conjugate vaccines** against *H. influenzae* type b that have been licensed for routine use in all children beginning at 2 months of age (see sec. **VII.B.1.b**) [28].

2. *Neisseria meningitidis. N. meningitidis* most commonly causes meningitis in children and young adults, isolated in 14–20% of cases of bacterial meningitis in the United States with an overall mortality of 10–13% [22, 25]. Serotype B strains account for 51% or so of meningeal isolates, usually occurring in sporadic outbreaks. Disease caused by serogroups A and C may occur in epidemics, and type Y strains may be associated with pneumonia. **Patients with deficiencies in the terminal complement components** (C5, C6, C7, C8, and perhaps C9), the so-called membrane attack complex, **have a markedly increased incidence of neisserial infections,** including that caused by *N. meningitidis,* although case fatality rates in meningococcal disease are lower than in patients with an intact complement system (3% versus 19% in the general population) [29].

3. **Streptococcus pneumoniae.** Pneumococcal meningitis is most frequently observed in adults, accounting for 13–17% of total cases in the United States and carrying a mortality of 19–26% [22, 25]. Patients often have contiguous or distant foci of pneumococcal infection such as pneumonia, otitis media, mastoiditis, sinusitis, and endocarditis. Serious infection may be observed in patients with various underlying conditions, including splenectomy or asplenic states, multiple myeloma, hypogammaglobulinemia, alcoholism, malnutrition, chronic liver or renal disease, malignancy, and diabetes mellitus [30, 31]. The pneumococcus is the most common etiologic agent of meningitis in patients who have suffered a basilar skull fracture with CSF leak [32].

4. **Listeria monocytogenes.** L. monocytogenes causes only 2–3% of cases of bacterial meningitis in the United States but carries a high mortality (22–29%) [22, 25]. Serotypes Ia, Ib, and IVb have been implicated in up to 90% of meningitis cases caused by this organism. Listerial infection is **most common in neonates** (up to 10% of cases); pregnant women may harbor the organism asymptomatically in their genital tract and rectum and transmit the infection to their infants. **Other predisposing conditions include** the elderly, alcoholics, cancer patients, immunosuppressed adults (e.g., renal transplant recipients), and patients with diabetes mellitus, liver disease, chronic renal disease, collagen vascular diseases, and conditions associated with iron overload [33, 34]. *Listeria* meningitis is found only infrequently in patients with HIV infection [35, 36], despite its increased incidence in patients with deficiencies of cell-mediated immunity. Meningitis can also occur in previously healthy adults [37].

5. **Streptococcus agalactiae.** The group B streptococcus is a **common** cause of meningitis **in neonates** [38]. In the United States, this organism accounts for 3–6% of cases of bacterial meningitis, with a mortality ranging from 12 to 27% [22, 25]. The risk of transmission from the mother to her infant is increased when the inoculum of organisms and number of sites of maternal colonization is high; the group B streptococcus has been isolated from vaginal or rectal cultures of 15–40% of asymptomatic pregnant women [39]. Horizontal transmission has also been documented from the hands of nursery personnel to the infant. Most cases of neonatal meningitis are caused by subtype III organisms and occur after the first week of life. The group B streptococcus can also cause meningitis in adults and appears to be increasing in frequency [40, 41]. Risk factors for adults include age beyond 60 years, diabetes mellitus, parturient women, cardiac disease, collagen vascular diseases, malignancy, alcoholism, hepatic failure, renal failure, and corticosteroid therapy; no underlying illnesses were found in 43% of patients [41].

6. **Aerobic gram-negative bacilli.** The aerobic gram-negative bacilli (e.g., *Klebsiella* spp., *Escherichia coli, Serratia marcescens, Pseudomonas aeruginosa, Salmonella* spp.) have become increasingly important etiologic agents in patients with bacterial meningitis [42, 43]. Meningitis caused by these agents has occurred **following head trauma or neurosurgical procedures** and may also be found **in neonates, the elderly, immunosuppressed patients, and patients with gram-negative septicemia.** Some cases have been associated with disseminated strongyloidiasis in the hyperinfection syndrome, in which meningitis caused by enteric bacteria occurs secondary to seeding of the meninges during persistent or recurrent bacteremias associated with the migration of infective larvae [44]. Alternatively, the larvae may carry enteric organisms on their surfaces or within their own GI tracts as they exit the intestine and subsequently invade the meninges.

7. **Staphylococci.** Meningitis caused by *Staphylococcus aureus* usually is found in early postneurosurgical or posttrauma patients as well as in those with CSF shunts [45, 46]. Rarely, *S. aureus* meningitis has occurred as an infectious complication of a temporary epidural catheter [46a]. Other underlying conditions include diabetes mellitus, alcoholism, chronic renal failure requiring hemodialysis, injection drug abuse, and malignancies. Thirty-five percent of cases are observed in the setting of head trauma or after neurosurgery, and an additional 20% of patients have underlying infective endocarditis or paraspinal infection. Other sources of community-acquired *S. aureus* meningitis include patients with sinusitis, osteomyelitis, and pneumonia. Mortality from *S. aureus* meningitis has ranged from 14 to 77% in various series. *Staphylococcus epidermidis* is the most common cause of meningitis in patients with CSF shunts [46].

8. **Other bacteria.** *Nocardia* **meningitis** usually occurs in the setting of certain predisposing conditions, including immunosuppressive drug therapy, malignancy, head trauma, CNS procedures, chronic granulomatous disease, and sarcoidosis [47]. **Enterococci** are unusual pathogens [47a]. **Anaerobic meningitis** is unusual and generally is associated with contiguous foci of infection (e.g., otitis, sinusitis, pharyngitis, brain abscess, head and neck malignancy, recent head and neck surgery or wound infection, posttrauma, postneurosurgery) [48, 49]. In many cases, more than one organism may be recovered. **Diphtheroids** have become important etiologic agents of meningitis in patients with CNS shunt infections [46]. Streptococcal meningitis has occurred after diagnostic myelography [49a].

C. **Tuberculosis.** Virtually all mycobacterial infections of the CNS are caused by the tubercle bacillus, *Mycobacterium tuberculosis*. Tuberculous meningitis accounts for approximately 15% of extrapulmonary cases or approximately 0.7% of all clinical tuberculosis in the United States [50]. A disproportionately increased rate of CNS tuberculosis occurs in the U.S. homeless population and in nonwhite Americans. Most cases have been reported in children during the first 5 years of life, although infection is uncommon among those younger than 6 months. Other factors such as advanced age, immunosuppressive drug therapy, lymphoma, gastrectomy, pregnancy, diabetes mellitus, and alcoholism also compromise the immune response, leading to reactivation in patients with smoldering chronic organ tuberculosis [51].

HIV infection has influenced the epidemiology of tuberculosis in the United States. Extrapulmonary disease occurs in more than 70% of patients with AIDS (or AIDS is discovered soon after the diagnosis of tuberculosis) but in only 24–45% of patients with tuberculosis and less advanced HIV infection [52].

D. **Spirochetes**

1. ***Treponema pallidum.*** *T. pallidum* disseminates to the CNS during early infection. The organism can be isolated from the CSF of patients with primary syphilis, and CSF laboratory abnormalities are detected in 5–9% of patients with seronegative primary syphilis [53]. However, the actual rate of invasion of the CNS during these early stages is likely to be considerably higher. Clinical neurosyphilis can be divided into four distinct syndromes: syphilitic meningitis, meningovascular syphilis, parenchymatous neurosyphilis, and gummatous neurosyphilis. The incidence of syphilitic meningitis is greatest in the first 2 years following initial infection and is estimated to occur in only 0.3–2.4% of patients with syphilis. In contrast, meningovascular syphilis is found in 10–12% of individuals with CNS involvement, occurring months to years after syphilis acquisition (peak incidence is at approximately 7 years) [53, 54]. Parenchymatous neurosyphilis has two variants, general paresis and tabes dorsalis, which are relatively rare today and do not become apparent until 10–20 years following acquisition of infection [53]. Gummata are late manifestations of tertiary syphilis and may occur anywhere, although gummatous neurosyphilis is rare.

   The overall incidence of neurosyphilis has recently increased in association with HIV infection [55, 56]. In one report, 44% of all patients with neurosyphilis had AIDS and 1.5% of AIDS patients were found to have neurosyphilis at some point during the course of their disease [57]. See related discussions of syphilis in Chaps. 13 and 19.

2. ***Borrelia burgdorferi.*** *B. burgdorferi* is the major etiologic agent of Lyme disease. The nervous system eventually is involved clinically in at least 10–15% of patients with Lyme disease [58, 59], either while erythema migrans is still present or 1–6 months later. Utilizing polymerase chain reaction (PCR), spirochetal DNA was detected in CSF samples from 8 of 12 patients with acute (< 2 weeks) disseminated Lyme borreliosis [60], indicating that *B. burgdorferi* usually invades the CNS early in infection (see Chap. 23).

E. **Fungi**

1. ***Cryptococcus neoformans.*** *C. neoformans* is associated with bird droppings but can also be found in fruits, vegetables, milk, and soil [61]. *C. neoformans* is the most common fungal cause of clinically recognized meningitis, usually occurring in persons who are immunosuppressed. Those who are immunosuppressed include patients with reticuloendothelial malignancies (e.g., lymphoma), sarcoidosis, collagen vascular diseases (e.g., systemic lupus erythematosus), diabetes mellitus, chronic hepatic failure, or chronic renal failure, patients

who have undergone organ transplantation, and patients receiving corticosteroids [62]. *C. neoformans* meningitis has also been documented in apparently healthy individuals. **Patients with AIDS currently constitute the highest-risk group for cryptococcal meningitis;** 6–13% of AIDS patients eventually develop cryptococcal meningitis [63–65].

2. *Candida. Candida* species are normal commensals of humans. Tissue invasion usually occurs in persons with altered host defenses, including patients with malignancies, neutropenia, chronic granulomatous disease, diabetes mellitus, thermal injuries, or a central venous catheter, and in those receiving corticosteroid therapy, broad-spectrum antimicrobial agents, or hyperalimentation [66]. *Candida* meningitis is uncommon, occurring in fewer than 15% of patients with CNS candidiasis [67–69]. *C. albicans* is the species most commonly isolated in CNS disease.

3. *Coccidioides immitis. C. immitis* is endemic in the semiarid regions and the desert areas of the southwestern United States (California, Arizona, New Mexico, Texas), where approximately one-third of the population is infected. Fewer than 1% of patients will subsequently develop disseminated disease, usually within the first 6 months after initial infection. Of the patients who develop disseminated disease, one-third to one-half have meningeal involvement [70, 71]. Disseminated disease has been associated with extremes of age, male gender, nonwhite race, pregnancy, and immunosuppression (e.g., corticosteroid therapy, organ transplantation, and HIV infection).

F. **Protozoa and helminths**

1. **Amebae.** *Naegleria fowleri* is the main protozoan causing primary amebic meningoencephalitis in humans [72, 73]. Strains have been recovered from lakes, puddles, pools, ponds, rivers, sewage, sludge, tap water, air-conditioner drains, and soil. Sporadic cases of primary amebic meningoencephalitis occur when persons, usually children and young adults, swim or play in water containing the amebae, or when swimming pools or water supplies have become contaminated, often through failure of chlorination. Several cases (often caused by *Acanthamoeba* species or leptomyxid amebae) have recently been reported in HIV-infected patients [74–76], all with advanced HIV disease at the time of amebic infection.

2. *Angiostrongylus cantonensis.* Infection of humans by the larvae of the nematode *A. cantonensis* can lead to development of an eosinophilic meningitis [44, 77]. *A. cantonensis* is widespread, and human infections are fairly common, reported from many parts of the world (e.g., Thailand, India, Malaysia, Vietnam, Indonesia, Papua New Guinea, and the Pacific Islands including Hawaii). The definitive hosts for the worm are rats. The parasites may spread to many countries as rats move freely from port to port on ships. The larvae invade the brain either directly from the bloodstream or after migrating through other organs before reaching the CNS. Once there, the larvae mature into adult worms that migrate through the brain.

II. **Clinical presentation**

A. **Viral meningitis**

1. **Enteroviruses.** The clinical manifestations of enteroviral meningitis depend on host age and immune status [2].

a. **In neonates** (≤ 2 weeks old), fever is a ubiquitous finding and usually is accompanied by vomiting, anorexia, rash, or upper respiratory symptoms and signs. Neurologic involvement may be associated with nuchal rigidity and a bulging anterior fontanelle, although infants younger than 1 year are less likely to demonstrate meningeal signs. Mental status may be altered, but focal neurologic signs are uncommon.

b. **In contrast,** the clinical findings of enteroviral meningitis **beyond the neonatal period** (> 2 weeks) are rarely those of severe disease and poor outcome [2, 78]. The onset of illness usually is sudden, with fever present in 76–100% of patients. More than half of the patients have nuchal rigidity. Headache (often severe and frontal in location) is nearly always present in adults; photophobia also is common. Nonspecific symptoms and signs include vomiting, anorexia, rash, diarrhea, cough, upper respiratory findings (especially pharyngitis), and myalgias. Other clues to the presence of enteroviral disease, in addition to time of year and known epidemic disease in the community, include the presence of exanthems, myopericarditis, conjunctivitis, and specifically recognizable enteroviral syndromes such as pleurodynia, herpangina, and hand-foot-and-mouth disease [1]. The duration of illness in enteroviral meningitis is usually less than 1 week, with many patients reporting improvement after the lumbar puncture [79], probably as a result of reduction of intracranial pressure.

c. In children and adults with absent or deficient humoral immunity (e.g., agammaglobulinemia), which impairs clearance of enteroviruses, chronic enteroviral meningitis or meningoencephalitis may develop and might last several years, often with a fatal outcome [80].

2. **Mumps virus.** The most frequent clinical presentation of mumps CNS infection is the nonspecific triad of fever, vomiting, and headache [9]. The fever usually is high and lasts for 3–4 days. Salivary gland enlargement is present in only 50% or so of patients. Other findings include neck stiffness, lethargy or somnolence, and abdominal pain. Most patients have signs of meningitis without evidence of cortical dysfunction. Following defervescence, there usually is clinical recovery and, in uncomplicated cases, the total duration of illness is 7–10 days. Mumps virus rarely causes encephalitis, seizures, polyradiculitis, polyneuritis, cranial nerve palsies, myelitis, Guillain-Barré syndrome, and fatality.

3. **Lymphocytic choriomeningitis virus.** Lymphocytic choriomeningitis virus infection begins with nonspecific viral symptoms and, following a brief period of improvement, approximately 15% of patients develop severe headache, photophobia, lightheadedness, lumbar myalgias, and pharyngitis [1]. Late manifestations such as orchitis, arthritis, myopericarditis, and alopecia are also seen occasionally.

4. **Herpesviruses.** Meningitis caused by HSV type 2 usually is characterized by stiff neck, headache, and fever [12]. In one review of 27 patients with HSV type 2 meningitis [13], neurologic complications were found in 37% of cases and consisted of urinary retention, dysesthesias, paresthesias, neuralgia, motor weakness, paraparesis, concentration difficulties of nearly 3 months' duration, and impaired hearing. All neurologic findings, however, subsided within 6 months in all patients. Recurrent meningitis was documented in five patients. Pharyngitis, lymphadenopathy, and splenomegaly should suggest Epstein-Barr virus infection. A diffuse vesiculopustular rash may be seen in patients with meningitis caused by varicella-zoster virus.

5. **Human immunodeficiency virus.** HIV-infected patients may present with a typical aseptic meningitis syndrome that is associated with the acute retroviral infection syndrome [19–21]. In addition, some patients may present with an atypical aseptic meningitis syndrome that often is chronic, tends to recur, and often is associated with cranial neuropathies (usually cranial nerves V, VII, and VIII) or long tract findings. The most common clinical features are headache, fever, and meningeal signs. The illness is self-limited or recurrent rather than progressive. HIV may occasionally cause a dramatic self-limited encephalitis or encephalopathy during the acute phase of infection.

B. **Bacterial meningitis**
1. **Clinical presentation.** More than 85% of patients with bacterial meningitis classically present with fever, headache, meningismus, and signs of cerebral dysfunction (i.e., confusion, delirium, or a declining level of consciousness ranging from lethargy to coma) [30, 81].

2. **Meningismus** may be subtle, marked, or accompanied by Kernig's or Brudzinski's signs. It is important to note, however, that these signs are elicited in only 50% or so of adult patients with bacterial meningitis, and their absence does not rule out the diagnosis.
   a. **Kernig's sign** is elicited with the patient in the supine position. The thigh is flexed on the abdomen, and the knee is flexed as well. The leg then is passively extended and, in the presence of meningeal inflammation, the patient resists leg extension.
   b. **Brudzinski's sign.** The best known sign described by Brudzinski is the nape-of-the-neck sign, in which passive flexion of the neck results in flexion of the hips and knees.

3. **Cranial nerve palsies** (especially involving cranial nerves III, IV, VI, and VII) and **focal cerebral signs** are seen in 10–20% of cases. **Seizures** occur in approximately 30% of patients.

   With disease progression, patients may develop signs of increased intracranial pressure including coma, hypertension, bradycardia, and palsy of cranial nerve III.

Papilledema is seen in fewer than 1% of cases early in infection, and its presence should suggest an alternative diagnosis.

4. **A specific etiologic diagnosis in patients with bacterial meningitis may be suggested by certain symptoms or signs.**
   a. **Characteristic skin rash.** For example, nearly 50% of patients with meningococcemia, with or without meningitis, present with a prominent rash located principally on the extremities [81]. The rash is typically **erythematous and macular early** in the course of illness, but quickly **evolves into a petechial phase** and then further coalesces into a purpuric form. (See Plate I A–D.) The rash often matures rapidly, with new petechial lesions appearing during the physical examination. A similar rash may also be seen in patients who have undergone splenectomy with rapidly overwhelming sepsis caused by *S. pneumoniae* or *H. influenzae* type b.
   b. **Rhinorrhea or otorrhea due to a CSF leak** may occur in patients who have suffered a basilar skull fracture in which a dural fistula is produced between the subarachnoid space and nasal cavity, the paranasal sinuses, or middle ear. In these patients, meningitis may be recurrent and is most commonly caused by *S. pneumoniae.*
   c. Patients with *L. monocytogenes* meningitis have an increased tendency to experience seizures and focal deficits early in the course of infection, and some patients may present with ataxia, cranial nerve palsies, or nystagmus due to rhomboencephalitis, although there may be no evidence of parenchymal brain involvement.

5. **Some patients may not manifest many of the classic symptoms and signs of bacterial meningitis. For example, elderly patients** with bacterial meningitis, especially those with underlying conditions (e.g., diabetes mellitus or cardiopulmonary disease), may present insidiously with lethargy or obtundation, no fever, and variable signs of meningeal inflammation [82]. **In patients with head trauma,** the symptoms and signs of meningitis may be present as a result of the underlying injury and not meningitis [32]. In all these subgroups of patients, an altered or changed mental status should not be ascribed to other causes until bacterial meningitis has been excluded by CSF examination.

C. **Tuberculous meningitis**
   1. **Children** with tuberculous meningitis commonly **present with** nausea, vomiting, and behavioral changes [50]. Headache is observed in fewer than 25% of cases. Seizures are infrequent (10–20% of cases) in children prior to hospitalization, although more than 50% may develop seizures during hospitalization. Some children develop an encephalitic course, characterized by stupor, coma, and convulsions without signs of meningitis.
   2. **Adults.** In contrast, the clinical presentation of tuberculous meningitis in adults is usually **more indolent,** with an insidious prodrome characterized by malaise, lassitude, low-grade fever, intermittent headache, and changing personality [82a]. A meningitic phase develops within 2–3 weeks, characterized by protracted headache, meningismus, vomiting, and confusion. **A history of prior clinical tuberculosis is obtained in fewer than 20% of cases** [83]. However, adult patients may also present with a rapidly progressive acute meningitis syndrome indistinguishable from pyogenic bacterial meningitis [51].
   3. **On physical examination,** fever is an inconstant finding, observed in 50–98% of cases of tuberculous meningitis [50, 84]. Meningismus and signs of meningeal irritation are also not uniform findings, being absent in 25–40% of children and adults with tuberculous meningitis. Up to 30% of patients have focal neurologic signs on presentation, most frequently consisting of unilateral or, less commonly, bilateral cranial nerve palsies. The most frequently affected is cranial nerve VI, followed by cranial nerves III, IV, and VIII. Hemiparesis may result from ischemic infarction, most commonly in the territory of the middle cerebral artery. Less frequently, abnormal movements such as chorea, hemiballismus, athetosis, myoclonus, and cerebellar ataxia may be seen on neurologic examination. Choroidal tubercles may be observed on funduscopic examination (~10% of cases).
   4. **Coexisting HIV infection.** The clinical manifestations of tuberculous meningitis do not seem to be modified significantly by HIV infection [85, 86]. Fever, headache, and altered mentation are the most frequent presenting symptoms; meningeal signs are absent in up to 50% of patients.

D. Spirochetal meningitis

1. ***Treponema pallidum.*** Patients with syphilitic meningitis usually present with complaints of headache, nausea, and vomiting. In one series these were present in 91% of patients [53]. Meningismus was seen in 59% and fever in fewer than half of patients. Seizures occurred in 17% of patients, whereas cranial nerve palsies were found in 45% of cases (most commonly cranial nerves VII and VIII, followed by II, III, V, and VI). Focal abnormalities such as hemiplegia, aphasia, or mental status changes were seen less commonly.

   Meningovascular syphilis is distinguished clinically from syphilitic meningitis temporally and on the basis of focal neurologic findings as a result of focal syphilitic arteritis, which almost always occurs in association with meningeal inflammation [53, 87]. Most patients experience weeks to months of episodic prodromal symptoms and signs that include headache or vertiginous episodes, personality changes (e.g., apathy or inattention), behavioral changes (e.g., irritability or memory impairment), insomnia, or occasional seizures. Focal deficits may also occur and, if untreated, may progress to a stroke syndrome with attendant irreversible neurologic deficits.

   Coinfection with HIV may modify the clinical course of syphilis [55–57]. Case reports and small series have suggested that patients with HIV infection are more likely to progress to neurosyphilis and to show accelerated disease courses. However, in one study of HIV-infected and noninfected patients with syphilis at sexually transmitted disease clinics in Baltimore [88], no significant differences were observed in clinical stage or in disease progression.

2. ***Borrelia burgdorferi.*** Meningitis is the most important neurologic abnormality of acute disseminated Lyme disease. Headache is the single most common symptom (30–90% of patients) in Lyme meningitis, whereas neck stiffness is seen in only 10–20% of cases [58]. Photophobia, nausea, and vomiting are intermediate in frequency between headache and neck stiffness. Approximately two-thirds of patients have accompanying systemic symptoms, including malaise, fatigue, myalgias, fever, arthralgias, and involuntary weight loss. In untreated patients, the duration of symptoms ranges from 1 to 9 months. Patients typically experience recurrent attacks of meningeal symptoms lasting several weeks, alternating with similar periods of milder symptoms.

   Approximately half of all patients with Lyme meningitis have mild cerebral symptoms, usually consisting of somnolence, emotional lability, depression, impaired memory and concentration, and behavioral symptoms [58]. These symptoms may fluctuate in severity in untreated patients before they resolve. Transverse myelitis, spastic paraparesis or quadriparesis, disturbances of micturition, and Babinski's signs also are reported rarely during this stage. Approximately 50% of patients have cranial neuropathies, facial nerve palsy being the most common (80–90%). Facial nerve palsy occurs with rapid onset (often over 1–2 days), frequently accompanied by slight ipsilateral facial numbness or tingling or ipsilateral ear or jaw pain. It is bilateral in 30–70% of cases, although the two sides are affected asynchronously in most cases. Other cranial nerves affected less commonly are cranial nerves II and III, the sensory portion of nerves V and VI, and the acoustic portion of nerve VIII. Recovery usually occurs within 2 months.

E. Fungal meningitis

1. ***Cryptococcus neoformans.*** Cryptococcal meningitis **presents differently in non-AIDS and in AIDS patients** [62–65, 89].

   a. **In non-AIDS patients,** the clinical **presentation** is typically **subacute** after days to weeks of infection. The most frequent complaint is headache; fever, meningismus, and personality changes also may occur. Approximately 50% of patients experience confusion, irritability, and other personality changes reflecting meningoencephalitis. Ocular abnormalities (e.g., papilledema and cranial nerve palsies) occur in nearly 40% of cases; direct invasion of the optic nerve also may occur.

   b. In contrast, the clinical **presentation** of cryptococcal **meningitis in AIDS** patients may be very subtle with minimal, if any, symptoms. The only clinical findings may be headache, fever, and lethargy. Meningeal signs occur in a minority of patients. Photophobia and cranial nerve palsies often are absent.

2. ***Candida.*** The onset of symptoms in *Candida* meningitis may be abrupt or insidious [67–69]. The most common symptoms are fever, headache, and menin-

gismus. Depressed mental status, confusion, cranial nerve neuropathies, and focal neurologic signs may also be seen.

3. *Coccidioides immitis.* Meningeal infection with *C. immitis* may present acutely, although it most often follows a subacute or chronic course [70, 71]. Complaints include headache, low-grade fever, weight loss, and mental status changes. Approximately 50% of patients develop disorientation, lethargy, confusion, or memory loss. Signs of meningeal irritation usually are absent, although they have been reported in as many as one-third of cases. Nausea, vomiting, focal neurologic deficits, and seizures may also occur.

F. **Protozoal and helminthic meningitis**
   1. **Amebae.** Primary amebic meningoencephalitis presents in two forms [72, 73].
      a. **Acute form.** Following an incubation period of 3–8 days, there is the sudden onset of high fever, photophobia, headache, and progression to stupor or coma. This is usually indistinguishable from acute bacterial meningitis, although focal signs and seizures are more common in amebic meningoencephalitis. Early symptoms of abnormal smell or taste may be reported because of early involvement of the olfactory area. Confusion, irritability, and restlessness progress to delirium, stupor and, finally, coma. Death in untreated patients generally occurs within 2–3 days from the onset of symptoms.
      b. **Subacute or chronic form.** Patients present more insidiously with low-grade fever, headache, and focal signs (e.g., hemiparesis, aphasia, cranial nerve palsies, visual field disturbances, diplopia, ataxia, seizures); the olfactory bulbs usually are spared. Deterioration occurs over a period of 2–4 weeks until death. However, longer durations of illness have also been reported (range, 5–18 months).
   2. *Angiostrongylus cantonensis.* Symptoms of meningitis begin 6–30 days after ingestion of raw mollusks or other sources of the parasite [44, 77]. Findings include severe headache (90%), stiff neck (56%), paresthesias (54%), and vomiting (56%). Moderate fever is present in approximately half of the cases.

III. **Diagnosis.** The diagnosis of meningitis ultimately is based on the findings in the CSF.
A. **Viral meningitis**
   1. **Enteroviruses.** CSF pleocytosis is almost always present in enteroviral meningitis [1, 2]. The cell count is usually 100–1,000/mm^3, although counts in the several thousands have also been reported; higher CSF white blood cell counts have been associated with a greater likelihood of isolating the causative enterovirus. **Neutrophils may dominate the CSF profile early in infection, although this quickly gives way to a lymphocytic predominance over the first 6–48 hours.** An elevated CSF protein and decreased CSF glucose, if present, are usually mild, although extremes of both have been reported. A specific virologic diagnosis of enteroviral meningitis depends on isolation of the virus from the CSF in tissue culture, although the sensitivity for enteroviral serotypes is only 65–75%. Isolation of a nonpolio enterovirus from the throat or rectum of a patient with aseptic meningitis is suggestive of an etiologic diagnosis, but the mean shedding periods from those sites following infection are 1 week and several weeks, respectively, so shedding from a past infection cannot be ruled out. In addition, viral shedding can occur in 7.5% of healthy controls during enterovirus epidemics [2]. Rapid diagnosis of enterovirus infections by immunoassay techniques has been hampered by the lack of a common antigen among the various serotypes and the low concentrations of virus in body fluids. Use of the PCR for detecting enteroviral RNA has also been studied, with positive results in 100% (12 of 12 subjects) in one study of patients with a clinical diagnosis of aseptic meningitis [90]. Recent advances in PCR technology promise to greatly facilitate the diagnosis of enteroviral infection [2a].
   2. **Mumps virus.** In patients with mumps meningitis, there is almost always a **CSF pleocytosis** (usually < 500/mm^3), **that is primarily mononuclear cells** (> 80% lymphocytes in 80–90% of patients) [9]. The CSF protein may be normal in more than half of patients with mumps meningitis. The CSF glucose is normal in most patients, but it may be decreased in up to 25% of cases. The most reliable serologic tests for the diagnosis of mumps are complement fixation and hemagglutination inhibition on serum specimens; testing of paired acute and convalescent sera should demonstrate a diagnostic fourfold rise in mumps antibody titer. Mumps virus can be grown from CSF in tissue culture for at least a week following the onset of disease, but sensitivity of this technique is

highly variable (30–50% if collected from CSF early during the course of mumps CNS infection). There are no rapid detection methods.

3. **Lymphocytic choriomeningitis virus.** The CSF of patients with meningitis caused by lymphocytic choriomeningitis virus typically shows a lymphocytic pleocytosis (usually $< 750/mm^3$, although counts up to several thousand may be seen) [1, 91]. Hypoglycorrhachia is seen in up to 25% of cases. No rapid detection method is available. The virus may be cultured from blood and CSF early in infection and later from urine. The diagnosis usually is made by a fourfold rise from acute to convalescent sera.

4. **Herpesviruses.** In patients with HSV type 2 meningitis, there is a lymphocytic meningitis ($< 500/mm^3$) and a normal glucose [1]. The virus has been cultured from the CSF and buffy coat of some patients. In initial studies, PCR on cerebrospinal fluid specimens appeared promising for the diagnosis of CNS infections caused by herpes simplex virus [92]. In a recent report, **PCR of CSF is now viewed as the standard for the diagnosis of herpes simplex encephalitis** [92a]. (See sec. III.A under Encephalitis.)

5. **Human immunodeficiency virus.** The CSF in HIV-infected patients typically shows a mild lymphocytic pleocytosis ($20–300/mm^3$), mildly elevated protein, and normal or slightly decreased glucose [21]. HIV has been isolated from the CSF in some patients with neurologic disease, although it can be isolated from HIV-infected patients without neurologic symptoms or signs as well [93, 94]. A few mononuclear cells and elevated protein in CSF are commonly documented in HIV-positive patients throughout the course of infection.

B. **Bacterial meningitis**

1. **Cerebrospinal fluid examination. The diagnosis of bacterial meningitis rests on CSF examination by lumbar puncture** [81, 95]. The opening pressure is elevated in virtually all cases, with values exceeding 600 mm H_2O, suggesting the presence of cerebral edema, intracranial suppurative foci, or communicating hydrocephalus.

   a. **The WBC count usually is elevated in untreated bacterial meningitis**—commonly 1,000–5,000/mm^3 (range of < 100 to $> 10,000/mm^3$) **with a neutrophilic predominance**—although approximately 10% of patients with acute bacterial meningitis present with a lymphocytic predominance in CSF. This is more common in neonatal gram-negative bacillary meningitis and meningitis caused by *L. monocytogenes* (approximately 30% of cases). Patients with very low CSF white blood cell counts ($0–20/mm^3$), despite high CSF bacterial concentrations, tend to have a poor prognosis. **In up to 4% of cases of bacterial meningitis, CSF pleocytosis will be absent [96]. CSF pleocytosis most commonly is not observed in premature neonates** (up to 15% of cases) **and in infants younger than 4 weeks** (17% of cases). **Therefore, a Gram stain and culture should be performed on all spinal fluid specimens even if the WBC count is normal.** A decreased CSF glucose concentration (< 40 mg/dl) is found in approximately 60% of patients and a CSF–serum glucose ratio of less than 0.31 in nearly 70% of patients [97]. The CSF protein is elevated in virtually all patients. Elevated CSF lactate concentrations (> 35 mg/dl) may be useful in differentiating bacterial from nonbacterial meningitis in patients who have not received prior antimicrobial therapy [98].

   b. **Gram staining of CSF** permits a rapid, accurate identification of the causative microorganism in 60–90% of patients with bacterial meningitis; the specificity is nearly 100% [97]. The likelihood of detecting the organism by Gram stain correlates with the specific bacterial pathogen and with the concentration of bacteria in CSF: Concentrations of 10^3 colony-forming units (CFU) per milliliter or fewer are associated with positive Gram stains approximately 25% of the time, whereas CSF concentrations of 10^5 CFU/ml or more lead to positive microscopy in up to 97% of cases [99]. The probability of identifying the organism may decrease in patients who have received prior antimicrobial therapy (40–60% and < 50% positivity on Gram stain and culture, respectively). In studies of infants and children with bacterial meningitis, initially positive CSF cultures became sterile in 90–100% of patients within 24–36 hours of administration of "appropriate" antimicrobial therapy [96].

   c. Several **rapid diagnostic tests** have been developed to aid in the diagnosis of bacterial meningitis [100]. **Counterimmunoelectrophoresis** (CIE) may detect specific antigens in CSF when meningitis is caused by meningococci (serogroups A, C, Y, or W135), *H. influenzae* type b, pneumococci (83 serotypes), type III group B streptococci, and *E. coli* K1. The sensitivity of CIE ranges from 50 to 95%, although the test is highly specific.

However, newer tests (i.e., staphylococcal coagglutination and latex agglutination) are now available that are more rapid (≤ 15 minutes) and 10-fold more sensitive than CIE. Currently available **latex agglutination techniques** detect the antigens of *H. influenzae* type b, *S. pneumoniae*, *N. meningitidis*, *E. coli* K1, and the group B streptococci. However, many of the kits do not include tests for group B meningococcus, and other kits probably are poor detectors of this antigen because of the limited immunogenicity of group B meningococcal polysaccharide.

One of these rapid diagnostic tests should be performed on all CSF specimens from patients with presumed bacterial meningitis, especially in cases with a negative CSF Gram stain, although it must be emphasized that a negative test does not rule out infection by a specific meningeal pathogen. PCR has been utilized to amplify DNA from patients with meningitis caused by *N. meningitidis* and *L. monocytogenes* [101–103]. In one small study of CSF samples from patients with meningococcal meningitis [102], the sensitivity and specificity of PCR were both 91%. Further refinements in PCR may demonstrate its usefulness in the diagnosis of bacterial meningitis, particularly when the CSF Gram stain, bacterial antigen tests, and cultures are negative.

2. **Radiography.** Cranial CT scanning and MRI do not aid in the diagnosis of acute bacterial meningitis but should be considered during the course of illness in patients who have persistent or prolonged fever, clinical evidence of increased intracranial pressure, focal neurologic findings or seizures, enlarging head circumference (in neonates), persistent neurologic dysfunction, or persistently abnormal CSF parameters or cultures [38, 95]. Radiographic studies may be particularly useful in the subset of patients with meningitis as a result of a basilar skull fracture with CSF leak [32, 46]. CT scanning may detect air-fluid levels, opacification of the air sinuses, or intracranial air; CT scanning with reconstruction can also be used to document or localize fracture sites. Radioisotope cisternography, with cottonoid pledgets placed at the outlet of the sinuses within the nasal passage, can be used to document a CSF leak, although high-resolution CT scanning with water-soluble contrast enhancement of the CSF (metrizamide cisternography) is the best currently available test for defining the site of leakage.

C. **Tuberculous meningitis.** Routine peripheral blood laboratory tests are not helpful in the diagnosis of tuberculous meningitis. A **syndrome of inappropriate antidiuretic hormone secretion** has been observed, resulting in hyponatremia, hypochloremia, and elevated urine osmolality and sodium; this syndrome recently was documented in 17 of 24 children with tuberculous meningitis [104]. **Chest radiographic abnormalities** (usually reflecting primary tuberculosis) are common in children with CNS tuberculosis, whereas in adults the changes usually include apical scarring, calcified Ghon complexes, and nodular upper lobe disease [50]. Chest radiographic evidence of miliary disease has been documented in 25–50% of adult patients with tuberculous meningitis. Children with CNS tuberculosis usually have reactive tuberculin skin tests (positivity rates of 85–90%), although in adults 35–60% of persons thought to have tuberculous meningitis do not react to first- or second-strength tuberculin tests [83, 84]. The rates of tuberculin reactivity are low in HIV-infected patients with active disease, ranging from 33 to 71% [52].

1. **Cerebrospinal fluid examination.** The CSF appearance in patients with tuberculous meningitis is typically clear or opalescent. When the CSF is permitted to remain at room temperature or in a refrigerator for a short time, however, a cobweblike clot, the classic **"pellicle" of tuberculosis,** may form secondary to the high fibrinogen content and presence of inflammatory cells in CSF [50]. A **moderate CSF pleocytosis** is present with counts of more than 5 cells/mm³ in 90–100% of patients, although the counts seldom exceed 500/mm³ [84]. The initial differential count contains both lymphocytes and neutrophils, with conversion to a lymphocytic predominance over several weeks.

Conversely, in patients with tuberculous meningitis receiving antituberculous chemotherapy, an initial lymphocytic predominance may become neutrophilic on subsequent CSF examinations [51], the so-called therapeutic paradox. The **CSF glucose concentration usually is modestly depressed** (median value, 40 mg/dl); hypoglycorrhachia has correlated with more advanced clinical stages of disease. Most patients have elevated CSF protein concentrations with median values of 150–200 mg/dl; values in excess of 1,000–2,000 mg/dl have been reported, usually in association with spinal block. In contrast, one recent review of 37 HIV-infected patients with tuberculous meningitis revealed normal CSF protein concentrations in 43% of cases [85].

Because of the small population of tuberculous organisms in CSF, identification by specific stains is difficult. In many series, fewer than 25% of specimens are smear-positive [50, 83]. The yield may be increased by staining the pellicle (if present), layering the centrifuged sediment of large CSF volumes onto a single slide with repeated applications until the entire pellet can be stained at once, and obtaining repeated specimens. One study demonstrated an 87% rate of acid-fast smear positivity when up to four separate CSF specimens were examined for each patient [84], although this rate has not been duplicated consistently in the literature. False negative CSF cultures are also common in patients with tuberculous meningitis and, even with as many as four CSF specimens, almost 20% of patients have persistently negative CSF cultures.

Based on the inadequate yield of CSF stains and cultures, several newer diagnostic modalities are being developed for the rapid diagnosis of tuberculous meningitis [50]. Some tests utilize biochemical assays to measure some feature of the organism or the host response to it (e.g., bromide partition test, adenosine deaminase assay), whereas other modalities are immunologic tests that detect mycobacterial antigen or antibody in CSF [e.g., tuberculostearic acid antigen, enzyme-linked immunosorbent assay (ELISA), latex agglutination]. Despite the promise of these immunodiagnostic tests for the rapid and sensitive diagnosis of tuberculous meningitis, there are problems with the presence of cross-reacting antibodies against nonpathogenic mycobacteria and with the presence of bacterial or fungal antigenic moieties. Use of **PCR** to detect fragments of mycobacterial DNA in CSF specimens appears to be an equally promising tool [105]; this test can be obtained on CSF through the CDC. The usefulness of these tests in the diagnosis of tuberculous meningitis requires large-scale confirmatory studies.

2. **Radiography.** There are **no radiologic changes that are pathognomonic** for a diagnosis of tuberculous meningitis [50]. On CT scanning of the head, hydrocephalus frequently is present at diagnosis or develops during the course of infection. Enhancement of the basal cisterns, following the intravenous administration of contrast material, with widening and blurring of the basilar arterial structures, may also be seen. Periventricular lucencies, reflecting the presence of tuberculous exudate and tubercle formation adjacent to the choroid and ependyma, may be evident. MRI may be superior to CT scanning in identifying basilar meningeal inflammation and small tuberculoma formation, although experience with MRI is minimal.

D. **Spirochetal meningitis**
  1. *Treponema pallidum.* For diagnosis of CNS involvement in patients with syphilis, no single routine laboratory test is definitive. CSF abnormalities are common in patients with syphilitic meningitis but are nonspecific. Findings include a mononuclear pleocytosis (> 10 cells/mm^3 in most patients), elevated CSF protein concentrations (78% of patients), and mild decreases in CSF glucose concentrations (< 50 mg/dl in 55% of patients) [53]. Oligoclonal bands and intrathecally produced antitreponemal antibodies frequently are present.

  Serologic testing has been used to aid in the diagnosis of neurosyphilis, although testing of CSF specimens in patients with syphilis is problematic [56, 106]. For example, CSF collected by lumbar puncture is subject to blood contamination in approximately 10% of patients, which may lead to contamination of CSF and, therefore, a false positive serologic test result; the likelihood of a false positive test depends on the relative amount of contamination, the antibody titer in blood, and the sensitivity of the test. For patients with a serum VDRL of less than 1:256, sufficient blood contamination to be visible to the naked eye is required to cause false positive cerebrospinal fluid VDRL results. **The specificity of the cerebrospinal fluid VDRL for the diagnosis of neurosyphilis is high, but the sensitivity is low (reactive tests in only 30–70% of patients).** Therefore, a reactive cerebrospinal fluid VDRL test in the absence of blood contamination is sufficient to diagnose neurosyphilis, and a nonreactive result does not exclude the diagnosis. The CSF fluorescent treponemal antibody absorption (FTA-ABS) test has also been examined as a possible diagnostic test for neurosyphilis. It appears that a nonreactive test effectively rules out the likelihood of neurosyphilis, although the specificity of the test is much less than the cerebrospinal fluid VDRL because of the possibility of leakage of small amounts of antibody from the serum into CSF. Furthermore, there are no compelling data that define the significance of a reactive cerebrospinal fluid FTA-ABS as a useful tool for the diagnosis of neurosyphilis. **PCR** has been used to detect *T. pallidum* DNA in CSF samples in patients with acute symptomatic neurosyphilis [107], although further large-scale studies are needed to determine the sensitivity and specificity of this technique. Based on the difficulties in the diagnosis of neurosyphilis, elevation of CSF concentrations of WBCs or protein in the appropriate clinical and serologic setting should lead to initiation of appropriate antimicrobial therapy. (**See related discussion in Chap. 13.**)

2. *Borrelia burgdorferi.* Typical CSF changes in patients with Lyme meningitis are a pleocytosis (usually < 500 cells/mm³), with more than 90% lymphocytes in 75% of cases [58]; plasma cells may also be present. There is usually an elevated CSF protein (up to 620 mg/dl) and a normal CSF glucose, although the glucose can be low in patients with illness of longer duration.

The best currently available laboratory test for the diagnosis of Lyme disease is demonstration of specific serum antibody to *B. burgdorferi*, in which a positive test in a patient with a compatible neurologic abnormality is strong evidence for the diagnosis [58, 59]. Specific antibody against *B. burgdorferi* also appears in CSF, and calculation of a specific antibody–IgG index for serum and CSF may indicate intrathecal antibody synthesis. However, it should be noted that available antibody tests are not standardized, and there is marked variability between laboratories [108]. The technique of PCR on CSF samples has also been used successfully to identify *B. burgdorferi* DNA in patients with Lyme neuroborreliosis [109]. See related discussions in Chap. 23.

E. **Fungal meningitis**

1. *Cryptococcus neoformans.* Most non-AIDS patients with cryptococcal meningitis have a CSF pleocytosis (range, 20–500 cells/mm³), with the proportion of neutrophils usually lower than 50% [62, 89]. **AIDS patients may have very low or even normal CSF leukocyte counts during active infection; as many as 65% have fewer than 5 WBCs/mm³** [63–65]. CSF protein concentrations usually are elevated, with concentrations in excess of 1,000 mg/dl suggesting subarachnoid block. CSF glucose concentrations often are reduced but may be normal in two-thirds of AIDS patients. CSF India ink examination is a rapid, effective test (if the laboratory has significant experience interpreting India ink preparations), which proves positive in 50–75% of patients with cryptococcal meningitis. This yield increases up to 88% in AIDS patients. Cases with completely normal CSF parameters have been described in AIDS patients with cryptococcal meningitis [110]. The yield of CSF culture is excellent in both non-AIDS and AIDS patients.

The **diagnosis of cryptococcal meningitis** may also be **aided by the latex agglutination test** for detection of cryptococcal polysaccharide antigen [62–65, 89]. The test is both sensitive and specific when samples are first heated to eliminate rheumatoid factor. The cryptococcal polysaccharide antigen may be positive in early infection even when the CSF culture is negative. In smaller laboratories, it may be a more reliable test than the India ink examination. A presumptive diagnosis of cryptococcal meningitis is indicated by a CSF titer of 1:8 or higher. **Serum cryptococcal polysaccharide antigen may also be detected, particularly in severely immunosuppressed patients** (i.e., those with AIDS) [65], although the value of the serum polysaccharide antigen for screening patients suspected of having meningeal disease has not been established. Antigen titers generally are higher in serum than in CSF of patients with cryptococcal meningitis. Furthermore, extremely high CSF polysaccharide antigen titers have been reported in AIDS patients; early reports suggested that titers of 1:10,000 or higher predicted a poor outcome [64], although some patients have responded well to antifungal therapy despite high initial titers.

2. *Candida.* Patients with *Candida* meningitis usually have a CSF pleocytosis, with a mean of 600 cells/mm³; lymphocytes or neutrophils may predominate [67, 68]. Direct microscopy of CSF detects yeast cells in approximately 50% of

cases. Detection of D-arabinitol in CSF may be useful. Organisms are readily grown from CSF in the majority of cases.

3. *Coccidioides immitis.* CSF pleocytosis is seen also in coccidioidal meningitis. CSF examination may occasionally reveal a prominent eosinophilia [71, 111]. Only approximately 25–50% of patients have positive CSF cultures. The best indication of disseminated disease is elevated serum concentrations of complement-fixing antibodies; titers in excess of 1:32 to 1:64 suggest dissemination [70, 71]. CSF complement-fixing antibodies are present in at least 70% of cases of early meningitis and from virtually all patients as disease progresses. In fact, the antibody titers appear to parallel the course of meningeal disease, although in patients who relapse, CSF pleocytosis, elevated protein, or decreased glucose usually develop before detectable CSF antibody recurs. Complement-fixing antibodies may fail to develop in serum or CSF in patients with immunodeficiencies.

F. **Protozoal and helminthic meningitis**
   1. **Amebae**
      a. **Acute form.** The CSF formula in patients with the acute form of primary amebic meningoencephalitis reveals a neutrophilic pleocytosis, low glucose, elevated protein, and RBCs [72, 73]. The Gram stain is always negative. However, examination of fresh, warm specimens of CSF can reveal the ameboid movements of the motile trophozoites.
      b. **Subacute or chronic form.** In patients with the subacute or chronic form of the illness, the CSF inflammatory response is less florid with a predominant mononuclear leukocytosis [72]. The CSF protein concentration is elevated, and the glucose is often normal or slightly reduced. Because amebae are not found in CSF, the diagnosis usually requires examination of a biopsy or necropsy specimen revealing the characteristic cysts. The value of serologic tests is variable. Serum immunofluorescence, amebic immobilization titers, and complement-fixing antibodies support the diagnosis, although demonstration of rising titers is necessary to establish the diagnosis as some normal persons have circulating antibodies.
   2. *Angiostrongylus cantonensis.* The combination of history of ingesting suspected food, moderate to high peripheral eosinophilia, and CSF eosinophilia leads to the suspicion of angiostrongyloidiasis [72]. The CSF leukocytosis is moderate, with 16–72% eosinophils and increased protein concentration; larvae are found occasionally in CSF.

IV. **Approach to the patient with meningitis.** Initial management of a patient with presumed bacterial meningitis includes performance of a lumbar puncture to determine whether the CSF formula is consistent with that diagnosis [81, 95, 96, 112]. If purulent meningitis is present, empiric antimicrobial therapy should be instituted based on results of Gram staining or rapid bacterial antigen tests. However, if no etiologic agent can be identified by these means or if there is a delay (i.e., longer than 30 minutes) in performance of the lumbar puncture, empiric antimicrobial therapy should be instituted based on the patient's age and underlying disease status. In most patients, antimicrobial therapy should be ordered on initial clinical impression; in critically ill patients, the first dose may even precede lumbar puncture. In patients who present for a focal neurologic examination or who have papilledema but in whom bacterial meningitis is suspected, a CT scan of the head should be performed prior to lumbar puncture to rule out the presence of an intracranial mass lesion because of the potential risk of herniation [97]. The true incidence of this problem is unclear but has been suggested to be much lower than 1.2% in patients with papilledema and approximately 12% in patients without papilledema but with elevated intracranial pressure. However, the time involved in waiting for a CT scan significantly delays initiation of antimicrobial therapy, with the potential for increased morbidity and mortality in patients with bacterial meningitis. Therefore, **emergent empiric antimicrobial therapy should be initiated before sending the patient to the CT scanner. Blood cultures should be obtained before empiric antibiotic therapy.** Although CSF cultures may be sterile after initiation of antimicrobial therapy, pretreatment blood cultures and the CSF formula, Gram stain, or bacterial antigen tests will likely provide evidence for or against a diagnosis of bacterial meningitis. Our choices of **empiric antimicrobial therapy** based on age and underlying disease status of the patient are shown in **Table 5-2**. Once the infecting meningeal pathogen is isolated and susceptibility testing is known, antimicrobial therapy can be modified for optimal treatment (Table 5-3). Recommended dosages of antimicrobial agents in adults for

Table 5-2. Empiric therapy for purulent meningitis[a]

Predisposing factor	Common bacterial pathogens	Antimicrobial therapy
Age		
0–4 wk	*Streptococcus agalactiae, Escherichia coli, Listeria monocytogenes, Klebsiella pneumoniae, Enterococcus* spp., *Salmonella* spp.	Ampicillin plus cefotaxime; *or* ampicillin plus an aminoglycoside (see Chap. 3)
4–12 wk	*S. agalactiae, E. coli, L. monocytogenes, Haemophilus influenzae, Streptococcus pneumoniae, Neisseria meningitidis*	Ampicillin plus a third-generation cephalosporin[b]
3 mo–18 yr	*H. influenzae, N. meningitidis, S. pneumoniae*	Third-generation cephalosporin[b]; *or* ampicillin plus chloramphenicol
18–50 yr	*S. pneumoniae, N. meningitidis*	Third-generation cephalosporin[b] ± ampicillin[c]
> 50 yr	*S. pneumoniae, N. meningitidis, L. monocytogenes,* aerobic gram-negative bacilli	Ampicillin plus a third-generation cephalosporin[b]
Immunocompromised host	*S. pneumoniae, N. meningitidis, L. monocytogenes,* aerobic gram-negative bacilli (including *Pseudomonas aeruginosa*)	Vancomycin + ampicillin + ceftazidime
Basilar skull fracture	*S. pneumoniae, H. influenzae,* group A beta-hemolytic streptococci	Third-generation cephalosporin[b]
Head trauma; postneurosurgery	*Staphylococcus aureus, Staphylococcus epidermidis,* aerobic gram-negative bacilli (including *P. aeruginosa*)	Vancomycin + ceftazidime
Cerebrospinal fluid shunt	*S. epidermidis, S. aureus,* aerobic gram-negative bacilli (including *P. aeruginosa*), diphtheroids	Vancomycin + ceftazidime

[a]Vancomycin should be added to empiric therapeutic regimens when highly penicillin-resistant or cephalosporin-resistant strains of *S. pneumoniae* are suspected; see text for details.
[b]Cefotaxime or ceftriaxone.
[c]See text for details.

infections of the CNS are shown in Table 5-4; dosages for infants and children are shown in Table 5-5.

V. Antimicrobial therapy

A. Viral meningitis. Currently, **there is no specific antiviral chemotherapy for the enteroviruses; treatment is supportive** [1, 2]. Antiviral drugs for enteroviral infection are under development [2a]. Recovery of patients with HSV type 2 meningitis usually is complete without neurologic sequelae; it is not clear whether antiviral treatment alters the course of mild HSV type 2 meningitis. However, treatment with acyclovir generally is indicated for primary genital herpes infection [11]. Specific antiretroviral therapy (e.g., zidovudine, didanosine, zalcitabine) is not indicated for the aseptic meningitis of acute HIV infection, although later neurologic involvement may respond to therapy and should be administered to patients with absolute CD4 lymphocyte counts of fewer than 500/mm^3 [113].

B. Bacterial meningitis

Table 5-3. Specific antimicrobial therapy for meningitis

Microorganism	Standard therapy	Alternative therapies
Bacteria		
Haemophilus influenzae		
Beta-lactamase-negative	Ampicillin	Third-generation cephalosporin[a]; chloramphenicol; aztreonam
Beta-lactamase-positive	Third-generation cephalosporin[a]	Chloramphenicol; aztreonam; fluoroquinolone
Neisseria meningitidis	Penicillin G or ampicillin	Third-generation cephalosporin[a]; chloramphenicol; fluoroquinolone
Streptococcus pneumoniae		
Penicillin MIC ≤ 0.1 μg/ml	Penicillin G or ampicillin	Third-generation cephalosporin[a]; chloramphenicol; vancomycin
Penicillin MIC 0.1–1.0 μg/ml	Third-generation cephalosporin[a]	Vancomycin; imipenem[b]
Penicillin MIC ≥ 2.0 μg/ml	Vancomycin[c] + a third-generation cephalosporin[a]	Imipenem[b]; meropenem[d]
Enterobacteriaceae	Third-generation cephalosporin[a]	Aztreonam; fluoroquinolone; trimethoprim-sulfamethoxazole
Pseudomonas aeruginosa	Ceftazidime[e]	Aztreonam[e]; fluoroquinolone[e]
Listeria monocytogenes	Ampicillin or penicillin G[e]	Trimethoprim-sulfamethoxazole
Streptococcus agalactiae	Ampicillin or penicillin G[e]	Third-generation cephalosporin[a]; vancomycin
Staphylococcus aureus		
Methicillin-sensitive	Nafcillin or oxacillin	Vancomycin
Methicillin-resistant	Vancomycin	
Staphylococcus epidermidis	Vancomycin[c]	
Mycobacteria		
Mycobacterium tuberculosis	Isoniazid + rifampin + pyrazinamide	Ethambutol[f]; ethionamide[f]; streptomycin[f]
Spirochetes		
Treponema pallidum	Penicillin G	Doxycycline[g]; ceftriaxone[g]
Borrelia burgdorferi	Third-generation cephalosporin[a]	Penicillin; doxycycline
Fungi		
Cryptococcus neoformans	Amphotericin B[h]	Fluconazole; itraconazole[g]
Candida spp.	Amphotericin B[h]	Fluconazole[g]
Coccidioides immitis	Amphotericin B[i]	Fluconazole

Table 5-3 (continued)

Microorganism	Standard therapy	Alternative therapies
Protozoa and helminths		
Naegleria fowleri	Amphotericin B[i] + rifampin + doxycycline	

MIC = minimum inhibitory concentration.
[a]Cefotaxime or ceftriaxone.
[b]Use is associated with an increased incidence of seizures.
[c]Addition of rifampin should be considered.
[d]Currently under investigation in patients with pneumococcal meningitis.
[e]Addition of an aminoglycoside should be considered.
[f]Add to standard therapy in cases of suspected drug resistance; see text for details.
[g]Value of these antimicrobial agents has not been established.
[h]Addition of 5-flucytosine should be considered.
[i]Intravenous and intraventricular administration.

1. **Haemophilus influenzae**
   a. Therapy for meningitis caused by *H. influenzae* type b has been markedly altered by the emergence of beta-lactamase-producing strains. Resistance of *H. influenzae* to chloramphenicol has also been described, although more commonly from areas such as Spain (> 50% of isolates) than from the United States (< 1% of isolates) [114, 115]. Even in patients with meningitis caused by chloramphenicol-sensitive isolates, a recent prospective study found chloramphenicol to be bacteriologically and clinically inferior to ampicillin, ceftriaxone, or cefotaxime in the treatment of childhood bacterial meningitis caused predominantly by *H. influenzae* type b [116]. Several studies have documented that the third-generation cephalosporins (particularly cefotaxime or ceftriaxone) are as effective as the combination of ampicillin plus chloramphenicol for bacterial meningitis, leading to a recommendation for use of the **third-generation cephalosporins (cefotaxime or ceftriaxone) as empiric antimicrobial therapy for children with bacterial meningitis** [112].
   b. Although cefuroxime, a second-generation cephalosporin, was initially believed to be as efficacious as the combination of ampicillin plus chloramphenicol for childhood bacterial meningitis, recent studies have questioned this finding. Several comparative trials have documented a slower rate of CSF sterilization and a higher incidence of hearing impairment in patients receiving cefuroxime for bacterial meningitis [117, 118]. Furthermore, there have been cases of *H. influenzae* meningitis in patients receiving cefuroxime for nonmeningeal *H. influenzae* disease [119]. Therefore, **cefuroxime cannot be recommended** as a first-line drug for the treatment of bacterial meningitis. In addition, there have been single case reports of delayed CSF sterilization in patients with *H. influenzae* meningitis treated with ceftizoxime or ceftazidime [120]. However, in vitro resistance of *H. influenzae* to the third-generation cephalosporins and fluoroquinolones has not yet been described.
2. **Neisseria meningitidis.** The antimicrobial agents of choice for meningitis caused by *N. meningitidis* are **penicillin G or ampicillin,** although these recommendations may change in future years [112]. Meningococcal strains have recently been reported from several areas (particularly Spain) that are relatively resistant to penicillin G, with a minimum inhibitory concentration (MIC) range of 0.1–1.0 µg/ml. This resistance has been reported to be mediated by a reduced affinity of the antibiotic for penicillin-binding proteins 2 and 3 [121]. The clinical significance of these isolates is unclear, however, because patients with meningitis caused by these organisms have recovered with standard penicillin therapy. Such strains are very rare in the United States, where the geometric mean MIC has remained 0.03 µg/ml or less for the last decade [122]. If an alternative agent is chosen for therapy of meningococcal meningitis caused

Table 5-4. Maximum recommended dosages of antimicrobial agents for central nervous system infections in adults with normal renal and hepatic function[a]

Antimicrobial agent	Total daily dose	Dosing interval (hr)
Amikacin[b]	15 mg/kg	8
Amphotericin B[c]	0.6–1.0 mg/kg	24
Ampicillin	12 g	4
Aztreonam	6–8 g	6–8
Cefotaxime	8–12 g	4–6
Ceftazidime	6 g	8
Ceftriaxone	4 g	12
Chloramphenicol[d]	4–6 g	6
Ciprofloxacin	800–1,200 mg	8–12
Doxycycline	200–400 mg	12
Ethambutol[e,f]	15–25 mg/kg	24
Ethionamide[e]	1 g	12
Fluconazole	400 mg	24
Flucytosine[e,g]	100–150 mg/kg	6
Gentamicin[b]	3–5 mg/kg	8
Imipenem	2 g[n]	6
Isoniazid[e,h]	300 mg	24
Metronidazole	30 mg/kg	6
Miconazole	1.5–3.0 g	8
Nafcillin	9–12 g	4
Oxacillin	9–12 g	4
Penicillin G	24 million units	4
Pyrazinamide[e,i]	15–30 mg/kg	24
Rifampin[e]	600 mg	24
Streptomycin[j,k]	15 mg/kg	24
Tobramycin[b]	3–5 mg/kg	8
Trimethoprim-sulfamethoxazole[l]	10 mg/kg	12
Vancomycin[b,m]	2–3 g	8–12

[a]Unless otherwise indicated, therapy is administered intravenously.
[b]Need to monitor serum concentrations to ensure adequate peaks. See Chap. 28H.
[c]Can increase dosage to 1.5 mg/kg/day in severely ill patients.
[d]Higher dose recommended for pneumococcal meningitis.
[e]Oral administration.
[f]Maximum daily dosage of 2.5 g.
[g]Maintain serum concentrations of 50–100 µg/ml.
[h]Initiate therapy at a dosage of 10 mg/kg/day (up to 600 mg/day).
[i]Maximum daily dosage of 2 g.
[j]Intramuscular administration.
[k]Maximum daily dosage of 1 g.
[l]Dosage based on trimethoprim component.
[m]May need to monitor cerebrospinal fluid concentrations in severely ill patients.
[n]In a patient with normal renal function, some clinicians may consider a higher dose. See Chap. 28G.

Table 5-5. Recommended dosages of antimicrobial agents for central nervous system infections in infants and children with normal renal and hepatic function[a,b]

Antimicrobial agent	Total daily dose in infants and children (dosing interval in hours)
Amikacin[c]	20–30 mg/kg (8)
Amphotericin B	0.25–1.0 mg/kg (24)
Ampicillin	200–300 mg/kg (6)
Cefotaxime	200 mg/kg (6–8)
Ceftazidime	125–150 mg/kg (8)
Ceftriaxone	80–100 mg/kg (12–24)
Chloramphenicol	75–100 mg/kg (6)
Ethambutol[d,e]	15–25 mg/kg (24)
Ethionamide[d,f]	10–20 mg/kg (12)
Flucytosine[d,g]	100–150 mg/kg (6)
Gentamicin[c]	7.5 mg/kg (8)
Isoniazid[d,h,i]	10–20 mg/kg (12–24)
Metronidazole	30 mg/kg (12)
Nafcillin	200 mg/kg (6)
Penicillin G	0.25 mU/kg (4–6)
Pyrazinamide[d,j]	15–30 mg/kg (12–24)
Rifampin[d,k]	10–20 mg/kg (12–24)
Streptomycin[l]	20–40 mg/kg (12)
Tobramycin[c]	7.5 mg/kg (8)
Trimethoprim-sulfamethoxazole[m]	10 mg/kg (12)
Vancomycin[c]	50–60 mg/kg (6)

[a]Unless otherwise indicated, therapy is administered intravenously.
[b]See Table 3-2 for neonate dosages.
[c]Need to monitor peak and trough serum concentrations.
[d]Oral administration.
[e]Maximum daily dosage of 2.5 g.
[f]Maximum daily dosage of 1 g.
[g]Maintain serum concentrations of 50–100 μg/ml.
[h]Some clinicians initiate therapy at 30 mg/kg for the first several weeks.
[i]Maximum daily dosage of 300 mg.
[j]Maximum daily dosage of 2 g.
[k]Maximum daily dosage of 600 mg.
[l]Intramuscular administration.
[m]Dosage based on trimethoprim component.

by these relatively resistant strains, ceftriaxone is recommended based on in vitro susceptibility data.

3. *Streptococcus pneumoniae*
   a. **The therapy for meningitis caused by pneumococci has recently been modified based on current pneumococcal susceptibility patterns.** Numerous reports from throughout the world have now documented strains of pneumococci that are relatively resistant to penicillin, with a MIC range of 0.1–1.0 µg/ml, as well as strains that are highly resistant to penicillin (MIC ≥ 2.0 µg/ml) [112, 123–125]. The overwhelming majority of resistant strains are serotypes 6, 14, 19, and 23. The mechanism of this resistance is alterations in the structure and molecular size of penicillin-binding proteins. Most of the multiresistant strains isolated in the United States have disseminated from a multiresistant serotype 23F clone of *S. pneumoniae* that was isolated in Spain as early as 1978 [126]. See Chap. 28C.

   Based on these antimicrobial susceptibility trends and because sufficient CSF concentrations of penicillin are difficult to achieve with standard high parenteral dosages (initial CSF penicillin concentrations of approximately 1 µg/ml), **penicillin can no longer be recommended as empiric antimicrobial therapy when *S. pneumoniae* is considered a likely infecting pathogen in patients with purulent meningitis. For patients in whom relatively resistant strains are found, a third-generation cephalosporin (ceftriaxone or cefotaxime) should be used [112, 127, 128]; vancomycin plus a third-generation cephalosporin should be utilized when highly resistant strains are suspected or isolated.** (See related discussions in Chap. 28C.)

   Pneumococcal resistance to the third-generation cephalosporins in the United States (MIC range, 4–32 µg/ml) and South Africa has also been reported [129–132]. Of three patients in the United States with pneumococcal strains that were highly resistant to the third-generation cephalosporins, two responded to initial antimicrobial therapy with vancomycin plus chloramphenicol, followed by chloramphenicol alone. However, clinical failures with chloramphenicol have been reported in patients with penicillin-resistant isolates [133], likely due to the poor bactericidal activity of chloramphenicol against these strains. In one study, 20 of 25 children had an unsatisfactory outcome (i.e., death, serious neurologic deficit, poor clinical response). Chloramphenicol alone cannot be recommended as a suitable regimen for empiric therapy. **These data indicate the need to perform susceptibility testing of all pneumococcal isolates,** at which time antimicrobial therapy can be modified for optimal treatment. See Chap. 25.
   b. Furthermore, **vancomycin may not be optimal therapy for patients with pneumococcal meningitis.** In a recent report of 11 consecutive patients with CSF culture–proven pneumococcal meningitis caused by relatively resistant strains who were treated with intravenous vancomycin, all patients improved and 10 were eventually cured of their infection, but 4 patients experienced a therapeutic failure with vancomycin, necessitating a change in therapy [134]. Reasons for failure may have included variability in serum vancomycin concentrations or impaired CSF vancomycin penetration as a result of adjunctive dexamethasone administration. **Nevertheless, these data indicate the need for careful monitoring of, and perhaps even measurement of CSF vancomycin concentrations in, adult patients receiving vancomycin therapy for pneumococcal meningitis.** Infectious disease consultation is advised. The addition of intrathecal or intraventricular vancomycin should be considered for treatment of unresponsive cases. Some investigators have recommended the addition of rifampin to vancomycin for treatment of meningitis caused by highly resistant pneumococcal strains, although there are no firm data to support this recommendation. Meropenem, a new carbapenem with less proconvulsive activity than imipenem, is currently under investigation in patients with pneumococcal meningitis; initial results appear promising. Some fluoroquinolones are active in animal models of penicillin-resistant pneumococcal meningitis [135], but the currently available fluoroquinolones are not recommended in humans with this disease. (See related discussions of vancomycin therapy in Chap. 28O.)

4. *Listeria monocytogenes.* Despite the broad range of in vitro activity of the third-generation cephalosporins, they are inactive in meningitis caused by *L. monocytogenes.* Therapy for patients with *Listeria* meningitis should con-

sist of ampicillin or penicillin G [33, 34]; the addition of an aminoglycoside should be considered in proven infection based on documented in vitro synergy and enhanced killing in vivo as documented in a variety of animal models of *Listeria* infection. In the penicillin-allergic patient, trimethoprim-sulfamethoxazole, which is bactericidal against *Listeria* in vitro, should be used. Chloramphenicol has been associated with an unacceptably high failure rate in patients with *Listeria* meningitis. Vancomycin is also unsatisfactory for *Listeria* meningitis, despite favorable in vitro susceptibility results. However, intraventricular administration of vancomycin was successful in one case of recurrent *L. monocytogenes* meningitis [136]. Meropenem is active in vitro and in experimental animal models of *L. monocytogenes* meningitis and may be a useful alternative in the future.

5. **Streptococcus agalactiae.** Standard therapy for meningitis caused by the group B streptococcus is the combination of ampicillin plus an aminoglycoside [38]. This combination is recommended due to documented in vitro synergy and recent reports detailing the presence of penicillin-tolerant strains [41]. Alternative agents are the third-generation cephalosporins. Vancomycin is reserved for penicillin-allergic patients in whom cephalosporins are contraindicated.

6. **Aerobic gram-negative bacilli**
   a. The treatment of bacterial meningitis caused by enteric gram-negative bacilli has been revolutionized by the availability of the **third-generation cephalosporins** [112], with cure rates of 78–94%. One particular third-generation cephalosporin, ceftazidime, has enhanced in vitro activity against *P. aeruginosa* and resulted in the cure of 19 of 24 patients in one study of *P. aeruginosa* meningitis when administered alone or in combination with an aminoglycoside [137]. In another study of 10 pediatric patients with *Pseudomonas* meningitis, 7 patients were cured clinically and 9 were cured bacteriologically when treated with ceftazidime-containing regimens [138]. Concomitant intrathecal or intraventricular aminoglycoside therapy should be considered in patients with gram-negative meningitis who are not responding to conventional parenteral therapy, although this mode of administration rarely is needed at present and was associated with a higher mortality than systemic therapy alone in infants with gram-negative meningitis and ventriculitis.
   b. **Other antimicrobial agents** used in patients with meningitis caused by aerobic gram-negative bacilli include aztreonam, which attains excellent CSF concentrations and has been shown to be efficacious in the treatment of gram-negative meningitis [139]. Imipenem was found to be effective in one case of *Acinetobacter* meningitis and in bacterial eradication from CSF in a recent study of 21 children with bacterial meningitis (most cases caused by *H. influenzae* type b and *N. meningitidis*) [140], although a high rate of seizure activity (33%) limits its usefulness in therapy for bacterial meningitis. High-dose meropenem (2 g q8h) given for 18 weeks was successful in a lymphoma patient with *P. aeruginosa* meningitis in whom therapy with ceftazidime plus gentamicin had failed [141].

   The fluoroquinolones (e.g., ciprofloxacin, pefloxacin) have been used successfully in some patients with gram-negative meningitis [142]. The primary area of usefulness of these agents is for treatment of multidrug-resistant gram-negative organisms (e.g., *P. aeruginosa*) or when the response to conventional beta-lactam therapy is slow (e.g., meningitis caused by *Salmonella* spp.). These agents should never be used as first-line empiric therapy in patients with meningitis of unknown etiology because of their poor in vitro activity against pneumococci and *L. monocytogenes*.

7. **Staphylococci.** *S. aureus* meningitis should be treated with nafcillin or oxacillin [45], with vancomycin reserved for patients allergic to penicillin or when methicillin-resistant organisms are suspected or isolated. The addition of rifampin should be considered in patients not responding to therapy. Meningitis caused by coagulase-negative staphylococci, the most commonly encountered organism in CSF shunt infections, should be treated with vancomycin; rifampin should be added if the patient fails to improve [46]. Removal of the shunt often is necessary to optimize therapy. Teicoplanin, an investigational glycopeptide antimicrobial agent, was also found to be successful following intraventricular administration in seven patients with staphylococcal neurosurgical shunt infection [143].

8. **Duration of therapy.** Traditionally, the duration of antimicrobial therapy in patients with bacterial nonmeningococcal meningitis has been 10–14 days [144, 145]. Several studies, however, have documented that 7 days of therapy is safe and effective for *H. influenzae* type b meningitis, although treatment must be individualized and some patients may require longer courses. Meningococcal meningitis can be treated for 7 days with intravenous penicillin, though some authors have suggested that 4 days of therapy are adequate. In adults with meningitis caused by enteric gram-negative bacilli, treatment regimens should be continued for 3 weeks due to the high rate of relapse in patients treated with shorter courses of therapy. Ten to fourteen days is the recommended course for treatment of meningitis caused by *S. pneumoniae,* and 14–21 days for *L. monocytogenes, S. aureus,* and the group B streptococci, although these regimens are based more on tradition and anecdotes than on rigidly standardized clinical trials.

   In carefully selected pediatric patients, completion of IV therapy for bacterial meningitis may be accomplished in the outpatient setting if patients meet several criteria: inpatient therapy for 6 days, afebrile 24–48 hours before discharge, no significant neurologic dysfunction, no seizure activity, clinically stable, taking all fluids by mouth, received at least one dose of the outpatient antibiotic in the hospital, daily examination by a physician, and reliable follow-up [145a].

C. **Tuberculous meningitis.** Until the advent of effective chemotherapy, CNS tuberculosis was a uniformly fatal disease. Even now, the optimal drug regimen, dosage, route of administration, and duration of therapy remain undefined (for recommendations, see Tables 5-3 through 5-5). Therapy for tuberculous meningitis should be initiated on the basis of a strong clinical suspicion and should not be delayed until proof of infection is obtained because of the problems with rapid organism identification. The principles of therapy for tuberculous meningitis are similar to those for treatment of tuberculosis in other locations [50, 51, 146]. Isoniazid and rifampin are the mainstays of treatment. In addition, many regimens have taken advantage of the merits of pyrazinamide, which has rapid intracellular mycobactericidal activity. All these agents have very good CSF penetration; in the presence of meningeal inflammation, the peak CSF concentrations of isoniazid, rifampin, and pyrazinamide are approximately 90%, 20%, and 100%, respectively, of peak serum concentrations. (See Chap. 9 under Tuberculosis.)

   1. **For isoniazid-rifampin-susceptible strains.** In nonimmunocompromised patients with tuberculous meningitis, a 6-month treatment regimen is recommended, consisting of isoniazid, rifampin, and pyrazinamide for the first 2 months, and isoniazid and rifampin for an additional 4 months. Several studies have demonstrated the efficacy of this short-course regimen in patients with tuberculous meningitis [147, 148]. However, some authors recommend a treatment duration of 9 months, and we favor this approach [51]. Furthermore, HIV-infected patients usually require longer courses of therapy [52]. Several studies have reported similar outcomes in patients with or without HIV infection who have tuberculous meningitis.

   2. **Multidrug-resistant strains and empiric therapy.** Clinical tuberculous disease with resistant organisms has been appearing with increasing frequency [50]. Patient populations with resistant organisms include immigrants from countries in Asia, Africa, and the Americas; known contacts of drug-resistant cases; homeless and impoverished individuals; and residents of certain geographic areas in the United States, particularly adjacent to the Mexican border. In addition, secondary resistance may develop during chemotherapy if compliance with a multiple drug regimen is poor. (See further discussion in Chap. 9.) In cases of suspected drug resistance, **ethambutol or streptomycin should be added to the three-drug regimen outlined in sec. 1 until susceptibility results have been obtained. This is the current recommendation (by the American Thoracic Society) for empiric therapy of tuberculosis until susceptibility test results are available.**

   Of greater concern are the recent reports of outbreaks of multidrug-resistant tuberculosis, especially in HIV-infected patients [149, 150]. Most strains in these outbreaks have been resistant to both isoniazid and rifampin, as well as many other first-line agents. The majority of cases have been reported from Florida and New York and have been characterized by high mortality (70–90%), with a median of 4–16 weeks from diagnosis to death. The optimal therapeutic regimen for these strains is unknown but should be guided by susceptibility testing. However, some patients who have received drugs to which their organisms were susceptible according to conventional testing did not respond clinically. In patients who have tuberculous meningitis caused by resistant organisms, therapy should also be guided by drug penetration into CSF [50]. Ethambutol penetrates poorly into CSF except when the meninges are inflamed. There is good evidence, however, that ethionamide crosses both healthy and inflamed meninges, with peak CSF concentrations comparable to those achieved in serum. The fluoroquinolones (e.g., ciprofloxacin and ofloxacin) also penetrate well into CSF and may have good in vitro activity against *M. tuberculosis;* sparfloxacin is a newer fluoroquinolone with excellent in vitro activity. Amoxicillin-clavulanate or imipenem has been used in individual cases of meningitis caused by multidrug-resistant *M. tuberculosis.* Meningitis suspected to be caused by multidrug-resistant *M. tuberculosis* should be treated with at least five drugs until susceptibility studies are performed. Infectious disease consultation is advised.

D. **Spirochetal meningitis**
  1. *Treponema pallidum.* For patients with clinical neurosyphilis syndromes, the goal may be to reverse clinical symptoms and signs or to arrest disease progression [53]. In patients with syphilitic meningitis, clinical findings other than cranial nerve abnormalities usually resolve without therapy. In patients with meningovascular syphilis, the prognosis after therapy is very good, generally. The exception may be patients with larger clinically apparent neurologic deficits prior to therapy; in this situation, therapy may halt progression and prevent further ischemic events caused by neurosyphilis.

  The preferred antimicrobial regimen for treatment of CNS syphilis is aqueous crystalline penicillin G at a dose of 12–24 million units IV daily in divided doses q4h for 10–14 days [53, 56, 56a]. Alternatively, procaine penicillin, at a dose of 2.4 million units IM daily, plus probenecid (500 mg PO qid) for 10–14 days can be utilized. Some experts also recommend follow-up therapy with three weekly injections of benzathine penicillin G, although there are no data to support this recommendation [53, 56, 56a]. No large studies have been performed to evaluate alternative antimicrobial agents for neurosyphilis. On the basis of case reports, clinical experience, and extrapolations from experimental animal studies, other antimicrobial agents with potential clinical utility in the penicillin-allergic patient include the tetracyclines, chloramphenicol, and ceftriaxone. Erythromycin is not recommended based on failures in erythromycin-treated patients. In HIV-infected patients with neurosyphilis, careful monitoring for response to therapy is needed [55, 151]. Follow-up lumbar puncture should be performed every 6 months in all patients until the CSF changes have normalized. There have been several reports of failures in HIV-infected patients receiving standard therapy for neurosyphilis, probably because the patient's immunologic response plays an important role in controlling the infection even in the presence of apparently adequate antimicrobial therapy. (**See related discussion of the therapy of neurosyphilis in Chap. 13.**)
  2. *Borrelia burgdorferi.* Parenteral antimicrobial therapy [i.e., high-dose (20–24 million units/day) IV penicillin G for 21 days] usually is needed to treat the neurologic manifestations of Lyme disease, including meningitis [58, 59]. The meningeal and systemic reactions tend to improve within days, whereas radicular pains and motor deficits improve over many weeks. CNS abnormalities are arrested by treatment and may slowly improve, but some residual deficit is common. Some patients have also responded to treatment with other regimens. A randomized trial comparing intravenous doxycycline (200 mg for 2 days, followed by 100 mg daily for 8 days) to intravenous penicillin G (20 million units daily for 10 days) found both treatments to be equally efficacious. Patients who have failed to respond to intravenous penicillin have responded to therapy with intravenous cefotaxime, ceftriaxone, or chloramphenicol. In one prospective randomized trial, ceftriaxone was superior to penicillin in the therapy of late Lyme borreliosis [152]. The current recommendation is to treat most patients with Lyme meningitis with intravenous ceftriaxone at a dosage of 2 g/day for 2–4 weeks [58, 59]; the literature contains no agreement on the duration of therapy or on the minimal adequate dose of the antimicrobial. At present, there is no evidence to support treatment durations of longer than 4 weeks. However, no regimen has proven to be universally effective. (See related discussion in Chap. 23.)

E. Fungal meningitis
  1. *Cryptococcus neoformans*
    a. Before the clinical availability of **amphotericin B,** cryptococcal meningitis
       was nearly always fatal. With the use of amphotericin B, the prognosis
       improved dramatically, although morbidity, mortality, and relapse rates
       remained high, especially in immunocompromised patients (cure rates
       ≤ 52% after the first course of therapy). Subsequently, it was discovered
       that amphotericin B had in vitro synergistic activity with another antifun-
       gal agent, 5-flucytosine. This led to a large prospective collaborative trial
       in patients (in the pre-AIDS era) with acute cryptococcal meningitis to
       compare combination therapy with amphotericin B (0.3 mg/kg/day) and 5-
       flucytosine (150 mg/kg/day) for 6 weeks to amphotericin B (0.4 mg/kg/day)
       alone for 10 weeks [153]. The results indicated that combination therapy
       produced fewer failures, fewer relapses, more rapid CSF sterilization, and
       less nephrotoxicity than therapy with amphotericin B alone; cure or im-
       provement occurred in 67% of patients receiving combination therapy ver-
       sus 41% of patients receiving only amphotericin B. Mortality between the
       two groups was not statistically different.
         However, this study has been criticized because of the low dose of ampho-
       tericin B used in the single-agent arm of the study. A subsequent study of
       patients with acute cryptococcal meningitis compared a 4-week to a 6-
       week regimen of amphotericin B plus 5-flucytosine therapy [154]. It was
       determined that a 4-week combination regimen could be used in the subset
       of patients who, at presentation, had no neurologic complications, no under-
       lying diseases, no immunosuppressive therapy, a pretreatment CSF white
       blood cell count of more than 20/mm^3, and a serum cryptococcal antigen
       titer of less than 1:32; and who, at 4 weeks, had a negative CSF India ink
       test and a CSF cryptococcal antigen titer of less than 1:8. Patients treated
       with combination therapy were noted to experience a high rate of toxicity
       due to 5-flucytosine (38% of cases), mainly hematologic, indicating that 5-
       flucytosine concentrations need to be monitored during therapy (maintain
       serum concentrations of 50–100 μg/ml) [155].
         In a retrospective analysis of AIDS patients with cryptococcal meningitis,
       no differences in survival were noted whether patients were treated with
       amphotericin B alone or amphotericin B plus 5-flucytosine [65]. However,
       in more than half of the patients receiving 5-flucytosine, therapy had to
       be discontinued due to toxicity, primarily cytopenias. **The role of the addi-
       tion of 5-flucytosine to amphotericin B in the treatment of AIDS patients
       with cryptococcal meningitis is currently being studied.**
    b. Despite the availability of amphotericin B, there has been a poor response
       to antifungal therapy in AIDS patients with cryptococcal meningitis. The
       availability of **fluconazole, a new triazole** antifungal agent, **holds promise**
       for the management of this condition. Fluconazole has excellent oral bio-
       availability, a long serum half-life (approximately 30 hours), and very good
       CSF penetration (approximately 70–80% of peak serum concentrations).
       Initial enthusiasm for the use of fluconazole in cryptococcal meningitis in
       patients with AIDS was based on small, uncontrolled studies. However,
       two recent studies have compared fluconazole to standard antifungal ther-
       apy for cryptococcal meningitis in AIDS [156, 157]. In the first trial, flucona-
       zole (400 mg/day) was compared to the combination of amphotericin B (0.7
       mg/kg/day) plus 5-flucytosine (150 mg/kg/day) [156]. In the fluconazole
       group, 8 of 14 patients (57%) failed, but there were no failures among 6
       patients receiving amphotericin B plus 5-flucytosine. In this study, combi-
       nation therapy had superior mycologic and clinical efficacy. In a second
       trial conducted by the Mycoses Study Group, fluconazole (initial dose of
       400 mg, followed by 200 mg/day) was compared to amphotericin B (at least
       0.3 mg/kg/day) for acute cryptococcal meningitis in AIDS patients [157].
       No significant differences were found in the number of patients who were
       cured or improved in either treatment group. There were also no significant
       differences in the overall case fatality rates, although there was a trend
       to early mortality (within the first 2 weeks) in the patients treated with
       fluconazole. In addition, in a post hoc analysis of the data, it appeared that
       fluconazole was inferior to amphotericin B only in patients with certain
       negative prognostic signs such as a positive blood culture for *C. neoformans,*

a CSF cryptococcal antigen titer in excess of 1:128, a positive CSF India ink smear, and altered mentation. This study has been criticized, however, because the drug dosages utilized in both arms of the study may have been too low for optimal treatment of cryptococcal meningitis. **Although the optimal therapeutic regimen for cryptococcal meningitis in AIDS patients is not known, the preceding data support the initial use of amphotericin B, with or without 5-flucytosine, for a period of approximately 2 weeks; this period may need to be prolonged in patients who are severely ill. This initial treatment period then is followed by fluconazole (400 mg/day) to complete a 10-week course. Pending further data, non-AIDS patients with cryptococcal meningitis should continue to receive standard amphotericin B plus 5-flucytosine for 4–6 weeks.**

Another important concern in AIDS patients with cryptococcal meningitis is the high rate of relapse once antifungal therapy is discontinued [63, 64]. The prostate gland may represent a sequestered reservoir from which systemic relapse can occur. Long-term suppressive therapy in AIDS patients using either ketoconazole or amphotericin B has been associated with improved survival (238 versus 141 days) [65]. In addition, several recent studies have examined the utility of fluconazole for preventing relapse in AIDS patients with cryptococcal meningitis. A placebo-controlled trial determined that the rate of relapse was markedly diminished in patients receiving fluconazole suppressive therapy (3% versus 37% in patients receiving placebo) [158]. In addition, a subsequent trial revealed that fluconazole (200 mg/day) was superior to amphotericin B (1 mg/kg/wk) in preventing relapse (2% versus 18%) in AIDS patients with cryptococcal meningitis [159]. These data indicate that **fluconazole (200 mg/day) is the antifungal agent of choice for prevention of relapse of cryptococcal meningitis in patients with AIDS; therapy must be continued for life.** Maintenance therapy with itraconazole is currently being studied. Dosages of fluconazole up to 800 mg/day have been used beneficially in some AIDS patients with cryptococcal meningitis who failed primary therapy or who experienced a relapse [160].

Primary prevention of cryptococcal meningitis by using oral fluconazole is undergoing evaluation [160a]. Potential problems with primary prevention with fluconazole are not only the cost of this regimen (see Chap. 18) but also concern that prolonged use of fluconazole may help select out resistant fungi.

See Chaps. 18 and 19 for further discussions of the prevention and therapy of cryptococcal meningitis.

2. *Candida.* The treatment of choice for *Candida* meningitis is amphotericin B with or without 5-flucytosine [67, 68]. Although there are no studies comparing the efficacy of single and combination therapy, some investigators recommend combination therapy based on more rapid CSF sterilization and possible reduction of long-term neurologic sequelae in newborns. Cure rates with amphotericin B alone have ranged from 67 to 89% in adults and 71 to 100% in neonates with *Candida* meningitis. However, as many as 56% of surviving neonates had psychomotor retardation, and hydrocephalus was seen in 50% [67, 68]. Increased mortality in adult patients with *Candida* meningitis has been associated with a delay of more than 2 weeks from the onset of symptoms to diagnosis, a CSF glucose concentration of less than 35 mg/dl, development of intracranial hypertension, and focal neurologic deficits.

3. *Coccidioides immitis.* Until further data on the use of fluconazole are available, coccidioidal meningitis should be treated with amphotericin B, usually administered both intravenously and intrathecally [70, 71]. Intrathecal administration may be via the lumbar, cisternal, or ventricular routes (i.e., through an Ommaya reservoir); the usual dosage is 0.5 mg 3 times weekly for 3 months, although 1.0–1.5 mg combined with hydrocortisone can be used. Mortality of 50% has been reported, although one study found a survival rate of 91% over a follow-up period of 75 months if larger doses of intrathecal amphotericin B (1.0–1.5 mg) were used [161]. Antifungal therapy is discontinued once the CSF has been normal for at least 1 year on an intrathecal regimen of once every 6 weeks. However, intrathecal amphotericin B is poorly tolerated, often leading to arachnoiditis.

Fluconazole and itraconazole have been used to treat coccidioidal meningitis.

Initial results appeared promising, although most of the patients were treated previously or concurrently with amphotericin B. A recent collaborative study examined the efficacy of fluconazole in the treatment of coccidioidal meningitis [162]. Fifty consecutive patients with active coccidioidal meningitis (including 9 patients coinfected with HIV) received fluconazole (400 mg once daily) for up to 4 years (median of 37 months) in responding patients. Of the 47 evaluable patients, 37 (79%) responded to treatment, with the most improvement occurring within 4–8 months of drug initiation. However, 24% of patients exhibited a persistent CSF pleocytosis despite the relative absence of symptoms, indicating the need for careful follow-up. In nonresponding patients, the authors suggested that increasing the dose of fluconazole (commonly done by physicians in the endemic area) or instituting intrathecal amphotericin B might be required. If utilized, fluconazole therapy may need to be continued indefinitely. Further studies are needed to optimize the use of fluconazole in patients with coccidioidal meningitis.

F. Protozoal and helminthic meningitis

1. **Amebae.** Many antimicrobial agents have in vitro activity against free-living amebae [73]. These include amphotericin B, the tetracyclines, the imidazoles, qinghaosu, and rifampin. Only four patients reported in the literature have survived after therapy for primary amebic meningoencephalitis [72, 73, 163]. All received amphotericin B along with various other antimicrobial agents. The best-documented survivor received amphotericin B and miconazole intravenously and intrathecally, as well as rifampin, sulfizoxazole, and dexamethasone. However, no effective regimen has been established. Therapy with parenteral and intracisternal amphotericin B combined with rifampin and tetracycline has been suggested. Treatment is continued over 2–3 weeks if the clinical response is good and no complications occur.

2. *Angiostrongylus cantonensis.* Symptomatic treatment for headache, nausea, and vomiting, and the like is indicated for eosinophilic meningitis caused by *A. cantonensis* [72]. Most patients recover within 1–2 weeks. Thiabendazole has been used in the early stages of migration of the larvae of *A. cantonensis,* but the drug fails as soon as the worm reaches the CNS.

VI. Adjunctive therapy

A. **Viral meningitis.** Because of the lack of effective antiviral therapy against the enteroviruses, other adjunctive measures have been employed in seriously ill patients with enteroviral meningitis [2]. Administration of gamma globulin by multiple routes (including directly into the CNS) has led to stabilization or improvement of agammaglobulinemic patients with chronic enteroviral meningitis or meningoencephalitis. Neonates with overwhelming enteroviral sepsis and meningitis have received intravenous gamma globulin, maternal plasma, and exchange transfusions, with occasional successes. This topic has recently been reviewed [163a].

B. **Bacterial meningitis**

1. **Antiinflammatory agents.** Despite the availability of effective bactericidal antimicrobial agents, morbidity and mortality from bacterial meningitis remain unacceptably high.

   a. **Animal model studies.** Studies in experimental animal models have demonstrated that development of a subarachnoid space inflammatory response is a major factor contributing to morbidity and mortality in bacterial meningitis [112, 164, 165]. Therefore, investigators have examined whether attenuation of this response would improve outcome in this disorder. For example, the inflammatory response induced by either live pneumococci or pneumococcal cell wall in an **experimental rabbit model** was reduced by agents (e.g., methylprednisolone, oxindanac) that inhibited the cyclooxygenase pathway of arachidonic acid metabolism [166]. Other studies revealed that methylprednisolone administration led to a significant reduction in the mass of leukocytes within the meninges of rabbits with pneumococcal meningitis [167]; CSF outflow resistance also was reduced by methylprednisolone therapy and to a greater extent than in untreated or penicillin-treated rabbits with pneumococcal meningitis [168]. In further studies that examined the effects of corticosteroids (methylprednisolone and dexamethasone) on brain water content, CSF pressure, and CSF lactate in rabbits with pneumococcal meningitis, it was determined that both agents completely reversed the development of brain edema, but only dexamethasone led to a reduction in CSF pressure and lactate [169].

In another study utilizing an experimental rabbit model of *H. influenzae* type b meningitis, treatment with ceftriaxone versus ceftriaxone plus dexamethasone revealed that combination therapy consistently reduced the brain water content, CSF pressure, and CSF lactate to a greater degree than ceftriaxone alone [170], although the differences were not statistically significant. However, it was suggested that adjunctive dexamethasone might be more beneficial if administered early, or even before the occurrence of antibiotic-induced bacterial lysis and release of microbial products. In a subsequent analysis using the same animal model [171], ceftriaxone administration led to a significant increase in CSF endotoxin concentrations followed by a rise in CSF tumor necrosis factor (TNF) concentrations. Simultaneous administration of dexamethasone and ceftriaxone did not affect release of endotoxin into CSF but markedly attenuated CSF concentrations of TNF. Adjunctive dexamethasone therapy also resulted in a significant decrease in CSF leukocytosis and a trend toward earlier improvement in CSF concentrations of glucose, lactate, and protein. These parameters improved without any apparent decrease in the rate of bacterial killing within the CSF in vivo [171].

b. Clinical trials. Based on these observations in experimental animal models, several clinical trials were undertaken in the late 1980s and early 1990s to determine the effects of adjunctive corticosteroids on outcome in patients with bacterial meningitis.

(1) In one double-blind, placebo-controlled trial of adjunctive dexamethasone therapy in infants and children with bacterial meningitis [172], patients were treated with antibiotic (cefuroxime or ceftriaxone) and either dexamethasone or placebo. The patients who received adjunctive dexamethasone became afebrile sooner, had a more rapid normalization of CSF parameters (glucose, protein, and lactate), and were significantly less likely to acquire moderate to severe bilateral sensorineural hearing loss (15.5% versus 3.3%). However, these findings were significant only for patients with meningitis caused by *H. influenzae* type b, and the benefits in terms of morbidity (i.e., sensorineural hearing loss) were statistically significant only in patients receiving cefuroxime and not ceftriaxone. Four patients who received adjunctive dexamethasone developed GI hemorrhage, two of whom required blood transfusions.

(2) In a second clinical trial from the same authors, 31 infants and children with bacterial meningitis were treated with cefuroxime and dexamethasone, whereas 29 patients received cefuroxime and placebo [173]. No statistically significant differences in neurologic abnormalities or hearing impairment were noted between the two groups at 6 weeks, although when the data from these two studies were combined, overall support for the benefit of adjunctive dexamethasone was suggested.

(3) In a third published trial conducted in Egypt, children and adults with bacterial meningitis were randomized to receive antibiotics (intramuscular ampicillin plus chloramphenicol) with or without adjunctive dexamethasone therapy [174]. The patients with pneumococcal meningitis who received adjunctive dexamethasone had a significant reduction in mortality (from approximately 40% to 13%) and overall neurologic sequelae. No differences in mortality were noted in patients with meningococcal or *H. influenzae* meningitis. Important findings were that no significant differences were noted between groups in time to afebrility or improvement in CSF parameters, possible adverse effects were not documented, and an extraordinarily high percentage of patients presented in a comatose state.

(4) A fourth published placebo-controlled, double-blind trial from Costa Rica randomized infants and children with bacterial meningitis to receive cefotaxime with either dexamethasone or placebo [175]. In this study, the dexamethasone or placebo was administered 15–20 minutes before the first dose of cefotaxime in an attempt to attenuate maximally the potential bacteriolytic antibiotic-induced CSF inflammatory response. Meningeal inflammation and CSF concentrations of TNF and platelet-activating factor had decreased more rapidly in patients who received adjunctive dexamethasone 12 hours after initiation of therapy. In follow-up for a mean of 15 months, patients who had received adjunctive dexamethasone had a significantly decreased incidence of one or more neurologic sequelae, although there was only a trend toward reduction of audiologic impairment. No differences in mortality were observed.

(5) In a recent prospective, multicentered, placebo-controlled trial of 173 children 8 weeks to 12 years old, patients were randomized to receive ceftriaxone with or without dexamethasone (given after the first dose of antibiotic but always within 4 hours of the first IV dose of antibiotic) [175a]. Dexamethasone did not demonstrate statistically significant reductions in the frequency of hearing loss or persistent neurologic abnormalities, with the exception of the frequency of bilateral hearing deficits in those with *H. influenzae* type b meningitis [175b]. A beneficial effect was not evident among the 33 children with meningitis caused by *S. pneumoniae* or among the 24 with meningitis caused by *N. meningitidis* [175a, 175b]. Auditory brainstem responses were measured within 24 hours of admission and serially; when hearing loss was documented, it occurred early after the onset of meningitis, unrelated to antibiotic or dexamethasone therapy [175a].

(6) In addition, in a review of the records of 97 infants and children with pneumococcal meningitis [176], the patients treated with adjunctive dexamethasone had a significantly reduced adverse long-term neurologic outcome, including hearing impairment. Although there were similarities in the demographics and clinical characteristics between the groups that received antibiotics alone and antibiotics plus dexamethasone, the study was retrospective, and no data on the use of specific antimicrobial agents were presented.

Finally, another published prospective, placebo-controlled, double-blind study of adjunctive dexamethasone in 115 children with acute bacterial meningitis in Switzerland revealed that neurologic sequelae (at 3, 9, and 15 months) were lower in the dexamethasone group (5% versus 16%; $p = 0.066$) [177].

c. **Summary.** Several points deserve emphasis.

(1) **Based on the preceding studies, the data support the routine use of adjunctive dexamethasone (0.15 mg/kg q6h for 4 days) in infants and children with bacterial meningitis caused by *H. influenzae* type b.** Administration of dexamethasone before or concomitant with antimicrobial therapy is recommended for optimal attenuation of the subarachnoid space inflammatory response; patients should be carefully monitored for the possibility of GI hemorrhage.

However, with the introduction and use of effective vaccination against *H. influenzae* type b in infancy, the incidence of serious infections due to *H. influenzae* type b has decreased more than 90%. Therefore, most cases of bacterial meningitis likely to be seen in the U.S. in the future will be caused by bacteria for which there are only limited data regarding the benefit of adjunctive steroid therapy [175b].

(2) **In adults or in patients with meningitis caused by other bacterial organisms, the routine use of adjunctive dexamethasone is not recommended pending results of ongoing studies.** However, some authors recommend its use in all cases of meningitis with a likely bacterial etiology (i.e., demonstrable bacteria on CSF Gram stain, which may predict the patients at greatest risk of bacteriolysis-induced exacerbation of inflammation) [164], although there are no clinical data to support this recommendation. In adults with severely impaired mental status (stupor or coma), documented cerebral edema (e.g., by CT scan), or markedly elevated intracranial pressure (i.e., high opening pressure on lumbar puncture, palsy of cranial nerve VI), dexamethasone may be beneficial. The use of adjunctive dexamethasone is of particular concern in patients with pneumococcal meningitis who are treated with vancomycin, as a diminished CSF inflammatory response may significantly reduce CSF vancomycin penetration.

(3) **In neonates,** clinical trials on the role of corticosteroids in meningitis have not been performed. Therefore, the use of these agents is not suggested. (See Chap. 3 for related discussion.)

(4) Penetration of antibiotics into the CSF is becoming a greater concern in treating meningitis caused by penicillin-resistant *S. pneumoniae* (see sec. **V.B.3** and Chap. **28C**). In particular, although vancomycin is active against virtually all strains of *S. pneumoniae*, it penetrates the CSF quite poorly. Furthermore, in an experimental rabbit model of meningitis, penetration of vancomycin into the CSF is reduced with concomitant dexamethasone therapy, with resulting delayed CSF sterilization. Therefore, in areas where high level penicillin-resistant strains of *S. pneumoniae* are prevalent and empiric vancomycin is used, steroid therapy may prove harmful [175b].

d. The 1994 "Red Book" [177a] makes the following recommendations which have been supported by recent reviews in 1995 [175a, 175b].

(1) Dexamethasone therapy should be considered when bacterial meningitis in infants and children 6 weeks and older is diagnosed or strongly suspected on the basis of the CSF tests, including Gram-stained smears, after the physician has weighed the benefits and possible risks and before the etiology has been established.

(2) Dexamethasone is recommended for treatment of infants and children with *H. influenzae* meningitis.

(3) Dexamethasone should be considered for the treatment of infants and children with pneumococcal or meningococcal meningitis. However, its efficacy for these infections is unproven, and some experts do not recommend its use.

(4) The recommended dexamethasone regimen is 0.6 mg/kg/day in four divided doses IV for the first 4 days of antibiotic treatment. A recent placebo-controlled trial indicates that a 2-day regimen of dexamethasone is also effective.

(5) If dexamethasone is given, it should be administered as early as possible, preferably at the time of, or shortly after, the first dose of antibacterial therapy. Dexamethasone therapy when initiated more than 12 hours after the start of parenterally administered antimicrobial therapy is unlikely to be effective.

(6) Dexamethasone should not be used for suspected or proven nonbacterial meningitis. If dexamethasone was started before the diagnosis of nonbacterial meningitis was made, it should be discontinued.

(7) "Partially treated" meningitis with negative cultures is not an indication for continued dexamethasone therapy.

(8) If dexamethasone is used, all patients, not just those with severe disease, should be treated.

(9) No data currently are available on which to base a recommendation concerning the use of dexamethasone for treatment of bacterial meningitis in infants younger than 6 weeks, or of meningitis in those with congenital or acquired abnormalities of the CNS, with or without a prosthetic device.

(10) Measurements of hemoglobin concentrations and examinations of stool for blood should be performed regularly during dexamethasone therapy. If gross blood is found, dexamethasone therapy should be stopped and the patient should be observed closely for possible transfusion therapy.

2. Reduction of intracranial pressure. Several methods are available to reduce intracranial pressure [178], including elevation of the head of the bed to 30 degrees to maximize venous drainage with minimal compromise of cerebral perfusion; the use of hyperosmolar agents (e.g., mannitol) to make the intravascular space hyperosmolar to the brain, thereby permitting movement of water from brain tissue into the intravascular compartment; and the use of corticosteroids. In a recent report from Finland, oral glycerol was studied and appeared to help prevent neurologic sequelae [178a]. In addition, hyperventilation to maintain the $PaCO_2$ between 27 and 30 mmHg, which causes cerebral vasoconstriction and reduction in cerebral blood volume, has also been employed, although some experts have questioned the routine use of hyperventilation to reduce intracranial pressure in patients with bacterial meningitis [179]. Infants and children with bacterial meningitis who have initially normal CT scans of the head can be treated with hyperventilation to reduce elevated intracranial pressure safely because it is unlikely that cerebral blood flow would be reduced to ischemic thresholds. However, in children with cerebral edema on head CT scanning, cerebral blood flow is more likely to be normal or reduced. Therefore, hyperventilation might decrease intracranial pressure at the expense of cerebral blood flow, possibly reducing the latter to ischemic thresholds. These patients would likely benefit more from early use of diuretics, osmotically dehydrating agents (provided that intravascular volume is protected), and corticosteroids, although controlled trials exploring these issues have yet to be performed.

Patients in whom elevated intracranial pressures continue despite these measures may be treated with high-dose barbiturate therapy to decrease cerebral metabolic demands and cerebral blood flow [178]. Vasoconstriction in normal tissue also occurs during barbiturate therapy, thereby shunting blood to ischemic tissue and protecting the brain from ischemic insult. This mode of treatment for meningitis and elevated intracranial pressure is of unproven benefit, however, and must be considered experimental.

3. **Basilar skull fracture.** Patients who have suffered a basilar skull fracture with CSF leak may have persistent dural defects associated with recurrent episodes of bacterial meningitis. Although many leaks will cease spontaneously, surgery is indicated for leaks that persist for several weeks or in patients who present with delayed or recurrent infection [32]. Surgery is not indicated in the acute phase (< 7 days) of leakage because there is no difference in outcome when patients with acutely repaired leaks are compared to those whose leaks stop spontaneously within 7 days.

4. **Cerebrospinal shunt infections.** In patients with infected CSF shunts, all components of the shunt should be removed at the beginning of antimicrobial therapy [46] and an external ventriculostomy placed to clear the ventriculitis and monitor CSF parameters. The ability of many organisms to adhere to the prostheses and survive antimicrobial therapy precludes effective treatment in situ. Furthermore, the propensity for the entire shunt to become contaminated when one portion becomes infected argues against partial revisions. This topic has recently been reviewed elsewhere [179a].

C. **Tuberculous meningitis.** Despite the availability of effective antituberculous chemotherapy, persistent morbidity and mortality continue to exist in patients with tuberculous meningitis. Chemotherapy may halt mycobacterial growth, but inflammation often continues at the base of the brain, with subsequent organization of necrotic tissue and exudate, fibroblastic proliferation, and formation of dense fibrocollagenous tissue compressing adjacent structures and impeding circulation of CSF. This has led to the search for adjunctive agents for treatment of tuberculous meningitis.

The most commonly advocated adjunctive agents for the treatment of tuberculous meningitis are **corticosteroids** [50, 51, 82a]. These agents have been shown to abrogate the symptoms and signs of disease; patients frequently defervesce, with clearing of sensorium and improvement in well-being even after only a few doses. The primary value of corticosteroids may be their ability to treat or avert the development of spinal block, possibly by lowering the CSF protein content; an improvement in overall mortality has been ascribed to their specific activity on this poor prognostic sign. Despite a reduced mortality, however, a concomitant, almost compensatory, increase in significant neurologic sequelae has been observed in survivors of tuberculous meningitis who have received corticosteroids. In contrast, a recent study from Egypt found reduced neurologic complications and reduced case fatality rates in patients who received dexamethasone in conjunction with antituberculous chemotherapy [180].

Despite the **controversy surrounding the role of corticosteroids** in the treatment of tuberculous meningitis, most authorities advocate the use of these agents in selected cases with extreme neurologic compromise, elevated intracranial pressure, impending herniation, or impending or established spinal block [50, 51]. Some authors also recommend adjunctive corticosteroids in patients with CT evidence of either hydrocephalus or basilar meningitis. Therapy with prednisone (approximately 1 mg/kg/day initially, then tapered over 1 month) often is recommended, although varying doses of dexamethasone or hydrocortisone have also been used.

D. **Fungal meningitis.** Patients with cryptococcal meningitis may have several complications despite antifungal therapy. Increased intracranial pressure has been noted in some AIDS patients with cryptococcal meningitis, possibly due to increased CSF outflow resistance [181]. Hydrocephalus has also been reported as a complication of cryptococcal meningitis. Therapeutic modalities utilized for these complications have included ventriculoperitoneal shunting, frequent high-volume lumbar punctures, acetazolamide, and corticosteroids. However, the precise roles of these adjunctive measures (particularly corticosteroids) in the treatment of cryptococcal meningitis remain to be established.

VII. Prevention

A. Viral meningitis.
The cornerstone of prevention of mumps is **active immunization** with the live, attenuated mumps vaccine [9]. Widespread use of the mumps vaccine has greatly reduced the incidence of mumps and mumps meningoencephalitis. Mumps meningitis has been reported in children 11 days to 2 months after vaccine administration [182], although it is not clear whether these cases represented vaccine failure or meningitis due to the vaccine strain of mumps virus.

B. Bacterial meningitis

1. Haemophilus influenzae

a. **Chemoprophylaxis.** Several studies have documented the transmission of *H. influenzae* type b from patients with meningitis to household contacts. Most secondary cases (75%) occur within 6 days of onset of the index case, although untreated household contacts remain at increased risk for *H. influenzae* type b disease for at least 1 month after onset in the index case. The risk is markedly age-dependent, highest for children younger than 2 years. Daycare outside the home may be another risk factor for transmission [183].

The **rationale for the use of chemoprophylaxis** to prevent secondary disease is eradication of nasopharyngeal colonization of *H. influenzae* type b, thereby preventing transmission to young, susceptible contacts and the subsequent development of invasive disease in those already colonized [183]. The chemoprophylactic agent of choice is rifampin (20 mg/kg/day, with a maximum dose of 600 mg, for 4 days) for all individuals, including adults, in households with at least one child younger than 48 months. Chemoprophylaxis is not currently recommended for daycare contacts 2 years or older unless two or more cases occur in the daycare center within a 60-day period. For children younger than 2 years, the determination of whether to administer prophylaxis needs to be individualized and should be considered more strongly in daycare centers that resemble households where children have prolonged contact. Rifampin is not recommended for pregnant women who are contacts of infected infants, as the risk of rifampin to the fetus has not been established.

The index patient with meningitis should also receive rifampin prophylaxis because some antibiotics (e.g., ampicillin) given for invasive *H. influenzae* type b disease do not necessarily eliminate nasopharyngeal colonization.

b. **Immunoprophylaxis.** The Immunization Practices Advisory Committee [184] recommends that all children be vaccinated with one of the conjugate vaccines licensed for infant use: *H. influenzae* type b conjugate vaccine (diphtheria CRM$_{197}$ protein conjugate, HbOC) or *H. influenzae* type b conjugate vaccine (meningococcal protein conjugate, PRP-OMP). Three doses of HbOC or two doses of PRP-OMP are administered 2 months apart beginning at 2 months of age. Unvaccinated children older than 60 months should be vaccinated based on their disease risk (e.g., patients with asplenia, sickle cell disease, or an immunosuppressive malignancy). These vaccines are discussed further in Chap. 22. Use of the vaccine does not preclude recommendations for rifampin chemoprophylaxis in the appropriate clinical setting.

2. Neisseria meningitidis

a. **Chemoprophylaxis.** Chemoprophylaxis is also necessary for contacts of patients with invasive meningococcal disease. **Chemoprophylaxis is recommended for close contacts of the index case, defined as** household contacts or daycare center members who sleep or eat in the same dwelling, close contacts in a closed community such as a military barracks or boarding school, and medical personnel performing mouth-to-mouth resuscitation [81, 177a]. Chemoprophylaxis may also need to be administered to the index case prior to hospital discharge because certain antimicrobial agents (e.g., high-dose penicillin or chloramphenicol) do not reliably eradicate meningococci from the nasopharynx of colonized patients.

b. Regimens

    (1) Rifampin. The CDC currently recommends administration of **rifampin** at 12-hour intervals for 2 days in the following dosages [81]: adults, 600 mg; children beyond the neonatal period, 10 mg/kg; and infants younger than 1 month, 5 mg/kg. However, there are several problems with rifampin chemoprophylaxis, including nasopharyngeal eradication rates of only 80% or so, adverse events, necessity for multiple doses over 2 days, and emergence of resistant organisms (up to 10–27% of isolates).

    (2) Alternatives. Ceftriaxone (250 mg IM in adults and 125 mg in children) was shown to eliminate the meningococcal serogroup A carrier state in 97% of patients in one study for up to 2 weeks [185], although parenteral administration is required. A single dose of **oral ciprofloxacin** (500 or 750 mg in adults) has also been demonstrated to be very effective in eliminating the nasopharyngeal carriage of *N. meningitidis* [142]; ciprofloxacin may well supplant rifampin for chemoprophylaxis in adults. Ciprofloxacin is not recommended for persons younger than 18 years because of concerns regarding cartilage damage [177a]. **In pregnant patients, ceftriaxone is probably the safest alternative agent for chemoprophylaxis.**

c. Immunoprophylaxis. Vaccination with the quadrivalent meningococcal vaccine (active against serogroups A, C, Y, and W135) is currently recommended for patients in certain high-risk groups including those with terminal complement component or properdin deficiency or dysfunction; asplenia; those who travel to areas with hyperendemic or epidemic meningococcal disease (e.g., Nigeria); military recruits; and those who are close contacts of the primary case as an adjunct to chemoprophylaxis [183], although this is controversial and of unproven efficacy. The vaccine is not recommended for routine use in the United States because of the overall low risk of infection, the inability to protect against serogroup B disease, and the inability to provide lasting immunity to young children. The major use of the meningococcal vaccine is during outbreaks of disease caused by the serogroups represented in the vaccine preparation.

3. *Streptococcus pneumoniae*

a. Chemoprophylaxis. The risk of secondary pneumococcal disease in contacts of infected patients has not been defined, although outbreaks have been described in closed populations such as gold miners, military recruits, and jail inmates [183]. Further studies are needed before chemoprophylaxis is recommended for contacts of patients with pneumococcal meningitis. Some authors do recommend prophylaxis with oral penicillin in patients with sickle cell disease in whom therapy has been shown to reduce the incidence of pneumococcal septicemia and meningitis; however, this practice is not universally accepted.

b. Immunoprophylaxis. The use of the current 23-valent pneumococcal vaccine is recommended for prevention of bacteremic pneumococcal disease in certain high-risk groups; studies of blood and CSF isolates from the United States, Sweden, and South Africa revealed that from 77 to 96% of the organisms were represented in the 23-valent vaccine [183, 186]. However, the efficacy of the vaccine in preventing pneumococcal meningitis has never been documented, although it would seem prudent to administer the vaccine to certain persons older than 2 years who are at increased risk for bacteremic pneumococcal disease: those older than 65 years; patients with diabetes mellitus, congestive heart failure, hepatic disease, renal disease, and other cardiopulmonary conditions; chronic alcoholics; patients with asplenia, multiple myeloma, or the Wiskott-Aldrich syndrome; patients with a CSF fistula or leak; and HIV-infected patients. Vaccination for persons traveling to an area with a significant incidence of resistant pneumococci may also be warranted. See further discussion of the pneumococcal vaccine in Chap. 9.

4. Basilar skull fracture. A number of studies have reported on the administration of prophylactic antibiotics in patients with basilar skull fractures and CSF leak [32, 46]. This is based on the premise that in patients with a dural defect, the CSF is exposed to pathogenic organisms from the nasopharynx, nasal or mastoid sinuses, or external auditory canal. Despite conflicting studies, the **use of prophylactic antibiotics is not recommended** for patients with basilar skull fracture and CSF leak because this practice does not appear to change the incidence of posttraumatic bacterial meningitis and may result in selection and growth of resistant organisms. See related discussion in Chap. 28B.

Encephalitis

The syndrome of acute encephalitis shares many features with acute meningitis, although the likelihood of mental status changes early in disease prior to the onset of obtundation or coma is more common in encephalitis. Clinically, seizures are more likely to occur with encephalitis, and associated systemic illness is more prominent [187–190]. Numerous infectious as well as noninfectious agents have been reported to cause acute encephalitis (see Table 5-1 for agents of meningitis that may also cause encephalitis). Here **we will concentrate on encephalitis caused by the herpesviruses, especially herpes simplex virus, as these represent the most common and only treatable forms of viral encephalitis.**

For a general review of viral encephalitis, see reference [190]; for a discussion of CMV infections of the CNS (which can include an encephalitis) in patients with AIDS, see reference [18a].

I. **Epidemiology and etiology**

   A. **Herpes simplex virus.** HSV infections of the CNS are among the most common (10–20% of encephalitic viral infections in the United States) and most severe of all human viral infections of the brain and are associated with significant morbidity and mortality (> 70% with ineffective or no therapy) [187]. HSV encephalitis occurs throughout the year (i.e., is nonseasonal) and in patients of all age groups, with whites accounting for 95% of patients with biopsy-proven disease.

   B. **Varicella-zoster virus.** The actual incidence of CNS involvement during active varicella infection is unknown, although the observed incidence has ranged from 0.1 to 0.75% in some series [188]. Herpes zoster is a consequence of reactivation of latent varicella zoster virus (VZV); a direct correlation exists between cutaneous dissemination and visceral involvement, including meningoencephalitis. In general, the CNS complications of herpes zoster are associated with a higher morbidity and mortality than those of acute varicella, possibly due to the patient's advanced age and underlying disease status.

II. **Clinical presentation**

   A. **Herpes simplex virus.** Most patients with biopsy-proven HSV encephalitis present with a focal encephalopathic process characterized by **altered mentation and decreasing levels of consciousness with focal neurologic findings,** including dysphasia, weakness, and paresthesias [187]. **Fever and personality changes** are uniformly present. Approximately two-thirds of patients with biopsy-proven disease develop either focal or generalized **seizures.** The clinical course of HSV encephalitis may progress slowly or with alarming rapidity; commonly, there is progressive loss of consciousness leading to coma. Although clinical evidence of a temporal lobe lesion often is believed to be a result of HSV encephalitis, a variety of other diseases have been shown to mimic this condition, including various infections (abscess/subdural empyema), tuberculosis, cryptococcosis, toxoplasmosis, CMV; tumor; and subdural hematoma [189].

   With the availability of an easier diagnostic test for HSV encephalitis (see sec. **III.A.2**), milder cases of HSV encephalitis are anticipated to be diagnosed more readily, expanding the clinical spectrum of HSV encephalitis [92a].

   B. **Varicella-zoster virus.** The most common neurologic abnormality associated with VZV is cerebellar ataxia; although meningoencephalitis and cerebritis are less common, they frequently are more severe complications [187]. Headache, fever, and vomiting often are accompanied by an altered sensorium, with seizures occurring in 29–52% of patients. Focal neurologic abnormalities, including cranial nerve dysfunction, aphasia, and hemiplegia, have also been described. Encephalitis is the most common abnormality associated with herpes zoster, seen most commonly in patients of advanced age, following immunosuppression, and in those with disseminated cutaneous zoster. Some patients with ophthalmic zoster sometimes present with a distinctive CNS process, which is contralateral hemiplegia; this finding is seen in up to one-third of CNS abnormalities in herpes zoster. The zoster ophthalmicus usually precedes the hemiplegia by several weeks or more, although it has been reported to occur as late as 6 months after the rash has resolved.

III. **Diagnosis**
   A. **Herpes simplex virus**
      1. **Routine studies of CSF** in patients with HSV encephalitis are **not diagnostic** [187, 190]. The CSF white blood cell count is elevated (mean of 100 cells/mm^3) in 97% of patients with biopsy-proven disease, with a lymphocytic predominance. The presence of RBCs in CSF **suggests** the diagnosis in the appropriate clinical setting but is not definitively diagnostic. The CSF protein is elevated also (averaging approximately 100 mg/dl). Approximately 3.5% of patients with HSV encephalitis have normal CSF studies. Virus is isolated from CSF only 4% or so of the time.
      2. **Polymerase chain reaction.** Recent studies suggest that **detection of herpes simplex virus DNA by PCR is highly sensitive and specific for** the diagnosis of HSV encephalitis [92, 92a]. This test may be obtained through the laboratory of Fred Lakeman at the University of Alabama at Birmingham (205-934-6750) and through other reference laboratories. **The PCR test for HSV in CSF is now the optimal way to diagnose HSV encephalitis** [92a].
      3. **Noninvasive studies may be useful to support the diagnosis** of HSV encephalitis [187, 190].
         a. A sensitive test (approximately 84%) is **electroencephalography** (EEG), which reveals characteristic spike–and–slow wave activity and periodic lateralizing epileptiform discharges (PLEDs), which are located predominantly over the temporal and frontotemporal regions.
         b. **CT scans** show low-density areas with mass effect localized to the temporal lobe in 50–75% of patients at sometime during the course of their illness.
         c. **MRI scans** have recently been considered to be more sensitive than CT for the detection of HSV encephalitis lesions and is considered by some experts to be the most important and specific imaging technique [191].
            HSV encephalitis typically affects the temporal lobes, predominantly their inferior aspects. Involvement is usually asymmetric, and the deep white matter may demonstrate the earliest abnormalities. Some reviewers believe it would be very unusual to have a normal MRI even in early HSV encephalitis [191].
         d. **Radionuclide brain scans** may reveal increased uptake in both temporal lobes; brain scan is more sensitive than CT scan early in the disease course.
         e. However, despite the availability of these diagnostic modalities, **none** are uniformly **satisfactory for the diagnosis of HSV encephalitis.**
      4. In the past, the most specific means of diagnosing HSV encephalitis was a **brain biopsy** [187, 192]. The presence of Cowdry type A intranuclear inclusions supports the diagnosis of viral infections, although these are found only in approximately 50% of cases. Brain tissue should also be subjected to immunofluorescence, which is a rapid, sensitive, and reliable method for detecting herpes antigen; virus can also be isolated from brain tissue. With the availability of PCR studies on CSF, brain biopsy now is seldom indicated (see sec. **2**).
   B. **Varicella-zoster virus.** The CSF often is abnormal in varicella-associated encephalitis with a lymphocytic pleocytosis and elevated protein [187]. The EEG usually reveals diffuse abnormalities (e.g., diffuse slowing), although focal abnormalities may occur even without seizure activity. In patients with herpes zoster–associated encephalitis, the CSF also usually reveals a lymphocytic pleocytosis and elevated protein; however, up to 40% of patients with uncomplicated herpes zoster (i.e., without CNS involvement) may have a mild CSF pleocytosis or elevated protein. The virus has been cultured from brain tissue and CSF in a number of cases, and viral inclusions are well-described in autopsy series. In patients with zoster ophthalmicus with contralateral hemiplegia, a unilateral arteritis or thrombosis of involved vessels may be seen on cerebral angiography, and cerebral infarction may be seen on CT scan.

IV. **Approach to the patient with viral encephalitis.** Despite the number of viral organisms that may cause encephalitis, herpes simplex remains the only viral CNS infection for which therapy (i.e., acyclovir) has been proven to be beneficial in controlled clinical trials. Based on the ease of administration and good safety profile of acyclovir, an empiric course should be administered for patients with presumed viral encephalitis

[190]. In unusual cases, a brain biopsy may be indicated. With the availability of PCR, this will eliminate the need for biopsy in most instances. Infectious disease consultation is advised in these difficult cases. MRI is an important imaging study to obtain when encephalitis is suspected [191].

V. Antimicrobial therapy

A. **Herpes simplex virus.** Initial antiviral therapy for HSV encephalitis was idoxuridine, although severe toxicity (e.g., bone marrow suppression and secondary bacterial infections) limited this drug's usefulness [193]. Subsequent studies demonstrated the efficacy of vidarabine in biopsy-proven HSV encephalitis, with reduction of mortality at 1 and 6 months after disease onset [194, 195]. **Acyclovir** has been demonstrated to be superior to vidarabine for the treatment of biopsy-proven HSV encephalitis, with a reduction in mortality with acyclovir compared to vidarabine (19% versus 55%) [196]. Furthermore, 38% of patients in the acyclovir group returned to a normal level of functioning compared to only 15–20% of patients in the vidarabine group. Acyclovir should be administered at a dosage of 10 mg/kg q8h in patients with normal renal function and should be continued for 10–14 days. Although many patients have been treated for 10–14 days, many experts now prefer a more protracted course of 14–21 days [197].

B. **Varicella-zoster virus.** Intravenous acyclovir is also the drug of choice for patients with VZV-associated CNS infection who are at high risk for progressive disease [198]. Although no clinical trial has established the value of an antiviral agent for therapy of herpes zoster–associated encephalitis, we believe acyclovir should be used in this setting.

C. **Other viruses.** Although ganciclovir or foscarnet commonly is given to HIV-infected patients with CNS symptoms, proof of efficacy against cytomegaloviral CNS disease is lacking. No therapy is of proven benefit for Epstein-Barr virus disease. The treatment of arboviral infections (e.g., Eastern or Western equine encephalitis, St. Louis encephalitis), is supportive.

Brain Abscess

I. Epidemiology and etiology

A. **Bacteria.** The likely bacterial species responsible for brain abscess formation depends on the pathogenic mechanism involved [199–200]. The most commonly isolated bacteria are the streptococci (aerobic, anaerobic, and microaerophilic), isolated in 60–70% of abscesses. These bacteria, particularly the *S. milleri* (also called *S. intermedius*) group, are normal inhabitants of the oral cavity, appendix, and female genital tract, and have a proclivity for abscess formation. *S. aureus* is isolated in 10–15% of patients with brain abscess, usually in those with endocarditis or cranial trauma. The isolation of anaerobes has increased with use of proper isolation techniques: *Bacteroides* species are isolated in 20–40% of cases, often in mixed culture. The enteric gram-negative bacilli (e.g., *E. coli, Klebsiella* species, *Pseudomonas* species) are isolated in 23–33% of cases; these usually are seen in patients with otitic foci of infection or in the immunocompromised patient. Other bacterial species are isolated much less frequently in patients with brain abscess (< 1% of cases). These include *H. influenzae, S. pneumoniae,* and *L. monocytogenes*. In addition, *Nocardia* species are more often isolated in patients with defects in cell-mediated immunity, as in patients receiving corticosteroid therapy, in organ transplant recipients, and in patients with neoplastic disorders; some *Nocardia* cases have also been described in patients with AIDS.

B. **Fungi.** Many of the etiologic agents of fungal meningitis (see sec. I.E under Meningitis) may also cause brain abscesses [201, 202]. For example, although *Candida* species may produce meningitis, focal CNS disease is more common. Indeed, *Candida* is the most common fungal species to cause brain abscess (often multiple, not macroscopic). However, several other fungal species need to be considered in the differential diagnosis, especially in the immunocompromised host. For further discussion see Chap. 18.

1. ***Aspergillus* species.** Intracranial seeding of *Aspergillus* species occurs during dissemination of the organism from the lungs or by direct extension from a site anatomically adjacent to the brain [201, 202]. Of patients with disseminated disease, the brain is involved in 40–70% of cases. Most patients with *Aspergillus* brain abscesses are neutropenic and have an underlying hematologic malig-

nancy. Other risk groups include patients with Cushing's syndrome, diabetes mellitus, hepatic disease, and chronic granulomatous disease. Injection drug abusers, postcraniotomy patients, organ transplant recipients, HIV-infected patients, and patients receiving chronic corticosteroid therapy are also at risk.

2. **Mucormycosis.** Mucormycosis is one of the most fulminant fungal infections known [200, 202]. Predisposing conditions include diabetes mellitus (70% of cases), usually in association with acidosis; acidemia from profound systemic illness; hematologic neoplasia; renal transplantation; injection drug abuse; and use of deferoxamine. Fewer than 5% of cases involve otherwise normal healthy patients. CNS disease may result from direct extension (i.e., the rhinocerebral form) or by hematogenous dissemination from other primary sites of infection. Most infections are caused by the genus *Rhizopus,* and the genera *Absidia* and *Mucor* have also been isolated.

3. *Pseudallescheria boydii.* CNS disease may occur in both normal and immuno-compromised hosts. The organism may enter the CNS by direct trauma, by hematogenous dissemination from a primary site of infection, via an intravenous catheter, or by direct extension from infected sinuses [202, 203]. Due to the presence of *P. boydii* in contaminated water and manure, there is an association between near-drowning and subsequent illness [204].

II. **Clinical presentation**
A. **Bacterial brain abscess.** Patients with bacterial brain abscess may present with an indolent or fulminant course [199, 200].

1. **The clinical manifestations occur secondary to the presence of a space-occupying mass lesion** rather than the systemic signs of infection. Clinical findings include **headache** (70%), which may be moderate to severe and hemicranial or generalized; **nausea and vomiting** (50%), presumably due to increased intracranial pressure; **seizures** (25–35%), which usually are generalized; and nuchal rigidity and papilledema (25%). The majority of patients also have mental status changes, ranging from lethargy to coma. **Focal neurologic deficits** are seen in approximately 50% of cases and will vary depending on the location of brain involved.

2. **Fever is observed in only 45–50% of cases.** Only approximately half of patients with bacterial brain abscess present with the triad of headache, fever, and focal neurologic deficit.

3. The clinical **presentation of brain abscess also depends on the intracranial location** [199, 200]. For example, patients with frontal lobe abscess often present with headache, drowsiness, inattention, and deterioration of mental status; hemiparesis with unilateral motor signs and a motor speech disorder also are commonly seen. Patients with cerebellar abscesses present with ataxia, nystagmus, vomiting, and dysmetria. Temporal lobe abscesses may cause headache, aphasia, or a visual field defect (e.g., upper homonymous quadrantanopia). Patients with abscesses of the brain stem usually present with facial weakness, fever, headache, hemiparesis, dysphagia, and vomiting [205].

B. **Fungal brain abscess.** The clinical presentation of fungal brain abscess is similar to that caused by bacteria and depends on the intracranial location of the abscess and the fulminant nature of the organism [200, 202]. However, patients with certain fungal pathogens may present with specific symptoms and signs.

1. *Aspergillus* **species.** Patients most commonly present with signs of a stroke referable to the area of involved brain. Headache, encephalopathy, and seizures have also been described. Fever is not a constant finding, and meningeal irritation is rare.

2. **Mucormycosis.** Symptoms in patients with rhinocerebral mucormycosis are referable to the eyes or sinuses and include headache (often unilateral), facial pain, diplopia, lacrimation, and nasal stuffiness or discharge; fever and lethargy have also been described [200, 202]. Signs include development of a nasal ulcer, facial swelling, nasal discharge, proptosis, and external ophthalmoplegia. Orbital involvement is seen in two-thirds of patients. Cranial nerve abnormalities are also common. Because of the proclivity of the organism for blood vessel invasion, thrombosis is a striking feature of disease. Focal neurologic findings (e.g., hemiparesis, seizures, monocular blindness) suggest far-advanced disease. Invasion and occlusion of the cavernous sinus and carotid artery can occur as the disease progresses.

3. *Pseudallescheria boydii.* CNS infection with *P. boydii* usually becomes manifest 15–30 days after an episode of near-drowning [203, 204]. Clinical presen-

tation depends on localization in the CNS and includes seizures, altered consciousness, headache, meningeal irritation, focal neurologic deficits, abnormal behavior, and aphasia.

III. **Diagnosis**

A. **Bacterial brain abscess. The diagnosis of brain abscess has been revolutionized by the availability of CT scanning,** which is excellent for examining the brain parenchyma as well as the paranasal sinuses, mastoids, and middle ear [199]. Typically, the CT scan reveals a hypodense lesion with a peripheral uniform ring enhancement following the injection of contrast material. This may also be surrounded by a hypodense area of brain edema. Preliminary results indicate that MRI may offer significant advantages over CT in the diagnosis of brain abscesses [205], including the early detection of cerebritis, detection of cerebral edema with greater contrast between edema and brain, more conspicuous spread of inflammation into the ventricles and subarachnoid space, and earlier detection of satellite lesions. Administration of the paramagnetic agent gadolinium diethylenetriamine penta-acetic acid permits clear differentiation of the central abscess, surrounding enhancing rim, and cerebral edema.

B. **Fungal brain abscess.** Noninvasive studies (e.g., CSF examination, CT, MRI) for the diagnosis of fungal brain abscess usually are nonspecific, although some exceptions do exist [200, 202]. For example, the finding of a cerebral infarct in a patient with risk factors for invasive aspergillosis suggests that diagnosis; such an area of infarction typically develops into either single or multiple abscesses. In patients with rhinocerebral mucormycosis, CT and MRI typically show sinus opacification, erosion of bone, and obliteration of deep fascial planes; cavernous sinus involvement may also be seen on MRI. In injection drug abusers with cerebral mucormycosis, the most frequent site of CNS disease is the basal ganglia.

   Definitive diagnosis of fungal brain abscess requires biopsy with appropriate stains for fungal organisms [200, 202]. The mucicarmine stain will specifically identify the cells of *C. neoformans. Aspergillus* species appear as septate hyphae with acute-angle, dichotomous branching, whereas typical nonseptate hyphae with right-angle branching are seen in mucormycosis. *P. boydii* appears as septate hyphae in clinical specimens, although the hyphae are narrower and do not show the dichotomous branching seen in aspergillosis. Fluorescent antibody staining is also a sensitive method for identifying *P. boydii.*

IV. **Approach to the patient with brain abscess**

A. **Microbiologic diagnosis.** When a diagnosis of brain abscess is made presumptively by radiologic studies, a microbiologic diagnosis ideally should be made. CT scanning has made it possible to perform stereotactically guided aspiration of the abscess to facilitate microbiologic diagnosis and guide antimicrobial therapy. At the time of aspiration, specimens should be sent for Gram stain, aerobic and anaerobic cultures, Ziehl-Neelsen stain for *Mycobacteria,* modified acid-fast stain for *Nocardia* [205a], and silver stains for fungi. Cultures for *Mycobacteria, Nocardia,* and fungi should also be performed.

B. **Empiric antibiotic therapy.** In patients with bacterial brain abscess, once a diagnosis is made either presumptively by radiologic studies or by CT-guided aspiration of the lesion, antimicrobial therapy should be initiated [199, 200]. If an aspiration cannot be performed or if Gram staining is unrevealing, **empiric therapy should be initiated based on the presumed pathogenic mechanism of abscess formation** (Table 5-6).

   1. **Streptococci.** Because of the high rate of isolation of streptococci, especially the *S. milleri* group, from brain abscesses of different etiologies, high-dose intravenous **penicillin G** or another drug active against these organisms (e.g., a third-generation cephalosporin—either cefotaxime or ceftriaxone) should be included as initial therapeutic regimens.

   2. **Anaerobes.** Although penicillin G is active also against most anaerobic species, *Bacteroides fragilis* is a notable exception. This organism may be isolated in a high percentage of brain abscess cases. **Metronidazole** is the antimicrobial agent of choice against *B. fragilis* in this setting. Metronidazole also attains high concentrations in brain abscess pus, and its entry into brain abscesses is not altered by concomitant administration of corticosteroids.

   3. **Enterobacteriaceae. A third-generation cephalosporin** or trimethoprim-sulfamethoxazole should be used when members of the Enterobacteriaceae family are suspected. Ceftazidime is the agent of choice for *P. aeruginosa* brain abscess.

Table 5-6. Empiric antimicrobial therapy for bacterial brain abscess

Predisposing condition	Usual bacterial isolates	Antimicrobial regimen
Otitis media or mastoiditis	Streptococci (anaerobic or aerobic), *Bacteroides* spp., Enterobacteriaceae	Penicillin + metronidazole + a third-generation cephalosporin[a]
Sinusitis (frontoethmoidal or sphenoidal)	Streptococci, *Bacteroides* spp., Enterobacteriaceae, *Staphylococcus aureus, Haemophilus* spp.	Vancomycin + metronidazole + a third-generation cephalosporin[a]
Dental sepsis	Mixed *Fusobacterium* and *Bacteroides* spp., streptococci	Penicillin + metronidazole
Penetrating trauma or postneurosurgery	*S. aureus*, streptococci, Enterobacteriaceae, *Clostridium*	Vancomycin + a third-generation cephalosporin[a]
Congenital heart disease	Streptococci, *Haemophilus* spp.	Penicillin + a third-generation cephalosporin[a]
Lung abscess, empyema, bronchiectasis	*Fusobacterium, Actinomyces, Bacteroides* spp., streptococci, *Nocardia asteroides*	Penicillin + metronidazole + a sulfonamide[b]
Bacterial endocarditis	*S. aureus*, streptococci	Vancomycin + gentamicin *or* nafcillin + ampicillin + gentamicin

[a]Cefotaxime or ceftriaxone; ceftazidime is used if *Pseudomonas aeruginosa* is suspected.
[b]Trimethoprim-sulfamethoxazole; include if *N. asteroides* is suspected.

4. ***S. aureus.*** Nafcillin should be used when *S. aureus* is considered a likely infecting pathogen (e.g., staphylococcal endocarditis, cranial trauma); vancomycin is reserved for patients allergic to penicillin or when methicillin-resistant organisms are suspected or isolated.

5. ***Nocardia.*** When a brain abscess caused by *Nocardia* species [205a] is suspected or proven, trimethoprim-sulfamethoxazole should be utilized. Alternative agents include minocycline, amikacin, imipenem, and the fluoroquinolones. (See discussion of *Nocardia* in Chap. 18.)

C. **Modification of antibiotics after culture data.** If positive cultures are obtained, antimicrobial therapy can be modified for optimal treatment (Table 5-7) [200]. Dosages of antimicrobial agents for CNS infections are shown in Tables 5-4 and 5-5.

D. **Surgical therapy**

1. **Most patients with bacterial brain abscess require surgical excision for optimal therapy** (see sec. **2,** below, for exceptions) [199, 200, 206, 207]. Abscess aspiration can be performed by stereotactic CT guidance, affording the surgeon rapid, accurate, and safe access to virtually any intracranial location and allowing for swift relief of increased intracranial pressure. However, aspiration has the major disadvantage of incomplete drainage of multiloculated lesions. Complete abscess excision after craniotomy can be employed when aspiration is unsuccessful and when abscesses exhibit gas on radiologic evaluation. Emergent surgery is indicated in patients developing worsening neurologic deficits. Excision is contraindicated in the early stages of abscess formation before a capsule is formed.

2. **Although surgical intervention usually is needed for optimal therapy, certain subsets of patients may require only medical therapy** [208, 209]. Among these are patients with medical conditions that increase risk of surgery, multiple abscesses, abscesses in a deep or dominant location, concomitant meningitis

Table 5-7. Antimicrobial therapy for brain abscess

Organism	Standard therapy	Alternative therapies
Actinomyces spp.	Penicillin G	Clindamycin
Aspergillus spp.	Amphotericin B[a]	Itraconazole[b]
Bacteroides fragilis	Metronidazole	Chloramphenicol, clindamycin, ampicillin-sulbactam
Candida spp.	Amphotericin B[a]	Fluconazole[b]
Cryptococcus neoformans	Amphotericin B[a]	Fluconazole
Enterobacteriaceae	Third-generation cephalosporin[c]	Aztreonam, trimethoprim-sulfamethoxazole, fluoroquinolone
Fusobacterium spp.	Penicillin G	Metronidazole
Haemophilus spp.	Third-generation cephalosporin[c]	Aztreonam, trimethoprim-sulfamethoxazole
Listeria monocytogenes	Ampicillin or penicillin G[d]	Trimethoprim-sulfamethoxazole
Nocardia asteroides	Trimethoprim-sulfamethoxazole or sulfadiazine	Minocycline, imipenem, a third-generation cephalosporin,[c] fluoroquinolone[b]
Pseudallescheria boydii	Miconazole	Fluconazole[b]
Pseudomonas aeruginosa	Ceftazidime[d]	Aztreonam,[b] fluoroquinolone[b]
Staphylococcus aureus		
Methicillin-sensitive	Nafcillin or oxacillin	Vancomycin
Methicillin-resistant	Vancomycin	
Streptococcus milleri, other streptococci	Penicillin G	Third-generation cephalosporin,[c] vancomycin

[a]Addition of flucytosine should be considered.
[b]Efficacy not yet proven in brain abscess due to this organism.
[c]Cefotaxime or ceftriaxone.
[d]Addition of an aminoglycoside should be considered.

or ependymitis, early abscess reduction with clinical improvement after antimicrobial therapy, and an abscess measuring less than 3 cm.

- **E. Duration of antibiotic therapy.** High-dose intravenous antimicrobial therapy should be continued for 4–6 weeks; this often is followed by oral antimicrobial therapy if appropriate agents are available. A shorter course of therapy (i.e., 3–4 weeks) may be appropriate for patients who have undergone surgical excision of the abscess.

  Nocardial brain abscess should be treated for 3–12 months [210]. Surgical excision should also be performed for optimal therapy.

- **F. Fungal brain abscess.** A combined medical and surgical approach usually is required for optimal treatment of fungal brain abscesses.

  1. ***Aspergillus* species.** Medical therapy for *Aspergillus* brain abscess is amphotericin B (0.6–1.0 mg/kg/day, with doses up to 1.5 mg/kg/day depending on the clinical response) [200, 211], although few instances of survival have been reported despite antifungal therapy. Total doses of 3 g or more of amphotericin B are required. The addition of 5-flucytosine may increase success rates, although no controlled trials have demonstrated the efficacy of this approach. Despite the in vitro activity of itraconazole against *Aspergillus* species, there are no reports of its clinical use in CNS disease. Successful management includes excisional surgery or drainage in combination with antifungal therapy.

  2. **Mucormycosis.** Therapy of mucormycosis includes amphotericin B, correction of underlying metabolic derangements, and aggressive surgical debridement [200, 202]. Surgery is essential because of the propensity of this organism to invade blood vessels and impede delivery of antifungal agents to the site of infection. A possible adjunct to therapy is hyperbaric oxygen, although no prospective, controlled studies have been performed to assess its efficacy.

3. **Pseudallescheria boydii.** *P. boydii* exhibits in vitro resistance to amphotericin B. Miconazole is the antifungal agent of choice [203, 204], although intravenous or intrathecal administration is required and relapses are common. A partial response to fluconazole (600–800 mg/day) has been reported in a case report [200]. Surgical drainage is the cornerstone of effective therapy.

References

1. Connolly, K.J., and Hammer, S.M. The acute aseptic meningitis syndrome. *Infect. Dis. Clin. North Am.* 4:599–622, 1990.
2. Rotbart, H.A. Viral Meningitis and the Aseptic Meningitis Syndrome. In W.M. Scheld, R.J. Whitley, and D.T. Durack (eds.), *Infections of the Central Nervous System.* New York: Raven, 1991. Pp. 19–40.
2a. Rotbart, H.A. Enteroviral infections of the central nervous system. *Clin. Infect. Dis.* 20:971, 1995.
    Nice review of pathogenesis, clinical presentation, diagnosis, and potential therapy. Notes that focal encephalitis is increasingly recognized as a complication of enterovirus infection. Patients at greatest risk for sequelae of CNS enteroviral disease include neonates and those who are immunocompromised.
    See also related reference [163a] and A. Thoren and A. Widell. PCR for the diagnosis of enteroviral meningitis. Scand. J. Infect. Dis. *26:249, 1994.*
3. Melnick, J.L. Enteroviruses: Polioviruses, Coxsackieviruses, Echoviruses, and Newer Enteroviruses. In B.N. Fields and D.M. Knipe (eds.), *Virology.* New York: Raven, 1990. Pp. 549–605.
4. Strikas, R.A., Anderson, L.J., and Parker, R.A. Temporal and geographic patterns of isolates of nonpolio enterovirus in the United States, 1970–1983. *J. Infect. Dis.* 153:346–351, 1986.
5. Rantakallio, P., Leskinen, M., and von Wendt, L. Incidence and prognosis of central nervous system infections in a birth cohort of 12,000 children. *Scand. J. Infect. Dis.* 18:287–294, 1986.
6. Monath, T.P. Flaviviruses. In B.N. Fields and D.M. Knipe (eds.), *Virology.* New York: Raven, 1990. Pp. 763–814.
7. Goodpasture, H.C., et al. Colorado tick fever: Clinical, epidemiologic, and laboratory aspects of 228 cases in Colorado in 1973–1974. *Ann. Intern. Med.* 88:303–310, 1978.
8. Wolinsky, J.S., and Waxham, M.N. Mumps Virus. In B.N. Fields and D.M. Knipe (eds.), *Virology.* New York: Raven, 1990. Pp. 989–1011.
9. Gnann, J.W., Jr. Meningitis and Encephalitis Caused by Mumps Virus. In W.M. Scheld, R.J. Whitley, and D.T. Durack (eds.), *Infections of the Central Nervous System.* New York: Raven, 1991. Pp. 113–125.
10. Dykewicz, C.A., et al. Lymphocytic choriomeningitis outbreak associated with nude mice in a research institute. *J.A.M.A.* 267:1349–1353, 1992.
11. Corey, L., and Spear, P.G. Infections with herpes simplex viruses (second of two parts). *N. Engl. J. Med.* 314:749–757, 1986.
12. Corey, L., et al. Genital herpes simplex virus infection: Clinical manifestations, course, and complications. *Ann. Intern. Med.* 98:958–972, 1983.
13. Bergström, T., et al. Primary and recurrent herpes simplex virus type 2–induced meningitis. *J. Infect. Dis.* 162:322–330, 1990.
14. Mayo, D.R., and Booss, J. Varicella zoster–associated neurologic disease without skin disease. *Arch. Neurol.* 46:313–315, 1989.
15. Barnes, D.W., and Whitley, R.J. CNS diseases associated with varicella zoster virus and herpes simplex virus infection. Pathogenesis and current therapy. *Neurol. Clin.* 4:265–283, 1986.
16. Yamamoto, L.J., et al. Herpes simplex virus type 1 DNA in cerebrospinal fluid of a patient with Mollaret's meningitis. *N. Engl. J. Med.* 325:1082–1085, 1991.
17. Graman, P.S. Mollaret's meningitis associated with acute Epstein-Barr virus mononucleosis. *Arch. Neurol.* 44:1204–1205, 1987.
18. Huang, L.M., et al. Meningitis caused by human herpesvirus-6. *Arch. Dis. Child.* 66:1443–1444, 1991.
18a. McCutchan, J.A. Cytomegalovirus infections of the nervous system in patients with AIDS. *Clin. Infect. Dis.* 20:747, 1995.
    Includes discussion of CMV diffuse micronodular encephalitis, which may be associ-

ated with dementia, and ventriculoencephalitis. At this point, treatment issues for CNS disease, except retinitis in AIDS, due to CMV infection are unresolved.

19. Evans, B.K., Donley, D.K., and Whitaker, J.N. Neurological Manifestations of Infection with the Human Immunodeficiency Viruses. In W.M. Scheld, R.J. Whitley, and D.T. Durack (eds.), *Infections of the Central Nervous System.* New York: Raven, 1991. Pp. 201–232.

20. McArthur, J.C. Neurologic manifestations of AIDS. *Medicine* (Baltimore) 66:407–437, 1987.

21. Hollander, H., and Stringari, S. Human immunodeficiency virus–associated meningitis. Clinical course and correlations. *Am. J. Med.* 83:813–816, 1987.

21a. Tunkel, A.R., and Scheld, W.M. Acute meningitis. In G.L. Mandell, J.E. Bennett, and R. Dolin (eds.), *Principles and Practice of Infectious Diseases* (4th ed.). New York: Churchill Livingstone, 1995. Pp. 831–865.

22. Schlech, W.F., III, et al. Bacterial meningitis in the United States, 1978 through 1981. The national bacterial meningitis surveillance study. *J.A.M.A.* 253:1749–1754, 1985.

23. Bryan, J.P., et al. Etiology and mortality of bacterial meningitis in northeastern Brazil. *Rev. Infect. Dis.* 12:128–135, 1990.

24. Durand, M.L., et al. Acute bacterial meningitis in adults. A review of 493 episodes. *N. Engl. J. Med.* 328:21–28, 1993.

25. Wenger, J.D., et al. Bacterial meningitis in the United States, 1986: Report of a multistate surveillance study. *J. Infect. Dis.* 162:1316–1323, 1990.

26. Spagnuolo, P.J., et al. *Haemophilus influenzae* meningitis: The spectrum of disease in adults. *Medicine* (Baltimore) 61:74–85, 1982.

27. Farley, M.M., et al. Invasive *Haemophilus influenzae* disease in adults. A prospective, population-based surveillance. *Ann. Intern. Med.* 116:806–812, 1992.

28. Murphy, T.V., et al. Declining incidence of *Haemophilus influenzae* type b disease since introduction of vaccination. *J.A.M.A.* 269:246–248, 1993.

29. Ross, S.C., and Densen, P. Complement deficiency states and infection: Epidemiology, pathogenesis and consequences of neisserial and other infections in an immune deficiency. *Medicine* (Baltimore) 64:243–273, 1984.

30. Geiseler, P.J., et al. Community-acquired purulent meningitis: A review of 1,316 cases during the antibiotic era, 1954–1976. *Rev. Infect. Dis.* 2:725–745, 1980.

31. Musher, D.M. Infections caused by *Streptococcus pneumoniae:* Clinical spectrum, pathogenesis, immunity, and treatment. *Clin. Infect. Dis.* 14:801–809, 1992.

32. Tunkel, A.R., and Scheld, W.M. Acute Infectious Complications of Head Trauma. In R. Braakman (ed.), *Handbook of Clinical Neurology, Head Injury.* Amsterdam: Elsevier Science, 1990. Pp. 317–326.

33. Gellin, B.G., and Broome, C.V. Listeriosis. *J.A.M.A.* 261:1313–1320, 1989.

34. Cherubin, C.E., et al. Epidemiological spectrum and current treatment of listeriosis. *Rev. Infect. Dis.* 13:1108–1114, 1991.

35. Decker, C.F., et al. *Listeria monocytogenes* infections in patients with AIDS: Report of five cases and review. *Rev. Infect. Dis.* 13:413–417, 1991.

36. Berenguer, J., et al. Listeriosis in patients infected with human immunodeficiency virus. *Rev. Infect. Dis.* 13:115–119, 1991.

37. Zuniga, M., Aguado, J.M., and Vada, J. *Listeria monocytogenes* meningitis in previously healthy adults: Long-term follow-up. *Q. J. Med.* 85:911–915, 1992.

38. Saez-Llorens, X., and McCracken, G.H., Jr. Bacterial meningitis in neonates and children. *Infect. Dis. Clin. North Am.* 4:623–644, 1990.

39. Regan, J.A., et al. The epidemiology of group B streptococcal colonization in pregnancy. *Obstet. Gynecol.* 77:604–610, 1991.

40. Farley, M.M., et al. A population-based assessment of invasive disease due to group B streptococci in nonpregnant adults. *N. Engl. J. Med.* 328:1807–1811, 1993.

41. Dunne, D.W., and Quagliarello, V. Group B streptococcal meningitis in adults. *Medicine* 72:1–10, 1993.

42. Cherubin, C.E., et al. *Listeria* and gram-negative bacillary meningitis in New York City, 1972–1979. *Am. J. Med.* 71:199–209, 1981.

43. Unhanand, M., et al. Gram-negative enteric bacillary meningitis: A twenty-one-year experience. *J. Pediatr.* 122:15–21, 1993.

44. Cameron, M.L., and Durack, D.T. Helminthic Infections of the Central Nervous System. In W.M. Scheld, R.J. Whitley, and D.T. Durack (eds.), *Infections of the Central Nervous System.* New York: Raven, 1991. Pp. 825–858.

45. Schlesinger, L.S., Ross, S.C., and Schaberg, D.R. *Staphylococcus aureus* meningitis: A broad-based epidemiologic study. *Medicine* (Baltimore) 66:148–156, 1987.

46. Kaufman, B.A., et al. Meningitis in the neurosurgical patient. *Infect. Dis. Clin. North Am.* 4:677–701, 1990.
46a. Pegues, D.A., et al. Infectious complications associated with temporary epidural catheters. *Clin. Infect. Dis.* 19:970, 1994.
47. Bross, J.E., and Gordon, G. Nocardial meningitis: Case reports and review. *Rev. Infect. Dis.* 13:160–165, 1991.
47a. Fazal, B.A., et al. Community-acquired enterococcal meningitis in an adult. *Clin. Infect. Dis.* 20:725, 1995.
    In prior reports, this unusual infection has usually occurred in patients with predisposing factors and has been reported in neonates, in parturients after administration of epidural anesthetics, and in patients with anatomic defects of the CNS or in those who have undergone prior neurosurgical interventions as well as those with endocarditis and urinary tract infections.
48. Heerema, M.S., et al. Anaerobic bacterial meningitis. *Am. J. Med.* 647:219–227, 1979.
49. Law, D.A., and Aronoff, S.C. Anaerobic meningitis in children: Case report and review of the literature. *Pediatr. Infect. Dis. J.* 11:968–971, 1992.
49a. Gelfand, M.S., and Abolnik, I.Z. Streptococcal meningitis complicating diagnostic myelography: Three cases and review. *Clin. Infect. Dis.* 20:582, 1995.
50. Zugar, A., and Lowy, F.D. Tuberculosis of the Central Nervous System. In W.M. Scheld, R.J. Whitley, and D.T. Durack (eds.), *Infections of the Central Nervous System.* New York: Raven, 1991. Pp. 425–456.
51. Leonard, J.M., and Des Prez, R.M. Tuberculous meningitis. *Infect. Dis. Clin. North Am.* 4:769–787, 1990.
52. Barnes, P.F., et al. Tuberculosis in patients with human immunodeficiency virus infection. *N. Engl. J. Med.* 324:1644–1650, 1991.
53. Hook, E.W., III. Central Nervous System Syphilis. In W.M. Scheld, R.J. Whitley, and D.T. Durack (eds.), *Infections of the Central Nervous System.* New York: Raven, 1991. Pp. 639–656.
54. Simon, R.P. Neurosyphilis. *Arch. Neurol.* 42:606–613, 1985.
55. Musher, D.M., Hamill, R.J., and Baughn, R.E. Effect of human immunodeficiency virus (HIV) infection on the course of syphilis and on the response to treatment. *Ann. Intern. Med.* 113:872–881, 1990.
56. Hook, E.W., III, and Marra, C.M. Acquired syphilis in adults. *N. Engl. J. Med.* 326:1060–1069, 1992.
56a. Centers for Disease Control. 1993 Sexually transmitted diseases treatment guidelines. *M.M.W.R.* 42(RR-14):36, 1993.
    For additional discussion, including the background papers for the above recommendations, see R.T. Rolfs. Treatment of syphilis, 1993. Clin. Infect. Dis. 20(Suppl. 1):S23, 1995. See also related discussion in Chap. 13.
57. Katz, D.A., and Berger, J.R. Neurosyphilis in acquired immunodeficiency syndrome. *Arch. Neurol.* 46:895–898, 1989.
58. Reik, L., Jr. Lyme Disease. In W.M. Scheld, R.J. Whitley, and D.T. Durack (eds.), *Infections of the Central Nervous System.* New York: Raven, 1991. Pp. 657–689.
59. Steere, A.C. Lyme disease. *N. Engl. J. Med.* 321:586–596, 1989.
60. Luft, B.J., et al. Invasion of the central nervous system by *Borrelia burgdorferi* in acute disseminated infection. *J.A.M.A.* 267:1364–1367, 1992.
61. Levitz, S.M. The ecology of *Cryptococcus neoformans* and the epidemiology of cryptococcosis. *Rev. Infect. Dis.* 13:1163–1169, 1991.
62. Sabetta, J.R., and Andriole, V.T. Cryptococcal infection of the central nervous system. *Med. Clin. North Am.* 69:333–345, 1985.
63. Kovacs, J.A., et al. Cryptococcosis in the acquired immunodeficiency syndrome. *Ann. Intern. Med.* 103:533–538, 1985.
64. Zugar, A., et al. Cryptococcal disease in patients with the acquired immunodeficiency syndrome. Diagnostic features and outcome of treatment. *Ann. Intern. Med.* 104:234–240, 1986.
65. Chuck, S.L., and Sande, M.A. Infections with *Cryptococcus neoformans* in the acquired immunodeficiency syndrome. *N. Engl. J. Med.* 321:794–799, 1989.
66. Crislip, M.A., and Edwards, J.E., Jr. Candidiasis. *Infect. Dis. Clin. North Am.* 3:103–133, 1989.
67. Bayer, A.S., et al. *Candida* meningitis. Report of seven cases and review of the English literature. *Medicine* (Baltimore) 55:477–486, 1976.
68. Lipton, S.A., et al. Candidal infection in the central nervous system. *Am. J. Med.* 76:101–108, 1984.

69. Walsh, T.J., Hier, D.B., and Caplan, L.P. Fungal infections of the central nervous system: Comparative analysis of risk factors and clinical signs in 57 patients. *Neurology* 35:1654–1657, 1985.
70. Bouza, E., et al. Coccidioidal meningitis. An analysis of thirty-one cases and review of the literature. *Medicine* (Baltimore) 60:139–172, 1981.
71. Ampel, N.M., Wieden, M.A., and Galgiani, J.N. Coccidioidomycosis: Clinical update. *Rev. Infect. Dis.* 11:897–911, 1989.
72. Niu, M.T., and Duma, R.J. Meningitis due to protozoa and helminths. *Infect. Dis. Clin. North Am.* 4:809–841, 1990.
73. Cegielski, J.P., and Durack, D.T. Protozoal Infections of the Central Nervous System. In W.M. Scheld, R.J. Whitley, and D.T. Durack (eds.), *Infections of the Central Nervous System*. New York: Raven, 1991. Pp. 767–800.
74. Gardner, H.A.R., et al. Granulomatous amebic encephalitis in an AIDS patient. *Neurology* 41:1993–1995, 1991.
75. Di Gregorio, C., et al. *Acanthamoeba* meningoencephalitis in a patient with acquired immunodeficiency syndrome. *Arch. Pathol. Lab. Med.* 116:1363–1365, 1992.
76. Gordon, S.M., et al. Culture isolation of *Acanthamoeba* species and leptomyxid amebas from patients with amebic meningoencephalitis, including two patients with AIDS. *Clin. Infect. Dis.* 15:1024–1030, 1992.
77. Koo, J., Pien, F., and Klıks, M.M. *Angiostrongylus (Parastrongylus)* eosinophilic meningitis. *Rev. Infect. Dis.* 10:1155–1162, 1988.
78. Wilfert, C.M., and Lehrman, S.N. Enteroviruses and meningitis. *Pediatr. Infect. Dis.* 2:333–341, 1983.
79. Jaffe, M., et al. The ameliorating effect of lumbar puncture in viral meningitis. *Am. J. Dis. Child.* 143:682–685, 1989.
80. McKinney, R.E., Jr., Katz, S.L., and Wilfert, C.M. Chronic enteroviral meningoencephalitis in agammaglobulinemic patients. *Rev. Infect. Dis.* 9:334–356, 1987.
81. Roos, K.L., Tunkel, A.R., and Scheld, W.M. Acute Bacterial Meningitis in Children and Adults. In W.M. Scheld, R.J. Whitley, and D.T. Durack (eds.), *Infections of the Central Nervous System*. New York: Raven, 1991. Pp. 335–409.
82. Gorse, G.J., et al. Bacterial meningitis in the elderly. *Arch. Intern. Med.* 149:1603–1606, 1989.
82a. Kent, S.J., et al. Tuberculous meningitis: A 30-year review. *Clin. Infect. Dis.* 17:987, 1993.
     Review of 58 cases from Australia. Corticosteroids were administered to 56 patients and authors felt their use may have contributed to the comparatively good outcome in these cases.
83. Ogawa, S.K., et al. Tuberculous meningitis in an urban medical center. *Medicine* (Baltimore) 66:317–326, 1987.
84. Kennedy, D.H., and Fallon, R.J. Tuberculous meningitis. *J.A.M.A.* 241:264–268, 1979.
85. Berenguer, J., et al. Tuberculous meningitis in patients infected with the human immunodeficiency virus. *N. Engl. J. Med.* 326:668–672, 1992.
86. Dube, M.P., Holtom, P.D., and Larsen, R.A. Tuberculous meningitis in patients with and without human immunodeficiency virus infection. *Am. J. Med.* 93:520–524, 1992.
87. Holmes, M.D., Zawadzki, B., and Simon, R.P. Clinical features of meningovascular syphilis. *Neurology* 34:553–555, 1984.
88. Hutchinson, C.M., et al. Characteristics of patients with syphilis attending Baltimore STD clinics: Multiple, high-risk subgroups and interactions with human immunodeficiency virus infection. *Arch. Intern. Med.* 151:511–516, 1991.
89. Patterson, T.F., and Andriole, V.T. Current concepts in cryptococcosis. *Eur. J. Clin. Microbiol. Infect. Dis.* 8:457–465, 1989.
90. Rotbart, H.A. Diagnosis of enteroviral meningitis with the polymerase chain reaction. *J. Pediatr.* 117:85–89, 1990.
91. Ratzan, K.R. Viral meningitis. *Med. Clin. North Am.* 69:399–413, 1985.
92. Rowley, A., et al. Diagnosis of herpes simplex encephalitis by DNA amplification of cerebrospinal fluid cells. *Lancet* 335:440–441, 1990.
92a. Lakeman, F.D., et al. and Infectious Diseases Collaborative Antiviral Study Group. Diagnosis of *Herpes simplex* encephalitis: Application of polymerase chain reaction to cerebrospinal fluid from brain-biopsied patients and correlation with disease. *J. Infect. Dis.* 171:857, 1995.
     Report of PCR analyses done to detect HSV DNA in CSF specimens from patients whose HSV encephalitis status was based on brain biopsy. HSV DNA was detected by PCR in CSF of 53 (98%) of 54 patients with biopsy-proved HSV encephalitis and

was detected in all 18 CSF specimens obtained before brain biopsy from patients with
proven HSV encephalitis. Thus, PCR detection of HSV DNA should be the standard
for diagnosis of HSV encephalitis. See related report by J.P. DeVincenzo et al.
Mild herpes simplex encephalitis diagnosed by polymerase chain reaction: A case report
and review. Pediatr. Infect. Dis. J. *13:662, 1994. Authors point out that the use of PCR*
may uncover mild cases of HSV encephalitis to have warranted definitive diagnostic
procedures and may begin to reveal a wider spectrum of HSV encephalitis. See related
report by Y. Schlesinger et al. Expanded spectrum of herpes simplex encephalitis in
childhood. J. Pediatr. *126:234, 1995.*

93. Hollander, H., and Levy, J.A. Neurologic abnormalities and recovery of human immunodeficiency virus from cerebrospinal fluid. *Ann. Intern. Med.* 106:692–695, 1987.

94. Chalmers, A.C., Aprill, B.S., and Shephard, H. Cerebrospinal fluid and human immunodeficiency virus. Findings in healthy, asymptomatic, seropositive men. *Arch. Intern. Med.* 150:1538–1540, 1990.

95. Feigin, R.D., McCracken, G.H., Jr., and Klein, J.O. Diagnosis and management of meningitis. *Pediatr. Infect. Dis. J.* 11:785–814, 1992.

96. Bonadio, W.A. The cerebrospinal fluid: Physiologic aspects and alterations associated with bacterial meningitis. *Pediatr. Infect. Dis. J.* 11:423–432, 1992.
    See recent report by J.G. Elmore et al., Acute meningitis with a negative Gram's stain:
    Clinical and management outcomes in 171 episodes. Am. J. Med. *100:78, 1996.*

97. Marton, K.I., and Gean, A.D. The spinal tap: A new look at an old test. *Ann. Intern. Med.* 104:840–848, 1986.

98. Genton, B., and Berger, J.P. Cerebrospinal fluid lactate in 78 cases of adult meningitis. *Intens. Care Med.* 16:196–200, 1990.

99. La Scolea, L.J., Jr., and Dryja, D. Quantitation of bacteria in cerebrospinal fluid and blood of children with meningitis and its diagnostic significance. *J. Clin. Microbiol.* 19:187–190, 1984.

100. Gray, L.D., and Fedorko, D.P. Laboratory diagnosis of bacterial meningitis. *Clin. Microbiol. Rev.* 5:130–145, 1992.

101. Kristiansen, B.E., et al. Rapid diagnosis of meningococcal meningitis by polymerase chain reaction. *Lancet* 337:1568–1569, 1991.

102. Ni, H., et al. Polymerase chain reaction for diagnosis of meningococcal meningitis. *Lancet* 340:1432–1434, 1992.

103. Jaton, K., Sahli, R., and Bille, J. Development of polymerase chain reaction assays for detection of *Listeria monocytogenes* in clinical cerebrospinal fluid samples. *J. Clin. Microbiol.* 30:1931–1936, 1992.

104. Cotton, M.F., et al. Plasma arginine vasopressin and the syndrome of inappropriate antidiuretic hormone secretion in tuberculous meningitis. *Pediatr. Infect. Dis. J.* 10:837–842, 1991.

105. Kaneko, K., et al. Rapid diagnosis of tuberculous meningitis by polymerase chain reaction (PCR). *Neurology* 40:1617–1618, 1990.

106. Hart, G. Syphilis tests in diagnostic and therapeutic decision making. *Ann. Intern. Med.* 104:368–376, 1986.

107. Noordhoek, G.T., et al. Detection by polymerase chain reaction of *Treponema pallidum* DNA in cerebrospinal fluid from neurosyphilis patients before and after antibiotic treatment. *J. Clin. Microbiol.* 29:1976–1984, 1991.

108. Corpuz, M., et al. Problems in the use of serologic tests for the diagnosis of Lyme disease. *Arch. Intern. Med.* 151:1837–1840, 1991.

109. Keller, T.L., Halperin, J.J., and Whitman, M. PCR detection of *Borrelia burgdorferi* DNA in cerebrospinal fluid of Lyme neuroborreliosis patients. *Neurology* 42:32–42, 1992.

110. Shaunak, S., Schell, W.A., and Perfect, J.R. Cryptococcal meningitis with normal cerebrospinal fluid. *J. Infect. Dis.* 160:912, 1989.

111. Schermoly, M.J., and Hinthorn, D.R. Eosinophilia in coccidioidomycosis. *Arch. Intern. Med.* 148:895–896, 1988.

112. Tunkel, A.R., Wispelwey, B., and Scheld, W.M. Bacterial meningitis: Recent advances in pathophysiology and treatment. *Ann. Intern. Med.* 112:610–623, 1990.

113. Volberding, P.A., et al. Zidovudine in asymptomatic human immunodeficiency virus infection. A controlled trial in persons with fewer than 500 CD4-positive cells per cubic millimeter. *N. Engl. J. Med.* 322:941–949, 1990.

114. Campos, J., et al. Multiply resistant *Haemophilus influenzae* type b causing meningitis: Comparative clinical and laboratory study. *J. Pediatr.* 108:897–902, 1986.

115. Givner, L.B., Abramson, J.S., and Wasilauskas, B. Meningitis due to *Haemophilus influenzae* type b resistant to ampicillin and chloramphenicol. *Rev. Infect. Dis.* 11:329–334, 1989.
116. Peltola, J., et al. Randomised comparison of chloramphenicol, ampicillin, cefotaxime, and ceftriaxone for childhood bacterial meningitis. *Lancet* 1:1281–1287, 1989.
117. Lebel, M.H., Hoyt, M.J., and McCracken, G.H., Jr. Comparative efficacy of ceftriaxone and cefuroxime for treatment of bacterial meningitis. *J. Pediatr.* 114:1049–1054, 1989.
118. Schaad, U.B., et al. A comparison of ceftriaxone and cefuroxime for the treatment of bacterial meningitis in children. *N. Engl. J. Med.* 322:141–147, 1990.
119. Arditi, M., Herold, B.C., and Yogev, R. Cefuroxime treatment failure and *Haemophilus influenzae* meningitis: Case report and review of the literature. *Pediatrics* 84:132–135, 1989.
120. Hatch, D.L., and Overturf, G.D. Delayed cerebrospinal fluid sterilization in infants with *Haemophilus influenzae* type b meningitis. *J. Infect. Dis.* 160:711–715, 1989.
121. Saez-Nieto, J.A., et al. Epidemiology and molecular basis of penicillin-resistant *Neisseria meningitidis* in Spain: A 5-year history (1985–1989). *Clin. Infect. Dis.* 14:394–402, 1992.
122. Jackson, L.A., et al. Prevalence of *Neisseria meningitidis* relatively resistant to penicillin in the United States, 1991. *J. Infect. Dis.* 169:438–441, 1994.
123. Appelbaum, P.C. Antimicrobial resistance in *Streptococcus pneumoniae:* An overview. *Clin. Infect. Dis.* 15:77–83, 1992.
124. Caputo, G.M., Appelbaum, P.C., and Liu, H.H. Infections due to penicillin-resistant pneumococci. Clinical, epidemiologic, and microbiologic features. *Arch. Intern. Med.* 153:1301–1310, 1993.
125. Centers for Disease Control and Prevention. Drug-resistant *Streptococcus pneumoniae*—Kentucky and Tennessee, 1993. *M.M.W.R.* 43:23–25, 1994.
126. McDougal, L.K., et al. Analysis of multiply antimicrobial-resistant isolates of *Streptococcus pneumoniae* from the United States. *Antimicrob. Agents Chemother.* 36:2176–2184, 1992.
127. Friedland, I.R., and Istre, G.R. Management of penicillin-resistant pneumococcal infections. *Pediatr. Infect. Dis. J.* 11:433–435, 1992.
128. Viladrich, P.F., et al. Characteristics and antibiotic therapy of adult meningitis due to penicillin-resistant pneumococci. *Am. J. Med.* 84:839–846, 1988.
129. Bradley, J.S., and Connor, J.D. Ceftriaxone failure in meningitis caused by *Streptococcus pneumoniae* with reduced susceptibility to beta-lactam antibiotics. *Pediatr. Infect. Dis. J.* 10:871–873, 1991.
130. Sloas, M.M., et al. Cephalosporin treatment failure in penicillin- and cephalosporin-resistant *Streptococcus pneumoniae* meningitis. *Pediatr. Infect. Dis. J.* 11:622–626, 1992.
131. Figueiredo, A.M.S., et al. A pneumococcal clinical isolate with high-level resistance to cefotaxime and ceftriaxone. *Antimicrob. Agents Chemother.* 36:886–889, 1992.
132. Friedland, I.R., et al. Dilemmas in diagnosis and management of cephalosporin-resistant *Streptococcus pneumoniae* meningitis. *Pediatr. Infect. Dis. J.* 12:196–200, 1993.
133. Friedland, I.R., and Klugman, K.P. Failure of chloramphenicol therapy in penicillin-resistant pneumococcal meningitis. *Lancet* 339:405–408, 1992.
134. Viladrich, P.F., et al. Evaluation of vancomycin for therapy of adult pneumococcal meningitis. *Antimicrob. Agents Chemother.* 35:2467–2472, 1991.
135. Friedland, I.R., et al. Evaluation of antimicrobial regimens for treatment of experimental penicillin- and cephalosporin-resistant pneumococcal meningitis. *Antimicrob. Agents Chemother.* 37:1630–1636, 1993.
136. Richards, S.J., Lambert, C.M., and Scott, A.C. Recurrent *Listeria monocytogenes* meningitis treated with intraventricular vancomycin. *J. Antimicrob. Chemother.* 29:351–353, 1992.
137. Fong, I.W., and Tomkins, K.B. Review of *Pseudomonas aeruginosa* meningitis with special emphasis on treatment with ceftazidime. *Rev. Infect. Dis.* 7:604–612, 1985.
138. Rodriguez, W.J., et al. Treatment of *Pseudomonas* meningitis with ceftazidime with or without concurrent therapy. *Pediatr. Infect. Dis. J.* 9:83–87, 1990.
139. Kilpatrick, M., et al. Aztreonam for treating meningitis caused by gram-negative rods. *Scand. J. Infect. Dis.* 23:125–126, 1991.
140. Wong, V.K., et al. Imipenem/cilastatin treatment of bacterial meningitis in children. *Pediatr. Infect. Dis. J.* 10:122–125, 1991.

141. Donnelly, J.P., et al. High-dose meropenem in meningitis due to *Pseudomonas aerugi-nosa. Lancet* 339:1117, 1992.
142. Tunkel, A.R., and Scheld, W.M. Treatment of Bacterial Meningitis. In J.S. Wolfson and D.C. Hooper (eds.), *Quinolone Antimicrobial Agents.* Washington, D.C.: American Society for Microbiology, 1993. Pp. 481–495.
143. Cruciani, M., et al. Evaluation of intraventricular teicoplanin for the treatment of neurosurgical shunt infections. *Clin. Infect. Dis.* 15:285–289, 1992.
144. Radetsky, M. Duration of treatment in bacterial meningitis: A historical inquiry. *Pediatr. Infect. Dis. J.* 9:2–9, 1990.
145. O'Neill, P. How long to treat bacterial meningitis. *Lancet* 341:530, 1993.
145a. Waler, J.A., and Rathore, M.H. Outpatient management of pediatric bacterial menin-gitis. *Pediatr. Infect. Dis.* 14:89, 1995.
     Complications of meningitis occur most frequently in the first 2–3 days and serious adverse complications are exceedingly rare after 3–4 days of therapy, especially in children who are clinically well and afebrile.
146. Humphries, M. The management of tuberculous meningitis. *Thorax* 47:577–581, 1992.
147. Alarcon, F., et al. Tuberculous meningitis. Short course of chemotherapy. *Arch. Neurol.* 47:1313–1317, 1990.
148. Jacobs, R.F., et al. Intensive short course chemotherapy for tuberculous meningitis. *Pediatr. Infect. Dis. J.* 11:194–198, 1992.
149. Dooley, S.W., et al. Multidrug-resistant tuberculosis. *Ann. Intern. Med.* 117:257–259, 1992.
150. Snider, D.E., Jr., and Roper, W.L. The new tuberculosis. *N. Engl. J. Med.* 326:703–705, 1992.
151. Hook, E.W., III. Management of syphilis in human immunodeficiency virus–infected patients. *Am. J. Med.* 93:477–479, 1992.
152. Dattwyler, R.J., et al. Treatment of late Lyme borreliosis—randomised comparison of ceftriaxone and penicillin. *Lancet* 1:1191–1194, 1988.
153. Bennett, J.E., et al. A comparison of amphotericin B alone and combined with flucyto-sine in the treatment of cryptococcal meningitis. *N. Engl. J. Med.* 301:126–131, 1979.
154. Dismukes, W.E., et al. Treatment of cryptococcal meningitis with combination ampho-tericin B and flucytosine for four as compared with six weeks. *N. Engl. J. Med.* 317:334–341, 1987.
155. Stamm, A.M., et al. Toxicity of amphotericin B plus flucytosine in 194 patients with cryptococcal meningitis. *Am. J. Med.* 83:236–242, 1987.
156. Larsen, R.A., Leal, M.A.E., and Chan, L.S. Fluconazole compared with amphotericin B plus flucytosine for cryptococcal meningitis in AIDS. A randomized trial. *Ann. Intern. Med.* 113:183–187, 1990.
157. Saag, M.S., et al. Comparison of amphotericin B with fluconazole in the treatment of acute AIDS-associated cryptococcal meningitis. *N. Engl. J. Med.* 326:83–89, 1992.
158. Bozette, S.A., et al. A placebo-controlled trial of maintenance therapy with fluconazole after treatment of cryptococcal meningitis in the acquired immunodeficiency syn-drome. *N. Engl. J. Med.* 324:580–584, 1991.
159. Powderly, W.G., et al. A controlled trial of fluconazole or amphotericin B to prevent relapse of cryptococcal meningitis in patients with the acquired immunodeficiency syndrome. *N. Engl. J. Med.* 326:793–798, 1992.
     For a nice review of this topic, see related article by W.G. Powderly. Cryptococcal meningitis and AIDS. Clin. Infect. Dis. *17:837, 1993. In this "AIDS Commentary" series, Dr. Powderly clearly outlines the progress made through clinical investigations and the problems that remain to be resolved. See related discussion and references in Chap. 18.*
160. Berry, A.J., Rinaldi, M.G., and Graybill, J.R. Use of high-dose fluconazole as salvage therapy for cryptococcal meningitis in patients with AIDS. *Antimicrob. Agents Chemo-ther.* 36:690–692, 1992.
160a. Quagliarello, V.J., et al. Primary prevention of cryptococcal meningitis by fluconazole in HIV-infected patients. *Lancet* 345:548, 1995.
     Fluconazole reduces the risk of a first episode of cryptococcal meningitis in those with CD4 counts < 250/mm³. The optimal dose is not defined, but a daily dose may not be necessary. See editorial comment in the same issue.
161. Labadie, E.L., and Hamilton, R.H. Survival improvement in coccidioidal meningitis by high-dose intrathecal amphotericin B. *Arch. Intern. Med.* 146:2013–2018, 1986.
162. Galgiani, J.N., et al. Fluconazole therapy for coccidioidal meningitis. *Ann. Intern. Med.* 119:28–35, 1993.

163. Brown, R.L. Successful treatment of primary amebic meningoencephalitis. *Arch. Intern. Med.* 151:1201–1202, 1991.

163a. Abzug, M.J., et al. Neonatal enterovirus infection: Virology, serology, and effects of intravenous immune globulin. *Clin. Infect. Dis.* 20:1201, 1995.
    Larger controlled studies are needed to determine the role of IV immunoglobulin. Until data are available, these authors do not recommend widespread use of immunoglobulin for neonates with suspected or proven enterovirus infection.

164. Quagliarello, V., and Scheld, W.M. Bacterial meningitis: Pathogenesis, pathophysiology, and progress. *N. Engl. J. Med.* 327:864–872, 1992.

165. Tunkel, A.R., and Scheld, W.M. Pathogenesis and pathophysiology of bacterial meningitis. *Clin. Microbiol. Rev.* 6:118–136, 1993.

166. Tuomanen, E., et al. Nonsteroidal anti-inflammatory agents in the therapy for experimental pneumococcal meningitis. *J. Infect. Dis.* 155:985–990, 1987.

167. Nolan, C.M., et al. Experimental pneumococcal meningitis: IV. The effect of methylprednisolone on meningeal inflammation. *J. Lab. Clin. Med.* 91:979–988, 1978.

168. Scheld, W.M., et al. Cerebrospinal fluid outflow resistance in rabbits with experimental meningitis. Alterations with penicillin and methylprednisolone. *J. Clin. Invest.* 66:243–253, 1980.

169. Täuber, M.G., Khayam-Bashi, H., and Sande, M.A. Effects of ampicillin and corticosteroids on brain water content, cerebrospinal fluid pressure, and cerebrospinal fluid lactate levels in experimental pneumococcal meningitis. *J. Infect. Dis.* 151:528–534, 1985.

170. Syrogiannopoulos, G.A., et al. Dexamethasone in the treatment of experimental *Haemophilus influenzae* type b meningitis. *J. Infect. Dis.* 155:213–219, 1987.

171. Mustafa, M.M., et al. Modulation of inflammation and cachectin activity in relation to treatment of experimental *Haemophilus influenzae* type b meningitis. *J. Infect. Dis.* 160:818–825, 1989.

172. Lebel, M.H., et al. Dexamethasone therapy for bacterial meningitis. Results of two double-blind, placebo-controlled trials. *N. Engl. J. Med.* 319:964–971, 1988.

173. Lebel, M.H., et al. Magnetic resonance imaging and dexamethasone therapy for bacterial meningitis. *Am. J. Dis. Child.* 143:301–306, 1989.

174. Girgis, N.I., et al. Dexamethasone treatment for bacterial meningitis in children and adults. *Pediatr. Infect. Dis. J.* 8:848–851, 1989.

175. Odio, C.M., et al. The beneficial effects of early dexamethasone administration in infants and children with bacterial meningitis. *N. Engl. J. Med.* 324:1525–1531, 1991.

175a. Wald, E.R., et al., for the Meningitis Study Group. Dexamethasone therapy for children with bacterial meningitis. *Pediatrics* 95:21, 1995.
    See editorial comment in reference [175b]. See related report by S.M. King et al. Dexamethasone therapy for bacterial meningitis: Better never than late? Can. J. Infect. Dis. 5:210, 1994.

175b. Prober, C.G. The role of steroids in the management of children with bacterial meningitis. *Pediatrics* 95:29, 1995.
    Nice editorial/commentary on the study in reference [175a] and prior studies using dexamethasone. Prober concurs with the 1994 Red Book recommendations for steroid use in meningitis (see text, p. 163).
      See related discussion of the pros and cons of this topic in U.B. Schaad, S.I. Kaplan, and G.H. McCracken, Jr. Steroid therapy for bacterial meningitis. Clin. Infect. Dis. 20:685, 1995.

176. Kennedy, W.A., Hoyt, M.J., and McCracken, G.H., Jr. The role of corticosteroid therapy in children with pneumococcal meningitis. *Am. J. Dis. Child.* 145:1374–1378, 1991.
    See also G.Y. Kandra et al. Beneficial effects of dexamethasone in children with pneumococcal meningitis. Pediatr. Infect. Dis. J. 14:490, 1995. Report from Turkey. Dexamethasone was thought to be beneficial with regard to hearing impairment. Also see S.M. Bhatt et al. The impact of dexamethasone on hearing loss in experimental pneumococcal meningitis. Pediatr. Infect. Dis. J. 14:93, 1995. In a rabbit model, steroid therapy appears to prevent profound deafness.

177. Schaad, U.B., et al. Dexamethasone therapy for bacterial meningitis in children. *Lancet* 342:457–461, 1993.

177a. Peter, G., et al. (eds.). *Report of the Committee on Infectious Disease: 1994 Red Book* (23rd ed.). Elk Grove, IL: American Academy of Pediatrics, 1994. P. 559.

178. Lyons, M.K., and Meyer, F.B. Cerebrospinal fluid physiology and the management of increased intracranial pressure. *Mayo Clin. Proc.* 65:684–707, 1990.

178a. Kilpi, T., et al., and the Finnish Study Group. Oral glycerol and intravenous dexameth-asone in preventing neurologic and audiologic sequelae of childhood bacterial meningi-tis. *Pediatr. Infect. Dis. J.* 14:270, 1995.
   In this small study, oral glycerol prevented neurologic sequelae in infants and children more effectively than IV dexamethasone. Authors conclude that additional data from placebo-controlled, double-blinded studies are needed before its use can be routinely recommended.
179. Ashwal, S., et al. Bacterial meningitis in children: Pathophysiology and treatment. *Neurology* 42:739–748, 1992.
179a. Bisno, A.L., and Sternau, L. Infections of Central Nervous System Shunts. In A.L. Bisno and F.A. Waldvogel (eds.), *Infections Associated with Indwelling Medical Devices* (2nd ed.). Washington, D.C.: ASM Press, 1994. Pp. 91–109.
180. Girgis, N.I., et al. Dexamethasone adjunctive treatment for tuberculous meningitis. *Pediatr. Infect. Dis. J.* 10:179–183, 1991.
181. Denning, D.W., et al. Elevated cerebrospinal fluid pressures in patients with crypto-coccal meningitis and acquired immunodeficiency syndrome. *Am. J. Med.* 91:267–272, 1991.
182. Forsey, T., et al. Mumps vaccines and meningitis. *Lancet* 340:980, 1992.
183. Lieberman, J.M., Greenberg, D.P., and Ward, J.I. Prevention of bacterial meningitis. Vaccines and chemoprophylaxis. *Infect. Dis. Clin. North Am.* 4:703–729, 1990.
184. Immunization Practices Advisory Committee. *Haemophilus* b conjugate vaccines for prevention of *Haemophilus influenzae* type b disease among infants and children two months of age and older. *M.M.W.R.* 40(RR-1):1–7, 1991.
185. Schwartz, B., et al. Comparative efficacy of ceftriaxone and rifampicin in eradicating pharyngeal carriage of group A *Neisseria meningitidis. Lancet* 1:1239–1242, 1988.
186. Immunization Practices Advisory Committee. Update on adult immunization. *M.M.W.R.* 40(RR-12):1–94, 1991.
187. Whitley, R.J., and Schlitt, M. Encephalitis Caused by Herpesviruses, Including B Virus. In W.M. Scheld, R.J. Whitley, and D.T. Durack (eds.), *Infections of the Central Nervous System.* New York: Raven, 1991. Pp. 41–86.
   For a related review, see update by R.J. Whitley and F. Lakeman, Herpes simplex virus infections of the central nervous system: Therapeutic and diagnostic considera-tions. Clin. Infect. Dis. 20:414, 1995.
188. Barnes, D.W., and Whitley, R.J. CNS diseases associated with varicella zoster virus and herpes simplex virus infection: Pathogenesis and current therapy. *Neurol. Clin.* 4:265–283, 1986.
189. Whitley, R.J., et al. Diseases that mimic herpes simplex encephalitis: Diagnosis, presentation, and outcome. *J.A.M.A.* 262:234–239, 1989.
   For two related diagnoses which may mimic HSV encephalitis, see D.R. Johns et al. MELAS syndrome masquerading as herpes simplex encephalitis. Neurology 43:2471, 1993 *(mitochondrial encephalopathy, lactic acidosis, and strokelike episodes: These patients may have seizures and focal abnormalities on MRI and EEG that raise the question of HSV encephalitis. However, patients with MELAS syndrome usually have no fever or alteration in consciousness or CSF pleocytosis; their seizures may also be separated by several months). See also A.P. Sempere et al. Q fever mimicking herpetic encephalitis.* Neurology 43:2713, 1993.
190. Whitley, R.J. Viral encephalitis. *N. Engl. J. Med.* 323:242–250, 1990.
   For a related update, see D.E. Griffin. Encephalitis, Myelitis, and Neuritis. In G.L. Mandell, J.E. Bennett, and R. Dolin (eds.), Principles and Practice of Infectious Dis-eases (4th ed.). New York: Churchill Livingstone, 1995. Pp. 874–880.
191. Bleck, T.P. Imaging for Central Nervous System Infections. In G.L. Mandell, J.E. Bennett, and R. Dolin (eds.), *Principles and Practice of Infectious Diseases: Update* 4(1):1–13, 1995.
   Recent excellent review. Published as an update to the 4th edition of this excellent text. MRI has revolutionized the diagnostic approach to suspected encephalitis.
192. Garcia, J.H., et al. Diagnosis of viral encephalitis by brain biopsy. *Semin. Diagn. Pathol.* 1:71–80, 1984.
193. Boston Interhospital Virus Study Group and the NIAID-Sponsored Cooperative Anti-viral Clinical Study. Failure of high dose 5-iodo-2'-deoxyuridine in the therapy of herpes simplex virus encephalitis: Evidence of unacceptable toxicity. *N. Engl. J. Med.* 292:599–603, 1975.
194. Whitley, R.J., et al. Adenine arabinoside therapy of biopsy-proved herpes simplex encephalitis: National Institute of Allergy and Infectious Diseases Collaborative Anti-viral Study. *N. Engl. J. Med.* 297:289–294, 1977.

195. Whitley, R.J., et al. Herpes simplex encephalitis: Vidarabine therapy and diagnostic problems. *N. Engl. J. Med.* 304:313–318, 1981.

196. Whitley, R.J., et al. Vidarabine versus acyclovir therapy of herpes simplex encephalitis. *N. Engl. J. Med.* 314:144–149, 1986.
See related article by B. Skolderberg et al. Acyclovir versus vidarabine in herpes simplex encephalitis: A randomized multicentre study of consecutive Swedish patients. Lancet 2:707–711, 1984.

197. Medical Letter. Drugs for non-HIV viral infections. *Med. Lett. Drugs Ther.* 36:27, 1994.
For HSV encephalitis suggests intravenous acyclovir, 10 mg/kg q8h for 14–21 days. See related discussion of therapy for 14–21 days by K.E. VanLandingham et al., J.A.M.A. 259:1051, 1988.

198. Shepp, D., Dandliker, P.S., and Meyers, J.D. Treatment of varicella-zoster virus in severely immunocompromised patients: A randomized comparison of acyclovir and vidarabine. *N. Engl. J. Med.* 314:208–212, 1986.

199. Wispelwey, B., Dacey, R.G., Jr., and Scheld, W.M. Brain Abscess. In W.M. Scheld, R.J. Whitley, and D.T. Durack (eds.), *Infections of the Central Nervous System.* New York: Raven, 1991. Pp. 457–486.

199a. Wispelwey, B., and Scheld, W.M. Brain Abscess. In G.L. Mandell, J.E. Bennett, and R. Dolin (eds.), *Principles and Practice of Infectious Diseases* (4th ed.). New York: Churchill Livingstone, 1995. Pp. 887–899.
See also E.A. Rosenfeld and A.H. Rowley. Infectious intracranial complications of sinusitis, other than meningitis in children: 12 year review. Clin. Infect. Dis. *18:750, 1994 (complications can include epidural abscess, subdural abscess, and cerebral abscess) and C.R. Woods, Jr. Brain abscess and other intracranial suppurative complications.* Adv. Pediatr. Infect. Dis. *10:41, 1995.*

200. Tunkel, A.R., and Scheld, W.M. Central Nervous System Infection in the Immunocompromised Host. In R.H. Rubin and L.S. Young (eds.), *Clinical Approach to Infection in the Compromised Host* (3rd ed.). New York: Plenum, 1994. Pp. 163–210.

201. Salaki, J.S., Louria, D.B., and Chmel, H. Fungal and yeast infections of the central nervous system: A clinical review. *Medicine* (Baltimore) 63:108–132, 1984.

202. Sepkowitz, K., and Armstrong, D. Space-Occupying Fungal Lesions of the Central Nervous System. In W.M. Scheld, R.J. Whitley, and D.T. Durack (eds.), *Infections of the Central Nervous System.* New York: Raven, 1991. Pp. 741–764.

203. Berenguer, J., et al. Central nervous system infection caused by *Pseudallescheria boydii. Rev. Infect. Dis.* 11:890–896, 1989.

204. Dworzack, D.L., et al. *Pseudallescheria boydii* brain abscess: Association with near-drowning and efficacy of high-dose, prolonged miconazole therapy in patients with multiple abscesses. *Medicine* (Baltimore) 68:218–224, 1989.

205. Zimmerman, R.D., and Haimes, A.B. The Role of MR Imaging in the Diagnosis of Infections of the Central Nervous System. In J.S. Remington and M.N. Swartz (eds.), *Current Clinical Topics in Infectious Diseases.* Boston: Blackwell, 1989. Pp. 82–108.
For an update of this topic, see reference [191].

205a. Mameiak, A.N., et al. Nocardial brain abscess: Treatment strategies and factors influencing outcome. *Neurosurgery* 35:622, 1994.

206. Stephanov, S. Surgical treatment of brain abscess. *Neurosurgery* 22:724–730, 1988.

207. Mampalam, T.J., and Rosenblum, M.L. Trends in the management of bacterial brain abscesses: A review of 102 cases over 17 years. *Neurosurgery* 23:451–458, 1988.
See related report by A.N. Mameiak et al. Improved management of multiple brain abscesses: A combined surgical and medical approach. Neurosurgery 36:76–86, 1995.

208. Carpenter, J.L. Brain stem abscesses: Cure with medical therapy, case report, and review. *Clin. Infect. Dis.* 18:219–226, 1994.

209. Boom, W.H., and Tuazon, C.U. Successful treatment of multiple brain abscesses with antibiotics alone. *Rev. Infect. Dis.* 7:189–199, 1985.

210. Filice, G.A., and Simpson, G.L. Management of *Nocardia* Infections. In J.S. Remington and M.N. Swartz (eds.), *Current Clinical Topics in Infectious Diseases.* New York: McGraw-Hill, 1984. Pp. 49–64.

211. Denning, D.W., and Stevens, D.A. Antifungal and surgical treatment of invasive aspergillosis: Review of 2,121 published cases. *Rev. Infect. Dis.* 12:1147–1201, 1990.

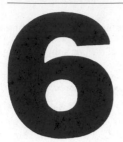

Eye Infections

Marlene L. Durand,
Gregory J. Riley,
and Ann Sullivan Baker

Although inflammatory eye conditions may be due to a variety of diseases, infectious agents play a major role in both acute and chronic eye disease. The primary care doctor is often the first physician to see the patient with an eye infection, and his or her role extends beyond the management of simple eyelid pustules and infectious conjunctivitis. He or she must be able to recognize more serious conditions, such as corneal ulcers, retinitis, or endophthalmitis, as well as provide initial emergency treatment of rapidly progressive bacterial eye infections.

Eyelid Infections

I. **Anatomy.** Each eyelid contains glands of Zeis (sebaceous) and Möll (sweat) adjacent to eyelash follicles (Fig. 6-1) and meibomian glands (sebaceous) within the tarsal plate (Fig. 6-2). The tarsal plate is the fibrous "skeleton" of each eyelid.

II. **Hordeolum**
   A. **Clinical characteristics.** A hordeolum is an acute infection of either a meibomian gland (internal hordeolum) or a gland of Zeis (external hordeolum, also called a *stye*). Both are painful, red swellings: A stye points to the lash margin. The most common pathogen is *Staphylococcus aureus*.
   B. **Treatment**
      1. Warm compresses should be applied every 4–6 hours.
      2. Topical antibiotic ointment (e.g., bacitracin) should be used daily at bedtime.
      3. If no response, incision and drainage may be required.

III. **Chalazion**
   A. **Clinical characteristics.** A chalazion is a chronic granuloma in a meibomian gland. It may begin with an acute inflammation, due to either infection (internal hordeolum or staphylococcal blepharitis) or a tissue reaction to inspissated sebum. It may become a chronic, painless lump in the eyelid. Although most resolve within 1 month, some recur. A chalazion usually points through the inside surface of the eyelid rather than anteriorly through the skin. It is noteworthy that a sebaceous cell carcinoma of the eyelid may be mistaken for a recurrent chalazion.
   B. **Treatment**
      1. In the **acute phase,** use warm compresses and topical antibiotic ointment (e.g., erythromycin) daily at bedtime. Oral antibiotics are not necessary unless there is surrounding cellulitis.
      2. In the **chronic phase,** intralesional steroids (triamcinolone acetonide) or surgical excision is required.

IV. **Marginal blepharitis.** Marginal blepharitis is a diffuse inflammation of the eyelid margins. It may be acute but is more typically chronic, waxing and waning over years, and may be associated with seborrheic dermatitis and rosacea. It is believed to be due to excessive secretions of the sebaceous glands of the eyelid as well as to superinfection with *S. aureus*. The latter has not been proven, however, as some studies have found that *S. aureus* colonizes normal eyelids as often as lids with blepharitis [1].
   A. **Clinical characteristics**
      1. **Irritation (burning and itching)** of the eyelid margins is the primary symptom.
      2. **Inflammation of the lid** may be mild, consisting of hyperemia of the lid margin with scaling of the skin (squamous or seborrheic blepharitis), or more severe, with destruction of the lash follicles and tiny eyelid ulcerations (staphylococcal or ulcerative blepharitis). In the milder form, seborrhea and infection coexist, and the patient may show other signs of seborrhea in the scalp, brow, and ears.

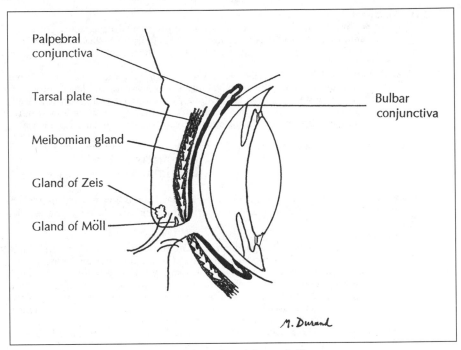

Fig. 6-1. Sagittal section of the eyelids and anterior eyeball.

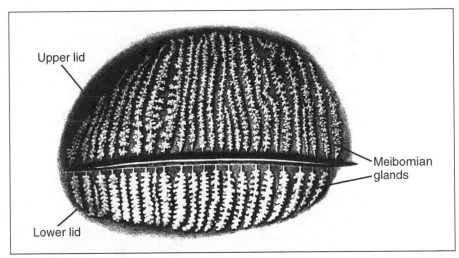

Fig. 6-2. The meibomian, or tarsal, glands of the eyelids. (From R. J. Last, *Eugene Wolff's Anatomy of the Eye and Orbit*. Edinburgh: Churchill Livingstone, 1976.)

B. **Treatment**
   1. **Acute.** Wash eyelids with warm water. Apply topical bacitracin ophthalmic ointment to the base of the eyelashes 2–4 times daily for 1–2 weeks (depending on severity), gradually decreasing frequency to once nightly for several more weeks.
   2. **Chronic.** Gently scrub eyelids with a washcloth with warm water 2–3 times daily to remove scales. Wash lashes and eyebrows with the lather of a baby shampoo twice weekly (when the scalp is washed) to control seborrhea. Apply topical bacitracin ointment to eyelid margins nightly. If there is associated rosacea, oral tetracycline, 250 mg once daily for several months, may be useful.

Infections of the Lacrimal System

I. **Anatomy.** Tears are produced primarily by the **lacrimal gland** (Fig. 6-3), drain through **canaliculi** into the **lacrimal sac,** and then drain into the nose beneath the inferior turbinate.

II. **Dacryoadenitis**
   A. **Clinical characteristics.** Dacryoadenitis, or inflammation of the lacrimal gland, is rare. Acute suppurative dacryoadenitis presents as a tender, warm, red swelling of the lateral portion of the upper eyelid. It usually is due to *S. aureus,* although some cases may be due to streptococci, *Chlamydia trachomatis* or, rarely, *Neisseria gonorrhoeae* [2]. Chronic dacryoadenitis presents as a painless swelling of the gland. It is most often caused by viruses (e.g., mumps, Epstein-Barr virus, cytomegalovirus, coxsackievirus) but may be due to tuberculosis or syphilis. The differential diagnosis of chronic dacryoadenitis includes autoimmune disorders (e.g., Sjögren's syndrome or sarcoidosis) and tumors.

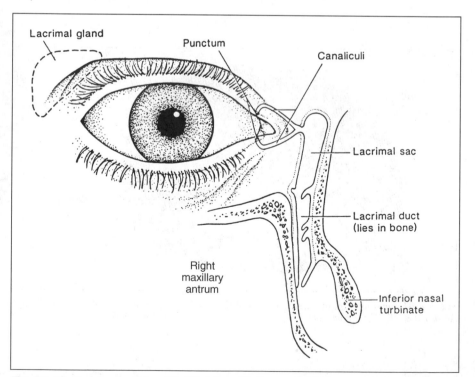

Fig. 6-3. The lacrimal system. (Modified from M. Barza and J. Baum, Ocular infections. *Med. Clin. North Am.* 67:131–152, 1983.)

    B. Treatment. For acute infections, intravenous antibiotics active against staphylococci and streptococci (e.g., nafcillin) should be given for several days, followed by oral dicloxacillin for a total of 7–14 days of therapy.

III. Canaliculitis

    A. Clinical characteristics. Canaliculitis is an inflammation of the canaliculi. The area of the punctum is swollen and red, and the patient complains of itching and burning of the area and excessive tearing. The most common pathogen is *Actinomyces israelii*. Often with pressure over the punctum, yellow "sulfur granules" may be expressed. The material expressed should be sent for Gram stain (which may show the delicate gram-positive branching filaments of this bacterium) as well as for anaerobic and aerobic cultures.

    B. Treatment. Expression of material and probing through the punctum (performed by an ophthalmologist) to remove infected material usually is curative. Some ophthalmologists also irrigate the outflow tract with penicillin ophthalmic solution.

IV. Dacryocystitis

    A. Clinical characteristics. Dacryocystitis is the most common infection of the lacrimal system and occurs as a result of outflow obstruction in the nasolacrimal duct. There usually is **epiphora** (excessive tearing) in both acute and chronic forms.

        1. Acute. Symptoms of acute dacryocystitis are pain, swelling, redness, and tenderness in the nasal corner of the eye. The pathogens involved are *S. aureus* and *Streptococcus pyogenes*, as well as *Streptococcus pneumoniae* (in infants) and *Haemophilus influenzae* (in children).

        2. Chronic. Epiphora and local swelling may be the only symptoms of chronic infection. Many bacteria (e.g., *Actinomyces*) and fungi (e.g., *Aspergillus* and *Candida*) have been implicated in the chronic form. Gram stains and cultures of the material expressed from the tear duct will aid in making a specific diagnosis.

    B. Treatment

        1. Acute

            a. Apply warm compresses every 2–4 hours.

            b. Give systemic antibiotics active against gram-positive organisms and, in children, also active against *H. influenzae*. (For example, in adults use intravenous nafcillin for severe infections or oral dicloxacillin for mild ones; in children use cefuroxime.)

            c. Consult an ophthalmologist: Surgical drainage may be required.

            d. Watch for signs of orbital cellulitis, an infrequent but dangerous complication of acute dacryocystitis.

        2. Chronic

            a. Establish adequate drainage of the lacrimal sac. In infants, this may be accomplished by massage alone. Adults require probing or possibly dacryocystorhinostomy, a surgical procedure to allow adequate drainage into the nose.

            b. Use topical antibiotic drops or, in adults, local irrigation with antibiotics through the punctum (performed by an ophthalmologist). Antibiotics should be selected on the basis of culture results.

Red Eye

Red eye is a sign rather than a clinical entity, but it is the most common ocular condition presenting to primary physicians. Although it may be attributable to nonspecific conjunctivitis, occasionally red eye is the first sign of serious ocular or systemic disease. **Table 6-1 lists the differential diagnosis of an inflamed eye. Note that the redness of conjunctivitis, due to dilation of the superficial conjunctival vessels, is most intense peripherally.** Redness that is most intense centrally around the corneal edge (paralimbal injection or "ciliary flush") is due to dilation of a deeper episcleral vascular plexus and always indicates serious eye disease. **A patient who has a red eye with ciliary flush, eye pain, unilateral photophobia, visual impairment, pupillary asymmetry, or loss of corneal clarity requires immediate ophthalmologic referral.**

Table 6-1. Differential diagnosis of the common causes of a red eye

	Acute conjunctivitis	Acute iritis[a]	Acute glaucoma[b]	Corneal trauma or infection
Incidence	Extremely common	Common	Uncommon	Common
Discharge	Moderate to copious	None	None	Watery or purulent
Vision	No effect on vision	Slightly blurred	Markedly blurred	Usually blurred
Pain	None	Moderate	Severe	Moderate to severe
Conjunctival injection	Diffuse; more toward fornices	Mainly circum-corneal	Diffuse	Diffuse
Cornea	Clear	Usually clear	Steamy	Change in clarity related to cause
Pupil size	Normal	Small	Moderately dilated and fixed	Normal
Pupillary light response	Normal	Poor	None	Normal
Intraocular pressure	Normal	Normal	Elevated	Normal
Smear	Causative organisms	No organisms	No organisms	Organisms found only in corneal ulcers due to infection

[a]Acute anterior uveitis.
[b]Angle-closure glaucoma.
Source: From D. Vaughan, T. Asbury, and P. Riordan-Eva (eds.), *General Ophthalmology* (13th ed.). Norwalk, CT: Appleton & Lange, 1992.

Conjunctivitis

Infectious conjunctivitis is the most common ocular infection seen by the primary physician. Distinguishing viral from bacterial conjunctivitis can be difficult. Most important is distinguishing both from other causes of red eye, as noted earlier. Conjunctival inflammation may be a manifestation of systemic disease. It is the most common ocular complication of Lyme disease (see Chap. 23), with an incidence of approximately 10%. In most cases, a specific etiologic diagnosis may be difficult to determine.

In children with acute conjunctivitis, one study found that three microorganisms account for the majority of cases: *H. influenzae, S. pneumoniae,* and adenoviruses. Approximately, one-half to two-thirds of cases of acute conjunctivitis are bacterial in etiology. The concurrent presence of acute otitis media increases the likelihood of a bacterial infection, whereas concurrent pharyngitis makes adenovirus the most likely cause [2a].

Chlamydiae are considered special types of intracellular bacteria [3] but, for purposes of clarity, chlamydial and bacterial infections are considered separately below.

I. **Anatomy.** The conjunctiva (see Fig. 6-1) is a thin, translucent mucous membrane that lines the eyelids (palpebral conjunctiva) and covers the anterior sclera, or "whites of the eyes" (bulbar conjunctiva). It does not cover the cornea but is continuous with the corneal epithelium at the **limbus** (corneal-scleral border). Goblet cells scattered in the conjunctiva add mucus to the tear film that lubricates the eye.

II. **General clinical characteristics.** Symptoms are similar for conjunctivitis of various etiologies. Initially, there is mild to moderate unilateral discomfort—itching, burning, and discharge—which spreads to the other eye within a few days (except in hyperacute conjunctivitis, when symptoms progress rapidly).

A. **Significant pain is not present.** A painful red eye suggests a different diagnosis.
B. **True visual impairment is not present.** A thick conjunctival discharge may cloud vision, but this clears with blinking.
C. **Table 6-2 lists features that help distinguish bacterial, viral, and chlamydial conjunctivitis.**
   1. **Follicles** are foci of lymphoid hyperplasia within the palpebral conjunctiva that give it a pebbly appearance. They are typical of viral or chlamydial infections but may also be seen as a reaction to eye drops such as idoxuridine and miotics [4]. Follicle formation does not occur in children younger than 3 years, who lack conjunctival lymphoid tissue.
   2. **Papillae** may be similar to follicles in appearance, but each has a central tuft of blood vessels that may be seen with magnification (each follicle, in contrast, is encircled by a blood vessel). Fine papillae, characteristic of bacterial or chlamydial infection, give the palpebral conjunctiva a smooth, red, velvety appearance [4]. Giant papillae suggest a type of allergic conjunctivitis (vernal keratoconjunctivitis) or a reaction to contact lenses.

III. **Viral conjunctivitis**
   A. **Clinical characteristics.** Viral conjunctivitis is more common than bacterial conjunctivitis in developed countries. Nearly all viruses causing human disease may affect the conjunctiva, but adenovirus is the most common cause of viral conjunctivitis. **Preauricular lymphadenopathy, conjunctival follicles, and a thin, watery discharge are characteristic of viral conjunctivitis.**
   1. **Adenovirus,** especially type 3, may be transmitted in poorly chlorinated swimming pools, causing summertime "swimming pool conjunctivitis" and fever and sore throat in children (**pharyngoconjunctival fever**). Infections with adenovirus types 8, 19, 29, and 37 may be complicated by a painful, centrally located corneal epithelial ulcer (**epidemic keratoconjunctivitis**) that usually develops after the conjunctivitis has been present for 6–10 days and may persist for months. These highly contagious viruses may be transmitted by hands, contaminated instruments, or contaminated eye-drop bottles.
   2. **Herpes simplex virus** (HSV) is an uncommon cause of follicular conjunctivitis but, when present, frequently involves the cornea. Herpetic vesicles may be

Table 6-2. Features that distinguish the common causes of conjunctivitis

Feature	Bacterial conjunctivitis	Viral conjunctivitis	Chlamydial conjunctivitis
Conjunctival injection	Moderately severe	Minimal	Absent or minimal
Exudate	Moderate to profuse (polymorphonuclear)	Minimal (usually mononuclear)	Minimal in adults, copious in newborns
Sticking of lids on awakening	Yes	No	Absent in adults, present in newborns
Papillae (palpebral conjunctiva)	Present	Usually absent	May be present
Follicles (palpebral conjunctiva)	Usually absent	Present	Present in adults, absent in newborns
Preauricular lymphadenopathy	Absent	Present	Present in adults, absent in newborns
Response to antibiotic therapy	Yes	No	Yes
Duration of untreated disease	Up to several weeks	Several weeks	Persistent

Source: From J. Baum and M. Barza, Infections of the Eye. In S. L. Gorbach, J. G. Bartlett, and N. R. Blacklow (eds.), *Infectious Diseases.* Philadelphia: Saunders, 1992.

found on the eyelids and lid margins (see sec. **III** under Infectious Keratitis and Chap. 4).

3. **Acute hemorrhagic conjunctivitis** is a disease of crowding and poor hygiene that is caused primarily by highly contagious enterovirus type 70 and coxsackievirus type A24. It has a short incubation period (8–48 hours) and lasts 5–7 days. It is characterized by subconjunctival hemorrhages and marked eyelid edema in addition to the usual signs and symptoms of viral conjunctivitis. It was more common in the 1970s than it is now [5].

4. **Miscellaneous.** Conjunctivitis may be a component of other viral infections, such as influenza, varicella, rubella, rubeola, infectious mononucleosis, or herpes zoster ophthalmicus. The conjunctival inflammation in these conditions, however, is usually a minor manifestation of a more generalized infection.

B. **Diagnosis is based on clinical features (see Table 6-2), although distinguishing viral from bacterial conjunctivitis may be difficult.** Viral cultures may be helpful in the presence of corneal involvement.

C. **Treatment.** Except for HSV conjunctivitis, viral conjunctivitis without corneal involvement warrants no specific therapy. These conditions usually are self-limited, lasting 7–10 days unless bacterial superinfection occurs. Patients should be advised to return immediately if symptoms worsen or if any eye pain develops. They should also be educated about the importance of good hand-washing in preventing spread of the disease to others.

   HSV conjunctivitis may last 2–3 weeks, and patients with this diagnosis should be followed by an ophthalmologist. Topical antiviral therapy (e.g., trifluridine drops q2h) is indicated to prevent corneal involvement (see sec. **III.A** under Infectious Keratitis).

IV. **Bacterial conjunctivitis**
   A. **Hyperacute (purulent)**
      1. **Clinical characteristics.** Hyperacute bacterial conjunctivitis is the most severe form of conjunctivitis and most often is caused by pathogenic *Neisseria*, especially *N. gonorrhoeae*. Other causes, such as *N. meningitidis* and *Corynebacterium diphtheriae,* are rare. There is usually marked eyelid edema, chemosis (conjunctival edema), a copious, purulent exudate, and tender, preauricular nodes. Untreated, it may lead to keratitis and corneal perforation. Toxic iritis may occur in gonococcal infections and can be recognized by the presence of pain, photophobia, and unilateral pupillary constriction [6].
      2. **Diagnosis.** Gram stain of conjunctival exudate shows gram-negative diplococci, many intracellular. For recovery of *Neisseria*, exudate should be plated directly onto chocolate and Thayer-Martin plates and these placed in a 5% carbon dioxide atmosphere as soon as possible. If delay in transport is anticipated, use a "Jembec" Thayer-Martin plate, which creates a microenvironment with the addition of a carbon dioxide–generating tablet.
      3. **Treatment.** For treatment of neonates, see sec. **VI.** For gonococcal conjunctivitis in adults, the Centers for Disease Control (CDC) [7] recommends a single 1-g dose of ceftriaxone (IM or IV). For highly penicillin-allergic patients, single-dose therapy with either 500 mg PO ciprofloxacin or 400 mg PO ofloxacin will treat most cases of genital and pharyngeal gonococcal infection; 2 g IM spectinomycin will treat genital but not pharyngeal infection. Any of these alternatives would presumably be adequate therapy for conjunctival disease in adults as well, although efficacy data are not available. Saline eye drops may be given to clear the exudate. We would also culture and treat for possible coexisting chlamydiae with either doxycycline (100 mg bid) or erythromycin (500 mg qid) in adults.
   B. **Acute (mucopurulent)**
      1. **Clinical characteristics.** With acute bacterial conjunctivitis, the patient complains of lids sticking together in the morning and has a thick, mucopurulent exudate. Symptoms usually begin in one eye but are bilateral 1–2 days later. The most common etiologies are *S. aureus, S. pneumoniae, H. influenzae* (especially in children), *S. pyogenes,* and *H. aegyptius* (in warm climates). Gram-negative bacillary infections are rare except in patients with abnormal corneas or those who are in intensive care units; *Pseudomonas* is particularly destructive (see sec. **IV** under Infectious Keratitis).
      2. **Diagnosis.** Pretreatment bacterial cultures and Gram stains are useful, particularly if the conjunctivitis fails to respond to initial empiric therapy.

3. Treatment. Except for *Pseudomonas* (see sec. **IV** under Infectious Keratitis), treatment is topical only [8]. Some commercially available ophthalmic ointments and solutions (eye drops) are listed in Table 6-3. Ointments can be given less frequently (q4–6h) than eye drops (q2–4h) and therefore are useful at bedtime but may transiently blur vision after each application during the day. Therapy may be stopped 48–72 hours after clearing of signs and symptoms (usually 7–10 days). Patients should be advised to avoid contamination of the ointment tube or dropper tip and to return if they are no better in 2–3 days.

    a. Empiric. Begin broad-spectrum topical therapy while awaiting culture results. **Sulfonamides are used most often** [9] (e.g., 10% sulfacetamide or 4% sulfisoxazole): Both are available as eye drops and ophthalmic ointment. Sulfa-allergic patients can be treated with combination products such as Polysporin ointment (bacitracin and polymixin B) or Polytrim eye drops (trimethoprim and polymixin B) for broad-spectrum coverage, or with erythromycin or bacitracin ointments for mild infection in adults (these cover only gram-positive organisms).

    b. Gram-positive infections. Use bacitracin (500 units/g) or erythromycin (0.5%) ophthalmic ointments. Cephalosporin or vancomycin eye drops can also be used but must be constituted by the pharmacy as they are not commercially available.

    c. Gram-negative infections. Use ciprofloxacin (see sec. **d**) or an aminoglycoside such as gentamicin or tobramycin (both available as a 3-mg/ml ointment or solution). Because of local concentrations achieved by topical application, aminoglycosides also provide some coverage of *S. aureus* (but not streptococci).

    d. Ciprofloxacin, 0.3% ophthalmic ointment or solution (Ciloxan), has recently become available and is well tolerated. It provides broad-spectrum coverage, although it more reliably treats gram-negative than gram-positive organisms. Some strains of streptococci may be resistant, and some strains of staphylococci and *Pseudomonas* may develop resistance during therapy. Ciprofloxacin is discussed further in sec. **IV** under Infectious Keratitis.

C. Chronic

    1. Clinical characteristics. *S. aureus* is the most common etiology; *Moraxella lacunata* is another cause. Both may be associated with a chronic blepharitis. Gram-negative organisms and anaerobes have also been reported.

Table 6-3. Some commercially available antibiotic eye drops and ophthalmic ointments

Antibiotic	Trade name[a]	Concentration
Bacitracin[b]	AK-TRACIN	500 units/g
Ciprofloxacin[c]	Ciloxan	0.3%
Erythromycin[b]	—	0.5%
Gentamicin[b,c]	Genoptic, Gentacidin	0.3%
Sulfacetamide sodium[b]	AK-SULF, Cetamide	10%
Sulfacetamide sodium[c]	Ocu-Sul-10,-15,-30	10%, 15%, 30%
Sulfisoxazole diolamine[c]	Gantrisin	4%
Tetracycline[b,c]	Achromycin	1%
Tobramycin[b,c]	Tobrex	0.3%
Combinations		
Bacitracin and polymyxin B[b]	Polysporin	—
Neomycin, polymyxin B, and bacitracin[b] *or* gramicidin[c]	Neosporin	—
Trimethoprim and polymyxin B[c]	Polytrim	—

[a]The trade name list is not all-inclusive. In addition, most of these antibiotics are available also as generic preparations.
[b]Ointment available.
[c]Solution (eye drops) available.

    2. **Diagnosis.** Gram staining and cultures (including anaerobic) will identify the underlying pathogen.

    3. **Treatment** should be guided by culture results (see sec. **B.3**). Eyelid hygiene is important if there is blepharitis. Evaluation of the lacrimal system (for organism reservoir) is indicated if symptoms recur.

V. Chlamydial conjunctivitis. *Chlamydia trachomatis* is responsible for two distinct ocular syndromes: trachoma, a blinding disease, and inclusion conjunctivitis, a relatively benign infection. Trachoma is caused by serotypes A–C, inclusion conjunctivitis by types D–K. Inclusion conjunctivitis occurs in sexually active adults and neonates; the neonatal disease is discussed in sec. **VI.**

  A. Trachoma

    1. **Clinical characteristics.** Trachoma is a leading cause of blindness in endemic areas of North Africa, the Middle East, and northern India. Blindness results only after many years of infection and reinfection. In hyperendemic areas, nearly all children acquire the infection by age 2 [10] and are the main reservoir for infection in the community. Vector (flies) and fomite (e.g., clothing) as well as person-to-person transmission occurs. Initial infection may heal spontaneously, but repeated reinfections lead to corneal vascularization and scarring. Women are much more likely to have severe trachoma than men, probably because of their closer contact with children.

        Trachoma has four stages: conjunctivitis, corneal vascularization, scarring, and scar retraction. A chronic and recurrent follicular conjunctivitis, which involves the upper eyelid and has corneal extension, is found to be typical of trachoma and is rare in other ocular conditions.

    2. **Diagnosis. Gram stain will not show the organism,** but Giemsa stain shows typical basophilic cytoplasmic inclusion bodies in conjunctival epithelial cells. However, the method of choice is now the more sensitive (87–100%) direct fluorescent monoclonal antibody stain [11] (e.g., MicroTrak), enzyme immunoassay (e.g., Chlamydiazyme), or DNA probe. Organisms may also be cultured.

    3. **Treatment** with an oral tetracycline (e.g., doxycycline, 100 mg bid) or sulfonamides should be directed by an ophthalmologist. Erythromycin and rifampin may also be used. Treatment of 3–6 weeks' duration is generally very effective. Treatment of chronic trachoma in hyperendemic areas is difficult because of the likelihood of reinfection.

  B. Adult inclusion conjunctivitis

    1. **Clinical characteristics.** Occurring in sexually active adolescents and adults, adult inclusion conjunctivitis is typically a low-grade, chronic, bilateral follicular conjunctivitis with a minimal mucopurulent discharge. It begins 2–19 days after exposure to infected genital or urinary tract secretions [10] and occurs in approximately 1 in 300 patients with genital chlamydial infections [4]. Indirect transmission in poorly chlorinated swimming pools may occur [12]. Conjunctival follicles are present as in trachoma, but there is greater involvement of the **lower palpebral conjunctiva,** and preauricular adenopathy is more common. Moreover, the macropannus and scarring of trachoma are not present.

    2. **Diagnosis.** See sec. **V.A.2.** If these studies are negative, adenovirus and HSV infections should be considered.

    3. **Treatment.** Use oral erythromycin (500 mg qid) or a tetracycline (doxycycline, 100 mg bid) for 2 weeks in adults. Azithromycin has been used as single-dose therapy for genital infections, but efficacy data for treating conjunctivitis are unavailable. Untreated inclusion conjunctivitis may lead to chronic follicular conjunctivitis lasting 3–12 months and to subepithelial corneal infiltrates.

VI. Ophthalmia neonatorum. Ophthalmia neonatorum (ON) refers to any conjunctival inflammation in the newborn. Most cases occur in the first 2 weeks of life. Chlamydiae are the most common infectious cause of ON [13], but gonococci are the most serious. Silver nitrate eye drops, tetracycline ointment, or erythromycin ointment all are equally effective in preventing gonococcal ON (incidence, 0.06% of all newborns given prophylaxis) and equally poor at preventing chlamydial ON (15% of newborns given prophylaxis who are born to infected women) [14]. In a recent study from Kenya, a 2.5% ophthalmic solution of povidone-iodine as prophylaxis against ophthalmia neonatorum was more effective than treatment with silver nitrate or erythromycin, and it was less toxic and costs less [14a].

  A. General guidelines. Because gonococcal infections are rapidly destructive, **consider conjunctivitis in the newborn as an ophthalmic emergency and obtain prompt ophthalmologic consultation.** Do not rely on the timing of the infection or the clinical appearance alone to make a specific diagnosis: There is too much overlap with other conditions. Obtain Gram stain, immunofluorescent stain for chlamydiae, routine cultures, and culture on chocolate and Thayer-Martin media for *N. gonorrhoeae.* If the stains are not diagnostic, begin topical erythromycin empirically while awaiting culture results.

B. Chlamydial conjunctivitis (neonatal inclusion conjunctivitis)
1. **Clinical characteristics.** Onset is classically 5–14 days after birth. There may be unilateral or bilateral involvement, with conjunctival hyperemia, eyelid edema, and profuse exudate. Newborns lack lymphoid tissue and fail to develop an acute follicular conjunctivitis, which is typical of the adult infection. *Chlamydia trachomatis* types D–K are responsible (as is true for adult inclusion conjunctivitis).
2. **Diagnosis.** See sec. **V.A.2.**
3. **Treatment.** Oral erythromycin (50 mg/kg/day) for 10–14 days is effective, well tolerated, and is the preferred agent as it eradicates nasopharyngeal carrier states. Topical erythromycin therapy may be omitted if it is not tolerated by the infant. Parents should be treated for presumed chlamydial genital infection.

C. Gonococcal conjunctivitis
1. **Clinical characteristics.** Onset is on days 2–5. This disease frequently is bilateral, with marked purulence and chemosis. Initially, the exudate may be serosanguineous. Complications are rare with adequate therapy but include corneal ulceration and endophthalmitis.
2. **Diagnosis.** If the Gram stain shows gram-negative diplococci (many intracellular), the infant should be hospitalized, immediately evaluated for systemic disease (arthritis, meningitis, sepsis), and started on therapy as soon as cultures are obtained.
3. **Treatment.** Although a single dose of ceftriaxone (25–50 mg/kg IM or IV; maximum 125 mg) is effective therapy for gonococcal ON [15], we recommend continuing daily therapy at this dose for at least 72 hours to ensure that CSF and blood cultures are negative. Cefotaxime (50–100 mg/kg/day divided q12h) may be used instead of ceftriaxone in neonates with hyperbilirubinemia. Prompt ophthalmologic consultation should be obtained in all cases. Parents should be evaluated and treated for genital disease.

D. Other infections. *S. aureus* infection has a variable onset (usually days 4–7) and results in an acute purulent conjunctivitis that is diagnosed by culture and Gram stain (in the absence of other detectable ocular pathogens). Topical erythromycin generally is effective for minor infections. For more serious infections, a systemic semisynthetic penicillin (e.g., oxacillin) for 7 days is suggested. See Table 3-2 (in Chap. 3) for dosages of systemic antibiotics in neonates. **HSV type 2** may cause a bilateral conjunctivitis in 15–20% of infected infants and may precede or follow dissemination [16]. Onset occurs on days 2–14 postpartum. Treatment is with systemic acyclovir and topical antiviral therapy.

E. Chemical conjunctivitis is the most common noninfectious cause of ON, occurring in 90% of infants treated with prophylactic silver nitrate drops. It is diagnosed by the appearance of inflammation (eyelid edema, conjunctival hyperemia, watery discharge) within 24 hours of prophylaxis, with negative smears and cultures. It resolves (without treatment) in 24–48 hours.

Infectious Keratitis
(Corneal Ulcers)

Infectious keratitis, or infection of the cornea, usually refers to the presence of a corneal ulcer. Corneal ulcers can lead to loss of vision either because of the resulting corneal scarring or because of progression to perforation and endophthalmitis. These infections **should be managed by an ophthalmologist.** Recognition of corneal disease is the primary function of the generalist.

I. **Anatomy.** The cornea is the 1-mm-thick clear "window" of the eye that has a major role in focusing light: It accounts for almost three-fourths of the total refractive power of the eye [17]. It has no blood vessels but has many sensory nerve fibers (cranial nerve V). The corneal epithelium is 5 cell layers thick and is continuous with the conjunctiva. It serves as a barrier to infection. Breaks in the epithelium may lead to bacterial invasion of the corneal stroma.

II. **General principles.** As in other eye infections, there may be considerable clinical variability, depending on the invasiveness of the infecting organisms. These infections may be acute (adenovirus type 8) or chronic (fungi), relatively indolent (herpes simplex) or rapidly destructive (*Pseudomonas* spp.). HSV is the most common cause of infectious keratitis in developed countries, whereas bacteria and fungi predominate in underdeveloped countries [5]. Infection in eyes that have undergone penetrating keratoplasty (i.e., that have corneal grafts) is usually bacterial.

The **major signs and symptoms** of acute keratitis are a **unilateral red eye** with moderately severe **pain, photophobia, tearing, decreased vision, and a corneal defect.** A **hypopyon** (visible layer of pus in the anterior chamber) may be present and, in keratitis but not endophthalmitis, more often represents a sterile inflammatory response than deeper invasion of bacteria. Fluorescein staining will assist in identifying a corneal ulcer but, with proper illumination, a corneal defect may often be recognized simply by the loss of corneal luster and transparency. Some corneal ulcers, however, can be seen only with a slit lamp.

III. **Viral keratitis**

A. **Herpes simplex.** HSV is the most common cause of corneal ulcers in the United States. HSV keratitis may be primary or recurrent. It is almost always unilateral and may affect any age group.

   1. **Clinical characteristics**

      a. **Primary** HSV infections usually are subclinical but, when symptomatic, manifest as a unilateral **conjunctivitis** with a vesicular eruption of the eyelid that resembles herpes zoster. Approximately two-thirds of these patients develop corneal lesions, usually 7–10 days later.

      b. **Recurrent** ocular HSV infections are more common than primary infections, especially in acutely ill, hospitalized patients whose immune mechanisms are compromised. Patients usually present with anterior eye involvement alone. Repeated attacks are the rule. Bilateral lesions develop in 4–6% of cases [18]. The initial minute epithelial vesicles rupture and give rise to the **typical branchlike (dendritic) ulcers.** Patients complain of mild irritation (foreign-body sensation) and photophobia, and the vision may be slightly impaired. However, there is less discomfort than expected because diminished corneal sensation is part of this condition. In some patients, recurrences may involve the corneal stroma rather than the epithelium and may lead to stromal keratitis.

   2. **Diagnosis.** The typical morphologic appearance of a dendritic ulcer (seen best with fluorescein dye) will usually allow a diagnosis, but its absence does not exclude HSV infection (especially in children). Viral cultures may be helpful.

   3. **Treatment.** With either HSV conjunctivitis or keratitis, **the patient should be followed by an ophthalmologist.** Topical antiviral agents, such as 1% solution of trifluridine (Viroptic eye drops q2h), idoxuridine (Herplex eye drops q1h), and vidarabine (Vira-A 3% ointment [5 times daily]), hasten recovery and reduce the risk of visual impairment. Therapy is given for 7–10 days. Trifluridine is suggested rather than idoxuridine or vidarabine [19]. Topical 3% acyclovir ophthalmic ointment, not yet available in the United States, appears to be as effective as trifluridine. Oral acyclovir is indicated for HSV epithelial keratitis [20]. Topical steroids are contraindicated in epithelial keratitis but, when used with topical trifluridine, may be helpful in treating HSV stromal hepatitis [20a].

B. **Herpes zoster ophthalmicus** is defined as herpes zoster involvement of the first (ophthalmic) division of the trigeminal nerve. It is due to reactivation of latent varicella and is most often seen in the elderly. Involvement of the eye occurs in approximately 75% of cases, corneal involvement in 55% [21].

   1. **Clinical characteristics.** In 25% of cases, the disease begins with severe, unilateral neuralgia. This is followed by typical skin lesions along the distribution of the first division of the trigeminal nerve. A rash on the tip of the nose (Hutchinson's sign) signifies involvement of the nasociliary branch of this division. This is said to increase the risk of corneal involvement, although this has not been substantiated by some studies [21]. Involvement of the cornea is often stromal (deep), unlike HSV, which primarily involves the corneal epithelium. Pseudodendrites may occur and may be confused with HSV dendrites. The keratitis often is accompanied by an anterior uveitis (inflammatory cells in the anterior chamber; see under Uveitis, sec. III). Loss of corneal sensa-

tion is common and may persist for months. Herpes zoster and varicella-zoster virus (VZV) infections are discussed further in Chap. 4 (see under Mucocutaneous Vesicles).

2. **Treatment.** As with other corneal infections, the primary care physician must recognize the disease and refer the patient promptly. Oral acyclovir for 10 days decreases the incidence of keratitis and uveitis in patients with herpes zoster ophthalmicus while also decreasing the duration of skin lesions [22]. We recommend acyclovir, 800 mg PO 5 times daily (i.e., q4h while awake) in adults; this dosage regimen assumes normal renal function. Acyclovir is discussed further in Chap. 26 as are the newer agents, famciclovir and valacyclovir (see p. 980). The role of topical antiviral agents in herpes zoster ophthalmicus is unclear. Topical steroids should not be used except under the supervision of an ophthalmologist.

IV. **Bacterial keratitis**

A. **Etiology.** Many of the bacteria that cause conjunctivitis may invade the cornea following minor trauma and a break in the corneal epithelium. In one recent multicenter trial in the United States [23], gram-positive organisms were isolated in nearly three-fourths of the cases, gram-negatives in one-fourth. The most common organisms in this study were coagulase-negative staphylococci (29%), S. aureus (17%), Pseudomonas aeruginosa (12%), S. pneumoniae (7%), and viridans streptococci (7%): Percentages are of culture-positive bacterial cases and include organisms in mixed bacterial infections.

Contact lens wear is a major predisposing factor for corneal ulcers [24–25a], especially soft contact lenses worn overnight (associated with a 10- to 15-fold excess risk of keratitis compared to daily wear only [26, 27]). Pseudomonas aeruginosa is the most frequent pathogen in contact lens–related cases. Gram-negative organisms, including Pseudomonas, are frequent causes of corneal ulcers in comatose, respirator-dependent patients in intensive care units.

B. **Clinical characteristics.** Most bacterial corneal ulcers present acutely with pain and deep conjunctival hyperemia, which is most intense at the limbus rather than peripherally as in conjunctivitis. Usually, the ulcer is readily apparent as a gray-white, well-circumscribed corneal lesion.

C. **Diagnosis.** When bacterial keratitis is suspected, **an ophthalmologist should see the patient immediately** and scrape the cornea (under slit-lamp visualization) for Gram stain and culture (aerobic, fungal, and anaerobic, if possible). Because of the paucity of material, scrapings should be planted at the bedside (rather than transported). In the elderly, contaminated eye medications (e.g., for glaucoma) may be a source of infection, and cultures of these bottles may be helpful.

A substantial proportion of keratitis cases are culture-negative but presumed bacterial (almost 25% in one study [23]), and many will respond to broad-spectrum antibacterial therapy. However, **failure of response to therapy in culture-negative cases warrants repeat corneal scrapings or biopsy** for culture of organisms including aerobes, anaerobes, fungi, mycobacteria, and Acanthamoeba [28].

D. **Treatment.** When bacterial keratitis is suspected, **obtain an emergency ophthalmologic referral** to secure corneal scrapings for Gram stain and cultures. The patient should be admitted and started on empiric broad-spectrum antibiotic eye drops. Antibiotic drops are given q30min (after a loading dose of one drop per minute × 5) around the clock for the first 24–48 hours (severe cases may require drops q15min). As the patient improves subsequently, drops are given less frequently (especially at night to allow sleep, e.g., q2h at night). If two different antibiotic drops are used, the second should be given 5 minutes after the first to prevent washout.

Nearly all antibiotic eye drops used for treating keratitis must be made up by the hospital pharmacy, as they are more concentrated than commercially available preparations (Table 6-4). For initial empiric therapy, we recommend using two antibiotics, such as vancomycin or cefazolin, plus tobramycin or ciprofloxacin. Recently, monotherapy with ciprofloxacin (Ciloxan) drops has been used with a success rate (approximately 90%) equal to that of standard (typically combination) therapy [23]. The new topical quinolones have demonstrated safety and efficacy in adults [29]; safety in children younger than 12 years has not been established. However, we prefer initial combination therapy as ciprofloxacin-resistant bacterial keratitis cases have been reported [30]. Once cultures are positive, therapy can be tailored to the organism (Table 6-5).

Table 6-4. Concentration of fortified topical antibiotic solutions (eye drops) used to treat bacterial corneal ulcers (keratitis)

Antibiotic[a]	Concentration
Amikacin	20 mg/ml
Bacitracin	10,000 units/ml
Cefazolin	33, 50, or 133 mg/ml
Chloramphenicol[b]	5 mg/ml (0.5%)[c]
Clindamycin	20 mg/ml
Ciprofloxacin[b]	3 mg/ml (0.3%)
Gentamicin	14 mg/ml
Penicillin G	100,000 units/ml
Sulfacetamide[b]	10%, 15%, 30%
Sulfisoxazole[b]	4%
Ticarcillin	6 mg/ml
Tobramycin	14 mg/ml
Vancomycin	14 or 25 mg/ml

[a]Start with a loading dose of 1 drop/min for 5 minutes, then 1 drop q30min.
[b]Available commercially at this concentration. All others must be made up by the hospital pharmacist.
[c]Concentrations may be expressed either as milligrams per milliliter or as a percentage: 10 mg/ml = 1%.

Parenteral antibiotics (e.g., a cephalosporin or ticarcillin-clavulanate or piperacillin-tazobactam plus a quinolone or an aminoglycoside combination) may be needed for deep corneal ulcers with impending perforation or extension into the sclera.

V. Fungal keratitis

A. **Etiology.** Fungal keratitis is rare, comprising less than 2 percent of infectious keratitis cases [31]. Many different fungi, often soil saprophytes, have been described as causes of keratitis. *Aspergillus, Candida,* and *Fusarium* have been most commonly reported, with *Candida* predominating in northern climates and *Fusarium* in the southern United States [31]. Filamentous fungi (e.g., *Aspergillus*) are more likely etiologies after corneal trauma with vegetable matter, whereas yeasts are more likely causes in abnormal corneas (e.g., keratoconjunctivitis sicca), where they may be predominant colonizers. Topical steroid usage is a major predisposing factor for fungal keratitis and may account for this condition's increasing incidence. Other common risk factors are topical antibiotic usage, preexisting dendritic keratitis, and corneal trauma (especially from use of nylon-line lawn trimmers) [32].

B. **Clinical characteristics.** Fungal ulcers are indolent. Typically, there is a gray, plaquelike infiltrate with an irregular edge in the cornea. Smaller satellite lesions may surround the central lesion, and there often is superficial ulceration of the cornea as well as a hypopyon.

C. **Diagnosis.** It may be difficult to isolate the causative organism. A fungal stain (e.g., calcofluor) should be performed. If initial cultures are negative, repeat scrapings must be done, and a corneal biopsy may be necessary.

D. **Treatment. Topical antifungal therapy** should be coordinated with the ophthalmologist (Table 6-6). For *Aspergillus* and *Candida,* topical amphotericin is the drug of choice. For *Fusarium,* the topical antifungal drug natamycin (Pimaracin) has significantly improved outcome. Itraconazole, both oral and topical, may be useful for therapy of *Aspergillus* keratitis. Oral fluconazole achieves excellent corneal penetration, and both oral and topical therapy may be useful in treating *Candida albicans* keratitis.

If lesions progress on topical and systemic therapy, corneal transplantation (keratoplasty) may be considered early by the corneal specialist.

Table 6-5. Suggested therapeutic regimen for bacterial corneal ulcers

Etiology	Topical drops (q30min)	Systemic (IV)
Empiric therapy	Cefazolin or vancomycin *plus* ciprofloxacin or tobramycin	If spread into sclera
S. aureus S. pyogenes S. viridans S. pneumoniae	Cefazolin or vancomycin	
N. gonorrhoeae	Ceftriaxone (50 mg/ml)	Ceftriaxone
Pseudomonas	Ciprofloxacin or ticarcillin *plus* tobramycin	Ceftazidime or ticarcillin *plus* tobramycin (if no improvement after 24 hours of topical therapy)
Moraxella	Gentamicin	
Nocardia	Sulfacetamide	

Table 6-6. Topical treatment of fungal corneal ulcers

Organism	Drug	Topical concentration
Candida	Amphotericin Flucytosine	1.5 or 3 mg/ml (0.15 or 0.3%) 10 mg/ml
Aspergillus	Amphotericin	1.5 or 3 mg/ml
Fusarium	Natamycin	5%

VI. **Parasitic keratitis**
   A. **Etiology.** *Acanthamoeba* is the most common cause of parasitic keratitis in industrialized countries. Most (85%) cases are in contact lens wearers [33]: Patients who wear soft contact lenses or use homemade storage solutions (e.g., saline tablets and distilled water) are especially at risk. The keratitis is usually chronic: Typically, the patient has been treated over weeks to months with various antibiotic regimens for "culture-negative" keratitis before the diagnosis is considered. Hallmarks of *Acanthamoeba* keratitis include (1) a ring corneal infiltrate, (2) a lack of corneal neovascularization despite chronicity, and (3) pain out of proportion to clinical findings [10].
   B. **Diagnosis.** A slide with corneal scrapings should be stained with calcofluor white and viewed with a fluorescent microscope to see the *Acanthamoeba* cysts. The organisms will grow (usually within 48 hours) on nonnutrient agar that has an *Escherichia coli* "lawn," and the agar plate may be viewed under a light microscope to see both cysts and amebae. If these techniques fail, a corneal biopsy should be obtained and examined [34].
   C. **Treatment.** *Acanthamoeba* is resistant to most medications, and advanced infections may fail medical therapy. Surgical replacement of the cornea (keratoplasty) may be necessary, but the prognosis for graft survival in inflamed eyes is poor [35]. Some patients have been treated successfully with hourly triple therapy using topical Brolene drops (propamidine isethionate 0.1%), Neosporin drops (neomycin-polymixin-gramicidin), and miconazole 1% drops, as well as dibromopropamidine isethionate 0.15% ointment at bedtime [36]. Brolene is investigational in the United States but is available over the counter in Great Britain.
VII. **Interstitial (stromal) keratitis.** This is a nonulcerative corneal inflammation. Herpes simplex and syphilis are the most common infectious etiologies. About 90% of syphilitic keratitis cases are due to congenital syphilis. In cases due to acquired syphilis, HIV testing should be considered as the incidence of ocular syphilis may be higher in HIV-positive patients than in others with syphilis. Tuberculosis, leprosy, and Lyme disease [37] may also cause interstitial keratitis.

Endophthalmitis (Infection of the Vitreous)

Endophthalmitis, or infection involving the vitreous, **is the most urgent and severe of any primary ocular infection.** Despite appropriate treatment, approximately 30–60% of affected eyes are left with worse than 20/400 vision [38]. With virulent organisms, such as *S. aureus, S. pneumoniae,* or *Clostridia,* extension to the outer coats of the eye (**panophthalmitis**) and surrounding orbital tissues may occur.

I. **Anatomy.** The vitreous body is a clear gel, rather than a liquid, that supports the posterior portion of the eye and helps keep the neural part of the retina attached to the pigmented part (Fig. 6-4). It has a volume of approximately 6 ml.

II. **Etiology.** A recent compilation of published large series found that 62% of all endophthalmitis cases occur after intraocular surgery, 20% after penetrating trauma, and 10% after filtering blebs; the other 8% are endogenous [38].

   A. **Postoperative.** The most common predisposing factor is **recent intraocular surgery** [25a]. Postoperative endophthalmitis occurs in nearly 0.1% of cataract extraction and intraocular lens implantation procedures (the most frequently performed eye surgery). It may also occur after penetrating keratoplasty (replacement of the cornea) or placement of a filtering bleb for glaucoma therapy [39], as well as other types of intraocular surgery.

   B. **Exogenous/traumatic** [39a]. Other exogenous causes of endophthalmitis include **trauma** to the eye and **penetrating corneal ulcer.**

   C. **Bloodstream infections.** The eye may also be seeded by bacteria or fungi **via the bloodstream,** causing endogenous endophthalmitis.

III. **Postoperative endophthalmitis**

   A. **Clinical characteristics.** Patients complain of ocular "ache" or discomfort (often denying pain) and decreasing vision and may also have supraorbital headache and photophobia. Clinical signs include conjunctival injection and cells in the aqueous or vitreous (view of the retina often is obscured by a haze of cells). There may be a **hypopyon** or visible layer of pus in the aqueous humor. Almost all patients are afebrile; most have a normal WBC count.

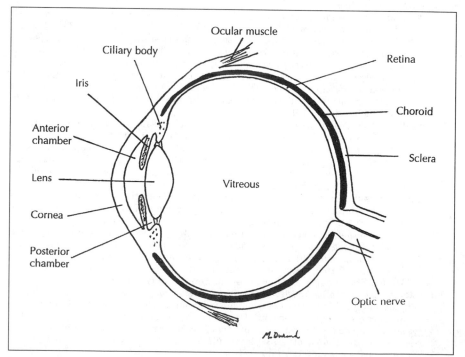

Fig. 6-4. The globe of the eye.

Most patients present 1–3 days after cataract surgery (77% within 1 week [25a, 40]), although "pseudophakic" (artificial lens) patients with *Propionibacterium acnes* endophthalmitis may have mild, chronic symptoms that persist for months to years, and their condition may be misdiagnosed as having "toxic lens syndrome" [41, 42]. Endophthalmitis after filtering bleb surgery typically presents with acute infection months to years postoperatively.

B. **Diagnosis. Patients with suspected endophthalmitis must be seen by an ophthalmologist** (preferably a retina specialist) **immediately.** At surgery, a vitreous aspirate or vitrectomy specimen will be sent for culture and Gram stain. Reading a vitreous Gram stain is similar to reading a CSF Gram stain: **Even a few neutrophils and one or two bacteria on the entire slide represent significant infection.** A word of caution: The vitreous or aqueous may contain **pigment granules** (a "dust" believed to come from the posterior surface of the iris in inflammation or trauma), and these may **closely resemble gram-positive cocci on Gram staining.** They appear more refractile than bacteria, however, and although they may be abundant on a slide, they usually are seen singly (rather than in pairs or chains).

C. **Bacteriology.** Coagulase-negative staphylococci (e.g., *S. epidermidis*) cause approximately 60% and *S. aureus* approximately 30% of cases after cataract extraction and lens implantation surgery [40]. Gram-negative bacilli may rarely be isolated. In contrast, streptococci (including pneumococci) and *H. influenzae* are the most common pathogens in late-onset endophthalmitis associated with filtering blebs [43].

D. **Treatment.** Although there is consensus that intravitreal antibiotics are essential, other aspects of therapy (e.g., the need for vitrectomy or for subconjunctival, topical, or intravenous antibiotics) are controversial. A recent multicenter trial attempted to answer some of these questions [44]. In addition, there is little information on the intraocular penetration of systemic antibiotics in the inflamed human eye. In general, antibiotics that cross the blood-brain barrier will also achieve good intraocular concentrations (although aminoglycosides and first-generation cephalosporins have been used with apparent success in treating endophthalmitis). The third-generation cephalosporins (see Chap. 28F) and quinolones (such as ofloxacin and ciprofloxacin [45]) achieve good intraocular penetration and are especially useful for treating gram-negative endophthalmitis. Vancomycin may be important in treating endophthalmitis due to coagulase-negative staphylococci, and a recent study in rabbits found that intravenous vancomycin achieved therapeutic vitreous levels in aphakic eyes [45a].

At present, **we recommend the following** for treating postoperative endophthalmitis:

1. **Emergency vitreous aspirate or vitrectomy** (surgical cutting or suctioning of the vitreous). A vitreous aspirate, rather than a vitrectomy, may be sufficient for patients with postoperative endophthalmitis who present with a visual acuity of hand-motion or better [44].

2. **Intravitreal antibiotics.** These should be injected into the anterior vitreous at the end of vitrectomy surgery. Table 6-7 lists the usual intravitreal antibiotic dosages (these must be made up by the pharmacist prior to surgery). For empiric therapy, we recommend intravitreal vancomycin (1 mg) and amikacin (400 μg). Some specialists recommend intravitreal ceftazidime in place of amikacin because of concern for the retinal toxicity of aminoglycosides [46]. Some retina surgeons also inject dexamethasone (400 μg) in addition to the intravitreal antibiotics.

3. **Intravenous antibiotics based on the Gram stain and culture results.** Empiric therapy with vancomycin and a third-generation cephalosporin (e.g., ceftazidime) will provide broad-spectrum coverage until culture results are available. Duration of therapy depends on the organism and the patient's clinical response: Typically, we give 5–7 days IV therapy for coagulase-negative staphylococcal infection, 10–14 days for *S. aureus*, streptococci, or gram-negative bacilli.

4. **Topical antibiotic drops** (e.g., vancomycin plus tobramycin) q2–4h for the initial few days, then taper (see Table 6-4 for concentrations).

5. In postcataract and lens implantation endophthalmitis, the implanted lens does **not** need to be removed. The one exception is in late-onset *P. acnes* endophthalmitis, where both the lens and the capsule may need to be removed.

IV. **Posttraumatic endophthalmitis**

A. **Clinical characteristics.** Symptoms and signs are the same as for postoperative endophthalmitis (see sec. **III.B**). Onset is usually in the first 3 days for virulent

Table 6-7. Intravitreal antibiotics (total volume 0.1 ml)

Antibiotic	Dose
Aminoglycosides	
Amikacin	0.2 or 0.4 mg
Gentamicin	0.1 or 0.2 mg
Tobramycin	0.1 or 0.2 mg
Cephalosporins	
Cefazolin	1.0 or 2.0 mg
Cefuroxime	1.0 mg
Ceftazidime	1.0 or 2.0 mg
Miscellaneous	
Chloramphenicol	2.0 mg
Clindamycin	1.0 mg
Vancomycin	1.0 mg
Antifungal	
Amphotericin B	0.005–0.01 mg (5–10 μg)

organisms (*Bacillus,* gram-negative bacilli) but may be weeks to months for fungi. *Bacillus cereus* typically produces a ring-shaped corneal infiltrate and causes a fulminant endophthalmitis with poor visual prognosis.

B. Diagnosis. See sec. **III.A.**

C. Bacteriology. *Bacillus* **species are uniquely important in posttraumatic endophthalmitis.** They were pathogens in 30% of cases in one series [47], 14.7% in a more recent series [39a], and were the second most commonly isolated organisms in several other series, after coagulase-negative staphylococci [48]. Gram-negative bacilli and fungi usually cause fewer than 20% of cases [49].

D. Treatment. See sec. **III.C.** Vancomycin should be one of the antibiotics used (both for intraocular injection and intravenously), because it will cover *Bacillus* species as well as *S. epidermidis. Bacillus* is also sensitive to clindamycin but usually resistant to penicillins and cephalosporins.

V. Endogenous endophthalmitis

A. Clinical characteristics. Patients with endogenous **bacterial** endophthalmitis complain of eye discomfort and decreased vision; 17% [50] have bilateral eye involvement. Although endophthalmitis may be the initial manifestation of bacteremia, there are often signs and symptoms related to the source of the bacteremia as well (e.g., endocarditis, urinary tract infection, gastrointestinal abscess, cellulitis, meningitis). However, systemic symptoms (fever, chills, weight loss, malaise) were present in only about half of the patients in one recent series [50]. Endocarditis was the most common source of infection (approximately 40% of cases) in this series. **Fungal** endophthalmitis, usually caused by *Candida,* may start as an asymptomatic chorioretinitis (see under Uveitis, sec. **IV**).

B. Diagnosis. Multiple **blood cultures** should be drawn. Unlike postoperative or posttraumatic endophthalmitis, blood cultures are frequently positive (in 72% of cases [50]).

C. Bacteriology. The single most common bacterial pathogen in a recent series [50] was *S. aureus,* causing one-fourth of cases, whereas streptococci (including pneumococci) and gram-negative bacilli each caused nearly one-third of cases. *Candida* is the most common cause of fungal endophthalmitis.

D. Treatment

   1. Bacterial. The type and duration of intravenous antibiotic therapy will be determined by the underlying infectious disease (e.g., endocarditis, meningitis). The need for additional therapy for the endophthalmitis is controversial, but we believe that early vitrectomy and intravitreal antibiotic injection (e.g., vancomycin and amikacin, as outlined previously) are indicated to preserve vision.

   2. Fungal. Systemic fungal infections will usually require intravenous amphotericin therapy. In addition, we recommend vitrectomy and intravitreal amphotericin (5–10 μg in 0.1 ml) in endophthalmitis due to filamentous fungi, such as *Aspergillus.*

In *Candida* endophthalmitis (but *not* for chorioretinitis alone), we also recommend vitrectomy and intravitreal amphotericin in addition to systemic amphotericin therapy. Systemic flucytosine may be added, as it achieves better intraocular levels than systemic amphotericin. The efficacy of fluconazole is being studied currently, and preliminary reports are encouraging [50a].

Infectious disease consultation is advised for this problem since the optimal approach is evolving.

Uveitis

I. **Anatomy.** The eye has three concentric coats (Fig. 6-4): (1) a fibrous, protective outermost coat composed of sclera (posterior five-sixths) and cornea (anterior one-sixth); (2) the highly vascular **uvea**, composed of iris, ciliary body, and choroid; and (3) the retina. The retina is in direct contact with the choroid, and inflammation of the choroid often involves the retina as well (chorioretinitis).

II. **Classification.** Uveitis classification is confusing because, although the retina is not part of the uveal tract, **retinitis** usually is considered a subset of posterior uveitis. **Posterior uveitis,** therefore, usually includes inflammation of the choroid (choroiditis) or retina (retinitis) or both (chorioretinitis). **Anterior uveitis** refers to inflammation of the iris (iritis) or iris and ciliary body (iridocyclitis). Most diseases predominantly cause either an anterior uveitis, which is usually acute and painful, or a posterior uveitis, which is usually subacute or chronic and painless. Intermediate uveitis, an inflammation of part of the choroid body called the *pars plana,* is almost never due to infection and will not be discussed here.

III. **Anterior uveitis (iritis, iridocyclitis)**
   A. **Clinical characteristics.** In acute cases, patients present with a **red eye, deep ocular pain** with a tender eyeball, **pupillary constriction, photophobia,** and **tearing.** On eye examination, there is a cellular reaction in the anterior chamber. This condition must be distinguished from conjunctivitis, which has minimal eye discomfort and no pupillary changes, and from acute glaucoma, which usually results in a cloudy cornea and a moderately dilated pupil.
   B. **Common viral etiologies**
      1. **Herpes simplex virus** type I is the virus most often associated with anterior uveitis and usually is accompanied by a dendritic keratitis. Treatment of herpetic keratouveitis includes oral acyclovir, 400 mg 5 times daily for 2 weeks with subsequent taper. The virus may cause recurrent anterior chamber inflammation without active corneal disease. See Chap. 26.
      2. **Herpes zoster virus** may cause an anterior chamber inflammation from iridocyclitis as part of **herpes zoster ophthalmicus,** and treatment is the same as for keratitis (see under Infectious Keratitis).
      3. **Cytomegalovirus** (CMV) may cause an iridocyclitis along with CMV retinitis (see Chap. 19).
   C. **Bacterial etiology.** Syphilis in the acquired form may cause an anterior uveitis and is seen more commonly now, especially in HIV-positive patients. It is usually bilateral and associated with secondary syphilis. **This diagnosis should be considered in any patient with uveitis and a positive rapid plasma reagin (RPR).** A lumbar puncture is indicated in such patients to rule out neurosyphilis. Treatment for ocular syphilis is 2 weeks of high-dose intravenous penicillin (20 million units/day) (see also Chap. 13).
   D. **Noninfectious etiologies,** either idiopathic or autoimmune, **account for more than 90% of cases of anterior uveitis.** Reiter's syndrome and ankylosing spondylitis are the major autoimmune causes [51].

IV. **Posterior uveitis (including retinitis)**
   A. **Clinical characteristics.** The onset is often gradual. Visual impairment is the predominant symptom and is the result of direct retinal damage and extension of inflammation to the vitreous. Pain and other signs of inflammation are absent. Retinal lesions and vitreal cloudiness are usually apparent on funduscopic examination.
   B. **Viral etiologies**
      1. **CMV** produces a retinitis in immunocompromised patients [52] and affects as many as 30% of patients with AIDS. It has been discussed in detail in Chap. 19.
      2. **Other herpesvirus infections.** HSV and VZV can cause a retinitis, but more typically they cause a keratouveitis (see sec. **III.B**). A member of the Herpes-

viridae family is believed to cause **acute retinal necrosis** (ARN). Only first described approximately 20 years ago, ARN often starts as an iritis and then causes a fairly rapid (days to weeks) destruction of the retina. The retinal destruction characteristically starts in the periphery. In one-third of patients, the other eye will become involved [49]. High-dose intravenous acyclovir (10 mg/kg q8h for 2–3 weeks) is the treatment of choice (see Chap. 26). HIV-positive patients who get ARN should be maintained on oral acyclovir for the rest of their lives. HIV-positive patients may also get a variant of ARN, "outer retinal necrosis," that has responded poorly to acyclovir therapy [53].

C. **Bacterial etiologies**

1. **Syphilis** was the leading cause of chorioretinitis in the early 1900s but is now uncommon. The most common ocular finding in congenital syphilis is a bilateral chorioretinitis, whereas a patchy neuroretinitis with retinal hemorrhage is most common in acquired syphilis (seen mainly in latent or tertiary stages). Treatment is as described for syphilitic anterior uveitis (see sec. **III.C**).

2. **Tuberculosis** was also a once-common cause of posterior uveitis that is now rare. It produces a granulomatous choroiditis, especially in the setting of miliary disease. Treatment is the same as for systemic diseases (see Chap. 9).

D. **Fungal etiologies**

1. *Candida* **caused a chorioretinitis in 28% of patients with candidemia in a recent prospective study** [54]. Risk factors for candidemia include an indwelling central venous access catheter and recent prolonged treatment with broad-spectrum antibiotics. Treatment of the candidemia (see Chap. 18) will also treat the chorioretinitis. However, because of the difficulty in achieving adequate vitreous amphotericin levels, flucytosine may be added for its greater penetration. The use of fluconazole is being investigated. Finally, if vitreous opacification (endophthalmitis) occurs, vitrectomy and intraocular instillation of amphotericin may be necessary (see under Endophthalmitis).

2. *Cryptococcus* may cause a chorioretinitis. This is almost always seen in patients who also have cryptococcal meningitis (see Chap. 18).

3. **Presumed ocular histoplasmosis syndrome** (POHS) is a syndrome of bilateral chorioretinal scars ("histo spots"), peripapillary atrophy, and maculopathy seen predominantly in patients who live in the Ohio and Mississippi River valleys of the United States. Although presumed to be due to *Histoplasma capsulatum,* there is no proof of this. No antifungal therapy is indicated.

4. *Histoplasma* may produce a chorioretinitis in AIDS patients. These patients have systemic infections and should be treated with IV amphotericin, 0.5–1.0 mg/kg/day, until a cumulative dose of 10–15 mg/kg is reached. This should be followed by chronic suppression for life (e.g., IV amphotericin, 50–80 mg once or twice weekly, or 400 mg/day of itraconazole or fluconazole). The role of itraconazole or fluconazole as primary therapy in treating these infections has not yet been determined.

E. **Parasitic etiologies**

1. *Toxoplasma gondii* was the leading cause of posterior uveitis and retinitis in one recent series [51]. It produces a retinochoroiditis, usually as a result of reactivation of latent infection. In immunosuppressed patients, especially patients with AIDS, the retinal lesions are multifocal and often bilateral, and there may be associated CNS lesions. The diagnosis is clinical (i.e., by the appearance of the retinal lesions). Serology is helpful only if negative, which essentially excludes the diagnosis. Treatment for vision-threatening lesions in adults includes sulfa drugs (e.g., sulfadiazine; see Chap. 28K), pyrimethamine (25–50 mg/day PO) with folinic acid "rescue" (5 mg PO 3 times/wk), and high-dose oral clindamycin (300–900 mg qid). Sulfadiazine probably is superior to trimethoprim-sulfamethoxazole, although the latter (one Bactrim DS tablet PO bid) has been used successfully in immunocompetent patients [55]. Note that patients should have frequent blood tests (especially CBC) while on pyrimethamine. See further discussion of this agent in Chap. 28U and further discussion of toxoplasmosis in Chaps. 17 (in normal hosts) and 19 (in HIV-infected patients).

   In patients with AIDS, maintenance therapy for ocular involvement with toxoplasmosis must be continued for life. Because side effects of medications are common in such patients, investigational uses of drugs such as atovaquone (formerly 566C80) [56] are being studied.

2. *Pneumocystis carinii* can cause yellow, plaquelike choroid lesions in HIV-positive patients. A search for *Pneumocystis* elsewhere in the body should be made. Treatment is the same as for systemic infection (see Chap. 24).

3. *Toxocara canis,* the dog roundworm, can cause posterior ocular inflammation, especially after death of a migrating larva. Most patients are younger than 8 years. What constitutes appropriate therapy is controversial. This infection has been mistaken for retinoblastoma.

F. **Noninfectious etiologies.** As with anterior uveitis, the majority of posterior uveitis cases are idiopathic or autoimmune. Sarcoidosis is the major autoimmune cause and produces a granulomatous choroiditis.

Orbital and Periorbital Infections

I. **Anatomy.** The orbit is surrounded by the paranasal sinuses (Fig. 6-5) and has bones in common with them (e.g., the medial wall of the orbit is the very thin lateral wall of the ethmoid sinus). The globe of the eye fills most of the anterior portion of the orbit, whereas loose fatty tissue and muscle fill most of the posterior part. The **orbital septum** is a fascial layer extending from the orbital rim periosteum to the tarsal plates in the eyelids, and it is a major barrier preventing superficial (**preseptal**) infection from extending posteriorly into the orbit. The orbital veins drain into the cavernous sinus. They have no valves so can freely communicate with the veins of the face and paranasal sinuses.

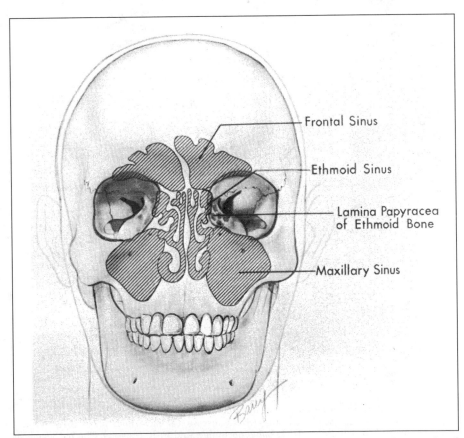

Frontal Sinus

Ethmoid Sinus

Lamina Papyracea of Ethmoid Bone

Maxillary Sinus

Fig. 6-5. The paranasal sinuses. (Modified from A. Lessner and G. A. Stern, Preseptal and orbital cellulitis. *Infect. Dis. Clin. North Am.* 6:933–952, 1992.)

II. Etiology. Most orbital infections (50–80%) are secondary to sinusitis, usually involving the ethmoid or frontal sinuses. Other orbital infections may follow trauma, surgery, dacryocystitis, or eyelid infections. Figure 6-6, adapted from the classic paper by Chandler, Langenbrunner, and Stevens [57] illustrates the five main categories of orbital infection described next. With the exception of cavernous sinus thrombosis, ocular findings are nearly always unilateral.

III. Preseptal ("periorbital") cellulitis

    A. Definition. Preseptal cellulitis is an infection that **involves the entire eyelid and surrounding tissues anterior to the orbital septum** but does not extend to the deeper contents of the orbit. Infection is secondary to sinusitis or upper respiratory infection in more than 50% of patients and to eye trauma in 25% [58]. Most patients are children younger than 10. *H. influenzae, S. aureus,* and streptococci are the most common pathogens.

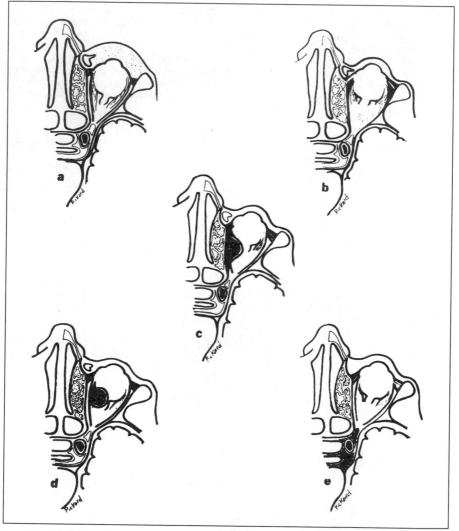

Fig. 6-6. The five main categories of orbital infection. (a) Preseptal cellulitis. (b) Orbital cellulitis. (c) Subperiosteal abscess. (d) Orbital abscess. (e) Cavernous sinus thrombosis. (Modified from J. R. Chandler, D. J. Langenbrunner, and F. R. Stevens, The pathogenesis of orbital complications in acute sinusitis. *Laryngoscope* 80:1414, 1970.)

B. **Clinical characteristics. Pain, swelling, and erythema of the eyelid** and low-grade fever are typical, although one-third of patients remain afebrile [58]. The distensibility of the periorbital tissues results in severe eyelid edema, making examination of the eye difficult. Often the conjunctiva is inflamed. There is no proptosis (anterior displacement of the eye), ophthalmoplegia (limitation of eye movement), pain with eye movement, or change in visual acuity.

   1. *H. influenzae* **preseptal cellulitis** primarily affects children younger than 5 years and results in a sharply demarcated purple discoloration of the involved area. It is commonly preceded by an upper respiratory infection. (See Chap. 4 under Cellulitis.)

   2. **Anaerobic cellulitis** is suggested by a history of trauma, especially a human or animal bite, and the presence of toxemia, foul-smelling discharge, necrotic tissue, and gas formation.

C. **Diagnosis.** Blood, conjunctival, and wound (if present) cultures should be obtained. If there is no obvious source, sinus disease should be excluded by x-rays or CT scan. An ophthalmology consultation should be obtained.

D. **Treatment.** In all but the mildest cases, intravenous antibiotics should be given initially.

   1. **Posttraumatic** (eyelid scratches, puncture wounds, etc.). Semisynthetic penicillin (e.g., nafcillin) or a first-generation cephalosporin (e.g., cefazolin).

   2. After **bite wounds or anaerobic infection.** Ampicillin-sulbactam is the preferred agent. See related discussion in Chap. 4 under Animal Bites.

   3. **Sinusitis-related** (or nontraumatic). Agents active against *S. aureus, S. pyogenes,* and *H. influenzae,* such as ampicillin-sulbactam or cefuroxime. See Chaps. 28E and 28F for detailed discussions of and dosages for these agents.

IV. **Orbital cellulitis**

A. **Definition.** Orbital cellulitis is **diffuse infection of the orbital contents.** Most infections follow sinusitis, but they may occur after trauma, preseptal cellulitis (and its etiologies) or, rarely, surgery.

B. **Clinical characteristics** [58, 58a]. In addition to the eyelid swelling, redness, warmth, and tenderness seen in preseptal cellulitis, there is **proptosis and pain with eye movement.** There is often orbital pain, conjunctival hyperemia, and chemosis (swelling of the conjunctiva). Most patients are febrile and have elevated WBC counts. As the infection progresses, there is limitation of ocular motility. **Orbital abscess or subperiosteal abscess should be considered if there is inferior and lateral displacement of the globe** (i.e., the eye looks downward and outward).

   The major pathogens are *S. aureus,* group A streptococci, *H. influenzae,* and *S. pneumoniae.* Anaerobic infections may follow bite wounds or chronic sinusitis. Common nosocomial pathogens (*S. aureus* and gram-negative rods) may be the etiology of postsurgical infections.

   1. **"Posterior" orbital cellulitis** is secondary to sphenoethmoiditis and produces an **orbital apex syndrome,** with marked visual loss and ophthalmoplegia but with minimal proptosis or signs of periorbital inflammation [59]. It is rare but should be considered in patients with sphenoid sinusitis who develop these findings. Pressure at the orbital apex may produce blindness from occlusion of the central retinal artery and vein.

   2. **Mucormycosis** (see Chap. 18) is a rapidly progressive, necrotizing fungal infection of the paranasal sinuses that may extend into the orbit, initially mimicking bacterial orbital cellulitis. It is an uncommon, frequently fatal disease of poorly controlled diabetics with ketoacidosis, but it may occur in overtly healthy patients with mild unsuspected diabetes as well as in any debilitated host. The fungus invades blood vessels, causing ischemic necrosis of tissues. It spreads rapidly (in days) from its sinus focus to involve the orbit and, frequently, the CNS. The **diagnosis** is made histologically by finding the characteristic nonseptate hyphae in a biopsy specimen of a necrotic area (**black eschar**) of the skin, nasal mucosa, or palate. Aggressive surgical debridement and intravenous amphotericin B therapy may be lifesaving.

   3. **Noninfectious diseases** that can mimic orbital cellulitis are rapidly enlarging orbital neoplasms such as rhabdomyosarcoma or malignant melanoma.

C. **Diagnosis.** Cultures of blood, conjunctiva, and wounds (if present) should be obtained. Needle aspiration of the orbital soft tissues is **not** indicated. A lumbar puncture should be performed if there is any clinical suspicion of meningitis. A cranial CT scan to look at the sinuses and orbit is helpful to determine whether sinusitis or an abscess is present. **An ophthalmologist should be consulted**, as well as an otolaryngologist if sinusitis is present.

D. **Treatment.** Delay in treatment or inadequate antibiotics may result in loss of vision or even death. Intravenous antibiotics should be started as soon as initial cultures are obtained. Antibiotics that penetrate the CSF should be chosen even in the absence of signs of meningitis.

   1. **Posttraumatic.** A semisynthetic penicillin (e.g., nafcillin)
   2. **Postsurgical.** Broad-spectrum coverage (e.g., nafcillin and cefotaxime)
   3. After **bite wounds or anaerobic infection.** Ampicillin-sulbactam is suggested. See related discussion in Chap. 4 under Animal Bites.
   4. **Sinusitis-related** (or nontraumatic). Nafcillin plus a third-generation cephalosporin (e.g., cefotaxime or ceftriaxone).

V. **Subperiosteal abscess**

   A. **Definition.** A subperiosteal abscess is a collection of pus between the periosteal lining and the bony wall of the orbit. If pus ruptures into the orbit itself, it is an orbital abscess (see sec. VI). A subperiosteal abscess **usually results from the extension of an infection within a sinus.**

   B. **Clinical characteristics.** As in orbital cellulitis, there is redness and swelling of the eyelids, proptosis, orbital pain, and usually a fever and an elevated WBC count. In addition, there is ophthalmoplegia and **displacement of the globe.** Because the ethmoid or frontal sinuses are most commonly involved, displacement tends to be downward and laterally ("down and out"). Staphylococci, streptococci, *H. influenzae*, and anaerobes are the most common pathogens.

   C. **Diagnosis.** Blood cultures should be obtained and a lumbar puncture performed if there are clinical signs of meningitis. **Emergency consultations with an ophthalmologist and an ear, nose, and throat (ENT) surgeon should be obtained as well as an emergency CT scan** (the relative merits of CT versus MRI in this setting have not been defined). Sinus cultures obtained endoscopically may be helpful if surgery is delayed. At the time of surgery, aerobic and anaerobic cultures should be obtained and the material should be Gram stained. In an immunocompromised (e.g., HIV-positive) patient, cultures and smears for fungi and mycobacteria should also be obtained.

   D. **Treatment.** As in orbital cellulitis, delay in treatment may result in loss of vision. In most patients, immediate surgical drainage of the subperiosteal abscess and involved sinus should be performed. Intravenous antibiotics should include a semisynthetic penicillin and a third-generation cephalosporin (e.g., nafcillin and cefotaxime or ceftriaxone) and should be started as soon as initial blood and sinus cultures have been taken.

VI. **Orbital abscess**

   A. **Definition.** An orbital abscess is a collection of pus within the orbit. It results either from a consolidation of infection in orbital cellulitis or from rupture of a subperiosteal abscess. Progression of infection in the patient with orbital cellulitis despite adequate intravenous antibiotics, or a decrease in either visual acuity or extraocular movement, suggests development of an intraorbital abscess.

   B. **Clinical characteristics.** The eyelids are red, warm, and swollen, and there is often marked chemosis. As in subperiosteal abscess, the **globe often is displaced downward and laterally. Eye mobility is severely limited,** and there is usually a marked decrease in vision. Fever and leukocytosis are common. *S. aureus* and streptococci are the most common pathogens. The distinction between orbital and subperiosteal abscess may be difficult to make clinically.

   C. **Diagnosis.** Blood cultures should be drawn and, if clinically indicated, a lumbar puncture performed. **An emergency CT scan and emergency consultations with an ophthalmologist and an ENT surgeon** should be obtained. At surgery, the abscess material should be sent for Gram staining and aerobic and anaerobic cultures. In immunocompromised patients, smears and cultures for acid-fast bacilli and fungus should also be done. Of note, an orbital abscess due to *Pneumocystis carinii* has been reported in a patient with AIDS who was on aerosolized pentamidine therapy [60].

   D. **Treatment.** Delay in treatment may result in loss of vision. After blood cultures have been taken, empiric intravenous therapy with a semisynthetic penicillin and a third-generation cephalosporin (e.g., nafcillin and cefotaxime) should be started. Antibiotics should be adjusted when culture results are available. In almost all patients, **immediate surgical drainage** of the abscess is indicated.

VII. Cavernous sinus thrombosis

A. Definition. Cavernous sinus thrombosis is a **rare but life-threatening complication of orbital infection** that can occur when a septic phlebitis of the veins draining the orbit leads to thrombosis of the cavernous sinus. Because the cavernous sinus drains **both** orbits, thrombosis leads to **bilateral eye findings** (proptosis, periorbital edema, ophthalmoplegia). Because of the proximity of the cavernous sinus to the meninges, meningeal signs and frank **meningitis can also occur.**

B. Clinical characteristics. The patient with cavernous sinus thrombosis usually is severely ill with headache, fever, and altered consciousness. There may be meningeal signs. There are usually bilateral findings of periorbital edema and erythema, proptosis, and ophthalmoplegia, although these findings may be much more prominent on one side than the other. Funduscopic examination may reveal venous engorgement and hemorrhages or papilledema.

The major pathogen is *S. aureus,* although streptococci (including *S. pneumoniae*) and, rarely, gram-negative bacilli may be involved.

C. Diagnosis. A lumbar puncture may be indicated to rule out meningitis. **High-resolution CT and high-field MRI** have supplanted invasive phlebography as the diagnostic imaging procedures of choice [61].

D. Treatment. Meningeal doses of CSF-penetrating antibiotics should be used (e.g., nafcillin and cefotaxime or ceftriaxone). The use of anticoagulants is controversial, although a literature review suggested that early anticoagulant therapy reduced morbidity but not mortality [62]. Steroids may be useful [63]. Infectious disease and ophthalmologic consultations should be obtained in these difficult cases.

References

1. Groden, L.R., et al. Lid flora in blepharitis. *Cornea* 10:50, 1991.
2. Boruchoff, S.A., and Boruchoff, S.E. Infections of the lacrimal system. *Infect. Dis. Clin. North Am.* 6:925, 1992.
2a. Gigliotti, F., et al. Etiology of acute conjunctivitis in children. *J. Pediatrics* 98:531, 1981.
   See also *F. Gigliotti, Management of the child with conjunctivitis.* Pediatr. Infect. Dis. 13:1161, 1994.
3. Jones, R.B. Chlamydial Diseases. In G.L. Mandell, J.E. Bennett, and R. Dolin (eds.), *Principles and Practice of Infectious Diseases* (4th ed.). New York: Churchill Livingstone, 1995. Pp. 1676.
4. Schwab, I.R., and Dawson, C.R. Conjunctiva. In D. Vaughan, T. Asbury, and P. Riordan-Eva (eds.), *General Ophthalmology* (13th ed.). Norwalk, CT: Appleton & Lange, 1992. P. 96.
   This textbook provides a concise summary of ophthalmology that is especially helpful for the nonophthalmologist.
5. Baum, J., and Barza, M. Infections of the Eye. In S.L. Gorbach, J.G. Bartlett, and N.R. Blacklow (eds.), *Infectious Diseases.* Philadelphia: Saunders, 1992. P. 1134.
6. Wan, W.L., et al. The clinical characteristics of the course of adult gonococcal conjunctivitis. *Am. J. Ophthalmol.* 102:575, 1986.
7. Centers for Disease Control. 1993 sexually transmitted diseases treatment guidelines. *M.M.W.R.* 42(RR-14):60, 1993.
8. McCloskey, R.V. Topical antimicrobial agents and antibiotics for the eye. *Med. Clin. North Am.* 72:717, 1988.
9. Ellis, P.P. Commonly Used Eye Medications. In D. Vaughan, T. Asbury, and P. Riordan-Eva (eds.), *General Ophthalmology* (13th ed.). Norwalk, CT: Appleton & Lange, 1992. P. 63.
10. Adamis, A.P., and Schein, O.D. *Chlamydia* and *Acanthamoeba* Infections of the Eye. In D.M. Albert and F.A. Jakobiec (eds.), *Principles and Practice of Ophthalmology.* Philadelphia: Saunders, 1994. P. 179.
   This recently published, five-volume text is an invaluable resource, with comprehensive discussions of each topic, many photographs, and extensive reference lists.
11. Rapoza, P.A., et al. Assessment of neonatal conjunctivitis with a direct immunofluorescent monoclonal antibody stain for *Chlamydia. J.A.M.A.* 255:3369, 1986.
12. Tabbara, K.F. Chlamydial Conjunctivitis. In K.F. Tabbara and R.A. Hyndiuk (eds.), *Infections of the Eye.* Boston: Little, Brown, 1986. P. 421.
13. Sandstrom, K.I., et al. Microbial causes of neonatal conjunctivitis. *J. Pediatr.* 105: 706, 1984.

14. Hammerschlag, M.R., et al. Efficacy of neonatal ocular prophylaxis for the prevention of chlamydial and gonococcal conjunctivitis. *N. Engl. J. Med.* 320:769, 1989.

14a. Isenberg, S.J., et al. A controlled trial of povidone-iodine as prophylaxis against ophthalmia neonatorum. *N. Engl. J. Med.* 332:562, 1995.
   Povidone-iodine deserves consideration as prophylaxis against ophthalmia neonatorum, especially in developing countries. It was also more effective in preventing chlamydial conjunctivitis, and povidone-iodine turns the surface of the eye brown, which indicates the medication has been properly administered. See editorial comment.

15. Laga, M., et al. Single dose therapy of gonococcal ophthalmia neonatorum with ceftriaxone. *N. Engl. J. Med.* 315:1382, 1986.

16. Flach, A.J. Ophthalmia Neonatorum. In K.F. Tabbara and R.A. Hyndiuk (eds.), *Infections of the Eye.* Boston: Little, Brown, 1986. P. 461.

17. Buckley, R.J. The Cornea. In S. Miller (ed.), *Clinical Ophthalmology.* Bristol, Engl.: Wright/IOP Publishing Ltd, 1987. P. 129.

18. Biswell, R. Cornea. In D. Vaughan, T. Asbury, and P. Riordan-Eva (eds.), *General Ophthalmology* (13th ed.). Norwalk, CT: Appleton & Lange, 1992. P. 125.

19. Medical Letter. Trifluridine (Viroptic) for herpetic keratitis. *Med. Lett. Drugs Ther.* 22:46, 1980.
   See also Drugs for non-HIV viral infections. Med. Lett. Drugs Ther. 36:27, 1994.

20. Schwab, I.R. Oral acyclovir in the management of herpes simplex ocular infections. *Ophthalmology* 95:423, 1988.

20a. Wilhelmus, K.R., et al. Herpetic eye disease study: A controlled trial of topical corticosteroids for herpes simplex stromal keratitis. *Ophthalmology* 101:1883, 1994.

21. Womack, L.W., and Liesegang, T.J. Complications of herpes zoster ophthalmicus. *Arch. Ophthalmol.* 101:42, 1983.

22. Cobo, L.M., et al. Oral acyclovir in the treatment of acute herpes zoster ophthalmicus. *Ophthalmology* 93:763, 1986.

23. Leibowitz, H.M. Clinical evaluation of ciprofloxacin 0.3% ophthalmic solution for the treatment of bacterial keratitis. *Am. J. Ophthalmol.* 112:34S, 1991.

24. Cohen, E.J., et al. Corneal ulcer associated with cosmetic extended-wear soft contact lenses. *Ophthalmology* 94:109, 1987.

25. Poggio, E.C., et al. The incidence of ulcerative keratitis among users of daily-wear and extended-wear soft contact lenses. *N. Engl. J. Med.* 321:779, 1989.

25a. Baker, A.S., and Schein, O.D. Ocular Infections. In A.L. Bisno and F.A. Waldvogel (eds.), *Infections Associated with Indwelling Medical Devices* (2nd ed.). Washington, D.C.: ASM Press, 1994. Pp. 111–134.
   Contains nice discussion of contact lens-associated infections and endophthalmitis associated with cataract surgery.

26. Schein, O.D., et al. The relative risk of ulcerative keratitis among users of daily-wear and extended-wear soft contact lenses: A case-control study. *N. Engl. J. Med.* 321:773, 1989.

27. Schein, O.D., et al. The impact of overnight wear on the risk of contact lens–associated ulcerative keratitis. *Arch. Ophthalmol.* 112:186, 1994.

28. Ficker, L., et al. Microbial keratitis—the false negative. *Eye* 5:549, 1991.

29. Borrmann, L.R., and Leopold, I.H. The potential use of quinolones in future ocular antimicrobial therapy. *Am. J. Ophthalmol.* 106:227, 1988.

30. Snyder, M.E., and Katz, H.R. Ciprofloxacin-resistant bacterial keratitis. *Am. J. Ophthalmol.* 114:336, 1992.

31. Foster, C.S. Fungal Keratitis. In D.M. Albert and F.A. Jakobiec (eds.), *Principles and Practice of Ophthalmology.* Philadelphia: Saunders, 1994. P. 171.

32. Clinch, T.E., et al. Fungal keratitis from nylon lawn trimmers. *Am. J. Ophthalmol.* 114:437, 1992.

33. Stehr-Green, J.K., Bailey, T.M., and Visvesvara, G.S. The epidemiology of *Acanthamoeba* keratitis in the United States. *Am. J. Ophthalmol.* 107:331, 1989.

34. Wilhelmus, K.R., et al. Rapid diagnosis of *Acanthamoeba* keratitis using calcofluor white. *Arch. Ophthalmol.* 104:1309, 1986.

35. Ficker, L.A., Kirkness, C., and Wright, P. Prognosis for keratoplasty in *Acanthamoeba* keratitis. *Ophthalmology* 100:105, 1993.

36. Berger, S.T., et al. Successful medical management of *Acanthamoeba* keratitis. *Am. J. Ophthalmol.* 110:395, 1990.

37. Baum, J., et al. Bilateral keratitis as a manifestation of Lyme disease. *Am. J. Ophthalmol.* 105:75, 1988.

38. D'Amico, D.J., and Noorily, S.W. Postoperative Endophthalmitis. In D.M. Albert and F.A. Jakobiec (eds.), *Principles and Practice of Ophthalmology.* Philadelphia: Saunders, 1994. P. 179.

39. Puliafito, C.A., et al. Infectious endophthalmitis: Review of 36 cases. *Ophthalmology* 89:921, 1982.

39a. Alfaro, D.V., et al. Posttraumatic endophthalmitis: Causative organisms, treatment, and prevention. *Retina* 14:206, 1994.
   Concludes that prompt diagnosis and early treatment with intraocular and systemic antibiotics are important. The most common isolates were Staphylococcus *spp. (26.5%),* Streptococcus *spp. (20.6%), and* Bacillus *spp. (14.7%).*

40. Weber, D.J., et al. Endophthalmitis following intraocular lens implantation. Report of 30 cases and review of the literature. *Rev. Infect. Dis.* 8:12, 1986.

41. Winward, K.E., et al. Postoperative *Propionibacterium* endophthalmitis. *Ophthalmology* 100:447, 1993.

42. Omerod, L.D., et al. Anaerobic bacterial endophthalmitis. *Ophthalmology* 94:799, 1987.

43. Mandelbaum, S., et al. Late onset endophthalmitis associated with filtering blebs. *Ophthalmology* 92:964, 1985.

44. Endophthalmitis Vitrectomy Study Group. Results of the Endophthalmitis Vitrectomy Study: A randomized trial of immediate vitrectomy and of intravenous antibiotics for the treatment of postoperative bacterial endophthalmitis. *Arch. Ophthalmol.* 113: 1479, 1995.
   This study randomized 420 patients who developed endophthalmitis within 6 weeks of cataract surgery into four groups: vitrectomy vs. vitreous tap only, and IV amikacin plus ceftazidime (or PO ciprofloxacin if penicillin-allergic) vs. no IV antibiotics. All patients received intravitreal and subconjunctival antibiotics. The study found that vitrectomy improved outcome only for patients who presented with very poor (light perception only) vision. The study authors also concluded that IV antibiotics did not affect outcome. However, we believe that no conclusion regarding the value of systemic antibiotics can be drawn from this study, as 68% of culture-positive study cases (17% of all study cases) were due to coagulase-negative staphylococci, organisms not likely to be susceptible to the study antibiotics.

45. Lesk, M.R., et al. The penetration of oral ciprofloxacin into the aqueous humor, vitreous, and subretinal fluid of humans. *Am. J. Ophthalmol.* 115:623, 1993.

45a. Meredith, T.A., et al. Vancomycin levels in the vitreous cavity after intravitreous administration. *Am. J. Ophthalmol.* 119:774, 1995.

46. Campochiaro, P.A., Lim, J.I., and the Aminoglycoside Toxicity Study Group. Aminoglycoside toxicity in the treatment of endophthalmitis. *Arch. Ophthalmol.* 112:48, 1994.
   See commentary in same issue by B.H. Doft and M. Barza. Ceftazidime or amikacin: Choice of intravitreal antimicrobials in the treatment of postoperative endophthalmitis. Arch. Ophthalmol. *112:17, 1994. Authors state that since the side effects of amikacin have not clearly been shown to be greater than those of ceftazidime, the investigators of the Endophthalmitis Vitrectomy Study continue to recommend amikacin with vancomycin as the standard choice for empiric treatment of postoperative endophthalmitis.*
   See also related papers in this same issue: T.M. Aaberg Jr. et al. Intraocular ceftazidime as an alternate to the aminoglycosides in the treatment of endophthalmitis. Arch. Ophthalmol. *112:18, 1994, which includes a discussion of the limited data on this topic; and S.P. Donahue et al. Empiric treatment of endophthalmitis: Are aminoglycosides necessary.* Arch. Ophthalmol. *112:45, 1994, which concludes that for empiric therapy vancomycin with an aminoglycoside or ceftazidime can be used.*

47. Affeldt, J.C., et al. Microbial endophthalmitis resulting from ocular trauma. *Ophthalmology* 94:407, 1987.

48. Davey, R.T., and Tauber, W.B. Posttraumatic endophthalmitis: The emerging role of *Bacillus cereus* infection. *Rev. Infect. Dis.* 9:110, 1987.

49. Hibberd, P.L., Schein, O.D., and Baker, A.S. Intraocular infections: Current therapeutic approach. *Curr. Clin. Top. Infect. Dis.* 11:118, 1991.
   Excellent discussion of uveitis and endophthalmitis, with extensive reference list.

50. Okada, A.A., et al. Endogenous bacterial endophthalmitis: Report of a ten year retrospective study. *Ophthalmology* 101:832, 1994.
   The best article on this topic in recent years.

50a. Akler, M.E., et al. Use of fluconazole in the treatment of candidal endophthalmitis. *Clin. Infect. Dis.* 20:657, 1995.
   Review of experience in Toronto and literature to date. Endophthalmitis was cured in 15 of 16 cases (94%), including 5 infections that were complicated by vitreitis. Successful treatment required the administration of fluconazole (100–200 mg PO) daily for about 2 months. Prospective evaluation is required to more clearly define the

role of this antifungal agent in the management of ocular infections due to Candida *spp.*
For a related report see J.K. Luttrull et al. Treatment of ocular fungal infections with oral fluconazole. Am. J. Ophthalmol. *119:477, 1995. Describes four patients with endogenous candida endophthalmitis who responded well to oral fluconazole.*

51. Rosenbaum, J.T. Uveitis: An internist's view. *Arch. Intern. Med.* 149:1173, 1989.

52. Bloom, J.N., and Palestine, A.G. The diagnosis of cytomegalovirus retinitis. *Ann. Intern. Med.* 109:963, 1988.

53. Dunn, J.P., and Holland, G.N. Human immunodeficiency virus and opportunistic ocular infections. *Infect. Dis. Clin. North Am.* 6:909, 1992.
The December 1992 issue of Infectious Disease Clinics of North America *is devoted to ocular infections and provides the internist or infectious disease specialist with a good overview of the subject.*

54. Brooks, R.G. Prospective study of *Candida* endophthalmitis in hospitalized patients with candidemia. *Arch. Intern. Med.* 149:2226, 1989.

55. Opremcak, E.M., Seales, D.K., and Sharpe, M.R. Trimethoprim-sulfamethoxazole therapy for ocular toxoplasmosis. *Ophthalmology* 99:920, 1992.

56. Lopez, J.S., et al. Orally administered 566C80 for treatment of ocular toxoplasmosis in a patient with the acquired immunodeficiency syndrome [letter]. *Am. J. Ophthalmol.* 113:331, 1992.

57. Chandler, J.R., Langenbrunner, D.J., and Stevens, F.R. The pathogenesis of orbital complications in acute sinusitis. *Laryngoscope* 80:1414, 1970.
The classic paper on this topic.

58. Jackson, K., and Baker, S.R. Periorbital cellulitis. *Head Neck Surg.* 9:227, 1987.

58a. Obrien, T.P., and Green, W.R. Periocular Infections. In G.L. Mandell, J.E. Bennett, and R. Dolin (eds.), *Principles and Practice of Infectious Diseases* (4th ed.). New York: Churchill Livingstone, 1995. P. 1129.
See also related clinical summary by K.R. Powell. Orbital and periorbital cellulitis. Pediatr. Rev. *16:163, 1995.*

59. Slavin, M.L., and Glaser, J.S. Acute severe irreversible visual loss with sphenoethmoiditis—"posterior" orbital cellulitis. *Arch. Ophthalmol.* 105:345, 1987.

60. Friedberg, D.N., et al. *Pneumocystis carinii* of the orbit [letter]. *Am. J. Ophthalmol.* 113:595, 1992.

61. Ellie, E., et al. CT and high-field MRI in septic thrombosis of the cavernous sinuses. *Neuroradiology* 34:22, 1992.

62. Levine, S.R., Twyman, R.E., and Gilman, S. The role of anticoagulation in cavernous sinus thrombosis. *Neurology* 38:517, 1988.

63. Southwick, F., Richardson, E.P., and Swartz, M.N. Septic thrombosis of the dural venous sinuses. *Medicine* (Baltimore) 65:82, 1986.

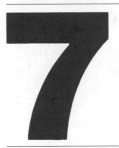

Infections of the Upper Respiratory Tract

Paula W. Annunziato
and Keith R. Powell

Upper respiratory tract infections (URIs) are the most common human affliction throughout life. Most people are familiar with the clinical characteristics of upper respiratory tract illnesses, such as the common cold and pharyngitis; some experience such infections 2 or more times yearly. These maladies result in a major share of the time lost from work and school and are the most common cause of antibiotic abuse.

Common Upper Respiratory Syndromes

I. **General tenets of viral respiratory tract infections.** Despite their variety and abundance, viral respiratory agents and syndromes appear to have certain common characteristics.
   A. Each respiratory tract syndrome is caused by more than one agent and usually by many. Each syndrome, however, has but a few major contributors, which depend partly on geography, season, and the age of the host.
   B. Each virus also is able to cause more than one syndrome, but each has a predilection to produce a particular type of illness. The personality of each viral respiratory pathogen may be described by (1) its preference of clinical expression, (2) its propensity for a certain age group or population, and (3) often its partiality for a certain season.

II. **Etiologic agents.** More than 200 distinct viruses produce acute respiratory illness (Tables 7-1, 7-2). They are members of six major families: Orthomyxoviridae, Paramyxoviridae, Picornaviridae, Coronaviridae, Adenoviridae, and Herpetoviridae.

   The epidemiologic pattern of a few of these viruses bestow on them particular distinction and importance. The influenza viruses, parainfluenza viruses, and respiratory syncytial virus (RSV) are epidemic in their occurrence. Outbreaks of influenza and RSV usually occur in the winter to early spring, whereas those from parainfluenza virus type 1 occur biennially in the fall.

III. **Acute viral rhinitis (common cold)**
   A. **Etiology.** The common cold is invariably a viral infection. The variety of associated viruses listed in Tables 7-1 and 7-2 probably account for at least 70% of common colds. Rhinoviruses account for the major proportion of colds, especially in adults. In young children, RSV, the parainfluenza viruses, and some of the adenoviruses and coronaviruses contribute an appreciable proportion.
   B. **Epidemiology.** Common colds occur worldwide. The incidence of colds in temperate climates is greater in winter than in summer months, but there is no evidence that exposure to a cold environment lowers host resistance or influences the course of common colds.
      1. **Frequency.** In the United States, illnesses restricting daily activity or requiring medical attention occur at an average rate of 1.4 per person per year, and milder illnesses occur more often. The frequency is age-related, with schoolchildren having the greatest number, usually between three and eight per year.
      2. **Transmission** is from person to person, requires close contact, and **probably involves transfer of virus from the hands of an infected person to an intermediate surface or directly to the hands of a susceptible person.** Psychosocial stressors, in addition to prior exposure, may influence host susceptibility [1]. Infection then results from self-inoculation of eyes or nose with virus on the fingers. **Good hand-washing, therefore, can help decrease the spread of these viral infections.** Under different experimental conditions, the aerosol transmission of rhinovirus has also been demonstrated [2].

Table 7-1. Viruses associated with respiratory syndromes in adults

Virus	Common cold	Pharyngitis		Tracheobronchitis	Pneumonia	
		Civilian	Military		Civilian	Military
Rhinovirus, 89 types	4+	2+	+	+	+	+
Influenza virus type A	+	2+	+	3+	2+	2+
Influenza virus type B	+	2+	+	2+	+	+
Coronavirus	+	+	+	+	+	+
Adenovirus types 4 and 7	+	+	4+	+	+	4+
Adenovirus types 1, 2, 3, and 5	+	+	+	+	+	+
Herpes simplex virus	–	2+	+	+	–	–
Epstein-Barr virus	–	+	+	–	+	+
Respiratory syncytial virus	+	+	+	+	–	–
Parainfluenza virus types 1, 2, and 3	+	2+	+	+	–	–
Group A coxsackievirus	+	+	+	+	+	+
Group B coxsackievirus	+	+	+	+	+	+
Echovirus	+	+	+	+	+	+
Poliovirus	+	+	+	+	–	–

Symbols for relative frequency: + = occasional case; 2+ = small proportion of cases; 3+ = substantial proportion of cases; 4+ = majority of cases; – = does not cause syndrome in immunocompetent host.

Source: From R. G. Douglas, Jr., Respiratory Diseases. In G. J. Galasso, T. C. Merigan, and R. A. Buchanan (eds.), *Antiviral Agents and Viral Diseases of Man* (2nd ed.). New York: Raven, 1984.

Table 7-2. Viruses associated with respiratory syndromes in children

	Relative importance for indicated syndrome					
	Common cold	Pharyngitis	Tracheobronchitis	Laryngotracheobronchitis (croup)	Pneumonia	Bronchiolitis
Respiratory syncytial virus	3+	2+	3+	2+	4+	4+
Parainfluenza virus type 3	3+	2+	3+	2+	3+	2+
Parainfluenza virus type 2	3+	2+	−	+	+	+
Parainfluenza virus type 1	3+	2+	2+	4+	2+	+
Influenza virus type A	+	2+	2+	2+	2+	+
Adenovirus types 1, 2, 3, and 5	2+	2+	+	+	+	+
Influenza virus type B	+	2+	2+	+	+	+
Rhinovirus, 89 types	2+	2+	+	+	+	+
Coronavirus	2+	+	+	+	−	−
Group A coxsackievirus	+	2+	+	+	+	−
Group B coxsackievirus	+	+	+	+	+	−
Echovirus	+	2+	+	+	+	−
Poliovirus	+	+	−	−	−	−

Symbols for relative frequency: + = occasional case; 2+ = small proportion of cases; 3+ = substantial proportion of cases; 4+ = majority of cases; − = does not cause syndrome in immunocompetent host.
Source: From R. G. Douglas, Jr., Respiratory Diseases. In G. J. Galasso, T. C. Merigan, and R. A. Buchanan (eds.), *Antiviral Agents and Viral Diseases of Man* (2nd ed.). New York: Raven, 1984.

C. **Clinical manifestations.** Acute rhinitis is a self-limited, **usually afebrile** illness. The incubation period is 2–5 days.

1. **The syndrome** is characterized by nasal discharge, obstruction, sneezing, pharyngeal discomfort, cough, malaise, and mild headache. A low-grade fever lasting fewer than 24 hours occurs in approximately 10% of adults but more frequently in children. Chills, marked sore throat, or prominent cervical adenopathy are not a part of this syndrome.

2. **Duration.** The median duration of illness is **7 days,** with peak symptomatology occurring on the second and third days. After the second or third day of illness, secretions from the nasopharynx decrease in volume, become viscous, and frequently appear purulent. A dry, nonproductive cough of a mild nature commonly begins at this time. Children in daycare may experience symptoms of uncomplicated URI for more than 10 days [3], but when symptoms remain prominent for more than 10–14 days, one must consider other diagnoses, such as *Mycoplasma* infections, secondary bacterial infections, or the complications discussed in the next section.

D. **Complications.** Upper respiratory tract infections with the common pathogens (influenza viruses, RSV, parainfluenza viruses, adenoviruses, and rhinovirus) result in morphologic ciliary abnormalities, which could cause compromised mucociliary clearance [4]. These dysmorphic findings may last for 2–10 weeks.

   In children, **acute otitis media** or **sinusitis** (or sometimes both) may follow a cold, usually on the fourth to seventh day of illness. In adults, otitis media is less common, but sinusitis occurs and, in mild cases, is manifested only by persistent nasal discharge. Occasionally, frank purulent sinusitis may occur, with chills, fever, erythema over malar eminences, and leukocytosis. (See further discussions under Otitis Media and Acute Sinusitis later in this chapter.)

E. **Laboratory findings.** No laboratory test is diagnostic or even helpful in the common cold. With some viral agents, the WBC count may initially be slightly elevated; however, counts rarely exceed 13,000 and are not accompanied by a left shift.

F. **Diagnosis.** The classic syndrome is easily recognized by both physicians and laypersons. Because of the multiple viral etiologies, the expense involved, and the absence of specific therapy, viral cultures are not warranted.

   The **differential diagnosis** includes prodromes of other infections, such as pertussis (the catarrhal stage), measles, streptococcosis, congenital syphilis, and diphtheria. Allergic rhinitis, structural abnormalities, foreign body, and vascular and neoplastic processes are more likely if symptoms are prolonged. Hay fever may closely mimic the common cold. However, the season of the year, allergic history, occurrence of tearing, itching of the eyes, lack of sore throat, progression from serous to purulent nasal discharge, and presence of eosinophils on a nasal smear stained with Wright's or Giemsa stain (in allergic rhinitis) may serve to distinguish allergic from viral rhinitis.

G. **Treatment.** The combination of intranasal interferon-alpha 2b (3 million units q8h), intranasal ipratropium (8 µg q8h), and oral naproxen (500 mg in one dose followed by 250 mg q8h) reduced the duration of viral shedding and symptoms by approximately 1 day in adults challenged with rhinovirus [5]. Given the expense of interferon therapy and the limited clinical effect, **specific antiviral therapy is not warranted.**

1. **Symptomatic therapy.** Symptomatic therapy should be designed to alleviate major symptoms. Most over-the-counter common cold remedies contain combinations of drugs of dubious value and should be avoided.

   a. **Analgesics.** For adults, aspirin, 0.6 g q4h, and for children, acetaminophen, 5–10 mg/kg q4–6h, are effective in reducing headache and myalgias.

   b. **Cold-water vaporization or normal saline drops** may help relieve nasal obstruction.

   c. **Nasal sprays or drugs** may help relieve nasal congestion, but they should be used for **short periods** (3–5 days) to avoid the rebound nasal obstruction seen with long-term usage.

   d. **Antihistamines** may help decrease nasal discharge but do not alter the course of the illness and are associated with frequent side effects, such as dryness and drowsiness. The use of oral decongestants and antihistamimes has been advocated for treating children, in an attempt to prevent otitis media. Such therapy has not been beneficial and may be harmful.

     e. **Cough suppressants** commonly are used (e.g., dextromethorphan, 15 mg/ 5 ml, 5–10 ml PO q2–3h in adults).

  2. **Antibiotics.** Antibiotics are not antiviral and therefore **should be reserved for documented or strongly suspected bacterial superinfections.** There is a risk that should bacterial superinfection occur when antibiotics are used during an acute viral episode, the superinfection may be associated with a resistant organism. Antibiotics are used in the early treatment of purulent complications of viral infections such as otitis media and sinusitis. Tracheobronchitis and pneumonia accompanying colds usually are viral or mycoplasmal in etiology in children. **Signs and symptoms of viral infection usually resolve in 10–14 days. Purulent nasal discharge occurring after that time may indicate bacterial sinusitis.**

 H. Prevention. Vaccines are not available. Isolation of patients is impractical, although care in disposing of tissues containing secretions and careful hand-washing may decrease the likelihood of virus transmission. **Vitamin C** in large doses (1–2 g/day) has been recommended by some to decrease the frequency or severity of colds, but data to support this contention are not conclusive, and the side effects of chronic long-term administration of such doses are unknown. **Recurrent colds have not been associated with any known immunologic deficiency** or disorder, and such illnesses are not more severe in immunosuppressed patients.

IV. Acute pharyngitis and tonsillitis

 A. Etiology. In contrast to the common cold, *Mycoplasma pneumoniae,* beta-hemolytic streptococci, *Neisseria gonorrhoeae, Chlamydia pneumoniae,* and *Arcanobacterium* (formerly *Corynebacterium*) *haemolyticum* contribute to the etiology of pharyngitis (see Tables 7-1 and 7-2). No single virus or group of viruses is responsible for a major segment of the illnesses, as is the case for common colds.

     Group A beta-hemolytic streptococci are the major cause of pharyngitis and tonsillitis, particularly **exudative** tonsillitis [6]. The frequency of streptococcal pharyngitis is closely related to age. **In children younger than 3 years, pharyngitis is almost always caused by viruses.** By contrast, in a large study of school-aged children (4–18 years), group A streptococci were isolated from 41% of patients and viruses from 16%. *M. pneumoniae* was isolated from 16% of the patients but was found also in 18% of the controls [7]. In private pediatric practices, group A streptococcal respiratory illness has been shown to be responsible for 11% of all office visits, for 24% of all acute infections, and for approximately 40–50% of pharyngitis in children from 6 to 15 years of age. The attack rate in children, according to several longitudinal studies, is 0.20–0.35 per person per year [6]. In university students, 15–26% of pharyngitis cases have been noted to be streptococcal. **Nevertheless, at any age, the majority of cases of pharyngitis, particularly if the milder nonexudative ones are included, are nonbacterial (usually > 70%) and largely viral.**

     In a study from Finland of the etiology of pharyngitis in adults (15–65 years old), 25% of cases were due to viruses (RSV, influenza A and B, adenovirus, Epstein-Barr virus [EBV], and herpes simplex virus [HSV]), 23% were due to beta-hemolytic streptococci (but only 5% of all cases were group A), 9% were due to *M. pneumoniae*, and 8% were presumably due to *Chlamydia pneumoniae* (TWAR strain), whereas in 31% the agent was not identifiable [8]. Huovinen and colleagues [8] question the importance of group C streptococci as a pathogen but suggest that group G streptococci can cause pharyngitis in some patients (see sec. **D.4**).

 B. Epidemiology

  1. **Group A beta-hemolytic streptococcal (GABHS) pharyngitis.** In temperate climates, streptococcal respiratory illness is much more frequent in the cooler months. The incidence begins to **rise in September, with the peak occurring in late winter to early spring** (usually in March), and with the nadir reached in the summer [6]. This is in contrast to the pattern of group A streptococcal impetigo, which peaks in the summer.

     Transmission of group A streptococci requires close contact with an infected person by direct inoculation of large droplets or by physical transfer of infectious respiratory secretions. Contagion is greatest during the acute phase of illness, and carriers are much less likely to transmit infection. Streptococci in the nose are more apt to be transmitted than those in the throat, but persistent nasal carriage is unusual in contrast to throat carriage. Group A streptococcal respiratory illness has also been spread by anal carriers, by impetigo, and by contaminated food. Spread within families is common, with approximately 20% of family members of infected persons also becoming infected.

2. **Nonbacterial pharyngitis.** The epidemiology of viral pharyngitis depends on both the agent and the age of the patient (see Tables 7-1 and 7-2). Parainfluenza, influenza, and respiratory syncytial viruses cause respiratory illness with pharyngitis in outbreaks in the fall and winter. Influenza affects all ages, whereas parainfluenza and RSV primarily affect children. Most of the other major viral agents are not epidemic. **EBV and HSV, which may mimic group A streptococcal pharyngitis, are major causes of exudative pharyngitis in college-aged students** throughout the year. Adenoviruses, the major viral agents isolated in exudative pharyngitis in younger children, are endemic. In military populations, adenovirus type 4 and, to a lesser extent, types 3, 7, and 21, cause the major share of pharyngitis.

3. *M. pneumoniae* can also cause pharyngitis, particularly in teenagers and young adults, throughout most of the year.

4. *Chlamydia pneumoniae* also causes pharyngitis in adolescents and adults, often infecting the lower respiratory tract as well. It appears to be uncommon in children younger than 5 years [9].

C. **Clinical manifestations.** For the majority of cases of pharyngitis, especially those that are mild or nonbacterial, the clinical findings are not distinctive or indicative of the etiology. In a study in adults, clinical manifestations (e.g., exudates, adenopathy, or fever) did not correlate with microbiologic findings [8].

1. **Nonbacterial pharyngitis.** The throat may be infected or normal in appearance, and the degree of erythema may not correlate with the degree of soreness. The presence of rhinitis, conjunctival injection, cough, and an enanthema of ulcers, vesicles, and macular papules on the soft palate or pharynx all suggest a virus, particularly an enterovirus, whereas ulcers anteriorly suggest HSV. Fever may be present with any of these agents and is more common and often higher in children than in adults.

2. **Exudative pharyngitis.** Exudative pharyngitis can be bacterial or nonbacterial in origin. The clinical signs according to the agent are shown in Table 7-3. In general, the exudate of viral agents tends to be whiter than that from group A streptococci, and the petechiae associated with infectious mononucleosis tend to be confined to the soft palate.

Table 7-3. Signs in exudative pharyngitis compared according to agent

Agent	Appearance			
	Redness	Exudative	Follicular	Petechial
Bacterial				
Streptococci	4+	3+	2+	3+
Diphtheria	3+	4+		
Meningococci	2+	+		
Gonococci	2+	2+		
Arcanobacteria	2+	2+		
Viral				
Adenoviruses	4+	2–3+	4+	
Influenza	3+			
Enteroviruses	3+	1–2+	±	
Epstein-Barr virus	3+	4+	+	2+
Herpes simplex virus	2+	2+		
Measles	3+			+
Rubella	+			2+
Mycoplasma				
M. pneumoniae	2+	+	+	
M. hominis	+	±		
Fungal				
Candida	+	4+		

Symbols for relative frequency: + = occasional case; 2+ = small proportion of cases; 3+ = substantial proportion of cases; 4+ = majority of cases; ± = etiology may or may not be associated with appearance.

3. **Group A streptococcal pharyngitis.** In a recent review of this topic, the **classic clinical features** of acute streptococcal pharyngitis **are:** onset in winter or spring; school-age child (5–15 years old); abrupt onset of fever, sore throat, headache, abdominal pain; pharyngeal/tonsillar inflammation, often with exudates; tender anterior cervical lymph nodes; scarlatiniform rash; and absence of symptoms of viral illness (rhinorrhea, cough, hoarseness, and diarrhea). However, since most patients with acute streptococcal pharyngitis lack some of these classic manifestations, a diagnostic test is also necessary (i.e., a throat culture or rapid antigen test) to separate out acute nonstreptococcal pharyngitis [9a].

   Group A streptococcal pharyngitis usually has an abrupt onset and is associated with fever, dysphagia, and a thick or muffled, but not hoarse, voice. Exudate is frequently, but not always, present and appears yellowish. The pharynx tends to be bright or beefy red and may have petechiae. **"Doughnut lesions" (red, raised, or hemorrhagic lesions with a yellow center) are highly diagnostic of streptococcal pharyngitis** but occur in only approximately 10% of cases. Aside from these lesions, the most useful physical findings for diagnosing streptococcal pharyngitis are an edematous beefy red uvula, tender anterior cervical nodes, and an exudate that appears serosanguineous or yellowish on throat swabs [6].

4. **Scarlet fever** [10] is similar in all respects to typical pharyngitis and tonsillitis due to beta-hemolytic streptococci except that in patients with scarlet fever, the tongue is red with large papillae **(raspberry tongue) or** is coated with protruding red papillae **(strawberry tongue)**. In addition, there is a **fine, sand-papery** scarlet **erythema** (often called a *boiled lobster* appearance) that is generalized, with accentuation in the skin folds **(Pastia's lines)**. The face is also involved, but circumoral pallor is present. The palms and soles are spared. The rash is characteristically followed by a fine desquamation, which often starts and is most prominent on the hands. In patients with similar symptoms in whom streptococci are not isolated, the mucocutaneous lymph node syndrome (Kawasaki disease) must be considered [11].

5. *Arcanobacterium haemolyticum* (formerly called *Corynebacterium haemolyticum*), a less common cause of exudative pharyngitis in teenagers and young adults, may also be associated with a scarlatiniform rash on the extremities and trunk but is not associated with a strawberry tongue or palatal petechiae [12–14]. This organism is not detected on media for routine throat culture and yet may respond to appropriate antimicrobial therapy (erythromycin) once it is accurately identified [12].

6. **Other diagnostic considerations.** When a patient presents with a sore throat, other specific diagnoses should be considered.

   a. **Peritonsillar abscess.** Patients may present with sore throat, drooling, hoarseness, **trismus,** and asymmetric tonsillar enlargement. Leukocytosis is common. These patients need evaluation by an otolaryngologist, intravenous antibiotics (e.g., penicillin), and, often, surgical drainage.

   b. **Epiglottitis.** Children typically have high fever, toxic appearance, drooling, and absence of spontaneous cough [12]. Adults may present with a severe sore throat, dysphagia, and fever (see Chap. 8).

   c. **Infectious mononucleosis.** This disease should be considered especially in young adults. (See Chap. 17 for further discussion.)

   d. **Parapharyngeal space** infections. Such infections, with neck swelling after a sore throat, are uncommon. CT scanning of the neck is useful [13]. **See the discussion of Infections of Deep Spaces of the Neck in Chap. 4.**

7. **Nonsuppurative complications** of group A beta-hemolytic streptococcal infections have appeared to be diminishing in the United States during the past two decades. The risk of acute rheumatic fever following an untreated streptococcal pharyngitis has been estimated to be 3% in epidemic situations and approximately 0.3% in endemic situations. A resurgence of rheumatic fever is of concern, with outbreaks reported in a number of states during the 1980s [15]. Rheumatic fever appears to follow streptococcal pharyngitis only and not pyoderma and occurs an average of 19 days after the onset of the pharyngitis. Acute glomerulonephritis may follow pharyngitis or pyoderma, and the risk depends on whether the infecting strain is nephritogenic; if so, the risk appears to be 10–15%. The streptococcal M serotype associated with most cases of acute

glomerulonephritis occurring after pharyngitis is type 12, but types 1, 3, 4, and 25 are also nephritogenic and are associated with pharyngitis.

D. Diagnosis and laboratory findings

1. **Isolation of the agent is generally the only means of specific diagnosis.** Other laboratory tests, such as the WBC count, may be helpful in differentiating streptococcal from nonbacterial infections. An elevated WBC count ($> 15,000$), particularly if associated with a left shift, supports the diagnosis of streptococcal pharyngitis. In viral pharyngitis, the WBC count initially may be slightly elevated without a left shift, followed by a decrease to fewer than 5,000 cells after 4–7 days of illness in approximately 50% of cases. An atypical lymphocytosis frequently is associated with a viral agent and may be especially helpful in the initial diagnosis of EBV infection (see Chap. 17) for diagnosis of EBV and infectious mononucleosis).

2. Specific viral diagnosis usually requires viral isolation from respiratory secretions. For most cases of pharyngitis, this is not warranted. In one study, the rapid viral antigen detection tests were not sensitive enough to be useful [8].

3. **Group A beta-hemolytic streptococcal infections.** A throat swab for culture has generally been the most reliable and practical means of diagnosing streptococcal pharyngitis [9a]. The accuracy of a single, well-taken throat culture compared with serial cultures is approximately 95%, although it may be lower in the office setting. Culture on trimethoprim-sulfamethoxazole blood agar incubated anaerobically is more sensitive than aerobic culture on blood agar for detecting group A streptococci [16]. The streptococci on the agar plate may be identified as being group A by their susceptibility to bacitracin; however, approximately 5% of beta-hemolytic non–group A streptococci may also be susceptible to the bacitracin disc. New rapid tests can detect group A streptococci on throat swabs within hours in the office setting. However, **when a rapid test is negative, a throat culture should be obtained** because false negative results occur.

   Clinical evaluations of rapid antigen detection tests, while showing high specificity, have demonstrated variable sensitivity—in some studies, as low as 30–70%—with no test clearly showing superior performance [16]. It remains unproved at present whether the recently introduced optical immunoassay method is associated with improved performance characteristics, particularly sensitivity, when compared to the enzyme immunoassay–based tests [9a]. Because of the poor sensitivity of the rapid antigen detection tests, the American Academy of Pediatrics and the Committee on Rheumatic Fever, Endocarditis, and Kawasaki Disease of the American Heart Association recommend culture confirmation for a negative antigen detection test result for a child suspected of having group A streptococcal pharyngitis. Thus, **the throat culture serves as the standard by which other diagnostic tests have been measured** [16]. Another concern with the rapid antigen tests is that surveys have demonstrated that routine quality control activities to ensure the reliability of these tests are frequently not carried out in physicians' offices [9a].

   If a diagnostic test (e.g., culture, rapid antigen test) is done on a patient with signs and symptoms of viral illness (e.g., rhinorrhea, hoarseness, cough, and/or diarrhea), any identified group A streptococci are much more likely to represent a chronic carrier of streptococci A rather than a true case of acute streptococcal pharyngitis [9a, 16a]. **Throat cultures and/or rapid antigen detection tests should be limited to those patients who are likely to have a bacterial streptococcal pharyngitis (see sec. C.3) rather than a viral illness [9a, 16a].**

   Antibody studies (ASO, streptozyme) generally are helpful only in the retrospective diagnosis of streptococcal pharyngitis (e.g., in a case of possible poststreptococcal glomerulonephritis or rheumatic fever).

4. **Throat swabs for other bacteria.** Throat swabs for *N. gonorrhoeae* should be obtained if the setting is consistent with a diagnosis of gonococcal pharyngitis (see Chap. 13). If *A. haemolyticum* is suspected, the diagnostic laboratory should be informed as this agent generally is not recognized on routine cultures of throat-swab specimens.

   Pneumococci, *Haemophilus* spp. and, occasionally, staphylococci are isolated from such throat-swab specimens. Gram-negative rods may be isolated in pure culture of throat-swab specimens from hospitalized patients with sore throats.

However, there are no convincing data that these organisms are involved in the pathogenesis of pharyngitis; treatment, therefore, is not warranted. Non–group A streptococci, such as group C, may rarely be associated with pharyngitis but are not rheumatogenic or nephritogenic.

E. **Treatment of pharyngitis.** As is the case for common colds, no specific antiviral treatment exists for acute viral pharyngitis except for that due to influenza A virus. Streptococcal pharyngitis may be treated effectively with penicillin G or erythromycin or a first-generation cephalosporin (e.g., cephalexin or cephradine) in patients who have histories of penicillin allergy [6].

Some causes of viral pharyngitis (e.g., HSV, EBV, or adenovirus) sometimes cannot be distinguished clinically from streptococcal pharyngitis and, if a rapid diagnostic test is negative, bacterial culture results will not be available for up to 24 hours. Therefore, **treatment of more severely ill patients or patients with known underlying rheumatic heart disease is warranted after one has obtained throat-swab specimens. In less severely ill patients, one can obtain the specimen and wait for the culture results.**

The object of therapy is primarily (1) to eliminate streptococci from the pharynx and prevent rheumatic fever (one can wait up to 4–5 days after onset of symptoms and still effectively accomplish this goal), (2) to prevent suppurative complications (e.g., peritonsillar abscess), and (3) to hasten clinical recovery. In moderately ill patients, antibiotic therapy produces a significantly more rapid decline in symptoms and fever [17–19]. Most patients become afebrile within 24 hours of the start of treatment. **Family members are not usually treated [20] unless they exhibit symptoms or they have rheumatic heart disease.** However, in cases with frequent relapses, throat cultures from family members may be obtained in an attempt to determine the source of reinfection.

1. **Group A streptococcal pharyngitis.** Controversy exists over whether patients with streptococcal pharyngitis need to have a repeat throat culture after treatment and whether the presence of group A streptococci on throat culture in an asymptomatic patient requires treatment [20, 21]. The 10-day bacteriologic failure rate with penicillin and many other antibiotic regimens is 5–30% [22, 23]. The carrier rate of group A streptococci in school-aged children may be as high as 5–25% during the peak season, and it may be difficult to differentiate clinically between the carrier with nonstreptococcal pharyngitis and the patient with acute streptococcal pharyngitis. Most experts would treat the patient with a positive throat culture and symptoms compatible with streptococcal pharyngitis but are less likely to treat the asymptomatic patient with a positive culture if the patient is normal with no family history of rheumatic fever [20, 21]. **Routine posttreatment throat cultures are not recommended** [22, 24].

   Penicillin remains the standard for therapy [24a].

   a. **Benzathine penicillin G,** 1.2 million units IM in a single dose, can be used in adults. In children who weigh less than 60 pounds, 600,000 units of benzathine penicillin IM is well tolerated [25]. This route of administration **eliminates the problem of patient compliance** with pill-taking over 10 days, which may be an important factor in some cases. The combination of 900,000 units of benzathine penicillin and 300,000 units of procaine penicillin G is satisfactory for most children; the efficacy of this combination for heavier patients such as teenagers or adults requires further study [25].

   b. **Penicillin V administered orally** usually is preferred over parenteral penicillin because of its greater acceptance by patients. There has been concern that bacteriologic treatment failures have been increasing with penicillin [23]. **Recent literature reviews found no difference in failure rates reported before 1979 compared with reports after 1980** [16a, 26]. Because of its low cost, safety, and efficacy, **penicillin V remains the recommended treatment option** [26a]. As eradication has been found to occur with **twice-daily dosing** and this will likely improve patient compliance, doses of 250 mg PO bid for children younger than 12 years and 500 mg PO bid for older children have been adopted [24, 25]. A 10-day course of therapy is necessary for optimal eradication. **Penicillin is the most cost-effective regimen.**

   In the *1994 Red Book* [26a], this point is further emphasized by the following statement:

   Although some studies suggest that beta-lactamase-producing upper respiratory tract flora may interfere with the efficacy of penicillin in treatment of GAS [group A streptococcal] pharyngitis [27], antibiotic therapy of GAS pharyngitis directed against these organisms remains controversial and **is usually not necessary in patients with acute pharyngitis**. However, beta-lactamase-resistant and antistaphylococcal drugs, such as amoxicillin-clavulanate, narrow-spectrum cephalosporins, dicloxacillin, and clindamycin, can be beneficial in the retreatment of patients with recurrent GAS pharyngitis who have failed penicillin treatment.

See also sec. **e.**

c. **In penicillin-allergic patients,** erythromycin for 10 days has commonly been used in the United States. Although *S. pyogenes* strains resistant to erythromycin have been prevalent in some areas of the world (e.g., Asia and Finland) and have resulted in treatment failures, they remain uncommon in most areas of the United States [24, 26a].

In children, erythromycin estolate, 20–40 mg/kg/day in two to four divided doses, is suggested. (If erythromycin ethyl succinate is used, 40–50 mg/kg/day, usually in four divided doses, is the suggested regimen. The maximum dose is 1 g/day [24, 26a].) The expensive, newer macrolides clarithromycin (twice-daily dosing) and azithromycin are reviewed in Chap. 28M [28–30].

In adults, the erythromycin estolate preparation is not advised (see Chap. 28M). The usual adult erythromycin dose is 500 mg bid (or 250 mg qid) for 10 days. The more expensive new macrolides (clarithromycin and azithromycin) are reviewed in Chap. 28M. These agents have fewer GI side effects. In adults, clarithromycin 250 mg bid for 10 days, and in children over 6 months of age, clarithromycin 15 mg/kg/d divided q12h for 10 days has been used (see Chap. 28M). Azithromycin (in those > 15 years of age) 500 mg on the first day, and 250 mg once daily for 4 days after, is considered an option [24a, 25]; a pediatric suspension is available (see Chap. 28M).

If a patient cannot tolerate erythromycin and has a delayed penicillin allergy, an oral cephalosporin (e.g., a first-generation agent such as cephalexin) can be used. Clindamycin is another option. Tetracycline and sulfonamides are not recommended because many streptococcal strains are resistant to these agents.

d. **Routine cephalosporin use in the nonallergic patient is not suggested** [24, 26a] (see sec. **b**).

(1) In the patient with a delayed penicillin allergy, a first-generation agent can be used (e.g., cephalexin [Keflex], 25–50 mg/kg/day in divided doses q6–12h in children and 500 mg bid [or 250 mg qid] in adults).

(2) A number of cephalosporins and related agents compare favorably with oral penicillin [23, 27]. **Disadvantages of routine cephalosporin therapy include high cost and a broad antimicrobial spectrum.** A limited number of studies have found treatment courses of fewer than 10 days to be efficacious, reducing the cost of therapy [27]. It is premature to recommend these shorter courses at this time.

(3) Cephalosporins have been used in recurrent streptococcal pharyngitis in patients who have presumably failed penicillin therapy. Usually, however, this is not necessary as discussed in sec. **e.** Various agents have been used, including cefuroxime axetil (Ceftin), 20 mg/kg/day in divided doses q12h in children or 250 mg q12h in adults; cefprozil (Cefzil), 30 mg/kg/day in divided doses q12h in children or 500 mg q24h in adults; or cefpodoxime (Vantin), 10 mg/kg/day in divided doses q12h in children or 100 mg q12h in adults. **These cephalosporin regimens are very expensive compared with penicillin, typically being 10–20 times more expensive than oral penicillin** (see Table 28A-5).

e. **Patients with recurrent pharyngitis who have apparently failed a course of antibiotic** for previous GABHS pharyngitis. This is a common concern yet complex issue which has recently been reviewed [16a].

(1) The fundamental question is whether this patient is having repeated episodes of GABHS pharyngitis or is, more likely, a streptococcal carrier experiencing repeated episodes of a concurrent viral pharyngitis. See Table 7-4 and reference [16a] for a detailed discussion.

(2) The specific reasons for possible treatment failures have been reviewed [16a], and the following summary is pertinent. Penicillin-resistant strains of group A streptococci have not been identified in the United

Table 7-4. Streptococcal carrier versus repeated episodes of group A
beta-hemolytic streptococcal (GABHS) pharyngitis

Streptococcal carrier
  Signs and symptoms of viral infection
  Wrong season
  Little clinical response to antibiotics
  GABHS present between episodes
  No ASO or ADB response
  Same serotype of GABHS
Repeated episodes of GABHS pharyngitis
  Signs and symptoms consistent with GABHS
  Seasonal clustering
  Marked clinical response to antibiotics
  No GABHS between episodes
  ASO or ADB response
  Different serotypes of GABHS

ASO = antistreptolysin O; ADB – antideoxyribonuclease B.
Source: M. A. Gerber, Treatment failures and carriers: Perception or problem? *Pediatr. Infect. Dis. J.* 13:576, 1994.

States. The clinical role of penicillin tolerance or bacterial interference, to explain "treatment failures" with penicillin, has not been established. It has been suggested that a variety of normal pharyngeal flora produce beta-lactamases that may contribute to penicillin treatment failures by inactivation of the penicillin in the upper respiratory tract. Although several investigators have addressed this issue, the findings have been inconsistent and inconclusive [16a]. Therefore, it is not advised to routinely treat these patients, who often are streptococcal carriers with a viral URI, with a beta-lactamase–stable cephalosporin. Finally, there has been no substantial increase in bacteriologic treatment failure rates with oral penicillin over the past 40 years [16a].

(3) Since streptococcal carriers are unlikely to spread GABHS to their close contacts and are at very low risk, if any, for developing suppurative (e.g., peritonsillar abscess) or nonsuppurative (e.g., acute rheumatic fever) complications, **most of these patients do not require antibiotic therapy** [16a].

(4) Although most streptococcal carriers require no medical intervention, there are specific situations in which identification and eradication of the streptococcal carrier is desirable. These would include the following: (a) when there is a family history of rheumatic fever; (b) when "ping-pong" spread has been occurring within a family; (c) when a family has an inordinate amount of anxiety about GABHS; (d) when outbreaks of GABHS pharyngitis occur in closed or semiclosed communities; (e) when outbreaks of acute rheumatic fever or poststreptococcal acute glomerulonephritis occur; and (f) when tonsillectomy is being considered only because of chronic carriage of GABHS [16a]. In the unusual patient in whom one desires to eradicate the carrier state [16a], the addition of rifampin, 20 mg/kg (not to exceed 600 mg) given once daily for the last 4 days of a 10-day course of another antibiotic, is highly effective in eradicating streptococci from the pharynx [31]. Clindamycin alone, 20 mg/kg/day in three divided doses, has also been effective [32].

2. **Non–group A streptococcal pharyngitis** is rare and usually does not require antibiotic treatment. More commonly, non–group A streptococci are colonizers, which need no therapy.
3. **Gonococcal pharyngitis.** See Chap. 13.
4. ***A. haemolyticum*** is susceptible to the antibiotics used to treat group A streptococci.
5. The benefits of therapy for *M. pneumoniae* and *Chlamydia pneumoniae* need further clinical study [8].

F. **Complications of group A streptococcal pharyngitis**
  1. **Otitis media, sinusitis,** and **cervical adenitis** can occur.

2. Acute streptococcal pharyngitis may lead to **peritonsillar abscess (quinsy)**, which appears as brawny edema of the affected side with movement of the tonsil toward the midline. Because the pus obtained when the abscess drains usually does not contain streptococci, it is believed that the abscess results from secondary infection with anaerobic mouth organisms. Surgical incision and drainage is the treatment of choice. Intravenous penicillin also is given.

3. Streptococcal pharyngitis can extend to involve the paranasal sinuses, middle ear, mastoid air cells, cervical lymph nodes and, rarely, the lungs. These complications are rare today due to the prompt antimicrobial therapy given in most cases.

4. The principal **nonsuppurative complications** are glomerulonephritis and acute rheumatic fever.

G. **Rare causes of pharyngitis**

1. **Vincent's angina.** This condition is an exudative tonsillitis usually due to *Fusobacterium necrophorum* or other anaerobic bacteria. Occasionally, infection spreads to the soft tissues of the neck.

2. **Diphtheria.** Infection with *Corynebacterium diphtheriae* still is seen occasionally in the United States, and 25% of the cases occur in adults.

   a. **Signs and symptoms** [33]. The onset of illness is sudden, with fever, malaise, and sore throat. A thick, gray tonsillar exudate is present and may spread rapidly to the tonsillar pillars, uvula, soft palate, posterior pharyngeal wall, and larynx. The exudate is not easily removable (as is streptococcal exudate). Toxemia is present with pallor, lethargy, prostration, and weakness.

   b. **Diagnosis.** It is important to make the diagnosis early because mortality increases with delay in diagnosis. **The diagnosis should be considered in an unimmunized patient with a rapidly spreading tonsillar exudate.** Stridor may occur. A pharyngeal swab should be cultured on a Loffler's slant, a tellurite, and a blood agar plate, to recover *C. diphtheriae*.

   c. **Treatment** often must be started empirically in the clinical setting just described. Infectious disease consultation is advised. When diphtheria is suspected on clinical grounds, 20,000–40,000 units of **equine antitoxin** should be injected intramuscularly. (If a history of sensitivity to horse serum is obtained, one should perform conjunctival or skin tests with a 1:10 dilution of antitoxin). In addition, aqueous **penicillin G**, 10 million units/day IV (in adults), should be given for 10 days. Erythromycin, 30–40 mg/kg/day, should be used in the allergic patient.

   d. **Complications** include cranial and peripheral nerve paralysis. Other important complications are airway obstruction [33] and myocarditis, which carry a high mortality.

3. **Secondary syphilis.** Ulceromembranous tonsillitis and pharyngitis may occur in secondary syphilis. If these are the only manifestations of syphilis, the syphilis is difficult to distinguish from pharyngitis and tonsillitis due to other causes (see Chap. 13).

4. **Mucositis.** Patients with **agranulocytosis often complain of sore throat,** which is **not due** to known viral, mycoplasmal, or bacterial agents.

Otitis Media

Otitis media is the most frequent diagnosis for illness in office practices that care for children. In surveys of diagnoses made by the Centers for Disease Control in office practices in the United States, 24.5 million office visits at which the principal diagnosis was otitis media were made in 1990 [33a]. For reasons that are uncertain, diagnoses of otitis media increased from 9.91 million office visits in 1975 to 24.5 million visits in 1990, possibly due in part to exposure of children to group daycare and/or increased interest in the disease. The annual cost of medical and surgical treatment of otitis media in the United States is estimated at between $2.5–4.0 billion annually [34, 34a]. It is estimated from market surveys, that in the late 1980s, one-fourth of the prescriptions written in the United States were to treat otitis [34]. In a recent review, otitis media was noted to be the most frequent reason for prescription of antimicrobial drugs for American infants and children [33a].

I. **Definitions.** Infections of the ear are a spectrum of diseases involving the structures of the outer ear (otitis externa), the middle ear (otitis media), the mastoid process (mastoiditis), and inner ear (labyrinthitis) [34a].

 A. **Acute otitis media** (AOM) is an inflammation of the middle ear that presents with a rapid onset of signs and symptoms (see sec. **III**).

 B. **Otitis media with effusion** is characterized by the presence of an asymptomatic middle-ear effusion, although it can be associated with a "plugged-ear" feeling.

 C. **AOM that is unresponsive to a treatment** is characterized by clinical signs and symptoms and otoscopic findings of inflammation that continue beyond 48 h of therapy.

 D. **Otitis media with residual effusion** is characterized by the presence of asymptomatic middle-ear effusion, without otoscopic signs of inflammation, 3–16 weeks after the diagnosis of acute otitis.

 E. **Otitis media with persistent effusion** involves the above (see sec. **D**), lasting more than 16 weeks.

 F. **Recurrent acute otitis media** often deserves consideration of an antibiotic prophylaxis and is considered to exist when three new episodes of AOM occur within a 6 month period.

 G. **Otitis media with complications** refers to damages to the structures of the middle ear (e.g., perforations, ossicular erosions), and cholesteatoma, as well as other intratemporal and intracranial problems.

II. **Incidence**

 A. The incidence of otitis media varies greatly with age and population. Of children followed 7 or more years in a private pediatric practice, otitis media was diagnosed at least once in 84%, and almost 50% of these patients had four or more episodes. The incidence is greatest in the first few years of life, becoming less frequent by 6 years of age. Children in the first several years of life appear to be particularly prone to developing otitis media because of the high incidence of URIs in their age group and because their relatively short and straight eustachian tubes allow reflux from the nasopharynx.

 B. **Otitis-prone child.** Approximately one-third of American children are "otitis-prone," which is defined as at least three episodes of acute otitis media (AOM) by age 3 years. **Risk factors include** [33a, 35]: (1) **male gender;** (2) **certain racial groups and locations** (native Americans, Alaskan and Canadian Eskimos, aboriginal settlements, Nigerian settlements, some developing countries); (3) **early occurrence** of infection (within first few months of age) is associated with recurrent episodes (in contrast, children with few episodes of AOM before age 3 are unlikely to have subsequent AOM); (4) **sibling history** of recurrent AOM; and (5) **those not breast-fed** (breast-feeding helps reduce respiratory infections). Therefore, the middle-ear system appears to be analogous to the urinary tract in that infection early in life signals an underlying disability. The predisposition of the infant to otitis media is caused by ill-defined features of eustachian tube anatomy, physiology, and immunology [33a]. Environmental and potentially reversible risk factors are also discussed in sec. **IX.D.**

III. **Signs and symptoms.** The clinical findings accompanying otitis media may be varied and nonspecific, especially in infants. Otitis media may be present as the sole manifestation of infection, or it may be part of a more generalized systemic disease.

 A. **Respiratory symptoms** (i.e., symptoms of a URI) are commonly present. Otitis media commonly accompanies bronchiolitis and pneumonia in infants younger than 6 months.

 B. **Pain** in the infant may be manifested only by irritability or, occasionally, by ear pulling.

 C. **Fever** may or may not be present and, in most series, 30–60% of the children with acute otitis media are afebrile. Particularly in infants younger than 2 months, fever is uncommon. A high fever accompanying otitis is more likely to occur as part of a systemic illness, and other sources for the fever, such as pneumonia or meningitis, should be ruled out.

IV. **Diagnosis.** Criteria for the diagnosis of otitis media are controversial.

 A. **Myringotomy.** Diagnosis may be made most specifically by myringotomy (i.e., incision of the tympanic membrane) or tympanocentesis. Generally, neither procedure is done in the office setting, and neither is warranted in most cases of otitis media.

 B. **Tympanic membrane appearance.** Diagnosis must be made on the basis of the clinical appearance of the tympanic membrane. Redness alone is not a reliable indication of acute infection, but bulging is. Some have proposed that the finding of immobility of the tympanic membrane is sufficient for diagnosis, but differentiation from secretory otitis media by this criterion alone is difficult.

   C. **Tympanometry.** Tympanic membrane compliance may be determined by tympanometry, with the use of an electroacoustic impedance bridge to detect middle-ear effusion objectively [35a]. The feasibility of this method of diagnosis in general practice has not been evaluated.

   D. **Aspiration.** In the **neonate,** clinical diagnosis is particularly difficult, as the tympanic membrane generally has a dull gray appearance but is sometimes erythematous. The light reflex often is diminished in the normal state. Aspiration of the middle ear is the best method of diagnosis in the neonate, and ideally it should be used because the infection in this age group may have different etiologies and more serious complications [36, 37]. Middle-ear aspiration is warranted also in children with persistent bulging of the tympanic membrane or in those who appear to be treatment failures (see Chap. 3).

V. **Etiology.** Otitis media can be caused by bacteria, mycoplasmas, and viruses, either alone or in combination. Bacteria are isolated in approximately 50–60% of the cases, and viruses, especially RSV, rhinoviruses, influenza A, and parainfluenza A, have recently been identified in 24–39% of cases [35, 38–39a].

   A. **Bacteria in acute otitis media**
      1. *Streptococcus pneumoniae* is the most commonly identified agent in children and adults.
      2. *Haemophilus influenzae* is the second most frequently identified organism, and more than 95% of the *H. influenzae* strains recovered are nontypeable. Several older studies suggested that the incidence of an *H. influenzae* otitis media is age-related and that it occurs most frequently in children younger than 5 years. However, more recent studies indicate that *H. influenzae* remains the second most frequent cause of otitis media in all age groups, comprising approximately 12–23% (or more) of cases.
      3. *Moraxella catarrhalis* (formerly *Neisseria* and then *Branhamella catarrhalis*) is currently the third most frequently identified organism in middle-ear fluid. More than 75% of strains of *M. catarrhalis* produce beta-lactamase [40].
      4. **Other bacterial agents** are seen less frequently, but these include group A beta-hemolytic streptococci (3% of cases) and *Staphylococcus aureus* (< 2%) [35]. In the neonate [36, 37], gram-negative bacilli and *S. aureus* are more frequently isolated than in older patients, but otherwise the bacteria are similar to those in older patients.

   B. *M. pneumoniae* seldom is a cause of either acute otitis media or bullous myringitis.

   C. **Viruses.** A variety of respiratory viruses have been associated with otitis media and appear to be able to play both primary and secondary roles. Recent studies have shown that the incidence of otitis media is related mostly to outbreaks of viral respiratory agents such as RSV, influenza, and adenovirus in the community [39a, 41]. In the winter, RSV infection in infants is particularly associated with the development of otitis media.

VI. **Treatment of acute otitis media.** Therapy, in most instances, must be initiated without knowledge of the exact organism and therefore must be aimed especially at covering pneumococci, *H. influenzae,* and *M. catarrhalis.* Although oral decongestants and antihistamines commonly are prescribed, they have been shown to be of no benefit [42, 43]. Such treatment is frequently associated with side effects and may even result in a greater frequency of persistent middle-ear effusions in children with an allergic history [42, 43].

   The precise role for antibiotics continues to be debated and is reviewed elsewhere [34a, 35]. About 70% of children have a bacterial etiology of AOM (and prior data suggest that 40% of these patients have a spontaneous bacteriologic cure). The other 30% of patients have primarily a viral etiology and do not require antibiotics. Therefore, of 100 patients with AOM of all etiologies, it is estimated that about 60% would have spontaneous resolution of infection [35]. In a recently published metaanalysis of outcome for AOM in 5,400 children enrolled in 33 randomized studies, spontaneous clinical resolution was thought to have occurred in 81% of patients [43a], but the high rate of spontaneous resolution may be spurious because of the inherent limitations of metaanalyses, the relatively late evaluation time of 7–14 days used in that analysis to determine clinical response, and the highly variable criteria used for diagnosis in the individual studies [35]. Studies conducted principally in the preantibiotic era show that about 1 in 5 untreated patients developed mastoiditis [35]. In his thoughtful review of this debate, Dr. George H. McCracken, Jr., concludes: ". . . because it is impossible to determine which infant or child requires antibiotic therapy and which can be treated expectantly, physicians must prescribe antimicrobial agents for acute otitis media when a bacterial agent etiology is suspected. On the other hand, many children with low-grade or no fever and minimal or early signs of middle-ear involvement can be treated symptomatically with follow-up evaluation in 24–48 h" [35].

A. **Neonates.** Ideally, tympanocentesis is performed either initially or when the patient has not responded to initial therapy. (See additional discussion in Chap. 3, sec. **II,** under Selected Specific Infections in the Newborn, and refs. [36, 37].)

B. **Infants and children.** In his excellent recent review, McCracken emphasizes that there is no one preferred therapeutic agent for all children with acute otitis media [35]. The regimen that has been advocated most commonly (and that seems reasonable) is either ampicillin or amoxicillin orally for a period of 7–10 days [35]. See Table 7-5. In some communities, however, where beta-lactamase–producing organisms account for a sizeable percentage of the otitis pathogens, alternative agents, such as amoxicillin-clavulanate, cefaclor, or trimethoprim-sulfamethoxazole (TMP-SMX) are used. Clinical failure is not necessarily caused by antibiotic failure, because in patients who fail to respond to treatment, organisms recovered from tympanocentesis are often susceptible to the antibiotic prescribed. Conversely, disease caused by resistant pathogens may respond satisfactorily to an inappropriate drug as in the case of beta-lactamase–producing *M. catarrhalis* when amoxicillin is given [35]. Other antibiotic issues are reviewed further by McCracken [35].

Although in recent years penicillin-resistant *S. pneumoniae* problems have increased in the United States, middle-ear disease due to these organisms overall accounts for fewer than 5% of all patients with otitis media [35]. (See related discussion in Chap. 28C.) Disease caused by resistant pneumococci should be considered in a child who continues to have signs of acute middle-ear inflammation despite one or more courses of antibiotic therapy [35], which includes activity against beta-lactamase–producing organisms. In this setting a myringotomy for drainage and culture of middle-ear fluid is prudent, to provide relief of symptoms and define the etiology and susceptibility of the pathogen. Therapy is tailored to the results of these studies [35].

1. **Ampicillin and amoxicillin still are the initial drugs of choice for uncomplicated otitis media in the nonallergic patient** [35, 44]. In general, the incidence of *H. influenzae* (typeable or nontypeable strains) resistant to ampicillin or amoxicillin is approximately 30–40%, although in some geographic areas of the United States a lower incidence may be seen. Because *H. influenzae* is the primary pathogen in 10–25% of cases of otitis media in children and because, in most areas, only a small proportion of such cases are resistant

Table 7-5. Antimicrobial agents for treatment of acute otitis media[a]

Group	Agent
I	Amoxicillin (Amoxil, others)
II	Amoxicillin + clavulanate (Augmentin)
	Cefaclor (Ceclor)
	Erythromycin-sulfa (Pediazole, others)
	Trimethoprim-sulfamethoxazole (Bactrim, Septra, and others)
III	Cefixime (Suprax)
	Cefpodoxime proxetil (Vantin)
	Cefprozil (Cefzil)
	Ceftriaxone (Rocephin)[b]
	Cefuroxime axetil (Ceftin)
	Loracarbef (Lorabid)

[a]Antibiotics are grouped on the basis of record of clinical effectiveness and safety (Group I = longest, Group III = shortest).
[b]Not approved by Food and Drug Administration for use in otitis media.
Source: G. H. McCracken, Jr. Considerations in selecting an antibiotic treatment of acute otitis media. *Pediatr. Infect. Dis. J.* 13:1054, 1994.

to ampicillin, most authorities believe that either ampicillin or amoxicillin should be used as the initial agent of choice for uncomplicated otitis media [35, 45].

The same logic can be used for *M. catarrhalis*. Furthermore, otitis media caused by beta-lactamase-positive *M. catarrhalis* usually is cured when treated with amoxicillin.

No clear advantage exists for ampicillin over amoxicillin. Because of the 3-times-daily dosage schedule of amoxicillin, this agent often is preferred. **Amoxicillin also is a cost-effective agent** (Table 7-6).

    a. Amoxicillin, 40 mg/kg/day, is given in divided doses q8h. (An oral suspension is available with 125 mg/5 ml or 250 mg/5 ml.) In children weighing more than 20 kg, the usual adult dose (250 mg q8h) is given.

    b. Ampicillin, 50–100 mg/kg/day, is given in divided doses q6h. Oral suspensions with 125 mg/5 ml and 250 mg/5 ml are available. In children weighing more than 20 kg, the usual adult dose can be given (250 mg q6h).

  2. Amoxicillin-clavulanate (Augmentin). The addition of a beta-lactamase antagonist, clavulanic acid, to amoxicillin creates a combination active against ampicillin-resistant *H. influenzae* and *M. catarrhalis*. The dosage of the fixed combination is based on the amoxicillin content. Amoxicillin-clavulanate is more expensive than amoxicillin alone and results in a higher incidence of diarrhea. A suspension is available for children, and the usual dose is 40 mg/kg/day, based on the amoxicillin component, in divided doses q8h. **The role of this alternative agent is summarized** in sec. **5.** (See Chap. 28E for further discussion.)

Table 7-6. Some antimicrobials for acute otitis media

Drug	Daily dosage	Cost[a]
Amoxicillin: average generic price	40 mg/kg in 3 doses	$ 6.02
Amoxil (SmithKline Beecham, Philadelphia)		6.10
Amoxicillin-clavulanate	40 mg/kg amoxicillin–10 mg/kg clavulanic acid in 3 doses	
Augmentin (SmithKline Beecham, Philadelphia)		48.10
Cefaclor: *Ceclor* (Lilly, Indianapolis)	40 mg/kg in 2 or 3 doses	51.78
Cefixime: *Suprax* (Lederle)	8 mg/kg in 1 or 2 doses	45.66
Cefprozil: *Cefzil* (Bristol, Princeton, NJ)	30 mg/kg in 2 doses	45.59
Cefuroxime axetil: *Ceftin*[b] (Allen/Hanburys, NC)	500 mg in 2 doses	62.84
Cefpodoxime: *Vantin* (Upjohn, Kalamazoo, MI)	10 mg/kg in 2 doses	54.00
Erythromycin-sulfisoxazole: average generic price	50 mg/kg erythromycin–150 mg/kg sulfisoxazole in 4 doses	22.77
Pediazole (Ross/Abbott, Columbus, OH)		30.08
Loracarbef—*Lorabid* (Lilly, Indianapolis)	30 mg/kg in 2 doses	56.40
Trimethoprim-sulfamethoxazole: average generic price	8 mg/kg TMP–40 mg/kg SMX in 2 doses	3.43
Bactrim (Roche, Nutley, NJ)		12.83
Septra (Burroughs Wellcome, NC)		12.26
Clarithromycin: *Biaxin*[c]	15 mg/kg in 2 doses	24.00

[a]Cost to the pharmacist as packaged for 10 days' treatment of a 15-kg child, according to average wholesale price listings in *Red Book* 1993 and February 1994 *Update*.
[b]Also available as a suspension; daily dose is 30 mg/kg in 2 divided doses. See Chap. 28F.
[c]Approved for use in otitis media August 1994. See discussion of agent in Chap. 28.
Note: Trade names of agents are provided in italic type.
Source: Modified from Medical Letter. Drugs for the treatment of acute otitis media. *Med. Lett. Drugs Ther.* 36:20, 1994.

3. **In penicillin-allergic patients, alternative agents** (see Table 7-6) **include:**
    a. **Erythromycin.** Erythromycin (30–40 mg/kg/day in children), like penicillin alone, often is inadequate for the eradication of *H. influenzae.* However, a combination of erythromycin and sulfisoxazole (Pediazole) is effective against both ampicillin-sensitive and ampicillin-resistant forms of *H. influenzae.* **Erythromycin, 50 mg/kg/day, and sulfisoxazole, 150 mg/kg/day,** in four divided doses is commonly used. **Some experts advocate this regimen in the penicillin-allergic patient** [35]. The new macrolide **clarithromycin** was approved for use in otitis media by the U.S. Food and Drug Administration in August 1994. This twice-daily agent has fewer GI side effects than erythromycin. **Azithromycin** has recently been approved for AOM in children over 6 months old. These agents are reviewed in detail in Chap. 28M.
    b. **Trimethoprim-sulfamethoxazole** (TMP-SMX). This combination agent is an alternative, as approximately 80–90% of *H. influenzae* infections (both ampicillin-sensitive and ampicillin-resistant strains) and most *S. pneumoniae* and *M. catarrhalis* infections are susceptible. In some areas, however, 20–40% of *S. pneumoniae* isolates are resistant to TMP-SMX [44]. In addition, some studies have shown a higher failure rate among patients treated with this drug compared with patients treated with ampicillin or erythromycin with a sulfonamide [45]. In children older than 2 years, the recommended dose for acute otitis media is TMP, 8 mg/kg/day, and SMX, 40 mg/kg/day. The drug is given in two divided doses q12h for 10 days. A cherry-flavored oral suspension containing the equivalent of 40 mg TMP and 200 mg SMX in each teaspoonful (5 ml) is available. Regular tablets contain 80 mg TMP and 400 mg SMX. This agent is not advised if there is an associated streptococcal pharyngitis, as it is not consistently effective against group A streptococci [35].
    c. **Oral cephalosporins.** In patients with delayed penicillin (or ampicillin) or sulfa allergies, oral cephalosporins are commonly used (Tables 7-5 and 7-7).
        (1) **Cefaclor** is an oral cephalosporin active against *S. pneumoniae* as well as *H. influenzae* (ampicillin-sensitive and ampicillin-resistant strains) (see Chap. 28F), but some strains of *H. influenzae* are resistant to it. Cefaclor has been less effective than some of the other alternative agents studied [44]. In otitis media in children, the recommended dose is 40 mg/kg/day PO (maximum, 1 g/day) divided on a q8h schedule. An oral suspension (125 mg/5 ml) is available. The usual adult dose is 250 mg q8h.
        (2) **Cefuroxime axetil** (Ceftin), an oral cephalosporin, is reviewed in Chap. 28F. It is active against *S. pneumoniae,* beta-lactamase-positive and beta-lactamase-negative *H. influenzae,* and *M. catarrhalis.* For otitis media, 125 mg bid for those younger than 2 years and 250 mg bid for those older than 2 years is suggested. Tablets come in 125-mg and 250-mg strengths. A suspension comes in 125 mg/5 ml and 250 mg/5 ml strengths (see Table 7-6).
        (3) **Cefprozil** is reviewed in detail in Chap. 28F. It can be given in a convenient twice-daily dosing regimen.
        (4) **Cefixime** is a so-called third-generation cephalosporin and is reviewed in Chap. 28F. Although it is very active against *H. influenzae* and *M. catarrhalis,* cefixime has the disadvantage of relatively poor activity against *S. pneumoniae* [44] and therefore is not an initial agent of choice for otitis media.
        (5) **Loracarbef and cefpodoxime** are potential alternative cephalosporins that are reviewed in Chap. 28F, but neither has any properties that make it uniquely useful in the therapy for otitis media.
        (6) See Tables 7-6 and 7-7 for cost and summary data.
4. **Other considerations**
    a. **Penicillin** alone has been suggested as adequate therapy by some physicians. However, in carefully performed studies, penicillin did not provide adequate levels in the middle ear to treat many *H. influenzae* strains. Therefore, **penicillin alone is not recommended.**
    b. **In areas where the incidence of ampicillin-resistant *H. influenzae* strains is appreciable, several alternatives are possible.** Amoxicillin may be used initially; if response is not prompt, the therapy is altered. It may be reason-

Table 7-7. Characteristics of oral cephalosporins for the treatment of otitis media

Cephalosporin	Dose		Comments
	Children	Adults	
Cefadroxil (Duricef)	30 mg/kg/day ÷ q12h	500 mg q8h	Less active than other comparable cephalosporins against *H. influenzae*.
Cefaclor (Ceclor)	40 mg/kg/day ÷ q8–12h	250–500 mg q8h	Some *H. influenzae* are resistant; 1–2% incidence of serum sickness.
Cefuroxime axetil (Ceftin)	30 mg/kg/day ÷ q12h	500 mg q12h	Oral suspension dose shown for children.
Cefixime (Suprax)	8 mg/kg/day ÷ q12–24h	400 mg/day	Less active than other comparable cephalosporins against *S. pneumoniae*.
Cefprozil (Cefzil)	30 mg/kg/day ÷ q12h	250–500 mg q12h	More active than cefaclor against *H. influenzae*.
Cefpodoxime (Vantin)	10 mg/kg/day ÷ q12h	200 mg q12h	Suspension tastes bitter.
Loracarbef (Lorabid)	30 mg/kg/day ÷ q12h	200 mg q12h	Similar activity to cefaclor but with greater activity against beta-lactamase–producing *H. influenzae* and fewer reports of serum sickness. Suspension does not require refrigeration.

able to switch to amoxicillin-clavulanate, erythromycin plus a sulfonamide, or TMP-SMX in the follow-up treatment of a patient who does not respond to ampicillin or amoxicillin initially. Oral cephalosporins such as cefaclor, cefuroxime axetil, cefixime, loracarbef, cefpodoxime, or cefprozil are other options (see Tables 7-5 and 7-7, sec. **5**, and Chap. 28F).

    c. Adults. Many of the pathogens active in childhood otitis media are seen also in the otitis media of adults. Although penicillin often is used effectively, it seems more reasonable to use amoxicillin or ampicillin. In the penicillin-allergic patient, erythromycin plus a sulfonamide, TMP-SMX, or an oral cephalosporin is reasonable.

  5. Summary of use of alternative agents. The following situations have been suggested as those in which alternative agents (e.g., TMP-SMX, amoxicillin-clavulanate, cefaclor, or cefuroxime axetil) for treatment or prevention of recurrent acute otitis media or otitis media with effusion might be used [35]:

    a. Culture-positive resistant organism isolated from otorrhea or tympanocentesis or myringotomy, such as beta-lactamase–producing *H. influenzae* or *M. catarrhalis*.

    b. History of allergic reaction to the penicillins.

    c. Initial treatment failure while on amoxicillin (i.e., failure to improve progressively or worsening of symptoms and signs of the acute infection).

    d. History of prior initial amoxicillin treatment failure in the recent past.

    e. Persistent middle-ear infection after a 10-day course of amoxicillin for acute otitis media.

    f. Recurrence of acute middle-ear infection within several weeks after a course of amoxicillin for acute otitis media.

    g. Presence in the community of a high incidence of resistant bacteria.

VII. Treatment of acute otitis media not responding to initial therapy, recurrent otitis media, and otitis media with residual effusion has been reviewed in detail elsewhere [34a] and is summarized in Fig. 7-1. A few points will be emphasized.

  A. Follow-up of acute otitis media. Children should be reexamined at the end of the course of antibiotics. At this time, up to 50% of those treated with antibiotics will have a persistent middle-ear effusion. This is a common finding and is not sufficient grounds for performing surgery such as myringotomy and tympanostomy tube insertion [35]. See Fig. 7-1 for suggestions of follow-up.

  B. AOM unresponsive to therapy. In these patients, clinical symptoms and otoscopic findings of membrane inflammation persist after 48 h of antibiotic therapy. This may occur in about 10% of children on antibiotics and raises concern that an underlying pathogen is not being eradicated [34a]. Often these patients have coexisting bacterial-viral middle-ear infections.

    When amoxicillin is initially used, changing to agents active against beta-lactamase–positive organisms is typically undertaken: amoxicillin-clavulanate, TMP-SMX, or a second- or third-generation cephalosporin. See sec. **VI.B.5.**

  C. Recurrent acute otitis media often is managed effectively with a **prophylactic antibiotic regimen,** particularly in children younger than 2 years. Infants whose first episode of acute otitis media occurred prior to 6 months of age and children who have had three or more episodes of otitis media during a 6-month period are at risk for recurrence and may benefit from daily antibiotics. Effective prophylaxis includes sulfisoxazole, 75 mg/kg/day in one or two divided doses, or amoxicillin, 20 mg/kg once daily. After 3–6 months, the antibiotic is discontinued and the child reevaluated [34a]. Children who continue to have recurrent episodes may require surgical intervention (see sec. **E**) [34].

  D. Otitis media with residual effusion. The persistence of abnormal appearance of the tympanic membrane 2 weeks after the initiation of therapy is common, occurring in 20–30% of patients, and does not necessarily imply relapse. An unsatisfactory response to the initial course of therapy may be expected in approximately 10–20% of cases, suggesting that an alternate therapy should be chosen [39].

    A concern about the negative effects of conductive hearing impairment on language development is the main reason to treat otitis media with residual effusion. The presence of an effusion is associated with a mild-to-moderate conductive hearing impairment of 20 dB or more. There is a causal relationship between severe (usually sensorineural) hearing loss, either congenital or acquired, and language development. A causal relation between the conductive hearing loss associated with otitis media and subsequent language development and learning has not been established [34a]. See related discussion in sec. **E.**

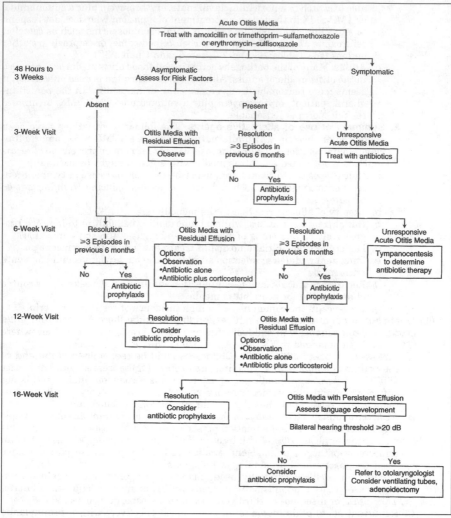

Fig. 7-1. An algorithm for the diagnosis and management of otitis media in children. Risk factors for the failure of treatment are an age of less than 15 months, a history of recurrent otitis media in the patient or a sibling, and antibiotic treatment of otitis media within the previous month. (Reprinted by permission of *The New England Journal of Medicine,* from S. Berman, Otitis media in children. *N. Engl. J. Med.* 332:1560. Copyright 1995, Massachusetts Medical Society.)

1. Management options for effusions that persist from 6 weeks to 4 months include observation, antibiotics alone, and antibiotics and corticosteroid [34a].
2. If combination therapy is selected, prednisone (1 mg per kg of body weight per day, given orally in two divided doses) can be given for 7 days along with an antibiotic (e.g., TMP-SMX or an alternative) for 14–21 days [34a]. Crushed prednisone tablets can be added to jelly to camouflage their bitter taste.

E. **Otitis media with persistent effusion (> 4 months) and documented bilateral hearing impairment** of 20 dB or more. In this setting ventilating tubes are often considered [34a, 46, 47].

1. The long-term sequelae of otitis media have been discussed elsewhere [47]. This summary reviews the clinical practice guidelines for otitis media published by the Agency for Health Care Policy and Research.

    2. The panel concluded that many fundamental questions of optimal therapy remain unanswered. Interim conclusions included:

        a. Sufficient data exist to suggest that there may be mild-to-moderate delay or impairment of speech and/or language stemming from persistent effusions early in life.

        b. Some medical interventions are supported by suitable studies.

        c. Definitive short-term intervention (myringotomy and tube insertion) is warranted for children in the first 3 years of life who have bilateral middle-ear effusions for at least 3 months and a bilateral hearing loss of at least 20 dB [47].

F. Surgical interventions are further reviewed elsewhere [46].

    1. **Tympanocentesis** is a needle aspiration of the middle ear when a middle-ear effusion is present and there is need to identify the causative organism. **Myringotomy** is performed when drainage of the middle ear (and mastoid air cells) is required. Indications for these procedures are shown in Table 7-8. Routine myringotomy for uncomplicated AOM is unnecessary [43a].

    2. **Myringotomy and tympanostomy tube insertion.** Insertion of tympanostomy tube into a myringotomy incision is indicated when long-term ventilation or drainage, or both, is desired. Indications for tympanostomy tube insertion are listed in Table 7-9. For recurrent AOM, often a trial of prophylactic antibiotics is initially undertaken (see sec. **B**). For those who fail a 2–3 month trial of prophylactic antibiotics, tympanostomy tubes can then be recommended.

    3. The role of adenoidectomy and tonsillectomy is reviewed elsewhere [43a].

VIII. Miscellaneous issues

  A. Suppurative complications such as **mastoiditis** are very rare since the advent of antibiotics. This topic is reviewed elsewhere [47a].

  B. Cholesteatoma is a complication that can lead to bony erosion and requires surgical management.

IX. Prevention of otitis media

  A. Vaccines. The potential role of vaccines in preventing otitis media has recently been reviewed [48]. Since otitis media is a disease of infancy, vaccines will be most effective if they are administered at 2 months of age and are fully effective by 4–6 months of age.

Table 7-8. Indications for myringotomy and tympanostomy tube placement

Chronic otitis media with effusion, unresponsive to medical management

Recurrent acute otitis media, especially antimicrobial prophylaxis failures

Frequently recurrent otitis media with effusion, e.g., 6 cumulative months of previous 12

Eustachian tube dysfunction, associated with one or more of the following: hearing loss, otalgia, vertigo, or tinnitus

Retraction pocket of the tympanic membrane

At time of tympanoplasty for retraction pocket/cholesteatoma when eustachian tube function is poor

Suppurative complications of otitis media, such as acute mastoiditis

Source: C. D. Bluestone, Surgical management of otitis media: Current indications and role-related increasing bacterial resistance. *Pediatr. Infect. Dis. J.* 13:1058, 1994.

Table 7-9. Indications for tympanocentesis and myringotomy

Tympanocentesis	Otitis media in patients who are seriously ill or toxic
	Unsatisfactory response to antimicrobial therapy
	Onset of otitis media in patients receiving antimicrobial agents
	Otitis media in newborns and immunologically deficient patients
	Presence of suppurative complications or when one is suspected
Myringotomy	Relief of severe otalgia
	Whenever tympanocentesis is performed, in selected patients

Source: C. D. Bluestone, Surgical management of otitis media: Current indications and role-related increasing bacterial resistance. *Pediatr. Infect. Dis. J.* 13:1058, 1994.

1. Currently available pneumococcal vaccines have not been effective and pneumococcal conjugate vaccines are being studied.
2. Nontypeable *H. influenzae* vaccines are also being studied. Since *H. influenzae* isolated from infected middle ears are almost always nontypeable, the currently available *H. influenzae* type b vaccine (see Chap. 22) is not useful in this setting.
3. **Viral vaccines.** RSV, adenovirus, and influenza viruses are strongly associated with symptomatic otitis media. Only influenza vaccine is currently available.

B. Although host factors cannot be modified in the "otitis-prone child" (see sec. **II.B**), **environmental factors** associated with severe and recurrent otitis media **may be modified** [33a].
1. **Breast-feeding** for a period as short as 3 months was associated with decreased risk of AOM for the first year of life [33a].
2. **Large group daycare centers** (≥ 7 children) attendees appear to be at increased risk of AOM. Therefore, a smaller daycare setting may be beneficial [33a].
3. Passive smoking may play a role.
4. Since fall, winter, and early spring are associated with more episodes of AOM, presumably related to an increased incidence of viral respiratory tract infections at these times, aggressive therapeutic interventions (e.g., surgery) at times may be reasonable to reassess after the current or after the next respiratory viral season.

Acute Sinusitis

Acute sinusitis is a common problem and one often seen in the outpatient setting [49, 50]. It presumably is an occasional complication of viral URIs. The most commonly involved sinus is the maxillary, but the others also may be involved.

I. **Etiology.** Some of the best studies have been performed on the etiology of acute maxillary sinusitis **in adults,** by using aspiration techniques and by careful culturing of the sinus contents.
A. **Bacteria**
1. *S. pneumoniae* **and nontypeable** *H. influenzae* are the **most common** pathogens and are seen in the majority of cases in which bacteria are isolated.
2. Anaerobes (penicillin-sensitive) and aerobic streptococci are common in adults.
3. *S. aureus* **is uncommon** and was seen in only 2% of cases in the series reported by Hamory and coworkers [50]. Prior studies probably have exaggerated the role of this pathogen because of poor techniques used in obtaining sinus content cultures.
B. **Viruses** (e.g., rhinovirus, influenza, parainfluenza) are seen in approximately 20% of carefully studied culture specimens.
C. Sterile cultures are not uncommon, despite a clinical presentation that is consistent with an acute process.
D. Wald [51] has conducted aspiration studies of acute maxillary sinusitis **in children.** The **most common** bacteria isolated were *S. pneumoniae, H. influenzae,* **and** *M. catarrhalis.* Viruses were infrequently recovered, and anaerobes were not isolated.

II. **Clinical findings**
A. **General.** In the setting of a viral URI, the development of facial pain, fever, and persistent purulent nasal discharge should suggest acute sinusitis. Headache, nasal obstruction, and loss of smell may be present. Because many of these symptoms may be present during a common cold, a valuable general rule is that **most symptoms due to uncomplicated viral URI should abate within 7–10 days.** Clinical characteristics do not distinguish patients who are clearly infected with bacteria.
In children, cough and nasal discharge are common. Fever may be absent. Facial pain and swelling may occur. In some cases, parents noted malodorous breath in preschoolers who did not have obvious pharyngitis or poor dental hygiene.
B. **More specific clinical criteria** have been suggested in the hope of assisting the clinician to make a more precise diagnosis.
1. Williams et al. [52], using four-view sinus radiographs to confirm cases, concluded maxillary toothache, history of a colored nasal discharge, poor response to nasal decongestants, abnormal sinus transillumination, and purulent secretions on examination were associated with acute sinusitis, especially when 3–5 of these findings were in a given patient.

      2. Another series emphasizes purulent nasal or pharyngeal discharge and coughing lasting more than 7 days [53].
III. **Diagnosis** is often heavily based on clinical findings noted in sec. II.
    A. **Nasal swabs** for cultures are **not helpful,** as the organisms isolated may not reflect the true pathogens causing disease in the involved sinus.
    B. **Transillumination** of the maxillary and frontal sinuses is often suggested in adults but may be difficult to perform reliably when done intermittently or without careful instruction in this technique. If light transmittance is normal, acute bacterial sinusitis is not likely. Dull transillumination is less specific. Transillumination in recurrent disease also is less helpful. Transillumination should be performed in a completely darkened room using a sinus transilluminator.
    C. **Sinus roentgenograms** (Waters' view) are often very helpful [49, 50] but are, unfortunately, expensive. In young children, the diagnosis may be difficult to establish because the sinuses are not fully developed [54]. Sinus radiographs are less useful in diagnosing active infection in patients with chronic sinus disease because of persistent radiographic abnormalities in such patients [52].
      1. An **air-fluid level implies acute infection,** whether or not it is associated with mucosal thickening.
      2. **Complete opacity** of the sinus is consistent with an acute infection, although with recurrent disease this may be hard to assess.
      3. **Mucosal thickening** (> 5 mm in adults or 4 mm in children) is suggestive of acute disease but may also be seen in chronic problems.
    D. **CT scans are not indicated** in most cases of acute sinusitis. CT scans provide exquisitely detailed views of all the paranasal sinuses and reveal many acute changes that are not detected by standard radiography. In some hospitals, the cost of limited CT scans of the sinuses has become equivalent to that of standard sinus radiographs [53]. CT scans are particularly useful in the patient with chronic sinusitis who is not responding to standard therapy, in those with underlying immunocompromised status, or in patients in whom an intracranial complication is suspected [55] or orbital complication (see Chap. 6) is a concern.
      The major deficiency of any imaging technique currently available for diagnosing acute sinusitis is the inability to distinguish bacterially infected sinuses from those with inflammation due to a viral infection or nonbacterial cause. Recent data have shown acute reversible CT abnormalities in the sinus cavities of patients with early and presumed uncomplicated colds; most of these findings, however, resolve or markedly improve on follow-up exam at approximately 2 weeks, the time when acute sinusitis is likely to develop [53].
    E. **Nasal endoscopy** is useful in selected cases, especially in the patient with prolonged symptoms despite presumed adequate therapy and the patient with repeat episodes of acute sinusitis. It is not indicated for the uncomplicated case of acute sinusitis.
    F. **Direct sinus aspiration** can provide excellent material for Gram stain and for both aerobic and anaerobic cultures. The procedure is therapeutic as well as diagnostic and should be considered particularly in patients who do not respond to initial therapy, who are immunocompromised and at risk for sinusitis due to unusual pathogens, and those with nosocomial sinusitis when it is not possible to predict or identify the susceptibility of the causative pathogen(s) [53].
IV. **Therapy**
    A. **Antibiotics are given empirically** to cover common sinus pathogens. **The optimal duration of therapy is unclear. Usually antibiotics are given for 10–14 days for acute sinusitis** [53]. In one study, 3 days of TMP-SMX appeared as effective for carefully selected acute maxillary sinusitis as did a 10-day regimen (see sec. 2).
      1. **Amoxicillin and ampicillin** are commonly recommended. For older children and adults, 500 mg PO tid for 3 or 4 days, and then 250 mg tid for an additional 7 days, may be given. (If ampicillin is used, 500 mg PO qid can be given for 3–4 days, followed by 250 mg qid for another 7 days.) In children, 40 mg/kg/day of amoxicillin in three divided doses for 10 days has been shown to produce a clinical cure rate of approximately 80% [51].
      2. **Penicillin-allergic patients** can be treated effectively with **trimethoprim-sulfamethoxazole** (80-mg and 400-mg regular tablets: two regular tablets bid or one double-strength tablet bid in adults). TMP-SMX also would cover *H. influenzae,* which may be resistant to ampicillin (although this is not considered a major problem in sinusitis). In the patient with ampicillin and sulfa drug allergies, an oral cephalosporin (e.g., cefaclor, cefprozil, or cefuroxime) can be used.

Cefixime is a consideration, but this agent is less active than the others against *S. pneumoniae*. (See Chap. 28F.)

In one report, selected patients with acute maxillary sinusitis appeared to respond as well to a 3-day course of TMP-SMX as did those treated for 10 days [56[. Patients with prolonged symptoms (over 30 days), prior sinus surgery, antibiotics within the prior week, and immunocompromised patients and children were excluded. Also patients who had prominent symptoms of frontal sinusitis (e.g., pronounced frontal headache or tenderness) were excluded; these patients probably deserve a longer course of antibiotics because the posterior wall of the frontal sinus provides a relatively thin barrier to central nervous system infection.

3. **Other regimens** have been used in the allergic patient and/or when it is desirable to provide activity against beta-lactamase–producing sinus pathogens. These include the following, usually for 14 days [53].

   a. Amoxicillin-clavulanate 250–500 mg/125 mg q8h (see Chap. 28E).

   b. Cefaclor 500 mg q6h, cefuroxime axetil 250 mg q12h, and cefixime 200 mg q12h. (See Chap. 28F on cephalosporins for a detailed discussion.)

4. **New macrolides.** Although the exact role of these agents for acute sinusitis is still evolving, preliminary studies suggest both clarithromycin and azithromycin are as effective for uncomplicated acute maxillary sinusitis as is amoxicillin [57]. See detailed discussion of these agents in Chap. 28M.

   Some authors are concerned about the level of activity of these agents against *H. influenzae* [53].

B. **Decongestants** usually are given.

1. **Oxymetazoline hydrochloride** nasal spray (e.g., Afrin), 3 times daily for 48–72 hours, commonly is used as a topical vasoconstricting agent for the nasal mucosa.

2. **Pseudoephedrine hydrochloride** can be used as a decongestant. In adults, one 60-mg tablet can be given tid–qid.

C. **Topical nasal steroids** (e.g., beclomethasone AQ) for 2–3 weeks may be beneficial, especially in those patients who do not respond initially to the preceding measures or in severe cases.

D. **Follow-up** generally is indicated. In patients who do not respond to therapy, careful consideration should be given to an ear, nose, and throat (ENT) consultation.

V. **Chronic sinusitis** is often a complication of allergies or, at times, inadequately treated acute sinusitis. It is more difficult to treat than acute sinusitis. Aspiration studies in adults and children commonly reveal a mixture of aerobes and anaerobes. **Patients with chronic symptoms often need referral to an otolaryngologist** for nasal endoscopy or CT studies (without contrast) and consideration of a drainage procedure. Acute exacerbation of symptoms may be due to superimposed acute infections. In general, along with the otolaryngology follow-up, the same principles of antibiotic therapy are applied as described in sec. **IV.** The optimal duration of antibiotic therapy is unclear, and some experts suggest protracted courses of 3–4 weeks.

VI. **Sinusitis in HIV-infected patients** is a common problem, particularly as their degree of immunodeficiency becomes more profound. In addition to the common etiologies, *S. epidermidis, P. aeruginosa, Streptococcus viridans, P. acnes,* gram-negative enteric organisms, *Mycobacterium avium* complex, and *Aspergillus* can cause sinusitis in these patients. Clinical signs and symptoms can be few, despite extensive sinus disease, especially in patients with CD4 counts of less than 200 and chronic sinusitis. The most common symptoms are headache and fever [54]. Most patients respond, at least partially, to antibiotics, but many will require surgical drainage. In one retrospective series, only 29% of the patients had complete resolution of symptoms, whereas 60% had recurrent or persistent symptoms over 12 or more weeks [58].

External Otitis

The common, relatively **benign forms of external otitis must be distinguished from a severe form of external otitis called** *malignant external otitis.*

I. **External otitis** [59] is a superficial infection of the external auditory canal that is frequently initiated by moisture. It is most commonly caused by *Pseudomonas* spp. Patients complain of pain, itching, and a sensation of fullness in the ear, and they may experience pain on examination. Exudate, erythema, and edema may be seen in the canal. Although the drum may be involved, it moves well with the pneumatic otoscope, in contrast to the immobility observed with otitis media. **Topical treatment usually suffices.** Often, the condition responds to careful cleaning of the canal by gentle suction or irrigation. In other instances, antibiotic drops (polymyxin, neomycin, and hydrocortisone [e.g., Cortisporin otic]) or dilute acetic acid or boric acid solutions suffice. If there is extensive edema in the canal, some ENT specialists insert a cotton wick saturated in 50% Burow's solution. If the infection has spread to cause cellulitis of surrounding tissues, systemic antibiotics may be necessary.

II. **Malignant external otitis** is a **very serious infection** and is associated with a high mortality (20%) [60]. Infection can spread from the external canal to the adjacent deep soft tissue and bony structures.

A. **Setting.** This disease occurs usually in **elderly diabetics.** It is unclear why these patients are so predisposed to this devastating infection.

B. **Symptoms and signs.** Patients complain of pain and tenderness of the tissues around the ear and in the mastoid region. Often, there is **persistent drainage** from the external canal. The presence of granulation tissue at the junction of the osseous and cartilaginous portions of the external ear is a highly suggestive finding. **Neurologic complications can occur** and are discussed in sec. **F.**

C. **Etiology.** Almost all cases have been due to *P. aeruginosa.*

D. **Diagnosis** often is difficult; one must have a high index of suspicion. The diagnosis must be considered in any diabetic with an external otitis (due to *P. aeruginosa*) who does not respond to topical therapy. Systemic manifestations of fever and leukocytosis usually are absent. As routine roentgenograms may be unremarkable, CT scanning is preferred over MRI for initial diagnosis [60a].

E. **Therapy.** Most patients require hospitalization and, at least initially, combination parenteral antibiotics to achieve synergy against *P. aeruginosa.* In this severe infection, ticarcillin or piperacillin often is combined with tobramycin or another aminoglycoside to which the pathogen is susceptible. In the penicillin-allergic patient, ceftazidime can be combined with an aminoglycoside (see Chap. 28 for details). Extensive surgical debridement is not necessary, but ENT consultation is advised.

Because of the presumed or documented bone-related infection, protracted antibiotic therapy is used (e.g., 4–6 weeks). If the pathogen is susceptible to ciprofloxacin, the oral agent may be very useful in the completion of a full course of antibiotics [61], and infectious disease consultation is advised for these difficult cases.

In a mild and early case of malignant external otitis, where careful compliance and follow-up can be assured, oral ciprofloxacin is a useful agent (see Chap. 28S). Infectious disease consultation is advised.

F. **Complications.** A **facial nerve palsy** can be seen in up to 50% of cases. Presumably, this is due to soft-tissue infection at the site of the seventh cranial nerve's exit from the stylomastoid foramen. Occasionally, there is osteomyelitis of the bony canal. Later, cranial nerves X, XI, and XII can be involved. Hoarseness, dysphagia, aspiration, and choking can be seen. Meningitis is rare.

References

1. Cohen, S., Tyrrell, D.A.J., and Smith, A.P. Psychological stress and susceptibility to the common cold. *N. Engl. J. Med.* 325:606–612, 1991.
2. Dick, E.C., et al. Aerosol transmission of rhinovirus colds. *J. Infect. Dis.* 156:442, 1987.
3. Wald, E.R., Guerra, N., and Byers, C. Upper respiratory tract infections in young children: Duration of and frequency of complications. *Pediatrics* 87:129–133, 1991.
   See related articles by T.A. Walker et al., Viral respiratory tract infections. Pediatr. Clin. North Am. *41:1365, 1994; and V.G. Hemming, Viral respiratory diseases in children: Classification, etiology, epidemiology, and risk factors.* J. Pediatr. *124: S13, 1994.*
4. Carson, J.L., Collier, A.M., and Hu, S.S. Acquired ciliary defects in nasal epithelium of children with acute viral upper respiratory infections. *N. Engl. J. Med.* 312:463, 1985.
5. Gwaltney, J.M. Combined antiviral and antimediator treatment of rhinovirus colds. *J. Infect. Dis.* 166:776–782, 1992.
6. Breese, B.B., and Hall, C.B. *Beta-Hemolytic Streptococcal Diseases.* Boston: Houghton Mifflin, 1978.
   Excellent color photographs of cases of pharyngitis with detailed discussions of this complex issue.

7. McMillan, J.A., et al. Viral and bacterial organisms associated with acute pharyngitis in a school-aged population. *J. Pediatr.* 109:747, 1986.
    Prospective study of 317 patients and 301 controls.
8. Huovinen, P., et al. Pharyngitis in adults: The presence and co-existence of viruses and bacterial organisms. *Ann. Intern. Med.* 110:612, 1989.
9. Grayston, J.T., et al. A new respiratory tract pathogen: *Chlamydia pneumoniae* strain TWAR. *J. Infect. Dis.* 161:618–625, 1990.
    For a recent related review, see M.R. Hammerschlag. Antimicrobial susceptibility and therapy of infections caused by Chlamydia pneumoniae. Antimicrob. Agents Chemother. *38:1873, 1994. Therapy of this pathogen may require 2–3 weeks of erythromycin or tetracycline. Shorter courses of azithromycin are feasible.*
9a. Shulman, S.T. Streptococcal pharyngitis: Diagnostic considerations. *Pediatr. Infect. Dis. J.* 13:567, 1994.
    See related articles in this journal, which contains a special series of articles on group A streptococcal infections in the 1990s.
10. Kaplan, E.L., and Krugman, S. Streptococcal Infections, Group A. In S. Krugman et al. (eds.), *Infectious Diseases of Children* (9th ed.). St. Louis: Mosby, 1992. P. 474.
11. Yanagihara, R., and Todd, J.K. Acute febrile mucocutaneous lymph node syndrome. *Am. J. Dis. Child.* 134:603, 1980.
    Excellent review of Kawasaki's disease.
12. Todd, J.K. The sore throat: Pharyngitis and epiglottitis. *Infect. Dis. Clin. North Am.* 2:149, 1988.
13. deMarie, S., et al. Clinical infections and nonsurgical treatment of parapharyngeal space infections complicating throat infection. *Rev. Infect. Dis.* 11:975, 1989.
14. Miller, R.A., Brancato, F., and Holmes, K.K. *Corynebacterium hemolyticum* as a cause of pharyngitis and scarlatiniform rash in young adults. *Ann. Intern. Med.* 105:867, 1986.
    Study and review with color photos of rash and Gram stain.
    The name of this organism has been changed to Arcanobacterium haemolyticum. *For a recent update on this topic see A. Mackenzie et al., Incidence and pathogenicity of* Arcanobacterium haemolyticum *during a 2-year study in Ottawa.* Clin. Infect. Dis. *21:177, 1995. In this July 1995 report, this organism appeared to be a pathogen in patients with pharyngitis, especially in 15–18-year-old patients. The organism is highly susceptible to erythromycin and less susceptible to penicillin.*
15. Dajani, A.S. Current status of nonsuppurative complications of Group A streptococci. *Pediatr. Infect. Dis. J.* 10:525–527, 1991.
16. Wegner, D.L., Witte, D.L., and Schrantz, R.D. Insensitivity of rapid antigen detection methods and single blood agar plate culture for diagnosing streptococcal pharyngitis. *J.A.M.A.* 267:695–697, 1992.
    See related article by B. Schwartz et al., Physicians' diagnostic approach to pharyngitis and impact of CLIA 1988 on office diagnostic tests. J.A.M.A. *271:234, 1994.*
16a. Gerber, M.A. Treatment failures and carriers: Perception or problems? *Pediatr. Infect. Dis. J.* 13:576, 1994.
    This is an excellent summary of a complex topic.
17. Pichichero, M.E., et al. Adverse and beneficial effects of immediate treatment of group A beta-hemolytic streptococcal pharyngitis with penicillin. *Pediatr. Infect. Dis. J.* 6:635, 1987.
    Patients treated early had a significantly higher recurrence rate.
18. Hall, C.B., and Breese, B.B. Does penicillin make Johnny's strep throat better? *Pediatr. Infect. Dis.* 3:7, 1984.
19. Krober, M.S., Bass, J.W., and Michels, G.N. Streptococcal pharyngitis: Placebo controlled double-blind evaluation of clinical response to penicillin therapy. *J.A.M.A.* 253:1271, 1985.
    Excellent study proving that penicillin results in a significantly faster clinical improvement.
20. Kaplan, E.L. The group A streptococcal upper respiratory tract carrier state: An enigma. *J. Pediatr.* 97:337, 1980.
    In-depth analysis of carrier state and clinical implications.
21. Breese, B.B., et al. Consensus: Difficult management problems in children with streptococcal pharyngitis. *Pediatr. Infect. Dis.* 4:10, 1985.
22. Gerber, M.A., and Markowitz, M. Management of streptococcal pharyngitis reconsidered. *Pediatr. Infect. Dis.* 4:518, 1985.
    Good review of streptococcal pharyngitis.

23. Pichichero, M.E. The rising incidence of penicillin treatment failures in Group A streptococcal tonsillopharyngitis: An emerging role for the cephalosporin? *Pediatr. Infect. Dis. J.* 10:S50–S55, 1991.
    See also reference [16a], which suggests that penicillin "failures" are often misinterpreted.
24. Bass, J.W. Antibiotic management of Group A streptococcal pharyngotonsillitis. *Pediatr. Infect. Dis. J.* 10:S43–S49, 1991.
24a. Klein, J.O. Management of streptococcal pharyngitis. *Pediatr. Infect. Dis. J.* 13: 572, 1994.
25. Dajani, A.S., et al. Treatment of acute streptococcal pharyngitis and prevention of rheumatic fever: A statement for health professionals by the committee on rheumatic fever, endocarditis, and Kawasaki disease of the council on cardiovascular disease in the young, the American Heart Association. *Pediatrics* 96:758, 1995.
26. Markowitz, M., Gerber, M.A., and Kaplan, E.L. Treatment of streptococcal pharyngotonsillitis: Reports of penicillin's demise are premature. *J. Pediatr.* 123:679–685, 1993.
    See also related reference [16a].
26a. Peter, G. et al. (eds.). *Report of the Committee on Infectious Diseases: 1994 Red Book* (23rd ed.). Elk Grove Village, IL: American Academy of Pediatrics, 1994. Pp. 434–436.
27. Pichichero, M.F. Cephalosporins are superior to penicillin for treatment of streptococcal tonsillopharyngitis: Is the difference worth it? *Pediatr. Infect. Dis. J.* 12:268–274, 1993.
28. Bachand, R.T., Jr. A comparative study of clarithromycin and penicillin VK in the treatment of outpatients with streptococcal pharyngitis. *J. Antimicrob. Chemother.* 27(Suppl. A):75–82, 1991.
29. Stein, G.E., Christensen, S., and Mummaw, N. Comparative study of clarithromycin and penicillin V in the treatment of streptococcal pharyngitis. *Eur. J. Clin. Microbiol. Infect. Dis.* 10:949–953, 1991.
30. Hooton, T.M. A comparison of azithromycin and penicillin V for the treatment of streptococcal pharyngitis. *Am. J. Med.* 91(Suppl. 3A):23S–26S, 1991.
31. Chaudhary, S., et al. Penicillin V and rifampin for the treatment of group A streptococcal pharyngitis: A randomized trial of 10 days penicillin vs 10 days penicillin with rifampin during the final 4 days of therapy. *J. Pediatr.* 106:481, 1985.
    There were no bacteriologic failures in patients who received rifampin.
32. Tanz, R.R., et al. Clindamycin treatment of chronic pharyngeal carriage of group A streptococci. *J. Pediatr.* 119:123–128, 1991.
33. Dobie, R.A., and Tobey, D.N. Clinical features of diphtheria in the respiratory tract. *J.A.M.A.* 242:2197, 1979.
    Forty-four cases are reviewed. Airway obstruction was the most common cause of death. Tracheostomy should be considered when laryngeal membrane is present on indirect laryngoscopy.
33a. Klein, J.O. Lessons from recent studies on the epidemiology of otitis media. *Pediatr. Infect. Dis. J.* 13:1081, 1994.
34. Bluestone, C.D. Current therapy for otitis media and criteria for evaluation of new antimicrobial agents. *Clin. Infect. Dis.* 14(Suppl. 2):S197–S203, 1992.
34a. Berman, S. Otitis media in children. *N. Engl. J. Med.* 332:1560, 1995.
    This June 1995 "current concepts" is an excellent summary. See also S. Berman, Otitis media in developing countries. Pediatrics 96:126, 1995.
35. McCracken, G.H., Jr. Considerations in selecting an antibiotic for treatment of acute otitis media. *Pediatr. Infect. Dis. J.* 13:1054, 1994.
    Nice summary of the natural history of AOM, clinical efficacy of therapy with antibiotics, choosing an antibiotic regimen, and preferred regimens.
35a. Klein, J.O., Bluestone, C.D., and McCracken, G.H., Jr. New perspectives in management of otitis media. *Pediatr. Infect. Dis. J.* 13:1030, 1994.
    Excellent symposium about the microbiology, pathophysiology, diagnosis, treatment, and prevention of otitis media.
36. Shurin, P.A., et al. Bacterial etiology of otitis media during the first six weeks of life. *J. Pediatr.* 92:893, 1978.
37. Tetzlaff, T.R., Ashworth, C., and Nelson, J.D. Otitis media in children less than 12 weeks of age. *Pediatrics* 59:827, 1977.
38. Klein, B.S., Dollete, F.R., and Yolken, R.H. The role of respiratory syncytial virus and other viral pathogens in acute otitis media. *J. Pediatr.* 101:16, 1982.
    Evidence that viral pathogens are important in otitis media.

39. Chonmaitree, T., Howie, V.M., and Truant, A.L. Presence of respiratory viruses in middle ear fluids and nasal wash specimens from children with acute otitis media. *Pediatrics* 77:698, 1986.
    Study demonstrating presence of viruses in middle ear fluid and nasal secretions.
39a. Ruuskanen, O., and Heikkinen, T. Viral-bacterial interaction in acute otitis media. *Pediatr. Infect. Dis. J.* 13:1047, 1994.
    Respiratory viruses are important in the pathogenesis of AOM. Viruses may predispose the middle-ear epithelium to bacterial infection and cause dysfunction of the eustachian tube. In particular, AOMs have been associated with RSV, rhinovirus, influenza A virus, adenovirus, and parainfluenza virus outbreaks. See related article by X. Saez-Llorens, Pathogenesis of acute otitis media. Pediatr. Infect. Dis. J. *13:1035, 1994.*
40. Bluestone, C.D., Stephenson, J.S., and Martin, L.M. Ten-year review of otitis media pathogens. *Pediatr. Infect. Dis. J.* 11:S7–S11, 1992.
41. Henderson, F.W., et al. A longitudinal study of respiratory viruses and bacteria in the etiology of acute otitis media with effusion. *N. Engl. J. Med.* 306:1377, 1982.
    Excellent, prospective long-term study of otitis media correlated with etiology and epidemiology.
42. Cantekin, E.I., et al. Lack of efficacy of decongestant-antihistamine combination for otitis media with effusion ("secretory" otitis media) in children. *N. Engl. J. Med.* 308:297, 1983.
43. Olson, A.L., et al. Prevention and therapy of serous otitis media by oral decongestant: A double-blind study in pediatric practice. *Pediatrics* 61:679, 1978.
43a. Rosenfeld, R.M., et al. Clinical efficacy of antimicrobial drugs for acute otitis media: Metaanalysis of 5400 children from thirty-three randomized trials. *J. Pediatr.* 124:355, 1994.
44. Medical Letter. Drugs for treatment of acute otitis media in children. *Med. Lett. Drug. Ther.* 36:19, 1994.
45. Howie, V.M., Dillard, R., and Lawrence, B. In vivo sensitivity test in otitis media: Efficacy of antibiotics. *Pediatrics* 75:8, 1985.
    Excellent summary of well-designed and well-controlled studies on the therapy of otitis media with etiology determined by tympanocentesis.
46. Bluestone, C.D. Surgical management of otitis media: Current indications and role-related increasing bacterial resistance. *Pediatr. Infect. Dis. J.* 13:1058, 1994.
    Nice review of current surgical options.
    With the increasing rise in the rate of resistant bacteria being isolated from the middle ears of some children with otitis media, prolonged antibiotic therapy is a potential concern, and surgical intervention may be useful, especially in some settings (e.g., large daycare centers). Culture at the time of tube placement is advised.
47. Teele, D.W. Long-term sequelae of otitis media: Fact or fancy? *Pediatr. Infect. Dis. J.* 13:1069, 1994.
    Includes a summary from a multidisciplinary group of experts entitled, Otitis media with effusion in young children. Clinical practice guideline No. 12. July 1994. Rockville, MD: U.S. Dept. of Health and Human Services, 1994.
47a. Nadol, J.B., Jr., and Eavey, R.D. Acute and chronic mastoiditis: Clinical presentation, diagnosis, and management. *Curr. Clin. Top. Infect. Dis.* 15:204, 1995.
48. Giebink, G.S. Immunology: Promise of new vaccines. *Pediatr. Infect. Dis. J.* 13:1064, 1994.
    A supplemental issue on this important topic.
49. Evans, F.O., et al. Sinusitis of the maxillary antrum. *N. Engl. J. Med.* 293:735, 1975.
50. Hamory, B.H., et al. Etiology and antimicrobial therapy of acute maxillary sinusitis. *J. Infect. Dis.* 139:197, 1979.
    Study of ampicillin, amoxicillin, and trimethoprim-sulfamethoxazole in sinusitis. See also reference [49].
51. Wald, E.R. Acute sinusitis in children. *Pediatr. Infect. Dis.* 2:61, 1983.
    A good review of sinusitis in children. For an update, see E.R. Wald, Sinusitis in children. Pediatr. Infect. Dis. J. *7:S150, 1988.*
52. Williams, J.W., Jr., et al. Clinical evaluation for sinusitis: Making the diagnosis by history and physical examination. *Ann. Intern. Med.* 117:705, 1992.
53. Gwaltney, J.M., Jr. Sinusitis. In G.L. Mandell, J.E. Bennett, and R. Dolin (eds.), *Principles and Practice of Infectious Diseases* (4th ed.). New York: Churchill Livingstone, 1995. Pp. 585–590.
54. Godofsky, E.W., et al. Sinusitis in HIV-infected patients: A clinical and radiographic review. *Am. J. Med.* 93:163–170, 1992.

55. Rosenfeld, E.A., and Rowley, A.H. Infectious intracranial complications of sinusitis, other than meningitis, in children: 12-year review. *Clin. Infect. Dis.* 18:750, 1994.

56. Williams, J.W., Jr., et al. Randomized controlled trial of 3 vs. 10 days of trimethoprim/ sulfamethoxazole for acute maxillary sinusitis. *J.A.M.A.* 273:1015, 1995.
    The daily dose of TMP-SMX was one double-strength tablet bid. For those who fail the 3-day regimen (about 25%), the authors suggest a 10–14-day course of broad-spectrum antibiotics active against beta-lactamase–producing organisms and sinus radiographs to confirm the diagnosis. If this therapy also fails, the patient should be referred to an otolaryngologist.

57. Eisenberg, E., and Barza, M. Azithromycin and clarithromycin. *Curr. Clin. Top. Infect. Dis.* 14:52, 1994.

58. Zurlo, J.J., et al. Sinusitis in HIV-1 infection. *Am. J. Med.* 93:157–162, 1992.

59. Farmer, H.S. A guide for the treatment of external otitis. *Am. Fam. Physician* 21: 96, 1980.
    Otolaryngologist's view of this common problem. Practical approach.

60. Johnson, M.P., and Romphal, R. Malignant external otitis: Report on therapy with ceftazidime and review of therapy and prognosis. *Rev. Infect. Dis.* 12:173–180, 1990.

60a. Grandis, J.R., Curtin, H.D., and Yu, V.L. Necrotizing (malignant) external otitis: Prospective comparison of CT and MR imaging in diagnosis and follow-up. *Radiology* 196:499, 1995.
    This study concludes that CT is preferred at initial diagnosis, as small cortical erosions are better seen. Either modality can be used to follow-up soft-tissue evolution. MRI may be better for evaluation and follow-up of meningeal enhancement and changes within the osseous cavity.

61. Lang, R., et al. Successful treatment of malignant external otitis with oral ciprofloxa-cin; report of experience with 23 patients. *J. Infect. Dis.* 161:537–540, 1990.
    See related paper by P. Gehanno, Ciprofloxacin in the treatment of malignant external otitis. Chemotherapy 40(Suppl. 1):35, 1994.

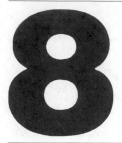

Influenza and Infections of the Trachea, Bronchi, and Bronchioles

John J. Treanor
and Caroline Breese Hall

Influenza

Influenza is a relatively specific syndrome resulting from infection with any influenza A or B virus. Infection with other respiratory viruses occasionally may result in influenzalike illness, but other viruses do not cause epidemics that affect all age groups. Infection with influenza A or B virus may result in any of the other viral syndromes discussed in this chapter. Influenza C virus infection results in only a small proportion of common cold illnesses and will not be discussed in this chapter.

I. **Etiology.** Influenza viruses are medium-sized enveloped viruses with a segmented RNA genome and are classified into types A, B, and C [1, 2]. The envelope of influenza A and B viruses contains two glycoproteins, the hemagglutinin (H) and the neuraminidase (N). Multiple subtypes of H and N exist for influenza A viruses. Thus, standard nomenclature for these viruses includes the type, location, and year of isolation, strain designation, and H and N subtype for influenza A viruses. For example, a specific strain of influenza A virus isolated in Beijing, China, in 1992, with subtype H3 hemagglutinin and N2 neuraminidase might be termed *influenza A/Beijing/32/92 (H3N2) virus.*

II. **Epidemiology** [3, 4]. Influenza virus infection occurs in yearly epidemics, with occasional worldwide epidemics referred to as *pandemics.* In a given community, an epidemic lasts 5–6 weeks and may be associated with attack rates as high as 10–20% of the population. Attack rates are generally highest in young children, whereas hospitalization rates are highest in the elderly. **Influenza is unique in that yearly epidemic activity is manifested by increases in school absenteeism, visits to health care facilities, admissions to hospitals for pneumonia, and deaths. Influenza viruses have a high degree of antigenic variability,** which allows for recurrent epidemics despite widespread prior exposure to influenza viruses in the population [5]. Two forms of this antigenic variation are recognized—antigenic drift and antigenic shift.

A. **Antigenic drift** refers to relatively **minor antigenic change** within the H or N due to the accumulation of point mutations. The antigenically variant virus is able to infect individuals and spread within the population despite the presence of antibody to previous strains of virus, and epidemics of variable extent result. Antigenic drift occurs in both influenza A and B viruses.

B. **Antigenic shift** refers to **major antigenic change** within the H or N, resulting in a new subtype. Antigenically shifted viruses enter a population that is essentially immunologically naive, and worldwide pandemics are the result (Table 8-1). Antigenic shift is likely the result of genetic reassortment between animal and human influenza viruses and occurs only with influenza A viruses.

III. **Clinical manifestations** [1, 6–9]. Characteristically, the onset of influenza is abrupt after an **incubation period** of 1–2 days. Many patients can recall the hour of onset.

A. **Symptoms. Systemic symptoms** predominate and include feverishness; chilliness or, occasionally, frank shaking chills; headaches; myalgias; malaise; and anorexia. Malaise and fatigue may be quite prolonged. Headache is a common complaint. Myalgias may involve the extremities or the long muscles of the back, and arthralgias, but not frank arthritis, are observed. **Respiratory symptoms,** particularly dry cough or nasal discharge, also are usually present at the onset, but they are

Revised from C. Breese Hall and R. Gordon Douglas, Jr. Influenza and Infections of the Trachea, Bronchi, and Bronchioles. In R.E. Reese and R.F. Betts (eds.), *A Practical Approach to Infectious Diseases* (3rd ed.). Boston: Little, Brown, 1991.

Table 8-1. Major antigenic shifts and pandemic influenza

Year	Interval (years)	Designation	Changes in indicated surface proteins	Results
1889	—	H3N2	—	Moderate pandemic
1918	29	H1N1	H, N	Most severe pandemic
1957	39	H2N2	H, N	Severe pandemic
1968	11	H3N2	H	Moderate pandemic
1977	9	H1N1	H, N	Mild

H = hemagglutinin; N = neuraminidase.

overshadowed by the systemic symptoms. Nasal obstruction, hoarseness, and dry or sore throat may be present as well, and these symptoms tend to become more prominent as the disease progresses. **Ocular symptoms,** although less commonly present, are helpful diagnostically and include photophobia, tearing, burning, and pain on moving the eyes. **In the young infant,** influenza may mimic sepsis, with fever and no localizing findings. Even in older children, influenza may be manifest occasionally as an undifferentiated febrile illness without respiratory or localizing symptoms.

   B. **Signs.** Early in the course of illness, the patient appears toxic, the face is flushed, and the skin is hot and moist. Eyes are watery and reddened.
      1. **Fever** is the most important finding. It usually rises rapidly to a peak of 100°–106°F (38°–41°C) within 12 hours of onset of systemic symptoms. It usually is continuous but may be intermittent, especially if antipyretics are administered. On the second and third days of illness, the fever is usually 0.5°–1.0°F (0.5°C) lower and, as the fever subsides, the systemic symptoms disappear. Classically, the duration of fever is 3 days, but it may last from 1 to 5 or more days.

      Illness appears to be similar at any age except that fever is more common and higher in childhood than in elderly patients.
      2. **Nasal and other respiratory findings.** Clear **nasal discharge** is common, but nasal obstruction is less frequent. The mucous membranes of the nose and throat are hyperemic, but exudate is not observed. Small, tender cervical lymph nodes may be present. Transient, scattered rhonchi or localized areas of rales are found in fewer than 20% of cases.

      As systemic signs and symptoms diminish, respiratory complaints and findings become more apparent. **Cough** is the most frequent and troublesome symptom and may be accompanied by substernal discomfort or burning. Nasal obstruction and discharge and pharyngeal pain and injection also are common. Such symptoms and signs usually persist 3–4 days after fever subsides, and cough commonly persists longer. Cough, lassitude, and malaise may last 1–2 weeks after disappearance of other manifestations.

IV. **Laboratory findings** are nonspecific. Leukocytosis of up to 15,000 cells/mm^3 is commonly observed early in the illness, usually without a shift to the left. Mild leukopenia may be observed later. Pulmonary findings seen on roentgenograms are described in sec. **VII.A.**

V. **Diagnosis**
   A. **Viral cultures. Specific diagnosis is best made by viral culture techniques.** The rapid diagnostic methods such as immunofluorescence or enzyme-linked immunosorbent assay (ELISA) are less reliable. **Swap specimens of throat and nose are ideal and need to be plunged into viral transport media** for good results. In cases of tracheobronchitis or pneumonia, sputum constitutes the best specimen in adults, whereas in children a nasal wash is best. Specimens should be tested in cell cultures or embryonated chicken eggs, and they may yield positive results as early as 3 days. For isolated or complicated cases, viral diagnosis is essential. (For further discussion of viral culture techniques, see Chap. 25.)
   B. **Influenza A direct antigen tests** have become available (e.g., Directogen Flu A, Becton Dickinson, Cockeysville, MD) in which nasopharyngeal secretions can be tested for the viral antigen. When positive, this test provides a useful technique

for rapid diagnosis; when negative, viral cultures are suggested because of the low sensitivity of the test. This test is discussed in Chap. 25.

C. **Epidemiologic data are sufficient to make the diagnosis in most uncomplicated cases** [10]; that is, when it is established that influenza A virus is prevalent in the community, most persons with acute febrile respiratory or acute febrile undifferentiated illness can safely be assumed to have influenza A virus infection. On the other hand, in hospitalized patients with complications of influenza, specimens for viral cultures should be obtained, especially if other nonviral processes are being considered in the differential diagnosis. For hospitals without viral diagnostic facilities, specimens often can be sent to the state health department laboratory, and these should be shipped on wet ice.

D. **Serologic studies** of acute and convalescent sera can be useful in making a retrospective diagnosis. Convalescent serum should be obtained at least 2 weeks after onset of illness. Complement fixation tests are used commonly.

VI. **Treatment**

A. **Symptomatic.** Symptomatic therapy such as that described for common colds, pharyngitis, and tracheobronchitis may be advised for fever, headache, myalgias, and cough. **Salicylates and salicylate-containing medications are not advised for children with influenza** [11]. **The use of salicylates in children has been associated with Reye's syndrome.** (Acetaminophen and ibuprofen are commonly used as antipyretic agents.)

B. **Antiviral agents**

1. The chemically related antiviral drugs **amantadine** and **rimantadine** [12, 13] are both **active only against influenza A virus** at clinically achievable levels. Both drugs are effective in the treatment of influenza A when administered within 48 hours of the onset of symptoms. Most studies have shown more rapid reductions in symptoms and fever and reduced levels and duration of virus shedding when compared to placebo or to aspirin or acetaminophen [14, 15]. The drugs should be administered during the period of acute illness only and for no longer than 5–7 days. Controlled studies of the efficacy of these drugs in the treatment of complicated influenza (e.g., hospitalized patients or those with pneumonia; see sec. **VII**) have not been reported. In most cases, such patients will be seen relatively later in the course of illness, and antiviral drug therapy may not be as effective. However, most authorities would support the use of amantadine or rimantadine in the treatment of complicated influenza A. Influenza viruses resistant to the antiviral effects of these drugs frequently are isolated from treated individuals. Where possible, individuals being treated with amantadine or rimantadine should not be in close contact with those receiving chemoprophylaxis, to reduce the chances of selection and transmission of resistant viruses.

    For further discussion of these agents see Chap. 26.

2. **Ribavirin** is active against both influenza A and B virus in vitro. Controlled studies of ribavirin aerosol therapy of uncomplicated influenza A and B in young adults have shown modest activity. See related discussion in Chap. 26.

C. **Antibiotics. Antibiotics should not be used in uncomplicated influenza: They are of no benefit and will alter the flora of the upper respiratory tract, allowing superinfection with a resistant bacterium to occur.** Treatment of bacterial pneumonia complicating influenza should be directed toward the most likely pathogen or pathogens.

VII. **Complications.** The great majority of influenza cases are not associated with any significant complications. However, a variety of well-recognized complications do occur [6].

A. Two kinds of **pulmonary complications** are well recognized: primary influenza viral pneumonia and secondary bacterial pneumonia [16].

1. **Primary influenza viral pneumonia.** Primary influenza viral pneumonia occurs predominantly in persons with cardiovascular disease (especially rheumatic heart disease with mitral stenosis) or in pregnant women. Cases rarely occur in young healthy adults, however.

    a. **Clinical manifestations.** Following a typical onset of influenza, there is usually rapid progression of fever, cough, dyspnea, hypoxemia, and cyanosis. Physical examination and chest roentgenogram reveal bilateral findings that often are consistent with pulmonary edema, but no consolidation is seen. There are no pathognomonic findings. (Dyspnea, hypoxemia, and bilateral infiltrates are commonly seen in the adult respiratory distress syndrome, which is due to many causes, including influenza.)

Bacteriologic examination of the sputum fails to reveal significant bacteria, whereas viral cultures yield high titers of influenza virus.

b. **Course and prognosis.** These patients often show **a progressive downhill course. They do not respond to antibiotics** because bacteria play no role. Serial arterial blood gases show progressive hypoxemia. Despite supportive care with artificial ventilation (including extracorporeal oxygenation), mortality is high. At autopsy, findings consist of tracheitis, bronchitis, diffuse hemorrhagic pneumonia, hyaline membrane lining alveolar ducts and alveoli, and a paucity of inflammatory cells within the alveoli.

c. In addition, **a relatively mild form of viral interstitial pneumonia may occur in young children** that is clinically similar to the lower respiratory tract disease produced by other common respiratory viruses in infants, such as respiratory syncytial and parainfluenza viruses. These infants may present with a fever, mild cough, and upper respiratory tract symptoms, and may be admitted with the diagnosis of possible sepsis. The chest roentgenogram typically shows interstitial infiltrates in one or more lobes. In such situations, the involvement of the lower respiratory tract is part of the acute influenza syndrome rather than a secondary complication. Comparative features of the secondary pulmonary complications of influenza are shown in Table 8-2.

2. **Secondary bacterial pneumonia occurs more commonly** than primary viral pneumonia and often presents as a characteristic syndrome.

   a. **Clinical manifestations.** These patients, who very often are elderly or have pulmonary disease, have a classic influenza illness, often followed by a period of improvement lasting 1–4 days. They then appear to have a relapse. Recrudescence of fever is associated with such symptoms and signs of bacterial pneumonia as cough, sputum production, and possibly an area of consolidation on physical examination and chest roentgenogram. However, the period of improvement may not occur, and the course is variable. Gram stains and cultures of sputum reveal predominance of a pathogen, most often *Streptococcus pneumoniae* and *Haemophilus influenzae*. Mixed bacterial pneumonias can occur. *Staphylococcus aureus* secondary pneumonia can occur.

   b. **Course and prognosis.** These patients **will respond to specific antibiotic therapy** and supportive measures.

   c. **Therapy.** Except for young infants with mild interstitial pneumonia as a component of the acute influenza syndrome, antibiotic therapy probably is indicated in most patients because of the difficulty of making a definitive diagnosis of pure viral pneumonia. **Where possible, therapy should be guided by the results of sputum Gram stain and culture.** Initial empiric therapy is directed against the organisms described in **a,** and monotherapy with cefuroxime (750 mg–1.5 g q8h), IV ceftriaxone (1 g q24h), or IV ampicillin-sulbactam (3 g q6–8h) is commonly used in this setting in adults with normal renal function.

3. **Other pulmonary complications.** During an outbreak of influenza, **many cases are observed that do not fit clearly into either of the preceding categories.** The disease is not relentlessly progressive, and yet the fever pattern may not be biphasic. **Many of these patients have mixed viral and bacterial infection** of the lung (see Table 8-2), and most of these mixed infections will respond to antibiotics. In addition, milder forms of influenza viral pneumonia involving only one lobe or segment have been described, which do not invariably lead to death and are more likely to be confused with pneumonia due to *Mycoplasma pneumoniae* than to that produced by bacterial infection.

B. **Reye's syndrome** is an often fatal hepatic and CNS complication. This has been seen most often **after influenza B** viral infection, but it can occur also after varicella and influenza A. Most patients are younger than 16 years, and the mortality is 20–40%. After several days of acute upper respiratory infection, the patient develops some degree of CNS manifestations such as lethargy or drowsiness. CNS manifestations may progress rapidly. The liver often is enlarged, and liver function tests are abnormal. There is **no known treatment.**

   Prior ingestion of aspirin and other salicylates is associated with an increased risk of Reye's syndrome [11] (see sec. **VI.A**). **Dissemination of warnings against the use of salicylates in children for influenza and febrile illnesses has resulted in a dramatic decline in the occurrence of Reye's syndrome.**

Table 8-2. Comparative features of pulmonary complications of influenza

Clinical parameter	Primary viral pneumonia	Secondary bacterial pneumonia	Mixed viral-bacterial pneumonia	Localized viral pneumonia
Setting	Cardiovascular disease; pregnancy; young adult (Hsw1N1)	Elderly age; pulmonary disease	Same as for primary viral or secondary bacterial pneumonia	?Normal host
Clinical history	Relentless progression from classic 3-day influenza	Improvement, then worsening after 3-day classic influenza	Picture of A or B	Continuation of cough after classic 3-day syndrome
Physical examination	Bilateral findings, no consolidation	Consolidation	Consolidation	Area of rales
Sputum ⎫ Bacteriologic ⎬ evaluation ⎭	Negative	Pneumococci Staphylococci, *H. influenzae*	Pneumococci Staphylococci, *H. influenzae*	Negative
Chest roentgenogram	Bilateral findings	Consolidation	Consolidation	Segmental infiltrate
WBC count	Leukocytosis with shift to left	Leukocytosis with shift to left	Leukocytosis with shift to left	Usually normal
Isolation of influenza virus	Yes	No	Yes	Yes
Response to antibiotics	No	Yes	Yes	No
Mortality	High	Low	Low	Very low

C. **Myositis and myoglobinuria** with tender leg muscles and elevated serum creatine phosphokinase (CPK) levels have been reported (mostly in children) after influenza A and influenza B infection, most commonly the latter. Symptoms may be sufficiently severe to prevent walking, but neurologic changes are not evident.

D. **Guillain-Barré syndrome (GBS)** has been reported to occur after influenza A infection, as it has after numerous other infections. In addition, cases of transverse myelitis and encephalitis have occurred rarely. Etiologic association with influenza virus infection has rarely been proved, and influenza infection accounts for only a small proportion of cases of each of these syndromes.

E. Both **myocarditis** and **pericarditis** have been associated rarely with influenza A and B viral infection. However, neither myocarditis nor pericarditis is observed commonly on autopsy of those dying of primary influenza viral pneumonia.

F. **Neurologic complications** besides Reye's syndrome may also occur with influenza, such as encephalopathy and ataxia. Febrile convulsions are a relatively frequent complication of influenza in preschool children.

VIII. **Prevention**

A. **Inactivated influenza vaccines.** Prospective, controlled trials in healthy adults have shown inactivated influenza vaccines to be safe and immunogenic and to have 70–90% efficacy in the prevention of influenza when a good antigenic match exists between the vaccine and the epidemic virus [17, 18]. Similar trials have not been reported in high-risk individuals or the elderly, but numerous retrospective case-control studies have shown that inactivated vaccine is effective in such individuals, particularly in the prevention of lower respiratory tract disease and complications [19, 19a]. Recent studies have also shown that vaccination of the elderly is cost-effective [19b].

1. **Formulation.** Inactivated influenza vaccines consist of inactivated whole virus, disrupted virus (split-product), or purified H and N (subunit) vaccines. The immunogenicity of each is similar. Because of the antigenic variability of influenza, the specific virus strains to be included in the vaccine are reviewed each year by the Bureau of Biologics of the US Food and Drug Administration. Over the last several years, a trivalent formulation, containing one H3N2, one H1N1, and one B virus, has been used, reflecting the recent epidemiology of influenza.

2. **Indications.** Target groups for influenza vaccination include those who are at increased risk for influenza-related complications and individuals who can transmit influenza to high-risk persons **(Table 8-3)**. In addition, vaccine may be used in any individual who wishes to avoid an unpleasant influenza illness.

3. **Administration. A single dose of vaccine is sufficient for most individuals, but two doses of vaccine are required in those who have not been primed**

Table 8-3. Target groups for influenza vaccination

Groups at increased risk for influenza-related complications
  Persons ≥65 years of age
  Residents of nursing homes and other chronic care facilities that house persons of any age with chronic medical conditions
  Adults and children with chronic disorders of the pulmonary and cardiovascular systems, including children with asthma
  Adults and children who have required regular medical follow-up or hospitalization during the preceding year because of chronic metabolic diseases (including diabetes mellitus), renal dysfunction, hemoglobinopathies, or immunosuppression (including immunosuppression caused by medications)
  Children and teenagers requiring long-term aspirin therapy
Groups that can transmit influenza to high-risk persons
  Physicians, nurses, and other personnel in both hospital- and outpatient-care settings
  Employees of nuring homes and chronic-care facilities who have contact with patients or residents
  Providers of home care (e.g., visiting nurses and volunteer workers) to persons at high risk
  Household members (including children) of persons in high-risk groups

Source: Adapted from the *Recommendations of the Advisory Committee on Immunization Practices (ACIP): Prevention and control of influenza. M.M.W.R.* 44(RR-3):1–22, 1995.

by previous infection or vaccination with similar antigen type, such as children, or in the event of antigenic shift. Whole virus vaccine should not be used in children younger than 12 years because of increased local reactions. Because the duration of protective immunity afforded by influenza vaccine appears to be limited and vaccine formulations change frequently, annual vaccination, usually in the late fall (e.g., late October or November) is recommended. Vaccine may be administered at the same visit as pneumococcal vaccine, which, although not give yearly, is also recommended for many of the same groups of individuals.

4. **Side effects** of influenza vaccine **are minimal,** consisting of mild soreness at the injection site in a minority of recipients. Systemic symptoms following vaccination are rare and occurred at approximately the same rate in vaccine and placebo recipients in controlled trials [17]. GBS has not been associated with influenza vaccine since the 1976 swine influenza program.

   Although some patients may believe they acquired influenza infection from a prior influenza vaccination and therefore do not want to receive future influenza vaccinations, this is impossible as a killed virus is used. Most likely such individuals had another respiratory illness occurring coincidentally with the vaccination. If these persons are at high risk for the development of influenza (see Table 8-3), they should be carefully educated and encouraged to receive future influenza vaccinations.

B. **Chemoprophylaxis** with amantadine or rimantadine has been shown to be effective **in the prevention of influenza A** in several controlled prospective trials [12, 17]. The two drugs appear to be equally effective, but rimantadine is associated with a lower frequency of CNS side effects, such as insomnia, than is amantadine [20].

1. **Indications.** Chemoprophylaxis is not an acceptable substitute for vaccination but may be useful in certain special circumstances. These include rare high-risk patients in whom influenza vaccination is absolutely contraindicated; such individuals should receive chemoprophylaxis for the duration of influenza A virus epidemic activity, generally 5–6 weeks. In addition, chemoprophylaxis should be used when vaccine is not available or when vaccination has been delayed and influenza A virus epidemic activity has already begun. In these cases, drug should be administered until approximately 2 weeks after vaccination, at which time effective immunity has developed. In the event of institutional outbreaks of influenza A, such as in nursing homes, chemoprophylaxis of both residents and employees has also been recommended.

2. **Administration.** The dose of both amantadine and rimantadine in individuals with normal renal function is 100 mg PO twice daily. A dose of 100 mg/day of amantadine has been shown to be as effective as 200 mg/day in preventing experimentally induced influenza A in young adult volunteers (see Chap. 26). Amantadine dosage should be adjusted in the presence of renal dysfunction, and both drugs should be used at a maximum dose of 100 mg/day in individuals older than 65. For children aged 9 years or younger, or for older children weighing less than 40 kg, the recommended dose for amantadine and rimantadine is 5 mg/kg/day in one or two divided doses given orally, not to exceed 150 mg/day. Little information is available on the use of amantadine or rimantadine in children younger than 1 year.

   For additional discussion of these agents, see Chap. 26.

Laryngitis and Croup (Acute Laryngotracheobronchitis)

I. **Acute viral laryngitis** is an afebrile, self-limited illness characterized by **hoarseness** or, in more severe cases, loss of voice. Visualization of the larynx reveals erythema and some edema, but the pharynx and nose frequently appear normal. As an isolated syndrome, acute viral laryngitis occurs much less frequently than does acute viral rhinitis or pharyngitis. However, some degree of laryngitis occurs in 10–20% of patients with common colds, and a somewhat higher incidence exists in patients with acute viral pharyngitis. The viruses most frequently isolated are parainfluenza virus types 1, 2, and 3. While presumably all the remaining respiratory viruses occasionally may be involved, none of these has been isolated regularly. **Bacteria are not a cause** of this syndrome. There is **no specific treatment,** but resting the voice and inhalation of steam or cold-water vapor often are helpful.

II. **Acute viral laryngotracheobronchitis (croup)** [21]. Acute laryngotracheobronchitis, or viral croup, is a clinically distinctive syndrome that occurs predominantly in children of a few months to 3 years of age. It is characterized by respiratory distress, inspiratory stridor, and subglottic swelling.

A. **Etiology** [22, 23]. As is shown in Table 7-2, parainfluenza virus type 1 is the most frequent cause of croup. Parainfluenza viruses types 2 and 3 and influenza A also are major agents. Influenza A is particularly important, for although it is a less frequent cause of croup than parainfluenza 1, it tends to cause more severe disease. Less common causes of croup are respiratory syncytial virus, influenza B virus, rhinoviruses, the low-numbered serotypes of adenoviruses, enteroviruses, and rubeola virus. Overall, viruses may be recovered from croup cases more frequently (40–75%) than from other types of respiratory illnesses. *M. pneumoniae* occasionally can cause laryngotracheobronchitis.

B. **Epidemiology.** The epidemiology of croup mirrors that of its major viral agents [22, 24]. Therefore, the major outbreaks of croup occur when parainfluenza type 1 is prevalent, which often is in the fall of every other year. Fewer upsurges of croup are seen with parainfluenza type 2 activity which, while less predictable than type 1, also occurs in the fall. The number of croup cases may increase with influenza A outbreaks (which usually occur between December and April). Recently, parainfluenza type 3 virus has changed in some areas of the United States from being endemic throughout most of the year to causing outbreaks of infection in spring [25].

C. **Clinical manifestations** [21, 23]. An upper respiratory tract infection usually precedes the onset of croup, which is heralded by a **distinctive cough** with a deep, brassy tone, called a *seal's bark*. Laryngitis and fever are common, particularly with influenza A and parainfluenza viral infections.

1. **Stridor.** The development of **inspiratory** stridor is usually abrupt, often occurring at night, and it is associated with respiratory distress. Obstruction of air flow occurs during both inspiration and expiration but is greater on inspiration because the negative inspiratory pressure tends to further narrow the subglottic area.

2. **Respiratory findings.** Retractions of the accessory muscles of the chest wall are common, and the **respiratory rate is increased** but usually to no more than 50–60 per minute. Inspiration is prolonged and, on auscultation, rales, wheezes, and rhonchi may be heard. With increasing obstruction, the breath sounds may diminish and cyanosis may appear. The course of croup is variable and fluctuating.

3. **Hypoxemia** is present in 80% of hospitalized patients with croup and arises from involvement of the lung parenchyma [26, 27]. This is commonly not appreciated. Although the subglottic inflammation is most evident clinically, it does not contribute to the hypoxemia until fatigue and hypercapnia ensue.

D. **Diagnosis** [23, 27]. The diagnosis is made on the basis of the characteristic clinical features and is confirmed by a posteroanterior roentgenogram of the neck, which, in viral croup, shows the narrowing of the tracheal air shadow in the subglottic region. Viral cultures can be performed on respiratory secretions.

E. **Treatment** [21, 22a, 23, 23a, 28]. Many and varied therapies have become legendary, their success being based on grandmothers' trials and the characteristic fluctuating course of croup!

1. **Oxygen is the mainstay** of treatment for the severely affected and should be given to all hypoxemic patients.

2. **The value of mist therapy has not been proved.** Water from the standard home-use vaporizer cannot reach the lower respiratory tract because of the large particle size.

3. **Nebulized racemic epinephrine** gives symptomatic relief, but one should observe the following cautions in its use: (1) The apparent clinical improvement is transitory (less than 2 hr); (2) the clinical improvement is not associated with an improvement in the arterial oxygen saturation; and (3) side effects, such as tachycardia, may occur.

4. **Corticosteroids.** Several studies have shown that **adrenocorticosteroids given at the time of hospital admission are beneficial in moderate to severe croup** [22a, 23, 28, 29], at doses of 0.3–0.6 mg/kg of dexamethasone (or its equivalent) once or repeated q6h for two to four doses. At this point, the data from multiple

studies suggest that for children with moderately severe to severe croup, who are sick enough to be hospitalized, steroids are reasonable to use and may result in significant clinical improvement and fewer intubations [23, 23a]. However, **because the disease is generally self-limited, routine use of steroids probably is not indicated.**

In a recent report, a randomized, double-blind trial compared nebulized budesonide (27 children) versus nebulized saline (27 children). Children 3 months to 5 years of age were eligible. The authors showed that nebulized budesonide leads to a prompt and important clinical improvement in children with mild-to-moderate croup who come to the emergency department [29a]. The role of steroids in mild croup awaits further clinical study; it may be reasonable to use inhaled steroids for those who do not improve rapidly [23a].

5. Croup is largely a viral illness, so **antibiotics are of no benefit** and should not be administered unless there is evidence of concomitant bacterial infection [23].

6. **Ventilatory support** may be necessary for some hospitalized patients with significant obstruction.

Epiglottitis

Epiglottitis is an acute and severe cellulitis of the epiglottis and surrounding tissues usually caused by *H. influenzae* type b [22a, 27, 30, 30a, 30b]. Its **rapidly progressive course** and potentially fatal outcome dictate that **this disease be recognized immediately** and differentiated from viral croup and other diseases causing dyspnea and stridor. Rarely, epiglottitis may be caused by other bacteria such as *Haemophilus parainfluenzae* or beta-hemolytic streptococci spread from a nearby major focus of infection.

H. influenzae epiglottitis occurs most commonly in children between the ages of 3 and 7 years but is also recognized in adults, including those with AIDS. The incidence of invasive *H. influenzae* disease has decreased dramatically in children since the introduction of the *H. influenzae* b (Hib) conjugate vaccines [30a]. The incidence in adults appears to be stable in recent years [30b].

I. **Pathogenesis** [27]. Infection with *H. influenzae* type b produces inflammation and edema of the epiglottis, the arytenoids, the arytenoepiglottic folds, and the surrounding area, often including the subglottic area. The edema and inflammation obstruct the flow of air, which is greater during the negative intrathoracic pressure generated on inspiration. The edematous epiglottis, often termed a *red cherry*, may be pulled into the larynx during inspiration and completely occlude the airway. Even without complete occlusion of the airway, the inflammatory reaction, the profuse secretions, and the exudate may produce severe dyspnea.

II. **Clinical manifestations.** The **onset** of epiglottitis is characteristically **abrupt,** with sore throat, fever, and toxicity.

A. **Symptoms.** The symptoms in children usually progress rapidly in such a manner that **dysphagia, drooling, and respiratory distress with stridor** become apparent. At the onset of the illness, stridor may not be evident. In adults, patients commonly complain of only a severe sore throat and odynophagia and typically do not have signs or symptoms of airway obstruction [30b].

B. **Signs**
1. **Retractions** of the chest wall are usually present, and the child typically seeks a **sitting position,** leaning forward with the characteristic facies of an open mouth, protruding tongue, and drooling.
2. **The pharynx** is usually edematous and filled with secretions. The beefy-red epiglottis often may be seen by examination of the pharynx. This, however, should **not** be attempted, for even with the use of a tongue depressor, fatal occlusion of the airway may occur.
3. **Auscultation** reveals inspiratory stridor and expiratory rhonchi and, as the patient's condition worsens, the breath sounds may diminish.
4. In adults, the oropharyngeal examination may be normal. The patient may have a muffled voice and drooling [30b].

III. **Diagnosis.** Because this disease is a **potential medical emergency,** the initial diagnosis must be made with a high index of suspicion on the basis of the history and clinical findings. If the diagnosis is suspected, the child or adult should be sent immediately to the hospital.

A. **Visualization of the epiglottis. With trained personnel and equipment available for maintaining an airway, the diagnosis may be confirmed by visualization of the epiglottis.** In adults, inflammation is often not confined to the epiglottis, and the condition may be referred to as supraglottitis with inflammation of contiguous structures [30b].

B. **Lateral neck roentgenograms** may be useful in early, less toxic patients who are not in respiratory difficulties. The epiglottis will be seen as an enlarged, rounded shadow resembling an adult's thumb (the "thumb sign"). In comparison, the normal epiglottis appears as the shadow of an adult's little finger viewed laterally. In the patient who is acutely ill, valuable time may be unnecessarily wasted obtaining roentgenograms: Ensuring an adequate airway must take priority.

C. **Leukocyte count.** The total WBC count usually is elevated to more than 15,000/ mm^3, often with a pronounced left shift.

D. **Blood cultures should be obtained.** Sepsis is concurrently present, and cultures of the blood and of the upper respiratory tract secretions usually will yield *H. influenzae* type b. Counterimmunoelectrophoresis (CIE) may identify the capsular polysaccharide antigen of the organism within hours in the blood, urine, and sometimes the secretions.

IV. **Differential diagnosis.** It is essential that viral croup be distinguished from epiglottitis. The salient differentiating features are the abrupt onset and rapid progression of epiglottitis and the **toxic appearance** of the child, especially the **drooling and dysphagia.** The barking cough of viral croup is absent. Bacterial tracheitis may appear similar (see Bacterial Tracheitis). Other syndromes, such as diphtheria and aspiration of a foreign body, should sometimes be considered, depending on the history.

If a child has been appropriately vaccinated in the past with Hib vaccine, the diagnosis of invasive *H. influenzae* disease would be less likely [30a] (see earlier discussion).

V. **Therapy.** Swift and careful management are essential in this disease and directly correlate with the outcome.

A. **Adequate airway.** Once the diagnosis has been established, an adequate airway must be obtained. In most centers, management of these patients entails the immediate establishment of an artificial airway. Nasotracheal intubation is the procedure of choice if experienced personnel are available. Complications are few with nasotracheal intubation, and extubation can usually be accomplished within 1–3 days.

In adults, upper airway obstruction was suggested by stridor or sitting straight upright. Patients without signs or symptoms of upper airway obstruction can be treated medically in a hospital unit where they can be observed closely with equipment and personnel available for prompt airway intervention, if it becomes necessary [30b].

B. **Antibiotics.** Parenteral antibiotic therapy should be initiated immediately. In this life-threatening disease, which is usually caused by *H. influenzae* type b, ampicillin-resistant forms (10–30% of isolates) must be treated adequately until susceptibility data are known. The usual antibiotic of choice is either a cephalosporin that is effective against ampicillin-resistant *H. influenzae* or chloramphenicol if a cephalosporin is contraindicated. The total duration of therapy should be 10–14 days in uncomplicated cases.

1. **Cephalosporins**
   a. **Second-generation agents.** Cefuroxime has good in vitro activity against *H. influenzae* strains that are sensitive to, as well as those that are resistant to, ampicillin, but it should not be used if there is a chance of CNS involvement (ceftriaxone is preferred in CNS infections). (See Chap. 28.)
   b. **Third-generation agents.** Several of these newer agents (e.g., cefotaxime and ceftriaxone) cover both sensitive and resistant *H. influenzae* and have excellent penetration into the CNS. (For a discussion of third-generation cephalosporins, see Chap. 28.)

2. **Chloramphenicol** (50–100 mg/kg/day divided into q6h intervals) was commonly used before the availability of the very active cephalosporins (e.g., ceftriaxone) and still is an option in patients in whom a cephalosporin is contraindicated. Serum levels should be monitored if chloramphenicol is continued.

C. **Corticosteroids** may be used briefly to help reduce the postintubation edema that develops. Although frequently given, corticosteroids have not been proven in a prospective controlled study to reduce the need for airway intervention or to hasten recovery in acute adult epiglottitis [30b].

Bacterial Tracheitis

I. **Bacterial tracheitis** is a relatively rare syndrome that mimics epiglottitis or severe viral croup [31]. Although this syndrome has been recognized only recently, and has been described mostly in children, it may occur at any age. It is important to differentiate bacterial tracheitis from viral croup because of its potential for rapid progression that necessitates intubation and because of the need for prompt antibiotic therapy.

II. **Etiology.** Bacterial tracheitis usually is caused by *S. aureus* and *H. influenzae* type b. Other bacteria, including group A streptococci and *S. pneumoniae,* have also been associated with this syndrome.

III. **Clinical manifestations.** Bacterial tracheitis tends to affect patients who have had previous tracheal injury or compromise, such as by intubation or sometimes by a preceding viral infection. The onset is acute, with fever that may be high, and with stridor and dyspnea. Abundant purulent sputum or secretions are usually evident and may cause rapid airway obstruction as in epiglottitis.

IV. **Diagnosis.** The diagnosis may be **made by direct laryngoscopy,** which shows localized inflammation and membranous exudate in the subglottic area, and sometimes by a lateral soft-tissue roentgenogram of the neck, demonstrating the subglottic narrowing with a shaggy, exudative membrane. The epiglottis is usually normal, however. Blood cultures are generally negative.

V. **Treatment.** Therapy should be initiated as soon as possible with intravenous antibiotics for the most likely organisms, such as ceftriaxone. Cultures of the exudative membrane should subsequently allow the antibiotic regimen to be narrowed to cover the isolated pathogen.

Acute Viral Tracheitis and Tracheobronchitis

Acute viral tracheitis and **tracheobronchitis** result from viral infection of the trachea or bronchi (see Tables 7-1, 7-2), especially influenza A and B viruses.

I. **Tracheitis.** The clinical findings in tracheitis include nonproductive, paroxysmal **cough;** substernal discomfort on inhalation, especially of cold air; and **tracheal tenderness,** which is elicited by gentle thumb pressure on the anterior trachea just below the thyroid cartilage. Diffuse rhonchi may be heard on auscultation of the chest, but these are variably present. Systemic symptoms, such as feverishness, headache, myalgias, and malaise, may be present. Only symptomatic therapy is indicated.

II. **Acute tracheobronchitis**

A. **Symptoms** include a **dry cough** that often is paroxysmal and is much **more severe at night.** Later in the course of illness, small amounts of clear or whitish sputum may be produced. Fever, headache, myalgias, malaise, and anorexia are frequent. Substernal discomfort is a frequent complaint and, after several days of coughing, the abdominal and chest wall musculature may become sore and tender. This muscle pain may be aggravated by breathing and thus may mimic pleuritis.

B. **Physical examination.** Coughing is easily stimulated, and its paroxysmal nature can be observed readily. **Tracheal tenderness** is present. The throat may be erythematous. Examination of the chest may reveal no adventitious sounds, but more commonly one hears diffuse rhonchi and occasional wheezes. There are no areas of dullness to percussion, and neither rales nor friction rubs are heard.

C. **Diagnosis.** Because coughing is a frequent manifestation of upper respiratory tract illness, the presence of cough alone is not sufficient evidence for the diagnosis of this syndrome (or tracheitis or bronchitis). **The diagnosis should be restricted to individuals who exhibit at least one of the following signs:** paroxysmal cough, tender trachea, or abnormal signs on auscultation. **The chest roentgenogram is normal.**

D. **Treatment** in adults is best effected by prescribing rest; aspirin, 0.6–0.9 g PO q3–4h, for headache and fever; cold-water vapor inhalation; and a cough syrup such as guaifenesin with 15 mg dextromethorphan per 5 ml (10 ml PO q3–4h). If coughing is particularly bothersome at night and interferes with sleep, a sedative such as flurazepam hydrochloride, 15–30 mg, together with one or two 10-ml doses of cough syrup often is effective. For children, a cough suppressant, such as guaifenesin with 15 mg dextromethorphan per 5 ml, may be helpful.

Acute Bronchitis and Acute Exacerbations of Chronic Bronchitis in Adults

I. **Acute bronchitis** is a common clinical problem that accounts for an estimated 12 million physician visits per year in the United States. The findings in bronchitis include cough, sometimes productive of small amounts of whitish sputum, and diffuse rhonchi on chest examination. Systemic symptoms also may be present. **Chest roentgenography reveals no infiltrate.** This topic has been reviewed [32].

   A. **Etiology**

      1. **Viral infections** account for more than half the diagnoses (see Tables 7-1, 7-2). The most common viral causes are probably rhinoviruses, influenza A and B, parainfluenza, and adenoviruses. (In children, respiratory syncytial virus is a common cause of tracheobronchitis.)

      2. *M. pneumoniae* is common in young adults (especially those younger than 40–45 years) and may account for 10–20% of cases (see Chap. 9).

      3. **Bacteria** play a role in some patients, although routine sputum culture may often reveal normal flora. *S. pneumoniae, H. influenzae,* and *Moraxella* (formerly *Branhamella*) *catarrhalis* are potential pathogens.

      4. *Chlamydia* spp., including *C. pneumoniae* (the so-called TWAR strain), can cause bronchitis (see Chap. 9).

   B. **Diagnosis** usually is based on the history of an acute productive cough, low-grade temperature, and no evidence of a pneumonia on physical examination or chest roentgenography.

   C. **Therapy** for acute bronchitis is largely empiric and, because **many cases** of acute bronchitis are **self-limited,** the role of antibiotics is still controversial [33]. In otherwise healthy patients who have no systemic symptoms, it is reasonable not to use antibiotics, especially if symptoms have been present only a few days. In those patients with underlying disease (e.g., congestive heart failure) or those with systemic symptoms, antibiotics often are used. In addition, in patients having symptoms for more than 7–10 days, *Mycoplasma* infection is a consideration (see Chap. 9). There has been increasing recognition that some adults with prolonged cough may have mild forms of pertussis.

      1. **Erythromycin.** In recent years, this agent has become particularly useful in this setting, especially if mycoplasmas are a concern. Typically, adults are given 250–500 mg for 10–14 days. In those patients who have excessive GI side effects from erythromycin, the more expensive similar agent clarithromycin (250–500 mg bid) can be used. Azithromycin is another consideration. (See Chap. 28M for a discussion of these macrolides.)

      2. If *Mycoplasma* and *Chlamydia* are not a concern, **other options** include ampicillin or amoxicillin, trimethoprim-sulfamethoxazole, tetracycline, and cefuroxime axetil, as described in sec. II.B.

II. **Acute exacerbations of chronic bronchitis** occur frequently. **Chronic bronchitis** is defined as the production of sputum on most days for at least 3 months per year for more than 2 years [32]. An acute exacerbation of chronic bronchitis is a clinical syndrome associated with an increase in cough, an increase of sputum (both in amount and purulence or a change in color), and increased breathlessness without evidence of pneumonia either clinically or by chest roentgenography. Wheezing is common. Most patients do not have systemic symptoms.

   A. **Causes** of acute exacerbations

      1. **Environmental factors,** such as exposure to cigarette smoke, pollutants, fumes, pollens, and the like, **are important** cofactors.

      2. **The precise role of microorganisms is less well understood.** As discussed earlier, respiratory viruses, *M. pneumoniae,* and bacteria such as *S. pneumoniae* and *H. influenzae* contribute to the etiology of acute exacerbations of bronchitis in patients with chronic obstructive pulmonary disease. Rhinoviruses have been recovered from 10 to 25% of such cases. In addition, respiratory syncytial virus, the influenza viruses, and the parainfluenza viruses have been associated with smaller proportions of cases. **Overall, respiratory viruses appear to play a more important role in these acute illnesses than do M. pneumoniae or bacteria.** Furthermore, some studies have suggested that these viral infections contribute to the deterioration of lung function that occurs in such patients.

B. Therapy. The precise role of antibiotics in flare-ups of chronic bronchitis is still unclear [32]. Because bacterial, mycoplasmal, and viral etiologies cannot be distinguished clinically, the physician is forced to make a decision regarding use of antimicrobial therapy on statistical grounds. It is probable that up to 25% of such episodes are due to treatable infections. Therefore, in a patient with chronic lung disease who presents with increased cough and sputum production, increased sputum purulence (thicker, darker color), and often increased dyspnea, but without evidence of pneumonia, it would seem wise to begin antimicrobial therapy [34].

The role of a routine sputum culture before starting therapy is debated. Cultures obtained after therapy is begun often are misleading.

Therapy is directed against *H. influenzae, S. pneumoniae*, M. catarrhalis* and, to a lesser extent, *M. pneumoniae,* which appears less frequently in older patients (see Chap. 9). Various regimens have been recommended for adults.

1. Amoxicillin, 250 mg PO tid for 7–10 days, is commonly used.

2. Trimethoprim-sulfamethoxazole has been approved for use in flare-ups of chronic bronchitis. This agent provides good sputum levels and is active against *S. pneumoniae* and *H. influenzae.* It is another alternative treatment for the penicillin-allergic patient. The dose is two regular tablets (or one double-strength tablet) bid for 7–10 days.

3. Erythromycin, 250 mg qid for 7–10 days, will provide adequate therapy for *S. pneumoniae* but is not as active against *H. influenzae* as the agents already listed. It is active against mycoplasmas. For patients who cannot tolerate the GI side effects of erythromycin, clarithromycin (250–500 mg bid) is a reasonable alternative, although it is more expensive. It also provides some increased activity against *H. influenzae.* Azithromycin (500 mg on day 1, followed by 250 mg on days 2–5) has been shown to be effective as well. (See Chap. 28M for a discussion of these macrolides.)

4. Tetracycline hydrochloride, 250 mg PO qid on an empty stomach for 7–10 days, can be used. It is also active against mycoplasmas. Doxycycline can be used.

5. Oral cefuroxime axetil, 250–500 mg bid for 7–10 days, can be used.

6. Oral fluoroquinolones (e.g., ciprofloxacin) **are not agents of choice** as many acute exacerbations of bronchitis, due to bacteria, are caused by pneumococci that are less susceptible to these agents (see Chap. 28S).

C. Prevention. These patients are prone to recurrent infection.

1. Prophylactic and chronic antibiotic use are controversial. We generally prefer to use antibiotics intermittently for episodes of increased purulent sputum, as discussed in sec. **II** earlier. However, in some patients, antibiotics given routinely 1 week per month, especially during the winter months, may be helpful. The antibiotics listed in sec. **B** can be rotated each month unless allergies preclude the use of some agents.

2. Pneumococcal vaccine should be given to these patients (see Chap. 9).

3. Influenza vaccinations should be given to these patients annually (see Influenza, sec. **VIII**).

4. Early therapy of mild bronchitis episodes may help prevent more serious lower respiratory infections, especially pneumonia.

5. If the patient can stop smoking or avoid smoke and other environmental irritants, this will be very beneficial.

Bronchiolitis

Bronchiolitis is a syndrome confined to young children (mainly ages 1–24 months) and is **due primarily to infection with respiratory syncytial virus.** It may be seen, however, with other viruses (see Table 7-2) [35–36a].

I. Symptoms. After several days of typical upper respiratory tract illness, the infant develops a deepening cough and the onset of dyspnea and wheezing.

II. Signs. The infant's respiratory rate increases, and retraction of the intercostal muscles is seen due to respiratory obstruction. On auscultation, rales, rhonchi, and expiratory

---

*The role of penicillin-resistant *S. pneumoniae* and implications for therapy in this setting have not been well studied. See related discussion in Chap. 28C.

wheezing are present and may fluctuate in intensity. Cyanosis may be present; even without overt cyanosis, however, hypoxemia is commonly present [37].

III. The **chest roentgenogram** shows hyperaeration with or without infiltrates. The infiltrates result either from the atelectasis, which is part of the pathology of bronchiolitis, or from a concomitant viral pneumonia, which is frequently also present.

IV. **Diagnosis.** Viral diagnosis can be made by testing respiratory secretions. **Rapid diagnostic tests** to detect respiratory syncytial virus are widely available (see Chap. 25). If viral studies are unavailable, the diagnosis can be made clinically, particularly during an outbreak of respiratory syncytial viral infections, by the characteristic findings of acute respiratory signs with wheezing and hyperaeration in a child younger than 3 years. The major entities in the differential diagnosis are asthma, gastroesophageal reflux, and aspiration of a foreign body.

V. **Therapy.** The antiviral agent **ribavirin** offers specific therapy for hospitalized patients with bronchiolitis and other lower respiratory tract infections from respiratory syncytial virus [38]. The drug is administered as a small-particle aerosol for approximately 12–20 hr/day for 3–5 days or longer if necessary. Ribavirin may be administered effectively to children on mechanical ventilation [39]. **See Chap. 26 for further discussion of this agent.** The indications for ribavirin in RSV have been reviewed recently [38a].

Antibiotics are not warranted and bacterial suprainfections are rare. The mainstay of supportive therapy is the monitoring and maintenance of adequate oxygenation. An aerosolized bronchodilating agent may be tried, for a small subset of infants with bronchiolitis appear to benefit from such therapy. Corticosteroids are of no benefit.

VI. **Prevention.** An effective **vaccine** to prevent respiratory syncytial virus infection is **not currently available.** However, prophylactic therapy with intravenous immunoglobulin preparations containing high titers of antibody to respiratory syncytial virus may prevent significant lower respiratory tract disease due to this virus in high-risk infants, such as those with bronchopulmonary dysplasia or congenital heart disease [40].

Viral Pneumonia

Pneumonia is covered in more detail in Chap. 9. However, because **viral pneumonia** [41] is due to the same viruses responsible for other respiratory tract syndromes, its etiology is included in Tables 7-1 and 7-2.

I. **Infants and children.** In infants and children younger than 5 years (especially under age 2), **viruses are the most common cause of pneumonia.** Respiratory syncytial virus, the parainfluenza viruses, and influenza A virus are the most important pathogens [38].

II. **Adults** seldom have true viral pneumonia.
   A. **Young adults.** *M. pneumoniae* is the most common cause of pneumonia in persons 5–40 years of age who do not have underlying human immunodeficiency virus (HIV) infection. **Viruses other than influenza only occasionally cause true pneumonia in this age group** [6].
   B. **Older adults** are much more likely to have bacterial pneumonia, although influenza virus can cause pneumonia, and respiratory syncytial virus has recently been associated with pneumonia and exacerbations of chronic lung disease in the elderly [38].
   C. **HIV-infected patients.** Cytomegalovirus often is isolated from the respiratory secretions (or lung biopsies) of these patients. How often cytomegalovirus is a primary pathogen (if ever) in this setting is unclear (see Chap. 19).
   D. **Other immunosuppressed patients** (specifically bone marrow transplant patients) may have interstitial infiltrates due to cytomegalovirus infection (see Chaps. 9, 19, and 20). Herpes simplex virus is a rare cause of pneumonia even in the immunocompromised patient.

References

1. Kilbourne, E.D. *Influenza.* New York: Plenum, 1987.
2. Murphy, B.R., and Webster, R.G. Orthomyxoviruses. In B.N. Fields et al. (eds.), *Virology* (2nd ed.). New York: Raven, 1990. Pp. 1091–1152.

An exhaustive review of the virology, immunology, epidemiology, and clinical presentation of influenza.

3. Glezen, W.P. Serious morbidity and mortality associated with influenza epidemics. *Epidemiol. Rev.* 4:25, 1982.
   Excellent description of the epidemiologic indicators and impact associated with influenza epidemics.

4. Glezen, W.P., et al. Acute respiratory disease associated with influenza epidemics in Houston 1981–83. *J. Infect. Dis.* 155:1119, 1987.
   Detailed study of age-associated attack rates, outpatient visits, and risk of hospitalization during influenza A and B viral epidemics.

5. Palese, P., and Young, J.F. Variation of influenza A, B, and C viruses. *Science* 215: 1468, 1982.
   Genetic explanation of the changing influenza viruses.

6. Betts, R.F. Influenza Virus. In G.L. Mandell, J.E. Bennett, and R. Dolin (eds.), *Principles and Practice of Infectious Diseases* (4th ed.). New York: Churchill Livingstone, 1995.
   For a recent related paper, see Centers for Disease Control, Pneumonia and influenza death rates, United States, 1979–1994. M.M.W.R. *44:535, 1995, which documents increasing mortality rates with this complication of influenza.*

7. Jordan, W.S., et al. A study of illness in a group of Cleveland families: XVII. The occurrence of Asian influenza. *Am. J. Hyg.* 68:190, 1958.

8. Monto, A.S., Koopman, J.S., and Longini, I.M., Jr. Tecumseh study of illness: XIII. Influenza infection and disease, 1976–1981. *Am. J. Epidemiol.* 121:811, 1985.

9. Wright, P.F., Bryant, J.D., and Karzon, D.T. Comparison of influenza B/Hong Kong virus infection among infants, children, and young adults. *J. Infect. Dis.* 141:430, 1980.

10. Marine, W.M., McGowan, J.E., Jr., and Thomas, J.E. Influenza detection: A prospective comparison of surveillance methods and analysis of isolates. *Am. J. Epidemiol.* 104:248, 1976.
    Good study of influenza detection.

11. Hurwitz, E.S., et al. Public health service study on Reye's syndrome and medications. *N. Engl. J. Med.* 313:849, 1985.

12. Centers for Disease Control. Prevention and control of influenza: Part II, antiviral agents. Recommendations of the Advisory Committee on Immunization Practices. *M.M.W.R.* 43(RR-15):1–10, 1994.

13. Douglas, R.G.J. Prophylaxis and treatment of influenza. *N. Engl. J. Med.* 322:443–450, 1990.
    Detailed discussion, especially of the use of amantadine and rimantadine.

14. Wingfield, W.L., Pollack, D., and Grunert, R.R. Therapeutic efficacy of amantadine HCI and rimantadine HCL in naturally occurring influenza A2 respiratory illness in man. *N. Engl. J. Med.* 281:579, 1979.

15. Hall, C.B., et al. Treatment of children with influenza A infection with rimantadine. *Pediatrics* 80:275, 1987.
    Shows efficacy of rimantadine treatment for ambulatory children with influenza, but reports also that resistant viruses may develop in treated patients.

16. Louria, D.B., et al. Studies on influenza in the pandemic of 1957–1958: II. Pulmonary complications of influenza. *J. Clin. Invest.* 38:213–265, 1959.
    The classic article describing primary and secondary viral pneumonia and mixed bacterial-viral pneumonia during the severe pandemic of that year.

17. Centers for Disease Control. Prevention and control of influenza: Recommendations of the Immunization Practices Advisory Committee (ACIP). *M.M.W.R.* 44(RR-3):1–22, 1995.

18. Peter, G., et al. (eds.). *Report of the Committee on Infectious Diseases: 1994 Red Book* (23rd ed.). Elk Grove Village, IL: American Academy of Pediatrics, 1994. Pp. 275–283.

19. Barker, W.H., and Mullooly, J.P. Influenza vaccination of elderly persons: Reduction in pneumonia and influenza hospitalizations and deaths. *J.A.M.A.* 244:2547–2549, 1980.
    Although not a prospective study, a fairly convincing demonstration of the efficacy of influenza vaccines in preventing influenza complications in high-risk adults when there is a good antigenic match.

19a. Govaert, T.M.E., et al. The efficacy of influenza vaccination in elderly individuals: A randomized double-blind placebo-controlled trial. *J.A.M.A.* 272:1661, 1994.
     Dutch study of patients over 60 years of age not belonging to a high-risk group. Data showed that influenza vaccination may halve the incidence of serologic and clinical influenza in a period of antigenic drift. See accompanying editorial by P.A. Patriarea, A randomized controlled trial of influenza vaccine in the elderly: Scientific scrutiny and

ethical responsibility, which comments on this study and the importance of universal vaccination of the elderly; it also summarizes prior studies of vaccinations of the elderly.

19b. Nichol, K.L., et al. The efficacy and cost effectiveness of vaccination against influenza among elderly persons living in the community. *N. Engl. J. Med.* 331:778, 1994.
Study of patients 65 years of age or older in a large health maintenance organization in the Minneapolis–St. Paul area. Data showed that vaccination against influenza is associated with reductions in the rates of hospitalization and death from influenza and its complications, as compared with respective rates in unvaccinated elderly persons, and that vaccination produces direct dollar savings. Direct savings per year averaged $117 per person vaccinated. See editorial comment in same issue by A.S. Monto, Influenza vaccines for the elderly. See also related report by J.P. Mullooly et al., Influenza vaccination programs for elderly persons: Cost-effectiveness in a health maintenance organization. Ann. Intern. Med. *121:947, 1994.*

20. Dolin, R., et al. A controlled trial of amantadine and rimantadine in the prophylaxis of influenza A in humans. *N. Engl. J. Med.* 307:580–584, 1982.
A direct comparison of the two drugs in a large, carefully controlled study, showing that both drugs were effective at a dose of 200 mg/day but that rimantadine was associated with fewer side effects.

21. Hall, C.B., and McBride, J.T. Upper Respiratory Tract Infections: The Common Cold, Pharyngitis, Croup, Bacterial Tracheitis, and Epiglottitis. In J.E. Pennington (ed.), *Respiratory Infections: Diagnosis and Management.* New York: Raven, 1988. Pp. 97–118.

22. Denny, F.W., et al. Croup: An 11-year study in a pediatric practice. *Pediatrics* 7: 871, 1983.

22a. Cressman, W.R., and Myer, C.M., III. Diagnosis and management of croup and epiglottitis. *Pediatr. Clin. North Am.* 41:265, 1994.
Recent clinical summary of these topics.

23. Hall, C.B. Acute Laryngotracheobronchitis (Croup). In G.L. Mandell, J.E. Bennett, and R. Dolin (eds.), *Principles and Practice of Infectious Diseases* (4th ed.). New York: Churchill Livingstone, 1995. Pp. 573–578.

23a. Landau, L.I., and Geelhoed, G.C. Aerosolized steroids for croup. *N. Engl. J. Med.* 331:322, 1994.
Although this is primarily an editorial comment on reference [29a] and steroid use in croup, it also has a nice clinical summary of croup. The results of metaanalyses support the use of steroids to treat hospitalized children with croup; corticosteroids certainly appear to be effective in those with moderately severe disease. Corticosteroids' mechanism of action is not known.
Further studies are now needed to determine the criteria that identify the patients more likely to benefit from steroids, determine optimal doses and optimal regimens.

24. Glezen, W.P., et al. Epidemiological patterns of acute lower respiratory disease of children in a pediatric group practice. *J. Pediatr.* 78:397, 1971.
Shows distribution of viral etiology for different respiratory syndromes.

25. Glezen, W.P., et al. Parainfluenza virus type 3: Seasonality and the risk of infection and reinfection in young children. *J. Infect. Dis.* 150:851, 1984.

26. Newth, C.J.L., Levison, H., and Bryan, A.C. The respiratory status of children with croup. *J. Pediatr.* 81:1068, 1972.
Classic study of pathophysiology of croup, showing the frequency and importance of the parenchymal lung involvement.

27. Newth, C.J.L., and Levison, H. Diagnosing and managing croup and epiglottitis. *J. Respir. Dis.* 2:22, 1981.
Good description of differentiation of croup and epiglottitis and physiologic basis of management in this issue.

28. Skolnik, N.S. Treatment of croup: A critical review. *Am. J. Dis. Child.* 143:1045–1049, 1989.
Careful review of controlled studies evaluating the use of inhaled epinephrine, steroids, and other measures.

29. Saper, D.M., et al. A prospective randomized double-blind study to evaluate the effect of dexamethasone in acute laryngotracheitis. *J. Pediatr.* 115:323–329, 1989.
In this small study, the authors concluded that a single injection of dexamethasone reduced the severity of moderate to severe croup in the first 24 hours. See also the accompanying editorial (D.S. Smith, J. Pediatr. 115:256–257, 1989) and S.W. Kairys et al., Am. J. Dis. Child. 143:1045–1049, 1989.

29a. Klassen, T.P., et al. Nebulized budesonide for children with mild-to-moderate croup. *N. Engl. J. Med.* 331:285, 1994.

See also reference [23a] for editorial comment.

Nebulized budesonide, a synthetic glucocorticoid with relatively strong topical anti-inflammatory effects and low systemic activity as compared with beclomethasone, was selected for the study because it can be administered without the discomfort of an intramuscular injection and because it begins to act as early as 1 hour after administration. A single dose of 2 mg (4 ml) was used.

30. Molteni, R.A. Epiglottitis. Incidence of extra-epiglottic infection: Report on 72 cases and review of the literature. *Pediatrics* 58:526, 1976.
    Good clinical study of epiglottitis.

30a. Centers for Disease Control. Progress toward elimination of *Haemophilus influenzae* type b disease among infants and children—United States, 1987–1993 and 1993–1994. *M.M.W.R.* 43:144, 1994 and 44:545, 1995.
    Summarizes data showing that since the introduction of the Hib conjugate vaccines in 1988, even though there is incomplete coverage of children with the vaccine, there is more than a 95% decrease in the incidence of invasive disease. An unexpected additional advantage of the Hib vaccine appears to be elimination of carriage resulting in reduced exposure to the pathogen and a decrease in disease incidence, even among unvaccinated persons.
    Related articles include T.V. Murphy et al., Declining incidence of Haemophilus influenzae *type b disease since introduction of vaccination. J.A.M.A. 269:246, 1993, and others in same issue.*

30b. Frantz, T.D., et al. Acute epiglottis in adults: Analysis of 129 cases. *J.A.M.A.* 272:1358, 1994.
    In multivariate analysis, factors associated with airway intervention were stridor and sitting erect. Only 12% of blood cultures yielded H. influenzae type b. Antibiotics should be aimed at this pathogen as well as S. aureus, group A streptococci, and S. pneumoniae. Cefuroxime or ceftriaxone are appealing agents.
    See also related paper by M.F. Mayo Smith et al., Acute epiglottitis in adults: An eight-year experience in the state of Rhode Island. N. Engl. J. Med. 314:1133, 1986, and editorial response in the same issue.

31. Donnelly, B.W., McMillan, J.A., and Weiner, L.B. Bacterial tracheitis: Report of eight new cases and review. *Rev. Infect. Dis.* 12:729–735, 1990.
    Excellent review of clinical and microbiologic findings in this relatively rare entity. Tracheoscopy is diagnostic, and Gram stain and culture of tracheal secretions should be done to guide therapy.

32. Rodnick, J.E., and Gude, J.K. The use of antibiotics in acute bronchitis and acute exacerbations of chronic bronchitis. *West. J. Med.* 149:347, 1988.
    Practical clinical summary of this important primary-care medical topic. For related discussion and more recent review, see H.A. Gallis, Acute bronchitis and acute exacerbations of chronic bronchitis: The role of new antimicrobial agents. Infect. Dis. Clin. Pract. 3:81, 1994.

33. Orr, P.H., et al. Randomized placebo-controlled trials of antibiotics for acute bronchitis: A critical review of the literature. *J. Fam. Pract.* 36:507–512, 1993.
    Metaanalysis of the few reported clinical trials of antibiotics in acute bronchitis. The value of antibiotic therapy in otherwise healthy adults is unclear.

34. Anthonisen, N.R., et al. Antibiotic therapy in exacerbations of chronic obstructive pulmonary disease. *Ann. Intern. Med.* 106:196–204, 1987.
    Reports a randomized placebo-controlled study in which a 10-day course of either trimethoprim-sulfamethoxazole, ampicillin, or doxycycline was shown to be superior to placebo in the treatment of selected patients with stable obstructive pulmonary disease experiencing acute exacerbations. Exacerbations were defined in terms of increased dyspnea, sputum production, and sputum purulence.

35. Henderson, F.W., et al. The etiologic and epidemiologic spectrum of bronchiolitis in pediatric practice. *J. Pediatr.* 95:183, 1979.

36. Kim, H.W., et al. Epidemiology of respiratory syncytial virus infection in Washington, D.C.: I. Importance of the virus in different respiratory tract disease syndromes and temporal distribution of infection. *Am. J. Epidemiol.* 98:216, 1973.
    Importance of respiratory syncytial virus infection.

36a. Isaacs, D. Bronchiolitis. *B.M.J.* 310:4, 1995.
    Concise summary of the importance of and approach to this problem, which is usually due to respiratory syncytial virus.

37. Wohl, M.E.B., and Chernick, V. Bronchiolitis. *Am. Rev. Respir. Dir.* 118:759, 1978.
    Excellent review with a pathophysiologic bent.

38. Hall, C.B., and McCarthy, C.A. Respiratory Syncytial Virus. In G.L. Mandell, J.E. Bennett, and R. Dolin (eds.), *Principles and Practice of Infectious Diseases* (4th ed.). New York: Churchill Livingstone, 1995. Pp. 1501–1519.

38a. Committee on Infectious Diseases, American Academy of Pediatrics. Reassessment of the indications for ribavirin therapy in respiratory syncytial virus infections. *Pediatrics* 97:137, 1996.

   Reviews recent data suggesting ribavirin may not be as effective for RSV as previously shown. Therapy needs more study. See Chap. 26.

39. Smith, D.W., et al. A controlled trial of aerosolized ribavirin in infants receiving mechanical ventilation for severe respiratory syncytial virus infection. *N. Engl. J. Med.* 325:24–29, 1991.

40. Groothuis, J.R., et al. Prophylactic administration of respiratory syncytial virus immune globulin to high-risk infants and young children. *N. Engl. J. Med.* 329:1524–1530, 1993.

   Administration of high doses of RSV immunoglobulin was an effective means of preventing lower respiratory tract infection due to this virus in high-risk infants and children. See also related article by M.L. Levin, Treatment and prevention options for respiratory syncytial virus infection. J. Pediatr. 124:S22, 1994.

41. Greenberg, S.B. Viral pneumonia. *Med. Clin. North Am.* 64:491–506, 1991.

   Good general review of syndromes of viral pneumonia.

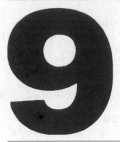

Lower Respiratory Tract Infections (Including Tuberculosis)

Robert L. Penn and Robert F. Betts

Pneumonia can be caused by virtually any type of infectious agent. This infection can develop when the host is confronted by a virulent organism for which he or she has no specific defense or when confronted with less virulent organisms at the same time that the usual defense mechanisms are impaired.

Most pneumonias occur when the microorganism gains access to the lung through the endobronchial tree. This can occur by inhalation of microorganisms in small-particle aerosols, by aspiration of minute quantities of virulent organisms, or by aspiration of larger quantities of less virulent organisms. In addition, aspiration of gastric contents or inhalation of toxic fumes, even without associated bacteria, can produce the inflammatory changes of chemical pneumonitis. In this setting there is a predisposition to secondary bacterial infection and, when this occurs, it may be difficult to detect.

Occasionally, microorganisms can reach the lung through the bloodstream. Embolic pneumonia is most likely to occur from right-sided endocarditis or when a noncardiac infected site is drained by the superior or inferior vena cava. Infections at sites whose main drainage is through the portal vein are less likely to lead to embolic pneumonia. Pneumonia arising from embolic spread often develops without obvious evidence of airway disease.

General Concepts of Organism-Host Interaction

I. **The organism**
   A. **Availability.** The presence, either endogenous or exogenous, of the organism in the environment is an essential precondition to the development of pneumonia due to that organism. Therefore, *Yersinia pestis* and *Bacillus anthracis* seldom cause disease in the United States.
   B. **Virulence.** The virulence of most bacteria that cause pneumonia is mediated primarily by the bacteria's **ability to resist phagocytosis** coupled, in some instances, with another feature. For example, the ability of the pneumococcus to resist phagocytosis allows the organism to replicate to high titer in the alveolus, even though only a few organisms initially may be inoculated (i.e., aspirated) into the lower respiratory tract. No other major pathogenic factor has been identified for the pneumococcus.
      1. **Importance of the capsule.** *Streptococcus pneumoniae* is the prime example. All the species that cause disease are encapsulated, and the types with the greatest quantity of capsule are most frequently associated with disease. Encapsulated *Haemophilus influenzae* type b is the most virulent strain. Nonencapsulated *H. influenzae,* although associated with exacerbations of bronchitis and, in some instances, bronchopneumonia, rarely are recovered from the bloodstream or from pleural fluid. The presence of a capsule probably explains why *Klebsiella pneumoniae* is one of the most important gram-negative rods associated with pneumonia. *Klebsiella* spp. also elaborate enzymes that destroy tissue and therefore propagate infection once the organism is established.
      2. **Inoculum effect.** Organisms that lack a capsule can cause pneumonia if the inoculum of organisms is sufficiently high, such as when an individual with poor dentition harbors high titers of anaerobic bacteria. Factors that hinder mechanical removal of inoculum include loss of ciliary activity, which may occur as a part of a viral infection of the lower respiratory tract; drugs, such

as alcohol; airway obstruction, as from a tumor or a foreign body; and chronic exposure to an irritant such as cigarette smoke.

II. Host defense mechanisms [1]

A. Upper airways defenses

1. **Mechanical defenses** are the first major barrier protecting the lower airway. These consist of air filtration, the epiglottic reflex, patency of the conducting airways, upper air-flow turbulence, cough, and mucociliary clearance. Neurologic diseases, inhaled or ingested toxins, abnormal bronchial secretions (e.g., cystic fibrosis), prior viral infections, endobronchial tumors or foreign bodies, and endotracheal or tracheostomy tubes all predispose to pneumonia by impairing one or more of these mechanical defenses.

2. **Secretory IgA** in the upper airways may contribute by impairing microbial adherence to the mucosal surface and by viral neutralizing activity.

B. Lower respiratory defenses

1. **IgG antibodies** diffuse relatively freely into mucosal secretions and the alveolar milieu [2]. Their importance is emphasized by the effectiveness of vaccines stimulating specific antibody formation and by the increased incidence of pneumonia in patients with immunoglobulin deficiencies (e.g., multiple myeloma, agammaglobulinemia). In addition, deficiencies of IgG_2 and IgG_4 predispose to recurrent sinus and bronchial infections, and this may be worsened if combined with IgA deficiency.

2. **Complement** activation generates opsonins, chemotactic molecules, and lytic activity. The functional absence of complement in sickle cell disease and certain inherited deficiency states is associated with an increased incidence of sinopulmonary infections.

3. **Phagocytic defenses consist of alveolar macrophages and neutrophils.** Either a quantitative or a qualitative defect in phagocytes may contribute to pyogenic infection. Pneumonia is common and often fatal in neutropenic patients. Impaired migration of phagocytes to sites of invasion may contribute to pneumonia. High alcohol concentrations impair neutrophil migration, which may contribute to the frequency of pneumonia among alcoholics. Certain organisms such as *Legionella* and *Mycobacterium* spp. can survive within nonimmune alveolar macrophages. Optimal defense against these and other facultative intracellular pathogens requires activation of macrophages through specific T-lymphocyte immunity.

Clinical Approach to Pneumonia

A definitive diagnosis of pneumonia depends on isolation of the infecting organism from a site not usually colonized (e.g., blood, pleural space, or lower respiratory tract) or the demonstration of a significant serologic change to a suspected infecting agent. However, historic data may be very useful in reaching a tentative diagnosis.

I. Importance of epidemiologic data

A. Family history.
Respiratory syncytial virus that produces bronchiolitis or pneumonia in an infant is almost always acquired from family members who may have only a mild respiratory illness. If an adult has pneumonia and a family member has had respiratory illness (pharyngitis, or even pneumonia) 18–21 days previously, *Mycoplasma pneumoniae* is a major consideration. If other family members (or friends) are currently ill and if influenza has been documented in the community, influenza-related pneumonia is likely (see Chap. 8).

B. Travel history.
A history of travel to certain areas of the country is essential for acquisition of coccidioidomycosis, histoplasmosis, or blastomycosis (see Chap. 18). Travel to Southeast Asia or the South Pacific at any time should raise the possibility of *Pseudomonas pseudomallei,* for illness can develop years after exposure.

C. Unusual contact.
Contact with animals and birds or their excreta suggests such entities as tularemia, hantavirus pulmonary syndrome, Q fever, plague, psittacosis, and histoplasmosis. Contact with excavations raises the question of the latter as well as Legionnaires' disease.

D. Recent hospitalization or institutionalization or antibiotic therapy.
Gram-negative pneumonias are much more frequent in hospitalized patients or those cared for in nursing homes.

E. **Heterosexuals and homosexuals who engage in "unsafe" sexual practices, intravenous drug abusers, and hemophiliacs** are at increased risk for AIDS (see Chap. 19).

II. **Frequency of various etiologies**
   A. **Community-acquired pneumonias** [3–3b]
      1. **Age** is an important factor.
         a. In the **neonatal period,** *Streptococcus agalactiae* is an important cause of pneumonia. It is acquired through contact in the birth canal (see Chap. 3).
         b. **The infant**
            (1) **Respiratory syncytial virus** (RSV), which is common in infancy, occurs in epidemics during the winter months. Bronchiolitis is a major manifestation of RSV infection, and significant hypoxemia can develop. Data suggest that infection occurs repeatedly but that each time the manifestations are less severe [4].
            (2) **Influenza** produces croup or pneumonia in infants and also occurs in epidemics (see Chap. 8). Infection in adults usually is a prominent part of these epidemics.
            (3) **Encapsulated bacteria.** Both *S. pneumoniae* and *H. influenzae* type b cause pneumonia in children 5–18 months of age. This is related both to loss of maternal antibody and to the failure of children in this age group to form antibody to polysaccharide antigens. (These encapsulated bacteria cause systemic infection and meningitis as well as pneumonia.) Since the introduction of the *H. influenzae* type b (Hib) conjugate vaccines in 1988, the incidence of invasive Hib infections in the United States has declined among infants and children. (See related discussion in sec. **III** under Special Considerations and Specific Therapy.)
         c. **Children** (3 months old to teenagers) occasionally develop pneumonia that may be diagnosed on the basis of helpful clues.
            (1) **Bacterial pneumonia** is particularly suspect when lobar consolidation or pneumonia with effusions develops. Staphylococcal pneumonia may occur in this age group.
            (2) **Viruses** (influenza, RSV, and other respiratory viruses) can cause diffuse bronchopneumonias.
            (3) *M. pneumoniae* is a major cause of pneumonias in children older than 5 years. (This type of pneumonia is discussed in sec. **V.B** under Special Considerations and Specific Therapy.)
         d. In **young adults** (18–45 years of age) *Mycoplasma* spp. and *Chlamydia pneumoniae* (formerly called *TWAR*) are the most common causes of pneumonia year-round, but influenza predominates during a community epidemic.
         e. **Older adults** are likely to have pneumococcal, *Legionella,* or aspiration pneumonias.
         f. **Institutionalized older adults,** most of whom require some help with the activities of daily living, are colonized with gram-negative rods much more frequently than are young individuals in the same environment. Therefore, when pneumonia develops, it is more likely to be gram-negative, although pneumococcal disease still is prevalent. Staphylococci (including methicillin-resistant strains), viruses, and *Mycobacterium tuberculosis* also may cause pneumonia in this group.
      2. **Predisposing conditions**
         a. **In alcoholics,** *S. pneumoniae* is the most prevalent organism, but anaerobes, *H. influenzae, K. pneumoniae,* and *M. tuberculosis* also cause disease in this setting.
         b. **Aspiration pneumonia** occurs in patients with mental obtundation or swallowing problems, esophageal disorders, seizure disorders, or poor dentition.
         c. **Chronic obstructive pulmonary disease** (COPD) is associated with a high frequency of *H. influenzae, S. pneumoniae,* and *Moraxella catarrhalis* pneumonias.
         d. **Cystic fibrosis** predisposes to staphylococcal and pseudomonal infection, the latter usually after administration of antibiotics. Thymidine-dependent staphylococcal infection may develop if trimethoprim-sulfamethoxazole (TMP-SMX) is used.
         e. **Postinfluenza bacterial pneumonias** are commonly caused by staphylococci, *H. influenzae,* or *S. pneumoniae* (see Chap. 8, sec. **VII** under Influenza).

B. Hospital-acquired pneumonias. Colonization of the oropharynx with gram-negative organisms, especially *Klebsiella* spp., is increased in the infirm elderly and by severe acute illness, prolonged hospitalization, diabetes, renal failure, intubation, or prior antibiotic exposure. **Gram-negative organisms must be considered when pneumonia develops in these settings.** Other important pathogens causing nosocomial pneumonia include *Staphylococcus aureus,* anaerobes from aspiration, *Legionella* species, and some viruses.

III. History. For pneumonias developing outside the hospital, the individual often has had a recent, mild, upper respiratory tract infection and then suddenly develops chills, fever, cough associated with pleuritic chest pain, and purulent sputum. However, the complete spectrum of these symptoms may be lacking, depending on the host and the organism.

A. Host considerations

1. **Neonates** with *Chlamydia* pneumonia characteristically do not have fever. Their symptoms are mild and prolonged (see Chap. 3).

2. **Young infants** with viral pneumonia almost always present with respiratory distress and fever but, at times, infants may appear septic.

3. **Elderly** patients often develop a change in eating habits or mental function with a minimum of respiratory symptoms. Other important clues to pneumonia in this population include unexplained diminished activity or fall, new incontinence, and the decompensation of a stable underlying medical problem. Fever may be minimal or absent. The chest roentgenogram may be the first objective evidence of pulmonary involvement.

4. **Patients with chronic bronchitis** may exhibit a change in the quantity and type (color and general appearance) of sputum as the first sign of pneumonia.

B. Special considerations by organism

1. Anaerobic pulmonary infections, tuberculosis, and pulmonary mycoses may be associated with a more gradual onset of symptoms than pyogenic bacterial pneumonias.

2. Some pneumonias characteristically have scant and nonpurulent sputum production (i.e., few polymorphonuclear leukocytes on Gram staining). (See secs. **V** and **VI** under Special Considerations and Specific Therapy.)

   a. *Mycoplasma* and *Chlamydia pneumoniae* usually have a gradual onset characterized by fever, protracted cough, and minimal sputum.

   b. **Legionnaires' disease** characteristically causes only a modest amount of sputum production and may be associated with relative bradycardia, renal abnormalities, delirium, at times diarrhea, and other findings [5, 6].

   c. **Q fever, psittacosis, and viral pneumonias** are nonbacterial pneumonias discussed in sec. **V** under Special Considerations and Specific Therapy. A history of occupational or other exposure to animals and birds or a local epidemic of influenza may help increase one's index of suspicion for these diagnoses.

IV. Physical examination. A complete description of physical findings associated with pneumonia may be found in standard texts of physical diagnosis. In addition to examination of the chest, special emphasis should be placed on a search for such signs of nonpneumonic infection as endocarditis, meningitis, and salpingitis. Specific evidence of an associated pleural effusion that may require a diagnostic or therapeutic thoracentesis should be sought. Other anomalies that may lead to an intrapulmonary process (e.g., deep venous thrombosis leading to pulmonary embolism, lymphadenopathy, or clubbing suggesting neoplasia) should be identified.

The compromised host, the very young, and the very old pose special diagnostic problems. In some, the physical findings may be minimal but the roentgenogram may clearly reveal the pneumonia. In others, particularly neutropenic patients, the initial roentgenogram may fail to show any infiltrates despite clinical findings of pneumonia.

V. Radiologic evaluation. Whenever pneumonia is suspected, even in an outpatient setting, a chest roentgenogram is indicated. The x-ray film yields useful clues, although it is **seldom possible to reach a specific etiologic diagnosis by roentgenography alone.**

A. Location of infiltrates

1. Infiltrates in the **apical segment of the lower lobe** or in the inferior segment of the **right upper lobe** suggest aspiration. However, during episodes of obtundation or unconsciousness that are associated with various postures, the resulting aspiration pneumonia may occur in other locations.

2. **Upper-lobe** involvement can occur in any pneumonia, but it is particularly common **in tuberculosis,** *Klebsiella* infection, and melioidosis. Lower-lobe infiltrates make tuberculosis less likely, although one should not exclude this possibility. The involvement of the anterior segment of an upper lobe by itself usually is considered nontuberculous and possibly related to other infection or tumor.

B. **Cavitation.** Cavities must be distinguished from pneumatoceles or infiltration around a bulla. Comparison to the normal lung can be helpful in the latter instance.

1. Cavities **without air-fluid levels** are **suggestive of tuberculosis,** but they occur also in fungal infections.

2. Cavities **with air-fluid levels** suggest abscess formation from staphylococci, anaerobes, gram-negative bacilli, coccidioidomycosis, nocardiosis, or melioidosis. **Occasionally, a loculated pleural effusion in association with a bronchopleural fistula can mimic an abscess.**

C. **Volume loss.** Early in infection, if there is evidence of volume loss in conjunction with an infiltrate, atelectasis is present. Under these circumstances, correctable bronchial obstruction must be excluded.

D. **Pleural fluid.** The presence of fluid in the pleural space carries diagnostic and therapeutic implications. Sampling the fluid may lead to a specific diagnosis and may mandate chest tube drainage if the fluid proves to be infected. In addition, the presence of an effusion is suggestive of certain pathogens. (See the discussion on pleural effusions later in this chapter under Pleural Effusion Versus Empyema.)

1. Pleural effusion without pneumonia may suggest tuberculosis, tumor, or a subdiaphragmatic process.

2. *Mycoplasma* and *C. pneumoniae* infections may be associated with pleural fluid, but usually the volume is not great and the effusion is not readily detected.

3. Pneumococcal pneumonia frequently is associated with effusion. The fluid may be sterile or may represent a frank empyema. Thoracentesis should be performed if the volume of effusion is significant or to exclude an associated empyema.

4. Anaerobic organisms, *Streptococcus pyogenes,* and *Escherichia coli,* as well as staphylococcal pneumonia in children, commonly produce pleural fluid.

5. *M. tuberculosis* that has produced cavities, *K. pneumoniae,* and *P. pseudomallei* may be associated with pleural fluid.

6. Influenza viral infections rarely are associated with effusion.

7. Bronchopneumonia, bilateral disease, and even abscess have been noted in Legionnaires' disease. Large effusions are uncommon [5].

E. **Mediastinal adenopathy.** Among the many causes of mediastinal adenopathy in association with acute pneumonia are *M. pneumoniae* in children, tuberculosis, fungal infections, tularemia, and lung cancer.

F. **Miscellaneous findings.** Pericardial effusion, widening of the mediastinum, evidence of a bronchopleural fistula, and free air under the diaphragm have specific implications for further evaluation. Noninfectious processes such as **chemotherapy, radiation,** and **drug reactions** also may alter the roentgenographic appearance acutely, and other disorders can mimic community-acquired pneumonia [7–9].

G. **Follow-up chest roentgenograms. Rapid changes in pulmonary infiltrates or sudden improvement** (e.g., over 8–36 hours) **seldom occurs in pneumonia. If rapid changes do occur, pulmonary congestion or atelectasis is the usual cause.** Although radiologic evaluation may assist in following a patient with pneumonia, serial roentgenography often is overused.

1. **Patients clinically improving. Pulmonary infiltrates due to pneumonia often take a month to clear completely [10, 11]. In elderly patients,** clearing may take **even longer** (1–12 weeks). Therefore, it is wise to postpone a follow-up radiographic examination in the patient who is responding appropriately. In patients in whom radiographic clearing does not occur after 1 month (or in whom pneumonias recur in the same location), neoplasia must be ruled out using bronchoscopy.

   In the late follow-up film, if volume loss is recognized after the infiltrate has cleared, either destruction of lung or fibrosis and scarring are responsible. Fibrosis is seen after aerobic gram-negative or anaerobic infection, and scarring often is associated with tuberculosis and histoplasmosis.

2. **Patients not improving** [10, 11]. In patients who are not clinically responding or in those who develop new fever, increasing pulmonary symptoms, or sputum

production, **follow-up roentgenograms are important** to determine the possible presence of (1) bronchial obstruction, (2) a superimposed, new pulmonary infection, (3) an associated effusion that may be infected, or (4) an abscess.

VI. **Recovery of the organism.** Identification of a pathogenic organism in a patient with pneumonia is the cornerstone of diagnosis and is of primary importance in further management. **Every effort should be made to obtain diagnostic specimens before initiating antibiotic therapy.** Obtaining specimens should not be left to the untrained. Blood cultures, a good sputum for smear and culture, aspiration and culture of pleural fluid if such is present, and cerebrospinal fluid (CSF) if meningitis is a possible complication should be obtained.

A. **Normal mouth flora.** The mouth contains both anaerobic and aerobic bacteria in concentrations of 10^7–10^9 organisms per milliliter. These are readily observed on Gram staining, and the aerobic organisms are recovered on routine cultures.

Common, normal colonizers of the oropharynx are listed in Table 9-1. At times, these normal colonizers are the pathogens in a lower respiratory tract infection [12]. However, as Table 9-1 emphasizes, **the mere isolation of these organisms from expectorated sputum does not prove they are pathogens in the lower respiratory tract.** (See the discussion of colonization versus infection in sec. **IX.**)

B. **Methods of sputum collection** [13, 14]
   1. **Coughed specimens.** The inherent problem in obtaining sputum specimens with coughing is that the specimens often are contaminated by oropharyngeal colonizers. To minimize such contamination, **sputum from a deep cough,** not saliva, must be studied. Even with careful attempts to obtain a proper sputum specimen, in approximately at least 20–30% of cases, sputum for culture typically is not available.
   2. **Nasotracheal aspirations** may provide a sputum sample, but they are always contaminated with some oral colonizers. However, the procedure may stimulate deep expectorations that produce an adequate specimen.
   3. **Bronchoscopy.** When the bronchoscope initially is passed into the upper airway, upper airway colonizers may contaminate the specimen collection unless special techniques are used. A protected (plugged) brush catheter (PBC) has been devised to reduce this problem but is best used in conjunction with quantitative cultures [13, 14]. (See further discussion in sec. **VII.**)
   4. **Transtracheal aspiration.** Transtracheal aspiration (TTA), direct lung aspiration, and lung biopsy bypass normal oropharyngeal colonizers. Thus, these specimens are suitable for anaerobic cultures. **Organisms seen in or cultured from these specimens usually represent lower respiratory tract pathogens.** (See further discussion in sec. **VII.**)

C. **Gram staining of sputum.** The technique and interpretation of Gram stains is discussed in Chap. 25, sec. **I,** under Smear and Stain Techniques. We believe that this helpful procedure should be performed in every case of pneumonia, although this view is not held by all [3]. The sputum Gram stain will assist in several ways.

Table 9-1. Common colonizers of the oropharynx

Organism	Incidence range (%)
Staphylococcus aureus	35–40
Streptococcus pyogenes (group A)	0–9
Streptococcus pneumoniae	0–50
Neisseria meningitidis	0–15
Haemophilus influenzae	5–20
Gram-negative bacteria	2*

*Approximate percentage isolated by using routine culture techniques. With special broth cultures, more than 10% of normals may have gram-negative colonizers. Of elderly nursing home patients, 6–40% may be found to be colonized with gram-negatives (as revealed by routine culture techniques). With special broth cultures, up to 60% of these elderly patients are found to be colonized [12].

Source: Adapted from H. M. Sommers, The Indigenous Microbiota of the Human Host. In G. P. Youmans et al. (eds.). *The Biologic and Clinical Basis of Infectious Diseases* (2nd ed.). Philadelphia: Saunders, 1980.

1. Gram staining will help to **assess the adequacy of the sputum specimen** that is obtained for culture. **If more than 10 squamous epithelial cells are seen per low-power field, the sputum sample is contaminated with oral secretions.** In such cases, a repeat sputum should always be obtained for Gram staining and culture, or an invasive method of specimen collection should be considered.

2. Gram staining will help **indicate whether unsuspected gram-negative organisms are present.** A specific agent may not be obvious on the Gram stain, but the presence or absence of gram-positive cocci or gram-negative bacilli may be very helpful.

3. Gram staining of pleural fluid, TTA, protected brush specimens, or percutaneous lung aspirates are even more valuable, because normal colonizers are not present in these samples.

D. **Acid-fast smears and cultures** should be obtained when upper-lobe disease is present or in other situations where tuberculosis is suspected, such as in alcoholics, in patients with pneumonias of unclear etiology, or in compromised hosts with pneumonias. The methods are described in Chap. 25, sec. **II,** under Smear and Stain Techniques.

E. **Sputum: special cultures.** Under certain circumstances, attempts to isolate certain pathogens should be considered.

1. During epidemics, virus isolation should be attempted in the infant with pneumonia and in seriously ill adults.

2. When pneumonia occurs in the young adult who is otherwise well, attempts at isolation of viruses and *M. pneumoniae* are reasonable if the facilities are available. Viruses other than influenza rarely are implicated in adult pneumonia unless the host is compromised.

3. The compromised host with a nonbacterial pneumonia merits viral studies, particularly of lung tissue specimens.

4. *Legionella* cultures and direct fluorescent antibody studies should be performed on appropriate specimens from patients in whom there is no obvious diagnosis. (See sec. **VI** under Special Considerations and Specific Therapy.)

F. **If no sputum is available for culture** and the patient is not ill enough for an invasive procedure (see sec. **B** and sec. **VII**), the clinician often is forced to use empiric antibiotics. Infrequently, blood cultures may be positive in these patients. Empiric antibiotic therapy is a particular problem in nosocomial pneumonias in which the risk for gram-negative infections is significant.

VII. **Invasive procedures [15].** The invasive procedures most widely used to collect lower respiratory specimens are fiberoptic bronchoscopy with a PBC and bronchoalveolar lavage (BAL). These are discussed in more detail later. **The diagnostic value of each is significantly reduced by prior antibiotic therapy.**

Percutaneous thin-needle lung aspiration is required only rarely in adults to diagnose infection. It is best reserved for enigmatic lesions that can be localized and are peripheral. Open lung biopsy in the diagnosis of pneumonia usually is considered only in immunocompromised hosts.

A. **Indications.** There are no firm criteria for the use of these invasive procedures to diagnose pulmonary infection [3]. It must be emphasized, however, that **most patients with community-acquired pneumonia are successfully managed without an invasive procedure** [3, 16, 17]. Thus, **noninvasive evaluations should always be performed first.** Pulmonary consultation is advised. **Consider an invasive procedure if the severity of the illness or its rate of progression is significant enough to warrant the risks of the procedure, and in the presence of all the following circumstances:**

1. Adequate specimens are unobtainable using noninvasive techniques.

2. The resulting specimens will be properly and quickly processed.

3. There are no absolute contraindications present.

B. **Transtracheal aspiration.** TTA is used only infrequently at present. Risks are associated with TTA, and in some patients the risks are significant, so **TTA should be performed only by experienced personnel.**

C. **Fiberoptic bronchoscopy with PBC.** Fiberoptic bronchoscopy has become a more frequently performed procedure than TTA to diagnose acute pulmonary infections. This is because fiberoptic bronchoscopy is widely available and PBCs plus appropriate culture techniques have been perfected.

1. **Fiberoptic bronchoscopy alone is unable to provide specimens that are free of oral contamination,** which occurs when the bronchoscope passes through the nasal or oral cavity and also during suctioning as the bronchoscope is inserted. To minimize contamination, the PBC was devised.
2. The **PBC** consists of a double-sheathed tube sealed at the distal end [14]. After the bronchoscope is positioned, the whole PBC is pushed through the inner channel several centimeters beyond the bronchoscope. The inner sheath then is pushed beyond the plug, and a sterile brush is advanced through the open inner sheath into the secretions being sampled. The steps are reversed, and the brush is withdrawn.
3. **Quantitative cultures are necessary** because some degree of contamination is inevitable even using a PBC and because the brush holds only approximately 0.001 ml of secretions. Organisms, including anaerobes, growing in concentrations of 10^3 or more per milliliter are considered significant [15, 18, 19]. The detection of antibody-coated bacteria is not uniformly helpful and is not routinely recommended [20, 21].
4. **This procedure has proved especially useful in diagnosing acute nosocomial pneumonia in the mechanically ventilated patient** [15, 18, 19, 21–23].
5. The **risks** of fiberoptic bronchoscopy with PBC brushing are low and include pneumothorax, transient fever or infiltrates, and decreased oxygenation.
   D. **Bronchoalveolar lavage** [14, 15]. BAL is performed by wedging the fiberoptic bronchoscope in a distal airway and injecting and aspirating 100–250 ml of sterile normal saline through the bronchoscope. The value of protected BAL has not been established [3, 18]. BAL samples a larger amount of the involved lung than the PBC and thus offers a theoretic advantage in the diagnosis of bacterial pneumonias. However, **contamination of BAL specimens with oropharyngeal or nasopharyngeal organisms is very common** (see sec. **C.1**). Quantitative cultures of BAL fluid may help to distinguish infecting from contaminating bacteria [18, 19, 23, 24]. Recently, BAL has proven useful in the diagnosis of anaerobic infections [25]. At present, it is a promising but often unnecessary method for diagnosing routine bacterial pneumonias. **BAL is most useful in evaluating immunocompromised patients with pulmonary infiltrates** [14, 15, 17, 26].
   E. **Alternatives to bronchoscopic BAL** in mechanically ventilated patients are undergoing study. For example, in one report the Ballard BAL catheter (Ballard Medical Products, Draper, UT), a disposable, flexible coude-tip device (which can be attached to the endotracheal tube without loss of positive end-expiratory pressure and allows supplemental oxygen delivery) that does not require bronchoscopy to insert, provided BAL samples equivalent to conventional bronchoscopy BAL samples [26a]. This technique is limited to patients in whom there is a diffuse process in at least one lung and in whom direct visualization is not required [26a].
VIII. **Other laboratory studies.** Most other laboratory studies generally are not helpful in the early diagnosis of pneumonia.
   A. **WBC count.** Detection of leukocytosis will help confirm the presence of infection, but it is otherwise fairly nonspecific. A markedly depressed WBC count has been linked to poor prognosis in patients with pneumonia. In the alcoholic, a decreased WBC count seems to be related to high blood alcohol levels.
   B. **Liver function tests.** Abnormal liver function tests have been associated with many different types of infection, both bacterial and nonbacterial. Therefore, this too is a nonspecific finding.
   C. **Cold agglutinins.** In approximately half of the patients infected with *M. pneumoniae,* cold agglutinins will be positive, with a titer of 1:32 or greater. If initially negative, the titer should be repeated in 5 days. Positive reactions, however, are not specific for *Mycoplasma,* as is discussed in sec. **V.B.2** under Special Considerations and Specific Therapy.
   D. **Serologic studies**
   1. **Mycoplasmal pneumonia.** Antibody demonstrated by enzyme-linked immunosorbent assay (ELISA) or complement-fixing antibodies often are present in high titer in acute disease. The rise in antibody may occur quickly, and a convalescent specimen should be obtained early (within 10–14 days of the onset of the illness). This is discussed further in sec. **V.B.2** under Special Considerations and Specific Therapy.
   2. **Influenza.** A retrospective diagnosis of influenza pneumonia can be made by observing changes in antibody titers between acute and convalescent serum specimens. Several antibody tests have been used. Other viral infections may

be documented by a fourfold rise in antibody titer. A convalescent titer usually is obtained 2–3 weeks after obtaining the acute sample. (See Chaps. 8 and 25.)

3. **Legionnaires' and other diseases.** Indirect fluorescent antibody assay, or ELISA testing, is useful for diagnosing Legionnaires' disease. The titer, however, develops only during or after the recovery period. (See sec. **VI.F.7** under Special Considerations and Specific Therapy.)

Other diagnoses often made serologically are those of Q fever and psittacosis.

4. **Fungal serologic studies.** These may help to support a diagnosis of a pulmonary mycosis, especially in patients with a chronic pneumonia [27] (see Chap. 18). Tests to detect fungal antigens, in addition to cryptococcal antigen, hold promise for the rapid diagnosis of pulmonary mycoses [28].

E. **Antigen detection. Latex agglutination** has generally replaced counterimmunoelectrophoresis (CIE) as the most readily available technique to detect bacterial antigens. Studies have shown that the **urine and serum are less frequently positive in patients with pneumonia than in patients with meningitis.** Detection of antigen in pleural fluid is most helpful. Although a positive test establishes a specific etiology, a negative test does not exclude a possible etiology. (See Chap. 25 for discussion of these techniques.)

F. **Tuberculosis skin test.** The tuberculosis skin test to detect evidence of delayed hypersensitivity **is not particularly helpful in a patient with pneumonia,** and the results can be misleading. First, delayed hypersensitivity persists for life; therefore, a positive reaction does not mean that the infection is recent. Second, the leukocytosis that accompanies bacterial pneumonia may be associated with transient anergy. If the skin test is repeated after an individual has recovered, the result will be positive, and the interpretation (i.e., recent conversion) will be incorrect. **For the diagnosis of active tuberculous pulmonary infection, concentrated sputum specimens are much more useful.** (See sec. **IV.A** under Tuberculosis: Basic Concepts for additional discussion of skin testing.)

IX. **Colonization versus infection (superinfection).** *Colonization* **refers to the presence of organisms that are not causing disease.** Gram-negative bacilli, staphylococci, and *Candida* spp. are all common colonizers of the oropharynx and, therefore, of the sputum (see Table 9-1).

The oropharynx of hospitalized individuals commonly becomes colonized with gram-negative bacteria. In patients receiving antibiotics, colonizers may be resistant to the antibiotic being administered [29]. Elderly patients in the nursing home setting also become colonized with gram-negative bacteria [12]. The determination that these organisms are causing a significant pulmonary infection or superinfection (i.e., a new pneumonia superimposed on a partially treated pneumonia) rests on clinical grounds. **It is crucial to make the distinction between colonization and actual infection** so as not to withhold necessary treatment or commit a patient inappropriately to prolonged antibiotic therapy. Three settings commonly confront the clinician.

A. **Elderly patients with pneumonia.** Elderly patients (not institutionalized) have an increased incidence of nasopharyngeal colonization by *S. aureus* and by gram-negative organisms, especially *Klebsiella.* Thus, if these patients develop pneumonia due to *S. pneumoniae,* sputum culture may reveal *S. pneumoniae* and one or more gram-negative rods. It is often very difficult to ascertain which bacterial species is responsible for the pneumonia, but two points are useful.

1. **Patients on antibiotics.** If an antibiotic (e.g., penicillin or ampicillin) has been administered that has no activity against the gram-negative bacterium or staphylococcus isolated from sputum, and the patient is nevertheless clinically improving, the gram-negative bacterium or staphylococcus can be ignored.

2. **Adequate sputum but light bacterial growth.** If the sputum is adequate (based on microscopic characteristics) and only small quantities of gram-negative organisms are isolated, such organisms generally can be ignored. Gram-negative organisms causing endobronchial pneumonia usually are isolated from sputum in large numbers. The exception is embolic pneumonia, for which blood cultures are positive.

B. **Debilitated hospitalized patients.** A second clinical situation in which respiratory colonization must be differentiated from infection involves the patient who is hospitalized for another reason (e.g., surgery or myocardial infarction) or who is debilitated enough to require intensive care monitoring or nursing.

1. **Fever not due to pneumonia is frequent.** Patients develop fever for a variety of reasons, none of which may be related to bacterial bronchopulmonary infection.

Such nonpulmonary sources as phlebitis, urinary tract infections, wound infections, drug fever, and myocardial infarction need to be assessed carefully.

2. **The chest roentgenogram often is abnormal but not because of a pneumonia.** Atelectasis or congestive heart failure (CHF) is common, and the roentgenographic differentiation from pneumonia is not always possible.

3. The major **findings that support colonization are** (1) a clinical course that is stable or improving without specific antibiotics (as evidenced on serial observations) [29], (2) an absence of marked sputum production, (3) nonpurulent sputum on Gram staining, and (4) only modest or light growth of bacteria.

C. **After primary pneumonia.** The most common problem facing the clinician is the patient recovering from acute pneumonia in whom gram-negative organisms or staphylococci or both are isolated from a sputum sample and who develops a fever. Here, the differentiation between colonization and superinfection imposed on the resolving primary pneumonia presents a challenge. In these cases, there is sufficient sputum volume and the sputum cultures reveal heavy growth. Therefore, clinical and laboratory data must be analyzed in toto. **Culture data cannot be analyzed in an isolated manner.**

1. **Interpretation of signs, symptoms, and laboratory data.** Three components commonly are present in the patient with superinfection: fever, leukocytosis, and increased respiratory signs and symptoms [29].

   a. **Fever and leukocytosis often occur in association with other problems.** If the individual recovering from pneumonia develops fever or leukocytosis and yet has stable respiratory signs and no increase in sputum, there will almost always be a reason other than pulmonary superinfection to explain these findings.

   b. **Respiratory changes are the important findings in diagnosing true superinfection.**

      (1) **Ventilatory status.** Because the initial pneumonia has compromised the ventilatory capacity, even minor additional pulmonary infection can greatly infringe on the minimal reserve, precipitating respiratory deterioration [29]. Because the patient with superinfection has no more pulmonary reserve, it is of paramount importance to begin appropriate therapy as soon as there is clinical evidence of disease. By contrast, if the patient has no increase in respiratory symptoms or no increase in purulent sputum, it is very unlikely that he or she has pulmonary superinfection, and every effort should be made to uncover another cause of the fever.

      A similar exacerbation of respiratory symptoms often will occur in the patient with underlying chronic lung disease who develops a superimposed pneumonia. These patients often have minimal reserve as well.

      (2) **Purulent sputum.** In the patient with a superinfection or with initial true infection rather than colonization, the **sputum Gram stain can be very helpful.** If an adequate specimen is examined, **many polymorphonuclear leukocytes are seen in superinfection or true infection.** If the sputum appears nonpurulent on the Gram stain and the patient is not leukopenic, a lower respiratory tract infection is less likely [29].

   c. A new infiltrate on the chest roentgenogram helps to differentiate between bronchitis and pneumonia in a patient with increased respiratory symptoms. However, the **roentgenogram is of limited value** in monitoring patients for superinfection. New infiltrates of superinfection may lag behind the increase in pulmonary symptoms. An increase in density of the initial infiltrate may occur in patients who are responding appropriately, or a definite infiltrate may be difficult to visualize in the patient with coexisting CHF.

2. **Specific diagnosis.** When infection or superinfection becomes apparent clinically, sputum smears and cultures and blood cultures should be obtained. If not contraindicated, an invasive procedure may help to differentiate between upper tract colonization and lower tract infection [13–15]. Culture results will allow further modifications of the antibiotic regimen, often to a less toxic therapeutic course.

D. **Summary.** For therapeutic decisions, it is important to separate colonization from true infection, whether the latter is an initial infection or a superinfection. **If colonization is present, the patient can be observed. However, if the patient has definite infection, therapy must be initiated.** Because the therapy may be prolonged and associated with toxic side effects (e.g., renal failure with aminoglycosides), unnecessary therapy for colonization must be avoided.

X. **General concepts of therapy.** Specific antibiotic dosages and durations of therapy for various types of pneumonias are discussed under Special Considerations and Specific Therapy. There are some general concepts that apply to patients with pneumonia when the etiology is not yet known.

   A. **When to hospitalize patients with pneumonia.** Except for young patients with apparent mycoplasmal pneumonia, initial hospitalization generally is indicated for patients with pneumonia. **Certain factors associated with a poor outcome from community-acquired pneumonia are listed in Table 9-2. When present, particularly if multiple factors are present together, hospitalization should be strongly considered** [3]. In addition, initial hospital care may be indicated if there is inadequate home support or follow-up. Need for oxygen, intubation, and assisted ventilation can be monitored closely while the patient is in the hospital.

   Furthermore, during the influenza season we often admit young patients with the clinical diagnosis of postinfluenza pneumonia because some of these patients may have mixed bacterial or *S. aureus* pneumonia or, infrequently, a primary influenza pneumonia. (See Chap. 8, sec. **VII** under Influenza.)

   In children, many pneumonias are of viral origin and, when these cases are mild, they can be carefully followed in the outpatient setting. If a bacterial process is suspected or if a complication (e.g., empyema) is present, or if the viral process leads to respiratory distress, the child will need hospitalization. (See further discussion of pneumonia in children in sec. **XIII** under Special Considerations and Specific Therapy.)

Table 9-2. Risk factors for a poor outcome from pneumonia*

Advanced age (≥65 years)

Serious underlying conditions
   Chronic lung, heart, liver, or renal disease
   Diabetes mellitus
   Malnutrition
   Recurrent aspiration
   Alcoholism
   Cystic fibrosis
   Immunodeficiency (including splenectomy)

Hospitalization for pneumonia within 1 year

Physical findings
   Tachypnea >30 breaths/min
   Hypotension
   Fever >38.3°C (101°F)
   Distant sites of infection
   Altered level of consciousness

Laboratory findings
   Leukocytosis >30,000 cells/mm^3
   Leukopenia <4,000 cells/mm^3
   Neutropenia <1,000 cells/mm^3
   Hypoxemia or hypercapnia
   Anemia
   Renal insufficiency

Complications
   Mechanical ventilation required
   Adult respiratory distress syndrome
   Sepsis syndrome

Radiographic findings
   Two or more lobes involved
   Significant pleural effusion
   Cavitation
   Rapid spread

*These factors have been associated with either death or a complicated course, particularly if multiple ones are present simultaneously [3].

B. **Antibiotic principles** [3, 30]

1. **Narrow-spectrum versus broad-spectrum coverage.** Initial therapy should be chosen to cover the types of organisms seen on Gram stains of sputum and pleural fluid, and those suspected from the clinical presentation. Antibiotics with narrow coverage are indicated for patients who are only mildly ill and at least risk. If a specific etiology is found, then specific therapy should be given based on susceptibility data. Broader empiric coverage may be necessary for severely ill patients, those at greatest risk for complications (see Table 9-2), or those with nondiagnostic smears and infection of uncertain etiology. Antibiotics should be modified after the results of cultures are available, taking into account the response to initial therapy. (Bronchoscopy to document *Pneumocystis* infection should be carried out in patients who are at risk for HIV infection if sputum is negative for *Pneumocystis*.) In addition, these patients should be placed in respiratory isolation pending the results of an evaluation for mycobacterial infection. Table 9-3 summarizes the effectiveness of various empiric regimens.

   The following modified guidelines [3] exclude patients at risk for HIV infection. These patients are discussed in Chap. 19.

   a. **Outpatient treatment for patients from 18–50 or 55 years of age without significant underlying disease**

      (1) If the Gram stain of sputum suggests pneumococci, oral amoxicillin, 500 mg q8h, is an option in areas with a known low incidence of penicillin-resistant *S. pneumoniae* (see Chap. 28C). (Because oral amoxicillin is better absorbed than oral penicillin, amoxicillin is preferred.) Erythromycin can be used in the allergic patient.

      (2) If the clinical presentation is highly suggestive of mycoplasma pneumonia (see pp. 281–282), erythromycin or tetracycline is suggested.

      (3) When a sputum Gram stain is not available, and the presentation is not highly suggestive of mycoplasma, empiric therapy is indicated. The agent chosen should be active against the most commonly identified pathogens: *S. pneumoniae,* mycoplasma, and *C. pneumoniae.* Other important but less frequently involved organisms include *Legionella pneumophila* and *H. influenzae* (probably an infrequent cause of true invasive pneumonia). In this setting, oral erythromycin (500 mg qid) has become a commonly used agent for an early community-acquired pneumonia. For patients with a prior history of gastrointestinal intolerance with erythromycin or a history of GI upset with oral antibiotic use, oral clarithromycin (500 mg bid) and azithromycin are options. These newer macrolides have fewer GI side effects and have somewhat greater activity against *H. influenzae* but are more expensive than erythromycin (see discussion in Chap. 28M).

      (4) If the patient develops a postinfluenza pneumonia, then *S. pneumoniae, H. influenzae,* or *S. aureus* (or a mixed bacterial infection of these) are more of a concern and hospitalization should be considered (see Chap. 8, sec. **VII** under Influenza).

      (5) A screening history to rule out HIV risk factors and the potential of exposure to *M. tuberculosis* should be routinely done.

      (6) In geographic regions with endemic fungal infections (e.g., histoplasmosis, blastomycosis), fungal pneumonias need to be considered (see Chap. 18).

   b. **Outpatient therapy for patients older than 50–55 years or those patients with underlying medical disease (comorbidity)**

      (1) **Note: The elderly patient or patient with significant underlying disease usually is admitted for initiation of therapy for pneumonia.**

      (2) In very early, mild illness, outpatient therapy may be reasonable if careful compliance with therapy and outpatient follow-up can be ensured.

      (3) If the Gram stain of sputum suggests pneumococcal infection, amoxicillin is suggested if the infection was acquired in geographical areas with a low incidence of penicillin-resistant *S. pneumoniae* [see sec. **a.(1)**].

      (4) **If no sputum is available, or the Gram stain is nondiagnostic, the optimal agent in this setting is unclear.** Empiric antibiotic activity should be directed against *S. pneumoniae* and, if the patient is from a nursing home, common community-acquired gram-negative bacteria.

Table 9-3. Initial empiric regimens for pneumonia in adults[a]

Setting or presumed type of pneumonia	Penicillin	Advanced cephalosporin	Beta-lactam plus an aminoglycoside	Tetracycline	Erythromycin	TMP-SMX
Community-acquired						
Gram-positive cocci[b]	1[c]	2[d]	2	3	[d]	2
Gram stain, other[b]	3	1–2[e,f]	2	3 or 4	3	2
Presumed nonbacterial or *Legionella*[g]	4	4	4	3[h]	1[h]	4
High risk for or known HIV infection[i]	3	3[j]	3	3	3[j]	1[j]
Hospital-acquired						
Gram-positive cocci[b]	3[k]	1[k]–2	2	4	3	2
Gram stain, other[b]						
Mild, early illness	4	1	1–2	4	4	2
Moderate to severe illness	4	3	1[l]	4	4	2

TMP-SMX = trimethoprim-sulfamethoxazole; COPD = chronic obstructive pulmonary disease.

Note: the number indicates the effectiveness of the **initial** regimen in the instance in which the pneumonia is found to be due to the type of pathogen listed in the far left column: **1 = drug of choice; 2 = effective, but not choice because of toxicity, cost, or unnecessarily broad spectrum; 3 = effective only in some instances; 4 = ineffective.**

[a]Many adults with a pneumonia should be admitted to the hospital (see text). **This table suggests empiric therapy. Once sputum culture data are available, antibiotic therapy can and should be modified based on culture data.** Unnecessary use of broad-spectrum agents may increase the risk of resistant pathogens colonizing the patient over time or may increase the risk of resistant pathogens in a given hospital over time. **For the critically ill patient, broad-spectrum antibiotics commonly are used.**

[b]Based on highly suggestive Gram stains of a well-obtained sputum. "Gram stain, other" implies gram-negative organisms, mixed gram-positive and gram-negative organisms, or gram-negative coccobacillary forms.

[c]During the influenza season (known or suspected), the possibility of penicillinase-producing *Staphylococcus aureus* should be treated with oxacillin or nafcillin. Some clinicians prefer a cephalosporin (e.g, cefuroxime) for postinfluenza pneumonia. See also text discussion of penicillin-resistant *S. pneumoniae* issues in this chapter, pages 274–275, and Chap. 28C. In areas with moderate to high frequency of high-level penicillin-resistant *S. pneumoniae*, penicillin/ampicillin cannot be used.

[d] In a patient with a delayed penicillin-allergic history, a first-generation cephalosporin can be used (e.g., cefazolin). Erythromycin is another option.

[e] In the mildly ill patient without a predisposition to COPD, a first-generation cephalosporin often is a reasonable initial agent. In the patient with COPD or a Gram stain suggestive of *Haemophilus influenzae*, cefuroxime or a third-generation cephalosporin is commonly used pending cultures.

[f] The resistance of *H. influenzae* to ampicillin varies in different institutions and geographic areas but is usually in the range of 10–35%. In areas of known high ampicillin resistance or in the moderately to very ill patient with underlying COPD, the possibility of resistant *H. influenzae* must be considered at admission, and cefuroxime or a third-generation cephalosporin often is used. (Other alternatives include TMP-SMX and chloramphenicol.)

[g] Not typical age group of bacterial pneumonia (e.g., healthy young patient younger than 45 years), scant sputum; patient with possible *Legionella* or *Mycoplasma* infection; or a patient with negative bacterial cultures and negative mycobacterial sputum smears and not responding to antibiotics.

[h] Tetracycline is active against *Mycoplasma pneumoniae* (psittacosis, Q fever and chlamydia), but not *Legionella* species, whereas erythromycin is active against *M. pneumoniae*, *Legionella*, and *Chlamydia* species. For patients with gastrointestinal side effects from oral or intravenous erythromycin, oral clarithromycin may be an alternative. See Chap. 28M. **Sputum for mycobacterium stains and cultures should routinely be done in these patients to rule out tuberculosis; respiratory isolation is recommended until mycobacterial disease has been excluded.**

[i] TMP-SMX is the agent of choice for *P. carinii* pneumonia (usually a diffuse process), but it would also be active against most strains of community-acquired *S. pneumoniae*, *H. influenzae*, *S. aureus*, and gram-negative bacilli. See Chap. 24. For more focal infiltrates, cefuroxime and erythromycin are often preferred (see Chap. 19).

[k] If Gram stain highly suggests staphylococci, a semisynthetic penicillin (e.g., oxacillin) or first-generation cephalosporin (e.g., cefazolin) would be reasonable if no gram-negatives are seen on the Gram stain. In a patient with mild, early illness and a Gram stain highly suggestive of *Streptococcus pneumoniae*, penicillin alone may be reasonable.

[l] If *Pseudomonas* infection is likely and the patient is moderately to severely ill, combination therapy with piperacillin and an aminoglycoside is indicated. In the critically ill patient, triple antibiotics may be reasonable until culture data are back (e.g., cefazolin, piperacillin, and an aminoglycoside). If the patient has a delayed penicillin allergy, ceftazidime can be combined with an aminoglycoside in the very ill patient to provide synergy against *P. aeruginosa*. If the patient has a very early, mild pneumonia, ceftazidime alone may be reasonable monotherapy (see Chap. 28F).

Source: From R. E. Reese and R. F. Betts (eds.), *Handbook of Antibiotics* (2nd ed.). Boston: Little, Brown, 1993. Pp. 613–615.

Other potential pathogens include *M. catarrhalis, H. influenzae,* and *L. pneumophila.*

TMP-SMX, a second-generation cephalosporin (e.g., cefuroxime, cefprozil) or amoxicillin-clavulanate are options for empiric initial therapy. We do not routinely add a macrolide to cover for *Legionella* in the outpatient setting.

(5) See secs. **a.(4)–(6).**

c. **Therapy for patients who require hospitalization (adults)**

(1) Although the trend is to use broader antimicrobial agents [3] than in the past for these patients, if **the patient is only mildly ill,** has not been on antibiotics or hospitalized recently, is not allergic to penicillins, is not from a nursing home, is from an area with a low incidence of penicillin-resistant *S. pneumoniae,* does not have a predominance of gram-negative bacilli or coccobacillary forms or has gram-positive diplococci on Gram stain, and can be watched carefully, we may still initiate therapy with intravenous ampicillin (1.5 g q6h) or aqueous penicillin (1.5–2.0 million units q4h) to provide activity against *S. pneumoniae,* mouth anaerobes, and most *H. influenzae.*

(2) **For patients with** penicillin allergy, those who clinically worsen after a trial of oral antibiotics in the outpatient setting, or those from a nursing home, or who are moderately ill, we commonly will use cefuroxime (750 mg q8h IV) when the Gram stain does not suggest *S. pneumoniae* or is not available. This agent will cover community-acquired gram-negative bacteria as well as *S. pneumoniae* and essentially all *H. influenzae* and *M. catarrhalis.* It is also very good for postinfluenza bacterial pneumonias (see sec. **VII** under Influenza in Chap. 8). In the nonallergic patient, ampicillin-sulbactam or piperacillin-tazobactam can be used (see Chap. 28E). If the Gram stain of sputum (when available) does not show gram-negative bacilli or if no sputum is available, we generally would not use a broad-spectrum third-generation cephalosporin in this setting, although some do advocate their use [3, 3a]. We prefer to use a second-generation cephalosporin (e.g., cefuroxime), which is narrower in its spectrum of activity than the third-generation cephalosporins and, therefore, presumably less likely to select out resistant bacteria. (See related discussions in Chaps. 28A and 28F.)

If *Mycoplasma* or *Legionella* spp. are a concern clinically, erythromycin can be added [3]. We do not routinely use erythromycin, but this agent can be added if the patient does not respond to the initial regimen.

d. **Therapy for critically ill adult patients requiring hospitalization** for community-acquired pneumonia. Specific therapy is available for a variety of agents including *S. pneumoniae, H. influenzae, S. aureus,* and *M. catarrhalis* and atypical organisms (e.g., *Mycoplasma, C. pneumoniae,* and *Legionella* spp.).

(1) A common combination to use is cefuroxime (750 mg q8h IV) and erythromycin (500–1,000 mg q6h IV). Alternatives include ampicillin-sulbactam, ticarcillin-clavulanate, or piperacillin-tazobactam, or a third-generation cephalosporin, **along with** erythromycin.

(2) *Pseudomonas* spp. are an unusual community-acquired pathogen. In the critically ill patient who had gram-negative bacilli on Gram stain or in someone we would want to cover for the possibility of *Pseudomonas* infection, we would add an aminoglycoside (e.g., tobramycin) to cefuroxime and erythromycin or use the combination of an antipseudomonal penicillin (e.g., piperacillin) along with an aminoglycoside and erythromycin.

We would not rely on ceftazidime alone for the critically ill patient with a possible underlying *Pseudomonas aeruginosa* pneumonia. (See Chap. 28F.)

(3) For severe postinfluenza pneumonia, see the detailed discussion in Chap. 8, sec. **VII** under Influenza.

(4) See secs. **a.(5)–(6).**

2. **Reevaluation of initial regimens**

a. **Pneumonia of known etiology.** Organisms isolated from blood, pleural fluid, or lower respiratory tract secretions are presumed to be etiologic agents. Once a specific cause of pneumonia has been identified, **therapy**

should be adjusted to the best narrow-spectrum regimen, taking into account the relative efficacies, toxicities, and costs of possible alternatives. Usually, there is no reason to continue a patient on a multidrug regimen simply because of response to that regimen [31].

b. **Pneumonia of unclear etiology.** Many times sputum cultures fail to reveal an etiology. The following data help interpret this result.

   (1) Both pneumococci and *H. influenzae* have been recovered from blood, TTA, lung puncture, or pleural fluid when the sputum cultures do not reveal the organism. Thus, there is a significant number of cases in which sputum cultures do not yield a definite pathogen, yet the patient responds to therapy directed at one or both of these potential pathogens.

   (2) If the patient has endobronchial gram-negative pneumonia, a well-collected sputum sample usually will reveal the pathogen. Prior studies have shown that gram-negative organisms recovered from TTAs also are found in the sputum. These organisms readily grow on laboratory media. **Therefore, if gram-negative bacteria are not isolated from well-collected sputum of a patient who is not on antibiotics directed at gram-negatives, one has essentially excluded the diagnosis of a gram-negative pneumonia.** In these patients, broad-spectrum therapy may safely be stopped after only a few days [31]. The exceptions are neutropenic patients and those with embolic gram-negative pneumonia. In embolic pneumonia, the blood cultures are positive.

c. **Pneumonia and no sputum available.** Empiric therapy is used in this setting.

3. **Duration of therapy.** This is discussed in more detail under the individual pneumonias reviewed under Special Considerations and Specific Therapy. Pneumococcal pneumonia is treated for at least 72 hours after the patient's temperature returns to normal and longer if there is an associated extrapulmonary focus of infection. For gram-negative pneumonia other than that due to *H. influenzae,* recommended duration of therapy is 2–3 weeks, depending on clinical improvement. Often this can consist of intravenous followed by oral therapy.

Special Considerations and Specific Therapy

I. **Acute community-acquired pneumonia in adults.** In prior series, 50–90% of these cases were said to be caused by *S. pneumoniae.* However, more recent surveys suggest that pneumococci account for 16–60% of cases of acute community-acquired pneumonia. Nevertheless, **pneumococcus remains the leading cause** of acute community-acquired pneumonia in virtually all series [3b] (see sec. **A**).

An estimated 4–15% of community-acquired pneumonia cases are due to *H. influenzae,* although the exact incidence of this pathogen is unclear because of difficulties in isolating it from sputum and distinguishing colonization from true infection (see sec. **III**). Aerobic gram-negative bacilli may cause 7–18% of community-acquired pneumonia cases and are often cited as particularly important pathogens in the elderly [3b]. *S. aureus* may account for 2–10% of cases, especially during the influenza season (see Chap. 8). Again, the distinction between colonization and true infection can at times be difficult with *S. aureus.*

The incidence of atypical pneumonia varies considerably depending in part on the age group studied and/or the vigor and sophistication of the methods used to confirm the diagnosis (see sec. **V**). A review of several series suggests that at least 2–4% of cases of community-acquired pneumonia are due to *Legionella* spp. (see sec. **VII**). The incidence of oropharyngeal-dental aspiration pneumonias is not well established (see sec. **II**).

Because a reliable sputum culture may be difficult to obtain or unavailable and blood cultures are positive in only a minority of adult patients, **many adults have community-acquired pneumonia of unknown etiology,** which requires empiric therapy (see sec. **B**).

In contrast to adults, in young children, viruses are the most common cause of pneumonia (see sec. **XIII**).

A. **Pneumococcal pneumonia** is the most common bacterial pneumonia in adults. Transient bacteremia occurs in 20–30% of patients (see Chap. 2).

  1. **Prognosis.** Pneumococcal pneumonia in the antibiotic era still has a significant mortality. In the study by Austrian and Gold [32], overall mortality in bacteremic pneumococcal pneumonia exceeded 15%. Those patients with preexisting systemic disease (cardiac disease, carcinoma, cirrhosis, and hematologic malignancies) had a mortality of approximately 30%, compared with a 7% mortality in those without preexisting disease. In addition to underlying disease, patients older than 50 years and those with more than one lobe involved were at greater risk.

  2. **Clinical manifestations.** Pneumococcal pneumonia is the prototype of acute lobar pneumonia, although a subacute presentation may be more common [33]. The onset of classic pneumococcal pneumonia is usually very abrupt, although symptoms of a prior viral upper respiratory infection are common. Many patients will recall the exact time their pneumonia began. They initially experience chills, rigor, fever, dyspnea, dry cough, and pleuritic chest pain. The rigor usually consists of a single episode, unless altered by intermittent antipyretics. Cough becomes productive of purulent sputum within the first 6–24 hours; a pinkish or rusty coloration indicates alveolar bleeding and is common. Examination reveals an acutely ill patient in obvious respiratory distress, with splinting of the involved chest and signs of consolidation with or without a friction rub. Radiographs show alveolar filling with air bronchograms in the affected lobes. Patients with underlying emphysema may not have frank consolidation. Subsegmental infiltrates are less common and indicate bronchopneumonia.

     a. **Complications** include shock, respiratory failure, empyema, meningitis, septic arthritis, purulent pericarditis, and endocarditis.

     b. **The differential diagnosis** consists of those bacteria that commonly cause acute lobar pneumonia, including *H. influenzae, K. pneumoniae,* and other gram-negative bacilli, *S. aureus,* and *S. pyogenes.* The setting, host factors, and Gram stains of respiratory secretions and pleural fluid will identify the most likely organism(s) before culture results are available [30].

  3. **Antibiotic therapy. Penicillin-resistant pneumococci are increasing in frequency in the United States,** as they have become a worldwide problem [34–36a]. Alterations in pneumococcal penicillin-binding proteins correlate with the degree of resistance to penicillins. **Intermediate-level resistance, defined as a minimum inhibitory concentration (MIC) of penicillin of 0.1–1.0 μg/ml, is found in 10–18% of US strains [33, 36]. High-level** resistance (a MIC > 1.0 μg/ml) **is less frequently encountered** in this country but is often associated with resistance to cephalosporins, chloramphenicol, TMP-SMX, erythromycin, and clindamycin [36].

     Infections with resistant pneumococci are common in children and are increasing in adults. Factors associated with their occurrence include prior antibiotic exposure and an institutional setting, although sporadic cases also occur. **The topic of penicillin-resistant *S. pneumoniae* is reviewed in detail in Chap. 28C.**

     Optimal recommendations for the treatment of infections caused by penicillin-resistant pneumococci are still evolving [36a]. Nonmeningeal infections caused by intermediately resistant *S. pneumoniae* may be successfully treated with a penicillin by raising the dose to provide higher levels of drug. Cefuroxime is effective against intermediately resistant *S. pneumoniae.* Either cefotaxime or ceftriaxone is a better choice when CNS involvement is likely or proven [33, 35, 36a]. Infections caused by highly resistant *S. pneumoniae* are best treated with vancomycin.

     a. **Outpatient therapy** is discussed on page 269.

     b. **For hospitalized patients** in whom the diagnosis of pneumococcal pneumonia has been made by classic Gram-stain of purulent sputum, and/or blood culture, and/or sputum culture (adult regimens):

        (1) **For initial therapy while awaiting susceptibility data,** higher intravenous doses of penicillin have recently been suggested to ensure activity against susceptible as well as intermediately resistant *S. pneumonia.* Therefore, IV aqueous penicillin 1.5–2.0 million units q4h is suggested (see Chap. 28C).

    (2) **For known penicillin-susceptible strains,** IV aqueous penicillin in conventional doses (i.e., 2.4 million units per day) seems rational and less likely to be associated with selecting out resistant bacteria.

    (3) **For penicillin-allergic patients.** In the patient with a history of delayed reaction, an intravenous cephalosporin is commonly used (see Chap. 27).

        (a) **For initial therapy** while awaiting susceptibility data, cefuroxime 750 mg q8h is commonly used, and this covers both penicillin-susceptible and intermediately resistant *S. pneumoniae.*

        (b) **For known penicillin-susceptible strains of *S. pneumoniae,*** cefazolin (500 mg q12h) would be a more cost-effective and narrower spectrum agent.

        (c) Erythromycin and vancomycin are alternate agents for patients with severe or immediate penicillin allergy.

  c. For therapy of a sustained bacteremia, see Chap. 2. For therapy of an associated meningitis, see Chaps. 5 and 28C.

4. Prevention. Despite use of antibiotics and vigorous supportive care, some patients with pneumococcal pneumonia die. Because of the frequent occurrence of this disease and its associated mortality, there has been a keen interest in the pneumococcal vaccine as a preventive measure.

  a. Rationale for pneumococcal vaccine. The currently available vaccine is the product of decades of study. *S. pneumoniae* (formerly called *Diplococcus pneumoniae*) contains a capsule of highly polymerized polysaccharides that interfere with phagocytosis.

    (1) **Capsular types.** There are more than 80 distinct antigenic capsular types. **Immunity or recovery** in the untreated host **occurs, in part, when the host forms an antibody specific for the capsular polysaccharide involved.** This type-specific antibody combines with the capsular material on the bacterium and neutralizes the antiphagocytic activity of the capsular polysaccharide. This was the basis for using type-specific serum. It is also the basis for the current pneumococcal vaccine, which stimulates the production of type-specific antibodies.

    (2) **Important serotypes.** The currently available pneumococcal vaccine contains 23 polysaccharides (25 μg each) [33]. These 23 serotypes of pneumococci have been shown to cause approximately 87% of bacteremic pneumococcal pneumonias.

    (3) **Patients at increased risk for pneumococcal infection.** Patients with certain chronic conditions are at a recognized increased risk for developing pneumococcal pneumonia and more severe disease [37]. This group includes patients with AIDS and other immunosuppressed patients [38] and those with asplenia, sickle cell disease, multiple myeloma, cirrhosis, renal failure, and transplants. Elderly patients, particularly those who are institutionalized, are at increased risk, as are alcoholics and those with poorly controlled diabetes, CHF, and COPD. In addition, influenza often is complicated by pneumococcal pneumonia in these same high-risk patients (see Chap. 8).

  b. Effectiveness. The overall clinical effectiveness of the vaccine in immunocompetent persons is approximately 60–64% [37]. A large case-control study found that protection varied markedly within certain populations [39, 40]. Highest efficacy was in immunocompetent adults younger than 55 years (93% protective) and declined significantly with age at vaccination and time since vaccination [39]. However, a protective effect in immunocompromised patients was difficult to measure [39].

  c. Antibody response. Antibody response, with presumed partial protection for pneumococcal disease, has been demonstrated in patients with asplenia, nephrotic syndrome and other forms of chronic renal failure, COPD, well-controlled diabetes, and asymptomatic HIV infection [41].

  d. Poor or partial antibody response observed in the following patients:

    (1) **Hodgkin's disease patients** who have had a splenectomy and have undergone radiation therapy and chemotherapy exhibit poor antibody response [41]. If patients with Hodgkin's disease are vaccinated at least 2 weeks **before** treatment for Hodgkin's disease, they manifest a good antibody response, although it declines somewhat with subsequent therapy [34].

    (2) Multiple myeloma patients have a poor antibody response after vaccination.

    (3) Renal transplant and hemodialysis patients show a partial antibody response and a more rapid decline of antibody levels.

    (4) HIV-infected patients with symptoms (AIDS and AIDS-related complex [ARC]) and those with depressed helper T cells respond poorly to vaccination [42]. Antibody responses to the vaccine are improved by at least 1 month of zidovudine (formerly azidothymidine, AZT) therapy [43]. **Thus, persons with HIV should be vaccinated as soon as possible in the natural course of their infection. Delay of vaccination for at least 4 weeks after starting zidovudine therapy may be considered [43].**

e. Side effects. The **safety** of this vaccine has been **well established** [41].

    (1) Local reactions of erythema or discomfort occur in approximately 30–40% of recipients. Local swelling is seen only occasionally.

    (2) Systemic reactions are rare and self-limited. Chills, fever to 40°C (104°F), and weakness may occur transiently.

    (3) The preceding reactions have been observed more frequently in some patients revaccinated after the first dose. However, serious local reactions are rare when current guidelines for repeat vaccination are followed.

f. Contraindications

    (1) In children younger than 2 years, the vaccine is not recommended because children in this age group do not develop an adequate antibody response.

    (2) In pregnant women, the safety of the vaccine has not been adequately studied. Therefore, the vaccine should be given to high-risk women prior to pregnancy.

g. Recommendations for use. The recommendations for pneumococcal vaccine use are based on its proven efficacy in immunocompetent persons and known risk factors for serious pneumococcal infection [37, 38, 41]. **Recipients should be informed that the vaccine will not entirely eliminate the risk of pneumococcal pneumonia.**

    (1) Vaccination is recommended for patients who are capable of producing an antibody response to the vaccine and who are at increased risk either of developing bacteremic pneumonia or of death if bacteremia or pneumonia does occur. These include the following:

        (a) Splenectomized patients, including autosplenectomy as in those with sickle cell anemia. Ideally, vaccination should be performed at least 2 weeks prior to an elective splenectomy.

        (b) Patients with alcoholism, COPD, CHF, cirrhosis, diabetes, nephrotic syndrome, or renal failure.

        (c) Asymptomatic or symptomatic HIV-infected patients (see sec. **4.d**).

        (d) In **special settings or populations** with a known increased risk, such as certain **Native American populations** [37] and those with **CSF leaks** [38].

    (2) Healthy elderly patients (> 65 years) may benefit from vaccination. The vaccine's efficacy is diminished in the elderly [39]. However, because of its safety and the increased incidence of bacteremic infection in the elderly, these patients may benefit from the vaccine and so **its use is advocated** [44].

    (3) Ideally, patients with Hodgkin's disease (and other patients about to undergo immunosuppression) should be vaccinated at least 2 weeks before immunosuppressive therapy is initiated (see sec. **4.a**).

    (4) When vaccinating patients with altered immune states, both the physician and the patient must recognize that the response to the vaccine may be limited, with a range of 30–60% reported [41] (see sec. **4**).

    (5) If an acute outbreak of pneumococcal disease occurs in a closed population (e.g., a nursing home, the military), vaccination of those at risk should be considered.

h. Use in children after splenectomy. Because the vaccine does not contain all the antigenic types of pneumococci and is only partially protective, the splenectomized child may still be at risk of an overwhelming pneumococcal infection. Therefore, in addition to the use of pneumococcal vaccine, continued prophylaxis with antimicrobial drugs seems reasonable (see Chap. 28B).

i. **Dosage and duration**

   (1) **Initial dose.** The usual dose is a single 0.5-ml IM or SC injection given at any time during the year. **The pneumococcal vaccine may be given simultaneously with influenza vaccination.** Injections should be made at separate sites. Studies have revealed adequate antibody response to both antigens, with no increase in side effects.

   (2) **Revaccination** is not routinely advised but **should be considered for highest-risk patients** [37]. The optimal interval between vaccinations is unknown; every 6 years is currently suggested, although 3–5 years has been proposed for some patient populations [33, 44], including:

   (a) Those at high risk previously given the 14-valent vaccine.

   (b) High-risk older children and adults vaccinated 6 or more years previously.

   (c) Older children and adults with an expected rapid decline in antibody, including those with asplenia, nephrotic syndrome, renal failure, organ transplants, and perhaps the elderly [44].

   (d) Children with nephrotic syndrome, asplenia, or sickle cell anemia vaccinated 3–5 years previously, if not older than 10 years at revaccination.

B. **Pneumonia of unclear etiology.** In many patients, despite careful efforts of the nursing staff and/or respiratory care therapists, no purulent sputum is available for culture. As previously discussed in this chapter, because of the limitation of sputum cultures, blood cultures, and other diagnostic approaches, empiric therapy is undertaken in these patients (see sec. **IV** under General Concepts of Organism-Host Interaction).

   The rationale and specific suggestions for this empiric therapy are discussed in detail in sec. **X** under General Concepts of Organism-Host Interaction.

II. **Aspiration pneumonia.** Although the pathogenesis of most pneumonias is through microaspiration, some pneumonias are related to macroaspiration. This is particularly common in the obtunded patient or in the patient with a defective cough epiglottic reflex.

   Often, however, when a patient is noted to develop gastric acid aspiration, no therapy is required; only institution of pulmonary drainage and careful observation are indicated. If an infection develops, usually several days later, therapy can be initiated at that time. Earlier therapy does not prevent infection but instead selects for resistant organisms.

   A. **Community-acquired aspiration pneumonia.** The typical patient population for this type of pneumonia has been discussed previously. These pneumonias generally are caused by oral anaerobes usually sensitive to penicillin [45]. However, penicillin resistance is increasingly common among **non–*Bacteroides fragilis* species, fusobacteria,** and certain other oral anaerobes [46–49]. There are no studies to suggest the proper dosage of penicillin in this setting. Experts suggest aqueous penicillin G in doses ranging from 10 to 15 million units/day IV, divided q4h. Clindamycin is a good alternative agent for the penicillin-allergic patient. Because of potential penicillin resistance, clindamycin may be considered the drug of choice. It definitely is indicated in patients who do not respond to penicillin, as well as for the initial therapy of patients seriously ill with an overwhelming anaerobic pulmonary aspiration pneumonia [50]. (See sec. **V** under Lung Abscess.)

   B. **Hospital-acquired aspiration pneumonia.** If hospitalized patients aspirate, they are at risk of developing a gram-negative pneumonia because of oropharyngeal colonization with these organisms. **Gastric and pharyngeal colonization by gram-negative bacilli and *S. aureus* is important in the pathogenesis** of nosocomial aspiration pneumonias [12, 51–53]. This occurs in patients given continuous gastric feedings or prophylaxis for stress ulcers with antacids or H_2-blockers. In these settings, the normal gastric acid barrier is overcome, permitting bacterial growth in the stomach that may be the source of subsequent oropharyngeal colonization or may be aspirated directly into the lungs. Stress-ulcer prophylaxis with sucralfate, as compared to agents that raise gastric pH, appears to lower the incidence of nosocomial pneumonia, although this is not the finding in all studies [54, 55]. See sec. **XII** for further discussion of nosocomial pneumonias.

It is often difficult to separate colonization from infection in these patients. The approach to this problem is discussed in detail in sec. **IX** under Clinical Approach to Pneumonia. The **therapy** for gram-negative pneumonias is discussed later in sec. **IV.D.**

III. ***H. influenzae*** may be associated with bronchitis in patients with chronic lung disease (see Chap. 8). In recent years, primary pneumonias due to *H. influenzae* in adults appear to be increasing in frequency. These usually occur in the elderly, in patients with chronic lung diseases, and in patients with HIV infection. Rapidly fatal pneumonia in younger adults with normal immune systems and ventilator-associated nosocomial pneumonia also have been described [56, 57]. These infections may be caused by both type b and nontypeable or other non–type b strains, including those complicated by bacteremia [58, 59]. The efficacy of the newer Hib vaccines in these high-risk groups of adults is unknown. In children younger than 5 years, the incidence of invasive Hib disease has decreased since the introduction and use of the Hib vaccines [59a].

  A. Diagnosis. A positive blood culture for *H. influenzae* in a patient with pneumonia confirms the diagnosis. Chocolate agar is required for isolation of the organism from sputum. Latex agglutination to detect type b antigen in serum and urine is specific when positive, but a negative test does not eliminate *H. influenzae* as a possible pathogen.

  B. Therapy. Ampicillin resistance of *H. influenzae* is of potential concern and, because it is seen in up to 36% of strains [59], beta-lactamase production should be tested.

  1. Known ampicillin-susceptible strains. When an isolate is known to be susceptible to penicillin or ampicillin, either of these agents is satisfactory. Most authorities recommend ampicillin because of clinical experience. Ampicillin, 1–2 g IV q4h, is recommended in adults. Therapy usually is continued for a total of 10–14 days, and the course may be completed with oral amoxicillin. (See Chap. 28E for pediatric doses.)

  In the patient with a delayed reaction to penicillin, cefuroxime (a second-generation cephalosporin) and ceftriaxone and cefotaxime (third-generation cephalosporins) are very active against *H. influenzae*. If cephalosporins cannot be used, clarithromycin, azithromycin, TMP-SMX, and chloramphenicol are alternative agents. See further discussion of these other options in Chap. 28.

  2. Unknown ampicillin susceptibility or known ampicillin-resistant organism. If the initial workup of the pneumonia yields information strongly suggestive of *H. influenzae* (e.g., a well-obtained sputum showing pleomorphic gram-negative rods on the Gram stain), an antibiotic that is active against beta-lactamase-positive *H. influenzae* type b should be used, especially in the very ill patient. Currently, 10–36% of *H. influenzae* type b strains are beta-lactamase-positive (i.e., ampicillin-resistant). For non–type b strains, this percentage is somewhat higher.

  Cefuroxime or a third-generation cephalosporin (e.g., ceftriaxone, cefotaxime) is the drug of choice for highly suspect or known ampicillin-resistant *H. influenzae* pneumonia in the seriously ill patient. Therapy can be modified when cultures become available.

  C. Prognosis. In bacteremia, mortality may approach 36% in older adults [59]. Infection during pregnancy is usually survived by the mother, but fetal loss is common [59].

IV. Gram-negative pneumonias are occurring with increased frequency [60, 61]. The **majority** of these pneumonias are **hospital-acquired,** although community-acquired gram-negative pneumonias do occur.

  A. Etiology. The common aerobic gram-negative bacilli include the Enterobacteriaceae (*Klebsiella, Enterobacter,* and *Serratia*), and *P. aeruginosa* and other *Pseudomonas* spp., as well as relatively uncommon pathogens such as *Acinetobacter calcoaceticus*. *K. pneumoniae* is the most common gram-negative pathogen [62], although both *Acinetobacter* and *P. aeruginosa* are occasionally responsible for community-acquired pneumonias.

  B. Setting

  1. Community-acquired gram-negative pneumonias usually occur in patients with underlying lung disease, other underlying disease such as alcoholism, or chronic debilitating disease [61]. Elderly patients from nursing homes are also at risk.

2. **Hospital-acquired** gram-negative pneumonias are common. If hospitalized patients have marked aspiration, they may develop a gram-negative pneumonia (see sec. **II**). The compromised host is at high risk.

C. **Diagnosis.** Diagnosis can be difficult. Because **gram-negative organisms are common colonizers, one must distinguish colonization from true infection with such organisms.** This distinction is crucial, as has been discussed in detail previously in sec. **IX** under Clinical Approach to Pneumonia.

   If a well-obtained sputum culture does not reveal gram-negative organisms, infection with these organisms is unlikely, as they are usually present in adequate numbers and are easy to culture when they are causing the disease.

D. **Therapy.** Antibiotics of the appropriate spectrum are essential. When aminoglycosides are used to treat gram-negative pneumonias, chances for a successful outcome are optimized by achieving high therapeutic peak blood levels [63]. Although definitive studies are lacking to determine whether more than a single antibiotic is required, most authorities use two agents known to be synergistic in vitro [64] (see Chap. 28H). We believe this is essential for patients with necrotizing infections, indicated by elastin fibers in the sputum (see later in sec. **XII.D.2.b** and sec. **III** under Lung Abscess), formation of multiple small cavities, or abscess formation. Partially because of difficulties with adequate sputum concentration of antibiotics, **these pneumonias usually are treated for 2–3 weeks with antibiotics.** (See also sec. **XI.F.**)

   1. *Klebsiella.* The **third-generation cephalosporins** (e.g., ceftriaxone, cefotaxime) are very active against *K. pneumoniae* in vitro. A single well-tolerated agent can be used, and these agents are viewed as potentially **the antibiotic of choice** for pneumonias due to *K. pneumoniae* [64]. The 1994 *Medical Letter* lists these as first-choice agents for *Klebsiella* [64a].

      Because of the potential necrotizing and severe pneumonias caused by community-acquired *Klebsiella* spp. and the typically excellent in vitro activity and anticipated high tissue level of bactericidal activity of the third-generation cephalosporins, we favor the use of these agents in this setting even when isolates may be susceptible to earlier-generation cephalosporins. Other potentially useful agents include aztreonam and the quinolones. We favor the use of these agents. Nosocomial *Klebsiella* spp. can be resistant to third-generation cephalosporins; imipenem is often very active against these isolates. See related discussion in Chap. 28F.

   2. *Pseudomonas.* **Combination intravenous therapy commonly is used** to achieve synergy. Therefore, ticarcillin or piperacillin and an aminoglycoside (gentamicin, tobramycin, or amikacin) are used together. In adults, many experts favor piperacillin (e.g., 3 g IV q4h or 4 g q6h) and tobramycin (1.5–1.7 mg/kg/dose) for known *P. aeruginosa* pulmonary infections. (See Chaps. 28E and 28H.) A third-generation cephalosporin, imipenem-cilastatin, or a quinolone alone is not optimal initial therapy even for susceptible *Pseudomonas* spp. (see related discussions in Chap. 28). Once a *Pseudomonas* pneumonia is under good control (e.g., after 7–10 days of intravenous combination antibiotics), we often complete a total of 3 weeks of therapy by using oral ciprofloxacin, assuming the organism is susceptible.

      Because of the serious nature of *Pseudomonas* infections, serum aminoglycoside levels should be monitored carefully, as much to ensure adequate levels as to avoid nephrotoxicity [63].

   3. **Gram-negative pneumonia of unclear etiology**

      a. **Community-acquired** gram-negative pneumonias are more likely to be due to cephalosporin-susceptible organisms than to cephalosporin-resistant ones (e.g., *Pseudomonas* spp.).

         In the very ill patient, a cephalosporin and aminoglycoside combination is appropriate for taking advantage of potential synergy and for covering *Pseudomonas* spp. that can occur uncommonly in this setting (see Table 9-3).

      b. **Hospitalized setting.** If the hospitalized patient develops a serious gram-negative pneumonia (as demonstrated by the Gram stain or suggested by the clinical setting) while cultures are pending, broad-spectrum antibiotics should be initiated that will cover *Pseudomonas* strains as well as more susceptible organisms. A cephalosporin and aminoglycoside combination often is used (doses are those described in sec. **1**); alternatively, one might select an expanded-spectrum penicillin (e.g., piperacillin) and an amino-glycoside. (See sec. **XII.F** for further discussion.) The potential role of aztreonam, imipenem-cilastatin, and the quinolones are discussed in detail in Chap. 28, as is the potential for monotherapy with ceftazidime.

4. **Other gram-negative pneumonias.** Therapy must be individualized, based on susceptibility studies. For *A. calcoaceticus,* a piperacillin and aminoglycoside combination is effective. Again, the potential role of aztreonam, imipenem, and fluoroquinolones in this setting is discussed in Chap. 28.

5. **Compromised hosts with pneumonia** are discussed separately in sec. **XI.**

V. **Atypical pneumonia**

A. **Overview.** Classic, or typical, lobar pneumonia had been described and associated with the pneumococcus at the turn of the century. Still, many atypical pneumonias remained that were clinically distinct from bacterial lobar pneumonia. These eventually came to be referred to as *nonbacterial pneumonias* (among other terms), in part because they did not respond to sulfonamides or penicillin. Epidemics resulted in the definition of the etiologies of psittacosis and influenza by the 1930s.

Mycoplasmal pneumonia was proven to be the cause of cold agglutinin-positive atypical pneumonia in 1962. In the decades since, the general syndrome of atypical pneumonia has been more clearly defined, and several new etiologies have been discovered.

1. The **atypical pneumonia syndrome** is marked by the following:
   a. **A subacute illness,** with onset over several days.
   b. **Nonspecific systemic manifestations early** in the illness, including fever, headache, and myalgias.
   c. **Cough, which often is the most prominent early respiratory symptom and is initially nonproductive.** Dyspnea and pleuritic chest pain are rare.
   d. **Initially scant** and mucoid **sputum,** which may become purulent as illness progresses.
   e. **Physical findings** in the lungs that often underestimate substantially the extent of chest roentgenographic changes.
   f. **Leukocytosis** ($\leq 15,000/mm^3$)

2. The etiologies of atypical pneumonia are numerous. **Clues to the differential diagnosis** have recently been reviewed [65-67]. The following organisms cause the syndrome much more frequently than others:
   a. *Mycoplasma pneumoniae* is the most commonly recognized atypical pneumonia (see sec. **B**).
   b. *Chlamydia pneumoniae* is probably the next most common offending organism (see sec. **C**).
   c. *Chlamydia psittaci* causes psittacosis. Psittacosis (or ornithosis) is a **systemic infection acquired from contact with infected birds,** including parrots, parakeets, turkeys, and others. Contact may be by occupational exposures as well as by pet ownership. The onset of psittacosis may be abrupt, and the illness is potentially fatal. Diagnosis depends on serologic studies, and acute and convalescent sera should be obtained. Tetracyclines are the agents of choice [64a] and may be given for 1-2 weeks after clinical improvement to minimize relapses.
   d. *Coxiella burnetii* causes **Q fever.** This pneumonia is endemic to certain regions in Canada and elsewhere but is infrequently recognized in the United States (see sec. **D**).
   e. **Viral pneumonia** [68] **commonly occurs in infants and children.** Influenza, RSV, parainfluenza viruses, adenoviruses, and varicella-zoster virus (VZV) are the most frequent agents. **In adults, influenza is the most important viral pneumonia.** Adenovirus may cause outbreaks of lower respiratory tract infections in military recruits. Respiratory tract infections due to RSV occur more frequently in the elderly and in adults who come in contact with children with RSV infection (e.g., adult family members and hospital personnel). In addition, nursing home outbreaks of RSV illness have been documented. For further discussion of these viral syndromes, see Chap. 8.
   f. *Pneumocystis carinii* **pneumonia** in patients with HIV infection may present like an atypical pneumonia. Therefore, it is important to take a careful history to exclude HIV risk factors (see Chap. 19).
   g. *Legionella* **infections** may present as atypical pneumonia (see sec. **VI**) but more commonly present as typical bacterial pneumonia with a negative Gram stain.

B. *Mycoplasma pneumoniae.* Of the recognized causes of atypical pneumonia, *M. pneumoniae* is the most common. The illness tends to spread in families and has an incubation period of 2–3 weeks. **Those at greatest risk for infection are 5–20 years old. However,** *M. pneumoniae* infection **occurs in all age groups, including the very young and the elderly** [69–71]. Outbreaks occur at intervals of 4–7 years [70, 72]. **Only partial immunity follows infection** and, over time, repeated infections in the same patient have been clearly documented. In addition, patients with hypogammaglobulinemia have an increased susceptibility to *Mycoplasma* infections [70, 73].

1. **Clinical manifestations [74]. A history of illness** (often pharyngitis, cough, or earache) **in a family member can be elicited if carefully sought. Pharyngitis** is much more prominent than rhinitis and may be the earliest symptom. **Protracted cough with minimal sputum production is the most common symptom,** although occasional individuals will produce significant quantities of sputum. Bullous myringitis is a traditional clue in the diagnosis, but it is infrequent and may be present in other pneumonias. Pleurisy and easily demonstrable pleural effusions are unlikely to be due to mycoplasmal pneumonia.

    The classic symptom complex of low-grade fever, protracted cough, pulmonary infiltrate, and normal WBC count with a negative bacterial workup was formerly called **primary atypical pneumonia.** However, it is now recognized that this syndrome may be due to other agents and that the spectrum of disease due to *M. pneumoniae* is more extensive. **Occasionally,** *M. pneumoniae* will **produce severe illness,** especially in patients with sickle cell disease. In addition, **a variety of nonpneumonic manifestations have been recognized,** either with or without the respiratory component [69]. These include vomiting or diarrhea, morbilliform skin rashes, erythema multiforme, arthritides, and a variety of CNS syndromes, including aseptic meningitis.

2. **Diagnosis.** Because the organism grows slowly and is difficult to culture, most laboratories do not attempt to culture *Mycoplasma.* The diagnosis often is made serologically; other tests are still undergoing clinical evaluation [75–77].

    a. Although the presence of **cold agglutinins** in approximately half of patients overall may be helpful, they are **not specific.** Cold agglutinins have been seen in influenza, mononucleosis, other infections, and lymphoproliferative diseases. A titer of 1:64 or more is suggestive of *Mycoplasma* infection. Hemolytic anemia is an uncommon complication.

    b. **Enzyme-linked immunosorbent assay** and **complement fixation** (CF) testing of acute and convalescent sera probably are the best serologic tests [65, 75]. A major disadvantage to serodiagnosis is that clinically useful information frequently is delayed and unavailable during the acute illness. Because of the prolonged incubation period, an acute serologic response may have begun by the time the patient comes to the physician. Those with a single CF titer in excess of 1:32 are more likely to have acute disease, as high titers do not persist for long periods of time. Ideally, a fourfold antibody rise may occur between acute and convalescent sera samples (the convalescent serum being drawn 10–14 days after the acute sample).

        False positive CF tests are, however, also common. Western blot analysis or antigen-specific ELISA may help detect those persons with true antimycoplasma antibodies [75, 77].

    c. **Rapid diagnostic techniques** have been undergoing evaluation [75–77]. These include antigen capture assays, nucleic acid hybridization tests for mycoplasmal mRNA, and polymerase chain reaction (PCR). Further studies are needed to clarify their usefulness, in part because their sensitivity can detect the prolonged carrier state that may exist in the absence of disease [70, 77].

3. **Differential diagnosis.** In some patients, it may not be possible to exclude other infections, such as *C. pneumoniae,* Legionnaires' disease, and even atypical presentations of bacterial pneumonia. Certain features, however, are helpful in distinguishing *Mycoplasma* from other infections [65]. Clinically, these include spread in family members or close contacts, the extrapulmonary findings cited previously, and absence of pleuritic symptoms. Radiographic features suggesting mycoplasmal pneumonia include the absence of consolida-

tion, limited progression, relatively rapid resolution and, in some reports, hilar adenopathy [74, 78].

4. **Therapy.** Either erythromycin or tetracycline will shorten the duration of illness, although the organism may be shed for up to 4 months even with therapy. Tetracycline should not be used during pregnancy, in nursing mothers, or in young children. In adults, **erythromycin or tetracycline,** 250 mg qid or 500 mg tid, are equally effective regimens. The usual duration of therapy is 14 days to reduce the frequency of relapse, but severely ill patients may be treated for 3 weeks. For the woman who may be pregnant, erythromycin is preferred. In children also, erythromycin should be used. The dose is 30–50 mg/kg/day for those weighing less than 25 kg and 1 g/day (divided q6h) for those who weigh more than 25 kg (see Chap. 28). If Q fever or psittacosis is a significant consideration, then tetracycline is preferred.

There is less clinical experience with the newer macrolides clarithromycin and azithromycin, but preliminary results show them to be effective alternatives [79].

In the patient with a history of GI intolerance to erythromycin, clarithromycin often is useful as it generally causes fewer GI side effects. In adults, clarithromycin, 250–500 mg bid, can be used. In children, a clarithromycin suspension (7.5 mg/kg q12h, up to the adult dose) is available but, as of spring 1996, the US Food and Drug Administration had not approved the use of this agent for pediatric lower respiratory tract infections. Although preliminary studies suggest that a 5-day course of azithromycin is effective for *Mycoplasma,* the exact role of this agent awaits further clinical experience. For a detailed discussion of these new macrolides, see Chap. 28M.

Although they are active in vitro against *Mycoplasma,* the quinolones' role as a therapeutic alternative awaits further clinical study.

C. ***Chlamydia pneumoniae.*** *C. pneumoniae* **may prove to be the second most common cause of atypical pneumonia.** It occurs year-round, is worldwide in its distribution, and may cause military and civilian outbreaks [80]. Antibodies to *C. pneumoniae* are rare in preschool-age children but increase rapidly in prevalence through adolescence and young adulthood. Seropositivity is high—up to 60%—among adults. Transmission is predominantly from human to human via the aerosol route, but environmental contamination and fomite spread also is possible [81].

1. **Clinical manifestations.** Our understanding of *C. pneumoniae* infections is expanding. Pneumonia, bronchitis, pharyngitis, otitis, and sinusitis are the most common syndromes [80]. However, the **majority of infections are asymptomatic or produce only mild illness.** Pneumonia is more likely with increasing age [80]. *C. pneumoniae* accounts for **approximately 10% of community-acquired pneumonias** and has been the third or fourth most commonly identified etiology [80]; nosocomial pneumonia is also possible [82]. Most studies have found the illness to be nonspecific. Initial symptoms may include a sore throat and pharyngitis. Although nonproductive cough almost always occurs, it may be delayed by several days to weeks and thus suggest a "biphasic" illness [80]. Fever is part of the early phase and may not be present when the patient eventually seeks medical care.

Bronchitis may occur with or without pneumonia, may be subacute in onset, and may have a prolonged recovery phase. Pharyngitis and sinusitis, with or without otitis, also may occur by themselves or as part of pneumonia [80]. An elevated erythrocyte sedimentation rate (ESR) and a normal WBC count are the rule. The most common radiographic picture of pneumonia is a unilateral subsegmental or segmental infiltrate that is indistinguishable from mycoplasmal infection and that resolves rapidly. Convalescence may be prolonged, but most patients recover. Severe illness and death from chlamydia pneumonia have been described, but this is most likely in the elderly or those with underlying illness.

C. pneumoniae has been implicated in several other clinical syndromes. These include bronchospastic disease, endocarditis, myocarditis, and atherosclerosis [80].

2. **Diagnosis.** There are **no readily available means for diagnosing** *C. pneumoniae* infection. Cultures for *Chlamydia* are not available in most centers and hence usually are not performed.

Serologic diagnosis is based on the microimmunofluorescence test for *C. pneumoniae* IgM and IgG antibodies [80]. Difficulties interpreting results of antibody titers may result from the fact that prior infection is common and reinfections may occur [80]. The older chlamydial CF test (e.g., for psittacosis) is nonspecific and insensitive and is not useful except perhaps in young people with primary infection. Tests to diagnose infection rapidly by detecting chlamydia antigen or DNA in respiratory secretions are currently being developed [80].

3. **Differential diagnosis.** As noted previously, prospective studies have not identified any feature distinctive of *C. pneumoniae* infection. Hoarseness and sore throat may be a consistent finding with illness from chlamydia, but many other prevalent respiratory agents also cause these symptoms.

4. **Therapy**

   a. In a cell culture assay, *C. pneumoniae* is inhibited by very low concentrations of tetracycline and erythromycin but is resistant to sulfonamides [80]. Clarithromycin, azithromycin, ofloxacin, and sparfloxacin are also active in vitro [83, 84].

   b. Clinical experience suggests that **erythromycin and tetracycline** are effective therapies when given in the doses and duration (10–14 days) recommended for mycoplasmal pneumonia (see sec. **B.4**) [80]. We favor tetracycline in adults, 500 mg qid for 10–14 days, because relapses may be greater with erythromycin [80]. **In the patient with an atypical pneumonia who does not respond to erythromycin, a course of tetracycline (if not contraindicated) may be reasonable;** doxycycline can also be used (see Chap. 28N). There is only very limited clinical experience with the newer macrolides and quinolones, and their roles in treating *C. pneumoniae* infections must await the results of further studies.

   c. Treatment failures and relapses occur, and excretion of the organism for up to 1 year after therapy has been described [85]. Either tetracycline or doxycycline is currently recommended for the treatment of relapses [80].

D. *Coxiella burnetii.* This obligate intracellular rickettsial parasite causes Q fever [86]. Although Q fever is considered rare in the United States, its true prevalence probably is substantially underestimated [87]. Although *C. burnetii* is found on 5 continents and in at least 51 countries, the rates of Q fever vary widely from region to region [86, 88]. **Q fever is endemic to Nova Scotia, Canada,** where it accounted for 20% of identified causes of pneumonia in hospitalized patients [88]. Overall, however, reviews of community-acquired pneumonia have identified Q fever in only 1.6% of cases [88].

C. *burnetii* infects many species of domestic and wild animals, including cattle, sheep, and goats. **Human infections occur most commonly after exposure** (often occupational) **to infected aerosols originating from contaminated products of conception or from contaminated materials** (e.g., milk, wool, or fresh cheese) **from infected animals.** Several outbreaks of acute Q fever have occurred that were unrelated to traditional animal reservoirs for *C. burnetii* [86, 88]. These cases have involved exposure to stillborn kittens or parturient cats, sheep used in research, wild rabbits, and manure, and living along a road used for a sheep drive.

1. **Clinical manifestations. Acute Q fever is a systemic illness** that may include atypical pneumonia, hepatitis, or both. Illness begins abruptly after an incubation period of approximately 20 days (range, 2–6 weeks). The most prominent symptoms are rigors, fever, headache, and myalgias. Nonproductive cough is present in at least half of the patients with **pneumonia.** Chest pains are noted in fewer than one-fifth of patients overall but are more frequent in those requiring hospitalization. Patients with Q fever may appear acutely ill and diaphoretic. The patient's pulse may be lower than predicted for the degree of fever. Examination of the chest often is unremarkable despite obvious radiographic infiltrates. Hepatomegaly accurately indicates liver involvement; splenomegaly is much less frequent. Importantly, skin rashes are seen in fewer than 5% of patients.

   Radiographic infiltrates usually are subsegmental or segmental and may have a pleural base; they are most often indistinguishable from those of other types of atypical pneumonia. However, rounded opacities may be seen and should suggest the possibility of Q fever pneumonia. Small pleural effusions are found in up to one-third of cases. Other laboratory findings are equally nonspecific. Only one-third of patients will have a leukocytosis, but the sedimentation rate usually is elevated. Thrombocytosis, thrombocytopenia, and microscopic hematuria also have been described [88].

Hepatitis is the major extrapulmonary manifestation of acute *C. burnetii* infection and, in some series, was more common than clinical pneumonia [86]. Most often hepatic involvement is detected biochemically, with fewer than 10% of patients having jaundice. Other uncommon findings outside of the lungs include thrombophlebitis, uveitis, meningitis, and spontaneous abortion.

Acute Q fever is almost always a self-limited illness, resolving within several weeks even without specific therapy. Rarely, endocarditis develops as the predominant manifestation of **chronic Q fever.** It may appear from months to years after the primary *C. burnetii* infection (which itself may have been asymptomatic) and is often accompanied by hepatosplenomegaly and typical signs of subacute endocarditis.

2. **Diagnosis. Serologic methods are the mainstay of diagnosis because isolation of *C. burnetii* from clinical specimens is difficult and extremely hazardous.** CF, indirect fluorescent antibody (IFA), and ELISA tests are most commonly used [86]. ELISA and IFA tests are more sensitive, and they can be used to determine specific IgM responses. In acute Q fever, IgM antibodies to phase II antigens are found by the second week of illness and usually decrease by the third month. Peak IgG antibody titers to *C. burnetii* are found 4–8 weeks after initial infection using IFA tests and after approximately 12 weeks using CF tests. It is important to remember that seropositivity, including IgM response, persists for a prolonged period after infection, so that a single positive titer must be interpreted with caution. Titers to phase I antigens are higher than titers to phase II antigens only in chronic Q fever.

3. **Differential diagnosis.** The signs and symptoms of Q fever pneumonia are nonspecific and may not reliably distinguish the illness from other acute systemic infections. Headache, fatigue, chills, and sweats were more common, and cough and sore throat less common, among 51 cases of Q fever pneumonia when compared with 102 controls having other community-acquired pneumonias [89]. **Exposure to cattle, sheep, goats, stillborn kittens, or parturient cats strongly supports the diagnosis. Hepatitis in a patient with atypical pneumonia** should suggest Q fever, Legionnaires' disease, and tularemia. A rounded infiltrate on roentgenography may also favor Q fever in the diagnosis of an atypical pneumonia.

4. **Treatment** [90]. Treatment **is suggested** for all symptomatic acute *C. burnetii* infections because of the potential for later chronic Q fever. Despite the fact that acute Q fever will resolve spontaneously in almost all patients, early therapy may shorten the duration of fever and other prominent symptoms [86, 90]. **In adults,** 2 weeks of oral **tetracycline,** 500 mg qid, or doxycycline, 100 mg bid, is the regimen of choice. TMP-SMX, rifampin, chloramphenicol, erythromycin, the newer quinolones, and ceftriaxone are active in vitro against *C. burnetii,* but their effectiveness in therapy is less clear than for the tetracyclines [90]. Chloramphenicol has been an accepted alternative to the tetracyclines in the past. Results with erythromycin for pneumonia have been mixed [90], but rifampin has been effective [89]; this lends further support to erythromycin plus rifampin as empiric treatment for moderate to severe atypical pneumonia [88].

VI. **Legionnaires' and related diseases.** Since the dramatic outbreak of the serious pulmonary infections in Philadelphia in July 1976 at the convention of the American Legion, a great deal has been learned about Legionnaires' disease and the organism that causes it (*Legionella pneumophila*). In addition, related organisms have been identified in this new genus *Legionella,* in the family Legionellaceae. Although these organisms have only recently been identified and named, they have caused unrecognized infections for years [5].

A. **Nomenclature and microbiology.** In addition to the bacteria that causes Legionnaires' disease, other *Legionella*-like organisms were identified that caused infections which were poorly understood in the past [6]. These infections formerly were believed to be due to *Rickettsia*-like organisms and were variously designated (e.g., WIGA, Tatlock, and HEBA organisms). The currently proposed names for these organisms have recently been reviewed [6]. Although the clinical pneumonias caused by these organisms are similar, the species do differ in their ability to produce beta-lactamase, a fact that may influence the choice of antibiotic therapy. The clinical aspects of *L. pneumophila* will be stressed as this organism is more commonly associated with recognized disease and is better understood. In surveys conducted in the 1980s, *L. pneumophila* serogroups were responsible for 80–85% of all the *Legionella* pneumonia in the United States [91, 92].

1. **L. pneumophila** is an aerobic, gram-negative, fastidious organism that grows on special media (e.g., charcoal yeast extract agar supplemented with alpha-ketoglutarate) containing cysteine [93]. It grows best in an atmosphere of 2.5–5.0% carbon dioxide, and growth may not occur for up to 10 days. Although this is a gram-negative bacillus, it does not stain well with ordinary Gram stain. **Special silver stains** (e.g., Dieterle) **are used to demonstrate the organism in tissue.** High-performance liquid chromatography is useful in the identification of *L. pneumophila* and other *Legionella* spp. [93].

   a. The organism produces a beta-lactamase and is resistant to penicillins and currently available cephalosporins.

   b. **At least 14 serologic types,** based on antigenic differences, have been identified [93].

   c. The organism contains an endotoxin (although it is not highly active biologically), hemolysins, proteases, acid phosphatase, and at least one toxin [94].

2. **Legionella micdadei** is the bacteria now recognized as causing so-called Pittsburgh pneumonia (see sec. **VII**) and infections previously believed to be due to *Rickettsia*-like organisms (i.e., the Tatlock and HEBA organisms) [6]. These organisms grow on charcoal yeast extract agar.

3. **L. bozemanii** is the current name of the *Rickettsia*-like organism, WIGA, that causes a Legionnaires'-like syndrome.

4. **Other Legionella spp.** causing disease in humans continue to be retrieved from new infections and identified and studied or recovered from samples of previously unidentified pneumonias. Those implicated in respiratory infections include *L. dumoffii, L. gormanii, L. longbeachae, L. jordanis, L. feeleii, L. wadsworthii, L. maceachernii, L. birminghamensis, L. cincinnatiensis, L. oakridgensis, L. anisa, L. cherrii,* and *L. sainthelensi* [6].

B. **Incidence.** The exact incidence of infections due to *L. pneumophila* and related species is **unknown;** estimates show wide variation with locale and time. Overall, **perhaps 2–6% or more of previously undiagnosed community-acquired pneumonias** are (or have been) due to these bacteria. **The rates of hospital-acquired pneumonias** caused by *Legionella* also **vary,** depending on the medical center and the patient population [95]. One literature review found that *Legionella* organisms were reported to cause from 0 to 32% of community-acquired pneumonias requiring hospitalization, from 0 to 47% of nosocomial pneumonias, and from 1 to 7% of pneumonias at autopsy [96].

C. **Epidemiology of L. pneumophila.** *L. pneumophila* is an **aquatic organism transmitted by water and air** [93, 96]. Environmental reservoirs frequently contain certain algae that provide nutrients and amebae and protozoa that support their intracellular multiplication; growth in artificial water sources is further favored by elevated temperatures, iron, and limited bacterial competition.

Epidemiologic data have suggested that soil excavation, air-conditioning systems, water evaporative condensers, and potable water have been point sources for outbreaks that have occurred, especially in summer months. However, sporadic cases occur year-round [5]. For those exposed to the organism in the environment, the attack rate (i.e., actual development of disease) is low and in the range of 1–7% [97].

The predominant mode of spread of *Legionella* has heretofore been believed to be through airborne droplets. Newer observations suggest that microaspiration may be more important, with potable water being the vehicle leading to colonization [97, 98]. **Human-to-human transmission does not occur.**

There have been outbreaks of *Legionella* infections, including *L. micdadei,* in health care facilities [95, 97, 98]. It is noteworthy that nursing personnel in these institutions have been infected, as demonstrated by serologic conversion, but have not been ill. The patients, especially the older or more compromised patients, developed serious pneumonias that often ended in death.

D. **Host factors.** Although Legionnaires' disease is seen in any age group, including the pediatric population, serologic data from outbreaks have revealed that when most young healthy individuals become infected, they develop no (or few) symptoms. In contrast, **elderly or compromised patients may develop a severe infection that may be fatal.** Patients at risk appear to be the following [96]:

1. **Immunocompromised patients,** including organ transplant patients (particularly during antirejection treatment), and persons receiving certain chemotherapeutic agents, radiation therapy, or corticosteroids. **Immunocompromised patients are at risk for acquiring nosocomial *Legionella* infection.** Legionellosis has been uncommon in HIV-infected individuals.

2. **Dialysis patients.**

3. **Late-middle-aged to elderly men.**

4. **Hosts with chronic underlying disease** (e.g., organic heart disease, lung disease, renal disease, and diabetes).

5. **Alcoholics and smokers.**

E. **Clinical manifestations.** There is a **broad spectrum** of disease due to *L. pneumophila* [5].

1. **Asymptomatic infection** is well described.

2. **Pontiac fever** is a nonpneumonic disease named after the outbreak in Pontiac, Michigan, in 1968. After a short 1- to 2-day incubation period, there is an abrupt onset of fever, headache, myalgias, and malaise. Acute symptoms usually last less than a week, the illness being self-limited even without specific therapy. It may be caused by *L. pneumophila, L. micdadei, L. feeleii,* or *L. anisa.*

3. **Pneumonia** is the most common problem for which the patient seeks and needs medical care.

   a. **Pulmonary manifestations.** The spectrum of disease is **highly variable** [5]. Patients may have mild to moderate illness (e.g., bronchitis or an atypical pneumonia syndrome) or moderate to severe pneumonia. Adult respiratory distress syndrome may occur [99]. Illness usually begins with nonspecific symptoms of malaise, myalgias, headache, and fever, after an incubation period of 2–10 days. Cough is present in approximately 90% of patients. It is initially a dry, nonproductive cough but may become productive or purulent in up to 75% [5]. Temperatures in the range of 39°–40°C (102°–104°F) are common, as are shaking chills. Pulmonary symptoms steadily progress over several days; chest pain and hemoptysis may appear in up to one-third of patients. Physical findings are often nonspecific early in the illness and may include a pulse-temperature deficit. Over time, signs of consolidation become evident, but pleural friction rubs are uncommon. There are **no pathognomonic radiologic findings.** Infiltrates that are initially unilateral and patchy frequently progress to consolidation, often bilateral. Nodular lesions or diffuse alveolar patterns may be seen. Cavitation and abscess formation have occurred. Small pleural effusions may develop, but large effusions are uncommon.

   b. **Other manifestations** of pneumonic infections are listed here, but their absence should not be used to eliminate the possibility of legionellosis [5]. In fact, the initial clinical presentation of Legionnaires' disease often is indistinguishable from other common pneumonias [5].

      (1) **Nausea and vomiting** are relatively common. **Diarrhea** is reported in up to 50% of cases but frequently also accompanies pneumonia of other causes [5].

      (2) **Relative bradycardia** may be seen.

      (3) **Neurologic findings** include headache, confusion, disorientation, delirium and, although rare, focal neurologic findings. Lumbar puncture studies are normal.

      (4) **Renal abnormalities,** including proteinuria, hematuria, hyponatremia, and renal failure, can occur.

      (5) **Myalgia** and **arthralgias** are seen.

      (6) **Miscellaneous findings.** Hepatomegaly and liver function test abnormalities, disseminated intravascular coagulation, hypophosphatemia, and the syndrome of inappropriate antidiuretic hormone have been described.

4. **Extrapulmonary infections** due to *L. pneumophila* [5, 95] have included bacteremia, lymphadenitis, **prosthetic valve endocarditis,** sinusitis, osteomyelitis, hemodialysis shunt infections, peritonitis, pancreatitis, pericarditis,

myocarditis, cellulitis, wound infection, and abscesses in organs and soft tissues. These can result from hematogenous seeding (with or without clinical pneumonia) or from direct inoculation with contaminated water [95]. An intestinal origin following ingestion of *Legionella* in water also has been proposed but not proven [5].

F. **Diagnosis is difficult.** There are no pathognomonic abnormalities early in the disease. **The fastidious causative organism rarely is isolated from routine sputum cultures and special media are required** to isolate the organism from sputum or other bodily fluids.

1. **Radiologic findings are nonspecific.**

2. **Routine Gram stains of sputum** frequently show moderate to large numbers of polymorphonuclear leukocytes (and monocytes), often with no bacteria.

3. **Cultures for *Legionella*** have a diagnostic specificity of 100%, and should be performed whenever possible [5, 93]. They **require special media and take several days to grow,** so the laboratory should be alerted to the possibility of these organisms. Cultures of respiratory secretions, bronchial washings, and lung tissue have a sensitivity of 80–99% [5]; the yield from pleural fluid probably is lower. *Legionella* organisms have also been isolated from blood, with a sensitivity of 10–30% [5]. Cultures may remain positive for an undetermined length of time after antibiotic therapy is begun, although their sensitivity is reduced over time.

4. **Direct fluorescent antibody** (DFA) **examination** of respiratory secretions, pleural fluid, or lung tissue, if properly performed, is a useful test for rapid diagnosis. Unfortunately, results may not be reliable in inexperienced laboratories or when monoclonal antibodies specific for *L. pneumophila* are not used [5, 93]. The sensitivity of this test on sputum or BAL specimens has therefore ranged from 25% to 75% [5]. Organisms may remain detectable by DFA for several days after starting antibiotics [5]. False positive DFA of sputums can be seen when *Pseudomonas* spp. or *Bacteroides* spp. are cultured in the sputum.

5. **DNA probe** tests using nucleic acid hybridization to detect *Legionella* are commercially available. This method is equivalent to DFA tests for rapid diagnosis, but some laboratories may be more experienced in this technique than in immunofluorescence microscopy [5, 93]. DNA probe assay has been 50–70% sensitive, and also may remain positive for a few days after therapy has begun [5]. DNA amplification using **PCR** is promising but remains **experimental** [5, 93]. Theoretically, DNA probes and PCR should be capable of detecting any *Legionella* spp.

6. **Antigen detection in urine** is commercially available in kits using radioimmunoassay and enzyme immunoassay (EIA) methods to diagnose *L. pneumophila* serogroup 1 infections rapidly [99a]. These tests have high specificity and sensitivity and may be positive well into the patient's illness or even after therapy has been started. Unfortunately, antigenuria may be prolonged, so that a positive test may result from an unrelated prior infection [5]. Also, false negative results may be obtained from infection with a serogroup not detected by the test. Latex agglutination kits are not recommended because of relatively poor performance [5, 93]. See Chap. 25.

7. **Indirect fluorescent antibody** (IFA) or ELISA **serologic studies** can lead to a retrospective diagnosis. Because serum antibody does not develop until the patient is well into the illness, **serial studies should be obtained** (e.g., samples every 2–3 weeks for 3–9 weeks). Serologic diagnosis is further complicated by the many serotypes of *L. pneumophila* that have been identified [96]. These serotypes do not cross-react completely, and regional laboratories may not be able to test for all serotypes or other *Legionella* spp. Thus, **yield is highest for *L. pneumophila* serogroup 1,** and results for other *Legionella* spp. should be interpreted with caution [5].

Serologic cross-reactions with *Mycoplasma* spp., tularemia, leptospirosis, and plague have been suggested. Other infectious causes for false positive results include *E. coli, B. fragilis, S. pneumoniae,* and *M. tuberculosis,* as well as *Pseudomonas, Citrobacter, Haemophilus, Campylobacter,* and *Bordetella* spp. [5, 93].

With paired sera, a fourfold rise in titer of IFA to 1:128 or more is considered diagnostic of recent exposure and disease, with a sensitivity of 75% [5]. A single titer of 1:256 or more in a patient with a compatible clinical illness has been presumptive evidence of a recent infection, although this has a low positive predictive value [99a] and should not be used for diagnosis in an individual patient.

G. **Therapy.** Standard in vitro antibiotic susceptibility tests of *Legionella* do not reliably predict clinical efficacy [5]. Thus, most of the evidence regarding effective therapeutic agents has been gleaned from empiric clinical experience or a guinea pig model. In that model, erythromycin, rifampin, TMP-SMX, and the fluoroquinolones are effective, whereas most penicillins, cephalosporins, and aminoglycosides are ineffective. Additional in vitro studies using cell culture monolayers have suggested that antibiotics must penetrate macrophages to be effective [5, 96].

Clinical efficacy is best established for erythromycin with or without rifampin but is also reported for TMP-SMX and tetracyclines. Ciprofloxacin, ofloxacin, perfloxacin, and imipenem have been used successfully in a few reported cases. However, ciprofloxacin and ofloxacin treatment failures have been reported [100–102]. The penicillins, cephalosporins, clindamycin, and aminoglycosides are ineffective. In fact, a pneumonia that progresses during treatment with these agents should suggest the possibility of *Legionella* infection.

1. **Indications for therapy**
   a. **Empiric therapy often is necessary because of the limitations in making a definitive early diagnosis.** When other causes of pneumonia have been excluded by careful clinical evaluation, including routine Gram stains and culture, and when the patient is in the proper clinical setting (see secs. **D** and **E**), empiric therapy is reasonable. One should particularly be alerted to the possibility of this diagnosis in the following:
      (1) Certain **high-risk hosts** (see sec. **D**).
      (2) **Patients with unexplained pneumonia** with diarrhea, relative bradycardia, and other **extrapulmonary manifestations** of Legionnaires' disease (see sec. **E.3.b**).
      (3) Patients with initial Gram stains of sputum that reveal moderate to large numbers of polymorphonuclear leukocytes yet few or no predominant organisms.
   b. **Specific therapy** is indicated for all patients with positive cultures or DNA probe tests. In the appropriate clinical setting, treatment also should be given to patients with a positive urine antigen test or diagnostic serologic tests (see sec. **F.7**).
   c. **Therapy** is indicated **for patients with progressive pneumonia** not responding to prior antibiotics **and when the diagnosis of Legionnaires' disease has not been initially considered.** Attempts to establish the diagnosis should be undertaken as discussed in sec. **F**, and obstructing lesions also should be ruled out.

2. **Drugs and dosages**
   a. **Erythromycin is the treatment of choice** [5, 64a]. In moderate to severe infections in adults, it should initially be given intravenously in a dose of 500–1,000 mg q6h. **Very severe or life-threatening infections may be treated with full doses of intravenous erythromycin plus 600-mg rifampin** PO or IV q12h; rifampin should not be used alone. Because peripheral intravenous erythromycin causes phlebitis, a central intravenous line usually is indicated for the 1-g dose regimen and patients should be monitored closely for arrhythmias [5]. If definite clinical improvement occurs after 5–10 days of intravenous erythromycin, use of oral erythromycin, 500 mg qid, may be substituted to complete a total of 3 weeks of therapy, and the rifampin may be stopped. Mild infections may be treated with 3 weeks of erythromycin in a dose of 500 mg PO qid. Lower doses or shorter treatment courses than those outlined result in an increased frequency of relapses or prolonged convalescence [5, 96]. For dosages in children, see Chap. 28M.
   b. Many patients are unable to tolerate full doses or a protracted course of oral erythromycin. Although there is less experience with **clarithromycin** [5], it causes fewer GI side effects than erythromycin and is administered on a twice-daily schedule. We believe clarithromycin is a useful agent in this setting and favor it in adults (500 mg bid) to complete a 3-week course of therapy (see Chap. 28M).
   c. Further clinical experience with **azithromycin** (500 mg the first day, fol-

lowed by 250 mg every day for 4 more days) is needed to determine how this agent fits in with more conventional 3-week therapies. Azithromycin is, however, a potential alternative to standard regimens [5]. See Chap. 28M for a more detailed discussion of the new macrolides.

d. **Other alternatives** to erythromycin are not as well established but include TMP-SMX given to adults in a dose of 320-mg trimethoprim and 1,600-mg sulfamethoxazole q12h, or doxycycline given in a dose of 100 mg IV q12–24h after a single 200-mg loading dose. One authority does not favor TMP-SMX and recommends adding rifampin whenever it is used [5].

e. **Fluoroquinolones.** The role of these agents for *Legionella* infections is evolving, although they show in vitro activity (see Chap. 28S). Ciprofloxacin (400 mg IV q12h or 500 mg PO q12h) or ofloxacin (400 mg IV or PO q12h) were recommended as substitutes for erythromycin plus rifampin, particularly in transplant patients receiving cyclosporine [5].

3. **Isolation.** There appears to be no conclusive evidence of human-to-human spread, and special precautions are not required.

4. **Prognosis** is related to the underlying disease and the early institution of appropriate therapy. In nonimmunosuppressed patients, the case-fatality rate was 7% in those treated with erythromycin, compared with 25% in those not receiving erythromycin. In immunosuppressed patients, those who received erythromycin had a fatality rate of 24%, compared with 80% in those who did not [96].

VII. *Legionella micdadei.* This organism, also called the **Pittsburgh pneumonia agent** and *Tatlockia micdadei,* was serendipitously identified in 1979 as a cause of pneumonia in immunocompromised hosts [6]. Retrospective analysis has established that it was first isolated decades earlier as the *Rickettsia*-like Tatlock and HEBA organisms [6]. *L. micdadei* is weakly acid-fast in clinical specimens but rapidly loses this characteristic on in vitro culture; an exception has been reported when acid-fast *L. micdadei* were isolated from BACTEC liquid mycobacteria media [103]. Other *Legionella* spp. are not acid-fast. *L. micdadei* is a fastidious organism but grows on the same special media used to isolate *L. pneumophila;* the addition of albumin may increase yield [93]. Unlike *L. pneumophila,* it does not regularly produce beta-lactamases. Environmental reservoirs for *L. micdadei* and *L. pneumophila* are similar, perhaps accounting for the many reported cases of simultaneous infection with both organisms.

A. **Clinical manifestations.** *L. micdadei* is the second most common cause of *Legionella* pneumonia [6]. **Although community-acquired infections occur, they are much less frequent than nosocomial infections** in the compromised host. Patients at greatest risk have been transplant recipients, those with hematologic malignancies, and anyone on high doses of corticosteroids. Previous surgery and underlying chronic lung disease or other serious illness are additional predisposing factors. The clinical features of *L. micdadei* infections generally are indistinguishable from those of *L. pneumophila* infections and even from those of other common nosocomial pneumonias [6, 104]. The disease may be mild and resolve without therapy in normal hosts. In contrast, disease in high-risk patients may begin abruptly with high fever, pleuritic chest pain, dyspnea, and cough; several authors have noted a **presentation mimicking acute pulmonary embolism** [6]. Common extrapulmonary manifestations include confusion, abdominal pain, diarrhea, and hyponatremia. At least two cases of soft-tissue infections caused by *L. micdadei* have been reported [105].

Radiographic findings in normal hosts include segmental or lobar infiltrates that rarely advance [106]. In compromised patients, there is more often rapid progression, and nodular and cavitary infiltrates may occur; small pleural effusions are common [6, 106].

B. **Diagnosis.** The methods of diagnosis are similar to those described earlier for *L. pneumophila.* Definitive diagnosis is established by isolation of the organism from respiratory secretions, pleural fluid, or lung tissue. Weakly acid-fast organisms may be seen in tissue, but there is acute inflammation involving neutrophils and alveolar macrophages and not granulomas. Reagents are available for DFA stains; at present, other techniques for rapid diagnosis are not available. However, most cases can be diagnosed by using DFA staining together with cultures. A presumptive diagnosis may be made retrospectively by demonstrating a fourfold or greater rise in antibody titer against *L. micdadei;* the specificity of this response has not been fully established [5].

C. **Therapy.** The optimal therapy remains undefined. Currently, **erythromycin** with or without rifampin is the treatment of choice for presumed or proven *L. micdadei* infections [6, 64a]. TMP-SMX is an acceptable alternative. Dosages and special considerations are similar to those for Legionnaires' disease (see sec. **VI.G**). Early therapy improves survival, which may be as low as 36% in untreated compromised patients. Penicillins, cephalosporins, and aminoglycosides are clinically ineffective agents, despite the fact that *L. micdadei* does not produce beta-lactamases. The therapeutic role of doxycycline, imipenem, and the fluoroquinolones has yet to be established.

VIII. **Melioidosis** [107–109]. This illness, caused by *Pseudomonas pseudomallei*, is **endemic to Southeast Asia and the South Pacific.** Although uncommon in North America, its recognition is important because untreated it is a potentially fatal disease.

A. **Microbiologic features.** *P. pseudomallei* (Whitmore's bacillus) is a small, gram-negative, obligately aerobic, mobile bacillus. It is a facultative intracellular parasite, a feature not shared by any other pseudomonad.

Smears may show a "safety-pin" morphology due to bipolar staining. The organism has a distinctive putrid odor on initial isolation, and a characteristic wrinkling of the colony surface usually occurs after 48–72 hours of incubation. Biochemical reactions distinguish this organism from other *Pseudomonas* spp.

B. **Incidence. More than 300 cases have been reported in American Vietnam War veterans.** Evidence suggests that approximately 1 in 20 individuals who reside in an endemic area has serologic evidence of infection. Apparently, there is an incidence of illness of 1:4,000 at risk, based on studies done during Indochina's occupation by French troops. It has been estimated that **approximately 250,000 of those who served in Vietnam became infected by *P. pseudomallei* and are at risk for recrudescent disease.**

C. **Epidemiology.** Although there is worldwide endemicity, most cases occur in individuals who have visited or resided in Southeast Asia or the South Pacific islands. **Illness can occur during residence or as long as 26 years after leaving the area.** Diabetes, many other intercurrent diseases, and surgery appear to trigger melioidosis reactivation. *P. pseudomallei* is widely distributed in soil and water. Transmission most often occurs from direct contact in the environment or from inhalation, but nosocomial and laboratory infections also have been described. Human-to-human spread has been reported only once. Asymptomatic carriage of the organism has not been identified [110].

D. **Clinical manifestations**
   1. There is a high incidence of **asymptomatic and mild** infection.
   2. **Pulmonary infections** occur in acute, subacute, and chronic forms [107, 109]. Each form may result either from an initial exposure to the organism or from reactivation of latent infection.
      a. **Acute pneumonia** begins abruptly with fever, myalgias, cough, and chest pain; septicemia may develop in some patients. The most common radiographic pattern is **upper-lobe consolidation, progressing to cavitation,** which may be thin-walled. In one series, pleural effusions were seen in 16% of pneumonia patients overall but were most commonly found in the acute form [109]. Empyema and purulent pericarditis are rare complications.
      b. **Subacute and chronic pneumonias** present with a prodrome lasting weeks to months. The clinical and **radiographic picture may be confused with tuberculosis.** Radiographs usually show confluent upper-lobe cavities, but the apices often are spared.
   3. **Acute septicemic melioidosis** is a systemic illness with a short prodrome. The lungs may be involved by hematogenous spread, but respiratory symptoms are not predominant. Initial findings usually include high fever, headache, myalgias, malaise, abdominal pain, hepatosplenomegaly, and diarrhea [109]. In those with a secondary pneumonia, radiographs most often show disseminated nodular infiltrates that coalesce and cavitate with progression.
   4. **Localized suppurative infections** outside the lungs may be acute or chronic in presentation. Skin and regional lymphatics are most commonly involved in the former, and illness may progress to the septicemic form. Chronic suppuration may involve skin, brain, liver, spleen, bones, lymph nodes, or prostate; these patients are chronically ill but may or may not be febrile.
   5. Melioidosis is an important cause of **fever of unknown origin** in those who recently resided in endemic regions.

E. Diagnosis
  1. **Gram stains** of respiratory secretions, exudate, or pus may show poorly stain-
     ing, small gram-negative bacilli. Wright's or methylene blue stain may accen-
     tuate the bipolar staining of the organism.
  2. **Cultures** on routine media may become positive at 24 hours, but colonies may
     take 72 hours to develop their typical morphologic appearance. Biochemical
     tests are helpful in identification.
  3. **Serologic tests** for antibody are available through state laboratories and the
     Centers for Disease Control (CDC) in Atlanta. Results must be interpreted
     with caution, however, because many patients with active disease will have
     negative serologic tests, and false positive reactions also occur. Indirect
     hemagglutination (IHA) is the method most widely used in endemic areas; a
     single IHA titer of 1:640 or greater is strongly supportive of melioidosis
     [107].
F. Therapy [107]. Treatment is reserved **for clinically active infections,** so that
  asymptomatic seropositive patients should not be treated. The usual therapeutic
  regimen consists of antibiotics, singly or in combination, which are selected based
  on the result of susceptibility tests and are given for at least 1 month. Infectious
  disease consultation is advised.
  1. **Drugs.** Tetracycline, chloramphenicol, TMP-SMX, sulfadiazine, sulfisoxazole,
     kanamycin, amikacin, and ceftazidime are among the active antibiotics that
     have been used successfully. Amoxicillin-clavulanate, ampicillin-sulbactam,
     ticarcillin-clavulanate, piperacillin, piperacillin-tazobactam, imipenem, and
     ciprofloxacin also are active against *P. pseudomallei,* but clinical experience
     with these drugs is limited. Ciprofloxacin and ofloxacin are less active than
     ceftazidime and exhibit relatively high MIC_{90} values. Many of these agents
     are not bactericidal in vitro, even in combination [111]. Some experts suggest
     that ceftazidime may be a preferred agent [64a].
  2. **Pneumonia.** The average time required to sterilize the sputum is 6 weeks.
     a. **Nonsepticemic infections** may be treated orally for 2–6 months. Mild
        illness may be treated with a single agent. Tetracycline, 2–3 g/day; TMP-
        SMX 2 mg/kg of trimethoprim component bid; and chloramphenicol, 3 g/day,
        are effective regimens in adults. Moderate illness may also be treated
        orally by combining TMP-SMX with either tetracycline or chloramphenicol
        (in the doses just cited) for the first month, followed by TMP-SMX alone
        for a minimum of another month.
     b. **Severe and septicemic illnesses** should initially be treated parenterally.
        The traditional therapy for adults is to combine tetracycline (4–6 g/day)
        or doxycycline (400 mg/day) with chloramphenicol (4–6 g/day) and add
        either TMP-SMX (8–12 mg/kg/day of the TMP component, up to a maxi-
        mum of 800 mg/day of TMP or kanamycin in standard doses or both.
        However, a recent prospective comparison indicates that the combination
        of **ceftazidime and TMP-SMX is now the regimen of choice** for severe
        disease [64a, 112]. Therapy may be narrowed and switched to oral drugs
        as clinical improvement occurs. If chloramphenicol is used, blood cell
        counts must be carefully monitored (see Chap. 28J).
  3. **Localized suppurations** are treated medically as described for pneumonia,
     except that antibiotics should be given for 6–12 months. Surgical drainage
     should be employed when needed but only after antibiotics have been
     started [107].
  4. **Mortality** may be as high as 87% in disseminated, septicemic infections; death
     usually occurs within the initial 3–5 days of treatment. The regimen of ceftazi-
     dime plus TMP-SMX results in significantly better survival than traditional
     combinations for patients with disseminated, septicemic melioidosis but not
     with other forms of the disease [112].
  5. **Relapses** are common in all varieties of melioidosis. Factors associated with
     relapse include immunosuppression, severity of illness, treatment for less
     than 2 months, the use of amoxicillin-clavulanate, and the absence of paren-
     teral ceftazidime from the initial regimen [107, 113].
IX. **Hantavirus pulmonary syndrome.** In May 1993, an outbreak of unexplained adult
  respiratory distress syndrome (ARDS) in otherwise healthy adults was reported in
  the Four Corners area of Arizona, Colorado, New Mexico, and Utah [114, 115, 115a].
  Intense investigation revealed the cause to be a newly discovered hantavirus, originally named the *Muerto Canyon virus* and recently renamed the *Sin Nombre* virus

[116, 118a]. It has since become evident that this syndrome also is present in other areas of the United States and is caused by at least two other new hantaviruses.

A. Etiology and epidemiology. The hantaviruses are enveloped negative-sense RNA viruses in the family Bunyavirudae and are found worldwide. Older viruses are associated with rodent vectors, although only a few cause human disease. Previously described hantavirus illnesses are most common in Asia and Europe and include syndromes of hemorrhagic fever with renal failure (e.g., Korean hemorrhagic fever) and nephropathia epidemica.

1. **The deer mouse** (*Peromyscus maniculatus*) **is the primary rodent reservoir** for Sin Nombre virus [116]. The Four Corners outbreak has been linked to an explosion in the deer mouse population during the prior year; this may have resulted from ecological changes that led to proliferation of their piñon nut and insect food supplies [117].

   As of a report in July 1995, confirmed cases of hantavirus pulmonary syndrome have occurred in 22 states, including many states west of the Mississippi River, Indiana, Florida, Rhode Island, and Virginia [115, 116, 118, 118a]. A few of these cases are outside of the known distribution of the deer mouse, suggesting that **other reservoirs and hantaviruses are also involved.** In fact, related but unique hantaviruses have been identified from patients in Florida and Louisiana. The cotton rat (*Sigmodon hispidus*) has been implicated as the reservoir for the Florida strain, but the animal reservoir for the Louisiana strain has not yet been identified [118]. The predominant **mode of transmission** of the hantavirus to humans has not been identified but may include aerosols of rodent urine or other fluids, disruption and inhalation of dried rodent excreta, food contamination, and direct contact with rodents, rodent excreta, or rodent saliva. **Human-to-human spread has not occurred.**

2. Almost all cases of hantavirus pulmonary syndrome have occurred in a **rural setting** or after a recent visit to such an area [114–116]. Most patients have become ill in the months between spring and early fall, with most of those in the original Four Corners outbreak presenting between April and July of 1993. There is an equal distribution of male and female patients. The median age of patients identified in 1993 was 31 years, but ranged from 12 to 69 years [116]. In Baltimore, Maryland, this is an uncommon cause of community-acquired pneumonia [118b].

B. Clinical manifestations [114, 115, 115a, 119]

1. A **brief prodrome** has included fever, chills, and myalgias; cough has also been noted but is less likely to be prominent initially.

2. **Additional early symptoms** may include headache, dizziness, abdominal discomfort, nausea, and vomiting.

3. **Adult respiratory distress syndrome** rapidly follows, with no obvious explanation. This phase is characterized by fever, hypoxia, hypotension, volume depletion, and thrombocytopenia. Invasive monitoring has revealed evidence of **noncardiogenic pulmonary edema** and depressed myocardial function [114, 115].

4. **Other laboratory abnormalities** have included leukocytosis with early myeloid forms and atypical lymphocytes, proteinuria, microscopic hematuria, hypoalbuminemia, and lactic acidosis.

5. Pharyngitis and coryza are not common features of this syndrome.

6. **Pathologic findings** at autopsy have included pleural effusions, pulmonary edema with hyaline membranes, and mononuclear cell infiltration. Similar atypical mononuclear cells have also been found in the spleen and lymph nodes. Neutrophils have not been prominent. Although most evident in the lungs, hantavirus antigen has been identified in the endothelium of many organs.

C. Diagnosis. Because there are no distinguishing features early in the hantavirus pulmonary syndrome, diagnosis **must rest on clinical suspicion. A potential case is currently defined as** unexplained ARDS in an otherwise healthy person, with no predisposing condition or acute illness that may provide an alternative reason for the respiratory failure [116]. **Physicians** caring for such patients **should contact their state health authorities and the CDC** to arrange for testing to confirm a hantavirus etiology.

1. Sin Nombre virus has been isolated in **culture,** but this is difficult and not readily available.

2. Recombinant nucleoprotein antigen expressed in *E. coli* is being made available by the CDC for use in **serologic tests** [116]. IgM and IgG against Sin Nombre virus may be detected with these assays, and preliminary Western blot analysis has shown these assays to be sensitive and specific. Antibodies often cross-react with older hantaviruses, particularly Prospect Hill and Puumala viruses. Serologic tests are not commercially available at this time.
3. **Immunohistochemical staining** of tissue may detect hantavirus antigen in biopsy or necropsy specimens.
4. **PCR** was able to identify the virus in patient and animal specimens before it was cultured. This technique also has proven invaluable in distinguishing Sin Nombre virus from the other hantaviruses responsible for the hantavirus pulmonary syndrome. Tissues, serum, and blood may all be positive very early in the illness.

D. **Prognosis and therapy**
   1. **Mortality** was 60% among the cases identified in 1993 [116].
   2. Rapid institution of **supportive therapy** in an intensive care unit has been critical to survival [114, 115].
   3. **Ribavirin** is active in vitro against older hantaviruses and has been used successfully in Korean hemorrhagic fever. Based on this information, intravenous ribavirin was made available from the CDC through an investigational protocol for use in patients who met the clinical definition of hantavirus pulmonary syndrome [114, 116]. **However,** at present there is **no evidence that ribavirin is effective therapy** for this illness.

E. **Prevention** is based on minimizing exposure to rodents and their excreta [120]. Persons engaged in outdoor activities, such as camping or hiking, should take precautions to reduce contact with rodents [118a].

X. **Pulmonary infiltration associated with therapeutic agents** [7]
A. **Antimicrobials**
   1. **Nitrofurantoin.** Two patterns of pulmonary disease are caused by nitrofurantoin. (For further discussion, see Chap. 28T.)
      a. **Acute reactions** occur within 1 month of drug therapy and account for 90% of the cases of nitrofurantoin-related pulmonary reactions. Most patients have taken the drug previously without problems. However, the more prior exposures, the shorter is the interval to symptoms, which may begin within hours of restarting nitrofurantoin therapy. The mechanism is unknown but is believed to involve hypersensitivity to the drug. Common clinical findings include dyspnea, nonproductive cough, fever, arthralgias, crackles in the lungs, an elevated ESR, and eosinophilia that may be delayed in appearance. Rash, wheezing, and pleural manifestations are much less common.

      Radiographic findings include interstitial or alveolar infiltrates in the bases. Unilateral pleural effusion may be present in a minority of patients, and in others the roentgenogram will be normal. Lung biopsy often shows an eosinophilic infiltration and inflammation.

      b. **Chronic reactions** occur after at least several months of therapy and account for only 10% of nitrofurantoin-induced pulmonary disease. The mechanism is believed to involve oxidant injury to the lung. Clinical illness begins slowly, with dyspnea, a nonproductive cough, and bilateral lung crackles. Fever, rash, and eosinophilia are not seen in chronic reactions. Radiographic findings are present in all patients; bilateral interstitial fibrosis is most common, with or without pleural effusion.

      c. **Treatment** for both acute and chronic reactions consists of **rapid withdrawal of the drug** and supportive care. Corticosteroids have no proven role in either the acute or chronic reaction. Prognosis in the acute form is excellent. In contrast, up to 10% of patients with chronic nitrofurantoin-induced pulmonary toxicity will have a fatal outcome, and many of the remaining patients will have persistent radiographic or clinical abnormalities.

   2. **Sulfonamides.** Sulfasalazine, used to treat inflammatory bowel disease, and other sulfonamides rarely may cause hypersensitivity lung disease. Treatment is immediate cessation of the drug, and prognosis is excellent.
   3. **Amphotericin B.** There has been an unconfirmed suggestion that amphotericin B given concomitantly with WBC transfusion induces pulmonary toxicity associated with dyspnea, hypoxia, and hemoptysis (see sec. **X.C.3**).

B. **Antiarrhythmic drugs. Amiodarone** has been associated with fibrosing alveolitis in approximately 1–6% of recipients. Pulmonary toxicity most often develops after 5–6 months of therapy with doses of at least 400–800 mg/day but less commonly can appear after 1 month or after years of therapy. Clinical illness usually presents slowly over 2–3 months, with fever, nonproductive cough, dyspnea on exertion, malaise, and bibasilar rales. Radiographs initially show diffuse interstitial infiltrates but, with progression, also may include patchy alveolar infiltrates. Some evidence suggests that the drug induces an acquired lysosomal storage disease, and other studies implicate immune-mediated mechanisms.

C. **Cytotoxic drugs.** A very confusing situation in immunocompromised hosts receiving chemotherapy occurs when pulmonary infiltrates develop. The differential diagnosis in such circumstances includes drug-related disease, infection, hemorrhage, and the primary disease. (See sec. **XI.C.3** for more details.)

XI. **Pneumonia in the compromised host.** Pneumonia is a relatively common problem in the compromised patient population [121–123]. When pneumonia occurs, the patient can become critically ill. Mortality in the range of 30–50% is frequently reported. A careful clinical approach to these patients is essential. The compromised host population includes patients on immunosuppressive chemotherapy or moderate-dose to high-dose corticosteroids; those with transplants; patients with congenital or acquired immune deficits; HIV-infected patients; and those with malignancy, especially myeloproliferative or lymphoproliferative disorders (see Chaps. 19 and 20).

A. **The clinical dilemma**
   1. **Urgent problem.** Rapid evaluation is necessary because these patients can deteriorate quickly.
   2. **Multiple etiologies.** Almost any infectious agent can cause pneumonia in the compromised patient. There are no pathognomonic features that allow one to determine from the clinical presentation the etiology of the pneumonia. Noninfectious etiologies can present with lung infiltrates and fever. An invasive procedure often is necessary to make a definite diagnosis.
   3. **Routine laboratory data often are nonspecific.** Many of the infectious agents causing the pneumonia cannot be diagnosed from routine sputum samples. Roentgenography cannot provide specific diagnoses.
   4. **Multiteam approach.** Management of pneumonia in the compromised host often requires the cooperative efforts of subspecialists in oncology, infectious disease, pulmonary disease, thoracic surgery, and pathology. If facilities are not available for such a multiteam approach, consideration should be given to transferring such patients to another institution.

B. **Host factors**
   1. **Humoral deficiencies** include hypogammaglobulinemias and hypocomplementemias. They may be congenital or acquired as the result of an underlying disease or its therapy. For example, humoral deficiencies commonly accompany multiple myeloma, chronic lymphocytic leukemia, bone marrow transplantation, and cancer chemotherapies. Patients with humoral deficiencies are at highest risk for lung infections caused by *S. pneumoniae* and *H. influenzae*, among other pyogenic bacteria.
   2. **Neutropenia** may result from a variety of causes, including immunologic and malignant diseases, drugs, and radiation. **The neutropenic host with pneumonia may not (1) produce sputum, (2) exhibit the expected findings on physical examination, or (3) initially demonstrate radiographic abnormalities.** Frequent pathogens in this group of patients include streptococci, staphylococci, Enterobacteriaceae, *P. aeruginosa, Aspergillus* spp., and Zygomycetes, the latter two often manifesting after prolonged antibiotic therapy.
   3. **Impaired cell-mediated immunity** may be part of a congenital immunodeficiency or may be acquired as a result of lymphomas, cytotoxic drugs, steroids, radiation therapy, HIV infection, and malnutrition. Defective cellular immunity predisposes to a diversity of infections, including those caused by *Nocardia* spp., *Legionella* spp., mycobacteria, *Cryptococcus neoformans, Histoplasma capsulatum,* cytomegalovirus (CMV), varicella-zoster virus, *Pneumocystis carinii,* and *Strongyloides stercoralis*. **Corticosteroids** are an important predisposing factor for many pathogens but particularly for *Nocardia, L. micdadei, M. tuberculosis,* most fungi, *P. carinii,* and *S. stercoralis*.
   4. **Renal and other organ transplant patients** are at high risk for pulmonary complications. Important factors in determining the type of infection include time interval since transplantation, type of immunosuppressive therapy, and the presence or absence of the spleen (see Chap. 20).

5. **Combinations** of the conditions cited in secs. **1–4,** in addition to impairments to nonimmune pulmonary defenses, are commonly present. Such impairments frequently occur as the underlying malignancy or other disorder is treated and predispose the patient to a variety of opportunistic bacterial, mycobacterial, fungal, viral, and protozoal infections.

C. **Differential diagnosis.** The differential diagnosis of a pulmonary infiltrate in the compromised host is extensive. The major considerations include the following:

1. **Infection.** With the exception of some viruses, most infections can be treated specifically if a particular organism or agent can be demonstrated.

   a. **Bacteria.** The gram-negative bacteria (*Klebsiella* spp., *E. coli, Pseudomonas* spp.) are common pathogens. *S. aureus* may occasionally be involved, as may gram-positive diphtheroids. *L. pneumophila* (Legionnaires' disease; see sec. **VI**) and *L. micdadei* (see sec. **VII**) also must be considered.

   b. **Tuberculosis.** Reactivation of tuberculosis can occur in patients on immunosuppressive therapy. (See separate discussion under Tuberculosis: Basic Concepts, later in this chapter.)

   c. *Pneumocystis carinii.* *P. carinii* pneumonia (PCP) is **most commonly seen in** two groups—**newborns with agammaglobulinemia and individuals with AIDS—but** it **also** occurs in individuals with **lymphocytic disorders** (specifically children with acute lymphocytic leukemia and adults with Hodgkin's disease) **and** with systemic **lupus** erythematosus. Except for AIDS patients and newborns, these individuals have received steroids, and usually cytotoxic agents as well, prior to the development of *P. carinii* infection. Infection results when a latent organism is reactivated, probably due in part to the immunosuppressive therapy for the neoplasia. For most of these patients, the disease becomes active when their underlying disease is in remission. Early clues are fever and shortness of breath with cough and no specific other localizing symptoms. The rapidity with which disease progresses is variable, but it can take a full week for full-blown manifestations to develop. AIDS patients typically experience subacute progression over 2–3 weeks (see Chap. 19). By contrast, in patients with underlying lymphoproliferative diseases, the picture can evolve within 24–48 hours. Sputum production is scant, and extrapulmonary disease, including pleural involvement, is rare. A variety of radiologic changes can be seen. **(See Chap. 24 for a complete discussion of PCP in HIV-infected patients.)**

   d. **Fungi**

      (1) *Aspergillus* spp. and members of the Phycomycetes (now called Zygomycetes), which include the *Mucor* spp., occur in this setting.

         (a) **Most patients are granulocytopenic and often are febrile despite broad-spectrum antibiotic therapy.** Other clues to the diagnosis include pleuritic chest pain, bloody sputum, nasal and sinus abnormalities, and rapidly progressive nodular or cavitary infiltrates on the chest roentgenogram.

         (b) Fungal elements invade vascular channels and cause thrombosis; thus, these infections may present as pulmonary infarction. In addition, dissemination to other organ systems, particularly the CNS, occurs.

         (c) The use of sputum cultures to diagnose pulmonary aspergillosis is complex; aspergilli may be commensals in the airways, particularly if there is underlying chronic lung disease. In addition to this difficulty in distinguishing colonization from infection, cultures often are falsely negative. Although BAL has been used to identify pulmonary aspergillosis, **demonstration of invasion of tissue by transbronchial biopsy or open lung biopsy usually is necessary to establish a definitive diagnosis.**

         (d) Early therapy, including amphotericin B and surgical debridement, is essential to increasing survival. Thus, therapy should be instituted in the appropriate clinical setting if sputum cultures are positive for aspergilli, pending the results of invasive tests. (See related discussion in Chap. 18.)

      (2) Other fungi, such as *C. neoformans,* can cause pulmonary infection but are less common (see Chap. 18).

   e. **Viruses. CMV** also causes pulmonary infection and is commonly reactivated in the compromised host. With CMV, asymptomatic reactivation is far more common than symptomatic reactivation. Thus, the vast majority of individuals who shed this virus are asymptomatic. CMV is unique in that it can be transmitted by fresh-blood transfusion, WBC transfusion, or allografts. If an individual has no previous immunity, a primary infection develops. Mixed infections with CMV and *Pneumocystis* occur. (See Chaps. 17, 19, 20, 24, and 26 for further discussion of CMV.)

CMV pneumonia is most common in recipients of allogeneic bone marrow transplants (see Chap. 20). Varicella-zoster virus, herpes simplex virus, and adenoviruses are other causes of viral pneumonias in compromised patients.

   f. *Nocardia* has been a cause of pulmonary infection in patients undergoing cardiac transplantation and in other compromised patients (see Chap. 18).
   g. **Other infectious agents.** *Toxoplasma gondii* (see Chaps. 17 and 19) and certain roundworms, especially *S. stercoralis,* may cause pneumonia in the compromised host.
 2. **Tumor** spread can mimic an infectious lung problem. This is particularly true of lymphomas and alveolar cell carcinoma.
 3. **Drug-induced infiltrates** must be considered [7]. Drugs that can induce lung disease include bleomycin, busulfan, methotrexate, mitomycin (with or without vinca alkaloids), the nitrosoureas (e.g., BCNU) and, occasionally, cyclophosphamide. The use of intravenous cytosine arabinoside may be associated with rapid development of pulmonary edema. Clinically, these patients developed tachypnea, hypoxemia, and pulmonary infiltrates. Because the patients often are febrile, this complication of cytosine arabinoside may mimic the development of an acute pneumonia.

   Leukocyte transfusions and amphotericin B have been associated with acute pulmonary infiltrates, particularly when the amphotericin and granulocytes have been infused at the same time; reactions were more likely early in the course of amphotericin B treatment. However, these observations have not been confirmed. When both leukocytes and amphotericin B therapy must be used in a patient, it may be best to leave as much time as possible between the infusion of amphotericin B and the leukocyte transfusion.
 4. **CHF** may, at times, be difficult to distinguish from diffuse interstitial pneumonia.
 5. **Hemorrhage** in the thrombocytopenic patient may cause an infiltrate and predispose the patient to develop a superimposed bacterial pneumonia.
 6. **Nonspecific interstitial pneumonitis** (NIP) may be present in 20–30% of patients undergoing lung biopsies. This diagnosis requires that all routine and special cultures be negative. Thus, if NIP is established as the only . diagnosis, empiric antimicrobial therapy may be discontinued (although we will sometimes continue erythromycin empirically because it is difficult to exclude *Mycoplasma* infection).
 7. **Radiation pneumonitis** may mimic an infectious process [8].
 8. **Pulmonary embolism with infarction** may be very difficult to distinguish from acute infection in this setting.
 9. **Collagen vascular diseases.** Pulmonary involvement mimicking pneumonia is most common in systemic lupus erythematosus, Goodpasture's syndrome, and Wegener's granulomatosis [122]. Therefore, in a patient with one of these underlying conditions who may also be receiving immunosuppressive therapy, worsening of the underlying condition with progressive pulmonary changes may occur, and it may be difficult to differentiate disease progression from an evolving opportunistic infection.
D. **Initial clinical approach.** The possibility of an infectious process should be thoroughly assessed initially, as early effective therapy may be lifesaving.
   1. **Diagnostic studies** have recently been reviewed [123a].
      a. **Spontaneous or induced sputum smears and cultures** should be performed routinely for bacteria, mycobacteria, fungi, and *Legionella.* Smears and stains for *Pneumocystis* should be performed.
      b. **An invasive procedure** to obtain lower respiratory tract secretions may be required (see discussion in sec. **VII** under Clinical Approach to Pneumonia).
      c. **Blood cultures** should be obtained for every patient and, for some (e.g., AIDS patients), special media for mycobacteria and fungi may be included.
      d. **Pleural fluid** should be examined when present if it can safely be obtained.

e. **Mucocutaneous lesions** should be examined for microorganisms by scraping or biopsy.

f. **Other specimens** such as bone marrow, joint fluid, CSF, and urine may be helpful in some patients.

g. **Serologic studies** may be obtained for *Legionella* and *Mycoplasma* organisms, fungi, and viruses, but rarely are these helpful in choosing initial therapy.

h. **Serial evaluations** of respiratory status should be monitored, including chest roentgenograms and arterial blood gases or oximetry. Progressive hypoxia may be the only early clue to the presence of *Pneumocystis* infection or other interstitial pneumonias.

2. **Host factors and the setting** in which the infection arose can help to narrow the possible etiologies [30]. The specific underlying disease may predispose to specific pathogens, as discussed in sec. **B.** In addition, the state of the disease process, recent cytoreductive and radiation therapies, and the setting all contribute to determining likely pathogens. For example, a leukemic patient with neutropenia and a nosocomial pneumonia during treatment is most likely infected with an organism such as *P. aeruginosa* or other gram-negative bacilli, *Legionella*, fungi, or parasites. However, the same patient prior to any therapy or while in remission with an acute community-acquired pneumonia is now at greater risk for pneumococcal, *Mycoplasma*, or *Haemophilus* infection, or aspiration pneumonia.

3. **The tempo of the illness and the type of radiographic abnormality** may be of some help in narrowing the diagnostic possibilities. An acutely progressive illness favors gram-positive and gram-negative bacteria, pulmonary edema, embolism, hemorrhage, and leukoagglutinin reactions. A subacute to chronic illness should suggest CMV, *Pneumocystis*, *Mycoplasma*, *Nocardia*, and *Mycobacterium* spp. and fungi, among other infections; radiation pneumonitis and drug toxicity would be among the noninfectious possibilities. Radiographic patterns (e.g., consolidative, nodular, or diffuse infiltrates) may help support certain infectious and noninfectious etiologies, but many pathogens are associated with more than one pattern. Thus, the roentgenographic appearance is best used in conjunction with an assessment of the tempo of the illness. A "wedge defect" or nodular defects in a febrile leukopenic patient, despite broad-spectrum antibiotics, raise the possibility of an invasive fungus, especially *Aspergillus* spp.

E. **Initial therapy.** Because the combinations of therapeutic agents necessary to treat all these potential infections can be highly toxic and virtually impossible to administer, it is imperative that a specific diagnosis be reached as quickly as possible.

1. **For the mildly to moderately ill patient,** empiric antibiotic therapy should be started while one awaits the results of sputum and blood cultures. If sputum stains and other rapid diagnostic studies are negative, antimicrobial therapy should be directed against the most likely pathogens, based on the evaluation of host factors, setting, tempo of illness progression, and radiographic pattern [121].

   Neutropenic patients will most often require combination therapy with ticarcillin or piperacillin plus an aminoglycoside, or a cephalosporin plus an aminoglycoside (see sec. **IV.D**). Alternatively, monotherapy with ceftazidime or imipenem may be substituted for combination antibiotics. Vancomycin may be added in those centers with a high incidence of methicillin-resistant staphylococci. If the patient responds rapidly to the initial regimen, a more invasive procedure may be avoided. When a causative organism is identified, specific therapy should be substituted.

   A more specific, pathogen-directed initial approach is sufficient for patients without neutropenia [121].

2. **In the very ill patient with diffuse infiltrates,** we empirically add TMP-SMX for *P. carinii,* and erythromycin for *Legionella* infections, to an antibiotic combination directed against common bacteria. If the infiltrate is focal and the patient is very ill, erythromycin alone for *Legionella* infections is more often added to the double-antibiotic combination outlined in sec. 1; amphotericin B may also be given if *Aspergillus* or other fungal infections are likely.

   An invasive procedure ideally should be planned within the first 24–48 hours. Most centers prefer fiberoptic bronchoscopy initially to obtain BAL specimens, PBC brushings, and biopsies, if possible. However, another procedure may be preferred in some circumstances, such as a transthoracic needle biopsy for a peripheral focal infiltrate.

Occasionally, if a biopsy is clinically contraindicated, empiric therapy for *P. carinii* and *Legionella* spp. for a full therapeutic course is undertaken.

F. **Modification of management plan.** If the initial studies are nondiagnostic and there is no response to empiric therapy within 48–72 hours, then lung biopsy is recommended if not contraindicated. An early multidisciplinary approach will help prevent unnecessary delays in this evaluation. Whether to perform an open lung biopsy initially, rather than begin with a transthoracic or transbronchial biopsy and then proceed to an open lung biopsy if negative, requires case-by-case assessment. The open lung biopsy provides a greater yield than transbronchial biopsy but still may not reveal a specific diagnosis. Therefore, one often proceeds from one biopsy to the next. The physician must try to predict whether the patient will be able to tolerate open lung biopsy at the time the results become available from transbronchial biopsy. If not, it is reasonable to perform the open lung biopsy first and bypass the transbronchial biopsy. In AIDS patients, bronchoscopy with BAL is preferred initially. **(See Chaps. 19 and 24 for further discussion of PCP and other pneumonias in patients infected with HIV.)**

1. **Bronchoscopy with transbronchial biopsy** provides a specific diagnosis in many patients (15–45%); yield is further increased (60–90%) when BAL and PBC specimens are obtained at the same procedure [121]. The procedure is contraindicated in patients with severe hypoxemia or those requiring mechanical ventilation and in those with bleeding diatheses. Major complications are hemorrhage and pneumothorax and occur in fewer than 10% of cases.

    Another consideration is **thoracoscopic lung biopsy,** which often can provide more lung tissue for cultures and histopathology than a transbronchial biopsy. Consultation with a thoracic surgeon is advised. This procedure may allow one to avoid an open lung biopsy and is often a safer procedure than an open lung biopsy if the patient has no coagulopathy.

2. **Open lung biopsy provides the highest diagnostic yields.** This procedure may be preferred for patients with focal infiltrates not accessible by transthoracic biopsy or in whom the latter is contraindicated, in patients suspected of having certain noninfectious diagnoses (e.g., NIP or drug reactions), in those with a rapidly advancing illness, in patients whose pneumonia developed while receiving broad-spectrum empiric antibiotics, and in patients in whom other biopsies (e.g., transbronchial) were nondiagnostic. Open lung biopsy provides a larger tissue sample, permits control of ventilation and bleeding, and is associated with low morbidity and mortality (less than 5%) in centers experienced with this approach. In some patient populations, however, the results have infrequently influenced therapy or improved the eventual outcome.

3. **Appropriate processing of specimens should be assured before the procedure is done,** including touch preparations, histopathologic analysis, and cultures. Cultures should include (1) aerobic and anaerobic bacteria, including fastidious organisms such as *L. pneumophila;* (2) mycobacteria; (3) fungi; and (4) viruses, if the proper facilities are available. Laboratory studies have recently been reviewed [123a]. In addition to regular stains, special stains should be done for fungi, acid-fast bacteria, and *Legionella* and *Pneumocystis* spp.

4. **The specifics of therapy for biopsy-proven infections** are discussed elsewhere (see under Tuberculosis: Basic Concepts in this chapter and Chaps. 18, 19, and 24).

5. **Continuing empiric therapy without an invasive procedure is inappropriate for most patients.** It is acceptable, however, if patients have clearly and quickly responded to the initial regimen and an alternative noninfectious diagnosis (e.g., pulmonary edema) is not established. It may also be appropriate for patients with far-advanced underlying disease expected to be rapidly fatal even in the absence of infection, for patients in whom invasive procedures are contraindicated, or in patients who refuse the procedures.

G. **Prevention.** Prevention of pneumonia in the compromised host generally has involved strategies to prevent colonization, prophylactic antibiotics to prevent clinical infection, immunoprophylaxis, and modulation of the immune system [121]. Avoidance of situations that may lead to aspiration also are of value.

1. **Hand-washing** is the most important measure to prevent colonization in hospitalized immunocompromised hosts. Total protected environments with HEPA (high-efficiency particulate air) filtration of room air are useful for bone marrow transplant patients and others with prolonged neutropenia.

2. It has been more difficult to establish that **antibacterial prophylaxis** is reliably effective. Selective GI decontamination with TMP-SMX is not effective [124]. However, the quinolones are the newest drugs showing promise for this purpose [125].

3. **Antifungal prophylaxis** with oral or topical agents may not affect the incidence of invasive infections, although mucosal disease is reduced [121]. The appearance of resistant yeasts and *Aspergillus* infections has been a problem with this approach. TMP-SMX prophylaxis, however, has been shown to be of value in preventing PCP in HIV-infected patients and in children with lymphatic leukemia (see Chap. 24).

4. **Antiviral agents** are effective as prophylaxis in certain specific populations such as kidney and bone marrow transplant recipients. (See Chap. 20 for further discussion of infections in transplantation.)

5. **Immunization** is an important preventive measure. For pneumococcal pneumonia, pneumococcal vaccine is indicated for elderly, asplenic, and other compromised hosts. Influenza vaccines, by reducing the frequency of influenza, should help prevent the secondary complication of pneumonia. Immunoglobulin may be given to patients with immunoglobulin deficiency or impairment.

6. **Growth factors**, such as G-CSF or GM-CSF, speed recovery from cytopenias and can reduce the frequency of infections by shortening the period of neutropenia.

XII. **Nosocomial pneumonia** [126, 127]. Nosocomial pneumonias are **those pneumonias that develop after at least 72 hours of hospitalization.** They are the second or third most common nosocomial infections, result in substantial costs and prolonged hospitalization, and have the highest mortality of all hospital-acquired infections.

A. **Etiologies.** The potential causative organisms are diverse, including unusual or multidrug-resistant bacteria, fungi, and viruses.

1. **Bacteria** are the most frequent cause of nosocomial pneumonia, and many infections are polymicrobial. Aerobic gram-negative bacilli are found in at least 60% and gram-positive aerobes in 20–25% of cases [127]. *E. coli, P. aeruginosa, S. aureus,* and *Klebsiella, Enterobacter, Serratia,* and *Proteus* spp. account for approximately two-thirds of episodes. *H. influenzae* is isolated in approximately 6% of cases overall and particularly from pneumonias that develop in the first 48–96 hours of intubation. *S. pneumoniae* also has been recognized as a cause of early nosocomial pneumonia [127].

Anaerobic bacteria have been found in 0–35% of cases, usually in patients not being mechanically ventilated [126]. These probably are underdiagnosed because specimens appropriate for anaerobic cultures are not routinely obtained. The incidence of *Legionella* infections varies from 0–14%, depending on the hospital and patient population [127]. (See secs. **VI** and **VII** for a discussion of legionellosis.)

2. **Fungi** are found in fewer than 1% of nosocomial pneumonias [127]; however, they are more frequent in immunocompromised hosts. *Aspergillus* species, *Candida albicans,* and other yeasts are the most common fungal isolates.

3. **Viral** etiologies for nosocomial pneumonia often are unrecognized because special studies for their detection are performed only infrequently. Influenza A and B, RSV, parainfluenza, and adenovirus account for at least 70% of viral cases [126].

B. The **pathogenesis** of bacterial pneumonias will be discussed as these are the most common. Nosocomial bacteria gain access to the lungs most often through aspiration of oropharyngeal flora or by inhalation of contaminated aerosols; hematogenous spread and direct inoculation also occur but are less frequent.

1. **Colonization of the pharynx by gram-negative bacilli** is more common in aged, debilitated, or institutionalized patients [12], and this accounts for the high incidence of these organisms in nosocomial pneumonias (see also sec. **II.B**).

Clinical conditions that increase the pharyngeal carriage of gram-negative bacilli include coma, acidosis, alcoholism, uremia, diabetes mellitus, prior antimicrobial therapy, and nasogastric or endotracheal intubation [126]. An increase in the adherence of gram-negative bacilli to oropharyngeal and tracheal cells may accompany many of these conditions; this can arise in part from antibiotic-induced reduction in normal flora, reduced salivary flow, increased salivary protease content, and decreased fibronectin on cellular surfaces [128]. The ability to bind to respiratory mucins and extracellular matrix proteins may be important for *P. aeruginosa* colonization [128].

2. **Gastric colonization** may also be an important reservoir for gram-negative bacilli and *S. aureus* [51–55, 126, 127, 129, 130]. This is **associated with conditions that raise intragastric pH over 4.0, including** aging, achlorhydria, enteral feedings, antacids, and H_2-blockers.

3. **Aerosols containing bacteria** may be directly inhaled into the lower airways. These bacteria-containing aerosols have been generated by contaminated nebulizers, certain types of humidifiers, and anesthesia equipment.

C. **Risk factors** for bacterial nosocomial pneumonia have been identified [126, 127]. Many of these factors increase the chances for **aspiration** or **impair lung defenses.**

1. **Host-related factors** include age over 65–70 years, obesity, smoking, underlying illnesses such as COPD, alcoholism, and malnutrition, and prior immunosuppression.

2. The **type of acute illness** also influences the risk for nosocomial pneumonia. **Surgery,** particularly thoracic and abdominal procedures, are important predisposing events. Other characteristics of the acute illness that have been related to nosocomial pneumonia include a depressed level of consciousness, need for an intracranial pressure monitor, admission to an intensive care unit, shock, and **mechanical ventilation.**

Endotracheal tubes impair coughing and provide access to the lung. They also become coated with a biofilm of organisms that may be a reservoir for potential pathogens.

3. Certain **management practices and devices** may also predispose to the development of pneumonia. These include **stress-ulcer prophylaxis** that increases intragastric pH, insertion of a **nasogastric tube,** large-volume **tube feedings,** reflux of **ventilator tube** condensate into the trachea, the changing of ventilator tubing on a daily basis, improper care of **respiratory devices, breaks in common infection-control practices** that carry organisms from one patient to another, and inappropriate use of antibiotics.

D. **Diagnosis.** The steps needed to diagnose a nosocomial pneumonia reliably differ depending on whether there is underlying lung disease present and whether the patient is intubated. **A diligent effort must be made to search for noninfectious causes of fever and pulmonary infiltrates,** particularly in ventilated patients [18].

1. Clinical criteria often are used in **nonintubated patients,** as discussed earlier under Clinical Approach to Pneumonia. These include the presence of fever, leukocytosis, cough, purulent sputum, and a new or progressive radiographic infiltrate. Caution must be used when applying these clinical criteria to patients with underlying lung diseases, because the criteria are nonspecific. A positive culture from blood or pleural fluid increases the specificity but is insensitive [126].

2. The **diagnosis of ventilator-associated pneumonias may be very difficult,** particularly in patients with accompanying ARDS. Clinical criteria, even when used with routine sputum or tracheal cultures, have very low specificity (30% or less) in this setting [18, 22, 126, 127]. Thus, other methods have been applied to help identify patients with true infections.

a. **Quantitative cultures of tracheal aspirates** have been evaluated to distinguish colonizers from true lung pathogens. Direct (routine nonquantitative) tracheal aspirate cultures, which cannot make this distinction, are of limited value in the diagnosis of ventilator-associated nosocomial pneumonia. Using a threshold concentration of 10^5 organisms per milliliter or greater, quantitative tracheal aspirate cultures have a positive predictive value of only 50–60% and a negative predictive value of 72–95% [18, 131]. Because of the problems with false positive and false negative results and an incomplete understanding of the effects of antibiotic therapy on interpreting results, quantitative cultures should be reserved for problem cases when other diagnostic techniques are not available.

b. The presence of microscopic **elastin fibers** in sputum has been associated with pathogens that cause lung necrosis [18, 132]. Elastin fibers have been found in nosocomial pneumonias caused by gram-negative bacilli and *S. aureus.* Unfortunately, noninfectious causes of lung necrosis may be present in these patients that also may yield elastin fibers in respiratory secretions. For example, in the presence of ARDS, the positive predictive value for pneumonia of elastin fibers is only 50% [18]. It is our impression that this approach is only occasionally used in centers with a special interest in this technique, which we routinely do not study.

c. **Quantitative cultures of PBC or BAL specimens** offer the most promise. In the absence of prior antibiotic therapy, they have been 70–100% sensitive and 60–100% specific [126]. Concomitant use of microscopic evaluations may result in the best yield, but this is not standardized [18]. Techniques are available to obtain these specimens with or without bronchoscopy [18, 126]. The effects of antibiotics on these quantitative methods are incompletely understood. Prior antibiotics may result in a false negative culture by suppressing growth of true pathogens, an accurate diagnosis of resistant pathogens present in high concentrations, or a false positive culture of resistant colonizers [18]. **Further studies are needed to clarify this issue and to determine the appropriate role for these procedures in the routine management of ventilator-associated pneumonia [126].**

d. **Open lung biopsy** is almost never necessary to diagnose ventilator-associated pneumonia. It should be reserved for patients with a deteriorating clinical course and negative results using the preceding techniques, or with such rapid disease progression that the most definitive diagnostic study is deemed appropriate from the outset [18]. Such patients usually are immunosuppressed.

E. **Therapy.** Effective therapy for nosocomial pneumonia involves ensuring patency of the airway and adequate oxygenation, using pressors and other supportive measures, draining secretions, and administering antibiotics. **Empiric antibiotics** should be chosen on the basis of the patient's risk factors, severity of illness, previous cultures, and local resistance patterns [127]. Gram stains of reliable specimens are useful to help direct initial therapy. Whenever possible, **specific antibiotics should be substituted as specific pathogens become known.**

The **following general guidelines** apply to choosing initial empiric therapy for suspected bacterial nosocomial pneumonia when smears are unavailable or are not reliable (e.g., tracheal aspirates in the ventilated patient). Most regimens should have activity against *S. pneumoniae, H. influenzae,* and the gram-negative bacilli noted in sec. **A.** (See sec. **IV.D** for further discussion of gram-negative pneumonia.)

1. **Early illness** may be treated with either monotherapy or a combination regimen [127, 133]. Ceftazidime, cefotaxime, and imipenem have been shown to be useful when used alone [133], but if these agents are overused in a hospital or specific area within a hospital (e.g., the intensive care unit), the development of resistant bacteria is a concern (see Chaps. 28A and 28F). It is likely that ticarcillin-clavulanate and piperacillin-tazobactam are effective as well. The fluoroquinolones as monotherapy must be used with caution because they are relatively less active against pneumococci and anaerobes. Imipenem and the fluoroquinolones may offer an advantage in institutions where aerobic gram-negative bacilli with inducible beta-lactamase resistance are prevalent.

2. **Severe, established illness** should be treated **with a combination regimen.** Traditionally, this has included an antipseudomonal penicillin plus an aminoglycoside. Any of the drugs suitable for monotherapy may be substituted for the antipseudomonal penicillin, and aztreonam may be substituted for the aminoglycoside. Clindamycin plus either an aminoglycoside or aztreonam or a fluoroquinolone may be used for patients with significant penicillin allergy.

3. We prefer a combination regimen (antipseudomonal penicillin and an aminoglycoside) for *P. aeruginosa* or for any necrotizing aerobic pneumonia.

4. Nafcillin or vancomycin should be included when *S. aureus* is suspected. Vancomycin is preferred if methicillin-resistant *S. aureus* infection is possible.

5. Metronidazole should not be used alone when anaerobes are suspected from aspiration (see sec. **V.B.1.c** under Lung Abscess). See sec. **II.B** for additional discussion of hospital-acquired aspiration pneumonia.

   6. Erythromycin should be added whenever *Legionella* organisms are possible. See secs. **VI** and **VII** for further discussions of legionellosis.
 F. **Prevention.** Strategies to prevent nosocomial pneumonias are based on an understanding of their pathogenesis and risk factors (see secs. **B** and **C**). This discussion will focus on the prevention of bacterial infections, although guidelines for preventing *Legionella, Aspergillus,* and viral infections also are available [126]. **Detailed guidelines for the prevention of nosocomial pneumonia have recently been published** [126].
   1. **The use of systemic antibiotics for pneumonia prophylaxis, or topical antimicrobials for selective decontamination, is not recommended.**
   2. **Hand-washing and other routine infection-control practices are essential** to prevent cross-contamination among patients.
   3. Whenever possible, **elevate the head of the bed** to 30–45 degrees to prevent aspiration. Discontinue tube feedings, nasogastric tubes and endotracheal tubes as soon as possible. Continuous aspiration of subglottic secretions in intubated patients also should be considered [133a].
   4. **Effective pain control and chest physiotherapy** (e.g., coughing, deep breathing, incentive spirometry) **should be priorities in postoperative patients.**
   5. **An agent that does not elevate gastric pH** (e.g., sucralfate) **is preferred** for stress-ulcer prophylaxis.
   6. **Immunizations** should be **updated** and smoking discouraged, particularly prior to elective surgery.
   7. **Sterile equipment and water** should be used for procedures that contact mucous membranes. The internal parts of mechanical ventilators do not need to be sterilized.
   8. **Ventilator tubing should be changed** no more frequently than every 48 hours, and tubing condensate should not be allowed to drain into the patient's airway.
   9. Small-volume nebulizers should be filled with sterile fluids and not used for more than one patient unless sterile. Water for bubbling humidifiers should be sterile. Large-volume nebulizers, room-mist humidifiers, and mist tents are discouraged; when used, they must be filled only with sterile fluids and sterilized or high-level-disinfected every day and between patients.
   10. Lateral rotational therapy has not yet been proven to be effective [126].
XIII. **Pneumonia in children** (1-month-olds to teenagers). Many of the principles discussed earlier in this chapter under General Concepts of Organism-Host Interaction can be applied to pneumonia in children [134–138]. However, certain aspects of childhood pneumonia warrant emphasis. Pneumonia in neonates is discussed in Chap. 3.
 A. **Age and setting.** Age is of great importance in the likely etiologies and their mode of presentation [134–138].
   1. **Infants aged 1–3 months** are most likely to have pneumonia of viral origin. Occasionally, the etiology will be bacterial, including group B streptococci, *H. influenzae, S. pneumoniae, S. aureus, S. pyogenes,* and *Bordetella pertussis.*
      Afebrile pneumonia in young infants between 1 and 3 months of age usually is caused by *Chlamydia trachomatis.* These patients usually present with an indolent illness marked by poor feeding, failure to thrive, and a chronic cough. Examination may reveal conjunctivitis, tachypnea, and diffuse rales. The differential diagnosis for this syndrome includes infections caused by *P. carinii, Ureaplasma urealyticum,* and CMV, but these are much less common than *C. trachomatis.*
   2. **Between the ages of 3 months and 5 years,** the most common etiologies are *S. pneumoniae, H. influenzae,* and respiratory viruses. Other bacteria and *Mycoplasma* are occasional pathogens in this age group.
   3. In contrast, the causes of pneumonia **in children older than 5 years** are more like those in adults so that pneumococcal, mycoplasmal, and viral etiologies predominate. Other bacteria and mycobacteria should also be considered in the older child.
   4. The very young child will have few symptoms or signs, except fever and tachypnea, and rarely will produce sputum, whereas the older child may have the more classic features.
   5. If the child is a **compromised host** [139], see the discussion in sec. **XI.**
 B. **Organisms**
   1. **Viruses** are very common among children from 1 month to 3 years old, with RSV, parainfluenza virus, and influenza types A and B being the most important.

2. **Bacteria.** The encapsulated organisms *S. pneumoniae, H. influenzae,* and *Neisseria meningitidis* more frequently produce pneumonia in children older than 3 months as maternal antibodies wane. *H. influenzae* type b is more often associated with other organ system infection than with pneumonia, but it can also produce pneumonia. **The frequency of serious *H. influenzae* type b infections should continue to decline as vaccination beginning at 2 months of age becomes the standard practice** (see sec. **III**). Pneumonia often coexists with meningitis in disease caused by *N. meningitidis.* As in adults, anaerobic pneumonias usually occur in patients prone to aspiration. Group A streptococci, *M. catarrhalis,* and *Legionella* spp. are less common in childhood pneumonias.

3. ***Mycoplasma*** may cause infection, particularly in children older than 5 years.

4. ***Chlamydia*** can cause pneumonia at different ages, depending on the species. *C. trachomatis* predominates in young infants (see Chap. 3, sec. **III.D** under Selected Specific Infections in the Newborn), and *C. pneumoniae* increases in frequency as children age into adolescence (see sec. **V.C**).

C. **Roentgenographic clues** [138, 140]
   1. **Pneumonia with effusion.** When an effusion is present on the x-ray film, the process is **usually bacterial,** unless the tuberculin skin test is positive or there is a contact history (i.e., with tuberculosis).
   2. **Lobar consolidation** implies a **bacterial process.** *S. pneumoniae* is the most likely pathogen, although *S. pyogenes* and *K. pneumoniae* may produce a similar picture.
   3. **Abscesses** are associated with staphylococci or, if putrid, with anaerobic infection. In the latter instance, a foreign body may have precipitated the process. Pneumatoceles may be found in staphylococcal pneumonia and in newborns with gram-negative infections [138].
   4. **Bronchopneumonias** (diffuse, patchy infiltrates) usually cause mild illnesses. More than 90% of these infections are **nonbacterial** in origin. The few **bacterial** infections have a much more acute onset, with progressive roentgenographic changes over hours.

D. **Therapy often is empiric** because of the problems in defining the etiology in this age group [134, 135, 138, 141]. For diagnosis, percutaneous lung puncture is highly specific and sensitive but not advisable in most instances [134, 137]. Cultures of blood and pleural fluid are also specific, but they are infrequently positive. Tests to detect bacterial antigens in the urine are not useful because they lack both sensitivity and specificity [138, 141]. Rapid diagnostic tests are unavailable for most viral pathogens except influenza and RSV. Furthermore, **the clinical, laboratory, and radiographic features often will not distinguish among the possible etiologies** [141].
   1. **Hospitalization.** The decision to hospitalize a child with pneumonia often is difficult. In general, hospital care should be considered when the child is very young, is immunocompromised, has a serious underlying disease, is toxic in appearance or is hypoxemic, has a bacterial infection with multilobar involvement or significant pleural effusion, has inadequate oral intake, is failing outpatient management, and when the family is unable to cope [137, 138].
   2. **Antibiotics.** If the onset is insidious and viral infection is suspected, antibiotics are of no value and may be detrimental. In circumstances in which bacterial infection is suspected, selection of an antibiotic agent is based on the appearance of the chest roentgenogram, the age of the child, and the Gram stain of any pleural fluid or other available material, such as that obtained by lung puncture [137, 138]. *Chlamydia* and *Mycoplasma* pneumonias will respond to erythromycin (see Table 9-3 and Chap. 28M for dosages).
   3. **Other therapeutic measures.** If infected pleural fluid is present, it should be drained by repeated aspiration or by insertion of a chest tube. Bronchoscopy followed by postural drainage should be carried out for abscess, obstruction, or suspected foreign body.
   4. **After improvement occurs,** the child may need to be evaluated for presence of an immunologic defect, particularly if he or she has recurrent severe bacterial infections or infection with an unusual organism.

E. **Miscellaneous**
   1. **Bronchiolitis** is particularly common in infants younger than 6 months and in neonates. These patients can exhibit prominent respiratory symptoms (e.g.,

tachypnea, wheezing, and hypoxia). Roentgenograms reveal no infiltrates in uncomplicated cases. These infections are due primarily to viruses, **most commonly RSV.** Therefore, routine antibiotics are not indicated unless bacterial superinfection is well documented. Oxygen supplementation commonly is required. (**For further discussion** of bronchiolitis, **see Chap. 8.**)

2. **Neonatal pneumonia,** including *C. trachomatis* pneumonia, is discussed in Chap. 3.

XIV. **Embolic pneumonia.** Most pneumonias are caused by the aspiration of oropharyngeal pathogens. Occasionally, pneumonias may result from septic emboli.

A. **Setting and organisms involved.** Four organisms are recognized as major causes of embolic pneumonia.

1. *S. aureus* is most commonly seen in drug addicts and in patients with acute bacterial endocarditis.

2. *Fusobacterium necrophorum* first causes an anaerobic infection of the oropharynx and then can invade the jugular vein and thereby gain access to the bloodstream [142]. (See Chap. 4, p. 121).

3. *Bacteroides fragilis* may be responsible in patients with pelvic or intraabdominal infections (particularly women).

4. *E. coli* can embolize to the lung from urinary, biliary, or GI tract infections.

B. **Signs and symptoms.** In the individual with embolic pneumonia, respiratory symptoms vary from minimal to severe. Because the vascular supply is compromised by the embolus, symptoms may suggest pulmonary embolism. Frequently, there is no sputum production, and often the etiologic agent is not recovered from the sputum, even when blood cultures are positive.

C. **Roentgenographic changes.** The infiltrate often will have a circular appearance and may go on to cavitate centrally. A characteristic feature of this disease, especially disease due to *E. coli,* is that in the course of the process a pleural effusion develops. This fluid usually is an exudate, generally will yield the causative organism, and has been referred to as **metapneumonic empyema.**

D. **Therapeutic approach.** In addition to administering systemic antibiotic and draining the pleural fluid, the source of the embolic pneumonia (i.e., the primary infection) should be sought. For example, in the drug addict, either the brachial veins or the heart valve can be a site of the initial staphylococcal infection. Antibiotics are adjusted according to the most likely site from which the infection has embolized, and peripheral sites may require surgical excision (e.g., in the case of a phlebitis with a localized vascular infection not responding to antibiotics alone). The use of anticoagulation must be individualized to the extent of the underlying thrombotic process.

XV. **Staphylococcal pneumonia** is fairly uncommon but very serious, with mortality ranging from 32 to 84% in recent series [143, 144]. It is particularly likely to be seen in certain settings, which deserve emphasis.

A. **Settings**

1. Most cases of **community-acquired staphylococcal pneumonia** occur as a complication of influenza [145] (see Chap. 8). This may be related to an increase in the colonization rate with *S. aureus* in individuals with influenza.

   In the absence of influenza, *S. aureus* is an infrequent cause of community-acquired pneumonia. When this does occur, it is usually in an older person with significant underlying pulmonary or other illness, and some patients may be nursing home residents [143].

2. **Nosocomial pneumonia.** Superinfection with *S. aureus* may occur in hospitalized, debilitated patients. Many are on respirators or have tracheostomies, have had surgery, or have had a prolonged and complicated hospitalization [143].

B. **Radiographic manifestations** of staphylococcal pneumonia are varied. Children with bacterial pneumonia and **pneumatoceles or macroabscesses** on roentgenography are likely to have staphylococcal infections. In adults, infiltrates are often bilateral and multilobar. Abscess formation varies from 16 to 70% [143], and an air-crescent sign has been reported in an immunocompromised host [146]. Pleural effusions are common, as are empyemas.

C. **Therapy** involves high-dose parenteral antistaphylococcal antibiotics for 2–3 weeks. Oxacillin or nafcillin (9–12 g/day) can be used in the adult. In children, 200 mg/kg/day divided into q4–6h doses can be given.

In a penicillin-allergic patient, a cephalosporin may be used if it is not contraindicated (see Chap. 27). A first-generation cephalosporin (e.g., cefazolin) is preferred. If a cephalosporin is contraindicated, vancomycin is the agent of choice.

   D. Isolation. Usually these patients are placed in a private room and their caregivers use gowns, gloves, and masks until at least 48 hours after a clinical response to antibiotic therapy to prevent nosocomial spread of staphylococcal infections.
XVI. *Candida* **in sputum cultures.** Sputum cultures often reveal *Candida* on Gram stains and on cultures. This is particularly common in patients on broad-spectrum antibiotics or in debilitated patients. Fortunately, *Candida* is usually a colonizer and **rarely causes pneumonia** with invasive tissue disease. To diagnose true pulmonary infection with *Candida*, a lung tissue biopsy showing tissue invasion is necessary. Actual tissue invasion is most likely to occur in the compromised host and does not necessarily represent widespread disease [147] (see Chap. 18).

Pleural Effusion
Versus Empyema

When a patient's chest roentgenogram reveals evidence of pleural fluid, a thoracentesis usually is indicated to determine whether the fluid is a transudate or an exudate. If the possibility exists that infection is the underlying cause, a thoracentesis will be necessary to exclude an empyema (infected fluid) or complicated parapneumonic effusion, which would require drainage.
  I. Pleural effusions. Well-established standardized criteria exist for separating exudates from transudates [148]. More recent proposals for identifying exudates include pleural fluid cholesterol of less than 60 mg/dl, a gradient of less than 1.2 g/dl between pleural fluid and serum albumin, and a pleural fluid–to–serum bilirubin ratio of 0.6 or greater. However, routine use of these methods is not recommended until they have been validated in larger populations of patients [148]. Presence of an exudate implies the need for further evaluation.
  A. Characteristics of exudative fluid. Pleural fluid is most likely to represent an exudate if **any one** of the following criteria are met [148, 149]:
    1. The ratio of pleural fluid protein to serum protein is greater than 0.5.
    2. Pleural fluid lactate dehydrogenase (LDH) exceeds two-thirds of the normal value in serum.
    3. The ratio of pleural fluid LDH to serum LDH is greater than 0.6.
  B. Differential diagnosis of exudates includes the following major categories:
    1. Malignancy. Common tumors include carcinoma of the lung, breast, or ovary; GI tumors; hypernephromas; and lymphoproliferative disorders.
    2. Pneumonia. Bacterial pneumonias can be associated with infected pleural effusions. *Mycoplasma, Legionella,* and viral pneumonias can have associated effusions that are exudative. *Nocardia, Actinomyces,* fungal, and parasitic infections also may produce exudative pleural effusion.
    3. Tuberculosis. Tuberculous pleurisy is discussed in sec. **V.B** under Tuberculosis: Basic Concepts.
    4. Pancreatitis and esophageal perforation. These are commonly associated with pleural effusions. With pancreatitis, often there is an elevated amylase of the pleural fluid. Exudative effusion also may follow abdominal surgery and may accompany **subphrenic abscess.**
    5. Miscellaneous. Other causes of exudative effusions include pulmonary infarction, rheumatoid arthritis, trauma, Dressler's syndrome, drug reactions, uremia, and collagen vascular diseases.
  C. Transudates are commonly seen in patients with CHF, cirrhosis, nephrotic syndrome, and hypothyroidism. Transudates may be seen with peritoneal dialysis.
  D. Diagnostic studies of pleural fluid. Certain studies are performed routinely on pleural fluid samples [148].
    1. Cell counts. Infected fluid may have high counts of polymorphonuclear leukocytes. A high percentage of lymphocytes may be seen in tuberculosis and malignancies. Uncommonly, 5–20% eosinophils can be seen, but this often is a nonspecific finding associated with pneumothorax, hemothorax, Hodgkin's disease, Churg-Strauss syndrome, benign asbestos effusion, drug reactions,

and paragonimiasis [149a]. A majority of small lymphocytes indicates the possibility of malignancy or tuberculosis. Mesothelial cells are uncommon in tuberculous effusions.

2. **Chemistries.** Protein and LDH levels are important, as discussed earlier. **Glucose** levels may be reduced in effusions associated with pneumonia, malignancy, tuberculosis, hemothorax, paragonimiasis, and Churg-Strauss syndrome; they may be very low in effusions from rheumatoid arthritis. Tuberculous effusions may, on occasion, have normal glucose levels. Amylase may be high in pleural effusions associated with pancreatitis or esophageal perforation.

3. **pH.** The pH of the pleural fluid may help distinguish complicated from benign effusions (see sec. **III**). Pleural fluid samples should be placed in wet ice, transported to the laboratory, and processed immediately. **A pleural fluid pH of less than 7.2 is seen in** effusions associated with bacterial infections, tuberculosis, esophageal rupture, malignancy, rheumatoid arthritis, hemothorax, urinothorax, paragonimiasis, Churg-Strauss syndrome, and systemic acidosis. The cause of pleural fluid acidosis is primarily leukocyte metabolism, but bacterial metabolism also may contribute. In empyemas caused by some *Proteus* spp., the pH may be normal or high because of the urea-splitting activity of the bacteria.

4. **Cytologic studies.** Cytologic studies should be performed on the cell pellet obtained from centrifuging larger volumes of fluid.

5. **Cultures.** Aerobic and anaerobic cultures should be performed routinely. If tuberculosis and fungal infections are considered, one should obtain and centrifuge large volumes (300–1,000 ml) of fluid and then culture the sediment.

6. **Needle biopsy.** This is useful when malignant, tuberculous or fungal effusions are being considered. (See sec. **V.B.2** under Tuberculosis: Basic Concepts.)

E. **Loculated fluid versus fibrosis.** At times, it is difficult to determine whether the fluid is loculated or whether pleural fibrosis has occurred. Thoracic CT scanning is now preferred to ultrasonography for localizing fluid for drainage procedures and for assessing the underlying lung [148].

II. **Empyema.** An empyema is **pus in the pleural space** [150]. Although some patients may be very toxic with an empyema, other patients may have only a low-grade fever. A diagnostic thoracentesis usually demonstrates an exudative, purulent fluid; it also provides material for cultures and Gram staining. Most of the special studies discussed in sec. **I.D** (e.g., pH, LDH, and protein) will not be needed to plan further management when frank pus is found in the pleural cavity.

A. **The underlying causes** for empyemas include the following:

1. **Pulmonary infections** (most commonly pneumonia, aspiration pneumonia, and lung abscess).

2. **Postthoracotomy.**

3. **Direct spread of infection** (e.g., from an abdominal or orofacial source).

4. **Esophageal rupture.**

5. **Idiopathic,** most of which empyemas are believed to be the result of a pneumonia that has since resolved.

6. **Hematogenous spread** to the pleural cavity (uncommon in adults but more frequent in children).

B. **Bacteriology.** The bacteria causing empyema vary with age and predisposing conditions [151–153]. Mixed infections are commonly encountered, and organisms producing beta-lactamases have been isolated with increasing frequency.

1. **Anaerobes** play a significant role in empyemas complicating aspiration pneumonia and lung abscess. They are found in approximately 75% of these cases and are the only isolate in approximately 33%. The anaerobes most commonly isolated include *Bacteroides* spp., *Prevotella* spp., *Fusobacterium nucleatum,* and *Peptostreptococcus* spp. More than one anaerobic organism often is isolated from the same patient, whereas mixed aerobic and anaerobic infections are nearly half as common.

2. **Aerobic bacteria** are more often seen in other settings. Although once common, *S. pyogenes* is now less frequently isolated. In contrast, pneumococci continue to be an important cause of empyema [152]. *S. aureus* and aerobic gram-negative bacilli are important pathogens in postthoracotomy patients and in patients with nosocomial pneumonias. Staphylococcal and *H. influenzae* empyemas are common in children. Because these are caused by pneumonias, the frequency of *H. influenzae* type b empyemas should decline as more young children become vaccinated.

C. Management [150, 154]. The principles of empyema management are to control infection, minimize morbidity and hospitalization, and maximize resultant lung function.

   1. Adequate drainage. Because pus in the pleural cavity represents an infection in an enclosed space (i.e., an abscess), drainage **is always necessary.** Only rarely will adequate drainage be achieved by daily thoracentesis; usually, the fluid becomes too thick or loculated and a chest tube is necessary. The initial step for drainage of free-flowing fluid without loculations is insertion of a single chest tube. If this is inadequate and the patient is clinically stable, then multiple chest tubes, often placed under CT guidance, may be tried. In some cases, despite appropriate chest tubes, adequate drainage cannot be achieved. Early surgical drainage and decortication procedures have been promoted for such patients [154, 155].

   A **new technique of video thoracoscopy** (also called *pleuroscopy*) may help break down loculations, provide for thorough irrigation, and allow visual placement of drainage tubes [156–158]. In some patients with acute empyema, this procedure may obviate the need for open thoracotomy, but surgery should not be delayed when decortication and pleurectomy are needed [158].

   The pleural instillation of fibrinolytic agents (streptokinase or urokinase) also may be used to lyse adhesions and promote closed drainage [150]. The appropriate patient population for these methods, the best time at which to apply such methods, and their use in combination must await further studies.

   2. Antibiotics are initiated on the basis of the Gram stain findings and the clinical setting. The regimen can be altered on the basis of culture results of the aspirated fluid. Empiric regimens for empyemas associated with pneumonia should provide aerobic and anaerobic coverage. Postthoracotomy empyemas should be treated for *S. aureus, P. aeruginosa,* and other aerobic gram-negative bacilli [159]. In general, if adequate drainage can be achieved, the authors will use high-dose parenteral antibiotics for approximately 10–14 days. However, the actual duration of therapy will depend on the underlying source, causative organisms, clinical response, and duration of significant pleural drainage or effusion. Bioavailability of aminoglycosides and some beta-lactams in empyema fluids is poor [159]. Thus, it probably is best that aminoglycosides not be used alone, at least initially, to treat gram-negative empyemas.

III. Parapneumonic effusions. Pleural effusions are found in approximately 40% of patients with pneumonia [160]. Most of these are small in volume, remain uncomplicated, and will resolve spontaneously. Complicated effusions and empyemas occasionally develop, depending on the infecting organisms and the duration of illness. **A complicated parapneumonic effusion is one that requires drainage** for resolution or that is culture-positive [160].

   A. Indications for chest tube drainage of parapneumonic effusions are any one of the following [150, 160]:

   1. Empyema (i.e., gross pus in the pleural cavity).
   2. Positive Gram stain of pleural fluid.
   3. Glucose level of less than 40 mg/dl in pleural fluid.
   4. pH of less than 7.0 in pleural fluid.

   B. Other considerations

   1. Serial thoracentesis should be **considered for** patients whose effusions have a pH between 7.0 and 7.2–7.3 or a pleural fluid LDH in excess of 1,000 IU/liter and who do not meet the preceding criteria [150, 160]. If the pH and glucose level fall and the LDH level rises, then tube drainage is indicated. If these values normalize, then the patient probably will not need a chest tube.

   2. Tube drainage also should be considered if the pleural fluid culture proves positive, particularly if an organism other than the pneumococcus is present, the effusion is large, or there are loculations [160].

   3. Strict reliance on chemical criteria alone for chest tube placement is not accepted by all authors [150, 160]. Nonetheless, we believe that these tests, when interpreted in the whole clinical context, help guide management of parapneumonic effusions. A thorough evaluation for persistent infection in the lung or other sites should be performed.

   C. Bronchopleural fistula may occur in association with empyemas or complicated effusions. Adequate percutaneous drainage is essential to obtaining a cure and to prevent escape of purulent material into the bronchial tree. Empyemas resulting from breakdown of a bronchial stump are particularly difficult to manage because the pleural space can never be completely drained and obliterated [150].

The initial clue to the presence of a bronchopleural fistula is an air-fluid level in the pleural cavity. Other causes of an air-fluid level in infected pleural fluid include a ruptured esophagus and rupture of an underlying lung abscess. Gas formation from microbial growth is less commonly the cause, so that another source should be sought. CT scans may be helpful in separating pleural from intraparenchymal air-fluid levels. The presence of a bronchopleural fistula will be confirmed by placing the chest tube to water seal, which will confirm an air leak (i.e., bubbling is seen). Thoracic surgical consultation is advised in these cases.

D. **Management** of complicated parapneumonic effusions entails adequate drainage and antibiotics, as described for empyemas.

Lung Abscess

A lung abscess is a suppurative lesion in the lung parenchyma consisting of a 1-cm or larger cavity surrounded by inflammation and necrosis. A necrotizing pneumonia is defined by multiple small (<1-cm) cavities within areas of acute consolidation. Thus, these entities represent different manifestations of the same pathophysiologic process. Their diagnosis usually is suspected because of the findings on the chest roentgenogram rather than because of a characteristic clinical presentation. Mycobacteria and fungi (e.g., histoplasmosis and coccidioidomycosis) can cause tissue necrosis and cavitating lung disease. Tuberculosis is discussed later in this chapter, and fungal infections are discussed in Chap. 18.

I. **Types of lung abscesses.** Two types of lung abscesses are recognized. The primary type (also known as *nonspecific* or *simple*) is due to a mixed anaerobic infection. The secondary type follows a specific, usually aerobic, pneumonia. Lung abscesses can be separated clinically into the following categories:

A. **Mixed anaerobic** lung abscesses are **due to aspiration** of oropharyngeal organisms, of which the majority are anaerobes [49]. Therefore, if the inoculum of bacteria is sufficient and not adequately cleared, an aspiration pneumonia may develop that progresses to abscess formation. Most infections involve two to three anaerobic species, and a significant minority also include a nonanaerobic species. Anaerobes most commonly isolated include *Bacteroides* spp., *Prevotella intermedia, P. melaninogenica,* other *Prevotella* spp., *F. nucleatum, Veillonella,* and peptostreptococci [48, 49]. Common nonanaerobes include *Streptococcus intermedius* and other microaerophilic and aerobic streptococci.

B. A **specific** lung abscess **follows a necrotizing pneumonia** caused by a single, usually **aerobic,** organism. This includes abscesses due to *K. pneumoniae, P. aeruginosa,* other gram-negative bacilli, *Legionella* spp., *S. aureus, Nocardia* spp., and *Actinomyces. S. pneumoniae* only rarely causes a lung abscess [161]. Melioidosis and paragonimiasis are more important causes of lung abscess in parts of the world other than the United States.

C. **Septic emboli** to the lung may result in abscess formation. Important sources include intravascular, pelvic, orofacial, gastrointestinal, and urinary infections. Embolic pneumonias are discussed earlier in this chapter, in sec. **XIV** under Special Considerations and Specific Therapy.

D. **Infected lung bullae** pose a special clinical problem [162]. In this setting, infection is a secondary phenomenon and is not responsible for lung necrosis. These patients tend to present with a milder illness than patients with lung abscess; duration of symptoms is shorter, putrid sputum is rare, and normal leukocyte counts are common [162]. The radiographic hallmark is the development of an air-fluid level in a preexisting emphysematous bulla, with minimal infiltrate in the adjacent parenchyma. A specific pathogen usually is not present, and often these patients respond to penicillin, which suggests that oral anaerobic and aerobic bacteria are the most important causative organisms. Response to oral antibiotics and chest physiotherapy is prompt, and bronchoscopy and other invasive procedures are not indicated [162].

E. **Nonbacterial** causes include lung tumors, which may undergo tissue necrosis and form cavities. Cavitary lung lesions also can be seen in Wegener's granulomatosis and periarteritis of the lung.

II. **Clinical setting and presentation.** Distinction between these various types of lung abscesses usually is made on the basis of clinical setting and culture data.
   A. **Anaerobic lung abscesses** are most likely to occur in patients with **poor dental and oral hygiene** and a **predisposition to aspiration.**
      1. The **poor oral and dental hygiene** allows for the development of a heavy inoculum of bacteria in the gingival crevices [49]. Because a high inoculum of anaerobes is required to cause disease, **lung abscess due to anaerobes is uncommon in the edentulous patient** unless there is an underlying pulmonary disorder, such as an obstructing bronchogenic carcinoma.
      2. **Predisposing conditions that lead to aspiration** should be sought in the history. In particular, has the patient had episodes of impaired consciousness or swallowing difficulties? High-risk patients include those with alcoholism, seizure disorders, cerebrovascular accidents, drug abuse, recent general anesthesia, trauma, esophageal disease (e.g., scleroderma), tracheoesophageal fistula, feeding tubes, tracheotomy, and other serious underlying diseases. After an episode of significant aspiration, it takes 7–16 days for chest roentgenographic evidence of an abscess to appear.
         Underlying pulmonary disorders also predispose to anaerobic lung abscess [49]. These include bronchogenic carcinoma or other bronchial obstructions, bronchiectasis, and pulmonary infarction. Although infection in a preexisting emphysematous bulla often involves anaerobes, overall COPD does not predispose to anaerobic lung infections.
      3. **Symptoms** of cough, production of sputum (which often has a foul odor), weight loss, and malaise may be present for several days to weeks or months. The symptoms generally are **insidious and prolonged** compared with those of the typical bacterial pneumonia.
      4. The patient with a lung abscess on roentgenography that does not fit the preceding description may have one of the secondary forms of lung abscess discussed next.
   B. **Aerobic lung abscesses** most often occur in the setting of an acute specific necrotizing pneumonia. The clinical manifestations of S. aureus and gram-negative pneumonias have been discussed previously. These patients are usually acutely ill, and the infection may be nosocomial in origin. Occasionally, an aerobic lung abscess will have an indolent presentation similar to that described in sec. **A** for anaerobic abscesses.
   C. **Embolic pneumonias** were discussed earlier in this chapter (see sec. **XIV** under Special Considerations and Specific Therapy). Serial blood cultures and the clinical setting provide clues for this diagnosis.
   D. **Nonbacterial causes** should be suspected, particularly in patients who do not appear to fit into the preceding categories; that is, there is no underlying condition predisposing them to aspiration, and they have, for instance, good oral hygiene, no necrotizing pneumonia, negative blood cultures, and no acid-fast bacteria on smear.
III. **Diagnosis.** The diagnosis of lung abscess is made when the **chest roentgenogram** reveals a cavity surrounded by a variable degree of infiltrate or consolidation and usually an air-fluid level in the cavity. Anaerobic abscesses that follow aspiration involve the right lung more often than the left, and most frequently are found in the dependent segments. These are the posterior segments of the upper lobes and the superior segments of the lower lobes when supine and the basal segments of the lower lobes when upright. Multiple round cavities in the lower lobes suggest hematogenous or embolic abscesses. Atelectasis, a mass, or a foreign body suggests obstruction of the airway. Parapneumonic effusions, empyemas, and bronchopleural fistulas commonly are present.
   At times, serial roentgenograms will be available that demonstrate the evolution of acute infiltrates through necrotizing pneumonia and into abscess formation. At present there is no means of reliably predicting which pneumonia will lead to a lung abscess. Preliminary studies, however, suggest that the **presence of elastin fibers** in sputum may be more sensitive than the chest roentgenogram in detecting necrotizing infections [18, 132]. Elastin fibers are detected by digesting sputum with 40% potassium hydroxide and examining wet preparations with a light microscope. Refractile fibers found at $100\times$ magnification must be observed at $400\times$ magnification to detect the split ends characteristic of elastin fibers [132]. A clump or clumps of elastin fibers

are regarded as significant, whereas one or more isolated fibers are an insignificant finding [132]. (See related discussion earlier in this chapter, page 301.)

IV. **Determining the type of abscess.** Further clinical evaluation is necessary to determine the type of abscess so that appropriate therapy can be planned.

  A. **Clinical setting.** The clinical setting provides clues, as discussed in sec. **II.**

  B. **Sputum collection and evaluation**

   1. **Expectorated sputum.** Sputum and breath often have a **foul odor** in anaerobic lung abscess. Sputum Gram stain findings suggestive of this diagnosis include the presence of many neutrophils, a mixture of gram-positive and gram-negative forms, and no predominant morphologic features. Routine cultures of these specimens reveal predominantly normal flora and minimal or no organisms commonly associated with an aerobic abscess (e.g., *S. aureus* or gram-negative bacilli).

   2. **Invasive procedures.** Transtracheal aspirates, fiberoptic bronchoscopy with PBC or BAL specimens for quantitative cultures, and percutaneous abscess puncture [163] provide specimens suitable for both anaerobic and aerobic cultures (see sec. **VII** under Clinical Approach to Pneumonia). Rapid transport to the laboratory using appropriate methods is essential to optimize yield from anaerobic cultures of these specimens.

   Most often, invasive procedures are unnecessary in the evaluation of anaerobic lung abscess because the clinical diagnosis is reliable and the microbiologic picture is predictable. An invasive procedure for microbiologic purposes may be helpful if an adequate spontaneous or induced expectorated specimen is unobtainable, if a delay in specific therapy due to inaccurate diagnosis would be life-threatening, or if an unusual or resistant organism is suspected. Pulmonary consultation is advised in these special settings.

  C. **Blood cultures** should be obtained in the febrile patient or in the setting of a possible embolic pneumonia (e.g., in addicts, in patients with acute bacterial endocarditis, or in those with intraabdominal or pharyngeal space infections).

  D. **Acid-fast smears** are useful to exclude *Mycobacterium,* although air-fluid levels are less frequent in tuberculosis. In addition, some patients (e.g., alcoholics) who are predisposed to aspiration and anaerobic infections may also have *Mycobacterium* infections.

   The diagnosis of fungal pneumonia is discussed in Chap. 18.

  E. **Thoracentesis** should be performed whenever sufficient quantities of pleural fluid are detected.

  F. **Bronchoscopy** is indicated to evaluate suspected cavitating carcinoma, the possibility of bronchial obstruction (cancer or a foreign body), and significant hemoptysis. Fiberoptic bronchoscopy should not be part of the routine evaluation of lung abscess [164].

V. **Therapy** depends on the type of underlying lung abscess.

  A. **Adequate drainage** is important, and this usually occurs through the tracheobronchial tree. If the patient is raising sputum and is improving clinically and radiologically, drainage is adequate. Cautious postural drainage and other respiratory therapy maneuvers are useful for patients having difficulty with their secretions. If the clinical situation is worsening or if sputum production abruptly ceases, a therapeutic bronchoscopy is indicated.

  B. **Antibiotics** are the mainstay of initial therapy.

   1. **Anaerobic abscess.** In these infections, **clindamycin is now considered the drug of choice** as it has been shown to be superior to penicillin in prospective, randomized comparative trials [49, 165, 166]. (Adult doses shown.)

    a. Although oral regimens may be effective in carefully selected cases, **the authors initially treat most patients intravenously** with clindamycin, 600 mg q8h. After the patient has become afebrile for at least 3–5 days, one can switch to oral clindamycin (e.g., 300–450 mg qid). The optimal duration of total antibiotic therapy is uncertain, but these patients usually require at least 4 additional weeks of antibiotics [166]. Therapy must be individualized; we continue antibiotics until there is no longer any surrounding parenchymal infiltrate, and the cavity is either gone or there is only a stable residual lesion.

    b. **Penicillin G** was accepted, in the past, as the traditional drug of choice based on extensive clinical experience [49]. However, many oral anaerobic gram-negative bacilli have become less susceptible to penicillin in association with penicillinase production. This is believed to explain, in part, the results of recent comparative trials that show a higher failure rate for penicillin than for clindamycin [165, 166]. If penicillin G is chosen for initial therapy, we suggest a dose of 12–18 million units/day to cover organisms that have a relatively high MIC; when appropriate, oral therapy may follow using penicillin V, 750 mg qid.

c. **Metronidazole should not be used alone** for these infections because of a high failure rate [49]. Penicillin plus metronidazole is acceptable and, because this combination can be administered both intravenously and orally, is potentially advantageous. However, long-term administration of metronidazole is complicated by its disulfuram-like interaction with alcohol and the occasional peripheral neuropathy it induces (see Chap. 28P).

d. **Alternative agents** that also should be effective, based on in vitro activity and some clinical experience, have not been as well studied [49]. For intravenous use, these include ampicillin-sulbactam, ticarcillin-clavulanate, piperacillin-tazobactam, cefoxitin, imipenem, and chloramphenicol. Oral alternatives include amoxicillin-clavulanate and chloramphenicol. However, these drugs are overly broad in coverage, are more expensive, or have a greater potential for unusual but serious toxicity (e.g., seizures with imipenem, and aplasia with chloramphenicol).

e. **Drugs that have limited activity** against some or most anaerobes commonly involved in lung abscess include the antistaphylococcal penicillins, ceftazidime, erythromycin and other macrolides, the fluoroquinolones, TMP-SMX, aztreonam, and the aminoglycosides [49].

f. **Successful treatment is initially indicated by** a rapid decrease in any foul odor to the sputum, an improved appetite, and the return of a subjective sense of well-being. Fever should abate within the first week [49, 166], but a minority of patients may take up to 2 weeks to become afebrile. On chest roentgenography, there is first a reduction in the surrounding infiltrate and a decrease in the fluid within the cavity. Initially, the cavity may enlarge as necrotic lung is expectorated. Large amounts of purulent sputum may be produced for several weeks, but Gram stains should reveal a marked decrease in the numbers of organisms. **Antibiotics are continued until** there is a return to the usual state of health, sputum is minimal and not purulent, there is no infiltrate surrounding the cavity, the cavity size has stabilized, and the ESR is normalized.

2. **Aerobic lung abscesses** are difficult to treat. Because prolonged parenteral antibiotic therapy will be necessary (e.g., 4–6 weeks), it is essential to know whether one is dealing with a true lower respiratory pathogen or just a sputum colonizer. Therefore, culture identification and susceptibility data must be interpreted carefully in this setting.

   Antibiotics and dosages were discussed earlier in this chapter (in secs. **IV** and **XV** under Special Considerations and Specific Therapy).

3. **Embolic pneumonia** therapy is discussed in sec. **XIV** under Special Considerations and Specific Therapy. Prolonged therapy (e.g., 6 weeks) often is indicated. These patients may need surgical drainage.

C. **Special problems**
1. An **empyema** can complicate a lung abscess, with or without a bronchopleural fistula. The approach to these complications is discussed in sec. **II** under Pleural Effusion Versus Empyema. Brain abscess and amyloidosis as complications of lung abscess are much less common than in the preantibiotic era.

2. **Obstruction to drainage should be suspected if sputum production abruptly diminishes,** fever recurs, and the amount of fluid in the cavity increases.

3. **Suspected cavitary lung cancer is an indication for bronchoscopy** [164]. The absence of any risk factors for aspiration, systemic symptoms, fever, leukocytosis, or an infiltrate surrounding the cavity should suggest this diagnosis.

4. **Surgery** for lung abscess is required in only a few circumstances. Lobectomy has been the procedure of choice. The most important indications include significant and persistent hemoptysis, suspected or proved lung cancer, and the failure of intensive medical therapy. A relative indication for surgery is a very large, fluid-filled abscess ($\geq$ 6 cm) with a significant risk of asphyxia from aspiration of cavity contents into the bronchial tree. Persistence of a thin-

walled stable cavity on the chest roentgenogram is no longer an indication for surgery.

Recent experience has suggested that **percutaneous catheter drainage may be preferred in selected patients** [167, 168]. This is particularly suitable for those failing medical therapy, those needing urgent drainage, or when the risk of surgical intervention is too great. CT guidance permits placement to avoid uninvolved pleura and lung, the detection of loculated abscess cavities, and an assessment of the extent of drainage.

5. Patients who do not seem to be responding may need a diagnostic or therapeutic bronchoscopy.

VI. **Outcome.** The prognosis in cases of lung abscess will depend on the underlying conditions and etiologic agents. In anaerobic lung abscess, survival has been up to 96% in the antibiotic era; the average time to maximum cavity closure is estimated at 65 days [49]. Risk factors for a worse outcome include multiple or large abscesses, prolonged symptoms, obstruction, old age, and debilitating chronic disease. An important cause of death from lung abscess has been asphyxia from aspiration of cavity contents.

Tuberculosis: Basic Concepts

Due to a variety of factors, including the HIV epidemic, tuberculosis has been increasing in frequency since 1985 [169–171a]. Thus, it remains fairly common and presents with sufficient variability that it causes confusion [172, 173]. The four major patterns of pulmonary tuberculosis (pneumonia, pleurisy, cavitary disease, and miliary disease) are discussed briefly in this chapter. In addition, the major extrapulmonary manifestations, therapeutic agents and their toxicity, and chemoprophylaxis are discussed.

I. **Epidemiology**

A. The incidence of tuberculosis in the United States was declining even before the introduction of specific chemotherapy, perhaps because patients were isolated in sanitoriums or other institutions [174]. A steady fall in the numbers of tuberculosis cases continued after antituberculous drugs were introduced until 1985. Since that time, **there has been a reemergence of tuberculosis in this country,** especially from 1985 to 1992. This has resulted in approximately 51,700 more cases of tuberculosis between 1985 and 1992 than would have been expected had the earlier rate of decline continued [174]. Much of this increase has been concentrated in urban centers and has disproportionately affected racial and ethnic minorities, foreign-born immigrants, children, and young adults aged 25–44 years [174].

Although from 1985 to 1992 the number of tuberculosis cases reported annually in the United States increased 20%, from 1992 to 1994 the number of tuberculosis cases reported annually decreased 8.7%, in part reflecting the impact of federal resources to assist state and local tuberculosis control efforts, including directly observed therapy (DOT), tuberculin screening and preventive therapy for persons at high risk for tuberculosis infection, and support for programs to prevent tuberculosis among HIV-infected persons [174a]. Of note, in 1994 the number and proportion of foreign-born persons with tuberculosis increased substantially; approximately one-third of these persons were in the United States less than 1 year prior to diagnosis [174a].

B. **Factors contributing to increased tuberculosis incidence in the United States** include a prior decline in public health efforts, poverty, homelessness, substance abuse, immigration from countries where tuberculosis is prevalent, the HIV epidemic, and multidrug resistance [169, 174, 174a]. Nonetheless, almost one-third of tuberculosis cases in the United States continue to occur in middle-class or higher-income individuals [175]. See related discussion in sec. **X.B.**

C. **Tuberculosis remains a tremendous problem throughout the world.** One-third of the world's population, 1.7 billion people, is estimated to be infected with *Mycobacterium tuberculosis* [170]. From this reservoir come 8 million new tuberculosis patients and 2.9 million deaths due to tuberculosis each year. In developing countries, tuberculosis causes 6.7% of all deaths, 18.5% of deaths in the age group 15–59 years, and 26% of avoidable deaths in adults [169]. This is further accentuated by concomitant HIV infection in Africa and many other parts of the world.

II. Pathogenesis of tuberculosis
A. Overview
1. **Reservoir.** The vast majority of tuberculosis in the United States today is due to *M. tuberculosis*. Only rarely is *Mycobacterium bovis* isolated. Although some animals are susceptible to *M. tuberculosis* infection, **humans** are the only important natural reservoir for this organism.
2. **Transmission.** Spread of *M. tuberculosis* is almost exclusively **by small-particle aerosols** and very rarely by contaminated dust or fomites. Airborne particles bearing organisms may be generated by coughing, sneezing, and even speaking or singing [169]. The most efficient aerosols, droplet nuclei, are of sufficiently small size (1–5 μm) so that they are inhaled and deposited into the alveolar space [169]. In animals, a single organism may be sufficient to yield infection; this is theoretically the case for humans, but most infections follow exposures to many more droplet nuclei and bacilli.

   Initial host defense against *M. tuberculosis* in the lung is the alveolar macrophage. The outcome from inhaling *M. tuberculosis* depends on the numbers of organism reaching the alveoli, their relative virulence, and the inherent capability of the macrophages to eliminate or contain the inoculum. Potential virulence factors for the organism include sulfatides, cord factor, cell wall constituents, and protein antigens. The organism also is able to impair phagosome acidification in the macrophage, perhaps by inhibiting fusion with lysosomes containing the proton-ATPase pump [176]. Genetic factors may underlly natural host resistance to infection, and this may be expressed in part in the intrinsic ability of macrophages to control organisms [177]. The exact nature of macrophage tuberculocidal activity is unknown [169].
3. **Initial infection** in previously uninfected immunocompetent persons results from significant exposure to airborne organisms produced by someone with active pulmonary tuberculosis. In most instances, the organism is able to multiply intracellularly in lung macrophages. **After a short period of replication,** an estimated 14–21 days, **the organism spreads through regional lymphatics to the hilar lymph nodes and then through the bloodstream to all sites in the body [178]. This dissemination usually is silent** and is accompanied almost simultaneously by the onset of cell mediated immunity and delayed hypersensitivity to the organism. **At the sites to which it disseminates, the organism usually is prevented from further replication, but it is not killed.** Consequently, organisms that have been dormant can become reactivated. **In approximately 5%, the host cannot contain the original infection, and clinical disease develops within the first year** [178]. However, in 95% the original infection is controlled by the host and remains subclinical.
4. **Reactivation infection.** Clinical disease develops in another 5% of immunocompetent persons at a time remote from the initial infection, as a result of endogenous reactivation of a previously established quiescent focus [178]. The **preferential sites at which the organism becomes reactivated are generally those of persistently high oxygen tension. These include the upper lung zones,** kidneys, bones, and CNS.

B. The role of cellular immunity in disease. The major host defense that controls *M. tuberculosis* is the macrophage-lymphocyte system [169]. Important targets of protective immunity remain controversial but include the dominant heat-shock protein and secreted and export proteins of *M. tuberculosis* [179]. Interleukins 1, 2, 4, 6, 8, and 10, gamma interferon, and tumor necrosis factor (TNF) are all involved in the response to infection [169, 179–181]. TNF may have an essential role in containing infection through granuloma formation [169]. Some of the cytokines and calciferol may activate macrophages to inhibit or kill the organism, as may neutrophils recruited to sites of inflammation. In addition, infected macrophages may be killed by natural killer cells, cytotoxic lymphocytes, CD4+ cells, CD8+ cells, and gamma-delta T cells. **Impairments of cellular immunity predispose the host to the development of clinical disease** from either progressive primary infection or from reactivation of a latent infection.

   Cell-mediated immunity also is responsible for many of the clinical findings in tuberculosis [169]. Fever, anorexia, and weight loss may be mediated by cytokines induced by the infection. Most of the tissue destruction, including caseous necrosis, is caused by the cell-mediated response to the organism, which has no important endotoxins or exotoxins [181].

III. **Skin-test reactivity** [175, 178, 182]. The presence of cellular immunity can be inferred from delayed-type hypersensitivity to an intracutaneous antigen. Histologically, a positive reaction is due to infiltration by a large number of mononuclear cells. These begin to accumulate 24 hours later and usually are fully manifest between 48 and 72 hours after injection of the antigen. The mechanism of the accumulation of cells at the site is initially antigen stimulation of one or a few memory cells, which elaborate factors that attract uncommitted mononuclear cells to the area. This presumably is the mechanism by which the cells control the infection at sites of bacterial replication and that also results in the detrimental effects of tuberculosis [181].

A. **Clinical materials available for skin testing.** There are a number of systems by which skin tests for tuberculosis can be done. The recommended method is intradermal inoculation of purified protein derivative of tuberculosis (PPD), which is available in three different strengths. In the United States and Canada, these are measured in tuberculin units (TU) and are based on achieving a biologic equivalence to the standard PPD preparation, PPD-S. Multiple puncture devices should be reserved for screening of large populations and should not be used for routine diagnostic purposes [182].

   1. **First-strength PPD** is very rarely available in hospitals. One TU is contained in the 0.1 ml PPD injected. It was used as initial inoculation in patients in whom tuberculosis was very likely. Use of this small dose might avoid an accelerated local reaction, but it is not standardized and **has little clinical utility** [182].

   2. **Intermediate-strength PPD** contains a concentration of 5 TU in the 0.1 ml injected. **All recommendations for interpreting skin testing are based on using this strength.**

   3. **Second-strength PPD (250 TU)** seldom is helpful. Reactivity can be due to infection with atypical mycobacteria or, because it is always administered after the intermediate strength, to a booster effect. In a patient who is not anergic, a negative second-strength test is additional evidence against tuberculosis in that patient. However, 10% of cases of pulmonary tuberculosis have a negative second-strength test as well as a negative intermediate PPD [183]. Thus, **the second-strength test should not be used for diagnostic purposes,** although it is occasionally helpful in assessing patients' immunologic status [178, 182].

B. **Reading the reaction. The test is read at 48–72 hours by recording the maximum diameter of induration.** The most reliable technique for this is to palpate the area gently with the index finger [182].

C. **Interpreting the reaction** [175, 178, 182]. The use of 5 TU (intermediate strength) was arrived at by the observation that most individuals in a tuberculosis sanitorium reacted to 5 TU and most normal individuals did not. However, **there are false negative responses and, in pulmonary tuberculosis, 10–25% of patients may have a negative intermediate PPD** [182, 183]. False positive reactions may result from infection with nontuberculous mycobacteria or from BCG vaccination.

   1. **A 5-mm or more induration is considered positive in** close contacts of infectious tuberculosis patients, in those with radiographic findings consistent with old healed tuberculosis, and in HIV-infected patients or those at risk for HIV infection but with unknown HIV status.

   2. **A 10-mm or more induration is considered positive in** those who do not meet the preceding criteria but who are at high risk for tuberculosis. These include foreign-born immigrants from countries where tuberculosis is prevalent; HIV-negative intravenous drug users; members of racial and ethnic minorities with an increasing incidence of tuberculosis; medically underserved low-income persons; residents of long-term care facilities, including prisons, mental institutions, and nursing homes; persons with predisposing underlying medical conditions, such as silicosis, gastrectomy, jejunoileal bypass, malnutrition (assessed as being at least 10% below one's ideal body weight), diabetes, chronic renal failure, and immunosuppressive diseases or treatment; and those in settings such as health care facilities, hospital microbiology laboratories, schools, and daycare facilities that put them or others at greater risk.

   3. **A 15-mm or more induration is considered positive in anyone.**

D. **Booster effect.** An enhancing or boosting phenomenon has been recognized with repeated tuberculin skin testing [175, 178, 184–187]. It is defined as an increase in induration from a negative to a positive interpretation (see **C**) because of an immunologic boost provided by a prior skin test in a previously sensitized individual; it thus mimics skin-test conversion from a recent infection. **The clinician**

needs to be aware of the booster effect when attempting to interpret skin-test conversion, especially after serial testing. It rarely occurs in children and becomes more important with increasing age. This booster effect may be seen within 1 week of the initial test, and the effect may persist for 1 year or longer.

The settings in which the clinician needs to be particularly aware of the booster effect include (1) new hospital employee screening programs involving serial skin tests, (2) serial skin tests done for diagnostic or other purposes, and (3) annual screening tests in nursing homes or other institutions. It may occur in individuals who have previously received the BCG vaccine. If the initial skin test is negative but is positive when repeated, it may be a positive test due to the booster effect rather than true conversion.

To avoid this problem, a two-step skin test has been suggested for use in screening programs. If the initial intermediate PPD skin test is negative, a repeat skin test is performed in 1–3 weeks. Interpretation of the second skin test serves as the baseline response. Studies have indicated that a three-step skin-test program may detect a significant number of additional booster reactions [184]. It is not clear, however, whether this is worth the effort in large-scale screening efforts. The interpretation of booster reactions is complicated by the fact that they may reflect prior infection with any mycobacterial species or BCG vaccination. In populations at low risk for tuberculosis, such as many young adults in North America, a positive booster reaction has a low positive predictive value for *M. tuberculosis* infection [187]. Thus, serial testing to detect the booster phenomenon is best applied to groups at greater risk of exposure to tuberculosis [182].

E. **Causes of negative skin-test reactions [178, 182]**
   1. The most common cause of a negative skin-test reaction is the absence of infection with *M. tuberculosis.*
   2. There are a wide variety of causes for a false negative skin test in a person with *M. tuberculosis* infection. A partial list of patient-related causes includes recent or overwhelming tuberculosis; tuberculous pleurisy; acute nontuberculous infections (especially acute viral infection); live virus vaccinations; malignancy; renal disease; poor nutrition; newborn or advanced age; immunosuppressive diseases or drugs; surgery; burns; and poor skin elasticity (which results in nonretention of the antigen in the skin site so that the host response cannot be manifested at the site). Other causes include inadequate technique in applying or interpreting the skin test and use of impotent tuberculin preparations.
   3. **To help identify false negative responses due to anergy, simultaneous intracutaneous (0.1-ml) skin testing with at least two other antigens is performed.** Recommended preparations include mumps, *Candida,* and tetanus toxoid (diluted 5:1 in phenol buffer); *Trichophyton* spp. have been less useful because of low rates of response to this antigen [188]. Second-strength PPD should not be used to assess anergy. **Any induration in response to one of these antigens indicates that cutaneous delayed hypersensitivity is intact [188]. However, patients with active tuberculosis may have an absent skin-test response to tuberculin and a positive skin test to other antigens.**
      Although we do not test for anergy in all patients undergoing skin testing (e.g., routine screening), we will test for anergy when skin testing is done in an ill, immunocompromised, or complex patient.
   4. Previously positive skin tests may revert to insignificant reactions over relatively brief periods of time in some patient groups. Perez-Stable and colleagues [185] administered a two-step skin-test program to 495 nursing home residents in 1982 and detected 258 patients with significant (>10-mm) reactions; the booster effect accounted for 21 of these. When these same 258 skin-test reactors were retested with a three-step program in 1985, a total of 64 (24.8%) had reverted to insignificant (<10-mm) reactions [185]. The reversions included 16 (76.2%) of the 21 previously identified booster reactions [185]. The clinical implications of such an instability of tuberculin skin-test reactions over time remain to be determined.

F. **Skin-test conversion.** Recent conversion from a negative PPD skin-test reaction is defined as an **increase within a 2-year period of** 10-mm or greater induration for patients younger than 35 years and a 15-mm or greater increase for patients 35 years or older [186]. There are a number of problems in interpreting skin-test conversion.
   1. The booster effect may mimic skin-test conversion (see sec. **D**).

2. Infection caused by other intracellular organisms can result in nonspecific enhancement of tuberculin skin-test reactivity. This has been observed with *Brucella* infection.

3. A number of the conditions that cause false negative skin-test reactions can be reversed. A negative skin test found when one of those conditions is present may prove positive if repeated after the condition is corrected, giving the false impression of skin-test conversion even though there has simply been a return to baseline skin-test reactivity.

4. If improper technique or test material is used in the first test and then proper technique or material is used in the second test, skin-test conversion will appear to have occurred.

G. **Skin testing is indicated** for populations identified by the American Thoracic Society and CDC as being at high risk for tuberculosis [175]. These include those with clinical findings compatible with tuberculosis, recent contact with active tuberculosis, HIV infection, radiographic changes suggestive of past tuberculosis, and medical conditions that place them at greater risk (see sec. **C.2**). Individuals in groups known to have a higher incidence of tuberculosis also should be skin-tested. Examples in the United States are recent immigrants from Asia, Africa, Latin America, and Oceania; the poor or medically underserved; and residents and employees of hospitals, nursing homes, prisons, and mental institutions (see sec. **I**).

IV. **Diagnosis.** The cornerstone of the diagnosis of tuberculosis is the demonstration of acid-fast bacilli (AFB) with characteristics of *M. tuberculosis* by culture. In many instances, demonstration of AFB on smear of a body fluid is strong circumstantial evidence that tuberculosis infection is present. Diagnostic methods have recently been reviewed [188a, 189].

A. **Smears and cultures.** Because *M. tuberculosis* is a slow-growing pathogen, **the traditional method for rapid presumptive diagnosis is the acid-fast smear. Early-morning sputum is best, and three specimens should suffice for almost all cases.**

"Concentrated sputum" smears often are examined in the microbiology laboratory (see Chap. 25).

1. **Sputum induction using nebulized saline** is helpful for patients unable to provide adequate coughed samples.

2. **Fiberoptic bronchoscopy** with biopsy or BAL may be needed when spontaneous or induced sputums fail to provide diagnostic specimens. Expectorated sputums should be collected in the immediate postbronchoscopy period because they may be the only smear-positive samples. One review suggests that sputum specimens obtained within the first 2 days after bronchoscopy is performed are highly diagnostic [188a].

3. **AFB smears** are discussed in Chap. 25. At least three acid-fast bacteria must be seen to consider a single smear positive, whether stained using a fluorochrome or a carbol-fuchsin method. The **fluorochrome stain is preferred,** however, because it is easier and faster to read [189].

   Sputum must contain 5,000–10,000 bacilli/ml before smears are reliably positive [189]. The bacillary burden in fibronodular lesions is estimated at 10^2–10^4 organisms, whereas that of cavitary lesions is 10^7–10^9 organisms. Thus, **cavitary disease is more likely to be smear-positive and contagious.**

4. **Gastric aspirates and urine specimens for smear and culture.** It is not always possible on smears to distinguish saprophytic from pathogenic mycobacteria. Because of this, it had been held that acid-fast smears of gastric aspirates and urine specimens could not be used as indicators of mycobacterial disease. This may not be true, however.

   Klotz and Penn [190] retrospectively reviewed a 10-year experience with gastric aspirate and urine specimens in their hospital and found only one possible false positive urine smear and no false positive smears of gastric aspirates. In this study, *M. tuberculosis* accounted for 86% of infections, *M. avium-intracellulare* was not isolated, and no patient had AIDS. It was concluded that because of their high specificity, positive acid-fast smears of gastric aspirate or urine specimens are helpful to the clinician as reliable indicators of mycobacterial disease [190]. (See Chap. 25 for further discussion of smear and culture methods.)

   Aspiration of gastric contents in the early morning before the patient has arisen from bed may be used for children and adults from whom sputum cannot be obtained. Prior studies have shown that a properly obtained gastric lavage specimen is equal to about three induced sputum specimens for the diagnosis of pulmonary tuberculosis [188a].

5. **Cultures may be positive when smears are negative** because cultures require only 10–100 viable organisms to become positive. Presumably, in patients with three negative, properly collected sputum smears but positive cultures, the level of infectivity (i.e., the likelihood of transmission) is low.

6. **Time delay of cultures**
   a. **Solid media.** It takes approximately **3–4 weeks** for visible growth to be detected using solid media, and often an additional 2–4 weeks for susceptibility test results with conventional techniques.

      In a recent review, for smear-positive cultures, the median number of days of incubation required before the culture results were reported was 18.5; for smear-negative specimens, the corresponding number was 27.5 [188a].

   b. **In contrast,** the **radiometric liquid BACTEC system reduces average detection time to 10–14 days** [189]. This system also may be used for susceptibility testing to commonly used drugs, with results available in approximately 4–7 days. Thus, the BACTEC system may provide essential information in a much shorter period of time [171].

7. **DNA probes.** Rapid identification of acid-fast growth is accomplished using DNA probes to hybridize with mycobacterial ribosomal RNA. Probes are commercially available that specifically identify *M. tuberculosis, M. avium, M. intracellulare, M. kansasii,* and *M. gordonae* [189]. However, by themselves these probes are currently of insufficient sensitivity to be used directly on clinical specimens (e.g., expectorated sputum) [189].

B. **Newer rapid diagnostic methods** include nucleic acid amplification techniques, immunologic techniques to detect antibodies to mycobacteria or mycobacterial antigens, and tests to detect mycobacterial cellular components [170, 171, 189, 191]. Some of these methods have been very helpful in the rapid diagnosis of tuberculous meningitis and are more sensitive than acid-fast smears [192].

A unique problem in interpretation arises when a nucleic acid amplification test is positive but cultures are negative in a patient without obvious clinical tuberculosis. Although such a result may be a false positive, it also may be a true positive representing early infection with very low mycobacterial populations. Further studies will require long-term follow-up to determine the frequency of each possibility.

1. **Polymerase chain reaction** tests have been developed to detect *M. tuberculosis* DNA directly in clinical specimens and yield results in 2–3 days. At present, the PCR tests are less sensitive on smear-negative specimens than on smear-positive specimens, and some samples may contain inhibitors [170, 171, 189]. In addition to needed technical improvements, there are significant problems in obtaining reliable PCR results when the test is performed in clinical laboratories [193]. This topic was reviewed in early 1996 [193a].

2. Another approach to direct testing is **ribosomal RNA amplification,** which is potentially advantageous because there are several thousand copies per cell. One manufacturer uses enzymatic rRNA amplification followed by a proprietary probe test: A recent evaluation on respiratory specimens revealed a sensitivity of between 94 and 97% and a specificity of approximately 97% [194]. Results in this study were available within 1 day [194].

3. **Immunoassays for both antigens and antibodies** use the ELISA technique [170, 192]. Antigen tests on CSF are promising, but such tests are less successful with sputum. Antibody tests are not standardized; are less sensitive with smear-negative, pleural, and miliary disease; and are of limited usefulness in HIV-infected or immunosuppressed patients [170, 192]. In a recent review, some encouraging results have been reported with ELISA or solid-phase radioimmunoassays [188a]. In the future, these approaches may be particularly useful in situations in which examination of sputum smears was not possible [188a].

4. **Detecting the mycobacterial products tuberculostearic acid and mycolic acid** requires expensive equipment and technology, which are not readily available. **Detection of tuberculostearic acid shows promise** on sputum and CSF, whereas there is little experience with mycolic acid detection [170]. For difficult

cases, tuberculostearic acid assays conducted at the CDC may be arranged through local or state health departments.

V. Clinical manifestations of different forms of pulmonary tuberculosis. There are four forms of pulmonary tuberculosis: tuberculous pneumonia, pleurisy, cavitary disease, and miliary disease. Some of these can appear in combination. Therapy is discussed in sec. **VII.**

A. Tuberculous pneumonia. After *M. tuberculosis* is inhaled, it replicates in the middle or lower lung lobes at the site of inhalation. In most instances, infection is controlled before clinical manifestations occur. On occasion, particularly at the extremes of age, infection continues unchecked to produce a progressive **primary pneumonia.** Although this form of disease can appear by itself, it also may be associated with hilar adenopathy, cavitation, or upper-lobe pulmonary disease [178, 195, 196].

1. **Clinical manifestations.** Patients with tuberculous pneumonia may be very ill, with high fever, cough, and inanition. Sputum volume is large and often contains abundant polymorphonuclear leukocytes. Similar cells can be seen on lung biopsy of these patients. Some patients with lower-lobe tuberculosis may be only mildly ill.

2. **Diagnosis.** When the sputum is stained for acid-fast organisms, it often is found to be teeming with these agents. Thus, **such individuals are highly infectious and should be placed on proper respiratory isolation.** Although delayed hypersensitivity may have developed at the onset of tuberculous pneumonia, in many instances it has not. **Skin tests often are negative and may not be helpful.** Radiographic features are varied and include lobar consolidation, simultaneous appearance of apical cavitary disease with lobar infiltration, hilar adenopathy, and atelectasis [178, 195, 196].

3. **Communicability is very high** because of the large numbers of organisms in the sputum of these patients.

B. Tuberculous pleurisy. A second form of tuberculosis is tuberculous pleural effusion. This can occur either alone or with simultaneous effusions in the pericardial and peritoneal spaces (tuberculous polyserositis). In the past, this disease was seen more commonly in younger than in older individuals but, in recent years, older individuals have been the most prominent group to develop this infection [197]. It usually occurs in the early period after a primary infection with *M. tuberculosis* but may also be a manifestation of reactivated disease [197–199]. Tuberculous pleural effusions are due to the breakdown of a granuloma releasing its contents into the pleural cavity, followed by acute inflammation from a local cell-mediated hypersensitivity reaction. In contrast, tuberculous empyema results when a bronchopleural fistula spills the contents of a parenchymal cavity into the pleural space.

1. **Clinical manifestations.** Mild or low-grade temperature accompanied by low-grade pleuritic pain is common. Usually, the patient is well except for these manifestations and complains merely of a "heaviness" of the chest. Occasionally, patients are very ill. Cough and sputum production generally are minimal or absent. When the underlying pulmonary parenchyma can be examined by roentgenogram, there is classically no evidence of parenchymal disease. However, patients with reactivation disease tend to have more chronic illness and often have a productive cough with radiographic changes [199].

   Tuberculous pleural effusions are self-limited, resolving spontaneously within several months. The risk of subsequent clinical tuberculosis is high, developing in up to two-thirds of patients within the next 5 years. Antituberculous chemotherapy may not shorten the illness, but a short course of concomitant corticosteroids may hasten improvement [200].

2. **Diagnosis**

   a. **Pleural fluid.** Diagnostic thoracentesis usually reveals an exudate with a predominance of lymphocytes; neutrophils may be prominent, however, particularly early in the illness [197]. Mesothelial cells should not constitute more than 5% of the total cell count. Glucose levels are most often normal but may be low. **Acid-fast smears of the pleural fluid are almost always negative,** and the results from cultures will be available only after several weeks. The yield from pleural fluid cultures varies with the amount of fluid processed but is usually less than 50%. If possible, several hundred milliliters or more of fluid should be submitted to the microbiology laboratory for culture.

b. **Pleural biopsy.** Before all the fluid has been removed, a needle biopsy of the parietal pleura should be performed. Histopathologic evaluation, acid-fast stains, and cultures should be performed on biopsy specimens. A single biopsy procedure (collecting three or four tissue samples) will provide positive findings in approximately 67% of cases of proven tuberculosis, and this increases to approximately 90% after a second biopsy [197]. A combination of pleural fluid studies plus histopathologic examination, acid-fast stains, and cultures of two pleural biopsies should establish the diagnosis in 90–95% of patients.

Directed biopsy using pleuroscopy has been proposed as a means of increasing yield [201]. At present, this procedure shows promise as a way of avoiding open biopsy when traditional percutaneous procedures have not established a diagnosis.

c. **Skin tests.** The **intermediate PPD** is usually positive but **may be negative in up to 30% of patients** [199]. However, most patients with an initial negative test eventually will develop a positive reaction during therapy.

d. **Biochemical tests** for adenosine deaminase levels in pleural fluid as an adjunct to diagnosis have been reviewed, with a sensitivity of 93–100% and a specificity of 76–100% [202]. In contrast, testing for tuberculostearic acid is less useful [203]. The value of combining these and other tests is uncertain at present.

3. **Communicability is low,** but skin-test conversion occasionally occurs in contacts.

C. **Cavitary tuberculosis.** A third form of pulmonary tuberculosis is **upper-lobe** cavitary disease [196]. Following inhalation and dissemination of *Mycobacterium*, the infection usually is controlled. Upper-lobe disease with cavitation may follow quickly if host immunity is insufficient, either with or without lower-lobe involvement (see sec. **V.A**).

More commonly, however, infiltrates and cavities in the upper lobes **represent endogenous reactivated tuberculosis** that occurs many months or years after the primary infection. Chest roentgenograms may appear normal in the intervening period prior to reactivation. Infiltration is most common in the apical and posterior segments of the upper lobes and the apical segments of the lower lobes. These infiltrates usually evolve to include air-filled cavities; noncavitary nodules or infiltrates are more common in the elderly and the immunosuppressed [178]. At this stage, the process almost never resolves spontaneously and will steadily progress unless treated. Bronchogenic spread of infection may involve lower and middle lobes and may be bilateral.

1. **Clinical manifestations.** Most individuals are moderately ill, with productive cough, night sweats, fever, weight loss, and weakness. Sputum may be blood-streaked. In some, the illness can be very severe, whereas in others with extensive parenchymal involvement, symptoms are minimal or nonexistent. Physical findings are nonspecific, and abnormalities in the chest may be minimal, despite extensive disease. Large cavities may produce amphoric breath sounds.

2. **Diagnosis.** Although very helpful, the chest roentgenogram cannot provide a specific diagnosis. A first-morning sputum sample should be sent for acid-fast smear and cultures (see Chap. 25); if the initial smear is negative, then a total of three (but no more than five) specimens should be examined. Sputum should be induced using nebulized hypertonic saline when spontaneous specimens are not produced. If this is unsuccessful, then fiberoptic bronchoscopy with BAL and biopsy should be considered. If bronchoscopy is not an option, then gastric aspirates should be sent. Gastric aspirates must be obtained before the patient wakens and empties the gastric contents. Three first-morning urine specimens for acid-fast smear and culture should also be obtained from most patients with suspected tuberculosis.

3. **Communicability is high** before the initiation of therapy because there usually are large numbers of organisms in cavitary disease. **These patients should be placed on respiratory precautions.**

D. **Miliary and generalized infection [204–209].** Generalized tuberculosis implies widespread disease due to hematogenous dissemination of the virulent tubercle bacilli. The resulting disease can have an **acute or insidious onset.** Acute disease (i.e., acute miliary tuberculosis) can occur shortly after the primary infection, when the infection is not contained and there is early massive dissemination of the bacilli. Disseminated disease can also occur at a time far removed (i.e., years to decades) from the primary or postprimary period of tuberculosis; this is known as *late generalized tuberculosis* [204]. If late generalized tuberculosis is associated with massive bacteremia, an acute miliary type of illness may occur. More commonly, the tuberculous bacteremia is low-grade, and patients have an indolent and insidious presentation [204]. In these patients, previously infected and yet contained foci (e.g., in the lung, lymph nodes, bone, adrenal glands, CNS, or genitourinary tract) break down and allow hematogenous dissemination. The breakdown may occur with advancing age or immunosuppression due to underlying diseases or drug therapy (see sec. II.A). **Factors predisposing to dissemination include** malnutrition, measles, and pertussis in children, and AIDS, alcoholism, diabetes, malignancies, and immunosuppressive therapies in adults.

1. **Clinical aspects.** There are no pathognomonic features of the acute or indolent forms of miliary disease. The onset of illness may be abrupt or very insidious. Although respiratory symptoms often are a prominent manifestation of acute miliary disease, in some cases such symptoms are not marked. Constitutional symptoms usually predominate, but between episodes of fever the patient may feel well. It is not uncommon for a patient with miliary tuberculosis who appears stable to have a sudden calamitous turn of illness and to deteriorate quickly, even before the chest roentgenogram becomes abnormal.

   Focal symptoms may be absent in disseminated tuberculosis. Patients may simply exhibit fever, night sweats, and weight loss [204–208]. Prominent headache suggests meningitis, and abdominal pain suggests peritonitis. Physical findings often are nonspecific, but abnormalities may occur in almost any site. The presence of lymphadenopathy, skin lesions, and scrotal or genital masses should be sought. Choroidal tubercles may be seen on funduscopy and are very supportive of the diagnosis (see Chap. 6).

2. **Diagnosis**
   a. **Chest roentgenogram**
      (1) **Acute miliary disease.** Miliary tuberculosis is so named because of the anatomically small millet seed–like lesions that develop in areas of high blood flow [178]. These are seen on the chest roentgenogram as diffuse, 2- to 4-mm nodular lesions. However, they may not be visible initially and take at least 2½ weeks to appear [205, 208]. Thus, repeat serial chest roentgenograms should be obtained (e.g., at 7- to 14-day intervals, once or twice at least) if the initial film is unremarkable.
      (2) **Late generalized tuberculosis (with indolent disease). Patients commonly have normal x-ray films.** In one study, 50% of patients had nonspecific chest roentgenograms [204]. These patients have nonpulmonary foci (e.g., nodes, prostate, bone) that caseate. In addition to miliary lesions, the chest film may reveal infiltrates, cavities, pleural effusion, or pneumothorax [205, 208].
   b. **Acid-fast smears and cultures.** Multiple cultures should be obtained as the yield is variable in disseminated disease. The details of mycobacterial culture are given in Chap. 25.
      (1) **Sputum AFB smears are positive in a minority of cases** (approximately 33%) and, at best, sputum cultures are positive in only 50–76% of patients with miliary disease [204–208]. Transbronchial biopsy and BAL should be considered in patients with abnormal chest roentgenograms but negative sputums.
      (2) **Gastric cultures** are positive in from 33 to 75% of patients [207].
      (3) **Urine cultures** are positive in 25 to 59% of patients, even in the absence of urinary abnormalities [205, 207].
      (4) **Bone marrow biopsy** for cultures may be positive in up to 33% of patients (some authorities suggest that 10 ml of aspirate be cultured). Histopathologic examination may reveal granulomas in more than 80% [208].
      (5) **Liver biopsy cultures are very helpful, as is the histologic appearance** [204, 205]. Supportive diagnostic material usually is found, provided there is some abnormality suggesting hepatic involvement prior to biopsy.
      (6) **Lymph node biopsy** should be considered whenever accessible adenopathy is present. This procedure is associated with very little morbidity

and frequently will confirm the diagnosis rapidly by revealing caseating granulomas or positive acid-fast smears.

   (7) CSF examination should be performed in patients with headaches or neurologic symptoms suggestive of tuberculous meningitis and may be considered in asymptomatic patients with suspected late generalized tuberculosis (see Chap. 5).

  c. **Histologic study** of biopsied organs may be very helpful. Typical granulomas with central necrosis may be seen, and organisms may be visible on acid-fast stains. However, the more common finding of smear-negative, noncaseating granulomas is nonspecific and may be seen in a variety of conditions.

  d. **Skin tests** are **often negative** in these patients.

  e. **Blood tests.** The WBC count can range from marked leukopenia to a leukemoid reaction [208]. Monocytosis, lymphopenia, and severe thrombocytopenia also may be present. Liver function tests may reveal an elevated alkaline phosphatase level or mild transaminase elevations. However, jaundice is uncommon. Hyponatremia can be found with meningeal involvement or adrenal insufficiency.

 3. **Relationship to fever of unknown origin** (FUO). As indicated, miliary tuberculosis and late generalized tuberculosis should be considered in the evaluation of FUO. If a patient has FUO and ill-defined hematopoietic or liver abnormalities suggesting cholestasis, some authorities would consider an antituberculous therapeutic trial if a thorough evaluation of the FUO has yielded no explanation (see Chap. 1).

 4. **Communicability.** Miliary tuberculosis is **relatively noninfectious** (in the absence of significant pulmonary involvement) and, like tuberculous pleurisy, represents a very low risk.

VI. Extrapulmonary tuberculosis [205, 206, 210]. Tuberculosis may occur in many organs and usually becomes manifest in one of three ways. First, extrapulmonary infection occurs **in the miliary process** but, usually, generalized signs and symptoms of disease are more important than the manifestation of symptoms or signs of specific organ infection. More commonly, **organ involvement** can occur **simultaneously with the reactivation process in the lung** and thus be manifest at that time. Equally common is the occurrence of extrapulmonary tuberculosis **in the absence of obvious clinical disease in the lung,** and this often results in an excessive delay in arriving at an accurate diagnosis. Extrapulmonary tuberculosis did not decline in frequency when pulmonary disease was declining [210]. The highest proportions of extrapulmonary tuberculosis are found in children, ethnic and racial minorities, women, and the foreign-born [210].

 A. **Clinical presentation**

 1. **Symptoms or signs of localized disease.** Patients with extrapulmonary tuberculosis usually present with localized symptoms or signs and minimal or absent constitutional symptoms. Often the diagnosis is reached when the patient is being evaluated for another problem (such as pyuria, peritonitis, pericardial effusion, or lymphadenopathy).

 2. **Systemic illness associated with a localized problem.** A small percentage of patients have constitutional symptoms associated with extrapulmonary disease. For the most part, these patients have more widespread disease or, in addition to the extrapulmonary focus, have pulmonary involvement as well.

 3. **Associated chest roentgenographic changes.** From the foregoing discussion, it is obvious that **roentgenographic evidence of pulmonary disease is not always seen** when active infection is present in an extrapulmonary focus. Analysis of most series of lymph node, renal, CNS, or bone tuberculosis reveals that fewer than 50% of patients demonstrate acute chest roentgenographic changes when they present with their extrapulmonary disease.

 B. **Forms of extrapulmonary disease**

 1. **Meningitis** [211]. See Chap. 5.

 2. **Pericarditis** [212]. See Chap. 10 under Pericarditis and Myocarditis.

 3. **Renal disease.** See Chap. 12 under Genitourinary Tuberculosis.

 4. **Bone disease.** See Chap. 16 under Special Forms of Osteomyelitis.

 5. **Lymph node disease.** Lymphatic tuberculosis is found in all age groups, although it is most common in children younger than 15 years [210]. It is also more common in women, and in the foreign-born [210].

a. Clinical manifestations depend on the extent of nodal involvement and underlying host characteristics [213].

(1) Localized lymph node disease. There is a well-recognized form of tuberculosis in which lymph nodes alone are the major organ system involved. Single complexes of lymph nodes can develop. The common sites are in the cervical lymph nodes (scrofula) or in the retroperitoneal area. In addition, bilateral or unilateral hilar adenopathy can develop without obvious parenchymal disease. When cervical lymph node disease is present, breakdown and drainage can occur with either minimal or no constitutional symptoms.

(2) Generalized lymph node involvement. This appears to represent a disease process lying between the phase of complete containment of primary infection and miliary disease. It is also present as part of miliary disease. Patients with this syndrome very commonly have constitutional symptoms, fever, and weight loss, and the initial impression clinically is of a lymphoreticular neoplastic process.

(3) Lymph node involvement due to drainage of an infected organ. This is a more common cause of lymph node infection than is primary lymph node disease. Hilar nodes may develop bilaterally as part of pulmonary infections, with or without detectable infiltrates [195, 196].

(4) Lymph node involvement with atypical mycobacteria. This is more common today than is node involvement with *M. tuberculosis*. Specifically, submandibular or cervical adenopathy due to *Mycobacterium scrofulaceum* in young children or to *M. avium-intracellulare* in older children is recognized. This is distinct from the lymph node involvement seen with disseminated *M. avium-intracellulare* infections in patients with AIDS (see Chap. 19).

b. Diagnosis. The standard for diagnosis in accessible nodes has been excisional biopsy, in order to avoid chronic draining fistulas. **Fine-needle aspiration biopsy** now is advocated as the initial procedure, because it frequently may support a presumptive diagnosis with limited risk for complications when combined with modern chemotherapy [214].

(1) Histologic features. Biopsy and culture of the lymph nodes often reveal the diagnosis. Although the lymph nodes may reveal epithelioid cells and granuloma, nonspecific changes with necrosis also may be present. Organisms can be very difficult, if not impossible, to see by staining and sometimes are recovered only with great difficulty.

(2) Tuberculin skin test. Lymph node disease is more common in younger than in older patients, and the skin test often is positive [214]. Thus, in a young individual with localized or generalized lymphadenopathy and a positive tuberculin skin test, *M. tuberculosis* should be considered as etiologic until proof of another cause is demonstrated.

6. Serous surface involvement (pleural effusion, pericardial effusions, and peritonitis) usually results from breakdown of a contiguous granuloma and discharge of its contents into the serous cavity of a previously sensitized individual. Thus, a significant inflammatory reaction may ensue despite the presence of relatively few intact organisms.

a. Clinical manifestations. Serous surface involvement in tuberculosis can mimic serositis of unexplained etiology. The peritoneum, the pericardial sac and, as already mentioned, the pleura may be involved either singly or in any combination. Serous tuberculosis can be highly exudative and associated with large effusions or with minimal fluid production.

(1) Pleural effusions are discussed in sec. **V.B.**

(2) Pericardial effusions are discussed in Chap. 10 under Pericarditis and Myocarditis.

(3) Peritonitis. Patients with tuberculous peritonitis usually present with insidious onset of fever, abdominal pain or mass, weight loss, and an exudative ascites [215]. The ascitic protein content usually exceeds 3 g/100 ml, with fewer than 3,000 WBCs and a predominance of lymphocytes. Many patients with tuberculous peritonitis have cirrhosis of the liver [216]. Cirrhotic patients may have atypical presentations and an increased mortality, and the disease process may be difficult to diagnose [216].

b. **Spontaneous resolution.** Serous effusions that develop in tuberculosis may resolve spontaneously and, at least temporarily, leave no evidence of overt disease. However, very frequently (usually within a few months but occasionally as long as a few years) additional focal disease develops. This can become manifest in the lung as cavitary disease, in the pericardium as progressive constrictive pericarditis, and in the peritoneum as extramural small-bowel compression. In women, peritoneal tuberculosis can lead to pelvic tuberculosis, with tuboovarian masses and seeding of the uterine cavity.

c. **Diagnosis**
(1) **Pleural effusions.** See sec. **V.B.**
(2) **Pericardial effusions.** See Chap. 10 under Pericarditis and Myocarditis.
(3) **Peritonitis.** Organisms are seldom seen on smears of peritoneal fluid. Large volumes of fluid can be centrifuged and cultured, but even this method results in a suboptimal yield [215]. The diagnosis depends on demonstration of caseous granulomas in peritoneal tissue. Blind peritoneal biopsy, laparotomy, or laparoscopy (peritoneoscopy) can be performed to obtain peritoneal biopsy specimens; many consider laparoscopy the procedure of first choice [215]. Associated pulmonary parenchymal abnormalities are seen in fewer than 50% of patients, although coexisting pleural effusions are not uncommon. Liver function tests usually are normal, and liver biopsies generally are not helpful. The PPD skin test often is positive. Therefore, **tuberculous peritonitis should be considered in any unexplained exudative ascites in a patient with a positive PPD** or even a negative PPD test. In elderly patients in particular, the skin test may be negative. Adenosine deaminase activity in ascitic fluid has been shown to be a useful adjunct to the diagnosis of tuberculous peritonitis [215].

7. **Skin.** Miliary involvement of the skin is rare and usually occurs in infants in association with tuberculous meningitis, or in the immunosuppressed.

VII. **Tuberculosis and HIV infection.** Latent infection with *M. tuberculosis* is estimated to be present in 10 million US residents and almost 2 billion people worldwide [170]. HIV-infected and other immunosuppressed patients are at increased risk for both reactivation of these infections and progressive primary infection. Thus, it is not surprising that clinical tuberculosis increased as the number of AIDS patients increased [169]. However, **most often tuberculosis appears even before any other manifestations of HIV infection develop,** with important epidemiologic and clinical consequences [217, 217a]. **Counseling and HIV antibody testing should be considered for almost all patients diagnosed with *M. tuberculosis* infection [217].** This is particularly true for patients with extrapulmonary or unusual manifestations of pulmonary tuberculosis. Furthermore, documentation of a positive PPD test in an asymptomatic patient should serve as a stimulus to assess the risk for HIV infection and to offer HIV education, counseling, and antibody testing [217]. **See Chap. 19 for a further discussion of mycobacterial infections in HIV-infected patients.** See also sec. **X.B.**

VIII. **Tuberculosis in the elderly.** The large and growing elderly segment of our population contains a significant reservoir of individuals previously exposed to tuberculosis when the disease was more prevalent. Reactivation of these infections contributes to the steady incidence of tuberculosis in the elderly [218, 219]. In some parts of the United States, the rate of tuberculosis in persons older than 65 years is as high as 150–200 cases per 100,000 population [219].

A. Several **risk factors** for active tuberculosis may be present in the elderly. These include declining cell-mediated immunity with aging, gastrectomy, diabetes mellitus, cancer and other debilitating diseases, immunosuppressive drug therapy, malnutrition, and perhaps smoking and alcoholism [218, 219]. Another risk factor is confinement in a nursing home, where reactivation tuberculosis will occur in 2–3% of previously skin-test-positive individuals. Such reactivated disease may, in turn, infect the 70–80% of residents with a negative skin test and thus no prior exposure to *M. tuberculosis* [219]. Among elderly nursing home residents with skin-test conversion, the rate of clinical tuberculosis over the next 2 years is 8% in women and 12% in men [219].

B. **Atypical clinical manifestations and delayed diagnosis are common in the elderly. Awareness of the possibility of tuberculosis is essential to prompt diagno-**

sis. Symptoms often are poorly articulated, and coexistent illness may provide alternative explanations for anorexia, cough, and weight loss. Radiographic findings also are frequently misinterpreted as supporting a diagnosis of bronchopneumonia or bronchogenic carcinoma. Other confusing radiographic appearances of active tuberculosis in the elderly have been upper-lobe scarring and apical pleural reaction, which often are misread as inactive disease [178], and midlung or basal infiltrates [196, 218, 219]. Miliary disease and many of the forms of extrapulmonary tuberculosis are more frequent in the elderly than in younger patients, and the mortality is higher in the elderly.

IX. **Tuberculosis in pregnancy** poses special problems. It is current opinion that pregnancy does not increase the risk for active tuberculosis, alter the manifestations of infection, change the outcome from clinical infection, or change the response to chemotherapy; in turn, tuberculosis does not alter the course of the pregnancy or its outcome [220, 221]. Thus, tuberculosis during pregnancy is not an indication for therapeutic abortion. Congenital tuberculosis is possible, however, when the placenta is infected. Nonetheless, most neonates with tuberculosis acquire their infection in the postpartum period from an adult with undiagnosed disease.

Skin testing is the mainstay of screening during pregnancy because of the need to avoid radiographic studies. Pregnancy does not significantly alter the skin-test response to tuberculin, and tuberculin is safe during gestation [220, 221]. A chest radiograph with appropriate shielding is indicated if the skin test is positive. Considerations about preventive therapy and drug treatment will be discussed in sec. **X.**

X. **Antituberculous therapy.** Treatment of tuberculosis is an area of ongoing investigation, the goal being to reduce the duration of therapy while retaining effectiveness, preventing relapse, overcoming drug resistance, minimizing toxicity, and maximizing patient acceptance. The current recommendations and basic principles of antituberculous therapy will be reviewed briefly [222, 222a]. These recommendations are based on the observations that certain combinations of agents given for shorter periods of time are as effective as older regimens, intermittent dosing is an effective alternative to daily therapy, and **directly observed therapy is important to achieve compliance** and reduce the risk of developing drug resistance.

A. **Mutations causing resistance to antituberculous agents are infrequent,** and they are unlinked phenomena [223, 224]. The rate of resistance is approximately 1 in 10^6 organisms for isoniazid (INH) and 1 in 10^8 organisms for rifampin, so that spontaneous resistance to both drugs is only 1 in 10^{14} organisms [223]. This explains, in part, the efficacy of combination regimens. Resistance rates are 1 in 10^4 organisms for ethambutol and 1 in 10^6 organisms for streptomycin [223]. **Multidrug resistance technically refers to organisms resistant to two or more first-line agents** but is more commonly used to mean resistance to both INH and rifampin (see sec. **B.1**).

   1. **Factors favoring the development of resistance** include the use of a single agent to treat active infection, erratic compliance with proper therapy, suboptimal drug dosing, malabsorption of drugs, or the failure to include enough active agents for partially resistant organisms [223].

   2. **Detecting resistance** traditionally depends on the use of solid media and takes many weeks. With such a system, resistance is defined as the growth on drug-containing media of 1% or more of the number of organisms growing on control media [178]. The BACTEC system may be used to speed up the process [171, 189]. Although we are beginning to understand the genetics of resistance [224–226], there are no available PCR or other nucleic acid–based methods for the rapid detection of resistance.

      A newer technique still being developed relies on a luciferase gene used as a reporter and inserted into a mycobacteriophage [227]. *M. tuberculosis* cells are infected with the mycobacteriophage, and resistance is detected when light is produced in the presence of the test drug. Such a luciferase reporter mycobacteriophage assay may be able to provide results within hours or a few days [171, 227].

B. **Multiple-drug-resistant (MDR) tuberculosis is increasing in the United States** [228–231a].

   1. **Definitions.** MDR *M. tuberculosis* is caused by a strain that is resistant to two or more antituberculous drugs. Many investigators require that the strain be resistant to isoniazid and rifampin to qualify for MDR status. In **primary resistance,** the patient from whom the isolate is obtained has never received any of the antituberculous drugs involved. In **secondary resistance,** the patient

has been treated for tuberculosis with the specific drug(s) to which the isolate was resistant. Some investigators have proposed a new term, *transmitted drug resistance,* to refer to the recovery of resistant strains from patients who are infected by contact with high-risk individuals who are known to be shedding drug-resistant strains with a comparable susceptibility pattern [231a].

2. **Epidemiology.** Contributing to the trend toward MDR strains are poor compliance with therapy, homelessness, crowding in jails and other institutions, the HIV epidemic, diminished public health efforts at tuberculosis control, and immigration from areas with high rates of drug resistance (e.g., Southeast Asia). Outbreaks of MDR tuberculosis have occurred in hospitals, prisons, congregate settings (e.g., homeless shelters), and other facilities [174, 228, 231a]. Nosocomial MDR tuberculosis in major urban areas has centered around HIV-infected patients. Mortality has ranged from 43 to 93%, and infections in health care workers have been documented [228]. Failure to identify rapidly those patients who may have tuberculosis, failure to implement isolation procedures promptly, and premature discontinuation of isolation have contributed to these outbreaks [175].

   a. **The most significant predictor** of MDR tuberculosis in all of the early studies was a **history of treatment with antituberculous drugs.** Inadequate therapy remains the most common mechanism by which resistant organisms develop. In the United States, **patients previously exposed to antituberculous medications are presumed to harbor MDR strains of *M. tuberculosis* until proven otherwise** [231a].

   b. Cavitary tuberculosis is another risk factor, presumably because of the greater number of organisms that exist in the cavitary lesions [231a].

3. There is no evidence that patients with MDR tuberculosis are more or less likely to transmit tuberculosis than are patients with drug susceptible strains [231a].

4. **The risk of disease due to *M. tuberculosis* (susceptible and MDR strains) in patients coinfected with HIV is enhanced.** It is estimated that coinfected patients have a 7–10% chance **per year** of developing active tuberculosis, as opposed to a 5–10% risk **per lifetime** for an adult with an intact immune system [231a].

   The lifetime risk of tuberculosis disease is 170 times higher for a patient with AIDS, 113 times higher for an HIV-infected patient, and 3.6–16.0 times higher for a patient immunocompromised by some other condition than for an individual with no known risk factors [231a]. MDR outbreaks have most frequently been described in HIV-positive patients (e.g., in hospital HIV wards, HIV hospice centers, etc.). See related discussion in Chap. 19.

C. **Two or more active antituberculous agents must be used** in order to minimize the risk of treatment failure associated with the selection of resistant organisms. The latest guidelines take into account the increasing prevalence of drug resistance by increasing the number of drugs used for initial therapy [223, 224].

   The choice of agents will depend on the local incidence of drug resistance. A four-drug regimen is used initially for the first 8 weeks of therapy when INH resistance is 4% or greater [223]. An initial regimen containing five or six drugs is recommended in areas where resistance to INH and rifampin or other agents is prevalent [224]. The continuation phase of therapy may involve two bactericidal agents (isoniazid and rifampin) when resistance is not a problem. Recommended treatment regimens are effective for pulmonary and extrapulmonary forms of tuberculosis.

   ***M. tuberculosis* isolates should routinely undergo susceptibility studies to help plan long-term drug regimens.**

   1. **Regimens for initial empiric therapy**

      a. **Four drugs are preferred** [222, 223]. Isoniazid, rifampin, pyrazinamide, and either ethambutol or streptomycin are given for the first 8 weeks.

      b. **Three drugs** may be used when local INH resistance rates are lower than 4% [222, 223], although some believe that resistance rates should be lower than 2% before the three-drug regimen is appropriate [224]. Isoniazid, rifampin, and pyrazinamide are given for the first 8 weeks.

      c. **When resistance to multiple agents is prevalent,** five or six drugs should be used based on the known patterns of susceptibility in the community.

   2. **Options to continue therapy for susceptible organisms** (i.e., organisms susceptible to INH, rifampin, and standard drugs) [222, 223].

      a. Isoniazid and rifampin may be used for the remaining 4 months of a minimum 6-month regimen. See sec. **E.2** for the use of intermittent therapy.

b. Intermittent therapy with the initial four-drug regimen may be used to complete a minimum of 6 months of treatment (see sec. **E.2**).

3. Continuation therapy when susceptibilities are unavailable is based on the clinical response to initial treatment and the probability for resistance. If after 8 weeks the patient is improving but has risk factors for resistance, or the prevalence of INH resistance is 4% or greater, then pyrazinamide may be stopped and ethambutol or streptomycin should be continued with INH and rifampin for the remaining course [223].

4. Treatment for resistant organisms must be individualized. In general, four to six drugs should be used and, initially, patients should be monitored in the hospital [224]. Ofloxacin and ciprofloxacin have proven to be useful adjuncts to oral retreatment regimens, but higher doses are required [224]. **Resistance to both INH and rifampin poses particular difficulties.** A recent review of 171 such cases found that resistance included a median of six drugs, patients required more than 7 months in the hospital, 65% had an initial response to retreatment, and relapses occurred in the follow-up period to bring the final response rate down to only 56% [232].

Consultation with an expert in the therapy of MDR tuberculosis is advised.

5. Use of a single drug. For therapy, a single drug is virtually never indicated. The major problem with single-drug therapy is emergence of resistance, which can occur very rapidly (weeks). The use of a single drug is essentially limited to prophylaxis, which must be distinguished from therapy. Chemoprophylaxis is discussed separately in sec. **XI**.

6. Addition of drugs to an existing regimen. Whenever antituberculous drugs are to be added to a regimen, as when there is concern about an inadequate response or resistant mycobacteria, at least two, and preferably three, new drugs should be added together [224]. The addition of only one drug to a regimen to which resistance has occurred may result in resistance to the new drug as well. Use of two or three new drugs should circumvent this problem. Susceptibility studies are particularly important in these patients.

D. Directly observed therapy (DOT) is optimal for all patients [223, 233, 233a]. It is particularly recommended for patients not adhering to daily self-medication regimens, those receiving intermittent treatment regimens, and for those with INH or rifampin resistance [223]. **DOT requires that a health care worker or other reliable person observe the patient while he or she takes the medications.** This strategy is effective in increasing compliance, increasing treatment completion rates, and reducing the emergence of resistance.

E. Frequency of drug administration

1. Daily therapy was the standard for many years. Oral agents usually are given once daily in the fasting state in the morning.

2. Intermittent therapy may be given 2 or 3 times weekly. Because fewer doses of medications are used, **all patients receiving intermittent regimens must be carefully supervised using DOT to ensure compliance.** This approach may be particularly suited to noncompliant patients, although some have advocated its routine use even in compliant patients [223, 233, 234]. Intermittent regimens decrease the number of doses required for therapy without sacrificing sputum conversion or cure rate [233]. The toxicities of intermittent regimens and daily regimens appear similar. Because fewer doses and less monitoring for efficacy are needed, the cost of these regimens usually is less than that of standard daily therapy [233]. The current recommendations offer three options for the use of intermittent therapy [222, 223].

a. After daily therapy for the first 8 weeks with three or four drugs (see sec. **C.1**), INH and rifampin may be given 2 or 3 times weekly for a minimum of 16 weeks. This regimen is suitable only when isolates are known to be susceptible to both of these drugs.

b. After daily therapy for the first 2 weeks, the four-drug regimen may be given twice weekly for the next 6 weeks. Twice-weekly INH and rifampin may be continued for a minimum of 16 more weeks, when isolates are known to be susceptible to both of these drugs.

c. The four-drug regimen may be given 3 times per week for a minimum of 6 months when isolates are known to be susceptible to INH and rifampin.

F. Duration and type of therapy

1. Short-course regimens. These regimens have replaced traditional longer courses and are regarded as the **treatments of choice for tuberculosis for**

organisms susceptible to INH and rifampin. The success of any regimen of less than 12 months' duration depends on the addition of rifampin to isoniazid and to other drugs as well if intermittent therapy is used. The optimal use of short-course therapy requires familiarity with those situations for which it is **not** suitable (see sec. **2**).

   a. **Six-month therapy.** The American Thoracic Society and the CDC have adopted minimum 6-month regimens as standard therapy for pulmonary tuberculosis in the United States and Canada [222, 223]. This duration also is suggested for most cases of extrapulmonary tuberculosis (see **b**). Treatment is given for a minimum of 6 months and for at least 3 months after sputum cultures become negative.

   b. **Nine-month therapy.** Experience with the 9-month regimen has shown it to be effective for pulmonary and most extrapulmonary tuberculoses [218]. It is used for susceptible organisms when INH and rifampin must be given alone or without the initial use of pyrazinamide.

2. **Exceptions. Standard regimens should not be used in the following circumstances:**

   a. **Suspected or proved isoniazid resistance.** This may include patients from countries with a high incidence of primary isoniazid resistance, those failing standard therapy, those who relapse after taking isoniazid without rifampin, and those who were close contacts of a patient with documented isoniazid-resistant tuberculosis [222].

   b. **When rifampin is not used.** An older regimen should be chosen for these patients when isolates are susceptible (see sec. **4**).

   c. **When isoniazid is not used.** Rifampin plus ethambutol for a minimum of 12 months is recommended for susceptible organisms [222].

   d. **When neither isoniazid nor rifampin is used.** Three or four drugs to which the organism is susceptible may be required for 18 months.

   e. **In the presence of significant hepatic disease.** In such a case, ethambutol plus either isoniazid or rifampin may be chosen. However, studies to date indicate minimal additive hepatic toxicity when patients with lesser degrees of liver disease are treated with isoniazid plus rifampin [222].

   f. **With severe renal insufficiency.** Measurement of blood levels of isoniazid or ethambutol may be required in patients with severe renal insufficiency [222]. Pyrazinamide is not recommended in such patients. Drugs to be avoided in patients with any impairment of renal function include streptomycin, kanamycin, capreomycin, and cycloserine.

   g. **When symptoms persist or sputum smears or cultures remain positive after 2 months of therapy.** This is an indication of treatment failure, and patients should be assessed for compliance and the presence of drug resistance. Expert consultation is advised [222].

   h. **When severe illness, miliary tuberculosis, tuberculous osteomyelitis, or lymphadenitis are present.** In the event that any of these is being treated, treatment often is extended to a minimum of 9–12 months [222, 223]. However, a recent evaluation of lymph node tuberculosis found that treatment for 6 months was as efficacious as treatment for 9 months [235]. Infants and children with miliary, bone and joint, or meningeal tuberculosis should be treated for at least 12 months [236]. Infectious disease consultation is advised.

   i. In **immunosuppressed patients.** These patients may receive any of the preceding options for initial and follow-up therapy, including intermittent regimens [223]. However, the **duration of therapy must be determined by the individual response to treatment [223]. In general, treatment should be given for a minimum of 9 months and for at least 6 months after sputum conversion** [223]. See Chap. 19 for therapy for HIV-infected patients.

3. **MDR tuberculosis** is treated for longer periods, depending on the extent of resistance and the clinical response. Some suggested regimens for various patterns of resistance have been published [224]. It may be necessary in some cases to continue therapy for 24 months after the last positive sputum culture was obtained [232].

4. **Older (traditional) regimens.** Combinations were used for susceptible organisms before the advent of the short-course regimens just outlined, but the combinations must be used for longer periods of time. Previously, traditional therapy consisted of isoniazid and ethambutol given for 18 months; streptomycin was added for the first 1–2 months. Isoniazid and streptomycin given for

the full 18 months of treatment is an acceptable alternative but is potentially more toxic and requires many injections. Either of these regimens may be administered daily or twice weekly.

5. **Pregnancy.** The 9-month regimen should be chosen to treat tuberculosis in a pregnant patient, and ethambutol is added initially to INH and rifampin. Pyridoxine should be given with any isoniazid-containing regimen. Pyrazinamide is not advised for use during pregnancy because its teratogenic potential is undefined [222, 223]. Streptomycin has documented harmful effects on the fetus and should not be used (see Chap. 28H). Kanamycin, capreomycin, cycloserine, and ethionamide should also be avoided because of their potential risk to the fetus [222]. Breast-feeding is permissible during treatment of tuberculosis. In addition, steps should be taken to prevent and detect transmission of maternal tuberculosis to the neonate [220–222].

G. **Infection control aspects.** Transmission of *M. tuberculosis* is a recognized risk to patients and health care workers (HCWs) in health care facilities. Transmission is most likely to occur from patients who have unrecognized or laryngeal tuberculosis, are not on effective antituberculous therapy, and have not been placed in tubercular (respiratory) isolation. Patients who have MDR tuberculosis can remain infectious for prolonged periods, which increases the risk for nosocomial and/or occupational transmission of *M. tuberculosis,* especially to HIV-infected patients or HCWs [236].

1. **Guidelines for preventing the transmission of *M. tuberculosis* in health care facilities** have recently been reviewed and discussed in detail elsewhere [236].

   Implementation of a tuberculosis infection-control program requires (1) risk assessment and development of a tuberculosis infection plan; (2) early identification, treatment, and isolation of infectious patients; (3) effective engineering controls (e.g., to provide negative airflow for respiratory isolation); (4) an appropriate respiratory protection program; (5) HCW tuberculosis training, education, counseling, and screening; and (6) evaluation of the program's effectiveness [236].

2. **Duration of isolation** [236]
   a. Isolation can be discontinued if the diagnosis of TB can be ruled out.
   b. The length of time required for a patient to become noninfectious after starting antituberculous therapy varies considerably. Isolation should be discontinued only when the patient is on effective therapy, is improving clinically, and has had three consecutive negative sputum smears collected on three separate days [236].

H. **Specific agents** [222, 222a]

1. **Isoniazid** remains the single most important antituberculous agent. It is bactericidal and penetrates tissue well, including the CNS. It is metabolized primarily by the liver. Doses are not reduced in patients with renal dysfunction, except in advanced renal failure when dosing may be guided by monitoring serum levels.

   a. **Dosage.** The usual adult dosage is 5 mg/kg up to 300 mg PO given once daily. An intramuscular form is available. In life-threatening disease (e.g., meningitis or miliary disease), dosages of 10 mg/kg/day (up to 600 mg/day) often are recommended. The usual dosage in children is 10 mg/kg/day (300-mg maximum), although higher doses in meningitis may be used.

      Doses for both the 2- and 3-times-weekly regimens are 15 mg/kg for adults and 20–40 mg/kg for children, up to a maximum of 900 mg [222].

   b. **Side effects**
      (1) **Hepatitis.** The major side effect is isoniazid-related hepatitis. Ten percent or more of patients on isoniazid will have transaminase elevations, but only approximately 1% overall will have significant hepatitis (deaths have been reported). Which patients will develop progressive hepatotoxicity is somewhat unpredictable, but serial SGOT levels greater than 5 times normal may correlate. Alcoholics and older patients are at risk for the development of hepatitis. It is rarely seen in patients younger than 30 years but is reported in more than 2% of patients older than 50 years [237]. There is no increased risk of hepatitis for most patients when isoniazid and rifampin are used together [238], as is discussed in sec. **2.**

      Any patient on isoniazid should be warned about the symptoms of hepatitis. Liver function tests should be obtained when suggestive symptoms occur and the drug discontinued if hepatitis is present. Whether routine serial liver function tests should be monitored is unclear. Most experts advocate testing only symptomatic patients and those with abnormal tests prior to the start of therapy. Isoniazid should be stopped if the patient develops symptoms or jaundice or if the transaminases are more than 5 times normal in the absence of symptoms [237].

Mild hepatic dysfunction (e.g., alcoholism) does not preclude the use of isoniazid (and rifampin), although serial monitoring is suggested. Elevations of the SGOT or SGPT to 3–5 times normal should lead to reassessment of the regimens. If baseline SGOT or SGPT is 6–8 times the normal level, isoniazid (and rifampin) should be avoided.

  (2) Neurologic toxicity can occur but is uncommon at the usual isoniazid dose of 5 mg/kg [222]. The peripheral neuropathies usually can be prevented by the concomitant administration of pyridoxine, 10–25 mg/day. After an isoniazid-induced neuropathy has occurred, pyridoxine, 50–100 mg/day, can be used as treatment. Thus, the routine prophylactic use of pyridoxine with isoniazid should be reserved for patients predisposed to neurologic toxicity because of higher INH doses, pregnancy, diabetes, uremia, alcoholism, malnutrition, or prior seizures [222]. Rarely, seizures, optic neuritis, encephalopathies, and the hand-shoulder syndrome may occur.

  (3) Hypersensitivity reactions with fever, rash, and rheumatoid syndromes can occur. Positive antinuclear antibodies and lupus erythematosus cell preparations may be seen.

  (4) Concomitant phenytoin use. Doses of phenytoin may have to be reduced when isoniazid is used, as isoniazid delays renal clearance of phenytoin sodium. Drug levels of phenytoin should be measured and doses adjusted as needed [222].

2. Rifampin has excellent in vitro and in vivo activity against *M. tuberculosis*. It is a bactericidal agent against this mycobacterium, and it penetrates tissues well, including the CNS. The spectrum of activity, pharmacokinetics, and adverse reactions are discussed in detail in Chap. 28Q; the reader is referred to this discussion.

  a. Dosages

    (1) The usual daily adult dosage is 10 mg/kg up to 600 mg once daily (two 300-mg tablets), 1 hour before or 2 hours after meals. In children, the daily dose is 10–20 mg/kg/day, not to exceed 600 mg/day. The same doses are used in the intermittent regimens.

      Patients should be warned in advance that their urine, tears, sweat, and saliva may have a red-orange, harmless discoloration; soft contact lenses may become permanently discolored [222]. (Rifampin is red-orange in the crystalline state.) In renal failure, the dose is not reduced.

    (2) Fixed-dose combinations. A combination of rifampin 120 mg, isoniazid 50 mg, and pyrazinamide 300 mg (Rifater; Marion Merrell Dow, Kansas City, MO) was recently approved by the FDA for the initial 2 months of daily tuberculosis therapy. The dosage is 4 tablets each day for patients weighing 44 kg or less, 5 tablets for patients 45–54 kg, and 6 tablets for patients weighing 55 kg or more. By simplifying compliance and preventing errors in self-administration, rifater may decrease acquired drug resistance during unsupervised therapy. Rifamate (rifampin 300 mg and isoniazid 150 mg; Marion Merrell Dow) has been licensed in the United States since 1975. The combined formulations are more expensive than the individual drugs purchased separately [222a].

  b. Adverse reactions. These are discussed in detail in Chap. 28Q, under Rifampin and will only be listed in brief here: They are (1) hepatotoxicity, which is the major concern; (2) adverse drug interactions with a variety of agents [239]; (3) immunologic reactions, including hypersensitivity reactions and a flulike illness with sporadic use; (4) renal failure, thrombocytopenia, and hemolysis, which can occur rarely; and (5) more frequent conversion of the skin test to negative.

  c. Role of rifampin. The **potential for hepatotoxicity** deserves special comment. Rifampin can cause mild liver function abnormalities and, at times, severe hepatitis. Nonetheless, accumulated experience has shown no increased hepatotoxicity from using isoniazid and rifampin together in most patients, including alcoholics without prior clinically significant liver dysfunction [238]. Risk probably is increased, however, in patients with preexisting liver disease of any cause.

If hepatitis develops in patients on isoniazid and rifampin, both agents must be stopped. A primarily cholestatic pattern is most likely caused by rifampin, whereas either drug may cause transaminase elevations.

3. **Ethambutol** is an oral agent that penetrates tissue well, except the CNS (even when the meninges are inflamed). Ethambutol is bacteriostatic against *M. tuberculosis.*

   a. **Dosages.** Tablets are available in 100-mg and 400-mg strengths. In prolonged therapy, 15 mg/kg/day to a maximum of 2.5 g, given once daily, usually is recommended. Some authorities use 25 mg/kg/day for no longer than the first 2 months of therapy and then reduce the dose to 15 mg/kg/day. The dose given twice weekly is 50 mg/kg and that for 3 times per week is 25–30 mg/kg, up to a maximum of 2.5 g [223].

   Because ethambutol is excreted by the kidney, doses must be reduced in renal failure. Precise guidelines are not available, but each dose may be reduced [240] or the interval between doses prolonged [241] or, ideally, serum drug levels may be monitored (levels available from the manufacturer).

   b. **Side effects.** Ethambutol can cause optic neuritis. The first manifestation may be loss of color vision. Thus, ethambutol should be avoided when possible in children too young to assess color discrimination ($<$6 years old) [223]. This appears to be dose-related and rarely occurs when the 15-mg/kg/day dose regimen is used. Hypersensitivity reactions, hyperuricemia, and GI intolerance can occur.

4. **Streptomycin** is a parenteral agent still used in some triple-drug regimens. It is bactericidal at an alkaline pH but, like other aminoglycosides, it provides only fair penetration into the CNS.

   a. **Dosages.** The average dose is 15 mg/kg for adults and 20–30 mg/kg for children, up to 1 g/day IM; 10 mg/kg up to a maximum of 500–750 mg/day is used for patients older than 60 years. Intermittent doses for children and adults are 25–30 mg/kg up to a maximum of 1.5 g for both twice-weekly and thrice-weekly regimens [222]. Attempts should be made to keep the total amount administered to less than 120 g [222]. Doses should be reduced in renal failure, usually by prolonging the dose interval [241]. The drug should be used with caution and in reduced doses in patients older than 60 years [222].

   b. **Side effects.** Hypersensitivity reactions can occur. Renal toxicity is less common than with other aminoglycosides, but ototoxicity may occur. (See Chap. 28H.)

5. **Pyrazinamide** has been studied in both initial therapy and retreatment regimens. It is bactericidal and works well in an acid environment and intracellularly [222].

   a. **Dosages.** Pyrazinamide is well absorbed orally and penetrates the CNS when the meninges are inflamed. The usual daily dosage is 15–30 mg/kg/day, up to a maximum of 2 g/day. Intermittent doses for children and adults are 50–70 mg/kg up to a maximum of 4 g for a twice-weekly regimen and up to a maximum of 3 g for use 3 times weekly [223].

   b. **Toxicity.** Hepatotoxicity can occur, but serial liver function tests should be monitored only in high-risk patients (see sec. **2.c**) or during long-term therapy. Pyrazinamide does not significantly increase the risk for hepatotoxicity when used for the first 2 months in short-course regimens [222]. In patients with preexisting liver disease, this agent should be avoided when possible (see discussion of isoniazid, sec. **1**). Hyperuricemia is common and may be used as an indication of compliance; acute gout is uncommon [222].

6. **Second-line drugs.** Paraaminosalicylic acid (PAS), cycloserine, ethionamide, capreomycin, kanamycin, and amikacin are all useful drugs under appropriate circumstances [222]. Some of these are particularly useful in resistant forms of tuberculosis. These agents also are used in treating atypical mycobacterial infections. Because side effects are common, the reader is advised to seek consultation before using these agents.

I. Therapy for specific problems. For complicated problems or in the case of a physician with little prior experience with tuberculosis, pulmonary or infectious disease consultation (or both) is advisable.

1. Pulmonary tuberculosis. Based on recent extensive studies, short-course chemotherapy now is generally recommended (for susceptible strains) unless a special exception exists (see sec. **F**).

    a. After the initial phase of daily four-drug therapy (see sec. **C.1**), isoniazid and rifampin (with or without other drugs) are continued for at least a total of 6 months.

    b. Either a daily or an intermittent regimen may be used. The twice-weekly regimen is particularly useful in patients who require supervision to ensure compliance (e.g., alcoholic, senile, and other unreliable patients) (see sec. **E.2**). Compliance is extremely important if the patient is going to follow either the daily or the twice-weekly regimens on his or her own. **Other antituberculous agents cannot be substituted for either isoniazid or rifampin in the standard regimens.**

    c. Smear-negative, culture-negative pulmonary tuberculosis poses special problems in management [242–244]. Patients with such disease present with clinical and radiographic tuberculosis and a positive PPD skin test but negative smears and cultures despite appropriate diagnostic efforts (e.g., bronchoscopy). Although their mycobacterial burden is low, these patients, if untreated, have a high rate of disease progression over the ensuing 5 years [242–244]. The role of PCR studies of sputum in these patients remains unclear and awaits further study.

        The results of two recent studies done in different parts of the world strongly support the notion that these patients benefit from treatment and that 4 months of therapy may be all that is necessary when drug resistance is not a concern [242–244]. We suggest that patients suspected of having active pulmonary tuberculosis despite negative smears be started on a standard therapy while awaiting culture results [242]. If cultures are negative, the patient is compliant, there is a good clinical response, and there is no concern about drug resistance, then it is appropriate to continue isoniazid and rifampin for a total of 4 months of therapy [222, 242–244].

2. Extrapulmonary disease. Most large studies of extrapulmonary disease were conducted prior to the availability of the newer antituberculous drugs. In many series, patients received three drugs and were treated for 2 years.

    Based on recent reviews, most experts now believe that extrapulmonary tuberculosis due to susceptible organisms can be treated in the same way as pulmonary tuberculosis if isoniazid and rifampin can be used [222, 223]. (If alternate drugs must be used, expert consultation is advised.) Extrapulmonary sites usually contain smaller numbers of bacilli than do pulmonary sites, and isoniazid and rifampin penetrate these sites well. Therefore, short-course regimens appear to be acceptable practice for extrapulmonary disease. The exceptions may be tuberculous osteomyelitis and extrapulmonary disease in immunosuppressed hosts; whether lymphadenitis requires longer therapy is unclear [223, 235]. The authors emphasize the following:

    a. CNS (tuberculous meningitis). Isoniazid, often at twice the usual dose, and rifampin are drugs that penetrate the inflamed meninges. For the first 2 months of four-drug therapy, pyrazinamide probably is preferable to streptomycin as pyrazinamide better penetrates the CNS. Although a total of 6–9 months of therapy may be adequate for adults, infants and children should be treated for 12 months [222, 236]. Infectious disease consultation is advised for determining the optimal total duration of therapy for this difficult problem (see Chap. 5).

    b. Disseminated and miliary disease presumably involves a failure of host defenses (see sec. **V.D**). Therefore, a conservative approach may be to rely on a 9-month course for adults and a 12-month course for infants and children that includes isoniazid and rifampin if the patient is responding well and the organism is susceptible. Infectious disease consultation is advised.

    c. Tuberculous osteomyelitis may be particularly difficult to eradicate [222, 223]. More prolonged courses of therapy may be indicated, and infectious disease consultation is advised. **Lymphadenitis** may respond to standard therapy [235].

   d. HIV infection should be considered in any patient presenting with extrapulmonary tuberculosis (see Chap. 19).
3. **Drug-resistant cases.** Drug resistance should be suspected in patients who relapse after receiving a regimen not containing both isoniazid and rifampin [222]. At least two, and preferably three, new agents should be used, pending the results of susceptibility tests. If isolated isoniazid resistance is found after beginning the standard four-drug regimen, then isoniazid should be discontinued and ethambutol, rifampin, and pyrazinamide continued for a minimum of 6 months [222]. If pyrazinamide has not been used, then ethambutol plus rifampin for a minimum of 12 months is recommended [222]. Relapses that follow isoniazid with rifampin in short-course therapy for susceptible organisms often are caused by susceptible organisms and are retreated using the same regimen [222]. Complicating the decision regarding treatment options is evidence that reinfection may occur, particularly in immunosuppressed patients [245, 246]. Treatment of patients who are close contacts of persons with proven drug-resistant tuberculosis, those who contracted the disease in countries with a high incidence of drug resistance, and those who fail therapy is best guided by the results of susceptibility tests. At least two active drugs must be given, and the total duration of therapy must be individualized [222, 224]. Some patients with MDR tuberculosis benefit from the addition of surgery [224, 232].
4. **HIV-infected patients.** Therapy for tuberculosis should be started whenever acid-fast bacilli are found in patients with HIV infections, because it is impossible to distinguish between *M. tuberculosis* and *M. avium-intracellulare* organisms without cultures. The use of rifampin will increase the methadone dose needed to prevent withdrawal symptoms in patients on methadone maintenance. **See Chap. 19 for a further discussion of this problem.**
5. **Tuberculosis in pregnancy.** The risks from active tuberculosis during pregnancy to the mother and fetus far outweigh the risks from chemotherapy. Isoniazid, rifampin, and ethambutol cross the placenta but have not been shown to be teratogenic [222]. Pyrazinamide, streptomycin, kanamycin, capreomycin, cycloserine, and ethionamide should be avoided because of documented or potential fetal risk. See important related discussion in sec. **F.5.**
6. **Tuberculosis in children.** Following the principles in adult therapy, short-course therapy has been recommended for use in children [222, 223].
7. **Therapy in renal failure.** Antituberculous medications cleared by the kidney include streptomycin, kanamycin, capreomycin, ethambutol, and cycloserine. If one needs to use these drugs, blood levels should be monitored.
J. **Miscellaneous issues related to therapy**
1. **Corticosteroids** have been used in tuberculous meningitis, peritonitis, pleuritis, and pericarditis, and in patients with adrenal insufficiency [247]. These drugs have also been given to severely toxic patients with disseminated tuberculosis, including those with concomitant HIV infection. Their precise role remains **controversial,** and consultation about their use in individual cases is suggested.
2. **Hospitalization may be necessary** for diagnostic evaluation and initiation of therapy, particularly for patients with severe disease or suspected drug resistance. Usually, uncomplicated pulmonary disease can be managed entirely as an outpatient problem because the patient probably has already exposed anyone in his or her immediate environment. Proper instructions about coughing into a tissue can be given to the compliant patient. Hospitalization is necessary in severe drug reactions, life-threatening infections, coexisting illnesses requiring hospitalization, and the rare social circumstance in which there is a special threat to the community.
   After 2 weeks of appropriate therapy, sputum infectivity is no longer apparent in most patients with susceptible organisms (see sec. **G** for a discussion of the duration of isolation).
3. **Follow-up cultures.** Guidelines for follow-up often are available from state or county health departments. Usually sputum smears and cultures are done monthly until three specimens are negative. Cultures can then be monitored at 2- to 3-month intervals during therapy and at 6 months (and perhaps 12 months) after completion of the 6-month regimen. Patients successfully completing a standard regimen of isoniazid and rifampin for susceptible organisms do not need routine follow-up [222].

4. **Follow-up roentgenograms.** A repeat chest roentgenogram after 2–3 months of therapy can be helpful to assess response to treatment. More frequent films may be needed to follow adequately patients whose initial sputum smears were negative. In addition, a film taken at completion of therapy provides a useful baseline for future comparison. Obtaining routine annual x-ray films is not recommended for patients who remain well. If there is a clinical suspicion of disease reactivation, then repeat roentgenography is indicated.

5. **Public health follow-up.** The local public health department should be involved in the screening of contacts of index cases, arrangements for DOT, and follow-up of discharged patients.

XI. **Chemoprophylaxis with isoniazid** is considered in patients with a positive intermediate PPD but without active disease that would require double- or triple-drug therapy. Isoniazid is the only carefully studied drug proven to be effective for prophylaxis. The positive skin test without active disease is interpreted to mean that a few dormant, but viable, bacilli are present with the potential for reactivation. There are certain settings in which the risk for reactivation is significant, as in recent PPD converters, children and adolescents with positive skin tests, immunologically impaired hosts, and patients with a history of tuberculosis that was inadequately treated by current standards [186, 222].

Only the basic concepts of isoniazid chemoprophylaxis are summarized here. The detailed recommendations for isoniazid chemoprophylaxis are published elsewhere [186, 222]. **An excellent summary of this topic is given in reference [171a].**

A. **Isoniazid-related hepatitis.** Before one initiates chemoprophylaxis with isoniazid, the potential risks of isoniazid-related hepatitis must be considered [see sec. **X.H.1.b.(1)**]. Hepatotoxicity is rare in patients younger than 20 years. The observed frequency in other age groups is as follows: ages 20–34, up to 0.3%; 35–49, up to 1.2%; 50 years and older, up to 2.3% [222]. Primarily because of this age-related risk of hepatitis, prophylaxis has not been recommended after the age of 35 unless other factors indicate a high risk of developing active tuberculosis (see sec. **B.5**).

Patients with currently active liver disease or a documented history of isoniazid-related hepatotoxicity should not be given preventive therapy with isoniazid [222].

B. **Current recommendations call for isoniazid preventive therapy** in the following populations regardless of age [186, 222]:

1. **Certain household members and other close associates of persons with potentially infectious tuberculosis**
   a. **Contacts** should be examined. Those with evidence of active disease will need therapy (e.g., short-course therapy) rather than simply chemoprophylaxis with isoniazid.
   b. **Contacts** without active disease should have intermediate PPD skin tests.
      (1) **Positive reactors.** Patients **with reactions of 5 mm or more** of induration should receive isoniazid because they must be assumed to have recently acquired their *M. tuberculosis* infection.
      (2) **Negative reactors. Because the risk of infection is especially high in children,** administration of isoniazid is recommended for 3 months in child contacts with a negative PPD test, and a repeat skin test should be performed at that time. If the test is positive when repeated, a full course of isoniazid is recommended. If the test is negative on follow-up, isoniazid usually is discontinued unless the person remains exposed to a contagious source.

      In adults, the approach is individualized. If the skin test initially is negative, the significance of the exposure (e.g., infectiousness of the index case) must be weighed against the risk of isoniazid therapy [186, 248]. If chemoprophylaxis is not used, the PPD test should be repeated in 3 months and, if positive, a full course of isoniazid chemoprophylaxis is indicated.

2. **Positive tuberculin skin test reactors** (skin test ≥5 mm) **with abnormalities on the chest roentgenogram** consistent with nonprogressive tuberculous disease (excluding calcified granulomas as the sole abnormality). Presuming there are no positive bacteriologic findings and no risk for isoniazid resistance (negative history of prophylaxis), treatment with isoniazid plus rifampin for 6 months is a possible approach. This is controversial in patients older than 35 years [248]. (See sec. **X.I.1.c** on p. 331.)

3. **Skin test converters** (i.e., ≥10-mm increase if younger than 35 years of age; ≥15-mm increase if 35 years or older). In the event that skin test conversion has been well documented within the last 2 years (implying recent infection) and if no clinical disease is obvious, prophylaxis is given for 6–12 months [186]. This approach is taken because of the high frequency of disease that occurs after documented skin test conversion. Approximately 5% of converters may develop active disease within the first year after conversion, a fact that outweighs the risk of potential isoniazid hepatitis. The booster effect must be considered (see sec. **III.D**).

4. **Tuberculin reactors in special situations.** In general, persons with a positive PPD test who are in the following groups should be considered for preventive therapy because they are at increased risk of developing tuberculosis (see secs. **III.C** and **G** for a complete list of risk factors) [186, 222]:

   a. **Patients on immunosuppressive therapy,** including high-dose corticosteroids (equivalent to >15 mg prednisone daily) for longer than 2–3 weeks with skin test ≥10 mm.

   b. **Patients with certain underlying diseases** (with skin tests >10 mm) that increase the risk for tuberculosis (see sec. **III.C**), including lymphoproliferative disorders, diabetes mellitus, end-stage renal failure, and silicosis. However, 4 months of isoniazid plus rifampin is preferred for patients with silicosis [222].

   c. **Postgastrectomy patients,** after intestinal bypass surgery for obesity, and any circumstance associated with prolonged malnourishment or rapid weight loss (with skin test ≥10 mm).

   d. **HIV-infected patients and those with risk factors for HIV infection before their status is known** (≥5 mm; see sec. **III.C**).

   e. **Intravenous drug users.** This population had a high incidence of tuberculosis even before the HIV epidemic. HIV infection further increases the risk for clinical tuberculosis and is rapidly spreading among intravenous drug users. Thus, isoniazid chemoprophylaxis currently is recommended for all HIV-seronegative intravenous drug users with 10 mm or more of induration to an intermediate PPD skin test, regardless of age.

   f. **Staff of long-term care facilities** (e.g., prisons, nursing homes, mental institutions). These persons also may benefit from prophylaxis regardless of age because of the potential spread of tuberculosis within the institution [222, 249].

5. **Other positive reactors.** If no recent skin-test results are known and a routine intermediate PPD test is positive (see sec. **III.C** for interpretation of the PPD based on risk factors), the following guidelines apply:

   a. Preventive therapy is mandatory in positive reactors through the age of 5 years [186, 222].

   b. The official recommendation is isoniazid for all patients younger than 35 years with or without other risk factors. For this age group, a 6- to 12-month course of chemotherapy is indicated whether or not there are other risk factors [186].

   c. For those older than 35 years, the potential benefit must be weighed against the risks of isoniazid-related hepatitis, but routine prophylaxis is not recommended.

C. **Preventive dosages.** Isoniazid is given orally once daily. In children, 10 mg/kg/day (maximum, 300 mg) is recommended. In adults, the usual daily dose is 300 mg isoniazid given for 6–12 months [186, 222]. Children should be treated for 9 months [222]. Pyridoxine (10 mg/day) may be given simultaneously to selected patients (see sec. **X.H.1**). **Twelve months of continuous INH therapy is used for persons with HIV infection or who are immunocompromised and for persons with stable abnormal chest radiographs consistent with past tuberculosis. Six months of continuous therapy appears effective in other groups** [186]. A twice-weekly, higher-dose (15 mg/kg/dose up to 900 mg), DOT regimen for 6–12 months is helpful in high-risk individuals [186].

Studies suggest that 6–12 months of preventive isoniazid therapy reduces the risk of subsequent infection up to 50–80% [222], and the effect persists for at least 20 years.

D. **Monitoring patients**

1. **Patients should be cautioned about the symptoms of hepatitis** (anorexia, malaise, jaundice, etc.) **and the need for medical evaluation if these symptoms**

develop. This is especially important in patients older than 35 years and in those who drink alcoholic beverages daily.

2. Liver function tests should be checked in patients with hepatitis-like symptoms.
3. Whether routine serial monitoring should be performed in all patients on preventive therapy is still unclear. Current guidelines recommend checking transaminase levels monthly in patients older than 35 years, and suggest that the drug be discontinued if levels in excess of 5 to 6 times normal occur [222]. This may be particularly true for those with a history of liver disease, pregnancy, daily alcohol use, and substance abuse, as well as for black and Hispanic women [222].

E. **Chemoprophylaxis for isoniazid-resistant organisms** is unclear. One recommendation is rifampin in standard doses for 12 months, if rifampin resistance is unlikely [222]. Prophylaxis decisions for MDR organisms have been outlined [236, 250]. Preventive treatment with at least two drugs is recommended for patients at high risk of developing infection; 6–12 months is suggested in the absence of more definitive data [250].

In a 1995 Medical Letter summary, it was suggested that tuberculin-positive persons exposed to patients infected with organisms resistant only to INH should be treated with rifampin (600 mg daily) with or without ethambutol for 6–12 months. For those with a known exposure to MDR tuberculosis, pyrazinamide (25–30 mg/kg/day) administered concurrently with ethambutol (15–25 mg/kg/day), ofloxacin (400 mg bid), or ciprofloxacin (750 mg bid) may be effective [222a].

F. **BCG vaccine.** The precise role and efficacy of the BCG vaccine remains controversial. In the United States and Canada, BCG has very limited usefulness because most cases of tuberculosis represent reactivation of old infections. It is considered only for children with negative skin tests who are repeatedly exposed to infectious cases of tuberculosis [222]. BCG is contraindicated in AIDS patients, other immunosuppressed hosts, and pregnant women [222].

Arguments against the use of BCG have been the inability, at least temporarily, to follow PPD skin test status and perhaps a false sense of security for health care workers if they received BCG. This topic has recently been reviewed elsewhere [250a].

XII. **Atypical mycobacteria.** The atypical mycobacteria are less virulent than *M. tuberculosis.* Before the 1950s, they usually were considered to be saprophytes. However, they can produce disease. Their importance has been highlighted by the frequent occurrence of *M. avium-intracellulare* infections in patients with AIDS (see Chap. 19).

It often is difficult for the clinician to determine whether the isolation of these mycobacteria is clinically significant. More detailed reviews of infections due to these organisms have been published elsewhere [251–255]. A few general points warrant emphasis.

A. **Incidence.** Approximately 2–10% of all mycobacterial infections in the United States are due to the atypical mycobacteria. A higher incidence may be observed in patients with malignancy and in AIDS patients (see Chap. 19).

B. **Classification.** Special bacteriologic methods have been established to identify and classify (e.g., Runyon group) these mycobacteria. The tests should be performed in reference laboratories or laboratories that are very familiar with these identification procedures.

From a clinical standpoint, the organisms can be classified according to their virulence. They include bacilli that are:

1. **Pathogenic** (e.g., *M. bovis, M. leprae* [the cause of leprosy], and *M. ulcerans*).
2. **Usually pathogenic** (e.g., *M. marinum [M. balnei], M. kansasii,* and *M. avium-intracellulare* [Battey]).
3. **Sometimes pathogenic** (e.g., *M. scrofulaceum, M. fortuitum,* and *M. chelonae*).
4. **Usually nonpathogenic** (e.g., *M. xenopi* and *M. gordonae*).
5. **Nonpathogenic** (e.g., *M. gastri, M. terrae,* and *M. smegmatis*).

C. **Epidemiology and pathogenesis**

1. **Sources.** The precise sources of these organisms are unclear but the pathogenic forms have been cultured from the environment (e.g., soil, dust, animals, aerosols from sea water).
2. **Transmission. Person-to-person spread does not occur.** With known disease, patients do not require special isolation procedures when hospitalized. Humans presumably acquire disease by inhalation or aspiration, which leads to pulmonary disease; local inoculation, which causes skin or subcutaneous infections; and, presumably, mucosal entry with cervical adenitis.

D. Diagnosis can be difficult because the special cultures and identification procedures take time (weeks) and, as stated previously, it sometimes is difficult to determine whether these organisms are merely saprophytes or true pathogens.

1. **Skin tests.** Antigens similar to the PPD have been prepared for some of the species but are not readily available. There is considerable cross-reactivity among the species, however. Most experts believe that the skin tests are useful in epidemiologic studies only and that they are **not useful in the individual patient.**

2. **Acid-fast smears.** One cannot reliably distinguish *M. tuberculosis* from the atypical mycobacteria; nor can one identify the atypicals by smear characteristics.

3. ***Mycobacterium* cultures.** These should be performed as discussed in Chap. 25.

4. **Serologic tests.** These are not available.

5. **Criteria.** Criteria for the diagnosis of true infection by mycobacteria have been suggested and include the following:

   a. **Repeated isolation** of a potentially pathogenic species. This is particularly important in sputum samples. From tissue (e.g., lymph node), one culture is usually sufficient.

   b. **Absence of other pathogens.**

   c. **A compatible clinical, radiologic, or pathologic picture.**

E. Clinical syndromes. These are briefly summarized to alert the physician to the variety of possible clinical presentations. More detailed discussions and specific references about individual infections are found elsewhere [251–255].

1. **Lymphadenitis** has been caused by *M. scrofulaceum* and, more recently, *M. avium-intracellulare* and less often by other species [255]. Cervical lymphadenitis will mimic tuberculous lymphadenitis (scrofula).

2. **Pulmonary infections** can mimic tuberculosis; therefore, clinically, one cannot distinguish *M. tuberculosis* infections from those due to other mycobacteria— cultures are necessary. *M. kansasii* and *M. avium-intracellulare* are most frequently involved.

3. **Cutaneous infections** can present with slowly enlarging papules or verrucae, which may go on to ulcerate. The swimming-pool granuloma due to *M. marinum* is the most common example.

4. **Disseminated disease** similar to miliary tuberculosis may occur and is more likely to be seen in immunocompromised patients. This is especially true in patients with AIDS in whom *M. avium-intracellulare* can be isolated from blood cultures.

5. **Miscellaneous.** Prosthetic device infections (e.g., heart valve or mammary implants) and unusual nosocomial infections are reported.

F. Therapy must be individualized. In general, atypical mycobacteria are very resistant to standard antituberculous agents, although *M. kansasii* and *M. marinum* are more susceptible than the other species. Localized disease (e.g., a single lymph node or skin nodule) usually is treated by surgical excision alone. Documented pulmonary infections may require multidrug regimens. Consultation is advisable for these and other infections in which disease is documented and therapy is being considered. Treatment of *M. avium-intracellulare* in AIDS patients is discussed in Chap. 19.

References

1. Reynolds, H.Y. Host defense impairments that may lead to respiratory infections. *Clin. Chest Med.* 8:339, 1987.
   Excellent recent review of pulmonary defense mechanisms and how their impairment may predispose to pulmonary infections.

2. Reynolds, H.Y. Immunoglobulin G and its function in the human respiratory tract. *Mayo Clin. Proc.* 63:161, 1988.
   Thorough overview of the importance of IgG in the respiratory tract and its pathophysiology.

3. Niederman, M.S., et al. Guidelines for the initial management of adults with community-acquired pneumonia: Diagnosis, assessment of severity, and initial antimicrobial therapy. *Am. Rev. Respir. Dis.* 148:1418, 1993.
   This framework for the initial management of community-acquired pneumonia is an official statement of the American Thoracic Society.

3a. Marrie, T.J. Community-acquired pneumonia. *Clin. Infect. Dis.* 18:501, 1994.
A state-of-the-art review from an authority in pulmonary infections.
3b. Donowitz, G.R., and Mandell, G.L. Acute pneumonia. In G.L. Mandell, J.E. Bennett, and R. Dolin (eds.), *Principles and Practice of Infectious Diseases* (4th ed.). New York: Churchill Livingstone, 1995. Pp. 619–637.
See related summaries by D.Y. Sue, Community-acquired pneumonia in adults. West. J. Med. 161:383, 1994, and B.A. Cunha, The antibiotic treatment of community-acquired, atypical, and nosocomial pneumonia. Med. Clin. North Am. 79:581, 1995.
4. Henderson, F.W., et al. Respiratory-syncytial-virus infections, reinfections, and immunity. A prospective, longitudinal study in young children. *N. Engl. J. Med.* 300: 530, 1979.
5. Edelstein, P.H. Legionnaires' disease. *Clin. Infect. Dis.* 16:741, 1993.
State-of-the-art review emphasizing recent clinically relevant developments.
6. Fang, G-D., Yu, V.L., and Vickers, R.M. Disease due to the Legionellaceae (other than *Legionella pneumophila*). *Medicine* 68:116, 1989.
Review of the microbiological and clinical features of these organisms.
7. Cooper, J.A.D., Jr. Drug-Related Pulmonary Disease. In R.C. Bone (ed.), *Pulmonary and Critical Care Medicine*. St. Louis: Mosby, 1993.
8. Phillips, T.L. Radiation Fibrosis. In A.P. Fishman (ed.), *Pulmonary Diseases and Disorders* (2nd ed.). New York: McGraw-Hill, 1988. Pp. 773–792.
9. Lynch, J.P., and Sitrin, R.G. Noninfectious mimics of community-acquired pneumonia. *Semin. Respir. Infect.* 8:14, 1993.
Review of the wide range of diseases that may be confused with acute pneumonia.
10. Fein, A.M., et al. When the pneumonia doesn't get better. *Clin. Chest Med.* 8:529, 1987.
Review of the clinical and radiographic progression and resolution of common pneumonias.
11. Marrie, T.J. Normal resolution of community-acquired pneumonia. *Semin. Respir. Infect.* 7:256, 1992.
12. Valenti, W.M., Trudell, R.G., and Bentley, D.W. Factors predisposing to oropharyngeal colonization with gram-negative bacilli in the aged. *N. Engl. J. Med.* 298:1108, 1978.
Colonization rates can vary from 6% to more than 40%, with higher colonization rates in those patients who require a higher level of care.
13. Bartlett, J.G. Diagnosis of bacterial infections of the lung. *Clin. Chest Med.* 8:119, 1987.
The infectious diseases perspective.
14. Tobin, M.J. Diagnosis of pneumonia: Techniques and problems. *Clin. Chest Med.* 8:513, 1987.
The pulmonary perspective.
15. Middleton, R.M., Kirkpatrick, M.B., and Bass, J.B., Jr. Invasive Techniques for the Diagnosis of Lower Respiratory Tract Infections. In M.S. Niederman, G.A. Sarosi, and J. Glasroth (eds.), *Respiratory Infections: A Scientific Basis for Management*. Philadelphia: Saunders, 1994. Pp. 499–507.
16. Levy, M., et al. Community-acquired pneumonia. Importance of initial noninvasive bacteriologic and radiographic investigations. *Chest* 92:43, 1988.
17. Ekdahl, K., et al. Bronchoscopic diagnosis of pulmonary infections in a heterogeneous, nonselected group of patients. *Chest* 103:1743, 1993.
Therapeutically important results were obtained infrequently in immunocompetent patients, in contrast to immunocompromised patients.
18. Meduri, G.U. Diagnosis of ventilator-associated pneumonia. *Infect. Dis. Clin. North Am.* 7:295, 1993.
19. Baselski, V. Microbiologic diagnosis of ventilator-associated pneumonia. *Infect. Dis. Clin. North Am.* 7:331, 1993.
This and [18] are two excellent reviews in the same issue.
20. Vereen, L., Smart, L.M., and George, R.B. Antibody coating and quantitative cultures of bacteria in sputum in bronchial brush specimens from patients with stable chronic bronchitis. *Chest* 90:534, 1986.
21. Wunderink, R.G., et al. The diagnostic utility of the antibody-coated bacteria test in intubated patients. *Chest* 99:84, 1991.
22. Fagon, J-Y., et al. Detection of nosocomial lung infection in ventilated patients. *Am. Rev. Respir. Dis.* 138:110, 1988.
The clinical diagnosis was incorrect most of the time, and use of a protected telescoping cannula brush with quantitative cultures was very useful in distinguishing infected from uninfected patients.
23. Chastre, J., et al. Diagnosis of nosocomial bacterial pneumonia in intubated patients undergoing ventilation: Comparison of the usefulness of bronchoalveolar lavage and the protected specimen brush. *Am. J. Med.* 85:499, 1988.

Quantitative cultures of bronchoalveolar lavage (BAL) specimens were not useful, but quantitation of intracellular bacteria in BAL sediments was helpful in identifying infected patients.

24. Cantral, D.E., et al. Quantitative culture of bronchoalveolar lavage fluid for the diagnosis of bacterial pneumonia. *Am. J. Med.* 95:601, 1993.
Most patients found to have pneumonia were immunosuppressed, and the sensitivity of quantitative cultures was decreased by prior antibiotics.

25. Henriquez, A.H., Meendoza, J., and Gonzalez, P.C. Quantitative culture of bronchoalveolar lavage from patients with anaerobic lung abscess. *J. Infect. Dis.* 164:414, 1991.

26. Pisani, R.J., and Wright, A.J. Clinical utility of bronchoalveolar lavage in immunocompromised hosts. *Mayo Clin. Proc.* 67:221, 1992.
Large series highlighting the strengths and weaknesses of BAL in this population.

26a. Levy, H. Comparison of Ballard catheter bronchoalveolar lavage with bronchoscopic bronchoalveolar lavage. *Chest* 106:1753, 1994.

27. Kaufman, L., and Reiss, E. Serodiagnosis of Fungal Infections. In N.R. Rose et al. (eds.), *Manual of Clinical Laboratory Immunology* (4th ed.). Washington, DC: American Society for Microbiology, 1992. Pp. 506–528.

28. Klotz, S.A., Penn, R.L., and George, R.B. Antigen detection in the diagnosis of fungal respiratory infections. *Semin. Respir. Infect.* 1:16, 1986.

29. Tillotson, J.R., and Finland, M. Bacterial colonization and clinical superinfection of the respiratory tract complicating antibiotic treatment of pneumonia. *J. Infect. Dis.* 119:597, 1969.

30. Penn, R.L. Choosing initial antibiotic therapy in pneumonia patients. *J. Crit. Illness* 1:57, 1986.
Practical guidelines concisely presented.

31. McGehee, J.L., et al. Treatment of pneumonia in patients at risk of infection with gram-negative bacilli. *Am. J. Med.* 84:597, 1988.
Broad-spectrum therapy given to patients at risk for community-acquired gram-negative pneumonia may be stopped if cultures are negative and the patient improved.

32. Austrian, R., and Gold, J. Pneumococcal bacteremia with special reference to bacteremic pneumococcal pneumonia. *Ann. Intern. Med.* 60:759, 1964.
A classic reference. Includes data on high-risk patients with bacteremia.

33. Musher, D.M. Infections caused by *Streptococcus pneumoniae:* Clinical spectrum, pathogenesis, immunity, and treatment. *Clin. Infect. Dis.* 14:801, 1992.

34. Applebaum, P.C. Antimicrobial resistance in *Streptococcus pneumoniae:* An overview. *Clin. Infect. Dis.* 15:77, 1992.

35. Jacobs, M.R. Treatment and diagnosis of infections caused by drug-resistant *Streptococcus pneumoniae. Clin. Infect. Dis.* 15:119, 1992.

36. Hofmann, J., et al. The prevalence of drug-resistant *Streptococcus pneumoniae* in Atlanta. *N. Engl. J. Med.* 333:481, 1995.
Over a 10-month period, 25% of invasive isolates were resistant to penicillin; 64% of the resistant isolates were from adults. See also accompanying editorial.

36a. Friedland, I.R., and McCracken, G.H., Jr. Management of infections caused by antibiotic-resistant *Streptococcus pneumoniae. N. Engl. J. Med.* 331:377, 1994.
Preliminary review of available therapeutic options, emphasizing the importance of ongoing local surveillance.

37. Centers for Disease Control. Update on adult immunization. *M.M.W.R.* 40(RR-12): 42, 1991.

38. Centers for Disease Control. Recommendations of the Advisory Committee on Immunization Practices: Use of vaccines and immune globulins in persons with altered immunocompetence. *M.M.W.R.* 42(RR-4):8, 1993.

39. Shapiro, E.D., et al. The protective efficacy of polyvalent pneumococcal polysaccharide vaccine. *N. Engl. J. Med.* 325:1453, 1991.

40. Broome, C.V., and Breiman, R.F. Pneumococcal vaccine—past, present, and future. *N. Engl. J. Med.* 325:1506, 1991.
Editorial comment on [39], emphasizing the importance of using the current vaccine now while waiting for a better product to be developed.

41. Centers for Disease Control. Pneumococcal polysaccharide vaccine. *M.M.W.R.* 38: 64, 1989.

42. Janoff, E.N., et al. *Streptococcus pneumoniae* colonization, bacteremia, and immune response among persons with human immunodeficiency virus infection. *J. Infect. Dis.* 167:49, 1993.

43. Glaser, J.B., et al. Zidovudine improves response to pneumococcal vaccine among

persons with AIDS and AIDS-related complex. *J. Infect. Dis.* 164:761, 1991.

44. Musher, D.M., et al. Antibody to capsular polysaccharide of *Streptococcus pneumoniae:* Prevalence, persistence, and response to revaccination. *Clin. Infect. Dis.* 17:66, 1993.

45. Mier, L., et al. Is penicillin G an adequate initial treatment for aspiration pneumonia? *Intensive Care Med.* 19:279, 1993.
    Protected catheter brush specimens done within 48–60 hours of suspected aspiration in patients admitted to an intensive care unit supported the use of penicillin as early empiric therapy for patients without risk factors for gram-negative colonization. Interestingly, the pneumococcus was isolated in 5 of 52 patients.

46. Finegold, S.M., and Wexler, H.M. Therapeutic implications of bacteriologic findings in mixed aerobic-anaerobic infections. *Antimicrob. Agents Chemother.* 32:611, 1988.
    Excellent review of the microbiology of these infections and its importance in clinical practice.

47. Applebaum, P.C., Spangler, S.K., and Jacobs, M.R. β-Lactamase production and susceptibilities to amoxicillin, amoxicillin-clavulanate, ticarcillin, ticarcillin-clavulanate, cefoxitin, imipenem, and metronidazole of 320 non–*Bacteroides fragilis* isolates and 129 fusobacteria from 28 US centers. *Antimicrob. Agents Chemother.* 34:1546, 1990.

48. Marina, M., et al. Bacteriology of anaerobic pleuropulmonary infections: Preliminary report. *Clin. Infect. Dis.* 16(Suppl. 4):S256, 1993.

49. Bartlett, J.G. Anaerobic bacterial infections of the lung and pleural space. *Clin. Infect. Dis.* 16(Suppl. 4):S248, 1993.
    An excellent updated overview of these infections.

50. Finegold, S.F. Aspiration pneumonia. *Rev. Infect. Dis.* 13(Suppl. 9):S737, 1991.

51. Daschner, F., et al. Stress ulcer prophylaxis and ventilation pneumonia: Prevention by antibacterial cytoprotective agents? *Infect. Control Hosp. Epidemiol.* 9:59, 1988.
    Gram-negative and gram-positive bacterial colonization in the stomach increased as gastric pH rose above 2.5, and this preceded tracheal colonization by 1 2 days in one-third of patients.

52. Craven, D.E. Nosocomial pneumonia: New concepts of an old disease. *Infect. Control Hosp. Epidemiol.* 9:57, 1988.

53. Heyland, D., and Mandell, L.A. Gastric colonization by gram-negative bacilli and nosocomial pneumonia in the intensive care unit patient. Evidence for causation. *Chest* 101:187, 1992.

54. Cook, D.J., et al. Nosocomial pneumonia and the role of gastric pH. A meta-analysis. *Chest* 100:7, 1991.

55. Hamer, D.H., and Barza, M. Prevention of hospital-acquired pneumonia in critically ill patients. *Antimicrob. Agents Chemother.* 37:931, 1993.

56. Eveloff, S.E., and Braman, S.S. Acute respiratory failure and death caused by fulminant *Haemophilus influenzae* pneumonia. *Am. J. Med.* 88:683, 1990.

57. Rello, J., et al. Pneumonia due to *Haemophilus influenzae* among mechanically ventilated patients. *Chest* 102:1562, 1992.

58. Murphy, T.F., and Apicella, M.A. Nontypeable *Haemophilus influenzae:* A review of clinical aspects, surface antigens, and the human immune response. *Rev. Infect. Dis.* 9:1, 1987.
    From their review, the authors consider nontypeable H. influenzae *as the second most common cause of community-acquired bacterial pneumonia in adults.*

59. Farley, M.M., et al. Invasive *Haemophilus influenzae* disease in adults. *Ann. Intern. Med.* 116:806, 1992.
    A large prospective survey of H. influenzae *isolated from normally sterile sites. Bacteremic pneumonia accounted for 70% of adult cases; important underlying diseases included chronic lung disorders, HIV infection, cancers, alcoholism, splenectomy, and pregnancy. Only half of tested isolates were serotype b.*

59a. Centers for Disease Control. Progress toward elimination of *Haemophilus influenzae* type b disease among infants and children—United States, 1993–1994. *M.M.W.R.* 44:545, 1995.
    See related discussions in Chaps. 8 and 22.

60. Levison, M.E., and Kaye, D. Pneumonia caused by gram-negative bacilli: An overview. *Rev. Infect. Dis.* 7(Suppl. 4):S656, 1985.
    Very good review.

61. Karnad, A., Alvarez, S., and Berk, S.L. Pneumonia caused by gram-negative bacilli. *Am. J. Med.* 79(Suppl. 1A):61, 1985.
    Review emphasizing frequent occurrence of gram-negative pneumonia in elderly patients and in those with serious underlying illness.

62. Carpenter, J.L. *Klebsiella* pulmonary infections; occurrence at one medical center and review. *Rev. Infect. Dis.* 12:672, 1990.
63. Moore, R.D., Smith, C.R., and Lietman, P.S. Association of aminoglycoside plasma levels with therapeutic outcome in gram-negative pneumonia. *Am. J. Med.* 77:657, 1984.
   Successful outcome was associated with mean peak serum levels of at least 6 μg/ml for gentamicin and tobramycin or at least 24 μg/ml for amikacin.
64. Collins, T., and Gerding, D.N. Aminoglycosides versus beta-lactams in gram-negative pneumonia. *Semin. Respir. Infect.* 6:136, 1991.
   Thoughtful review highlighting the paucity of studies that would help define the optimal antibiotic choices for this problem.
64a. Medical Letter. The choice of antibacterial drugs. *Med. Lett. Drugs Ther.* 36:53, 1994.
65. Douglas, R.G., Jr. Atypical pneumonias today: Clues to the differential diagnosis. *J. Respir. Dis.* 10:52, 1989.
66. Martin, R.E., and Bates, J.H. Atypical pneumonia. *Infect. Dis. Clin. North Am.* 5: 585, 1991.
67. Lynch, D.A., and Armstrong, J.D., II. A pattern-oriented approach to chest radiographs in atypical pneumonia syndromes. *Clin. Chest Med.* 12:203, 1991.
68. Ruben, F.L., and Nguyen, M.L.T. Viral pneumonitis. *Clin. Chest Med.* 12:223, 1991.
69. Mansel, J.K., et al. *Mycoplasma pneumoniae* pneumonia. *Chest* 95:639, 1989.
   Review of 148 patients seen at the Mayo Clinic over a 14-year period with proven mycoplasmal infection.
70. Foy, H.M. Infections caused by *Mycoplasma pneumoniae* and possible carrier state in different populations of patients. *Clin. Infect. Dis.* 17(Suppl. 1):S37, 1993.
71. Marrie, T.J. *Mycoplasma pneumoniae* pneumonia requiring hospitalization, with emphasis on infection in the elderly. *Arch. Intern. Med.* 153:488, 1993.
   Clinical findings were nonspecific, and mortality was low even in older patients.
72. Centers for Disease Control. Outbreaks of *Mycoplasma pneumoniae* respiratory infection—Ohio, Texas, and New York, 1993. *M.M.W.R.* 42:931, 1993.
73. Roifman, C.M., et al. Increased susceptibility to mycoplasma infection in patients with hypogammaglobulinemia. *Am. J. Med.* 80:590, 1986.
74. Clyde, W.A., Jr. Clinical overview of typical *Mycoplasma pneumoniae* infections. *Clin. Infect. Dis.* 17(Suppl. 1):S32, 1993.
75. Jacobs, E. Serologic diagnosis of *Mycoplasma pneumoniae* infections: A critical review of current procedures. *Clin. Infect. Dis.* 17(Suppl. 1):S79, 1993.
76. de Barbeyrac, B., et al. Detection of *Mycoplasma pneumoniae* and *Mycoplasma genitalium* in clinical samples by polymerase chain reaction. *Clin. Infect. Dis.* 17(Suppl. 1):S83, 1993.
77. Marmion, B.P., et al. Experience with newer techniques for the laboratory detection of *Mycoplasma pneumoniae* infection: Adelaide, 1978–1992. *Clin. Infect. Dis.* 17(Suppl. 1):S90, 1993.
78. MacFarlane, J.T., et al. Comparative radiographic features of community-acquired Legionnaire's disease, pneumococcal pneumonia, mycoplasma pneumonia, and psittacosis. *Thorax* 39:28, 1984.
79. Bébéar, C., et al. Potential improvements in therapeutic options for mycoplasmal respiratory infections. *Clin. Infect. Dis.* 17(Suppl. 1):S202, 1993.
80. Grayston, J.T. Infections caused by *Chlamydia pneumoniae* strain TWAR. *Clin. Infect. Dis.* 15:757, 1992.
   A state-of-the-art clinical review. See related minireview by M.R. Hammerschlag, Antimicrobial susceptibility and therapy of infections caused by Chlamydia pneumoniae. Antimicrob. Agents Chemother. *38:1873, 1994.*
81. Falsey, A.R., and Walsh, E.E. Transmission of *Chlamydia pneumoniae*. *J. Infect. Dis.* 168:493, 1993.
82. Grayston, J.Y., et al. Community- and hospital-acquired pneumonia associated with *Chlamydia* TWAR infection demonstrated serologically. *Arch. Intern. Med.* 149: 169, 1989.
83. Hammerschlag, M.R., Hyman, C.L., and Roblin, P.M. In vitro activity of five quinolones against *Chlamydia pneumoniae*. *Antimicrob. Agents Chemother.* 36:682, 1992.
84. Hammerschlag, M.R., Qumei, K., and Roblin, P.M. In vitro activity of azithromycin, clarithromycin, L-ofloxacin and other antibiotics against *Chlamydia pneumoniae*. *Antimicrob. Agents Chemother.* 36:1573, 1992.
85. Hammerschlag, M.R., et al. Persistent infection with *Chlamydia pneumoniae* following acute respiratory illness. *Clin. Infect. Dis.* 14:178, 1992.

86. Reimer, L.G. Q fever. *Clin. Microbiol. Rev.* 6:193, 1993.
    Comprehensive review. See also state-of-the-art clinical review by R. Didier and T. Marrie, Q fever. Clin. Infect. Dis. J. 20:489, 1995.
87. Sienko, D.G., et al. Q fever. A call to heighten our index of suspicion. *Arch. Intern. Med.* 148:609, 1988.
88. Marrie, T.J. Q fever pneumonia. *Semin. Respir. Infect.* 4:47, 1989.
    This review contains excellent illustrations of the radiographic findings associated with Q fever pneumonia.
89. Marrie, T.J., et al. Exposure to parturient cats: A risk factor for acquisition of Q fever in Maritime Canada. *J. Infect. Dis.* 158:101, 1988.
90. Raoult, D. Treatment of Q fever. *Antimicrob. Agents Chemother.* 37:1733, 1993.
91. Reingold, A.L., et al. *Legionella* pneumonia in the United States: The distribution of serotypes and species causing human disease. *J. Infect. Dis.* 149:819, 1984.
92. Reingold, A.L. Role of *Legionella* in acute infections of the lower respiratory tract. *Rev. Infect. Dis.* 10:1018, 1988.
    Legionella spp. have accounted for fewer than 1% to more than 30% of pneumonias reported in the literature, suggesting the possibility of geographic and temporal differences in incidence, and most of these have been L. pneumophila.
93. Winn, W.C., Jr. *Legionella* and the microbiologist. *Infect. Dis. Clin. North Am.* 7: 377, 1993.
94. Dowling, J.N., Saha, A.K., and Glew, R.H. Virulence factors of the family Legionellaceae. *Microbiol. Rev.* 56:32, 1992.
95. Lowry, P.W., and Tompkins, L.S. Nosocomial legionellosis: A review of pulmonary and extrapulmonary syndromes. *Am. J. Infect. Control* 21:21, 1993.
    Useful review; emphasis on the extrapulmonary manifestations of nosocomial infections.
96. Finegold, S.M. Legionnaires' disease—still with us. *N. Engl. J. Med.* 318:571, 1988.
97. Yu, V.L. Could aspiration be the major mode of transmission for *Legionella? Am. J. Med.* 95:13, 1993.
    Editorial commentary stimulated by [98], reviewing the evidence that aspiration, and not aerosolization, is the primary mode of transmission of both sporadic and epidemic legionellosis.
98. Blatt, S.P., et al. Nosocomial Legionnaires' disease: Aspiration as a primary mode of disease acquisition. *Am. J. Med.* 95:16, 1993.
    This case-control study of nosocomial Legionnaires' disease showed that nasogastric tubes, bed bathing, and immunosuppression, but not shower use, were significant risk factors. The outbreak organism was isolated from the water system and not from cooling towers.
99. Falcó, V., et al. *Legionella pneumophila,* a cause of severe community-acquired pneumonia. *Chest* 100:1007, 1991.
99a. Plouffe, J.F., et al. Reevaluation of the definition of Legionnaire's disease: Use of the urinary antigen assay. *Clin. Infect. Dis.* 20:1286, 1995.
    Single antibody titers ≥1:256 were not predictive of proven Legionella *infection. In contrast, a positive urinary antigen assay was 80% sensitive and 99% specific for* L. pneumophila *serogroup 1 infection.*
100. Kurz, R.W., et al. Failure of treatment of *Legionella* pneumonia with ciprofloxacin [letter]. *J. Antimicrob. Chemother.* 22:389, 1988.
101. Meyer, R.D. Role of the quinolones in the treatment of legionellosis. *J. Antimicrob. Chemother.* 28:623, 1991.
102. Salord, J.-M., et al. Unsuccessful treatment of *Legionella pneumophila* infection with a fluoroquinolone. *Clin. Infect. Dis.* 17:518, 1993.
    This patient, who had AIDS and was receiving corticosteroids, developed Legionnaires' disease while receiving 400 mg ofloxacin per day.
103. Schwebke, J.R., Hackman, R., and Bowden, R. Pneumonia due to *Legionella micdadei* in bone marrow transplant recipients. *Rev. Infect. Dis.* 12:824, 1990.
104. Rudin, J.E., and Wing, E.J. A comparative study of *Legionella micdadei* and other nosocomial acquired pneumonia. *Chest* 86:675, 1984.
105. Kilborn, J.A., et al. Necrotizing cellulitis caused by *Legionella micdadei. Am. J. Med.* 92:104, 1992.
    Infection occurred in a renal transplant patient and led to amputation of the affected limb; several color illustrations.
106. Muder, R.R., Yu, V.L., and Parry, M.F. The radiologic manifestations of *Legionella* pneumonia. *Semin. Respir. Infect.* 2:242, 1987.
    Well-illustrated and useful review.

107. Leelarasamee, A., and Bovornkitti, S. Melioidosis: Review and update. *Rev. Infect. Dis.* 11:413, 1989.
Thorough review from an endemic area.

108. Dance, D.A.B. Melioidosis: The tip of the iceberg? *Clin. Microbiol. Rev.* 4:52, 1991.
This review emphasizes the historical and geographic distribution of the disease.

109. Dhiensiri, T., Puapairoj, S., and Susaengrat, W. Pulmonary melioidosis: Clinical-radiologic correlation in 183 cases in northeastern Thailand. *Radiology* 166:711, 1988.
Useful analysis of a large number of cases from an endemic region.

110. Kanaphun, P., et al. Serology and carriage of *Pseudomonas pseudomallei:* A prospective study in 1000 hospitalized children in northeast Thailand. *J. Infect. Dis.* 167: 230, 1993.

111. Sookpranee, T., et al. *Pseudomonas pseudomallei,* a common pathogen in Thailand that is resistant to the bactericidal effects of many antibiotics. *Antimicrob. Agents Chemother.* 35:484, 1991.

112. Sookpranee, M., et al. Multicenter prospective randomized trial comparing ceftazidime plus co-trimoxazole with chloramphenicol plus doxycycline and co-trimoxazole for treatment of severe melioidosis. *Antimicrob. Agents Chemother.* 36:158, 1992.

113. Chaowagul, W., et al. Relapse in melioidosis: Incidence and risk factors. *J. Infect. Dis.* 168:1181, 1993.

114. Duchin, J.S., et al. Hantavirus pulmonary syndrome: A clinical description of 17 patients with a newly recognized disease. *N. Engl. J. Med.* 330:949, 1994.
A thorough clinical and pathologic description of 17 early cases seen in the Four Corners area.

115. Wenzel, R.P. A new hantavirus infection in North America. *N. Engl. J. Med.* 330: 1004, 1994.
Editorial comment on [114].

115a. Butler, J.C., and Peters, C.J. Hantaviruses and hantavirus pulmonary syndrome. *Clin. Infect. Dis.* 19:387, 1994.
A "state of the art" clinical review series article. For a related summary, see C.J. Peters and K.M. Johnson, California encephalitis viruses, hantaviruses, and other bunyaviridae. In G.L. Mandell, J.E. Bennett, and R. Dolin (eds.), Principles and Practice of Infectious Diseases (4th ed.). New York: Churchill Livingstone, 1995. Pp. 1567–1572. See also H. Levy and S.Q. Simpson, Hantavirus pulmonary syndrome. Am. J. Respir. Crit. Care 149:1710, 1994.

116. Centers for Disease Control. Hantavirus pulmonary syndrome—United States, 1993. *M.M.W.R.* 43:45, 1994.

117. Stone, R. The mouse–piñon nut connection. *Science* 262:833, 1993.

118. Centers for Disease Control. Newly identified hantavirus—Florida, 1994. *M.M.W.R.* 43:99, 1994.

118a. Centers for Disease Control. Hantaviruses pulmonary syndrome—Virginia, 1993. *M.M.W.R.* 43:876, 1994.

118b. Auwaerter, P.G., et al. Hantavirus serologies in patients hospitalized with community-acquired pneumonia. *J. Infect. Dis.* 173:237, 1996.

119. Centers for Disease Control. Update: Hantavirus pulmonary syndrome—United States, 1993. *M.M.W.R.* 42:816, 1993.

120. Centers for Disease Control. Hantavirus infection—southwestern United States. Interim recommendations for risk reduction. *M.M.W.R.* 42:1, 1993.

121. Shelhamer, J.H. (moderator). Respiratory disease in the immunosuppressed patient. *Ann. Intern. Med.* 117:415, 1992.
Summary of a National Institutes of Health (NIH) conference, including outlines of the diagnostic approach to pneumonia in various categories of immunosuppressed patients. See also reference [123a].

122. Rosenow, E.C., III, Wilson, W.R., and Cockerill, F.R., III. Pulmonary disease in the immunocompromised host. *Mayo Clin. Proc.* 60:473, 610, 1985.
Excellent review article.

123. Fishman, J.A. Diagnostic approach to pneumonia in the immunocompromised host. *Semin. Respir. Infect.* 1:133, 1986.

123a. Shelhamer, J.H., et al. The laboratory evaluation of opportunistic pulmonary infection. *Ann. Intern. Med.* 124:585, 1996.
Excellent NIH review of recent microbiological advances.

124. Ward, T.T., et al. Trimethoprim-sulfamethoxazole prophylaxis in granulocytopenic patients with acute leukemia: Evaluation of serum antibiotic levels in a randomized, double-blind, placebo-controlled Department of Veterans Affairs cooperative study. *Clin. Infect. Dis.* 17:323, 1993.

TMP-SMX prophylaxis had no significant effect on survival, rate of bacteremia, overall infections, or use of systemic antimicrobials. Serum drug levels were significantly related to afebrile periods, suggesting that drug absorption may be critical to the efficacy of this strategy.

125. Bow, E.J., and Ronald, A.R. Antibacterial chemoprophylaxis in neutropenic patients—where do we go from here? *Clin. Infect. Dis.* 17:333, 1993.
     Editorial stimulated by the study reported in [124].

126. Tablan, O.C., et al. Guidelines for prevention of nosocomial pneumonia: Parts I and II. *Am. J. Infect. Control* 22:247, 267, 1994.
     This is a detailed report from the Hospital Infection Control Practices Advisory Committee.

127. Craven, D.E., Steger, K.A., and Duncan, R.A. Prevention and Control of Nosocomial Pneumonia. In R.P. Wenzel (ed.), *Prevention and Control of Nosocomial Infections* (2nd ed.). Baltimore: Williams & Wilkins, 1993. Pp. 580–599.

128. Niederman, M.S. Microbial Flora of the Respiratory Tract: Normal Inhabitants and Abnormal Colonization. In R.C. Bone (ed.), *Pulmonary and Critical Care Medicine.* St. Louis: Mosby, 1993.

129. Ferrer, M., et al. Utility of selective digestive decontamination in mechanically ventilated patients. *Ann. Intern. Med.* 120:389, 1994.
     Topical polymyxin, tobramycin, and amphotericin plus systemic cefotaxime for 4 days were compared to placebo in a randomized, double-blind, prospective design. Treatment decreased detectable gram-negative and Candida *colonization but had no effect on the incidence of pneumonia or mortality.*

130. Prod'hom, G., et al. Nosocomial pneumonia in mechanically ventilated patients receiving antacid, ranitidine, or sucralfate as prophylaxis for stress ulcer. *Ann. Intern. Med.* 120:653, 1994.
     The risk for late-onset, but not early-onset, nosocomial pneumonia in ventilated patients was lower with sucralfate. This difference was apparent only in patients with gastric pH of less than 4.0; however, half of the sucralfate patients had a gastric pH in excess of 4.0. Gastric and tracheal colonization by the eventual pathogen preceded pneumonia in two-thirds of the late-onset cases.

131. El-Ebiary, M., et al. Quantitative cultures of endotracheal aspirates for the diagnosis of ventilator-associated pneumonia. *Am. Rev. Respir. Dis.* 148:1552, 1993.
     Quantitative cultures of endotracheal aspirates were less sensitive and specific than similar cultures of BAL and PCB specimens.

132. Schlaes, D., et al. Sputum elastin fibers and the diagnosis of necrotizing pneumonia. *Chest* 85:763, 1984.
     Finding elastin fibers in sputum (well illustrated) may be more sensitive than chest roentgenogram in detecting necrotizing infections.

133. LaForce, F.M. Systemic antimicrobial therapy of nosocomial pneumonia: Monotherapy versus combination therapy. *Eur. J. Clin. Microbiol.* 8:61, 1989.

133a. Vallés, J., et al. Continuous aspiration of subglottic secretions in preventing ventilator-associated pneumonia. *Ann. Intern. Med.* 122:179, 1995.
     This simple procedure significantly reduced early-onset pneumonias and lowered mortality attributed to ventilator-associated pneumonia by 2.5-fold. See also the thoughtful editorial by D.E. Craven on P. 229 of this reference.

134. Gilsdorf, J.R. Community-acquired pneumonia in children. *Semin. Respir. Infect.* 2: 146, 1987.
     Excellent review article in an issue devoted to pediatric pulmonary infections.

135. Denny, F.W., and Clyde, W.A., Jr. Acute lower respiratory tract infections in nonhospitalized children. *J. Pediatr.* 108:635, 1986.

136. Boyer, K.M., and Cherry, J.D. Nonbacterial Pneumonia. In R.D. Feigin and J.D. Cherry (eds.), *Textbook of Pediatric Infectious Diseases* (3rd ed.). Philadelphia: Saunders, 1992. Pp. 254–265.

137. Klein, J.O. Bacterial Pneumonias. In R.D. Feigin and J.D. Cherry (eds.), *Textbook of Pediatric Infectious Diseases* (3rd ed.). Philadelphia: Saunders, 1992. Pp. 299–309.

138. Schutze, G.E., and Jacobs, R.F. Management of community-acquired bacterial pneumonia in hospitalized children. *Pediatr. Infect. Dis. J.* 11:160, 1992.

139. Feigin, R.D., and Matson, D.O. The Compromised Host. In R.D. Feigin and J.D. Cherry (eds.), *Textbook of Pediatric Infectious Diseases* (3rd ed.). Philadelphia: Saunders, 1992. Pp. 960–989.

140. Condon, V.R. Pneumonia in children. *J. Thorac. Imaging* 6:31, 1991.

141. Isaacs, D. Problems in determining the etiology of community-acquired childhood pneumonia. *Pediatr. Infect. Dis.* 8:143, 1989.

142. Sinave, C.P., Hardy, G.T., and Fardy, P.W. The Lemierre syndrome: Suppurative thrombophlebitis of the internal jugular vein secondary to oropharyngeal infection. *Medicine* 68:85, 1989.
143. Kaye, M.G., et al. The clinical spectrum of *Staphylococcus aureus* pulmonary infection. *Chest* 97:788, 1990.
144. Watanakunakorn, C. Bacteremic *Staphylococcus aureus* pneumonia. *Scand. J. Infect. Dis.* 19:623, 1987.
145. Woodhead, M.A., Radvan, J., and MacFarlane, J.T. Adult community-acquired staphylococcal pneumonia in the antibiotic era: A review of 61 cases. *Q. J. Med.* 64:783, 1987.
146. Gold, W., Velland, H., and Brunton, J. The air crescent sign caused by *Staphylococcus aureus* lung infection in a neutropenic patient with leukemia. *Ann. Intern. Med.* 116:910, 1992.
147. Haron, E., et al. Primary *Candida* pneumonia. Experience at a large cancer center and review of the literature. *Medicine* 72:137, 1993.
148. Light, R.W. Pleural Diagnostic Procedures. In R.C. Bone (ed.), *Pulmonary and Critical Care Medicine.* St. Louis: Mosby, 1993.
149. Kinasewitz, G.K. Pleuritis and Pleural Effusions. In R.C. Bone (ed.), *Pulmonary and Critical Care Medicine.* St. Louis: Mosby, 1993.
   Two thorough reviews by leading authorities in the area.
149a. Adelman, M., et al. Diagnostic utility of pleural fluid eosinophilia. *Am. J. Med.* 77:915, 1984.
150. Strange, C., and Sahn, S.A. Management of parapneumonic effusions and empyema. *Infect. Dis. Clin. North Am.* 5:539, 1991.
   Thorough and practical review.
151. Alfageme, I., et al. Empyema of the thorax in adults. *Chest* 103:839, 1993.
152. Brook, I., and Frazier, E.H. Aerobic and anaerobic microbiology of empyema. *Chest* 103:839, 1993.
153. Bartlett, J.G. Bacterial infections of the pleural space. *Semin. Respir. Infect.* 3:308, 1988.
   Excellent review.
154. Pothula, V., and Krellenstein, D.J. Early aggressive surgical management of parapneumonic empyemas. *Chest* 105:832, 1994.
   Surgical intervention was successful in most patients who failed 48 hours of chest tube drainage, with a mortality of 8%.
155. Hoover, E.L., et al. Reappraisal of empyema thoracis. Surgical intervention when the duration of the illness is unknown. *Chest* 90:511, 1986.
   Surgical intervention should be considered early in hospitalization, particularly if 24–48 hours of tube drainage is ineffective.
156. Ridley, P.D., and Braimbridge, M.V. Thoracoscopic debridement and pleural irrigation in the management of empyema thoracis. *Ann. Thorac. Surg.* 51:461, 1991.
157. Kern, J.A., and Rodgers, B.M. Thoracoscopy in the management of empyema in children. *J. Pediatr. Surg.* 28:1128, 1993.
158. Ferguson, M.K. Thoracoscopy for empyema, bronchopleural fistula, and chylothorax. *Ann. Thorac. Surg.* 56:644, 1993.
159. Hughes, C.E., and Van Scoy, R.E. Antibiotic therapy of empyema. *Semin. Respir. Infect.* 6:94, 1991.
160. Light, R.W. Management of parapneumonic effusions. *Chest* 100:892, 1991.
   Editorial response to an article in the same issue (R.H. Poe et al., pp. 963–967) that questioned the value of chemical criteria for tube thoracostomy in parapneumonic effusions. This expert's approach is outlined here and updated in Chest *108:299, 1995.*
161. Penner, C., Maycher, B., and Long, R. Pulmonary gangrene. A complication of bacterial pneumonia. *Chest* 105:567, 1994.
162. Peters, J.I., et al. Lung bullae with air-fluid levels. *Am. J. Med.* 82:759, 1987.
   This is a milder illness than lung abscess. Invasive procedures are not needed, and response to oral penicillin is prompt.
163. Griban, N.P., et al. Yield of percutaneous needle aspiration in lung abscess. *Chest* 97:69, 1990.
   These investigators used a 22-gauge lumbar puncture needle and fluoroscopic guidance. Yield was reduced by prior antibiotic therapy. Pneumothorax occurred in 14 (14%), 10 of whom required a chest tube.
164. Sosenko, A., and Glassroth, J. Fiberoptic bronchoscopy in the evaluation of lung abscess. *Chest* 87:489, 1985.
   The major usefulness is to distinguish cavitary neoplasm from lung abscess.
165. Levison, M.E., et al. Clindamycin compared with penicillin for the treatment of anaerobic lung abscess. *Ann. Intern. Med.* 98:466, 1983.

166. Gudiol, F., et al. Clindamycin vs penicillin for anaerobic lung infections. *Arch. Intern. Med.* 150:2525, 1990.
     Patients treated with penicillin had a significantly higher failure rate and longer duration of putrid sputum; penicillin-resistant anaerobic Bacteroides *(now* Prevotella*) were associated with treatment failure.*
167. Ball, W.S., Bisset, G.S., and Towbin, R.B. Percutaneous drainage of chest abscesses in children. *Radiology* 171:431, 1989.
168. vanSonnenberg, E., et al. Lung abscess: CT-guided drainage. *Radiology* 178:347, 1991.
169. Bloom, B.R., and Murray, C.J.L. Tuberculosis: Commentary on a reemergent killer. *Science* 257:1055, 1992.
170. Barnes, P.F., and Barrows, S.A. Tuberculosis in the 1990s. *Ann. Intern. Med.* 119: 400, 1993.
171. Ellner, J.J., et al. Tuberculosis symposium: Emerging problems and promise. *J. Infect. Dis.* 168:537, 1993.
171a. U.S. Department of Health and Human Resources, Public Health Services, Centers for Disease Control and Prevention, Division of Tuberculosis Elimination, *Core Curriculum on Tuberculosis: What the Clinician Should Know* (3rd ed.). Atlanta, 1994. *(To order call CDC Fax Information Service at 404-332-4565.)*
     An excellent summary including INH chemoprophylaxis.
172. Snider, D.E., Jr. Recognition and elimination of tuberculosis. *Adv. Intern. Med.* 38:169, 1993.
     For related discussions on tuberculosis in children see H.S. Schaaf et al., Respiratory tuberculosis in childhood: The diagnostic value of clinical features and special investigations. Pediatr. Infect. Dis. J. *14:189, 1995, and C.R. Driver et al., Tuberculosis in children younger than five years old: New York City.* Pediatr. Infect. Dis. J. *114: 112, 1995.*
173. Mathur, M., et al. Delayed diagnosis of pulmonary tuberculosis in city hospitals. *Arch. Intern. Med.* 154:306, 1994.
     This retrospective review of hospitalized patients found that diagnosis of tuberculosis often was delayed or missed entirely (20%). Age older than 65 years and minimal respiratory findings were among the features associated with misdiagnosis.
174. Centers for Disease Control. Tuberculosis morbidity—United States, 1992. *M.M.W.R.* 42:696, 1993.
     The latest figures available at the time of this writing.
174a. Centers for Disease Control. Tuberculosis morbidity—United States, 1994. *M.M.W.R.* 44:387, 1995.
175. American Thoracic Society. Control of tuberculosis in the United States. *Am. Rev. Respir. Dis.* 146:1623, 1992.
     An official statement issued jointly from the American Thoracic Society, the American Academy of Pediatrics, and Centers for Disease Control, and the Infectious Diseases Society of America. See also Screening for tuberculosis and tuberculosis infection in high-risk populations: Recommendations of the Advisory Council for the Elimination of Tuberculosis. MMWR 44 (No. RR-11):19–34, 1995.
176. Sturgill-Koszycki, S., et al. Lack of acidification in *Mycobacterium* phagosomes produced by exclusion of the vesicular proton-ATPase. *Science* 263:678, 1994.
177. Stead, W.W. Genetics and resistance to tuberculosis. *Ann. Intern. Med.* 116:937, 1992.
178. American Thoracic Society and Centers for Disease Control. Diagnostic standards and classification of tuberculosis. *Am. Rev. Respir. Dis.* 142:725, 1990.
179. Orme, I.M., Andersen, P., and Boom, W.H. T cell response to *Mycobacterium tuberculosis. J. Infect. Dis.* 167:1481, 1993.
180. Rom, W.N., and Zhang, Y. The rising tide of tuberculosis and the human host response to *Mycobacterium tuberculosis. J. Lab. Clin. Med.* 121:737, 1993.
181. Dunlap, N.E., and Briles, D.E. Immunology of tuberculosis. *Med. Clin. North Am.* 77:1235, 1993.
182. Heubner, R.E., Schein, M.F., and Bass, J.B., Jr. The tuberculin skin test. *Clin. Infect. Dis.* 17:968, 1993.
     Excellent recent review.
183. Nash, D.R., and Douglas, J.E. Anergy in active pulmonary tuberculosis: Comparison between positive and negative reactors and evaluation of 5 TU and 250 TU test doses. *Chest* 77:32, 1980.
     Twenty-five percent of patients with active pulmonary tuberculosis failed to respond to intermediate purified protein derivatives. See editorial comment in the same issue. Nonresponders are not necessarily anergic to other skin tests.
184. Gordin, F.M., et al. Evaluation of a third sequential tuberculin skin test in a chronic care population. *Am. Rev. Respir. Dis.* 137:153, 1988.

Significant booster reactions occurred in 13.8% of 1,146 second skin tests and in 8.7% of 769 third skin tests.

185. Perez-Stable, E.J., et al. Conversion and reversion of tuberculin reactions in nursing home residents. *Am. Rev. Respir. Dis.* 137:301, 1988.
    Of 258 patients with significant reactions, 24.8% had reverted to insignificant reactions when tested 3 years later.

186. Centers for Disease Control. The use of preventive therapy for tuberculosis infection in the United States. *M.M.W.R.* 39(RR-8):9, 1990.
    Summary of preventive INH therapy. See early portion of this supplement discussing high-risk groups, including intravenous drug users known to be HIV-negative, foreign-born persons from high-prevalence countries, and medically underserved low-income populations, including high-risk racial or ethnic minorities, especially blacks, Hispanics, and native Americans. See also related discussion in references [171] and [236].

187. Menzies, R., et al. The booster effect in two-step tuberculin testing among young adults in Montreal. *Ann. Intern. Med.* 120:190, 1994.

188. Centers for Disease Control. Purified protein derivative (PPD)–tuberculin anergy and HIV infection: Guidelines for prevention and management of anergic persons at risk for tuberculosis. *M.M.W.R.* 40(RR-5):27, 1991.
    In contrast to the above recommendations, a recent review concluded that anergy tests do not add to the interpretation of a standard skin test (Pesanti, E.L. The negative tuberculin skin test. Tuberculin, HIV, and anergy panels. Am. J. Respir. Crit. Care Med. 149:1699, 1995).

188a. Wolinsky, E. Conventional diagnostic methods for tuberculosis. *Clin. Infect. Dis.* 19:396, 1994.

189. Shinnick, T.M., and Good, R.C. Diagnostic mycobacteriology laboratory practices. *Clin. Infect. Dis.* 21:291, 1995.

190. Klotz, S.A., and Penn, R.L. Acid-fast staining of urine and gastric contents is an excellent indicator of mycobacterial disease. *Am. Rev. Respir. Dis.* 136:1197, 1987.
    Smears of these specimens have a high specificity for mycobacterial disease and a low but acceptable sensitivity.

191. Daniel, T.M. The rapid diagnosis of tuberculosis: A selective review. *J. Lab. Clin. Med.* 116:277, 1990.
    One of the foremost investigators in the area offers his perspective.

192. Watt, G., et al. Rapid diagnosis of tuberculous meningitis by using an enzyme-linked immunosorbent assay to detect mycobacterial antigen and antibody in cerebrospinal fluid. *J. Infect. Dis.* 158:681, 1988.

193. Noordhoek, G.T., van Embden, J.D.A., and Kolk, A.H.J. Questionable reliability of the polymerase chain reaction in the detection of *Mycobacterium tuberculosis*. *N. Engl. J. Med.* 329:2036, 1993.

193a. Haas, D.W. Current and future applications of polymerase chain reaction for *Mycobacterium tuberculosis*. *Mayo Clin. Proc.* 71:311, 1996.

194. Pfyffer, G.E., et al. Direct detection of *Mycobacterium tuberculosis* complex in respiratory specimens by a target-amplified test system. *J. Clin. Microbiol.* 32:918, 1994.

195. Agrons, G.A., Markowitz, R.I., and Kramer, S.S. Pulmonary tuberculosis in children. *Semin. Roentgenol.* 2:158, 1993.

196. Miller, W.T., and Miller, W.T., Jr. Tuberculosis in the normal host. *Semin. Roentgenol.* 2:109, 1993.
    This and [195] emphasize radiographic features and are among several in this issue devoted to tuberculosis.

197. Epstein, D.M., et al. Tuberculous pleural effusions. *Chest* 91:106, 1987.

198. Seibert, A.F., et al. Tuberculous pleural effusion. *Chest* 99:883, 1991.
    In this 20-year retrospective review, the mean age of patients was 47 years, and half had infiltrates and half had only effusions.

199. Antoniskis, D., Amin, K., and Barnes, P.F. Pleuritis as a manifestation of reactivation tuberculosis. *Am. J. Med.* 89:447, 1990.

200. Lee, C-H., et al. Corticosteroids in the treatment of tuberculous pleurisy. A double-blind, placebo-controlled, randomized study. *Chest* 94:1256, 1988.
    Prednisolone therapy hastened the relief of symptoms and resolution of effusions.

201. Sarkar, S.K., et al. Pleuroscopy in the diagnosis of pleural effusion using a fiberoptic bronchoscope. *Tubercle* 66:141, 1985.

202. Babales, J.L., et al. Adenosine deaminase in the diagnosis of tuberculous pleural effusions. *Chest* 99:355, 1991.

203. Yew, W.W., et al. Diagnosis of tuberculous pleural effusion by the detection of tuberculostearic acid in pleural aspirates. *Chest* 100:1261, 1991.

204. Slavin, R.E., Walsh, T.J., and Pollack, A.D. Late generalized tuberculosis: A clinical pathologic analysis and comparison of 100 cases in the pre-antibiotic and antibiotic eras. *Medicine* 59:352, 1980.
   An important article emphasizing the fact that even patients without HIV infection may have occult disseminated tuberculosis, no pulmonary symptoms, and a normal-appearing chest roentgenogram.
205. Alvarez, S., and McCabe, W.R. Extrapulmonary tuberculosis revisited: A review of experience at Boston City and other hospitals. *Medicine* 63:25, 1984.
   Excellent overview of the authors' recent experience at large city hospitals, including a thorough review of the literature.
206. Wier, M.R., and Thornton, G.F. Extrapulmonary tuberculosis. Experience of a community hospital and review of the literature. *Am. J. Med.* 79:467, 1985.
   Review of the recent experience at a community hospital found that 37% of all new cases of tuberculosis involved extrapulmonary sites.
207. Kim, J.H., Langston, A.A., and Gallis, H.A. Miliary tuberculosis: Epidemiology, clinical manifestations, diagnosis, and outcome. *Rev. Infect. Dis.* 12:583, 1990.
   Most of 38 patients had a predisposing underlying condition other than AIDS, and mortality was 21%.
208. Maartens, G., Willcox, P.A., and Benatar, S.R. Miliary tuberculosis: Rapid diagnosis, hematologic abnormalities, and outcome in 109 treated adults. *Am. J. Med.* 89:291, 1990.
   Forty-two percent of patients had a predisposing condition, and mortality was 24%.
209. Hussey, G., Chisholm, T., and Kibel, M. Miliary tuberculosis in children: A review of 94 cases. *Pediatr. Infect. Dis. J.* 10:832, 1991.
   The mean age was 10.5 months, most were malnourished, and miliary infections were almost eightfold more frequent in children than adults.
210. Rieder, H.L., Snider, D.E., and Cauthen, G.M. Extrapulmonary tuberculosis in the United States. *Am. Rev. Respir. Dis.* 141:347, 1990.
211. Kent, S.J., et al. Tuberculous meningitis: A 30-year review. *Clin. Infect. Dis.* 17:987, 1993.
212. Fowler, N.O. Tuberculous pericarditis. *J.A.M.A.* 266:99, 1991.
213. Shriner, K.A., Mathisen, G.E., and Goetz, M.B. Comparison of mycobacterial lymphadenitis among persons infected with human immunodeficiency virus and seronegative controls. *Clin. Infect. Dis.* 15:601, 1992.
214. Lee, K.C., et al. Contemporary management of cervical tuberculosis. *Laryngoscope* 102:60, 1992.
215. Marshall, J.B. Tuberculosis of the gastrointestinal tract and peritoneum. *Am. J. Gastroenterol.* 88:989, 1993.
   Excellent clinical review of all aspects of tuberculous involvement of the gastrointestinal tract.
216. Aguado, J.M., et al. Tuberculous peritonitis: A study comparing cirrhotic and noncirrhotic patients. *J. Clin. Gastroenterol.* 12:550, 1990.
217. Centers for Disease Control. Tuberculosis and human immunodeficiency virus infection: Recommendations of the Advisory Committee for the Elimination of Tuberculosis (ACET). *M.M.W.R.* 38:236, 1989.
217a. Haas, D.W., and Desprez, R.M. Tuberculosis and acquired immunodeficiency syndrome: A historical perspective on recent developments. *Am. J. Med.* 96:439, 1994.
218. Couser, J.I., Jr., and Glassroth, J. Tuberculosis an epidemic in older adults. *Clin. Chest Med.* 14:491, 1993.
219. Dutt, A.K., and Stead, W.W. Tuberculosis in the elderly. *Med. Clin. North Am.* 77:1353, 1993.
   For a related paper see Y.S. Liaw et al. Clinical spectrum of tuberculosis in older patients. J. Am. Geriatr. Soc. 43:256, 1995.
220. Hamadeh, M.A., and Glassroth, J. Tuberculosis and pregnancy. *Chest* 101:1114, 1992.
221. Vallejo, J.G., and Starke, J.R. Tuberculosis and pregnancy. *Clin. Chest Med.* 13:693, 1992.
222. American Thoracic Society and Centers for Disease Control. Treatment of tuberculosis and tuberculosis infection in adults and children. *Am. J. Respir. Crit. Care Med.* 149:1359, 1994.
   Latest recommendations. Revision of 1986 guidelines. Includes therapy for multidrug resistant tuberculosis. This article has been reprinted in its entirety in the July 1995 issue of Clin. Infect. Dis. 21:9, 1995. The article is the official statement of the American Thoracic Society (ATS) and was adopted by the ATS Board of Directors in March 1993; it is a joint statement of the ATS and the Centers for Disease Control and

Prevention. This statement was endorsed by the American Academy of Pediatrics in April 1993.

222a. Medical Letter. Drugs for tuberculosis. *Med. Lett. Drugs Ther.* 37:67, 1995.

223. Centers for Disease Control. Initial therapy for tuberculosis in the era of multidrug resistance. Recommendations of the Advisory Council for the Elimination of Tuberculosis. *M.M.W.R.* 42(RR-7):1, 1993.

224. Iseman, M.D. Treatment of multidrug-resistant tuberculosis. *N. Engl. J. Med.* 329: 784, 1993.
Timely and important review.

225. Banarjee, A., et al. *inhA,* a gene encoding a target for isoniazid and ethionamide in *Mycobacterium tuberculosis. Science* 263:227, 1994.

226. Zhang, J., et al. The catalase-peroxidase gene of *Mycobacterium tuberculosis. Nature* 358:591, 1992.

227. Jacobs, W.R., Jr., et al. Rapid assessment of drug susceptibilities of *Mycobacterium tuberculosis* by means of luciferase reporter phages. *Science* 260:819, 1993.

228. Kent, J.H. The epidemiology of multidrug-resistant tuberculosis in the United States. *Med. Clin. North Am.* 77:1391, 1993.

229. Bloch, A.B., et al. Nationwide survey of drug-resistant tuberculosis in the United States. *J.A.M.A.* 271:665, 1994.
The overall resistance rate was 14.2% (13.4% in new cases and 26.6% in recurrent disease). Importantly, 9.5% of cases were resistant to INH or rifampin. See also the editorial comment in the same issue.

230. Sepkowitz, K.A., et al. Trends in the susceptibility of tuberculosis in New York City, 1987–1991. *Clin. Infect. Dis.* 18:755, 1994.

231. Frieden, T.R., et al. The emergence of drug-resistant tuberculosis in New York City. *N. Engl. J. Med.* 328:521, 1993.
For related papers see D.S. Swanson and J.R. Starke, Drug-resistant tuberculosis in pediatrics. Pediatr. Clin. North Am. 42:553, 1995, and J.J. Ellner, Multidrug-resistant tuberculosis. Adv. Intern. Med. 40:155, 1995.

231a. Jacobs, R.F. Multiple-drug-resistant tuberculosis. *Clin. Infect. Dis.* 19:1, 1994.
One of the series of "state of the art" clinical articles. Nice review with summary of data as of July 1994.

232. Goble, M., et al. Treatment of 171 patients with pulmonary tuberculosis resistant to isoniazid and rifampin. *N. Engl. J. Med.* 328:527, 1993.

233. Iseman, M.D., Cohn, D.L., and Sbarbaro, J.A. Directly observed treatment of tuberculosis. *N. Engl. J. Med.* 328:576, 1993.
A plea for widespread use of short courses of directly observed therapy from experienced experts.

233a. Weis, S.E., et al. The effect of directly observed therapy on the rates of drug resistance and relapse in tuberculosis. *N. Engl. J. Med.* 330:1179, 1994.
A total of 407 episodes in which patients received traditional therapy for tuberculosis (1980–1986) were compared with 581 episodes of directly observed therapy (1986–1992). Despite higher rates of intravenous drug use and homelessness and an increasing rate of tuberculosis during this 13-year period, the frequency of primary drug resistance decreased from 13% to 6.7% after institution of directly observed therapy, and the incidence of acquired resistance declined from 14% to 2.1%. The relapse rate decreased from 20.9% to 5.5% and the number of multiple-drug-resistant organisms decreased from 25 to 6. (All differences were significant at p < 0.001.)
See related summary by R. Bayer and D. Wilkinson, Directly observed therapy for tuberculosis. History of an idea. Lancet 345:1545, 1995.

234. Dutt, A.K., Moers, D., and Stead, W.W. Short-course chemotherapy for tuberculosis with mainly twice-weekly isoniazid and rifampin: Community physician's seven-year experience with mainly outpatients. *Am. J. Med.* 77:233, 1984.

235. Campbell, I.A., et al. Six months versus nine months chemotherapy for tuberculosis of lymph nodes: Final results. *Respir. Med.* 87:621, 1993.

236. Centers for Disease Control. Guidelines for preventing the transmission of *Mycobacterium tuberculosis* in health-care facilities, 1994. *M.M.W.R.* 43(RR-13):1–132, 1994.
This extensive document updates and replaces prior CDC guidelines for the prevention of M. tuberculosis in health care facilities. For related papers see also (1) S.A. Maloney et al., Efficacy of control measures in preventing nosocomial transmission of multidrug-resistant tuberculosis to patients and health care workers. Ann. Intern. Med. 122:90, 1995, which suggests that control measures help; (2) W.R. Jarvis et al., Respirators, recommendations, and regulations: The controversy surrounding protection of health care workers from tuberculosis. Ann. Intern. Med. 122:142, 1995, which reviews the

evolution of CDC recommendations; and (3) H.M. Blumberg et al., Preventing the nosocomial transmission of tuberculosis. Ann. Intern. Med. *122:658, 1995, which again concludes that infection control measures work.*

237. Stead, W.W., et al. Benefit-risk considerations in preventive therapy for tuberculosis in elderly persons. *Ann. Intern. Med.* 107:843, 1987.
The risk of active tuberculosis was clearly greater than the risk of significant drug toxicity for recent skin test converters.

238. Kucers, A., and Bennett, N.M. (eds.), Isoniazid. *The Use of Antibiotics* (4th ed.). Philadelphia: Lippincott, 1987. Pp. 1351–1393.

239. Baciewicz, A.M., Self, T.H., and Bekemeyer, W.B. Update of rifampin drug interactions. *Arch. Intern. Med.* 147:565, 1987.
Useful review of rifampin's clinically significant drug interactions.

240. Kucers, A., and Bennett, N.M. (eds.), Ethambutol. *The Use of Antibiotics* (4th ed.). Philadelphia: Lippincott, 1987. Pp. 1400–1411.

241. Bennett, W.M., et al. *Drug Prescribing in Renal Failure* (3rd ed.). Philadelphia: American College of Physicians, 1994. P. 35.

242. Dutt, A.K., Moers, D., and Stead, W.W. Smear- and culture-negative pulmonary tuberculosis: Four-month short-course chemotherapy. *Am. Rev. Respir. Dis.* 139: 867, 1989.
INH and rifampin for 4 months in patients with negative smears and cultures gave results similar to 9 months of therapy in patients with positive smears and cultures.

243. Hong Kong Chest Service, Tuberculosis Research Centre, Madras/British Medical Research Council. A controlled trial of 3-month, 4-month, and 6-month regimens of chemotherapy for sputum-smear-negative pulmonary tuberculosis. *Am. Rev. Respir. Dis.* 139:871, 1989.
Four months of therapy with isoniazid, rifampin, pyrazinamide, and streptomycin was equivalent to 6 months of therapy whether or not cultures were positive.

244. Sbarbaro, J. To treat or not to treat, that was the question. *Am. Rev. Respir. Dis.* 139:865, 1989.
Editorial comment on [214] and [215].

245. Nardell, E., et al. Exogenous reinfection with tuberculosis in a shelter for the homeless. *N. Engl. J. Med.* 315:1570, 1986.

246. Small, P., et al. Exogenous reinfection with multi-drug-resistant *Mycobacterium tuberculosis* in patients with advanced HIV disease. *N. Engl. J Med.* 328:1137, 1993.

247. Alzeer, A.H., and FitzGerald, J.M. Corticosteroids and tuberculosis: Risks and use as adjunct therapy. *Tuber. Lung Dis.* 74:6, 1993.

248. Rose, D.N., Schechter, C.B., and Silver, A.L. The age threshold for isoniazid chemoprophylaxis. A decision analysis for low-risk tuberculin reactors. *J.A.M.A.* 256:2709, 1986.
The authors' analysis supports isoniazid chemoprophylaxis in patients older than 35 years. See editorial in this same issue.

249. Centers for Disease Control. Prevention and control of tuberculosis in correctional institutions. *M.M.W.R.* 38:313, 1989.

250. Centers for Disease Control. Management of persons exposed to multidrug-resistant tuberculosis. *M.M.W.R.* 41(RR-11):61, 1992.
See related paper by M.R. Passannante et al., Preventive therapy for contacts of multi-drug-resistant tuberculosis. A Delphi survey. Chest 106:431, 1994, in which this panel of experts agreed that some form of preventive therapy was warranted; however, they were not able to reach a defined consensus on what regimen should be used, although a regimen of pyrazinamide 1,500 mg daily, with ciprofloxacin 750 mg bid for 4 months, was considered somewhat appropriate. More clinical data are needed. See updated discussion of this topic in reference [236].

250a. Colditz, G.A., et al. Efficacy of BCG vaccine in the prevention of tuberculosis: Meta-analysis of the published literature. *J.A.M.A.* 271:698, 1994.
See related paper by T.F. Brewer and G.A. Colditz, Bacille Calmette-Guérin vaccination for the prevention of tuberculosis in health care workers. Clin. Infect. Dis. 20:136, 1995. Review suggests BCG is effective in reducing tuberculosis among health care workers.

251. Woods, G.L., and Washington, J.A., II. Mycobacteria other than *Mycobacterium tuberculosis:* Review of microbiologic and clinical aspects. *Rev. Infect. Dis.* 9:275, 1987.

252. Davidson, P.T. The diagnosis and management of disease caused by *M. avium* complex and other mycobacteria. *Clin. Chest Med.* 10:431, 1989.

253. American Thoracic Society. Diagnosis and treatment of disease caused by nontuberculous mycobacteria. *Am. Rev. Respir. Dis.* 142:940, 1990.

254. Wolinsky, E. Mycobacteria other than tuberculosis. *Clin. Infect. Dis.* 15:1, 1992.

255. Wolinsky, E. Mycobacterial lymphadenitis in children: A prospective study of 105 nontuberculous cases with long-term follow-up. *Clin, Infect. Dis.* 20:954, 1995.

10 Cardiac Infections

Deborah E. Sentochnik
and Adolf W. Karchmer

Infective Endocarditis

The term *infective endocarditis* denotes bacterial, fungal, rickettsial, chlamydial, and possibly viral infection of heart valves or mural endocardium. Infections of vascular endothelium that occur with patent ductus arteriosus, arteriovenous fistulas, or coarctation of the aorta present a similar clinical syndrome and are included in this broadly defined condition. Bacterial endocarditis (BE) is the most commonly recognized form of the disease and often is characterized as acute (ABE) or subacute (SBE) on the basis of its clinical presentation. Fungal endocarditis is seen primarily in intravenous drug users (IVDUs) or in patients with prosthetic valves. Endocarditis in addicts or in association with prosthetic heart valves presents special clinical and microbiologic features and is discussed separately in this chapter.

I. **Pathogenesis** [1, 2]. SBE almost always occurs in a previously damaged endothelium. Endocardial damage may be initiated by inflammatory conditions such as rheumatic valvulitis and by trauma from turbulent blood flow. Sterile platelet-fibrin thrombi form on the damaged or denuded endothelial surface and, in turn, become a nidus for bacterial invasion in the course of bacteremia from whatever source. In SBE, the bacteria are most frequently those of low inherent virulence such as viridans streptococci. In contrast, in ABE the organism usually is highly virulent, such as *Staphylococcus aureus*. In approximately half the cases of ABE, there is no apparent underlying heart disease. In these cases, it is possible that invasive bacteria are able to establish infection directly on the normal endocardial surface.

Most likely, the incidence of endocarditis will increase in the future because, despite the decline in rheumatic heart disease, the number of patients with prosthetic heart valves and the use of indwelling catheters and pacing wires are increasing. Moreover, IVDUs and patients with immunosuppression or immunodeficiency constitute an enlarging population [2a].

A. **Location of infection.** The hydrodynamics of flow through an orifice from a high-pressure to a low-pressure area favor deposition of bacteria immediately beyond the low-pressure side of the orifice or at the site where a jet stream strikes the opposing endocardial surface. Thus, in mitral insufficiency, BE typically involves the atrial surface of the mitral valve. In aortic insufficiency, the ventricular surface of the aortic valve typically is involved, and the chordae tendineae may also become infected; in a ventricular septal defect, the right ventricular surface of the defect and the right ventricular wall opposite it are involved. Endocarditis is much less common in association with low-pressure flow abnormalities such as isolated atrial septal defect or pure mitral stenosis.

B. **Adherence of bacteria** [3]. The ability of bacteria to adhere to the endocardial surface may play an important role in the pathogenesis of infection. Streptococci and staphylococci, the organisms most commonly involved in BE, adhere far more readily to valve surfaces in vitro than do gram-negative enteric bacilli such as *Escherichia coli* and *Klebsiella,* which rarely cause BE, despite the frequency of bacteremia with these organisms. The propensity to cause BE has also been related to the capacity of bacteria to produce extracellular dextran, to aggregate platelets, and to bind to fibronectin.

Revised from M.W. Brandriss and J.S. Lambert, Cardiac Infections. In R.E. Reese and R.F. Betts (eds.), *A Practical Approach to Infectious Diseases* (3rd ed.). Boston: Little, Brown, 1991.

II. Clinical presentation
A. Patient population
1. **Underlying heart disease.** The type of underlying heart disease in patients with BE has varied widely among reports and has changed in frequency over the years [4, 5]. Some of the variability is due to different criteria and diagnostic techniques, referral bias [5], and inclusion of IVDUs or patients with prosthetic valves. Rheumatic valvular damage, once the most common type of underlying heart disease, is found in fewer than 15% of patients in many recent series, whereas mitral valve prolapse [6, 7] has been identified in 10–50% of patients and is the single most common disease in some studies. Congenital heart disease is identified in approximately 10% of patients and degenerative heart disease in 10–20%. From one-fourth to one-half of all patients have had no definitely identifiable underlying disease. Some of these are IVDUs, and it is likely that others have minimal degenerative changes that elude diagnosis.
2. **Other underlying diseases.** A substantial number of cases of nosocomial endocarditis associated with bacteremia from intravenous catheters, postoperative wound infections, genitourinary manipulation, hyperalimentation lines, hemodialysis shunts, and pacemakers have been described in patients hospitalized or treated for a variety of other illnesses [8–10]. In a recent report, bacteremia associated with intravenous catheterization and instrumentation of a diseased urogenital tract were the most common predisposing factors [10a].
3. **Age.** Currently, the mean and the median age of patients with BE is older than 50 years. This is a significant increase in mean age from the preantibiotic era, which may reflect a larger number of older persons at risk and a smaller number of young people with rheumatic heart disease.

B. Signs and symptoms.
The presenting signs and symptoms of BE are variable and often nonspecific. The possibility of this diagnosis should be considered whenever a patient presents with **fever** of more than several days' duration with no other apparent cause and in association with a significant heart murmur. The **type of clinical presentation** can have practical implications in regard to probable bacterial etiology and the degree of urgency in instituting therapy; it is therefore useful to attempt to classify suspected BE as acute or subacute.

1. **SBE.** Patients with typical SBE have an insidious and poorly defined onset of a variety of symptoms that may include weakness, fatigue, anorexia, night sweats, weight loss, arthralgias, myalgias, fever, and neurologic symptoms. Symptoms may be present for weeks or months at the time of presentation. The onset may be related to antecedent events such as dental work, although in most cases no definite antecedent event is apparent.
2. **ABE.** In contrast, patients with ABE usually have a more circumscribed and acute onset of chills, fever, back pain, arthralgia, and myalgia, and often look acutely ill. The patient may be seen within several days to a week from the onset of illness. Infections that antedate the onset of endocarditis may be identified, although, as in SBE, they often are not apparent. Some patients fall between these extremes and cannot be classified easily.
3. **Peripheral signs** [11] of BE, many of which are immunologically mediated, can include splenomegaly, petechiae, clubbing, and retinal and subungual hemorrhage. Janeway lesions are small hemorrhagic or erythematous, nontender macules on the palms and soles due to septic emboli. They occur more often in ABE. Osler's nodes are small, subcutaneous, tender nodules found on the pulp of digits and are due to septic emboli or, possibly, vasculitis. Roth spots are pale-centered, oval, retinal hemorrhages, usually near the optic disc. More common in the preantibiotic era, these signs, which increase in incidence with increasing duration of untreated illness, are now seen in fewer than 20% of cases of BE.
4. **Fever.** Because fever is almost always present in the patient who is not on antipyretics or antiinflammatory agents, a normal temperature pattern under reliable observation makes the diagnosis doubtful. Occasional exceptions to this rule occur in elderly patients or those with debilitating illness.
5. **Cardiac signs**
   a. **Murmurs.** A heart murmur is apparent in 85% or more of cases, and the absence of both fever and murmur makes the probability of BE very slight, although it does not rule out the possibility entirely.
      (1) **Valvular lesions.** The distribution of valvular lesions, as expected, will vary with the type of underlying heart disease reported. If IVDUs are

excluded, the vast majority of patients will have either aortic or mitral valve involvement (in approximately equal proportions), or both. Tricuspid involvement is rare except in IVDUs, where it is common. Occasional cases of right-sided endocarditis have been described secondary to infected central venous catheters or pulmonary artery catheterization [9, 12].

(2) **Changing murmurs.** The appearance of new murmurs or of striking changes in the intensity of murmurs is the **exception** rather than the rule in patients with BE. Some change in intensity due to tachycardia, anemia, or fever is fairly common. If new murmurs or very significant changes in murmur intensity occur, they are likely to represent either aortic or mitral insufficiency and are frequently associated with congestive heart failure (CHF).

(3) **BE without a murmur** tends to be seen (1) early in the course of acute endocarditis that involves previously normal valves, (2) with infection that involves mural endocardium rather than valves, (3) with congenital bicuspid aortic valves, (4) in isolated tricuspid valve involvement, and (5) in some elderly patients.

b. **Other cardiac signs**
(1) **CHF** results primarily from progressive valvular insufficiency, although associated myocarditis also may contribute.
(2) **Heart block and arrhythmias** might occur if there is involvement of the conducting system.
(3) **Pericarditis** rarely complicates BE but can result from extension of a mural or valvular ring abscess.

6. **Embolic phenomena.** In either ABE or SBE, signs and symptoms of embolic phenomena may occur. These are manifested as episodes of vascular occlusion that cause pain in the abdomen (mesenteric or splenic arterial involvement), chest (coronary or pulmonary emboli), or extremities. Hematuria may result from emboli to the kidneys, blindness from retinal artery involvement, and acute neurologic symptoms (including stroke) from cerebrovascular involvement. These signs and symptoms in combination with fever or a murmur should always suggest the strong possibility of underlying BE.

7. **Central nervous system. Approximately one-third of patients with BE exhibit neurologic disturbances as a major presenting symptom or as a later complication of BE** [13, 14]. Stroke is a common presenting neurologic problem, and toxic encephalopathy manifesting as a variety of severe mental disturbances without focal neurologic defects also is common. Meningitis, headache, visual impairment, mononeuritis, convulsions, brain abscess, mycotic aneurysm, and intracerebral bleeds also are seen. **The possibility of BE should be considered in patients of any age when fever or a murmur accompany these neurologic signs or symptoms.**

8. **Rheumatologic manifestations.** From 25 to 40% of patients with BE will have myalgias, especially low back pain, or arthralgias as a presenting or predominant symptom [15]. Arthritis is less common and is typically a nonspecific inflammatory response. Septic arthritis can be seen in ABE, especially with *S. aureus* infection.

9. **The elderly.** Within this large group of patients, the diagnosis of BE is particularly prone to be missed or inordinately delayed. CNS or cardiac signs and symptoms frequently are ascribed to progression of underlying arteriosclerotic disease, and the possibility of BE thus is overlooked. The onset of symptoms often is insidious, fever may not be prominent, and a murmur may be absent [9]. The systolic murmurs that are common in elderly individuals may be erroneously regarded as insignificant.

III. **Laboratory studies.** With the exception of microbiologic studies, laboratory findings are variable, nonspecific, and of little definitive value in the diagnosis of endocarditis.
A. **Nonspecific findings**
1. **Erythrocyte sedimentation rate** is elevated in almost all patients with SBE who are not in CHF.
2. A mild to moderate normocytic-normochromic **anemia** is common. The severity tends to be related to the duration of the illness, and patients with ABE often are not anemic.
3. **Peripheral leukocyte counts** usually are normal or moderately elevated, although prominent leukocytosis may be seen in acute infection.

4. **Thrombocytopenia** may be seen in patients with ABE and in those with spleno-megaly accompanying more chronic infections.
5. On **urinalysis,** microscopic hematuria and proteinuria are common, whereas RBC casts may appear if glomerulonephritis complicates the course.

B. **Blood cultures and bacteremia.** Blood cultures must be obtained whenever the diagnosis of BE is suspected; they will be positive in 85–95% of cases. (See Chap. 25 for the technique of obtaining blood cultures.) Culture media should be capable of supporting both aerobic and anaerobic growth. In endocarditis, as in other intravascular infections, bacteremia (when present) is persistent in the great majority of cases; large numbers of cultures therefore are not necessary, and their timing is not critical. The finding of intermittent bacteremia in a suspected case of endocarditis should suggest some other focus as a source.

1. **In suspected ABE.** When acute endocarditis is suspected and prompt therapy is believed to be indicated, three blood cultures, taken from separate venipuncture sites at 15- to 30-minute intervals over 1–2 hours, are adequate for identifying more than 90% of bacteremic patients with ABE; at the same time, they provide enough samples to minimize confusion over possible contamination.
2. **In suspected SBE.** When the presentation of endocarditis is subacute and the need for therapy is not so urgent, three blood cultures over a 24-hour period are sufficient. If these cultures remain negative after 24–48 hours, another two or three sets should be obtained [16, 17]. Culture of arterial blood or bone marrow offers no advantage over culture of venous blood.
3. **Recent antibiotic therapy.** In the presence of active disease, blood cultures are usually positive even if the patient has been receiving inadequate antibiotics in the previous 2 weeks; exceptions do occur, however. Therefore, if therapy is not urgently required, it is advisable to take blood cultures for at least several days after antibiotic treatment is stopped.
4. **Special culture techniques.** If blood cultures are negative after a few days (whether or not the patient has been on antibiotics) and endocarditis is still suspected, various special techniques may be of value. These are discussed in Chap. 25. Because some organisms grow very slowly, the laboratory should be asked to hold blood cultures for at least 3 weeks in suspected cases of endocarditis.

C. **Resected emboli.** Resection of large emboli may be of diagnostic, as well as therapeutic, value in patients with suspected endocarditis and with negative blood cultures. Resected emboli should be cultured and examined histologically for bacteria and fungi.

D. **Spinal fluid.** Purulent meningitis is rare in BE but can be seen in ABE due to a virulent organism such as *S. aureus* or *Streptococcus pneumoniae.* Spinal fluid in BE due to other organisms with signs of meningeal irritation typically has an aseptic profile, albeit with a slight predominance of polymorphonuclear cells, and cerebrospinal fluid (CSF) cultures are typically negative. With neurologic involvement, the CSF may show a mild pleocytosis (predominantly leukocytic), elevated protein level, and normal glucose level.

E. **Echocardiography.** Among patients with clinical and microbiologic evidence of endocarditis, two-dimensional echocardiography (2D echo) used across the chest wall (transthoracic echo, or TTE) identifies vegetations in approximately 65% of patients. In contrast, 2D echo with biplane imaging from the esophagus (trans-esophageal echo, or TEE) visualizes vegetations in 85–90% of these patients [18].

The ability to identify vegetations varies with vegetation size and location as well as body habitus and underlying diseases. TEE is particularly useful in pa-tients with suboptimal TTE (e.g., those with pulmonary disease, obesity, chest wall deformities, and ventilator dependency). Furthermore, TEE is the approach of choice for evaluating the tricuspid and pulmonic valves and a prosthesis in the mitral position. In a recent editorial, Jamieson concludes that TEE is better than TTE in finding evidence of vegetations, quantifying valvular dysfunction, and diagnosing the spread of infection; this advantage is especially noted in patients with prosthetic valve endocarditis [2a]. Nevertheless, 2D echo, regardless of the approach, cannot distinguish between marantic and infective endocarditis (healed versus actively infected vegetations) or thrombus and vegetation. Furthermore, in some patients, 2D echo may not distinguish between vegetations and noninfective valve abnormalities (i.e., valve thickening or calcification). Given its less than 100% sensitivity for detecting vegetations as well as these other limitations, 2D echo **cannot be used to exclude BE** [18]. It also is generally an inadequate approach to screening for BE among patients in whom the clinical index of suspicion is not high. Whereas 2D-echo-demonstrated vegetations are not required to establish the diagnosis of BE in a patient with positive blood cultures and a clinical syndrome indicative of endocarditis, the echocardiogram may provide clinically useful information among patients with a BE syndrome and negative blood cultures. Furthermore, 2D echo supplemented by pulsed, continuous, and color flow Doppler may provide information regarding intracardiac complications of BE and cardiac hemodynamic status that is important in assessing prognosis and the role of surgical intervention in therapy [18, 19] (see sec. **VIII.G**). See related discussions in sec. **IV.D** and sec. **V.H,** under Endocarditis Associated with Prosthetic Valves.

F. **Diagnostic criteria.** Recently there has been renewed interest in diagnostic criteria for infective endocarditis. Reviewers have emphasized that it is important to have reliable diagnostic criteria for infective endocarditis in order to establish accurate statistics and epidemiological information and to design effective new clinical trials for treatment and prevention of infective endocarditis [19a]. Furthermore, for complex cases, diagnostic criteria might help the clinician make a more precise diagnosis of infective endocarditis.

1. **In 1981 von Reyn and colleagues** published a set of criteria to help diagnose "definite," "probable," "possible," and "rejected" cases of infective endocarditis. The potential limitations of these criteria have recently been reviewed [19a, 19b]. The limitations include the criteria's retrospective nature and lack of prospective validation, the lack of inclusion of echocardiographic findings, the nonrecognition of intravenous drug use as an important predisposing condition for infective endocarditis, and the requirement for histopathologic confirmation of infective endocarditis [19a]. Because of these limitations, investigators from Duke University Medical Center have recently proposed new clinical criteria for the diagnosis of infective endocarditis.

2. **Duke criteria for infective endocarditis** are summarized in Tables 10-1 and 10-2, and a detailed discussion is reviewed elsewhere [19b]. The precise role of these criteria for the clinician (versus their use in helping clinical studies) awaits further experience with their use. However, when used carefully over the entire clinical evaluation period (i.e., not limited to initial findings only), the criteria appear to be sensitive and specific [19b].

    a. We do not believe that every patient needs cardiac echocardiography in order to diagnose infective endocarditis. For example, in the proper setting (e.g., underlying valve disease, periodontal disease) in a patient with com-

Table 10-1. Duke criteria for diagnosis of infective endocarditis

Definite infective endocarditis
  Pathologic criteria
    Microorganisms: demonstrated by culture or histology in a vegetation, *or* in a vegetation that has embolized, *or* in an intracardiac abscess, *or*
    Pathologic lesions: vegetation or intracardiac abscess present, confirmed by histology showing active endocarditis
  Clinical criteria, using specific definitions listed in Table 10-2
    2 major criteria, *or*
    1 major and 3 minor criteria, *or*
    5 minor criteria

Possible infective endocarditis
  Findings consistent with infective endocarditis that fall short of "definite," but not "rejected"

Rejected
  Firm alternate diagnosis for manifestations of endocarditis, *or*
  Resolution of manifestations of endocarditis, with antibiotic therapy for 4 days or less, *or*
  No pathologic evidence of infective endocarditis at surgery or autopsy, after antibiotic therapy for 4 days or less

Source: D. T. Durak et al., New criteria for diagnosis of infective endocarditis: Utilization of specific echocardiographic findings. *Am. J. Med.* 96:200, 1994.

Table 10-2. Definitions of terminology used in the Duke criteria

Major criteria
1. Positive blood culture for infective endocarditis
   a. Typical microorganism for infective endocarditis from two separate blood cultures
      (1) Viridans streptococci,[a] *Streptococcus bovis,* HACEK group, *or*
      (2) Community-acquired *Staphyloccus aureus* or enterococci, in the absence of a primary focus, *or*
   b. Persistently positive blood culture, defined as recovery of a microorganism consistent with infective endocarditis from:
      (1) Blood cultures drawn more than 12 hours apart, *or*
      (2) All of three or a majority of four or more separate blood cultures, with first and last drawn at least 1 hour apart
2. Evidence of endocardial involvement
   a. Positive echocardiogram for infective endocarditis
      (1) Oscillating intracardiac mass, on valve or supporting structures, *or* in the path of regurgitant jets, *or* on implanted material, in the absence of an alternative anatomic explanation, *or*
      (2) Abscess, *or*
      (3) New partial dehiscence of prosthetic valve, *or*
   b. New valvular regurgitation (increase or change in preexisting murmur not sufficient)

Minor criteria
1. Predisposition: predisposing heart condition *or* intravenous drug use
2. Fever: $\geq 38.0°C$ (100.4°F)
3. Vascular phenomena: major arterial emboli, septic pulmonary infarcts, mycotic aneurysm, intracranial hemorrhage, conjunctival hemorrhages, Janeway lesions
4. Immunologic phenomena: glomerulonephritis, Osler's nodes, Roth spots, rheumatoid factor
5. Microbiologic evidence: positive blood culture but not meeting major criterion as noted previously[b] *or* serologic evidence of active infection with organism consistent with infective endocarditis
6. Echocardiogram: consistent with infective endocarditis but not meeting major criterion as noted previously

HACEK = *Haemophilus* spp., *Actinobacillus actinomycetemcomitans, Cardiobacterium hominis, Eikenella* spp., and *Kingella kingae.*
[a]Including nutritional variant strains.
[b]Excluding single positive cultures for coagulase-negative staphylococci and organisms that do not cause endocarditis.
Source: D. T. Durak et al., New criteria for diagnosis of infective endocarditis: Utilization of specific echocardiographic findings. *Am. J. Med.* 96:200, 1994.

    munity-acquired sustained bacteremia with viridans streptococci (e.g., three positive blood cultures over 12–18 hours), the clinical diagnosis of infective endocarditis can be made without echocardiography.
    b. The criteria may be especially useful in patients with bacteremia in whom one is trying to determine the presence of infective endocarditis. While the medical community gains experience with the use of the criteria in clinical practice, it seems prudent to request infectious disease consultations in difficult cases (e.g., for bacteremia in a patient with a prosthetic valve, staphylococcal bacteremia).
    c. When using these criteria to guide therapy in an individual patient, patients who are categorized as having "possible infective endocarditis" should be treated as having infective endocarditis.
    d. See related discussion of echocardiography in sec. **E** and related discussions under Endocarditis Associated with Prosthetic Valves.

IV. **Microbiologic features**
    A. **Organisms**
        1. **Streptococci** account for approximately 55% of all cases of native valvular BE in the nonaddict population.
            a. Approximately 35% of all cases are due to viridans streptococci, the single most common organism.

      b. Approximately 10% are caused by enterococci (group D streptococci).

      c. Approximately 10% are caused by other nonhemolytic, microaerophilic, anaerobic, or nonenterococcal group D streptococci. Group A beta-hemolytic streptococci are a rare cause.

    2. Staphylococci (approximately 35% of cases). Most staphylococci causing BE are coagulase-positive. Coagulase-negative staphylococci are common in prosthetic valve endocarditis but are infrequent with nonprosthetic valves.

    3. Miscellaneous organisms (10% of cases). Infection with HACEK organisms (*Haemophilus, Actinomyces, Cardiobacterium, Eikenella, Kingella*), pseudomonads, gram-negative enteric bacilli [20], pneumococci [21], gonococci [22], and other organisms is responsible for the remaining cases of BE. Reports can be found of endocarditis caused by almost any bacterium [23, 24].

  B. Culture-negative endocarditis [25–26a]. A small proportion of patients with BE have persistently negative blood cultures. In some series, this comprised 15% or more of all patients; however, the true proportion is probably fewer than 5%. The diagnosis usually is suspected in patients with fever of undetermined cause who have underlying heart disease or a newly discovered murmur. The premortem diagnosis of BE with negative cultures is usually in doubt, so accurate figures are difficult to obtain.

    The usual cause is prior antibiotic therapy, because its effect can last for days and, if therapy was prolonged, even for weeks, rendering blood cultures negative. For example, in a recent review from France, 42 of 88 cases (48%) involved patients who had received antibiotics before the first blood culture was taken [26a]. Fungi and organisms that are difficult to culture might also be responsible. A search for pathogens such as *Coxiella burnetii* and *Chlamydia* spp. may be worthwhile in some situations [26a].

  C. Microbiologic and clinical correlations. Although some overlap exists, there is a correlation between clinical presentation and the infecting organism. Bacteria with low inherent virulence such as viridans streptococci usually infect previously damaged heart valves. Damage due to infection tends to progress slowly, and patients are likely to have a subacute or chronic course.

    More virulent organisms, such as *S. aureus,* may infect previously normal valves, and they tend to produce acute systemic toxicity as well as rapid valve destruction. *S. aureus* **is, at present, the most commonly isolated organism in patients presenting with typical ABE.**

V. Treatment: basic principles

  A. General considerations. Although recommendations regarding details of antibiotic therapy for BE differ among various authorities, there is general agreement, supported by clinical and experimental data, that prolonged administration of relatively high doses of bactericidal antibiotics is indicated. The ease of bacteriologic cure, other things being equal, tends to be related directly to the degree of antibiotic susceptibility of the infecting organism.

    With the exception of infection by highly resistant organisms, it generally is not difficult to obtain a response in terms of symptomatic improvement, sterilization of blood cultures, and decline of fever in cases of uncomplicated BE. Bacteriologic cure with permanent sterilization of lesions, however, is considerably more difficult. Bacteria in vegetations are surrounded by fibrin and are relatively inaccessible to phagocytic cells. This may explain the need for bactericidal, rather than bacteriostatic, drugs.

  B. Laboratory aids

    1. Minimum inhibitory concentration (MIC) and minimum bactericidal concentration (MBC) of antibiotics for selected organisms. The MIC and MBC of appropriate antibiotics relative to the infecting organism should be determined by tube dilution tests in addition to the usual disc susceptibilities. This information is of practical value in selecting antibiotics, in determining dosage and duration of therapy, and in determining the desirability of antibiotic combinations. (See Chap. 25, under Laboratory Guidance in Therapy.)

    2. Serum bactericidal levels. In some patients, it may be useful to monitor therapy by determining serum bactericidal activity against the infecting organism. It has commonly been suggested that antibiotic dosage be adjusted to achieve bactericidal activity at a serum dilution of 1:8 or greater at peak concentration, but this is largely empiric or based on experimental animal studies rather than on a clear correlation between bactericidal levels and outcome in patients with BE. (See related discussion in Chap. 25 under Monitoring Antimicrobial

Therapy.) Determination of serum bactericidal activity should not be necessary in patients who are receiving appropriate doses of penicillin for treatment of highly susceptible organisms such as sensitive viridans streptococci, for which bacteriologic cure is rarely a problem. Serum bactericidal levels may be worth evaluating in infection with more resistant organisms for which less conventional antibiotics or antibiotic combinations may be required or in patients whose response to therapy is not satisfactory. Although serum bactericidal tests **have not been able to predict clinical outcome,** one study indicated that peak bactericidal titers equal to or greater than 1:64 and trough titers equal to or greater than 1:32 **accurately predicted bacteriologic cure** [27]. Serum bactericidal levels, however, were **poor predictors of bacteriologic failure** [27]. A critical review of the subject is recommended [28]. Also see further discussion of this topic in Chap. 25.

3. **Saving blood isolates.** The infecting organisms should be stored in the laboratory for the duration of therapy and for a few months thereafter. This might be helpful should complications of antibiotic therapy arise, should the patient not do well on initial treatment, or should relapse occur. Bacterial susceptibility studies to alternative drugs or combinations of drugs can then be determined.

C. **Initiating treatment.** When a patient has suspected BE, a decision must be made as to the urgency of initiating therapy on a presumptive basis before blood culture results are available. In the severely ill patient in whom ABE is suspected, it is reasonable to take three blood cultures over a 1-hour period and to institute therapy promptly because of the rapid progression of this disease. In the patient who has a subacute or chronic illness and a nonspecific clinical picture, it often is best to await blood culture results before starting antibiotics. Therapy usually is not urgent in this situation; it may further complicate the clinical course and differential diagnosis. Judgment is required in determining the degree of urgency of instituting therapy in suspected cases of BE that fall between the two extremes.

VI. **Antibiotic therapy for specific types of endocarditis. The following recommendations assume normal renal function;** drug doses may have to be adjusted for renal insufficiency, as is described in Chap. 28. The doses given here are for adult patients. Treatment in penicillin-allergic patients is discussed in sec. **VII.** Consensus recommendations for therapy from the American Heart Association writing group have recently been published [29].

A. **Viridans streptococci.** The MICs of penicillin G for these streptococci vary widely but usually are less than 0.2 μg/ml. Occasionally, more resistant strains are seen. Most viridans streptococci are susceptible to less than 0.1–0.2 unit/ml, and this level has been used as a convenient (although somewhat arbitrary) dividing line between susceptible, or sensitive, streptococci and those that are regarded as relatively resistant (MIC ≥ 0.5 μg/ml).

1. **Sensitive viridans streptococci**

a. **Penicillin alone.** In more recent series, which report almost uniform bacteriologic success, most patients have been treated with penicillin, 12–18 million units/day IV, divided into q4h doses. The duration of therapy is 4 weeks. This regimen can be expected to achieve bacteriologic cure in up to 99% of patients [29]. It is not known whether doses in excess of 12 million units/day offer any advantage, but one might choose to use the larger doses for organisms with a MIC of 0.1–0.2 μg/ml.

b. **Penicillin plus an aminoglycoside.** In combination, penicillin plus an aminoglycoside synergistically kills viridans streptococci in vitro. Penicillin plus streptomycin (7.5 mg/kg q12h) or plus gentamicin (1 mg/kg q8h) for 2 weeks, followed by penicillin alone for an additional 2 weeks, has been used to treat patients with normal renal function and susceptible streptococcal BE of at least 3 months' duration or when the course of illness was complicated. Despite excellent results, it is doubtful that the outcome differs significantly from the results with penicillin alone [29–31], especially for illness of less than 3 months' duration. The added aminoglycoside for the first 2 weeks is optional in patients who have no relative contraindications to its use, but it should not be given to the elderly, those with renal insufficiency or auditory or vestibular disorders, or those who may not be in a condition to identify symptoms of eighth nerve toxicity should they occur.

Short-course (2-week) combination therapy with penicillin and streptomycin (or gentamicin) has been associated with bacteriologic cure rates as high as 98% in selected cases [29]. The 2-week regimen is appropriate for uncomplicated cases of endocarditis due to highly penicillin-susceptible viridans streptococci occurring in patients at low risk for aminoglycoside toxicity. The 2-week program is not recommended for patients with complications such as shock, intracardiac abscess, extracardiac foci of infection [29] and, possibly, patients who were ill for more than 3 months before therapy was initiated.

Although most clinical experience with two-drug regimens involves penicillin and streptomycin, **data suggest that it is reasonable to consider gentamicin as interchangeable with streptomycin in combination therapy** [29]. Physicians are currently more familiar with gentamicin, and serum gentamicin levels are more readily obtained.

   c. **Ceftriaxone once daily.** A 4-week course of ceftriaxone, 2 g IV or IM once daily, has been as efficacious as IV penicillin (see sec. **a**) and allows for easier completion of therapy as an outpatient with a once-daily antibiotic [29, 32, 33] in uncomplicated cases.

   A recent report from Europe and South America suggests that once-daily ceftriaxone and once-daily netilmicin may be equivalent to treatment with 2 weeks of penicillin and an aminoglycoside in daily divided doses [29, 29a].

   d. **Oral therapy.** For viridans streptococci, this is not recommended [29].
2. **Nutritionally deficient (variant) streptococci** [34]. A combination of penicillin and aminoglycoside for at least 4 weeks often is used, but bacteriologic cure may be difficult and relapse rates are high even with penicillin-sensitive strains.
3. **Resistant viridans streptococci.** For some viridans streptococci, the MIC for penicillin G falls between 0.2 and 0.4 μg/ml. Although no precise guidelines are available, treatment with penicillin, 20 million units/d for a total of 4 weeks, plus streptomycin or gentamicin, is advisable. Occasional viridans streptococci more resistant than this should be regarded as equivalent to enterococci.
B. **Group D streptococci.** Group D streptococci may be enterococcal or nonenterococcal.
   1. **Nonenterococcal *Streptococcus bovis*.** The MIC of penicillin G for most of these organisms is similar to that of susceptible viridans streptococci. When this has been demonstrated, patients with *S. bovis* endocarditis can be treated as for susceptible viridans streptococci. (See Chap. 2, under Positive Blood Cultures, for further discussion of the significance of *S. bovis* bacteremias; many of these patients have an underlying pathologic process of the bowel.)
   2. **Enterococci.** Ninety percent of enterococcal endocarditis [35–37] is due to *E. faecalis,* with the remainder due almost entirely to *E. faecium.* Enterococci are less susceptible to killing by penicillins alone than are other streptococci and are resistant to clinically applicable levels of gentamicin. Effective bactericidal therapy generally requires the use of a cell wall–active agent with an aminoglycoside to achieve synergy. A detailed discussion of therapy has recently been published [29].
      a. MICs to penicillin vary from 1 to 2 μg/ml, with most in the range of 1.0–4.0 μg/ml. Twenty to 24 million units of intravenous penicillin daily is appropriate when renal function is normal (see Chap. 28C). Peak gentamicin levels need only be in the range of 3 μg/ml for synergy to occur. Though there is ample in vitro evidence for the role of gentamicin, most clinical evidence comes from using streptomycin in combination with penicillin. However, the ototoxicity of streptomycin, the need for intramuscular administration, and the substantial percentage of in vitro resistance has led to the more standard use of gentamicin instead. The recommended duration of therapy is at least 4 weeks with both agents and 6 weeks if the symptoms were present for more than 3 weeks before appropriate antibiotic therapy was begun [29]. In patients with renal dysfunction, dosage modification of penicillin is necessary (see Chap. 28C).
      b. The incidence of **high-level gentamicin-resistant strains of enterococci** (MIC 2,000 μg/ml) [38] **warrants routine laboratory screening of clinically significant isolates.** Of isolates with this gentamicin resistance, 30–40% will be sensitive to streptomycin, whose resistance is mediated by a distinct genetic element. There are few well-documented cases of endocarditis due to aminoglycoside-resistant enterococci. Infectious disease consultation is advised. Optimal duration of antibiotic therapy is unknown. Successful therapy may include valve replacement.

c. **High-level penicillinase production,** especially among *E. faecium,* has been documented [39]. Screening for the production of this beta-lactamase should be undertaken if therapy is to include ampicillin or penicillin. Vancomycin activity is not influenced by the enzyme. Unfortunately, many penicillinase-producing strains are also highly resistant to aminoglycosides, thus precluding the use of a known synergistic combination.

d. **Enterococci resistant to vancomycin** and variably resistant to other glycopeptides are reported [40], as are isolates resistant to all available antibiotics. See related discussion in Chap. 28O.

C. **Staphylococci** [41]

1. **Penicillins.** MICs and MBCs should be determined. Prior to determination of susceptibilities, suspected or proved *S. aureus* endocarditis should be treated with one of the penicillinase-resistant semisynthetic penicillins, such as oxalin or nafcillin, in a dose of 2 g q4h. If the staphylococci subsequently are determined to be penicillin-susceptible, penicillin G, 20 million units/day, should be used.

2. **Combination therapy.** There is in vitro and experimental in vivo evidence that low-dose gentamicin in combination with a semisynthetic penicillin effects more rapid killing of staphylococci and sterilization of valves than does penicillin alone. This suggests that addition of gentamicin, 1 mg/kg q8h for the first few days of treatment, may be of value. Because clinical trials have failed to show an improved outcome with combined therapy [42], gentamicin generally should be omitted in patients with relative contraindications to its use, as is described for streptomycin use in cases of viridans streptococci (see sec. **A.1.b**).

    From a practical standpoint, it may be reasonable to use combination therapy (if not contraindicated) for the first 3–5 days, in an attempt to clear the bacteremia rapidly and minimize damage to the heart valve [29].

3. **Tolerant strains.** Some strains of *S. aureus* exhibit tolerance to the bactericidal effect of penicillins in that the MBC for the organism is considerably greater than the MIC. Although the clinical significance of this laboratory finding is not entirely clear, endocarditis due to tolerant *S. aureus* may be more difficult to treat than that with nontolerant strains.

    The addition of gentamicin (1 mg/kg q8h) or rifampin (300 mg PO q8h), or both, in patients who are not responding to a beta-lactam alone, whether or not they are infected with tolerant strains, has been suggested [42]. Determination of serum bactericidal levels may be useful in this circumstance.

4. **Methicillin-resistant *S. aureus*** (MRSA) BE is treated with vancomycin. The usual initial dose is 1.0 g q12h (see Chap. 28O).

5. **Coagulase-negative staphylococci** account for 1–3% of native valve endocarditis [43]. Therapeutic options are similar to those for *S. aureus.* Sensitivity testing should guide treatment decisions. There may be a role for combination therapy.

    See sec. **III** under Endocarditis Associated with Prosthetic Valves, for prosthetic valve endocarditis due to coagulase-negative staphylococci, which is far more common than native valve endocarditis caused by this organism.

6. **Duration of therapy.** Treatment should be continued for 4–6 weeks. The 6-week course often is suggested for patients with an initial delayed clinical response or complicated course.

    Shorter courses of therapy (e.g., 2 weeks of a penicillinase-resistant penicillin and an aminoglycoside) have been proposed for the therapy of uncomplicated, exclusively right-sided endocarditis caused by methicillin-susceptible *S. aureus* infections in injection drug users. (See sec. **III** under Endocarditis in Intravenous Drug Users.)

D. **Other forms of BE** [20, 44, 45]. Infectious disease consultation is recommended.

1. **HACEK** organisms usually are treated with ampicillin or ceftriaxone plus gentamicin for 4 weeks. Ceftriaxone alone can be used [29].

2. **Enteric gram-negative** BE is difficult to treat. The most potent agent, as determined by in vitro sensitivity testing, should be used and serum bactericidal levels followed. It is wise to combine most agents, especially the beta-lactams, with gentamicin. Duration of therapy is 4–6 weeks.

3. ***Pseudomonas aeruginosa*** endocarditis is seen almost exclusively in IVDUs. Tobramycin, 5–8 mg/kg/day, combined with an antipseudomonal penicillin (e.g., mezlocillin or piperacillin), ceftazidime, or ciprofloxacin for 6 weeks is usual therapy.

4. **Miscellaneous.** Antimicrobial therapy for other types of endocarditis should be guided by the same general principles previously outlined, and one should rely on determination of MBCs to select appropriate bactericidal drugs or drug combinations in each case. With more sensitive organisms, 4 weeks of therapy is considered adequate, whereas 6 weeks (and occasionally more) are desirable when one is dealing with more resistant bacteria.

E. **Initial treatment of suspected ABE prior to culture results.** Therapy should be directed to *S. aureus* because it is the most common organism in patients who have ABE. Vancomycin (1 g q12h) plus gentamicin (1 mg/kg q8h) is appropriate and will also provide coverage for possible enterococcal infection. Oxacillin or nafcillin, 2 g q4h, may be substituted for vancomycin in the patient at increased risk for nephrotoxicity. The antibiotic regimen should be simplified as soon as blood culture results are available, so that prolonged administration of unnecessary antibiotics does not continue. In addition, antibiotic therapy aimed at both staphylococci and enterococci will cover, with few exceptions, any other bacteria that are likely to be present. This approach does not commit one to a prolonged course of blind therapy. If blood cultures fail to confirm the diagnosis or if other diagnoses become apparent, management can be altered accordingly.

F. **Blood culture-negative endocarditis.** Presumed endocarditis presenting subacutely with negative blood cultures usually is treated with penicillin or ampicillin plus an aminoglycoside. If the presentation is acute, nafcillin or vancomycin may be added [25]. There are no good data correlating outcome with type of antibiotic therapy in these cases. If the patient becomes afebrile within a week of institution of therapy, a total of 4 weeks of treatment is appropriate. If the response to therapy is not good and if the diagnosis seems certain or highly probable, surgery should be considered. Infectious disease consultation is advised.

G. **Fungi.** Fungal endocarditis will almost always require a combined chemotherapeutic and surgical approach [46]. Amphotericin B is administered at 0.5 mg/kg/day. Most *Candida* and *Torulopsis* spp. are sensitive to flucytosine, and 150 mg/kg/day PO may be added to the amphotericin; flucytosine, however, should not be used alone. The best results have been reported with early surgical intervention and prolonged postoperative amphotericin therapy (see Chap. 18). There is little experience in this setting with newer oral agents such as fluconazole and itraconazole. Infectious disease consultation is advised.

VII. **Treatment of patients with a history of penicillin allergy.** If appropriate skin tests for penicillin allergy are performed properly and the results are negative, the chance of a serious immediate or accelerated reaction to penicillin administration is negligible. Most patients with a history of penicillin allergy will have negative skin tests and can receive penicillin. Cephalosporins are often a useful alternative in penicillin-allergic patients, but a possibility of cross-reactivity does exist. This subject is covered in detail in Chap. 27. The doses outlined here are for adults who have normal renal function.

A. **Sensitive viridans streptococci.** For some patients, it may be preferable to perform skin tests for penicillin allergy and to give penicillin G if the results are negative. If the patient has a history of a delayed penicillin allergy, cephalosporins can usually be administered (see Chap. 27). In these patients, ceftriaxone 2 g IV can be used [29] as discussed in sec. **A.1.c.** If the patient has a history of an immediate, severe reaction to penicillins, or if skin tests to a cephalosporin also are positive, or if one is waiting for skin tests to be performed, vancomycin, 0.5 g q6h or 1 g q12h, can be given. (See Chap. 28O for dosing regimens for vancomycin.) Therapy should continue for 4 weeks.

B. **Penicillin G–susceptible *S. aureus*.** Proceed in the same manner as for viridans streptococci. (A first-generation cephalosporin, e.g., cefazolin, can be used.)

C. **Penicillin G–resistant *S. aureus*.** Most patients can be treated with a semisynthetic penicillin after appropriate skin tests. If alternative drugs are necessary, either a first-generation cephalosporin, e.g., cefazolin 2 g q8h (in the patient with delayed allergy) [29] or vancomycin, 0.5 g q6h or 1 g q12h (see Chaps. 28F and 28O), can be used. Therapy should continue for 6 weeks if possible. Some clinical failures are observed when vancomycin has been used as an alternate therapy in *S. aureus* endocarditis [47]. Therefore, in the penicillin-allergic patient, infectious disease consultation is advised to help determine the optimal antibiotic regimen.

D. **Enterococcal and other resistant streptococci.** Every effort should be made, including appropriate skin testing and consideration of desensitization procedures if necessary (see Chap. 27), to give penicillin or ampicillin to patients with endocarditis due to these pathogens. If neither of these drugs can be given, vancomycin, 0.5 g q6h or 1 g q12h (see Chap. 28O for dosing regimens) for 6 weeks, is the best alternative. Although the MIC of vancomycin for enterococci averages approximately 3 μg/ml or less, it usually is not bactericidal in vitro against enterococci, and the addition of gentamicin or streptomycin is advisable. The toxic effects of vancomycin plus an aminoglycoside may be additive, and it is important to observe the patient closely for any evidence of renal or eighth nerve toxicity. Should these occur, the aminoglycoside should be stopped. Serum levels should be monitored (see Chap. 28H).

Because of a relatively high degree of resistance, cephalosporins are not useful alternative drugs in the treatment of enterococcal endocarditis. An occasional nonenterococcal streptococcus that is resistant to more than 0.1 unit/ml of penicillin might be sensitive enough to treat with a cephalosporin along with an aminoglycoside. Tube dilution MBCs should be performed; if results indicate that adequate serum levels are feasible, a cephalosporin plus streptomycin or gentamicin can be used. If not, the therapeutic regimen should be changed to vancomycin.

E. **Other infections.** The general principles outlined in **A–D** are applicable. The choice of alternative drugs should be guided by results of in vitro testing. Bactericidal antibiotics or antibiotic combinations should be used, and serum bactericidal levels should be monitored, if possible, when in vitro MBCs imply that it may be difficult to achieve adequate blood levels. For unusual or resistant bacteria, infectious disease consultation is advised.

VIII. **Role of surgery in endocarditis.** The need for surgical intervention in the course of endocarditis sometimes is clear but at other times is questionable; guidelines are not precise [2a, 48–50a]. Novel surgical approaches include homograft replacement of infected valves [51].

A. **Progressive or significant heart failure that does not resolve with medical therapy.** There is general agreement that valve replacement is indicated with minimal delay [52, 53]. With aortic valve disease especially, a striking reduction in mortality has been demonstrated with a combined medical-surgical approach. Severe CHF in this setting carries a very high mortality with medical therapy alone. Heart failure that resolves with medical therapy is not considered an absolute criterion for prompt surgical intervention, although in conjunction with other problems it may contribute to a decision for surgical intervention.

B. **Fungal endocarditis** was discussed previously (see sec. **VI.G**).

C. **Persistent bacteremia** (7–10 days) despite appropriate antibiotic therapy is considered a strong indication for surgery. Metastatic extracardiac foci of infection such as osteomyelitis, septic pulmonary emboli, and intraabdominal abscesses should be excluded. A TEE is indicated to look for a perivalvular or myocardial abscess [54].

D. **Emboli.** A single major embolic episode raises the question of surgery, and some have suggested that two major embolic episodes are a strong indication. However, the risk of further embolization in these patients is unknown, and precise recommendations are difficult.

E. **Relapse of infection.** Surgery may be indicated if relapse occurs after a single course of antibiotic therapy, and it is almost certainly indicated if relapse occurs after a second extended therapeutic course.

F. **Evidence of extension of infection. The development of persistent heart block or bundle branch block strongly suggests extension of infection** (see sec. **IX.C.2**); the onset of pericarditis suggests rupture of an annular abscess into the pericardial space. These, as well as detection of valvular ring or myocardial abscesses, left-to-right shunts with septal infection, ruptured chordae tendineae, or papillary muscle all suggest the need for surgery, although they may not individually be absolute indications. See related discussion of myocardial abscess in sec. **V.B.1** under Endocarditis Associated with Prosthetic Valves.

G. **Microbiologic considerations**

1. **Staphylococcus aureus** endocarditis often is complicated by heart failure and periannular abscess [47, 48]. It is also an independent predictor of in-hospital mortality [49]. Early surgery should be considered in the presence of CHF or a perivalvular abscess or if bacteremia fails to clear within 7–10 days.

2. **Pseudomonas aeruginosa** has been difficult to cure with medical therapy alone and has been regarded as an indication for early valve replacement

[55]. However, with the advent of more potent antipseudomonal antibiotics, particularly the fluoroquinolones, this tenet is no longer absolute.

H. Echocardiographic findings as indications for cardiac surgery. The echocardiogram can provide information regarding hemodynamic status and intracardiac complications of endocarditis, which is very useful in assessing the potential role of surgery in the therapy of BE [18, 19]. See related discussion under sec. **III.E.**

1. Echocardiographic quantitation of regurgitant flow across valves damaged by BE, combined with echocardiographic assessment of left ventricular function and clinical findings, allows accurate identification of patients who will benefit from surgical correction of valve dysfunction.

2. Similarly, judgment regarding the timing of surgical intervention is facilitated by echocardiographic findings. Simultaneous reading of the electrocardiogram and an M-mode image of the mitral valve can identify premature closure (before the onset of systole) of the valve, which is a sign of acute left ventricular overload and severe cardiac decompensation and indicates a need for prompt surgical intervention.

3. The Doppler studies can reveal aberrant flow through fistulous connections, thereby identifying patients with invasive extravalvular disease. Similarly, the TEE has been shown to be highly sensitive and specific, in comparison with TTE, for identifying paravalvular and septal myocardial abscesses [54] (see sec. **III.E**). Also, by identifying pericarditis and pericardial effusion in patients with aortic valve BE—a finding often associated with aortic ring abscess—the echocardiogram may call attention to this intracardiac complication. These findings suggest the need for surgical intervention.

4. The demonstration of vegetations, especially large ones in patients with BE, often raises anxiety about serious emboli and the advisability of valve replacement. In many studies, patients with vegetations detectable by echocardiography have had higher rates of CHF and systemic embolization than patients without detectable vegetations and, in some series, these rates are particularly increased when vegetations are greater than 10 mm in diameter.

   Vegetation mobility and valve location may also be important factors in the rate of embolization [56, 57]. However, studies relating imaged vegetations to embolic complications have not routinely distinguished whether complications preceded or followed echocardiography. Additionally, decision analyses that weigh the role of surgical intervention against the hazards of continued medical therapy are not available for these settings.

   As a result, there is no general agreement as to the predictive value of demonstrable vegetations, whatever the size or location, in terms of the need for prompt surgical intervention. Decisions for surgery are based primarily on assessment of valve dysfunction, hemodynamics, antibiotic efficacy, and intracardiac complications, although the presence, size, mobility, and location of vegetations may be important additional considerations when, despite the primary assessment, the role of surgery remains uncertain [58]. The reader is referred to two reviews that discuss the role of surgery in endocarditis [49, 50].

I. Postoperative antibiotics. Duration of antibiotic therapy following valve replacement is not clear-cut. It has been suggested that the full course of antibiotics be given postoperatively if cultures of the blood or the valve are positive at the time of operation or if Gram stains of resected tissue are positive. Otherwise, the usual course should be completed, but a minimum of 2 weeks of postoperative antibiotic therapy should be given.

J. Survival after surgery for culture-positive active endocarditis has recently been reviewed [2a, 50a]. Mortality rates of 20–30% or more have commonly been reported in the acute perioperative phase. However, the long-term outcome of hospital survivors is excellent. Subsequent reoperations for periprosthetic leak are common, but recurrent infection is uncommon [50a].

K. See related discussions about the indications for surgery in sec. **V.B** under Endocarditis Associated with Prosthetic Valves.

IX. Course and complications of BE [59, 60]

A. General. When appropriate antibiotic therapy is begun, symptomatic improvement, decline in fever, and reversion of blood cultures to negative are usually prompt. With very sensitive organisms, this is likely to occur in 24–48 hours, but with more resistant ones, such as *S. aureus,* it may take several days to a week before definite improvement is noted, and it may be 2 weeks or more before the patient is afebrile. Many patients who have become afebrile will continue to be so through a course of therapy, without further difficulty.

Anemia usually persists during the course of therapy, and it may take weeks or months for the hematocrit to return to normal. **Splenomegaly** also tends to resolve very slowly. Some patients will continue to have petechiae or Osler's nodes during or after a course of successful therapy. The occurrence of these does not necessarily reflect antibiotic failure. Significant arterial emboli also may occur up to months after completion of therapy, in the absence of any bacteriologically active disease.

B. **Fever.** One of the most common problems seen during the course of therapy is persistence or recurrence of fever after an afebrile period [61, 62]. If the infecting organism is known to be sensitive and appropriate doses of antibiotics are being administered, simple bacteriologic failure is rarely the cause.

1. **Causes of recurrent or persistent fever**
   a. **Failure to control infection.** If the infecting organism has a relatively high degree of antibiotic resistance, fever and positive blood cultures may persist despite optimal antimicrobial therapy. Failure to control infection in this circumstance indicates that valve replacement is necessary.

   In one study, extensive cardiac infection with discrete abscesses extending from the valvular ring or with widespread tissue destruction without localized abscesses was the most common cause of persistent or recurrent fever; valve replacement was required [62]. More than half the cases were caused by viridans streptococci, and most were not accompanied by pericarditis or conduction defects.
   b. **Intravenous-related phlebitis** (sterile or septic) can occur, particularly with indwelling catheters.
   c. **Metastatic abscess formation** is more likely to occur in staphylococcal infection than in infection by other organisms.
   d. **Recurrent emboli** from the endocardium or from deep venous thrombosis can occur.
   e. **Superimposed infections** involving the urinary tract, respiratory tract, or other sites are not uncommon.
   f. **Drug fever is a common cause of recurrent fever in this setting** (see Chaps. 1 and 27).

2. **Approach to the patient with recurrent or persistent fever**
   a. A careful **reevaluation of symptoms and physical findings**, aided by appropriate laboratory and other diagnostic procedures directed toward the possibilities listed in **1,** is indicated.
   b. **Drug fever** is reviewed in Chap. 1. Antimicrobial therapy can be stopped briefly if other potential causes of drug fever are excluded. If a patient is on more than one antimicrobial agent, the less essential one should be stopped first. For the patient on penicillin plus an aminoglycoside, the aminoglycoside should be stopped for 2–3 days. If fever persists, the penicillin can be stopped. If the organism is sensitive to a non-cross-reacting antibiotic such as vancomycin, this type of drug may be substituted temporarily. Drug fevers usually will clear in 24–48 hours, although longer periods occasionally are required (i.e., 72–96 hours).

   If the fever does not clear, antimicrobial therapy should be reinstituted while the patient is further evaluated for other causes. If the fever does clear and further antimicrobial therapy is necessary, one can either reinstitute the penicillin or change to an alternative non-cross-reacting drug such as vancomycin if the organism is sensitive. If the fever is not too severe and is the sole manifestation of a drug reaction, it may be reasonable to reinstitute the offending drug. However, marked and sustained fever sometimes is associated with vasculitis and, occasionally, reinstitution of the drug may be hazardous. This danger needs to be weighed against that of inadequately treated endocarditis.

   Infrequently, patients will continue to have unexplained fever through and beyond a course of therapy, even though they otherwise appear to be doing well. This tends to clear eventually, and the cause usually remains obscure.

C. **Cardiac effects**
   1. **CHF** occurring during or after treatment of endocarditis is the most common serious cardiac complication of the disease and the major cause of mortality.

CHF usually results from destruction of valves during the course of active disease or from subsequent shrinkage or scarring of valves or their supporting structures, although myocarditis may also contribute. Patients who develop aortic insufficiency are especially prone to rapid and severe cardiac decompensation. The role of surgery in these circumstances has been discussed previously.

2. **Conduction abnormalities** may occur. The appearance of new or changing conduction block suggests extension of infection to the myocardium and is associated with aortic valve involvement in most cases. It has been recommended that valve replacement be considered in patients who develop conduction abnormalities that persist for more than a week during medical therapy and that are not secondary to drugs or ischemic heart disease [63].

3. **Coronary embolization** with myocardial infarction can occur and may contribute to CHF.

4. **Valvular obstruction** due to large vegetations occasionally is seen and generally involves the mitral valve.

D. **Mycotic aneurysms** can be seen in 5–10% of cases of BE in autopsy series [64]. These can occur at any site in the arterial vasculature, usually at points of bifurcation. There is a 1–3% incidence of intracranial mycotic aneurysms [65]. There may be prodromal symptoms, such as headache before rupture [14], which warrant investigation such as arteriography. Management is controversial, but resection is indicated for accessible lesions that are clinically apparent and found to be enlarging or bleeding [65, 66]. Rupture is associated with significantly increased morbidity.

E. **Renal complications** [67]—specifically, focal or diffuse glomerulonephritis—may be seen in the course of endocarditis. Both types of glomerulonephritis are probably immunologically mediated by renal deposition of circulating immune complexes, often with decreased levels of serum complement.

1. **Focal glomerulonephritis** is the more common form and results in proteinuria and hematuria and rarely in renal insufficiency.

2. **Diffuse glomerulonephritis** can cause significant renal failure. The picture sometimes is complicated by concomitant administration of nephrotoxic antibiotics or by the possibility of interstitial nephritis from penicillins. The occurrence of diffuse glomerulonephritis is related to duration of disease and is less common today than in the preantibiotic era. Renal insufficiency secondary to diffuse glomerulonephritis is likely to improve with appropriate therapy, although it may not respond well after extensive damage has occurred.

F. **Complications of antibiotic therapy**

1. **Drug fever** is discussed in Chap. 1.

2. **Allergic drug reactions.** In addition to fever, prolonged administration of high-dose penicillins or cephalosporins results in a significant rate of allergic drug reactions (see Chap. 27).

3. **Aminoglycoside toxicity** is discussed in Chap. 28H.

4. **Acute interstitial nephritis,** often accompanied by renal insufficiency, may be seen with the use of almost any penicillin or cephalosporin, although the incidence is much higher with methicillin (see Chap. 28D).

X. **Sustained bacteremia in the patient without clinically apparent endocarditis.** Patients with repeatedly positive blood cultures are at some risk of having endocarditis, whether or not there are clinical findings suggestive of the diagnosis. This sometimes has implications for dose and duration of therapy. The degree of risk of endocarditis in this circumstance largely depends on the organism involved. (Also see more detailed discussions in Chap. 2, under Positive Blood Cultures.)

A. **Staphylococci.** Patients with *S. aureus* bacteremia are at some risk of having endocarditis, whether or not a heart murmur or other clinical evidence of BE is present. In recent studies, rates of BE in patients with *S. aureus* bacteremia have varied from approximately 5 to 25%, depending on the population studied, the number of community-acquired versus hospital-acquired bacteremias, the proportion of IVDUs, and other factors [68, 69].

When (1) bacteremia is prolonged at the time of presentation, (2) the duration of bacteremia is not known, (3) an extracardiac source is not identifiable, (4) a significant murmur or other evidence suggestive of BE is present, (5) there is persistent fever or bacteremia, or (6) the patient is immunosuppressed, a minimum of 4 weeks of treatment, as for staphylococcal endocarditis, is indicated. The risk of BE in nosocomial, intravenous catheter–induced bacteremia appears to be low if the catheter is removed promptly and antibiotics are given for 2 weeks [69].

B. *Staphylococcus epidermidis* and *viridans streptococci.* Sustained bacteremias involving these organisms usually are accompanied by heart murmurs and sometimes by other evidence of endocarditis. Affected patients are likely to have BE, whether or not the diagnosis is clinically apparent, and should be treated accordingly.

C. Enterococcal bacteremia. In a recent review, endocarditis was present in 12 of 34 cases of enterococcal bacteremia that were community-acquired but in only 1 of 118 cases that were nosocomial in origin [70]. Treatment for endocarditis should not be necessary in a patient with nosocomial enterococcal bacteremia who does not have evidence of endocarditis or underlying valvular disease, unless there is no identifiable focus for the bacteremia [70].

D. Bacteremia caused by enteric gram-negative rods. This type of bacteremia is common, but these organisms infrequently cause endocarditis. Unless clinical evidence of BE is present, prolonged therapy for BE usually is not indicated.

E. Other bacteria. For therapeutic purposes, patients with bacteremia occurring in the course of pneumococcal pneumonia, group A beta-hemolytic streptococcal cellulitis, or gonococcal or meningococcal sepsis also should be regarded as potentially having endocarditis if a significant murmur is present. Such cases need not be so regarded in the absence of heart disease or other evidence of BE.

The combination of pneumococcal pneumonia and meningitis increases the probability of concomitant endocarditis [71]. Patients with this disease combination should receive 4 weeks of treatment (see Chap. 2).

Endocarditis Associated with Prosthetic Valves

The incidence of prosthetic valve endocarditis (PVE) is highest during the initial 6–12 months after valve replacement but continues at a low rate thereafter. By 4–5 years postoperatively, as many as 3–6% of patients may have had PVE. In most series, the rate of infection in mechanical and bioprosthetic valves is similar. Rates of infection are similar for prostheses of the mitral or aortic [72] position.

I. Time of onset of PVE

A. PVE occurring within 12 months (especially that within 2 months) of valve replacement presumably is acquired at the time of operation or in the early postoperative period. Potential sources of contamination accounting for these cases are the heart-lung machine itself, coronary suction lines, other sources of intraoperative contamination, postoperative intravenous and urinary catheters, postoperative pneumonias, and sternal wound infections. In individual cases, however, a definite source of infection often is not identified.

B. PVE presenting more than 12 months postoperatively. Late infections presumably are caused by bacteremia unrelated to the initial surgical procedure and often occurring in a community setting.

II. Pathologic features. With mechanical valves, infection involves the valve annulus at the site of attachment, resulting in ring abscesses, with frequent extension to adjacent structures [72]. With **aortic valve** involvement, prosthetic detachment often leads to severe regurgitation, and extension of infection to conducting tissue may cause serious conduction defects. With **mitral prosthesis** involvement, severe regurgitation or conduction defects are less common, but obstruction by vegetative material may be encountered. With **bioprosthetic valves**, ring abscesses occur when infection arises in the year after valve replacement. Infection beginning later is more typically (but not always) confined to the valve leaflets. Infection may destroy the leaflets of bioprosthetic valves or may cause delayed-onset leaflet stiffness with later development of stenosis [72].

III. Microbiologic features. *S. epidermidis* and *S. aureus* together account for almost half the total cases of PVE. The microbiologic profile of PVE within 12 months of surgery differs from that of later onset.

A. In early PVE, *S. epidermidis* is the most common organism, with occasional infections by *S. aureus,* diphtheroids, gram-negative rods, and fungi.

B. In later-onset PVE, viridans streptococci, enterococci, *S. aureus,* and fastidious gram-negative coccobacilli often are encountered. Coagulase-negative staphylococci may cause 20% of these later infections. **Importantly, coagulase-negative staphylococci that cause PVE within 12 months of surgery often are methicillin-resistant (>75%),** whereas those causing later-onset PVE are less commonly methicillin-resistant (<30%) [72, 73].

C. **Culture-negative PVE** occurs occasionally. Most often, it is the result of recent antimicrobial therapy. However, PVE due to *Legionella* spp., mycelial fungi, *Coxiella burnetii, Mycoplasma* spp., mycobacteria, and occasional fastidious bacteria may cause PVE with negative routine blood cultures [72].

IV. **Diagnosis**

A. **Clinical features.** The clinical picture may be nonspecific or atypical, and precise diagnosis may be difficult, particularly during the initial weeks after surgery.

1. **Fever.** An unexplained and persistent fever in patients with prosthetic valves always raises the possibility of endocarditis. Therefore, serial blood cultures should routinely be drawn in febrile patients with prosthetic valves.

2. **Cardiac findings** of either a new regurgitant murmur (indicating a paravalvular leak) or unexplained refractory heart failure are important clues to the diagnosis of PVE.

3. **The presence of embolic phenomena** or immunologically mediated vasculitic lesions helps support the diagnosis, but their absence does not exclude the diagnosis.

B. As the time after surgery increases (>6 months), the clinical features usually are similar to those of BE in patients without prosthetic valves. However, the diagnosis of endocarditis in the early postoperative period often presents considerable difficulties, with multiple other nosocomial events confounding the evaluation of postoperative bacteremia. Patients with no cardiac or peripheral evidence of endocarditis are particularly problematic in this respect.

1. If sustained bacteremia is caused by relatively avirulent organisms that are not otherwise expected to be invasive (e.g., *S. epidermidis,* micrococci, or diphtheroids) or if there is no apparent extracardiac source for bacteremia, the patient should be treated for endocarditis.

2. Transient bacteremia, with gram-negative rods especially, may or may not indicate endocarditis in this setting. It has been suggested that the postoperative patient with gram-negative rod bacteremia associated with an obvious extracardiac focus of infection and no clinical evidence of endocarditis need not be placed on prolonged therapy for presumed valvular infection. If bacteremia recurs after a course of therapy sufficient to eradicate the extracardiac focus, endocarditis must be seriously considered.

   Some prefer to treat all valve recipients with bacteremia for presumed endocarditis. In one study, only 16% of valve recipients with nosocomial bacteremia (not due to PVE itself) went on to develop subsequent PVE [74]. Staphylococcal bacteremia and the presence of a prosthetic mitral valve was associated with an increased risk for PVE [74]. Infectious disease consultation is advisable.

3. Sustained *S. aureus* bacteremia should be treated as endocarditis.

C. **Blood cultures**

1. In the absence of antibiotic therapy, most patients with prosthetic valve BE (85–95%) have positive blood cultures [72].

2. With some causes of PVE, however, blood cultures may be negative (see sec. **III.C**). Infections with *Candida* spp. can result in intermittent fungemia or negative cultures. With *Aspergillus* or other mycelial fungi causing PVE, blood cultures are usually negative. Fungal PVE may result in emboli to large vessels, and the diagnosis often depends on the demonstration of fungi in resected large emboli (see Chap. 18).

3. It is important that the etiology of PVE not be obscured by premature antibiotic treatment [72].

   a. Indolent endocarditis, in the absence of hemodynamic instability that mandates surgical intervention, does not require immediate antimicrobial therapy. Antibiotics should be withheld briefly pending the isolation of an organism from blood culture [72].

   b. If oral antibiotics that might render initial blood cultures sterile have been given, this delay (3–5 days) is particularly important because it allows blood cultures to be repeated without the interference of additional therapy [72].

   c. Presentations of PVE that are acute or complicated by hemodynamic instability due to prosthetic valve dysfunction require that blood cultures be obtained and antibiotics administered promptly.

D. Other aids to diagnosis. Electrocardiographic demonstration of **conduction defects,** such as increasing P-R interval, complete heart block, or left bundle branch block, suggest infection involving the conduction system. **Echocardiography** may be useful in detecting large vegetations, prosthesis detachment, perivalvular abscess, or pericarditis. TEE, which is exceptionally useful in evaluating prostheses in the mitral position, is indicated when investigating patients with possible PVE. TEE provides excellent views of the posterior portion of the aortic prosthesis; the anterior aortic root area is better visualized from a transthoracic approach. In patients at high risk of PVE, repeat studies may detect abnormalities not noted on the initial echocardiogram. TEE is strikingly more sensitive in the detection of myocardial abscess in patients with PVE than is TTE [72]. Nondiagnostic TTE evaluations are insufficient to exclude the diagnosis of PVE [18, 19, 57].

V. Therapy for PVE

A. Antibiotic therapy follows the same general principles previously outlined for native valve endocarditis [72]. Bactericidal antibiotics are used and administered parenterally. Because antibiotics are often given for 6 weeks, recovery of the causative organism and careful determination of susceptibility data are essential [72] (see sec. **IV.C**).

1. *S. epidermidis.* Most *S. epidermidis* isolates from patients with PVE are resistant to semisynthetic penicillins such as methicillin (see sec. **III**), although this may not be apparent by routine disc diffusion tests or automated MIC tests using a low bacterial inoculum. Careful evaluation of these isolates using proper methods is necessary [72]. Strains that are resistant to methicillin are also resistant to cephalosporins and other beta-lactam antibiotics when studied carefully.

The best results have been obtained with a combination antimicrobial regimen that includes rifampin and gentamicin if the organism is sensitive to these agents.

The usual recommended dosages, assuming normal renal function, are vancomycin (see Chap. 28O for dosage regimens); rifampin, 300 mg PO q8h; and gentamicin, 1.0–1.3 mg/kg q8h. To prevent emergence of rifampin resistance, it has been suggested that vancomycin be adjusted to give peak levels of 25–35 µg/ml and trough levels of 10–15 µg/ml and that gentamicin dosage be adjusted to give a 5-µg/ml peak and 1-µg/ml trough [29, 72]. Additive nephrotoxicity may result from simultaneous vancomycin and gentamicin administration; therefore, renal function should be monitored carefully (see Chap. 28H).

Ideally, the vancomycin and rifampin are given for 6 weeks and the gentamicin (if the strain is susceptible) for the first 2 weeks. If a strain is resistant to gentamicin and other aminoglycosides, ciprofloxacin (if the strain is susceptible to it) may be used in lieu of the aminoglycoside [72]. **Most patients require valve replacement in addition to antibiotic therapy**

For treatment of PVE caused by methicillin-susceptible *S. epidermidis,* a beta-lactam antibiotic can be substituted for vancomycin in the combination regimen [29, 42, 72].

2. Other organisms are treated with high doses of intravenous antibiotics guided by sensitivities, as discussed earlier in sec. **VI** under Infective Endocarditis. Antibiotics usually are administered for at least 6 weeks; a longer course may be required for patients who do not respond promptly. **In the setting of PVE, every effort should be made to attain maximum bactericidal blood levels.** For example, it probably is best to add an aminoglycoside to penicillin for sensitive viridans streptococci infection, even though this may not be necessary for native valve infection.

3. Initial therapy while awaiting culture results. The decision to start antibiotic therapy before a microbiologic diagnosis has been established should be based on the clinical findings. Of particular importance is the possible need for urgent surgical intervention. In selecting antibiotics for empiric therapy, the clinical and epidemiologic circumstances must be weighed. The time that has elapsed since valve replacement may provide insight into potential causes of PVE (see sec. **III**) and should be carefully considered. In general, therapy should include vancomycin, gentamicin, and to provide coverage for HACEK organisms, either ampicillin or a third-generation cephalosporin.

Antibiotics are adjusted when culture results become available. If blood cultures remain negative, the causes of culture-negative PVE should be sought. For patients with culture-negative PVE who remain febrile during empiric therapy, surgery should be considered. Infectious disease consultation is advised.

B. Surgery

1. **Indications for surgery** in PVE are similar to those previously discussed for native valve endocarditis [49] (see sec. **VIII** under Infective Endocarditis).

   These **indications have been summarized in Table 10-3.** Some of these indications are not absolute but rather serve to prompt careful consideration of surgical therapy.

   Because invasive infection unlikely to respond to antibiotics alone is often a feature of PVE beginning within 12 months after valve implantation, these patients will often benefit from surgical intervention. Evidence of invasive disease even in the absence of CHF warrants surgery [72, 75]. PVE caused by *S. aureus* is unusually lethal, with low cure rates attributed to antibiotic therapy alone; affected patients should be considered for early surgical intervention [72]. Failure to achieve an afebrile status with appropriate antibiotic therapy, assuming drug fever and metastatic infection have been ruled out, is evidence of invasive disease and should prompt consideration of surgery.

   Similarly, relapse after appropriate medical therapy usually is due to invasive disease; patients who experience such a relapse should be treated surgically. Failure of a patient with culture-negative PVE to become afebrile in 10 days indicates either inappropriate empiric therapy or invasive disease. Such patients should undergo surgery to clarify the etiology of PVE and debride invasive infection. Surgical intervention is appropriate and probably beneficial in as many as 40–50% of patients with PVE [72].

2. **Results of PVE surgery** have been reviewed elsewhere and operative mortality rates range from 20–30% [50a]. However in a recent series, those who survived the surgical period had a good 5- to 10-year survival rate with about 70% at

---

Table 10-3. Indications for cardiac surgery in patients with PVE

1. Moderate to severe heart failure due to prosthesis dysfunction (incompetence or obstruction)
2. Invasive and destructive paravulvular infection
   a. Partial valve dehiscence
   b. New or progressive conduction system disturbances
   c. Fever persisting 10 or more days during appropriate antibiotic therapy
   d. Purulent pericarditis
   e. Sinus of Valsalva aneurysm or intracardiac fistula
3. Uncontrolled bacteremic infection during therapy
4. Infection caused by selected organisms
   a. Fungi
   b. *Staphylococcus aureus*[a]
   c. Coagulase-negative staphylococci[a]
5. Relapse after appropriate antimicrobial therapy
6. Persistent temperature during therapy for culture-negative PVE in absence of other causes of fever
7. Recurrent arterial emboli[b]
8. Renal failure with severe aortic regurgitation[c]

---

[a]While not a uniformly accepted indication for surgical treatment of PVE, several investigators favor surgical therapy for PVE caused by *S. aureus* or coagulase-negative staphylococci [72]. This may especially apply to patients who do not respond rapidly to antibiotic therapy.
[b]Rather than an indication for surgery, the potential for additional systemic emboli is often viewed as a factor that, in combination with other considerations, might help to justify surgery. Reviews suggest recurrent emboli are rare in patients who are receiving appropriate antibiotics [72].
[c]The presence of deteriorating renal function in patients with endocarditis associated with severe aortic regurgitation should, in itself, stimulate urgent operation [2a].
Source: Modified from A. W. Karchmer and G. W. Gibbons, Infections of Prosthetic Heart Valves and Vascular Grafts. In A. L. Bisno and F. A. Waldvogel (eds.), Infections Associated with Indwelling Medical Devices (2nd ed.). Washington, DC: American Society for Microbiology, 1994. Pp. 213–249; S. W. Jamieson, Surgical therapy for infective endocarditis. *Mayo Clin. Proc.* 70:598, 1995.

5 years and 60% at 10 years [50a]. There appears to be no striking difference in survival whether a valve replacement is with tissue or mechanical prostheses [2a, 50a].

In a recent report, operative mortality was related to the presence of an abscess at the time of operation. Formation of an abscess cavity was commonly associated with staphylococcal infections, PVE, and the aortic site [2a, 50a].

VI. Prevention of PVE. See Chap. 28B.

Endocarditis in Intravenous Drug Users

I. **Clinical characteristics and diagnosis.** Symptoms of endocarditis in IVDUs are usually of 1–2 weeks' duration at the time of presentation, and fever is almost always observed. Endocarditis often is difficult to predict on clinical grounds in the febrile IVDU, and it differs from that in nonaddicts in several respects [76–79].
   A. A history of prior heart disease is usually absent.
   B. The incidence of tricuspid valve involvement, otherwise very low, approximates 50%. Repeated injections of particulate foreign material may damage the tricuspid endothelium, predisposing it to infection during a bacteremic episode. With isolated tricuspid involvement, a murmur is often undetectable; neurologic and peripheral manifestations of endocarditis are relatively infrequent, whereas symptoms of cough, hemoptysis, dyspnea, and pleuritic chest pain associated with pneumonia or septic pulmonary emboli are common.
   C. Aortic or mitral valves are involved in 25–33% of patients, whereas pulmonic valve involvement is rare. With left-sided involvement, the clinical pattern of endocarditis is similar to that in nonaddicts.
   D. There is a high rate of recurrence, presumably due to continued parenteral drug use [80].

II. **Microbiologic features.** *S. aureus,* the single most common organism responsible for endocarditis in IVDUs, accounts for approximately 60% of the total isolates and 80% of isolates from cases of right-sided disease. Streptococci, including enterococci, comprise approximately 20% and cause left-sided endocarditis in the great majority of cases. *P. aeruginosa* and other aerobic gram-negative bacilli account for 10–15%, and fungi—mainly *Candida* spp., which cause left-sided endocarditis predominantly—account for approximately 5%. Polymicrobial blood cultures are reported in nearly 5% and negative blood cultures in fewer than 10%; many of these may result from prior antibiotic administration.
   A. **Regional variation.** Unexplained regional variations have been reported, with *P. aeruginosa* in Detroit and Chicago and enterococci in Cleveland being identified as common pathogens; an outbreak of *Serratia* endocarditis occurred in addicts in San Francisco.
   B. **Source of organisms.** Aside from staphylococcal skin, nose, or throat carriage, which has been shown to bear a close relationship to staphylococcal endocarditis in addicts, the source of infecting organisms has been difficult to identify. With a few exceptions, cultures of drugs themselves or of paraphernalia have failed to incriminate a source.

III. **Treatment.** Antimicrobial therapy for endocarditis in drug addicts follows the same principles outlined earlier for the nonaddict population, except that presumptive therapy (pending culture results) should include gram-negative coverage; indications for a surgical approach to left-sided disease also are similar. In one study, 2 weeks of nafcillin, 1.5 g q4h, and tobramycin, 1 mg/kg q8h, was reported to result in a 94% cure rate in right-sided BE caused by methicillin-sensitive *S. aureus* in drug users whose illness was not complicated by renal insufficiency, extrapulmonary infectious foci, or meningitis. Pregnant patients or those with any evidence suggesting the possibility of left-sided disease were excluded [81]. In a recent report, short course therapy was similarly found to be effective in uncomplicated cases due to methicillin-susceptible *S. aureus* [81a]. Patients with *S. aureus* tricuspid valve involvement usually do well, but occasional cases that are refractory to antimicrobial therapy require valvulectomy with or without valve replacement.

IV. **Prognosis.** The mortality of addicts with staphylococcal endocarditis is considerably lower than that of the general population. This probably reflects the younger population involved, a lower incidence of underlying heart or other serious diseases, and the frequency of tricuspid valve involvement. However, the mortality for repeated bouts of endocarditis and of gram-negative or fungal endocarditis remains high.

The course of BE in patients who are HIV-positive is similar to that in HIV-negative patients. However, mortality is increased for those in Centers for Disease Control category IV for HIV disease [82].

Pericarditis and Myocarditis

I. **Pericarditis** [83, 84]
  A. **Clinical characteristics.** Pericarditis, sometimes accompanied by clinically significant myocarditis, may present as the sole or major manifestation of an infectious illness, or it may occur as a minor or incidental finding. The patient is usually febrile, and the diagnosis is suggested by symptoms of substernal pain or discomfort, which sometimes is relieved by sitting up and leaning forward; the presence of a pericardial rub is confirmatory. Occasionally, pericarditis may present with signs and symptoms of cardiac tamponade. Roentgenographic findings of an enlarged cardiac silhouette may further suggest the diagnosis, although this is not always present. Typical electrocardiographic changes, which may be present in the early stages, are generalized ST segment elevations without reciprocal ST depression except in leads V_1 and aVR. Low-voltage QRS complexes may be seen with sizable pericardial effusions. Echocardiography is a sensitive and reliable noninvasive procedure for demonstrating the presence of significant amounts of pericardial fluid.
  B. The **etiology** often is difficult to establish. Numerous noninfectious as well as infectious causes must be considered.
    1. **Noninfectious causes.** Among these are uremia, neoplasm, trauma, myocardial infarction, postmyocardial infarction (Dressler's syndrome), connective tissue diseases (e.g., lupus erythematosus, rheumatoid arthritis), and rheumatic fever. History, physical examination, and appropriate laboratory studies should be directed toward ruling these out.
    2. **Infectious causes.** Although their true incidence is not known, viral agents probably are the most common cause of infectious pericarditis in the United States. Among proved or highly suspect viral agents, the most important are enteroviruses, especially coxsackievirus B, coxsackievirus A, and echovirus. Influenza, mumps, varicella, Epstein-Barr virus, and others have been implicated occasionally. Cytomegalovirus is an uncommon cause [84a]. The most common diagnosis, especially in young patients without other apparent cause, is idiopathic or nonspecific pericarditis. This is often equated with viral pericarditis although, in most cases, a definite viral etiology cannot be proved. Much less common are cases of pyogenic or tuberculous pericarditis; nonetheless, it is important to rule these out in suggestive clinical settings. Other infectious agents known or suspected to cause pericarditis are fungi, rickettsiae, chlamydiae, mycoplasmas, protozoa, and *Legionella pneumophila* [85].
  C. **Differential diagnosis.** Although the patient's history, physical findings, and ancillary diagnostic tests may help, specific diagnosis of presumed infectious pericarditis usually will depend on examination of pericardial fluid or on pericardial biopsy. However, these procedures may not be necessary, often are not diagnostic and, in most patients, are not indicated. In a case of pericarditis in which the cause is still unknown after the usual diagnostic studies, one often needs to decide whether pericardiocentesis or pericardial biopsy should be performed. This decision must be individualized. Should any evidence of impending tamponade appear, a procedure is necessary for therapeutic purposes, and diagnostic information can be obtained at the same time.

  In the case of the typical idiopathic pericarditis that appears to follow a relatively benign course, it usually is best to observe the patient and treat symptomatically. Should fever persist for more than a few weeks, or should the clinical course appear to be one of continued toxemia or deterioration, open drainage of the pericardium, with pericardial biopsy, may be indicated.

  In a recent report from Spain, between 1991 and 1993, 100 patients with primary acute pericarditis were reported. A general diagnostic protocol was performed in all patients, whereas only pericardiocentesis was performed in patients with clinical cardiac tamponade or an unfavorable course with antiinflammatory drugs. Surgical drainage and pericardial biopsy were performed in patients with tamponade relapse. A specific etiology was discovered in 22 patients (neoplasms in 7, tuberculosis in 4, other infection in 3, collagen diseases in 3, thyroid disorders in 4, and dissecting aortic aneurysm in 1). The general diagnostic protocol led to a specific diagnosis in 15 patients and pericardiocentesis of the other 7 patients [85a].

D. Specific infections

1. Viral, idiopathic, or nonspecific pericarditis

  a. Presentation. In the case of viral, idiopathic, or nonspecific pericarditis, the illness tends to present acutely. In some cases, a history is obtained suggesting a viral respiratory or GI infection that began 2–3 weeks previously. Signs and symptoms may be those of pericarditis alone, or there may be accompanying pleural effusions or pulmonary infiltrates.

  b. Course and complications. The illness usually follows a benign course, resolving in 2–6 weeks, but symptoms may recur in 15–30% or more of patients [86]. The latent period between the preceding viral infection and the first symptoms of pericarditis, as well as the continued relapsing course observed in some patients, suggests a postinfectious, immunologically mediated process. Associated myocarditis, reflected by electrocardiographic changes, is frequent and occasionally is severe enough to cause cardiomegaly and CHF. Chronic cardiomyopathies have been observed in some patients. Hemorrhagic pericardial effusions, cardiac tamponade, and chronic constrictive pericarditis, also have been described.

  c. Diagnosis. The diagnosis often is presumptive and depends on observation of the clinical course after specific etiologies have been ruled out as carefully as possible.

    (1) Cultures and serologic studies. Viral cultures of the pharynx, fecal specimens, and pericardial fluid may be done but, in most cases, they are negative. Examination of acute and convalescent sera for a fourfold or greater rise in antiviral antibody is most practical if a virus is isolated. Screening for antibody to all possible viruses is not practical in the absence of viral isolation.

    (2) Pericardial drainage and biopsy may be indicated in some patients for diagnostic purposes. Cardiac tamponade, or impending tamponade, occurs occasionally and requires drainage through an open surgical procedure or pericardiocentesis. Open drainage, which is preferred by many, offers an opportunity for examination of pericardial tissue. This is useful primarily in ruling out nonviral causes such as tuberculosis or tumor. The fluid and tissue can be cultured for virus and the tissue examined by histologic and immunofluorescent techniques. Histology is nonspecific, however, and viruses are isolated infrequently.

    (3) Treatment. Other than pericardial drainage when indicated, management for idiopathic pericarditis consists primarily of bed rest and administration of analgesic or antiinflammatory agents. The duration of treatment will be dictated by signs and symptoms of disease activity and by chemical evidence of any ongoing associated myocarditis. Aspirin (600–900 mg qid) may be given. Indomethacin (25–50 mg qid) is often useful in cases of persistent severe pain, toxemia, or large pericardial effusions. Prednisone, 60 mg/day (or its equivalent) for 3–5 days, followed by gradual tapering in 5- to 10-mg reductions every other day, has been used. There may be recrudescence of activity with steroid withdrawal, necessitating reinstitution of higher doses. Enthusiasm for steroids should be tempered by experimental demonstrations that cortisone enhances myocardial damage in coxsackievirus B–infected mice. Steroids should be reserved for severe cases that fail to respond to other therapeutic measures such as aspirin or indomethacin. In some patients with chronic recurrent pericarditis, pericardiectomy has been necessary to terminate the disease.

2. Purulent pericarditis [87]

  a. Presentation. Purulent pericarditis almost always occurs in the setting of other serious disease or a surgical procedure and results from postoperative infections after thoracic surgery (commonly open heart surgery); contiguous spread of infection from pleural, mediastinal, or pulmonary foci; contiguous spread from intracardiac infections (endocarditis, myocardial abscess); or hematogenous spread of infection from distant foci. Although the patient is obviously ill, specific signs of pericarditis such as chest pain, pericardial rub, or electrocardiographic changes often are absent. The disease is likely to follow a rapidly progressive course and carries a high mortality.

b. **Microbiologic features.** In the preantibiotic era, *Streptococcus pneumoniae,* usually associated with pneumonia, caused more than 50% of cases of purulent pericarditis; staphylococci and streptococci were the next most common causative agents. More recently, staphylococci and gram-negative bacilli account for the majority of cases, usually occurring after major surgery or in patients with uremic pericarditis, cancer, myocardial infarction, diabetes, and immunosuppressed states. Meningococci, streptococci, gonococci, *H. influenzae,* and a variety of other bacteria as well as fungi also are reported.

c. **Diagnosis and treatment. Prompt drainage of pericardial fluid is essential for diagnostic and therapeutic purposes.** This may be attempted with pericardiocentesis, but surgical intervention with drainage through a pericardial window usually is preferable due to the thick nature of the infected fluid and should not be delayed. Antibiotic therapy is guided by results of Gram stains and cultures of pericardial fluid or tissue. High doses of parenteral antibiotics, equivalent to endocarditis regimens, are used. The role of early pericardiectomy is controversial.

3. **Tuberculous pericarditis** [88–90]

a. **Presentation.** Tuberculous pericarditis may occur as the only clinically evident manifestation of tuberculosis, or it may be accompanied by pulmonary or other (extrapulmonary) disease. Tuberculous pericarditis has its origins in extension from adjacent pulmonary, bone, or lymph node disease; retrograde lymphatic spread from tracheobronchial nodes; or hematogenous dissemination. The presentation may be acute, subacute, or chronic. The acute disease may be productive and granulomatous, with little effusion, or it may present with abrupt accumulation of fluid and may cause tamponade. The presentation usually is insidious, however, with slow accumulation of pericardial fluid. Chronic constrictive pericarditis may result.

In patients with AIDS who present with large pericardial effusions, underlying mycobacterial infections should be considered [90a].

b. **Diagnosis.** If pericarditis occurs in association with proven active pulmonary or extrapulmonary tuberculosis, the presumptive diagnosis usually is made and the patient is treated accordingly. Otherwise, specific diagnosis depends on examination of pericardial fluid or on pericardial biopsy. Acid-fast organisms usually are not seen in pericardial fluid, and diagnosis is made mainly on the basis of cultures of fluid and pericardial tissue and histologic examination of biopsy material. Granulomatous pericarditis should be regarded as tuberculous if no other cause can be found, even if acid-fast bacilli are not demonstrable histologically.

c. **Treatment is with specific antituberculous agents.** Optimal regimens have not been clearly established. Data reviewed in Chap. 9 suggest that extrapulmonary tuberculosis due to susceptible organisms can be treated in the same way as pulmonary tuberculosis if isoniazid and rifampin are not contraindicated. (If alternate drugs must be used, infectious disease consultation is advised.) Short-course regimens appear to be acceptable practice for extrapulmonary tuberculosis. For additional discussion and specific dosage regimens, see Chap. 9 under Tuberculosis.

The indications for corticosteroid therapy and pericardiectomy remain controversial. A faster reduction in heart size and a reduced mortality have been reported in patients with tuberculous pericarditis who received steroids in addition to specific therapy [89]. Prednisone, 80 mg/day, or its equivalent can be given for 5–7 days and progressively reduced to discontinuation in 6–8 weeks. A reasonable generalization is that patients with hemodynamic deterioration should receive corticosteroids.

Pericardiectomy is required in some patients. Indications for pericardiectomy include (1) a persistently enlarged heart, (2) progressive CHF, (3) increasing or persistently elevated venous pressure, and (4) other evidence of hemodynamic compromise.

II. **Myocarditis**

A. **Etiology** [91, 92]

1. **Viral.** Most cases of acute myocarditis in the United States are believed to be

viral in origin. Although the etiology is rarely proven, coxsackievirus B, groups 1–5, as well as some coxsackievirus A and echovirus strains have been implicated.

2. **Human immunodeficiency virus (HIV)** [93, 94]. Although several autopsy series demonstrate an incidence of myocarditis of approximately 50% in AIDS patients, only a small percentage of patients have clinical evidence of myocardial dysfunction. The cause in most cases remains unclear. Diagnostic and therapeutic options are undefined. HIV may have a primary role in causing myocardial damage. The precise role of other viruses is unknown. In the 15–20% of autopsy cases where there seemed to be a specific cause, cryptococci, toxoplasma, and mycobacteria were the most common organisms found (see Chap. 19).

3. **Lyme disease** has recently been recognized as a significant cause of myocarditis in endemic areas [95]. See Chap. 23.

B. **Clinical presentation.** Cardiac involvement by the viruses cited in **A** may present with a clinical picture of pericarditis, myocarditis, or both. With myocarditis, **fatigue, dyspnea, palpitations, and precordial discomfort are common presenting symptoms.** Pericardial or pleuropericardial rubs are also common. Patients are usually febrile, and tachycardia often is disproportionate to the fever; arrhythmias and heart block may occur. The heart may be enlarged, and murmurs of mitral or tricuspid regurgitation may be associated with ventricular dilatation; hypotension or CHF may complicate the course. Cardiac problems in Lyme disease are reviewed in Chap. 23.

C. **Treatment.** Treatment is with bed rest and analgesics or antiinflammatory agents, similar to that for pericarditis.

D. **Prognosis.** It is probable that most patients recover completely, although some are believed to progress to a chronic dilated cardiomyopathy. In the acute stage, diagnostic viral studies such as those for acute pericarditis may be performed, but they are rarely definitive. Myocardial biopsy may be indicated in patients who develop or present with dilated cardiomyopathy [96, 97].

Infections of Permanent Cardiac Pacemakers and Implantable Cardioverter Defibrillators

---

I. **Permanent cardiac pacemaker infections.** Pacemaker systems consist of a generator, which sits in a surgically created pocket below the subcutaneous or subfascial tissue in the chest or abdominal wall, and electrode leads, which may be epicardial or, more commonly, transvenous (in which case the electrodes are attached to the endocardium). The generator pocket, as well as the intravascular and intracardiac portions of the leads, become encased in dense layers of endothelialized fibrous tissue. Treatment of infection is thereby complicated by the lack of penetration of antibiotics into this avascular matrix, thus generally necessitating removal of some or all of the components to eradicate infection. The incidence of pacemaker infections is approximately 3–6% [98, 98a].

A. **Predisposing factors**

1. **Early infection.** The term *early infection* generally refers to infection occurring within 6 months of pacemaker implantation and is most likely due to intraoperative contamination. However, factors usually associated with later-occurring infection (see **2** and **3**) can play a role at any time after implantation.

2. **Late infections** are those occurring beyond 6 months after implantation.

3. The **factors** listed here may be **associated with increased risk of infection** any time during the life of the pacemaker.

   a. **Skin necrosis** overlying the generator can predispose to infection. This is less common with subfascial than subcutaneous placement of the generator. Skin erosion can occur for multiple reasons, including body build, shift in generator placement, or poor nutrition [99].

   b. **Self-induced trauma,** such as from heavy lifting, repetitive movements involving the chest wall, or a direct blow to the generator pocket area, can occur.

    c. Bacteremia from a source other than an infected pacemaker can cause infection of the system in rare circumstances. The pacemaker is at greatest risk for infection associated with bacteremia during the first few weeks after insertion. The offending organisms would typically be staphylococci or streptococci from a remote site of infection. Therefore, it is important to treat promptly any infections, especially those of the skin or teeth, in patients with a pacemaker.

    d. Dermatologic conditions may predispose the patient to pacemaker infection if the skin overlying the generator is not intact as a consequence [100].

    e. Replacement or repositioning of the generator or electrodes appeared to be a predisposing factor for infection in older studies [99]. However, more recent studies have **not** borne this out, perhaps because current generators are smaller and lighter [99].

B. Location

1. The **generator pocket** is the most frequent site of infection.
2. **Leads** can become infected by contiguous spread from an infected generator. If the lead lies in uninflamed, culture-negative tissue, it is considered to be at least contaminated. If the lead is in culture-positive, inflamed tissue, or if there is bacteremia not attributable to a site remote from the pacemaker system, the lead is considered to be infected [101]. The distinction between infection and contamination can have bearing on decisions regarding removal of leads in the setting of a generator pocket infection [101].
3. **Myocardium and valves** become infected by contiguous spread from infected leads. Sustained bacteremia with infection of any portion of the pacemaker requires investigation for endocarditis [99] with TTE or TEE, or both.

C. Microbiologic features. A review of multiple series revealed that *S. aureus* and coagulase-negative *Staphylococcus* spp. accounted for 75% of pacemaker infections [102]. *S. aureus* alone may account for 75% of infections seen within the first 2 weeks of implantation [100]. Mixed infections, gram-negative rods, streptococci and, very rarely, fungi, can also cause infection [98, 100, 102].

D. Diagnosis [98] is based on the clinical picture as well as culture results from blood or a generator pocket abscess. Criteria include

1. Local inflammation or abscess of the pocket *or*
2. Secondary infection of the skin after erosion of the generator *or*
3. Fever and positive blood culture results in a patient with a pacemaker and no other identifiable source of infection. TEE may be a useful diagnostic tool [103].

E. Therapy

1. **Explantation.** The necessary extent of explantation is somewhat controversial. If pocket infection alone is present, some groups have treated with systemic antibiotics and local irrigation only, especially if the causative organism was coagulase-negative staphylococcus [99]. However, the highest cure rate involves removal of the entire pacing system [104] for a generator pocket infection, even in the absence of clear-cut lead infection, and this is the most widely advocated approach. Partial removal of the system (e.g., removal of the generator and retunneling but not removal of sterile proximal leads) is less successful [99, 104]. Lead infections require removal of the entire system [100, 104]. There are several techniques now available for removing an entire pacemaker system that do not involve thoracotomy [101].
2. **Timing of reimplantation.** In the absence of bacteremia, new permanent pacemaker generator can be implanted at a new site at the time of explantation of the infected system. Another option is to use either temporary or no pacing for several days after explantation before reinserting a system [101]. The latter approach may be preferable for infection due to a virulent organism such as *S. aureus*, if explantation is done while the patient is acutely ill, or if an entire new system is to be placed.
3. **Antibiotics.** Use of an antistaphylococcal drug is imperative. Vancomycin is a good empiric choice, unless *S. aureus* infection seems far more likely than coagulase-negative staphylococci, in which case an antistaphylococcal penicillin or a first-generation cephalosporin is adequate. If the patient is extremely ill, it is reasonable also to add coverage for gram-negative organisms while awaiting culture results.
4. **Duration of therapy.** Suggested guidelines are as follows [105]:
    a. Ten to fourteen days if all hardware is removed and there was no bacteremia.

    b. Four weeks if all hardware is removed and there was bacteremia.

    c. Six weeks if hardware cannot be completely removed. There may also be a role for lifelong suppressive therapy in this setting.

  F. Pacemaker endocarditis—characterized by continuous bacteremia originating from an infected focus located on the pacemaker electrode tip, the tricuspid valve, or fibrotic endocardial areas in contact with the electrode tip—is an unusual complication and has been reviewed elsewhere [105a].

II. Implantable cardioverter defibrillator (ICD) infections. The ICD system consists of sensing and shock-delivery electrodes inserted by thoracotomy or a transvenous approach, a pulse generator placed subcutaneously or submuscularly in the abdominal wall, and tunneled wires to connect these two components. The shocking portion of the system may consist of two mesh patches on the epicardium, or of one patch and a transvenously placed endocardial electrode. Placement often is done in conjunction with another open chest procedure, such as coronary artery bypass grafting or valve replacement. The incidence of infection is 2–6% [106, 107].

  A. Predisposing conditions [107]

    1. Prolonged operative time, such as occurs when ICD placement is done in conjunction with another procedure

    2. Reoperation or generator replacement

    3. Remote Infection during perioperative period

  B. Location. As in permanent cardiac pacemaker infections, some infections may involve only the generator pocket, though the entire system usually is infected. Bacteremia is sporadic and does not distinguish localized from more extensive infection [107].

  C. Clinical presentation. *S. aureus* infections of any portion of the system usually present with clinically apparent signs and symptoms of infection and pain over the generator site. Coagulase-negative staphylococcal infections may present indolently, with only increased induration noted over the generator pocket [107].

  D. Diagnosis. The diagnosis of ICD infection can be difficult. If evaluation is done more than 4 weeks after ICD placement, a chest roentgenogram may show patch deformity and a CT scan may demonstrate fluid collections that might indicate infection in the appropriate clinical setting [108].

  E. Therapy. There are no clear-cut guidelines for determining limited versus more extensive infection and thereby distinguishing those patients who may profit from removal of the generator only [109]. In those patients who would not tolerate removal of the entire system, reimplantation of the generator at a new site might be considered under the following conditions: normal radiologic studies; no bacteremia; coagulase-negative staphylococcal infection; no purulence in the pocket; and no ongoing sepsis [107]. Relapse after a prolonged course of antibiotics would demand removal of the entire system; long-term suppression after the initial course may be considered [107]. **Antibiotic choices and duration** of therapy are similar to those outlined for permanent cardiac pacemaker infections.

References

1. Sullam, P.M., Drake, T.A., and Sande, M.A. Pathogenesis of endocarditis. *Am. J. Med.* 78:110, 1985.
2. Livornese, L.L., and Korzienkowski, O.M. Pathogenesis of Infective Endocarditis. In D. Kaye (ed.), *Infective Endocarditis.* New York: Raven, 1992. P. 19.
2a. Jamieson, S.W. Surgical therapy for infective endocarditis. *Mayo Clin. Proc.* 70: 598, 1995.
3. Johnson, C.M. Adherence events in the pathogenesis of infective endocarditis. *Infect. Dis. Clin. North Am.* 7:21, 1993.
4. McKinsey, D.S., Ratts, T.E., and Bisno, A.L. Underlying cardiac lesions in adults with infective endocarditis. *Am. J. Med.* 82:681, 1987.
5. Steckelberg, J.M., et al. Influence of referral bias on the apparent clinical spectrum of infective endocarditis. *Am. J. Med.* 88:582, 1990.
6. Baddour, L.M., and Bisno, A.L. Infective endocarditis in mitral valve prolapse. *Rev. Infect. Dis.* 8:117, 1986.
7. Danchin, N., et al. Mitral valve prolapse as a risk factor for infective endocarditis. *Lancet* 8641:743, 1989.
8. Friedland, G., et al. Nosocomial endocarditis. *Infect. Control* 5:284, 1984.

9. Terpenning, M.S., Buggy, B.P., and Kauffman, C.A. Infective endocarditis: Clinical features in young and elderly patients. *Am. J. Med.* 83:626, 1987.

10. Terpenning, M.S., Buggy, B.P., and Kauffman, C.A. Hospital-acquired infective endocarditis. *Arch. Intern. Med.* 148:1601, 1988.

10a. Fernandez-Guerrero, M.L., et al. Hospital-acquired infectious endocarditis not associated with cardiac surgery: An emerging problem. *Clin. Infect. Dis.* 20:16, 1995.

11. Bush, L.M., and Johnson, C.C. Clinical Syndrome and Diagnosis. In D. Kaye (ed.), *Infective Endocarditis.* New York: Raven, 1992. P. 99.

12. Robbins, M.J., et al. Right-sided valvular endocarditis. *Am. Heart J.* 111:128, 1986.

13. Salgado, A.V., et al. Neurologic complications of endocarditis. *Neurology* 39:173, 1989.

14. Pruitt, A.A. Neurologic complications of infective endocarditis: A review of an evolving disease and its management issues in the 1990s. *Infect. Dis. Clin. Pract.* 5:101, 1996.

15. Thomas, P., et al. Rheumatological manifestations of infective endocarditis. *Am. Rheum. Dis.* 43:716, 1984.

16. Auckenhalter, R.W. Laboratory diagnosis of infective endocarditis. *Eur. Heart J.* 5(Suppl. C):49, 1984.

17. Washington, J.A. The role of the microbiology laboratory in the diagnosis and antimicrobial treatment of infective endocarditis. *Mayo Clin. Proc.* 57:22, 1982.

18. Mugge, A. Echocardiographic detection of cardiac valve vegetations and prognostic implications. *Infect. Dis. Clin. North Am.* 7:877, 1993.

19. Jaffe, W.M., et al. Infective endocarditis, 1983–1988: Echocardiographic findings and factors influencing morbidity and mortality. *J. Am. Coll. Cardiol.* 15:1227, 1990.

19a. Bayer, A.S. Infective endocarditis. *Clin. Infect. Dis.* 17:313, 1993.
    One of the "state-of-the-art" series. Addresses controversial issues including new diagnostic criteria, diagnosis, and therapy of S. aureus endocarditis, the role of echocardiography, therapy of PVE due to coagulase-negative staphylococci, and management of mycotic aneurysms.

19b. Durak, D.T., et al. New criteria for diagnosis of infective endocarditis: Utilization of specific echocardiographic findings. *Am. J. Med.* 96:200, 1994.
    Presents the Duke Criteria and results of the clinical use of these criteria in 369 patients. The sensitivity of the new criteria is superior to the von Reyn criteria. See related paper in same issue by A.S. Bayer et al., Evaluation of new clinical criteria for the diagnosis of infective endocarditis. Am. J. Med. *96:211, 1994, in which the Duke criteria were established to be superior to the von Reyn criteria for the clinical diagnosis of infective endocarditis in 63 patients. For other reports favoring the Duke criteria over the von Reyn criteria, see N. Uriel et al., von Reyn versus Duke criteria for the diagnosis of infective endocarditis in a non-drug abuse population (abstract K-129). 35th Interscience Conference on Antimicrobial Agents and Chemotherapy. San Francisco, CA. Sept. 19, 1995; and B. Hoen et al., Evaluation of the Duke criteria versus the Beth Israel criteria for the diagnosis of infective endocarditis.* Clin. Infect. Dis. *21:905, 1995.*

    See also editorial comments on the Duke criteria by C.F. von Reyn and R.D. Arbeit, Case definitions for infective endocarditis. Am. J. Med. *96:220, 1994, and related editorial comments by C.F. von Reyn et al., Criteria for the diagnosis of infective endocarditis.* Clin. Infect. Dis. *19:368, 1994, both of which raise concerns about the use of the Duke criteria.*

20. Geraci, J.E., and Wilson, W.R. Endocarditis due to gram-negative bacteria. *Mayo Clin. Proc.* 57:145, 1982.

21. Powderly, W.G., Stanley, S.L., Jr., and Medoff, L. Pneumococcal endocarditis. *Rev. Infect. Dis.* 8:786, 1986.

22. Wall, T.C., Peyton, R.B., and Corey, G.R. Gonococcal endocarditis. *Medicine* 68:375, 1989.

23. Fernandez-Guerrero, M.D. Zoonotic endocarditis. *Infect. Dis. Clin. North Am.* 7:135, 1993.

24. Siller, K.A., and Johnson, D.W., Jr. Unusual Bacterial Causes of Endocarditis. In D. Kaye (ed.), *Infective Endocarditis.* New York: Raven, 1992. P. 265.

25. Von Scoy, R.E. Culture-negative endocarditis. *Mayo Clin. Proc.* 57:149, 1982.

26. Tunkel, A.R., and Kaye, D. Endocarditis with negative blood cultures. *N. Engl. J. Med.* 326:1215, 1992.

26a. Hoen, B., et al. Infective endocarditis in patients with negative blood cultures: Analysis of 88 cases from a one-year nationwide survey in France. *Clin. Infect. Dis.* 20:501, 1995.

27. Weinstein, M.P., et al. Multicenter collaborative evaluation of a standard serum bactericidal test as a prognostic indicator in infective endocarditis. *Am. J. Med.* 78:262, 1985.

28. Vosti, K. Serum bactericidal test. *Curr. Clin. Top. Infect. Dis.* 10:43, 1989.
29. Wilson, W.R., et al. Antibiotic treatment of adults with infective endocarditis due to streptococci, enterococci, staphylococci, and HACEK microorganisms. *J.A.M.A.* 274:1706, 1995.
29a. Francioli, P., et al. Treatment of streptococcal endocarditis with a single daily dose of ceftriaxone and netilmicin for 14 days: A prospective multicenter study. *Clin. Infect. Dis.* 21:1406, 1995.
30. Tuason, C.U., Gill, V., and Gill, F. Streptococcal endocarditis: Single versus combination therapy and the role of various species. *Rev. Infect. Dis.* 8:54, 1986.
31. Wilson, W.R. Antimicrobial therapy of streptococcal endocarditis. *J. Antimicrob. Chemother.* 20(Suppl. A):147, 1987.
32. Francioli, P., et al. Treatment of streptococcal endocarditis with a single daily dose of ceftriaxone for four weeks. *J.A.M.A.* 267:264, 1992.
33. Francioli, P.B. Ceftriaxone and outpatient treatment of infective endocarditis. *Infect. Dis. Clin. North Am.* 7:97, 1993.
34. Stein, D.S., and Nelson, K.E. Endocarditis due to nutritionally deficient streptococci. *Rev. Infect. Dis.* 9:908, 1989.
35. Maki, D.G., and Agger, W.A. Enterococcal bacteremia: Clinical features, the risk of endocarditis and management. *Medicine* 67:248, 1988.
36. Rice, L.B., et al. Enterococcal endocarditis: A comparison of prosthetic and native valve disease. *Rev. Infect. Dis.* 13:1, 1991.
37. Morgan, D.W. Enterococcal endocarditis. *Clin. Infect. Dis.* 15:63, 1992.
38. Eliopoulos, G.M. Aminoglycoside resistant enterococcal endocarditis. *Infect. Dis. Clin. North Am.* 7:117, 1993.
39. Bush, L.M. High-level penicillin resistance among isolates of enterococci. *Ann. Intern. Med.* 110:515, 1989.
40. Spara, R.V., and Farber, B.F. Multiply-resistant *Enterococcus faecium.* *J.A.M.A.* 268:2563, 1992.
41. Esperson, F., and Frimoldt-Moller, N. *Staphylococcus aureus* endocarditis. *Arch. Intern. Med.* 146:1118, 1986.
42. Karchmer, A.W. Staphylococcal endocarditis: Laboratory and clinical basis for antibiotic therapy. *Am. J. Med.* 78(Suppl. 6B):116, 1985.
43. Caputo, G.M., et al. Native valve endocarditis due to coagulase-negative staphylococci. *Am. J. Med.* 83:619, 1987.
44. Baldasarre, J.S., and Kaye, D. Principles and Overview of Antibiotic Therapy. In D. Kaye (ed.), *Infective Endocarditis.* New York: Raven, 1992. P. 169.
45. Parker, S.W., Apicella, M.A., and Fuller, C.M. *Hemophilus* endocarditis. *Arch. Intern. Med.* 143:48, 1983.
46. Mayer, D.V., and Edwards, J.E., Jr. Fungal Endocarditis. In D. Kaye (ed.), *Infective Endocarditis.* New York: Raven, 1992. P. 299.
47. Karchmer, A.W. *Staphylococcus aureus* and vancomycin. *Ann. Intern. Med.* 115:739, 1991.
48. Dinubile, M.J. Surgery in active endocarditis. *Ann. Intern. Med.* 96:650, 1982.
49. Alsip, S.G., et al. Indications for cardiac surgery in patients with active infective endocarditis. *Am. J. Med.* 78:138, 1985.
50. Douglas, J.L., and Dismukes, W.E. Surgical Therapy of Infective Endocarditis on Natural Valves. In D. Kaye (ed.), *Infective Endocarditis.* New York: Raven, 1992. P. 402.
50a. Mullany, C.J., et al. Early and late survival after surgical treatment of culture-positive active endocarditis. *Mayo Clin. Proc.* 70:517, 1995.
51. Tuna, I.C., Orszulak, T.A., and Schaff, H.V. Results of homograft aortic valve replacement for active endocarditis. *Ann. Thorac. Surg.* 49:619, 1990.
52. D'Agostino, R.S., et al. Valve replacement in patients with native valve endocarditis. *Ann. Thorac. Surg.* 40:429, 1985.
53. Middlemost, S., et al. A case for early surgery in left-sided endocarditis complicated by heart failure. *J. Am. Coll. Cardiol.* 18:663, 1991.
54. Daniel, W.A., et al. Improvement in the diagnosis of abscesses associated with endocarditis by transesophageal echocardiography. *N. Engl. J. Med.* 324:795, 1991.
55. Reyes, M.P., and Lerner, A.M. Current problems in the treatment of infective endocarditis due to *Pseudomonas aeruginosa.* *Rev. Infect. Dis.* 5:314, 1983.
56. Sanfilippo, A.J., et al. Echocardiographic assessment of patients with infectious endocarditis: Prediction of risk for complications. *J. Am. Coll. Cardiol.* 18:1191, 1991.
57. Mugge, A., et al. Echocardiography in infective endocarditis: Reassessment of prognostic implications of vegetation size determined by the transthoracic and the transesophageal approach. *J. Am. Coll. Cardiol.* 14:631, 1989.

58. Parker, J.D., Sutton, M.G., and Karchmer, A.W. Echocardiography in the management of patients with suspected or proven endocarditis. *Curr. Clin. Top. Infect. Dis.* 11:248, 1989.
59. Weinstein, L. Life-threatening complications of infective endocarditis. *Arch. Intern. Med.* 146:953, 1986.
60. Mansur, A.J., et al. The complications of infective endocarditis: A reappraisal in the 1980's. *Arch. Intern. Med.* 152:2428, 1992.
61. Blumberg, E.A., et al. Persistent fever in association with infective endocarditis. *Clin. Infect. Dis.* 15:983, 1992.
62. Douglas, A., Moore-Gillon, J., and Eykyn, S. Fever during treatment of infective endocarditis. *Lancet* 8494:1341, 1986.
63. Dinubile, M.J. Cardiac conduction abnormalities complicating native valve active infective endocarditis. *Am. J. Cardiol.* 58:1213, 1986.
64. Weinstein, L., and Schlesinger, J.J. Pathoanatomic, pathophysiologic and clinical correlation in endocarditis. *N. Engl. J. Med.* 291:832, 1974.
65. Wilson, W.R., et al. Management of complications of infective endocarditis. *Mayo Clin. Proc.* 57:152, 1982.
66. Wilson, W.R., et al. The management of patients with mycotic aneurysm. *Curr. Clin. Top. Infect. Dis.* 2:151, 1981.
67. Feinstein, E.I., et al. Renal complications of bacterial endocarditis. *Am. J. Nephrol.* 5:457, 1985.
68. Bayer, A.S., et al. *Staphylococcus aureus* endocarditis. *Arch. Intern. Med.* 147:457, 1987.
69. Mylotte, J.M., McDermott, C., and Spooner, J.A. Prospective study of 114 consecutive episodes of *Staphylococcus aureus* bacteremia. *Rev. Infect. Dis.* 9:891, 1987.
70. Gullberg, R.M., Homan, S.R., and Phair, J.P. Enterococcal bacteremia. *Rev. Infect. Dis.* 11:74, 1989.
71. Grandsden, W.R., Eykyn, S.J., and Phillips, I. Pneumococcal bacteremia. *Br. Med. J.* 290:505, 1985.
72. Karchmer, A.W., and Gibbons, G.W. Infections of Prosthetic Heart Valves and Vascular Grafts. In A.L. Bisno and F.A. Waldvogel (eds.), *Infections Associated with Indwelling Medical Devices* (2nd ed.). Washington, DC: American Society for Microbiology, 1994. Pp. 213–249.
73. Calderwood, S.B., et al. Risk factors for the development of prosthetic valve endocarditis. *Circulation* 72:31, 1985.
74. Fang, A., et al. Prosthetic valve endocarditis resulting from nosocomial bacteremia. *Ann. Intern. Med.* 119:560, 1993.
75. Calderwood, S.B., et al. Prosthetic valve endocarditis: Analysis of factors affecting outcome of therapy. *J. Thorac. Cardiovasc. Surg.* 92:776, 1986.
76. Chambers, H.F., Korzeniowski, O.M., and Sande, M.A. *Staphylococcus* endocarditis: Clinical manifestations in addicts and non-addicts. *Medicine* 62:170, 1983.
77. Hecht, S.R., and Berger, M. Right-sided endocarditis in intravenous drug users. *Ann. Intern. Med.* 117:560, 1992.
78. Weiss, A.B., et al. The febrile parenteral drug user: A prospective study in 121 patients. *Am. J. Med.* 94:274, 1993.
79. Cherubin, C.E., and Sapira, J.D. The medical complications of drug addiction and the medical assessment of the intravenous drug user. *Ann. Intern. Med.* 119:1017, 1993.
80. Baddour, L.M. Twelve year review of recurrent native valve infective endocarditis. *Rev. Infect. Dis.* 10:1063, 1988.
81. Chambers, H.F., Miller, T., and Newman, M.D. Right-sided *Staphylococcus aureus* endocarditis in intravenous drug abusers: Two-week combination therapy. *Ann. Intern. Med.* 109:619, 1988.
81a. DiNubile, M.J. Short-course antibiotic therapy for right-sided endocarditis caused by *Staphylococcus aureus* in injection drug users. *Ann. Intern. Med.* 121:873, 1994.
82. Nahass, R.G., et al. Infective endocarditis in intravenous drug abusers: A comparison of HIV type-1-negative and -positive patients. *J. Infect. Dis.* 162:967, 1991.
83. Sternbach, G.L. Pericarditis. *Ann. Emerg. Med.* 17:214, 1988.
84. Shabetai, R. Acute pericarditis. *Cardiol. Clin.* 8:639, 1990.
84a. Campbell, P.T., et al. Cytomegalovirus pericarditis: A case series and review of the literature. *Am. J. Med. Sci.* 309:229, 1995.
85. Savoia, M.C., and Oxman, M.N. Myocarditis, Pericarditis and Mediastinitis. In G.L. Mandell, J.E. Bennett, and R. Dolin (eds.), *Principles and Practice of Infectious Disease* (4th ed.). New York: Churchill Livingstone, 1995. Pp. 799–812.

85a. Zayas, R., et al. Incidence of specific etiology and role of methods for specific etiologic diagnosis of primary acute pericarditis. *Am. J. Cardiol.* 75:378, 1995.

86. Fowler, N.O. Recurrent pericarditis. *Cardiol. Clin.* 8:621, 1990.

87. Park, S., and Bayer, A.S. Purulent pericarditis. *Curr. Clin. Top. Infect. Dis.* 12:57, 1989.

88. Ortbals, D.W., and Avioli, L.V. Tuberculous pericarditis. *Arch. Intern. Med.* 139: 231, 1979.

89. Quale, J.M., Lipschik, G.Y., and Heurich, A.E. Management of tuberculous pericarditis. *Ann. Thorac. Surg.* 43:653, 1987.

90. Sagrista-Sauleda, J., Permanyer-Miralda, G., and Soler-Soler, J. Tuberculous pericarditis: Ten-year experience with a prospective protocol for diagnosis and treatment. *J. Am. Coll. Cardiol.* 11:724, 1988.

90a. Reynolds, M.M., et al. Large pericardial effusions in the acquired immunodeficiency syndrome. *Chest* 102:1746, 1992.

91. Peters, N.S., and Poole-Wilson, P.A. Myocarditis—continuing clinical and pathological confusion. *Am. Heart J.* 121:942, 1991.

92. Maze, S.S., and Adolph, R.J. Myocarditis: Unresolved issues in diagnosis and treatment. *Clin. Cardiol.* 13:69, 1990.

93. Stansell, J.D. Cardiac, Endocrine and Renal Complications of HIV Infection. In M.E. Sande and P.A. Volberding (eds.), *The Medical Management of AIDS* (3rd ed.). Philadelphia: Saunders, 1992. P. 247.

94. Acierno, L.J. Cardiac complications in acquired immune deficiency syndrome. *J. Am. Coll. Cardiol.* 13:1144, 1989.

95. Rahn, D.W., and Malawista, S.E. Lyme disease. *Ann. Intern. Med.* 114:472, 1991.

96. Rezkella, S.H., and Kloner, R.A. Management strategies in viral myocarditis. *Am. Heart J.* 117:706, 1989.

97. Mason, J.W., and O'Connell, J.B. Clinical merit of endomyocardial biopsy. *Circulation* 79:971, 1989.

98. Heimberger, T.S., and Duma, R.J. Infections of prosthetic heart valves and cardiac pacemakers. *Infect. Dis. Clin. North Am.* 3:221, 1989.

98a. Waldvogel, F. Pacemaker Infections. In A.L. Bisno and F.A. Waldvogel (eds.), *Infections Associated with Indwelling Medical Devices* (2nd ed.). Washington, DC: American Society for Microbiology, 1994. Pp. 251–258.

99. Wade, J.S., and Cobbs, C.G. Infections in cardiac pacemakers. *Curr. Clin. Top. Infect. Dis.* 9:44, 1988.

100. Lewis, A.B., et al. Update on infections involving permanent pacemakers. *J. Thorac. Cardiovasc. Surg.* 89:758, 1985.

101. Myers, M.R., Parsonnet, V., and Bernstein, A.D. Extraction of implanted transvenous pacing leads. *Am. Heart J.* 121:881, 1991.

102. Bluhm, G. Pacemaker infections. *Acta Med. Scand.* (Suppl.) 699.1, 1985.

103. Vilacosta, I., et al. Infected transvenous permanent pacemakers: Role of transesophageal echocardiography. *Am. Heart J.* 125:904, 1993.

104. Harjula, A., et al. Pacemaker infections—treatment with total or partial pacemaker system removal. *Thorac. Cardiovasc. Surg.* 33:218, 1985.

105. Threlkeld, M.G., and Cobbs, C.G. Infectious Disorders of Prosthetic Valves and Intravascular Devices. In G.L. Mandell, J.E. Bennett, and R. Dolin (eds.), *Principles and Practice of Infectious Diseases* (4th ed.). New York: Churchill Livingstone, 1995. P. 783.

105a. Arber, N., et al. Pacemaker endocarditis: Report of 44 cases and review of the literature. *Medicine* 73:299, 1994.

106. Bakker, P.F., Hauer, R.N., and Wever, E.F. Infections involving implanted cardioverter devices. *P.A.C.E.* 15:654, 1992.

107. Spratt, K.A., et al. Infections of implantable cardioverter defibrillators. *Clin. Infect. Dis.* 17:679, 1993.

108. Goodman, L.R., et al. Complications of automatic implantable cardioverter defibrillators: Radiographic, CT, and echocardiographic evaluation. *Radiology* 170:447, 1989.

109. Taylor, R.L., et al. Infection of an implantable cardioverter defibrillator: Management without removal of the device in selected cases. *P.A.C.E.* 13:1352, 1990.

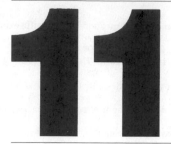

Gastrointestinal and Intraabdominal Infections

Richard E. Reese
and Jerome F. Hruska

Gastroenteritis and Food Poisoning

Acute onset of diarrhea is a common complaint. Whether a patient needs special evaluation, antibiotic therapy, or hospitalization must be routinely evaluated. Several reviews of this topic are available [1–7].

I. **Background**
  A. **Prevalence and impact**
    1. In **developing countries,** diarrheal illness is the most common infectious disease, estimated to cause 3–5 billion cases of infectious disease annually, with an associated 5–10 million deaths per year [2]. Children have 50–60 days of diarrhea per year, and approximately 10% of these episodes result in dehydration that requires therapy [6].
    2. In the **United States,** it is estimated that there are between 25 and 99 million cases of diarrhea or vomiting per year, with approximately 10,000 deaths. Each child has two to two and a half episodes of acute diarrhea annually [2, 6]. Approximately, 8.2 million patients seek medical advice, with 250,000 patients requiring hospitalization. If 50% of patients with diarrhea lose 1 day of activity, it is projected to cost $23 billion yearly in the United States (based on medical costs and loss of productivity) [2].
  B. **Definitions**
    1. **Acute diarrhea** is defined as illness of less than 2–3 weeks' duration. These episodes commonly are caused by infectious agents [6].
    2. **Mild diarrhea** is three or fewer stools per day without abdominal or systemic symptoms [4].
    3. **Moderate or severe diarrhea** is four or more loose stools per day, usually associated with abdominal symptoms (cramps, nausea, vomiting, tenesmus, or systemic symptoms of fever, malaise, dehydration) [4].
    4. **Dysentery** is a **generic term** that refers to any of a variety of disorders marked by inflammation of the intestines (especially the colon) and attended by pain in the abdomen, tenesmus, and frequent stools containing blood and mucus (e.g., amebic, bacillary, shigella dysentery) [8].
    5. **Tenesmus** refers to straining, especially painful or ineffectual straining with a bowel movement [8] or straining on defecation owing to postdefecation spasms of an inflamed rectal sphincter (e.g., in shigellosis) [9].
  C. **Mechanisms of pathogenesis in infectious diarrheas.** A detailed discussion of this topic is beyond the scope of this chapter and is reviewed elsewhere [1–6]. However, a **few basic points deserve emphasis** for understanding clinical presentations and evaluations of patients with acute bacterial diarrhea. **Many pathogens employ more than one mechanism** to overcome host defenses.
    1. **Adherence.** For bacteria to colonize the bowel, they must resist the clearing action of peristalsis, a major host-defense mechanism. Some pathogens circumvent this by attaching or adhering to the mucosal surface. Attachment may increase the toxicity of enterotoxins by decreasing the distance they have to travel to reach target intestinal cells [2].
      a. **Bacterial surface protein structures** (pili or fimbria) bind to specific ligands or receptors on intestinal epithelial cells. This is an **important mechanism for enterotoxigenic** *Escherichia coli* (ETEC) [2].
      b. **Adherence factor.** A distinctly different mechanism of enteroadherence is

seen with **enteropathogenic E. coli** (EPEC). Bacteria adhere to the intestinal cells based on a plasmid-conferred EPEC adherence factor (EAF). No extensive intracellular invasion occurs, and the exact mechanism of diarrhea with EPEC remains unclear but may be secondary to production of a Shiga-like toxin [2].

2. **Invasion.** Certain enteroinvasive organisms can adhere to and invade mucosal epithelial cells. Invasion and multiplication elicits an **intense inflammatory response followed by cell death.** The mucosal inflammatory reaction is not clearly understood but probably involves the release of inflammatory mediators including kinins, interleukins, leukotrienes, and other vasoactive agents. Clinically, one sees fever, abdominal cramps, malaise, and dysentery.

Shigella (which also forms a toxin called Shiga toxin) is the classic example. Enteroinvasive E. coli (EIEC) and Salmonella may employ similar mechanisms [2].

3. **Enterotoxin production.** Vibrio cholerae binds to the intestinal mucosa and produces **cholera toxin,** which stimulates an increased amount of intracellular adenosine 3′5′-monophosphate (cyclic AMP) through the adenylate cyclase system. In response, an active secretion of electrolytes and fluid into the intestinal lumen occurs. It is the classic prototype enterotoxin and stimulates production of voluminous quantities of watery stools (over several hours), leading to potentially life-threatening dehydration. The **intestinal mucosa appears morphologically intact** and is believed to be capable of absorbing electrolytes in a normal behavior because of the empiric observation that oral solutions supplemented with glucose can be used to treat these patients. The overall effect leads to marked increase in the luminal small bowel fluid that is delivered to the colon, and this fluid overwhelms colonic absorption capacity, thereby causing watery diarrhea [2]. **ETEC** has a similar mechanism.

4. **Cytotoxins.** Some organisms can secrete a toxin that causes cytotoxicity in cultured cell lines.
   a. **Shigella.** The **classic prototype** cytotoxin is the **Shiga toxin** produced by Shigella dysenteria [2].
   b. **Enterohemorrhagic E. coli** (EHEC) of **serotype 0157** produce Shiga-like toxins.
   c. **Enteropathogenic E. coli** and **Vibrio parahemolyticus** also secrete Shiga toxin.

D. **Intestinal factors** that may help prevent acquisition of diarrheal disease include gastric acidity and the normal bacterial flora.
   1. **Gastric acid** destroys enteric bacteria and may be an important factor in decreasing susceptibility to infection. Patients with gastric resections and achlorhydria have increased susceptibility to infection. In addition, bicarbonate taken orally has been documented to increase the attack rate of experimental Shigella, E. coli, and cholera infections.
   2. **Normal bacterial flora** of the bowel are believed to compete for space and nutrients with pathogenic organisms. In addition, short-chain fatty acids produced by many intestinal flora may be inhibitory of pathogens. It has been demonstrated that pretreatment with streptomycin lowers the required infective dose of experimental Salmonella typhi infections [1], presumably by changing bowel flora. See also the discussion of antibiotic-related diarrhea in Chap. 28A.

II. **Clinical approach to the patient with diarrhea**
   A. **History.** A careful history may provide clues to the type of infection involved.
      1. **High-risk groups or settings.** There are several settings in which patients are at greater risk than the general population for developing diarrhea [2, 3, 6].
         a. **Recent travel,** especially **international** travel and **camping** (e.g., using water from mountain streams), is a risk factor. For a discussion of travelers' diarrhea, see Chap. 21.
         b. **Infants in daycare centers, or family members of these infants,** are at risk because there is close contact between children who are not toilet-trained and who are unaware of the concepts of personal hygiene. The mode of transmission appears to be either from child to child or through fomites (e.g., toys, bathrooms, shared diaper-changing areas). Currently in the United States, it is estimated that more than 10 million children attend daycare centers [2]. Viruses commonly are identified in outbreaks.

    c. **Patients from chronic care facilities** (e.g., nursing homes, mental institutions, hospitals) appear to be at increased risk, often due in part to their debilitated state, fecal incontinence, or suppressed immune response [2].

    d. **Homosexuals and AIDS patients** are at especially high risk for infectious diarrheas. See Chap. 19 for a detailed discussion of diarrhea in AIDS patients.

    e. **Other family members or very close contacts of an index case** of acute infectious gastroenteritis are at risk for similar illness.

2. **Medication exposure**

    a. Antibiotic use currently or in the preceding 4–6 weeks can be associated with *Clostridium difficile* diarrhea, which is discussed in detail in sec. **I.B** under Miscellaneous Aspects of Antibiotic Use in Chap. 28A.

    b. Ascertain whether the patient uses excessive amounts of **laxatives, antacids, or alcohol.** Note whether the patient is on chemotherapy.

3. Inquire whether the patient may have been exposed to a potential **common-source outbreak** in which other individuals acquired similar illnesses (e.g., picnics, banquets, fast-food restaurants).

4. Ask the patient if he or she has a **pet** (e.g., turtle, iguana, dog) that is implicated in some cases of infectious diarrhea.

5. Ascertain whether the patient recently ate **seafood** or **shellfish** that may have been improperly handled or prepared.

6. **Certain symptoms may be helpful.** Even the number of episodes and type of diarrhea may provide clues to the pathogens involved (Table 11-1).

    a. **When vomiting is a predominant symptom,** viral gastroenteritis or a food-borne intoxication is suggested [4]. Food poisoning due to a preformed toxin frequently causes vomiting within 4 hours of ingesting the food [6]; this is discussed in sec. **IV.**

    b. **Mucus in the stool,** if in small amounts, raises the question of irritable bowel syndrome, but large amounts can be seen with invasive bacterial diarrheas [4].

    c. **Blood in the stool** indicates the possibility of inflammatory mucosal disease of the colon. Blood often is evident on gross examination of the stool. Occult blood testing is more sensitive but less specific [7]. Noninfectious etiologies, such as ischemic bowel disease, diverticulitis, ulcerative colitis, and radiation injury, are in the differential diagnoses [4].

Table 11-1. Clinical features of acute diarrhea

Clinical observation	Anatomic consideration	Pathogens to consider
Passage of few, voluminous stools	Diarrhea of small bowel origin	*Vibrio cholerae,* enterotoxigenic *Escherichia coli, Shigella* strains early in the infection, *Giardia*
Passage of many small-volume stools	Diarrhea of large bowel origin	*Shigella, Salmonella, Campylobacter, Entamoeba histolytica*
Tenesmus, fecal urgency, dysentery	Colitis	*Shigella, Salmonella, Campylobacter, E. histolytica*
Vomiting as the predominant symptom	Gastroenteritis	Viral agents (rotavirus, Norwalk virus) or intoxication (*Staphylococcus aureus, Bacillus cereus*)
Fever as a predominant finding	Mucosal invasion	*Shigella, Salmonella, Campylobacter,* viral agents (rotavirus, Norwalk virus)

Source: From J. C. Bandres and H. Dupont, Approach to the Patient with Diarrhea. In S. L. Gorbach, J. G. Bartlett, and N. R. Blacklow (eds.), *Infectious Diseases.* Philadelphia: Saunders, 1992. Pp. 572–575.

Organisms that produce enterotoxins and are invasive (e.g., *Campylobacter* spp., *Aeromonas* spp., *Shigella* spp., and *V. parahemolyticus*) may initially cause watery diarrhea followed by bloody diarrhea.

d. **Watery diarrhea** is more likely seen in those infections in which organisms adhere, infect, or colonize but do not destroy the epithelium (parasites, EPEC, enteric viruses) [6], and when the small bowel is affected.

e. **Fever** suggests a mucosally invasive pathogen [4].

f. **Systemic illness with hemolytic uremic syndrome,** characterized by acute hemolytic anemia, renal failure with uremia, and disseminated intravascular coagulation, occurs with shigellosis and EHEC [6].

7. **A prior history of inflammatory bowel disease** should be assessed in case the acute symptoms represent an exacerbation of this prior, more chronic problem.

B. **Physical examination.** The physical examination usually is of little help in determining the cause of the diarrhea.

1. **Fever** suggests an invasive bacterial organism.

2. **Signs of dehydration** should be assessed in severe cases, especially in children who may have dry mucous membranes, lethargy, postural hypotension, and tachycardia, sunken fontanelles, and dry skin [7]. This will help determine whether the patient needs hospitalization.

3. **Stool testing for occult blood.** In the patient with multiple episodes of diarrhea and mucosal irritation, occult blood might be present without representing a true invasive process.

C. **Laboratory aids** in diagnosis

1. **Gram staining** of the stool usually is not helpful because most pathogens cannot be differentiated from the normal gram-negative bowel flora. The exception is *Staphylococcus aureus* enterocolitis, which may be suggested on a Gram stain by findings of predominantly gram-positive cocci and fecal leukocytes. Stool cultures should also be done if this diagnosis is suspected. In recent years, this has been a very uncommon diagnosis to confirm. *Campylobacter* may be suggested by Gram stain findings in stool specimens (see sec. **IV.D.2**).

2. **Fecal leukocytes** (WBCs) are found in inflammatory diarrheal disease and give a clue as to the etiology. Mucus can be examined. The presence of a few leukocytes usually is considered an indeterminant result and does not help clarify the diagnosis [4].

   a. **Fecal leukocytes are present in** (1) **bacterial infections that invade the intestinal wall,** such as invasive *E. coli* and *Shigella* and *Salmonella* spp., (2) **ulcerative colitis and Crohn's disease,** and (3) **antibiotic-related diarrhea** (*C. difficile*), in which fecal leukocytes appear in nearly 50% of cases (see Chap. 28A).

   b. **Fecal leukocytes are not seen in** (1) **viral gastroenteritis** (the absence of fecal leukocytes helps support a diagnosis of this very common entity), (2) **parasitic diarrhea,** (3) **enterotoxigenic bacterial diarrheas** (*V. cholerae, Bacillus cereus,* ETEC, etc.), and (4) *Salmonella* **carrier states.**

3. **Stool cultures.** Special media are needed to culture many of the bacterial agents that cause diarrhea. **If one suspects a particular pathogen, it is helpful to discuss the diagnostic possibilities with the microbiology laboratory supervisor** so that proper handling of such a specimen can be carried out. In addition, one should carefully mark the suspected agents on the laboratory specimen sheet. When a laboratory receives a request to culture for enteric pathogens, *Salmonella* and *Shigella* will be sought by using appropriately selected media. Special enriching techniques or media will be necessary to isolate other agents such as *V. cholerae and V. parahemolyticus* (e.g., after exposure to coastal areas or seafood), *Yersinia enterocolitica,* and *Campylobacter jejuni.* The need for these special culture techniques emphasizes the importance of alerting the diagnostic microbiology laboratory in advance.

4. **Virus detection** is particularly useful in evaluating children younger than 3 years. **Rotavirus** can be identified with commercial kits (see sec. **VI**).

5. **Ova and parasite examination** are discussed in sec. **D** and in sec. **II.A** under Gastrointestinal Parasites. In patients with chronic diarrhea, international travelers, homosexual men, and contacts of daycare centers with protracted symptoms, these specimens are especially useful to examine.

6. *Clostridium difficile* **toxin** assay is useful in an attempt to diagnose *C. difficile*–related diarrhea and in patients who are on or who have been on antibiotics in the preceding 4–6 weeks (see Chap. 28A).

7. Proctosigmoidoscopy examinations seldom are indicated except as follows [4]:
   a. In homosexual men and in some cases of AIDS-related illness (see Chap. 19).
   b. In some cases of chronic or recurrent diarrhea in patients with possible inflammatory bowel disease.
   c. In some cases of *C. difficile* diarrhea in which an immediate answer is needed (see Chap. 28A).
   d. In a potential case of *Entamoeba histolytica,* as ulcerations of the intestinal wall may be characteristic in this setting. Rectal mucosal biopsy may also help [7].

8. Radiographic studies usually are not indicated.
   a. If toxic megacolon is a potential concern as a complication—for example, with *C. difficile* diarrhea—radiographic plain films are useful.
   b. In chronic diarrhea, pancreatic calcifications may be a clue that chronic pancreatitis exists.
   c. Barium contrast studies will render microscopical stool examinations (e.g., for ova and parasites) essentially useless [7].

9. Miscellaneous studies
   a. Peripheral WBC counts are nonspecific. Although it may be elevated in acute infectious diarrhea (e.g., *Salmonella* or *Shigella*), WBC count also may be falsely elevated in patients with significant dehydration due to nonbacterial processes.
   b. Blood cultures. In the febrile patient with gastroenteritis, blood cultures may be helpful. They may be positive when other sources, including stool cultures, are negative.
   c. Bone marrow cultures. Biopsy specimens often are positive in typhoid fever but are performed only in unusual circumstances (e.g., in the workup of an unclear chronic fever).
   d. Rose spots (the transient skin rash of typhoid fever) can be biopsied and cultured.
   e. Serologic studies. In acute gastroenteritis, serologic studies **offer little help.** Special circumstances in which serologic evaluation may be helpful include the following:
      (1) Amebiasis. Indirect hemagglutination (available through reference laboratories, state health departments, and the Centers for Disease Control, Atlanta) is a useful adjunct in the diagnosis of extraintestinal amebiasis (92–98% positive) or active intestinal infection (80–90% positive) but is of little assistance for the asymptomatic patient who is passing cysts (see sec. **IV.E** under Gastrointestinal Parasites).
      (2) *Salmonella* **O antigen titers.** Titers rise slowly to a peak at approximately 6 weeks. Of infected patients, 50% convert to seropositivity after 1 week, and only by the fourth week do 90–95% of patients show an elevated titer. Usually, a case of acute *Salmonella* gastroenteritis will remit spontaneously before there is any seroconversion. The usefulness of the antibody tests is limited by circumstances in which a persistent infection has allowed time for a host antibody response; they are unlikely to be useful for *Salmonella* gastroenteritis or acute bacteremia or in individuals with abnormal humoral responses. The carrier state produces very little response. The usual tests apply only to *S. typhi.* Other serologic tests are being investigated [10].
      Caution should be exercised in the interpretation of a single value without evidence of seroconversion. Previous seroconversion, typhoid immunization, and some cross-reaction with Enterobacteriaceae O antigens can cause an isolated elevation of antibody titer.

D. Diagnostic workup. Much has been written about the cost-effectiveness of stool cultures in a nonselective group of patients with diarrhea. Only 1–2% of samples will test positively for *Salmonella* or *Shigella* in unselected stool specimens. This translates into a cost of more than $1,000 per positive stool culture, an extremely cost-*in*effective workup. Approaches have been developed to improve the diagnostic yield and provide a rational cost-effective basis for evaluating stool specimens [1, 2] (Fig. 11-1).
   Even with a careful evaluation and laboratory workup, between 20 and 40% of all acute infectious diarrheas will remain undiagnosed [6].
   1. If the history suggests a foodborne toxin-related illness (i.e., symptoms occur within a few hours of a meal, with nausea and vomiting as prominent symp-

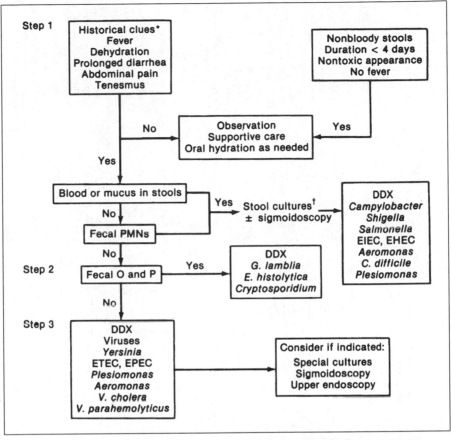

Fig. 11-1. An algorithm for diagnostic evaluation of acute infectious diarrhea. *PMNs* = polymorphonuclear leukocytes; *fecal O and P* = fecal ova and parasites; *EIEC* = entero-invasive *E. coli; EHEC* = enterohemorrhagic *E. coli; ETEC* = enterotoxigenic *E. coli; EPEC* = enteropathogenic *E. coli; DDX* = differential diagnosis; *recent use of antibiotics, recent travel, homosexual activity, camping, seafood ingestion, and history of local outbreak of diarrhea; †in homosexual population with proctitis on sigmoidoscopy, include cultures of *Neisseria gonorrhoeae, Chlamydia trachomatis,* herpes simplex virus, and *Mycobacterium avium-intracellulare.* (Modified from C. P. Cheney and R. K. H. Wong, Acute infectious diarrhea. *Med. Clin. North Am.* 77:1169, 1993.)

toms), see Table 11-2 for a summary of important pathogens and presentation. Foodborne toxins are discussed in sec. **IV.**

2. Afebrile stable patients with nonbloody diarrhea of short duration can be observed and treated conservatively with oral rehydration and no extensive laboratory workup.

3. **High-risk patients, as determined by history** (see sec. **II.A.1**), **and those who have fever, dehydration, prolonged diarrhea (more than 4 days), abdominal pain, or tenesmus deserve further evaluation** as follows.

   a. **Step 1: If the patient has mucus or blood in the stool or if fecal leukocytes are present,** a stool culture is indicated.

      According to Guerrant [1, 2, 6], this screening approach dramatically increased the yield of positive stool cultures and the cost of a positive stool culture decreased to only $30.

      Note: You must alert the microbiology laboratory to culture for *Campylobacter* or *Yersinia* if these are potential concerns, as these pathogens may not be routinely tested for in your laboratory (see sec. **II.C**).

Table 11-2. Clinical features of agent-specific foodborne disease with symptom onset of less than 12 hours

Organism or agent	Incubation period	Duration of illness (range)	Diarrhea	Fever	Vomiting	Enterotoxin	Invasion	Foods most commonly implicated	Comments
Staphylococcus aureus	1–8 hr	24 hr (8–48 hr)	+ (infrequent)	–	+++	++	–	Salads, cream-filled pastries, meats (pork, beef, poultry)	High attack rates (80–100%) Outbreaks most frequent during summer
Bacillus cereus Emetic illness	1–6 hr	9 hr (2–10 hr)	+	–	+++	++	–	Fried rice	Abdominal cramps often experienced Vomiting occurs more often than diarrhea
Diarrheal illness	6–14 hr	20 hr (16–48 hr)	+++	–	+	+	–	Meats, vanilla sauce, cream-baked goods, salads, chicken soup	Diarrhea occurs more often than vomiting Organism may be found in stool of healthy person
Clostridium perfringens	8–24 hr	24 hr (8–72 hr)	+++	–	±	++	–	Improperly stored beef, fish, or poultry dishes (after preparation); pasta salads, dairy products; Mexican foods	"Pig-bel" or necrotizing enterocolitis is a rare variant Stool has no white blood cells or blood Commercial kit available for detection of toxin in stool
Non 0:1 *Vibrio cholerae*	6–72 hr	2 days (2–12 days)	++	±	±	+ (a minority produce cholera toxin)	±	Seafood, grated eggs, potatoes	25% can have bloody diarrhea Illness similar to cholera but much less dehydration
Puffer fish	<2 hr	Variable	+	–	+	+ Tetrodotoxin (i.e., a neurotoxin)	–	Fugu (especially prepared Japanese puffer fish), other puffer fish, vividly colored frogs of South America, blue-ringed octopus	Symptoms include paresthesias, ataxia, hypotension, seizures, cardiac arrhythmias, respiratory and skeletal muscle paralysis Mortality 30–60% Treatment: gastric lavage and cardiorespiratory support

Paralytic shellfish	1–3 hr	3 days (0.5–7 days)	–	+	–	+ Saxitoxin (i.e., a neurotoxin)	–	Most bivalved mollusks (shellfish) especially from endemic waters experiencing red tide blooms	Prognosis greatly improves if patient survives first 6 hours. Symptoms and treatment similar to puffer fish poisoning. Mortality 5–18%. Etiology is concentration of toxic dinoflagellates in mollusks during "red tide" season (spring and fall)
Ciguatera	1–6 hr	Variable (can persist for months)	+	+	–	+ Ciguatoxin (i.e., a neurotoxin)	–	Barracuda, grouper, snapper, jacks, reef sharks	Most common form of fish intoxication in United States. Commonly seen in Florida, Hawaii, and the Caribbean. Symptoms similar to puffer fish poisoning. ELISA available for detection of toxin. Treatment suggested with amitriptyline
Scombroid fish	<2 hr	Variable (2–10 hr)	±	+	–	– (preformed histamine causes symptoms; *not* an allergic reaction)	–	"Blood fish" (tuna, albacore, mackerel, skip jacks) under spoiling conditions	Symptoms: flushing, generalized or localized erythema, vertigo, generalized burning sensation. Histamine levels can be assayed in implicated fish. Treatment with antihistamines very effective. Fish with unpleasant odor or clouded eyes should be avoided

Source: From A. G. Miranda and H. L. DuPont, Small Intestine: Infections with Common Bacterial and Viral Pathogens. In T. Yamada (ed.), *Textbook of Gastroenterology*. New York: Lippincott, 1991. Pp. 1452–1453.

If the patient has had a history of antibiotic use, either currently or in the preceding 4–6 weeks, a stool for *C. difficile* toxin should be sent to exclude this diagnosis. If this diagnosis is suspected and the patient is not toxic, it may be desirable to get *C. difficile* results before obtaining the stool culture.

b. **Step 2: If blood or mucus is not in the stools and no fecal leukocytes are seen, the ova and parasite examinations are suggested.**

   (1) It is usual to obtain three stools for ova and parasite examination.

   (2) If *Giardia* spp. are likely, the *Giardia* antigen test can be useful (see sec. **IV.A.2** under Gastrointestinal Parasites).

   (3) In children younger than 3 years in whom the fecal leukocyte test is negative and a viral etiology is possible, an early examination for **rotavirus** is suggested (see sec. **VI.A**).

c. **Step 3: If no parasites are found, then the differential diagnosis is narrowed to include viruses and certain difficult-to-culture bacteria** (e.g., *Yersinia, V. cholerae,* ETEC, EPEC, *Aeromonas hydrophila, Plesiomonas shigelloides*).

   (1) Special media can be used for *V. cholerae*.

   (2) Discuss the microbiology workup with your laboratory supervisor if routine cultures are negative.

III. **Therapy. In most cases of infectious diarrhea, therapy consists of supportive care.**
   A. **Fluid replacement**
   1. **Oral fluids** will suffice in most patients [11]. Because of the common occurrence of diarrhea worldwide, the World Health Organization (WHO) has developed an oral rehydration formula that is inexpensive, easy to administer, and effective in all types of diarrhea and all age groups. The WHO formula and all other oral rehydration formulas are based on the principal that carbohydrate absorption, especially that of glucose, in the small bowel facilitates sodium and water resorption of fluid from the intestinal lumen into the intravascular compartment [1, 2].

      a. The composition of the WHO oral rehydration fluid is shown in Table 11-3.

      b. Oral replacement therapy is contraindicated only in patients with uncontrolled vomiting, in the presence of an ileus, or in patients with severe fluid deficits [2] that require hospitalization and intravenous fluid.

      c. A commercially available oral electrolyte solution (Pedialyte) is available for use in infants and children with mild to moderate diarrhea. A comparable solution can be made with 4 tblsp. sugar, ³/₄ tsp. salt, and 1 tsp. sodium bicarbonate in 1 cup orange juice diluted with water to make 1 liter. If this mixture is not available, fruit juices, cola, ginger ale, or other carbonated beverages, with added salt, can be taken as an approximate equivalent. It is important to taste the solution before administering it to children to ensure that it is not too salty, because an accidental overdose of salt can cause hypernatremia. When there is associated nausea and vomiting, the patient can often be given small volumes of oral fluids on an hourly basis.

      d. Some authors have suggested saltine crackers may help replace some of the salt losses [4].

Table 11-3. Composition of World Health Organization oral rehydration solution (ORS) for diarrheal illness

Ingredient	Amount
Sodium chloride	3.5 g/L
Potassium chloride	1.5 g/L
Glucose	20.0 g/L
Trisodium citrate*	2.9 g/L

*An earlier formulation used sodium bicarbonate 2.5 g/L, had a shorter shelf-life, but was physiologically equivalent and may still be produced in some countries.
Source: Centers for Disease Control, *Health Information for International Travel 1994*. U.S. Department of Health and Human Services. Washington, DC: U.S. Government Printing Office. HHS Publication No. 94-8280.

2. **Intravenous fluids** (normal saline with potassium chloride supplementation or Ringer's solution) are used in patients who are severely dehydrated or in whom oral hydration is contraindicated.

B. **Antimotility agent use has been debated** and may be counterproductive in that such an agent may delay clearance of the pathogen or its toxin, causing prolonged illness [2]. One study demonstrated that diphenoxylate (Lomotil) prolonged the fever and illness in shigellosis [12]. These authors concluded that whenever fever or dysentery (bloody mucoid stool) occurs in acute diarrhea, drugs that reduce intestinal motility, such as belladonna or opium alkaloids, should not be employed because they may retard the natural purgative effect of diarrhea.

   Loperamide (Imodium) **commonly is used in adults in short-course therapy regimens for travelers' diarrhea** [13] (see Chap. 21). Although phenoxylate (Lomotil) and loperamide have been used in this setting, in recent years loperamide has been preferred in adults because it has a good safety record and is available over the counter. These agents are not advised for infants and young children.

   Diphenoxylate and loperamide should not be taken by patients who have fever or bloody stools as these agents may potentiate the effects of bacterial disease [6].

C. **Antibiotics. Most patients who present with acute diarrhea do not need antibiotics.** The need for antibiotics depends on (1) the patient's clinical course superimposed on his or her underlying medical problems and age and (2) the pathogen involved, though identification of this may take days [2].

   1. In the patient who is **toxic** and **profoundly dehydrated** without evidence of a self-limited process (e.g., fever, bloody stool, fecal leukocytes, all of which suggest a bacterial etiology), empiric antibiotics are indicated while awaiting cultures. Very young and very old patients deserve empiric therapy if they are toxic or significantly dehydrated. Antibiotics are essential for patients whose history suggest a bacteremia. Ceftriaxone and oral fluoroquinolones (if not contraindicated) are possible options for empiric therapy.

   2. For further discussion of therapy of individual pathogens, see sec. **V.**

D. **Miscellaneous agents**

   1. **Antisecretory agents.** The GI peptide **somatostatin** and its synthetic analogues (**octreotide** and **vapreotide**) are very powerful inhibitors of intestinal secretion. These agents have been used in controlling chronic AIDS-related diarrhea of unknown etiology or diarrhea caused by cryptosporidiosis [4] (see Chap. 19).

   2. **Absorbent agents.** Cholestyramine is a nonabsorbable exchange resin that has been used especially in *C. difficile* diarrhea (see Chap. 28A) as well as in other forms of chronic diarrhea [4].

E. **Bismuth subsalicylate** (Pepto-Bismol) has been used primarily in the prevention and therapy of travelers' diarrhea (see Chap. 21). It has also been used in conjunction with oral rehydration for diarrhea in young children [14].

F. **Antiemetics** sometimes are used orally, parenterally, or rectally, depending on the individual clinical situation. Some examples follow.

   1. **Prochlorperazine** (e.g., Compazine). For adults, the dose is one rectal suppository (25 mg) bid, or 5 mg or 10 mg tablets PO tid or qid; or 5–10 mg IM q4h not to exceed 40 mg/day when given IM.

   2. **Trimethobenzamide** (e.g., Tigan). For adults, the dose is one rectal suppository (200 mg) tid or qid; oral capsules, 250 mg tid or qid; or 200 mg IM tid or qid.

IV. **Clinical review of agents causing rapid onset of illness** (<12 hours after ingestion) (see Table 11-2)

A. **Staphylococcal food poisoning** occurs by **ingestion of a preformed enterotoxin** produced by *S. aureus,* that is heat-stable and is not destroyed by ordinary rewarming temperatures. **Foods commonly implicated are** cream-filled pastries, custards, milk products, and meats that have been improperly refrigerated.

   1. **Symptoms.** Severe nausea, vomiting, abdominal pain, diarrhea, and prostration occur 1–6 hours after ingestion of the preformed enterotoxin. The symptoms last less than 1 day and remit spontaneously.

   2. **Diagnosis** is suggested by the history and short incubation period. Actual diagnosis is made by demonstrating large quantities of *S. aureus* in the contaminated food.

   3. **Therapy is supportive.** No antibiotic is indicated for this self-limited disease.

B. *Bacillus cereus* **food poisoning** may resemble staphylococcal food poisoning. It is due to the ingestion of preformed enterotoxin in foods such as cereal (especially rice), dried foods, and dairy products. Illness is self-limited and not severe.

   1. **Two syndromes** [15]

  a. The emetic syndrome is mediated by a highly stable toxin that survives high temperatures. Fried rice subsequently held at room temperature is the leading cause.

  b. The diarrheal syndrome is mediated by a heat- and acid-labile enterotoxin.

 2. Diagnosis of *B. cereus* food poisoning can be confirmed by the isolation of at least 10^5 *B. cereus* organisms per gram from epidemiologically implicated food [15]. Special cultures are necessary.

C. *C. perfringens* **food poisoning** results from ingestion of foods harboring the organisms. The ingested *C. perfringens* multiply in the small intestine and produce the diarrhea-forming enterotoxin. **Treatment is supportive.** Anaerobic **cultures and Gram staining of the incriminated food will establish the diagnosis.**

D. Fish and shellfish poisoning are due to toxins present in the tissues of fish. A detailed discussion of this topic is beyond the scope of this book, but the topic has been reviewed elsewhere [16]. **See Table 11-2 for a summary.**

  In ciguatoxic fish (barracuda, red snapper, and grouper), the toxin is believed to be acquired in the food chain of the fish; large fish weighing more than 2.8 kg are more likely to be toxic. Scombroid fish poisoning (tuna, mackerel, bonito, skipjack) is due to toxin production by marine bacteria that grow when these fish are improperly refrigerated or preserved. Shellfish poisoning (mussels, clams, oysters, and scallops) occurs because toxic dinoflagellates usually associated with red tide are ingested by the mollusks and concentrated in their tissues. **All these toxic substances have no effect on the fish or shellfish, are heat-stable, and cannot be destroyed by cooking temperatures.**

 1. Symptoms occur within minutes to several hours after ingestion. The GI symptoms include abdominal cramps, nausea, vomiting, and diarrhea. Neurologic symptoms in ciguatera and shellfish poisoning may include numbness, paresthesias, and nerve palsies. Case fatalities, which in some series are as high as 10%, have been due to respiratory paralysis.

 2. Diagnosis is suggested by the epidemiologic features.

 3. Therapy is primarily symptomatic. Unabsorbed toxin should be removed by inducing emesis, performing gastric lavage, and administering a cathartic if vomiting and diarrhea have not occurred.

V. Clinical review of specific **diseases causing delayed onset** of GI symptoms (Table 11-4)

A. *Salmonella* **infections** [10]. Salmonellae are motile, flagellated, aerobic or facultatively anaerobic, gram-negative bacilli that do not ferment lactose or sucrose.

 1. Nomenclature and serotyping. Over the years, there have been many changes in the nomenclature, classification, and reporting of salmonellae bacteria. Recently, many experts have adopted a simplified nomenclature for routine use that considers all the serotypes of *Salmonella* as species. Thus, *Salmonella* serotype typhimurium is conveniently written as *Salmonella typhimurium* [17]. Salmonellae possess both somatic O antigens (lipopolysaccharide cell wall components) and flagellar H antigens (proteins), which allow for serotyping. More than 2,000 *Salmonella* serotypes are found in nature. Serotyping is relevant both clinically and epidemiologically. Certain serotypes are associated with specific clinical syndromes, and serotyping of isolates serves as an important tool in defining and controlling epidemics [10].

 2. Epidemiology. Salmonellosis is a reportable disease (to state health departments) [10]. In the United States, it is estimated that 2 million cases of salmonellosis occur each year, with a rise in cases in recent years, largely due to an increase in outbreaks associated with the mass production and distribution of food products and to an increase in reporting.

  a. More than 98% of isolates are nontyphoidal, with important sources of human food (e.g., chicken, eggs, egg products) **frequently contaminated with these organisms.**

   Chickens may transmit *Salmonella enteritidis* through infected oviducts that contaminate the inside of the egg before the shell is laid down [18]. It is estimated that 0.01% of all shell eggs contain *Salmonella enteritidis* although the percentage may be higher in the northeastern United States. When these eggs are used raw (such as in dressing for Caesar salad, hollandaise sauce, or homemade eggnog or ice cream) or are undercooked (such as in sunny-side-up eggs, "soft" scrambled eggs, or soft-boiled eggs with liquid centers), the *Salmonella* will not be killed and can proliferate in the food [19].

   b. Common serotypes include *S. typhimurium, S. enteritidis, S. heidelberg, S. newport, S. infantis,* and *S. agona* [10].
   c. The incidence of cases peaks during the summer and fall due to outbreaks of food poisoning in association with picnics. Contaminated food-processing equipment can spread disease [10] and, less commonly, person-to-person spread via the fecal-oral route can occur.
   d. Subtherapeutic concentrations of antibiotics commonly are put in the feed of animals as nonspecific growth factors. Such practices promote the emergence of antibiotic-resistant bacteria, including *Salmonella* spp. During slaughtering of the animals, this gut flora then will contaminate the animal meat, which is subsequently consumed by humans [10].
   e. *S. typhi* is the most frequent isolate in developing countries but is much less commonly isolated in the United States. Animals do not serve as a reservoir of *S. typhi*. Food is infectious only if contaminated by humans during processing. In developing countries, transmission occurs primarily by direct fecal-oral spread between individuals or by fecal contamination of drinking water or food. In the United States, transmission is primarily by contamination of foodstuffs with human feces. More than half of the nonepidemic cases in the United States occur in travelers returning from developing countries [10].
3. Clinical syndromes. Several different clinical presentations of *Salmonella* disease exist, each with its own symptoms: gastroenteritis, enteric fever, metastatic infection, and the carrier state.
   a. Gastroenteritis. Most infections due to *S. enteritidis, S. newport,* and *S. anatum* result in gastroenteritis. Salmonellae cause 10–15% of food poisoning cases in the United States [10]. There is an intestinal invasion with the production of fecal leukocytes and low-grade fever. In addition, an enterotoxin causes intestinal fluid secretion.
      (1) Symptoms develop 8–48 hours after ingestion of contaminated food; they include the sudden onset of colicky abdominal pain, nausea and vomiting, and then loose, watery diarrhea. There may be fever to 38°–39°C (100.4°–102.2°F). Symptoms usually subside spontaneously in 2–5 days, without sequelae. Certain underlying conditions—AIDS, achlorhydria, prior gastric surgery, and inflammatory bowel disease—predispose the patient to more severe disease [10].
      (2) Diagnosis is made by isolating the organism from the stool or the ingested food. Stool leukocytes (WBCs) often are seen.
      (3) Treatment of uncomplicated gastroenteritis due to nontyphoid *Salmonella* spp. is primarily supportive. The disease is self-limited. In fact, **antibiotic therapy may prolong the carrier state** [20].
         Furthermore, it has never been established that antibiotics improve the course of gastroenteritis. Their use should be limited to prophylaxis against bacteremia in high-risk groups who cannot tolerate bacteremia or focal metastatic infection. These groups include (1) newborn infants, probably up to 3 months of age [21], (2) the elderly, because of the high risk of atherosclerotic plaques or an aneurysm, and (3) patients who have lymphoproliferative disease, prosthetic joints or significant joint disease, transplant recipients, AIDS patients, and those with underlying sickle cell disease [10].
         (The ideal antibiotic to use is uncertain. In adults, a 1-week course of ciprofloxacin is reasonable. Susceptibility data should guide therapy in children.)
   b. Enteric fever usually is due to *S. typhi* (i.e., typhoid fever) but, infrequently, other salmonellae such as *S. paratyphi* or *S. choleraesuis* also may cause bacteremias and systemic disease.
      (1) Symptoms. Enteric fever is a systemic illness characterized by **sustained fever** (often 2–4 weeks' duration), headaches, abdominal tenderness, sustained bacteremia without endothelial or endocardial seeding, leukopenia, rose spots (2–4 mm in diameter, slightly raised, discrete, irregular, blanching pink macules, often on the anterior thorax), and hepatosplenomegaly. Metastatic seeding and immune complex deposition leading to multiorgan dysfunction can occur [10]. Intestinal hemorrhage or perforation may occur from the hyperplasia of the lymphoid tissue in the terminal ileum (Peyer's patches). A febrile systemic illness

Table 11-4. Clinical features of agent-specific foodborne disease with symptom onset of greater than 12 hours

Organism or agent	Incubation period	Duration of illness (range)	Diarrhea	Fever	Vomiting	Enterotoxin	Invasion	Foods most commonly implicated	Comments
Salmonella	8–48 hr	3 days (1–14 days)	+++	++	+	+	+ (little mucosal damage)	Eggs, poultry, beef, dairy products	Infection with some serotypes can lead to severe complications in certain patients (those with malignancy, atherosclerosis, and AIDS) Treatment not recommended except in severe or disseminated disease because it prolongs carriage of organism Stool contains white blood cells and may contain blood
Shigella	24–72 hr (up to 7 days)	3 days (1–14 days)	+++	+++	±	+	++	Salads (egg, tuna, poultry), milk	Low infective dose (10^2 organisms). Person-to-person transmission common Stools often contain blood, mucus, and pus Systemic symptoms (headache, malaise, lethargy) common

Organism	Incubation						Foods	Comments
Yersinia	24–72 hr (up to 6 days)	+++	++	±	+	+	Milk (raw or chocolate), tofu	Abdominal pain is a very prominent feature of illness and may be confused with appendicitis. Presence of pharyngitis common in children. Rheumatologic postinfectious complications have been reported (see text)
Campylobacter	2–11 days	+++	++	±	+	+	Raw milk, poultry, beef, clams, pet animals	Stool contains red and white blood cells. Mostly resistant to trimethoprim-sulfamethoxazole. Complications include meningitis and Guillain-Barré syndrome
Escherichia coli (enterotoxigenic)	24–72 hr	+++	+	–	+	–	Salads, peeled fruits, meat dishes, pastries	At least two toxins elaborated: heat-labile (similar to choleratoxin) and heat-stable. Most common bacterial agent of travelers' diarrhea
Vibrio parahemolyticus	4–96 hr	++	±	+	+	± (not documented in humans)	Oysters, crabs, shellfish, sea water, contaminated food	Antimicrobials do not shorten illness. Fecal white blood cells and blood uncommon

Table 11-4 (continued)

Organism or agent	Incubation period	Duration of illness (range)	Diarrhea	Vomiting	Fever	Enterotoxin	Invasion	Foods most commonly implicated	Comments
Clostridium botulinum	12–36 hr (may be as long as 8 days)	Weeks to months	±	±	–	++ (neurotoxin)	–	Raw honey (infants), improperly canned products	Neurologic symptoms are results of parasympathetic and neuromuscular blockade Fatality rate 15% Treatment is early administration of antitoxin Infants younger than 1 year should not be fed raw honey
Rotavirus	48–72 hr	5 days (3–14 days)	+++	++	+ (low grade)	–	– (superficial damage to mucosa)	Fresh water, seafood	Primarily an illness of infants and children Endemic in nature Respiratory symptoms common Can cause severe dehydration in children Vaccine under development
Norwalk	24–48 hr	1 day (1–3 days)	++	++	+ (low grade)	–	– (superficial damage to mucosa)	Shellfish, drinking water	Affects primarily older children and adults Endemic in nature Illness is milder than with rotavirus

Source: Modified from A. G. Miranda and H. L. DuPont, Small Intestine: Infections with Common Bacterial and Viral Pathogens. In T. Yamada (ed.), *Textbook of Gastroenterology*. New York: Lippincott, 1991. Pp. 1453–1455.

occurring in an individual who has returned from a developing area of the world should suggest the possibility of an early stage of enteric fever [10].

Surprisingly, **diarrhea occurs in as few as 50% of cases** and then only as an early symptom. **Constipation may be a frequent complaint later in the illness.**

(2) **Diagnosis** can be made by culturing *S. typhi* or other salmonellae from stool specimens, blood, bone marrow, or rose spots. Demonstration of a serologic rise of febrile agglutinins against the somatic or O antigen for group D salmonella is supportive evidence of enteric fever if the clinical syndrome is consistent. Serologic studies may be useful in epidemiologic evaluation.

(3) **Therapy.** The current agent of choice for *S. typhi* and *Salmonella* spp. is a third-generation cephalosporin (e.g., ceftriaxone or cefotaxime) [22]. Alternative agents include trimethoprim-sulfamethoxazole (TMP-SMX), a fluoroquinolone, and ampicillin, depending on susceptibility studies.

The duration of treatment for uncomplicated enteric fever is 12–14 days, with longer periods (i.e., 4 weeks) necessary for metastatic foci. Oral ciprofloxacin may allow one to avoid prolonged intravenous therapy (see Chap. 28S). Note that drug resistance is a recognized problem in infections acquired in some foreign countries such as Mexico.

(4) **Prevention.** An oral and parenteral typhoid vaccine is available to help prevent *S. typhi* infections in international travelers (see Chap. 21).

c. **Metastatic Infection.** Salmonellae, once they have entered the bloodstream, have a unique capability to metastasize particularly to intravascular lesions, the skeletal system, and the meninges [10].

(1) **High-grade bacteremia** strongly suggests focal **intravascular infection.** Salmonellae have a predilection for arterial atherosclerotic plaques and aneurysms (see Chap. 2). A combination of medical and surgical therapy provides the best opportunity for cure. Infectious disease consultation is advised.

(2) **Osteomyelitis** can occur at any skeletal site. Patients with sickle cell anemia or skeletal prostheses are predisposed to osteomyelitis [10]. Suppurative arthritis can occur.

(3) **Meningitis** occurs principally in young children, especially newborn infants. **Hence, in young children with salmonellae gastroenteritis, early therapy is indicated** [10].

(4) **Antibiotic** therapy is the same as for enteric fever except that therapy is prolonged for endocarditis or osteomyelitis.

d. **Chronic carriers.** The chronic carrier state **(i.e., positive stool cultures for more than 12 months)** develops in approximately 3% of adults with typhoid fever. In other *Salmonella* infections, the development of the carrier state occurs much less frequently 0.2–0.6% [10]. The carrier state may follow symptomatic disease or may be the only manifestation of infection; it may be the consequence of the ingestion of a small inoculum [10].

(1) The persistence of the organism, in many cases, is due to **biliary tract carriage.** If biliary calculi are present, cholecystectomy and a 10- to 14-day course of antibiotics most often is required to cure the carrier state. This invasive approach will eradicate infection in 90% of cases and may be appropriate for food handlers, medical personnel, and individuals with poor personal hygiene, and for other public health reasons. Antibiotics alone are unlikely to eradicate infection in patients with biliary calculi [10].

If normal gallbladder function is present, attempts to cure the carrier state may be made with a 4- to 6-week course of amoxicillin (6 g/day for 28 days) [23] or ciprofloxacin (500–750 mg PO bid for 28 days) [24]. Fluoroquinolones such as norfloxacin (400 mg PO bid for 28 days) or ofloxacin (200 mg bid) [25, 26] or TMP-SMX, one double-strength tablet bid, all have been tried [10]. However, even with use of the fluoroquinolones, eradication of the carrier state may be impossible (see Chap. 28S).

(2) **Chronic urinary tract** carriage can occur. Predisposing factors include obstructive uropathy from renal stones, strictures, hydronephrosis, tumors, and schistosomiasis [10].

e. Special considerations

(1) *Salmonella* causes severe infection with repeated recurrences in patients with AIDS (see Chap. 19).

(2) Other patients with an increased susceptibility to *Salmonella* infections include patients with leukemia, lymphoma, renal transplants, underlying inflammatory bowel disease, and underlying schistosomiasis.

B. Shigellosis (bacillary dysentery). Shigellae are nonmotile, gram-negative bacilli that do not ferment lactose. There are four serogroups: group A (*S. dysenteriae*), group B (*S. flexneri*), group C (*S. boydii*), and group D (*S. sonnei*). Most disease in the United States is produced by *S. sonnei* or *S. flexneri*.

1. Pathogenesis and epidemiology. Shigellosis represents the most highly communicable of the bacterial diarrheas; ingestion of as few as 200 viable bacteria will produce illness, and thus this organism is spread commonly between persons in a family setting or in confined settings, such as a daycare center. In the United States, most cases result from person-to-person spread [9].

Shigella strains invade mucosal epithelial cells (see sec. **I.C.2**). Characteristically, there is a descending intestinal infection in which small-bowel involvement is associated with fever and watery diarrhea followed by colitis [9]. The hemolytic uremia syndrome that occasionally follows infection by *S. dysenteriae* is due to production of *Shigella* toxin.

2. Symptoms. Approximately 24–48 hours after ingestion of the microbe, abdominal pain, high fever, and diarrhea develop. In a large percentage of cases, tenesmus and gross blood in the stool develop.

Nearly half of the patients will have the classic biphasic illness in which initially a small-bowel type of diarrhea occurs and small numbers of voluminous stools are passed, followed by large-bowel involvement, at which time many small-volume stools containing blood and mucus are passed [9].

3. Diagnosis usually is **made by stool cultures. Bacteremia is rare.** A sigmoidoscopic examination may be suggestive of this diagnosis when diffuse inflammation and shallow, well-documented ulcers are seen. Leukocytes often are seen in stool smears.

4. Therapy. Although mild disease has often responded to supportive care, **antibiotics are indicated** because they shorten the duration of illness and decrease the relapse rate. In vitro susceptibility tests should be performed because of the increasing problem of resistance to ampicillin.

Currently, the agents of choice are the fluoroquinolones [22] if these are not contraindicated (see Chap. 28S). Optimal duration of therapy is unclear (e.g., one dose versus 3 days versus 5 days of therapy) [27]. Ciprofloxacin, 500 mg bid, can be used in adults [9]. Alternative regimens include TMP-SMX (160 mg TMP and 800 mg SMX) twice daily in adults [9].

C. *Yersinia enterocolitica* is a gram-negative coccobacillus formerly classified as a *Pasteurella* species. Although first recognized in 1933 in New York State, disease caused by this organism is more frequently reported in Scandinavia, northern Europe, Japan, and Canada than in the United States. Because the organism requires special culture techniques, the incidence of disease in the United States probably is underestimated [28].

1. Symptoms. Fever, abdominal pain, and diarrhea commonly appear together. **Diarrhea, however, is present in only approximately 50% of the recognized infections.** Other symptoms associated with infection include erythema nodosum, reactive arthritis, exudative pharyngitis, septicemia, and terminal ileitis or mesenteric lymphadenitis. **The latter syndromes usually mimic appendicitis** clinically; however, at operation the appendix appears normal. Consequently, a clustering of cases of mesenteric lymphadenitis should lead to the suspicion of *Y. enterocolitica* infection.

The diarrheal illness is indistinguishable from that caused by other enteric pathogens, although symptoms commonly last 2 weeks on average [28].

2. Diagnosis often is missed because the normal bowel flora obscure these organisms in the stool culture. **Special cold-enrichment of cultures** are necessary to increase the possibility of isolating yersiniae but, even so, isolation of the organism may take several days with these special techniques. Special selective media are available to enhance isolation of these organisms. **The laboratory must be alerted** to set up these special cultures if they are not done routinely. Appendiceal tissue also can be cultured.

3. **Treatment.** In most cases, resolution occurs spontaneously. The value of antimicrobial agents in the treatment of *Y. enterocolitica* diarrhea or mesenteric adenitis has not been established.
   a. **Intestinal infection usually is self-limited,** and there have been few clinical studies of efficacy. Treatment of diarrhea should focus on appropriate management of fluid replacement. Therapy for mesenteric adenitis is symptomatic [28].
   b. **Treatment of extraintestinal disease or complications** should be based on in vitro susceptibility data. Most isolates have been shown to be sensitive to third-generation cephalosporins, aminoglycosides, fluoroquinolones, tetracyclines, and TMP-SMX [28]. In a retrospective review of 43 cases of bacteremic patients, Gayraud and colleagues [29] concluded fluoroquinolones alone or third-generation cephalosporins used in combination with aminoglycosides or fluoroquinolones constituted the best treatment.
4. **Epidemiology.** Little is known, but foodborne transmission has been suggested. The ability of *Yersinia* to grow at low temperatures also makes it a potential source of food contamination. One recent epidemic has shown that contaminated chocolate milk was the means of spread. However, isolates have also been cultured from meat, mussels, poultry, oysters, cheese, and ice cream [28]. Person-to-person transmission has been suggested.
D. *Campylobacter.* In the past decade, *Campylobacter* has been recognized as a human pathogen and probably causes 5–7% of cases of acute diarrhea in the United States, a higher rate than *Salmonella* (approximately 2.3%) and *Shigella* (approximately 1%) [30]. *C. jejuni* is the most frequently isolated species. Most cases of *Campylobacter* diarrhea are sporadic, but outbreaks can occur [30]. **Special techniques are required for the isolation** of this organism, and this fact may account for the failure in the past to discover the organism by routine culture.
   1. **Symptoms. Diarrhea,** abdominal pain, and constitutional symptoms (especially fever) predominate in this acute GI illness. **Grossly bloody stools or occult blood** may be seen in the majority of patients. Most patients are symptomatic only for a few days, although enteric symptoms may last up to 3 weeks. The incubation period is usually 48–72 hours after ingestion of the organism [30]. Occasionally, patients may have an associated bacteremia (see Chap. 2). The clinical presentation mimics other forms of acute bacterial diarrhea, and the diagnosis can be established only by culture.
   2. **Diagnosis.** A special selective medium is required to identify *Campylobacter fetus* from stool cultures (which may take 2–7 days), but routine blood cultures have grown the organisms in bacteremic patients. Methylene blue **fecal smears** commonly **show leukocytes.**
      Fresh stools can be screened for *Campylobacter* by direct microscopy. The finding of leukocytes and RBCs in the presence of bacteria with characteristic darting motility leads to a presumptive diagnosis. On Gram staining of stool, the presence of many small curved rods and reduced amounts of normal flora suggests *Campylobacter* [30].
   3. **Treatment.** Gastroenteritis is usually a self-limited illness, and it seems prudent not to treat most cases [30]. If treatment is required, in vitro antibiotic sensitivities usually show the organism to be susceptible to erythromycin, fluoroquinolones, the tetracyclines, the aminoglycosides, and chloramphenicol. The agent of choice is erythromycin or a fluoroquinolone [22]. In patients with protracted symptoms, treatment with antibiotics appear to shorten the illness and prevent relapses. Oral erythromycin (e.g., 250–500 mg qid for 7 days in adults) [30] or ciprofloxacin (500 mg bid for 7 days in adults) is suggested. Bacteremic patients deserve full therapeutic courses (see Chap. 2).
   4. **Epidemiology.** The organism is a known enteric pathogen in cattle, dogs, and fowl. Animals (symptomatic and nonsymptomatic) that have been identified as index cases for human disease include dogs, cows, and chickens. Undercooked or raw poultry is believed to be a major source of infection. Cross-contamination during food preparation can occur [30]. Fecal-oral contamination can occur and is a major route for acquiring the organism, whether in human-to-human spread, waterborne infection, or animal-related infection. Enteric precautions should be exercised.
E. *E. coli* 0157:H7. *E. coli* has emerged as an **important cause of both bloody diarrhea and hemolytic uremic syndrome** (HUS), the most common cause of acute

renal failure in children [31–33]. In the United States alone, *E. coli* 0157:H7 is estimated to cause more than 20,000 infections and as many as 250 deaths each year [32a]. The organism has been referred to as an enterotoxigenic *E. coli* (ETEC) as well as an enterohemorrhagic strain (EHEC) because of its frequent production of bloody diarrhea in infected patients [31a]. The *E. coli* serotype 0157:H7 is designated by its somatic (0) and flagellar (H) antigens.

1. **Pathogenesis.** These *E. coli* produce large amounts of toxins (Shiga-like) which are specified by bacteriophages that have infected the bacterial cells. A recent multistate epidemic in the western United States was traced to **contaminated hamburger** patties that were undercooked by a restaurant chain. Subsequent US Food and Drug Administration (FDA) recommendations call for increasing internal temperature for cooked hamburgers to 155°F such that the interior is no longer pink [31]. In addition to undercooked ground beef, foods such as roast beef, unpasteurized milk, and apple cider have been implicated, as well as municipal water, person-to-person transmission in child daycare centers [34], and swimming in a fecally contaminated lake [32a].

   These *E. coli* live in the intestines of healthy cattle and can contaminate meat during slaughter. Ground beef is likely to be internally contaminated [31].

2. **Clinical syndrome.** *E. coli* 0157:H7 **causes a spectrum of illness** from asymptomatic carriage: nonbloody diarrhea (about 10% of cases), bloody diarrhea (i.e., hemorrhagic colitis, in 90% of diagnosed cases), HUS (in 6–10% of patients <10 years of age), and at times thrombotic thrombocytopenia purpura (TTP) in adults (which in part is similar to HUS seen in children). These clinical syndromes have recently been reviewed [31a, 32a]. **Watery diarrhea,** often **bloody,** is the prominent symptom. Vomiting can occur, and fever is infrequent. The absence of fever or its low-grade nature may make some clinicians suspect a noninfectious etiology of the diarrhea [32a]. Abdominal cramps or pain can be severe in some patients. The incubation period usually is 24–48 hours, and most illness resolves in 5–7 days. HUS syndrome develops on average 1 week after the onset of diarrhea. Because patients clear the organism from the gastrointestinal tract rapidly, up to two-thirds of patients with HUS will not have *E. coli* 0157:H7 in their stools. Serologic tests for 0157 lipopolysaccharide antigen using monoclonal antibody are positive in the first several months after HUS [31a], although this is currently primarily performed in research laboratories [32a]. Children and the elderly are at the highest risk for **complications,** 5–10% of patients developing HUS, which is characterized by hemolytic anemia, thrombocytopenia, and renal failure. In children, the case-fatality rate of HUS is 3–5% [33].

3. **Diagnosis** is made by culture on special sorbitol-MacConkey agar that is commercially available. *E. coli* 0157:H7 does not ferment the sorbitol and can readily be picked and confirmed by serotyping with specific antisera [31]. **Most laboratories have not cultured routinely for this organism unless requested to do so.** Because of the increasing importance of this pathogen, microbiology laboratories now are encouraged to routinely culture for this organism in bloody and nonbloody diarrheal specimens [31a, 32a].

4. **Therapy is supportive.** Most strains of *E. coli* 0157:H7 are sensitive in vitro to common antibiotics used to treat infective gastroenteritis. However, several reports found no clinical benefit from antimicrobial therapy. In fact, the use of TMP-SMX may increase the frequency of HUS [32].

   a. **In recent reviews, experts suggest antibiotics not be used** [31a, 32a], and some data suggest that prior antibiotic use may be a risk factor for poor outcome of *E. coli* 0157:H7 infection [31a].

   b. **Antimotility agents or narcotics are not advised** because they may delay clearance of the pathogen, and use of an antimotility agent has been demonstrated to be a risk factor for the development of HUS [31a].

   c. **Intravenous rehydration** with isotonic saline is advised and may be useful to reduce the stress imposed by dehydration of the kidneys, which are at risk of sustaining toxemic injury. Oral intake appears to increase crampy abdominal pain, whereas IV fluid administration in lieu of feedings can reduce symptoms [31a].

5. **Prevention**

   a. Thorough cooking kills *E. coli* 0157:H7. The optimal food protection practice is to **cook ground beef thoroughly** until the interior is no longer pink and the juices are clear [31, 33].

    b. Patients infected with *E. coli* 0157:H7 should be considered **highly contagious** and should not return to group settings, such as daycare, unless it is certain hygienic practices are well maintained. The dose of *E. coli* 0157:H7 that leads to symptomatic infection is low as is that of shigellae [31a]. Some authorities have recommended that at least two negative stool cultures be obtained before infected children return to school. However, shedding of the organism may be intermittent [31a]. The most important preventive measure in childcare centers is supervised hand washing [32a].

    c. All cases of confirmed *E. coli* 0157:H7 infection should be reported immediately to appropriate public health authorities. Early detection can lead to measures that will help reduce additional cases from occurring [31a, 32a].

F. *Vibrio parahemolyticus* is a gram-negative, halophilic, marine organism that was isolated first in 1950 as a cause of self-limited gastroenteritis. It is very common in Japan (where it may account for up to 70% of recognized causes of gastroenteritis) and occurs rarely in the United States [35], in such coastal areas as eastern Maryland and Louisiana and on cruise ships sailing between Florida and the Caribbean.

    1. Symptoms. Diarrhea, cramps, weakness, nausea, chills, headache, fever, and vomiting occur 3–76 hours **after ingestion of contaminated raw or improperly cooked shellfish.** The mean duration of illness is approximately 3 days [35].

    2. Diagnosis is made by culture of stool specimens with use of special media. Stool specimens may be tinged with blood and contain fecal leukocytes indicative of invasive disease. Sigmoidoscopy demonstrates superficial ulceration in some cases.

    3. Treatment. Resolution occurs spontaneously in most cases. No studies on the efficacy of antibiotics in gastroenteritis have been reported, but most are sensitive to tetracycline and TMP-SMX [35].

G. *Clostridium difficile* (antibiotic-related) diarrhea is discussed in detail in Chap. 28A. **This diagnosis should be considered in any patient with the new onset of diarrhea while taking antibiotics or within 4–6 weeks after completing a course of antibiotics.** Fever, abdominal tenderness, leukocytosis, and fecal leukocytes are common findings.

H. Travelers' diarrhea is discussed in Chap. 21.

I. Miscellaneous

    1. Other *Vibrio* spp. can cause diarrhea and epidemiologically may be linked to the consumption of raw or undercooked shellfish [35].

    2. *Cholera*, infection due to *V. cholerae*, is rare in the United States. Domestically acquired cholera has been reported from an endemic Gulf Coast focus involving shellfish or imported foods; international travelers can also acquire cholera [35, 36].

    3. *Aeromonas hydrophila* may, at times, be pathogenic. These organisms are found in fresh water in the United States, coastal waters, shellfish, and even farm animals. Their clinical significance awaits further study [35].

    4. *Plesiomonas shigelloides* may also cause diarrhea in patients who eat contaminated shellfish (e.g., raw oysters). More study is required to confirm or exclude this as a true pathogen [35].

J. Parasitic disease may mimic bacterial gastroenteritis, *Giardia* spp., and *Entamoeba histolytica*. See related discussions under Gastrointestinal Parasites.

VI. Viral gastroenteritis occurs commonly [37]. Current estimates suggest that viral gastroenteritis produces **30–40% of the cases of infectious diarrhea in the United States.** A study of diseases affecting families in Cleveland over a 10-year period indicated that infectious nonbacterial gastroenteritis was second in frequency to the common cold and amounted for 16% of illnesses [38].

A. Etiology. Since the discovery of the Norwalk virus in 1972, five major categories of human gastroenteritis viruses have been defined. Rotavirus, enteric adenovirus, and Norwalk virus are well-established medically important pathogens. Calicivirus and astrovirus clearly produce gastroenteritis, but the extent of their medical importance is still being evaluated (Table 11-5). This topic has been well summarized in a review by Blacklow and Greenberg [38].

    Still, the etiology of many bouts of gastroenteritis cannot be explained.

    1. Rotavirus is the agent **responsible for 30–60%** of all **cases of severe watery diarrhea in children.** It is a double-stranded RNA virus that can undergo gene reassortment, leading to new serotypes. Group A rotavirus causes most diseases and is the **single most important cause of dehydrating diarrhea necessitating**

Table 11-5. Medical importance, clinical and epidemiologic characteristics, and diagnosis of human gastroenteritis viruses*

Virus	Medical importance demonstrated	Epidemiologic characteristics	Clinical characteristics	Laboratory diagnostic tests
Rotavirus				
Group A	Yes	Major cause of endemic severe diarrhea in infants and young children worldwide (in winter in temperate zone)	Dehydrating diarrhea for 5–7 days; vomiting and fever very common	Immunoassay, electron microscopy, PAGE
Group B	Partially	Large outbreaks in adults and children in China	Severe watery diarrhea for 3–5 days	Electron microscopy, PAGE
Group C	Partially	Sporadic cases in young children worldwide	Similar to characteristics of group A rotavirus	Electron microscopy, PAGE
Enteric adenovirus	Yes	Endemic diarrhea of infants and young children	Prolonged diarrhea lasting 5–12 days; vomiting and fever	Immunoassay, electron microscopy with PAGE
Norwalk virus	Yes	Epidemics of vomiting and diarrhea in older children and adults; occurs in families, communities, and nursing homes; often associated with shellfish, other food, or water	Acute vomiting, diarrhea, fever, myalgia, and headache lasting 1–2 days	Immunoassay, immune electron microscopy
Norwalk-like viruses (small, round, structured viruses)	Partially	Similar to characteristics of Norwalk virus	Acute vomiting, diarrhea, fever, myalgia, and headache lasting 1–2 days	Immunoassay, immune electron microscopy
Calcivirus	Partially	Usually pediatric diarrhea; associated with shellfish and other food in adults	Rotaviruslike illness in children; Norwalk-like in adults	Immunoassay, electron microscopy
Astrovirus	Partially	Pediatric diarrhea; reported in nursing homes	Watery diarrhea, often lasting 2–3 days, occasionally longer	Immunoassay, electron microscopy

PAGE = polyacrylamide-gel electrophoresis and silver staining of viral nucleic acid in stool.
*Laboratory diagnostic tests, other than those for rotavirus Group A, usually are available only in specialized research or diagnostic referral laboratories. Immunoassays are usually ELISAs or radioimmunoassays.
Source: From N. R. Blacklow and H. B. Greenberg, Viral gastroenteritis. *N. Engl. J. Med.* 325:252. Copyright 1991, Massachusetts Medical Society.

hospitalization in children younger than 2 years in both developed and less-developed countries. Mild disease is seen in older children and, at times, adults may acquire disease, especially after close contact with infected infants. Infants younger than 3 months seem less likely to be infected, presumably because of immunity by passive transplancental transfer of maternal antibody. Whether breast-feeding is protection is not clear [38].

  a. **Transmission** is probably by the **fecal-oral route.** Rotavirus is shed in large numbers in the feces, and fecal infiltrates are infectious to volunteers [38].

  b. **Infection is more common** in cooler, **winter** months in the United States, with spread typically from the Southwest to the Northwest annually. The basis for these observations is unclear [38].

  c. At least seven serotypes exist; four cause most infections [38].

  d. **Clinical syndrome.** Rotavirus infection frequently is asymptomatic. In symptomatic infection, the incubation period is 1–3 days, with illness lasting 5–7 days in normal hosts, but the course may be more protracted in the immunocompromised host. **It is not possible to differentiate rotavirus-associated gastroenteritis from illness caused by other enteric pathogens on the basis of clinical criteria. Vomiting is common,** as is dehydration [38].

  e. **Diagnosis.** Because large amounts of the rotavirus are in the stool, a wide variety of assays able to detect **rotavirus antigen in the stool** are available, sensitive, and specific [38].

  f. **Treatment** is symptomatic, preferably with oral rehydration fluids.

  g. **Vaccines** are undergoing careful evaluation and are anticipated in the next decade [38].

2. **Enteric adenovirus** is second to the rotavirus in causing pediatric gastroenteritis, especially in children younger than 1 year. Estimates suggest that this virus accounts for 4–10% of pediatric diarrhea in children younger than 2 years [38].

  a. **Transmission** is from person to person.

  b. No seasonal peak occurs.

  c. Serotypes 40 and 41 cause diarrheal disease, usually without respiratory symptoms.

  d. **Clinical syndrome.** Asymptomatic infection can be seen. The incubation period is 8–10 days, and watery diarrhea may last 5–12 days, with 1–2 days of vomiting. Low-grade fever can be seen, and dehydration can occur. Nosocomial outbreaks are possible, but spread to adults is uncommon.

  e. A presumptive **diagnosis** can be made if large numbers of adenoviral particles are seen on electron-microscopical examination of diarrheal stool and if the virus cannot be cultured with conventional cell culture. Immunoassays using carefully selected monoclonal antibodies specific for adenoviruses 40 and 41 are available.

  f. **Treatment** is symptomatic.

3. The **Norwalk virus** or serologically related viruses **cause approximately 40% of the outbreaks of gastroenteritis** that occur in recreational camps, on cruise ships, in communities or families, in elementary schools or colleges, in nursing homes, hospital wards, and cafeterias, and among sports teams, **or** that result from the ingestion of contaminated drinking or swimming water, poorly cooked clams and oysters from contaminated waters, and contaminated foods such as salads and cake frosting [38].

  a. **Transmission** is by the fecal-oral route.

  b. **Clinical syndrome.** The incubation period is 12–48 hours, and watery diarrhea is the main symptom. Nausea and vomiting are common. Mild degrees of small-intestinal malabsorption can persist for 2 weeks after the acute episode [38].

  c. **Diagnosis.** The Norwalk virus cannot be cultivated in cell culture and cannot induce disease in animals, so purified reagents are unavailable for diagnostic and research purposes. Stools and serum from volunteer studies are available for use in immunoassays that usually are restricted to research laboratories [38]. A promising new polymerase chain reaction assay will aid in further understanding infection with these agents.

  d. **Norwalk-like viruses** are named after the location of a diarrheal outbreak due to such viruses (e.g., Hawaii, Snow Mountain). They cause a clinical syndrome similar to that of the Norwalk virus.

4. **Calicivirus.** Human caliciviruses are less well understood than the viruses just discussed but can cause disease in infants and young children that is clinically indistinguishable from mild rotaviral illness. Approximately 3% of the cases of diarrhea among infants and young children at US daycare centers are due to this virus [38]. Detection of the virus in stool by electron microscopy has been the mainstay of diagnosis until an immunoassay was developed recently.

5. **Astrovirus** is a single-stranded RNA virus that causes diarrheal illness in children from infancy to 7 years of age. Although similar to rotavirus illness, it is less severe. The incubation period is 1–2 days, and watery diarrhea is the prominent symptom. Outbreaks have been described in residential homes for the elderly. Young adults may be protected by serum antibodies whose levels may decline with age [38].

In addition to electron-microscopical stool examination, an enzyme-linked immunosorbent assay (ELISA) recently has been developed that uses group-reactive monoclonal antibodies that detect all astroviral serotypes in stool. This is used primarily in epidemiologic studies.

B. **Diagnosis**
1. **In adults,** the diagnosis of viral gastroenteritis is, for all practical purposes, **a diagnosis of exclusion** because techniques are not routinely available to isolate the virus from stool.
   a. **History.** There is no obvious history suggesting a bacterial or parasitic process (e.g., no recent international travel, no high fever or rigors, no recent seafood ingestion). The patient may well have been exposed to a friend or family member with similar GI symptoms.
   b. **Stool examination.** The diagnosis of a viral process is supported, although not proven, by the absence of fecal leukocytes. Stools for culture or ova and parasite examination will be negative, and the decision of whether to order these must be individualized.
2. **In children,** similar principles hold, but stools can be examined for rotavirus and, at times, enteric adenovirus.

C. **Therapy is supportive** with fluid replacement.

Helicobacter pylori and Peptic Ulcer Disease

In the past few years, there has been intense interest and study of the possible role of *Helicobacter pylori* (formerly called *Campylobacter pylori*) in peptic ulcer disease [39–44]. In a thoughtful editorial review of this topic, Isenberg [41], in 1993, noted that in the preceding 3 years more than 1,200 articles related to *H. pylori* and its possible role in peptic ulcer disease were published. A detailed discussion of this topic is beyond the scope of this book, but several points warrant emphasis. The organism's clinical role has recently been reviewed [40, 42]. Most peptic ulcers not caused by nonsteroidal antiinflammatory drugs (NSAIDs) are now thought to be associated with *H. pylori* infection [40, 43, 44].

I. **The organism** [42]. *H. pylori* is a curved, motile, microaerophilic gram-negative bacillus, with flagella at one end, that is found in the mucous layer overlying the epithelium of the gastric mucosa.

A. In North America, more than 50% of asymptomatic persons older than 60 years showed evidence of active or past *H. pylori* infection. In developing countries, the prevalence of *H. pylori* colonization of gastric mucosa is nearly 80% by the age of 30. Patients with active or inactive peptic ulcer disease, especially duodenal but also gastric, have *H. pylori* infection more often than age-matched controls, with a relative risk of approximately 2–3:1 [42]. The only known reservoir of *H. pylori* is humans [40].

B. Virtually all who harbor *H. pylori* in their antral mucosa have focal epithelial cell damage and inflammation in the lamina propria [42].
1. *H. pylori* produces urease, which seems important in colonization and is cytotoxic to human epithelial cells [42].
2. *H. pylori* produces catalases, proteinases, and compounds that may damage epithelial cells and degrade mucus and produces chemotactic factors for monocytes and neutrophils, leading to an influx of these cells and the release of inflammatory cytokines, all of which exacerbate the inflammatory process.

   C. The high incidence of *H. pylori* infection in patients with peptic ulcer disease and the lower relapse rates of such disease after eradication of *H. pylori* suggest a role for this organism in the pathogenesis of peptic ulcer disease. **However, most people infected with this organism never develop an ulcer.** Overall, *H. pylori* appears to be a strong risk factor for ulcer development, but its presence is not sufficient to cause ulcers [42]. The mechanism whereby infection with *H. pylori* results in peptic ulcer disease is not well understood [40].

   D. The pathogenetic role of *H. pylori* duodenal-related ulcers still is being investigated. Perhaps once *H. pylori*–related mucosal changes occur, the presence of acid or pepsin will enhance mucosal injury. Concomitant smoking, the use of nonsteroidal antiinflammatory drugs (NSAIDs), and other factors may play synergistic roles [42].

II. Diagnosis of *H. pylori* infection [40, 42]

   A. Invasive techniques require endoscopy.

   1. Culture. Under normal circumstances, demonstration of an organism by culture is the criterion of infection. Culturing for *H. pylori* involves obtaining the sample by endoscopy, and culture techniques are tedious and difficult. Culture is no more sensitive than routine histologic analysis. For these reasons, cultures are **not indicated** for diagnosis [40].

   2. Endoscopy with biopsy

   a. The organism may have a patchy distribution, especially in the body and fundus of the stomach. Because the antrum is more uniformly involved, two biopsy specimens from the prepyloric antrum generally suffice. The yield may be increased further by sampling the fundus as well as the antrum [40].

   b. Routine hematoxylin and eosin staining may be unreliable for detecting *H. pylori* by microscopy. The Giemsa and Warthin-Starry stains permit easier visualization, especially by inexperienced observers [40].

   c. Endoscopy is an expensive procedure, and several days may be required to obtain the stain/biopsy results.

   3. Campylobacter-like organism (Clo) test on endoscopic biopsy samples

   a. Mucosal biopsy specimens may be directly inoculated into medium containing urea and phenol red, which turns pink if the pH rises above 6.0. This change occurs when urea in the gel is metabolized to ammonia by the urease produced by *H. pylori*.

   b. This test is commercially available and inexpensive and can provide a diagnosis within 1 hour of inoculation of the biopsy specimen. Its sensitivity and specificity have been reported as high as 98% and 100%, respectively, at 24 hours. **The low cost and excellent reliability of this test make it the endoscopic method of choice for diagnosis** [40].

   B. Noninvasive tests

   1. Serologic tests are available, based on ELISAs, which have a reported sensitivity of 99% and a specificity of 100% for detecting IgG antibody to diagnose infection [40].

   a. An elevated antibody titer to *H. pylori* indicates current infection, because spontaneous clearance is rare.

   b. There are **several limitations to use of serology to document eradication of infection** after therapy. Although the antibody titer falls after eradication, the rate of decline is uncertain. Titers must be followed for at least 6 months to determine a decline. Whether a 20% or 50% decline in IgG titer over 6 months suggests eradication is still undergoing evaluation [40].

   c. The excellent accuracy and low cost of serology make it the noninvasive method of choice to document infection with *H. pylori;* endoscopy is still required to diagnose ulcer disease [40].

   2. Urea breath tests have been developed because *H. pylori* has high urease activity. A solution containing urea labeled with carbon 13 or carbon 14 is ingested. If *H. pylori* is present in the stomach, labeled carbon dioxide is split off by urease, absorbed, and expired in the breath. These breath tests are **not yet commercially available.** They have the potential to be useful not only in the diagnosis but also very useful in following patients after therapeutic interventions [42].

III. Infectious nature of peptic ulcer disease. Although many questions remain unanswered, in his recent editorial on this topic, Isenberg [41] stresses several points. Other reviewers have emphasized similar points [40, 43].

A. *H. pylori* **is:**
   1. **A definite cause of acute and chronic active gastritis.**
   2. **A cofactor in the pathogenesis and recurrence of peptic ulcer diseases** (especially duodenal ulcer). Approximately 90–100% of patients with duodenal ulcers and nearly 70–90% of patients with gastric ulcers harbor *H. pylori*. However, many healthy people harbor *H. pylori* and are free of ulcer disease (see sec. **I.A**). **The strongest evidence for the pathogenic role of** *H. pylori* **in peptic ulcer disease is the marked decrease in recurrence rates of ulcers following the eradication of** *H. pylori* [43].
   3. Possibly a cofactor in the pathogenesis of gastric adenocarcinoma. However, there is no evidence at present to recommend treatment of *H. pylori* infection in patients to prevent subsequent development of gastric carcinoma.
   4. Not established as a factor in nonulcer dyspepsia. Eradication of *H. pylori* in these patients does not consistently result in resolution of troublesome symptoms.
B. How *H. pylori* directly **contributes to** the development of **peptic ulcers** is not entirely clear (see sec. **I.D**) [40, 41, 43, 43a].
C. Treatment to eradicate *H. pylori* **is suggested by the NIH Consensus Development Panel** [43], American College of Gastroenterology [43b], and by reviewers [40].
   1. **All patients with gastric or duodenal ulcers who are infected with** *H. pylori* should be treated with antimicrobials whether they are suffering from the initial presentation of the disease or a recurrence [43]. Before treatment both the organism and the ulcer need to be documented [40].
   2. *H. pylori*–infected patients with peptic ulcer disease who are receiving maintenance therapy with antisecretory agents or who have a history of complicated or refractory disease should be treated.
   3. **Note**
      a. Prophylactic antimicrobial therapy is **not** recommended for asymptomatic *H. pylori*–infected patients without ulcers, in order to prevent future ulcers or possible gastric neoplasia.
      b. Treatment is not advised for patients with nonulcerative dyspepsia.
IV. Treatment regimens. Optimal treatment regimens are still evolving [43, 43b].
   A. Attempts to eradicate *H. pylori* with single agents have not been effective and may lead to antimicrobial resistance [43].
   B. Multidrug regimens are suggested [22, 40, 43, 43b, 44]. **No optimal regimen has emerged [43b].**
      1. **A common triple-drug regimen** [22, 40, 43] includes 2 weeks of bismuth subsalicylate (Pepto-Bismol) tablets, 2 tablets (525 mg) qid, **plus** metronidazole, 250–500 mg tid, **plus either** tetracycline, 500 mg qid, or amoxicillin, 500 mg qid. Concomitant use of an H_2-blocker (e.g., ranitidine) or omeprazole (for duodenal ulcers) usually is advised (see sec. **C.2**).
         Side effects are common with a triple-drug regimen and occur in up to 30% of recipients [43]. **Nausea and vomiting** may be seen in 20%. Alcohol should be avoided. Oropharyngeal or vaginal fungal infections can occur and may require topical therapy. **Diarrhea** may be reduced if tetracycline is used instead of amoxicillin. **Rash** is seen in 5% or fewer patients receiving therapy and necessitates stopping the antimicrobials. *C. difficile* diarrhea has been seen in fewer than 1% of recipients. Triple-drug therapy has been associated with eradication rates of 80–85% [40].
      2. **Proton pump double therapy** has been suggested as a simpler regimen, often with fewer side effects. **Omeprazole** (Prilosec), 20 mg bid, **and amoxicillin,** 500 mg qid, both for 2 weeks, has been an effective regimen [40]. Pretreatment with omeprazole alone before instituting antibiotic therapy markedly attenuates the efficacy of dual therapy with amoxicillin and omeprazole and should be avoided [40]. Although clarithromycin and omeprazole have also been used [44a], recent recommendations have favored omeprazole with two antibiotics. These regimens have included [43b]: (1) omeprazole (20 mg bid), metronidazole (500 mg bid with meals), and clarithromycin (500 mg bid with meals) for 1 week; (2) omeprazole, clarithromycin, and amoxicillin (1 g bid with meals) for 1 week, or (3) omeprazole, metronidazole, and amoxicillin for 1–2 weeks. These regimens have had cure rates of approximately 80–90% [43b].
      3. **Other therapeutic regimens** are under evaluation including **clarithromycin and omeprazole** [44a]. See related discussion of clarithromycin use in this setting in Chap. 28M.

C. Miscellaneous therapeutic issues [43]
  1. The topical action of effective antibiotics is important.
  2. At increased gastric pH levels, the efficacy of many antibiotics is enhanced, which may help explain the higher rates of eradication of *H. pylori* when antimicrobial agents are combined with H_2-blockers or omeprazole.
  3. **Acquisition of resistance during antibiotic therapy is a concern,** especially with metronidazole, and may explain why in some patients eradication of *H. pylori* fails with standard regimens.
  4. **Compliance is important yet difficult** because of the high incidence of side effects with these regimens.
  5. Reinfection after eradication is uncommon and appears to occur at a rate of 1–3% annually [40].
V. Relationship of *H. pylori* to other gastrointestinal diseases
  A. Gastric carcinoma. Although *H. pylori* is hypothesized to be associated with an increased risk of gastric carcinoma, other factors are important in the pathogenesis of gastric carcinoma (see sec. **III.A.2**).
  B. Gastric non-Hodgkin's lymphoma is rare. Prior *H. pylori* infection is more common in these patients than in controls, perhaps because this infection causes chronic inflammation that results in lymphoid proliferation, thereby increasing the chance of mutation [40].
  C. Mucosa-associated lymphoid tissue tumors (MALT lymphomas). *H. pylori* is also associated with MALT lymphoma, a low-grade subtype of non-Hodgkin's lymphoma of the stomach. In one pilot study, eradication of *H. pylori* in six patients with MALT lymphoma was associated with complete regression of the lesion in five patients [40].

Gastrointestinal Parasites

The epidemiology and symptoms of intestinal parasitic infestation are too numerous to review in detail in this book. However, Table 11-6 lists the vectors, most common clinical symptoms, sites of involvement in the host, and laboratory tests commonly used to make the diagnosis of intestinal parasitic infestation. For details, the reader is referred to a text devoted to this topic [45].

I. Pathogenesis of symptoms usually is related to one of the following:
  A. Physical presence of organisms in the GI tract with loss of nutrients or blood (as in hookworm, ascaris, strongyloides, fluke, and protozoal infestations)
  B. Inflammatory reaction by the host to some parasite-related protein (as in schistosomiasis and trichinosis)
  C. Migration of parasite (as in creeping eruption and visceral larva migrans)
II. Diagnosis
  A. Stool examination is the most common means of identifying the pathogen.
    1. One should **contact the diagnostic parasitology or microbiology laboratory** if one does not know what tests to order or how to handle specimens.
    2. **Fresh stool specimens** are required to preserve the trophozoites of some parasites such as *E. histolytica*. The diagnostic laboratory often will reject a specimen unless it is fresh or placed in appropriate fixatives.
    3. **Many drugs and materials interfere** with the stool examination for parasites. Substances that can interfere up to 1 week after ingestion include **iron,** bismuth, castor oil or mineral oil, and particulate substances such as **Metamucil.** Materials such as **barium,** gallbladder dye, **antibiotics,** iodine preparations, bismuth, antiamebic drugs, and some antimalarial drugs may make the patient's stool difficult to examine correctly for as long as 3 weeks after ingestion.
    4. **Stool specimens should be collected before any medications or purgatives for radiologic procedures are given.**
    5. **Macroscopic examination** of the stool may reveal nematodes or proglottids. Adult worms may be washed in warm sodium chloride and examined fresh or fixed. Proglottids may be visualized clearly by mounting in 5% acetic acid [45].
    6. Saline and iodine **wet mounts** for microscopic examination are useful for trophozoites, cysts, ova, and certain helminth larvae.
    7. Three stool samples for ova and parasite examination are suggested, as a single examination may be negative. The specimen should be passed on a clean dry surface such as a bedpan or collection cup; the specimen should not be taken from the toilet or be contaminated with urine.

Table 11-6. Helminth infections of humans

	Common name of parasite or disease	Site in host	Source of infection, intermediate host, or vector	Most common clinical symptoms	Laboratory diagnosis	Remarks
Nemathelminths: Roundworms						
Ancylostoma duodenale[a]	Old world hookworm; ancylostomiasis	Small intestine (attached)	Infective filariform larvae in soil	Anemia, growth retardation, GI symptoms	Eggs in stool	Prophylaxis by excreta disposal. Iron therapy important in blood regeneration
Necator americanus[a]	New world or tropical hookworm; uncinariasis					
Ascaris lumbricoides[b]	Large roundworm	Small intestine	Eggs from soil or vegetables	Vague abdominal distress	Eggs in stool	Worms migrate into bile, pancreatic duct, and peritoneum. Intestinal obstruction
Enterobius vermicularis[b]	Pinworm, seatworm; Oxyuris	Large intestine, appendix	Eggs in environment; autoinfection	Anal pruritus	Eggs in perianal region, cellophane tape swab	Entire family frequently infected. Personal hygiene important
Strongyloides stercoralis[a]	Cochin, China diarrhea	In wall of small intestine	Larvae in soil	Abdominal discomfort, diarrhea	Larvae in stool	Autoinfection occurs
Trichinella spiralis[b]	Trichinosis	Intestinal wall; cyst in striated muscle	Infected pork, cyst (rarely bear)	Orbital edema, muscle pain, eosinophilia	Skin test, complement fixation, flocculation, biopsy	Thorough cooking of pork and pork products to kill cysts
Trichuris trichiura[b]	Whipworm, threadworm	Cecum, large intestine, ileum	Eggs from soil or vegetables	Abdominal discomfort, anemia, bloody stools	Eggs in stool	Worm lives many years. Frequently with hookworm and ascaris
Toxocara canis, T. cati[b]	Visceral larva migrans	Liver, lung, brain, eye	Eggs from soil	Pneumonitis, eosinophilia	Hemagglutination, flocculation tests	Eosinophilia, anemia, hyperglobulinemia

Platyhelminths: Tapeworms

Organism	Common name	Location	Source	Symptoms	Diagnosis	Remarks
Diphyllobothrium latum[b]	Fish or broad tapeworm	Small intestine	Plerocercoid in freshwater fish	Anemia very rare	Eggs in stool	Prophylaxis by excreta disposal. Cook fish well
Hymenolepsis nana[b]	Dwarf tapeworm	Adults and cysts in small intestine	Eggs from feces	Abdominal discomfort	Eggs in stool	Numerous worms, infection of children
Taenia saginata[b]	Beef tapeworm	Small intestine	Cysts in beef	Usually no symptoms	Eggs and segments in stool	Usually only one worm
Taenia solium[b]	Pork tapeworm	Small intestine	Cysts in pork	Usually no symptoms	Eggs and segments in stool	Uncommon in US. Frequent in Mexico, S. America, Central America
T. solium (cysts)[b]	Cysticercosis; verminous epilepsy	Muscle, brain eye	Eggs from feces	Intracranial pressure, epilepsy	Skin tests, roentgenography of calcified cysts	Autoinfection possible. Uncommon in US
Echinococcus granulosus[b]	Hydatid cyst	Liver, lungs, brain, bones	Eggs from dog feces	Pressure symptoms in various organs	Skin, complement fixation, hemagglutination tests, roentgenography	Uncommon in Native Americans

Platyhelminths: Flukes

Organism	Common name	Location	Source	Symptoms	Diagnosis	Remarks
Schistosoma haematobium[a]	Schistosomiasis (bilharziasis)	Veins of urinary bladder	Cercaria in fresh water, from snail	Urinary disturbances, hematuria	Eggs in urine, cystoscopy	Africa, Middle East
Schistosoma japonicum[a]	Schistosomiasis	Veins of small intestine	Cercaria in fresh water, from snail	Dysentery, hepatic cirrhosis	Eggs in stool, liver biopsy	China, Japan, Philippines
Schistosoma mansoni[a]	Schistosomiasis	Veins of large intestine	Cercaria in fresh water, from snail	Chronic dysentery, cirrhosis of liver	Eggs in stool, rectal or liver biopsy	Africa, South America, common in Puerto Ricans

Table 11-6 (continued)

Common name of parasite or disease	Site in host	Source of infection, intermediate host, or vector	Most common clinical symptoms	Laboratory diagnosis	Remarks
Protozoa					
Entamoeba histolytica[b] Intestinal amebiasis	Lumen and wall of large intestine	Cysts in food and water, from feces	Mild to severe GI distress, dysentery	Cysts in cold stool; trophozoites in purged stool	Consider possibility of hepatic infection
E. histolytica[b] Amebic hepatitis, amebic liver abscess	In liver	Cysts in food and water, from feces	Enlarged, tender liver; fever; leukocytosis	Roentgenography, complement fixation test, cysts or trophozoites in stool	Treat intestinal amebic infection
Giardia lamblia[b] Flagellate diarrhea	Upper small intestine	Cysts in food and water, from feces	Mild GI distress and diarrhea	Cysts and trophozoites in stool	More common in children than adults

[a] Portal of entry is the skin.
[b] Portal of entry is the mouth.
Source: Adapted from H. W. Brown, *Basic Clinical Parasitology* (4th ed.). New York: Appleton-Century-Crofts, 1975. Pp. 4–11.

8. **Artifacts or other objects can be mistaken for parasites.** This is especially true in old specimens. It is best to confirm one's observation by consulting with an expert.
9. **Diagrams of some common helminth eggs** are shown in Fig. 11-2 and Neva's text [45].

B. **Geographic distribution** of the parasite may be useful knowledge when one is considering the diagnosis. For example, hookworms survive poorly in cold, northern environments, and *Echinococcus* cysts are found primarily in sheepherders of Basque origin in the western United States.

The **relative prevalence** of various parasitic diseases in the general population can be estimated from a survey done by the Centers for Disease Control, of stool specimens examined by public health laboratories. A total of 363,567 specimens were examined [46]. The most commonly identified pathogenic parasites include *Giardia lamblia,* 4%; *E. histolytica,* 0.9%; *Trichuris trichiura,* 2.2%; *Ascaris lumbricoides,* 1.8%; *Enterobius vermicularis,* 1.5%; and *Strongyloides stercoralis,* 0.2%.

C. **Cellophane tape (Scotch tape) swab** or cellulose tape technique for **pinworms** is the test of choice for *E. vermicularis* infestations. A piece of clear (old-type) cellophane tape (the sticky side) is pressed against several areas of the perineum of a child with pruritus. Next, the tape is placed sticky side down onto a clean glass slide, smoothed out with a cotton gauze, and examined under the microscope. The tape may be held conveniently while obtaining the specimen if one end is attached to the slide as an anchor and then folded back on itself so that the sticky side is outward. A tongue depressor may be used between the slide and the tape to prevent any accidental cuts or abrasions from the slide.

D. **Eosinophilia** is seen in many, but not all, parasitic infestations. Its presence should raise one's suspicion of parasitic tissue infestation. **The following organisms usually elicit eosinophilia:** (1) *Trichinella* spp., (2) visceral larva migrans, (3) filaria, (4) hookworms, (5) *Schistosoma* spp., and (6) whipworms.

E. **Serologic tests**
1. Amebiasis serologic tests are discussed in sec. **IV.E.4.**
2. *Trichinella spiralis* infection can be confirmed by sending a blood specimen to the state or reference laboratory. (Usually, a complement fixation test is done.)

F. **Duodenal aspirates** have been useful in making the diagnosis in a small number of cases of giardiasis and strongyloidiasis when stool specimens were not positive for cysts, trophozoites, or larvae, and the diagnosis was strongly suspected.

G. *Giardia* **antigen** is discussed in sec. **IV.A.2.**

III. **Therapy.** A summary of the recommended drugs for treatment is given in Table 11-7.

IV. **Discussion of selected parasitic diseases**
A. **Giardiasis** [47, 48]. *Giardia lamblia* (also called *G. intestinalis* and *G. duodenalis*) is the most frequently isolated intestinal parasite in the United States. Although the most common mode of transmission has been through contaminated water (e.g., surface water contaminated by humans or animals and in which the cysts survive), person-to-person (e.g., daycare centers, male homosexuals, and persons in custodial institutions) and foodborne (e.g., after fecal contamination) transmission can occur [48]. Young children in daycare centers can be the source of infection in a parent or caregiver [48]. Large-scale outbreaks have occurred in Leningrad, Colorado, New Hampshire, upstate New York, Oregon, Utah, and Washington. These infections have been related to ingestion of contaminated municipal water supplies and untreated water.

1. **Symptoms and life cycle.** A week or two after the ingestion of contaminated water (chlorination does not destroy the cystic stage), the acute symptoms of explosive diarrhea, abdominal cramps, flatulence, nausea, vomiting, and low-grade fever may occur. Patients do not pass gross pus, blood, or mucus [48]. Chronic infections result in milder, intermittent symptoms and malaise. The **spectrum** of disease **varies widely,** from patients with acute symptoms to asymptomatic cyst-passing patients to patients with persistent steatorrhea and weight loss; weight loss may be seen in approximately 50% of patients with chronic symptoms and averages 10 pounds per person [48].

Lactase deficiency after infection is **common,** especially in children. Patients who recover from giardiasis should be counseled to avoid lactose-containing products for approximately 1 month after therapy [48].

Because hypogammaglobulinemic patients often have an associated *Giardia* infection, and because achlorhydric patients are more susceptible to infection, it is believed that IgG and stomach acid both play a role in host defense.

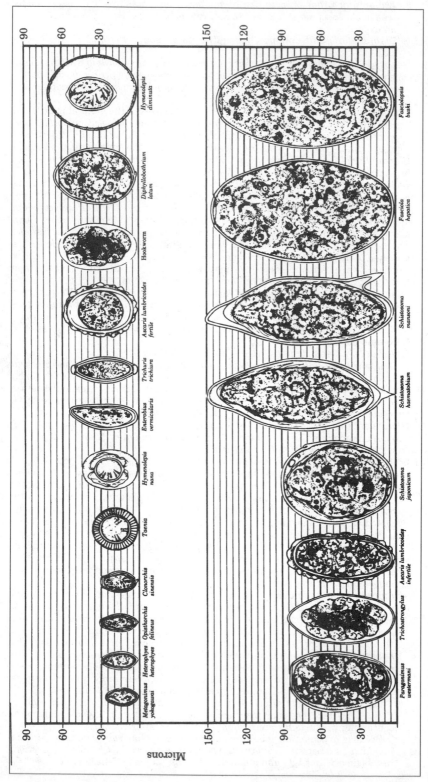

Fig. 11-2. Relative size of helminth eggs. (From M. M. Brooke and D. M. Melvin, *Morphology of Diagnostic Stages of Intestinal Parasites of Man.* Atlanta: U.S. Department of Health, Education, and Welfare, Publication No. (HSM) 72-8116, PHS, CDS, 1972.)

Table 11-7. Treatment of common parasitic infections

Organism	Drug choice	Adult dose	Pediatric dose
Giardia lamblia	Metronidazole[a]	250 mg tid × 5 d	15 mg/kg/d in 3 doses × 5 d
	Furazolidone	100 mg qid × 7–10 d	6 mg/kg/d in 4 doses × 7–10 d
	Paromomycin[b]	25–35 mg/kg/d in 3 doses × 7 d	
Trichuris trichiura	Mebendazole *or*	100 mg bid × 3 d	Same
	Albendazole[c]	400 mg once	Same
Ascaris lumbricoides	Mebendazole *or*	100 mg bid × 3 d	Same
	Pyrantel pamoate *or*	11 mg/kg once (max 1 g)	Same
	Albendazole	400 mg once	Same
Enterobius vermicularis	Pyrantel pamoate *or*	11 mg/kg once (max 1 g); repeat after 2 wk	Same
	Mebendazole *or*	100 mg once; repeat after 2 wk	Same
	Albendazole	400 mg once; repeat after 2 wk	Same
Entamoeba histolytica			
Asymptomatic	Iodoquinol[d] *or*	650 mg tid × 20 d	30–40 mg/kg/d in 3 doses × 20 d
	Paromomycin	25–35 mg/kg/d in 3 doses × 7 d	Same
Intestinal disease[g]	Metronidazole[e]	750 mg tid × 10 d	35–50 mg/kg/d in 3 doses × 10 d
Hepatic abscess[g]	Metronidazole[e]	750 mg tid × 10d	35–50 mg/kg/d in 3 doses × 10 d
Dientamoeba fragilis	Iodoquinol[d] *or*	650 mg tid × 20 d	40 mg/kg/d in 3 doses × 20 d
	Tetracycline[h] *or*	500 mg qid × 10 d	40 mg/kg/d in 4 doses × 10 d (max 2 g/d)
	Paromomycin	25–30 mg/kg/d in 3 doses × 7 d	25–30 mg/kg/d in 3 doses × 7 d
Blastocystis hominis[f]	Iodoquinol[d] *or*	650 mg tid × 20 d	—
	Metronidazole[e]	750 mg tid × 10 d	—

d = day.

[a]Contraindicated in patients younger than 8 years and in pregnancy.

[b]See discussion in Chap. 28H. May be useful in pregnancy.

[c]In heavy infection, it may be necessary to extend therapy for 3 days.

[d]Dosage and duration of administration should not be exceeded because of the possibility of causing optic neuritis. Maximum dose 2 g/d.

[e]Avoid in pregnant women, especially first trimester (see discussion of this agent in Chap. 28P).

[f]Whether this organism is a true pathogen is controversial. See text.

[g]Treatment should be followed by a course of iodoquinol or one of the other intraluminal drugs used to treat asymptomatic amebiasis.

[h]Approved drug but investigational in this condition.

Source: Adapted from The Medical Letter. Drugs for parasitic infections. *Med. Lett. Drugs Ther.* 37:99, 1995. (For details of drug use and regimens for less common parasites [summarized in Table 11-6], and for a summary of adverse effects of antiparasitic drugs, see this excellent source.)

2. **Diagnosis**
   a. **The patient's history** of prolonged diarrhea without blood or mucus, weight loss, surface water exposure, exposure to daycare children, or a homosexual lifestyle among men, and mild malabsorption or lactose intolerance should raise suspicion for this diagnosis.
   b. **Stool examination.** There are only two stages in the life cycle of this parasite: the trophozoite, which exists freely in the small bowel, and the cyst, which is passed into the environment [48]. **Fecal leukocytes are not present.**
      (1) **Ova and parasite examinations** are still the test of choice, especially if other parasitic infections are possible (e.g., assessing an international traveler). The literature suggests that if three serial liquid stools are examined properly, stool examinations will demonstrate the organism in 90% of cases [48]. Three stools over several days are preferred as cysts may be shed intermittently. Fresh and preserved specimens are examined.
         Because the organisms reside in the small bowel, early symptoms may precede stool positivity by 1–2 weeks in a minority of patients.
      (2) *Giardia* **stool antigen** tests have become commercially available. In these assays, a polyclonal or monoclonal antibody against cyst or trophozoite antigens is used in either an immunofluorescent antibody test or a capture ELISA. The sensitivity of such assays is 85–98%, and the specificity is 90–100%. The optimal use of this test is still undergoing clinical evaluation, but Hill [48] suggests use of these assays to rule out exclusive infection with *Giardia* (e.g., in an outbreak of *Giardia,* screening of children in daycare centers, or examining for test of cure in a patient who has been treated).
   c. **Duodenal sampling.** Occasionally, patients with persisting suggestive symptoms of *Giardia* infestation have negative serial stool examinations. In these patients, a string test or Entero-Test (HDC Corporation, San Jose, CA), duodenal aspirate, or duodenal biopsy may be considered; these are reviewed elsewhere [48].
   d. **Serum anti-***Giardia* **antibody** studies usually are not available and are used more **in epidemiologic studies.**
3. **Therapy. All symptomatic patients deserve treatment.** Although some cases resolve spontaneously over 3–4 days, most persist until treatment intervenes [48]. Formerly, either quinacrine or metronidazole was used for treatment in the United States. In 1992, Sanofi Winthrop Pharmaceuticals discontinued production of quinacrine [48] because of a shortage of raw materials, which persists as of spring 1996 and is expected to continue.
   a. **Metronidazole** is commonly used but, as of spring 1996, is not approved by the FDA. High-dose, short-course regimens have lower efficacy rates and are not tolerated as well as standard regimens (see Table 11-7).
   b. **Furazolidone** is an alternative agent for children, is available in liquid suspension, and is well tolerated. Because it is only about 80% effective, serial follow-up is important. It can cause mild hemolysis in patients deficient in glucose–6–phosphate dehydrogenase [48].
   c. **Tinidazole** (Fasigyn) is effective but not yet available in the United States.
   d. **Therapy in pregnancy** remains an unclear issue. Hill [48] suggests the following:
      (1) Avoid treatment altogether in the first trimester.
      (2) Women with mild disease may delay therapy until after delivery. Nutrition and hydration must be maintained.
      (3) For women with persisting symptoms of weight loss, nausea, or dehydration necessitating therapy, use of paromomycin, an oral aminoglycoside that is excreted in the feces nearly 100% unchanged, is advised, although its efficacy may be in the 60–70% range [48]. See Chap. 28H.
         The use of metronidazole in pregnancy remains debated (see Chap. 28P), but it is a potential option in the third trimester (see Table 11-7).
   e. **Persisting symptoms** may be due to lactose intolerance, and this warrants therapy as well as careful repeat stool examination.
4. **Therapy of asymptomatic infection** (asymptomatic cyst passer) is **controversial.** Therapy is indicated if reinfection is unlikely, such as in environments

where the level of sanitation is high. Asymptomatic food handlers should be treated [48].

5. **Empiric therapy** sometimes is used in situations where the clinical suspicion is h'gh but serial stool examinations are negative and endoscopy is not believed to be in the patient's best interest (see sec. **2.c**).

6. **Prevention** requires proper handling and treatment of community water supplies, appropriate disposal of human and animal waste, and good personal hygiene [48].

   a. **For wilderness hikers or international travelers,** attention must be paid to preparing drinking water [48]. Water needs to be boiled for at least 10 minutes or longer at higher altitudes. Water also needs to be halogenated, using Halozone tablets, Potable Aqua tablets, or saturated crystalline iodine treatment, for example. These may be more effective than chlorine treatment. Several portable filter systems are available, but the pore size should be 2 μm or less.

   b. Good personal hygiene after changing a diaper is important.

B. *Trichuris trichiura* **(whipworm) infestation**

   1. **Life cycle.** Infection occurs in humans by ingestion of embryonated eggs on contaminated hands, food, soil, or fomites. After a 10- to 30-day period in the small intestine, the larvae migrate to the large intestine (primarily cecum and appendix), where they imbed their anterior end into the mucosa, with the posterior end free to "whip" in the lumen. These mature adults lay eggs, which pass to the soil and repeat the cycle if conditions (temperature, humidity) are favorable. The distribution of whipworm is similar to that of *Ascaris lumbricoides*.

   2. **Symptoms** are correlated with the worm burden in the large bowel. Light infections may be asymptomatic. Infections produce their damage by mechanical and lytic damage to the mucosa, with petechial hemorrhages and disruption of integrity of the GI tract by bacteria. Heavy worm burdens produce diarrhea, abdominal pain, anemia, weight loss, weakness, and even rectal prolapse.

   3. **Diagnosis** is made **by examination of fecal specimens** by direct smear, formalin-ether centrifugal sedimentation, or flotation techniques. In some severe infections, adult worms may be observed attached to the colonic mucosa if sigmoidoscopy is performed.

   4. **Treatment** is summarized in Table 11-7. A stool examination should be performed 3 weeks after treatment to confirm the eradication of parasites, and a second course of therapy should be undertaken if necessary.

C. *Ascaris lumbricoides* **infestation**

   1. **Life cycle.** Infection results from ingestion of second-stage larvae that usually are contaminants of hands or soil (e.g., geophagia in children). The larvae hatch in the small intestine, penetrate the intestinal wall, and are carried to the lungs through the portal vein or, indirectly, through the lymphatics. In the lung, they live and molt in the alveoli for 10–14 days. Subsequently, they migrate up the respiratory tract to the pharynx, are swallowed, and mature sexually in the small intestine some 8–12 weeks after the initial ingestion of eggs. The adult phase persists for approximately 9 months. Eggs are laid daily during this period. To become infectious to humans, these eggs must be deposited in an external environment with adequate shade and moisture and a temperature conducive to hatching. **In the United States, the endemic areas include** southeastern parts of the Appalachian mountain range and areas of the southern and Gulf Coast states.

   2. **Symptoms are related** primarily to the **mechanical presence of the parasites.** During the transient pulmonary stage, **Loffler's syndrome** (pulmonary infiltrates with eosinophilia, dyspnea, cough, and fever) may occur. The adult worm's presence in the intestine usually is asymptomatic except in cases where the worm **migrates abnormally** and causes obstruction of various organs such as the common bile duct, pancreatic duct, appendix, or even the bowel itself if the mass of worms is large. At times, a patient, especially a child, may report having coughed up a worm or passed one per rectum.

   3. **Diagnosis.** Identification of ascaris **eggs in the stool** is the primary means of diagnosis. Direct smears usually are sufficient, although concentration techniques may have to be used occasionally.

      In the patient with partial bowel obstruction due to a mass of ascaris, an upper GI barium study may allow the diagnosis to be made when worms are visualized in the small bowel.

4. Treatment is summarized in Table 11-7.

D. *Enterobius vermicularis* **(pinworm) infestation**

  1. **Symptoms.** Intense **pruritus ani** and, occasionally, **pruritus vulvae** are caused by the presence of adult worms and embryonic eggs. The 15-day life cycle is initiated by the ingestion of eggs on contaminated hands or in food or drink. Because the eggs are infectious when laid, autoinoculation can occur after anal scratching for a current infection. The larvae emerge in the upper intestine, temporarily attach themselves, copulate in the lower small intestine, and then migrate to the anus to deposit their sticky eggs on the perianal skin. Irritability, restlessness, anorexia, and insomnia (in children) with enterobiasis have been attributed to a heavy worm infestation.

  2. **Diagnosis.** No eggs are found in the stool. The **cellophane tape test is used** (see sec. **II.C**) to make the diagnosis. Occasional worms may be seen on the perineum and identified.

  3. **Treatment** is summarized in Table 11-7. Often, pinworm is epidemic among the entire family, and it is judicious to **consider treating all members simultaneously.**

E. *Entamoeba histolytica* **infestation.** This entity has recently been reviewed [49].

  1. **Life cycle.** Amebiasis is **acquired by the ingestion of cysts in contaminated water or in food that has been soiled** by a cyst carrier or contaminated by houseflies or cockroaches that have fed on human feces. The cysts undergo excystation in the small bowel. The trophozoites reach the large bowel and divide by binary fission. Some trophozoites may invade the colon and produce the characteristic flask-shaped ulcers. Others may invade the portal vein, lodge in the liver, and form a hepatic abscess. The trophozoites metamorphose into cysts as they are passed in the stools. If the diarrhea is loose and intestinal transit short, trophozoites may be seen in the stool.

  2. **Pathophysiology.** Virulent strains of *E. histolytica* have significant cytopathic properties in vitro, consistent with their ability to cause invasive colitis in vivo. The majority of individuals infected with *E. histolytica* are asymptomatic. The difference between commensal and invasive *E. histolytica* infection is attributable to the existence of distinct pathogenic and nonpathogenic strains. Nonpathogenic strains have never been found to cause amebic colitis or liver abscess [49]. Nearly 10% of persons infected with *E. histolytica* harbor pathogenic strains. Although almost all these patients will mount a serum antibody response to pathogenic *E. histolytica* infection, only 1 of 10 patients with pathogenic strains have symptomatic disease [49].

  3. **Clinical symptoms** vary widely [49].

     a. *E. histolytica* infection has a number of diverse clinical presentations (Table 11-8).

     b. **The most common finding is asymptomatic intestinal infection without evidence of tissue invasion,** as defined by the absence of serum antibodies, blood in the stool, and mucosal ulcerations on colonoscopy.

     c. **Amebic colitis** has a subacute onset of bloody, mucoid diarrhea (onset over 7 days; duration, 3–4 weeks), with abdominal pain, tenesmus, **fecal leukocytes,** fever often, and positive serology for antiamebic antibodies (in 90% by day 7 of illness). **Fecal occult blood** tests are positive.

     d. **Liver abscess** classically presents with fever, right upper quadrant abdominal pain, and tenderness over the liver. Affected returning international travelers usually present within 5 months of their exposure. Diarrhea is seen in only 30–40% of those with liver abscess, and finding amebae in the stool is even less common [49].

  4. **Diagnosis of amebic colitis**

     a. **A freshly passed liquid stool is examined** to identify the motile **trophozoites** of *E. histolytica*. Refrigeration at 4°C or storage in a fixative may allow some preservation (check with the parasitology laboratory). Three separate specimens should be examined (see sec. **II.A.3**).

        Formed stools in saline and iodine preparations are examined for amebic cysts. The formalin-ether concentration technique may help increase the yield.

     b. **Serum antiamebic antibodies** develop only with pathogenic strains, and the absence of antibodies after 7 days of infection is strong evidence against invasive amebiasis.

     c. **Colonoscopy** with scraping or biopsy of mucosal ulcers provides definitive

Table 11-8. Clinical syndromes due to infection by *Entamoeba histolytica*

Intestinal
  Asymptomatic cyst passers (colonization)
  Symptomatic cyst passers
  Acute rectocolitis
  Fulminant colitis
    Toxic megacolon
    Perforation with peritonitis
  Chronic nondysenteric colitis
  Ameboma
Extraintestinal
  Liver abscess
  Lung abscess, empyema
  Pericarditis
  Brain abscess
  Venereal disease
  Cutaneous disease

Source: From J. N. Aucott and J. I. Ravdin, Amebiasis and "nonpathogenic" intestinal protozoa. *Infect. Dis. Clin. North Am.* 7:467, 1993.

diagnosis. Special stains (e.g., periodic acid–Schiff [PAS]) will demonstrate the organism. A tissue diagnosis is especially indicated if corticosteroid therapy is being considered for the patient who has inflammatory bowel disease.

  5. **Diagnosis of amebic abscess** [49]
     a. **Ultrasonography** of the liver and biliary tract is suggested. CT scanning can be used in those with nondiagnostic findings.
     b. **Serum antiamebic antibodies** are **present** in 99% of patients with amebic abscess within 7–10 days of their illness.
     c. If the clinical setting and evaluation are nondiagnostic, **fine-needle aspiration** under ultrasound or CT guidance can be performed. **Aspiration** of a liver abscess yields an "anchovy-paste" fluid containing neither polymorphonuclear leukocytes nor amebae. The amebae occasionally are seen in the wall of the abscess.
  6. **Therapy.** Treatment is summarized in **Table 11-7** and reviewed in detail elsewhere [49].
     a. **Asymptomatic *E. histolytica* infection.** It is unclear whether this condition routinely needs therapy. If serum antiamebic antibodies are positive in nonendemic areas, the patient has underlying human immunodeficiency virus (HIV) infection, or the patient is from a nonendemic area, therapy is suggested [49].
     b. If metronidazole is the preferred agent (see Table 11-7) but is contraindicated or not tolerated, alternative regimens are available [49].
     c. **Amebic abscess** usually will respond to metronidazole therapy without the need to drain the abscess. It should be noted that metronidazole has excellent antibacterial activity against anaerobes, and several reports have warned that a metronidazole therapeutic trial cannot be used to differentiate an amebic abscess from an anaerobic liver abscess. (See the discussion in sec. **V.C** under Intraabdominal Abscess.)
  7. **Prevention.** Avoiding fecal-oral contamination is the only effective means of preventing *E. histolytica* infection. Boiling is the only certain means of eradicating *E. histolytica* cysts in water [49].
 F. *Cryptosporidium, Isospora belli,* **cytomegalovirus, and atypical mycobacterial infections are causes of chronic diarrhea in AIDS patients** but rarely cause more than transient diarrhea in the immunocompetent host. These are discussed in Chap. 19.
   Infrequently, outbreaks of cryptosporidiosis have occurred due to water contamination, with *Cryptosporidium* affecting municipal water plants. This topic has recently been reviewed in detail [49a]. Some microbiology laboratories screen all *Giardia*-negative ova and parasite specimens for *Cryptosporidium* by enzyme-

linked immunosorbent assay (see related discussion in Chap. 19).

G. *Dientamoeba fragilis* is an intestinal protozoan parasite that formerly was believed to be a harmless commensal; however, more recent reviews have concluded that this organism is a pathogen [50, 51]. Only the trophozoite forms are found in stool samples, and the organism does not invade tissue. The mode of transmission is unknown. Symptoms have been reported more frequently in children than in adults [51].

1. **Clinical manifestations** [50]
   a. **Acute dysentery** with watery diarrhea, abdominal pain, anorexia, nausea, vomiting, occasional fever, and malaise can occur. Physical examination may reveal abdominal tenderness.
   b. **Chronic,** vague, nonspecific, **abdominal pain** that is dull, crampy, colicky, and usually in the lower abdomen can occur. It may occur postprandially and last for hours. Symptoms may last for months to years [50].

2. **Diagnosis**
   a. **Stool specimens.** The diagnosis can be made by staining a fresh stool specimen or by examining a stool specimen in a stool preservative such as polyvinyl alcohol (PVA). At least three stool samples should be examined before any barium studies are done.
   b. **Routine laboratory and radiographic studies are nonspecific.** No serologic test is available for diagnosis.

3. **Therapy** is summarized in Table 11-7. Stool specimens should be examined 3–4 weeks after therapy to determine whether the parasite has been eliminated.

H. *Blastocystis hominis.* Although *B. hominis* may be found in up to 25% of stool specimens examined, only occasional patients have mild diarrhea, and there is much controversy about whether *B. hominis* is sometimes or never a pathogen [51]. **Recent data favor the view that *B. hominis* is a commensal organism** [52–54].

Rarely, *B. hominis* has been implicated as a pathogen in immunocompromised individuals (e.g., AIDS patients, patients on corticosteroids). The role of *B. hominis* as an opportunistic pathogen requires further study [52]. A trial of therapy in this setting may be reasonable if no other pathogen has been demonstrated (see Table 11-7).

Intraabdominal Infection

I. **Initial approach.** In patients who present with abdominal pain, fever, abdominal tenderness, and leukocytosis, the question of an intraabdominal infection is raised. Although an exact diagnosis is an ultimate goal, antibiotic therapy often is started before a specific diagnosis is reached [55].

A. The **history and physical examination** provide important clues to the most likely clinical diagnosis, and the reader is referred to basic surgical texts for detailed information of this topic [56] as it is beyond the scope of this book. However, a few points deserve special emphasis.

1. **Percussion tenderness** on examination is a useful indicator of peritoneal inflammation or possible focal infection [56]. Therefore, right upper abdominal percussion tenderness may suggest biliary tract infection; right lower quadrant tenderness may suggest appendicitis or a focal pelvic infection in women; left lower quadrant tenderness may suggest diverticulitis; and so on. Diffuse abdominal percussion tenderness, often with rebound tenderness, may reflect a diffuse peritoneal irritation (i.e., peritonitis). Corticosteroids and analgesia may mask these findings.

2. **A rectal and pelvic examination** (in women) should routinely be performed, especially in patients with mid- to lower abdominal pain.

3. **Fever** may be modified by analgesics, NSAIDs, corticosteroids, and age (i.e., the elderly patient).

4. **Leukocytosis** and a left shift are commonly, but not always, present.

B. **Serial clinical evaluations and surgical evaluation are routinely indicated.**

C. **Empiric antibiotic therapy** often is started before a specific diagnosis has been established, to help contain the infection and prevent the clinical septic syndrome described in Chap. 2.

Knowledge of the normal flora of the colon helps determine empiric regimens for peritonitis (see sec. II). Knowledge of the flora in the obstructed biliary tract helps to determine antibiotic regimens for cholangitis (see sec. **I.C** under Biliary Tract Infections).

D. Cultures
   1. **Blood cultures** may sometimes be positive and should routinely be performed (e.g., two sets drawn at a 20- to 30-minute interval).
   2. **Peritoneal fluid cultures.** Adequate quantities of infected fluid (tissue) should be cultured aerobically and anaerobically. One surgical text appropriately emphasizes that immediately after the abdominal cavity has been opened, a syringe is used to take up as much pus and fluid free of air as can be obtained. If air bubbles are present, they should be injected into a sponge saturated with alcohol. **Pus is the best transport medium to maintain viability of bacteria. Dry or wet swabs should be used only if pus or fluid is not available** from the peritoneal cavity. The syringe containing pus can be taken immediately to the laboratory for processing, or 3–4 ml can be injected into the proper anaerobic culture tube (e.g., Port-a-Cult) and sent to the laboratory for both aerobic and anaerobic processing [56].
E. Diagnostic studies are reviewed later. See sec. **III.D.4** and sec. **IV.C.2** under Peritonitis for the role of abdominal CT scanning.

II. Principles of antibiotic therapy of intraabdominal infections have recently been reviewed [57–58a].
   A. Microbiologic features. The source of infecting microorganisms in most patients with intraabdominal infection is the microflora of the GI tract.
      1. **Normal gastrointestinal flora.** More than 400 different species of bacteria can be found in a single fecal specimen. Under healthy conditions, the stomach and small bowel harbor a sparse microflora generally not exceeding 10^5 bacteria per milliliter of contents. The number of bacteria increases in the middle and lower ileum, and there is an even greater augmentation across the ileocecal valve. **The colon harbors approximately 10^{11} organisms per milliliter, a number that approaches the theoretic limit that can fit into a given mass** [57].
      2. Damage to the intestinal wall (e.g., perforation with peritonitis, surgery with a later anastomotic leak) leads to contamination of the abdominal cavity and the structures within.
         a. **Cultures** typically **reveal a mixture of organisms**—on average, two aerobes and three anaerobes. Common bacterial isolates are shown in Table 11-9.
            (1) Animal model studies have shown that the aerobic flora, especially *E. coli*, was responsible for the initial peritonitis and septicemic phase that causes high mortality initially if not treated appropriately [57–58a].
            (2) **Abscesses** were caused primarily by the anaerobes in animal models.

Table 11-9. Bacteriology of intraabdominal infections

	Frequency of isolation (%)
Aerobes	
Escherichia coli	65
Proteus spp.	25
Klebsiella spp.	20
Pseudomonas spp.	15
Enterococci	15
Streptococcus spp. (other than groups A or D)	10
Anaerobes	
B. fragilis	80
Bacteroides spp. (other)	30
Clostridium spp.	65
Peptostreptococcus spp.*	25
Peptococcus spp.*	15
Fusobacterium spp.	20

*Sometimes grouped as anaerobic gram-positive cocci.
Source: From S. L. Gorbach, Treatment of intra-abdominal infections. *J. Antimicrob. Chemother.* 31(Suppl. A):67, 1993.

In particular, *Bacteroides* spp. have a virulence factor—the polysaccharide capsule—which could explain, at least in part, the selective advantage that facilitated the emergence of these organisms as important pathogens in abscess formation [58].

   b. The site of perforation of the GI tract is significant because an injury to the large bowel (releasing a high inoculum of bacteria) carries a higher risk of complications than injury to other parts of the intestinal tract [57].

B. Antibiotic therapy is directed at both aerobic and anaerobic bacteria [57, 58, 59]. If antibiotics are not aimed at both aerobic and anaerobic pathogens, clinical failure is common. As reviewed in sec. **I.C**, empiric antibiotic therapy typically is begun before an exact diagnosis is reached and before culture data are available.

   1. Aminoglycosides. Although historically aminoglycosides in combination with clindamycin or metronidazole or in triple-drug regimens (ampicillin, clindamycin, or metronidazole, and an aminoglycoside) were commonly used, **the current trend is to decrease the routine use of aminoglycosides** [56, 57, 57a, 58a].

      a. Limitations of aminoglycosides include their associated nephrotoxicity (especially in severely ill patients) and the potential for inadequate serum or tissue levels [57–59]. Aminoglycosides are susceptible to inactivation by low pH within abscess cavities [57a]. For details, see Chap. 28H. In addition, for community-acquired organisms, the expanded cephalosporins and broad-spectrum penicillin agents with beta-lactamase inhibitors offer options for monotherapy.

      b. In his review of the treatment of intraabdominal infection, Gorbach [58] concluded: **"There is now sufficient evidence to support the position that aminoglycosides are not needed and should not be used for the initial treatment of uncomplicated intra-abdominal infection."** This policy should apply to acute appendicitis, penetrating abdominal trauma, and spontaneous bowel perforation associated with diverticulitis or carcinoma [57]. The potent activity of aminoglycosides should be saved for special situations that involve resistant gram-negative bacilli [58]. Other reviewers have reached similar conclusions [59], and we concur with these recommendations.

      Other reviewers have recently emphasized the declining role of aminoglycosides for similar reasons [57a, 58a].

      c. Gorbach [57] emphasizes that **aminoglycosides still are indicated in the therapy for intraabdominal infection when resistant gram-negative bacilli are suspected.** These exceptions represent the minority of cases and include (1) previous use of antibiotics, especially broad-spectrum antibiotics, in the last 30 days; (2) isolation of resistant gram-negative bacilli (e.g., to cephalosporins) in initial abdominal cultures with susceptibility to aminoglycosides; (3) reoperation or recurrence of infection; and (4) prolonged hospitalization preoperatively or prolonged nursing home stays preoperatively, especially if these institutions have a background incidence of resistant gram-negative bacilli that may colonize or infect the patient.

   2. Clindamycin and metronidazole both have excellent anaerobic activity and have been **used** extensively **in combination** regimens (e.g., with aminoglycosides) for intraabdominal infection. In several comparative studies, both clindamycin and metronidazole performed equally well [58]. These agents are reviewed in detail in Chap. 28. Metronidazole may be a more cost-effective agent and possibly is associated with less *C. difficile* toxin diarrhea. Metronidazole is also more consistently active in vitro against *B. fragilis* than clindamycin [57a, 58a] (see Chaps. 28I and 28P). Metronidazole should be avoided in the first trimester of pregnancy and probably throughout pregnancy (see Chap. 28P).

      In the past, these agents have been combined with aminoglycosides commonly. More recently, they have been combined with a first-generation cephalosporin (cefazolin) or a third-generation cephalosporin (e.g., ceftriaxone, ceftazidime, or cefotaxime) or aztreonam, although some reviewers do not advocate the combination of aztreonam and metronidazole because of this combination's lack of activity against gram-positive organisms [57a]. See Table 11-10.

   3. Monotherapy has become increasingly popular [57, 58], especially among mild to moderately ill patients with community-acquired disease.

      a. Cefoxitin alone has been most widely studied. It has been compared with either an aminoglycoside-containing regimen or a single broad-spectrum antibiotic regimen in 13 studies, which show that cefoxitin alone is as effective as the comparative regimen [57, 58]. Thus, cefoxitin seems to be a **satisfactory initial treatment for uncomplicated intraabdominal infection** [57].

Fewer studies have been conducted with **cefotetan,** which presumably is a reasonable alternative to cefoxitin. See Chap. 28F for a detailed discussion of these two agents.

b. **Imipenem** in eight studies has been shown to be as good or even better than regimens containing an aminoglycoside [58]. Because of the broad-spectrum activity of this agent, it may be prudent to **save this agent for complex intraabdominal infections,** as discussed in Chap. 28G, rather than using it for community-acquired intraabdominal infection.

c. **Beta-lactam antibiotics in combination with a beta-lactamase inhibitor** have been studied as initial treatment of mixed infections [57, 58].

(1) **Ampicillin-sulbactam** (Unasyn) commonly is used in this setting. However, a significant percentage of community-acquired *E. coli* may be resistant to this agent and, in the very ill patient, it may be more appropriate to use combination therapy (e.g., metronidazole and ceftriaxone). Ampicillin-sulbactam is reviewed in detail in Chap. 28E.

(2) **Ticarcillin-clavulanate** (Timentin) has been used in this setting also. See the discussion of this agent in Chap. 28E.

(3) **Piperacillin-tazobactam** was approved for use in October 1993 and is another potential agent for use in this setting, although there is less experience with it. This may be the optimal β-lactamase inhibitor combination because these agents have a broader spectrum of activity against Enterobacteriaceae than do the other β-lactamase inhibitors [57a]. See the discussion of this agent in Chap. 28E.

4. **Determining whether to cover for enterococci in intraabdominal infection.** There is debate about whether empiric regimens should cover enterococci. If enterococci are isolated from an intraabdominal source in a mixed culture, is specific therapy needed?

a. Gorbach and others [57–58a] have recently reviewed these questions. Although enterococci are relatively common isolates (see Table 11-9), a review of multiple studies using combination therapy **without** specific activity against enterococci did not reveal clinical failure due to persistent enterococcal infection [57–58a].

Based on his review of accumulated studies, Gorbach [57, 58] concluded: **"There appears to be no justification for the inclusion of specific antienterococcal therapy in the initial treatment of mixed infections.** Furthermore, **even the isolation of enterococcus in mixed cultures initially does not necessitate specific enterococcal antibiotic therapy"** [58].

Triple antibiotic regimens (e.g., ampicillin, clindamycin, and an aminoglycoside) in the past were encouraged, in part because they were believed to be active against enterococci as well as other bowel flora, but this enterococcal therapy is not necessary. Gorbach [58] states that clinicians have "almost mythical adherence to the belief that this organism has some special pathogenic powers in intraabdominal infections" [58] and, therefore, it is hard not to want to "cover" for this pathogen.

b. **Specific antibiotic regimens aimed at enterococci isolated from intraabdominal infections are occasionally rational, but only in special settings** [57, 58], as follows:

(1) Patients with **persistent positive cultures** of these organisms in the absence of clinical improvement on nonenterococcal treatment regimens

(2) Patients with enterococcal bacteremia (see Chap. 2)

(3) Other reviewers suggest life-threatening intraabdominal sepsis with *Enterococcus* spp. isolated in pure culture or a predominance of gram-positive cocci in chains on the Gram's stain of peritoneal fluid [57a].

c. The role that vancomycin-resistant enterococci (VRE) may play in nosocomially acquired intraabdominal sepsis is not well defined but is of potential concern in the patient at risk for VRE (see related discussions in Chap. 28O).

5. **Isolation of *Candida* spp.** *Candida* is considered normal flora of the gastrointestinal tract and consequently is commonly isolated. Its precise role in infection has been debated and recently reviewed [57a, 58a].

    a. When *Candida* is the sole isolate, or *Candida* is isolated from cultures of both peritoneal (or abscess) fluid and blood, or *Candida* invasion is identified on histologic examination of tissue, antifungal therapy is essential [57a]. Other authors suggest that if *Candida* is isolated in high concentrations or increasing concentrations with sequential cultures, treatment is indicated, especially when host defenses are impaired [57a, 58a]. Isolation of *Candida* from the peritoneum of patients with acute pancreatitis also probably warrants specific therapy, as these patients are more likely to have invasive disease than simple contamination [57a].

    b. When *Candida* is identified as one of the multiple organisms contaminating the peritoneum after perforation of a viscus and its successful repair, antifungal therapy is generally not required [57a].

    c. Therapeutic options include amphotericin B or fluconazole (see Chap. 18). Infectious disease consultation is advised.

6. Significance of *Pseudomonas aeruginosa* isolated from appendiceal specimens or specimens collected after penetrating trauma. Rates of isolation vary from 5 to 20% [58]. Clinical significance of the data is unclear, as is the need for antipseudomonal antibiotic therapy. Further data are needed [58].

7. Summary. For empiric and initial antibiotic regimens for intraabdominal infection, many options are possible based on the previous principles and data. **See the summary in Table 11-10.**

    a. For mild to moderate community-acquired infection, monotherapy (e.g., cefoxitin, ampicillin-sulbactam) or a cost-effective combination (e.g., cefazolin and metronidazole) is rational.

    b. For severe community-acquired infection, a broader combination seems rational (e.g., metronidazole plus ceftriaxone) while awaiting culture data.

    c. For hospital-acquired infection or complex recurrent infections, aminoglycosides often are used in combination (see sec. **II.B.1**).

III. Peritonitis is a localized or general inflammation of the peritoneal cavity. It may be due to microorganisms (e.g., bacteria, fungi) or to irritating chemicals (bile salts, gastric contents, or talc).

  A. Classification. A classification system commonly used is shown in Table 11-11.

  B. The **pathogenesis** of peritonitis is complex. Some of the common ways it can occur are listed here.

    1. Primary peritonitis refers to inflammation of the peritoneum from a suspected extraperitoneal source, often via hematogenous spread.

      a. Spontaneous peritonitis usually occurs in patients with underlying ascites and is seen most frequently in patients with cirrhosis, nephrotic syndrome, and systemic lupus erythematosus (see sec. **F.1**).

      b. Peritonitis in patients with continuous ambulatory peritoneal dialysis (CAPD) is discussed in sec. **F.2.**

      c. Tuberculous peritonitis is discussed in Chap. 9 under Extrapulmonary Tuberculosis.

Table 11-10. Empiric antibiotics in intraabdominal infection, including peritonitis

Severity and setting	Antibiotic regimen (assumes normal renal function)
Community-acquired	
Mild–moderate	Cefazolin (1 g q8h) + metronidazole (500 mg q6h)*
	Cefoxitin (2 g q6–8h)
	Ampicillin-sulbactam (3 g q6h)
	Piperacillin-tazobactam (3.75 g q6h; see Chap. 28E)
Severe	Ceftriaxone (2 g q24h) + metronidazole (500 mg q6h)
	Clindamycin (600 mg q8h) + gentamicin (see Chap. 28H for dose)
	Ampicillin-sulbactam or piperacillin-sulbactam + gentamicin
	Imipenem (500 mg q6h or 1 g q8h)
Hospital-acquired	Piperacillin (3 g q4h or 4 g q6h) + metronidazole + an aminoglycoside
	Imipenem ± an aminoglycoside

*Cost-effective regimen.

Table 11-11. Classification of intraabdominal infections

I. Primary peritonitis
   A. Spontaneous peritonitis in children
   B. Spontaneous peritonitis in adults
   C. Peritonitis in patients with CAPD
   D. Tuberculous and other granulomatous peritonitis
   E. Other forms
II. Secondary peritonitis*
   A. Acute perforation peritonitis (acute suppurative peritonitis)
      1. Gastrointestinal tract perforation
      2. Bowel wall necrosis (intestinal ischemia)
      3. Pelvic peritonitis
      4. Other forms
   B. Postoperative peritonitis
      1. Anastomotic leak
      2. Leak of a simple suture
      3. Blind loop leak
      4. Other iatrogenic leaks
   C. Posttraumatic peritonitis
      1. Peritonitis after blunt abdominal trauma
      2. Peritonitis after penetrating abdominal trauma
      3. Other forms
III. Tertiary peritonitis
   A. Peritonitis without evidence for pathogens
   B. Peritonitis with fungi
   C. Peritonitis with low-grade pathogenic bacteria
IV. Other forms of peritonitis
   A. Aseptic or sterile peritonitis
   B. Granulomatous peritonitis
   C. Drug-related peritonitis
   D. Periodic peritonitis
   E. Lead peritonitis
   F. Hyperlipidemic peritonitis
   G. Porphyric peritonitis
   H. Foreign-body peritonitis
   I. Talcum peritonitis
V. Intraabdominal abscess
   A. Associated with primary peritonitis
   B. Associated with secondary peritonitis

CAPD = continuous ambulatory peritoneal dialysis.
*Secondary peritonitis is often defined as the presence of purulent exudate in the abdominal cavity from an enteric source.
Source: From D. H. Wittman, A. P. Walker, and R. E. Condon, Peritonitis and Intraabdominal Infection. In S. I. Schwartz et al. (eds.), *Principles of Surgery* (6th ed.). New York: McGraw-Hill, 1994. P. 1449.

2. **Rupture of viscus** can occur by innumerable means, including the following:
   a. **Traumatic injury** to the abdomen, including both sharp trauma (e.g., knives, bullets, surgical procedures) and blunt trauma (e.g., automobile steering columns)
   b. **Ulcerated lesions** from ulcerative colitis, typhoid fever, necrotizing enterocolitis, and perforation of gastric or duodenal peptic ulcers
   c. **Perforation** of colonic diverticula
   d. **Ischemic** necrotic **bowel** due to vascular insufficiency, incarcerated hernias, volvulus, intussusception, or neoplasia (adenocarcinoma)
   e. Ingestion of foreign bodies (e.g., toothpicks, bones, pins)
3. **Pelvic inflammatory disease,** including salpingitis and endometritis, can produce a localized lower-abdominal peritonitis indistinguishable from appendicitis. The related Fitz-Hugh-Curtis syndrome results from perihepatitis or localized peritonitis in the upper part of the abdomen due to gonococcal infection (see Chap. 13).

4. **Surgical postoperative** leaks and anastomotic breakdowns can occur.
5. **Tertiary peritonitis** is reviewed elsewhere [56]. In brief, it may be seen in patients in whom bacteria have been eliminated by successful antibiotic therapy but in whom the normally activated host defense systems continue to act through failure of autoregulation, resulting in an autoaggressive devastation of organ system functions. The clinical picture mimics occult sepsis, but no infection is active. There is no effective therapy [56].
6. **Noninfectious forms** of peritonitis are reviewed elsewhere [56].
7. **Rupture of an abscess** (e.g., hepatic, splenic, pancreatic) or rarely a distended gallbladder can cause peritonitis.

C. **Flora.** Bacterial peritonitis typically is caused by multiple organisms of the large bowel (see sec. **II** and Table 11-9).

D. **Diagnosis**
   1. **The patient's history,** remote and recent, is useful in delineating the present problem.
      a. **Remote medical history** may disclose previous episodes of a similar illness such as diverticulitis, gastric ulcers, pancreatitis, and past surgery.
      b. **Travel** and family history may disclose an exposure to typhoid fever or tuberculosis.
      c. **Accidents with blunt trauma** (e.g., recent automobile accident with the possibility of steering wheel–related injury) should be sought in the history. Such an accident may have caused a hematoma that later became infected.
      d. **Recent surgical procedures** should be noted.
      e. A surgical **history of appendectomy** will help eliminate the suspicion of a perforated appendix as the cause of the peritonitis.
   2. **Symptoms** can be grouped into two classes, **reflex** and **toxic** [60]. **Corticosteroid use by a patient may mask typical signs and symptoms.**
      a. **Reflex symptoms** include localized or generalized pain (usually the predominant symptom), nausea and vomiting (especially with an obstruction), and muscular rigidity. Rigidity commonly is seen in the early stages of an acute peritonitis, but it may be absent in peritonitis that progresses slowly (tuberculosis, primary spontaneous peritonitis) or when sterile bile, urine, or pancreatic juice leak into the peritoneal cavity.
      b. **Toxic symptoms** due to the accumulation of bacterial toxins, exudates, and intraperitoneal fluid include the following: distention, intestinal paresis, fever and general toxemia, and bacteremia. The sepsis syndrome can occur (see Chap. 2).
   3. **Physical examination** (see sec. **I**).
   4. **Laboratory tests** that should be evaluated are as follows:
      a. **Leukocyte count** usually is elevated but is nonspecific.
      b. **Liver function tests and a serum amylase level** may help localize sepsis or symptoms of the liver, gallbladder, or pancreas.
      c. **Roentgenographic examination of the abdomen** may reveal air under the diaphragm (in the case of ruptured viscus), paralytic ileus, intestinal obstruction, volvulus, or intussusception (barium enema). Findings suggestive of paralytic ileus are common [56]. A chest roentgenogram should be obtained to rule out any supradiaphragmatic process that may be causing peritoneal signs.
      d. **Scans.** Computed tomography is not required in the initial workup of acute peritonitis and may only delay needed operative management [56]. CT scanning is indicated early if there is a high suspicion of an underlying intraabdominal abscess.
      e. **Aspiration of peritoneal fluid** is usually a routine part of the workup of peritonitis in the setting of ascites or if trauma with hemorrhage into the peritoneal cavity is a concern. Fluid should be examined for leukocytes (with a differential count), bacterial and fungal organisms, amylase, gastric acid, and RBCs, as indicated by the particular case. The fluid **should be cultured both aerobically and anaerobically.**
      f. **Laparoscopy** is used by some institutions to eliminate unnecessary open surgery in some patients with superficial stab wounds, blunt trauma, or suspected pelvic inflammatory disease or appendicitis. It also may help localize an ectopic pregnancy or a ruptured spleen.
   5. The **differential diagnosis** of peritonitis is complex and reflects the many diagnoses raised in Table 11-11.

E. Treatment principles
1. **Supportive care** is necessary in the patient with peritonitis. Use of nasogastric suction and intravenous fluid are routine. The sepsis syndrome may occur (see Chap. 2).
2. **Cause of the peritonitis** should be found and eliminated. Surgical consultation is imperative.
   a. Surgical repair of a ruptured viscus is essential.
   b. Contaminating secretions, pus, or fecal material should be drained, and then the peritoneal cavity should be lavaged copiously with saline until the lavage fluid is clean.
3. **Systemic antibiotics** to cover coliforms and anaerobes should be started preoperatively; the rationale and alternative choices are reviewed in sec. **II. The optimal duration of therapy is not well defined** [58]. We have tended to treat nonbacteremic patients with 7–10 days of antibiotics, which can initially be administered intravenously and then orally. Shorter regimens may be effective in uncomplicated cases and, in penetrating trauma–related peritonitis, 2 days of treatment may sometimes be adequate [58].

   Another approach is to continue antibiotic therapy until all systemic signs of sepsis have resolved and the patient's appetite and sense of well-being have returned [56] and he or she has been afebrile for 48–72 hours. In bacteremic patients, we tend to use a total of 14 days of intravenous and oral therapy to prevent infectious complications at metastatic sites.

F. Special considerations
1. **Spontaneous bacterial peritonitis** (SBP). These patients do not have any evidence of rupture or contamination of the peritoneal cavity. The population affected and the spectrum of bacteria involved have changed over the last two decades [61]. Spontaneous peritonitis is now more common in adults than in children and shows no predilection for one gender or the other. **Formerly, children with nephrosis were the most commonly affected. Now SBP occurs more commonly in adults with cirrhosis or systemic lupus erythematosus** [56]. This topic has recently been reviewed [61a, 61b].

   Primary peritonitis of childhood usually occurs in girls younger than 10 years who have no preexisting cirrhosis. The organisms are almost always pneumococci or beta-hemolytic streptococci.
   a. **Adults.** Spontaneous peritonitis usually is seen in patients with ascites, primarily with underlying cirrhosis. Although formerly pneumococci were the most frequent organisms, coliforms are now the major pathogens in adults, accounting for 70% of infections, with *E. coli* being the most common isolate and *Klebsiella* spp. the next most common isolates. Gram-positive cocci may be seen in 10–20% and anaerobes in less than 5% [56, 61–61b]. Single organisms usually are isolated, in contrast to the polymicrobial nature of most forms of peritonitis [56]. (See sec. **II.**)
   b. **Pathogenesis.** Enteric organisms, primarily gram-negative bacilli, probably translocate to regional lymph nodes to produce bacteremia and seeding of ascitic fluid [61b]. There is a decreased ability to kill bacteria in low-protein ascites in these patients [61a]. At times a urinary tract infection may be the source of bacteremia [61a].
   c. **Clinical features of SBP** may be subtle, and **a high index of suspicion is necessary.** Ascites is uniformly present [61b].
      (1) Fever and abdominal pain are seen in 60–80% of patients.
      (2) Onset or worsening of hepatic encephalopathy is seen in about 60% of patients.
      (3) Only about half of patients may have abdominal tenderness or rebound tenderness, so clinical deterioration in both the presence and absence of peritoneal signs should raise the diagnosis of SBP.
   d. **Diagnosis.** A peritoneal tap is the most useful diagnostic test [56, 61a, 61b].
      (1) **Peritoneal fluid cell count. An absolute granulocyte count** (but not total leukocyte count) **of greater than 250 cells/mm^3 is a likely indication of peritoneal infection** in patients with uncomplicated alcoholic liver disease [62]. However, patients with other inflammatory disease of the abdomen, such as tuberculous peritonitis, pancreatitis, secondary bacterial peritonitis due to perforation, and even cancer, also will show elevated granulocyte counts. Thus, an increased count may be useful

in uncomplicated patients before culture results are available to help the clinician decide when to initiate empiric therapy.

   (a) **SBP classically has been defined** by an ascitic neutrophil count of at least 250 cells/mm^3, a positive ascitic fluid culture, and no obvious intraabdominal source of infection [61a].

   (b) **Culture-negative neutrocytic ascites** (CNNA) **is a variant** of SBP and is defined by an ascitic fluid neutrophil count of at least 500 cells/mm^3, negative ascitic cultures with no prior antibiotics in the preceding month, absence of an intraabdominal source of infection, and no alternative explanation of the elevated neutrophils in the ascitic fluid. CNNA may be seen in up to 35% of patients with suspected SBP [61a]. Analysis of clinical signs, symptoms, ascitic fluid measurements, response to antibiotic therapy, and mortality rates showed no statistically significant differences from SBP and CNNA. **Therefore, CNNA patients should be treated aggressively with IV antibiotics as would be done for SBP** [61a, 61b].

  (2) Ascitic fluid pH is low in spontaneous peritonitis, whereas in sterile ascitic fluid, the pH is the same as serum [56].

  (3) Gram stains of ascitic fluid. In only approximately one-third of patients will organisms be seen on centrifuged fluid that is subsequently culture-positive, reflecting a low concentration of bacteria [56]. If either gram-positive cocci or gram-negative rods are seen as single pathogen types, the diagnosis of spontaneous peritonitis is supported, although gram-negatives by themselves occur in secondary peritonitis. If mixed gram-positive and gram-negative bacteria are seen, an intestinal perforation is more likely [56].

  (4) Cultures of peritoneal fluid should routinely be performed aerobically and anaerobically: To maximize results, 10 ml of ascitic fluid should be routinely inoculated at the bedside in blood culture media [61a, 61b].

  (5) Blood cultures are also useful because they have been reported to be positive in about ⅓ of patients with spontaneous peritonitis [61, 61a]. **Urine cultures** are routinely suggested [61a] (see sec. **b**).

  (6) Protein content is not very useful in diagnosing spontaneous bacterial peritonitis because it is usually less than 2.5 g/dl. However, protein content may be a useful parameter in the differential diagnosis of pancreatic ascites and tuberculous peritonitis as these conditions generally are associated with ascitic protein levels of 3.0 g/dl or greater.

e. Therapy. Once the diagnosis of SBP is made or highly suspected, intravenous antibiotics are indicated.

  (1) Cefotaxime has been favored by recent reviewers [61a, 61b]. In adult patients with normal renal function, 2 g q8h is suggested [61a, 61b]. Ceftriaxone is also a reasonable agent (e.g., 1–2 g q24h). See Chap. 28F.

  (2) Aminoglycosides have recently been **avoided** because their use in patients with underlying liver disease is associated with excess nephrotoxicity. See Chap. 28H.

  (3) Other options include agents such as ampicillin-sulbactam and cefoxitin. Monotherapy with aztreonam is discouraged because this agent does not cover gram-positive organisms.

  (4) A repeat paracentesis 48 hours after antibiotic therapy has been initiated to confirm that cell counts have decreased and that the fluid has become sterile in culture-positive cases is often suggested [61a, 61b].

  (5) Duration of antibiotic therapy. Standard therapy has been 10–14 days of IV antibiotics. Recent reviewers emphasize that studies suggest a 5–7 day course of IV antibiotics is safe and effective [61a, 61b].

f. Prognosis. Currently, most studies show a mortality rate for SBP cases of 30–40%. After an initial episode of SBP, the probability of recurrence at 1 year is 70%, and recurrent episodes are associated with high mortality rates [61b]. Many patients with SBP may be candidates for liver transplantation.

g. Prevention of recurrent episodes of SBP is being evaluated. Norfloxacin (400 mg PO daily) has reduced the 1-year recurrence rate from 68% to 20% [61b]. TMP-SMX has also been used in this setting [62a]. Whether prophylactic agents should be routinely used, which one should be used, and for how long is still unclear. Infectious diseases consultation is advised.

2. **Peritonitis as a complication of CAPD** occurs commonly. This is reviewed in detail elsewhere [56, 63–65], but several points deserve emphasis.

  a. **Incidence.** An overall average is 1.3 episodes per patient per year [56].

  b. **Clinical presentation.** Patients typically complain of **abdominal pain,** have **abdominal tenderness** (often with rebound), and are aware of a **cloudy appearance of the drainage dialysate fluid.** This turbidity of the dialysate is often the earliest sign of infection and the only finding in one-fourth of cases in some reviews [56]. Fever is present in few patients.

  c. **Bacteriology.** Most patients have infection due to coagulase-negative staphylococci or *S. aureus*. Methicillin-resistant organisms are common. *Streptococci* spp. are isolated 10–15% of the time. Gram-negative bacteria are seen in patients with recurrent episodes of infections. A single organism usually is isolated. Gram stains of the effluent generally are negative [56], with 9–40% reported positive in several series [65]. When multiple organisms are isolated from a given patient or anaerobes are isolated, bowel perforation should be suspected [56, 64].

  d. **Diagnosis.** The peritoneal effluent should be cultured. Peritonitis can be assumed to be present when the dialysate drainage fluid contains more than 100 leukocytes/mm^3 [63]. Blood cultures usually are negative.

  e. **Therapy.** In recent years, studies have demonstrated the value of intraperitoneal instillation of antibiotics. This helps facilitate outpatient therapy. See Fig. 11-3, which summarizes a recent recommendation of experts [65].

  Because intravenous antibiotics penetrate the peritoneal fluid, some clinicians may prefer the intravenous route: For example, while awaiting cultures, a single intravenous dose of an aminoglycoside and vancomycin could be used. See Chap. 28 for dosing of these antibiotics in renal failure.

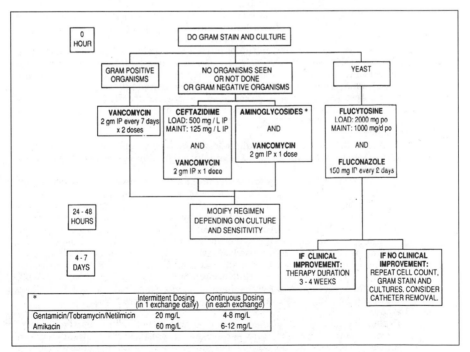

Fig. 11-3. Treatment of peritonitis, 1993 update. IP = intraperitoneal administration; MAINT = maintenance dose. (From the Ad Hoc Advisory Committee on Peritonitis Management, Peritoneal dialysis–related peritonitis treatment recommendations. *Periton. Dialysis Int.* 13:14, 1993.)

(1) Treatment of patients who fail on initial regimens or who have complex infections is reviewed elsewhere [65].

(2) Catheter removal indications include persisting peritonitis despite adequate therapy, fungal peritonitis, *Pseudomonas aeruginosa* peritonitis, and severe skin catheter site infection [56, 63–65].

f. **Sclerosing encapsulating peritonitis** can occur in patients with recurrent prior bouts of bacterial peritonitis, although the exact etiology is unknown. This complication may be seen in 1–5% of patients with chronically implanted catheters. Treatment is directed at such complications as bowel obstruction [56].

IV. General concepts of intraabdominal abscesses. Onset of intraabdominal abscesses may be insidious. Mortality with undrained hepatic, pancreatic, and retroperitoneal abscesses is reported to be 45–100%. Therefore, it is important always to consider the search for intraabdominal abscess in febrile patients without any obvious cause of fever, especially in those who have a potential predisposing cause such as inflammatory bowel disease, diverticulitis, or a history of abdominal surgery or abdominal trauma.

A. Etiology and pathophysiology. The GI lesions or events that typically predispose to secondary peritonitis and intraabdominal abscess include **organ perforation** (e.g., acute appendicitis, acute cholecystitis, diverticulitis, bowel neoplasm with perforation), **extension of preexisting infection** (e.g., suppurative cholangitis or cholecystitis, rupture of intraabdominal abscess as in the liver, secondary to pancreatitis), **surgical procedure or trauma** (e.g., anastomotic leak, stab wound, or blunt trauma) or **intraabdominal ischemia** (e.g., mesenteric vascular occlusion, colonic volvulus, intestinal obstruction). Some reviewers emphasize that most abscesses seen today are postoperative complications of biliary tract or GI surgery [66].

1. Abscess formation can be considered a host defense response as it limits the extent of disease. In doing so, it creates an environment that readily supports the proliferation of anaerobic bacteria and produces conditions that impair the microbial activity of infiltrating neutrophils as well as the effectiveness of humoral factors, such as complement. Antibiotic transport to the suppurative focus is inhibited, and drugs within the abscess often are inactivated by a reduced local pH (e.g., aminoglycosides) [66].

2. **Abscesses can be found virtually anywhere** within the abdomen, including the retroperitoneal space. Their location usually correlates with the original site of contamination, but they can develop at distant sites (e.g., a subphrenic abscess may be preceded by perforated appendicitis) [66] (Fig. 11-4).

B. Microbiologic evaluation of an intraabdominal abscess usually reflects both quantitative and qualitative aspects of the microflora of the intestinal tract. This was discussed earlier in sec. **II.A.**

C. Diagnosis

1. Fever, chills, anorexia, and weight loss may occur. Some patients may have abdominal pain. An unexplained fever may be the only sign of an occult intraabdominal abscess.

2. **An abdominal CT examination is the most efficient means of diagnosing an abscess** [56]. The once-popular gallium 67 scan seldom is used now because it is slower and not as specific as the indium 111–tagged leukocyte scan (^{111}In-WBC). The ^{111}In-WBC scan is performed by labeling the patients' leukocytes with indium. When rejected, these labeled WBCs concentrate in the abscess. Scanning is done at 18 and 48 hours. Because of the technical aspects and time delays, indium scans are used less frequently than CT scans. In an unusual setting (e.g., in the patient with an abnormal CT scan of the spleen in which multiple abscesses versus multiple infarcts is the major differential diagnosis), a gallium or indium scan may be helpful. A more detailed discussion of white blood cell labeling studies has been reviewed elsewhere [57a].

D. Therapy

1. **Drainage** either by percutaneously introduced catheters or operatively is the primary mode of therapy. Many series have emphasized that patients with an undrained abscess die [56, 66, 67]. The surgical texts state that once a localized collection of pus is formed, it must be drained. If not, the risk of complications due to delayed rupture of the abscess increases markedly [56], and the infection cannot be eradicated by antibiotics alone (see sec. **A.1**).

a. **Percutaneous needle aspiration and closed-catheter drainage, using CT and ultrasound guidance, is often preferred** to operative drainage of most

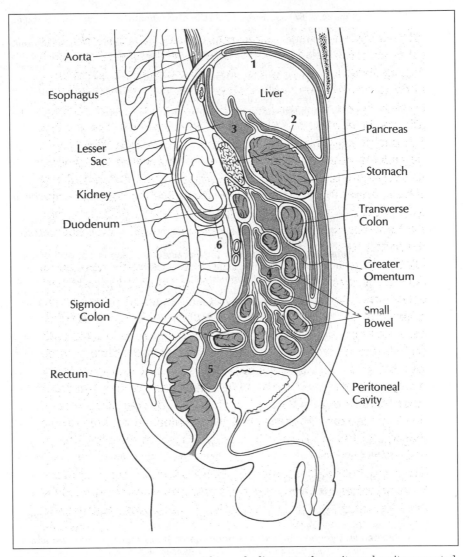

Fig. 11-4. Areas of abscess formation within and adjacent to the peritoneal cavity are noted. They include the subphrenic space (*1*) and the subhepatic space (*2*); the lesser sac (*3*); interstices between loops of the small and large intestine (*4*); and the pelvic space (*5*). In the retroperitoneal space, abscesses may be perinephric (*6*); they may also be adjacent to or involve the pancreas, duodenum, or rectum. Because of intraabdominal circulation of infected material, abscesses may develop far from the original site of contamination. (From H. W. Murray, Secondary peritonitis and intra-abdominal abscess. *Hosp. Prac.* 25:109. Copyright © 1990, The McGraw-Hill Companies. Illustration by Laura Duprey.)

intraabdominal abscesses [56, 57a, 58a, 67]. Percutaneous drainage of an intraabdominal abscess is **usually successful if the following criteria are met:** (1) There is a well-established, unilocular fluid collection; (2) a safe percutaneous route of access is available (this often means location of the abscess adjacent to the body wall); (3) joint evaluation by a surgeon and a radiologist is done so that correct judgments and decisions are made; and (4) there is immediate operative backup available in case of failure or complications [56]. After aspiration is complete, the catheter often is placed for drainage via gravity on low suction until the drainage volume is minimal

(<10 ml/24h). Repeat scanning at this time should show complete collapse of the abscess cavity [57a].

b. **Open surgical drainage** is indicated when (1) percutaneous drainage cannot be accomplished safely; (2) percutaneous drainage fails; (3) infected pancreatic necrosis or carcinomatous abscess is present; (4) the abscess is associated with a bowel fistula; (5) multiple isolated, interloop abscesses are present [56]; or (6) there is a coagulopathy. Pelvic abscesses usually are drained through the rectum or vagina [56] (see Chap. 14).

c. **Carefully obtained cultures.** Cultures should be taken carefully at the time of drainage, with special attention to culturing anaerobically as well as aerobically.

2. **Empiric antibiotics.** Antibiotics are used primarily to prevent metastatic infection from bacteremia and to treat nondrainable cellulitis around the abscess. When an intraabdominal abscess is diagnosed, drained, and cultured, empiric therapy should be started with antibiotics that cover most of the common abdominal flora, until the culture results return. **Several regimens have been summarized previously** (sec. II.B and **Table 11-10**). Even if the sometimes difficult-to-culture anaerobes are not isolated, most experts would continue to administer antibiotics active against anaerobes as well as gram-negative aerobes [56–58].

The optimal duration of therapy for a drained abscess is not well defined [58]. Antibiotic administration should continue until all systemic signs of sepsis have resolved and the patient's appetite and sense of well-being have returned. It is not necessary to continue antibiotic therapy simply because drains remain in place [56]. After initial intravenous antibiotic therapy (see Table 11-10) and clinical improvement, oral therapy can commonly be used to complete a course of therapy and not prolong the hospital stay.

Some surgical reviews suggest that in uncomplicated cases, antibiotics can be stopped 48–72 hours after drainage has been established [56]. We would tend to treat patients with a combination of intravenous and oral antibiotics for at least 10 days after drainage to ensure that contiguous soft-tissue cellulitis has been adequately treated. In bacteremic patients, we use at least a 14-day course of total therapy to prevent metastatic infections.

3. **Nutritional support.** Many patients with protracted illnesses or underlying debilitating conditions are nutritionally depleted and may need parenteral or enteral nutrition [56]. The enteral route is preferred, if possible.

E. **Special issues.** Uncommon intraabdominal abscesses are discussed in sec. V.

F. **Pancreatic abscess** is discussed under Acute Necrotizing Pancreatitis, Pancreatic Abscess, and Infected Pancreatic Pseudocyst.

V. **Special types of intraabdominal abscess**

A. **Diverticulitis-related abscess** (see pages 434–437).

B. **Pancreatic abscess** (see pages 446–448).

C. **Hepatic abscesses** are related to *E. histolytica* (see page 444) **and pyogenic bacteria** (discussed below).

1. **Incidence. Pyogenic abscess is uncommon.** Its incidence in hospital admissions ranges from 0.013% to 0.035% in reported series [68].

2. **Pathogenesis.** Liver abscesses usually develop by spreading infection from an intraabdominal source to the liver. Historically, the appendix and colon were the major sources of pyogenic abscesses, seeding the liver via the portal vein [69]. Recent reviews implicate the biliary tract (e.g., cholecystitis, obstruction with infection) in 20–35% of cases or gastrointestinal foci with hematogenous spread (e.g., appendicitis, diverticulitis) in approximately 25%; cryptogenic causes (i.e., no obvious focal infection) are implicated in 30–35%, with other hematogenous spread from urinary tract infection, pneumonia, or endocarditis in 3–25% [68–70].

3. **Clinical presentation.** Many reviews emphasize that **symptoms are nonspecific** or secondary to the original pyogenic source for the liver abscess: **fever, chills, anorexia,** nausea and vomiting, and weight loss. Signs associated with liver abscess may include an enlarged liver, right upper quadrant tenderness, jaundice, and pleural effusion [68–73].

4. **Diagnosis**

a. Leukocytosis, elevated alkaline phosphatase, and other liver function tests are commonly done but nonspecific.

b. Roentgenographic chest examinations may suggest hepatic abscess by an elevation or paralysis of the right hemidiaphragm or right pleural effusion.

    c. **CT scanning usually is** considered the **procedure of choice,** with a sensitivity of 100% in some series [69]. **Ultrasonography is useful,** having a sensitivity of 82–96% [68, 69]. In some reviews, it may be the preferred initial diagnostic test as it often will identify associated biliary tract abnormality [69].

    d. **The potential of amebic abscess needs to be assessed.** Amebic abscesses are seen more frequently in young Hispanic men and international travelers, and these patients tend to have more focal right upper quadrant abdominal pain and less leukocytosis and left shift of the leukocyte count [74]. A serologic workup will help (e.g., amebic hemagglutination test). (See further discussion of amebic abscess in sec. **IV.E** under Gastrointestinal Parasites.)

    e. **Blood cultures** may be positive in up to 60% of patients but may not reflect all the bacterial pathogens involved when compared with liver abscess aspirates [69].

    f. **Aspiration of the abscess** with good aerobic and anaerobic cultures provides both diagnostic and therapeutic roles.

5. **Microbiologic workup.** Either CT- or ultrasound-guided needle (catheter) aspiration will provide material that should be cultured aerobically and anaerobically. As might be expected with an abdominal source of infection, the organisms recovered from liver abscesses include aerobic and anaerobic organisms in mixed and pure cultures [68–71]. The most common aerobic gram-negative rods are *E. coli, Klebsiella, Enterobacter,* and *Proteus* spp., and *P. aeruginosa.* The streptococci involved include enterococci, viridans streptococci, and microaerophilic species. *Streptococcus milleri* is an important pathogen [75], *S. aureus* also can be isolated, usually in bacteremic patients. The recent emphasis on the study of anaerobic organisms has made it apparent that as many as 45% of liver abscesses may involve infections with anaerobes [69–72, 76]. Commonly involved anaerobes include *Fusobacterium* and *Bacteroides* spp.

6. **Treatment.** Drainage of the abscess is critical, and antibiotic use is primarily adjunctive therapy.

    a. **Drainage of abscess.** The **optimal approach** (i.e., aspiration versus percutaneous drainage versus an open surgical procedure) is **still debated,** and the approach sometimes must be individualized [68–70, 77, 78]. Consultation with a surgeon and radiologist is essential. In recent years, ultrasound- or CT-guided percutaneous catheter drainage has been favored, but some groups prefer open drainage in selected patients [78] and in patients who fail aspiration or catheter drainage.

        The mortality associated with multiple small abscesses continues to be high as compared to that associated with a solitary large abscess. It is recommended that attempts be made to drain all abscesses, with drainage of the small satellite abscesses through the larger ones, if feasible. Multiple small abscesses may have to be treated with antibiotics alone.

    b. **Antibiotics.** Initial empiric therapy involves regimens aimed at mixed aerobic-anaerobic GI-biliary flora. See options in Table 11-10.

        For protracted therapy, antibiotic regimens should be individually fashioned according to the results of the cultures and sensitivities. Many authors recommend prolonged therapy (1–2 months) for a drained solitary abscess and no less than 4 months' therapy for multiple liver abscesses, to prevent relapses [69, 71]. Many of these patients may be candidates for home intravenous antibiotic regimens if a good oral agent is not available. Infectious disease consultation is advised for these difficult problems.

7. **Prognosis.** Mortality rates for hepatic abscesses have been reported to be in the 10–20% range, depending on underlying conditions, with a recent report of 11% [68].

D. **Splenic abscesses** are **rare** [79–83]. The incidence quoted in several autopsy series ranged from 0.2 to 0.7% [80].

1. **Pathogenesis.** The causes can be divided into (1) metastatic infections associated with bacteremias, (2) contiguous infection, (3) embolic noninfectious events causing ischemia and subsequent superinfection (including hemolytic and sickle cell anemias, which tend to obstruct free blood flow and oxygen delivery to the spleen on the microscopic level), (4) trauma with subsequent infection of a hematoma, and (5) immunodeficiency [80].

2. **Clinical presentation** often is **subtle,** regardless of the cause. **Fever** (93% of cases), **vague abdominal pain** (58%), and pain in the left hypochondrium (40%) is seen; pleuritic pain may occur. Splenomegaly is seen in slightly more than half of the patients [82]. Recent series have shown an increased incidence in immunocompromised patients (e.g., status postchemotherapy or postcorticosteroid use, AIDS) [80].

   Unexplained thrombocytosis in a septic intensive care unit patient with persistent left pleural effusion is suggestive of splenic abscess [83].

3. **Diagnosis**
   a. **Leukocytosis** usually is seen but is nonspecific.
   b. The **chest radiograph** is surprisingly sensitive, showing abnormalities in 82% of patients independent of the type of abscess or predisposing condition. Findings include left pleural effusion, elevation of the left hemidiaphragm, left lower-lobe infiltrate, and mass effect in the left upper quadrant [80].
   c. **Blood cultures** may identify a pathogen in patients with a bacteremia causing the splenic abscess.
   d. **Scans. CT scanning is the procedure of choice** and has a sensitivity of 96%, which proved significantly superior to ultrasonography (76% sensitivity) and gallium scanning (71%) [80].
   e. The entity of hepatosplenic candidiasis is reviewed in Chap. 18.

4. **Microbiologic features.** In recent reviews [80, 82], approximately 30% of cases are due to gram-positive aerobes (staphylococci, streptococci); up to 25% are due to fungi (usually *Candida*), depending on the number of immunocompromised hosts in the series; 20–30% are due to gram-negative bacteria, including *Salmonella,* and about 20% are due to anaerobes. Even with improved anaerobic cultures, up to 10% of specimens may be sterile [80].

5. **Treatment**
   a. **Splenectomy is the treatment of choice** [80–82] **for pyogenic abscesses.** Radiologically guided percutaneous drainage has been used in selected cases, but treatment failure occurred in 30% in one series [80], though it was more successful in other small series [84].

      The treatment of fungal abscesses (e.g., **hepatosplenic candidiasis**) involves long-term systemic antifungal therapy (see Chap. 18). Treatment of disseminated *Mycobacterium avium-intracellulare* (MAI) infections in AIDS patients is discussed in Chap. 19.
   b. **Antibiotic therapy** should be directed against the organisms cultured from the splenic abscess and blood (approximately 50% of blood cultures are positive). Duration of therapy should be sufficient to treat the original source of the bacteremia (e.g., endocarditis, pyelonephritis).

6. **Potential complications.** The most frequent complication of splenic abscess is rupture into the peritoneal cavity that causes an acute peritonitis [80, 82].

E. **Retroperitoneal abscesses** are uncommon [85, 86]. Because of their insidious presentation and delays in diagnosis and therapy, mortality in modern series ranges from 25 to 45% [86].

1. **Etiology and pathogenesis.** The kidneys, ureters, pancreas, abdominal aorta, and inferior vena cava are wholly contained in the retroperitoneum. The ascending and descending colon and duodenum are contiguous with it. The bladder, uterus, and rectum are located in the pelvic extraperitoneal space.

   The most common causes of isolated retroperitoneal space abscess in recent series were renal infections and postoperative infections. Other known causes include osteomyelitis of the spine with rupture into the retroperitoneal space, seeding of posttraumatic pelvic hematomas, acute cholecystitis, perforated appendicitis, diverticulitis, perforated colon carcinoma, ischiorectal abscess with penetration to the pelvic retroperitoneum, and a cryptogenic origin [86]. Tuberculosis is now uncommon.

2. **Clinical presentation is nonspecific,** with nonlocalized abdominal pain and variable GI symptoms in the majority of patients. A history of chills is seen in approximately 20% of cases; fever is documented in nearly 80%. Abdominal tenderness is noted in the majority of cases [86].

3. **Diagnosis** [86]
   a. **Routine laboratory tests are not specific.** Even with a renal origin, urinalysis often is normal.

b. **Blood cultures** may be positive in approximately 25% of cases, *E. coli* and *Bacteroides* spp. being the most common isolates.

c. **CT scanning** is the **most useful test.** The role of MRI awaits further clinical experience.

4. **Microbiologic** evaluation reflects the primary process.

5. **Treatment** involves drainage and intravenous antibiotics.

    a. The retroperitoneal approach (flank incision) and the pelvic approach (presacral) were reported as more effective surgical approaches than the transperitoneal approach [86].

    b. **Percutaneous drainage may be the preferred** approach [87] for drainage.

    c. **Antibiotic coverage** is based on blood culture data, clinical setting, and drainage culture results. Careful aerobic and anaerobic cultures should be performed on any percutaneous or surgical specimens. Infectious disease consultation is advised for these difficult cases.

F. **Psoas abscesses** are uncommon [88–90]. These were formerly synonymous with tuberculous disease of the spine or sacroiliac joint. In recent years, the incidence of this entity as a result of tuberculosis has become rare in the United States; now most cases are a complication of intestinal disorders [88]. **The psoas muscle is closely associated with and is subject to any infectious process of** the ureters, renal pelvis, spine, appendix, and ascending colon [90].

1. **Etiology.** In the United States, the cause **in adults** of psoas abscess is an underlying intestinal disease, **especially Crohn's** disease, but also diverticulitis, osteomyelitis, intraabdominal abscess and, in fewer than 10%, a primary staphylococcal psoas abscess [88]. **In children,** there is a much higher incidence of primary staphylococcal psoas abscess (up to 75% of cases) [89]. Children are more likely to have a history of preceding trauma or cutaneous abscess, which may predispose them to seeding with staphylococci.

2. **Pathogenesis.** Organisms may enter the retrofascial space **directly by extension** from adjacent infection (e.g., in Crohn's disease). In primary psoas abscess, hematogenous spread of staphylococci is most likely, with trauma playing a role in at least some patients [89].

    For a discussion of anatomic considerations, see Bresee and Edwards [89].

3. **Clinical presentation**

    a. **In adults,** symptoms often are nonspecific, but pain in the iliac fossa, groin, or hip, and tenderness of the iliac fossa are clues. Fever and leukocytosis may not be present. A positive psoas sign (pain on extension and elevation of the leg) is common, especially if there is underlying Crohn's disease. The patient may complain of a limp. Frequently, the patient will lie with the hip flexed at all times. Weight loss is common [88, 90]. Psoas abscess rarely occurs in the elderly, and secondary abscesses usually are seen in 10- to 40-year-old patients [90].

    b. **In children,** often there is hip or abdominal pain, more on the right than the left side. Many have fever and a limp or decreased use of the affected leg, and some have malaise, anorexia, or history of trauma. Usually there is no discomfort on flexion or rotation of the hip. Children present similarly to adults (see **a**) [89].

4. **Diagnosis.** **CT and ultrasound** examination are the most accurate tests for diagnosis, though neither reliably differentiates abscess in the muscle from hematoma or neoplasm. Clinical correlation and ultrasound- or CT-guided **aspiration** of the mass with culture (aerobic and anaerobic) is useful diagnostically and therapeutically [88–90]. The role of MRI awaits definition by further clinical experience.

5. **Treatment**

    a. **Open or percutaneous drainage** is necessary. An open surgical procedure is required if the underlying pathogenesis is gastrointestinal (e.g., Crohn's) [89]. A primary psoas abscess responds well to ultrasound- or CT-guided percutaneous drainage [90].

    b. **Antibiotics.** For known or highly suspected primary abscesses, antibiotics aimed at *S. aureus* are used (see Chap. 28). If it is unknown whether the abscess is primary or secondary or if a secondary abscess is present, broad-spectrum antibiotics for the underlying condition can be used until specific culture results are available [90]. For example, if an underlying GI source is suspected or known, Table 11-10 suggests antibiotic options.

6. **Prognosis.** With appropriate therapy, the prognosis is generally good, espe-

cially with a primary psoas abscess. Secondary psoas abscesses have been associated with a mortality as high as 18%, primarily because of delayed or inadequate therapy [90].

VI. Appendicitis and perforation. Appendicitis is best treated by surgical removal of the appendix before perforation occurs. Diagnosis is made primarily on clinical grounds. It is of interest that the incidence of acute appendicitis in the United States has decreased significantly in the last two to four decades. The reasons for this are unclear [91].

   A. Pathogenesis. Obstruction is believed to be one of the major mechanisms that predisposes the appendiceal wall to bacterial invasion by intraluminal bacteria. The common obstructions include fecaliths, enlarged lymphatic follicles, tumors, inspissated barium, and other foreign bodies such as worms. With distention, the mucosal lining is susceptible to impairment of its blood supply, and bacterial invasion of deeper tissues occurs. As this sequence worsens, tissue infarction can occur, with the potential for perforation at the antimesenteric border [91].

   B. Microbiologic features. Cultures reveal polymicrobial involvement, with 5–10 different species typically isolated. *Bacteroides fragilis* and *E. coli* are almost universally isolated. *Pseudomonas* spp. may be seen in up to 40% of cultures [91] (see sec. **II.A**).

   C. Clinical presentation and differential diagnosis are reviewed elsewhere [91]. In recent years, ultrasonography has been used to complement the clinical diagnosis. An inflamed appendix is visualized in 86% of cases. Ultrasonography reportedly has reduced the unnecessary appendectomy rate to 7% and the delay in operation beyond 6 hours to 2% [91]. Enlarged mesenteric nodes and mural thickening of the ileum suggest bacterial enteritis due to *Y. enterocolitica* and *C. jejuni*. Laparoscopy can be used to distinguish gynecologic disease and ileitis from appendicitis [91].

   Acute appendicitis in pregnancy does not occur frequently, but diagnosis can be difficult, in part because of displacement of the appendix by the gravid uterus [91].

   Acute appendicitis in AIDS patients may not be associated with leukocytosis. Diagnostic laparoscopy is helpful in establishing the diagnosis. (Appendectomy is the treatment and is not associated with increased morbidity or mortality in this group [91].)

   D. Complications. The **major complication is appendiceal rupture** with 20–30% of charity hospital patients having ruptured appendicitis on admission versus approximately 15% in private hospitals. The incidence of rupture is higher in the pediatric and geriatric populations [91].

   1. The use of antibiotic therapy in an attempt to avoid or postpone operative therapy ignores the obstructive origin of acute appendicitis, is dangerous, and is ill-advised [91].

   2. **Patients with appendiceal rupture tend to be quite ill,** toxic, and dehydrated, with persisting abdominal pain due to local peritonitis. Usually there is obvious percussion and rebound tenderness of the right lower quadrant [91].

   3. **Acute appendicitis is a more serious disease in infants and children** than in adults, because the rupture rate is higher, which in turn produces higher morbidity and fatality rates. Diagnostic accuracy for acute appendicitis is considerably lower than in adults, and the disease progresses more rapidly. Rupture is more frequently followed by diffuse peritonitis and distant intraabdominal abscesses than in adults.

   4. **Acute appendicitis in the elderly is similarly a much more serious disease:** From 60 to 90% of elderly patients are found to have a ruptured appendix at operation. Fewer than 10% of patients operated on for acute appendicitis are older than 60 years of age, but more than 50% of all deaths from appendicitis are in this age group. This is due to the delay in definitive treatment, greater frequency of progressive uncontrolled infection, and the high incidence of concomitant disease. The clinical presentation may be subtle, and fever or leukocytosis may be blunted in the elderly [91].

   E. Therapy

   1. **Surgical intervention is routinely indicated** for acute appendicitis and its complications. Schwartz [91] cautions that to attempt to treat appendicitis with antibiotics alone is misguided because it ignores the obstructive causation of appendicitis and so is to be condemned. The timing of surgical intervention is discussed elsewhere [91].

   2. **Antibiotics**

  a. **For acute appendicitis without rupture,** short courses of antibiotics to prevent wound infection are recommended by many experts [58, 91]. For example, either a single dose of cefoxitin (2 g in adults) [92] or three doses are adequate in uncomplicated cases [58].

  b. **For appendiceal rupture with local peritonitis,** a full therapeutic course is suggested. For antibiotic options, see sec. II. The optimal duration of therapy is unclear [58], but it seems prudent that the patient be treated until he or she is afebrile for 47–72 hours and is clinically improving. Oral antibiotics can be used to complete the course so that hospitalization does not have to be prolonged.

VII. **Intraabdominal infections in the immunocompromised host** (e.g., acute abdomen) have been reviewed elsewhere [57a, 93]. Certain issues deserve special emphasis.

  A. **Processes that can occur in any host** (e.g., appendicitis) may be seen. Peptic ulcer disease after renal transplantation is common if excess corticosteroids are used or H_2-blockers are not used. Acalculous cholecystitis (see sec. III under Biliary Tract Infections) and acute cholecystitis with perforation appear with increased frequency in immunocompromised hosts [93]. Diverticulitis or cytomegalovirus (CMV) infection with colon perforation can be seen more frequently after renal transplantation. Appendicitis infrequently occurs in the immunocompromised host, except perhaps in children [93].

  B. **Special conditions in immunocompromised hosts**

   1. **Neutropenic enterocolitis** is a rare but well-recognized GI complication during therapy for acute and chronic leukemia, lymphoma, and solid tumors. It is the most **common cause of** the **acute abdomen in patients with acute leukemia** [93].

   The diagnosis is based on a high index of suspicion in patients with profound neutropenia, abdominal pain, and fever. Plain abdominal roentgenograms may show thickened air-filled loops of bowel, an obstructive pattern, or pneumatosis intestinalis (see sec. **8**). In most patients the condition does not progress to necrosis, perforation of the bowel, or peritonitis. Medical management consists of bowel rest, intravenous fluids, and broad-spectrum antibiotics. Indications for operation include persistent or worsening abdominal tenderness or a worsening clinical course.

   2. **Acute graft-versus-host disease** [93] **may present as an acute abdomen** in bone marrow recipients. The syndrome of acute graft-versus-host disease usually starts 3–4 weeks (range, 2–10 weeks) after marrow transplantation and consists of dermatitis (a red maculopapular rash on the trunk, palms, soles, and ears), crampy abdominal pain that may be aggravated by food, and profuse watery diarrhea. Abdominal features usually follow skin manifestations, but they can precede them.

   Patients may have abdominal distention and peritoneal signs on examination, probably due to transmural edema of the small intestine. Free perforation is rare.

   The treatment is increased doses of immunosuppressive agents.

   3. **Venoocclusive disease.** See Chap. 20.

   4. **Hepatitis** with right upper quadrant abdominal pain can occur. Hepatitis C virus, CMV, and Epstein-Barr virus may be seen in these patients.

   5. **Cytomegalovirus GI disease** can occur [94].

   6. **Hepatosplenic candidiasis** is discussed in Chap. 18 and is associated with persisting fever, despite broad-spectrum antibiotics and resolution of leukopenia.

   7. **Liver transplantation** recipients may suffer surgical technical complications (see Chap. 20).

   8. **Pneumatosis intestinalis** is an uncommon problem consisting of multiple gas-filled cysts in the wall of the small or large intestine. Radiologically, translucencies are found parallel to and just outside the gas-filled bowel lumen. Pneumoperitoneum can result if the cysts burst into the intestinal cavity. The patient is asymptomatic as no peritonitis results from the sterile gas. This condition is associated with a variety of conditions including GI infections, lymphoma, leukemia, ischemic bowel disease, and intestinal obstruction. Surgical consultation is advised.

   9. **Polymicrobial sepsis** in the immunocompromised host suggests possible intraabdominal pathology (e.g., abscess), and a CT scan is advised.

Diverticulitis and Related Complications

Diverticulosis is very common and afflicts approximately 30% of the population older than 45 years and 60% of those older than 70. It is estimated that approximately 10–20% of these people with diverticulosis have symptoms of either hemorrhage or diverticulitis. Thus, it is a problem of increasing significance as the average age of our population increases [95–97].

I. **Pathogenesis** [95, 96]
  A. **Diverticula form as outpouchings** (herniations) of mucosa through weak portions of the colonic wall. The inherent weak spots exist where branches of the marginal artery penetrate the colonic tunica muscularis, which consists of an inner layer of circular smooth muscle and a thin outer layer of three longitudinal bands (teniae coli).
  B. **The precise pathogenesis** of diverticular disease **is unknown:** Aging, elevation of colonic intraluminal pressure, and decreased dietary fiber appear to be related. An increased consumption of beef fat may also be related. Decreased luminal fiber lowers stool volume and requires more colonic segmentation to propel the material aborally. Segmentation generates greater intraluminal pressures and may predispose to the formation of diverticula [96]. Genetic or other environmental factors may be important, because diverticula are seen in the right colon of Asians and the sigmoid and left colon of Occidentals [96].
  C. **Forms of the disease**
    1. **Simple diverticulosis** is generally asymptomatic. Although there may be shortening and narrowing of the bowel, there is no muscle thickening, and the diverticula frequently are reducible.
    2. **Spastic colon diverticulosis** and **painful diverticular disease** are names given to symptomatic diverticulosis. Pathologic findings show a thickened sigmoid wall but no inflammation. The longitudinal muscle bundles are thickened and shortened, whereas the circular muscle is corrugated like a concertina.
    3. **Diverticulitis,** in contrast, **results from a perforation in the fundus** (not the neck) **of the diverticulum, which produces pericolic inflammation.** The perforation may be large or small. Pathologic examination of colons resected for diverticulitis supports the conclusion that some of these perforated diverticula proceed to spontaneous healing, with fibrosis and granuloma formation next to a diverticulum.

II. **Clinical presentation and evaluation.** A practical approach to the patient with suspected acute diverticulitis is shown in Table 11-12.
  A. **Clinical presentation.** Diverticulitis often is called *left-sided appendicitis* because of its similarity of symptoms to appendicitis. However, inflammation can occur anywhere that diverticula are found, so inflamed diverticula of the transverse colon may simulate ulcer pain, whereas diverticulitis of the cecum and redundant sigmoid may mimic appendicitis.
    1. The severity of pain, persistence of symptoms, and the signs of inflammation (fever, leukocytosis, and elevated erythrocyte sedimentation rate) help to distinguish diverticulitis (with inflammation) from diverticulosis. At times, it may be difficult to distinguish mild diverticulitis from irritable bowel syndrome with coincidental diverticula [96].
    2. True diverticulitis in patients younger than 40 years can occur and may be severe.
    3. Abdominal findings may be minimal in the elderly and in those on corticosteroids.
    4. Patients with diverticulosis can have GI hemorrhage, but **bleeding usually is not seen in patients with diverticulitis** [96].
    5. **Signs** of diverticulitis include left lower quadrant tenderness, tenderness on rectal examination in the left cul-de-sac and, occasionally, a tender mass if an abscess or phlegmon has formed.
  B. **Diagnosis.** Often the diagnosis is made clinically. If a patient has a history of diverticulitis or diverticula on a prior barium enema and now presents with fever, leukocytosis, left lower quadrant abdominal pain and tenderness, leukocytosis, and an elevated sedimentation rate, then a clinical diagnosis can often be made.

Table 11-12. A practical approach to the evaluation and diagnosis of acute diverticulitis

Clinical history and physical examination
Usually > 60 years of age
LLQ localized tenderness and unremitting abdominal pain
Fever
Leukocytosis

DDx	Elderly	Middle-aged and younger
	Ischemia	Appendicitis
	Carcinoma	Salpingitis
	Volvulus	Inflammatory bowel
	Obstruction	Penetrating ulcer
	Penetrating ulcer	Urosepsis
	Nephrolithiasis or urosepsis	

Qualifiers
Extremes of age (more virulent), oriental ancestry (right-sided symptoms), corticosteroids, immunosuppressives, and chronic renal failure (abdominal examination insensitive)

Evaluations
Plain roentgenograms   Good initial first step; may show ileus, obstruction, mass effect, ischemia, perforation

Contrast enema   For mild to moderate cases of diverticulitis when the diagnosis is in doubt, water-soluble contrast examination is safe and helpful; otherwise, delay examination for 6–8 weeks

Endoscopy   Acute diverticulitis is a relative contraindication to endoscopy—must exclude perforation first. Examination only when the diagnosis is in doubt (rectal bleeding, anemia) to exclude the possibility of ischemic bowel, Crohn's disease, carcinoma

CT scan   Very helpful in staging the degree of complications and evaluating for other diseases. Should be considered in all cases of diverticulitis with a palpable mass or clinical toxicity, failure of medical therapy, orthopedic complications, and corticosteroid use. The test of choice to evaluate acute diverticulitis in most centers

Ultrasonography   Can be a safe and helpful noninvasive test to evaluate acute diverticulitis. Examinations suboptimal due to intestinal gas in 15%, very institution-dependent

LLQ = lower left quadrant; DDx = differential diagnosis.
Source: From S. R. Freeman and P. R. McNally, Diverticulitis. *Med. Clin. North Am.* 77:1149–1167, 1993.

However, a clinical diagnosis is not always confirmed by histopathologic examination of surgical colon specimens (see sec. **I.C**).
1. The **WBC count** and **sedimentation rate** may be elevated but are not always.
2. **Plain films of the abdomen** are useful to exclude extracolonic air in an abscess or evidence of colonic obstruction. Dr. Schoetz [98], from the Lahey Clinic, suggests that when the clinical diagnosis is reasonably secure, additional radiographic testing is of no benefit. He would avoid routine use of CT scanning, which can be associated with a high false negative rate (see sec. **3**).
3. **CT scanning** has recently become the **radiographic test of choice, especially if the clinical diagnosis is not clear or a complication is suspected** [95, 96] or if the patient is not responding to medical care [98]. **Any patient with a palpable abdominal mass should have a CT scan.** CT criteria used for diagnosis of acute diverticulitis include localized colonic wall thickening (> 5 mm) and inflammation of pericolic fat (poorly marginated, stranding, increased attenuation) or localized wall thickening and presence of periodic abscess [95, 96].
    CT scanning has the additional advantage of delineating extraluminal complications of diverticulitis and suggesting other diseases: tuboovarian abscess, colonic ischemia, mesenteric thrombosis, and pancreatitis which may, at times, present like diverticulitis.

4. **Contrast enema.** The **safety and utility** of a contrast enema to evaluate acute diverticulitis is **controversial.** Barium contrast is avoided because a free leak would leave contaminated intraperitoneal foreign-body material in the peritoneum. A water-soluble contrast enema can be safe and a useful adjunct in the evaluation of patients with suspected mild to moderate diverticulitis [96].

   No preparation of the bowel should precede a water-soluble contrast enema. Communication with the radiologist to limit the study to the segment of colon in question, with careful attention to the amount of pressure being applied, is essential [98].

5. **Endoscopy.** Colonoscopy often is used in patients with diverticulosis when bleeding is present and when a stricture or a malignancy is suspected [96]. However, most authorities consider uncomplicated diverticulitis a general contraindication to colonoscopy or flexible sigmoidoscopy because of the risk of diverticular perforation with insufflation of the bowel during the procedure [96].

6. **Ultrasonography.** The role of ultrasonography has not been fully clarified. In one series, false negative results were seen in 15% of the 54 patients examined. The effectiveness of this examination is very examiner-dependent [96].

7. **Blood cultures** should be obtained in hospitalized patients to exclude a bacteremia.

C. **Complications**
   1. **Fistulas.** With repeated attacks of diverticulitis, a fistulous tract can form among the bowel, bladder, integument, pelvic floor, and vagina [96].
   2. **Obstruction** is reported in a number of hospitalized patients with diverticulitis. With repeated episodes of subclinical diverticulitis, the colon becomes fixed, fibrotic, and stenosed. It is important to rule out other causes of colonic stricture such as carcinoma, Crohn's disease, and ischemia [96].
   3. **Perforation** of a diverticulum may cause peritonitis. Free peritoneal air seen on plain roentgenograms of the abdomen is uncommon in diverticulitis, as the perforations usually are microscopic and walled-off by surrounding structures.
   4. **Abscess.** Failure of any patient with acute diverticulitis to respond to medical therapy within 24–48 hours or the palpation of an abdominal mass should raise the suspicion of an intraabdominal mass [95, 96]. CT scanning is helpful to clarify this finding.
   5. Note that **frank rectal bleeding is not seen with diverticulitis,** and so if bleeding is present, other etiologies should be sought [96].

D. **Microbiologic evaluation** of diverticulitis and related abscesses is reflective of colon flora (see sec. **II.A** under Intraabdominal Infection, page 417).

E. **Therapy** varies depending on the severity of symptoms, duration of illness, and comorbid disease [96, 98].
   1. **Asymptomatic diverticulosis** probably is best treated by use of a high-fiber diet (which increases bulk), because evidence suggests that this type of diet reduces intraluminal pressure and produces a satisfactory subjective response in many patients. Foods with high-fiber content are seedless raisins, grapes, peaches, oranges, bananas, apples, peas, carrots, turnips, lettuce, and unrefined wheat. Unprocessed, or miller's, bran can be purchased separately and added to water, cereal, or milk. Constipation should be prevented by a high-fiber diet and bulk laxatives (such as Metamucil) and other measures such as prune juice. Harsh laxatives and high enemas should be avoided.
   2. **The mildest cases of acute diverticulitis can often be handled on an outpatient basis.** Typically, these involve patients with recurrent mild symptoms [96].
      a. **Clear liquid diets** are suggested until symptoms improve.
      b. **Oral antibiotics** are useful. Although we have found amoxicillin useful in some patients, a more rational regimen based on GI flora (see Table 11-9) would be TMP-SMX and metronidazole. In the sulfa-allergic patient, ciprofloxacin and metronidazole (or clindamycin) is an alternative combination. A 1-week course often is effective.
   3. **Moderately to severely ill patients are hospitalized for various reasons:**
      a. **Provide GI rest** (nothing by mouth) for 48–72 hours or until symptoms improve. The diet can be advanced to liquid and semisolid foods as tolerated. Nasogastric suctioning is used if the patient is vomiting or has abdominal distention or obstruction.
      b. **Intravenous fluids**
      c. **Broad-spectrum antibiotics** aimed at mixed aerobic-anaerobic abdominal

flora (see options in Table 11-10). Monotherapy is used often. For example, in a recent randomized, prospective, multicenter study, cefoxitin was as effective in treating patients with moderately severe diverticulitis as the combination of gentamicin and clindamycin [99]. The optimal duration of intravenous antibiotics is unclear, but some authors suggest 1 week [98].

d. **Pain control.** Initially, severe pain may require meperidine, but morphine should be avoided because it may increase intracolonic pressure.

e. **Serial observation. Most patients** in whom diverticulitis is correctly diagnosed and treated medically **will improve in 48–72 hours,** with a decrease in abdominal pain, leukocytosis, and fever. **Failure to improve or worsening in this initial period of maximal medical therapy is an indication for possible surgical intervention.** If not done initially, a **CT scan** is suggested for the patient who does not improve in this time period, to determine whether an abscess is present that might lend itself to percutaneous drainage [98].

f. **Surgery.** Most series of hospitalized patients with acute diverticulitis show that 20–30% require operation at the time of the initial attack. The **indications for surgery** are reviewed elsewhere [96, 98] but **include** failure to improve with medical therapy; clinical deterioration despite medical therapy; complications of uncontrolled abscess-related sepsis, fistula, or obstruction; and recurrent disease. Surgery often is recommended early for patients younger than 40 years (often with severe disease), immunocompromised patients (e.g., those on corticosteroids, transplant patients), and those with presumed right-sided diverticulitis [96].

Biliary Tract Infections

I. **Introduction.** The anatomy of the gallbladder and the extrahepatic biliary system and the microbiology of the obstructed biliary system are important to the understanding of biliary tract infections.

A. **Anatomic considerations** are reviewed in detail elsewhere [100], but we will highlight a few important features (Fig. 11-5).

1. **The gallbladder** lies in a fossa on the undersurface of the liver and in close proximity to the duodenum, pylorus, hepatic flexure of the right colon, and right kidney [100]. Therefore, diseases of these adjacent organs may clinically mimic some diseases of the gallbladder–biliary system. The wall of the gallbladder is richly innervated with sympathetic and parasympathetic nerve fibers [100].

2. The **cystic duct** is the tubular structure connecting the gallbladder to the common bile duct. Its configuration, length, and course are quite variable, and anomalies in this structure are common [100].

3. **Bile ducts.** The biliary tract has its origin within the small **intrahepatic ducts.** Using the classic definitions, the extrahepatic biliary tree begins with the **right and left hepatic ducts,** which exit the liver in the shape of a Y and join the hilum of the liver to form the single, **common hepatic duct.**

   The common bile duct is approximately 8 cm long and courses from the juncture of the cystic duct with the common hepatic duct through the substance of the pancreas and ultimately drains into the duodenum. In many patients, the bile duct actually lies within the substance of the pancreas, and this intrapancreatic portion of the duct can be the site of significant involvement by benign and malignant disease.

   The common bile duct empties into the duodenum at the papilla of Vater. Typically, there is a common channel, created by the joining of the pancreatic and the distal common bile duct, which empties through a single orifice into the duodenum. This common channel is believed to be important in the pathogenesis of gallstone pancreatitis [100].

4. **Related terminology**
   a. **Cholelithiasis:** the presence of gallstones in the gallbladder.
   b. **Choledocholithiasis:** the presence of stones in the common bile duct.

B. **Diagnostic tests** [100–102]
   1. **Plain roentgenograms** of the abdomen are of limited value in assessing either patients with gallstones or those who are jaundiced. Supine and upright films of the abdomen may be useful in excluding other causes of abdominal pain,

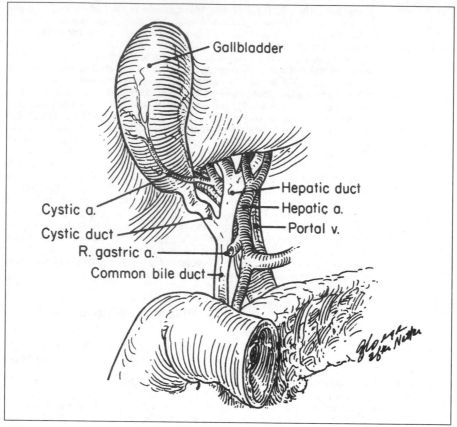

Fig. 11-5. Normal anatomy. The diagram depicts the relationships in the porta hepatis. The triangle of Calot is bordered by the edge of the liver, the cystic duct, and the hepatic duct. (From J. J. Roslyn and M. J. Zinner, Gallbladder and Extrahepatic Biliary System. In S. I. Schwartz et al. (eds.), *Principles of Surgery* (6th ed.). New York: McGraw-Hill, 1994. P. 1368.)

such as a perforated viscus or bowel obstruction. Only 15–20% of gallstones comprise enough calcium to show up on routine films [100].

2. **Oral cholecystography** commonly was used to demonstrate gallstones in the past but has largely been replaced by ultrasonography [100].

3. **Noninvasive imaging**
    a. **Abdominal ultrasonography** (US). In most institutions, abdominal US can replace the oral cholecystogram as the **procedure of choice when evaluating patients for gallstones.** In this setting, ultrasonography has a diagnostic accuracy of 95% [100, 101]. The patient should fast for at least 6 hours before the examination. Obesity may interfere with adequate visualization.
        (1) **US** is useful in identifying intrahepatic and extrahepatic ductal dilatation as well as masses that may cause biliary obstruction [100].
        (2) **Sonographic signs of acute cholecystitis** include the presence of gallstones (possibly impacted in the neck or cystic duct), a thickened gallbladder wall, and intraluminal sludge. A positive Murphy sign (i.e., maximum tenderness over the US-localized gallbladder) in combination with gallstones may have a positive predictive value of more than 90% for acute cholecystitis [101].
            The efficacy of abdominal US in diagnosing acute cholecystitis is not as great as for stones [100], and the presence of stones does not diagnose acute cholecystitis. This is reviewed in detail elsewhere [101, 102]. HIDA scans can be more helpful in this situation (see sec. **4**).

   b. CT scanning is not particularly sensitive in identifying gallstones but provides much information regarding the extent, nature, and location of biliary dilatation and masses in and around the biliary tract and pancreas. In general, the CT scan provides more useful information than does ultrasonography when evaluating the jaundiced patient [100].

   c. MRI. The role of MRI in evaluating patients with hepatobiliary disease is still being evaluated [100].

4. **Biliary scintigraphy.** The use of intravenous radioisotope-labeled substances that are rapidly excreted into the bile **offers an excellent opportunity to assess cystic duct patency and is sensitive in diagnosing acute cholecystitis** [100–102]. The most commonly used scintigraphic substance is technetium 99–labeled iminodiacetic acid (**HIDA scan**).

   a. The patient should fast for at least 2–4 hours before the examination. In the nonfasted state, as many as two-thirds of normal persons have an abnormal scan, in part due to the contracted state of the postprandial gallbladder, which causes decreased flow of tracer into the gallbladder [102].

   b. Various **patterns** may be seen [102].

   (1) Normal. The gallbladder, common bile duct, and duodenum are all visualized in 60 minutes, confirming the patency of the cystic and common bile ducts.

   (2) Nonvisualization of the gallbladder (i.e., the gallbladder is not seen even on delayed views or after morphine sulfate administration. This is **strongly associated with acute cholecystitis** in the appropriate clinical setting because it implies cystic duct obstruction. The gallbladder may not be visualized 60–90% of the time, even if it is **not** diseased, in patients who are alcoholic, receiving parenteral nutrition, or severely ill. This apparently is due to the prolonged fasting state. Active hepatitis or pancreatitis may also give a false positive scan [102].

   (3) Delayed gallbladder visualization (the gallbladder is visualized at 1–4 hours despite intestinal visualization at 1 hour). This is most **suggestive of chronic cholecystitis,** although such a test is fairly insensitive in this setting and is abnormal only 45% of the time. This pattern can also be seen in acute cholecystitis.

   (4) Persistent hepatocyte phase (nonvisualization of the gallbladder and common bile duct and absent or delayed bowel activity). This is seen most commonly with common duct obstruction [102].

   c. Biliary scintigraphy is a functional test, whereas US is an anatomic test [100].

5. **Cholangiography.** The previous method to visualize the anatomy of the biliary tract was by intravenous cholangiography. This has been replaced by endoscopic retrograde cholangiopancreatography (ERCP) and percutaneous transhepatic cholangiography.

   a. ERCP employs a side-viewing endoscope, permitting the biliary tract and pancreatic duct to be intubated and visualized. This technique has been especially useful in benign (and malignant) common duct disease (e.g., evaluating obstructive jaundice) [100].

   b. Percutaneous transhepatic cholangiography is useful in patients with more complex problems, including duct strictures or tumors [100].

C. Microbiologic features of biliary tract infection [103–105]. The biliary tract of healthy people usually does not harbor bacteria. In acute cholecystitis, infection of the gallbladder appears to be a secondary phenomenon, most bile cultures testing positively for a mixture of organisms usually [103]. The frequency of bacteria isolation is higher with long-term obstruction, in the elderly, in the jaundiced patient, in acute cholecystitis (as opposed to chronic cholecystitis), and when the common bile duct is obstructed [104].

1. **Organisms found in the biliary tract are commonly the same as the normal intestinal flora** (see Table 11-9). Polymicrobial infections are the rule [104, 105]. Anaerobes may be more frequently isolated in patients with common duct manipulations or complex prior biliary procedures (especially biliary-intestinal anastomosis) and in the elderly.

2. **The source of bacteria** is unknown but has been assumed to be the duodenum, and spread is assumed to occur via an ascending route [104].

D. Antibiotic therapy. Although many antibiotics concentrate in the bile when there is no obstruction, obstruction of either the hepatic ducts or the common bile duct

markedly reduces the levels of such agents, often below therapeutic values. No antibiotic alone has been determined to be effective in sterilizing an infected **obstructed** biliary tree. Antibiotics should be regarded as adjunctive to surgical therapy; they are useful in curtailing the progression of infection and preventing possible septicemia and liver abscesses.

1. **Empiric antibiotic regimens.** Therapy in most cases is **aimed primarily at gram-negative bacteria.** Whether specific therapy needs to be directed at enterococci in these mixed infections is unclear and less well studied than in intraabdominal infections, in which specific therapy aimed at enterococci is not essential (see page 419). Consequently, **in most biliary tract infections, we do not specifically aim therapy at enterococci** unless the patient is critically ill with sepsis.

   Although anaerobes commonly are isolated from biliary cultures, they are in a relatively low inoculum compared with the high concentrations of bowel anaerobes associated with colon perforations. Prior experience with intraabdominal infections suggest that a fairly high inoculum of anaerobes appears necessary for abscess formation. Therefore, in mild to moderately ill patients, we often do not use antibiotics with optimal bowel anaerobic activity. In the elderly or critically ill patient and the patient with prior common bile duct or complex biliary procedures (and, therefore, with distorted anatomy), we will select a therapeutic regimen that includes anaerobic activity (Table 11-13).

2. Once blood cultures or biliary operative culture data are available, antibiotic regimens can be designed more specifically on the basis of susceptibility data.

II. **Acute cholecystitis**

　A. **Pathogenesis**

　　1. **Calculi** are associated with inflammation of the gallbladder in 85–95% of cases. The proposed pathogenesis includes obstruction of the neck of the cystic duct by impacted stones. Pressure on the mucosa by a calculus presumably causes sudden distention of the gallbladder, with edema and impairment of venous return and the possible development of ischemia, necrosis, ulceration, gangrene, and perforation.

　　2. **Bacteria** have been cultured from 50 to 70% of acute cholecystitis cases. The origin of inflammation in the 30% or so without bacteria is believed to be chemical or physical. Culture positivity is greater in acute cholecystitis as opposed to chronic cholecystitis and is also greater in patients older than 50 years (see sec. **I.C**).

　B. **Clinical presentation.** Acute onset of right upper quadrant abdominal pain, nausea, vomiting, and fever are the most frequently presenting symptoms. Right upper abdominal tenderness, fever, leukocytosis, and elevated liver function tests (obstructive pattern) are common.

Table 11-13. Empiric antibiotic therapy in biliary tract infections (when renal function is normal)

Setting	Antibiotic regimen
Mild–moderate	Cefazolin (1 g q8h) + metronidazole (500 mg q6h) Cefoxitin (2 g q6–8h) Ampicillin-sulbactam (3 g q6–8h) Piperacillin-tazobactam (3.75 g q6h) Ceftriaxone (2 g/day) + metronidazole
Severe[a]	Ceftriaxone + metronidazole[b] Ampicillin-sulbactam + gentamicin Piperacillin-tazobactam + gentamicin Ampicillin, gentamicin, + metronidazole or clindamycin Imipenem (500 mg q6h or 1 g q8h)
Complex nosocomial	Piperacillin, an aminoglycoside, + metronidazole or clindamycin; imipenem + an aminoglycoside

[a]For very severe infection, we usually will cover enterococci.
[b]No enterococcal coverage.

C. **Diagnosis.** Even though hepatobiliary scintigraphy is the most specific test for diagnosing acute cholecystitis (see sec. **I.B.4**), **abdominal US is usually the preferred initial study** as it is easy to obtain and provides additional information [100]. Many institutions reserve cholescintigraphy for patients with a normal ultrasound scan despite a strong clinical suspicion [106] or when uncertainty remains after ultrasound examination [102].

D. **Therapy** [106]
1. **Initial therapy** is conservative, consisting of intravenous fluids, nothing by mouth, parenteral analgesics, and broad-spectrum antibiotics. Antibiotic therapy is aimed at mixed flora (see sec. **I.D**). If the patient is vomiting or has evidence of gastric distention or ileus on plain radiographs of the abdomen, a nasogastric tube should be inserted. Most patients respond to this treatment in 24–48 hours.
2. Surgical cholecystectomy remains the treatment of choice for patients with acute cholecystitis. The timing and potential role of laparoscopic cholecystectomy are reviewed elsewhere [100, 106].

III. **Acute acalculous cholecystitis.** Acute inflammation of the gallbladder can occur without stones (approximately 5–15% of all cases of cholecystitis) [106–108]. This entity has been recognized with increased frequency in recent years. **Persons at risk include debilitated hospitalized patients** who have had major surgical procedures, major trauma, burns, sepsis, multiple transfusions, hyperalimentation, prolonged intensive care stays with inadequate nutrition or multiorgan failure, or associated underlying disease such as diabetes or malignancy.

A. **Etiology and pathogenesis.** The etiology is unclear but may involve bile stasis, cholecystoparesis, or gallbladder ischemia [106]. Histologically, there is intense injury to the blood vessels of the tunica muscularis and serosa of the gallbladder, possibly related to activation of factor XII (Hageman factor), which can occur after multiple transfusions, in endotoxemia, after trauma, and so forth [107, 108].

B. The **symptoms and findings** are similar to those of calculous cholecystitis.

C. **Diagnosis.** The imaging procedure of choice remains controversial; HIDA scanning, ultrasonography, and CT scanning are suggested. Because each test has certain limitations in establishing this diagnosis, the use of multiple complementary imaging techniques may be necessary [108].

   Preoperative diagnosis is difficult, and therapeutic intervention often is delayed [100] with subsequently high morbidity and mortality [106].

D. **Therapy.** Urgent cholecystostomy or, preferably, cholecystectomy is advised [100]. Broad-spectrum antibiotics are used. Percutaneous transhepatic cholecystostomy has also been used as a temporary alternative.

E. **Prognosis.** Higher mortality may result from underlying disease in these critically ill patients with multiorgan failure and sepsis.

IV. **Acute cholangitis** (acute biliary sepsis) occurs because of infection of the biliary duct system. It is a **serious and potentially lethal disorder requiring prompt recognition and treatment** [106]. This topic has recently been reviewed [108a].

A. **Etiology**
1. **Choledocholithiasis.** The most common cause of acute cholangitis in the United States is obstruction and infection associated with stones in the common bile duct. Usually these stones have migrated from the gallbladder.
2. **Other causes** of biliary tract obstruction include **malignant obstruction** of the bile duct due to pancreatic cancer, cholangiocarcinoma, cancer of the papilla of Vater, and portahepatic metastases. Biliary stricture, pancreatitis, and *A. lumbricoides* infection can cause obstruction at times.

B. **Pathogenesis.** Acute cholangitis is caused by the infected bile, which is under pressure because of the obstruction. Although the exact site of origin of the bacteria is not well-known, bacteria can enter the bile duct from the GI tract through the bloodstream or lymphatics; bile in the obstructed biliary tree can be quickly infected, whereas bile in the nonobstructed, normal-pressure bile duct is difficult to infect [106, 109].

C. **Clinical presentation.** The most common symptoms are abdominal pain, fever, and jaundice. The so-called Charcot's triad of fever, right upper quadrant pain, and jaundice occur in only 50–60% of patients. Septic shock and obtundation are common, especially if therapy is delayed [110].

D. **Diagnosis**
1. Leukocytosis and elevated liver function tests (obstructive pattern) are common but nonspecific.

2. Blood cultures should be drawn.
3. **Ultrasonography** provides a rapid test to evaluate the gallbladder and bile duct and to differentiate extrahepatic obstruction from intrahepatic cholestasis, but detection rates of choledocholithiasis are poor [106]. **CT scanning** may detect stones in some patients and also may define the level and cause of obstruction if from tumor [106].

E. Therapy

1. **Supportive care,** including nothing by mouth, intravenous fluids, and evaluation for or treatment of sepsis (see Chap. 2).
2. **Broad-spectrum antibiotics** with optimal regimens in these very ill patients (see pages 418–420).
3. **Surgical consultation** for consideration of **biliary decompression.** Approximately 85–90% of patients will respond to antibiotics and supportive care alone. Those who fail to respond or who deteriorate on medical therapy may require urgent bile duct decompression. Even patients who respond to medical therapy will require a semielective approach to biliary decompression. Options for decompression include the following [100, 106]:
   a. **Surgical decompression** with bile duct exploration, with or without cholecystectomy, T-tube drainage, or biliary-enteric anastomosis.
   b. **Percutaneous transhepatic biliary drainage** (PTBD), which is not definitive treatment and is associated with significant complications including bleeding, bile leak, fistulous communications between the biliary tree and vascular tree, and sepsis.
   c. **Endoscopic decompression** with endoscopic sphincterotomy (ES) or biliary drainage with a nasobiliary catheter or endoprosthesis when endoscopic extraction of a stone has failed.
   d. **Summary.** Nonsurgical drainage (PTBD, ES) is believed to be the treatment of choice in the seriously ill and high-risk patient. Elective surgery can be performed at a later date once the patient has stabilized; endoscopy treatment may be definitive in patients with previous cholecystectomy and retained common bile duct stones [106].

V. Miscellaneous infections

A. **Gallstone pancreatitis.** See the discussion under Acute Necrotizing Pancreatitis, Pancreatic Abscess, and Infected Pancreatic Pseudocyst.
B. **Emphysematous cholecystitis** [100, 111]. This potential fatal complication of acute cholecystitis is characterized by gas within the wall or lumen of the gallbladder. Its pathogenesis remains unclear, but obstruction of the cystic duct with subsequent development of acute ischemia and proliferation of gas-forming bacteria may occur [100]. The disease affects primarily diabetic men. Patients are acutely ill and septic-appearing. The diagnosis may be suggested on plain abdominal radiographs by the presence of gas bubbles in the right upper quadrant or outlining the biliary tract. Whereas US may provide clues to this diagnosis, CT scans may be the most accurate study [100]. Early surgical intervention is indicated to control sepsis and avoid perforation of the gallbladder.
C. **Perforation of the gallbladder** [100] can occur as a complication in 3–10% of cases of acute cholecystitis. Local ischemia, advanced age, and immunosuppression may be contributing factors.
   1. **With free perforation** (a rare occurrence), an acute abdomen and septic presentation can occur.
   2. **With pericholecystic abscess** formation, subacute presentation is common.
   3. **With fistula formation,** a communication between the fundus of the gallbladder and duodenum can occur, especially in chronic cholecystitis. This may be asymptomatic unless a gallstone (which enters the GI tract via the fistula) causes obstruction, usually in the terminal ileum, referred to as **gallstone ileus.** The combination of small-bowel obstruction and air in the biliary tract is characteristic. Treatment consists of enterotomy proximal to the obstruction, removal of the impacted stone, and cholecystectomy [100].
D. **Acute cholecystitis as a postoperative complication** has been reported many times in the surgical literature. The antecedent operations are numerous and need not be bowel procedures. The mechanism proposed is bile stasis leading to concentration and inspissation of the bile in the gallbladder and asymptomatic gallstones resulting in obstruction. The onset of the disease has been correlated by several authors with the resumption of oral feedings; this supports the hypothesis that contractions of the gallbladder in response to food may be a contributing

factor. A high percentage of acalculous cholecystitis (30–35%) is seen; this has been discussed in sec. **III.**

E. **Post-ERCP cholangitis** can occur [112]. Presumably, the procedure may introduce bacteria along with contrast media. The risk for sepsis is higher in patients with malignant causes of biliary obstruction. Antibiotic use is similar to cases of acute cholangitis unless the patient has had recent ERCP and, if so, therapy for *P. aeruginosa* and other nosocomial pathogens may be warranted while awaiting culture data [112].

F. **Ceftriaxone** (Rocephin) **causing cholecystitislike syndrome.** Ceftriaxone can cause sludge in the gallbladder and symptoms suggesting cholecystitis. Symptoms resolve after ceftriaxone therapy is discontinued. See Chap. 28F for a complete discussion.

Acute Necrotizing Pancreatitis, Pancreatic Abscess, and Infected Pancreatic Pseudocyst

---

Acute pancreatitis is usually a sterile inflammatory process caused by autodigestion of the pancreas. This discussion emphasizes the infectious complications of acute pancreatitis; reviews of pancreatitis appear elsewhere [113–116].

I. **Etiology.** Identification of the etiology of an attack is important to help prevent recurrences and possible complications. In up to 10% of cases, the cause may not be recognized [113].

A. **Alcohol.** Pancreatitis usually is seen in patients who have been drinking quantities of alcohol for 7–10 years.

B. **Gallstones.** Gallstones are seen as the cause more frequently in private hospitals, whereas alcohol is overwhelmingly more common in public and Veterans' Administration hospitals. The procedure of choice to visualize gallstones is US [113]. Biliary sludge has recently been demonstrated to be associated with acute pancreatitis [115].

C. **Miscellaneous causes**
1. **Hypertriglyceridemia.** Pancreatitis is associated with triglyceride levels usually in excess of 1,000 mg/dl [113]. It is important to recognize this relationship because appropriate therapy can prevent recurrences.
2. **Abdominal trauma** (e.g., automobile accident) can result in pancreatitis.
3. **Postoperative pancreatitis** can be seen especially after upper abdominal, renal, or cardiovascular surgery, although it is not related to pancreatic trauma. Perioperative medications are strongly implicated.
4. **Hypercalcemia** has been associated with pancreatitis.
5. **Pregnancy.** In the third trimester and in the first 6 weeks postpartum, pancreatitis can occur and probably is related to alcohol abuse or gallstone disease [113].
6. **Anatomic causes.** Among the anatomic causes are tumors of the ampulla or pancreas, pancreatic or ampullary strictures, and periampullary diverticula. The initial clinical presentation of 3% of patients with pancreatic cancer is acute pancreatitis. Conversely, 1.3% of patients with acute pancreatitis are found to have pancreatic carcinoma. Therefore, in patients with so-called idiopathic pancreatitis, pancreatic duct visualization is mandatory, especially in patients with more than one episode or those older than 45 years [113].
7. **Infections.** Viruses (including mumps, rubella, coxsackie B virus, Epstein-Barr virus, CMV, and acute hepatitis A, B, and C), parasites (e.g., *Ascaris*), and *Mycoplasma pneumoniae* have been associated with pancreatitis. Acute pancreatitis in patients with AIDS is most often secondary to drug use [113] (see sec. **9**).
8. **Complication of ERCP**
9. **Drugs.** NSAIDs, erythromycin, thiazides, didanosine (ddI), pentamidine, estrogens, sulfonamides, and L-asparaginase are among the agents that can cause pancreatitis [113].
10. **Systemic vasculitis** can be the cause of pancreatitis.

II. **Assessing the prognosis of acute pancreatitis.** Criteria have been developed [e.g., Ranson's criteria, APACHE (Acute Physiology and Chronic Health Evaluation II) criterial to help predict the survival of a given patient based on the severity of acute pancreatitis. A discussion of those is beyond the scope of the text, but they are reviewed elsewhere [113, 114, 116]. Patients with more than two Ranson signs usually are considered to have severe pancreatitis or to be at risk for severe disease [116]. However, certain related points deserve special emphasis.

A. **Approximately 80% of patients with acute pancreatitis have a mild form;** most of these patients recover uneventfully. Pancreatic and peripancreatic necrosis are rarely or minimally present in these patients [113].

B. **Approximately 20% of patients have severe pancreatitis** with sterile or infected pancreatic or peripancreatic **necrosis or pancreatic fluid collections** [116]. **Necrosis of either the duct system or the pancreatic parenchyma is the initiating event in most of the complications of acute pancreatitis and occurs in the absence of bacteria** [116]. Necrosis occurs early in the clinical course, typically on the first day of onset of symptoms.

   1. Nearly 10% of all patients have fluid collections due to extravasation of fluid from the pancreatic ductal system.

   2. Another 10% of the total group have extensive necrosis (>10–15% of the gland) and, of these, nearly 50% will become infected. Infections rarely occur in the absence of pancreatic or peripancreatic necrosis. The more extensive the necrosis, the higher is the risk for infection. Consequently, **of all patients with acute pancreatitis, approximately 5% develop pancreatic infections, but 80% of all deaths from pancreatitis result from these difficult-to-treat infections** [116].

   The incidence of infection increases over the first 3 weeks and peaks during the third and fourth week of the illness. High mortality is seen especially with early infection, typically with extensive necrosis, and in the very ill patient [116].

III. **Assessing infection**

A. The **CT scan with vascular enhancement** is the most useful study for predicting or anticipating **who is at risk for the development of infection. Poorly enhanced pancreatic tissue,** as shown by dynamic contrast-enhanced CT, **correlates well with the presence of pancreatic necrosis** [117]. Between 40 and 70% of those with more than 30% necrosis will become infected [116]. If gas bubbles are seen in the region of the pancreas on the scan, infection may be presumed to be present [117].

B. Because sterile pancreatic necrosis and peripancreatic necrosis may cause leukocytosis and fever even without infection, it is difficult to determine clinically whether a patient's course is complicated by superimposed infection. Also, 50% of patients with infection may not show clinical signs of an active infection [117].

   CT scan–guided aspirations of necrotic tissue for Gram stains and aerobic and anaerobic cultures will clarify whether infection actually exists [116]. Commonly isolated organisms are shown in Table 11-14 [118]. Organisms resemble intestinal flora.

   The mechanism by which colonic bacteria arrive at the pancreatic tissues injured by the catabolic and cytolytic consequences of acute pancreatitis is unclear. Infection of the injured pancreatic tissues appears to be a secondary phenomenon, thus raising the possibility that prophylactic antibiotics can prevent or limit the extent of infection [119].

Table 11-14. Frequency of bacteria in pancreatic infection

Escherichia coli	25.9%
Pseudomonas spp.	15.9%
Staphylococcus aureus	15.3%
Klebsiella spp.	10.1%
Proteus spp.	10.1%
Streptococcus faecalis	4.4%
Enterobacter spp.	2.5%
Different anaerobes	15.6%
Total	100.0%

Source: From M. Buchler et al., Human pancreatic tissue concentration of bactericidal antibiotics. *Gastroenterology* 103:1903, 1992.

IV. **Effect of early prophylactic antibiotics on later infectious complications.** The data are still unclear regarding whether early prophylactic antibiotics can prevent later infectious complications [116].
   A. **Early studies** in the mid-1970s indicated that early therapy in acute pancreatitis was not beneficial [120–122], especially in alcohol-induced or idiopathic pancreatitis. **Reviewers** have questioned the validity of these early studies. For example, ampicillin does not adequately penetrate pancreatic tissue and may not be active against some of the common pathogens and, therefore, would not be expected to be effective. In 1989, Bradley [119] concluded, "It is currently unknown whether prophylactic antibiotics in acute pancreatitis are useful at all, or if they are useful, whether they are more useful in acute pancreatitis due to gallstones or acute pancreatitis due to alcohol abuse." Antibiotics probably are not clinically useful in most patients (mild pancreatitis) as the incidence of infection is minimal in this group. Bradley [119] indicates that if prophylactic antibiotics are to be useful in pancreatitis, they should be used at an early stage of tissue damage, before secondary infection has developed.
   B. **Studies**
      1. **Antibiotic penetration into pancreatic tissue** and activity against common pancreatic infection isolates has recently been reviewed [118].
         a. **Aminoglycosides** typically do not penetrate pancreatic tissue well in usual dosage regimens and therefore are **not preferred agents.**
         b. **Imipenem** penetrates pancreatic tissue and is active against common bacterial isolates. The **fluoroquinolones** (e.g., ciprofloxacin, ofloxacin) penetrate well and are active against the colonic gram-negative bacteria but not the anaerobic isolates.
         c. Piperacillin, cefotaxime, and ceftizoxime penetrate pancreatic tissue and are active against many gram-negative bacteria but may not provide adequate activity against anaerobes or enterococci.
         d. Metronidazole shows good penetration into pancreatic tissue. Because it is active against anaerobes, it is an appealing agent to combine with an antibiotic effective against the gram-negative bacteria (e.g., fluoroquinolones, cefotaxime).
         e. Clinical trials of the efficacy of antibiotics in severe pancreatitis are suggested [118].
      2. **Imipenem** recently was studied in a randomized multicenter clinical trial of antibiotic prophylaxis in severe necrotizing pancreatitis with a Ranson mean score of 3.7 [123]. Acute pancreatitis originated in the biliary tract in 37 patients, was caused by alcoholism in 24, and issued from miscellaneous causes in 13. CT scanning was performed routinely. Forty-one patients received medical therapy plus 500 mg of imipenem q8h for 14 days, beginning at the time of CT demonstration of pancreatic necrosis. The other 33 patients received medical therapy alone. Pancreatic infection was detected by percutaneous CT or ultrasound-guided needle aspiration or intraoperative cultures. The incidence of pancreatitis-related sepsis was much lower in treated patients (12.2 versus 30.3%, $p < .01$). Therefore, the authors recommend prophylactic use of imipenem in patients with severe acute necrotizing pancreatitis [123].
         Neither the incidence of multiorgan failure observed in 25 patients nor the mortality or the need for surgical intervention was affected by antibiotic therapy; however, several medical centers were involved, possibly with different surgical expertise. The authors note that their conclusions on mortality data are incomplete and that larger additional studies are needed [123].
   C. **Commentary.** The preliminary report from Italy about the potential usefulness of prophylactic imipenem is interesting, but further clinical studies are needed before one can conclude that this is an effective agent of choice in this setting.
      Because patients with severe necrotizing pancreatitis with infectious complications are prone to have protracted courses and possibly serial surgical interventions, they may acquire infections due to resistant bacteria [124]. Hence, one might want to save a broad-spectrum antibiotic such as imipenem for later use rather than early use in these high-risk patients.
      While the results of further clinical studies and experience with prophylactic antibiotics are awaited, infectious disease consultation is suggested for consideration of initial and serial antibiotic use in patients with severe acute pancreatitis.
      A compromise approach may be to use prophylactic antibiotics (e.g., a third-

generation cephalosporin and metronidazole) in severe cases of necrotizing pancreatitis for 7–10 days and save imipenem for future infectious complications when resistant bacteria may be a problem. Biliary-associated pancreatitis, because of the obstruction involved, may be a particularly good setting in which to use antibiotics, but whether these patients may benefit more is unclear.

V. **Related issues**

A. **When infection occurs, surgical intervention is indicated.** The optimal approaches are still being evaluated [113, 116, 117], and serial surgical evaluation is essential in the management of patients with severe acute pancreatitis. Typically, a surgical team directs the management of these patients. Aggressive surgical debridement (often requiring serial procedures) with open drainage in selected patients with extensive pancreatic and peripancreatic necrosis is advised. Serial CT scanning with vascular enhancement is very useful [116].

Percutaneous drainage of an area of infected necrosis, as a primary therapy, is believed by some to be an exercise in futility [116]. Further discussion of surgical indications is published elsewhere [117].

B. **Large fluid collections** can occur early in the course of acute pancreatitis, within days or weeks of the onset of symptoms. These fluid collections, unlike a pseudocyst, lack a wall of granulation or fibrous tissue. More than 50% of these collections will disappear spontaneously. Therefore, aspirating these before 4–6 weeks is mettlesome and unnecessary [116]. Percutaneous CT-guided aspiration of fluid is a useful technique if infection is a concern [116].

C. **Fluid resuscitation** is important. The hyperdynamic cardiovascular state is similar to that seen in patients with the septic syndrome (see Chap. 2), and patients with severe pancreatitis have diminished peripheral vascular resistance and decreased intravascular volume. Blood flow to the pancreas is known to be reduced during pancreatitis. It is believed that trypsin released into the surrounding tissues and the circulation triggers the complement cascade, kinins, and so forth. Acute renal failure is a common consequence of poor fluid resuscitation in pancreatitis. Monitoring with a Swan-Ganz catheter often is essential in the care of the severely ill patient [116].

The use of furosemide to maintain urinary output in patients with severe pancreatitis is to be condemned. Organ hypoperfusion results, and multiple organ failure is the inevitable consequence in some experts' opinions [116].

D. **Biliary pancreatitis.** The role of surgery in these patients continues to undergo clinical evaluation. In their recent editorial, Reber and McFadden [117] conclude that in those few patients with severe biliary pancreatitis and persistent signs and symptoms of obstruction or if cholangitis is present, endoscopic or surgical relief of the biliary obstruction is indicated within the first 48 hours. These authors prefer the endoscopic approach if skilled personnel are available [117]. Some authors feel that ERCP is indicated in all cases of biliary pancreatitis.

VI. **Local infectious complications** have been reviewed [125, 125a].

A. **Infected pancreatic necrosis** occurs in at least 40% of patients with severe acute pancreatitis and necrosis of more than 50% of the pancreas demonstrated by CT scan [125a].

1. **The assessment** of this early infection, most often seen during or after the second week of an episode of acute pancreatitis, **has been reviewed in sec. III.**

2. **Surgical drainage is necessary** for definitive management. Percutaneous drainage is almost always inadequate, and open drainage with wide debridement of the necrotic material is necessary. Serial reoperation to drain persistent or recurrent infection is often required [125a].

3. Sometimes it may be difficult to distinguish between infected necrosis and early abscess formation.

4. Associated complications such as fistulas from the bowel or pancreas, or bleeding from the retroperitoneal structures, are common [125a]. The overall mortality rate varies from 0–25% [125a]. Patients often are critically ill and very debilitated. Multiorgan system failure, often as a consequence of underlying sepsis, is a common complication and is frequently associated with a fatal outcome [125]. See Chap. 2.

B. **Pancreatic abscess.** A true pancreatic abscess is a collection of pus and necrotic pancreatic tissue surrounded by an ill-defined wall (capsule), which occurs either within the pancreatic parenchyma or expands into the lesser sac and retroperitoneum. Although not common, pancreatic abscesses are an important cause of death in patients with infectious complications of acute pancreatitis. A classic review was done by Altemeier and Alexander in 1963 [126] and a more recent review by Witt and Edwards in 1992 [125].

1. **Incidence** ranges between 2 and 5% in most series [116, 125].
2. **Etiology.** In multiple series, the cause of pancreatitis was alcohol in 32%, biliary tract disorders in 25%, postoperative complications in 19%, and miscellaneous causes in 25% [125].
3. **Pathogenesis.** Acute necrotizing pancreatitis is the most common antecedent event, with more extensive necrosis associated with an increased risk of abscess, presumably because a larger area of necrosis serves as a better culture medium (see sec. **II**). In most cases, the origin and route of bacterial seeding remain obscure but presumably there is direct transmural passage of bacteria from the nearby adjacent transverse colon [125]. Whether prophylactic antibiotics prevent this complication remains controversial (see sec. **IV**).
4. **Clinical presentation is nonspecific.** Pancreatic abscess should be suspected in any patient with an acute or resolving pancreatitis whose course is complicated by persistent fever, abdominal pain, and leukocytosis, especially about 3–4 weeks after onset of the initial attack [125a]. Initially, there is clinical improvement and then clinical deterioration. The presentation may be indolent, and some patients may not be febrile or have leukocytosis [127].
5. **Diagnosis**
   a. **CT scanning** is the best method to demonstrate the abscess [125, 128]. CT scans may reveal a fluid collection that may be indistinguishable from a pseudocyst. The presence of air within fluid collections or within the pancreas itself is strongly suggestive of a pancreatic abscess harboring gas-forming organisms such as gram-negative or anaerobic bacteria, and gas is seen in 20–90% of abscesses on CT [125].

   However, retroperitoneal gas or air within peripancreatic fluid collections may also be seen in uninfected patients who develop a fistulous tract between the pancreas or pseudocyst and an adjacent viscus, in the postoperative patient, or in patients with a perforated duodenal ulcer [125].
   b. **CT-guided percutaneous thin-needle aspiration** and culture of the fluid will clarify the diagnosis. Aerobic and anaerobic cultures should routinely be performed.
   c. The **role of MRI** is undergoing clinical evaluation. Only limited data are available with this technique [125].
   d. **Blood cultures** may occasionally be positive but are not diagnostic of abscess or its contents.
6. **Bacteriologic findings** in pancreatic abscess are only partially studied (Table 11-15). Many infections are polymicrobial, and the infrequency of anaerobic isolations may reflect poor culture technique [125].
7. **Therapy**
   a. **Surgical drainage is essential** for a true pancreatic abscess.

   In Altemeier's series in 1963 [126], 86% of the patients whose abscesses were diagnosed correctly, drained surgically, and treated with antibiotics survived. By contrast, if the diagnosis was missed and no surgical drainage was performed, 100% mortality was seen. More recent data confirm a near 100% death rate if surgical drainage is not performed [125, 128].

   The optimal surgical drainage remains controversial [125].
   (1) **Percutaneous catheter drainage** at times is regarded as a temporary maneuver until patients can tolerate definitive surgery [125]. However, if the abscess fluid is thin in consistency and there is little particulate matter in it, percutaneous drainage may be adequate treatment [125a].
   (2) **Open surgical drainage** is indicated if the abscess is thick, if rapid improvement does not occur after percutaneous drainage, or if there is CT evidence of considerable surrounding tissue necrosis in addition to the abscess [125a].
   b. **Nutritional support** with enteral or total parenteral nutrition is favored [125].

Table 11-15. Bacteriology of pancreatic abscesses*

Organism	No. of patients/total	Percentage	Range (%)
Escherichia coli	164/494	33	11–49
Enterobacter	60/284	21	7–43
Klebsiella	26/189	14	7–42
Proteus	50/430	12	5–21
Serratia	8/162	5	2–11
Pseudomonas	16/386	4	3–29
Enterococcus	57/260	22	6–48
Streptococcus	58/323	18	4–36
Staphylococcus	69/499	14	0–38
Bacteroides	31/285	11	5–29
Candida (yeast)	15/158	9	2–9
Polymicrobial	140/380	37	21–57
Monomicrobial	207/380	54	29–78

*Summary of 16 series from specimens obtained intraoperatively or by percutaneous needle aspiration. Anaerobic cultures may not have been optimal.
Source: From M. D. Witt and J. E. Edwards, Jr., Pancreatic abscess and infected pancreatic pseudocyst: Diagnosis and treatment. *Curr. Clin. Top. Infect. Dis.* 12:111, 1992.

   c. **Antibiotics** are useful to prevent bacteremia, aid in healing, and are used in conjunction with surgical drainage. The antibiotics should be selected on the basis of sensitivity testing against any organism that can be cultured from blood or the abscess cavity at the time of surgery or on the basis of prior aspiration culture data. In the absence of culture data, therapy should be instituted as outlined in sec. **IV.**
  8. **Prognosis.** Despite aggressive surgical therapy coupled with the use of antibiotics and nutritional support, mortality in patients with pancreatic abscess is still 20% or more [125, 125a]. See sec. **A.4.**
C. **Pancreatic pseudocysts.** Despite considerable information generated by CT scanning and ultrasonography over the past 20 years, the natural history of pancreatic pseudocysts remains poorly understood, their classification system remains vague, and their nomenclature is controversial. Classically, the term *pancreatic pseudocyst* has been used to refer to all intrapancreatic and peripancreatic fluid collections, usually within a nonepithelialized capsule, arising in the setting of acute or chronic pancreatitis [125].
   Once a fluid collection is diagnosed, it is important to define the functional behavior of the fluid collection, such as a change in size or the development of signs of infection, because these are the characteristics that will determine appropriate therapy [125].
  1. **Epidemiologic features.** Pseudocysts almost always arise in the setting of acute or chronic pancreatitis. In a summary of 11 series, the underlying condition was alcohol in 65%, biliary disease in 10%, alcohol and biliary disease in 9%, postoperative trauma in 9%, and miscellaneous conditions in 14% [125].
  2. **Pathogenesis.** The origin of the pseudocysts is not well understood. Presumably, they develop as a result of the disruption of the pancreatic ductal system, with subsequent leakage of activated pancreatic enzymes leading to necrosis of the gland and surrounding tissue, accompanied by the production of larger volumes of exudate. They can dissect along retroperitoneal planes. Multiple pseudocysts are seen in approximately 10% of patients [125].
  3. **Clinical presentation**
     a. Abdominal pain (60–100%), nausea or vomiting (20–70%), weight loss (30–60%), palpable abdominal mass (20–50%), jaundice (10–20%), and abdominal tenderness (10–60%) can be seen [125]. Probably 50% of cysts

are nonpalpable, and up to 50% of palpable masses in patients with pancreatitis simply represent inflammation and edema rather than a pseudocyst [125].

   b. Routine laboratory tests (WBC count, amylase levels, etc.) are nondiagnostic.
4. **Diagnosis. CT scanning** is the most accurate imaging technique, although the CT scan does not differentiate between a sterile and an infected fluid collection [125].
5. **Natural history of pancreatic cysts.** In reports of cases in which serial US or CT scanning is done, **8–43% of the pseudocysts underwent spontaneous resolution,** usually within 6 weeks after onset [125]. Collections of pancreatic secretions in the peripancreatic area are in a dynamic equilibrium as they usually maintain communication with the pancreas and fluid is continuously absorbed and replaced by pancreatic secretions [125].

   Therefore, it is suggested that drainage procedures be postponed until either the pseudocyst persists for more than 6 weeks or a complication arises [125]; some suggest prolonged observation unless the patient is symptomatic.
6. **Complications of pancreatic pseudocysts** [125]
   a. Obstructive jaundice. Pseudocysts at the head of the pancreas may obstruct the duodenum or compress the common bile duct.
   b. Chemical pancreatitis can occur if the pseudocyst ruptures acutely. This is associated with a high mortality.
   c. Pancreatic ascites can occur with a slow leak into the peritoneal cavity.
   d. Hemorrhage either within the cyst itself or as a result of the cyst eroding into a major artery or perforating into the GI tract can occur.
   e. Chronic pancreatic cysts may be drained internally (e.g., cystogastrostomy, Roux-en-Y cystojejunostomy, anastomosis, or cystoduodenostomy) [125].
   f. Secondary cyst infection can occur (see sec. **C**).
D. **Infected pancreatic pseudocyst** [125]
   1. **Incidence.** The exact incidence is unclear; from 0 to 25% of pseudocysts become infected. Further data gleaned from good aspiration culture studies are needed. Overall, this is believed to be an uncommon complication [125].
   2. **Pathogenesis.** Secondary infection presumably results from (1) hematogenous seeding, (2) direct transmural passage of bacteria from adjacent bowel, and (3) possibly, bacterial seeding after ERCP.
   3. **Diagnosis.** Although persisting fevers, abdominal pain, and an abdominal mass in a patient with a known pseudocyst may suggest the diagnosis, no data exist on unique features of patients with infected pancreatic pseudocysts. Routine laboratory tests are nondiagnostic.
      a. CT scanning will demonstrate whether a pseudocyst exists.
      b. CT-guided or ultrasound-guided percutaneous needle aspiration with aerobic and anaerobic cultures will clarify whether the fluid is infected.
   4. **Bacteriologic** data are limited. Polymicrobial infection with GI gram-negative and gram-positive organisms typically are isolated [125].
   5. **Therapy.** When planning appropriate therapy for an infected pancreatic fluid collection, it is critically important to differentiate an infected pseudocyst from a pancreatic abscess. Whereas an infected pseudocyst can be treated successfully by drainage alone, this intervention would be completely inadequate for an abscess, for which open drainage and extensive debridement often are necessary [125].
      a. External drainage is preferred if the cyst is infected. Traditionally, a large-bore catheter is placed into the infected cyst cavity and the catheter then is brought out the abdominal wall. In recent years, percutaneous drainage has been used as an alternative [125].
      b. Internal drainage may be a consideration in selected patients [129].
VII. **Pancreatic disease in AIDS** (see Chap. 19) [125]
   A. **Drug-induced pancreatitis** can occur (see sec. **I.C**).
   B. **Neoplasms** of the pancreas, including Kaposi's sarcoma and lymphoma, have been seen in up to 8% of patients in autopsy series.
   C. **Infectious agents** have been demonstrated at autopsy series, and microorganisms involved include CMV, cryptococci, *T. gondii, Candida* spp., and *M. tuberculosis.* These are typically seen in the setting of disseminated infections.

Acute Viral Hepatitis

Acute viral hepatitis is a common and potentially serious viral infection of the liver that leads to inflammation and necrosis. This topic has recently been reviewed [130–130b]. We will discuss some important clinical aspects of this problem. Discussion of chronic hepatitis is beyond the scope of this chapter, and the reader is referred elsewhere [131, 132].

I. **Introduction.** A practical approach to the patient with hepatitis is to consider those entities affecting primarily the liver (viral hepatitis) versus more systemic infections associated with a hepatitislike presentation versus noninfectious etiologies that cause hepatic inflammation [130].

A. **Acute viral hepatitis** due to the agents listed here results in hepatic inflammation and hepatocellular necrosis without major pathologic involvement of other organs. **Clinically, these syndromes usually cannot be distinguished from one another** and, therefore, an etiologic diagnosis depends on serologic assays [130]. These infections include:

1. **Hepatitis A virus (HAV),** formerly called *infectious hepatitis*
2. **Hepatitis B virus (HBV),** formerly called *serum hepatitis*
3. **Hepatitis C virus (HCV),** the cause of parenterally transmitted non-A, non-B hepatitis as well as a small number of cases transmitted by unknown routes.
4. **Hepatitis delta (D) virus (HDV),** which requires coinfection with or prior infection with HBV.
5. **Hepatitis E virus (HEV),** an enterically transmitted, epidemic, non-A, non-B hepatitis agent
6. Other viral agents that may be identified; e.g., hepatitis G; see **sec. VIII.**

B. **Viral systemic illnesses with a hepatitislike component.** Other viruses can infect the liver and produce a hepatitislike picture, but they do so in the context of a more widespread viral illness [130].

1. **Yellow fever virus** (see Chap. 21)
2. **Epstein-Barr virus** (see Chap. 17)
3. **Cytomegalovirus** (see Chap. 17)
4. **Miscellaneous:** herpes simplex virus, varicella-zoster virus, HIV, rubella, rubeola, coxsackie B virus, and adenovirus.

C. **Nonviral etiologies** are discussed in standard medical textbooks and include:

1. **Infectious** hepatitis: leptospirosis, toxoplasmosis.
2. **Drug-induced hepatitis** (e.g., halothane, isoniazid, acetaminophen, alpha-methyldopa). Also, a drug-induced cholestatic hepatitis can occur (e.g., erythromycin, chlorpromazine).
3. **Alcohol-induced** hepatitis.
4. **Obstructive** hepatitis (see prior discussion).
5. **Toxic** (e.g., carbon tetrachloride, phosphorus, mushroom poisoning).
6. **Hypoperfusion** (e.g., with hypotension or ischemia).

II. **Clinical approach to acute viral hepatitis.** There are no clinical features that unequivocally distinguish the individual types of acute viral hepatitis, although certain epidemiologic data may suggest a specific etiology.

A. **Clinical stages.** The following phases have been identified [130]:

1. The **incubation phase** is virus dependent (Table 11-16).
2. The **preicteric phase** typically lasts a few days and includes **nonspecific symptoms** such as malaise, fatigue, anorexia, nausea, vomiting, and dull right upper quadrant abdominal pain. Fever sometimes precedes the icteric phase but with the onset of jaundice, fever abates.
3. Approximately 5–15% of patients may have a serum sickness-like illness with urticarial rash, arthralgia, and/or arthritis accompanying fever. Some of these individuals do not develop frank hepatitis.
4. A significant proportion of infected individuals never develop clinical hepatitis and the nonspecific symptoms lead to the diagnosis of "flu-like" illness [130].
5. The icteric phase begins with the onset of dark urine and/or jaundice. These are the symptoms that lead the patient to seek medical attention. Pruritus often develops at this time, but fever is absent.

B. **Fulminant viral hepatitis** [130], defined as the development of severe acute liver failure with hepatic encephalopathy within 8 weeks of the onset of symptoms with jaundice, usually is due to hepatitis B, with or without HDV coinfection.

Table 11-16. Epidemiologic and clinical features of viral hepatitis

	Type A (infectious hepatitis)	Type B (serum hepatitis)	Type C	Type D	Type E
Incubation	15–45 days (avg 25–30)	50–180 days	8 wk (avg 5–12)	40–180 days	45 days (avg 2–9 wk)
Route of infection	Predominantly fecal-oral	Parenteral, sexual, and perinatal	Predominantly parenteral	Predominantly parenteral; requires simultaneous infection with HBV	Fecal-oral
Occurrence of viral antigen					
In blood	2 wk before to 1 wk after jaundice	Months to years	Months to years	Months to years	Unknown
In stool	2 wk before to approximately 2 wk after jaundice	Infrequent	Unknown		Yes
Carrier state in blood	No	Yes	—*	Yes	Unknown
Chronic active hepatitis	None	Occasional	Common	Yes	No evidence
Nucleic acid	RNA	DNA	RNA	RNA	RNA

*At least 50% and as many as 70–90% of infected individuals fail to clear the virus during the acute phase [144].

HAV is a rare cause of fulminant infection. Fulminant viral hepatitis is not described with HCV.

C. **Physical examination** findings are nonspecific unless there is evidence of serum sickness (e.g., rash) or unless hepatic encephalopathic changes are noted.

D. **Routine laboratory findings.** In clinically apparent hepatitis the following abnormalities occur.

1. **Elevations of hepatic enzymes.** The aminotransferases [aspartate aminotransferase (AST or SGOT) and alanine aminotransferase (ALT or SGPT)] usually are elevated at least 8 times above normal levels (often > 1000 U/L) at the appearance of jaundice [130].

2. Alkaline phosphatase and gamma-glutamyltransferase (markers typically of obstruction) are only minimally elevated (e.g., 1–3 times normal) [130].

3. Bilirubin levels range from 5 to 15 times normal. Patients with underlying hemolytic states (glucose-6-phosphate dehydrogenase deficiency or sickle cell disease) may have accelerated hemolysis with a viral infection [130].

4. The **prothrombin time** is usually normal and, if elevated, is a worrisome marker of potential or evolving hepatic failure.

5. The WBC count is normal to slightly low usually, although a mild leukocytosis can occur. The sedimentation rate generally is normal to minimally elevated. Serum albumin too is usually normal [130].

E. **Diagnosis** of the agent involved in acute viral hepatitis depends on serologic markers (Table 11-17).

F. **Isolation** [133, 134]. Routine universal precautions should protect the health care worker from hepatitis B. In hepatitis A infections, patients are most contagious before the onset of symptoms and jaundice. Once these symptoms appear, transmission risk declines rapidly. Universal precautions are important and sufficient to prevent transmission.

III. **Hepatitis A virus**

A. **Epidemiology**

1. Other names for this disease include *infectious hepatitis* and *short-incubation hepatitis* (because its incubation period is 15–45 days) (see Table 11-16). It is a 27-nm, spherical, nonenveloped particle with single-stranded RNA and four structural polypeptides. HAV bears many similarities to the picornaviruses such as poliomyelitis and other enteroviruses [135].

2. **Spread occurs almost exclusively by the fecal-oral route,** although viremic blood is capable of transmitting the infection. Parenteral transmission (e.g., in intravenous drug users or after blood transfusion) can occur but is uncommon because of the short duration of the viremic phase (see Table 11-16).

3. **HAV is highly contagious** and can spread rapidly to close contacts; outbreaks with a point source can often be identified, although some cases occur in which there is no known point source. HAV has been shown to be spread by the following means [130]:

   a. Contaminated water, milk, or food

   b. After the breakdown in usually sanitary conditions (e.g., broken pipes, mountain streams) or after floods or natural disasters

   c. By ingestion of raw or undercooked shellfish (oysters, clams, and mussels) from contaminated waters

   d. During international travel to areas with poor hygienic conditions where hepatitis A is endemic

   e. In institutionalized children and adults

   f. After exposure to recently imported chimpanzees or apes

Table 11-17. Diagnosis of acute viral hepatitis

Virus	Testing choice for acute infection
HAV	IgM anti-HAV
HBV	Anti-HBc (IgM) with positive HBsAg
HCV	Anti-HCV performed serially: see text
HDV	HBsAg-positive patient with rising anti-HDV titer
HEV	Research labs to test anti-HEV

g. Among attendees at daycare centers involving children who are not toilet trained

h. Among male homosexuals, with spread probably related to sexual practices

4. The virus is present in the stools of patients for as long as 1–2 weeks before the onset of jaundice and for a short time thereafter. Because fecal excretion primarily occurs early in the infection, **by the time the patient is hospitalized, he or she is excreting either no virus or only low titers of virus in the feces** [133].

5. Antibody to HAV is detectable at approximately the time jaundice appears. The early appearance of HAV antibody suggests a possible role in the pathogenesis of HAV infection. In developing countries and economically disadvantaged environments, HAV infection, often subclinical, occurs at an early age; in hygienically more advanced countries, viral infection takes place at a later age. Immunity appears to be lifelong, and chronic infection probably does not occur [130b].

Antibody to HAV (IgG) is found in approximately 20–80% of the US adult population, depending on socioeconomic status, thus indicating exposure to the virus and either clinical or subclinical disease in the majority of the adult population. Antibody is more likely to be present in lower socioeconomic classes (70–80%) than in middle and upper classes (18–30%). However, because the prevalence of antibody is highest in people 50 years of age and older, young adults are often susceptible to HAV in the United States.

6. HAV accounts for about 35% of cases of acute viral hepatitis in developed countries. In developing countries, HAV is endemic, the majority of the population is exposed during childhood, and nearly 90% of adults demonstrate immunity to HAV from childhood exposure [130a].

B. Diagnosis. A commercial radioimmunoassay test that detects antibody to HAV is available. Because many adults have this antibody, it is important to be able to separate acute infection from prior antibody response.

1. If the IgM antibody level to HAV is elevated, acute disease with a recent exposure is indicated. After 3–12 months, IgM anti-HAV disappears.

2. An elevated IgG antibody level is compatible with **prior infection,** for this antibody remains positive for years and is presumably lifelong.

C. Therapy. There is no current treatment available other than supportive care.

D. Prophylaxis. Two methods of immune protection (prophylaxis) are available, passive and active. Because a substantial proportion of the normal population has been infected in the past, pooled lots of **gamma globulin** (IG), contain substantial antibody that can be passively transferred. In addition, an immunogenic and safe **vaccine** recently has been approved and is available, but because antibody response takes 2 weeks to fully develop and hepatitis A immunization for postexposure protection has not been fully evaluated in clinical trials, **IG is important in providing immediate protection in postexposure situations.**

1. Postexposure prophylaxis. A single dose of IG, 0.02 ml/kg IM into the gluteus muscle, is recommended for those exposed if they have no prior history of HAV. There are no definite contraindications to the use of IG, and it even can be given to a pregnant woman. **To be effective, IG must be given within 2 weeks of the exposure.** Candidates for consideration of prophylaxis include those from the following groups [133].

a. Point source outbreak (e.g., food handler exposing a particular group). IG might be effective in preventing foodborne or waterborne HAV if exposure is recognized in time. However, IG is not recommended for persons exposed to a common source of hepatitis infection after cases have begun to occur in those exposed, because the 2-week period during which IG is effective will have been exceeded. This issue is reviewed in more detail elsewhere [133]. Usually local public health officials make specific recommendations in this setting.

b. Close personal contacts of index cases (e.g., family members and permanent and temporary household residents who have not had HAV) are at a particularly high risk of developing the disease and should receive IG. Sexual contacts also are at high risk and should receive IG.

c. Daycare center attendees and staff. If there is epidemiologic evidence of one or more cases of HAV among children or employees in a daycare center for children in diapers, or if cases are recognized in two or more households of center attendees, IG should be administered to all children and to the staff. When an outbreak (hepatitis cases in three or more families) at a daycare center occurs, IG should also be considered for members of households whose diapered children attend. In centers not enrolling children in diapers, IG need be given only to classroom contacts of an index case.

The role of giving hepatitis A vaccine in this setting is being evaluated and, pending additional studies, should be discussed with public health officials (see sec. **2**).

d. Institutional contacts, such as occur in prisons and facilities for the developmentally disabled, are similarly at high risk in an outbreak of HAV. In this setting, it would be reasonable to inoculate inmates or patients and staff with IG if they are exposed to an acute case of HAV and they are not known to have protective levels of HAV antibody.

High-risk groups are potential candidates for preexposure vaccination with hepatitis A vaccine (see sec. **2**).

e. Certain groups are at low-risk exposure **and are not candidates for IG,** including the following.

  (1) School contacts of sporadic cases of HAV are less likely to acquire the disease than are contacts who live in closer proximity. Routine use of IG is not indicated for teachers and pupils in contact with a patient. However, when epidemiologic study clearly shows the existence of a school- or classroom-centered outbreak, IG can be used to limit spread in such instances.

  (2) Office and factory workers. Routine IG administration is not recommended for persons exposed to a fellow worker with HAV under usual office or factory conditions. Experience shows that casual contact in the work setting does not result in HAV infection.

  (3) Hospital personnel. Routine use of IG prophylaxis for hospital personnel is not recommended. High-risk hospital workers are candidates for the hepatitis A preexposure vaccine, which is discussed in sec. **2**.

2. Preexposure prophylaxis involves either the new hepatitis A vaccine (when there is adequate time to develop an antibody response; i.e., at least 2 weeks) or IG when immediate protection is needed.

a. Hepatitis A vaccine (Havrix; SmithKline Beecham) was approved for use in the United States in the spring of 1995 [136–140]. This inactivated vaccine is prepared in human cell culture, and purified and inactivated with formalin. Each ml of the U.S. vaccine for adults contains 1,440 ELU (i.e., ELISA Units) of viral antigen; the pediatric formulation contains 720 ELU/ml [136b].

  (1) Protective levels of specific humoral **antibodies** are detectable in 80–98% of adult recipients 15 days after the first dose and in 96% after 1 month. After the booster dose, mean antibody titers increase to 40 to 80 times the protective level, and based on these levels protection against HAV would be expected to last 10 years or more after the booster. Immunosuppressed patients may not have a protective response to recommended doses of the vaccine and may need additional doses [136b].

  (2) Clinical trials. In a double-blind, randomized trial in about 40,000 children in Thailand, the new hepatitis A vaccine was about 90% effective in preventing hepatitis A [136b, 139].

  (3) Dosages

   (a) For adults 1 ml as an IM injection into the deltoid muscle, plus a 1-ml booster dose 6 to 12 months later.

   (b) For children, the pediatric formulation is used. For children 2–18 years old, two 0.5-ml doses IM 1 month apart, followed by a booster dose 6–12 months after the first dose, is advised.

   (c) Hepatitis A vaccine has been given at the same time (at separate injection sites) as other vaccines before travel without interference with immune response [136b].

   (d) Hepatitis A vaccine and IG can be given at the same time at separate injection sites. The resulting long-term antibody titers are lower than when the vaccine is given alone, but still manyfold higher than the minimal protective level [136a, 136b].

  (4) Indications for preexposure hepatitis A vaccine are evolving [136, 136a, 136b, 139a] and include

        (a) International travelers at risk who can receive the vaccine at least 2 weeks before travel (see Chap. 21).

        (b) Handlers of **nonhuman primates** that are known to carry HAV (e.g., chimpanzees).

        (c) Other **"high-risk" groups, including** (1) Native Americans living on reservations; (2) Alaskan natives living in small villages; (3) homosexual men; (4) intravenous drug users; (5) daycare center employees; and (6) military personnel. Other potential target groups include health care personnel, workers at institutions for people with mental retardation, and possibly sewage workers and dietary personnel [139a].

        (d) However, because 50% of persons who develop HAV have no risk factors, vaccination of targeted "risk groups" in the United States has little chance of lowering the overall incidence of infection in this country [136a]. Therefore, consideration is being given to universal childhood vaccination to eliminate susceptibility and reduce transmission of HAV in the United States [136a, 139a].

        (e) Further strategies and specific recommendations for hepatitis A vaccine are being developed by the Advisory Committee on Immunization Practices of the U.S. Public Health Service and by the Committee on Infectious Diseases of the American Academy of Pediatrics.

    (5) Costs. A 1-ml dose of the currently available hepatitis vaccine is $54.70. A single 2.0-ml IM dose of IG is under $5 and a test for anti-HAV costs $40 to $50 [136b].

  E. Prognosis. HAV is an acute, self-limited disease that only rarely causes death (2 per 1,000 icteric cases). Although 20,000–30,000 cases per year may be reported, it is estimated that as many as 200,000 cases per year may actually occur in the United States annually [136]. HAV does not lead to a chronic carrier state and never causes a chronic hepatitis [130]. In a recent symposium, it was estimated that in the United States approximately 10–15% of patients with acute HAV will require hospitalization and nearly 100 patients per year may die of acute liver failure from HAV infection [136].

IV. HBV also is known as serum hepatitis or long-incubation (50–180 days) hepatitis. Because HBV can lead to a chronic carrier state and chronic liver disease, it has far greater clinical impact worldwide than does HAV [130, 141].

  A. Epidemiology [130, 130b]

    1. The persistence of HBV. The maintenance of hepatitis B as an entity prior to the era of needle and parenteral transmission was for a time an enigma. However, it now is well understood that two critical factors explain the persistence of this virus:

      a. Chronic carrier state. The virus persists chronically in the infected individual in a potentially infectious form.

      b. Routes of transmission other than parenteral have been identified. Thus, even though the virus transmits inefficiently by casual contact, it has been maintained by this process.

    2. Groups with a high frequency of carrier state include intravenous drug users, hemodialysis patients, male homosexuals, Down's syndrome patients, and patients with leukemia and other hematologic malignancies.

    3. Method of spread. In HBV, this is strikingly different from HAV. There are two basic routes of transmission.

      a. Nonparenteral

        (1) The **most common mode** of transmission worldwide is from **mother to child during the perinatal period.**

          (a) If the mother initially is infected in the third trimester, the rate of transmission is very high.

          (b) If the mother is a chronic carrier, transmission is of higher frequency if the mother is hepatitis B e antigen (HBeAg) positive (vida infra), than if she is HBeAg negative.

        (2) Transmission occurs between heterosexual partners or between homosexual men. This also occurs more commonly if the carrier is HBeAg positive.

        (3) Casual-contact transmission does occur (e.g., children in long-term care institutions) but far less efficiently than does HAV; this may be related to intimate oral contact and bites. Point-source outbreaks are a rarity.

(4) **Infectious viral particles have been reported in saliva, feces, urine, bile, tears, semen, and many other bodily fluids.** The precise risk of infection these fluids pose is unknown, although saliva has been documented to transmit HBV from human to chimpanzee.

b. **Parenteral**

(1) **Via blood transfusion.** This is very uncommon in the developed world since the initiation of screening of blood donors for hepatitis markers and since the elimination of paid blood donations.

(2) **Needle sharing by drug addicts.**

(3) **Accidental needlesticks of health care workers.**

(4) **Sharing of razors, etc. This should be avoided.**

4. **Most patients recover** from their illness, but a certain percentage continue to carry the virus or other markers of active HBV infection in their blood for a long period of time, even a lifetime. These **chronic carriers** become a potential source of infection to others.

5. **Chronicity.** In a recent report, data indicate that **age is the primary determinant of chronic HBV infection** and that there is a pronounced inverse relationship between age and the risk of chronicity. The highest incidence of chronic infection (80–90%) was found among children infected at birth by HBeAg-positive carrier mothers. Of children infected after the perinatal period and before 6 years of age, chronic infection develops in about 30%. The risk of development of the carrier state for children infected between 6–15 years of age is less well understood but may be low following acute symptomatic HBV. For generally healthy adult populations, prospective studies found a relatively wide range of risk (1–12%), with most studies indicating a risk of less than 5% [141a]. Other factors associated with increased risk of chronic HBV include male gender and various causes of immunodeficiency [141a].

B. **Definition of terms used to describe HBV and HBV infection.** Many different terms have been used to describe HBV, and a glossary is provided here to facilitate understanding of them. Also, see Fig. 11-6 for the usual chronologic development of these markers. A more detailed discussion of these appears elsewhere [141].

1. **The Dane particle is believed to be the infectious virus particle.** It is a complex, double-layered, lipid-enveloped structure with a diameter of 42 nm.

a. **The outer layer** or envelope contains hepatitis B surface antigen (HBsAg) proteins (see sec. **2**), glycoproteins, and cellular lipid.

b. **The HBV core** is the 28-nm, electron-dense core of the Dane particle, which possesses the double-stranded circular DNA and the DNA polymerase associated with HBV. It can be recovered from Dane particles by treatment with mild detergents to disrupt the 42-nm particle.

(1) The **hepatitis core antigen (HBcAg)** is associated with the HBV core. It is detectable in infected liver tissue but does not circulate in the serum.

(2) The **hepatitis B e antigen (HBeAg)** is part of the virion core and is found as a soluble antigen in serum. HBeAg is released from infected liver cells in which HBV is replicating [141].

HBeAg has been considered a **marker of infectivity** in both acutely and chronically infected HBV patients. If the patient has HBeAg, the patient poses a greater risk to contacts. There is a strong correlation between the presence of HBeAg and the finding of a high serum concentration of Dane particles, HBsAg, and HBV-associated DNA polymerase activity.

(3) **HBV-associated DNA polymerase** synthesizes DNA using the Dane particle–associated double-stranded circular DNA as a template. Because it is associated with the Dane particle, HBV-associated DNA polymerase has been used as a marker of viral replication and possible infectivity.

HBV DNA is used in research studies and is a marker for acute viral replication. HBeAg-positive patients are typically positive for HBV DNA.

2. **HBsAG** is not only the principal protein component of the HBV viral envelope but also is released from infected cells as components of small spherical particles. These are heterogeneous in size and appearance (16–25 mm, and called

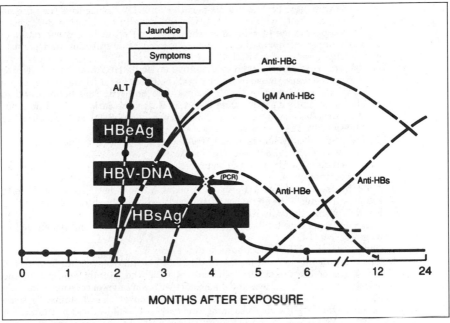

Fig. 11-6. The clinical, virologic, and serologic courses of a typical case of acute hepatitis B. *HBsAg* = hepatitis B surface antigen; *HBeAg* = hepatitis B e antigen; *HBV-DNA* = hepatitis B DNA; *anti-HBc* = antibody to hepatitis B core antigen; *anti-HBe* = antibody to hepatitis B e antigen; *anti-HBs* = antibody to hepatitis B surface antigen; *ALT* = alanine aminotransferase; *PCR* = polymerase chain reaction. (From H. H. Hsu, S. M. Feinstone, and J. H. Hoofnagel, Acute Viral Hepatitis. In G. L. Mandell, J. E. Bennett, and R. Dolin (eds.), *Principles and Practice of Infectious Diseases* (4th ed.). New York: Churchill Livingstone, 1995. Pp. 1136–1153.)

        22-mm particles) and are filamentous or rod-shaped. They are considered incomplete viral envelope proteins [141].
  a. A characteristic of HBV infection is the production of large amounts of viral antigen in the liver, which are detected in the blood. HBsAg in the blood remains the most useful marker of HBV viral infection.
  b. The concentrations of incomplete viral forms in the serum usually greatly exceed the concentrations of complete virions or Dane particles.
  c. High concentrations of viral antigens found during acute infection may be present continuously when HBV becomes a chronic infection.
  d. The tests available for HBsAg (radioimmunoassay, immunodiffusion, or complement fixation) cannot distinguish between HBsAg found on Dane particles and that on the small spherical or filamentous particles. Because the Dane particle is believed to be the infectious agent, it is conceivable that a patient may be HBsAg-positive (mostly spheres and filaments) and not be infectious. However, practically all **HBsAg-positive blood** should be considered **potentially infectious** because it may contain low and even undetectable levels of Dane particles.
3. **Anti-HBs is antibody to HBsAg.** It is **considered a protective antibody** and is monitored in the preparation of hepatitis B immune globulin (HBIG). Anti-HBs usually appears in the serum after HBsAg disappears (see Fig. 11-6). Anti-HBs develops 1–3 months after acute infection or immunization.
      Only rarely are both HBsAg and anti-HBs found together in the blood of a patient. When they are, these antigen-antibody complexes are believed to be the mechanisms of some of the unusual manifestations of HBV infection, such as polyarteritis nodosa, arthritis, and glomerulonephritis.
4. **Anti-HBc** is antibody to HBcAg. It develops shortly after the appearance of HBsAg and has been used diagnostically to identify a small number of HBV

infections that were both anti-HBs-negative and HBsAg-negative (i.e., the so-called core antibody window). Anti-HBc can usually be detected 3–5 weeks after the appearance of HBsAg in the blood and often before the onset of clinically apparent hepatitis. It also is detected after infection and persists even in the absence of anti-HBs.

   a. **IgM anti-HBc can be used to diagnose an acute HBV infection** as it rises during the acute phase of disease and then declines. Although most of the anti-HBc activity is in the IgG class, **IgM anti-HBc has been found in almost all patients with acute hepatitis B.** It rises early in the illness but then rapidly decreases in titer so that it declines 6–24 months after the illness [130, 141].

   b. IgG anti-HBc, by contrast, can be detected 5–6 years after acute infection in most patients [141] (see Fig. 11-6).

   c. Anti-HBc is now believed to be protective antibody [141]. It is not induced by vaccination.

5. **Anti-HBe** is antibody to HBeAg. It appears in most patients when HBeAg becomes undetectable. Presence of this antibody has been correlated with a low risk of infectivity in HBsAg-positive blood.

   Anti-HBe persists for 1–2 years after resolution of HBV and is believed to be protective [141].

C. **Diagnosis** of acute HBV infection (see Fig. 11-6).

1. HBsAg commonly is used for the confirmation of infection. It can be detected 2–7 weeks before the onset of clinical hepatitis and usually remains for the duration of the acute illness and disappears with convalescence. Approximately 95% of patients will be HBsAg-positive at the onset of symptoms. In some patients, the HBsAg is cleared rapidly and may be absent by the time the patient is tested. When present with IgM anti-HBc, HBsAg indicates acute infection.

2. **IgM anti-HBc** helps make an early diagnosis of acute disease as anti-HBc or anti-HBs may reflect prior infection (see sec. **B.4**).

3. **Markers of active viral replication** include the presence of HBeAg, HBV DNA (as detected by molecular hybridization or polymerase chain reaction) and DNA polymerase (the endogenous polymerase of this virus).

4. A detailed discussion of the serologic response to HBV is described elsewhere [141].

D. **Clinical manifestations and course**

1. **Infants and children**

   a. Acquired postnatally. Both have milder disease than adults; fulminant disease is rare.

   b. Acquired perinatally. Acute disease is rare but lifelong carriage and persistent hepatitis is common. This is an important target group for prevention (see sec. **A.4**).

2. **Adults.** Four possibilities exist following exposure to infection with HBV:

   a. No infection occurs.

   b. **Acute hepatitis** clinically indistinguishable from HAV develops [141], and antigen is cleared completely. A small proportion of these cases are more fulminant than HAV. Acute infection may result in fulminant liver failure in about 1% of patients, with a case fatality rate of 80% [130b].

   c. As in sec. **b,** but antigen is not cleared, and a chronic carrier state develops (i.e., HBsAg-positive for at least 6 months).

   d. No acute illness develops, but a chronic carrier state develops. The development of the chronic carrier state occurs less frequently after acute symptomatic illness than after asymptomatic HBV infection.

3. **Clinical consequences of infection.** Persistent HBV and hepatic disease is reviewed elsewhere [141].

   a. As in sec. **2.b,** except for the occasional case of postnecrotic cirrhosis, no obvious clinical problem persists.

   b. As in sec. **2.c,** chronic persistent or chronic active hepatitis ensues, often eventuating in cirrhosis and/or hepatoma.

      In a recent report, the risk for developing hepatocellular carcinoma may be increased by 10- to 300-fold among patients with chronic HBV infection. Hepatic cirrhosis is evident in more than 90% of patients with HBV-associated hepatocellular carcinoma [130b].

   c. As in sec. **2.d,** two possibilities exist.

(1) These patients proceed as do patients in sec. **2.c;** those whose serum contains HBeAg are more likely to do so.

(2) A persistent carrier state, usually without identifiable HBeAg, occurs, and liver function remains normal.

d. If hepatitis D is superimposed on a carrier state, severe disease can result (see sec. **VI**).

4. Risk of transmission. Those with chronic active liver disease and the associated HBeAg pose significant risk for sexual and perinatal transmission. All carriers can transmit parenterally.

5. Special manifestations

a. In addition to the general symptoms of hepatitis, HBV infection has a 16–20% incidence of serum sickness–like illness with urticaria, skin rash, or arthralgias.

b. Some patients develop frank arthritis, arteritis, or glomerulonephritis that is caused by HBsAg-antibody complexes.

c. HBV infection has been implicated as the cause of some cases of polyarteritis nodosa and cryoglobulinemia.

E. Therapy

1. Acute HBV. No therapeutic measure has been proven to have beneficial effect on the disease process in the liver [141]. Strict bed rest, special diets, and corticosteroids have shown no benefit.

2. Chronic HBV. For selected patients, **interferon** therapy may be useful. A detailed discussion of this is beyond the scope of this chapter, but the topic is reviewed elsewhere [141]. The hepatocellular injury caused by HBV appears to be largely immune related. Therapy with corticosteroids results in reduced hepatic inflammation but also in markedly increased viral replication. **Interferon-alpha exerts both antiviral and immunoregulatory effects** and has been useful in the treatment of chronic HBV infection [130b]. (See the detailed discussion of interferon in Chap. 26.) Also oral lamivudine once daily is undergoing clinical evaluation for therapy of chronic HBV [141b].

F. Prevention of HBV infection

1. Preexposure immunization with HBV vaccine is recommended for certain high-risk adults (e.g., health care workers, international travelers taking prolonged trips, hemodialysis patients, household contacts of HBV carriers) as **discussed in Chap. 22.** In addition, since 1991, the Centers for Disease Control have recommended **universal childhood vaccination against HBV** in an attempt to eliminate HBV in the United States.

2. Postexposure prophylaxis of HBV infection should be exercised in the following situations (in which the involved patient is anti-HBs-negative, has not been vaccinated with the HBV vaccine, or has failed to respond to the vaccine): (1) accidental percutaneous or permucosal exposure to HBsAg-positive blood, (2) sexual exposure to an HBsAg-positive person, and (3) perinatal exposure of an infant born to an HBsAg-positive mother (see Chap. 3 for details). Recent recommendations include the use of both HBIG and the HBV vaccine in persons known or suspected to be negative for anti-HBs. This affords an immediate passive immunity combined with long-lasting active immunization. The cost of this newer combined therapy is lower compared to previous recommendations, which called for two HBIG treatments at a total cost of approximately $300. In addition, HBIG alone is only approximately 75% effective.

For the details of postexposure prophylaxis, see Table 22-6 and the recommendations of the Centers for Disease Control [133]. If HBIG is not immediately available, Ig should be used. The latter contains low-level anti-HBs and, although not as good as HBIG, is better than no therapy.

3. Postexposure immunization of neonates. See Chap. 3.

4. Infection control measures [141]

a. Universal precautions should be followed.

b. Health care workers should receive the HBV vaccine.

c. Contaminated equipment or environmental surfaces should be disinfected or sterilized. The importance of thorough mechanical cleansing of any item (surface) before disinfection or sterilization cannot be overemphasized.

(1) Heat is the treatment of choice for materials that can tolerate the required conditions: boiling water for 10 minutes, autoclaving, or dry heat (160°F) for 2 hours.

(2) Presumably, solutions of sodium hypochlorite (Clorox) of 0.5–1.0% for 30 minutes, 40% aqueous formalin for 12 hours, or gas sterilization with ethylene oxide is effective.

(3) Very active detergents such as sodium dodecyl sulfate (1% SDS), which completely disrupts Dane particles, are cidal for most viruses and undoubtedly are cidal for HBV [141].

(4) All household members who are not HBsAg- or anti-HBs-positive should be vaccinated against HBV [141].

V. Hepatitis C virus. Until recently, the diagnosis of non-A, non-B hepatitis has been a diagnosis of exclusion [142] after the test results for HAV, HBV, the delta virus, CMV, and the Epstein-Barr virus were negative. The virus responsible for most cases of non-A, non-B hepatitis is HCV, a single-stranded RNA type of the togavirus family. HCV is a **common disease,** representing the **most common cause of nonalcoholic liver disease in the United States.** Approximately 150,000 individuals are acutely infected with HCV in the United States annually [143, 144]. Approximately 0.6% of volunteer blood donors in the United States have antibodies to HCV (anti-HCV) [145].

A. Epidemiology [143, 144]

1. **Risk factors** include **parenteral exposure,** in particular intravenous drug use and blood transfusions. In comparison to HBV, sexual exposure, especially homosexual exposure, and perinatal routes infrequently cause HCV. Data suggest that HCV is approximately 10 times less efficiently sexually transmitted than either the human immunodeficiency virus or HBV [143].

   As a result of improved donor selection criteria, volunteer donors, HBV testing, human immunodeficiency virus testing, and anti-HCV testing since May 1990, the incidence of HCV after transfusion has declined significantly in recent years (now accounting for fewer than 6% of cases of HCV) [143]. Anti-HCV is found in nearly 0.6% of blood donors in the United States [145].

2. **Sporadic cases** in which no identifiable risk factor is evident account for 40–50% of HCV infections in the United States [143].

3. The risk of a small parenteral exposure (e.g., needlestick) is unclear. In one report, there was a 3.7% transmission rate to medical personnel [143]. Repeated exposures (e.g., in dentistry or dialysis workers) presumably pose a risk.

4. Casual contact is unlikely to transmit infection. An increased prevalence of anti-HCV antibody in family members of HCV-infected patients has not been confirmed.

5. Perinatal transmission can occur but the predominant route (transplacental or perinatal) and the incidence of transmission are not known [143].

B. Pathogenesis

1. It is unclear whether HCV is directly cytopathic to hepatocytes, as in HAV, or causes damage by activating the immune destruction of infected cells, as in HBV [145].

2. The mean seroconversion time is 15 weeks after clinical hepatitis, with a range of 4–32 weeks. Seroconversion occurring more than 1 year after exposure has been reported. Patients with chronic disease have sustained levels of anti-HCV but, in those with self-limited disease, antibody response can decline and disappear over years.

C. Clinical course [143–145]

1. **Acute infection**

   a. **Asymptomatic infection is common** and occurs in approximately 75% of acute hepatitis cases. Cases may come to the clinician's attention when the patient is notified of anti-HCV after donating blood or as part of the workup of minor liver function test abnormalities.

   b. **Symptomatic** acute infection is clinically and biochemically indistinguishable from other forms of viral hepatitis. Extrahepatic complications such as glomerulonephritis, arthritis, or rash are unusual in HCV infection. Aplastic anemia can occur, and HCV may be a major viral cause of aplastic anemia. Fulminant hepatitis is rare (<1/1,000 cases) [143].

2. **Chronic hepatitis** usually is defined by elevated serum transferase levels for more than 6 months. **The major liability of HCV infection is the risk of developing chronic hepatitis, which occurs in at least 50% of cases of acute HCV infection.** This propensity of HCV to cause chronic infection is a unique feature of this virus [130].

   a. Most cases go unrecognized as patients are often asymptomatic. Mild fatigue can occur.

b. Although HCV is typically a clinically silent infection, it is histologically an insidiously progressive disease. Neither the symptoms nor the serum ALT elevation correlate with the histologic severity of disease [143].
   (1) Most patients will have histologic evidence of chronic active hepatitis.
   (2) Cirrhosis may develop over time in 20–50% of those with chronic active hepatitis.
c. Chronic HCV infection accounts for nearly 25% of adults referred for liver transplantation.
d. Infection may be more rapidly progressive in the elderly and immunosuppressed patient (e.g., human immunodeficiency virus or transplant patient). Chronic HCV is the major cause of morbidity that occurs more than 5 years after renal transplantation.
e. The risk of developing hepatocellular carcinoma [146] in HCV is significant and appears to be similar to that of HBV infection. The mechanisms by which HCV causes hepatocellular carcinoma are unclear.
f. Chronic HCV infection has been associated with cryoglobulinemia [147].
D. Diagnosis. Acute hepatitis due to HCV often remains a diagnosis of exclusion because it takes time to develop anti-HCV.
   1. Anti-HCV. The diagnosis of HCV is made by commercially available second-generation ELISA using hepatitis C viral proteins made in yeast by recombinant DNA technology (because the HCV has not been grown in tissue culture). The test detects antibody to HCV 6 weeks to 1 year from the date of infection. Therefore, it is recommended that the test be repeated at 3- and 6-month intervals from the onset of disease before concluding that the test is negative [148]. Anti-HCV testing performed serially will turn positive in more than 90% of patients within 6 months of exposure.
   2. False positive anti-HCV tests have been reported in autoimmune hepatitis and paraproteinemia. When anti-HCV is used as a universal screening test in blood donors, nearly 50% of those who test positively represent false positive results [143].
   Findings that support a true positive result include persistence of anti-HCV on serial testing, elevation of the serum ALT, an ELISA ratio (sample to cutoff) of greater than 2, confirmation of reactivity by either neutralizing (Abbott Laboratories) or immunoblot (RIBA, Ortho Laboratories), persistent positivity after urea treatment of the sample, presence of HCV RNA by the polymerase chain reaction, or risk factors for hepatitis C [143].
   3. The **polymerase chain reaction** detects HCV RNA. Using this test, HCV RNA can be demonstrated early in the course of the disease before seroconversion to anti-HCV occurs. This test currently is available only in research laboratories [148]. It may eventually help identify those patients actively infected.
E. Prevention
   1. Approximately 40–50% of cases have no obvious preventable risk factors.
   2. Intravenous drug use is potentially avoidable. Exposure to multiple sexual partners may increase the risk of HCV acquisition, but exposure to a spouse who is antibody-positive has a low transmission rate, and condom use may not be necessary in this setting [143, 149].
   3. Postexposure prophylaxis with immunoglobulin is not believed to be effective at this point [143].
   4. Careful blood bank donor criteria and screening processes have reduced the risk of HCV in posttransfusion hepatitis.
F. Therapy. A detailed discussion of therapy of HCV is beyond the scope of this book. The topic is reviewed elsewhere [150]. Corticosteroids and acyclovir are not useful agents. **Interferon-alpha is the most effective agent** (discussed in Chap. 26). Ideally, a gastroenterologist or a physician with special interest and expertise in liver disease should supervise the treatment and follow-up of patients who are receiving chronic interferon therapy. Whether famciclovir will have a role is undergoing evaluation, as is alpha-thymosine in combination with interferon-alpha, as well as oral ribavirin [130b] alone and in combination therapy.
VI. Delta virus or hepatitis D virus [151, 152]. The delta virus was discovered during analysis of the antigens of some hepatitis B patients. It is believed to be **a defective RNA virus that requires coinfection with HBV to replicate,** for it uses HBsAg for its structural protein shell [130]. **Delta virus is only observed in patients with HBV infection and not in those without it.**

In the case of simultaneous acquisition of HBV and HDV, two peaks of transaminase elevation are observed, separated by 2–3 weeks owing to the two individual infections. More commonly, chronic HBV carriers who are delta virus–negative may also acquire superinfection from exposure to delta virus and HBsAg-positive blood.

HDV infection is worldwide, the high areas of prevalence being the Amazon basin in South America, Central Africa, Southern Italy, and the Middle Eastern countries [130]. **Coinfection with HBV and HDV is associated with both a more severe course of hepatitis and progression to cirrhosis** [153–155].

A. **Epidemiology.** There are at least two distinct patterns.
   1. **In endemic areas** such as Mediterranean countries, transmission occurs by nonpercutaneous routes.
   2. **In nonendemic areas** such as North America and Europe, HDV infection is confined to groups with frequent percutaneous exposure (e.g., drug addicts, hemophiliacs, and persons who have had multiple transfusions [130]).
   3. **Epidemic** HDV can occur in sustained outbreaks, with coinfection in acutely HBV-infected persons or superinfection in chronically HBV-infected persons.

B. **Clinical manifestations.** Because HDV can occur only in the presence of HBV infection, the duration of HDV is determined by the duration of HBV infection. **The clinical importance of the delta virus lies in its association with the more severe outcomes of hepatitis B** (i.e., **fulminant hepatitis, chronic active hepatitis,** and **cirrhosis**).

   Simultaneous HDV and HBV coinfection leads to chronic hepatitis in fewer than 5% of cases. In contrast, HDV superinfection in an HBsAg carrier commonly leads to chronic delta hepatitis, which then develops over 10–15 years into chronic hepatitis, often with cirrhosis, in 70–80% of cases [130, 156].

C. **Diagnosis.** Delta antigen can sometimes be detected in the serum of the early phase of acute HDV infection; with disappearance of the antigen, anti-HDV develops. The appearance of anti-HDV may be delayed, short-lived, and in low titer and therefore, in acute infection, patients may test negatively for anti-HDV and will become positive in convalescence and then only in low titer [130].
   1. A radioimmunoassay for anti-HDV is commercially available [157], but anti-HDV tests are not always reliable for diagnosis of acute infection [130].
   2. High titers of anti-HDV (> 1:100) indicate ongoing delta viral infection.
   3. Using research techniques, demonstration of HDV antigen or HDV RNA in serum indicates acute viral infection. The polymerase chain reaction is more sensitive for detecting HDV RNA than is molecular hybridization [130].
   4. Rising titers of anti-HDV indicate acute infection, while sustained high titers indicate chronic infection.

D. **Prevention**
   1. In those susceptible to HBV infection, **hepatitis B vaccination** will prevent delta virus infection [151].
   2. In persons already chronically infected with HBV, prevention is limited to precautions to avoid intimate contact with those who have the delta virus.

E. **Therapy.** Interferon therapy inhibits delta replication and is associated with improvement in serum enzyme activity. The effect of therapy is not sustained once treatment is withdrawn.

VII. **Hepatitis E virus.** A different and distinct type of non-A, non-B hepatitis **acquired by the fecal-oral route** was first identified through investigations of large epidemics (and sporadic cases) in developing countries such as India, Asia, Africa, and Central America [130a, 142, 158]. The most commonly recognized cases occur after contamination of water supplies by natural events such as flooding. There have been no reported cases of HEV acquired in the United States [130a], but international travelers have acquired HEV. Virus particles measuring 27–32 nm in diameter have been identified from feces of patients with this hepatitis.

A. **Clinical manifestations.** The clinical features of this form of hepatitis are similar to other types of hepatitis. The incubation period ranges from 15 to 60 days [130a]. Enterically transmitted non-A, non-B hepatitis produces a high case-fatality rate in pregnant women and is one of the leading causes of acute viral hepatitis in young to middle-aged adults in developing countries (see Chap. 21).

B. **Diagnosis.** Serologic tests have been developed to detect antibody to HEV but are currently available only in research laboratories. Preliminary serologic testing has not documented any transmission in the United States, although cases have been reported in travelers to Mexico and India [158].

C. **Therapy.** No specific therapy is available.

D. Prevention. Because most U.S. citizens have not been exposed to HEV, the usual source of immune serum globulin would not be expected to have anti-HEV, which if present would be protective for an international traveler; therefore, there is no evidence that Ig will prevent HEV. Proper preparation of food and purification of water need to be emphasized (see Chap. 21).

VIII. A candidate **hepatitis F virus** [159] and **hepatitis G virus** [160–162] have been described.

References

1. Guerrant, R.L., and Bobar, D.A. Bacterial and protozoal gastroenteritis. *N. Engl. J. Med.* 325:327, 1991.
2. Cheney, C.P., and Wong, R.K.H. Acute infectious diarrhea. *Med. Clin. North Am.* 77:1169, 1993.
   This and the first reference summarize a logical and cost-effective workup of acute diarrhea. For a related discussion of the therapy of infectious diarrhea, see D.D. John and M.M. Levine, Treatment of diarrhea. Infect. Dis. Clin. North Am. *2:719, 1988.*
3. Blaser, M.J. Infectious diarrheas: Acute, chronic, iatrogenic. *Ann. Intern. Med.* 105:786, 1986.
4. Bandres, J.C., and DuPont, H. Approach to the Patient with Diarrhea. In S.L. Gorbach, J.G. Bartlett, and N.R. Blacklow (eds.), *Infectious Diseases.* Philadelphia: Saunders, 1992. Pp. 572–575.
5. Miranda, A.G., and DuPont, H.L. Small Intestine: Infections with Common Bacterial and Viral Pathogens. In T. Yamada (ed.), *Textbook of Gastroenterology.* New York: Lippincott, 1991. Pp. 1447–1472.
   Authoritative text. This chapter is written by two infectious disease experts.
6. Powell, D.W. Approach to the Patient with Diarrhea. In T. Yamada (ed.), *Textbook of Gastroenterology.* New York: Lippincott, 1991. P. 732.
   See related paper by C.W. Hedberg et al., Changing epidemiology of food-borne disease: A Minnesota perspective. Clin. Infect. Dis. *18:671, 1994.*
7. Guerrant, R.L. Principles and Syndromes of Enteric Infection. In G.L. Mandell, J.E. Bennett, R. Dolin, (eds.), *Principles and Practice of Infectious Diseases* (4th. ed.). New York: Churchill Livingstone, 1995. Pp. 945–961.
8. *Dorland's Illustrated Medical Dictionary* (27th ed.). Philadelphia: Saunders, 1988.
9. DuPont, H. Shigella. *Infect. Dis. Clin. North Am.* 2:599, 1988.
   See related paper by J. Tuttle and R. Tauxe. Antimicrobial-resistant shigella: The growing need for prevention strategies. Infect. Dis. Clin. Pract. *2:55, 1993.*
10. Goldberg, M.B., and Rubin, R.H. The spectrum of *Salmonella* infection. *Infect. Dis. Clin. North Am.* 2:571, 1988.
    See related paper by L.A. Lee et al., Increase in antimicrobial-resistant Salmonella infections in the United States, 1989–1990. J. Infect. Dis. *170:128, 1994.*
11. Avery, M.E., and Snyder, J.D. Oral therapy for acute diarrhea: The underused simple solution. *N. Engl. J. Med.* 323:891, 1990.
12. DuPont, H.L., and Hornick, R.B. Adverse effect of Lomotil therapy in shigellosis. *J.A.M.A.* 226:1525, 1973.
    Diarrhea due to invasive organisms may act as a defensive mechanism for the body.
13. Dupont, H.L., and Ericsson, C.D. Prevention and treatment of travelers' diarrhea. *N. Engl. J. Med.* 328:1821–1827, 1993.
14. Figueroa-Quintanilla, D., et al. A controlled trial of bismuth subsalicylate in infants with acute watery diarrheal disease. *N. Engl. J. Med.* 328:1653, 1993.
    See thoughtful editorial comment in the same issue, in which Dr. J.D. Snyder expresses concern that emphasizing the use of adjunctive antidiarrheal therapy may divert attention and resources away from the use of oral rehydration therapy and early appropriate therapy.
15. Centers for Disease Control. *Bacillus cereus* food poisoning associated with fried rice at two child day care centers. *M.M.W.R.* 43:177, 1994.
    See related paper by S. Luby et al., A large outbreak of gastroenteritis caused by diarrheal toxin-producing Bacillus cereus. J. Infect. Dis. *167:1452, 1993.*
16. Underman, A.E., and Leedom, J.M. Fish and shellfish poisoning. *Curr. Clin. Top. Infect. Dis.* 13:203, 1993.
17. Lennette, E.H., et al. *Manual of Clinical Microbiology* (6th ed.). Washington, DC: American Society for Microbiology. 1995. P. 453.

18. Mishu, B., et al. *Salmonella enteritidis* gastroenteritis transmitted by intact chicken eggs. *Ann. Intern. Med.* 115:190–194, 1991.
19. Centers for Disease Control. Outbreak of *Salmonella enteritidis* infection associated with consumption of raw shell eggs, 1991. *M.M.W.R.* 41:369–372, 1992.
20. Aserkoff, B., and Bennett, J.V. Effect of antibiotic therapy in acute salmonellosis on fecal excretion of salmonellae. *N. Engl. J. Med.* 281:636, 1969.
    Demonstration that antibiotics prolong the carrier state.
21. St. Geme, J.W., III, et al. Consensus: Management of *Salmonella* infections in the first year of life. *Pediatr. Infect. Dis. J.* 7:615, 1988.
22. Medical Letter. The choice of antimicrobial drugs. *Med. Lett. Drug Ther.* 36:53, 1994.
23. Nolan, C.M., and White, P.C., Jr. Treatment of typhoid carriers with amoxicillin: Correlates of successful therapy. *J.A.M.A.* 239:2352, 1978.
24. Ferreuio, C., et al. Efficacy of ciprofloxacin in the treatment of chronic typhoid carriers. *J. Infect. Dis.* 157:1235–1239, 1988.
25. Tigaud, S., et al. Use of ofloxacin for the treatment of enteric infections. *Rev. Infect. Dis.* 10(Suppl. 1):S207, 1988.
26. Asperilla, M.D., Smego, R.A., and Scott, L.K. Quinolone antibiotics in the treatment of *Salmonella* infections. *Rev. Infect. Dis.* 12:873–889, 1990.
27. Bannish, M.L., et al. Treatment of shigellosis: III. Comparison of one or two doses ciprofloxacin with standard 5-day therapy. *Ann. Intern. Med.* 117:727, 1992.
28. Black, R.E., and Slome, S. *Yersinia enterocolitica. Infect. Dis. Clin. North Am.* 2: 625, 1988.
29. Gayraud, M., et al. Antibiotic treatment of *Yersinia enterocolitica* septicemia: A retrospective review of 43 cases. *Clin. Infect. Dis.* 17:405–410, 1993.
30. Cornick, N.A., and Gorbach, S.L. *Campylobacter. Infect. Dis. Clin. North Am.* 2: 643, 1988.
    For a related discussion, see B.M. Allos and M.J. Blaser, Campylobacter jejuni *and the expanded spectrum of related infections.* Clin. Infect. Dis. *30:1092, 1995.*
31. Centers for Disease Control. Update: Multistate outbreak of *Escherichia coli* 0157:H7 infections from hamburgers—Western United States, 1992–1993. *M.M.W.R.* 42:258–263, 1993. [*See reprint of this in* J.A.M.A. *269:2194, 1993.*]
31a. Tarr, P.I. *Escherichia coli* 0157:H7: Clinical, diagnostic and epidemiologic aspects of human infection. *Clin. Infect. Dis.* 20:1, 1995.
    An excellent summary.
32. Swerdlow, D.L., et al. A waterborne outbreak in Missouri of *Escherichia coli* 0157:H7 associated with bloody diarrhea and death. *Ann. Intern. Med.* 117:812–818, 1992.
32a. Boyce, T.G., Swerdlow, D.L., and Griffin, P.M. *Escherichia coli* 0157:H7 and the hemolytic uremic syndrome. *N. Engl. J. Med.* 333:364, 1995.
    Recent review as of August 1995.
33. Centers for Disease Control. *Escherichia coli* 0157:H7 outbreak linked to home-cooked hamburger. *M.M.W.R.* 43:214, 1994.
34. Belongia, E.A., et al. Transmission of *Escherichia coli* 0157:H7 infection in Minnesota child day care facilities. *J.A.M.A.* 269:883, 1993.
35. Holmberg, S.D. *Vibrios* and *Aeromonas. Infect. Dis. Clin. North Am.* 2:655, 1988.
    See related paper by S.W. Lacey, Cholera: Calamitous past, ominous future. Clin. Infect. Dis. *30:1409, 1995.*
36. Webster, J.T., et al. Cholera in the United States, 1965–1991. *Arch. Intern. Med.* 154:551, 1994.
    See related article by D.L. Swerdlow and A.A. Ries, Cholera in the Americas: Guidelines for the clinician. J.A.M.A. *267:1495, 1992.*
37. Centers for Disease Control. Viral agents of gastroenteritis: Public health importance and outbreak management. *M.M.W.R.* 39(RR-5):1, 1990.
38. Blacklow, N.R., and Greenberg, H.B. Viral gastroenteritis. *N. Engl. J. Med.* 325: 252, 1991.
    Excellent review of this topic. See also related review by J.W. Burns and H.B. Greenburg, Viral gastroenteritis. Infect. Dis. Clin. Pract. *3:411, 1994.*
39. Blaser, M.J. Type B gastritis, aging, and *Campylobacter pylori. Arch. Intern. Med.* 148:1021, 1988.
40. Falk, G.W. Current status of *Helicobacter pylori* in peptic ulcer disease. *Cleve. Clin. J. Med.* 62:95, 1995.
    Nice concise clinical review.
41. Isenberg, J.I. Is peptic ulcer disease an infectious disease? *West. J. Med.* 159:616, 1993.
    Interesting editorial comment appearing in the November 1993 issue with commentary on reference [42].

42. Friedman, M., and Peterson, W.L. *Helicobacter pylori* and peptic ulcer disease. *West. J. Med.* 159:555, 1993.
43. National Institutes of Health Consensus Development Panel on *Helicobacter pylori* in Peptic Ulcer Disease. *Helicobacter pylori* in peptic ulcer disease. *J.A.M.A.* 272:65, 1994.
43a. Feldman, M. The acid test: Making clinical sense of the consensus conference on *Helicobacter pylori*. *J.A.M.A.* 272:70, 1995.
43b. Soll, A.H., for the Practice Parameters Committee of the American College of Gastroenterology. Medical treatment of peptic ulcer disease: Practice guidelines. *J.A.M.A.* 275:622, 1996.
44. Medical Letter. Drugs for treatment of peptic ulcers. *Med. Lett. Drugs Ther.* 36:65, 1994.
44a. Logan, R.P.H., et al. Eradication of *Helicobacter pylori* with clarithromycin and omeprazole. *Gut* 35:323, 1994.
     The MIC_{90} of clarithromycin for H. pylori is 0.03 µg/ml. A regimen of clarithromycin 500 mg tid and omeprazole 40 mg qd for 2 weeks was used. Therapy was associated with a 78% eradication rate. The majority of patients experienced a metallic taste, but only 5% of recipients could not complete the course due to side effects. This is an expensive regimen.
45. Neva, F.A. *Basic Clinical Parasitology* (6th ed.). New York: Appleton & Lange, 1994.
46. Centers for Disease Control. Intestinal Parasite Surveillance Annual Summary 1977. September 1978.
47. Panosian, C.B. Parasitic diarrhea. *Infect. Dis. Clin. North Am.* 2:685, 1988.
48. Hill, D.R. Giardiasis: Issues in diagnosis and management. *Infect. Dis. Clin. North Am.* 7:503, 1993.
     See related papers by E.J. Lengerich et al., Severe Giardia in the United States. Clin. Infect. Dis. 18:760, 1994, and editorial comment in same issue by D. Overturf, Endemic giardiasis in the United States: Role of the day care center.
49. Aucott, J.N., and Ravdin, J.I. Amebiasis and "nonpathogenic" intestinal protozoa. *Infect. Dis. Clin. North Am.* 7:467, 1993.
49a. Centers for Disease Control. Assessing the public health threat associated with waterborne cryptosporidiosis: Report of a workshop. *M.M.W.R.* 44(RR-6):1, 1995.
50. Frenkel, L.M. *Dientamoeba fragilis.* In R.D. Feigin and J.D. Cherry (eds.), *Textbook of Pediatric Infectious Diseases* (3rd ed.). Philadelphia: Saunders, 1992. P. 2016.
51. Healy, G.R., and Garcia, L.S. Intestinal and Urogenital Protozoa. In A. Balows et al. (eds.), *Manual of Clinical Microbiology* (6th ed.). Washington, DC: American Society for Microbiology, 1995. Pp. 1207–1208.
52. Frenkel, L.M. *Blastocystis hominis.* In R.D. Feigin and J.D. Cherry (eds.), *Textbook of Pediatric Infectious Disease* (3rd ed.). Philadelphia: Saunders, 1992. P. 2019.
53. Senay, H., and MacPherson, D. *Blastocystis hominis:* Epidemiology and natural history. *J. Infect. Dis.* 162:987, 1990.
     Concludes that B. hominis, though commonly seen in stool samples, is believed to be a commensal organism.
54. Udkow, M.P., and Markell, E.K. *Blastocystis hominis:* Prevalence in asymptomatic versus symptomatic hosts. *J. Infect. Dis.* 168:242, 1993.
     Found B. hominis is prevalent in healthy, asymptomatic people but could find no solid evidence that it is pathogenic.
55. Condon, R.E., and Wittman, D.H. Approach to the Patient with Intra-Abdominal Infection. In S.L. Gorbach, J.G. Bartlett, and N.R. Blacklow (eds.), *Infectious Diseases.* Philadelphia: Saunders, 1992. Pp. 654–660.
56. Wittmann, D.H., Walker, A.P., and Condon, R.E. Peritonitis and Intra-Abdominal Infection. In S.I. Schwartz et al. (eds.), *Principles of Surgery* (6th ed.). New York: McGraw-Hill, 1994. P. 1449.
57. Gorbach, S.L. Treatment of intra-abdominal infections. *J. Antimicrob. Chemother.* 31(Suppl. A):67, 1993.
     Nice review of this topic by a national expert. Good reference list. For the references on animal model studies, see W.M. Weinstein et al., Antimicrobial therapy of experimental intra-abdominal sepsis. J. Infect. Dis. 132:282, 1975, which reviews the rat model and illustrates the need to treat both aerobic and anaerobic bacteria; and F.P. Tally and S.L. Gorbach, Therapy of mixed anaerobic-aerobic infections. Lessons from studies of intra-abdominal sepsis. Am. J. Med. 78(Suppl. 6A):145, 1985.
57a. McClean, K.I., et al. Intraabdominal infection: A review. *Clin. Infect. Dis.* 19:100, 1994.
     Comprehensive review of this topic including microbiology, pathogenesis, antibiotic, and surgical therapeutic options.

58. Gorbach, S.L. Intra-abdominal infections. *Clin. Infect. Dis.* 17:961, 1993.
   State-of-the-art clinical article. Overview.
58a. Bartlett, J. Intraabdominal sepsis. *Med. Clin. North Am.* 79:599, 1995.
   Concise review of recent developments.
59. Ho, J.L., and Barza, M. Role of aminoglycoside antibiotics in the treatment of intra-abdominal infection. *Antimicrob. Agents Chemother.* 31:485, 1987.
60. Silen, W. (ed.). *The Early Diagnosis of the Acute Abdomen* (17th ed.). London: Oxford University Press, 1987.
   A classic discussion of signs, symptoms, and differential diagnosis.
61. Conn, H.O., and Fessel, J.M. Spontaneous bacterial peritonitis in cirrhosis. *Medicine* 50:161, 1971.
   Classic review of topic.
61a. Bhuva, M., Ganger, D., and Jensen, D. Spontaneous bacterial peritonitis. An update on evaluation, management, and prevention. *Am. J. Med.* 97:169, 1994.
61b. Gilbert, J.A., and Kamath, P.S. Spontaneous bacterial peritonitis: An update. *Mayo Clin. Proc.* 70:365, 1995.
62. Jones, S.R. The absolute granulocyte count in ascites fluid: An aid to the diagnosis of spontaneous bacterial peritonitis. *West. J. Med.* 126:344, 1977.
   When the absolute granulocyte count in ascitic fluid is greater than $250/mm^3$, infection is likely.
62a. Singh, N., et al. Trimethoprim-sulfamethoxazole for the prevention of spontaneous bacterial peritonitis in cirrhosis: A randomized trial. *Ann. Intern. Med.* 122:595, 1995.
   Patients were given 1 DS tablet daily, five times a week (Monday–Friday). TMP-SMX was efficacious, safe, and cost effective for the prevention of spontaneous bacterial peritonitis in this study.
63. Peterson, P.K., et al. Current concepts in the management of peritonitis in patients undergoing continuous ambulatory peritoneal dialysis. *Rev. Infect. Dis.* 9:604, 1987.
64. Vas, S.I. Infections of continuous ambulatory peritoneal dialysis catheters. *Infect. Dis. Clin. North Am.* 3:301, 1989.
   See update by S.I. Vas, Infections Associated with the Peritoneum and Hemodialysis. In A.L. Bisno and F.A. Waldvogel (eds.). Infections Associated with Indwelling Devices (2nd ed.). Washington, DC: American Society for Microbiology, 1994.
65. The Ad Hoc Advisory Committee on Peritonitis Management. Peritoneal dialysis–related peritonitis treatment recommendations, 1993 update. *Periton. Dialysis. Int.* 13:14, 1993.
   Excellent comprehensive summary.
66. Murray, H.W. Secondary peritonitis and intra-abdominal abscess. *Hosp. Pract.* 25:101, 1990.
67. Lurie, D.K., Plzak, L., and Deveney, C.W. Intraabdominal abscess in the 1980's. *Surg. Clin. North Am.* 67:621, 1987.
68. Georges, R.N., and Deitch, E.A. Pyogenic hepatic abscess. *South. Med. J.* 86:1233, 1993.
   Review of 37 patients, 38% with cryptogenic source.
69. Stain, S.C., et al. Pyogenic liver abscess: Modern treatment. *Arch. Surg.* 126:991, 1991.
   Broad-spectrum antibiotics and aspiration or percutaneous catheter drainage was used in most of the 54 patients.
70. Robert, J.H., et al. Critical review of the treatment of pyogenic hepatic abscess. *Surg. Gynecol. Obstet.* 174:97, 1992.
   Emphasizes surgical drainage considerations in 29 patients. Favors percutaneous drainage and surgical drainage over simple aspiration.
71. Rubin, R.H., Swartz, M.N., and Malt, R. Hepatic abscess: Changes in clinical, bacteriologic and therapeutic aspects. *Am. J. Med.* 57:601, 1974.
72. McDonald, M.I., et al. Single and multiple pyogenic liver abscesses. Natural history, diagnosis and treatment, with emphasis on percutaneous drainage. *Medicine* 63:291, 1984.
73. Miedema, B.W., and Dineen, P. The diagnosis and treatment of pyogenic liver abscesses. *Ann. Surg.* 200:328, 1984.
74. Barnes, P.F., et al. A comparison of amebic and pyogenic abscess of the liver. *Medicine* 66:472, 1987.
75. Chua, D., Reinhart, H.H., and Sobel, J. Liver abscess caused by *Streptococcus milleri.* *Rev. Infect. Dis.* 11:197, 1989.
   A positive blood culture with this organism should alert the physician of the possibility of hepatic suppuration.
76. Sabbaj, J. Anaerobes in liver abscess. *Rev. Infect. Dis.* 6(Suppl. 1):152, 1984.

77. Bak, S.Y., et al. Therapeutic percutaneous aspiration of hepatic abscesses: Effectiveness in 25 patients. *A.J.R.* 160:799, 1993.

78. Hansen, N., and Vargish, T. Pyogenic hepatic abscess: A case for open drainage. *Am. Surg.* 59:219, 1993.
    In a series of 24 patients reported from the University of Chicago, overall mortality was 25%. With open drainage in addition to a definitive procedure such as cholecystectomy or bowel resection, there were no deaths.

79. Chun, C.H., et al. Splenic abscess. *Medicine* 59:50, 1980.
    Review of published cases up to 1977.

80. Nelken, N., et al. Changing clinical spectrum of splenic abscess: A multicenter study and review of the literature. *Am. J. Surg.* 154:27, 1987.
    Reviews 170 previously published cases plus the authors' series of 19 cases from 1967 through 1986. An update of reference [79]. From San Francisco Hospital.

81. Alonso Cohen, M.A., et al. Splenic abscess. *World J. Surg.* 14:513, 1990.
    Reviews 227 cases from the world literature plus 7 of the authors' cases. Report from Spain.

82. Westh, H., Reines, E., and Skibsted, L. Splenic abscess: A review of 20 cases. *Scand. J. Infect. Dis.* 22:569, 1990.
    Still favors splenectomy as treatment of choice. Series from Denmark. See related review by J.D. Allan, Splenic abscess: Pathogenesis, clinical features, diagnosis, and treatment. Curr. Clin. Top. Infect. Dis. 14:23, 1994.

83. Ho, H.S., and Wisner, D.H. Splenic abscess in the intensive care unit. *Arch. Surg.* 128:842, 1993.

84. Hadas-Halpren, I., Hiller, N., and Dolberg, M. Percutaneous drainage of splenic abscesses: An effective and safe procedure. *Br. J. Radiol.* 65:968, 1992.
    Successful in 8 patients without complication.

85. Altemeier, W.A., and Alexander, J.W. Retroperitoneal abscess. *Arch. Surg.* 83:512, 1961.
    General review with good illustrations of the anatomy. A classic.

86. Crepps, J.T., Welch, J.P., and Orlando, R., III. Management and outcome of retroperitoneal abscesses. *Ann. Surg.* 205:276, 1987.
    A relatively recent review emphasizing the insidious presentation of these abscesses, drainage techniques, and importance of CT studies. Reviews 50 cases.

87. Sacks, D., et al. Renal and related retroperitoneal abscess: Percutaneous drainage. *Radiology* 167:447, 1988.
    Report of 18 cases: In 11, percutaneous drainage was the only drainage procedure necessary; in 7, after initial improvement with percutaneous drainage, a definitive elective nephrectomy was done with fewer complications.

88. Leu, S.Y., et al. Psoas abscess: Changing patterns of diagnosis and etiology. *Dis. Colon Rectum* 29:694, 1986.
    Review of 43 cases from 1976 through 1984 from the Mayo Clinic.

89. Bresee, J.S., and Edwards, M.S. Psoas abscess in children. *Pediatr. Infect. Dis. J.* 9:201, 1990.
    Describes 2 cases and reviews literature. Shows nice anatomical review. Emphasizes children.

90. Greenwald, I., Abrahamson, J., and Cohen, O. Psoas abscess: Case report and review of the literature. *J. Urol.* 147:1624, 1992.
    Report from Israel of a case due to Proteus mirabilis and literature review.

91. Schwartz, S.I. Appendix. In S.I. Schwartz et al. (eds.), *Principles of Surgery* (6th ed.). New York: McGraw-Hill, 1994. P. 1307.

92. Bauer, T., et al. Antibiotic prophylaxis in acute nonperforated appendicitis: The Danish multicenter study group III. *Ann. Surg.* 209:307, 1989.
    A single preoperative 2-g dose of cefoxitin reduced wound infections.

93. Nylander, W.A., Jr. The acute abdomen in the immunocompromised host. *Surg. Clin. North Am.* 68:457, 1988.

94. Goodgame, R.W. Gastrointestinal cytomegalovirus disease. *Ann. Intern. Med.* 119:924, 1993.
    Reviews spectrum of CMV GI disease in immunocompromised hosts.

95. Chappuis, C.W., and Cohn, I. Acute colonic diverticulitis. *Surg. Clin. North Am.* 68:301, 1988.
    Good review from a department of surgery.

96. Freeman, S.R., and McNally, P.R. Diverticulitis. *Med. Clin. North Am.* 77:1149–1167, 1993.
    Review by gastroenterologists.

97. Erton, A. Colonic diverticulitis. Recognizing and managing its presentations and complications. *Postgrad. Med.* 88:67–77, 1990.
98. Schoetz, D.J. Uncomplicated diverticulitis: Indications for surgery and surgical management. *Surg. Clin. North Am.* 73:965, 1993.
    Surgeon's view from Lahey Clinic. For a related discussion, see D.A. Rothenberger and D. Wiltz, Surgery for complicated diverticulitis. Surg. Clin. North Am. 73:975, 1993.
99. Kellum, J.M., and Sugerman, H.J. Randomized, prospective comparison of cefoxitin and gentamicin-clindamycin in the treatment of acute colonic diverticulitis. *Clin. Ther.* 14:376, 1992.
100. Roslyn, J.J., and Zinner, M.J. Gallbladder and Extrahepatic Biliary System. In S.I. Schwartz et al. (eds.), *Principles of Surgery* (6th ed.). New York: McGraw-Hill, 1994. P. 1367.
101. Cooperberg, P.I., and Gibney, R.G. Imaging of the gallbladder. *Radiology* 163:605, 1987.
    Still a useful review, including pitfalls of tests in acute cholecystitis.
102. Marton, K.I., and Doubilet, P. How to image the gallbladder in suspected cholecystitis. *Ann. Intern. Med.* 109:722, 1988.
    Excellent, clear review.
103. Williams, R.A., Kourtesis, G., and Wilson, S.E. Cholecystitis and Cholangitis. In S.L. Gorbach, J.G. Bartlett, and N.R. Blacklow (eds.), *Infectious Diseases*. Philadelphia: Saunders, 1992. P. 736.
104. Levison, M.E., and Bush, L.M. Peritonitis and Other Intra-Abdominal Infections. In G.L. Mandell, J.E. Bennett, R. Dolin (eds.), *Principles and Practice of Infectious Diseases* (4th ed.). New York: Churchill Livingstone, 1995. P. 705.
105. Brook, I. Aerobic and anaerobic microbiology of biliary tract disease. *J. Clin. Microbiol.* 27:2373, 1989.
    Approximately 25% of isolates were anaerobes. Enterococci were isolated nearly 15% of the time.
      See related paper by S.J. Van den Hazel et al., Role of antibiotics in the treatment and prevention of acute and recurrent cholangitis. Clin. Infect. Dis. 19:279, 1994, which includes a nice discussion of the bacteriology of acute biliary tract infections. Emphasizes that enterococcal bloodstream infections are unusual from acute cholangitis. See discussion of the use of preventive antibiotics for recurrent cholangitis in Chap. 28B.
106. Kadaskia, S.C. Biliary tract emergencies: Acute cholecystitis, acute cholangitis, and acute pancreatitis. *Med. Clin. North Am.* 77:1015, 1993.
107. Glenn, F., and Becker, C.G. Acute acalculous cholecystitis: An increasing entity. *Ann. Surg.* 195:131, 1982.
108. Frazee, R.C., Nagorney, D.M., and Mucha, P., Jr. Acute acalculous cholecystitis. *Mayo Clin. Proc.* 64:163, 1989.
108a. Hanau, L.H., and Steigbigel, N.H. Cholangitis: Pathogenesis, diagnosis, and treatment. *Curr. Clin. Top. Infect. Dis.* 15:153, 1995.
109. Huang, T., Bass, J.A., and Williams, R.D. The significance of biliary pressure in cholangitis. *Arch. Surg.* 98:629, 1969.
110. Welch, J.P., and Donaldson, G.A. The urgency of diagnosis and surgical treatment of acute suppurative cholangitis. *Am. J. Surg.* 131:527, 1976.
111. Jolly, B.T., and Love, J.N. Emphysematous cholecystitis in an elderly woman: Case report and review of the literature. *J. Emerg. Med.* 11:593, 1993.
112. Deviere, J., et al. Septicemia after endoscopic retrograde cholangiopancreatography. *Endoscopy* 22:72, 1990.
    Review of 55 patients.
113. Calleja, G.A., and Barkin, J.S. Acute pancreatitis. *Med. Clin. North Am.* 77:1037, 1993.
    Recent review by two gastroenterologists from the University of Miami. Good reference list. See related review by J.R. Potts (from the Department of Surgery at Vanderbilt), Acute pancreatitis. Surg. Clin. North Am. 68:281, 1988.
114. Steinberg, W., and Tenner, S. Acute pancreatitis. *N. Engl. J. Med.* 330:1198, 1994.
    Excellent medical progress summary from the gastroenterology unit at George Washington University. For related updates, see J.H.C. Ranson, The current management of acute pancreatitis. Adv. Surg. 28:93, 1995, and T.J. Howard et al, Classification and treatment of local septic complications in acute pancreatitis. Am. J. Surg. 170:44, 1995.
115. Lee, S.P., Nicholls, J.F., and Park, H.Z. Biliary sludge as a cause of acute pancreatitis. *N. Engl. J. Med.* 326:589, 1992.
    On careful study, many patients with so-called idiopathic pancreatitis may have biliary sludge as an underestimated cause of their pancreatitis. See accompanying editorial

comment in this same issue by Dr. William A. Steinberg, who discusses both a logical workup of biliary pancreatitis and the article.

116. Frey, C.F. Management of necrotizing pancreatitis. *West. J. Med.* 159:675, 1993.
     Excellent review from a surgeon at the University of California, Davis Medical Center. See the editorial comment in reference [117].

117. Reber, H.A., and McFadden, D.W. Indications for surgery in necrotizing pancreatitis. *West. J. Med.* 159:704, 1993.
     Editorial comment on reference [116]. From the Department of Surgery, University of California at Los Angeles.

118. Buchler, M., et al. Human pancreatic tissue concentrations of bactericidal antibiotics. *Gastroenterology* 103:1902, 1992.
     In a comparative analysis, human pancreatic tissue concentrations of 10 different bactericidal antibiotics were determined in 89 patients undergoing pancreatic surgery. Antibiotics studied were mezlocillin, piperacillin, cefotaxime, ceftizoxime, netilmicin, tobramycin, ofloxacin, ciprofloxacin, imipenem, and metronidazole. See related report by C. Bassi et al., Behavior of antibiotics during human necrotizing pancreatitis. Antimicrob. Agents Chemother. 38:830, 1994.

119. Bradley, E.L., III. Antibiotics in acute pancreatitis: Current and future directions. *Am. J. Surg.* 158:472, 1989.
     State-of-the-art review of this topic as of 1989.

120. Craig, R.M., Dordal, E., and Myles, L. The use of ampicillin in acute pancreatitis. *Ann. Intern. Med.* 83:831, 1975.
     Initially 1 g ampicillin q6h was used.

121. Howes, R., Zuidema, G.D., and Cameron, J.L. Evaluation of prophylactic antibiotics in acute pancreatitis. *J. Surg. Res.* 18:197, 1975.
     Compares intravenous ampicillin, 1 g q6h for 5 days, to no antibiotic.

122. Finch, W.T., Sawyers, J.L., and Schenker, S.A. A prospective study to determine the efficacy of antibiotics in acute pancreatitis. *Ann. Surg.* 183:667, 1976.
     This study shows that ampicillin (500 mg–1 g q6h) in acute pancreatitis was not beneficial in reducing infectious complications.

123. Pederzoli, P., et al. A randomized multicenter clinical trial of antibiotic prophylaxis of septic complications in acute necrotizing pancreatitis with imipenem. *Surg. Gynecol. Obstet.* 176:480, 1993.
     Report from the University of Verona, Italy, from six Italian centers. First such study in recent years.

124. Warshaw, A.L., and Gongliang, J. Improved survival in patients with pancreatic abscess. *Ann. Surg.* 202:408, 1985.
     Indiscriminate use of broad-spectrum antibiotics may select out resistant pathogens.

125. Witt, M.D., and Edwards, J.E., Jr. Pancreatic abscess and infected pancreatic pseudocyst: Diagnosis and treatment. *Curr. Clin. Top. Infect. Dis.* 12:111, 1992.

125a. Reber, H.A. Pancreas. In S.I. Schwartz et al (eds.), *Principles of Surgery* (6th ed.). New York: McGraw-Hill, 1994. Pp. 1412–1413.

126. Altemeier, W.A., and Alexander, J.W. Pancreatic abscess. *Arch. Surg.* 87:80, 1963.
     Classic initial study.

127. Fink, A.S., et al. Indolent presentation of pancreatic abscess: Experience with 100 cases. *Arch. Surg.* 123:1087, 1988.
     This series had a high incidence of abscess after alcoholic pancreatitis, but alcoholism was common in the reporting hospital's patient population.

128. McClave, S.A., et al. Pancreatic abscess: 10-year experience at the University of South Florida. *Am. J. Gastroenterol.* 81:180, 1986.

129. Mullins, R.J., et al. Controversies in the management of pancreatic pseudocysts. *Am. J. Surg.* 155:165, 1988.

130. Hsu, H.H., Feinstone, S.M., and Hoofnagle, J.H. Acute Viral Hepatitis. In G.L. Mandell, J.E. Bennett, and R. Dolin (eds.), *Principles and Practice of Infectious Diseases* (4th ed.). New York: Churchill Livingstone, 1995. Pp. 1136–1153.
     For a related paper, see M.J. Koziel, Immunology of viral hepatitis. Am. J. Med. 100:98, 1996.

130a. American Medical Association. Prevention, diagnosis, and management of viral hepatitis: A guide for primary care physicians. Chicago, IL: American Medical Association, 1995.

130b. Hirschman, S.Z. Current approaches to viral hepatitis. *Clin. Infect. Dis.* 20:741, 1995.
     Nice concise discussion of available antiviral therapy.

131. Krawitt, E.L. Chronic Hepatitis. In G.L. Mandell, J.E. Bennett, and R. Dolin (eds.), *Principles and Practice of Infectious Diseases* (4th ed.). New York: Churchill Livingstone, 1995. Pp. 1153–1159.

132. Maddrey, W.C. Chronic hepatitis. *Dis. Mon.* 39:53, 1993.
This Disease-a-Month *issue is devoted to this topic.*
133. Centers for Disease Control. Protection against viral hepatitis. *M.M.W.R.* 39(RR-2):1, 1990.
134. Centers for Disease Control. Update: Universal precautions for the prevention of transmission of human immunodeficiency virus, hepatitis B virus and other blood-borne pathogens in health-care settings. *M.M.W.R.* 37:377, 1988.
135. Coulepis, A.G., Anderson, B.N., and Gust, I.D. Hepatitis A. *Adv. Virus Res.* 32:129, 1987.
136. Margolis, H.S. Epidemiology of hepatitis A in the United States and strategies for the use of hepatitis A vaccine. Symposium on vaccines: On the move in 1994. The American Society for Microbiology's Thirty-Fourth Interscience Conference on Antimicrobial Agents and Chemotherapy. Orlando, Fla., Oct. 6, 1994.
136a. Margolis, H.S., and Alter, M.J. Will hepatitis A become a preventable disease? *Ann. Intern. Med.* 122:464, 1995.
136b. Medical Letter. Hepatitis A vaccine. *Med. Lett. Drugs Ther.* 37:51, 1995.
See also R. Clemens et al, Clinical experience with an inactivated hepatitis A vaccine. J. Infect. Dis. *171(Suppl. 1):S44, 1995, which summarizes many clinical trials.*
137. Wezberger, A., et al. A controlled trial of a formalin-inactivated hepatitis A vaccine in healthy children. *N. Engl. J. Med.* 327:453–457, 1992.
138. Tong, M.J., Co, R.L., and Bellak, C. Hepatitis A vaccination. *West. J. Med.* 158:602–605, 1993.
139. Innis, B.L., et al. Protection against hepatitis A by an inactivated vaccine. *J.A.M.A.* 271:1328, 1994.
In this study performed in Thailand, protective efficacy was 94% after two doses.
139a. Brewer, M.A., et al. Who should receive hepatitis A vaccine? *Pediatr. Infect. Dis. J.* 14:258, 1995.
140. Lemon, S.M. Inactivated hepatitis A vaccines. *J.A.M.A.* 271:1363, 1994.
Editorial comment on references [137, 139]. It is estimated that these vaccines will provide protection for 5–10 years, perhaps longer.
141. Robinson, W.S. Hepatitis B virus and hepatitis D virus. In G.L. Mandell, J.E. Bennett, and R. Dolin (eds.), *Principles and Practice of Infectious Diseases* (4th ed.). New York: Churchill Livingstone, 1995. Pp. 1406–1438.
141a. Hyams, K.C. Risks of chronicity following acute hepatitis B virus infection: A review. *Clin. Infect. Dis.* 20:992, 1995.
141b. Dienstag, J.L., et al. A preliminary trial of lamivudine for chronic hepatitis B infection. *N. Engl. J. Med.* 333:1657, 1995.
142. Alter, M.J. Non-A, non-B hepatitis: Sorting through a diagnosis of exclusion. *Ann. Intern. Med.* 110:583, 1989.
143. Davis, G.L. Hepatitis C Virus. In G.L. Mandell, J.E. Bennett, and R.G. Douglas, Jr. (eds.), *Principles and Practice of Infectious Diseases* (update 10, June). New York: Churchill Livingstone, 1991.
See next reference for an update.
144. Lemon, S.M., and Brown, E.A. Hepatitis C Virus. In G.L. Mandell, J.E. Bennett, and R. Dolin (eds.), *Principles and Practice of Infectious Diseases* (4th ed.). New York: Churchill Livingstone, 1995. Pp. 1474–1486.
For a related review by these same authors, see Hepatitis C and chronic liver disease. Curr. Clin. Top. Infect. Dis. *14:120, 1994.*
See also S. Iwarson et al., Hepatitis C: Natural history of a unique infection. Clin. Infect. Dis. *20:1361, 1995. For an interesting commentary, see Hepatitis C: An unsolved mystery.* Harvard Health Letter *21(No. 4):1–3, 1996.*
145. Tang, E. Hepatitis C virus: A review. *West. J. Med.* 155:164, 1991.
See related review by E.R. Schiff and N.J. Greenberger, The patient with chronic hepatitis C. Hosp. Pract. Aug. 15, 1993.
146. Resnick, R.H., and Koff, R. Hepatitis C–related hepatocellular carcinoma. *Arch. Intern. Med.* 153:1672–1677, 1993.
147. Agnello, V., Chung, R.T., and Kaplon, L.M. A role for hepatitis C virus infections in type II cryoglobulinemia. *N. Engl. J. Med.* 327:1490–1495, 1992.
148. Aledort, L.M. Consequences of chronic hepatitis C. *Am. J. Hematol.* 44:29–37, 1993.
149. Pachucki, C.T., et al. Low incidence of sexual transmission of hepatitis C virus in sex partners of seropositive intravenous drug abusers. *J. Infect. Dis.* 164:820, 1991.
150. Hoofnagle, J.H., DiBisceglie, A.M., and Shindo, M. Antiviral therapy of hepatitis C—present and future. *J. Hepatol.* 17(Suppl. 3):S130–S136, 1993.
151. Centers for Disease Control. Delta hepatitis. *M.M.W.R.* 33:493, 1984.

152. Sherlock, S. Landmarks in viral hepatitis. *J.A.M.A.* 252:402, 1984.
153. Bonino, F., and Smedile, A. Delta agent (type D) hepatitis. *Semin. Liver Dis.* 6:28, 1986.
     For an additional clinical summary, see W.S. Robinson, Hepatitis D (Delta) Virus. Curr. Clin. Top. Infect. Dis. *8:84, 1987.*
154. Farci, P., Barbara, C., and Navone, C. Infection with the delta agent in children. *Gut* 26:4, 1985.
155. Bortolotti, F., Calzia, R., and Cadrobbi, P. Liver cirrhosis associated with chronic HBV infection in childhood. *J. Pediatr.* 108:224, 1986.
156. Bonino, F., et al. The Natural History of Chronic Delta Hepatitis. In M. Rizzetto, J.L. Gerin, and R.H. Purcell (eds.), *Hepatitis Delta Virus and Its Infections.* New York: Alan R. Liss, 1987. Pp. 145–152.
157. Schnell, G.A., and Schubert, T.T. Delta hepatitis. *South. Med. J.* 81:952, 1988.
158. Centers for Disease Control. Hepatitis E among U.S. travelers. *M.M.W.R.* 42:1–4, 1993.
     See related paper by A. Zuckerman, Hepatitis E virus. B.M.J. 300:1475, 1990; and recent report by K.C. Hyams et al. Hepatitis E virus infection in Peru. Clin. Infect. Dis. *22:719, 1996.*
159. Bowden, D.S., et al. New hepatitis viruses: Are there enough letters in the alphabet? *Med. J. Australia* 164:87, 1996.
     An enteric agent isolated from human stool samples and transmitted experimentally to primates is a candidate hepatitis F virus. A provisionally designated bloodborne hepatitis G virus is associated with acute and chronic non-ABCDE hepatitis and has worldwide distribution.
160. Linnen, J., et al. Molecular cloning and disease association of hepatitis G virus: A transfusion-transmissable agent. *Science* 271:505, 1996.
     HGV is associated with acute and chronic hepatitis and is transfusion transmissable. It is present within the volunteer blood donor population in the United States. (Approximately 1.7% of blood donors were HGV RNA positive.)
161. Feucht, H. Vertical transmission of hepatitis G. *Lancet* 347:615, 1996.
     HGV infection can be detected by reverse-transcription polymerase chain reaction (RT-PCR). The risk of HGV seems to be increased in people who are also infected with HBV or HCV and in individuals with a history of intravenous drug use.
     Vertical transmission was shown in three of nine infants born to mothers with HGV viremia. During the mean of 13 months follow-up, none of the three infants became icteric or showed biochemical or clinical signs of hepatitis.
162. Jeffers, L.J., et al. Hepatitis G virus infection in patients with acute and chronic liver disease of unknown etiology. (Abstract 302). *Hepatology* 22(Part 2):182A, 1995.
     HGV RNA was detected (with RT-PCR) in 9% of patients with liver disease of unknown etiology. Thus, HGV may be an important agent contributing to acute and chronic liver disease and should be considered in the diagnostic evaluation of patients presenting with liver disease of unknown etiology.

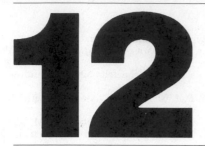

Genitourinary Tract Infections

Thomas T. Ward
and Stephen R. Jones

Urinary tract infections (UTIs) are the most prevalent infection of adults for which antimicrobials are used. UTIs are most often an infection of otherwise healthy people and usually are treated on an outpatient basis. In the United States, symptoms of dysuria, urgency, or frequency result in three to four clinic visits per 100 adult women, and 80% or more of such episodes lead to the use of laboratory tests or to the prescription of drug therapy, or both. In addition to the inconvenience and cost posed by UTIs, infections occasionally result in protracted illness and serious disease, including gram-negative sepsis and death.

General Approach to UTIs

I. **Terminology.** The term **urinary tract infection** is a general one, referring only to the presence of bacteria in the urine. More appropriate terminology should indicate the anatomic area actually involved in infection.
   A. **Lower UTIs.** In women, dysuria and increased urinary frequency may be seen with cystitis, urethritis, or vaginitis. As discussed later, attention to the patient's history, with detailed characterization of dysuric symptoms, may help differentiate the site of infection.
      1. **Cystitis** refers to infection of the bladder and is itself frequently called **lower UTI.** This most common site of UTI is a **superficial mucosal infection** and is much easier to eradicate than renal parenchymal infection.
      2. **Urethritis,** or inflammation of the urethra, frequently is caused by sexually transmitted pathogens.
         a. **Urethritis in men** is associated with urethral discharge or dysuria, or both, but without increased frequency. This entity is **discussed** in detail **in Chap. 13** under Urethritis.
         b. **Urethritis in women** is associated with the same symptoms as cystitis. These patients often complain of dysuria and increased frequency, but their urine cultures are sterile or show small numbers of bacteria.
      3. **Prostatitis and epididymitis.** Infections of the prostate may be associated with syndromes of acute and chronic disease. Chronic bacterial prostatitis is the principal cause of recurrent cystitis in men. Complications of prostatitis such as epididymitis may uncommonly occur.
   B. **Upper UTIs**
      1. **Acute pyelonephritis** refers to an **inflammatory process of the renal paren-chyma.** This is most often due to bacteria but occasionally may be caused by fungi. These tissue infections are more difficult to eradicate than bladder infections, which usually involve only the superficial mucosa.
      2. **Chronic pyelonephritis** refers to a histopathologic pattern of diffuse, interstitial inflammatory disease of the kidneys that is not specific for infection. When related to infection, it is not possible to differentiate changes of active disease from residuum of past infection. Although this term continues to be used, it has **little clinical meaning.** Relapsing infection from presumptive, silent, persistent renal parenchymal infection is better termed **subclinical pyelo-nephritis.**
   C. **Uncomplicated versus complicated UTI**
      1. **Uncomplicated UTI** generally refers to cystitis in nonpregnant young adult to middle-aged women without underlying anatomical (structural) abnormality or neurologic dysfunction. These patients represent the largest single group with UTI. They are characterized by the ease with which their infections

respond to antimicrobial therapy. Recently, sexually active young men with acute dysuria and uncomplicated cystitis have been described (see discussion under UTI in Adult Men).

2. **Complicated UTI** includes those UTIs that occur at sites other than the bladder (e.g., pyelonephritis), and those in children, most men, and pregnant women, as well as UTIs associated with obstruction, foreign body (e.g., catheter), elevated postvoiding residual volume (see sec. **II.C.3.a**), renal transplant recipients, and surgically created ileal loop [1, 1a]. Some have further suggested a **"high-risk" group,** which includes a patient with immunosuppression, pregnancy, diabetes mellitus, sickle cell anemia, or UTI caused by an organism resistant to most antibiotics [1a]. **Complicated UTIs** are characteristically more difficult to treat and may deserve radiographic or urologic investigation [1].

II. **Epidemiology and pathophysiology.** In early infancy (< 3 months of age), UTIs occur more frequently in boys than in girls, but the ratio reverses thereafter; elderly men and women have about the same prevalence of infection (Table 12-1).

The normal urinary tract in men and women is bacteriologically sterile, with the exception of the distal urethra, which may be colonized with a variety of gram-positive and gram-negative bacteria.

A. **Ascending infection.** Work by Stamey [2] has shown that the **ascending route of infection** (i.e., urethral organisms spreading to or invading the bladder) **is the most important** means by which the urinary tract becomes infected.

1. Microorganisms causing initial and recurrent infections in women are coliform bacteria that colonize the vaginal introitus, the urethra and, subsequently, the bladder.

2. **In men, the prostate plays a major role in recurrent UTIs.** These infections may or may not be associated with obstruction of the urinary tract.

B. **Hematogenous infection** is much less common. UTIs secondary to bacteremia may occur but are rare.

1. **Renal abscess.** The kidney may be the site of the UTI in patients with bacteremia or endocarditis due to *Staphylococcus aureus,* as discussed under Intrarenal and Perinephric Abscess later in this chapter.

Table 12-1. Overview of the epidemiology of UTI by age group

Age group (yr)	Females		Males	
	Period prevalence (%)	Risk factors	Period prevalence (%)	Risk factors
<1	1	Anatomic or functional urologic abnormalities	1.0	Anatomic or functional urologic abnormalities
1–5	4–5	Congenital abnormalities, vesicoureteral reflux	0.5	Congenital abnormalities, uncircumcised penis
6–15	4–5	Vesicoureteral reflux	0.5	None
16–35	20	Sexual intercourse, diaphragm use	0.5	Homosexuality
36–65	35	Gynecologic surgery, bladder prolapse	20.0	Prostatic hypertrophy, obstruction, catheterization, surgery
Over 65	40	As above, plus incontinence, chronic catheterization	35.0	As above, plus incontinence, long-term catheterization

Source: W. E. Stamm, Approach to the Patient with Urinary Tract Infection. In S. L. Gorbach, J. G. Bartlett, and N. R. Blacklow (eds.), *Infectious Disease.* Philadelphia: Saunders, 1992.

2. **Acute pyelonephritis** can occur by the hematogenous route as a result of gram-negative bacteremia, but this is rare.

C. **Determinants of infection.** The inoculum of bacteria present, virulence of the organism, and defense mechanisms inherent in the urinary tract will determine whether infection is established [4–5].

1. **Inoculum size.** Size of the inoculum is particularly important and has been best studied in hematogenous infections. Experimental evidence has shown that delivery of large numbers of organisms to the kidney is required to initiate infection.

2. **Virulence of the organism.** The ability of bacteria to establish infection within the urinary tract varies with the individual strain. Nearly any species of bacterium or fungus can produce lower UTI. Only certain species, however, are likely to cause pyelonephritis. These include Enterobacteriaceae, *Pseudomonas* spp., enterococci, and certain fungi.

   Fimbria-mediated adherence (i.e., the ability to attach to a mucosal surface) by uropathogenic *Escherichia coli* to vaginal and uroepithelial cells determines infectivity and, in some cases, the propensity to develop upper tract infection. Studies have characterized several specific bacterial protein ligands and host cell carbohydrate receptor sites. Cranberry juice has been purported to prevent adherence of uropathogens to uroepithelial cells and, in one study in elderly women, has been reported to decrease the frequency of bacteriuria [2a].

3. **Host defense mechanisms.** As many as one-third of patients with bacteriuria undergo spontaneous cure. Defense mechanisms are present throughout the urinary tract and contribute to resistance of the tract to infection. Some examples follow.

   a. **Complete bladder emptying** is one of the most important defense mechanisms. When residual urine volumes are high, large numbers of bacteria may remain in the urine. The ability to expel bacteria is complete when voiding is complete. This concept is important in understanding the association between urinary infection and neurologic or urologic diseases (e.g., diabetes with neurogenic bladder, or obstruction) that allow bacteria to grow in the residual urine [3]. A postvoiding residual urine volume of more than 100 ml is considered severe enough urinary retention to be associated with UTI [1a].

   b. **High fluid intake and frequent voiding** may also be important. These may allow for washout of bacteria and form the basis for recommendations that patients with UTI increase their fluid intake and void frequently. Theoretically, such advice seems sound, but there is no evidence that hydration improves the results of appropriate antibiotic therapy.

   c. **The vesicoureteral valve** also may provide a barrier to the spread of infection by preventing reflux of bacteria once bladder bacteriuria is established.

   d. **Length of the urethra.** The relatively long urethra is believed to protect against infection in men. The shorter female urethra probably allows entry of bacteria from urethra to bladder, and this, in part, may account for the higher frequency of UTI in women.

   e. **Vaginal flora.** Vaginal colonization with lactobacilli appears to prevent vaginal colonization and bacteriuria with *E. coli* and other uropathogens. **By altering the normal vaginal flora, contraceptive diaphragm and spermicide use, as well as postmenopausal vaginal atrophy,** increase introital colonization with Enterobacteriaceae and result in an increased likelihood of recurrent UTIs [6].

4. **Urinary tract abnormalities.** A number of urinary tract abnormalities interfere with the defense mechanisms just noted [4–5].

   a. **Obstruction** anywhere in the urinary tract increases susceptibility of the kidney to infection. The exact role of urinary stasis in obstruction-related infection, however, has not been defined. Specific types of obstruction include ureteral obstruction (ureteral calculi and congenital abnormalities such as stenosis and ureteral valves) and urethral obstruction (prostatic hypertrophy).

   b. **Vesicoureteral reflux** increases the susceptibility of the kidney to infection by providing a route for ascending infection and interfering with the normal flow of urine. Reflux can be either the cause of infection or its result. Endotoxin from gram-negative bacteria inhibits ureteral peristalsis. During acute lower tract infection in adults, reflux from bladder to ureter often is present and resolves as the acute infection resolves.

    c. **Incomplete bladder emptying.** Because urine acts as a culture medium for bacterial growth, residual urine can serve as a source of infection.

    d. **Foreign bodies** also serve as a nidus for infection. Renal **calculi** and **indwelling bladder catheters** are the foreign bodies implicated most frequently in UTI.

  5. **Diabetes mellitus in women** appears to increase the frequency of UTI, including upper tract infections and nosocomial infections [6a]. The cause of the high prevalence of UTI with upper tract involvement is speculative, and a combination of factors is probably involved, including bladder dysfunction as a result of diabetic neuropathy, structural abnormalities (e.g., cystocele, rectocele), recurrent vaginitis, and underlying vascular disease [6a].

III. **Clinical manifestations.** Localization studies make it clear that clinically it is very difficult, if not impossible, to distinguish upper from lower UTIs. Urinary frequency, dysuria, lower abdominal-suprapubic discomfort, and even costovertebral angle (CVA) or flank discomfort are nonspecific and may be seen both in upper and lower UTI [5].

  A. **Lower UTIs. Clinically, it is not possible to distinguish cystitis from urethritis in women; vaginitis may also cause dysuria. UTI symptoms in men should direct attention to excluding concurrent prostate disease.**

    1. **Acute cystitis**

      a. **Dysuria,** or burning during or just after urination, as well as urgency and increased frequency of urination, often are associated with cystitis. Suprapubic pain, fullness, or a sensation of pressure may also be present. Gross or microscopic hematuria occurs in approximately 50% of women with acute cystitis [1a] but is uncommon with other causes of dysuria. Obstructive symptoms may predominate in men. The patient may complain of CVA or flank discomfort, making these latter findings unreliable in distinguishing upper from lower UTI.

        Physical examination often is unremarkable; the patient may complain only of pain on suprapubic palpation. Patients should be examined for CVA tenderness. Inspection and palpation of the external genitalia along with rectal examination should be performed in men. In women, vaginal examination may be indicated.

        Ordinarily, no systemic symptoms are present in uncomplicated lower UTI. Fever generally is absent, although low-grade temperature elevations are not uncommon. In women, prior episodes of confirmed cystitis and diaphragm use suggest a diagnosis of cystitis [6].

      b. **Vaginitis** also must be considered as it may present with dysuria caused by irritation of the mucosal surface by the urine stream. **Vaginitis should be suspected when patients complain of perineal, labial, or external dysuria, which may be accompanied by odor, itching, or vaginal discharge.** Patients may describe the pain on urination as being more delayed than the discomfort that often begins before or at initiation of voiding with cystitis or urethritis. If these symptoms are present, a pelvic examination should be performed and appropriate vaginal, cervical, and urethral cultures obtained. See Chap. 13 for a discussion of vulvovaginitis.

    2. **Urethritis**

      a. **Urethritis in women** is a very common problem. Studies have shown that as many as **one-third of women presenting with symptoms of lower UTI have urethritis without cystitis.** These patients exhibit symptoms of increased frequency and dysuria and, therefore, the clinical presentation is identical to that in cystitis. Patients usually are afebrile. Urinalysis demonstrates pyuria but not bacteriuria. Clues in the history that suggest a sexually transmitted cause of urethritis include suspected or proved sexually transmitted disease (STD) in a sex partner or the presence of a new or multiple sex partners.

      b. **Urethritis in men** frequently is suggested by concurrent dysuria and urethral discharge. Urinalysis may demonstrate pyuria. Historic clues to STD, as discussed in **a,** should be sought. Urethritis in men is discussed in Chap. 13.

    3. **Prostatitis** symptoms may be those of cystitis, with dysuria, frequency, and urgency, or symptoms of bladder outlet obstruction may predominate, with

hesitancy, diminished stream, nocturia, or postmicturition dribbling. Perineal or low back pain may, on occasion, be the only manifestation. Physical examination findings that help differentiate acute from chronic prostatitis are discussed in sec. **III** under UTI in Adult Men. Examination should include inspection and palpation for evidence of urethral discharge, penile lesions, local epididymal or testicular disease, and inguinal adenopathy [7].

B. Upper UTIs. Clues from the medical history that suggest an increased likelihood of upper UTI include a prior history of pyelonephritis or structural abnormalities of the urinary tract, UTIs in childhood, diabetes, prolonged symptoms with the current episode (7 or more days), and failure to respond to single-dose or 3-day short-course therapy administered for presumed cystitis.

  1. **Pyelonephritis** [7a]. Some patients with **acute** pyelonephritis have characteristic findings of high fever (39.5°–40.5°C [103°–105°F]), shaking chills, and lumbar pain. Many authorities argue that **fever may be the most reliable clinical finding** in differentiating between upper and lower UTI. Presence of shaking chills implies that the UTI may be complicated by bacteremia. These findings may develop rapidly over a period of a few hours or 1–2 days and occur with or without antecedent or concurrent symptoms of lower UTI. Nausea, vomiting, and diarrhea or constipation also may be seen. Examination often reveals CVA and flank tenderness, but this may be a nonspecific finding. Urinalysis in most patients reveals significant pyuria (at least 10 leukocytes per cubic millimeter or per high-power field of the spun sediment), but 4–5% of cases of pyelonephritis do not involve pyuria [8].

    Some authors have subdivided syndromes of pyelonephritis [7a].

    a. **Uncomplicated pyelonephritis,** which usually refers to pyelonephritis in women, including many episodes of acute pyelonephritis, pyelonephritis in pregnancy, and silent (subclinical) pyelonephritis.

    b. **Complicated pyelonephritis** is generally the result of structural and functional abnormalities (e.g., obstruction, including prostate hypertrophy, calculi, reflux, neurogenic bladder) and/or urologic manipulations (catheters, renal transplantation) and those with underlying disease (e.g., diabetes, immunosuppression, cystic renal disease) and the elderly.

  2. **Renal abscesses** present with signs and symptoms identical to pyelonephritis and should be **considered** in the patient with upper UTI whose **fever persists beyond 48–72 hours despite appropriate antimicrobial therapy** [9].

IV. Laboratory diagnosis of UTI focuses on the determination of the presence or absence of pyuria and bacteriuria. Rapid tests for the detection of leukocytes and bacteria in urine are available. Comprehensive laboratory testing in every patient is not needed for clinical management; indiscriminate use of urine cultures results in unnecessary costs. The management of UTI, the most common infection for which adults receive antimicrobial agents, should emphasize cost-effective strategies.

A. Microscopic examination of urine. Laboratory diagnosis in the patient with suspected UTI should usually begin with microscopic examination for leukocytes in the urine sediment. **Pyuria still is considered a useful indicator of UTI, and its absence should suggest an alternative diagnosis.** Pyuria in the elderly may be a nonspecific finding, but its absence means that bacteriuria is unlikely (see sec. **V.C** under UTI in the Elderly).

  When a health care provider has a long-standing relationship with a reliable patient who has recurrent uncomplicated UTIs, it is reasonable and cost-effective not to do a urinalysis (or culture) but rather to treat empirically.

  1. **Pyuria.** Unspun or spun urine (2,000 rpm, for 5 minutes) can be used. The most accurate method for diagnosis is counting leukocytes in unspun urine using a chamber method [1a, 9a], although many clinical laboratories find this a cumbersome technique. Although different levels for pyuria have been proposed, a WBC count of 10 cells/mm³ by the counting chamber method seems to be the best diagnostic cutoff [1a].

    a. The **leukocyte esterase dipstick** is employed widely as a rapid, alternative office test for the detection of pyuria; it is 75–95% sensitive in detecting pyuria associated with infection. Although not as reliable as the chamber method to define pyuria, the leukocyte esterase dipstick is an acceptable alternative [9a]. (See related discussion in sec. **C.**)

    b. The WBC count may vary depending on urine flow, state of hydration, previous antibiotic treatment, and method of specimen collection.

    c. "Sterile pyuria" may be associated with acute urethritis, renal tuberculosis, foreign body or tumor of the urinary tract, nonbacterial infections in the genital tract [8], and a poorly understood entity called *interstitial cystitis,* which is typically seen in women with chronic dysuria and urgency. (The etiology and treatment of this problem remains unclear [9b].)

  d. The absence of pyuria in the symptomatic patient suggests that cystitis is not the cause of dysuria, and urethritis or vaginitis should be considered as alternative diagnoses.

2. **Bacteria** seen on microscopic examination, especially of the unspun urine, can be a useful test for the presumptive diagnosis of UTI [3]. Generally, bacteria counts of fewer than 10^5 colony-forming units (CFU) per milliliter cannot be seen microscopically. Falsely elevated numbers of bacteria may be noted if the specimen was improperly collected or if the specimen was allowed to stand at room temperature for long periods of time before centrifugation. Numbers of bacteria may be decreased by the same factors that cause low numbers of WBCs in urine.

  a. **A Gram stain** of one drop of fresh-voided, unspun urine can be done quickly and easily. The finding of 1 bacterium or more in each oil-immersion field suggests the presence of at least 10^5 CFU/ml urine. When several fields must be searched for the presence of bacteria, the quantitative counts are generally lower, ranging from approximately 10^4 to 10^5 CFU/ml. With experience in its use, this Gram stain technique has been shown to correlate well with the quantitative urine culture.

  Anecdotally, we suspect Gram stains of unspun urine are not done as often as in the past. **We believe they are still especially useful in the patient with presumed urosepsis,** severe pyelonephritis, and in patients at risk for enterococcal UTI (e.g., elderly men). If the Gram stain of the unspun urine shows gram-positive cocci, enterococci may be the pathogen, and empiric therapy should be active against enterococci. By contrast, if the Gram stain of unspun urine reveals gram-negative bacilli, empiric therapy aimed at enterococci is not necessary.

  b. **Microscopic examination of spun urine** for WBCs and bacteria can be done under high, dry power. With this method, the presence of more than 1 bacteria on a Gram stain correlates well with more than 10^4 bacteria/ml [10].

3. **Hematuria,** as detected by rapid dipstick methods within the office setting, occurs in approximately 50% of women with acute cystitis but is uncommon in urethritis or vaginitis. Thus, microscopic hematuria in acutely dysuric young women is a marker of cystitis.

B. **Urine culture.** Urine is normally a sterile body fluid. Care in urine collection for culture is important to prevent contamination from the urethra, vagina, or perineum. It is to be emphasized that obtaining a clean-catch, midstream, voided urine is cumbersome and difficult for many patients.

  In recent years it has become common practice and is more cost effective in women who have uncomplicated UTIs (i.e., symptoms of cystitis and urinalysis findings of pyuria) to prescribe treatment without an initial or follow-up urine culture [11, 12]. **Urine cultures still are advised in pyelonephritis, complicated UTI** (see sec. **I.C**), **and in recurrent UTI** (except in recurrent episodes of UTI that are clearly associated with sexual activity) [1a]. Cultures are also suggested to help assess for asymptomatic bacteriuria in certain settings, including (1) pregnancy, (2) before and after urological manipulation, and (3) after definitive removal of a chronic indwelling Foley catheter [1a].

1. **Clean-catch urine specimen.** Collection of the urine specimen should be done with care. The specimen can be split, with a portion being used for urinalysis and the rest for culture.

  a. **Female patients** can be instructed to wash their hands, straddle or squat over the toilet, and spread the labia with the nondominant hand. Then, using the dominant hand, they should swab the vulva three times, front to back, with sterile gauze pads soaked in sterile water or with a sponge soaked in a mild nonhexachlorophene soap. The first 10 ml of voided urine is the urethral specimen and is discarded, unless it is saved to help diagnose urethritis. The urine specimen collected in a sterile cup during the middle of voiding (midstream sample) is used for culture. It should be quickly processed or refrigerated [1a].

  b. **Male patients** can be instructed to retract the foreskin and clean the glans penis three times using gauze pads or sponges. However, some studies have questioned the necessity of these steps in a male, when only a midstream collection is necessary [1a]. (See related discussion under sec. **III.A.1** under UTI in Adult Men.)

   c. **Other collections. In the very obese, acutely ill, or infirm, a single, straight catheterization may be performed to obtain a clean sample for urinalysis and culture.** Suprapubic aspirations also can be performed and may be particularly useful in children.

2. **Urine culture interpretation.** Because microbiology laboratories vary in the degree to which they have adopted new criteria for what is significant bacteriuria, and because of ambiguities in the interpretation of newer guidelines, it is important for physicians and microbiology laboratory personnel to work together in interpreting how the bacteriologic workup of urine should be approached in the laboratory.

   a. **Clean-catch urine.** The older criterion proposed that urine counts exceeding 100,000 CFU/ml (i.e., $\geq 10^5$ bacteria/ml) were significant, and counts of 10,000 CFU/ml or less from clean-catch specimens were generally considered contaminants. Studies from Stamm and others [9a, 13, 14, 14a] have emphasized that approximately one-third of women with acute lower UTI have colony counts in midstream urine of between 10^2 and 10^4 CFU/ml. **In acutely dysuric women with confirmed pyuria, therefore, the threshold for significant bacteriuria should be 10^2 CFU/ml or more of a single or predominant uropathogen** (e.g., *E. coli, Pseudomonas aeruginosa, Staphylococcus saprophyticus*). Low colony counts of diphtheroids, lactobacilli, *Gardnerella vaginalis,* and *Staphylococcus epidermidis* are consistent with contaminants [9a].

   In men, only limited data on the significance of lower colony counts in voided urine are available; in one study comparing voided urine with bladder specimens, approximately one-third of men with bladder bacteriuria had colony counts in midstream urine of greater than 10^3 CFU/ml but less than 10^5 CFU/ml [15]. **In dysuric men, growth of 10^3 CFU/ml or more of a single or predominant uropathogen should be regarded as significant for presumptive UTI.**

   b. **Multiple isolates.** Voided urine cultures revealing two or more species of bacteria with no predominant organism are seen frequently. In people with normal urinary tracts, these usually represent contaminated urine samples; therefore, the culture should be repeated, with meticulous care in the collection of the specimen.

   c. **Straight catheter and suprapubic aspiration specimens.** Colony counts are considered to be significant if greater than 10^2 CFU/ml of a single or predominant uropathogen are cultured.

   d. **Indwelling catheter.** Culture of urine specimens obtained by indwelling catheter frequently yields multiple isolates that change rapidly over time. Identification and susceptibility testing is most commonly performed on the one or two organisms that are clearly predominant at 10^4 CFU/ml or more.

   e. **Limitations of urine culture** [8]

      (1) **Transport time.** Delays is transport from collection of the urine specimen to processing in the laboratory can affect colony counts considerably. In general, a urine culture should be processed as soon as possible after collection. Urine specimens may be stored at room temperature for 1 hour, or in a refrigerator for up to 48 hours, without appreciable changes in bacterial counts. **Storage at room temperature for 2 hours or more will result in significant increases in bacterial counts, and the results of such specimens cannot be reliably interpreted.**

      (2) **Fastidious microorganisms.** Standard urine culture procedures are directed toward routine uropathogens. Unusual microorganisms should be considered in patients with unexplained pyuria or when there is suspicion of STD. Mycobacteria, fungi, gonococci, chlamydiae, and viruses require special transport media or special culture techniques.

C. **Rapid diagnostic tests.** Multiple tests have become available to detect pyuria and bacteriuria more rapidly. The most reliable chemical measurement of pyuria is the leukocyte esterase dipstick test; although somewhat less sensitive than microscopic examination for leukocytes, it is a useful alternative for the detection of pyuria when urine microscopy is unavailable [16]. (See sec. **A.1.a.**)

Newer bacteriuria screening tests employ nephelometry, bioluminescence, or a colorimetric filtration system. They yield comparable results, and all have a sensitivity similar to the urine Gram stain; none of the tests detect fewer than 10^4 CFU/ml. Because a urine culture is often not done in young to middle-aged women with uncomplicated UTI, the need for these rapid culture screens has diminished. For recurrent UTI or complicated UTI, a urine culture with suscepti-bilities is advised (see sec. **B**).

D. Blood cultures. As many as 30–40% of patients with pyelonephritis will have positive blood cultures. In general, blood cultures should be obtained in those patients with a fever and a history of rigors, as well as in patients sufficiently ill to be hospitalized, especially if prior antibiotic therapy may have selected out resistant pathogens. The need for blood cultures has been debated by some in this cost conscious era. With the availability of good oral agents and the common practice to treat for 2 weeks the complex UTI (e.g., pyelonephritis) with or without bacteremia, the need for blood cultures may be superfluous [9b]. This is an unre-solved issue and the approach needs to be individualized.

V. Microbiologic features of UTIs. Organisms causing UTI are derived primarily from the aerobic members of the fecal flora. In women, these microorganisms colonize the perineum as a way station to the urinary tract and, in men, the prostate may be colonized or subclinically infected.

A. Bacteria. Bacteria involved include members of the family Enterobacteriaceae: *E. coli* and *Klebsiella, Enterobacter, Serratia, Proteus,* and *Providencia* spp. are most frequently seen in uncomplicated UTI. Of these, *E. coli* accounts for up to 80% of all infections. *Pseudomonas* spp. and group D streptococci account for approximately 5–10% of uncomplicated infections and are associated most often with instrumentation of the urinary tract.

Coagulase-negative staphylococci (e.g., *S. saprophyticus*) may be pathogenic more often than was previously realized. Formerly believed to be urinary contami-nants, *S. saprophyticus* have been documented in urine by suprapubic catheteriza-tion, ureteral aspiration, and renal biopsy culture. Generally, patients with UTI due to *S. saprophyticus* (1) are young female patients in the 16- to 25-year-old group, (2) have pyuria, and (3) have symptoms of lower UTI. *S. saprophyticus* is rarely the cause of UTI in hospitalized patients unless there has been instrumenta-tion of the genitourinary tract. Again, the organism will be recovered on serial cultures if it is a significant pathogen.

See Table 12-2 for a list of microbial species commonly associated with UTIs.

B. Fungi. The presence of fungi in the urine often presents a diagnostic dilemma.

Table 12-2. Microbial species most often associated with specific types of UTIs

	Acute uncomplicated cystitis (%)	Acute uncomplicated pyelonephritis (%)	Complicated UTI (%)	Catheter-associated UTI (%)
E. coli	79	89	32	24
S. saprophyticus	11	0	1	0
Proteus	2	4	4	6
Klebsiella	3	4	5	8
Enterococci	2	0	22	7
Pseudomonas	0	0	20	9
Mixed	3	5	10	11
Other	0	2	5	10
Yeast	0	0	1	28
S. epidermidis	0	0	15	8

Source: M. E. Falagas and S. L. Gorbach, Practical guidelines: Urinary tract infections. *Infect. Dis. Clin. Pract.* 4:242, 1995.

For the purpose of this and later discussions, the term **fungi** will refer to organisms such as *Candida albicans,* other *Candida* spp., and *Torulopsis glabrata (Candida glabrata).* Fungi are isolated most frequently in diabetics, in patients with indwelling bladder catheters, in those receiving antibiotics and, occasionally, in patients who have had previous instrumentation of the urinary tract.

C. **Viruses.** Viruria occurs in a variety of systemic illnesses such as measles, mumps, and infections with herpes simplex virus, cytomegalovirus, and adenovirus. There is indirect evidence to suggest that viruses may also be responsible for certain renal lesions, including glomerulonephritis. The role of varicella-zoster virus in hemorrhagic cystitis is well documented, and adenovirus has been strongly implicated as a cause of a similar syndrome. Adenovirus type 8 has been associated with hemorrhagic cystitis in children.

D. *Chlamydia trachomatis, Neisseria gonorrhoeae* **and herpes simplex virus.** These are the major causes of urethritis in women, an infection in which dysuria may falsely suggest a diagnosis of cystitis [13].

E. *Trichomonas vaginalis* **and** *Candida* **species.** These are the principal pathogens associated with vaginitis, an alternative cause of dysuria in young women that may be confused with UTI (see Chap. 13).

VI. **Indications for urologic workup.** In treating patients with UTIs, the question of when to perform a urologic evaluation often arises. The goals of radiologic imaging studies and urologic evaluation are to identify correctable anatomic abnormalities (e.g., obstruction) that may predispose to recurrent UTIs, and/or prevent adequate response without urologic intervention.

Although the intravenous pyelogram (IVP) was commonly used in the past [17], in recent years **renal ultrasound and abdominal CT scans have commonly replaced the IVP** [1a, 9a, 9b]. Renal ultrasound is very useful to assess noninvasively for obstructive neuropathy. CT scan will help identify renal abscesses.

A. **UTI in male patients.** UTIs in men are infrequent compared to their incidence in women, and bacteriuria in men may be the first sign of an anatomic or functional abnormality.

1. **In boys,** the first UTI warrants ultrasonographic evaluation of the kidneys (to detect malformation or scarring) and voiding cystography (to detect vesicoureteral reflux and urethral obstruction) [18]. See related discussion under UTI in Children.

2. **In young men,** there has been recent recognition that uncomplicated cystitis can occur and that urologic evaluation usually is unrewarding in those who respond to a 7-day course of therapy (see UTI in Adult Men). In older men, persistent or recurrent bacteriuria is frequently an indication of prostatic enlargement and obstruction or of chronic prostatitis. In addition to a physical examination of the prostate, intravenous pyelogram and cystoscopy may also be useful. For further discussion, see secs. **II** and **III** under UTI in Adult Men.

B. **UTI in female patients.** When to initiate investigation in female patients is controversial, particularly in the highly prevalent group of middle-aged to older women with recurrent UTIs, a group who rarely exhibit anatomic or functional abnormalities.

1. Imaging studies should be performed after the first UTI in girls younger than 5 years of age, older girls with recurrent UTIs, and in any child with pyelonephritis. As in boys, renal ultrasonography and voiding cystography are indicated; however, radionuclide voiding cystography can be substituted as a screening test to detect the presence of vesicoureteral reflux. If the facilities are available, radionuclide cystography greatly reduces ovarian radiation exposure in comparison to conventional fluoroscopic voiding cystourethrography. See related discussion under UTI in Children later in this chapter.

2. Most recurrent UTIs in adult women are exogenous reinfections rather than relapsing infections due to the same organism. Documented relapsing infections should prompt urologic evaluation to exclude a treatable anatomic defect. Postmenopausal women should be evaluated for increased postvoiding residual associated with bladder or uterine prolapse.

C. **Pyelonephritis.** Upper UTI should manifest a clinical response within 72 hours of initiation of appropriate antimicrobial therapy. If flank pain or fever persists for longer than 72 hours, ultrasonography or computed tomography should be performed to exclude unrecognized obstruction or intrarenal or perinephric abscess. Routine radiologic imaging studies for all cases of pyelonephritis is generally unrewarding and unnecessarily expensive. Patients with a prolonged clinical course, recurrent upper UTI, or a childhood history of infection should be evaluated for anatomic or functional abnormalities.

General Management
Principles of UTIs

I. **Nonspecific treatment** [19]

  A. **Hydration.** Forcing fluids has long been advocated in the initial treatment of UTI. There are theoretic reasons for and against it. The benefit of hydration has never been critically documented in clinical studies; it probably is not necessary once appropriate antimicrobial treatment has been instituted.

  B. **Urinary analgesics.** Such pain relievers as phenazopyridine hydrochloride (e.g., Pyridium, 200 mg PO tid after meals) may be useful to relieve symptoms of severe dysuria or urethral irritation but generally are necessary only for the first 24–48 hours of treatment if they are used at all. It is best to prescribe only a small number of tablets, for a 1- or 2-day period, as many patients mistakenly will use the drug as primary treatment and will avoid consulting a physician in the event of relapse or reinfection. It should be stressed to the patient that this drug is only adjunctive treatment and is not an antibiotic. Phenazopyridine should be avoided in pregnancy and probably in nursing mothers also.

  We suspect these agents are used less frequently in recent years with the availability of very effective antimicrobial regimens.

II. **General principles of antimicrobial therapy** [19]. The choice of therapy in UTI will depend on the patient's age and gender, on whether the infection is symptomatic or asymptomatic, on the presumed site of infection (upper versus lower), and on whether the UTI is recurrent. **Specific treatment guidelines based on these considerations are discussed in this section and are summarized in Table 12-3.** Factors such as whether the infection is community- or hospital-acquired and host considerations such as the presence of impaired renal function or abnormal collecting systems often influence the likely causative pathogen, the severity of illness, and the response to therapy, and therefore will influence the choice of antimicrobial agent.

  A. **Choice of antimicrobial agent.** Many antimicrobial agents with a broad gram-negative spectrum of activity are effective in the treatment of UTI. Most UTIs are localized to the collecting system, and active urine levels are achieved after oral administration of essentially all commonly used antimicrobial agents. Bacteriostatic and bactericidal drugs are of equal efficacy. Given the availability of several drugs microbiologically active against known or suspected uropathogens, considerations in choosing empiric antimicrobial therapy are the patient's history of drug allergy, relative drug toxicities, and cost of available agents.

    1. **Resistance to sulfonamides, ampicillin, and amoxicillin** is now present in 25–35% of *E. coli* strains causing outpatient cystitis, making these agents **no longer the standards for empiric therapy** of gram-negative UTIs.

      Although resistance to trimethoprim and trimethoprim-sulfamethoxazole (TMP-SMX) has been increasing nationwide, in most areas it still is sufficiently uncommon that these two antimicrobial agents remain the empiric therapies of choice on the basis of cost [20]. If a geographical area has a high incidence of TMP resistance to common urinary pathogens (e.g., > 15–20%), then a fluoroquinolone can be used. We would otherwise avoid using the fluoroquinolones routinely in this setting to avoid selecting out resistant pathogens (see sec. **2**). For a discussion of fluoroquinolones, see Chap. 28S.

    2. **UTIs** are the **most common indication** for which antimicrobial agents are prescribed. Small increments in cost of individual therapies have the potential for large aggregate expense. Because of cost and concern with emergence of resistance, the fluoroquinolones should be reserved for complicated UTIs in which resistance has been demonstrated or is likely. Fluoroquinolones are not the agents of choice for uncomplicated cystitis. This is discussed in detail in Chap. 28S.

    3. With **renal functional impairment,** dosage modification is necessary for agents that are primarily renally excreted. See Chap. 28 for details of dosage modifications.

      UTIs in patients with **end-stage renal disease** pose a therapeutic challenge because of the lack of the usual high concentration of antimicrobial agents in the urine. In general, the penicillins and cephalosporins have little nephrotoxicity,

Table 12-3. Antibiotic therapy for adults with symptomatic urinary tract infection (UTI)

Syndrome	Duration	Route	Medication	Dose[a] (mg)	Interval
Cystitis, females, uncomplicated[b]	3 days	PO	TMP[c]	100	q12h
			TMP-SMX[c]	160/800	q12h
			Amoxicillin + clavulanate	500	q8h
			Tetracycline	500	q6h
			Norfloxacin[d]	400	q12h
			Ciprofloxacin[d]	250	q12h
			Ofloxacin[d]	200	q12h
			Nitrofurantoin	100	q6h
	7 days (see text)		Cephalexin	500	q6h
Cystitis, complicated[e]	10–14 days[f]	PO	Same as 3-day regimens for uncomplicated cystitis (shown above) Also:		
			Lomefloxacin[d]	400	q24h
			Enoxacin[d]	400	q12h
Urethritis, female	See Chap. 13				
Urethritis, male	See Chap. 13				
Prostatitis, acute[g]	14 days[f,h]	PO	TMP[c]	100	q12h
			TMP-SMX[c]	160/800	q12h
			Ciprofloxacin[i]	500	q12h
			Ofloxacin[i]	300	q12h
Prostatitis, chronic[g]	6–12 wk[f]	PO	TMP[c]	100	q12h
			TMP-SMX[c]	160/800	q12h
			Ciprofloxacin[i]	500	q12h
			Ofloxacin[i]	500	q12h
Pyelonephritis, outpatient[j]	14 days[f]	PO	TMP[c]	Same as 3-day regimens for uncomplicated cystitis	
			TMP-SMX[c]		
			Amoxicillin + clavulanate		
			Cephalexin		
			Ciprofloxacin	500	q12h
			Ofloxacin	200	q12h
			Enoxacin	400	q12h
Pyelonephritis, hospitalized patient[j]	14 days[f] (IV + PO)[k]	IV	See footnote[l]		

TMP = trimethoprim; SMX = sulfamethoxazole.

[a]**See individual chapter discussions for dose modification in renal failure and details of intramuscular and intravenous regimens.**

[b]Short-course therapy (3 days) may be preferable to single-dose regimens [1]; therefore, the 3-day regimens are emphasized. **Uncomplicated** UTI is cystitis in nonpregnant adult women (young to middle-age), without genitourinary tract structural abnormality or bladder neurologic dysfunction.

[c]Preferred antibiotic selections on the basis of cost.

[d]**The fluoroquinolones are reserved for more resistant pathogens** (see Chap. 28). These agents should be avoided in pregnancy, nursing mothers, and adolescents younger than 17 years of age.

[e]See definition of uncomplicated UTI in footnote[b]. Other UTIs, including those in men, are, by definition, complicated.

[f]Susceptibility of pathogen to selected antibiotic must be confirmed with in vitro susceptibility testing.

[g]**In acute prostatitis,** symptoms included fever, acute perineal pain and discomfort and, usually, signs of an acute lower UTI such as dysuria, frequency, and urgency. The rectal examination reveals a swollen prostate that often is exquisitely tender on palpation, and prostatic massage may precipitate bacteremia. **In chronic prostatitis,** the prostate can remain a persistent source of UTI, with recurrent episodes of UTI. Symptoms are variable, including asymptomatic bacteriuria, perineal or low back discomfort, and relapsing UTI. For further discussion, see text.

Table 12-3 (continued)

[h]Some experts prefer to treat both acute and chronic prostatitis for protracted periods of time (e.g., 4–6+ weeks) to eradicate the infection clearly.
[i]Other fluoroquinolones (e.g., lomefloxacin and enoxacin) are potentially useful agents in this setting, but there is less experience with their use in prostatitis (see Chap. 28S).
[j]The decision regarding outpatient or in-hospital treatment of acute pyelonephritis is primarily one of clinical judgment. It is influenced by the patient's clinical condition, age, underlying disease, and potential compliance. In general, older or frail patients, bacteremic patients, toxic patients, and noncompliant patients will require inpatient therapy initially [5].
[k]Change from intravenous to oral therapy when the patient has clinically improved and is afebrile at least 24–48 hours.
[l]The optimal regimen for a patient admitted with acute pyelonephritis depends on many factors. Enterococci can be in part ruled out if a Gram stain of the urine shows no gram-positive cocci.
  In patients without prior UTI and only moderate illness, cefazolin, 1 g q6–8h, is reasonable.
  In patients who are very ill or who have a history of prior UTI infection (therefore the potential of a resistant gram-negative infection), ampicillin-sulbactam (3 g q6–8h) with or without an aminoglycoside or ampicillin (1.5 g q4h) and an aminoglycoside (see Chap. 28H) can be used, especially if enterococci are a concern.
  If *Pseudomonas aeruginosa* is a concern, an aminoglycoside should be used initially until culture data are available. Vancomycin (see Chap. 28O) can be used instead of ampicillin in the penicillin-allergic patient.
  In patients in whom enterococci is not a concern, a third-generation cephalosporin (e.g., ceftriaxone 2 g q24h) can be used. If *P. aeruginosa* is a consideration, ceftazidime, 2 g q8h, is another alternative.
  Intravenous TMP-SMX, fluoroquinolones, and aztreonam are options for the patient unable to receive the aforementioned regimens. Neither TMP-SMX nor aztreonam is active against enterococci.
  For activity against enterococci, ampicillin, ampicillin-sulbactam, or vancomycin is preferred. The fluoroquinolones also are active against many enterococci.
Sources: Adapted from R. E. Reese and R. F. Betts, *Handbook of Antibiotics* (2nd ed.). Boston: Little, Brown, 1993; and W. E. Stamm and T. M. Hooton, Management of urinary tract infections in adults. *N. Engl. J. Med.* 329:1328, 1993.

attain adequate urine levels despite severe renal functional impairment, and may be the agents of choice in renal failure.

4. **Oral and parenteral therapies** are equally effective in the treatment of UTI provided that the patient is able to take and absorb oral medication adequately. Most patients with pyelonephritis who are ill enough to require hospitalization should be treated initially with parenteral agents until there is symptomatic improvement and fever subsides. (See sec. **III.A** under UTI in Adult Women.) Then, therapy can be completed with an oral regimen.

B. **Duration of therapy.** This primarily depends on the presumed site of infection. **For cystitis** in women, short-course therapy, usually for 3 days, is preferable to the historic 7- to 14-day therapeutic regimen because it is equally efficacious, costs less, is associated with fewer side effects, has a lower incidence of emergence of resistant GI flora, and allows for better compliance. **Based on published studies [5], the authors favor 3-day regimens as more effective than single-dose therapy.** (For single-dose therapy, the best results have been observed with TMP-SMX, 320/1,600 mg, as a single dose. Single-dose therapy with drugs such as amoxicillin and the oral cephalosporins, which are excreted rapidly, has been less efficacious.) Short-course regimens of documented efficacy are shown in Table 12-3 and are discussed in sec. **II.D.2** under UTI in Adult Women. **For pyelonephritis,** typically a 2-week course of antibiotics is advised [7a].

  Extended-duration antimicrobial therapy may be indicated for recurrent infection (as discussed later) and in pyelonephritis failing a 14-day regimen. See sec. **III.A** under UTI in Adult Women.

III. **Determinants of specific antimicrobial therapy. Asymptomatic and symptomatic, acute and recurrent, upper and lower UTIs in children, in adult men and women, in the elderly, and in catheterized patients are discussed separately and in detail later in this chapter.** General comments regarding several of these major determinants of therapy follow.

A. **Age and gender.** Children with UTIs and severe vesicoureteral reflux are at high risk for progressive renal scarring and eventual functional impairment. Most UTIs in adult women represent cystitis, which is easily treated. UTI in adult men is usually related to prostatic enlargement or infection. Adult women have many more UTIs than men until approximately age 65, after which time the prevalence of bacteriuria rises with age and functional status in both men and women.

B. **Asymptomatic versus symptomatic bacteriuria.** Detection of asymptomatic bacteriuria is often the result of laboratory screening procedures because, as the term implies, such patients are indeed symptomless. Asymptomatic bacteriuria is likely to occur in patients with indwelling catheters, patients with urologic abnormalities, pregnant women, and approximately 5% of school-age girls.

Because of the problems of contamination of clean-catch specimens, this diagnosis should not be based on the results of a single urine culture.

1. **Criterion to establish the diagnosis of asymptomatic bacteriuria**
   a. Two consecutive clean-catch specimens having greater than 100,000 organisms per milliliter, with the same organism in both specimens.
   b. Alternatively, a single urethral catheter specimen with greater than 100 organisms per milliliter.

2. **Approach** to the treatment of asymptomatic bacteriuria depends on an appreciation of the prognosis of the untreated infection and the long-term results that are anticipated from therapy. The side effects and cost of therapy are of paramount importance.
   a. **Screening for asymptomatic bacteriuria in children is controversial.** Although bacteriuria can be associated with hypertension and renal insufficiency, these complications are rare, as is asymptomatic bacteriuria, occurring in only 1–2% of children. Although there is up to a 3% prevalence of asymptomatic bacteriuria in premature infants, the difficulties in obtaining a clean urine specimen make screening neonates impractical. (See related discussion in sec. **IV.D** under UTI in Children.)
   b. **Screening for asymptomatic bacteriuria in adults is of particular value in two situations: before urologic surgery and during pregnancy.** Postoperative infectious complications are reduced by treating bacteriuria preoperatively. The importance of routine screening during the first trimester is discussed in sec. **1.C** under UTI in Adult Women.

C. **Localization of the site of infection.** It is well recognized that upper UTI (pyelonephritis) requires longer-duration therapy than lower UTI (cystitis). As previously discussed, the clinical presentation may not be reliable enough to make an accurate distinction between upper and lower infection. Although several methods have been developed to help distinguish upper from lower UTI, such methods are either invasive, with resultant considerable patient discomfort, or are not widely available for clinical application. They are sometimes used in clinical research studies.

1. **Invasive techniques** include ureteral catheterization with direct culturing and the bladder washout technique with sequential sampling of bladder and ureteral urine. Both techniques are complex urologic and microbiologic procedures, requiring close cooperation between physicians and the clinical laboratory.

2. **The noninvasive technique** that has received most attention is the antibody-coated bacteria test [21]. The test detects antibodies against infecting bacteria that are believed to form when tissue infection (upper tract or prostatitis) is present (in contrast to cystitis). Because it is not widely available, the test has been used primarily as an epidemiologic and research tool and, to date, has not had a major role in influencing management of UTI in a given patient [22].

3. **In most clinical settings, therapy is based on clinical manifestations,** recognizing that most UTIs are lower tract infections. Patients with fever and flank pain are likely to have upper tract disease.

   The outcome of therapy has implications about whether upper versus lower tract infection may be present. **Relapse of infection following short-course therapy in adult women is associated with upper UTI.**

D. **Recurrent UTI.** Repeated episodes of UTI can be either **reinfection** (i.e., new infections with new organisms) or **relapse** (i.e., a recrudescence of a prior, partially treated infection). The distinction is an important one to make because it has implications both for the type and extent of workup indicated for therapy. **Reinfections** tend to occur more than 2 weeks after completion of therapy for the initial episode and are more frequent after uncomplicated cystitis. **Relapses** tend to occur within 2 weeks after completion of therapy of complicated UTI [1a].

1. **Reinfection** is more common than relapse in women; conversely, in men most recurrent infection is due to relapse. After successful therapy of a prior infection, recurrence of symptoms and evidence of **clinical infection with a new organism** (either a new bacterial species or a new serologic type of *E. coli*) indicates reinfection. In general, most reinfections occur within weeks to months of the preceding UTI.

   a. **Reinfection in adult women** (of childbearing age to middle age) is common. As discussed under UTI in Adult Women, it is recommended that women with three or more symptomatic lower UTIs within a 6-month period receive extended-duration (6- to 12-month) prophylactic therapy.
   b. **Reinfection in adult men** is a much less common cause of recurrent infection than is relapse and, as discussed under UTI in Adult Men, is most commonly related to prostatic enlargement causing partial urethral obstruction.
2. **Relapse** refers to the recurrence of symptoms and clinical infection after the cessation of treatment. Implied in this definition is that relapse involves the **same organism** or same serotype of *E. coli* that caused the initial infection. Most relapses occur shortly after the patient has completed a course of therapy (i.e., perhaps within a few days and certainly within 1 month).
   a. **Setting.** Relapse is likely to occur (1) if there is persistent infection in the renal parenchyma or prostate gland, (2) if the patient does not receive the proper antibiotic therapy, or (3) if there is an underlying renal pathologic process, such as renal calculi.
   b. **Implications. Relapse often implies underlying urologic abnormality.** Therefore, **urologic evaluation is mandatory,** particularly if previous antibiotic therapy was adequate on the basis of susceptibility data.
   c. The **approach** should be directed initially at defining the underlying urologic defect, if possible. **If no correctable urologic defect is found and the patient has failed conventional 10- to 14-day therapy, one may presume there is a deeply seated tissue infection. In this group of patients, prolonged therapy (e.g., 4–8 weeks) may eradicate the infection.**
   d. **Suppressive therapy.** If a prolonged course of therapy also fails, chronic suppressive therapy may be necessary. In vitro susceptibility results should be used to determine the choice of chronic suppressive antibiotic therapy. The agent should be administered in full therapeutic dose. In recurrent UTI, there are limited indications for this approach. The major group are patients with urologic abnormalities that cannot be corrected surgically. **This approach should not be taken in patients with indwelling urethral catheters.**

UTI in Adult Women

Adult women constitute the largest group of patients with UTI [5]. Most such UTIs represent cystitis, but the overlapping clinical symptoms of urethritis or vaginitis may cause confusion. **In most patients, short-course antibiotic therapy (3 days) may be administered empirically on the basis of symptoms along with urinalysis confirmation of pyuria, without the use of pretherapy or posttherapy urine cultures.** Recurrent UTI poses a not infrequent and troublesome problem.

I. **Asymptomatic bacteriuria**
   A. **Significance.** There are insufficient data regarding the long-term effects of asymptomatic bacteriuria in young or middle-aged, nonpregnant women. Many patients in this group will clear their bacteriuria spontaneously and will not require treatment.
   B. **Approach. The current consensus is that this entity in the nonpregnant adult patient does not require treatment,** provided there is no urinary tract obstruction.
   C. **Pregnancy.** It is important to screen for and treat asymptomatic bacteriuria in adult women only during pregnancy as morbidity associated with UTI in pregnant women has been clearly demonstrated [5, 22a]. Asymptomatic bacteriuria occurs in about 5% of pregnant women with the most common onset between weeks 9 and 17 of pregnancy. Approximately 40% of pregnant women with asymptomatic bacteriuria will develop acute pyelonephritis in their pregnancy if not treated [1a]. Pyelonephritis in the mother and low birth weight in the infant are sufficiently common complications to warrant mandatory screening for bacteriuria during gestation. Treating pregnant bacteriuric patients lowers the subsequent incidence of symptomatic UTIs by 80–90% [22a]. Increased rates of premature labor have been seen in pregnant women with symptomatic UTI. The mechanisms for premature labor developing in patients with symptomatic infection are not completely clear but may be related, in part, to microorganism production of phospholipase A_2. Human term labor is believed to be initiated by amniotic and chorionic phospholipase A_2 [22a].

1. **All pregnant women should be screened for the presence of bacteriuria** on the first prenatal visit and again at the twenty-eighth week in women with a history of frequent UTIs. If only a single cost-effective screening culture is done, the sixteenth gestational week may be an optimal time [22a]. Cultures with colony counts exceeding 10^5 bacteria warrant therapy. The significance of lower colony counts of clean-catch samples is less well defined [7].

2. **Treatment.** Because of the risk of pyelonephritis and subsequent stillbirth or prematurity, **asymptomatic bacteriuria in pregnant women should be treated. Oral antimicrobials that are safe to give during pregnancy** include amoxicillin, cephalosporins, nitrofurantoin, and sulfonamides. **(The use of sulfonamides should be avoided in the third trimester.) Recommended duration of therapy is 7–10 days** [22a].

3. **Follow-up. Eradication of bacteriuria is the goal.** This should be confirmed with follow-up cultures at 1 and 4 weeks after therapy ends.

    If infection returns with the same bacterium, a relapsing infection from an occult source should be suspected. In this setting, a second course of antibiotics for a longer duration and an agent based on susceptibility data, may be tried. If infection is present on further follow-up cultures, then a short course of antibiotics to which the bacterium is susceptible can be used to suppress the infection, followed by nitrofurantoin, 50–100 mg daily at bedtime, until delivery, with the hopes of suppressing recurrent infection. (For susceptible pathogens, chronic suppression with amoxicillin or a cephalosporin is also a potential regimen.) Serial urine cultures should be performed to detect the possibility of a resistant pathogen. Follow-up urine cultures should be performed after delivery, and urologic evaluation should be undertaken 3–6 months after delivery [22a].

4. See related discussion in sec. **V.**

D. **Diabetes mellitus in women.** Although studies are limited, many experts believe that asymptomatic bacteriuria in diabetics without obvious anatomic abnormalities should be treated when detected because of the frequency of upper UTI in diabetics when bacteriuria is present [6a].

II. **Lower UTI** [5, 23]. Women with dysuria but without fever constitute the largest group of UTI patients and the largest group of adults for whom antimicrobials are prescribed. With such women, the **first step is to exclude vaginitis from the differential diagnosis.** Women with vaginitis usually experience dysuria as an external discomfort, and those with cystitis have a deeper and more visceral dysuria. If vaginitis is suspected, a pelvic examination should be done. Clinical and laboratory evaluation of vaginitis or cervicitis should be performed as described in Chap. 13.

A. **Cystitis.** Women with lower UTIs form a homogenous group of patients who are appropriately managed as outpatients. As a common outpatient illness, this type of UTI presents a challenge to the primary care provider. Because a UTI generally is seen more as a nuisance and an inconvenience than a harmful state, the practitioner may be lulled into unwarranted indifference and may thus not acknowledge uncommon but significant events (e.g., the presence of occult or subacute pyelonephritis with or without mechanical or neurologic dysfunction). However, with confirmation of pyuria on urinalysis, there is an opportunity for use of cost-effective antimicrobial therapy. The absence of comorbidity and the limited extent of the infection makes this bacterial infection particularly appropriate for short-course therapy, now the standard of management for lower UTI (see sec. **D.2**). The **microbial agents responsible** include *E. coli* (60%), other Enterobacteriaceae organisms (20%), and *S. saprophyticus* (10%).

B. **Urethritis.** Acute onset of dysuria along with pyuria also occurs with urethritis. Previously discussed clues about the nature of the dysuria may help distinguish cystitis from urethritis (see sec. **III** under General Approach to UTIs). Recent onset of dysuria in patients who have a new coital partner in the month before onset of symptoms and who have not had symptoms of a UTI in the preceding 2 years may signal urethritis due to a sexually transmitted infection. *C. trachomatis,* trichomoniasis, gonorrhea, and herpes simplex virus may be the etiologic agent (see Chap. 13).

    Strong consideration should be given to performing a pelvic examination in sexually active women with dysuria.

    1. Obtain a culture or Gram stain for the gonococcus.
    2. If ulcerations are present, herpes simplex virus cultures should ideally be performed.

3. Although *Chlamydia* confirmation by culture is not widely available and does not give prompt results, a sensitive immunofluorescent test that gives more immediate results is now available. However, both tests are expensive and are not mandatory for initial management.

C. Vaginitis. Vaginitis as a cause of dysuria should be suspected in the patient who lacks pyuria; has vaginal discharge, odor, pruritus, or dyspareunia; relates external dysuria; or has dysuria without frequency or urgency.

D. Clinical approach to acute dysuria. If vaginitis is excluded, the next step is to examine the urine sediment for leukocytes.

1. Diagnostic clues

  a. A positive leukocyte esterase test or the presence of more than 10 WBCs within a high-power field of a spun urine is consistent with but not diagnostic of UTI or urethritis.

  b. In the patient with acute dysuria, if pyuria is not present the probability of infection is less than 5%. The diagnosis of vaginitis should be considered in the absence of pyuria.

  c. If pyuria is present, the unspun urine should be examined carefully using a Gram stain for bacteria, and if bacteria are seen in most fields under oil immersion, it is likely that the urine contains 100,000 bacteria or more per milliliter. If bacteria are not seen, then the infection may still be bacterial with low colony counts or it may be nonbacterial.

2. Therapy

  a. Most authorities advocate administering empiric, short-course antibiotic therapy for uncomplicated UTI without obtaining an initial urine culture. Indeed, treatment decisions are made and completed before culture results would be available, and this approach is supported by cost-effectiveness studies [12].

  b. There is a debate in the literature about the virtues of single-dose versus 3-day therapy, with many authorities favoring the latter [5]. **Not all antimicrobials have been shown to be effective in short-course therapy,** and only the doses and agents with proven efficacy should be employed (see Table 12-3). In one review, single-dose therapy was less effective than 10 days of therapy, especially with amoxicillin and, to a lesser extent, with TMP-SMX; therefore, the reviewers believe that 3 days of therapy may prove to be an optimal intermediate regimen [4]. **Overall, most experts favor the 3-day regimen over the single-dose regimen [1a, 9b].**

   (1) Short-course (3-day) therapy is indicated for only those adult women with uncomplicated infections.

   (2) Contraindications for short-course therapy include pregnancy, suspected upper UTI or known prior pyelonephritis, relapsing infection, recent antibiotic use or bladder instrumentation, suspected or known urinary tract structural abnormality, childhood UTIs, symptoms for longer than 7 days, recent diaphragm use [1a], and inability to provide follow-up. Because of the high rate of upper UTI in **diabetic women,** many experts do not recommend 3-day regimens for acute uncomplicated UTI in diabetic women; a 7-day regimen is preferred [1, 6a]. Furthermore, **use of the cephalosporins in 3-day regimens may be less effective** than other 3-day regimens (e.g., TMP-SMX, quinolones) and therefore some experts prefer 7- to 10-day courses of cephalosporins rather than use of a 3-day course, even for uncomplicated cystitis [9b, 19, 23a]. Macrodantin, likewise, may not be quite as effective in 3-day regimens when compared with TMP-SMX or the quinolones [9b].

3. Indications for urine culture

  a. Urine culture should be obtained in acutely dysuric women who lack pyuria, in situations when urethritis and cystitis are not clearly distinguished clinically, in patients with relapsing or frequent recurrent infections, in complicated UTIs, and in pregnant women.

  b. In women with sterile cultures, acute dysuria, and pyuria, chlamydial urethritis should be suspected. The sexually active woman should have a pelvic examination with appropriate urethral or cervical cultures. Empiric therapy with tetracycline, 500 mg PO q6h for 7 days (or doxycycline, 100 mg PO bid), or azithromycin, 1 g PO as a single dose (see Chap. 13) should be administered if not contraindicated (see Chap. 28), and test-of-cure cultures should be obtained as appropriate.

4. **Follow-up**
   a. **If symptoms resolve with short-course therapy, no follow-up culture is necessary.**
   b. If short-course therapy fails or symptoms recur, then a urine culture should be obtained.
      (1) Such patients should be suspected of having occult or subclinical pyelonephritis [1a]. See sec. **VI** under General Approach to UTIs for decisions on urologic evaluation.
      (2) Significant bacteriuria ($>10^2$ CFU/ml) should be treated with at least 14 days of antibiotics directed by susceptibility testing.
   5. It is unclear how to treat dysuric patients with negative cultures and with no pyuria. Vaginitis should be excluded in all such patients. Observation and a short course of phenazopyridine hydrochloride (e.g., Pyridium) may be reasonable.
E. **Recurrent cystitis** requires that urine cultures be obtained and susceptibility tests be performed.
   1. **Antibiotic therapy** directed by susceptibility test results should be administered for 7–14 days.
   2. **Follow-up urine cultures** should be obtained at 1 and 4 weeks after the end of therapy.
III. **Upper UTI**
A. **Pyelonephritis.** The syndrome of acute pyelonephritis includes dysuria and increased frequency accompanied by **fever** (temperature usually exceeds 102°F) or definite CVA tenderness; the patient may also appear septic. However, upper UTI may be difficult to distinguish from lower UTI or so-called silent (subclinical) pyelonephritis. Up to 30% of women in a primary-care setting and up to 80% of indigent patients suffering from clinically apparent cystitis in emergency rooms also have silent, invasive bacterial infections of renal parenchyma; this infection is indistinguishable from lower UTI because most patients have dysuria and pyuria but not back pain [7a]. (See sec. **III.B** under General Approach to UTIs.) **Women who fail short-course antibiotic therapy for presumed lower UTI should be assumed to have subclinical or occult pyelonephritis [9a].** Subclinical pyelonephritis is more common in pregnant women with UTI, in patients who have had a UTI before age 12, and those who have had previous pyelonephritis or more than three UTIs in the past year [7a]. Patients with UTI and positive blood cultures have pyelonephritis with invasive tissue infection.

   Painless complicated **pyelonephritis,** which in fact is a different entity than subclinical pyelonephritis, can be observed in diabetics, renal transplant patients, and alcoholics. These patients have minimal symptoms due to autonomic nervous system damage associated with underlying disease but often have severe pyelonephritis [7a].
   1. **Microbiologic features.** *E. coli* causes approximately 85% of all cases of community-acquired pyelonephritis. Other members of the family Enterobacteriaceae cause approximately 10%, and gram-positive bacteria such as *Streptococcus faecalis* or *S. saprophyticus* the remainder. More antibiotic-resistant gram-negative aerobes, including *P. aeruginosa,* should be anticipated in patients with hospital-acquired infection and in women who have had recurrent UTIs or who have recently failed antimicrobial therapy (see Table 12-2).
   2. **Principles of antibiotic therapy.** The best way to treat pyelonephritis is poorly defined in the literature and despite initial therapy with 2 weeks of an antibiotic effective in vitro, approximately 20% of patients may fail this therapy (i.e., patients may have relapsing infection) [7a].
      a. The relatively high failure rates reported may in part be due to the absence of sufficient levels of antibiotic in renal tissue to sterilize the infected medulla. Whether or not the antibiotic must reach inhibitory concentrations in the bloodstream as well as in the urine and renal tissue to be effective in pyelonephritis is debated and reviewed elsewhere, but some reviewers believe it is important for inhibitory levels to be attained in both the kidney tissue and urine of patients with pyelonephritis [7a].
      b. Laboratory studies have suggested that pyelonephritic and endotoxemic kidneys accumulate more aminoglycosides (e.g., gentamicin, tobramycin) and quinolones than beta-lactams (e.g., cephalosporins). TMP-SMX penetrates renal tissue adequately [7a]. Furthermore, renal tissue levels of

aminoglycosides are prolonged and their effectiveness in treating pyelonephritis is confirmed in the animal model [7a].

Therefore, especially while awaiting susceptibility data, when parenteral
therapy is needed for acute gram-negative bacilli pyelonephritis, **aminoglycosides are clinically effective and cost effective if not contraindicated**
(see Chap. 28H). Because of their prolonged tissue levels, even 48–72 hours
of initial aminoglycoside therapy may be effective; therapy can then be
narrowed based on susceptibility data [9a].

3. **Outpatient versus inpatient therapy.** The decision regarding outpatient or in-
hospital treatment of acute pyelonephritis is primarily one of clinical judgment.
It is influenced by the patient's clinical condition, age, underlying disease, and
potential for compliance. In general, patients who are older or more frail,
bacteremic, toxic, or immunocompromised will require inpatient therapy initially. In mild cases in which the actual diagnosis of upper or lower UTI may
be unclear, outpatient therapy is reasonable [24].

   a. **Outpatient therapy.** Empiric therapy with oral antibiotics should be started
      as outlined in Table 12-3 pending receipt of urine culture results and
      susceptibility data. **Antibiotics usually are given for 2 weeks** because
      renal parenchymal infections are more difficult to treat than superficial
      bladder infections.

   b. **Inpatient therapy** with empiric, parenteral, antimicrobial treatment is indi-
      cated for many patients with pyelonephritis.

      (1) Initial antibiotic therapy should include agents that are known to be
          active against anticipated pathogens. Doses should be appropriate to
          provide sufficient drug levels within the renal parenchyma and at dis-
          tant nonrenal sites, as indicated in Table 12-3. Intravenous ampicillin
          alone probably is inadequate. Up to 30% of organisms may be resistant,
          even in community-acquired infections [4].

      (2) However, ampicillin (or vancomycin in the penicillin-allergic patient)
          should be used when urine Gram staining suggests the possibility of
          enterococcal infection (i.e., gram-positive cocci).

      (3) Patients in whom multiple antibiotic-resistant isolates are anticipated
          (e.g., hospital-acquired infection) should be given agents that have
          broad gram-negative coverage, to include *P. aeruginosa*. Often, the
          most cost-effective agent is an aminoglycoside, unless contraindicated.
          Aztreonam, ceftazidime, and imipenem may be used as alternatives to
          an aminoglycoside. See Chap. 28 for a discussion of these agents.

      (4) Therapy should be modified to the narrowest-spectrum agent possible
          and to a less expensive antibiotic when the results of susceptibility
          tests are available.

      (5) Once the infection is well controlled with intravenous therapy, outpa-
          tient therapy with either oral or intravenous antibiotics is reasonable.

4. **Duration of therapy.** In pyelonephritis, antibiotics usually are given for a **total
   of 14 days** [25]. Because of the occasional difficulties in eradicating renal tissue
   infection in patients failing 14-day therapy, longer courses of therapy (e.g., 4–6
   weeks) should be employed. For the hospitalized patient, parenteral therapy
   usually is continued until the patient has clinically improved and is afebrile
   for 24–48 hours. Then the patient can be placed on oral antibiotics. This
   decision must be individualized, particularly in a patient with complications
   such as obstruction or bacteremia.

5. **Response to therapy.** It is important to recognize and treat the complications
   of acute pyelonephritis. Nearly all patients with uncomplicated acute pyelonephritis are afebrile after 3 days of effective antimicrobial therapy, and the
   remainder are afebrile by 4 days [9]. **The persistently febrile patient may have
   a collection of undrained pus in or around the kidney, a metastatic site of
   infection** [26], or obstruction with pyonephrosis, or she may have received
   ineffective therapy. If fever or toxicity persists beyond 48 hours of appropriate
   therapy, an obstructive uropathy or renal abscess should be excluded (e.g.,
   with renal ultrasonography). **Intrarenal and perinephric abscesses** are discussed later in this chapter. Diabetics have an increased incidence of these
   complications [6a].

6. **Follow-up.** Approximately 48 hours after initiation of therapy, results of susceptibility testing will be available. If the organism isolated is **not** susceptible to

the treatment given, treatment should be changed to the most appropriate drug.

   a. The urine should become sterile 2 or 3 days after initiation of appropriate therapy, with no bacteria noted in the urine sediment. Some authorities recommend routine culturing of the urine at 2–3 days to assess response to therapy. This rarely is done in outpatient settings but may be indicated in hospitalized patients, especially if there is a question of resistant organisms, if the infection is complicated by mechanical or neurologic obstruction, or if the patient is not responding clinically.

   b. Whereas antibiotic treatment may relieve or reduce the patient's symptoms, such treatment does not always result in bacteriologic cure. For this reason, follow-up after treatment is important. Recommendations of experts in the field vary with regard to the extent of follow-up, but the **minimum follow-up should be a repeat urine culture 1–2 weeks after completion of antimicrobial therapy** in all patients. In patients with frequent UTIs, repeat cultures at 4–6 weeks after treatment may be useful.

  7. Urologic evaluation generally is indicated for any patient with relapsing pyelonephritis.

B. Infection in patients with known urinary tract abnormalities. In patients with known renal calculi, obstructive uropathies, or other abnormalities, antibiotic therapy may suppress infection temporarily but may not eradicate it. Treatment of these patients, therefore, should be directed toward correction of the underlying abnormality if this is possible.

C. Miscellaneous. UTIs in patients with **polycystic kidney disease** are difficult to treat, in part because of the poor penetration of antibiotics (e.g., aminoglycosides) into cystic fluid [27]. Infectious disease consultation is advised in these difficult cases.

  UTI in the setting of **renal transplantation** is discussed in Chap. 20.

IV. Recurrent infections. The healthy young woman who has had two UTIs within the last 6 months and is now presenting with her third is a candidate for long-term prophylactic therapy to prevent recurrent symptomatic bacteriuria [28].

A. The **source** of the recurrent bacteriuria is usually reinfection from the periurethral flora or, less commonly, it may be the result of persistent or relapsing infection in the upper urinary tract—that is, smoldering pyelonephritis. Some women will clearly indicate sexual intercourse as a causal factor for recurrent infections [29].

B. Prophylactic therapy. In patients with reinfection, 6–12 months of continuous preventive or antibiotic therapy has been shown to decrease recurrences by 95% during the period of active treatment [30, 31]. **Prophylactic therapy should be initiated only after the acute episode is bacteriologically cured.** For individuals with reinfection immediately after discontinuation of prophylactic therapy, more extended duration of prophylaxis (2 or more years) has been shown to be effective.

C. Recommended prophylactic antibiotics of equal efficacy include TMP-SMX, one-half regular tablet at bedtime every other night; trimethoprim, 100 mg/day at bedtime; or nitrofurantoin, 50 or 100 mg/day at bedtime (see related discussions in Chap. 28).

D. Alternative approaches

  1. Some patients prefer **patient-administered short-course therapy** at the onset of symptoms, which may be more efficacious, economical, and desirable than conventional prophylactic therapy [32]. This approach probably is justified only for the highly motivated, compliant, and well-educated patient.

  2. Postintercourse, single-dose, prophylactic therapy can be effective in patients who identify intercourse as a precipitating factor [29].

  3. In postmenopausal women, topically applied intravaginal estradiol cream is a possible alternative to antimicrobial prophylaxis [32a].

  4. In one study with elderly women, drinking **cranberry juice** daily reduced the frequency of bacteriuria and pyuria [2a].

E. Behavioral changes may be important [9b]:

  1. Voiding after intercourse has been suggested as a way of reducing UTI episodes related to sexual intercourse.

  2. If a diaphragm and spermicide are used for contraception, an alternative method [6] may reduce the frequency of recurrent UTI.

  3. Voiding when the urge to void occurs rather than delaying may help some individuals (e.g., school teachers who postpone voiding during school hours).

F. Urologic evaluation

1. When accurate classification is possible, women with recurrent infections characterized as **relapse** should be examined at least once for the presence of mechanical (e.g., obstruction or stones) or neurologic dysfunction of the urinary tract. The role of suppressive long-term antibiotic therapy in these patients is discussed in sec. **III.D** under General Management Principles of UTIs.
2. Women with sporadic **reinfections** that respond to short-course therapy or low-dose prophylaxis usually do not have urologic abnormalities. Therefore, invasive evaluation is not warranted.

V. UTI in pregnancy [22a]

   A. The overall **prevalence of bacteriuria** in pregnancy ranges from 4 to 7% in most studies but is as high as 11% in socially indigent multiparas and as low as 2% in private patients [22a]. Pyelonephritis in pregnancy occurs in 3 to 7% of pregnant women who have asymptomatic bacteriuria [7a]. Sickle cell trait has been associated with bacteriuria also. Catheterization should be avoided in the pregnant patient because pregnancy sets the stage for the development of symptomatic infection [22a].

   B. Physiologic changes with pregnancy

      1. The most impressive changes involve dilatation of the collecting system, called **hydroureters of pregnancy.** This is a normal condition in pregnancy and extends to the level of the pelvic brim. The changes are more pronounced on the right side. Dilatation begins as early as the seventh week of gestation and gradually progresses until term.

         Although the precise explanation for the development of hydroureters is unclear, both mechanical and hormonal factors are involved.

      2. In the third trimester, the **bladder** undergoes a relative **change in position,** becoming an abdominal rather than a pelvic organ, and undergoes a progressive **decrease in tone** owing to hormonal changes.

      3. The net effect of these changes is to increase the risk of UTI, especially in the third trimester.

      4. After delivery, in the absence of infection, the hydroureters return to normal in 66% of patients by 1 month and in most patients by 2 months [22a].

   C. Therapy of UTI

      1. **Asymptomatic UTI.** See discussion in sec. **I.C** under UTI in Adult Women.

      2. **Symptomatic UTI** deserves 7–10 days of antibiotic therapy based on susceptibility data. (Antibiotic use in pregnancy is discussed in Chap. 28A.) Short 3-day courses are not recommended.

      3. **Pyelonephritis.** Hospitalization is usually advised. Empiric therapy with a broad-spectrum cephalosporin (e.g., ceftriaxone) is appealing until culture data are available that may allow one to use a narrower spectrum cephalosporin. Aztreonam is another possible parenteral beta-lactam antibiotic [1a, 7a]. There is some concern about using aminoglycosides in pregnancy because of the potential of ototoxicity for the fetus [7a] (see Chap. 28H). The duration of therapy for pyelonephritis has not been well studied. After a 2-week course of an appropriate antibiotic based on susceptibility data, suppression with nitrofurantoin until delivery is rational [22a] (see sec. **I.C** under UTI in Adult Women).

   D. Follow-up. See related discussion in sec. **I.C** under UTI in Adult Women.

UTI in Adult Men

UTI in adult men [33] occurs most commonly in men with prostatic hypertrophy and partial urethral obstruction or in association with persistent infection of the prostate gland. UTIs in children and the elderly are discussed separately.

I. Asymptomatic infections. Bacteriuria is uncommon without symptoms in the healthy adult man, although it is relatively common in the elderly male (see sec. **I** under UTI in the Elderly).

   A. Screening for bacteriuria in asymptomatic healthy men is not suggested.

   B. Therapy. If bacteriuria is found by chance, it should lead to an investigation to exclude predisposing structural or functional abnormalities of the urinary tract, especially chronic prostatitis. Routine antibiotic treatment in asymptomatic men is not supported by available data. Patients should be treated before genitourinary instrumentation.

II. Lower UTI

A. **It is important to recognize the concept of the relationship between lower UTI in men and prostatitis.** Prostatitis may cause symptomatic infection with or without bladder infection. Bladder infection in the man with a mechanically normal urinary system often is associated with bacterial prostatitis [34, 35]. However, uncomplicated cystitis alone can also occur (see sec. **B.1.c**). Instrumentation is the most common identifiable cause of infection but, in most cases, the events leading to infection are not clear. Obstruction is often coexistent with and inseparable from instrumentation.

B. **General approach to lower UTI in the adult man**

   1. **Clinical presentation.** The history is important.

   a. **Dysuria (with or without urethral discharge).** Initially, one should identify patients having **dysuria alone,** with or without a urethral **discharge,** because these patients usually have urethritis rather than a true UTI. Most men between the ages of 15 and 30 years will have either nonspecific urethritis or gonococcal urethritis. The clinical approach to this problem is discussed in Chap. 13 under Urethritis.

   b. **UTI.** Patients may have **dysuria, frequency, and urgency,** symptoms similar to those seen in uncomplicated UTI in women. Acute perineal pain and discomfort may occur in patients with prostatitis, as discussed in sec. **III.** **Prostatitis is particularly common in men between 40 and 45 years of age who present with a UTI.**

   c. **Cystitis.** It has recently been appreciated that **uncomplicated cystitis can occur in sexually active young men with acute dysuria.** Risk factors include homosexuality with anorectal intercourse, lack of circumcision, human immunodeficiency virus (HIV) infection with a CD4 lymphocyte count of less than 200 cells per cubic millimeter, or a sexual partner with vaginal colonization with uropathogens [1a, 23]. Urethritis should be excluded and/or treated (see Chap. 13).

   2. **Diagnosis**

   a. **Examination of any urethral discharge** should be performed if possible, as discussed in Chap. 13 under Urethritis. This will usually allow one to make the distinction between nonspecific urethritis and gonococcal urethritis.

   b. **Routine urinalysis and quantitative urine culture are essential** for proper evaluation of patients with no urethral discharge but with symptoms of a UTI.

   c. **Rectal examination.** If the prostate gland is swollen, firm, and exquisitely tender, an associated acute prostatitis is likely; this entity is discussed in sec. **III.**

   d. **Prostatic localization technique.** A technique for localizing the site of UTI in men is discussed in sec. **III.B.** This technique is seldom performed at present; however, it **may be useful in the diagnosis of chronic prostatitis** and in the evaluation of adult men with relapsing UTI [35]. It appears to be used with diminishing frequency, even by urologists. It is **not appropriate in acute prostatitis.**

   3. **Treatment**

   a. **Antimicrobial therapy**

   (1) **Urethritis alone.** The approach to and treatment of this problem is discussed in Chap. 13 under Urethritis.

   (2) **Prostatitis** therapy is discussed in sec. **III.**

   (3) **Initial therapy** in the adult man who presents with his first UTI (if the condition **is not believed** to be clearly **related to prostatic focus** after initial evaluation) is uncertain. (This may be a particular problem in the young or middle-aged man compared to the older man, who is more likely to have a prostatic focus.) A subclinical prostatic focus still is possible, as is an occult genitourinary structural problem. With **recurrent UTI,** the prostatic localization test (see sec. **III.B**) sometimes is performed to help localize the problem. It is reasonable to use TMP-SMX (which penetrates the prostate well) because of the possibility of a prostatic focus in all men with UTI. Alternatively, one may use TMP alone in the sulfa-allergic patient or a fluoroquinolone as these agents penetrate the prostate well (see Chap. 28).

   (4) For that subgroup of sexually active young males (see sec. **2.c**) a 7-day course of TMP-SMX, TMP, or fluoroquinolone is suggested [1a] once urethritis is excluded. Failure of this regimen necessitates more careful evaluation, including consideration of a prostatic focus [1a].

  b. Urologic evaluation. In addition to antimicrobial therapy, urologic evaluation to determine whether a urinary tract abnormality exists should be considered. It is reasonable to treat a first UTI in an adult man who has no history of prior genitourinary abnormalities, then watch closely, and eventually proceed with a urologic workup when and if a second UTI or relapse occurs. Cystoscopy usually is indicated in patients with recurrent infections. **In patients with a typical initial episode of cystitis or acute prostatitis responding to antibiotics, a complete urologic evaluation is not necessary.** The approach to patients with an enlarged prostate (compatible with benign prostate hypertrophy) is an evolving area, with the increased availability of medical therapy for some forms of benign prostate hypertrophy. Also, stents can be inserted in the prostatic urethra segment (instead of conventional prostatic surgery) only in carefully selected patients. Urological consultation is therefore important [9b].

III. Bacterial prostatitis [7, 33] can present as either an acute or a chronic disease. It has been estimated that prostatitis constitutes approximately 25% of annual office visits for genitourinary complaints by men. Unfortunately, many aspects of prostatitis have been poorly understood, and both patients and clinicians often become confused and frustrated in dealing with this condition [7].

The common forms of prostatitis are summarized in Table 12-4. Bacterial prostatitis is associated with a UTI, positive cultures localizing the bacterial pathogen to the prostatic fluid, and excessive numbers of inflammatory cells (WBCs and macrophages containing fat) in the prostatic secretion [7]. **Studies suggest that nearly 90% of patients with prostatitis symptoms have nonbacterial prostatitis or prostatodynia [7].**

  A. Acute bacterial prostatitis is an abrupt febrile illness. Symptoms include fever, chills, and low back and acute perineal pain and discomfort. In addition, symptoms of acute lower UTI such as dysuria, frequency, and urgency usually are present.

   1. Diagnosis. The signs and symptoms are sufficiently abrupt, severe, and typical that the clinician seldom has difficulty in making the diagnosis [7].

     a. Rectal examination often is not necessary, thereby avoiding the discomfort and potential risk of prostate massage, as symptoms and urinalysis usually support the diagnosis of acute bacterial prostatitis. If a single gentle rectal examination is performed, it reveals a swollen prostate that often is exquisitely tender on palpation.

     b. Urinalysis usually demonstrates pyuria and bacteriuria.

     c. Prostatic localization studies, as discussed later, require prostatic massage and are **unnecessary** to support the clinical diagnosis in patients with acute prostatitis. Massage may precipitate bacteremia and causes considerable patient discomfort.

     d. Clean-catch urine culture. Because acute cystitis usually is associated with acute prostatitis, **the infecting pathogen generally can be identified by routine culture of a clean-catch urine specimen.** Data suggest a clean-catch culture may not be necessary in men. Neither meatal cleansing nor midstream sampling generally is needed to obtain urine for culture [33].

   2. Therapy. The inflammation of acute bacterial prostatitis allows most antibiotics to achieve high prostatic concentration, and patients generally respond rapidly to antibiotic therapy. Most infections are caused by enteric gram-negative bacilli (75%), particularly *E. coli* (25%), although gram-positive infections occur in the other 25% [7, 33].

     a. Antibiotic choice. Currently, **TMP-SMX, or TMP alone, is the treatment of choice** for acute bacterial prostatitis because of cost and the good penetration of prostatic tissue by TMP (see Table 12-3) [7, 36]. Trimethoprim alone may be administered in the sulfa-allergic patient. Comparable results have been published with the fluoroquinolones, and these agents are the drugs of choice for TMP-SMX-resistant organisms or as another alternative in sulfa-allergic patients (see Chaps. 28K and 28S). There are few data to support the use of oral carbenicillin indanyl.

     b. Other antibiotics. Some patients with acute prostatitis are systemically ill and may require therapy with parenteral antibiotics initially. Ampicillin and aminoglycosides have commonly been used in combination while awaiting cultures, especially if enterococci are a concern. Broad-spectrum

Table 12-4. Clinical features of common prostatitis syndromes

Syndrome	History of confirmed UTI	Prostate abnormal on rectal examination	Excessive WBCs in EPS	Positive culture of EPS	Common causative agents	Response to antimicrobial treatment	Impaired urinary flow rate
Acute bacterial prostatitis	Yes	Yes	Yes	Yes	Coliform bacteria	Yes	Yes
Chronic bacterial prostatitis	Yes	±	Yes	Yes	Coliform bacteria	Yes	±
Nonbacterial prostatitis	No	±	Yes	No	None ? *Chlamydia* ? *Ureaplasma*	Usually no	±
Prostatodynia	No	No	No	No	None	No	Yes

UTI = urinary tract infection; WBCs = white blood cells; EPS = expressed prostatic secretions.
Source: From E. M. Meares, Jr., Prostatitis. *Med. Clin. North Am.* 75:497, 1991.

penicillins, cephalosporins, and aminoglycosides are effective in many patients with acute prostatitis, even though these drugs are generally not believed to penetrate the prostate well. The inflammation in acute prostatitis allows these drugs to penetrate the prostate to a greater extent in acute infections than in chronic prostatitis.

   c. **Duration of therapy.** The optimal duration of therapy is not well defined. Conventionally, the treatment spans a minimum of 14 days. However, continuing therapy for at least 30 days in an attempt to treat a focus of chronic prostatitis has often been advocated [7, 34]. If the antibiotic is well tolerated, we tend to treat these patients with a 3- to 4-week course.

3. **Prognosis.** Most patients recover from acute prostatitis with appropriate treatment. Relapse may occur in some cases, or the prostate may remain a persistent source of infection, as discussed next.

B. **Chronic bacterial prostatitis** is a more subtle condition than acute prostatitis. Bacterial organisms in this disease are **difficult to eradicate** despite antibiotic therapy, and the prostate can remain a persistent source of UTI. The prostatic focus can repeatedly infect the bladder urine and is believed to be responsible for most relapsing lower UTIs in men. Infection usually is due to gram-negative bacilli but occasionally may be due to gram-positive organisms (e.g., enterococci). The role of other gram-positive bacteria is unclear. *S. aureus* at times may be a pathogen, but *S. epidermidis,* micrococci, and diphtheroids probably are not pathogens [7].

   Infected prostate calculi that cannot be appreciated by rectal examination or simple plain-film radiographic studies may function as infected foreign bodies, explaining in part why it may be difficult to eradicate infection in chronic bacterial prostatitis.

1. **Symptoms** are highly variable, and some patients are detected because of asymptomatic bacteriuria. Many patients may not have a history of acute prostatitis. Some complain of perineal or low back discomfort. Periodic episodes of cystitis symptoms or irritative voiding dysfunction, such as urgency, frequency, nocturia, and dysuria, may occur. **The best clue to this diagnosis is that prostatitis is the most common cause of relapsing UTIs** (with the same pathogen) **in adult men.** Because many antibiotics penetrate the prostate poorly, the pathogen remains viable in the prostatic tissue. Some antibiotic regimens will eradicate concomitant cystitis and sterilize the patient's urine, temporarily providing relief of symptoms, but symptoms return when the antibiotic is discontinued, because the prostatic infection persists.

2. **Diagnosis**

   a. **Rectal examination** reveals no characteristic findings on prostatic palpation. An enlarged or slightly boggy prostate is a nonspecific finding.

   b. **Localization studies.** The classic method of confirming the diagnosis is to perform prostatic localization studies, with **careful microscopic and culture examination of the segmented urines and the prostatic fluid. Localization studies may not be necessary in bacteriuric patients in whom the causative agent is already identified;** the procedure is time-consuming, fairly expensive, and uncomfortable for patients, and therefore is infrequently performed by clinicians. A justifiable alternative to performing prostatic localization studies is to treat bacteriuric men with prolonged courses of antibiotics known to penetrate the prostate. Studies are important in the patient who is not bacteriuric, to distinguish bacterial from nonbacterial prostatitis, to confirm a prostatic focus of infection for patients in whom prostatic surgery is contemplated because of recurrent UTI, or to help confirm the diagnosis in patients with recurrent symptoms.

   The prostatic localization method requires that the patient be well hydrated and have a full bladder before starting. The glans must be cleaned as previously noted, and the foreskin must be fully retracted during the procedure. The specimens collected usually are examined microscopically and cultured immediately after collection, employing methods that allow quantitation of small numbers of bacteria. **Careful microscopic examination alone can provide useful information** (see sec. (6)).

   (1) The patient first voids 20 ml urine (VB$_1$) into one container.

   (2) A midstream specimen then is obtained in a second container (VB$_2$).

   (3) During prostatic massage, expressed prostatic secretions (EPS) are collected.

(4) Finally, 10 ml urine is collected after prostatic massage (VB$_3$).

(5) Interpretation. Meares [7] has reviewed the interpretation of this technique in detail, including illustrative cases; the reader is referred to this discussion. Briefly, if colony counts in specimen VB$_1$ exceed those in VB$_3$, the bacteria are localized to the anterior urethra. If VB$_1$ and VB$_2$ are negative or have low counts of bacteria, and the EPS and VB$_3$ have larger numbers of bacteria, bacterial prostatitis must be considered. If the specimens all yield more than 10^5 CFU/ml, interpreting the test is not possible. In this instance, the patient should be treated with a 2- to 3-day course of nitrofurantoin, which will eradicate bladder bacteriuria but will not penetrate the chronically inflamed prostate; then the four-specimen test should be repeated.

(6) In chronic prostatitis, the prostatic fluid (EPS) should reveal more than 15 WBCs per high-power field. Culture of prostatic fluid should reveal the offending organism. Colony counts of fewer than 100,000 CFU/ml generally are seen, with counts of 1,000 CFU/ml or fewer on occasion.

Provided that the urethral and midstream specimens show insignificant pyuria, more than 15 WBCs per high-power field in the prostate expressate is diagnostic of prostatic inflammation. The most convincing sign of prostatitis is the finding of both excessive WBCs and macrophages containing fat droplets (ovoid fat bodies) in EPS.

3. Treatment. Eradication of a persistent prostatic focus of infection often is difficult. Except for TMP (alone or in combination with SMX), erythromycin (for gram-positive bacteria), and the quinolones, most antibiotics useful against gram-negative bacteria diffuse poorly into the prostatic fluid. Therefore, despite prolonged 6- to 12-week courses of appropriate antibiotics, cure rates of only about 30–40% are reported [7], but these rates are better than those for short-course regimens.

a. TMP-SMX or a quinolone (see Table 12-3) has been reported to be most successful for chronic prostatitis when used for prolonged periods. Therapy with TMP-SMX (one double-strength tablet twice daily) should be continued for a minimum of 6 weeks and preferably for 12 weeks. Optimal duration of therapy with the quinolones awaits further study. Ciprofloxacin (500 mg bid), norfloxacin (400 mg bid), or ofloxacin (300 mg bid) for 30 days has been suggested [7].

b. Even prolonged courses of antibiotics may be unsuccessful, particularly if there are prostatic calculi. Further urologic evaluation and partial prostatectomy may be indicated in refractory cases. Complete prostatectomy may result in incontinence or sexual impotency and therefore is contraindicated. Chronic suppressive therapy with TMP-SMX (one tablet daily) or TMP alone is appropriate in patients who continue to relapse after a 12-week course of full-dose therapy. Nitrofurantoin (100 mg/day) has been used [7]. The quinolones also are used for chronic suppression, but these agents are far more expensive than TMP or TMP-SMX (see Chap. 28).

C. Nonbacterial prostatitis is far **more common than chronic bacterial prostatitis.** It is defined as symptomatic prostatic inflammation with negative culture of urine and prostatic secretions. It has also been referred to as **prostatosis** [37]. Some authorities believe that prostatosis is merely bacterial prostatitis caused by small numbers of organisms. The etiology remains unclear; it is an inflammatory condition of unknown cause [7].

1. Symptoms. Complaints are similar to those of patients with chronic bacterial prostatitis. The patient often has no prior history of a UTI.

2. Diagnosis. Physical examination generally is unremarkable, although some patients may complain of prostatic tenderness on palpation. **Expressed prostatic secretions show more than 10–15 WBCs per high-power field,** but routine urine cultures and prostatic localization cultures show no bacterial etiology.

3. Treatment. There is **no accepted approach** to therapy as the etiology of this disease is unknown. Empiric treatment directed toward chlamydiae, with a 2-week trial of tetracycline (500 mg qid), doxycycline (100 mg bid), or erythromycin (250–500 mg qid), may provide symptomatic relief, and a partial response in some patients may justify longer therapy with these agents (e.g., 4–6 weeks).

Other antibacterial agents are neither effective nor indicated [7]. Sitz baths, therapy with nonsteroidal antiinflammatory agents and, in some patients, prostatic massage also may provide symptomatic relief. Surgical intervention is not indicated. Some patients have greater relief from aspirin than from nonsteroidal antiinflammatory agents, which may aggravate the problem.

D. Prostatodynia. Patients with this condition have no associated UTI, noninflammatory prostatic secretions with negative cultures of EPS, and no excessive inflammatory cells in their prostatic secretions. This is a common condition [7].

1. **The typical patient** is a young to middle-aged man with irritative voiding symptoms (frequency, urgency, and nocturia) and symptoms of abnormal urinary flow (hesitancy, diminution of stream force and size, postvoid dribbling).

2. General physical and neurologic examinations are normal except that many patients have "tight" anal sphincters and tender prostates and paraprostate tissues on rectal examination [7].

3. Cystoscopic examination often suggests mild to moderate bladder neck obstruction and variable bladder trabeculation. Meares [7] believes that these patients have "spastic" dysfunction of the bladder neck and prostate urethra and therefore calls this the **bladder neck–urethral spasm syndrome.**

   Smooth-muscle spasm and high prostatic urethral pressures during voiding probably lead to intraprostatic reflux of urine and an associated chemical prostatitis. Alpha-blocking agents are beneficial in some patients [7].

4. Most men with this syndrome admit to stress and emotional tension. Whether stress is a cause or merely an effect of prostatodynia is unclear [7].

IV. Epididymitis. This condition is diagnosed readily by physical examination. Most infections in sexually active men are caused by *C. trachomatis* and *N. gonorrhoeae;* urethritis and prostatitis may occur concurrently [38, 39]. Infection in older men is caused by the usual uropathogens, gram-negative bacilli and, infrequently, enterococci; infection may occur as a complication of concurrent prostatitis. Etiologic agents generally are recovered from culture of the urethra, urine, or prostatic secretions; alternatively, direct aspiration of the epididymis may be required. Therapy is directed at the etiologic agent and, if present, concurrent sites of infections.

V. Upper UTI. The approach to pyelonephritis in the normal adult man does not differ from that in the normal adult woman. See sec. **III** under UTI in Adult Women.

VI. Recurrent infections. The definition of recurrent UTIs in men differs from that used for women. The defining, but arbitrary, time limit set for repeated infections in women is 6 months. For men, because UTIs are much less common and less likely to occur as a sporadic event, **two or more UTIs at any time within a 3-year period** has been used to define the syndrome [34].

A. Predisposing factors. The association of prostatitis and recurrent UTIs is even stronger than for sporadic lower UTIs. Unlike women, men with recurrent UTIs almost always have evidence of tissue-invasive disease. **Most men with recurrent UTIs will be found to have structural defects of the urinary tract.** In those without structural defects, most will be found to have chronic bacterial prostatitis. **Urologic evaluation is essential** in these patients.

B. Therapy

1. The ideal antimicrobial agent is one that penetrates the prostate-blood barrier. At this time, TMP and TMP-SMX are the agents with an appropriate antimicrobial spectrum. The dosages given in Table 12-3 are appropriate for recurrent infection. The best chance for cure is with 6 weeks of therapy. The quinolones are other commonly used agents and are discussed in more detail in Chap. 28S.

2. If recurrences are frequent and severe, it may be appropriate to give chronic suppressive therapy, as discussed in sec. **III.D** under General Management Principles of UTIs. Treatment should be with full therapeutic dosages (not the low-dose suppressive regimens used in women) in an attempt to eradicate the focus of tissue infection and, therefore, cause cessation of symptomatic episodes.

UTI in the Elderly

Although many of the basic principles in the understanding and treatment of UTI in the elderly are similar to those for younger patients, several differences are noted in the elderly, and these deserve emphasis [40–45].

I. **Asymptomatic bacteriuria** is much more common in the geriatric population than in younger patients [40, 41]. Among young to middle-aged women, the prevalence of bacteriuria is less than 5% and, among young to middle-aged men, less than 0.1%. By contrast, at least 20% of women and 10% of men who are older than 65 years and are living at home have bacteriuria. Some, but not all, studies suggest the incidence of bacteriuria in the elderly rises with increasing age [41].

   A. **Factors** [41]

   1. The **place of residence** is a major factor in determining the prevalence of bacteriuria. Approximately 25% of women and 20% of men living in nursing homes or extended-care facilities have bacteriuria; even higher percentages of hospitalized elderly patients have bacteriuria.

   2. **Debilitated state** (i.e., the frail elderly). The higher rates of bacteriuria are related to the more debilitated state of patients (e.g., after cerebrovascular accidents, presence of decreased functional status), perineal soiling, poor hygiene, less complete bladder emptying, and more frequent catheterization.

   B. Serial studies show that although at one point in time an elderly patient may not have bacteriuria, at another point in time he or she will. It seems likely that most elderly persons experience episodes of asymptomatic bacteriuria at some time [41].

   C. **Significance of asymptomatic bacteriuria** [41]

   1. **Therapy** of asymptomatic bacteriuria in the elderly **to prevent renal insufficiency is not justified.** No causal relationship between uncomplicated UTI and worsening of renal function has been shown.

   2. Therapy of asymptomatic bacteriuria is unlikely to result in improvement of incontinence when present; asymptomatic bacteriuria rarely, if ever, causes incontinence.

   3. **Bacteriuria and mortality.** Although it has been suggested that the elderly with asymptomatic bacteriuria die earlier than their noninfected cohorts, randomized, controlled trials have shown that therapy does not provide a permanently sterile urine and has no effect on mortality [43–45]. Further studies are under way.

   D. **Treatment.** In a recent review, the authors conclude that "it seems best to avoid adopting a vigorous approach to the treatment of asymptomatic bacteriuria" because the bacteriuria cannot usually be eradicated, therapy is associated with side effects, and treatment is not cost-effective [41].

   We concur: **Available data do not support routinely treating asymptomatic bacteriuria in the frail elderly** [45]. Asymptomatic bacteriuria may be treated, however, prior to perioperative urethral catheterization or genitourinary instrumentation.

II. **Pathogenesis.** The same principles for UTI in adults apply to the elderly. A few points warrant special emphasis. The vast majority of UTIs in the elderly follow invasion of the urinary tract with bacteria by the **ascending route.** The inoculum size probably is increased by a shift of the normal vaginal flora toward coliforms, by soiling of the perineum from fecal incontinence in women, and by catheterization. Lack of estrogen effect may be important in elderly women (see sec. **II.C** under General Approach to UTI). Prostatitis is a very important cause of recurrent UTI in men.

   Micturition with complete emptying of the bladder often is impaired in the elderly owing to prostate disease in men, bladder prolapse in women, and neurogenic bladder in either gender.

III. **Microbiologic features** [41]

   A. *E. coli* is still the **most common** pathogen infecting the elderly.

   B. *S. saprophyticus* is **uncommon** in the elderly compared to its incidence in young women.

   C. Elderly men have a higher incidence of gram-positive isolates (e.g., enterococci) for unclear reasons.

   D. Elderly patients have often had prior therapy for UTI or other infections and often are infected with other gram-negative bacteria (e.g., *Proteus, Klebsiella, Enterobacter, Pseudomonas* spp.). Frequently, these bacteria are more resistant to antibiotics than bacteria isolated from younger patients.

   E. The frequency of true polymicrobial infections is unclear.

IV. **Clinical presentation.** Catheter-related infections are discussed separately later in this chapter.

   A. **Lower UTIs.** These usually are easy to recognize as patients complain of dysuria, frequency, and urgency.

B. Upper UTIs. Acute pyelonephritis in the frail elderly, like other intraabdominal processes, may present in an atypical fashion. Elderly patients may not have the classic presentation of high fever, chills, flank pain, and symptoms of lower UTI. At times, GI (nausea or vomiting, abdominal tenderness) or respiratory symptoms may be the patients' initial complaint, even though they do not have another underlying GI or respiratory infection. **Clinicians must always exclude UTIs in the differential diagnosis of disease in septic-appearing elderly patients.** Because of the nonspecificity of pyuria in this age group and the coexistence of asymptomatic bacteriuria with other causes of sepsis, some ambiguity will always have to be accepted. The criteria for diagnosis, however, do not differ from those described earlier (see sec. **V**).

Absence of fever in the elderly does not exclude upper UTI as elderly patients may have difficulty mounting a fever. Peripheral leukocytosis may also be absent.

Bacteremia and shock are more common in the elderly with pyelonephritis than in young adults [41]. Blood cultures should be routinely obtained.

V. Diagnosis. In general, the same diagnostic principles that apply to younger patients apply also to the elderly, with a few noteworthy differences [41].

A. Urine collection. It may be difficult to obtain a reliable midstream clean-catch urine sample for culture in the elderly woman. A single straight-catheter sample is a reasonable approach in a symptomatic patient.

B. Significant urine culture colony counts (midstream collections)
  1. For symptomatic infections, Enterobacteriaceae in volumes of more than 10^2 CFU/ml probably are significant.
  2. For asymptomatic bacteriuria, more than 10^5 CFU/ml are needed.

C. Nonspecificity of pyuria. Unlike younger people, in the elderly the presence of pyuria does not correlate highly with bacteriuria. In a population-based study in Finland, 47% of residents had pyuria, but only half of those had bacteriuria [42]. Other studies have shown even higher rates of pyuria in elderly women.

The presence of pyuria is a poor predictor of the presence of bacteriuria, but the **absence of pyuria is a good indicator of the absence of bacteriuria.**

D. Necessity of routine urine culture [41]
  1. For **elderly women** with typical symptoms of lower UTI, urine **culture at the time of first presentation is not mandatory.** If pyuria is present, empiric therapy is rational; if the patient does not respond, a urine culture should be done as an aid to future antibiotic choices.
  2. In recurrent UTI in the elderly woman, urine cultures are advisable to help guide antibiotic therapy choices.
  3. In men, routine cultures are advised.

E. Blood cultures. Obtain blood cultures in febrile patients or in any elderly patient who may have pyelonephritis because bacteremia is relatively common in the elderly with upper urinary tract disease.

F. Urologic evaluation. Consider urologic evaluation in:
  1. **Men** to help assess for obstructive uropathy. (A residual urine volume or bladder sonogram is a useful screen.)
  2. **Women** with bacteremia or pyelonephritis that does not respond well to antibiotics.

VI. Therapy. Asymptomatic bacteriuria should not be treated, as previously discussed.

A. Lower UTI
  1. **Women.** Although some experts are recommending that elderly women be treated initially with 3-day regimens, others favor a more conventional 7- to 14-day regimen [41a]. Anyone who fails a 3-day regimen should be tried on a 2-week course for presumed upper UTI. Because of the drug's spectrum of activity and low toxicity, TMP alone, norfloxacin, or ciprofloxacin is favored by Baldassarre and Kaye [41]; others may still choose cephalosporins that are well tolerated. For elderly women with recurrent UTI, a trial of local vaginal topical estrogen therapy may be beneficial by normalizing vaginal flora (see sec. **IV.C.1** under UTI in Women).
  2. **Men** deserve at least the conventional duration of therapy (e.g., 10–14 days) and consideration of underlying structural abnormality or prostatitis, which may warrant protracted therapy, especially if recurrent infections occur.
  3. Long-term suppressive therapy may be indicated for patients with recurrent UTI.

B. Upper UTI. Elderly patients with pyelonephritis are more likely to have bacteremia and hypotension, and hospitalization usually is indicated [41].

Although *E. coli* remains the most common bacterium, more resistant bacteria are more often found in the frail elderly. For those patients who have acquired their infection in a long-term care facility, the likelihood of a multiple antibiotic-resistant bacterium is appreciable.

A **Gram stain of the unspun urine** will help guide therapy, in part by helping to determine whether enterococci are a concern. This is more likely in men.

1. **Empiric choice of an agent.** Most frail elderly will have some degree of renal impairment, whether recognized or covert (see Chap. 28A). If an aminoglycoside is used in a very ill patient, careful serum level monitoring is advised. Once susceptibility data are available, alternative safer agents may often be selected. Alternatives are indicated in Table 12-3. Careful attention to dosage modification of antibiotics for renal impairment is important (see Chap. 28).

   For empiric therapy of pyelonephritis with or without urosepsis, intravenous ampicillin and gentamicin have commonly been used, especially if enterococci are suggested on the Gram stain of an unspun urine or if urine Gram staining has not been performed. If only gram-negative bacilli are seen on a Gram stain, an aminoglycoside or a third-generation cephalosporin alone is a rational choice. If *P. aeruginosa* or a multiresistant gram-negative organism is a concern, an aminoglycoside can be used alone while awaiting culture data.

2. **Definitive therapy.** Once the bacterium is isolated, therapy can be modified based on the susceptibility data of the causative agent. Complete eradication of bacteriuria often is not a reasonable goal for the frail elderly and, in the absence of bacteremia, the authors sometimes employ a shorter course of therapy—that is, 3 days beyond the time the patient has become afebrile if the patient has responded well to therapy. Otherwise, a routine 2-week course of therapy seems prudent.

C. **Urologic evaluation.** An evaluation for the exclusion of obstructive disease is important for the man but is not cost-effective for the frail elderly woman who is responding to therapy. However, in both men and women, if the patient is not clinically responding after 72 hours of appropriate antibiotic therapy, renal ultrasonography is suggested to help rule out an obstructive uropathy (see under UTI in Adult Men). A CT scan would be indicated if renal abscess was a concern.

VII. **Recurrent infections.** Because they have not been studied in a focused manner, recurrent infections in the frail elderly should be managed as described in sec. **VI** under UTI in Adult Men and in sec. **IV** under UTI in Adult Women.

VIII. **Foley catheter–related infections.** These are discussed separately later in this chapter under Catheter-Associated UTI.

UTI in Children

Neonatal UTIs are discussed in Chap. 3 under Selected Specific Infections in the Newborn. Both acute and chronic UTIs in children are relatively common. Several points deserve special emphasis based on recent reviews of this topic [46–47].

I. **Incidence.** UTI occurs in as many as 5% of female and 1–2% of male children [3, 46].

II. **Pathogenesis.** Hematogenous spread of infection to the kidney is the most common mode of infection in neonates. In older children, the ascending route of infection is most common.

A. **Obstruction with urinary stasis predisposes to UTI.** Posterior urethral valve, obstruction at the ureteropelvic junction or ureterovesical junction, and ectopic ureterocele are the main causes of anatomic obstruction in children [46]. **Vesicoureteral reflux is the most common abnormality.** The likelihood of parenchymal scarring and renal damage is related to the severity of vesicoureteral reflux.

B. **Risk groups. Children who are at increased risk for bacteriuria or symptomatic UTI with subsequent renal damage include:**

1. Premature infants discharged from neonatal intensive care units (see Chap. 3).
2. Children with systemic or immunologic diseases.
3. Children with urinary tract abnormalities, renal calculi, neurogenic bladder, voiding dysfunction, constipation, or a family history of UTI with anomalies such as reflux.
4. Girls younger than 5 years with a previous history of UTI.
5. **Uncircumcised** males are at an increased risk for UTI [9b].

III. Etiology is essentially the same as in adults, with at least 80% of infections due to *E. coli.* Patients with underlying structural abnormalities and recurrent infections are more likely to demonstrate other pathogens (*Klebsiella, Proteus,* and *Pseudomonas* spp.) over time.

IV. Asymptomatic bacteriuria

   A. Incidence. Approximately 1% of preschool children, 1.2–1.8% of school-age girls, and 0.03% of school-age boys have asymptomatic bacteriuria [46].

   B. Diagnosis. Diagnosis is made when, in an asymptomatic child, cultures of two properly obtained, clean-voided, midstream urine specimens grow at least 10^5 organisms (of one bacterial type) per milliliter.

   C. Implications [46]. Asymptomatic bacteriuria in children is associated with increased risk of recurrent symptomatic infections that may result in renal scarring. Hypertension or renal insufficiency, however, is unusual.

   1. In 20–30% of school-age girls with asymptomatic bacteriuria, radiographic investigation will reveal upper tract damage, vesicoureteral reflux, or both. **Most of the kidney damage occurs before 5 years of age.**

   2. Most prospective studies of schoolgirls older than 5 years with asymptomatic bacteriuria have failed to demonstrate decreased glomerular filtration rates, impaired renal growth, or progressive parenchymal damage in kidneys that are normal at the start, even if the bacteriuria is left untreated.

   3. Bacteriuria in neonates and infants, and in boys beyond infancy, is associated with a high incidence of urinary tract abnormalities and necessitates prompt diagnosis and early treatment.

   D. Screening neonates and infants for asymptomatic bacteriuria is not practical because of the difficulties of obtaining a clean urine specimen in this age group. **The only group of children who should definitely be screened at 6- to 12-month intervals are children at high risk for bacteriuria and subsequent renal damage** (see sec. **II.B**).

   E. Radiographic studies. Appropriate imaging studies should be performed in boys of any age with bacteriuria, in girls younger than 5 years, and in older girls with recurrent episodes of bacteriuria. (See detailed discussion of this in sec. **V.E.**)

   F. Treatment of asymptomatic bacteriuria. Some have argued that therapy of asymptomatic bacteriuria may eradicate organisms of low virulence and facilitate UTI with more resistant bacteria or, alternatively, may be associated with unnecessary antibiotic side effects. Although this remains a controversial area, **we agree with recent reviewers who suggest the use of antibiotic therapy in children** (1) younger than 5 years, (2) with underlying structural abnormalities, and (3) who progress to symptomatic UTI. A 7- to 10-day course of therapy is suggested, and failure to respond suggests noncompliance, improper antibiotic therapy, or underlying structural defect requiring radiographic evaluation [46].

V. Symptomatic bacteriuria

   A. Clinical manifestations. The usual signs and symptoms of lower UTIs in adults (e.g., dysuria and frequency) often are not present, and patients may have a variety of symptoms depending on their age. Fever may not be present and, by history, examination, and routine tests, it often is difficult to distinguish upper from lower UTI in children.

   1. See Table 12-5.

   2. When fever is present in a child, the diagnosis of UTI should routinely be considered [47].

   3. Dysuria, especially without bacteriuria, when present may be attributable to other causes such as vaginitis, local perineal irritation, use of bubble baths, masturbation, and pinworm infections. At times, it may be a clue to sexual molestation [46, 47].

   B. Physical examination. A careful abdominal examination, gentle rectal examination, and inspection of the genitals is suggested [46]. Growth failure or hypertension may be present in a child with renal insufficiency.

   C. Diagnosis. A positive urine culture that is properly obtained **is essential** for the diagnosis [46].

   1. Pyuria ($\geq$ 5 WBCs per high-power field) may be absent in centrifuged urine sediment in 30–50% of children with UTI [46, 47]. If pyuria is present, it is strong supportive evidence of a UTI.

   2. The **leukocyte esterase** and **nitrite tests** on a urinalysis may be falsely negative or positive in 15–30% of childhood cases [46].

Table 12-5. Signs and symptoms of urinary tract infections in different age groups

Age	Presentation
Neonate and infant	Hypothermia, hyperthermia, failure to thrive, vomiting, diarrhea, sepsis, irritability, lethargy, jaundice, malodorous urine
Toddler	Abdominal pain, vomiting, diarrhea, constipation, abnormal voiding pattern, malodorous urine, fever, poor growth
School-age child	Dysuria, frequency, urgency, abdominal pain, abnormal voiding pattern (including incontinence or secondary enuresis), constipation, malodorous urine, fever
Adolescent	Dysuria, frequency, urgency, abdominal discomfort, malodorous urine, fever

Source: From J. R. Sherbotic and D. Cornfeld, Management of urinary tract infections in children. *Med. Clin. North Am.* 75:328, 1991.

3. **Urine culture** is advised. A properly collected sample may be difficult to obtain but is essential.
   a. **For neonates,** see Chap. 3.
   b. **For infants and toddlers,** either urethral catheterization (growth of $\geq 1,000$ CFU/ml is significant) or suprapubic bladder aspiration (any growth on culture is significant) is suggested.
      "Bagged" urine specimens frequently are contaminated and, when positive for growth, are difficult to interpret. A negative urine culture from a bagged sample is useful in ruling out a UTI [46].
   c. **For older and cooperative children,** clean-voided, midstream collection for urinalysis, Gram stain, and culture is suggested. Significant colony counts have already been reviewed under UTI in Adults and in sec. **IV.B.2** under General Approach to UTIs.
4. **Gram stain (or unstained examination) of unspun urine under a 40-power microscope lens.** If bacteria and leukocytes are seen, UTI is likely [46, 47].
D. **Antimicrobial therapy.** In general, children who appear ill or who are at significant risk of becoming seriously ill because of their age (e.g., young infants) or who have urinary tract abnormalities should be admitted to the hospital and treated aggressively.
   1. **Neonates.** See Chap. 3.
   2. **Infants** are at risk for serious sequelae of UTI (e.g., sepsis) and so should be treated with intravenous antibiotics. Initial therapy with intravenous ampicillin and gentamicin is suggested (Table 12-6).
      a. A repeat urine culture 48 hours after starting therapy is advised. It should prove negative.
      b. Intravenous antibiotics for 5–7 days commonly are used. If the patient improves rapidly, a switch may be made to oral antibiotics after 3–5 afebrile days; a total course of 10–14 days of antibiotics (IV plus oral) is advised. For the very ill infant, some suggest a full 1-week course of intravenous therapy followed by an additional 2 weeks of oral antibiotics [46, 47].
      c. Radiographic evaluation is advised as below.
      d. A repeat urine culture 1 week after completion of therapy is suggested.
   3. **Children**
      a. **Uncomplicated UTI.** Children older than 6–12 months of age with normal urinary tracts who are not toxic can be treated with oral outpatient regimens.
         (1) Ideally, a urine culture at 48 hours is suggested to ensure that the urine has become sterile.
         (2) A conventional 7- to 10-day course of therapy is advised [46, 47] (see Table 12-6). Ampicillin or amoxicillin still is commonly used in children with initial, uncomplicated UTI, as resistance to *E. coli* occurs less in childhood UTI than in adult UTI.
         (3) Single-dose regimens are not advised in children.

Table 12-6. Suggested antimicrobial therapy for urinary tract infections: dosages and alternatives

Parenteral therapy (suspected upper UTI or sepsis)
Neonates and infants <4–6 months old
  Ampicillin, 75–200 mg/kg/day divided into 4 doses
                      plus
  Gentamicin, 5–7.5 mg/kg/day divided into 2–3 doses
Older children
  Ampicillin, 100 mg/kg/day divided into 4 doses
                      plus
  Gentamicin, 7.5 mg/kg/day divided into 3 doses, *or* a cephalosporin (e.g.,
    cefotaxime, 100–200 mg/kg/day divided into 3–4 doses)

Oral therapy (acute cystitis, resolving upper UTI)
Neonates and infants <4–6 months old
  Amoxicillin, 40 mg/kg/day divided into 3 doses
                      or
  TMP-SMX,* 6–12 mg/kg/day TMP with 30–60 mg/kg/day SMX, divided into 2
    doses
                      or
  Cephalexin, 50 mg/kg/day divided into 3 doses
Older children
  TMP-SMX, 6–12 mg/kg/day TMP with 30–60 mg/kg/day SMX, divided into 2 doses
                      or
  Amoxicillin, 40 mg/kg/day divided into 3 doses

Prophylaxis (for recurrent infections)
TMP-SMX, based on 2 mg/kg/day of TMP as a single nighttime dose
                      or
Nitrofurantoin, 2 mg/kg/day as a single nighttime dose

UTI = urinary tract infection; TMP = trimethoprim; SMX = sulfamethoxazole.
*Sulfonamide agents (e.g., TMP-SMX) should not be used in children younger than 6 weeks. Antibiotic dosages should be adjusted for the level of renal function, and serum levels should be followed where appropriate.
Source: From J. R. Sherbotic and D. Cornfeld, Management of urinary tract infections in children. *Med. Clin. North Am.* 75:335, 1991.

(4) The use of short-course therapy for UTI in children remains controversial. Until further data are available, 3-day regimens should be reserved only for selected patients with asymptomatic bacteriuria and girls older than 5 years with clinical findings of lower UTI, a documented normal genitourinary tract, and poor compliance (in which case a short course would be beneficial) [46].

b. **Complicated UTI.** For patients with fever, chills, CVA tenderness, or GI upset (i.e., presumed pyelonephritis), those who have undergone recent instrumentation, or those with significant anatomic abnormalities, aggressive intravenous antibiotics are suggested [46, 47].

(1) Empiric therapy with ampicillin and gentamicin can be started (see Table 12-6). Regimens can be revised after susceptibility data are available.

(2) Clinical improvement with a decrease in the fever usually begins within 48 hours. If this does not occur, obstruction or a resistant pathogen should be sought.

(3) Intravenous therapy is continued until the patient improves clinically (3–5 days after the temperature normalizes), with completion of a 2- to 3-week total course based on susceptibility studies [46].

(4) A follow-up urine culture is advised 1 week after therapy and, when possible, 4–6 weeks after therapy.

E. **Radiographic evaluation.** In children with UTI, radiographic evaluation of the urinary tract is indicated to identify vesicoureteral reflux, obstruction, or other urinary tract abnormalities. In approximately 30–50% of young children with their first symptomatic UTI, structural abnormality will be found—most commonly, vesicoureteral reflux, which is rare in children without UTI. The indications for radiographic study have recently been reviewed [46, 47].

1. **Indications**
   a. **Any male or female child younger than 5 years** with asymptomatic UTI or asymptomatic bacteriuria.
   b. **Any male child** with a first episode of UTI or asymptomatic bacteriuria.
   c. Recurrent UTI or recurrent asymptomatic bacteriuria in female children older than 5 years who have not been previously evaluated. A sexually active adolescent girl with recurrent lower UTI does not need a radiographic evaluation generally.
   d. A child with his or her first UTI and a family history of urinary tract abnormalities (e.g., reflux) or recurrent UTI, and abnormal voiding pattern, poor growth, or hypertension.
   Recent data suggest that siblings of patients with known vesicoureteral reflux should have a screening study done for early detection of reflux, which may be found in as many as 45% of these children. This is a somewhat controversial recommendation [46].
   e. Any child with pyelonephritis.
2. **The choice of radiographic examinations depends on the facilities available, the skills and experience of the radiologist, and clinical findings** [46, 47]. The clinician should review options and plan studies after discussion with the radiologist.
   a. **Voiding cystourethrography (VCUG)** will detect vesicoureteral reflux, grade the severity of reflux, and provide anatomic as well as functional information of the lower urinary tract.
   b. **Intravenous urogram** has been the time-honored method to evaluate upper tract abnormalities but exposes the patient to more radiation than other options. In recent years, sonography and radionuclide scintigraphy may provide similar data more safely.
   c. **Renal ultrasonography** is noninvasive and free of ionizing radiation. It can reveal obstruction, renal size and contour, stones, size of the collecting system, and bladder anatomy. Upper tract infection may be associated with increases of renal volume of more than 30%.
   Therefore, ultrasonography provides anatomic information and must be combined with a functional study (e.g., special scan).
   d. **Radionuclide scans**
      (1) **Direct radionuclide voiding cystography** will detect reflux with a 50- to 100-fold decrease in gonadal radiation exposure when compared to VCUG, but anatomic detail is not sufficient enough to grade the severity of reflux [46]. **If this test is used as a screen and is abnormal, then a more definitive VCUG can be done.** Periodic radionuclide cystography examinations can be performed to assess the degree of reflux over time.
      (2) **Technetium penetrate** (diethylenetriamine-pentaacetic acid, **DTPA**), like inulin, is cleared by glomerular filtration and results in a dynamic radionuclide intravenous urogram equivalent. When combined with the administration of furosemide, excretory function can be quantitated.
      (3) **Iodohippurate sodium** (^{123}I or ^{131}I), which is secreted by the kidney, can help assess renal blood flow.
      (4) **Technetium succimer** accumulates in functional renal cortex and provides exquisite renal images. It is useful in demonstrating acute pyelonephritis and evaluating focal parenchymal scarring.
   e. **A reasonable approach** is the radiographic evaluation of UTI in children, as shown in Figure 12-1 [46].
      (1) Patients with abnormalities deserve careful evaluation by a specialist in this area.
      (2) The **optimal timing of radiographic studies** is **debated.** Because transient reflux can be masked or overestimated during an acute UTI, some suggest the ideal time of the VCUG is 4–6 weeks after antibiotic therapy is stopped; immediate sonography can be done in the acutely ill child to exclude obstruction [46].
      Others suggest that although a delay may be ideal, to ensure that the study is done, it is reasonable to conduct the radiographic study

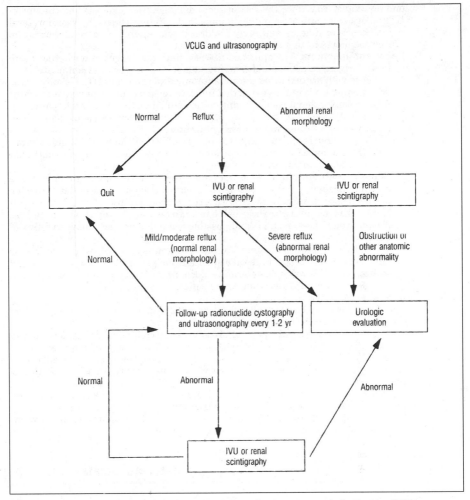

Fig. 12-1. The protocol for radiologic evaluation of urinary tract infection in children. IVU = intravenous urography; VCUG = voiding cystourethrography. (Reprinted by permission of the *Western Journal of Medicine*. From I. Zelikovic et al., Urinary tract infections in children: An update. *West. J. Med.* 157:558, 1992.)

during the initial hospital admission or while the patient is on antibiotic therapy. If radiographic studies are delayed, it probably is prudent to continue low-dose prophylactic agents until the urinary tract anatomy has been defined [47].

3. **Follow-up studies. Mild to moderate reflux usually disappears with increasing age.** The goal of management of reflux is to prevent recurrent UTI and the resultant potential for renal scarring. In patients with documented reflux, repeated ultrasonography every 1–2 years is indicated to follow renal growth, and radionuclide cystograms should be used (e.g., every 1–2 years) serially to determine the resolution of reflux so that antimicrobial prophylaxis can be discontinued when appropriate [47].

VI. **Sequelae** [46, 47]
   A. As many as 80% of children with uncomplicated UTI will have **recurrences.**
   B. **Renal parenchymal infection and renal scarring are well-established complications of UTI in children.** Parenchymal scarring is found in 10–15% of children with UTIs. It has been estimated that nearly 10% may develop hypertension and a smaller percent renal insufficiency [46]. **The risk is especially great in infants**

and neonates. To reduce the risk of renal damage, the diagnosis and therapy of UTI must be prompt. Most of the damage to the kidney caused by vesicoureteral reflux occurs in infancy and early childhood and, therefore, careful workup to prevent sequelae in this age group is essential.

C. Recurrent infections. The approach to these patients depends on whether there is an underlying structural abnormality and on the degree of symptomatology.

1. **Patients with normal urinary tract anatomy and recurrent UTI.** Usually, three documented UTIs in a 1-year period indicate the need for prophylactic therapy. After a conventional course of antibiotics aimed at the susceptible pathogen, either TMP-SMX (10 mg/kg/day of the sulfamethoxazole component, given nightly or every other night) or nitrofurantoin (1–2 mg/kg/day, given nightly) is administered [46]. These agents are very effective and have few side effects. Usually prophylactic antibiotics are given for 6–24 months and discontinued if the patient remains free of infection.

2. **Children with structural abnormalities,** especially vesicoureteral reflux, are best managed with continuous use of prophylactic antibiotics after the urine has been successfully sterilized with a conventional course of antibiotics. Antibiotic regimens similar to those listed in **1** can be used. A prophylactic antibiotic is employed to prevent UTIs and possible renal damage secondary to reflux of infected urine.

   Prophylaxis often is continued for 12–24 months or longer while waiting for mild to moderate reflux to resolve spontaneously. Serial ultrasonography and scanning studies will help determine optimum duration of prophylactic antibiotics for patients with vesicoureteral reflux.

VII. Surgical intervention

A. Mild to moderate vesicoureteral reflux will resolve spontaneously with growth of the child in the majority of patients [46, 47].

B. High-grade vesicoureteral reflux, nonresolving vesicoureteral reflux, or reflux in those children unable to take prophylactic antibiotic therapy may require surgical intervention. These patients should be carefully followed by an experienced pediatric urologist and pediatric nephrologist with a special interest and expertise in these problems.

   Even in patients with high-grade vesicoureteral reflux, conservative management with prophylactic antibiotics often is attempted and frequently is successful. Overall, in approximately 70% of patients with vesicoureteral reflux that is managed conservatively, the condition resolves spontaneously.

Catheter-Associated UTI

The most common nosocomial infections are of the urinary tract, accounting for approximately 40% of all nosocomial infections [47a–48a]. Most patients with nosocomial UTI have had genitourinary manipulation, usually urethral catheterization (approximately 80%) or urologic manipulation (about 20%) [48]. Foley catheters are commonly used in hospitalized patients and in aged nursing home residents.

I. Methods of catheterization and risk of UTI

A. **Single (straight) catheterization.** After this procedure, bacteriuria develops in approximately 1–5% or more (up to 20%) of patients. The risk of infection is lowest in healthy outpatients and greatest in certain high-risk patients such as diabetics, prepartum or postpartum patients, and especially in the elderly, debilitated, hospitalized patient [3, 48].

   Indications for single catheterization include (1) providing relief of temporary obstruction or inability to void; (2) obtaining urine from patients who are unable to provide a clean specimen because of weakness, debility, or other medical problems; (3) determining the amount of residual urine; and (4) conducting a urologic study of urethral anatomy.

B. **Intermittent catheterization.** This method has been helpful in avoiding long-term catheterization, **especially in young patients with spinal cord injuries** [49, 50]. The technique, as originally described after World War II, was a "no-touch" technique performed by a nurse or urologic technician wearing mask, sterile gown, and gloves. Using this technique, approximately 65% of male patients and 50% of female patients were discharged from the hospital with sterile urine [49]. In recent years, a "clean" (as opposed to "sterile") technique has been taught to paraplegic patients who have been able to learn the procedure rather easily. Quadriplegics have been successfully catheterized by a caregiver using a similar technique. This has become a very useful approach for treating spinal cord–injured patients [49, 50]. Intermittent catheterization might also be useful in the postoperative patient who is unable to void.

Intermittent catheterization should not be used in circumstances in which traumatic catheterization may be a problem, such as in obstruction of the urinary tract due to benign prostatic hypertrophy or carcinoma of the prostate. In these cases, an indwelling urethral or suprapubic catheter generally is indicated.

The role of prophylactic antibiotics in this setting is unclear. A preliminary study suggests that prophylactic antibiotics (e.g., TMP-SMX) can reduce bacteriuria and symptomatic UTIs. However, adverse reactions to TMP-SMX are relatively common, and the development of resistant pathogens occurred with prolonged prophylactic antibiotic regimens in this setting [50a]. This approach is likely only to delay episodes of bacteriuria and pose a concern for selecting resistant pathogens. Whether a regimen of mandelamine and ascorbic acid may work has not yet been tested [9b] but is a consideration (see Chap. 28T).

C. **Short-term catheterization.** This may be necessary for monitoring acutely ill patients who are unable to void or who are incontinent and in whom measurement of urine output is mandatory (e.g., postoperative patients or selected patients in intensive care areas). The catheter should be removed as soon as possible to avoid increasing the risks of nosocomial UTI.

1. **Risk factors** associated with catheter-related infection [48]
   a. **Unalterable factors** that increase the risk of infection include female gender, older or debilitated patients, and patients with meatal colonization.
   b. **Potentially alterable factors,** such as duration of catheterization, catheter care techniques, type of drainage system (a closed system is preferred), and whether the patient is receiving systemic antibiotics or not, affect infection rates.

2. The per-day risk of developing bacteriuria is approximately 3–6%, and the cumulative risk increases with duration of catheterization. Therefore, **nearly 50% of hospitalized patients catheterized for longer than 7–10 days develop bacteriuria** [48].

D. **Chronic catheterization.** The patient with a long-term indwelling catheter is at high risk of morbidity due to this procedure. The risk of bacteriuria increases with the duration of catheterization, at a rate of approximately 5% per day. **With protracted catheterization** (> 30 days) **bacteriuria** with at least one bacterial strain **is universal,** and many patients have at least two bacterial strains [47a].

1. **Indications for long-term bladder catheterization**
   a. Patients with atonic bladders, such as those with diabetes or other chronic neurologic disorders
   b. Patients with obstructive uropathy preoperatively, or patients who are not surgical candidates but who have benign prostatic hypertrophy, prostatic carcinoma, and the like

2. **Chronic catheterization should be avoided in the chronically ill, incontinent patient if at all possible.** When other methods of incontinent management such as nursing care, behavioral modification, medication, special clothes, and special bed linens are not successful, there may be no alternative to long-term urethral catheterization in an attempt to prevent skin maceration and resultant decubitus ulcers. Condom catheters are an option for the incontinent male patient.

II. **Pathogenesis of catheter-associated UTI.** Bacteria can enter the urinary tract by either the periurethral or the intraluminal route [47a–48a].

A. **Periurethral or transurethral route.** This route of entry is especially important in catheterized women, probably accounting for 70% of episodes of bacteriuria. Bacteria involved in UTI emanate from the rectal flora and organisms colonize the periurethral zone. Then organisms enter the urinary tract via the external surface of the catheter in the mucous sheath between the catheter and urethral mucosa, similar to the pathogenesis of UTI in noncatheterized women [47a, 48]. This route may be less important in men.

B. **Intraluminal route.** Microorganisms can ascend through the lumen of the urinary catheter into the bladder [47a–48a].

1. In approximately 15–20% of infected patients, the infecting organism appears in the collecting bag before entry into the bladder, which occurs 24–48 hours later.

2. Once in the bladder, small numbers of microorganisms (e.g., 100 organisms per milliliter) can increase to large numbers (e.g., $>10^5$) in 24–48 hours.

3. **Two populations of bacteria** exist in the catheterized urinary tract.

   a. **Planktonic growth** (bacteria growing in the urine itself). Particularly adherent strains of *E. coli* (to uroepithelial cells) may be more likely to cause UTI.

   b. **Biofilm growth** (those bacteria growing on the surface of the catheter). The growth of a bacterial biofilm progresses in an orderly fashion: Bacteria attach to the catheter and initiate a biofilm form of growth in which organisms coat the catheter and secrete an extracellular matrix of bacterial glycocalyces in which they become embedded. Host urinary proteins such as Tamm-Horsfall protein and urinary salts can be incorporated into this biofilm growth, which eventually leads to encrustation of the inner surface of the catheter [47–48a].

      (1) Certain bacteria (e.g., *Proteus* and *Pseudomonas* spp.) appear especially to contribute to biofilm growth.

      (2) In general, biofilm seen on the inner surface of the catheter is much thicker and of a different nature than that seen on the external surface [47a–48a].

      (3) **Implications of the biofilm** [47a]

         (a) **To prevent biofilm growth,** catheter materials that retard bacterial adherence and biofilm growth should be sought.

         (b) **Urine cultures** obtained from the catheter may not reflect bladder bacteriuria in patients who have organisms in a biofilm on the inner surface of the catheter. Bladder urine could be sterile, but organisms from the catheter biofilm may contaminate the aspirated urine culture.

         (c) Biofilms have been demonstrated to retard the activity of antimicrobials. **Therefore, if bacteriuria is treated in a given patient, it may be prudent to replace the catheter.**

4. Breaking the connection at the junction of the catheter and drainage tube or contamination by improper manipulation of the collection bag may facilitate retrograde migration.

C. **Catheter insertion.** Only occasionally do nosocomial UTIs result from direct introduction of urethral microorganisms at the time of catheter insertion, assuming proper technique is used [48].

III. **Complications arising in use of urinary catheters.** Before using indwelling catheters in a patient, one should be thoroughly familiar with the complications associated with their use. Whenever possible, an indwelling catheter should be avoided and, when used, it should be left in place for the shortest time possible.

A. **Bacteriuria.** The incidence of bacteriuria with a bladder catheter depends on the host and the method and duration of catheterization, as has been discussed previously [48].

   1. Most episodes of bacteriuria are asymptomatic. Criteria have not been established for differentiating asymptomatic colonization of the urinary tract from symptomatic infection [47a, 48].

   2. Pyuria accompanies most episodes of symptomatic infection, and its presence suggests host invasion rather than simple bladder colonization.

B. **Pyelonephritis.** The association between bacteriuria and subsequent pyelonephritis is well documented in both clinical and research settings.

   1. The incidence of bacteriuria associated with upper tract disease has not been well defined or studied.

   2. In studies using the antibody-coated bacterial test, as many as 25% of episodes of catheter-associated bacteriuria were positive, suggesting upper UTI [48]. Fever, flank pain, or other symptoms of pyelonephritis are uncommon in these patients.

   3. Patients with prolonged use of catheters (> 10 days) are at increased risk.

C. **Bacteremia or gram-negative sepsis.** In hospitalized patients, approximately 30–40% of all nosocomial gram-negative bacteremias originate from a UTI, usually catheter-associated [48]. It is estimated that 30,000 deaths per year occur as a result of catheter-related sepsis due to gram-negative bacilli [48].

D. **Increased mortality.** Epidemiologic studies have related nosocomial bacteriuria to an approximate threefold relative increase in death. The exact explanation for this is not known but may involve unrecognized episodes of bacteremia [47a, 48].

E. **Other complications** of prolonged urinary catheterization include urinary stones, vesicoureteral reflux, and local periurethral complications such as prostatitis, prostatic abscesses, epididymitis, and scrotal abscesses. The frequency of these infections remains ill-defined.

IV. **Catheter care.** Once the decision to use a catheter has been made, the following guidelines may be useful in decreasing or minimizing the risk of infection. **Catheters should be used only when absolutely necessary and then for the shortest time possible.**

A. For short-term use, two or three single straight catheterizations (every 6 hours) over a 24- to 72-hour period may be preferable to an indwelling catheter because of the lower risk of infection. Repeated straight catheterizations are not advisable in the patient who may be difficult to catheterize (e.g., patients with prostatic hypertrophy, prostatic cancer, or urethral strictures).

B. **Insertion** of the catheter should be **performed under aseptic conditions,** with the use of sterile gloves, sterile catheter, liquid antiseptic soap or an iodophor for perineal cleaning, and sterile, water-soluble lubricating jelly for the catheter. Studies of siliconized or silver ion–coated catheters in comparison to latex catheters have given mixed results. We believe that the limited value, if any, of newer catheters does not warrant their added cost.

C. **A sterile, closed drainage system** with a disposable plastic bag and connecting tubes should be used. The **junction of the catheter and drainage tube should not be disconnected** unless irrigation of an obstructed catheter is necessary, and irrigation should be done with sterile technique. Urine for culture should be aspirated from the aspiration port or distal-most portion of the catheter.

D. **Maintain adequate urine flow** at all times. Ideally, sufficient fluid to maintain a urine output of greater than 100 ml/hr should be given if it is not contraindicated by the patient's clinical condition. Such a urine flow may prevent the ascent of bacteria through the collecting system.

E. **Gravity drainage** should be maintained, with the collection bag lower than the level of the bladder at all times. The bag should never touch the floor and should have a valve adequate to prevent reflux of urine into the bladder if the bag is accidentally raised above the level of the bladder. Urine in the collection bag may have very high bacterial colony counts. The downward drainage will help prevent retrograde spread of bacteria to the patient's bladder. The catheter should not be clamped except when the patient must be separate from his or her drainage bag or temporarily when a culture specimen is being collected.

F. Although some have suggested routine catheter change every 2–3 weeks [1a], we concur with other experts [9b] who suggest that a chronic catheter should **not be changed on a routine schedule. Indications for catheter change include:** (1) malfunction or leakage; (2) obstruction of the catheter; (3) contamination of the system (e.g., breaking the connection between catheter and drainage tube); (4) concretions felt in the catheter lumen, which may precede obstruction of the catheter; and (5) bacteriuria requiring antibiotic therapy as previously discussed in sec. **II.B.3;** and (6) in candiduria, catheter-change may be associated with clearing of the candiduria [9b] (see related discussion in Chap. 18).

G. To minimize the risks of cross-contamination, **a patient with an indwelling catheter should not be placed in the same room** as another patient with an indwelling catheter. Likewise, it is important that **hospital personnel wash their hands** before and after handling any portion of the collection system. Gloves should be used whenever the collection bag is handled, as the bag may be contaminated.

H. After the catheter has been removed, a follow-up urine culture should be done. Symptomatic or persistent bacteriuria should be treated.

I. **Urinary catheters should not be used as a matter of convenience** for the nursing staff or physician.

J. Cleansing the periurethral area with povidone-iodine solution or daily cleansing with soap and water are no longer recommended. These forms of **meatal care** may, in fact, cause meatal irritation and increase the risk for retrograde extraluminal bacterial migration. In addition, they are expensive.

K. **Additional measures** have been employed. Attempts to prevent collection bag–related infection using a variety of bag antibacterial substances (e.g., hydrogen peroxide) have demonstrated no difference in the incidence of bacteriuria among patients whose bags were treated and those whose bags were not. Attempts to modify the catheter by incorporating a vent or by coating the catheter with various antibacterial substances require further study before they can be recommended for routine use.

L. **Condom catheters** are a preferred alternative in selected alert, cooperative patients who can receive meticulous skin care to prevent meatal ulceration. See discussion in sec. **VI.**

M. **Chronic catheterization.** Prevention of infection is very difficult in these patients, who universally develop bacteriuria over time.

V. **Management of catheter-associated bacteriuria.** While the catheter is in place, systemic antimicrobial **treatment of asymptomatic catheter-associated bacteriuria is not recommended** [47a, 48]. Because complications of long-term catheterization are primarily infectious in nature, there is a temptation to treat all patients with catheter-associated bacteriuria; such treatment during catheterization is not helpful in eradicating infection for prolonged periods of time and serves only to select populations of organisms that are resistant to the antibiotics being used. Therefore, **while the catheter is in place, antibiotic treatment is recommended only for symptomatic infection** (i.e., bacteremia, pyelonephritis, epididymitis) [47a, 48].

A. **Short-term catheterization.** In patients who have been catheterized for short periods of time, a urine culture should be obtained at the time the catheter is discontinued or within 24–72 hours of that event. Most patients who have bacteriuria immediately after catheter removal are asymptomatic and many patients, especially younger women, will have cleared the bacteria on repeat culture 1–2 weeks later. If symptomatic or persistent bacteriuria is present, appropriate antibiotic treatment based on susceptibility data should be instituted. The optimal antibiotic regimen in this setting is unclear. In one study of women, persistent bacteriuria after short-term catheterization (e.g., 4–6 days) that was asymptomatic or associated with lower UTI symptoms only was treated as effectively with single doses of TMP-SMX (320–1600 mg) as with a 10-day course of TMP-SMX (160–800 mg bid) in women younger than 65 years old [50b]. For older women, patients with upper tract symptoms, and males (with possible prostatic involvement), we favor conventional therapy (i.e., 10–14 days of antibiotic therapy based on susceptibility studies).

B. **Long-term catheterization.** Certain guidelines are helpful in monitoring and managing these patients.

1. **Urine cultures** in patients with chronic indwelling catheters often reveal multiple species of organisms, frequently with counts of 100,000 CFU/ml or more. These results are difficult to interpret and frequently change over short periods of time. **Routine urine cultures are not recommended if the catheter is draining properly.**

2. **Antibiotic irrigation** of the catheter and bladder have recently been shown to be of no advantage. Although bacteria can be suppressed, the beneficial effect is canceled by the contamination that occurs by periodically opening the collecting system.

3. **Asymptomatic bacteriuria should not routinely be treated.** This condition is very common, as was indicated previously. Because of the presence of a foreign body (i.e., the catheter), one cannot sterilize the bladder for prolonged periods of time. Unnecessary or prolonged use of antibiotics will only increase the likelihood of selecting out more resistant organisms.

4. **Systemic antibiotics should be used for catheterized patients who are febrile and ill-appearing, presumably from a UTI, with signs or symptoms suggesting a possible UTI-related bacteremia or pyelonephritis. Causes of fever other than a urinary tract source should be evaluated,** the catheter should be assessed for partial or complete obstruction, the patient should be examined for periurethral complication of urethral catheterization, and a urine culture should be aseptically obtained. **Because these are hospital-acquired infections, relatively resistant bacteria should be anticipated when selecting empiric antibiotic therapy.** Definitive antibiotic therapy should be adjusted based on susceptibility studies once they are available.

a. **Bacteremic patients.** If bacteremia is suspected or known, broad-spectrum antibiotics are indicated while one is awaiting results of urine and blood cultures. For the hospitalized patient, enterococcal bacteremia would be uncommon and could, for all practical purposes, be excluded if an unspun urine Gram stain showed no gram-positive cocci. While awaiting cultures, an aminoglycoside alone could then be used.

These patients usually require a full 10- to 14-day course of antibiotics because of the associated bacteremia. Once culture data are available, initial empiric therapy can be tailored based on susceptibility data.

b. **Nonbacteremic UTI.** If no bacteremia is suspected or documented, these patients can be treated with short courses of antibiotics (e.g., 3–5 days) based on susceptibility data. This will usually sterilize the urine without selecting out more resistant bacteria. The optimal duration of therapy for a UTI in a male with a chronic catheter is not established. Prolonged therapy may only select out resistant organisms. However, a 3-day course may allow a prostatic focus to persist. While awaiting further guidelines in this setting, a 7-day course may be a reasonable compromise.

For a patient who has just a low-grade temperature and is clinically stable, observation may be reasonable as the low-grade temperature may be transient.

c. **Catheter change.** When antibiotics are given for catheter-related infections, the catheter should be changed as discussed in sec. **II.B.3.**

5. **Chronic antibiotic suppressive therapy is not effective** in these patients. Because the catheter acts as a foreign body, the urine of these patients cannot be sterilized for a prolonged period. Therefore, there are no data to support the use of daily TMP-SMX or quinolones or other antibiotics in this group of patients. In addition, chronic use of methenamine and ascorbic acid is not effective in these patients. Methenamine requires 30–90 minutes to form formaldehyde, the active urinary suppressant. If the catheter is providing adequate drainage, the necessary "contact time" is not provided in the catheterized patient. (See methenamine discussion in Chap. 28T.)

6. **Follow-up therapy.** When the catheter is discontinued, the urine should be cultured and persistent or symptomatic bacteriuria should be treated (see sec. **V.A**).

VI. **Condom catheters.** To obtain adequate urinary outputs, to maintain dryness of the patient with urinary incontinence, or to prevent soiling of an adjacent wound of the sacrum or perineum, a condom catheter system is an excellent alternative to indwelling urethral catheters in the male patient without outlet obstruction. This avoids problems associated with having a catheter within the bladder; however, bladder bacteriuria may still develop in condom-catheterized patients [51].

A. The **risk for bladder bacteriuria** in condom-catheterized patients is increased in uncooperative patients who frequently manipulate their condom drainage system.

B. Other **complications** of condom catheterization include local skin maceration, breakdown, and ulceration.

C. These problems should not occur if (1) constriction by the condom roller ring is avoided; (2) kinking of the collection roller ring or the collection system, which would result in urine retention, is prevented; and (3) the condom is removed once or twice daily to wash and dry the skin. Circumcision may be necessary if the prepuce is macerated and inflamed.

D. Physicians should be aware of the potential for bladder distention and vesicoureteral reflux in some patients with neurogenic bladders, including spine-injured patients.

Fungal UTIs

The presence of fungi in the urine often presents a diagnostic dilemma. *Candida albicans* and other *Candida* spp. in the urine are seen most frequently in diabetics, in patients with indwelling bladder catheters, in patients receiving antibiotics, and occasionally in patients who have had previous instrumentation of the urinary tract. **The presence of fungi in the urine is most often due to colonization** of the bladder and does not represent true infection. **This topic is discussed in Chap. 18.**

Intrarenal and Perinephric Abscess

Intrarenal abscess occurs either as an uncommon consequence of ascending UTI, usually in patients with pyelonephritis and underlying obstructive urinary tract abnormalities, diabetes [6a], or from hematogenous spread of bacteria from an extrarenal primary focus of infection [52]. Intrarenal abscess also may result from spontaneous infection of preexisting renal cysts. Perinephric abscess usually is the result of rupture of an intrarenal abscess into the perinephric space [52]. These are uncommon complications of UTI and, because the onset of symptoms is **characteristically insidious,** they may be overlooked as a cause of fever and flank or abdominal pain.

I. **Clinical manifestations**
  A. **Setting.** Intrarenal and perinephric abscesses are most frequently associated with pyelonephritis in patients with underlying obstructive urinary tract abnormalities. Sometimes, intrarenal abscess is caused by *S. aureus*. Although one-third of patients with hematogenously derived *S. aureus* intrarenal abscesses will have no discernible primary focus of infection, the majority will have clinically apparent skin and soft-tissue infections due to *S. aureus;* predisposing conditions are those that increase the risk for *S. aureus* bacteremia, including hemodialysis, intravenous drug abuse, and diabetes mellitus. Renal cyst infection in patients with polycystic kidney disease usually follows ascending UTI; however, on occasion, infection may be iatrogenic, following cyst instrumentation.
  B. **Signs and symptoms.** Intrarenal and perinephric abscesses usually present with fever, chills, and flank or abdominal pain [52]. Confusion and resultant delay in diagnosis occur when no localized signs or symptoms are present, when nausea, vomiting, or abdominal symptoms predominate, and because of the usual insidious nature of the onset of symptoms. Flank and CVA tenderness are the most common physical findings, with a minority of patients demonstrating a tender flank or abdominal mass. Dysuria may or may not be present.

II. **Diagnosis**
  A. **Signs and symptoms.** Clinical findings of fever, chills, and back pain are nonspecific and may be seen with pyelonephritis, renal and perirenal abscesses and, occasionally, with renal tumor. An abscess or other space-occupying lesion and pyelonephritis complicated by obstruction **should be considered in the patient with UTI when fever persists beyond 48–72 hours despite appropriate antimicrobial therapy.**
  B. **Urinalysis.** Pyuria, proteinuria, bacteriuria, or hematuria usually are present in patients whose infections originate from ascending infection; however, **in one-third of patients, abscess collections will not be in communication with the collecting system and urinalysis will be normal** [52]. Patients with intrarenal abscesses due to *S. aureus* bacteremia and those with infected cysts often will have a normal urinalysis.
  C. **Urine culture.** Two-thirds of patients will have urine cultures positive for aerobic gram-negative bacilli, most commonly *E. coli, Klebsiella* spp., and *Proteus* spp. **However, urine cultures frequently are sterile in patients with infected renal cysts.** Low colony counts (10^2–10^4 CFU/ml) of *S. aureus* are present in one-half of patients with bacteremic intrarenal abscesses; **urine cultures positive for S. aureus in patients who have neither been catheterized nor treated by instrumentation should suggest an underlying S. aureus bacteremia** and, if clinical manifestations are present, possible secondary intrarenal abscess [52].
  D. **Blood cultures.** Bacteremia is confirmed in fewer than one-third of patients [52]. Sustained *S. aureus* bacteremia suggests concurrent endocarditis (see Chaps. 2 and 10).
  E. **Radiographic studies. Ultrasonography and CT scanning** are the imaging tests preferred for definite diagnosis. **Ultrasonography** can identify associated urinary obstruction, and **CT** scanning allows precise anatomic information on the extent of extrarenal soft-tissue extension. Both imaging procedures provide guidance for percutaneous aspiration and drainage. Infected intrarenal cysts may be identified by gallium scanning. Scan-guided percutaneous cyst aspiration and culture provide the definite diagnosis. Excretory urography is employed less frequently today for diagnosis; abnormalities suggestive of intrarenal or perinephric abscess include decreased renal mobility, diminished renal function, calyceal abnormalities, and displacement of the kidney or ureter.

III. Therapy

A. Intrarenal abscesses often respond to antimicrobial therapy alone, and surgical intervention generally is not required. Empiric antimicrobial therapy should be directed against aerobic gram-negative bacilli and *S. aureus*. An aminoglycoside (gentamicin or tobramycin) or aztreonam in combination with a semisynthetic, penicillinase-resistant penicillin (nafcillin or oxacillin) or a first-generation cephalosporin (cephalothin, cephapirin, or cefazolin) provide appropriate therapy pending the results of culture and susceptibility testing. Intravenous antibiotics are suggested in doses used for bacteremic patients, as high renal and extrarenal tissue levels of antibiotics are desirable.

Once susceptibility data are available, a conservative course of therapy of 6–8 weeks usually is begun; however, longer-term therapy may be necessary based on the clinical response.

Treatment of patients with polycystic disease is complicated by the unpredictable penetration of antibiotics into infected cysts [52a] and infectious disease consultation is advised. Percutaneous drainage is indicated in a patient with a large intrarenal abscess, persistent fever, and no clinical improvement after 5–7 days of appropriate antimicrobial therapy. Prompt percutaneous nephrostomy drainage of obstructive lesions should be performed acutely, with delayed permanent corrective surgery.

B. Perinephric abscesses usually require percutaneous or open drainage, and frequently nephrectomy is necessary for definitive therapy. Along with early drainage, empiric antibiotic therapy, as stated in **A**, should be instituted. Despite improved diagnostic and surgical techniques, the mortality for perinephric abscesses remains high [52]. Early urologic and infectious disease consultations are advised.

Genitourinary Tuberculosis

I. Renal tuberculosis.
As in most forms of extrapulmonary tuberculosis, renal tuberculosis is the result of bloodborne dissemination from a primary focus elsewhere in the body, usually the lung but occasionally the GI tract. The tubercle bacilli may be dormant for many years and may reactivate at a later time, with subsequent formation of caseous and cavitary necrosis of the kidney, prostate, or other genitourinary organs [53]. Tuberculosis is discussed in detail in Chap. 9.

A. Clinical presentation

1. Symptoms of dysuria, frequency, nocturia or urgency, and flank or back pain are frequently reported, but fever and constitutional symptoms generally are absent.

2. Approximately one-third of patients with renal tuberculosis have a history of tuberculosis elsewhere in the body that occurred many years previously. Sites of concurrent infection include the lung, bones, joints, other genitourinary organs, and adrenal glands.

B. The **tuberculin skin test** generally is positive in these patients.

C. The **urinalysis** frequently is abnormal, demonstrating the presence of pyuria or hematuria or both. Proteinuria also may be present. Routine bacterial cultures of urine are characteristically negative—hence, the so-called sterile pyuria that often is associated with renal tuberculosis.

D. Abnormal **chest roentgenograms** may be obtained in as many as 75% of such patients, most of whom have inactive pulmonary disease. Some patients have active pulmonary tuberculous infection concurrently.

E. Special studies

1. **Smears.** Urine smears for acid-fast bacilli may have false positive results because of saprophytic mycobacteria present in the urine of healthy patients (see Chap. 9).

2. **Acid-fast bacilli cultures.** Three first-morning clean-catch specimens of urine are preferred over 24-hour collections, which often are contaminated samples. The urine culture will be positive in as many as 90% of patients.

3. **IVP.** Autonephrectomy is common in renal tuberculosis, and often there is secondary calcification.

F. Therapy. Extrapulmonary tuberculosis has been treated in a manner similar to pulmonary tuberculosis if isoniazid and rifampin can be used. Even a short course

(9-month regimen) is reasonable. If isoniazid and rifampin cannot be used together, more protracted therapy (18–24 months) may be indicated (see Chap. 9).

Surgery was the mainstay of treatment before the advent of antituberculous chemotherapy. At present, surgery generally is reserved for complications of renal tuberculosis, such as hemorrhage, sepsis, pain, inability to sterilize the urine, or ureteral stricture.

G. **Prognosis** with chemotherapy is good, with few relapses occurring in patients completing a full course of chemotherapy. Complications may result even though bacteriologic cure has been achieved. Hypertension, bacterial UTI, and ureteral obstruction may be seen.

II. **Male genital tuberculosis.** Tuberculosis of other portions of the male genitourinary tract may be present concurrently with renal tuberculosis. This suggests that infection may occur directly from the urine itself, although hematogenous spread can occur. Epididymitis is the most common form of male genital tuberculosis. A palpable, painful lesion is characteristic of this disease, and the tuberculin skin test generally is positive. Diagnosis is made by biopsy and culture of the mass.

III. **Female genital tuberculosis.** Tuberculosis of the female genital tract is the result of hematogenous spread of tubercle bacilli. The **fallopian tubes** are most commonly involved. Common complaints are chronic pelvic and abdominal pain, menstrual disorders, and infertility. The tuberculin skin test generally is positive, and constitutional symptoms and fever are absent. The demonstration of tubercle bacilli is necessary for diagnosis. Endometrial curettage may reveal granulomas in half the patients with tuberculous endometritis. However, monthly sloughing of the endometrium in the menstruating patient may make histologic diagnosis difficult. Culdoscopy, laparoscopy, and laparotomy ultimately may be required to establish the diagnosis.

References

1. Preheim, L.C. Complicated urinary tract infections. *Am. J. Med.* 79:62, 1985.
1a. Falagas, M.E., and Gorbach, S.L. Practice guidelines: Urinary tract infections. *Infect. Dis. Clin. Pract.* 4:241, 1995.
   This is a nice concise summary of definitions, etiology, epidemiology, natural history, diagnosis, and therapy of UTI.
2. Stamey, T.A. *Pathogenesis and Treatment of Urinary Tract Infections.* Baltimore: Williams & Wilkins, 1980.
2a. Avorn, J., et al. Reduction of bacteriuria and pyuria after ingestion of cranberry juice. *J.A.M.A.* 271:751, 1994.
   Study in more than 150 elderly women and subjects randomly assigned to consume 300 ml daily of commercial cranberry juice versus a flavored placebo. Findings suggest cranberry juice reduces the frequency of bacteriuria and pyuria.
3. Kunin, C.M. *Detection, Prevention and Management of Urinary Tract Infections* (4th ed.). Philadelphia: Lea & Febiger, 1987.
   For a more recent textbook devoted to UTI, see H.L.T. Mobley and J.W. Warren, Urinary Tract Infections: Molecular Pathogenesis and Clinical Management. *Washington, D.C.: ASM Press [in press].*
4. Stamm, W.E., et al. Urinary tract infections: From pathogenesis to treatment. *J. Infect. Dis.* 159:400, 1989.
   Emphasizes that susceptibility data alone may not predict the success of an antibiotic in treating a UTI. The length of time that a therapeutic concentration of an antibiotic remains in the urine, whether significant vaginal fluid levels of the drug are achieved, and whether the drug accumulates in renal tissue also are important. Trimethoprim-sulfamethoxazole is superior to amoxicillin in many of these characteristics.
5. Kunin, C.M. Urinary tract infections in females. *Clin. Infect. Dis.* 18:1, 1994.
   One of the state-of-the-art clinical article series. For a review of 270 episodes of S. saprophyticus, see P. Hedman and O. Ringertz, Urinary tract infections caused by Staphylococcus saprophyticus. J. Infect. Dis. *23:145, 1991.*
6. Hooton, T.M., et al. *Escherichia coli* bacteriuria and contraceptive method. *J.A.M.A.* 265:64–69, 1991.
   Study concluded that use of the diaphragm with spermicidal jelly or use of a spermicidal foam with a condom markedly alters normal vaginal flora and strongly predisposes users to the development of vaginal colonization and bacteriuria with E. coli.
6a. Patterson, J.E., and Andriole, V.T. Bacterial urinary tract infections in diabetes. *Infect. Dis. Clin. North Am.* 9:25, 1995.

Includes nice discussion of complications of UTI: renal cortical abscesses, renal corti-
comedullary abscess, emphysematous complications, perinephric abscess, and renal
papillary necrosis.
7. Meares, E.M., Jr. Prostatitis. *Med. Clin. North Am.* 75:405, 1991.
    A good summary of prostatic infection from the investigator who has studied and
    written widely on the condition.
7a. Bergeron, M.G. Treatment of pyelonephritis in adults. *Med. Clin. North Am.* 79:
    619, 1995.
8. Stamm, W.E. Measurement of pyuria and its relation to bacteriuria. *Am. J. Med.*
    75:53, 1983.
    A critical analysis of the sensitivity and specificity of pyuria as it relates to bacteriuria.
9. Mears, E.M. Renal Abscess. In S.L. Gorbach, J.G. Bartlett, and N.R. Blacklow (eds.).
    Infectious Diseases. Philadelphia: Saunders, 1992.
9a. Stamm, W.E. Quantitative urine cultures in infectious disease diagnosis: Use and
    abuse. Symposium on quantitative cultures in infectious disease diagnosis: Use and
    abuse. 35th Interscience Conference on Antimicrobial Agents and Chemotherapy.
    San Francisco, CA: Sept. 19, 1995.
9b. Stamm, W.E., and Warren, J.E. Meet the Professor Session: Urinary Tract Infection.
    Infectious Disease Society of America 33rd Annual Meeting. San Francisco, CA: Sept.
    16, 1995.
10. Jenkins, R.D., Fenn, J.P., and Matson, J.M. Review of urine microscopy for bacteriuria.
    J.A.M.A. 255:3397, 1986.
11. Komaroff, A.L. Urinalysis and urine culture in women with dysuria. *Ann. Intern.*
    Med. 104:212, 1986.
    Neither pretherapy nor posttherapy urine cultures are necessary in dysuric women
    with presumed cystitis if pyuria is confirmed.
12. Stamm, W.E. When should we use urine cultures? *Infect. Control* 7:431, 1986.
    See also J.P. Patton, D.B. Nash, and E. Abrutyn, Urinary tract infections: Economic
    considerations. Med. Clin. North Am. *75:495–513, 1991.*
13. Stamm, W.E., et al. Causes of acute urethral syndrome in women. *N. Engl. J. Med.*
    303:409, 1980.
    A pivotal investigation for our current understanding of UTI symptoms in women.
14. Stamm, W.E., et al. Diagnosis of coliform infection in acutely dysuric women. *N. Engl.*
    J. Med. 307:463, 1982.
14a. Kunin, C.M. A reassessment of the importance of "low-count" bacteriuria in young
    women with acute urinary symptoms. *Ann. Intern. Med.* 119:454, 1993.
15. Lipsky, B.A., et al. Diagnosis of bacteriuria in men: Specimen collection and culture
    interpretation. *J. Infect. Dis.* 155:847–854, 1987.
16. Scheer, W.E. The detection of leukocyte esterase activity in urine with a new reagent
    strip. *Am. J. Clin. Pathol.* 87:86, 1987.
17. American College of Physicians. Common uses of intravenous pyelography in adults.
    Ann. Intern. Med. 111:83, 1989.
    See also A.I. Mushlin and J.R. Thornbury, Intravenous pyelography: The case against
    its routine use. Ann. Intern. Med. *111:58, 1989.*
18. Belman, A.B. Urinary imaging in children. *Pediatr. Infect. Dis. J.* 8:548, 1989.
19. Sobel, J.D., and Kaye, D. Urinary Tract Infections. In G.L. Mandell, J.E. Bennett,
    and R. Dolin (eds.), *Principles and Practice of Infectious Diseases* (4th ed.). New York:
    Churchill Livingstone, 1995. P. 662.
20. Medical Letter. The choice of antibacterial drugs. *Med. Lett. Drugs Ther.* 36:53, 1994.
    For acute, uncomplicated UTI, before the infecting organism is known, the drug of
    first choice is trimethoprim-sulfamethoxazole.
21. Jones, S.R., Smith, J.W., and Sanford, J.P. Localization of urinary tract infections
    by detection of antibody-coated bacteria in urine sediment. *N. Engl. J. Med.* 290:
    591, 1974.
22. Thomas, V.L., and Forland, M. Antibody-coated bacteria in urinary tract infections.
    Kidney Int. 21:1, 1982.
    A noninvasive technique for localizing the site of UTI, which has been primarily
    employed in research settings.
22a. Andriole, V.T., and Patterson, T.F. Epidemiology, natural history, and management
    of urinary tract infections in pregnancy. *Med. Clin. North Am.* 75:359, 1991.
23. Stamm, W.E., and Hooton, T.M. Management of urinary tract infections in adults.
    N. Engl. J. Med. 329:1328–1334, 1993.
23a. Norrby, S.R. Short-term treatment of uncomplicated lower urinary tract infections
    in women. *Rev. Infect. Dis.* 12:458, 1990.

24. Safrin, S., et al. Pyelonephritis in women: Inpatient vs. outpatient treatment. *Am. J. Med.* 85:793, 1988.
    When pyelonephritis occurs in otherwise healthy adult women who do not appear bacteremic, oral antibiotics are reasonable and very cost-effective.

25. Stamm, W.E., McKevitt, M., and Counts, G.W. Acute renal infection in women: Treatment with trimethoprim-sulfamethoxazole or ampicillin for two or six weeks. A randomized trial. *Ann. Intern. Med.* 106:341, 1987.
    Two weeks was as effective as 6 weeks. There were more recurrences with amoxicillin. Overall, these patients had mild illness allowing outpatient therapy. Trimethoprim-sulfamethoxazole therapy was preferred over amoxicillin therapy by the authors.

26. Sikorsky, M.B., et al. Metastatic infection secondary to genitourinary tract sepsis. *Am. J. Med.* 61:351, 1976.
    Although much less likely than Staphylococcus aureus *to cause metastatic infection, aerobic gram-negative uropathogens can cause vertebral osteomyelitis, splenic abscess, and other infections if bacteremia occurs during a UTI.*

27. Schwab, S.J., Bander, S.J., and Klahr, S. Renal infection in autosomal dominant polycystic kidney disease. *Am. J. Med.* 82:714, 1987.
    Trimethoprim-sulfamethoxazole is a potentially useful agent. See the related article by W.M. Bennett et al., Cyst fluid antibiotic concentrations in autosomal-dominant polycystic kidney disease. Am. J. Kidney Dis. *6:400, 1985.*

28. Nicolle, L.E., and Ronald, A.R. Recurrent urinary tract infection in adult women: Diagnosis and treatment. *Infect. Dis. Clin. North Am.* 1:793–806, 1987.
    A concise review of a common condition by an important investigative group.

29. Stapleton, A., et al. Postcoital antimicrobial prophylaxis for recurrent urinary tract infection: A randomized, double-blind, placebo-controlled trial. *J.A.M.A.* 264:703–706, 1990.

30. Stamm, W.E., McKevitt, M., and Toberts, N.J. Natural history of recurrent urinary tract infections in women. *Rev. Infect. Dis.* 13:77–84, 1991.
    A recent review of the pathogenesis and pattern of recurrent UTIs in women.

31. Stamm, W.E., et al. Antimicrobial prophylaxis of recurrent urinary tract infections. A double-blind, placebo-controlled trial. *Ann. Intern. Med.* 106:341–345, 1980.
    The single best clinical investigation of the response of recurrent UTIs to antimicrobial management.

32. Wong, E.S., et al. Management of recurrent urinary tract infections with patient-administered single-dose therapy. *Ann. Intern. Med.* 102:302–307, 1985.
    An approach to management of recurrent UTIs that may be used more often than clinicians either are aware of or admit. As per text discussion, in an educated, reliable patient, self-administration of a 3-day course of antibiotics probably is more appropriate.

32a. Raz, R., and Stamm, W.E. A controlled trial of intravaginal estriol in postmenopausal women with recurrent urinary tract infections. *N. Engl. J. Med.* 329:753–756, 1993.
    Study concluded that intravaginal estriol prevents UTIs in postmenopausal women probably by modifying vaginal flora. See editorial comment in same issue.
    The treated group received 0.5-mg estriol in vaginal cream, used nightly for 2 weeks followed by twice-weekly applications for 8 months.

33. Lipsky, B.A. Urinary tract infections in men. Epidemiology, pathophysiology, diagnosis and treatment. *Ann. Intern. Med.* 110:138–150, 1989.
    See related article by J.N. Krieger et al., Urinary tract infections in healthy university men. J. Urol. *149:1046, 1993. This study concludes that extensive evaluation of young college-age men with bacteriuria that responds to antimicrobial therapy seems unnecessary.*

34. Smith, J.W., et al. Recurrent urinary tract infections in men. Characteristics in response to therapy. *Ann. Intern. Med.* 91:544, 1979.
    Highlights the principal role of the prostate as the source for relapsing UTIs in men.

35. Meares, E.M., Jr., and Stamey, T.A. Bacteriologic localization patterns in bacterial prostatitis and urethritis. *Invest. Urol.* 5:492, 1968.

36. Meares, E.M., Jr. Prostatitis and Related Disorders. In P.C. Walsh et al. (eds.), *Campbell's Urology* (5th ed.). Philadelphia: Saunders, 1986. Pp. 868–887.

37. Meares, E.M., Jr. Bacterial prostatitis versus "prostatosis." A clinical and bacteriological study. *J.A.M.A.* 224:1372, 1973.

38. Ireton, R.C., and Berger, R.E. Prostatitis and epididymitis. *Urol. Clin. North Am.* 11:83–93, 1984.

39. Berger, R.E., Kessler, D., and Holmes, K.K. Etiology and manifestations of epididy-

mitis in young men: Correlations with sexual orientation. *J. Infect. Dis.* 155:1341–1343, 1987.

40. Vorland, L.H., Carlson, K., and Aalen, O. An epidemiological survey of urinary tract infections among outpatients in Northern Norway. *Scand. J. Infect. Dis.* 17:277–283, 1985.

41. Baldassarre, J.S., and Kaye, D. Special problems of urinary tract infection in the elderly. *Med. Clin. North Am.* 75:375, 1991.

41a. Nicolle, L.E. *Infection* 20(Suppl.4):S261, 1992.
Therapy of 7–14 days is suggested in elderly women, as short-course therapy is not as effective in these patients. A similar recommendation is made by J.D. McCue, Urinary tract infections in the elderly. Pharmacotherapy *13:51S, 1993. The reviewer emphasizes that relapse or recurrence is more common in the elderly, regardless of the duration of therapy.*

42. Heinamaki, P., et al. Urinary characteristics and infection in the very aged. *Gerontology* 30:403, 1984.
Pyuria in the elderly lacks specificity as a predictor for bacteriuria.

43. Yoshikawa, T.T. Unique aspects of urinary tract infection in the geriatric population. *Gerontology* 30:339–344, 1984.

44. Nicolle, L.E., et al. The association of bacteriuria with resident characteristics and survival in elderly institutionalized men. *Ann. Intern. Med.* 106:682–686, 1987.
Bacteriuria in the frail elderly is not associated with any reduction in survival. See related discussions by L.E. Nicolle, Urinary tract infection in the institutionalized elderly. Infect. Dis. Clin. Pract. *1:68, 1992, and E. Abrutyn et al., Does asymptomatic bacteriuria predict mortality and does antimicrobial treatment reduce mortality in elderly ambulatory women?* Ann. Intern. Med. *120:827, 1994. The latter concludes that screening and treatment of asymptomatic bacteriuria in ambulatory elderly women do not appear warranted to decrease mortality.*

45. Boscia, J.A., et al. Epidemiology of bacteriuria in an elderly ambulatory population. *Am. J. Med.* 80:208–214, 1986.
Attempts at eradication of asymptomatic bacteriuria in the elderly are frequently unsuccessful and not warranted. See also L.E. Nicolle, W.J. Mayhew, and L. Bryan, Prospective randomized comparison of therapy and no therapy for asymptomatic bacteriuria in institutionalized elderly women. Am. J. Med. *83:27 33, 1987.*

46. Zelikovic, I., Adelman, R.D., and Nancarrow, P.A. Urinary tract infections in children, an update. *West. J. Med.* 157:554–561, 1992.
A thoughtful review of the diagnosis and management of UTIs in children, including a discussion of appropriate imaging for vesicoureteral reflux.

47. Carmack, M.A., and Arvin, A.M. Urinary tract infections—navigating complex currents. *West. J. Med.* 157:587–588, 1992.
A concise review of the controversies in managing UTIs in children.

47a. Stamm, W.E. Catheter-associated urinary tract infections: Epidemiology, pathogenesis, and prevention. *Am. J. Med.* 91(Suppl. 3B):65–71, 1991.

48. Stamm, W.E. Nosocomial Urinary Tract Infections. In J.V. Bennett and P.S. Brachman (eds.), *Hospital Infections* (3rd ed.). Boston: Little, Brown, 1992. Pp. 597–609.

48a. Warren, J.W. The catheter and urinary tract infection. *Med. Clin. North Am.* 75:481, 1991.
See related review by J.W. Warren, Catheter-associated urinary tract infections. Infect. Dis. Clin. North Am. *1:823, 1987.*

49. Perkash, I., and Giroux, J. Clean intermittent catheterization in spinal cord injury patients: A follow-up study. *J. Urol.* 149:1068, 1993.
Study of 50 patients over time (average of 22 months) concluding that clean intermittent catheterization is a successful long-term option to drain bladders in spinal cord injury patients who can perform catheterization independently.

50. Kamitsuka, P.F. The pathogenesis, prevention, and management of urinary tract infections in patients with spinal cord injury. *Curr. Clin. Top. Infect. Dis.* 13:1, 1993.

50a. Gribble, M.J., and Putterman, M.L. Prophylaxis of urinary tract infection in persons with recent spinal cord injury: A prospective, randomized, double-blind, placebo-controlled study of trimethoprim-sulfamethoxazole. *Am. J. Med.* 95:141, 1993.

50b. Harding, G.K.M., et al. How long should catheter-associated urinary tract infections in women be treated? A randomized controlled study. *Ann. Intern. Med.* 114:713, 1991.

51. Hirsh, D.D., Fainstein, V., and Musher, D.M. Do condom catheter collecting systems cause urinary tract infection? *J.A.M.A.* 242:340, 1979.
Substantiates the risk of UTIs associated with condom catheters.

52. Patterson, J.E., and Andriole, V.T. Renal and perirenal abscesses. *Infect. Dis. Clin. North Am.* 1:907–926, 1987.
Also see H. Edelstein and R.E. McCabe, Perinephric abscess in pediatric patients: Report of six cases and review of the literature. Pediatr. Infect. Dis. *8:167, 1989. See also reference [9].*

52a. Andriole, V. Intrarenal and Perinephric Abscess. In P.D. Hoeprich, M.C. Jordan, and A.R. Arnold (eds.), *Infectious Diseases* (5th ed.). Philadelphia: Lippincott, 1994. P. 617.

53. Simon, H.B., et al. Genitourinary tuberculosis: Clinical features in a general hospital population. *Am. J. Med.* 63:410, 1977.
Though published nearly 20 years ago, this remains a useful article. For a recent series, see J.A. Garcia-Rodriguez et al., Genitourinary tuberculosis in Spain: A review of 81 cases. Clin. Infect. Dis. *18:557, 1994.*

Sexually Transmitted Diseases

John A. Jernigan
and Michael F. Rein

General Principles in Management

I. **Definition.** The sexually transmitted diseases (STDs) are infections with heterogeneous agents that are grouped together because sexual contact is epidemiologically significant, although it is not necessarily the only mechanism through which the diseases are acquired.

II. **Consequences**
   A. One can immediately identify a population of patients at high risk for each infection—namely the sexual partners of patients with the STD.
      1. Sexual partners must be evaluated.
      2. The risk of infection may be so high that such partners are treated when first evaluated, even if their infection has not yet been confirmed. Such treatment, on the basis of risk rather than diagnosis, is termed **epidemiologic treatment** and is a cornerstone of management of STDs [1].
      3. **Epidemiologic treatment** recognizes the following possibilities:
         a. Diagnostic tests are imperfect and may miss some (particularly early) stages of some infections.
         b. Some patients will fail to return for follow-up.
         c. Some patients will develop complications while awaiting the results of diagnostic tests.
         d. Some patients will infect other partners while awaiting the results of diagnostic tests.
         e. It may be considerably cheaper to treat a patient than to perform a diagnostic test.
   B. The **STDs are diseases of life-style.** Patients with more than one sexual partner, or whose partners have more than one sexual partner, are more likely to acquire STDs.
      1. **Patients with one STD are significantly likely to have others.** Thus, a patient in whom one STD has been diagnosed should be carefully evaluated for others that may be clinically silent but of much greater eventual medical consequence.
      2. Sexually active patients often present repeatedly with new infections. **Patient education regarding risk reduction** is an important aspect of management.
      3. Some patients appear to be members of **core groups,** populations manifesting an extremely high incidence of STD, and which account for most STD morbidity.
   C. **Management** of an STD **always involves dealing with more than one patient.**
      1. Cure rates usually are increased by treating sexual partners simultaneously, meaning that all have completed treatment before unprotected sexual contact is resumed.
      2. Several STDs [syphilis, gonorrhea, chancroid, lymphogranuloma venereum, AIDS and, in some states, asymptomatic human immunodeficiency virus (HIV) infection] must be reported to local health departments so that contact tracing can be undertaken.
      3. Many STDs are asymptomatic. Patients with an asymptomatic STD should be treated.

III. A careful and complete **sexual history** must be obtained for each patient.
   A. The history must be taken in terms understandable to the patient. Thus, the examiner must become desensitized to using street terms (e.g., "Do you take your

partner's penis into your mouth?" or "Do you give head?") rather than technical jargon (e.g., "Do you practice fellatio?").

B. **Never make assumptions regarding your patient's sexual orientation.** Obtain a sexual history in gender-neutral terms (e.g., "Have you had sex with any new partners in the past month?" rather than "Have you had sex with any new women [men] in the past month?") until the patient's sexual preferences have been defined explicitly.

IV. **A history of recent antibiotic use** is critical because antibiotics may mask clinical features of disease without producing a cure.

Urethritis

Urethritis is a common presenting syndrome. Initial evaluation requires differentiating gonococcal from nongonococcal urethritis.

I. **Epidemiology.** The major single specific etiology of acute urethritis is *Neisseria gonorrhoeae*, producing **gonococcal urethritis (GCU).** Urethritis of all other etiologies is collectively referred to as **nongonococcal urethritis (NGU).**

A. NGU is twice as common as GCU in the United States. NGU is the most common STD syndrome that occurs in men and accounts for an estimated 4 to 6 million physician visits annually [1a].

B. NGU appears disproportionately common in higher socioeconomic groups with acute urethritis, but this may be an artifact of health care behavior.

C. GCU is relatively more common among homosexual than it is among heterosexual men with acute urethritis [2].

II. **Clinical features in men.** (**Urethritis in women** is discussed in sec. **VI.**) Although the spectrum of clinical features of GCU and NGU differ, there is so much overlap that **differential diagnosis cannot be based reliably on clinical features alone.** A significant proportion of men with GCU or NGU may be asymptomatic.

A. **Incubation period.** This can sometimes be assessed if the patient has had a single sexual exposure or sex with a new partner within the preceding several weeks.
1. Seventy-five percent of symptomatic men with GCU develop symptoms within 4 days and 80–90% within 2 weeks [3].
2. Fifty percent of symptomatic men with NGU develop symptoms within 4 days, but the incubation period is much more variable, ranging from 2 to 35 days [3].
3. An incubation period of less than 1 week has no differential diagnostic significance.
4. Incubation periods can be prolonged by subcurative doses of antibiotics.

B. **Urethral discharge.** Discharge is described by 75% of men with GCU but only by 11–33% of men with NGU [3].
1. Discharge present at the meatus without stripping strongly suggests GCU.
2. Mucopurulent discharge (purulent flecks in a mucoid matrix) is seen in 50% of cases of NGU but also in 25% of cases of GCU.
3. A completely clear urethral discharge suggests NGU.
4. The discharge in NGU may be so slight as to be present only as a meatal bead or a crust noted when the patient first arises.

C. **Dysuria** is common in both GCU and NGU.
1. Urethral discomfort may occur at other times and be described as itching or irritation.
2. Urethral symptoms may mimic those of cystitis, particularly in women.

D. **Onset.** Symptoms usually begin fairly abruptly with GCU, whereas the onset of NGU may be less acute.

E. **Natural history.** The clinical features of acute urethritis eventually will resolve without treatment.
1. Ninety-five percent of patients with GCU will become asymptomatic within 6 months.
2. Chronic gonorrhea sometimes manifests as gleet, producing a thin discharge containing only small numbers of gonococci.
3. Of patients with NGU, 30–70% become asymptomatic over 1–3 months [3].

III. **Diagnosis and differential diagnosis in men.** A simple physical examination and Gram stain of the urethral specimen provide an extremely accurate guide to initial therapy.

A. **Examination of the patient.** Men should stand before the seated examiner, and the entire genital area should be examined.
  1. It is preferable that the patient be examined at least 2 hours after micturition.
  2. The underwear may reveal stains of discharge.
  3. Erythema around the meatus may indicate urethritis, but some degree of perimeatal blush is often a normal finding.
  4. Discharge spontaneously present at the meatus is easily recovered for examination.
  5. If discharge is not spontaneously present, the urethra should be gently stripped by placing the gloved thumb along the ventral surface of the penis with the fingers above, applying gentle pressure, and moving the thumb forward to deliver discharge.

B. **Examination of the urethral specimen**
  1. If no discharge is expressed from the meatus, urethral material must be recovered by inserting a small swab into the urethra.
    a. The patient should be warned about the brief discomfort that will result.
    b. **A calcium alginate or rayon swab on a metal shaft is preferred.** Cotton swabs, and particularly wooden shafts, may be toxic to some organisms. A 1- to 2-mm swab should be used rather than the larger cotton swabs.
    c. The swab is inserted approximately 1.5–2.0 inches into the urethra and removed while the shaft is being rotated.
  2. The swab is rolled across a microscope slide and then rolled across a plate of medium selective for *N. gonorrhoeae*. Media in common use include modified Thayer-Martin, Transgrow, Martin-Lewis, and NYC, among others.
  3. The slide is fixed and Gram-stained using standard methods.
  4. The slide is examined using the oil-immersion objective (950–1,000 ×).
    a. The urethra has a cuboidal epithelium, and sheets of such cells are seen in the normal smear.
    b. The distal urethra supports a **normal bacterial flora** consisting primarily of gram-positive cocci and rods. Such organisms, seen on Gram stain, have no clinical significance.
    c. **Spermatozoa** sometimes are present in physiologic secretions. The heads are gram-positive and characteristically fade out toward the achrosomal cap. Gram-negative tails sometimes are observed.
    d. Some authorities have suggested that one must observe five polymorphonuclear neutrophils (PMNs) per oil-immersion field to make a diagnosis of urethritis. In clinical practice, this criterion is too restrictive and insensitive, and 16–50% of men with acute urethritis will fail to show this number of PMNs in the densest portion of the slide [3]. The number of PMNs observed is reduced by recent micturition. **The presence of even small numbers of PMNs on a urethral smear provides objective evidence of urethritis,** especially if discharge can be expressed from the meatus.
    e. The **complete absence of PMNs** argues against urethritis. The discomfort of symptomatic patients may persist from adequately treated urethritis, psychosomatic symptoms, or perhaps discomfort resulting from excessive consumption of urethral irritants such as caffeine or alcohol. Such patients are best managed with reassurance and reexamination if symptoms persist.
    f. The presence of PMNs supports the diagnosis of urethritis. If, in addition, one sees characteristic **gram-negative, intracellular diplococci,** the diagnosis of gonorrhea is established. If the organisms are not observed, the patient is said to have NGU. This test is more than 95% accurate in men with symptomatic acute urethritis. The presence of extracellular organisms with the same morphology has no diagnostic significance [4, 5].
  5. **One cannot diagnose concurrent NGU by Gram staining in the presence of gonorrhea. However, because coincident infection with chlamydiae is very common in GCU, the examiner should assume that patients with gonorrhea are coinfected with nongonococcal pathogens** (see sec. V.A.5).

IV. **Microbiologic features in men**
  A. **Gonorrhea**
    1. *N. gonorrhoeae* is a gram-negative, kidney-shaped diplococcus with flattened opposed margins.
    2. **Growth requirements.** Optimum results are obtained when clinical specimens are plated directly [4] and incubated immediately at 35–37°C in an atmosphere containing 5–10% CO_2.

    a. Some strains of *N. gonorrhoeae* are susceptible to the vancomycin contained in selective media and will not grow thereon. **A negative culture in the face of a positive Gram stain does not rule out GCU.**

    b. **Growth of typical colonies that are oxidase-positive and consist of gram-negative diplococci strongly suggests gonorrhea.** Other *Neisseria* species will, however, grow on selective media, and cultures from other sites (e.g., conjunctiva, pharynx) should not be considered positive until the organisms have been conclusively identified biochemically or immunologically [4].

  3. Antimicrobial susceptibility. The gonococcus has developed resistance to antimicrobial agents by two mechanisms.

    a. Chromosomal mutations. Any of several mutations on the bacterial chromosome confer small increases in resistance to single or multiple antibiotics. The effect of such mutations is additive, and strains with relatively high resistance to many classes of antibiotics are now widely observed [6, 7].

    b. Plasmids. Gonococci bearing plasmids coding for **penicillinase production** were recognized in 1976 [8]. Data from a US surveillance system reveal that the proportion of penicillinase-producing isolates rose from 3.2% in 1988 to 11% in 1991 [7]. They are not eradicated by achievable doses of penicillins (unless accompanied by a penicillinase inhibitor). Penicillinase-resistant penicillins (e.g., nafcillin, cloxacillin) possess too little antigonococcal activity for clinical use. A plasmid coding for high-level **tetracycline resistance** and that is self-transmissible has been recognized and is widespread among gonococcal strains in the United States [7].

    c. Consequently, penicillins (e.g., procaine penicillin G, ampicillin, amoxicillin) **and tetracyclines** (e.g., tetracycline, hydrochloride, doxycycline, minocycline) **can no longer be considered reliable treatment for gonorrhea** [6, 9, 9a].

B. Nongonococcal urethritis

  1. NGU is caused by any of several organisms. The cause of perhaps 20% of cases has not been identified.

  2. *Chlamydia trachomatis* appears to cause 20–50% of cases of NGU in various studies [1a, 3, 9b, 10–14].

    a. The organism is an obligate intracellular parasite with a unique life cycle. It possesses both DNA and RNA and replicates by binary fission rather than by subunit assembly. It thus resembles bacteria (rather than viruses) and is, most importantly, **sensitive to a variety of antibiotics, principally the tetracyclines and the macrolides.**

    b. The organism can be grown only in tissue culture, an expensive and time-consuming procedure. The presence of the organism can be detected with new techniques including a commercially available **nucleic acid hybridization** test, which appears to be both sensitive and specific [15]. **Enzyme-linked immunosorbent assay (ELISA)** and **direct immunofluorescence** tests are also available [14]. These tests have somewhat lower sensitivity than tissue culture but are far more economical and may be used for screening.

    c. The spectrum of diseases caused by *C. trachomatis* closely parallels that caused by *N. gonorrhoeae,* and differential diagnosis usually involves these two organisms. **Coinfection with these two organisms is very common and affects management strategies.**

  3. *Ureaplasma urealyticum,* formerly known as the T-strain mycoplasma, causes some poorly defined fraction of the remaining cases, perhaps 15–30% of NGU [1a, 3, 10, 11, 13].

    a. Ureaplasmas are free-living agents that can be grown in broth or on culture plates. Cultures rarely are performed in clinical practice.

    b. Although most ureaplasmas are sensitive to the tetracyclines, some are resistant and must be treated with a macrolide (e.g., erythromycin) [16–18].

  4. *Trichomonas vaginalis* usually is carried asymptomatically by men but is believed to be an occasional cause of tetracycline-resistant NGU [19]. However, recent reviewers suggest it may be a more common pathogen in nonchlamydial NGU [1a].

  5. Herpes simplex virus can infect the urethra and cause dysuria, which is usually far more severe than the amount of discharge would suggest [20].

    a. The urethritis usually occurs in the setting of external lesions.

    b. Urethral smear shows relatively few PMNs.

  6. Other organisms are rare causes of NGU [3].

V. Treatment in men
  A. Gonorrhea. The frequency with which infection is caused by antimicrobial-resistant strains of *N. gonorrhoeae* forces abandonment of traditional treatment regimens based on penicillin, ampicillin, amoxicillin, or tetracyclines.
   1. According to data from a US national sentinel surveillance system established in 1986, the proportion of all isolates resistant to penicillins or tetracyclines has steadily increased, accounting for nearly one-third of all isolates in 1991 [7].
   2. Recommended for uncomplicated anogenital or pharyngeal gonococcal infection is a single dose of intramuscular ceftriaxone. Probenecid is not required [9, 9a].
     a. Although the recommended dose of ceftriaxone in the past has been **250 mg IM,** many authorities now recommend **125 mg IM** on the basis of economy and ease of administration (e.g., in the deltoid). Clinical experience suggests that either dose is safe and effective [9]. The larger dose has been advocated based on the supposition that its use may delay the onset of emergence of resistance.
     b. The 0.5- to 1-ml injection is less painful if made up in 1% lidocaine.
     c. The dose in children is 125 mg IM once.
   3. Several other regimens are effective against anogenital disease [9, 9a]. Of these, only ciprofloxacin and cefixime have demonstrated acceptable cure rates for pharyngeal infections, and so these should be used if pharyngeal infection is a concern.
     a. Parenteral regimens
       (1) Ceftizoxime 500 mg IM once
       (2) Cefotaxime 500 mg IM once
       (3) Spectinomycin 2 g IM once. Use of this drug should be limited because of the risk of resistance developing in populations [21].
     b. Oral regimens. Until 1992, virtually all strains of *N. gonorrhoeae* tested were susceptible to fluoroquinolones. However, strains with decreased susceptibilities to ciprofloxacin have been isolated sporadically from patients in the United States, with one bothersome report from Ohio indicating 5.6% of strains endemic to a community had decreased susceptibility to ciprofloxacin [21a]. Serum levels achieved with the recommended doses of ciprofloxacin suggest that these strains should respond to therapy, but treatment efficacy data are not available to confirm this interpretation [21a]. Resistant strains of *N. gonorrhoeae* also have been infrequently isolated from travelers to Southeast Asia and Australia. Strains with decreased susceptibilities to ciprofloxacin have decreased susceptibilities to all fluoroquinolones. Although at this time the CDC believes these findings do not justify changes in recommendations for the routine treatment of gonorrhea in the United States (i.e., fluoroquinolones are still viewed as acceptable initial agents), clinicians treating persons believed to have been infected in Southeast Asia or Australia should probably choose a regimen not involving a fluoroquinolone [21a]. For further discussion of the quinolones, see Chap. 28S.
       (1) Ciprofloxacin, 500 mg PO once (contraindicated in pregnancy or in children 16 years of age or younger)
       (2) Ofloxacin, 400 mg PO once (contraindicated in pregnancy or in children 16 years of age or younger)
       (3) Norfloxacin, 800 mg PO once (contraindicated in pregnancy or in children 16 years of age or younger)
       (4) Cefixime, 400 mg PO once
       (5) Cefpodoxime, 200 mg PO once
       (6) Cefuroxime axetil, 1 g PO, plus probenecid, 1 g, once
   4. Because 10–30% of heterosexual men and 40–60% of women with gonorrhea (in STD clinics) are also infected with *Chlamydia,* treatment for gonorrhea should include a second regimen effective against this organism (see sec. B).
  B. Nongonococcal urethritis (NGU). Because it is impossible to differentiate among the common etiologies of NGU, the condition is treated syndromically, including in the initial treatment regimen those drugs effective against the common causative agents.
   1. Recommended regimen [9, 9b]. Doxycycline, 100 mg PO bid for 7 days
     a. Patients should be warned not to take the medication with antacids, to

avoid excessive sun exposure, and to avoid taking the medication immediately before retiring (to prevent rare esophagitis).

b. One may also use tetracycline, 500 mg PO qid for 7 days. This regimen is more difficult to take than is the doxycycline; patient compliance is lower.

c. Minocycline is effective at a dose of 100 mg at bedtime for 7 days [13].

d. Regimens lasting longer than 7 days have no demonstrable advantage [22].

2. There are several **alternative regimens** [9].

a. **Azithromycin,** 1,000 mg **as a single PO dose,** offers the advantages of eliminating patient compliance as a therapeutic problem and being safe in pregnancy. Unfortunately, it is much **more expensive** than more traditional regimens.

In a recent report by Stamm et al., in a randomized, double-blind, multicenter trial comparing azithromycin (1.0-g single oral dose) versus doxycycline (100 mg bid for 7 days), the drugs were determined to be equally effective in 452 patients. Clinical cure rates were comparable with either regimen regardless of the presence or absence of *Chlamydia* or *Ureaplasma* infection. Adverse reactions were mild to moderate and occurred in 23% of azithromycin recipients and 29% of doxycycline recipients [22a]. **Because azithromycin can be given as a single dose and compliance ensured, it is a very appealing agent.** However, the azithromycin single dose is six to ten times more expensive than the usual 7-day course of doxycycline [1a, 22a]. **Therefore, for now it seems reasonable to use a single dose of azithromycin to treat patients with NGU who are considered likely to be noncompliant with doxycycline [1a].**

The Food and Drug Administration has recently approved a single-dose, 1-g oral suspension of azithromycin that will be available for $15 to wholesalers (about 50% cost reduction compared with the capsules) and $9.50 to public sexually transmitted disease clinics that are recipients of a grant from the Centers for Disease Control and Prevention [22a].

Further studies of the overall cost effectiveness of azithromycin for NGU are suggested [22a]. (Despite its higher initial acquisition costs, one recent report in women suggests that overall, in some settings, azithromycin may be more cost-effective therapy [22b].) Azithromycin is discussed in Chap. 28M.

b. **Erythromycin** base, 500 mg PO qid for 7 days, or erythromycin ethylsuccinate, 800 mg PO qid for 7 days, is another option.

(1) Equivalent regimens of other erythromycin salts can be substituted.

(2) Although both these regimens have the advantage of safety in pregnancy and effectiveness against tetracycline-resistant *Ureaplasma urealyticum,* they are less well tolerated than the tetracycline regimens.

(3) Patients not tolerating these regimens might be given half the cited doses on a regimen extended to 14 days.

c. **Ofloxacin,** 300 mg PO bid for 7 days, is very expensive and should be avoided in pregnancy or in children 16 years of age or younger.

d. Patients **known to be infected with** *C. trachomatis* can be treated with sulfisoxazole, 500 mg PO qid for 10 days (or with an equivalent sulfonamide regimen). This regimen is not effective against ureaplasmas and is thus less effective than the preceding regimens for syndromic treatment.

3. Test of cure

a. Patients should be reexamined to document the disappearance of urethral inflammation.

b. One should wait for approximately 3 weeks after treatment to test for cure of chlamydial infection.

4. Regimens for NGU are no longer reliably effective for gonococcal infections.

C. Management of recurrent disease. A careful sexual history regarding reexposure and adequate treatment of sexual partners is critical to the management of this condition. **Reinfection is the most common cause of recurrence.**

1. Gonorrhea. Patients returning for follow-up who report persistence or recurrence of symptoms should be reevaluated with urethral Gram stain and culture for *N. gonorrhoeae.*

a. Persistence of PMNs but the absence of gram-negative intracellular diplococci suggests a diagnosis of **postgonococcal urethritis (PGU).** This condition is observed when gonorrhea is treated with a regimen (e.g., single-dose beta-lactam or fluoroquinolone) that is ineffective against coincident chlamydial infection; it represents NGU following GCU. The syndrome should be treated as NGU (which is indeed what it is) as in sec. **B.** PGU is not seen if gonorrhea is treated with the recommended double regimen (see sec. **A.4**).

- **b.** Persistence of *N. gonorrhoeae* by smear or culture requires retreatment for gonorrhea. If the patient had been treated initially with a regimen ineffective against resistant strains, the patient should be retreated with ceftriaxone or one of the alternative regimens discussed in sec. **A.2–4**.
- **c.** Careful evaluation for untreated sexual partners is essential.

2. **Nongonococcal urethritis.** The pattern of recurrence can be of great value in deciding further management, particularly if cultures for specific pathogens are not available.

- **a. Response, reexposure, recurrence.** Initial response suggests infection with a tetracycline-sensitive agent. Reexposure followed by recurrence strongly suggests reinfection, supports retreatment with an effective regimen, and demands careful investigation of possible sources of reinfection.
  - **(1)** A woman, informed of NGU in a male partner, may consult her regular physician for evaluation but may fail to reveal the epidemiologic situation. A routine genital physical examination often fails to reveal clinical evidence of chlamydial infection, and the woman may go untreated, having been told that she is not infected.
  - **(2)** Such female partners should be treated on initial presentation (see sec. **II.A.3** under General Principles in the Management of Sexually Transmitted Disease).
- **b. Failure to respond.** Lack of response **to doxycycline** suggests infection with a tetracycline-resistant agent (see sec. **IV.B.3–4**) such as *U. urealyticum* or *T. vaginalis*.
  - **(1)** The persistence of urethritis should be documented by observing PMNs on a urethral smear. The absence of PMNs suggests resolution of the infectious process with a persistent pain syndrome that does not require further treatment with antimicrobials.
  - **(2)** Patients with documented persistent urethritis should be empirically treated for both organisms with metronidazole, 2 g PO as a single dose, and erythromycin or azithromycin (see sec. **V.B.2**).
- **c. Response with relapse** in the absence of reinfection is poorly understood. Such patients are disproportionately those men who are initially culture-negative for chlamydiae and ureaplasmas [22]. Treatment is uncertain.
  - **(1)** Of such patients, 50–75% may respond to a 3- to 6-week course of erythromycin or a tetracycline [23, 24].
  - **(2)** Patients relapsing after this treatment should probably be referred for urologic evaluation [25].
  - **(3)** These patients do not develop complications, and their sexual partners have no clinical evidence of infection.
  - **(4)** Patients who relapse after an initial 3- to 6-week treatment course may be rendered asymptomatic with a standard regimen and then placed on long-term suppressive doses of a tetracycline [24]. Tetracycline hydrochloride is preferred for the sake of economy, and one should use the lowest dose that keeps the patient free of symptoms, often 500 mg PO once daily. Treatment for 6–12 months is well tolerated and might be followed by discontinuation of the drug and reevaluation [24].

VI. Urethritis in women

A. Clinical features

1. **Women usually are unaware of urethral discharge, and urethritis presents as dysuria and frequency.**
2. Women with dysuria should be asked whether it is external or internal. Internal dysuria is associated with urethritis or cystitis, whereas external dysuria is more frequently associated with vulvovaginitis such as that caused by *Candida* spp. or herpes simplex virus.
3. Infected women usually manifest **pyuria.**
4. If routine urine cultures are negative, affected women are said to have the **acute urethral syndrome** [26, 27]. See related discussions in Chap. 12.

B. Etiology

1. Some women have cystitis caused by small numbers of Enterobacteriaceae [26].
2. Some patients have urethritis caused by Enterobacteriaceae [28].

3. Some patients have gonococcal or nongonococcal urethritis [26, 27].
    a. Such patients will respond initially to standard urinary tract treatments such as trimethoprim-sulfamethoxazole (TMP-SMX) or amoxicillin, either of which would be active against chlamydia or sensitive gonococci.
    b. Recurrence of such an apparently culture-negative urinary tract infection may reflect reinfection with sexually transmitted urethritis by an untreated and possibly asymptomatic sexual partner.

C. **Treatment of GCU or NGU in women is the same as treatment in men** (see secs. **V.A** and **V.B**). **Treatment in pregnancy involves the following:**
    1. Gonorrhea can be treated with a cephalosporin (see sec. **V.A**) or, in the setting of beta-lactam allergy, with spectinomycin (see sec. **V.A.3**).
    2. **Tetracyclines and fluoroquinolones are contraindicated in pregnancy.**
    3. **Chlamydial infection in pregnancy can be treated with** amoxicillin, 500 mg PO tid for 7 days [28a], or with clindamycin, 450 mg PO tid for 10 days [28b].

D. **Test of cure of gonococcal infection in women must include a rectal as well as a cervical culture** because almost half of women with gonorrhea are infected at the rectum as well as at the cervix, presumably by autoinoculation. Almost 20% of treatment failures are manifest only at the rectum. **Test of cure is unnecessary following treatment with ceftriaxone.**

VII. **Asymptomatic urethritis**
A. Both GCU and NGU can occur without symptoms.
B. Urethritis is prevalent among the male partners of women whose gonococcal or chlamydial infections are detected on routine screening or because these women present with symptoms or complications [29]. Up to 30% of these male partners will be asymptomatic [30]. **Asymptomatic male partners of infected women must be evaluated and probably should be treated on initial presentation.**
C. Many men with asymptomatic urethritis will have PMNs on Gram-stained smear of a urethral specimen [29–31].
D. The sensitivity of the urethral smear for gonococci in *asymptomatic* gonococcal urethritis probably is only 70% [29].
E. Most men harboring trichomonads are asymptomatic [19].

VIII. **Disseminated gonococcal infections** are discussed in sec. **V** under Genital Lesions.

Cervicitis

I. **Etiology.** The **etiologic spectrum** of mucopurulent cervicitis (MPC) is very **similar to** that of **urethritis in men.** The major pathogens include *N. gonorrhoeae, C. trachomatis,* and herpes simplex. However, most women with *N. gonorrhoeae* or *C. trachomatis* do not have MPC [9].
A. **Acute gonococcal cervicitis** has been known for hundreds of years. The endocervix is the site from which gonococci are most frequently isolated in women with uncomplicated gonococcal infections.
B. *C. trachomatis* can be recovered from the endocervix of 60–90% of the sexual partners of men with chlamydial urethritis [3, 32–34]. Cervical abnormalities, often subtle, have been observed in 80–90% of *Chlamydia*-positive women [32–34].
C. **Herpes simplex virus** is isolated from the cervix in 88% of women with primary infection but from only 12% of women with recurrent herpetic infection [35, 36]. **Herpetic cervicitis may be present without external lesions.**
D. **Human papillomavirus,** particularly certain subtypes, frequently infects the cervix [37]. It has been observed since 1837 that cancer of the cervix behaves epidemiologically as if it were an STD, and **now several types of human papillomavirus have been implicated as causes of cervical cancer** [37–39].
E. **Other organisms** [3] occasionally considered causes of cervicitis include adenovirus, measles virus, cytomegalovirus, *Enterobius vermicularis,* amebae, *Mycobacterium tuberculosis,* group B streptococci, *Neisseria meningitidis,* and actinomycetes, the last usually in association with the use of intrauterine contraceptive devices.

II. **Diagnosis.** The clinical features of specific cervical infections overlap too much to permit an accurate etiologic diagnosis without laboratory assistance [32, 40]. **Multiple infections are common [41] and may be missed if the diagnosis is attempted on clinical grounds alone.**
A. **Clinical features. Many women** with cervicitis may be completely **asymptomatic,** but nearly one-third note a discharge from the vagina that actually originates in the inflamed cervix. With herpetic cervicitis, there may be lower abdominal pain.

B. **Examination**
   1. **Erythema around the cervical os may indicate infection or may merely represent cervical ectropion** (previously called *erosion* or *eversion*), a term indicating migration of endocervical epithelium over the surface of the cervix. This lesion usually is symmetric about the os and is not particularly friable. It is often impossible on clinical grounds alone to differentiate ectropion from true infection. **Hypertrophic cervicitis,** on the other hand, is manifested as an intensely erythematous, raised, irregular lesion that bleeds easily. This lesion often is associated with chlamydial infection [32–34, 40].
   2. Normal cervical discharge is clear and mucoid. Purulent or mucopurulent discharge (MPC) is associated with gonococcal or chlamydial infection [40, 42–44].
   3. In typical cases of **gonococcal cervicitis,** the cervical os is reddened and produces a purulent discharge.
   4. **Chlamydiae** have been isolated from 50–90% of sexually active patients with hypertrophic cervicitis. Only 19–32% of women with chlamydial cervical infection manifest hypertrophic cervicitis, and only 30% or so have a mucopurulent or purulent cervical discharge [32, 33, 42]. On examination, **20–70% [42, 45] of infected women have a completely normal cervix. Therefore, physical examination never adequately excludes chlamydial infection, similar to the situation with gonococcal cervicitis.**
   5. **Cervicitis is seen on physical examination** in approximately 90% of women whose cervical cultures are positive for **herpes simplex virus** [35, 36]. The cervix usually displays diffuse friability and, less frequently, frank ulcers or necrosis [35]. Cervical discharge is usually mucoid, but it is occasionally mucopurulent and, in one series, herpetic cervical infection caused 8% of cases of MPC [40]. Inguinal adenopathy is rare unless the disease is accompanied by lesions of the external genitalia, because lymphatic drainage of the cervix involves the external iliac rather than the inguinofemoral nodes.

C. **Laboratory tests**
   1. **Microscopy**
      a. Observing 10–30 PMNs per oil-immersion field in the densest portion of a Gram-stained specimen of cervical discharge correlates statistically with the presence of gonococci or chlamydiae [40, 43, 46–49], but the sensitivity and positive predictive value of the observation (both 25–45% in a high-risk population) are far too low for a definitive diagnosis.
      b. In the setting of MPC, a Gram stain diagnosing gonorrhea mandates treatment for both gonococci and chlamydiae. A Gram stain negative for gonococci rules out the infection with a sensitivity of only 50%, and so such patients must still be treated for both gonococcal and nongonococcal cervicitis. **The cervical Gram stain has very limited utility in the management of MPC.**
   2. **Culture and other tests**
      a. **Gonorrhea.** The standard method for detecting *N. gonorrhoeae* is culture. The sensitivity of the endocervical culture is disputed but generally is held to be on the order of 90%. The presence of the organism can also be detected with a commercially available nucleic acid hybridization test [50].
      b. *C. trachomatis.* Culture of the organism is an expensive and time-consuming procedure. Chlamydiae can be identified in cervical specimens from 75–95% of infected women by using immunofluorescence microscopy [44, 45, 51–53]. Enzyme immunoassays are also 65–95% sensitive in women [53–56]. DNA probes detect chlamydial infection with a sensitivity of nearly 80% [57, 58].
      c. **Herpes simplex virus.** The diagnosis of herpetic cervicitis may be made cytologically by observing multinucleate giant cells, often with intranuclear inclusions. In the presence of severe necrosis, however, cellular architecture is so distorted that cytologic examination becomes insensitive, and the diagnosis is best made by recovering the virus in tissue culture (i.e., obtaining viral cultures) or by immunofluorescent staining.

III. **Therapeutic approach**
   A. Specifically diagnosed gonococcal or chlamydial cervicitis should be treated in the same manner as gonococcal and chlamydial urethritis, described in sec. **V** under Urethritis. **Because 30–60% of women with gonococcal cervicitis also have chlamydial infection, simultaneous treatment for both infections is advised when gonorrhea is diagnosed** [9].

B. **Mucopurulent cervicitis** in patients at risk for STD should be treated in symptomatic and asymptomatic patients with a regimen that is effective against both *N. gonorrhoeae* and *C. trachomatis*. In a patient whose history suggests she is at very low risk for STD and in whom compliance is good, one could await the results of the screening tests.

C. **Female partners of men with NGU should be epidemiologically treated** even before the diagnosis of chlamydial infection is confirmed by laboratory techniques. Likewise, sex partners of women with MPC should receive similar therapy, which is usually presumptive therapy in high-risk groups.

D. **Herpes simplex virus.** Management of cervicitis due to herpes simplex virus is identical to that of other genital herpes infections. The appropriate regimens are discussed in section **III.B.4** under Genital Lesions.

Pharyngeal Infections and Sexually Transmitted Pharyngitis

The oropharynx can be infected by *N. gonorrhoeae, C. trachomatis, Treponema pallidum,* or herpes simplex virus.

I. **Gonococcal pharyngeal infection** [59]

A. **Epidemiology.** The major risk factor is fellatio. Cunnilingus is less likely to transmit infection, and transmission by kissing is very rare.

B. **Most infected patients are asymptomatic,** although erythematous and exudative gonococcal pharyngitis does occur.

C. The identity of *N. gonorrhoeae* on culture must be confirmed by biochemical or immunologic testing because *N. meningitidis,* too, will grow on selective media and resembles gonococcus.

D. Pharyngeal infection has been linked with disseminated gonococcal infection in some older series, and so workup for disseminated gonococcal infection should include pharyngeal cultures.

E. **Treatment.** Several drugs are ineffective in treating pharyngeal infection even when the organisms are sensitive.

1. **Ineffective drugs include** ampicillin, amoxicillin, and spectinomycin.

2. **Recommended regimens** [9]

a. **Ceftriaxone, 125–250 mg IM as a single dose.**

b. For beta-lactam-allergic patients, ciprofloxacin (if not contraindicated), 500 mg PO as a single dose. Test of cure by culture should be performed 4–7 days after treatment.

c. **TMP-SMX,** 9 single-strength tablets daily for 5 days, may be effective therapy for a patient weighing more than 50 kg in whom cephalosporins and quinolones are contraindicated, but data are limited and patients' compliance may be a problem. (See Chap. 28K for a discussion of the use of TMP-SMX in pregnancy.)

II. **Chlamydial pharyngeal infection**

A. *C. trachomatis* occasionally is isolated from the pharynx of the patient who practices fellatio [60].

B. Such infection is usually asymptomatic, but symptomatic pharyngitis may be associated with infection with *Chlamydia pneumoniae* (see Chap. 9).

C. Regimens effective for genital chlamydial infection eradicate the organism from the pharynx as well.

III. **Pharyngeal herpetic infection** [20]

A. **Epidemiology.** In adults, this syndrome generally is associated with primary genital infection.

B. **Clinical features.** Patients usually are symptomatic, and one may see erythema or frank ulcers on the oropharynx. Fever and anterior cervical adenopathy are common.

C. **Treatment.** Primary disease is ameliorated with acyclovir, 200 mg PO 5 times daily for 10 days (see Chap. 26).

D. Herpetic pharyngitis **may recur** and be particularly severe in patients who are immunocompromised, including those with AIDS. Extension to the esophagus is frequent. Such patients may require considerably longer courses of acyclovir to control the infection. Intravenous acyclovir may be required, particularly if the patient cannot swallow oral medication (see Chaps. 19 and 26).

Genital Lesions

I. **Significance.** Genital lesions present problems in differential diagnosis because of clinical overlaps in presentation. The issue is further complicated by the frequency with which different infections coexist. Some data suggest that ulcerative genital lesions predispose to the transmission of HIV infection by acting as the portal of exit or entry for the virus [61–63]. The morphology of genital lesions may be greatly modified in AIDS.

II. **Initial approach.** The initial approach to genital lesions in the sexually active patient involves taking a careful history, including the following information [64]:
   A. The **incubation period** can be assessed by inquiring about new or recent sexual contacts.
      1. A very short incubation period of minutes to hours suggests trauma or an allergic reaction to a topical chemical used by a partner. Infectious diseases do not have such short incubation periods.
      2. An incubation period of 2–5 days is seen with most cases of chancroid or herpes simplex virus infection, although the mean incubation period for the latter is approximately 6 days [20].
      3. Longer incubation periods of 1–3 weeks are seen with syphilis, 4–12 weeks with venereal warts, and approximately 4 weeks for pubic lice and scabies.
      4. The incubation periods for some conditions such as molluscum contagiosum [65] and donovanosis [66] are poorly defined, but the latter may be 2 weeks.
   B. A **travel history** influences the likelihood of various etiologies. Lymphogranuloma venereum is far more common in Africa and the Far East than in the United States. Donovanosis is endemic in India, New Guinea, the West Indies, and some parts of Africa and South America, but it is distinctly rare in the United States. Chancroid has become more common in the United States, particularly in major metropolitan areas.
   C. **Pain** usually accompanies the lesions of herpes and chancroid. Although not classically painful, the lesions of primary syphilis cause some discomfort in up to 30% of patients [67]. **Pruritus** accompanies some cases of herpes but is characteristic of crabs and scabies.
   D. A **history of STD in a partner** is an important clue to the differential diagnosis.
   E. **Recurrence** at intervals is characteristic and highly suggestive of herpes.
   F. The **morphologic features of the lesions** are key to the differential diagnosis.

III. **Ulcerative lesions**
   A. **General principles**
      1. A clinical differential diagnosis of genital ulcers is the most challenging aspect of venereal dermatology.
      2. The most common error is the overdiagnosis of chancroid [68], which has been associated with some epidemics in this country. Often, in fact, the condition that is present is herpes.
   B. **Genital herpes simplex infection**
      1. **Epidemiologic considerations**
         a. Some 70–95% of genital herpes infections are caused by herpes simplex virus (HSV) type 2 [20]. Type 1 genital infections may result from orogenital sexual contact.
         b. Recent serologic studies suggest that 20% of young adults in the United States are infected with HSV type 2 [69].
         c. Initial infections are classified as **primary** if the patient has no prior exposure to HSV (either type 1 or type 2); otherwise the episode is referred to as **nonprimary initial infection.** Patients with prior exposure to HSV have milder initial episodes than do those patients suffering true primary genital infection.
         d. **Many patients (perhaps 70–90%) have asymptomatic initial genital infections [70–73], and many have asymptomatic recurrent infections as well.** This phenomenon is important as a possible explanation for the appearance of herpetic lesions in a patient who is in a long-term, stable, monogamous sexual relationship. Originally asymptomatic herpetic infection may finally

manifest symptoms, or an asymptomatically infected individual may shed virus in high enough concentration to produce symptomatic infection in a partner even after an extended sexual relationship wherein transmission has not occurred.

  e. Shedding of virus by asymptomatic individuals is intermittent and involves 100- to 1,000-fold less virus than does shedding by patients with lesions [73].

  f. Most infections appear to have been contracted from sexual partners who are asymptomatic shedders of virus.

  g. The rate of transmission of HSV type 2 from symptomatic to uninfected partners who have been advised not to have unprotected intercourse when the infected partner is symptomatic is approximately 10% per year (95% confidence interval, 5–14%) [74].

2. **Clinical features. The diagnosis can usually be made on clinical grounds alone.**

  a. Lesions appear 2–20 days after exposure, but the mean incubation period is approximately 6 days. The lesions are initially **vesicular,** and they often are grouped. Some vesicles are seen to be umbilicated, and they usually surmount an erythematous base. Particularly in women, the vesicles quickly rupture to form clean, shallow, markedly painful **ulcers,** which are generally all about the same size and are not indurated. Ulcers may coalesce (see Plate I).

  b. Lesions usually are located on the penis or on the labia or vulva. The adult vagina is involved in only 5% or so of cases [20]. The cervix is involved in nearly 90% of primary infections.

  c. Involvement of the urethra is common.

  d. **Regional lymphadenopathy,** usually tender, develops generally toward the end of the first week of illness.

  e. Lesions heal by **crusting** over. Primary disease often lasts 3 weeks.

  f. **Extragenital manifestations. Fever, malaise, and anorexia** are common in primary infection. A true **aseptic meningitis** without encephalitis accompanies some primary infections with HSV type 2. These manifestations are rare in recurrent disease.

  g. Within the first year after infection, **recurrent disease** is seen in approximately 90% of symptomatic patients with HSV type 2 genital infections but in only about 25–50% of those infected with HSV type 1 [75, 75a]. Recurrences with HSV type 2 appear 4–8 times per year, whereas recurrences with HSV type 1 are, on the average, nearly 10 times less frequent. The rate of recurrence varies dramatically from patient to patient. Many patients give a history of recurrences triggered by stress.

    (1) Recurrent disease may be preceded by a prodrome of itching, tingling, or burning that begins 6–24 hours before lesions appear [20].

    (2) Recurrences generally last 7–10 days and proceed through the same stages as primary disease. Systemic manifestations are far less common.

3. **Diagnosis** can usually be made clinically.

  a. A **dark-field examination** may be performed **if syphilis is suspected.** Multiple chancres may be seen in almost half of patients with primary syphilis [67, 76].

  b. The **Tzanck smear** is prepared by making a smear of a fresh vesicular lesion, which then is stained with Wright or Giemsa stain and examined for the presence of characteristic multinucleate giant cells. The test has only limited utility because the presence of vesicles is largely diagnostic by itself, and the sensitivity of the test is only 40% for ulcers, for which clinical differential diagnosis is more difficult [64].

  c. **HSV antigen detection tests,** such as direct immunofluorescence and ELISA, are now available [77, 78], although the ELISA kits vary in sensitivity and specificity [79]. Their role in clinical practice has not yet been established.

  d. At present, no commercially available serologic tests are able reliably to differentiate between HSV type 1 and HSV type 2 antibodies.

  e. **Culture remains the gold standard for diagnosis,** but its utility is limited by inconvenience and expense. It is the only method useful for diagnosis of asymptomatic shedding. The sensitivity of the culture rapidly diminishes in recurrent disease and is often negative if taken from lesions that are just a few days old [77].

4. **Treatment. Acyclovir** is the treatment of choice. **This agent is discussed in detail in Chap. 26,** but its use in genital herpes simplex infection will be covered here. (Oral valacyclovir is discussed in Chap. 26.) Many other treatments (e.g., photoactive dyes, 2-deoxy-D-glucose, topical ether) have failed in carefully controlled trials. Occlusive topical treatment increases the risk of maceration and delays healing. The lesions should be kept clean and dry.

   a. **Topical acyclovir** is available in a 5% ointment. It has a minimal [80] but statistically significant effect on duration of symptoms in initial infections and virtually no effect on recurrent disease. It is **not recommended for treatment [9] because** of its important disadvantages.

      (1) It has no effect on systemic manifestations.

      (2) It must be applied 6 times daily.

      (3) Incautious application involves the risk of autoinoculation.

   b. **Intravenous acyclovir** is used for serious infection, in immunocompromised patients, or when accompanying clinical problems make oral administration inadvisable. The drug is given as 5–10 mg/kg intravenously q8h for 5–7 days or until clinical resolution occurs [9]. Adequate hydration reduces the risk of nephrotoxicity caused by tubular precipitation.

   c. **Oral acyclovir is, in general, the regimen of choice.** It is used in three ways.

      (1) **Initial infection** with genital herpes is treated with 200 mg acyclovir PO 5 times daily for 7–10 days or until clinical resolution occurs [9]. Initial episodes of herpes proctitis are treated with 400 mg PO 5 times daily for 10 days or until clinical resolution occurs.

      (2) **Recurrent disease** may be treated with a 5 day regimen of 200 mg acyclovir PO 5 times per day, 800 mg PO bid, or 400 mg PO tid [9]. **The effect on recurrent disease is substantially less than that observed with initial infection,** and its value depends on starting the drug early in the course of the relapse, preferably during the prodrome. In this setting, the patient should keep a supply of the drug at home so that therapy can be started immediately.

      (3) **Frequently recurring disease** can be controlled with long-term **suppressive therapy** consisting of 200 mg acyclovir PO 3–5 times per day or 400 mg PO bid [9]. After 1 year of continuous daily therapy, the drug should be discontinued and the frequency and severity of recurrences should be reassessed. Approximately 75% of patients will be free of symptomatic recurrences while on this regimen [81, 82]. **Such suppressive therapy prevents symptomatic recurrences but does not completely prevent viral shedding.** Patients should be warned that they may be contagious without knowing it.

5. **Special considerations**

   a. **AIDS** patients suffer from chronic, necrotizing herpetic infection, and infection may disseminate. Longer-term, higher-dose, or intravenous therapy may be required. Resistance has developed and should be suspected if lesions persist among patients undergoing acyclovir therapy. An alternative regimen for resistant infections is foscarnet, 40 mg/kg body weight IV q8h until clinical resolution is obtained [9]. (See Chap. 26 for a discussion of foscarnet.)

   b. **Pregnancy** poses problems for mother and baby, and **management remains controversial.** The risk to the newborn is highest among women with the first episode of genital herpes near the time of delivery and is lower among women with recurrent herpes [83]. The likelihood that a completely asymptomatic individual is shedding virus at the time of delivery is probably as low as 1% [84]. Antepartum cultures are not useful [85], but women should be carefully examined for the presence of active lesions, which are considered by many to be an indication for cesarean section (see Chaps. 3 and 14).

C. **Syphilis** is, after some years, making a dramatic reappearance among heterosexuals, particularly among drug users.

   1. **Microbiologic features.** *T. pallidum* is a spirochete 5–15 μm long and less than 0.5 μm wide. Living organisms are visualized by reflected light using **dark-field** microscopy. The organism can also be identified by silver staining or by direct immunofluorescence [86].

2. Epidemiology

a. From 1986 to 1990, an epidemic of syphilis occurred in the United States. However, in 1991 the number of reported cases of primary and secondary syphilis declined for the first time since 1985 and has declined yearly since that time [87, 88]. The reasons for this are uncertain but may include the use of ceftriaxone for treatment of gonorrhea, HIV prevention education with personal protection measures being followed (e.g., condom use), or HIV partner notification (which may allow for early therapy of new cases of contacts).

b. Rates of infection remain high among lower-socioeconomic inner-city populations. Several studies have found a strong epidemiologic association between syphilis and crack cocaine use, probably due to crack cocaine–associated changes in sexual behavior such as sex-for-drugs prostitution [89–91].

c. Sexual transmission occurs by direct contact with a moist lesion (rather than by contact with the dry lesions of secondary syphilis), and transplacental transmission is the second major route of acquisition. Transfusion syphilis is no longer a problem.

3. Clinical manifestations. Syphilis is a chronic infection, usually latent, the course of which is punctuated by clinically apparent stages.

a. The **incubation period** averages approximately 3 weeks but is said to range from 10 to 90 days. During this interval, infected patients have, by definition, neither clinical nor serologic evidence of disease.

b. Primary syphilis consists of one or more **ulcerated lesions, called *chancres*,** which appear at the site of initial infection and multiplication by the spirochetes. There are multiple lesions in many cases. Chancres usually are minimally painful or tender (compared, most dramatically, to chancroid or herpes, both of which produce tender ulcers) and are usually clean ulcerations with distinctly indurated edges. Regional **adenopathy** develops within the first week and usually consists of several discrete nodes that are relatively nontender and rubbery. Inguinal adenopathy generally is bilateral. The cervix, proximal third of the vagina, and the glans penis are drained by deep iliac nodes, and regional lymphadenopathy is not detected on physical examination of patients infected at these sites. Although most chancres occur on the genitalia, the examiner must maintain a high index of suspicion for lesions about the mouth or anus as well. Untreated, the manifestations of primary syphilis usually resolve in 3–6 weeks.

Nontreponemal serologic tests for syphilis are positive in only approximately 50% of patients at the time the chancre first appears. A nonreactive test does not rule out syphilis in such patients.

c. Secondary syphilis. *T. pallidum* disseminates throughout the body even before the appearance of the chancre. Approximately 3–6 weeks after the appearance of the chancre—indeed, often after its resolution—this dissemination manifests as a generalized rash, commonly involving the palms and soles and almost always involving the oral mucous membranes and the genitalia.

The rash is highly variable, and differential diagnosis is often challenging [92, 93]. **The rash generally is maculopapular, bilaterally symmetric,** and nonpruritic or minimally pruritic, and is described classically as having a "sinister" coppery or boiled-ham color [94]. It may, however, be papular or, rarely, papulopustular. The rash may resemble pityriasis rosea. The dry lesions of secondary syphilis are not contagious for they contain very few organisms. Arguing against secondary syphilis in the adult is sparing of the mouth and genitalia, a markedly pruritic eruption, or bullous lesions [94].

(1) Secondary syphilis generally begins with a nonspecific, constitutional illness that commonly includes a sore throat and myalgias.

(2) Patchy alopecia is frequent.

(3) Generalized lymphadenopathy is observed in approximately 75% of patients.

(4) *Condylomata lata* are hypertrophic lesions, resembling flat warts, that occur in moist areas (e.g., around the anus) and are highly contagious.

(5) Painless shallow ulcers of the mucous membranes—**mucous patches—are highly contagious.**

(6) Serologic tests are almost always reactive in secondary syphilis, usually in high titer. Therefore, a negative test can be used to rule out secondary syphilis. Rarely, patients have such high levels of antibody that the nontreponemal tests are falsely negative, a so-called **prozone phenomenon.** One can avoid this by performing quantitative nontreponemal tests in which serial dilutions of serum are examined.

(7) The manifestations of secondary syphilis resolve without treatment.

(8) Nearly 25% of patients will again develop the manifestations of secondary syphilis, termed **mucocutaneous relapse,** during the first year of infection. Such patients are contagious to sexual partners.

d. **Latent syphilis** is clinically silent, and diagnosis can be made only on the basis of serologic tests.

e. **Late (tertiary) syphilis** eventually develops in approximately one-third of infected patients. A discussion of late syphilis is beyond the scope of this chapter, but good descriptions are available elsewhere [94–98]. Briefly, syphilis should be suspected in the following clinical settings:

  (1) **Lymphocytic meningitis** may be a manifestation of secondary syphilis or appear somewhat later as **meningovascular syphilis.** A cerebrovascular accident in a young person without other cause should raise suspicion. See further related discussions in Chap. 5.

  (2) **Destructive lesions of skin and bones** may represent so-called **late benign syphilis.**

  (3) **Dementia** may be due to **general paresis.**

  (4) **Posterior column disease** may result from **tabes dorsalis.** Stabbing (lightning) pains are suggestive.

  (5) Disease of the **aorta or incompetence of the aortic valve** for which other etiologies are not documented may represent **cardiovascular syphilis.**

  (6) The diagnosis of late syphilis is confounded by the lack of sensitivity of the nontreponemal tests in these conditions. **A nonreactive nontreponemal test should be confirmed with a treponemal test in the workup of patients with suspected late syphilis.**

f. Approximately one-third of patients will remain seroreactive but will not develop late manifestations of syphilis. Nearly one-third remain well and become nonreactive on nontreponemal testing.

4. **Serologic diagnosis.** Because syphilis is subclinical for much of its course, we have come to rely heavily on serologic diagnosis. **Potential pitfalls in serodiagnosis must be recognized.** These tests have recently been reviewed [98a].

  a. **Nontreponemal tests. Screening tests for syphilis** exploit the observation that patients with syphilis develop antibodies reactive with a variety of poorly defined lipids. These antibodies, termed **reagin,** are IgG and should not be confused with the immunologists' reagin, which refers to IgE. Nontreponemal tests include the **VDRL** (Venereal Disease Research Laboratory), **RPR** (rapid plasma reagin), and **ART** (automated reagin test), among others.

    (1) **Nontreponemal tests are nonspecific,** yielding false positive reactions in a variety of acute and chronic conditions such as acute viral illnesses, collagen vascular disease, pregnancy, intravenous drug use, and leprosy. A nontreponemal test is considered diagnostic in the setting of a highly suggestive clinical syndrome (e.g., chancre) but cannot be used to diagnose latent syphilis without confirmation by a treponemal test.

    (2) The tests **often are quantitated** and reported as the highest twofold dilution of serum eliciting a positive reaction. Titers of 1:8 or higher are unusual among false positives. The highest titers are seen in secondary syphilis; 1:256 or higher is not unusual.

    (3) The tests are **relatively insensitive in primary and late syphilis.** In these settings, it may be prudent to order a treponemal test even when the nontreponemal test is nonreactive.

    (4) **The titer of the test diminishes after adequate treatment of syphilis. A fourfold drop in titer is considered evidence of adequate treatment** [99] and should occur within 3 months of treatment of early syphilis and within 6 months of treatment of latent syphilis.

    (5) **After treatment, one should follow serologic tests at 3 and 6 months and then every 6 months thereafter until titers stabilize or disappear.**

    (6) The RPR converts to nonreactive within 2 years in only 72% or so of patients treated for primary syphilis and 56% or so of patients treated for secondary syphilis [100]. The VDRL is more likely to revert to nonreactive after treatment.

(7) A subsequent reappearance or fourfold rise in titer of nontreponemal tests is considered evidence of relapse or reinfection.

(8) It is essential that the same nontreponemal tests be used in follow-up as were used for the original testing, because the RPR can yield two- to eightfold higher titers on the same specimen than does the VDRL. Switching between tests invites confusion.

b. Treponemal tests. Confirmatory tests for syphilis use *T. pallidum,* or fractions thereof, as antigen. The fluorescent treponemal antibody absorption test (**FTA-ABS**) is the most sensitive test for syphilis. It requires a fluorescence microscope. More easily performed is the microhemagglutination test for antibody to *T. pallidum* (**MHA-Tp**), which requires no special equipment. The treponemal tests are **more specific and more sensitive** than the nontreponemal tests, **particularly in very early primary and late syphilis.**

(1) Treponemal tests are used to confirm a diagnosis of past or present treponemal infection in patients with reactive nontreponemal tests. The treponemal tests are not used for screening because of their cost and because they are most effective when used in the high-prevalence population already defined by a reactive nontreponemal test.

(2) The MHA-Tp is less sensitive (80%) than the FTA-ABS (90%) but more sensitive than the VDRL or RPR (75%) in primary syphilis.

(3) The treponemal tests are not quantitated but are reported as reactive or nonreactive.

(4) The treponemal tests remain positive for extended periods, probably for life, even after adequate treatment of syphilis in most patients. A persistently reactive treponemal test does not indicate inadequate treatment, relapse, or reinfection.

(5) Although they are highly specific, **the treponemal tests are reactive in other treponemal diseases** (e.g., yaws, pinta, bejel) and **in some other spirochetal diseases (e.g., Lyme disease)** [101].

c. Interpretation. Syphilis serology is an imperfect science, and the clinician is well advised to take all clinical and epidemiologic information into account before making decisions regarding treatment. Patterns of seroreactivity may be interpreted initially as follows:

(1) Nontreponemal test (NT) and treponemal test (TT) nonreactive: past or present treponemal infection highly unlikely; very early primary syphilis cannot be ruled out.

(2) NT reactive, TT nonreactive: classical biologic false positive reaction; treponemal infection extremely unlikely; consider host of other conditions yielding false positive reactions; will be seen in 1–2% of the general population [86]. See sec. **4.a.(1).**

(3) NT nonreactive, TT reactive: early primary syphilis; secondary syphilis with prozone; late syphilis; adequately treated syphilis or other treponemal disease; Lyme disease [101].

(4) NT reactive, TT reactive: syphilis, any stage; adequately treated latent or late syphilis; other treponemal disease; reinfection syphilis; inadequately treated syphilis.

(5) NT reactive with rising titer, TT reactive: relapse or reinfection syphilis; adequately treated syphilis with superimposed condition generating a false positive NT.

5. Treatment. Penicillin remains the drug of choice for all stages of syphilis, unless the patient is hypersensitive [9, 101a]. **All patients being treated for syphilis should be strongly advised to undergo testing for HIV antibody.**

a. Contact to syphilis (epidemiologic treatment, incubating syphilis). Infection is present in 25–50% of the sexual partners of patients with syphilitic lesions. Syphilis may take up to 90 days to become clinically or serologically manifest. Thus, **all patients presenting as contacts to syphilis within the past 90 days (the so-called critical period) are treated with a regimen effective for early syphilis.** Patients whose exposure was more than 90 days previously may be evaluated serologically to determine whether they need treatment.

b. Early syphilis (primary, secondary, and latent syphilis of < 1 year's duration)

(1) Recommended: benzathine penicillin G, 2.4 million units, IM, in one treatment.

      (2) In penicillin allergy: doxycycline, 100 mg PO bid for 2 weeks, **or** tetracycline, 500 mg PO qid for 2 weeks.

      (3) The pregnant woman with severe penicillin allergy ideally should be desensitized to penicillin so she can receive penicillin, because tetracyclines are contraindicated in pregnancy and erythromycin should not be used as it cannot be relied on to cure an infected fetus (see Chap. 27).

      (4) Ceftriaxone may be a suitable alternative in patients whose allergy to penicillin is not manifested by anaphylaxis [102]. It is not advised in pregnancy [9].

  c. Latent syphilis of unknown duration or of more than 1 year's duration, late benign syphilis, cardiovascular syphilis

      (1) Recommended: benzathine penicillin G, 7.2 million units total, administered as three doses of 2.4 million units IM, given 1 week apart for 3 consecutive weeks.

      (2) Alternatively **for penicillin-allergic, nonpregnant patients:** doxycycline, 100 mg PO bid for 4 weeks, **or** tetracycline, 500 mg PO qid for 4 weeks.

      (3) Management of the **penicillin-allergic pregnant woman** is uncertain and should probably involve desensitization to penicillin.

      (4) Examination of cerebrospinal fluid is recommended in the following situations [9]:

        (a) Neurologic signs or symptoms

        (b) Treatment failure

        (c) Serum nontreponemal titer greater than 1:16

        (d) Other evidence of active syphilis (e.g., aortitis, gumma, iritis)

        (e) Nonpenicillin therapy planned

        (f) Concurrent HIV infection

  d. Neurosyphilis (see related discussion in Chap. 5)

      (1) Recommended: aqueous crystalline penicillin G, 12–24 million units/day IV for 10–14 days, administered 2–4 million units q4h or by continuous drip. In the HIV-positive patient, neurosyphilis may be particularly difficult to treat, and failures of therapy can occur despite optimal therapy with high-dose IV aqueous penicillin [102a].

      (2) Alternatively, procaine penicillin G, 2.4 million units IM/day, and probenecid, 500 mg PO qid, both for 10–14 days.

      (3) An alternative for which data are severely limited: ceftriaxone, 1 g IM/day for 14 days [103]. This might be used in patients whose allergy to penicillin is not manifested by anaphylaxis.

      (4) Another alternative for which data are severely limited: doxycycline 200 mg, PO bid for 21 days [104]. This regimen might be used in the penicillin-allergic nonpregnant patient or when oral therapy must be given.

      (5) Yet another alternative for which data are severely limited: amoxicillin, 3 g PO, with probenecid, 1 g PO, both twice daily for 2 weeks [105]. This regimen might be used when an oral regimen is necessary.

      (6) It is believed by many workers that the benzathine penicillin G regimen formerly recommended for neurosyphilis is inadequate. However, because the currently recommended regimen is shorter than that recommended for late syphilis in the absence of neurosyphilis, **some experts administer one or more doses of benzathine penicillin, 2.4 million units IM, after completion of regimen (1) or (2)** [9].

  e. The **Jarisch-Herxheimer reaction** occurs 1–6 hours **after beginning treatment for syphilis** and is seen in approximately 50% of patients with primary syphilis and in almost all patients with secondary syphilis. It manifests as fever, increased rash, adenopathy, and sometimes hypotension. The mechanism is not fully defined, but it probably results from the release of treponemal antigens on lysis of the organisms. The Jarisch-Herxheimer reaction is self-limited and usually requires treatment only with antipyretics, but patients should be warned of its occurrence.

  f. Serologic follow-up. See sec. 4.a.

  g. Syphilis in pregnancy should be managed according to the maternal stage of syphilis. Monthly serologic follow-up is required to ensure that treatment has been effective and reinfection has not occurred. The tetracyclines are to be avoided in pregnancy.

h. The effect of **HIV infection** on the clinical course of syphilis is unclear. Anecdotal reports suggest that HIV infection may affect the serologic manifestations, the natural history, or the response to therapy in patients coinfected with *T. pallidum* [106], but the only controlled study of the issue to date failed to confirm this [107]. However, many clinicians remain particularly **concerned about reports suggesting that neurosyphilis may occur more rapidly in patients with HIV** [108, 109]. **Some experts recommend that cerebrospinal fluid examination be performed on all HIV-infected patients with syphilis,** regardless of clinical stage.

D. Chancroid is an infection with the gram-negative rod *Hemophilus ducreyi.* The incidence of chancroid has increased in the United States, and small epidemics have occurred, usually associated with prostitutes [110]. Chancroid is **a major public health problem in the developing world** [64], and its significance is compounded by its striking **association with HIV infection** [61–63, 111]. **Patients should be tested for HIV at the time of diagnosis.**
  1. Clinical manifestations [112, 112a]
    a. The incubation period is 4–7 days.
    b. Presentation is with painful, ragged ulcers on the genitalia. The ulcers often are dirty or necrotic-appearing, are not indurated, and may vary in size. So-called **kissing lesions** of the thighs may occur by autoinoculation. Painful inguinal adenopathy occurs in more than 50% of patients, and the nodes may become fluctuant and rupture. Occasionally, one sees superinfection with mixed anaerobic organisms.
  2. Diagnosis. The major differential diagnoses are herpes simplex genital infection and syphilis. Clinical differential diagnosis is notoriously unreliable [64]. Unfortunately, laboratory assistance usually is lacking.
    a. Dark-field examination helps to rule out syphilis. Serology is less helpful because the diseases may coexist, and nontreponemal tests are insensitive early in primary syphilis.
    b. Gram staining of the lesions may reveal chains of gram-negative streptobacilli, but the technique is insensitive and nonspecific and **is not recommended** [112].
    c. Culture of the organism is definitive but difficult [113] and, at best, may have a sensitivity of only 80%.
  3. Treatment [9, 113a] is complicated by recent development of resistance to traditional agents.
    a. Uniformly effective in all geographic areas are (1) ceftriaxone, 250 mg IM as a single dose; (2) erythromycin, 500 mg PO qid for 7 days; and (3) azithromycin, 1 g PO as a single dose.
    b. Alternative regimens with few supporting data [9] include (1) amoxicillin, 500 mg, plus clavulanic acid, 125 mg PO tid for 7 days, and (2) ciprofloxacin, 500 mg PO bid for 3 days (contraindicated in pregnancy).
    c. Patients coinfected with HIV may require longer courses of therapy [9].
E. Donovanosis (granuloma inguinale) is very rare in the United States although it is far more common in other parts of the world including India and Latin America. Caused by an intracellular gram-negative rod, *Calymmatobacterium granulomatis,* it manifests as **painless, destructive ulcers** characterized by exuberant tissue formation and healing with scarring. Diagnosis is made by biopsy of involved tissue. Initial treatment is with a tetracycline or an aminoglycoside [114–116].

IV. Papular lesions
  A. Pearly penile papules are regular white papules that form in one to five rows on the penile corona or in the coronal sulcus. They have no pathologic significance but sometimes precipitate a consultation.
  B. Molluscum contagiosum is seen frequently in children, among whom it is spread by contact. After an incubation period of 2–8 weeks, infected adults usually develop 1- to 5-mm lesions around the genitalia, thighs, and buttocks. The infection is caused by a poxvirus that has not been cultured. The **painless lesions** are easily identified clinically by their **central umbilications,** often filled with keratin plugs. Treatment is by curettage. Patients should be warned to avoid squeezing the lesions and touching other areas of the body, which presents the risk of autoinoculation. Disseminated cutaneous disease is seen in AIDS [117].
  C. Venereal warts (condylomata accuminata)
    1. Etiology. Warts are **caused by human papillomaviruses,** double-stranded DNA viruses that have not been cultured. Nearly 70 types have been identified.

Types 6 and 11 usually are associated with benign genital warts, but **types 16, 18, 31, 33, and 35 have been implicated as causes of cervical cancer** [39, 118]. Maternal human papillomavirus infection is associated with the development of laryngeal papillomatosis in vaginally delivered offspring.

2. **Clinical features.** The incubation period probably is approximately 4–6 weeks. Lesions appear as soft papules with irregular, verrucous surfaces. They are usually located around the external genitalia and may be found inside the urethra, inside the vagina, and on the cervix. Perianal warts in women may result from spread from a primary genital focus, but perianal warts in men strongly suggest receptive anal intercourse, and such patients should be evaluated for other anal infections such as gonorrhea or chlamydial infection as well as for HIV infection. Daughter lesions appear near older lesions. **Subclinical infection** is extremely important, with most infected patients having papillomavirus DNA identified in normal epithelium near visible lesions.

3. **Diagnosis of overt external lesions usually is made clinically. Warts in other locations,** including flat warts of the cervix, may require **biopsy**, which reveals characteristic koilocytosis, clear zones around the nuclei of infected cells. Subclinical infections may be detected by swabbing suspect epithelium with 3–5% **acetic acid,** which turns infected areas white. Usually applied to the vagina and cervix, this technique has been applied to the penis as well [119]. Acetic acid staining is nonspecific and requires histologic confirmation. Subsequent colposcopic examination reveals smaller lesions. **Cytologic studies** are useful; cervical cytology has high specificity but low sensitivity [120]. **DNA hybridization** kits are now commercially available.

4. **Treatment** is largely unsatisfactory and generally **controversial.** Subclinical infection may be widespread, and the benefit of treating such infections has not been demonstrated [9]. Thus, the goal of therapy is elimination of overt warts and relief of signs and symptoms.
   a. **Cryotherapy** with liquid nitrogen or cryoprobe is **preferred** because of its lack of toxicity (and usefulness in pregnancy) and its destruction of warts with a single treatment.
   b. **Podofilox 0.5% solution** has been approved for the treatment of genital warts. Its major advantage is that it is the only treatment approved for application by the patient. It is applied twice daily for 3 days followed by a 4-day rest interval. The cycle may be repeated up to 4 times. The response rate is essentially identical to that with podophyllin, but podofilox is much more expensive [121].
   c. **Trichloroacetic acid, 80–90%,** can be applied carefully to warts, followed by an application of sodium bicarbonate. Treatment can be repeated at weekly intervals. This regimen is safe in pregnancy.
   d. **Podophyllin, 10–25% in tincture of benzoin,** is widely used. It is applied directly to the warts at weekly intervals and washed off after about 6 hours. **Absorption occurs, and so the regimen is contraindicated in pregnancy.**
   e. The cervix should not be treated before cytologic studies have ruled out malignancy.
   f. The **relapse rate** with the treatments listed in this section approaches 75%.
   g. **Intralesional interferon** has been used to treat warts [122], but the technique is expensive and time-consuming and is inapplicable to patients with many warts.

V. **Pustular lesions (disseminated gonococcal infection).** Dissemination is reported to occur in approximately 1–3% of patients infected with gonococci and manifests most commonly as a rash and arthritis or tenosynovitis [123, 124].
   A. **Epidemiology**
      1. **Factors predisposing to dissemination** appear to include (1) female gender, (2) pregnancy or menstruation, (3) rectal carriage of *N. gonorrhoeae,* (4) pharyngeal carriage of *N. gonorrhoeae,* (5) asymptomatic urogenital infection, and (6) **complement deficiency states,** particularly of the terminal components, most frequently of C8. Such patients also are predisposed to disseminated meningococcal infection.
      2. **Organism.** It was at one time the case that disseminated gonococcal infection was caused by organisms highly sensitive to penicillin and other antimicrobials. This is no longer true [125–127]. Disseminated gonococcal infection can be caused by organisms with chromosome- or plasmid-mediated resistance to penicillin and other antimicrobial agents.

B. Clinical features [123, 124]

1. Bacteremia usually manifests as **fever,** accompanied by **pustular or hemorrhagic skin lesions,** usually distributed primarily **on the distal portions of the extremities.**

   a. The classic lesion is a tiny pustule, sometimes with a central eschar, surmounting a hemorrhagic base (see Plate I).

   b. Vesicular lesions sometimes are observed.

   c. Although most patients have few lesions, some have hundreds [128].

   d. **Differential diagnosis** includes such dangerous diseases as meningococcemia [128], staphylococcal endocarditis or, in geographically relevant areas, Rocky Mountain spotted fever or dengue. Sometimes all of the bacterial conditions must be treated simultaneously until the diagnosis is definite.

2. **Arthritis**

   a. Most patients, particularly early in their course, will have a **polyarthritis,** often accompanied by prominent tenosynovitis (which has differential diagnostic significance). Effusion usually is absent. Skin lesions are common and may continue to form in this type of presentation.

   b. Some patients present with involvement of one or very few joints manifesting effusion, a septic joint picture. Skin lesions are no longer forming at this stage. See Chap. 15.

   c. Differential diagnosis includes septic arthritis of other etiologies. One must consider **Reiter's syndrome,** which consists of urethritis, arthritis (usually asymmetric), dermatitis, and conjunctivitis, and is seen most frequently in sexually active individuals.

C. Diagnosis is initially made clinically.

1. **Cultures for *N. gonorrhoeae* should be obtained for all sites used for sexual contact** (urethra, anorectum, cervix, pharynx) even if the site is asymptomatic.

2. **Blood cultures** are positive in only 40% or so of patients.

3. **Joint effusions should be cultured** but will be positive only in approximately 20% of cases. Joint fluid can be directly plated to chocolate agar media or may be sent to the laboratory in an Anaport transport bottle.

4. Skin lesions are rarely positive by culture or by Gram stain. Direct fluorescent antibody staining may be useful.

5. In many patients, all cultures are negative, and diagnosis depends on clinical impression and response to therapy.

D. Treatment must take into account new patterns of gonococcal resistance [9, 125–128].

1. **Initial therapy** should consist of **any of the following:**

   a. Ceftriaxone, 1 g IM or IV q24h

   b. Ceftizoxime, 1 g IV q8h

   c. Cefotaxime, 1 g IV q8h

   d. In beta-lactam allergy, use ciprofloxacin, 500 mg PO or IV q12h, or spectinomycin, 2 g IM q12h (if not contraindicated; see Chaps. 28R and 28S).

   e. **If the organism is known to be penicillin-sensitive,** treatment can consist of ampicillin, 1 g IV q6h, or penicillin G, 10 million units/day IV. **Note:** Merely demonstrating that the organism is not penicillinase-producing does not indicate that a penicillin will be effective [126].

2. **Intravenous therapy may be discontinued 24–48 hours after symptoms resolve, and 1 week of total therapy may be completed with**

   a. Cefixime, 400 mg PO bid, or

   b. Ciprofloxacin, 500 mg PO bid (**contraindicated in pregnancy and in children younger than 16 years**).

3. **Special considerations**

   a. **Sexual partners** must be evaluated and treated. A diagnosis of gonorrhea in a sexual partner supports the diagnosis of disseminated gonococcal infection in those patients whose cultures were negative.

   b. Patients with disseminated gonococcal infection should also be treated for chlamydial infection.

   c. **Meningitis** or **endocarditis** rarely complicate this infection. These conditions require longer-duration treatment [9].

VI. Ectoparasites (see Plate II)

A. Pubic (crab) lice are *Phthirus pubis.* The infestation is markedly pruritic and appears with an incubation period of approximately 4 weeks [129, 130]. Signs include observation of the **lice,** 1- to 2-mm-long gray-brown organisms; **nits,** 0.5-

mm brown or white ovoids attached to the hair shafts; or **excreta,** tiny red dots on the skin among the hair. Infestation may include the pubic and perianal, abdominal, chest, axillary, and superciliary hair.

1. Various **treatment regimens** are equally effective [9, 130a].
   a. Permethrin (e.g., Nix) 1% creme rinse, applied to affected areas and washed off after 10 minutes
   b. Pyrethrins and piperonyl butoxide (e.g., RID) applied to affected areas and washed off after 10 minutes
   c. Lindane (gamma-benzene hexachloride) (e.g., Kwell) 1% shampoo applied for 4 minutes and then washed off. **Note:** This regimen is not recommended for pregnant or nursing women or children under 2 years old [9].
2. **Additional measures.** Clothing or bed linen contaminated within the past 48 hours should be washed before reuse.
3. **Follow-up.** Patients should be reevaluated after 1 week if they remain symptomatic. The presence of **any lice** or the presence of **nits at the base of the hair shafts is an indication for retreatment.**

B. **Scabies** is caused by infestation with the itch mite, *Sarcoptes scabiei* [130]. After an incubation period of approximately 4 weeks, most patients develop severe pruritus of the infected areas, usually worse at night or after bathing.
   1. **Diagnosis** is confirmed by **demonstrating the mite** in unexcoriated papules or burrows. The mites often are difficult to demonstrate. The female adult has a rounded body with four pairs of legs and is less than 0.5 mm long. See Plate II.
      a. A hand lens is used to identify suspicious lesions. The classic linear burrows, occurring most frequently in the interdigital spaces and on the penis, are the best sites from which to take the scrapings.
      b. With a needle or a scalpel blade, a superficial epidermal shave biopsy is performed.
      c. The specimen is suspended in immersion oil and covered with a glass coverslip.
      d. The mite or its products will be seen under the high dry lens of a light microscope (see Plate II).
      e. Exclusion of coexisting STDs should be part of the diagnostic evaluation of all patients with scabies.
   2. **Treatment for adults**
      a. **Recommended** [9, 130a]. **Permethrin 5% cream** applied to all areas of the body below the chin and washed off after 8–14 hours; **or**
      b. **Lindane (gamma-benzene hexachloride) 1% lotion or cream** applied to all areas of the body below the chin and washed off after 8 hours. **Application must be complete, including the interdigital spaces. Patients should be cautioned not to wash their hands after applying the medication** [86].
         Note: **This regimen should not be used by pregnant or nursing women or children under 2 years old [9].**
      c. **Alternatively,** one can use crotamiton 10%, applied to all areas of the body below the chin for 2 successive nights and washed off thoroughly 24 hours after the second application. Data on the effectiveness of this regimen are lacking.
   3. **Additional measures**
      a. Clothing or bed linens contaminated within the previous 48 hours should be washed before reuse.
      b. Sexual and close household contacts should be treated.
   4. **Follow-up.** Pruritus may persist for several weeks after adequate treatment. A single retreatment may be indicated if pruritus is not improved after 1 week.
   5. **HIV-infected patients,** especially those with advanced HIV disease, may present with **atypical and severe forms** of scabies that may not respond to first-line agents [131]. Management may include repeated applications and should be done in consultation with a dermatologist.

Vulvovaginitis

Vulvovaginitis is a common clinical syndrome and is diagnosed in more than one-fourth of women attending STD clinics. Its incidence appears to be increasing (Table 13-1) [132, 133].

Table 13-1. Typical features of common vaginal infections

	Trichomoniasis	Candidiasis	Bacterial vaginosis
Epidemiology			
Sexual transmission	Yes	Very rarely if ever	Often but not always
Symptoms			
Relation to menses	Often postmenstrual	Often premenstrual	None
Vulvar irritation	Mild to marked	Mild to marked	Absent to mild
Dysuria	Internal and external	External	Absent
Odor	Sometimes	Absent	Fishy, aminelike
Signs			
Labial erythema	Variable	Variable	No
Satellite lesions	No	Yes	No
Vaginal tenderness	Yes	Yes	No
Rugal hypertrophy	Yes	Sometimes	No
Adnexal tenderness	Occasionally	No	No
Discharge			
Consistency	Frothy 25%	Sometimes curdy	Homogeneous, frothy
Color	Yellow-green 25%	White	Gray, white
Adherent to vaginal walls	No	Yes	Yes
pH	Usually ≥ 4.7	≤ 4.5	≥ 4.7
Microscopy			
Epithelial cells	Normal	Normal	Studded with coccobacilli (clue cells)
Polymorphonuclear neutrophils	Usually increased	Variable	Not increased
Bacteria	Gram-positive rods	Gram-positive rods	Gram-variable coccobacilli
Pathogens	Trichomonads 70%	Yeasts or pseudohyphae 50%	Coccobacilli and short, motile rods

I. Differential diagnosis of vulvovaginitis
  A. Candidiasis
    1. Epidemiology
      a. Vulvovaginal candidiasis accounts for approximately one-third of the vaginitis cases seen in private practice. Some workers have estimated that 75% of adult women suffer at least one episode of vulvovaginal candidiasis during their lifetimes [134].
      b. *Candida albicans* is isolated from nearly 80–90% of cases of vulvovaginal candidiasis, and other species of *Candida* account for approximately 15% of cases [132, 135].
      c. Inhibition of normal bacterial flora by the **use of broad-spectrum antibiotics** favors the growth of yeasts and therefore predisposes to the development of vulvovaginal candidiasis.
      d. Overgrowth of yeast is favored by high estrogen levels [136]. This may explain the observation that vulvovaginal candidiasis is more common in **pregnancy;** it occurs in 10% of first-trimester gravidas and 36–55% of third-trimester gravidas [137]. In addition, some nonpregnant women note recurrent or increasing symptoms, **preceding each menstrual period.** The prevalence of vaginal carriage of *Candida* is higher among women using **oral contraceptives** compared to those using other methods of birth control [132, 138].
      e. There is some evidence that tight, insulating clothing predisposes to vulvovaginal candidiasis by increasing vulvar warmth and moisture [139].
      f. Patients with cell-mediated immune defects, such as in **AIDS,** may experience severe and recalcitrant disease.
    2. Clinical features
      a. Symptoms. Patients generally complain of **perivaginal pruritus,** often with little or no discharge. Dysuria occasionally is noted and is likely to be perceived as vulvar rather than urethral.
      b. Physical findings. The labia may be pale or erythematous, and excoriation often is present. **Shallow, linear ulcerations,** especially on the posterior portion of the introitus, are common. Tiny **satellite papules** or papulopustules just beyond the main area of erythema are helpful diagnostically. The vaginal walls may be erythematous. Candidal discharge is classically thick and adherent and contains curds. It may, however, be thin and loose and thus resemble the discharge of other vaginitides.
    3. Diagnosis
      a. A **wet mount** to which 10–20% KOH is added will reveal fungi in 50–70% of infected women. If negative, a presumptive diagnosis must be made on the basis of clinical features, pH, "whiff test," and microscopy negative for other pathogens.
      b. The **vaginal pH** generally is **normal** (approximately 4.5) in women with vulvovaginal candidiasis, in contrast to trichomoniasis and bacterial vaginosis, in which it is characteristically elevated. Thus, demonstrating a normal pH in a woman with signs and symptoms of vaginitis suggests that she has candidiasis.
      c. The **whiff test** (see sec. **II.B.2.b** on page 544) is characteristically **negative** in vulvovaginal candidiasis.
      d. The discharge usually contains relatively few PMNs.
      e. A commercially available latex agglutination test has a limited sensitivity of approximately 60% [140].
  B. Trichomoniasis. *Trichomonas vaginalis* is an anaerobic, flagellated, motile protozoan, approximately the size of a polymorphonuclear leukocyte.
    1. Epidemiology
      a. An estimated 3 million American women contract trichomoniasis every year. The incidence of trichomoniasis appears to be declining in the United States and Western Europe, possibly because of the widespread use of metronidazole for bacterial vaginosis [141].
      b. Trichomoniasis only occasionally is acquired nonvenereally. It is found with high prevalence in some institutionalized populations.
    2. Clinical features
      a. History. The incubation period in women ranges from approximately 5–28 days [142]. Infected women usually note **vaginal discharge and vulvovaginal soreness or irritation. Dysuria** and **dyspareunia** are common. Although

up to two-thirds of infected women complain of a disagreeable **odor,** this symptom may actually be more suggestive of bacterial vaginosis. Symptoms often begin or exacerbate during the menstrual period. **Abdominal discomfort** is described by only 5–12% of infected women and should prompt careful evaluation for a second process, such as pelvic inflammatory disease. Approximately 10–50% of infected women attending STD clinics carry the organism asymptomatically.

The majority of men infected with *T. vaginalis* are asymptomatic.

  b. Physical findings

    (1) Examination usually reveals a copious, rather loose **discharge** that pools in the posterior vaginal fornix and often is yellow or green. In the discharge of 10–33% of the cases, bubbles are observed. Up to half of the infected women have a relatively thick discharge that may be confused with vaginal candidiasis.

    (2) There is usually **inflammation of the vaginal walls** and the exocervix. Punctate hemorrhages (colpitis macularis), including the so-called **strawberry cervix,** are observed colposcopically in 45% of infected women but in only 2% by visual inspection alone [142, 143].

    (3) Vaginal discharge from 90% of women with trichomoniasis has a **pH level elevated above the normal value of 4.5.**

  c. Diagnosis. The accurate diagnosis of trichomoniasis depends on **demonstrating the organism** in genital specimens.

    (1) Trichomonads may be identified in vaginal secretions using the **wet-mount** technique, which will detect them in nearly 60% of infected women [142, 143]. *T. vaginalis* is most easily recognized by its **characteristic movements.** The wet mount generally also reveals large numbers of **white blood cells,** although asymptomatic women may have very few.

    (2) Direct fluorescent antibody staining [144], latex agglutination [145], and ELISA techniques [146] are more sensitive than a wet mount (80–90%) but less sensitive than culture.

    (3) Culture remains the most sensitive (<95%) technique for the diagnosis of trichomoniasis, and commercially available kits have increased the ease with which the organism can be cultured.

    (4) Serologic testing has no current role in the evaluation of the individual patient owing to the lack of sensitive and specific tests.

    (5) The Papanicolaou (Pap) smear is not a sensitive diagnostic tool. However, if a Pap smear reveals trichomonads, the patient and her sexual partners should be treated.

C. Bacterial vaginosis. Most women who consult their physicians with vaginal symptoms have a specific condition first described by Gardner and Dukes in 1955 [147]. Seen primarily in sexually active women, it is characterized by a **nonirritating, malodorous vaginal discharge.** Though previously called *nonspecific vaginitis* and originally attributed to infection with *Gardnerella vaginalis,* there is now considerable evidence that bacterial vaginosis is actually a **synergistic infection** involving not only *G. vaginalis* but also certain anaerobic bacteria [148].

  1. Epidemiology

    a. Bacterial vaginosis was described initially in sexually active women and is common in populations with a high prevalence of STDs. **The precise contribution of sexual transmission to the overall epidemiology of the condition remains controversial.**

    b. Recurrence in the absence of sexual reexposure is well described. **It is not demonstrably necessary to treat male sexual partners** of women with an initial diagnosis of bacterial vaginosis. Some women suffering from frequently recurring bacterial vaginosis can be cured, however, only if sexual partners are treated as well.

  2. Clinical features

    a. History. Affected women usually are sexually active and often **complain predominantly of vaginal odor.** Approximately 90% of patients also notice a **mild to moderate discharge.** Inflammation and perivaginal irritation are mild, if present. Dysuria and dyspareunia are rare. Abdominal discomfort is occasionally present, but it is usually mild and should prompt evaluation for coincident infections including salpingitis.

    b. Physical findings. Discharge often is present at the introitus and is visible on the labia minora. The labia and vulva generally are not erythematous or edematous. On speculum examination, the vaginal walls usually appear uninflamed. The vagina often contains a grayish white, thin, homogeneous discharge manifesting **small bubbles.** This discharge differs from normal physiologic discharge in that the latter has a floccular appearance and bubbles are absent. Because it is **relatively thin but adherent to the vaginal walls,** this discharge is often apparent only as an increased light reflex, giving rise to the impression that the vaginal walls are too wet. The endocervix is unaffected by the process, and cervical discharge should be physiologic and therefore mucoid.

3. **Diagnosis.** Bacterial vaginosis is perhaps most easily differentiated from trichomoniasis on the basis of direct microscopic examination of vaginal discharge.

   a. A **wet mount** of the discharge reveals **clue cells** (see sec. **II.C.1.c**), which are vaginal epithelial cells studded with tiny coccobacilli. Not all cells in the specimen are clue cells, but **some clue cells are seen in more than 90% of patients with bacterial vaginosis.**

   b. The **pH of vaginal discharge is elevated** above the normal of 4.5 in approximately 90% of women with bacterial vaginosis [147, 149, 150].

   c. A **positive whiff test** (see sec. **II.B.2.b** on page 544) is found in nearly 70% of cases.

   d. Bacterial flora can also be assessed on a wet-mount slide. In healthy women, the predominant morphotype is a large rod (presumably *Lactobacillus* spp.). In the discharge from a patient with bacterial vaginosis, these rods have been completely supplanted by **clumps of coccobacilli.**

   e. Discharge in bacterial vaginosis contains **few PMNs.**

   f. It has been suggested [151] that the clinician **look for (1) a pH greater than 4.5; (2) homogeneous, white, adherent vaginal discharge; (3) a positive whiff test; and (4) clue cells. Finding any three of these four signs strongly supports the diagnosis of bacterial vaginosis;** the finding of clue cells is the most specific of the criteria [148, 152].

   g. Culture for *G. vaginalis* is easily accomplished on a variety of media, but the mere presence of this organism does not prove that the patient has bacterial vaginosis or suggest a need for treatment as *G. vaginalis* is a common vaginal colonizer.

4. **Bacterial vaginosis and pregnancy.** Bacterial vaginosis has been associated with adverse outcomes of pregnancy (e.g., preterm labor, preterm delivery, premature rupture of membranes). The organisms found in increased concentrations in bacterial vaginosis are also commonly present in postpartum or post–caesarean section endometritis. Whether treatment of bacterial vaginosis among pregnant women would reduce the risk of adverse pregnancy outcomes is not clear [9] but preliminary studies suggest therapy may be beneficial [152a].

D. **Other vaginal conditions** to consider include vaginitis due to foreign bodies, herpes simplex virus, human papillomavirus and, much less commonly, *Mycobacterium tuberculosis,* salmonellae, actinomycetes, schistosomes, and pinworms. **N. gonorrhoeae and C. trachomatis can cause true vaginitis in prepubescent girls.**

E. **Noninfectious causes** of vulvovaginal complaints include genital neoplasms, chemical irritation, or vulvar vestibulitis. Physiologic vaginal fluid can sometimes be perceived by the patient as vaginal discharge.

II. **Approach to the patient with vaginal complaints.** The etiologic diagnosis of vaginitis depends on a careful evaluation of the history, physical examination, and immediate laboratory tests.

A. **Historical features** are relatively nonspecific, but they may direct clinical suspicion toward certain causes.

   1. **Age.** Prepubescent vaginal epithelium is not cornified, and the entire vagina is susceptible to infection with *N. gonorrhoeae* or *C. trachomatis.* Vaginal candidiasis is extremely rare in prepubescent girls [153]. Genital neoplasia is more common among older women, and postmenopausal women are more likely to have atrophic vaginitis.

   2. **Mode of onset.** An abrupt and identifiable time of onset of symptoms suggests infection. Symptoms beginning during or immediately after the menstrual period are somewhat suggestive of trichomoniasis, whereas a premenstrual onset more frequently accompanies candidiasis.

   3. **Quantity of discharge.** The amount of discharge is highly variable in all conditions. Patients with candidiasis often have scanty discharge or note no dis-

charge at all. Atrophic or neoplastic discharges are commonly scanty unless infection has supervened.

4. **Perineal irritation.** Pruritus with a scanty or absent discharge frequently is seen in candidiasis and is less common with trichomoniasis. Perineal discomfort is an infrequent complaint in bacterial vaginosis. Severe episodic perineal pain sometimes preventing urination strongly suggests herpes genitalis, which affects the labia but usually spares the vagina per se. **Chronic discomfort, often interfering with sexual activity, should prompt consideration of vulvar vestibulitis.**

5. **Abdominal pain.** Abdominal discomfort **is rare in uncomplicated vulvovaginitis** except for occasional cases of trichomoniasis. Women complaining of abdominal pain should be examined carefully for evidence of coincidental infections including cystitis and pelvic inflammatory disease.

6. **Medication. Antibiotic use** predisposes to candidal vaginitis. Patients taking **corticosteroids or oral contraceptives** are at increased risk for developing vulvovaginal candidiasis. Oral contraceptive use may also be associated with the development of a physiologic vaginal discharge.

B. **Examination of the female genitalia**
   1. A **complete pelvic examination** should be performed, including a careful examination of the external genitalia, a bimanual examination for adnexal masses or tenderness, and speculum examination of the vaginal mucosa and cervix.
   2. **Other bedside evaluation**
      a. After the speculum is withdrawn, the **pH of vaginal secretions** can be determined by inserting a strip of indicator paper into the material collected in the lower lip of the speculum. A normal pH of 4.5 is seen in most patients with vulvovaginal candidiasis, whereas a pH elevated to 5.0 or higher is associated with bacterial vaginosis or trichomoniasis.
      b. Several drops of 10% KOH then are added to the material on the speculum. A resultant pungent, fishy, aminelike odor constitutes a positive **whiff test.** The whiff test is positive in more than 90% of patients with bacterial vaginosis and in many patients with trichomoniasis. This test may also be evaluated on a slide that has been prepared for KOH microscopic examination.

C. **Laboratory examination**
   1. A **wet mount is of greatest value in the differential diagnosis of a vaginal discharge,** and the specimen may be prepared in several ways. A swab of vaginal discharge may be agitated in a tube containing approximately 0.5 ml of normal saline. One drop of the resulting suspension is put on a microscope slide, and a coverslip is applied. Alternatively, the examiner may place a drop of saline on the slide and mix in a loopful of vaginal material, after which a coverslip is applied. The slide is examined initially under low power ($100 \times$) and then under high power ($400 \times$) on a bright-field microscope with the substage condenser racked down and with the substage diaphragm closed to increase the contrast. Phase-contrast microscopy is becoming more widely available in clinical settings and provides an excellent means of evaluating vaginal wet mounts.
      a. **The relative numbers of epithelial cells and PMNs should be noted.** Finding more than one PMN per epithelial cell should raise the examiner's suspicion of cervical or vaginal inflammation. The relative absence of PMNs is characteristic of the discharge of bacterial vaginosis.
      b. The wet preparation should be **scanned for motile trichomonads.** Trichomonads are best recognized by their characteristic twitching motility. Trichomonad motility is improved by gently warming the preparation. Unfortunately, the wet mount is negative in approximately 30% of the women with trichomoniasis, and a negative wet mount does not rule out this infection, particularly in relatively asymptomatic women.
      c. Normal squamous epithelial cells have transparent cytoplasm and small nuclei. Epithelial cells covered with tiny coccobacillary forms are **clue cells** and are associated with bacterial vaginosis. Clue cells are best recognized by observing the edges of epithelial cells, which may be obscured by the adherent coccobacilli. Some cells are so heavily encrusted that the nuclei are obscured.
      d. The **bacterial flora can be assessed** on the wet mount. Normal vaginal flora consists primarily of rods. In bacterial vaginosis, the predominant flora is tiny coccobacilli.

    e. Combining a drop of 10% or 20% **KOH** with the vaginal material on a microscope slide, applying a coverslip, and gently heating will destroy cellular elements but leave the bacteria and fungi unscathed. Small numbers of yeast frequently are observed and do not necessarily indicate that the patient's vaginitis is of fungal origin.

  2. A **Gram stain of vaginal material** is somewhat **less useful for differential diagnosis than is the wet mount** because, although *G. vaginalis* and *Candida* species are readily recognized on the Gram-stained smear, trichomonads are very difficult to identify.

III. Treatment

  A. Candidiasis

    1. Topical therapy. Vulvovaginal candidiasis usually is treated with the topical application of an antifungal agent. Commercially available preparations are characterized by high patient acceptability and safety in pregnancy. The choice of an agent is based primarily on cost, the patient's preference for cream versus suppository, and the availability of agents. We prefer 3- or 7-day regimens.

    In a recent review of this topic, the Medical Letter noted ". . . imidazole creams, vaginal tablets, and suppositories are all effective for treatment of acute vulvovaginal candidiasis. No advantage in effectiveness has been demonstrated for any particular formulation, or for longer regimens over shorter ones. Nystatin vaginal tablets are somewhat less effective" [153a]. The cost of these various regimens, including the newly approved one dose of oral fluconazole, is shown in Table 13-2.

    a. One 14-day regimen is nystatin, a 100,000-unit suppository at bedtime. The cure rate exceeds 90%.

    b. Seven days of treatment with an imidazole yields cure rates ranging from 80 to 94% [137].

      (1) Miconazole (Monistat) 2% cream, 5 g daily at bedtime (available over the counter)

      (2) Miconazole, 100-mg vaginal suppository daily at bedtime

      (3) Clotrimazole, 100-mg vaginal suppository daily at bedtime

      (4) Clotrimazole (Gyne-Lotrimin) 1% cream, 5 g daily at bedtime (available over the counter)

      (5) Terconazole (Terazol) 0.4% cream, 5 g daily at bedtime

    c. Three-day regimens. Current interest centers on shorter courses of therapy. Newer, **3-day regimens** produce approximately equivalent cure rates, although some reviews suggest marginally better results with 7 days of therapy [154]. Because patients' compliance is likely to be better, it seems reasonable to recommend a 3-day regimen [155].

      (1) Miconazole, 200-mg vaginal suppository daily at bedtime

      (2) Clotrimazole, 200-mg suppository daily at bedtime

      (3) Butoconazole 2% cream, 5 g daily at bedtime

      (4) Tioconazole 2% cream, 5 g daily at bedtime

      (5) Econazole, 150-mg suppository daily at bedtime

      (6) Terconazole 0.8% cream, 5 g daily at bedtime

      (7) Terconazole, 80-mg suppository daily at bedtime

    d. A few studies have examined the efficacy of **single-dose regimens** with larger amounts of imidazoles. Such regimens may be preferred for the sake of convenience in the treatment of mild infections [153a]. Cure rates obtained in some of these studies have not quite matched those obtained with longer courses. Treatment in pregnancy is more often unsuccessful, and so the longer-course regimens may be preferred in this setting.

      (1) Clotrimazole, 500-mg vaginal tablet once

      (2) Tioconazole 6.5% ointment, 4.6 g at bedtime once

  2. Oral therapy. Several orally administered and well-absorbed imidazoles and triazoles appear to be of value in treating vulvovaginal candidiasis [156–168]. **Results do not appear to be substantially superior to those obtained with topical regimens, and the clinician must consider carefully the need for systemic therapy for vulvovaginal candidiasis in view of the potential toxicities and possible teratogenicity of the drugs. As of fall 1995, only the fluconazole single-dose regimen [153a] is approved for this use by the US Food and Drug Administration.**

    a. Single-dose fluconazole, 150-mg single oral dose, is at least as effective as intravaginal treatment of vulvovaginal candidiasis, and many patients

Table 13-2. Some drugs for vaginal candidiasis

Drug	Formulation	Dosage	Cost[a]
Butoconazole			
Femstat (Syntex; Palo Alto, CA)	2% cream	5 g at bedtime × 3 days	28 g— $18.35
Clotrimazole			
Gyne-Lotrimin (Schering; Kenilworth, NJ)[b]	100-mg vaginal tab[c]	1 tab at bedtime × 7 days	7 tab— 12.00
	1% cream	5 g at bedtime × 7 days	45 g— 12.00
Mycelex-7 (Miles; Westhaven, CT)[b]	100-mg vaginal tab	1 tab at bedtime × 7 days	7 tab— 11.77
	1% cream	5 g at bedtime × 7 days	45 g— 11.77
Mycelex-G (Miles)	500-mg vaginal tab[c]	1 tab once	1 tab— 12.71
Fluconazole			
Diflucan (Roerig; New York, NY)	150-mg oral tab	1 tab PO once	1 tab— 10.62
Miconazole			
Monistat 7 (Ortho; Raritan, NJ)[b]	2% cream	5 g at bedtime × 7 days	45 g— 12.85
	100-mg vaginal supp	1 supp at bedtime × 7 days	7 supp— 12.85
Monistat 3 (Ortho)	200-mg vaginal supp[c]	1 supp at bedtime × 3 days	3 supp— 23.22
Nystatin			
Average generic price	100,000-U vaginal tab	1 tab at bedtime × 14 days	15 tab— 6.44
Terconazole			
Terazol 7 (Ortho)	0.4% cream	5 g at bedtime × 7 days	45 g— 22.26
Terazol 3 (Ortho)	80-mg vaginal supp	1 supp at bedtime × 3 days	3 supp— 22.26
	0.8% cream	5 g at bedtime × 3 days	20 g— 22.26
Tioconazole			
Vagistat (Mead Johnson; Princeton, NJ)	6.5% ointment	4.6 g at bedtime once	4.6 g— 24.20

tab = tablet; supp = suppository.
[a]Cost to the pharmacist based on wholesale price (AWP) listings in *Red Book* 1994 and August *Update.*
[b]Available without a prescription.
[c]Also available in kit that includes cream (Gyne-Lotrimin Combination Pack, Mycelex-G Twin Pack, Monistat Dual-Pak).
Source: Medical Letter. Oral fluconazole for vaginal candidiasis. *Med. Lett. Drugs Ther.* 36:81, 1994.

may prefer the convenience of a single-dose oral regimen [153a, 157a].

  (1) In the 1995 report by Sobel et al. and the Fluconazole Vaginititis Study Group, in a multicenter, randomized, prospective, single-blinded study of 429 patients with acute candida vaginitis, a single dose of oral fluconazole (150 mg) was as safe and effective as 7-day clotrimazole 100 mg vaginal therapy [157a]. At the 14-day evaluation, clinical cure or improvement was seen in 172 of 182 (94%) of fluconazole-treated patients (73% cured, 21% improved) and 171 of 176 (97%) of the clotrimazole-treated patients (67% cured, 30% improved). The differences in responses were not statistically significant [157a].

  (2) Adverse effects. Even as a single dose, oral fluconazole can cause nausea, vomiting, diarrhea, abdominal pain, and headache [153a]. In the multicenter study discussed in sec. **(1)**, treatment-related side effects were reported for 59 of 217 (27%) of fluconazole recipients versus 37 of 212 (18%) of clotrimazole-treated patients. The most common complaints with fluconazole were headache (12%), abdominal pain (7%), and nausea (4%). The most common treatment-related side effects with vaginal clotrimazole were headache (9%), abdominal pain (3%), and pain on insertion (2%). Most of the side effects were mild to moderate in severity, and no patient discontinued therapy [157a]. An anaphylactic reaction to a single oral dose of fluconazole has been reported [153a]. See detailed discussion of fluconazole in Chap. 18.

  (3) Oral fluconazole's safety during pregnancy and breast-feeding are unknown [153a].

  (4) Cost. See Table 13-2.

  b. Other oral regimens include (1) ketoconazole, 200 mg PO bid for 3–5 days; (2) ketoconazole, 200 mg PO every day for 3 days (clinical data are limited); (3) itraconazole, 200 mg PO bid for 1 day (clinical data are limited); and (4) itraconazole, 200 mg PO every day for 3 days (clinical data are limited).

3. **Recurrent infection.** Recurrent symptomatic infection is a major problem, and other forms of chronic vulvovaginitis must be excluded [168a]. The mechanisms of recurrence remain obscure, but recurrence does not appear to result from the development of resistance to antifungals. Short courses of topical antifungal therapy administered on the fifth to eleventh days of the menstrual cycle [169] or immediately preceding [170, 171] or following [172, 173] menses reduce, but by no means eliminate, symptomatic recurrences. Likewise, 200 mg itraconazole PO on days 5 and 6 of the menstrual cycle suppresses symptoms for the duration of therapy [174]. Continuous daily treatment with ketoconazole [171] or fluconazole [138] prevents recurrences but only for the duration of treatment. In some cases of frequently recurrent vulvovaginal candidiasis, a switch to lower-dose oral contraceptives or even a discontinuation of oral contraceptives may be indicated. Also, underlying HIV infection should be considered in women with recurrent infections. See Chap. 19.

B. **Trichomoniasis.** The index case and all sex partners should be treated. Cure rates of 95% have been achieved when recommended metronidazole regimens are used [9].

1. The **standard treatment is metronidazole, 2 g, as a single oral dose.**

2. An **alternative regimen** is metronidazole, 250 mg PO tid or 500 mg PO bid for 7 days. **Note:** Metronidazole gel has been approved for treatment of bacterial vaginosis but it is **not** recommended for the treatment of trichomoniasis.

3. **Metronidazole probably is contraindicated in the first trimester of pregnancy.** In this case **clotrimazole,** which has some antitrichomonal activity, can be given intravaginally, although it produces cure in only about 20% of patients.

4. **Metronidazole resistance is increasing** in prevalence. Treating metronidazole-resistant trichomoniasis usually involves the administration of high doses of metronidazole, which can be associated with toxicity.

  Noncompliance of the patient with standard therapy or reinfection by an untreated partner should be considered.

  Usually, retreatment with metronidazole, 500 mg bid for 7 days, is tried. If repeated failure occurs, the patient can be treated with a single 2-g dose of metronidazole once daily for 3–5 days. Patients with culture-documented infection who do not respond to these regimens and in whom reinfection has been excluded should be referred for consultation with an expert, so that susceptibility of the *T. vaginalis* to metronidazole can be determined.

C. Bacterial vaginosis. Successful regimens have been aimed at the anaerobic bacteria that participate in the infection. The principal goal of therapy is to relieve vaginal symptoms and signs [9, 174a]. Because male sex partners of women with bacterial vaginosis are not symptomatic and because treatment of male partners has not been shown to alter either the clinical course of bacterial vaginosis in women during treatment or the relapse or reinfection rate, preventing transmission to men is not a goal of therapy. Therefore, male sexual contacts do not require therapy [9] for initial episodes. In women with recurrent episodes of bacterial vaginosis, it would be prudent also to treat sexual contacts.

1. Oral regimens

  a. Metronidazole, 500 mg PO bid for 7 days.

  b. Metronidazole, 250 mg PO tid for 7 days.

  c. Metronidazole, 2 g PO as a single dose. (The equivalence of this regimen to the 1-week courses remains somewhat controversial [175].)

  d. Clindamycin, 300 mg PO bid for 7 days. This regimen has the advantage of being safe in pregnancy [176].

  e. Cefadroxil, 500 mg PO bid for 7 days. This regimen is safe in pregnancy but is supported by very limited data [177].

2. Topical regimens appear to have acceptable cure rates, although data are limited.

  a. Clindamycin 2% vaginal cream, 5 g (one full applicator) vaginally at bedtime for 7 days. This may be the preferred treatment for bacterial vaginosis during pregnancy, especially the first trimester of pregnancy [9].

  b. Metronidazole 0.75% vaginal gel, 5 g (one full applicator) vaginally bid for 5 days. Although systemic absorption is limited, this regimen should probably be avoided in pregnancy.

Sexually Transmitted Intestinal Infections

Sexually transmitted intestinal infections (e.g., due to *Salmonella* spp., *Campylobacter jejuni*, *Shigella* spp., *Cryptosporidium* spp.) are discussed in Chaps. 11 and 19.

References

1. Rothenberg, R.B., and Potterat, J.J. Strategies for Management of Sexual Partners. In: K.K. Holmes et al. (eds.), *Sexually Transmitted Diseases*. New York: McGraw-Hill, 1990. Pp. 965–972.
   Covers a number of strategies. The definitive text on STDs.
1a. Schmid, G.P., and Fontanarosa, P.B. Evolving strategies for management of the nongonococcal urethritis syndrome. *J.A.M.A.* 274:577, 1995.
   Editorial comment in August 1995 on reference [22a].
2. Stamm, W.E., et al. *Chlamydia trachomatis* urethral infections in men. Prevalence, risk factors, and clinical manifestations. *Ann. Intern. Med.* 100:47, 1984.
3. Rein, M.F., and McCormack, W.M. Urethritis. In G.L. Mandell, J.E. Bennett, and R. Dolin (eds.), *Principles and Practice of Infectious Diseases* (4th ed.). New York: Churchill Livingstone, 1995. P. 1063.
4. Goodhart, M.E., et al. Factors affecting the performance of smear and culture tests for the detection of *Neisseria gonorrhoeae*. *Sex. Transm. Dis.* 9:63, 1982.
5. Kleris, G.S., and Arnold, A.J. Differential diagnosis of urethritis: Predictive value and therapeutic implications of the urethral smear. *Sex. Transm. Dis.* 8:110, 1981.
6. Centers for Disease Control. Antibiotic-resistant strains of *Neisseria gonorrhoeae*: Policy guidelines for detection, management, and control. *M.M.W.R.* 36(Suppl.):1–18, 1987.
   Recommendations for program design and implementation. Explains at what degree of resistance one should move to newer regimens.
7. Gorwitz, R.J., Moran, J.S., and Knapp, J.S. Sentinel surveillance for antimicrobial resistance in *Neisseria gonorrhoeae*—United States, 1981–1991. *M.M.W.R.* 42(SS-3): 29–39, 1993.
   Details the important results from a national surveillance system that document the substantial increase in prevalence of resistant strains in recent years.

8. Elwell, L.P., et al. Plasmid-mediated beta-lactamase production in *Neisseria gonorrhoeae. Antimicrob. Agents Chemother.* 11:528, 1977.
   The classic, initial description. Very frightening to those in the field.
9. Centers for Disease Control. 1993 Sexually transmitted disease treatment guidelines. *M.M.W.R.* 42(RR-14):1–102, 1993.
   The definitive and essential compendium of up-to-date management of STDs in the United States. The major background papers that were drafted by experts in the preparation of these guidelines in early 1993 have recently been published. See special symposium (April 1995) by W.C. Levine et al., 1993 sexually transmitted diseases treatment guidelines. Clin. Infect. Dis. 20(suppl. 1):S1, 1995, which emphasizes background information on the therapy of syphilis, chancroid, gonococcal infections, chlamydial infections, bacterial vaginosis, and vulvovaginal candidiasis.
9a. Moran, J.S., and Levine, W.C. Drugs of choice for treatment of uncomplicated gonococcal infections. *Clin. Infect. Dis.* 20(suppl. 1):S47, 1995.
   Summary of background information for recommendations in reference [9].
9b. Weber, J.T., and Johnson, R.E. New treatments for *Chlamydia trachomatis* genital infection. *Clin. Infect. Dis.* 20(suppl. 1):S66, 1995.
   Summary of background information for recommendations in reference [9].
10. Handsfield, H.H., et al. Differences in the therapeutic response of chlamydia-positive and chlamydia-negative forms of nongonococcal urethritis. *J. Am. Vener. Dis. Assoc.* 2:5, 1976.
   This article and the next are excellent, classic examples of defining an etiologic role without satisfying Koch's postulates.
11. Bowie, W.R., et al. Etiology of nongonococcal urethritis: Evidence for *Chlamydia trachomatis* and *Ureaplasma urealyticum. J. Clin. Invest.* 59:735, 1977.
   The definitive work.
12. Centers for Disease Control. *Chlamydia trachomatis* infections: Policy guidelines for prevention and control. *M.M.W.R.* 34(Suppl.):53, 1985.
13. Romanowski, B., et al. Minocycline compared with doxycycline in the treatment of nongonococcal urethritis and mucopurulent cervicitis. *Ann. Intern. Med.* 199:16, 1993.
   An effective once-daily regimen for NGU and MPC. At this dosage, minocycline caused fewer side effects than doxycycline.
14. Centers for Disease Control. Recommendations for the prevention and management of *Chlamydia trachomatis* infections, 1993. *M.M.W.R.* 42(RR-12):1, 1993.
   An up-to-date and thorough manual on prevention, diagnosis, and treatment.
15. Warren, R., et al. Comparative evaluation of detection assays for *Chlamydia trachomatis. J. Clin. Microbiol.* 31:1663, 1993.
16. Stimson, J.B., et al. Tetracycline-resistant *Ureaplasma urealyticum:* A cause for persistent nongonococcal urethritis. *Ann. Intern. Med.* 94:192, 1981.
   The initial description. Infected men did not respond to standard doses of tetracyclines.
17. Magalhaes, M. Persistent nongonococcal urethritis associated with a minocycline-resistant strain of *Ureaplasma urealyticum. Sex. Transm. Dis.* 10:151, 1983.
18. Arya, O.P., and Pratt, B.C. Persistent urethritis due to *Ureaplasma urealyticum* in conjugal or stable partnerships. *Genitourin. Med.* 62:329, 1986.
19. Krieger, J.N., et al. Clinical manifestations of trichomoniasis in men. *Ann. Intern. Med.* 118:844, 1993.
   An important study of a problem for which there are few data.
20. Corey, L., et al. Genital herpes simplex virus infection: Clinical manifestations, course, and complications. *Ann. Intern. Med.* 98:958, 1983.
   Excellent review article on all aspects of the disease.
21. Boslego, J.W., et al. Effect of spectinomycin use on the prevalence of spectinomycin-resistant and of penicillinase-producing *Neisseria gonorrhoeae. N. Engl. J. Med.* 317:272, 1987.
21a. Centers for Disease Control. Decreased susceptibility of *Neisseria gonorrhoeae* to fluoroquinolones—Ohio and Hawaii, 1992–1994. *M.M.W.R.* 43:325, 1994.
22. Bowie, W.R., et al. Therapy for non-gonococcal urethritis: Double blind, randomized comparison of two doses and two durations of minocycline. *Ann. Intern. Med.* 95:306, 1981.
22a. Stamm, W.E., et al. Azithromycin for empirical treatment of the nongonococcal urethritis syndrome in men: A randomized double-blind study. *J.A.M.A.* 274:545, 1995.
22b. Magid, D. Doxycycline compared with azithromycin for treating women with genital *Chlamydia trachomatis* infections: An incremental cost-effectiveness analysis. *Ann. Intern. Med.* 124:389, 1996.

23. Wong, E.S., et al. Clinical and microbiological features of persistent or recurrent nongonococcal urethritis in men. *J. Infect. Dis.* 158:1098, 1988.
24. Berger, R.E. Recurrent nongonococcal urethritis. *J.A.M.A.* 249:409, 1983.
    Explains current practices but provides no new data.
25. Krieger, J.N., et al. Evaluation of chronic urethritis: Defining the role for endoscopic procedures. *Arch. Intern. Med.* 148:703, 1988.
    Many of these patients have evidence of obstruction to urine flow, but not many have identifiable lesions that require surgical intervention.
26. Stamm, W.E., et al. Causes of the acute urethral syndrome in women. *N. Engl. J. Med.* 303:409, 1980.
    This is an important article that defines low-inoculum urinary tract infection as well as sexually transmitted urethritis.
27. Stamm, W.E. Etiology and management of the acute urethral syndrome. *Sex. Transm. Dis.* 8:235, 1981.
    Good review of current knowledge.
28. Fihn, S.D., Johnson, C., and Stamm, W.E. *Escherichia coli* urethritis in women with symptoms of acute urinary tract infection. *J. Infect. Dis.* 73:196, 1988.
28a. Cromblerhome, W.R., et al. Amoxicillin therapy for *Chlamydia trachomatis* infections in pregnancy. *Obstet. Gynecol.* 75:752, 1990.
28b. Campbell, W.F., and Dodson, M.G. Clindamycin therapy for *Chlamydia trachomatis* in women. *Am. J. Obstet. Gynecol.* 162:343, 1990.
29. Handsfield, H.H., et al. Asymptomatic gonorrhea in men: Diagnosis, natural course, prevalence, and significance. *N. Eng. J. Med.* 290:117, 1974.
    Classic description of the syndrome.
30. Kamwendo, F., et al. Gonorrhea, genital chlamydial infection, and nonspecific urethritis in male partners of women hospitalized and treated for acute pelvic inflammatory disease. *Sex. Transm. Dis.* 20:143, 1993.
31. Swartz, S.L., and Kraus, S.J. Persistent urethral leukocytosis and asymptomatic chlamydial urethritis. *J. Infect. Dis.* 140:614, 1979.
    Workup of an asymptomatic man for STD should include a urethral swab looking for polymorphonuclear neutrophils.
32. Tait, I.A., et al. Chlamydial infection of the cervix in contacts of men with nongonococcal urethritis. *Br. J. Vener. Dis.* 56:37, 1980.
33. Mardh, P.A., Moller, B.R., and Paavonen, J. Chlamydial infection of the female genital tract with emphasis on pelvic inflammatory disease. A review of Scandinavian studies. *Sex. Transm. Dis.* 8:140, 1981.
34. Paavonen, J., and Vesterinen, E. *Chlamydia trachomatis* in cervicitis and urethritis in women. *Scand. J. Infect. Dis.* 32(Suppl.):45, 1982.
35. Corey, L., et al. Genital herpes simplex virus infections. Clinical manifestations, course, and complications. *Ann. Intern. Med.* 98:958, 1983.
36. Pazin, G.H. Management of oral and genital herpes simplex viral infections: Diagnosis and treatment. *Dis. Mon.* 32:725–784, 1986.
37. Reid, R., et al. Sexually transmitted papillomavirus infections: I. The anatomic distribution and pathologic grade of neoplastic lesions associated with different viral types. *Am. J. Obstet. Gynecol.* 156:212–222, 1987.
38. Pfister, H. Relationship of papillomaviruses to anogenital cancer. *Obstet. Gynecol. Clin. North Am.* 14:349–362, 1987.
39. Koutsky, L.A., et al. A cohort study of the risk of cervical intraepithelial neoplasia grade 2 or 3 in relation to papillomavirus infection. *N. Engl. J. Med.* 327:1272–1278, 1992.
40. Brunham, R.C., et al. Mucopurulent cervicitis—the ignored counterpart in women of urethritis in men. *N. Engl. J. Med.* 311:1–6, 1984.
41. Wentworth, B.B., et al. Isolation of viruses, bacteria and other organisms from venereal disease clinic patients: Methodology and problems associated with multiple isolations. *Health Lab. Sci.* 10:75, 1973.
42. Spence, M.R., et al. A correlative study of Papanicolaou smear, fluorescent antibody, and culture for the diagnosis of *Chlamydia trachomatis*. *Obstet. Gynecol.* 68:691–695, 1986.
43. Paavonen, J., et al. Etiology of cervical inflammation. *Am. J. Obstet. Gynecol.* 154:556–564, 1986.
44. Harrison, H.R., et al. Cervical *Chlamydia trachomatis* infection in university women: Relationship to history, contraceptives, ectopy, and cervicitis. *Am. J. Obstet. Gynecol.* 153:224–251, 1985.

45. Quinn, T.C., Gupta, P.K., and Burkman, R.T. Detection of *Chlamydia trachomatis* cervical infections: A comparison of Papanicolaou and immunofluorescent staining with cell cultures. *Am. J. Obstet. Gynecol.* 157:394–399, 1987.
46. Moscicki, B., et al. The use and limitations of endocervical Gram stain and mucopurulent cervicitis as predictors for *Chlamydia trachomatis* in female adolescents. *Am. J. Obstet. Gynecol.* 157:65–71, 1987.
47. Nugent, R.P., and Hillier, S.L. Mucopurulent cervicitis as a predictor of chlamydial infection and adverse pregnancy outcome. *Sex. Transm. Dis.* 19:198–202, 1992.
48. Knud-Hansen, C.R., et al. Surrogate methods to diagnose gonococcal and chlamydial cervicitis: Comparison of leukocyte esterase dipstick, endocervical Gram stain, and culture. *Sex. Transm. Dis.* 18:211–216, 1991.
49. Katz, B.P., Caine, V.A., and Jones, R.B. Diagnosis of mucopurulent cervicitis among women at risk for *Chlamydia trachomatis* infection. *Sex. Transm. Dis.* 16:103–106, 1989.
50. Dolter, J., Bryant, L., and Janda, J.M. Evaluation of five rapid systems for the identification of *Neisseria gonorrhoeae*. *Diagn. Microbiol. Infect. Dis.* 13:265, 1990.
51. Stamm, W.E., et al. Diagnosis of *Chlamydia trachomatis* infections by direct immunofluorescence staining of genital secretions: A multicenter trial. *Ann. Intern. Med.* 101:638–642, 1984.
52. Hipp, S.S., Han, V., and Murphy, D. Assessment of enzyme immunoassay and immunofluorescence tests for detection of *Chlamydia trachomatis*. *J. Clin. Microbiol.* 25:1938–1943, 1987.
53. LeBar, W., et al. Comparison of the Kallstead Pathfinder EIA, cytocentrifuged direct fluorescent antibody, and culture for the diagnosis of *Chlamydia trachomatis*. *Diagn. Microbiol. Infect. Dis.* 14:17–20, 1991.
54. Coleman, P., et al. TestPack Chlamydia, a new rapid assay for the direct detection of *Chlamydia trachomatis*. *J. Clin. Microbiol.* 27:2811–2814, 1989.
55. Ferris, D.G., and Martin, W.H. A comparison of three rapid chlamydial tests in pregnant and nonpregnant women. *J. Fam. Pract.* 34:593–597, 1992.
56. Skulnick, M., et al. Comparison of the Clearview Chlamydia test, Chlamydiazyme, and cell culture for the detection of *Chlamydia trachomatis* in women with a low prevalence of infection. *J. Clin. Microbiol.* 29:2056–2058, 1991.
57. Nohara, M., Sugase, M., and Kawana, T. Evaluation of DNA probe for chlamydial and gonococcal infections of the uterine cervix. *Acta Obstet. Gynaecol. Jpn.* 43:459–464, 1991.
58. Mercer, L.J., et al. Comparison of chemiluminescent DNA probe to cell culture for the screening of *Chlamydia trachomatis* in a gynecology clinic population. *Obstet. Gynecol.* 76:114–117, 1990.
59. Wiesner, P.J., et al. Clinical spectrum of pharyngeal gonococcal infections. *N. Engl. J. Med.* 288:181, 1973.
    Classic description of all phases of the infection; treatment recommendations are now seriously outdated.
60. Jones, R.B., et al. *Chlamydia trachomatis* in the pharynx and rectum of heterosexual patients at risk for genital infection. *Ann. Intern. Med.* 102:757, 1985.
    A good epidemiological study.
61. Quinn, T.C., et al. AIDS in Africa: An epidemiological paradigm. *Science* 234:955, 1986.
62. Chamberland, M.E., Ward, J.W., and Curran, J.W. Epidemiology and Prevention of AIDS and HIV Infection. In G.L. Mandell, J.E. Bennett, and R. Dolin (eds.), *Principles and Practice of Infectious Diseases* (4th ed.). New York: Churchill Livingstone, 1995 Pp. 1174–1203.
    Excellent review.
63. Simonsen, J.N., et al. Human immunodeficiency virus infection in men with sexually transmitted diseases. *N. Engl. J. Med.* 319:274, 1988.
64. Rein, M.F. Genital Skin and Mucous Membrane Lesions. In G.L. Mandell, J.E. Bennett, and R. Dolin (eds.), *Principles and Practice of Infectious Diseases* (4th ed.). New York: Churchill Livingstone, 1995. P. 1055.
65. Brown, S.T., Nalley, J.F., and Kraus, S.J. Molluscum contagiosum. *Sex. Transm. Dis.* 8:227, 1981.
    A definitive review article in an area for which there is little literature.
66. Sehgal, V.N., and Shyam-Prasad, A.L. Donovanosis: Current concepts. *Int. J. Dermatol.* 25:8, 1986.
    A good review in an area for which there is even less literature than for molluscum contagiosum.

67. Chapel, T.A. The variability of syphilitic chancres. *Sex. Transm. Dis.* 5:68, 1978.
    An important accounting of recent experience. If you haven't made another diagnosis already, think of syphilis.

68. Sturm, A.W., Stolting, G.J., and Cormane, R.H. Clinical and microbiological evaluation of 46 episodes of genital ulceration. *Genitourin. Med.* 63:98, 1987.
    Contains some good practical advice.

69. Johnson, R.E., et al. A seroepidemiologic survey of the prevalence of herpes simplex virus type 2 infection in the United States. *N. Engl. J. Med.* 321:7, 1989.
    An eye-opening study that found the prevalence of HSV 2 infection among young American adults to be nearly 20%!

70. Koutsky, L.A., et al. Underdiagnosis of genital herpes by current clinical and viral-isolation procedures. *N. Engl. J. Med.* 326:1533, 1992.
    Suggests that our current strategies for diagnosing HSV 2 infection may greatly underestimate prevalence as 60% of infected women in this study never had symptoms.

71. Breinig, M.K., et al. Epidemiology of genital herpes in Pittsburgh: Serologic, sexual, and racial correlates of apparent and inapparent herpes simplex infections. *J. Infect. Dis.* 162:299, 1990.
    Another study suggesting that the vast majority of HSV 2 infections are subclinical.

72. Kulhanjian, J.A., et al. Identification of women at unsuspected risk of primary infection with herpes simplex virus type 2 during pregnancy. *N. Engl. J. Med.* 326:916, 1992.

73. Guinan, M.S., Wolinsky, S.M., and Reichman, R.C. Epidemiology of genital herpes simplex virus infections. *Epidemiol. Rev.* 7:127, 1985.
    Contains a wealth of information.

74. Mertz, G.J., et al. Double-blind, placebo-controlled trial of a herpes simplex virus type 2 glycoprotein vaccine in persons at high risk for genital herpes infection. *J. Infect. Dis.* 161:653, 1990.
    A very important study—not because of the vaccine (which did not work)—but because it prospectively measures rates of acquisition of infection in uninfected partners of persons with recurrent genital herpes.

75. Lafferty, W.E., et al. Recurrences after oral and genital herpes simplex virus infection. Influence of the site of infection and viral type. *N. Engl. J. Med.* 316:1444, 1987.

75a. Benedetti, J., Corey, L., and Ashley, R. Recurrence rates in genital herpes after symptomatic first-episode infection. *Ann. Intern. Med.* 121:847, 1994.
    Concludes that almost all persons with initially symptomatic HSV-2 infections have symptomatic recurrences. More than 35% of such patients have frequent recurrences. Recurrence rates are especially high in persons with an extended first episode of infection whether they received acyclovir or not. Men with genital HSV-2 have more recurrences.

76. Diaz-Mitoma, F., et al. Etiology of nonvesicular genital ulcers in Winnipeg. *Sex. Transm. Dis.* 14:33, 1987.
    Good study of etiologies in North America.

77. Lafferty, W.E., et al. Diagnosis of herpes simplex virus by direct immunofluorescence and viral isolation from samples of external genital lesions in a high prevalence population. *J. Clin. Microbiol.* 25:323, 1987.

78. Ashley, R. Laboratory techniques in the diagnosis of herpes simplex infection. *Genitourin. Med.* 69:174, 1993.
    A good general review of diagnostic techniques.

79. Gonik, B., et al. Comparison of two enzyme-linked immunosorbent assays for detection of herpes simplex virus antigen. *J. Clin. Microbiol.* 29:436, 1991.

80. Corey, L., et al. A trial of topical acyclovir in genital herpes simplex virus infections. *N. Engl. J. Med.* 306:1313, 1982.
    One of several similar trials showing beneficial effects that are statistically but not clinically significant.

81. Straus, S.E., et al. Suppression of frequently recurring genital herpes. *N. Engl. J. Med.* 310:1545, 1984.

82. Douglas, J.M., et al. A double blind study of oral acyclovir for suppression of recurrences of genital herpes simplex virus infections. *N. Engl. J. Med.* 310:1551, 1985.

83. Prober, C.G., et al. Low risk of herpes simplex virus infections in neonates exposed to the virus at the time of vaginal delivery to mothers with recurrent genital herpes simplex virus infections. *N. Engl. J. Med.* 316:240, 1987.
    The risk to the infant is less than 8%. See related papers by C.G. Prober et al., The management of pregnancies complicated by genital infections with herpes simplex

virus. Clin. Infect. Dis. *15:1031, 1992; and R.S. Gibbs et al., Management of genital herpes infection in pregnancy.* Obstet. Gynecol. *71:779, 1988. The latter contains recommendations from the Infectious Disease Society for Obstetrics and Gynecology for the management of pregnant women with genital herpes.*

84. Frenkel, L.M., et al. Clinical reactivation of herpes simplex virus type 2 infection in seropositive pregnant women with no history of genital herpes. *Ann. Intern. Med.* 118:414, 1993.

85. Arvin, A.M., et al. Failure of antepartum maternal cultures to predict infant's exposure to herpes simplex virus at delivery. *N. Engl. J. Med.* 315:796, 1986.

86. Larsen, S.A., Hunter, E.F., and Creighton, E.T. Syphilis. In K.K. Holmes et al. (eds.), *Sexually Transmitted Diseases* (2nd ed.). New York: McGraw-Hill, 1990. Pp. 927–934. *Contains the nitty-gritty of the techniques for performing diagnostic tests for syphilis.*

87. Centers for Disease Control and Prevention. Special focus: Surveillance for sexually transmitted diseases. *M.M.W.R.* 42(SS-3):13, 1993.

88. Centers for Disease Control and Prevention. Cases of selected notifiable diseases, United States, weeks ending January 1, 1994, and December 26, 1992 (52nd week). *M.M.W.R.* 42:1004, 1994.

89. Rolfs, R.T., Goldberg, M., and Sharrar, R.G. Risk factors for syphilis: Cocaine use and prostitution. *Am. J. Public Health* 80:853, 1990.

90. Greenberg, J., Schnell, D., and Conlon, R. Behaviors of crack cocaine users and their impact on early syphilis intervention. *Sex. Transm. Dis.* 19:346, 1992.

91. Finelli, L., Budd, J., and Spitalny, K.C. Early syphilis: Relationship to sex, drugs, and changes in high-risk behavior from 1987–1990. *Sex. Transm. Dis.* 20:89, 1993.

92. Chapel, T.A. The signs and symptoms of secondary syphilis. *Sex. Transm. Dis.* 7: 161, 1980.

93. Chapel, T.A. Physician recognition of the signs and symptoms of secondary syphilis. *J.A.M.A.* 246:250, 1981.

94. Stokes, J.H., Beerman, H., and Ingraham, N.R. *Modern Clinical Syphilology* (3rd ed.). Philadelphia: Saunders, 1944. *This is the classic clinical description of syphilis. A valuable resource. Treatment discussion is outdated; the authors suspect that the new drug, penicillin, will revolutionize therapy of syphilis. Buy this book if you find it at a used book sale!*

95. Swartz, M.N. Neurosyphilis. In K.K. Holmes et al. (eds.), *Sexually Transmitted Diseases* (2nd ed.). New York: McGraw-Hill, 1990. Pp. 231–246. *A superb discussion by one of the master clinicians and teachers of our generation.*

96. Healy, B.P. Cardiovascular Syphilis. In K.K. Holmes et al. (eds.), *Sexually Transmitted Diseases* (2nd ed.). New York: McGraw-Hill, 1990. Pp. 247–250. *Excellent discussion by a classmate of both the author of this chapter and the editor of this book.*

97. Kampmeier, R.H. Late Benign Syphilis. In K.K. Holmes et al. (eds.), *Sexually Transmitted Diseases* (2nd ed.). New York: McGraw-Hill, 1990. Pp. 251–262. *The author has many decades of experience with syphilis.*

98. Tramont, E.C. *Treponema pallidum* (Syphilis). In G.L. Mandell, J.E. Bennett, and R. Dolin (eds.), *Principles and Practice of Infectious Diseases* (4th ed.). New York: Churchill Livingstone, 1995. P. 2117. *Excellent discussion of all aspects of syphilis, including newest treatment recommendations and considerations in AIDS. See also E.C. Tramont, Syphilis in adults.* Clin. Infect. Dis. *21:1361, 1995; and J.L. Flores, Syphilis: A tale of twisted treponemes (review).* West J. Med. *163:552, 1995, with editorial comment.*

98a. Larsen, S.A., Steiner, B.M., and Rudolph, A.H. Laboratory diagnosis and interpretation of tests for syphilis. *Clin. Microbiol. Rev.* 8:1, 1995.

99. Brown, S.T., Zaidi, A., and Larsen, S.A. Serological response to syphilis treatment: A new analysis of old data. *J.A.M.A.* 253:1296, 1985.

100. Romanowski, B., et al. Serologic response to treatment of infectious syphilis. *Ann. Intern. Med.* 114:1005, 1991. *An important study that took advantage of a sustained outbreak of syphilis to better define the serologic response to treatment.*

101. Magnarelli, L.A., et al. Cross-reactivity in serological tests for Lyme disease and other spirochetal infections. *J. Infect. Dis.* 156:183, 1987. *Approximately 10% of Lyme disease patients will have reactive FTA-ABS tests, but they will not have reactive nontreponemal tests.*

101a. Rolfs, R.T. Treatment of syphilis, 1993. *Clin. Infect. Dis.* 20(suppl 1):S23, 1995. *Contains background information for recommendations in reference [9].*

102. Moorthy, T.T., et al. Ceftriaxone for treatment of primary syphilis in men. *Sex. Transm. Dis.* 14:116, 1987.
102a. Musher, D.M., and Baughin, R.E. Neurosyphilis in HIV-infected persons. *N. Engl. J. Med.* 331:1516, 1994.
      Editorial comment on two articles in this same issue that deal with the difficulties of treating neurosyphilis in the immunosuppressed HIV-positive patient. See related articles in this same journal.
103. Hook, E.W., III, et al. Ceftriaxone therapy for asymptomatic neurosyphilis. *Sex. Transm. Dis.* 13:185, 1987.
104. Yim, C.W., Flynn, N.M., and Fitzgerald, F.T. Penetration of oral doxycycline into the cerebrospinal fluid of patients with latent or neurosyphilis. *Antimicrob. Agents Chemother.* 28:347, 1985.
105. Faber, W.R., et al. Treponemacidal levels of amoxicillin in cerebrospinal fluid after oral administration. *Sex. Transm. Dis.* 10:148, 1983.
106. Musher, D.M., Hamill, R.J., and Baughn, R.E. Effect of human immunodeficiency virus (HIV) infection on the course of syphilis and on the response to treatment. *Ann. Intern. Med.* 113:872, 1990.
      A literature review on the topic. Unfortunately, there are not many controlled studies available.
107. Gourevitch, M.N., et al. Effects of HIV infection on the serologic manifestations and response to treatment of syphilis in intravenous drug users. *Ann. Intern. Med.* 118:350, 1993.
      The only controlled study of this problem. It found that HIV did not alter manifestations of syphilis in this cohort.
108. Musher, D.M. Syphilis, neurosyphilis, penicillin and AIDS. *J. Infect. Dis.* 163:1201, 1991.
      Another review on the subject.
109. Johns, D.R., Tierney, M., and Felsenstein, D. Alteration in the natural history of neurosyphilis by concurrent infection with human immunodeficiency virus. *N. Engl. J. Med.* 316:1569, 1987.
110. Schmid, G.P., et al. Chancroid in the United States, reestablishment of an old disease. *J.A.M.A.* 258:3265, 1987.
111. Jessamine, P.G., and Ronald, A.R. Chancroid and the role of genital ulcer disease in the spread of human retroviruses. *Med. Clin. North Am.* 64:1417, 1990.
      A very thorough review of chancroid and its relationship to transmission of HIV.
112. Ronald, A.R., and Albritton, W. Chancroid and *Haemophilus ducreyi*. In K.K. Holmes et al. (eds.), *Sexually Transmitted Diseases* (2nd ed.). New York: McGraw-Hill, 1990. Pp. 263–271.
      Definitive, up-to-date review.
112a. Marrazzo, J.M., and Handsfield, H.H. Chancroid: New developments in an old disease. *Curr. Clin. Top. Infect. Dis.* 15:129, 1995.
113. Nsanze, H., et al. Comparison of media for the primary isolation of *Haemophilus ducreyi*. *Sex. Transm. Dis.* 11:6, 1984.
      The vast majority of routine laboratories will not be able to culture the organism reliably. This article explains why.
113a. Schulte, J.M., and Schmid, G.P. Recommendations for treatment of chancroid, 1993. *Clin. Infect. Dis.* 20(Suppl 1):S39, 1995.
114. Hart, G. Donovanosis. In K.K. Holmes et al. (eds.), *Sexually Transmitted Diseases* (2nd ed.). New York: McGraw-Hill, 1990. Pp. 273–277.
115. Freinkel, A.L., and Counihan, R.J. Granuloma inguinale (donovanosis) in South Africa. *S. Afr. Med. J.* 63:599, 1983.
      One of the very few recent articles on this disease, which is very rare in the developed world.
116. Bassa, A.G.H., et al. Granuloma inguinale (donovanosis) in women: An analysis of 61 cases from Durban, South Africa. *Sex. Transm. Dis.* 20:164, 1993.
      Provides new clinical data regarding a disease for which there is little recent literature.
117. Schwartz, J.J., and Myskowski, P.L. Molluscum contagiosum in patients with human immunodeficiency virus infection. *J. Am. Acad. Dermatol.* 27:583, 1992.
      One of the biggest published case series in AIDS patients.
118. Campion, M.J., et al. Increased risk of cervical neoplasia in consorts of men with penile condylomata accuminata. *Lancet* 1:943, 1985.
      One of many recent articles establishing a strong epidemiological relationship.

119. Schultz, R.E., and Skelton, H.G. Value of acetic acid screening for flat genital condylomata in men. *J. Urol.* 139:777, 1988.
     One of several recent articles describing the technique. Diagnosis must be confirmed by biopsy.
120. Lorincz, A.T., et al. Correlation of cellular atypia and human papillomavirus DNA in exfoliated cells from the uterine cervix. *Obstet Gynecol.* 68:508, 1986.
     Eleven percent of normal smears contained human papillomavirus DNA.
121. Medical Letter. Podofilox for genital warts. *Med. Lett. Drugs Ther.* 33:115, 1991.
     The basics regarding this drug.
122. Eron, L.J., et al. Interferon therapy for condylomata accuminata. *N. Engl. J. Med.* 315:1059, 1986.
     Expensive, uncomfortable, and not for the faint of heart.
123. Eisenstein, B.I., and Masi, A.T. Disseminated gonococcal infections (DGI) and gonococcal arthritis (GCA): 1. Bacteriology, epidemiology, host factors, pathogen factors, and pathology. 2: Clinical manifestations, diagnosis, complications, treatment, and prevention. *Semin. Arthritis Rheum.* 10:155, 173, 1981.
     Superb review of all that was known about the condition at the time. Treatment recommendations are outdated. See Centers for Disease Control reference [9] for updated therapy.
124. O'Brien, J.P., et al. Disseminated gonococcal infection: A prospective analysis of 49 patients and a review of pathophysiology and immune mechanisms. *Medicine* 62:395, 1983.
125. Bush, L.M., and Boscia, J.A. Disseminated multiple antibiotic-resistant gonococcal infection: Needed changes in antimicrobial therapy. *Ann. Intern. Med.* 107:692, 1987.
126. Strader, K.W., et al. Disseminated gonococcal infection caused by chromosomally mediated penicillin-resistant organisms. *Ann. Intern. Med.* 104:365, 1986.
127. Pritchard, C., and Berney, S.N. Septic arthritis caused by penicillinase-producing *Neisseria gonorrhoeae. J. Rheumatol.* 13:719, 1988.
128. Rompalo, A.M., et al. The acute arthritis-dermatitis syndrome: The changing importance of *Neisseria gonorrhoeae* and *Neisseria meningitidis. Arch. Intern. Med.* 147:281, 1987.
129. Chapel, T.A., et al. Pediculosis pubis in a clinic for sexually transmitted diseases. *Sex. Transm. Dis.* 6:257, 1979.
130. Orkin, M., and Maibach, H.I. Current views of scabies and pediculosis pubis. *Cutis* 33:85, 1984.
130a. Brown, S., Becher, J., and Brady, W. Treatment of ectoparasitic infections: Review of the English-language literature, 1982–1992. *Clin. Infect. Dis.* 20(suppl. 1):S104, 1995.
     Background information for recommendations in reference [9].
131. Funkhauser, M.E., and Ross, A. Management of scabies in patients with human immunodeficiency virus disease. *Arch. Dermatol.* 129:911, 1993.
     Documents the unusual severity with which this infection can present in AIDS patients.
132. Sobel, J.D. Candidal vulvovaginitis. *Clin. Obstet. Gynecol.* 36:153–165, 1993.
     For a related paper, see A. Spirillo et al., Torulopsis glabrata vaginitis. Obstet. Gynecol. 85:993, 1995. Authors note T. glabrata was isolated in 10% of women with vulvovaginal candidiasis who attended a vaginitis clinic. This infection was associated with recurrent vaginitis in almost one-third of case patients presenting with symptoms.
133. Kent, H.L. Epidemiology of vaginitis. *Am. J. Obstet. Gynecol.* 165:1168–1176, 1991.
134. Sobel, J.D. Epidemiology and pathogenesis of recurrent vulvovaginal candidiasis. *Am. J. Obstet. Gynecol.* 1523:924–935, 1985.
     Important summary of a controversial field.
135. O'Connor, M.I., and Sobel, J.D. Epidemiology of recurrent vulvovaginal candidiasis: Identification and strain differentiation of *Candida albicans. J. Infect. Dis.* 154:358–363, 1986.
136. Larsen, B. Vaginal flora in health and disease. *Clin. Obstet. Gynecol.* 36:107–121, 1993.
137. Rein, M.F., and Holmes, K.K. "Nonspecific vaginitis," vulvovaginal candidiasis, and trichomoniasis. *Curr. Clin. Top. Infect. Dis.* 4:281, 1983.
138. Sobel, J.D. Pathogenesis and treatment of recurrent vulvovaginal candidiasis. *Clin. Infect. Dis.* 14(Suppl. 1):S148–153, 1992.
139. Heidrich, F.E., Berg, A.O., and Bergman, J.J. Clothing factors and vaginitis. *J. Fam. Pract.* 19:491–494, 1984.
     It really does appear that tight clothing increases the rate of genital colonization with yeasts.

140. Reed, B.D., and Pierson, C.L. Evaluation of a latex agglutination test for identification of *Candida* species in vaginal discharge. *J. Am. Board Fam. Pract.* 5:375–380, 1992.
141. Kent, H.L. Epidemiology of vaginitis. *Am. J. Obstet. Gynecol.* 165:1168–1176, 1991.
142. Wolner-Hanssen, P., et al. Clinical manifestations of vaginal trichomoniasis. *J.A.M.A.* 264:571–576, 1989.
    Good study defining current descriptions of the disease in women and role of colposcopy.
143. Rein, M.F. Clinical Manifestations of Urogenital Trichomoniasis in Women. In B.M. Honigberg (ed.), *Trichomonads Parasitic in Humans.* New York: Springer-Verlag, 1990. Pp. 225–234.
    See related summary by P. Heine and J.A. McGregor, Trichomonas vaginalis: A re-emerging pathogen. *Clin. Obstet. Gynecol. 36:137, 1993.*
144. Krieger, J.N., et al. Diagnosis of trichomoniasis: Comparison of conventional wet-mount examination with cytologic studies, cultures, and monoclonal antibody straining of direct specimens. *J.A.M.A.* 259:1223–1227, 1988.
145. Carney, J.A., et al. A new rapid agglutination test for the diagnosis of *Trichomonas vaginalis* infection. *J. Clin. Pathol.* 41:806–808, 1988.
146. Yule, A., et al. Detection of *Trichomonas vaginalis* antigen in women by enzyme immunoassay. *J. Clin. Pathol.* 40:566–568, 1987.
147. Gardner, H.L., and Dukes, C.D. *Haemophilus vaginalis* vaginitis: A newly defined specific infection previously classified "non-specific" vaginitis. *Am. J. Obstet. Gynecol.* 69:962, 1955.
    The classic description of this important disease.
148. Speigel, C.A. Bacterial vaginosis. *Clin. Microbiol. Rev.* 4:485–502, 1991.
    Excellent review emphasizing microbiological aspects.
149. Pheifer, T.A., et al. Nonspecific vaginitis: Role of *Haemophilus vaginalis* and treatment with metronidazole. *N. Engl. J. Med.* 298:1429, 1978.
    Classic study first calling attention to the role of anaerobic bacteria in the disease process and defining the value of metronidazole.
150. Chen, K.C.S., et al. Amine content of vaginal fluid from untreated and treated patients with nonspecific vaginitis. *J. Clin. Invest.* 63:828, 1979.
151. Amsel, R., et al. Nonspecific vaginitis: Diagnostic criteria and microbial and epidemiological associations. *Am. J. Med.* 74:14, 1983.
    The article that tells us to find three of four diagnostic criteria for clinical diagnosis.
152. Thomason, J.L., et al. Statistical evaluation of diagnostic criteria for bacterial vaginosis. *Am. J. Obstet. Gynecol.* 102:155–160, 1990.
    Update of reference [151].
152a. Morales, W.J., et al. Effect of metronidazole in patients with preterm birth in preceding pregnancy and bacterial vaginosis: A placebo-controlled, double-blind study. *Am. J. Obstet. Gynecol.* 171:345, 1994.
    Treatment of bacterial vaginosis with metronidazole was effective in reducing preterm births in patients with a history of prematurity in the preceding pregnancy. See related paper by H.M. McDonald et al., Bacterial vaginosis in pregnancy and efficacy of short-course oral metronidazole: A randomized controlled trial. Obstet. Gynecol. 84:343, 1994. Paper concludes that further studies are needed. See related editorial by M. Hack and I.R. Merkatz, Preterm delivery and low birth weight—A dire legacy. N. Engl. J. Med. 333:1772, 1995, and two related articles on bacterial vaginosis in the same issue.
153. Paradise, J.E., et al. Vulvovaginitis in premenarchal girls. Clinical features and diagnostic evaluation. *Pediatrics* 70:193, 1982.
153a. Medical Letter. Oral fluconazole for vaginal candidiasis. *Med. Lett. Drugs Ther.* 36:81, 1994.
    For related papers, see S.E. Reef et al., Treatment options for vulvovaginal candidiasis, 1993. Clin. Infect. Dis. 20(Suppl 1):S80, 1995, which provides background on the recommendations summarized in the text and in reference [9]. See also D.W. Denning, Working Group of the British Society for Medical Mycology, et al., Management of genital candidiasis. B.M.J. 310:1241, 1995, which discusses acute and recurrent candida vulvovaginitis.
154. Weisberg, M. Treatment of vaginal candidiasis in pregnant women. *Clin. Ther.* 8:563–567, 1986.
155. Nixon, S.A. Vulvovaginitis: The role of patient compliance in treatment success. *Am. J. Obstet. Gynecol.* 165:1207–1209, 1991.
156. Houang, E.T., et al. Fluconazole levels in plasma and vaginal secretions of patients after a 150-milligram single oral dose and rate of eradication of infection in vaginal candidiasis. *Antimicrob. Agents Chemother.* 34:909–910, 1990.

157. van Heusden, A.M., et al. Single-dose oral fluconazole versus single-dose topical miconazole for the treatment of acute vulvovaginal candidosis. *Acta Obstet. Gynecol. Scand.* 69:417–422, 1990.

157a. Sobel, J.D., et al. Single oral dose fluconazole compared with conventional clotrimazole topical therapy of *Candida* vaginitis. *Am. J. Obstet. Gynecol.* 172:1263, 1995.

158. Boag, F.C., et al. Comparison of vaginal flora after treatment with a clotrimazole 500 mg pessary or a fluconazole 150 mg capsule for vaginal candidosis. *Genitourin. Med.* 67:232–234, 1991.

159. Salem, H.T., et al. Oral versus local treatment of vaginal candidosis. *Int. J. Gynaecol. Obstet.* 30:57–62, 1989.

160. Osser, S., Haglund, A., and Westrom, L. Treatment of candidal vaginitis: A prospective randomized investigator-blind multicenter study comparing topically applied econazole with oral fluconazole. *Acta Obstet. Gynecol. Scand.* 70:73–78, 1991.

161. Brammer, K.W. (coordin.) et al. A comparison of single dose oral fluconazole with 3-day intravaginal clotrimazole in the treatment of vaginal candidiasis. Report of an international multicenter trial. *Br. J. Obstet. Gynecol.* 96:226–232, 1989.

162. Phillips, R.J., Watson, S.A., and McKay, F.F. An open multicentre study of the efficacy and safety of a single dose of fluconazole 150 mg in the treatment of vaginal candidiasis in a general practice. *Br. J. Clin. Pract.* 44:219–222, 1990.

163. Calderon-Marquez, J.J. Itraconazole in the treatment of vaginal candidosis and the effect of treatment of the sexual partner. *Rev. Infect. Dis.* 9(Suppl. 1):143–145, 1987.

164. Tobin, J.M., Loo, P., and Granger, S.E. Treatment of vaginal candidosis: A comparative study of the efficacy and acceptability of itraconazole and clotrimazole. *Genitourin. Med.* 68:36–38, 1992.

165. Stein, G.E., and Mummaw, N. Placebo-controlled trial of itraconazole for treatment of acute vaginal candidiasis. *Antimicrob. Agents Chemother.* 37(1):89–92, 1992.

166. Silva-Cruz, A., et al. Itraconazole versus placebo in the management of vaginal candidiasis. *Int. J. Gynecol. Obstet.* 36:229–232, 1991.

167. Roongpisuthipong, A., et al. Itraconazole in the treatment of acute vaginal candidosis. *J. Med. Assoc. Thailand* 75:30–34, 1992.

168. Wesel, S. Itraconazole: A single-day oral treatment for acute vulvovaginal candidosis. *Br. J. Clin. Pract. (Symp. Suppl.)* 71:S77–80, 1990.

168a. Ledger, W.L. Chronic vulvovaginitis. *Infect. Dis. Clin. Pract.* 2:60, 1993. *Includes a discussion of noninfectious problems causing vaginitis.*

169. Davidson, F., and Mould, R.F. Recurrent genital candidosis in women and the effect of intermittent prophylactic treatment. *Br. J. Vener. Dis.* 54:176, 1978.

170. Sobel, J.D. Management of recurrent vulvovaginal candidiasis with intermittent ketoconazole prophylaxis. *Obstet. Gynecol.* 65:435–440, 1985.

171. Sobel, J.D. Recurrent vulvovaginal candidiasis. A prospective study of the efficacy of maintenance ketoconazole therapy. *N. Engl. J. Med.* 315:1455–1458, 1986. *Works only for as long as one takes the drug.*

172. Roth, A.C., et al. Intermittent prophylactic treatment of recurrent vaginal candidiasis by postmenstrual application of a 500 mg clotrimazole tablet. *Genitourin. Med.* 66: 357–360, 1990.

173. Sobel, J.D., Schmitt, C., and Meriwether, C. Clotrimazole treatment of recurrent and chronic *Candida* vulvovaginitis. *Obstet. Gynecol.* 73:330–334, 1989.

174. van Heusden, A.M., and Merkus, J.M. Chronic recurrent vaginal candidiasis: Easy to treat, difficult to cure. Results of treatment with a new oral antifungant. *Eur. J. Obstet. Gynecol. Reprod. Biol.* 35:75–83, 1990.

174a. Joesoef, M.R., and Schmid, G.P. Bacterial vaginosis: Review of treatment options and potential clinical implications of therapy. *Clin. Infect. Dis.* 20(Suppl 1):S72, 1995. *Contains background information for recommendations in reference [9].*

175. Lugo-Miro, V.I., Green, M., and Mazur, L. Comparison of different metronidazole therapeutic regimens for bacterial vaginosis. *J.A.M.A.* 268:92, 1992.

176. Greaves, W.L., et al. Clindamycin versus metronidazole in the treatment of bacterial vaginosis. *Obstet. Gynecol.* 72:799, 1988.

177. Wathne, B., Hovelius, B., and Holst, E. Cefadroxil as an alternative to metronidazole in the treatment of bacterial vaginosis. *Scand. J. Infect. Dis.* 21:585, 1989.

Bibliography

Centers for Disease Control. 1993 Sexually transmitted disease treatment guidelines. *M.M.W.R.* 42(RR-14):1–102, 1993.

The definitive and essential compendium of up-to-date management of STD in the United States. For the background papers of these 1993 guidelines, see special symposium edited by W.C. Levine et al. Clin. Infect. Dis. *20(Suppl. 1):S1, 1995.*

Handsfield, H.H. (ed.). *Sexually Transmitted Diseases.* Philadelphia: Saunders, 1987.
Less encyclopedic than the preceding text, but what it covers, it does well.

Holmes, K.K., et al. (eds.). *Sexually Transmitted Diseases* (2nd ed.). New York: McGraw-Hill, 1990.
The newest and most complete textbook in the field; the next edition is anticipated in 1997.

Mandell, G.L., Bennett, J.E., and Dolin, R. (eds.). *Principles and Practice of Infectious Diseases* (4th ed.). New York: Churchill Livingstone, 1995.
Covers the entire field of infectious diseases; sections on the STDs are up-to-date but not as detailed as in Holmes et al.

Medical Letter. Drugs for sexually transmitted diseases. *Med. Lett. Drugs Ther.* 37:117, 1995.
This is the December 22, 1995 issue.

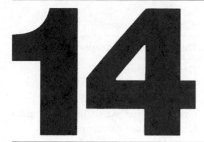

Gynecologic and Obstetric Infections

Harold C. Wiesenfeld
and Richard L. Sweet

Normal Microbial Flora of the Female Genital Tract

The normal cervical and vaginal microflora are complex and dynamic, changing over time according to a woman's age and hormonal status [1]. Up to 100 different species and species groups have been identified as components of the normal flora.

I. **Microbiologically sterile areas.** Certain anatomic areas are normally sterile, such as Bartholin's and Skene's glands, the uterine cavity, fallopian tubes, ovaries and other adnexal structures, and the pelvic peritoneum. Mechanisms that maintain the sterility of these areas include mechanical barriers, circulating and secretory immunoglobulins, and resident phagocytes.

II. **Normal flora versus pathogens.** The term **normal flora** refers to those organisms that can be demonstrated to colonize the female genital tract in the absence of disease. Such flora include bacteria, fungi, and occasionally viruses. **Those organisms present as normal flora at different stages of a woman's life are the same organisms that may cause obstetric and gynecologic infections in the appropriate setting.**

   A. **Determinants of the normal genital flora.** The following factors may determine, in part, which microorganisms colonize the female genital tract:
      1. **Adherence or penetration** capabilities of the organism
      2. Status of the **epithelial surfaces** of the cervix and vagina (which is hormonally determined and relates to the degree of cornification, amount of glycogen, pH, and mucous properties)
      3. Vaginal and cervical **secretory components,** such as IgG, IgA, and lysozymes
      4. **Established resident microflora** that may limit the growth of some bacterial species or provide substrates necessary for the proliferation of other species
      5. **Mechanical activities,** such as douching habits, the douche substance, and devices such as tampons and diaphragms that are inserted and left in place for variable lengths of time, all of which may influence the composition of the vaginal flora

   B. **Cervical and vaginal microbiology.** The average concentrate of bacteria is 10^8–10^9 colony-forming units (CFU) per gram or milliliter of secretions. A mixture of aerobes, facultative anaerobes, and strict anaerobes commonly is present.
      1. **Common isolates.** Table 14-1 lists, in descending order of frequency, the most commonly isolated organisms. Anaerobic species frequently outnumber the aerobic species. **Note that bacteria classically considered pathogenic may be a part of the normal flora.** Specifically, *Bacteroides fragilis* may be cultured from the normal vagina in approximately 10% of patients, enterococci in 25%, *Clostridium perfringens* in 10%, group B streptococci in 10–15%, *Gardnerella vaginalis* in 10–40%, and *Prevotella* (formerly *Bacteroides*) spp. in 25%.
      2. **Unusual isolates.** Noteworthy for their infrequent appearance are other facultative aerobes, found in fewer than 10% of patients. Among these are *Staphylococcus aureus* (5%), *Streptococcus pyogenes,* and *Haemophilus influenzae,* which are found rarely in the normal flora.
      3. *Mycoplasma. Mycoplasma hominis* and *Ureaplasma urealyticum* are frequently found in the cervices of sexually active women, and colonization rates increase with increasing number of sexual partners. Isolation of *Mycoplasma* spp. in the absence of illness does not warrant therapy.
      4. **Fungi.** Yeasts are the only fungi of importance regularly isolated from the normal genital tract. Of healthy women without vaginitis, 5–10% are found

Table 14-1. Microbial flora in normal menstruating women*

Microorganism	Gram stain appearance
Lactobacilli	Gram-positive rod
Staphylococcus epidermidis	Gram-positive coccus, clumps
Gardnerella vaginalis	Gram-negative pleomorphic rod
Diphtheroids	Gram-positive rod ("Chinese" characters)
Peptostreptococci	Gram-positive coccus, chains
Bacteroides spp.	Gram-negative rod (safety-pin appearance)
Aerobic streptococci (not group A)	Gram-positive coccus, chains
Escherichia coli	Gram-negative rod
Eubacterium spp.	Gram-positive pleomorphic rod
Veillonella spp.	Gram-negative coccus
Fusobacterium spp.	Gram-negative rod
Clostridium spp.	Gram-positive rod (bulbous ends)
Candida and *Torulopsis* spp.	Gram-positive yeast forms
Other aerobic gram-negative rods	Gram-negative rod
Staphylococcus aureus	Gram-positive coccus, clumps
Streptococcus agalactiae (group B streptococcus)	Gram-positive coccus, chains

*In decreasing order of frequency.

    to have yeast in the vagina. *Candida albicans* is the most common species, although *C. glabrata* and other *Candida* spp. occasionally are found.
    5. Viruses. Cytomegalovirus (CMV) has been recovered repeatedly from the healthy lower genital tract. Studies using cervical cultures or serologic testing show an association between CMV infection and sexual activity [2].
C. Dynamics of the microflora. The vaginal microflora varies not only from woman to woman but also in any given woman over the course of time [1]. Changes occur in the flora with changes in age, sexual activity, phase of menstrual cycle, gestational status, and drug therapy (Table 14-2).

Acute Salpingitis (Pelvic Inflammatory Disease)

The terms **acute salpingitis, acute adnexitis,** and **acute pelvic inflammatory disease** (PID) have been used synonymously in the gynecologic literature. This infection often is seen by the primary care physician in previously healthy women and in the ambulatory clinic or emergency department setting.
  I. Incidence. Acute salpingitis is not a reportable disease, and therefore the exact incidence in the United States is not known. However, it is **estimated** that **approximately 1 million cases** of acute PID are **diagnosed annually in the United States,** with an estimated treatment cost of more than $4 billion [3].
  II. Risk factors [4]
    A. Age. Teenage girls (15–19 years) have the highest rates of PID, even when adjusted for frequency of sexual activity.
    B. Multiple sexual partners. Multiple sexual partners (arbitrarily defined as more than two partners in a 30-day period) increases fourfold the risk of PID.
    C. Method of contraception. Although an association between the use of an intrauterine contraceptive device (IUD) and increased risk of PID has been documented for years, recent studies suggest that this association has been overestimated. Contamination of the endometrial cavity at insertion apparently results in a slightly increased risk of PID for the first 4 months of IUD use. Infections after this time are probably acquired by sexually transmitted pathogens rather than pathogens from the IUD itself [4a].

Table 14-2. Dynamic alterations in female microflora

Variable	Expected quantitative changes
Prepuberty	Coliforms predominate, lactobacilli infrequent
Menstrual cycle	↑ Anaerobes, coliforms, and group B streptococci in first half of cycle; ↑ lactobacilli and gram-positive aerobes in latter half of cycle
Pregnancy	↑ Lactobacilli, *Candida* spp.; ↓ anaerobes
After menopause	↑ Aerobic gram-negative rods, especially *Escherichia coli*
Contraception	↑ *E. coli* in diaphragm users; ↑ anaerobes and group B streptococci in intrauterine device users; ↑ lactobacilli and *Candida* spp. in oral contraceptive pill users
Antibiotic therapy	↑ Coliforms and yeast; ↓ lactobacilli
Gynecologic surgery	↑ Coliforms and *Bacteroides* spp.; ↓ lactobacilli

Oral contraceptive users appear to be at decreased risk of salpingitis. Use of barrier methods of contraception most likely affords the greatest degree of protection against the development of acute PID and the acquisition of sexually transmitted diseases (STDs).

D. Prior PID. Women who have had PID are twice as likely to present with acute PID than women who have never had the infection.

III. Pathophysiology. Of women with untreated gonococcal or chlamydial cervicitis, 10–40% will develop salpingitis [4a]. The documentation of histologic evidence of endometritis in more than one-third of women with chlamydial cervicitis is further evidence of the propensity for ascending infection with these pathogens. A relationship between bacterial vaginosis and the occurrence of PID has been noted [5, 5a].

The cause of the ascending, intraluminal spread of sexually acquired or endogenous lower genital tract pathogens into the normally sterile upper tract (endometrium, fallopian tubes, and peritoneal cavity) is not fully understood. Because most cases of gonorrheal and chlamydial salpingitis occur within 1 week of the onset of menses [6], it is postulated that the loss of cervical mucus at this time represents the loss of an important mechanical and bacteriostatic barrier to bacterial penetration. Other factors, such as differences in microbial adherence properties, variation in bacterial virulence according to strain, and degree of host response, appear also to play a role in determining the extent of infection. A popular but unproved hypothesis is that infection by gonorrhea or chlamydiae facilitates secondary invasion of the upper genital tract by the endogenous vaginal flora. However, it has been demonstrated in laparoscopic studies that nongonococcal, nonchlamydial organisms can be recovered from the upper genital tract of women with acute PID even in the absence of gonococcal or chlamydial cervical infection.

IV. Microbiologic features. Acute salpingitis is most often a **polymicrobial** infection. The usual practice of culturing from the cervix has made it difficult to assess accurately the causative role of organisms in tubal inflammation. However, the use of laparoscopy or culdocentesis has helped to clarify the bacteriologic nature of the infection [6a]. In the United States, the major causative organisms of PID include *N. gonorrhoeae* (25–50%), *C. trachomatis* (10–40%), and mixed aerobic-anaerobic bacteria (25–60%). The microorganisms associated with bacterial vaginosis include anaerobes such as *Prevotella bivia,* other *Prevotella* spp., and *Peptostreptococcus* spp. [5a]. The role of *M. hominis* and *U. urealyticum* in the pathogenesis of PID remains unclear. Microorganisms that can be part of the vaginal flora, such as anaerobes, *G. vaginalis, H. influenzae,* gram-negative bacilli, and *Streptococcus agalactiae,* also can cause PID [7].

V. Clinical characteristics. The diagnosis of acute PID on clinical grounds alone is notoriously inaccurate in that fewer than two-thirds of suspected cases are confirmed at laparoscopy [8]. A history of fever or chills was the only symptom that occurred significantly more frequently in women with PID than in women without PID in a controlled laparoscopic study by Jacobson and Westrom [8]. However, as **fever** occurred in only 40% of women with PID, it cannot be relied on when making a clinical diagnosis. Of the signs, **adnexal tenderness** on bimanual examination, **abnormal vaginal discharge,** temperature in excess of 38°C, and an **erythrocyte sedimentation rate (ESR) of 15 mm/hr or more were found significantly more frequently in women with laparoscopically confirmed PID** than in those without PID [8]. However, no one sign or symptom is pathognomonic; the classic triad of pelvic pain, increased vaginal discharge, and fever is found in only 20% of women with visually confirmed salpingitis [8]. Other symptoms include nausea, vomiting, dyspareunia, dysuria, and abnormal vaginal bleeding.

    Asymptomatic disease (or at least unrecognized disease) **may be common.** Reviews have shown that up to two-thirds of patients with evidence of tubal damage due to PID on laparoscopy or hysterosalpingography could not recall a history of PID. Similarly, only about 18% of women with ectopic pregnancies and detectable antichlamydial antibody or inflammatory tubal damage report a history of PID [4a].

VI. Sequelae of acute salpingitis. One-fourth of all women who have had acute salpingitis will experience one or more long-term sequelae: These include infertility, ectopic pregnancy, chronic pelvic pain, and recurrent episodes of salpingitis.

  A. Involuntary infertility occurs in up to 20% of women after an episode of PID [9, 10]. Risk of infertility is correlated with the severity of tubal inflammation during the acute episode, as determined by laparoscopy, and with the number of recurrent episodes of PID. In addition, the rate of infertility is approximately 3 times greater after nongonococcal salpingitis than after gonococcal salpingitis. An association between the presence of serum antibody to chlamydiae and infertility has been noted, and it is believed that latent chlamydial infection may cause progressive tubal damage over time. In one study, 30% of tubal cultures were positive for *C. trachomatis* in 160 women undergoing laparoscopy for evaluation of fallopian tube–related infertility; only 40% of women who tested positively had a history of PID [11]. Repeated episodes of PID increase the risk of infertility; for example, incidence rates of 13% after one episode, 25–35% after two episodes, and up to 50–75% after three or more episodes have been reported [4a].

  B. Ectopic (tubal) pregnancy. Risk of ectopic pregnancy increases by 6–10 times after an episode of acute PID and continues to rise proportionally with each subsequent episode of PID. Approximately 50% of women undergoing laparoscopy for ectopic pregnancy have evidence of prior PID.

  C. Recurrent PID. One in five women with PID will ultimately have recurrent salpingitis; more than half of these recurrences will take place within the first year of the initial episode.

  D. Chronic pelvic pain. Approximately 18% of women will develop complaints of chronic pelvic pain after an episode of acute PID [12]. Typically, this is attributable to tubal occlusion and intraabdominal adhesions.

  E. Tuboovarian abscess is the most common early complication, occurring in 5–10% of patients hospitalized for PID.

VII. Diagnosis. Because of the wide variation in many symptoms and signs among women with PID, a **clinical diagnosis of acute PID is difficult to make.** Although laparoscopic visualization of the pelvis is the gold-standard diagnostic test, it is usually impractical, will not detect endometritis, and may not detect subtle inflammation of the fallopian tubes [7]. A delay in diagnosis and effective treatment probably contributes to inflammatory sequelae in the upper reproductive tract [7]. **No single historical, physical, or laboratory finding is both sensitive and specific for the diagnosis of acute PID. Experts recommend that providers maintain a low threshold of suspicion for the diagnosis of PID [7].**

  A. The Infectious Diseases Society for Obstetrics and Gynecology has recommended the criteria listed below for the clinical diagnosis of acute salpingitis [13]. However, it should be noted that determination of the sensitivity and specificity of these suggested criteria awaits comparison with laparoscopic diagnosis of PID in clinical studies. **A diagnosis of PID is probable in the presence of** [13]:

    1. All three of the following:
      a. Direct lower abdominal tenderness
      b. Cervical motion tenderness
      c. Adnexal tenderness
    2. Plus one or more of the following:
      a. Temperature greater than or equal to 38°C
      b. WBCs in excess of 10,000/mm^3
      c. Purulent material from culdocentesis

       d. Pelvic abscess or inflammatory complex on bimanual examination or sonography

       e. Evidence of gonococcal or chlamydial cervicitis:

          (1) Gram stain of endocervix positive for gram-negative intracellular diplococci

          (2) Chlamydial infection by antigen detection testing

          (3) Purulent endocervical discharge with 10 WBCs or more per high-power field on a Gram-stained smear

  B. In the Center for Disease Control's (CDC's) *Sexually Transmitted Disease Treatment Guidelines* [7], the following guidelines for diagnosing PID are offered.

    1. Minimal criteria (see sec. **A.1**). **Empiric therapy of PID should be instituted** if all three of the minimal criteria for pelvic inflammation (i.e., lower abdominal tenderness, adnexal tenderness, and cervical motion tenderness) are present and if an established cause other than PID is absent.

    2. Additional criteria. For women with severe clinical signs, more elaborate diagnostic evaluation is warranted because incorrect diagnosis and management may cause unnecessary morbidity. These additional criteria may be used to increase the specificity of the diagnosis [7].

       a. Routine criteria for diagnosing PID:

          (1) Oral temperature greater than 38.3°C

          (2) Abnormal cervical or vaginal discharge

          (3) Elevated ESR

          (4) Elevated C-reactive protein

          (5) Laboratory documentation of cervical infection with *N. gonorrhoeae* or *C. trachomatis*

       b. Elaborate criteria for diagnosing PID:

          (1) Histopathologic evidence of endometritis on endometrial biopsy

          (2) Tuboovarian abscess (TOA) on sonography or other radiologic tests

          (3) Laparoscopic abnormalities consistent with PID

VIII. Differential diagnosis. Laparoscopic studies have demonstrated that the major differential diagnostic considerations include ectopic pregnancy, acute appendicitis, ovarian cyst (ruptured or hemorrhagic), endometriosis, and torsion of adnexal structures.

IX. Clinical approach

  A. Initial evaluation

    1. Historic points, such as risk factors, sexual contacts, menstrual status, and birth control method, are important to elicit.

    2. Abdominal and pelvic examinations provide evidence for involvement of the pelvic structures.

    3. Assessment of systemic signs includes obtaining temperature, peripheral WBC count, and ESR. A pregnancy test should be performed as an aid to exclude the possibility of ectopic pregnancy. Cervical specimens for culture for gonorrhea and testing for *C. trachomatis* should be performed. **Serologic workup to rule out syphilis and the human immunodeficiency virus (HIV) should be done routinely in all patients.**

  B. Further evaluation

    1. Once pelvic inflammation is confirmed, assessment of the severity of illness is important in determining the **necessity for hospitalization.** Clinical grading systems for acute salpingitis are found in other sources [13].

    2. Indications for hospitalization include the following [7]:

       a. Unclear diagnosis, particularly when surgical emergencies such as ectopic pregnancy or appendicitis cannot be excluded

       b. Adolescent patient (among adolescents, compliance with therapy is unpredictable)

       c. Pregnant patient

       d. Signs of peritonitis on examination

       e. Presence of an adnexal mass on examination or ultrasonography; suspicion of pelvic abscess

       f. Failure to respond to outpatient therapy in 48–72 hours

       g. Inability to tolerate oral medication (e.g., nausea and vomiting) or probability that patient will not comply with an oral regimen

       h. Presence of an IUD

       i. Patient with HIV infection

      j. Inability to arrange clinical follow-up within 72 hours of starting antibiotic treatment

   3. In addition, some authorities have recommended that *all patients* with acute PID **be hospitalized** for the initiation of supervised parenteral antimicrobial therapy [7].

   4. Outpatients should return 48–72 hours after the initiation of therapy for reassessment. Lack of improvement should prompt hospitalization for further diagnostic evaluation and initiation of intravenous antibiotics.

   5. An IUD, if present, **should be removed.**

   6. Contact tracing of all male sexual partners for empiric antibiotic therapy aimed at *C. trachomatis* and *N. gonorrhoeae* is imperative [7]. Empiric therapy is suggested because cultures and nonculture tests for *C. trachomatis* and *N. gonorrhoeae* are insensitive among male sex partners, especially those who are asymptomatic [7].

   7. Test-for-cure cervical cultures for *N. gonorrhoeae* and *C. trachomatis* should be performed 7–10 days after therapy is completed in every patient. Some experts also recommend rescreening for *C. trachomatis* and *N. gonorrhoeae* 4–6 weeks after the patients complete therapy [7].

   8. Preliminary data suggest that HIV-infected women with PID are more likely to require surgical intervention [14].

X. Antibiotic therapy. Early initiation of antibiotic therapy is important for optimal efficacy. In addition, the polymicrobial etiology of the disease should be considered when selecting antimicrobial therapy. Recent recommendations for therapy have reflected both the common simultaneous occurrence of gonorrhea and chlamydial infection and the increasing prevalence of penicillinase-producing *N. gonorrhoeae* [7]. In addition, as bacteria involved with bacterial vaginosis are likely pathogens in PID, antibiotic regimens should be active against anaerobic bacteria.

  A. Outpatient therapy. Clinical trials of outpatient regimens have provided little information regarding intermediate and long-term outcomes. The following regimens provide coverage against common etiologic agents of PID, but evidence from clinical trials supporting their use is limited. The second regimen (see sec. **2**) provides broader coverage against anaerobic organisms but costs substantially more than the regimen described in sec. **1** [7].

   1. Cefoxitin, 2 g IM, plus **probenecid,** 1 g PO, in a single dose concurrently, or **ceftriaxone,** 250 mg IM, or other parenteral third-generation **cephalosporin** (e.g., **ceftizoxime** or **cefotaxime**),

plus

   doxycycline, 100 mg PO bid for 14 days.

   2. Ofloxacin, 400 mg PO bid for 14 days,

plus

   either **clindamycin,** 450 mg PO qid, or **metronidazole,** 500 mg PO bid for 14 days.

   3. Patients who do not respond to outpatient therapy within 72 hours should be hospitalized to confirm the diagnosis and to receive parenteral therapy [7].

  B. Inpatient therapy

   1. One of two parenteral regimens should be used, as recommended by the CDC [7]: cefoxitin, 2 g IV q6h, or cefotetan, 2 g IV q12h, plus doxycycline, 100 mg IV or PO q12h; or clindamycin, 900 mg* IV q8h, plus gentamicin, loading dose of 2 mg/kg IV or IM followed by 1.5 mg/kg IV q8h (dose should be adjusted according to serial creatinine levels and serum gentamicin levels; see Chap. 28). These two regimens have been demonstrated to be of equal efficacy and have clinical cure rates in excess of 90% [3].

     The bioavailability of doxycycline administered orally is similar to that of the intravenous formulation, and so the agent may be administered orally (for more cost-effective therapy) if normal GI function is present [7].

   2. Intravenous drugs should be continued for at least 48 hours after the patient shows objective signs of improvement. Doxycycline (100 mg PO bid) in the first regimen and clindamycin (450 mg PO qid) in the second regimen should be continued on an outpatient basis to complete 14 total days of therapy.

---

*Note: In PID and gynecologic infections discussed later in this chapter, intravenous clindamycin typically is given as 900 mg q8h. In other infections (e.g., anaerobic soft-tissue wounds, intraabdominal infections), intravenous clindamycin usually is given as 600 mg q8h. (See discussion in Chap. 28I.)

3. All patients with TOAs should receive intravenous antibiotic therapy. Both inpatient regimens for PID appear to be equally effective in the treatment of TOAs. Patients with a TOA require careful monitoring; approximately 70% respond to medical therapy alone [15]. However, surgical intervention is required in 30% of cases and should be undertaken if there is no response to therapy within 48–72 hours or if there is clear-cut worsening at any point during therapy.

4. **PID in a pregnant patient may occur but is rare.** In such patients, use of intravenous clindamycin plus gentamicin is preferred for therapy. Doxycycline is contraindicated in pregnant or lactating women.

Pelvic Abscesses

Pelvic abscesses remain among the most serious complications of obstetric and gynecologic infections. They generally are categorized on the basis of etiologic origin [16]. The major types of pelvic abscesses include those that are an infectious complication of pelvic surgery; are secondary to infection in nongynecologic organs (i.e., appendiceal or diverticular abscess); occur secondary to ascending, intracanalicular spread of microorganisms from the cervix via the endometrial cavity to the adnexa (i.e., TOA); or arise after puerperal infections via lymphatic or hematogenous spread from the endometrium or myometrium to the parametrium, broad ligament, or adnexa.

I. **Postoperative abscess.** Although their frequency has been reduced by the use of prophylactic antibiotics, postoperative pelvic infections remain a significant problem. **Frequency is greatest after hysterectomy, particularly** that performed by the **vaginal** route. Postoperative abscesses can be divided into two major categories [16].
   A. The **vaginal apex cuff abscess** or infected hematoma usually presents between the fifth and seventh postoperative day. Patients generally have fever and a sensation of fullness or vague discomfort in the area of the rectovaginal septum. Painful defecation often is an accompanying symptom. Examination typically discloses an infected, foul-smelling hematoma; radiographs may demonstrate an adynamic ileus. **Antibiotic therapy alone is usually insufficient.** Antimicrobial therapy with anaerobic coverage, such as the regimens suggested for treatment of TOA (see sec. **II.D.1**) should be instituted pending surgical intervention. **Surgical drainage is mandatory** and can usually be accomplished easily via the vagina, with prompt response.
   B. **Pelvic or adnexal abscesses** usually occur after discharge from the initial hospitalization and most commonly follow vaginal hysterectomy. Overall incidence approximates 4%, and occurrence is an average of 18–20 days postoperatively [16]. Presenting characteristics are abdominal pain, fever, and a tender palpable pelvic mass. Antibiotic coverage should include an agent effective against the gram-negative anaerobes (including *B. fragilis*), such as clindamycin or metronidazole. Early surgical intervention may be indicated because rupture of an adnexal abscess carries a high mortality.

II. **Tuboovarian abscess.** TOA is a major complication of salpingitis and has been reported to occur in up to one-third of patients hospitalized for salpingitis [15].
   A. **Clinical characteristics**
      1. **Symptoms.** In a review of 232 patients with TOA, presenting symptoms were found to be nonspecific. Abdominal or pelvic pain was present in 89% of patients, a history of fever or chills in 50%, vaginal discharge in 28%, nausea in 26%, and abnormal vaginal bleeding in 21% [17].
      2. **Signs.** Although fever and leukocytosis are present in the majority of patients with TOA, their absence does not eliminate the possibility of the diagnosis of TOA. Fever may be absent in up to 40% of patients and leukocytosis may be absent in 32% [17].
   B. **Microbiology.** In general, the inciting organisms are the same as those outlined for acute salpingitis. In addition to the sexually transmitted pathogens *N. gonorrhoeae* and *C. trachomatis,* TOAs commonly are composed of mixed anaerobic and facultative or aerobic organisms. Anaerobes appear to play a particularly important role in the development of the abscess and, in one study, were recovered from 85% of positive cultures of material obtained by needle aspiration of TOA [17]. *Actinomyces israelii,* a gram-positive anaerobe, has also been reported in association with TOAs, particularly in women using IUDs [15].

C. **Diagnosis.** Clinical **evaluation** should **proceed as outlined under Acute Salpingitis, sec. VII–IX.** The **differentiation of patients with uncomplicated salpingitis from those with TOA requires the demonstration of an inflammatory mass.** If physical examination is inconclusive, a variety of noninvasive techniques are available, including sonography and CT scanning. Gynecologic consultation should be obtained early in the course of illness.

D. **Treatment.** Although there is general acceptance that rupture of a TOA is an indication for immediate surgical intervention, there is **controversy about the necessity of surgery in the management of unruptured TOA.** Preservation of fertility and ovarian function is of prime concern in therapy. Pregnancy rates following TOAs are reported to be less than 15%.

Improved response rates with the addition of anaerobic antibiotic coverage in recent years has led **most gynecologists to select closely supervised medical therapy as initial management** in patients with unruptured TOA. However, surgical intervention will be required in approximately 30% of patients and is particularly likely to be necessary in patients with adnexal masses larger than 8 cm or with bilateral adnexal involvement [18].

1. **Medical therapy.** Antimicrobial therapy must cover the major pathogens of salpingitis (i.e., *N. gonorrhoeae* and *C. trachomatis*) and the anaerobic and aerobic gram-negative organisms that are likely to be present. The combination of clindamycin (900 mg IV q8h) and gentamicin (1.5 mg/kg q8h in patients with normal renal function) has commonly been used in the past. Cefoxitin (2 g IV q6h) plus doxycycline (100 mg IV or PO q12h) is an alternative regimen that appears to be as effective [18] and appealing because it allows one to avoid an aminoglycoside. Presumably, ampicillin-sulbactam, piperacillin-tazobactam, or cefotetan could be used (as alternatives to cefoxitin) along with doxycycline. Intravenous therapy should be continued for at least 7 days; if improvement is substantial, then therapy may be completed on an outpatient basis. For completion of oral therapy, the regimens used for outpatient treatment of PID would be reasonable. A total course of therapy of 14 days is desirable, with close clinical monitoring throughout. Response rates to these regimens exceed 70% [15, 18].

2. **Surgical management.** Surgical intervention **is mandatory in patients with ruptured TOAs or in those who fail to respond to medical management,** suggested by failure to defervesce in 72 hours or an increase in the size of the mass [4a]. Options include unilateral or bilateral adnexectomy, with or without total abdominal hysterectomy. Laparoscopic and transabdominal, guided, percutaneous radiologic drainage techniques have been reported; however, randomized controlled trials are needed to determine their roles in the management of TOAs. Recently, endovaginal ultrasonographically guided transvaginal drainage has been reported and used to treat patients who failed intravenous antibiotics and whose abscesses were not amenable to percutaneous or colpotomy drainage [18a].

E. **Sequelae.** Infertility, ectopic pregnancy, and chronic pelvic pain can be late complications of tubal abscess [15].

Intraamniotic Infections

Intraamniotic infections (IAI) occur in 1–2% of all term pregnancies and in up to 20–25% of women with preterm labor [4a] and are a major cause of perinatal morbidity and mortality. **Chorioamnionitis** refers to the microscopic detection of inflammation of the umbilical cord, amniotic membranes, or placenta.

I. **Pathophysiology.** IAI is most often encountered following prolonged rupture of membranes or labor. Once the relatively efficient barrier of the cervix is disrupted, bacteria from the vagina gain entrance to the uterine cavity and establish infection. Most cases of IAI are due to this **ascending process.** Up to 30% of patients in preterm labor with intact membranes have positive amniotic fluid cultures [19, 20]. Hematogenous transmission occasionally is observed (e.g., *Listeria monocytogenes*). There is a small risk of IAI following obstetric procedures such as amniocentesis, cordocentesis, and cervical cerclage. Lengthy duration of membrane rupture and multiple vaginal examinations in labor are additional risk factors.

II. **Microbiology.** Most IAI are **polymicrobial.** The most frequently isolated organisms include anaerobes (*Prevotella* and *Peptostreptococcus* spp.), group B and viridans streptococci, *Escherichia coli, G. vaginalis,* and the genital mycoplasmas [21]. An association between bacterial vaginosis and infection of the chorioamnion has been reported [21a].

III. **Clinical characteristics.** Signs of IAI are varied, including maternal fever, maternal or fetal tachycardia, uterine tenderness, malodorous amniotic fluid, and leukocytosis. Patients may present with preterm labor or preterm rupture of fetal membranes. **A high index of suspicion** must be maintained for any patient with a fever in the third trimester. Gram stain and culture of amniotic fluid may be diagnostic. Amniotic fluid assays for the presence of leukocyte esterase or low glucose levels are less commonly used indirect markers.

IV. **Management.** The treatment of IAI is a **combination of antibiotics and delivery of the fetus.**
   A. Cesarean sections are performed for standard obstetric indications, not solely for the diagnosis of IAI.
   B. **Antibiotics** should be **administered at the time of diagnosis** (intrapartum) rather than after delivery [21].
      1. Most authorities [4a, 21] recommend **ampicillin** (2 g IV q4–6h) plus an **aminoglycoside** (see Chap. 28H for aminoglycoside dosing). Both ampicillin and gentamicin cross the placenta and obtain good levels in the fetal compartment.
      2. In patients with chorioamnionitis undergoing cesarean section, **clindamycin** should be added after cord clamping, providing additional anaerobic coverage.
      3. Other regimens may be successful, such as the extended-spectrum penicillins and cephalosporins and the penicillin–beta-lactamase inhibitor combinations [21].

V. **Complications.** Maternal complications of IAI include dysfunctional labor, increased cesarean section rate, postpartum endomyometritis, and bacteremia. Low-birth-weight infants are at risk of various infections, respiratory distress syndrome, and perinatal death.

Puerperal Endometritis

Puerperal endometritis is known also as **endomyometritis** and **endoparametritis.**

I. **Incidence.** At present, the rate of endomyometritis is estimated to be 5%, but this depends on the setting (see sec. **II.A**). Although the absolute risk of death from infection is small among postpartum women, sepsis remains a common cause of maternal death in the United States.

II. **Risk factors**
   A. **Method of delivery. Cesarean section,** particularly following labor or rupture of the membranes of any duration [4a], **is the major predisposing factor** for puerperal pelvic infection, increasing both the frequency and severity of such infections. Endometritis rates rarely exceed 3% after a vaginal delivery, whereas the rates after cesarean section have been 10–85% [21]. Possible explanations for this include increased intrauterine manipulation, foreign-body (suture) reactions, tissue necrosis at the suture line, hematoma-seroma formation, and wound infections [21]. Following cesarean section, endometritis ranges from 10% or less in most private services to 50% or more in large teaching services caring for indigent patients [4a].
   B. **Prolonged labor.** Duration of labor is the most significant variable related to postpartum morbidity after cesarean section.
   C. **Prolonged rupture of membranes.** The degree of bacterial colonization increases with time after rupture of membranes, and several studies have correlated positive amniotic fluid cultures after rupture of membranes with subsequent intrauterine infection [4a, 21].
   D. **Other.** The number of vaginal examinations and use of the internal fetal monitor have been proposed as risk factors for postpartum endometritis. Other purported risk factors for puerperal infection have included anemia, maternal colonization with group B streptococci, and low socioeconomic status. Bacterial vaginosis has been associated with endometritis after cesarean section [5, 21a, 22].

III. **Microbiologic features**
   A. **Common isolates.** Endometritis is most often a **mixed** infection of **aerobic and anaerobic** bacteria from the genital tract. Aerobic organisms are found in 50–70% of upper genital tract cultures, the most common being *G. vaginalis, E. coli,* and the streptococci. Group B and group D streptococci may each be found in 10–15%

of infections. Anaerobic organisms are isolated from 46–80% of properly collected and processed cultures; the most common are *Bacteroides* spp., *Prevotella* spp., and peptostreptococci.

    B. Other isolates. Although *C. trachomatis* infection in pregnancy has been linked to preterm delivery and premature rupture of membranes, the causative role of chlamydia has not been well documented and requires further study. Chlamydia may play a role in these mixed infections, especially with a so-called late form of endometritis that occurs 2 days to 6 weeks postpartum among women who delivery vaginally [4a]. Although *M. hominis* has been isolated from the bloodstream in cases of puerperal sepsis, clinical improvement has occurred in response to antibiotics not active against *Mycoplasma,* so that the role of this organism in postpartum infection also needs further elucidation. The significance of the microbiologic presence of clostridia is analogous to that discussed later under Infected Abortions, and the reader is referred to that discussion.

IV. Diagnosis. Low-grade fever or isolated temperature elevations occur commonly in the puerperium and often resolve spontaneously, especially after vaginal delivery.

    A. The diagnosis of endomyometritis is based on the clinical findings of fever, uterine tenderness, purulent or foul lochia, peripheral leukocytosis, and exclusion of another infected site.

        1. Nonspecific symptoms and signs such as malaise, abdominal pain, chills, leukocytosis, and tachycardia may be present.

        2. However, many febrile patients with group A or B streptococcal bacteremia have no localizing signs.

        3. Fever usually occurs in the first or second postpartum day and has been defined as an oral temperature of at least 38.5°C in the first 24 hours after delivery or of 38°C or higher for at least 4 consecutive hours 24 hours or more after delivery [4a].

    B. A bimanual pelvic examination is suggested to determine uterine size, consistency, and tenderness [4a]. **An endometrial culture** may be performed, although the exact role of transvaginally obtained endometrial cultures, and the best way to obtain them, remain controversial [4a]. However, the identification of a specific pathogen such as *N. gonorrhoeae, C. trachomatis,* or group A or B streptococcus will help to guide antibiotic therapy.

    C. Gram staining of the uterine smear may be helpful in guiding empiric therapy.

    D. Blood cultures. Of patients with puerperal uterine infection, 10–20% have bacteremia; therefore, **blood cultures should be obtained in all patients.** Isolation of a particular species, especially if it is an organism not covered by routine therapy (e.g., *S. aureus,* enterococcus) will aid in the selection of antimicrobial therapy.

V. Differential diagnosis. The major diagnostic considerations of fever in a postpartum woman include pyelonephritis, atelectasis, pneumonia, intravenous catheter–associated infections, surgical wound complications, complications of anesthesia, and mastitis.

VI. Treatment

    A. Epidemiologic measures. Isolation of group A streptococci is an indication for isolation of the mother. The nursery and infection control coordinator should be notified in cases of isolation of group A streptococci so that a search for the source of this predominantly nosocomial pathogen may be initiated. If group B streptococci are isolated, this is not necessary.

    B. Antibiotic therapy. Most uterine infections are polymicrobial, involving mixed aerobic and anaerobic organisms. Antibiotic coverage should therefore be broad, even in the case of isolation of a single species from the bloodstream.

        1. Clindamycin (900 mg IV q8h) in combination **with gentamicin** (1.5 mg/kg IV q8h) in patients with normal renal function results in a 90–95% cure rate and may be preferred by some experts in severe infection and/or infection after cesarean section [4a]. Most patients with endometritis and enterococci on uterine culture will respond to this regimen, although it is not active against enterococci.

        2. Alternatively, a broad-spectrum single agent with activity against aerobic and anaerobic bacteria (especially beta-lactamase-producing *Bacteroides* spp.) can be used, particularly in the patient with mild to moderate illness. Examples of such agents include (1) cefoxitin, 2 g IV q6h; (2) cefotetan, 2 g IV q12h; (3) ampicillin and sulbactam (2 g/1 g IV q6h); and (4) ticarcillin and clavulanic acid (3.1 g IV q4–6h). These agents have comparable cure rates to clindamycin plus gentamicin. The role of the new agent piperacillin-tazobactam in this setting awaits further clinical experience, but this should also be a useful agent in this setting (see Chap. 28E).

3. If group A streptococcal endometritis is suspected or confirmed, penicillin G (18–20 million units/day IV in divided doses) has been an agent of choice. However, in recent years, for severe and/or invasive group A streptococcal infections, many experts use clindamycin 600–900 mg IV q8h. (See related discussions in Chaps. 4 and 28I.) Alternatives in the patient with a delayed penicillin allergy include cefazolin (1–2 g IV q8h) or, in the patient with a history of immediate or anaphylactic allergy to penicillin, erythromycin (500–1,000 mg IV q6h) or vancomycin. Also, clindamycin, as above, can be used in patients with delayed or immediate reactions to penicillin, and clindamycin may be the preferred alternative (see Chaps. 4 and 28I).

4. **Antibiotics should be continued until patients are afebrile for 48 hours. If intravenous therapy is successful, further treatment with oral agents is unnecessary** [23].

C. **Obstetric and gynecologic consultation** is critical to the proper evaluation of patients with puerperal endometritis. Possible complications include uterine myonecrosis necessitating hysterectomy, adnexal abscess formation, and septic pelvic thrombophlebitis (SPT).

D. **Causes of antibiotic failure.** For the patient with persistent fever (48–72 hours) on appropriate antimicrobial therapy, a thorough examination, particularly of the wound, catheter sites, and pelvis, is essential. Antimicrobial susceptibilities of cultured organisms should be reviewed, as should dosages of antibiotics and, where suitable, serum concentration levels of antibiotics. Pelvic sonography or CT scanning should be performed in search of pelvic abscess, pelvic hematoma, or SPT. Pelvic abscesses or hematomas should be drained. Surgical intervention is indicated in patients with pelvic abscess, myonecrosis, or septic pelvic thrombophlebitis that has failed to respond to heparin plus antibiotics (see under Septic Pelvic Thrombophlebitis). If a wound infection is discovered, treatment consists of incision and drainage, with debridement as indicated. Drug fever should be excluded (see Chap. 1).

Septic Pelvic Thrombophlebitis

Septic pelvic thrombophlebitis is an uncommon but serious complication of puerperal, postabortion, and postoperative pelvic infections.

I. **Incidence.** Incidence estimates of SPT in association with delivery or pregnancy termination have been 0.05–0.20%. The frequency is higher in women with operative site infection (e.g., 1–2% in postcesarean endomyometritis) [24]. Recognition of the importance of including in the initial therapy for obstetric and gynecologic infections an agent effective against beta-lactamase-producing *Bacteroides* organisms has dramatically decreased the incidence of SPT [25, 26].

II. **Etiology.** Several of the physiologic alterations associated with pregnancy may be responsible for the fact that SPT is primarily an obstetric complication. These include stasis of venous blood flow in the pelvis, a relative hypercoagulability (due to increased clotting factors and tissue thromboplastin), and estrogen-induced changes in the pelvic veins that predispose them to injury. The significance of infection and trauma as antecedent factors in the bacterial invasion and suppuration of pelvic venous thrombi is apparent as well, in that cesarean section and septic abortion patients have a tenfold higher incidence of SPT than do patients delivered vaginally [25].

III. **Microbiologic features.** The pathogenic microorganisms are similar to those generally associated with female genital tract infections. Specifically, the bacteria associated with SPT are the **mixed aerobic and anaerobic organisms** that compose the normal flora of the vagina and cervix, particularly *Bacteroides* spp. (especially *B. fragilis*), anaerobic cocci (especially *Peptostreptococcus*), gram-negative facultative aerobes (e.g., *E. coli*), and gram-positive aerobes such as streptococci and staphylococci. *B. fragilis* infection particularly is associated with clot formation and SPT, perhaps because it is capable of heparinase production [25].

IV. **Clinical characteristics.** Cases may be divided into two distinct syndromes.

A. **Puerperal ovarian vein thrombosis** (POVT) is characterized by early onset (usually within 2–3 days of delivery), lower abdominal pain, a normal or elevated temperature, and **findings consistent with an acute abdomen.** Many patients will have previously been diagnosed with postcesarean endometritis, but infection may be absent. Patients appear ill [4a]. In approximately 50% of cases, there is a palpable abdominal mass; flank pain and costovertebral angle tenderness may also be present.

- **B. Enigmatic fever** is less dramatic, usually manifesting as fever that persists despite treatment with broad-spectrum antibiotics. Patients do not appear acutely ill in contrast to patients with POVT. This condition is almost always associated with a diagnosed operative site infection and typically has onset 4–8 days after surgery [4a]. Physical findings are minimal despite spiking temperatures. In particular, no mass suggestive of an abscess or hematoma can be appreciated. Rarely, cordlike induration is palpable on pelvic examination.

V. Systemic complications. Septic pulmonary embolization occurs in up to 30% of untreated cases, with the associated sequelae of pulmonary infarction, lung abscess, bronchopleural fistula, or empyema.

VI. Diagnosis. Early diagnosis depends on a **high index of suspicion.**

- **A. Fever.** It is important to recognize that persistent, **unexplained temperature elevation despite appropriate antibiotic treatment** of a pelvic infection in the puerperal, postabortion, or postoperative patient may be the only manifestation of SPT.
- **B. Abdominal pain.** Because the patient with POVT may have a dramatic clinical presentation (e.g., localized abdominal pain, rebound tenderness, and a palpable abdominal mass), differentiation from acute appendicitis or other intraabdominal process may require diagnostic laparotomy.
- **C. Septic pulmonary embolism rarely** may be the presenting manifestation.
- **D. Routine laboratory** parameters are nonspecific (e.g., CBC).
- **E. Blood cultures** should be obtained, as they will be positive in approximately 35% of patients with SPT but are usually sterile in POVT [4a].
- **F.** Computed tomography, duplex Doppler ultrasonography, and MRI have all been used to confirm POVT [4a]. Diagnosis of SPT is one of exclusion and is verified by defervescence of fever with heparinization [4a].
- **G.** The **use of heparin** in a therapeutic trial in suspected cases of SPT has been suggested by several authors. Prompt clinical improvement in the 24–36 hours following heparinization is viewed as a confirmatory sign [25].

VII. Treatment. Early presumptive diagnosis of SPT, early anticoagulation, and the institution of broad antimicrobial coverage have replaced the traditional surgical approach.

- **A. Antibiotic therapy.** Appropriate choices include a third-generation cephalosporin (e.g., cefotaxime, 2 g IV q8h, or ceftriaxone, 2 g q24h) plus clindamycin (900 mg IV q8h) or metronidazole (500 mg IV q6h); or clindamycin (900 mg IV q8h) plus an aminoglycoside. Therapy should continue for 10–14 days.
- **B. Intravenous heparin infusion** as a continuous drip is recommended, with the goal of maintaining the activated partial thromboplastin time at 2 times normal. The optimal duration of therapy with herapin is unclear, but most clinicians use 7–10 days [4a]. If pulmonary emboli have occurred, anticoagulation should be continued orally for a total of 3–6 months.
- **C. Surgical intervention** is reserved for instances in which medical treatment has failed. If the patient is not afebrile within 24–48 hours or continues to develop pulmonary emboli, surgical exploration is indicated for appropriate surgical extirpation of the infected site or ligation of the inferior vena cava and ovarian veins.

Infections of Bartholin's and Skene's Glands

Infections of Bartholin's and Skene's glands may be classified clinically as cellulitis, infected cysts, or abscess formation. A key element in establishment of infection seems to be ductal obstruction.

I. Anatomic considerations

- **A. Bartholin's glands** are the perineal vestibular glands of the woman and correspond to the bulbourethral glands of the man. These normally small and nonpalpable glands are located bilaterally, within the vestibule and close to the hymen. Bartholin's glands respond with secretory activity to sexual arousal but contribute little

to actual vaginal lubrication. Glandular elements predominate after puberty and involute with the menopause.
   B. **Skene's glands** are the periurethral glands of the woman and are believed to be analogous to the male prostatic glands. Skene's glands are located posterior to the urethral orifice, and their presence is not normally evident. Because of the contiguity to the female urethra, chronic infection of a Skene's gland and duct may result in recurrent urinary tract infection.
II. **Clinical characteristics**
   A. **Asymptomatic.** Most patients who are asymptomatic are not infected at the time and have simple ductal or glandular cysts. However, in the presence of the underlying ductal obstruction, a number of patients progress to develop cellulitis or abscess formation.
   B. **Cellulitis.** Bartholin's and Skene's glands may provide the focus for perineal cellulitides, respectively referred to as *bartholinitis* and *skenitis*.
      1. Signs and symptoms do not differ from those of cellulitis anywhere in the body, with pain, swelling, redness and, perhaps, purulent drainage present.
      2. **Systemic findings are unusual.** Most patients have little or no fever, no leukocytosis, and no bacteremia. Occasionally, regional adenopathy is found.
      3. **Synergistic necrotizing cellulitis.** In rare cases, the patient will progress from cellulitis localized to the gland to widespread involvement of adjacent tissue. Many such patients are diabetic. The progression of infection is rapid, with prominent tissue necrosis.
   C. **Abscess.** When ductal obstruction and infection occur, abscess formation may take place. Surrounding cellulitis may or may not be evident. Spontaneous drainage may occur externally or, with time, a firm induration may form, indicating a chronic abscess.
III. **Microbiologic features.** These infections are typically polymicrobial, and anaerobic organisms have, in fact, been predominant. The most commonly isolated anaerobic organisms are *B. fragilis, Prevotella (Bacteroides)* spp., and peptostreptococci [27]. *N. gonorrhoeae* is found in up to 20% of cases. Commonly isolated aerobic organisms include *E. coli* and *Proteus* and *Klebsiella.*
IV. **Treatment**
   A. **Localized infection.** The treatment of choice for the majority of these infections is **surgical.** The procedure chosen should provide wide drainage, because simple incision or aspiration is followed by a high incidence of relapse. Occasionally, total excision is necessary. Bed rest, analgesia, and other symptomatic measures (such as hot baths) also may prove useful.
   B. **Severe soft-tissue infection** may complicate some cases, particularly in diabetics. If such tissue necrosis is suspected, these patients should be evaluated in the hospital, seen early in surgical consultation, and given parenteral antibiotics. While one is awaiting the results of cultures, antibiotics are chosen initially for activity against anaerobes (e.g., clindamycin) and gram-negative aerobes (e.g., an aminoglycoside or a third-generation cephalosporin) in doses described in sec. **VII** under Septic Pelvic Thrombophlebitis and in Chap. 4 under Necrotizing Soft-Tissue Infections. Gram stain examination may be helpful in choosing appropriate antibiotics. In the patient in whom *N. gonorrhoeae* is highly suspected, appropriate therapy may be added while one is awaiting cultures.

Infected Abortions

Legalization of elective pregnancy termination and the application of advances in medical technology to abortion techniques have changed the character and frequency of infections complicating abortion. Nonetheless, infected abortions still occur, posing serious diagnostic and therapeutic problems for the physician. Prompt diagnosis and management are crucial to the prevention of pelvic abscesses, septic shock, and death [27a].
I. **Risk factors**
   A. **Gestational age.** Rates of postabortion infection rise incrementally with increased gestational age.
   B. **Procedure.** The use of termination procedures other than suction curettage or transcervical evacuation is associated with a higher rate of postabortion complica-

tion. Intraamniotic injection of saline or prostaglandin and hysterotomy in particular are associated with a higher incidence of postabortion infections. The use of dilatation and evacuation for termination of second-trimester pregnancies has been reported to decrease markedly the risk of postabortion infection.

C. Untreated infection. The presence of **untreated** endocervical **gonorrhea** has been associated with a threefold increased risk of postabortion endometritis. Untreated *C. trachomatis* infection of the cervix poses a similar risk of complication. These sexually transmitted organisms are recovered more frequently from women who are younger than 24 years, have multiple sexual partners, live in urban areas, are in a lower socioeconomic group, and do not use barrier contraception.

D. Intrauterine devices. All IUDs are associated with an increased risk of septic midtrimester abortion [28].

II. Pathogenesis. Postabortion infections are **ascending infections** caused by cervicovaginal flora. Three mechanisms of infection are postulated:

A. Retained products of conception. Necrotic tissue, such as retained products, serves as an ideal nidus for infection with vaginal and cervical microorganisms, which gain access to the uterine cavity at the time of the termination procedure.

B. Contamination during surgery. There may be introduction of a virulent pathogen into the operative site at the time of surgery, particularly when the clinician is the source of the organism, such as with group A beta-hemolytic streptococcus.

C. Uterine trauma. Surgically related uterine trauma results in damage to the myometrium, providing a favorable environment for bacterial growth and subsequent endomyometritis. If perforation is unrecognized at the time of surgery, such patients may present at a later date with extrauterine infections such as infected hematomas or pelvic abscesses.

III. Clinical characteristics. Patients with infected abortion usually present with tachycardia, fever, chills, lower abdominal pain, and pelvic tenderness. However, the clinical presentation varies according to the etiologic conditions. The onset of symptoms in most cases is within 4 days of the procedure. However, if patients present very shortly after the procedure (within 24 hours), the clinician should suspect involvement with group A beta-hemolytic streptococci or *S. aureus*.

A common feature in reported cases of death from septic abortion is delayed treatment: A young or unmarried woman may be reluctant to reveal that she has had an abortion and may delay seeking help until she is moribund [27a].

Septic shock has been reported in 5–15% of septic abortions.

IV. Microbiologic features. With the exceptions of *N. gonorrhoeae, C. trachomatis,* and group A beta-hemolytic streptococci, the microorganisms involved arise from the normal flora of the cervix and vagina. Access to the upper genital tract, particularly in the presence of traumatized tissue, retained necrotic tissue, or foreign bodies, allows these endogenous organisms to become pathogenic. **Most infections are polymicrobial** [27a].

A. Organisms most frequently involved are the **gram-negative facultative bacteria** (especially *E. coli*), **facultative streptococci, and anaerobic bacteria** (especially *Peptostreptococcus* and beta-lactamase-producing *Bacteroides* spp.). *N. gonorrhoeae* and *C. trachomatis* are often involved. Bacteremia due to gram-negative organisms results in septic shock in approximately 15–20% of cases, compared to 5% for gram-positive organisms.

B. Of special note is *C. perfringens,* a gram-positive, anaerobic, spore-forming rod capable of producing potent exotoxins. Although the incidence of clostridial septic abortions has decreased since the legalization of abortion, it is a potentially lethal infection for which the clinician must be on the alert. The full-blown syndrome of clostridial sepsis—characterized by hemolysis, jaundice, hypotension, renal failure, and disseminated intravascular coagulation—has been fatal in 50–85% of cases. (See Chap. 2 also.) In the United States, infection with *C. perfringens* is largely associated with illegal abortion [27a].

C. In developing countries, tetanus is a cause of mortality from septic abortion [27a].

V. Diagnosis

A. Clinical setting. A diagnosis of infected abortion should be considered when any woman of reproductive age presents with vaginal bleeding, lower abdominal pain, and fever [27a]. Additionally, chorioamnionitis and sepsis may occur in any pregnant woman who has an IUD in place and presents with fever or vague abdominal pain.

B. Physical findings. On initial abdominal examination, one may note abdominal tenderness, guarding, and rebound. One also should note whether the tenderness is limited to the lower abdomen (pelvic peritonitis) or is present throughout the abdomen (generalized peritonitis) [27a]. The diagnosis of septic abortion may be confirmed by the presence of (1) a tender, soft, enlarged uterus, (2) foul-smelling exudate from the cervix, and (3) an open cervical os with evidence of passage of the products of conception. There may be evidence of instrumentation, such as tenaculum marks on the cervix, or the presence of a foreign body. The patient usually is febrile but, with severe infection and septic shock, may be hypothermic. Leukocytosis with a shift to the left usually is present, but leukopenia may occur in severe endotoxemia.

C. **Laboratory findings**

1. **A complete blood cell count with platelet count, electrolytes, and creatinine should be obtained.** Hyperkalemia may be present secondary to the effects of myonecrosis, hemolysis, or renal failure.

2. **Gram stains of endometrial smears** should be made to provide a clue to the predominant pathogen. The diagnosis of clostridial infection is suggested by the identification of large gram-positive rods on the smear.

3. **Aerobic and anaerobic cultures of blood and uterine contents** should be routinely performed.

4. **Roentgenograms** of the abdomen should be obtained to determine the presence of intraperitoneal air. In severe clostridial myometritis, gas may be seen in the myometrium.

5. **A pregnancy test** may be useful in selected, atypical cases. A sensitive pregnancy test (capable of detecting 20–50 IU of the beta subunit of human chorionic gonadotropin per milliliter) usually is positive, as it takes 4–6 weeks for human chorionic gonadotropin to become undetectable after complete uterine evacuation [27a].

VI. **Therapy.** Patients with established infection as indicated by temperature greater than 38°C, pelvic peritonitis, or tachycardia, should be hospitalized to receive parenteral antibiotics and prompt uterine evacuation. In early mild illnesses, some patients can be managed in the clinic or emergency room with careful follow-up [27a].

A. **Antibiotics.** Institution of early antibiotic therapy is important to prevent the development of SPT, pelvic abscess, and septic shock. However, operative removal of necrotic tissue also is a critical factor in determining outcome.

1. **In mild to moderately severe infection,** single-agent therapy with cefoxitin (2 g IV q6–8h) or cefotetan (2 g IV q12h), or ampicillin and sulbactam (2 g/1 g IV q6h), or ticarcillin and clavulanic acid (3.1 g IV q4–6h) may be employed. Piperacillin and tazobactam (3.0 g/0.375 g q6h) is another option (see Chap. 28E).

The regimens of antibiotics used for the outpatient management of PID are appropriate for early postabortion infection limited to the uterine cavity [27a].

2. **In patients with suspected sepsis or septic shock,** a combination of agents that covers all the potential pathogens should be administered. Although a time-honored triple-drug regimen such as clindamycin (900 mg IV q8h) or metronidazole (500 mg IV q6h) in combination with an aminoglycoside and ampicillin (2 g IV q6h) has commonly been used and is still suggested [27a], an alternative regimen would be a third-generation cephalosporin (e.g., cefotaxime or ceftriaxone) and clindamycin or metronidazole. Because this latter combination would not be active against enterococci, some clinicians may elect to use a third-generation cephalosporin, plus clindamycin or metronidazole, plus ampicillin (or vancomycin in the penicillin-allergic patient). In communities where methicillin-resistant *S. aureus* is prevalent, vancomycin (1 g q12h) should be substituted for ampicillin. High-dose penicillin should be administered for known clostridial sepsis.

Another consideration would be monotherapy with imipenem. We would not use ampicillin-sulbactam or ticarcillin-tazobactam alone as monotherapy in the critically ill patient.

B. **Surgical management.** Ideal management often is immediate reevacuation in the ambulatory clinic or the emergency room as soon as antibiotic therapy and fluid resuscitation have been started [27a].

1. Septic abortion is most common secondary to retained products of conception, and removal of infected necrotic tissue is the cornerstone of treatment. Retained products are suggested by an open cervical os or bleeding per os. The uterus should be evacuated, preferably by suction curettage, once adequate serum levels of antibiotics have been achieved.

2. In patients in whom the onset of infection occurs within 24 hours of abortion and in whom the introduction of a virulent pathogen at the time of operation is likely, treatment with antibiotics alone may be sufficient. If after 24–48 hours of antibiotic therapy no response has occurred, dilatation and curettage should be performed to exclude retained products.
3. If radiographic studies of the pelvis and abdomen reveal intrauterine gas, intraperitoneal foreign body, or free air in the peritoneal cavity suggestive of uterine perforation, immediate exploratory laparotomy is indicated to determine the extent of damage. When infection extends beyond the uterus, hysterectomy and salpingo-oophorectomy often are necessary.
4. **Laparotomy** will be needed if there is no response to uterine evacuation and adequate therapy. Other indications for laparotomy are uterine perforation with suspected bowel injury, a pelvic abscess, and clostridial myometritis [27a].
5. Tissue obtained during endometrial biopsy or uterine aspiration provides a better specimen for culture than does cervical discharge [27a].

C. **Severe sepsis and septic shock** should be managed in an intensive care setting in collaboration with physicians and nurses trained in critical care medicine [27a].

Breast Infections

I. **Puerperal mastitis.** Mastitis in the nursing woman is the most common form of breast infection. Both epidemic and endemic forms of puerperal mastitis may occur. However, most reports are of the endemic form. **Epidemic mastitis** occurs primarily among hospitalized women in conjunction with staphylococcal nursing epidemics and primarily involves the lactiferous glands and ducts of the breast. Epidemic mastitis rarely is encountered in modern obstetrics. **Sporadic, or endemic, mastitis** occurs in nonhospitalized nursing women. It manifests mainly as a unilateral mammary cellulitis and usually is due to infection that has gained entrance through fissures, cracks, or irritation of the nipple [29].

A. **Pathogenesis.** Thomsen and colleagues [30] have described a continuum of disease of the mammary glands of nursing women.
1. **Milk stasis** is characterized by leukocyte counts of fewer than 10^6 per milliliter of milk and is limited in duration to a few days, regardless of treatment.
2. **Noninfectious inflammation** describes patients with a leukocyte count of more than 10^6 per milliliter of milk and cultures that are sterile or reflect skin contamination. Symptoms typically last for a mean of 7.9 days, and approximately half of patients will progress to infectious mastitis. Emptying of the breast as a therapeutic maneuver results in a significant decrease in the duration of symptoms and an improved outcome.
3. **Infectious mastitis is diagnosed on the basis of high leukocyte counts in conjunction with high bacterial counts in milk.** Although emptying of the breast shortens the duration of symptoms, abscesses will develop in 11% of women not treated with antibiotics.

B. **Clinical characteristics.** Sporadic mastitis most often begins in the weeks to months after delivery (mean, 5.5 weeks). Temperature may be mildly elevated or may be as high as 105°F. The onset of symptoms typically is abrupt, with chills and breast soreness. A V-shaped cellulitis of the periglandular connective tissue, representing the divisions between the lobes of the breast, is visible [29].

C. **Clinical evaluation.** The breast as the source of the illness will be readily apparent on examination.
1. **Samples of breast milk should be obtained for leukocyte count and culture.**
2. **If pus can be expressed from the nipple, it should be cultured and Gram-stained to guide therapy.**
3. **Blood cultures** should be performed if systemic signs are present.
4. In all cases, the neonate should be examined for evidence of infection.

D. **Microbiologic features.** *S. aureus* **is the most common isolate** from milk in women with puerperal mastitis, whether epidemic or sporadic. Other organisms less commonly isolated from breast milk in women with sporadic puerperal mastitis include *S. epidermidis,* beta-hemolytic streptococci, enterococci, and *E. coli* [30].

E. **Treatment.** A key principle in management is attention to maximal breast care and optimal nursing technique.

1. **Nursing.** There is **no contraindication to nursing,** in that no ill effects have been observed in infants of mothers with mastitis [29]. In fact, because effective breast emptying seems to be important in promoting healing, a breast pump should be employed if nursing from the infected breast is halted temporarily.
2. **Antibiotics.** Early antibiotic treatment is important to prevent the progression of endemic mastitis to abscess. While one is awaiting cultures, initial therapy should include antistaphylococcal coverage.
    a. **Oral regimens.** Dicloxacillin (250–500 mg PO qid) or a first-generation cephalosporin such as cephalexin or cephradine (500 mg PO qid) can be used.

       In the patient with an immediate penicillin-allergic reaction, erythromycin (500 mg qid) or clarithromycin (500 mg bid) are considerations. Another option is clindamycin (300 mg tid or qid). (See Chap. 28.)

       The usual duration of therapy is 10 days.
    b. **Parenteral antibiotics** are necessary for initial therapy of more severe infections: Oxacillin or nafcillin (1–1.5 g q4h), or cefazolin (1 g q8h) in the patient with a delayed penicillin allergy, can be used. In the patient with an immediate severe allergic reaction to penicillin, intravenous clindamycin (600 mg q8h) can be used for this soft-tissue infection (see Chap. 28I).

       Once the patient has responded to intravenous therapy and is afebrile, one can switch to an oral regimen (see sec. **a**).
3. **Local care** provides symptomatic relief and is important in preventing recurrences. Particular attention should be paid to the presence of fissures or cracks. Adjunctive measures such as ice packs, breast support, and analgesics have been suggested.
4. **Breast abscess.** In the unusual patient in whom an abscess has developed, nursing should be interrupted. In addition to therapy with parenteral or oral antibiotics as described earlier, prompt incision and drainage should be performed.

II. **Mastitis in the nonlactating breast.** Less commonly, breast infections can occur that are unrelated to the puerperium.
  A. **Breast abscess** may occur rarely in premenopausal and postmenopausal women. In postmenopausal women, these abscesses occur without inflammation, which may result in the misdiagnosis of carcinoma. These infections often are polymicrobial, and anaerobic organisms are commonly isolated [31]. Treatment consists of surgical incision or excision, in conjunction with antimicrobial therapy based on culture results.
  B. **Granulomatous mastitis** presents as firm, hard masses and may simulate carcinoma of the breast [32]. Biopsy and culture reveal the true etiology.
    1. **Chronic bacterial abscess** of the breast may result in a firm mass consisting of necrotic tissue, fibrosis, and granulomatous inflammation.
    2. **Tuberculous mastitis** rarely may be a component of extensive reactivated tuberculosis.
    3. In **fat necrosis,** the surrounding inflammation forms a firm mass and is granulomatous in nature. Infection does not play a role in this entity.
    4. An idiopathic form also exists, possibly due to an autoimmune mechanism. The best therapy of this rare entity is unclear; corticosteroids may be useful [32].

Infectious Vulvovaginitis and Cervicitis

These entities are discussed in Chap. 13.

References

1. Larsen, B. Vaginal flora in health and disease. *Clin. Obstet. Gynecol.* 36:107–121, 1993.
2. Chandler, S.H., et al. The epidemiology of cytomegaloviral infection in women attending a sexually transmitted disease clinic. *J. Infect. Dis.* 152(3):597–604, 1985.

Proposes that cytomegalovirus (CMV) infection is a sexually transmitted pathogen. Finds a significant correlation of seropositivity to CMV with the number of lifetime sexual partners and of cervical CMV shedding with cervical chlamydial infection.

3. Walker, C.K., et al. Pelvic inflammatory disease: Metaanalysis of antimicrobial regimen efficacy. *J. Infect. Dis.* 168:969–978, 1993.

4. McCormack, W.M. Pelvic inflammatory disease. *N. Engl. J. Med.* 330(2):115–119, 1994.

4a. Mead, P.B. Infections of the Female Pelvis. In G.L. Mandell, J.E. Bennett, and R. Dolin (eds.), *Principles and Practice of Infectious Diseases* (4th ed.). New York: Churchill Livingstone, 1995. Chap. 90.

5. Eschenbach, D.A. Bacterial vaginosis and anaerobes in obstetric-gynecologic infection. *Clin. Infect. Dis.* 16(Suppl. 4):S282–287, 1993.

5a. Sweet, R. Role bacterial vaginosis in pelvic inflammatory disease. *Clin. Infect. Dis.* 30(Suppl. 2):S271, 1995.

6. Sweet, R.L., et al. The occurrence of chlamydial and gonococcal salpingitis during the menstrual cycle. *J.A.M.A.* 255(15):2062–2064, 1986.
Eighty-one percent of chlamydial or gonococcal salpingitis occurred within 7 days of the onset of menses.

6a. Bevan, C.D., et al. Clinical, laparoscopic, and microbiological findings in acute salpingitis: report on a United Kingdom cohort. *Br. J. Obstet. Gynaecol.* 102:407, 1995.
A recent report on 104 women from an inner-city hospital with acute salpingitis confirmed at laparoscopy. C. trachomatis was identified in the genital tract of 38.5% and N. gonorrhoeae in 14.4%. A dual infection was in 7.7%. Serologic evidence suggested another 6.7% of women had acute chlamydial infection at the time of diagnosis.

7. Centers for Disease Control. 1993 Sexually transmitted diseases treatment guidelines. *M.M.W.R.* 42(RR-14):1–102, 1993.
Update of prior 1989 STD treatment guidelines.

8. Jacobson, L., and Westrom, L. Objectivized diagnosis of acute pelvic inflammatory disease. *Am. J. Obstet. Gynecol.* 105(7):1088–1098, 1969.
Landmark prospective study of the accuracy of the clinical diagnosis of acute pelvic inflammatory disease when compared with the gold standard of laparoscopy.

9. Westrom, L. Effect of acute pelvic inflammatory disease on fertility. *Am. J. Obstet. Gynecol.* 121(3):707–713, 1975.
The landmark prospective study of women with laparoscopically verified acute pelvic inflammatory disease, with assessment of the frequency of long-term complications through careful follow-up.

10. Sweet, R.L. Pelvic inflammatory disease and infertility in women. *Infect. Dis. Clin. North Am.* 1(1):199–215, 1987.
Thorough review.

11. Henry-Suchet, J., et al. Microbiologic study of chronic inflammation associated with tubal factor infertility: Role of *Chlamydia trachomatis. Fertil. Steril.* 47(2):274–277, 1987.
Demonstrates a strong correlation between infertility due to tubal factors and presence of chlamydial infection by culture or serologic study.

12. Westrom, L. Incidence, prevalence, and trends of acute pelvic inflammatory disease and its consequences in industrialized countries. *Am. J. Obstet. Gynecol.* 138:880–892, 1980.

13. Hager, W.D., et al. Criteria for diagnosis and grading of salpingitis. *Obstet. Gynecol.* 61(1):113–114, 1983.

14. Korn, A.P., et al. Pelvic inflammatory disease in human immunodeficiency virus–infected women. *Obstet. Gynecol.* 82(5):765–768, 1993.

15. Wiesenfeld, H.C., and Sweet, R.L. Progress in the management of tuboovarian abscesses. *Clin. Obstet. Gynecol.* 36(2):433–444, 1993.

16. Sweet, R.L., and Gibbs, R.S. Mixed Anaerobic-Aerobic Pelvic Abscess. In R.L. Sweet and R.S. Gibbs (eds.), *Infectious Diseases of the Female Genital Tract.* Baltimore: Williams & Wilkins, 1995. Pp. 189–230.

17. Landers, D.V., and Sweet, R.L. Tubo-ovarian abscess: Contemporary approach to management. *Rev. Infect. Dis.* 5:876–884, 1983.
Review of 232 patients with tuboovarian abscess and review of the literature.

18. Reed, S.D., Landers, D.V., and Sweet, R.L. Antibiotic treatment of tuboovarian abscess: Comparison of broad-spectrum β-lactam agents versus clindamycin-containing regimens. *Am. J. Obstet. Gynecol.* 164:1556–1563, 1991.
Study demonstrated that extended-spectrum antibiotic regimens, including single-agent broad-spectrum antibiotics such as cefoxitin, in conjunction with doxycycline

have efficacy equivalent to clindamycin-containing regimens. Medical treatment successful in 75% of cases.

18a. Nelson, A.L., et al. Endovaginal ultrasonographically guided transvaginal drainage for treatment of pelvic abscess. *Am. J. Obstet. Gynecol.* 172:1926, 1995.
In this report 26 of 31 women were successfully treated by drainage performed by gynecologists. Five required surgical drainage. Authors conclude that this approach should be the route of choice for draining collections not amenable to percutaneous or colpotomy drainage. Indwelling catheters were not routinely used.

19. Gibbs, R.S., et al. A review of premature birth and subclinical infection. *Am. J. Obstet. Gynecol.* 166:1515–1528, 1992.
Up to 30% of patients in "idiopathic" preterm labor have positive amniotic fluid cultures, but it is not clear whether infection preceded labor or occurred as a result of labor.

20. Gibbs, R.S., and Duff, P. Progress in pathogenesis and management of clinical intraamniotic infection. *Am. J. Obstet. Gynecol.* 164:1317–1326, 1991.

21. Faro, S. Postpartum endometritis. In J.G. Pastorek III (ed.), *Obstetric and Gynecologic Infectious Diseases.* New York: Raven, 1994. Pp. 427–434.

21a. Hillier, S.I., et al. The role of bacterial vaginosis and vaginal bacteria in amniotic fluid infection in women in preterm labor with intact fetal membranes. *Clin. Infect. Dis.* 20(Suppl. 2):S276, 1995.

22. Watts, D.W., et al. Bacterial vaginosis as a risk factor for post-cesarean endometritis. *Obstet. Gynecol.* 75:52–58, 1990.

23. Dinsmoor, M.J., Newton, E.R., and Gibbs, R.S. A randomized, double-blind, placebo-controlled trial of oral antibiotic therapy following intravenous antibiotic therapy for postpartum endometritis. *Obstet. Gynecol.* 77:60–62, 1991.

24. Sweet, R.L., and Gibbs, R.S. Postpartum Infection. In R.L. Sweet and R.S. Gibbs (eds.), *Infectious Diseases of the Female Genital Tract.* Baltimore: Williams & Wilkins, 1995.

25. Sweet, R.L. Septic Pelvic Thrombophlebitis. In L. Cibils (ed.), *Surgical Diseases in Pregnancy.* New York: Springer, 1989.

26. Sweet, R.L. Treatment of mixed aerobic-anaerobic infections of the female genital tract. *J. Antimicrob. Chemother.* 8:105–114, 1981.

27. Brook, I. Aerobic and anaerobic microbiology of Bartholin's abscess. *Surg. Gynecol. Obstet.* 169:32–34, 1989.

27a. Stubblefield, P.G., and Grimes, D.A. Septic abortion. *N. Engl. J. Med.* 331:310, 1994.
Concise, recent, current concepts review.

28. Cates, W., et al. The intrauterine device and deaths from spontaneous abortion. *N. Engl. J. Med.* 295:1155–1159, 1976.
Risk of death from spontaneous abortion was more than 50 times greater for women continuing their pregnancy with an intrauterine device (IUD) in place than for those without an IUD.

29. Niebyl, J.R., Spence, M.R., and Parmely, T.H. Sporadic (nonepidemic) puerperal mastitis. *J. Reprod. Med.* 20(2):97–100, 1978.
A case review of 20 women with acute puerperal mastitis forms the basis for much of our current knowledge about the microbiology and treatment of this entity.

30. Thomsen, A.C., Espersen, T., and Maigaard, S. Course and treatment of milk stasis, noninfectious inflammation of the breast, and infectious mastitis in nursing women. *Am. J. Obstet. Gynecol.* 149:492–495, 1984.
Inflammation of the breast was categorized on the basis of duration of symptoms, leukocyte and bacterial counts of breast milk samples, and requirement for antibiotic therapy in 213 nursing women.

31. Edminston, C.E., Jr., et al. The nonpuerperal breast infection: Aerobic and anaerobic microbial recovery from acute and chronic disease. *J. Clin. Microbiol.* 162(3):695–699, 1990.

32. Salam, I.M.A., et al. Diagnosis and treatment of granulomatous mastitis. *Br. J. Surg.* 82:214, 1995.

15

Joint Infections

Norbert J. Roberts, Jr.,
and David J. Mock

Septic (Infectious) Arthritis

Septic (infectious) arthritis usually begins acutely in a single joint. Symptoms of inflammation may include pain, erythema, tenderness, swelling, and limitation of motion of the joint. Occasionally, multiple joints are involved. **A noninfectious inflammatory joint process such as crystal-induced arthritis (gout or pseudogout) may mimic a septic joint.** Therefore, a careful approach is necessary to ensure an early diagnosis [1–4]. Appropriate and rapid therapy for a septic joint is essential to avoid unnecessary joint damage.

Smith and Piercy [2a] have succinctly described the pathogenesis. Most cases of infectious arthritis involve hematogenous spread of an organism from a distant site. Synovial tissue is highly vascular and lacks a basement membrane; thus, it is susceptible to hematogenous seeding by bacteria [2a]. Following infection of the synovial membrane, the influx of polymorphonuclear leukocytes results in the release of enzymes that are destructive to the ground substance of the articular surface. If appropriate therapy is not instituted, the cartilage erodes and the joint space narrows. For patients who do not have chronic arthritis, trauma is often antecedent to infection. Patients with underlying arthritis, especially those receiving intraarticular injections, are predisposed to joint infections [2a].

I. **Clinical presentation.** A history and physical examination are most important in searching for the presence of a **primary infection site elsewhere** or for the presence of **risk factors** such as rheumatoid arthritis, sickle cell disease, immunosuppressive disease or therapy, prior sexually transmitted diseases, narcotic use, or the presence of a prosthetic joint. Any such finding might modify expectations regarding microbial etiology and, thus, the initial therapy. Less common etiologies might be suggested by such an approach. For example, the possibility of *Pasteurella multocida* arthritis is raised by the history of a cat bite. More common etiologies also might be expected, such as gonococcal arthritis with the finding of tenosynovitis.

A. **History**

1. **Multiple joint involvement** can occur, as in disseminated staphylococcal infections, but potentially with any bacteremia [5]. Multiple joint involvement occurs in about 10% of patients with septic arthritis [2a].

2. **Prior joint damage** (whether by trauma or underlying disease such as rheumatoid arthritis, gout, or an implanted joint prosthesis) predisposes the joint to infection. It may be difficult to distinguish superimposed infection from underlying disease. **In a patient with rheumatoid arthritis, an inflamed joint that is out of phase with other joints** (i.e., especially tender or warm) **may be infected.**

3. The usual **signs of inflammation** (tenderness, erythema, and swelling) **may be minimal** in some patients (e.g., those with rheumatoid arthritis or in those on steroid therapy).

4. **Systemic symptoms** include fever usually, though it may be low-grade. In 5–10% of patients, fever may be absent. Chills occur in a minority of patients (25%). Patients who are immunosuppressed or who have rheumatoid arthritis may have minimal systemic symptoms, perhaps only low-grade fever.

5. **Duration of symptoms** is highly variable. In bacterial infections, the symptoms are usually relatively recent (days) but can be prolonged before the diagnosis is made in patients with preexisting joint disease. With mycobacterial or fungal infections, insidious symptoms often have been present for months to years [4].

6. The knee, elbow, wrist, shoulders, hip, or ankle **joints** are **most commonly involved,** but any joint can become infected. Joint infections in children occur primarily (79%) in the hip, knee, or ankle [6]. With hip infection, the presenting complaint may be only pain on motion. Localization of infection to the sacroiliac joint may be difficult [7]. Although heroin users seem to have a predilection for sternoclavicular and sacroiliac joint involvement, these sites may be involved in the absence of this risk factor.

7. **Prosthetic joint infections** are discussed in detail in a separate section in this chapter.

8. **Gonococcal disease is currently the most common cause of septic arthritis in the 15- to 40-year-old group.** Therefore, the physician should be highly suspicious of this etiology in this age group. (See related discussion in Chap. 13.) The disseminated gonococcal syndrome tends to occur in women during the second and third trimesters of pregnancy and during menstruation. (The microbiology of nongonococcal joint infections is age related, as is discussed in sec. **III.A.3.**)

9. **Viral syndromes**—particularly rubella infection, rubella vaccination, and hepatitis B infections—can be associated with arthritis [4, 8]. Therefore, associated symptoms should be sought in obtaining the initial history. **Erythema infectiosum** (also known as **fifth disease**) is generally a mild exanthematous disease of childhood, linked serologically to human parvovirus. **Joint involvement has been reported primarily in adults** during localized epidemics and affects both large and small joints [9]. See also sec. **III.C.1.**

10. **Joint tuberculosis** classically presents as a monoarthritis of subacute onset involving a weight-bearing joint, with pain, swelling, and limitation of movement [4, 10, 11]. Joint pain may be highly variable with **fungal infection,** which is often (but not always) of gradual onset.

11. **Postinfectious, or reactive, arthritis** has been associated with infection of the GI tract with *Shigella, Salmonella, Campylobacter,* and *Yersinia* spp. in patients with the HLA-B27 histocompatibility antigen [12]. See also sec. **III.B.**

12. **Lyme disease.** See Chap. 23.

B. **Physical examination**

1. **Joint inflammation** should be carefully sought. Many of the expected signs of inflammation (erythema, tenderness, and swelling) may be absent in the patient who is immunosuppressed by disease or chemotherapy.

2. **Decreased range of motion** usually is marked **(generally to less than 15 degrees)** if a septic process involves a nonprosthetic joint, because of the associated pain.

3. **Tenosynovitis** (inflammation of the tendon sheath) may be seen in rheumatoid arthritis, gout, and trauma. However, it is a common manifestation of gonococcal disease, and its presence in the sexually active young adult is very suggestive of this diagnosis. **Patients with tenosynovitis typically have pain when the involved joint is flexed** to stress the tendon or with active motion.

4. **Concurrent infections** at other sites are fairly common in patients with bacterial arthritis (50–75% of cases).

5. **Skin rashes** commonly occur in disseminated gonococcal infections. These macular, vesicular, or pustular skin lesions, often with a necrotic center, are most often seen in the bacteremic phase, when migratory arthralgias occur with variable signs of joint inflammation. The lesions are most commonly noted over the distal extremities (see Plate I). Joint cultures often are negative and blood cultures positive at this stage. Within a day or two, classic joint inflammation develops, and cultures and Gram stains of the purulent fluid from joint aspiration are positive in the minority of cases (see Chap. 13). Pyogenic nongonococcal arthritis tends not to be associated with migratory arthralgias, but skin lesions similar to those seen in disseminated gonococcal infection have been reported in streptococcal and meningococcal arthritis [4].

6. **Prosthetic joint** examination may not reveal an inflammatory process. A good range of passive joint motion may persist, but active movement is limited by pain. See Prosthetic Joint Infections.

7. **Joint tuberculosis** often involves a weight-bearing joint; there is swelling, limitation of movement, and adjacent muscle spasm. Erythema often is absent, but lymph nodes draining the involved joint often are enlarged [4, 10, 11]. In **fungal joint infections,** signs are more variable.

II. **Laboratory aids.** The most important test is the examination of the joint fluid.

A. **Direct joint aspiration.** This has both diagnostic and therapeutic value and should be performed in virtually every case of joint disease in which infection is suspected. As a therapeutic maneuver, aspiration of the joint fluid should be as complete as possible without manipulation of the needle and consequent trauma to the synovial lining. Orthopedic or rheumatologic consultation should be sought if there is difficulty in obtaining fluid or in cases of presumed prosthetic joint infection that may require aspiration. The characteristics of synovial fluid in pyogenic and other types of arthritis are shown in Table 15-1. There are no substantial differences in synovial fluid analysis among the different acute bacterial pyarthroses. **Joint fluid analysis should include the following:**

1. **The total differential cell (anticoagulated tube) and the leukocyte count appear to be both the most sensitive (84%) and most specific (84%) synovial fluid tests for pyarthrosis.** The total number of WBCs generally exceeds 40,000/mm³ with polymorphonuclear neutrophils comprising more than 75% of the total [13]. However, both crystal-induced and rheumatoid arthritis flares can cause a similar picture.

2. **Synovial fluid glucose level** (sensitivity, 20%; specificity, 84%) may be less than 50% of the blood glucose level, but it also may be normal, particularly in gonococcal arthritis [13]. Neither low synovial fluid glucose levels nor elevated protein levels are sensitive or specific indicators of bacterial arthritis [2a].

3. In approximately 35–65% of bacterially infected joints, the **Gram stain** will be positive [1–2a]. Gram stains may be helpful especially if the patient has received some antibiotic therapy before evaluation. The antibiotic therapy may affect the cultures, but organisms often remain detectable by Gram staining.

4. **Cultures and special stains** also are helpful. Routine aerobic and anaerobic cultures should be performed on all inflammatory joints. **Fluid can be directly plated to chocolate agar media** rather than to media with antimicrobial agents (e.g., Thayer-Martin) **to culture for gonococci** (see Chap. 13). **In chronic and ill-defined inflammatory joint problems,** mycobacterial and fungal cultures should be obtained. In these settings, smears for mycobacteria and fungi can be done. The synovial fluid smear may be positive in 20–25% of cases of tuberculous arthritis. Cultures can be positive in as many as 80% of cases.

5. **Counterimmunoelectrophoresis (CIE)** has been used successfully to detect antigens of *Haemophilus influenzae* type b, *Streptococcus pneumoniae,* and group B streptococcus in synovial fluid [14]. CIE may be of special help in a patient who has received antibiotics.

6. **Crystal examination** is important. Joint fluid should be examined under polarized light to see whether the characteristic crystals of gout or pseudogout are present. **Acute crystal-induced arthritis** can cause inflammation of the joints that may **mimic bacterial processes,** and both processes can occur simultaneously.

7. Although not yet established outside of research laboratories, the detection of a pathogen by polymerase chain reaction (PCR) may prove to be helpful. For example, PCR testing was shown to detect *Borrelia burgdorferi* DNA in synovial fluid from 85% of 88 patients with Lyme arthritis and none of 64 control patients [15]. Of note, PCR testing might be able to show whether Lyme arthritis that persists after antibiotic treatment is due to persistence of the spirochete [15].

B. **Blood cultures.** Two blood samples, drawn at least 20 minutes apart, should be obtained. Blood cultures have been reported to be positive in up to one-third of patients but are the only source of a causative organism for 10% of cases [2a].

C. **Cultures of other infected sites.** These may provide the clue to an associated infection. In the sexually active young adult, careful culturing for gonococci must be done (i.e., of the cervix, urethra, pharynx, and rectum, as appropriate) (see Chap. 13).

D. **Radiography**

1. **Early.** In most patients with pyogenic arthritis, roentgenograms early in the course will reveal only soft-tissue changes (e.g., swelling, fascial plane obliteration, or increased volume of the joint) that suggest the presence of synovial effusion [16].

Table 15-1. Examination of joint fluid

Measure	Normal	Group 1 (noninflammatory)	Group 2 (inflammatory)	Group 3 (septic)
Volume (ml) (knee)	<3.5	Often >3.5	Often >3.5	Often >3.5
Clarity	Transparent	Transparent	Translucent-opaque	Opaque
Color	Clear	Yellow	Yellow-opalescent	Yellow–green
Viscosity	High	High	Low	Variable
WBC/mm^3	<200	200–2,000	2,000–100,000	>100,000*
Polymorphonuclear leukocytes	<25%	<25%	≥50%	≥75%*
Culture	Negative	Negative	Negative	Often positive
Mucin clot	Firm	Firm	Firm	Friable
Glucose (mg/dl)	Nearly equal to blood	Nearly equal to blood	>25, lower than blood	<25, much lower than blood

*Lower with infections caused by partially treated or low-virulence organisms.
Source: From G. P. Rodnan, C. McEwen, and S. L. Wallace (eds.), Primer on the rheumatic diseases. *J.A.M.A.* 224(Suppl.):661, 1973. Copyright 1973, American Medical Association.

2. **Late.** Radiographic changes in contiguous bony structures rarely are evident before 10–14 days. Early and follow-up roentgenograms are **important in uncovering coexisting osteomyelitis that would modify the therapy** (see Chap. 16).

3. **Settings in which radiographs are particularly helpful** [16]:

   a. With infections of **deep-seated joints,** such as the **hip,** evidence of synovial inflammation can be hidden from direct examination.

   b. In **slowly developing infectious arthritis,** such as tuberculous arthritis, and in the setting of a joint effusion, synovial biopsies may not have been obtained and the diagnosis may have remained obscure.

   c. **In a patient with active underlying joint disease,** such as rheumatoid arthritis, more rapid and severe destruction may be noted in one or two joints, which is suggestive of infection in those sites.

   d. In a **prosthetic joint,** spontaneous loosening of the prosthesis can occur, and space between the glue and bone is not diagnostic of infection. An arthrogram is often useful. Joint aspiration at the time of the procedure, with appropriate studies of the fluid (especially cultures), would establish the presence of infection. Also see under Prosthetic Joint Infections.

4. **Radioisotope scans.** These scans (usually technetium 99m [^{99m}Tc]) may be useful in certain cases, especially in the early investigation of infections in deep-seated joints. Radioisotope scans provide the earliest evidence of septic arthritis at a time when the plain radiograph may be normal or show only nonspecific soft-tissue swelling. For example, **sacroiliac pyogenic arthritis** frequently can be demonstrated with scintigraphy, whereas the standard roentgenographic examinations often are normal initially and may actually remain normal, despite extensive joint involvement [17, 18]. Scintigraphy may also be useful for monitoring the progress of therapy. Gallium 67 (^{67}Ga) and indium 111 (^{111}In) WBC imaging are other highly sensitive means of detecting infection in both native and prosthetic joints [16, 19]. Neither the roentgenograms nor the radioisotope scans are specific for infection; joint aspiration is required to establish the presence of infection [20].

5. **CT scanning.** To date, CT scanning has no defined role in the evaluation of septic arthritis [16], except in detecting infections associated with osteomyelitis (see Chap. 16). CT scanning and particularly MRI scanning have proved useful in the evaluation of infections of the spine (see sec. **II.C** under Intervertebral Disc Space Infections). MRI has also been used to demonstrate extraarticular spread of infections (e.g., those in which sinus tract formation has occurred) [2a].

E. **Miscellaneous. Peripheral blood leukocytosis** is relatively common (60–75%) but may be absent in the case of an immunosuppressed patient or a prosthetic joint infection. An elevated **erythrocyte sedimentation rate** (ESR) generally is noted (85–90%), even in cases of prosthetic joint infection. However, bacterial, viral, or mycobacterial infections of the joint may cause ESR elevations [2a]. A **tuberculin skin test** is appropriate in the patient with an insidiously developing monarticular arthritis, particularly if destructive lesions are evident on radiography and routine cultures and evaluation are unremarkable.

F. **Synovial tissue biopsy,** with cultures and histologic examination, is indicated in **ill-defined, chronic processes** in which routine joint fluid study has been unrewarding [2a, 21]. This is particularly true when granulomatous disease (e.g., mycobacterial infection) is suspected. Such studies occasionally may be helpful in cases of pyogenic arthritis, but usually they are not necessary.

III. **Microbiologic features of septic joints**

A. **Bacterial infection.** Although almost any organism can cause infectious arthritis, select bacteria are implicated in most cases. Age and predisposing factors help predict likely pathogens [1, 4]. **In the 15- to 40-year-old group, gonococcal arthritis constitutes approximately 94% of cases and other pyogenic bacteria 6%.** In those younger than 15 or older than 40 years, gonococci cause approximately 13% and other agents 87% of cases [1, 4]. The gonococcal cases occur primarily in women (>75%), and arthritis due to other agents is seen primarily in men (>65%). Table 15-2 lists the most common nongonococcal bacterial causes of septic arthritis according to age group.

1. **Neonates.** In infants younger than 3 months, adjacent bone is involved in as many as two-thirds of cases of septic arthritis [22]. Group B streptococci and

Table 15-2. Percent incidence of common organisms in septic arthritis[a]

Organism	Age			Total pediatric	Total adult	Adult rheumatoid arthritis
	<3 months	3–24 months	2–15 years			
Staphylococcus aureus	34	5	27	18	68	67
Streptococci[b]	30	12	14	13	20	12
Haemophilus influenzae	3	0–41[a]	3	—	1	—
Gram-negative bacilli	11	6	6	7	10	7
Miscellaneous and mixed[c]	22	4	14	10	1	7
Unknown	—	32	36	33	—	7

[a]Excluding *Neisseria gonorrhoeae*; see text. Also see text regarding incidence of *H. influenzae* infection.
[b]Includes beta-hemolytic groups, viridans streptococci, and *Streptococcus pneumoniae*.
[c]Includes *Staphylococcus epidermidis*, *Neisseria meningitidis*, *Neisseria gonorrhoeae*, *Candida* spp., anaerobic bacteria, and so on.

gonococci have emerged as the most common community-acquired causes in this age group (95% of cases). In contrast, staphylococci have been responsible for 55% of hospital-acquired infectious arthritis cases, followed by *Candida* and gram-negative bacilli [22]. Pyogenic arthritis has a striking propensity to affect joints of the lower extremities, even before weight bearing occurs [23]. (See Chap. 3, sec. **VI**, under Selected Specific Infections in the Newborn, and Chap. 16 under Hematogenous Osteomyelitis.)

2. **Children** [23–27]. In pediatric patients, *Staphylococcus aureus, H. influenzae,* and streptococci are the most important pathogens. However, *H. influenzae* is uncommon after 5 years of age. **Since the introduction and use of the *H. influenzae* b conjugate vaccine, there has been a continuous and marked decline in the percent of cases due to this pathogen in young children** [27a]. Prior to the introduction of this vaccine, staphylococci caused as many as 40% of the cases of these infections [23–27], but in a recent series, in part due to the decline of *H. influenzae* b disease, staphylococci and streptococci accounted for 70% of culture-confirmed cases [27a]. Development of sequelae is significantly associated with (1) infection in infants younger than 6 months, (2) delay of 4 or more days in instituting medical or surgical treatment, (3) infection due to *S. aureus,* and (4) most strikingly, involvement of the hip or shoulder with concomitant presence of osteomyelitis [23–27].

3. **Adults with nongonococcal arthritis**
   a. ***S. aureus* is implicated in the majority of cases.** In some reported series, more than 90% of patients with underlying rheumatoid arthritis and septic arthritis had *S. aureus* infection [2]. **Local prevalence rates of oxacillin resistance** (i.e., oxacillin-resistant [ORSA], or methicillin-resistant *S. aureus* [MRSA]) **should be considered in choosing therapy** [28].
   b. ***Streptococcus* spp.** are important etiologically at all age levels. Reports have emphasized the importance of routine serologic typing of streptococcal isolates from joint fluid. The incidence of infections with groups G and B streptococci appears to be increased in patients with several chronic underlying conditions, such as cirrhosis and diabetes [2a, 28a]. Arthritis caused by these streptococci may be marked by a slow response to therapy, with persistent synovitis, and joint destruction [29, 30]. Enterococcal infections are unusual but have recently been reviewed [30a].
   c. **Gram-negative bacilli** are less commonly the cause, but they warrant **special consideration in certain patients,** such as those with malignancies, medical immunosuppression, narcotic use, underlying chronic debilitating diseases, especially in the elderly, or prior noninfectious joint disease [1, 2, 2a, 4]. However, gram-negative bacillary septic arthritis has

also been seen in young and generally healthy hosts [31]. *H. influenzae* is an uncommon etiology in adults (approximately a dozen reported cases). In heroin addicts with septic arthritis, *Serratia* and *Pseudomonas* spp. are relatively common. Brucella arthritis may be seen in immigrants to the United States who usually present with involvement of the sacroiliac, knee, or hip joint. The diagnosis is made either by blood cultures or serology [2a].

- d. **Anaerobic bacteria,** although uncommon, have received increasing recognition as etiologic agents in septic arthritis, with the predominant species being *Propionibacterium acnes,* anaerobic gram-positive cocci, and *Bacteroides* spp. [32]. Coinfection with facultative or aerobic organisms occurred in only 11% of cases. **Predisposing factors** include trauma, contiguous infection, prosthetic joint, prior surgical or needle entry into the joint, and diabetes. Such factors were present in 75% of cases.
- e. **Prosthetic joint infections** are associated with a wide spectrum of implicated bacteria. Although staphylococci (both *S. aureus* and *S. epidermidis*) may be involved in more than half the cases, streptococci, gram-negative enteric bacilli, and anaerobic bacteria often are isolated in this setting. See also Prosthetic Joint Infections.
- f. **Polyarticular septic arthritis** may occur in approximately 10% of adult patients with nongonococcal septic arthritis. **Many of these patients do poorly.** In a recent review [33] of 25 patients with nongonococcal polyarticular septic arthritis, all the patients were older than 50 years, 52% had concurrent rheumatic diseases (generally rheumatoid arthritis), blood cultures were positive in 86%, and the mortality was 32%. **At presentation, many patients were mistakenly believed to be manifesting flares in their underlying rheumatoid arthritis or systemic lupus erythematosus and 20% were afebrile.** *S. aureus* accounted for 80% of cases, and streptococci, including *S. pneumoniae,* and gram-negative organisms accounted for approximately 20%.
- g. **Bite wounds** with contiguous joint involvement may be associated with mixed flora (see detailed discussion in Chap. 4).
- B. **Reactive arthritis.** This is the term used to describe a sterile but inflammatory process of the synovium preceded or triggered by an infection occurring anywhere outside the joint. Infectious agents that have been implicated include *Salmonella, Shigella, Yersinia, Campylobacter,* group A beta-hemolytic streptococci, *Staphylococcus* and, most especially, *Chlamydia* [34–36]. The latter has been strongly associated with the subsequent development of Reiter's syndrome, and some reports suggest that effective long-term antimicrobial therapy of chlamydia may have a salutary effect on the course of the associated Reiter's syndrome [37].
- C. **Nonbacterial disease**
  1. **Viral infections generally are distinguished by the sudden onset of severe joint pain with or without swelling. Various types of skin rashes occur in almost all viral arthritides.** The most common viral causes of arthritis are **human parvovirus B19 (fifth disease),** natural **rubella** infection, rubella vaccination, **hepatitis B** virus, and the human immunodeficiency virus (HIV) [4, 8, 9, 38]. **In** outbreaks of **fifth disease,** women present with symmetric arthritis in late winter and in the spring. The onset of joint symptoms in adults occurs with the rash or shortly after the eruption; small joints of the hands are most frequently involved with a self-limited course [38a]. **With hepatitis B,** patients may have a history of urticaria 1 to 6 weeks along with the onset of joint symptoms, resolving commonly with the onset of jaundice. The arthritis is symmetrical: hands are affected most often, followed by knees and ankles; joint effusions are scanty [2a].

     Although active controversy continues regarding the role of the virus **HIV has been associated with a variety of arthritis syndromes including:** (1) an acute symmetric polyarthritis affecting the small joints of the hands and wrists; (2) a disabling subacute oligoarticular arthritis affecting mainly knees and ankles; and (3) a "painful articular syndrome," lasting fewer than 24–48 hours, involving the knees, elbows, or shoulders and characterized by severe, intermittent arthralgia without synovitis, often requiring narcotic analgesics. Psoriatic arthritis, Reiter's syndrome, and a variety of other miscellaneous syndromes may also be associated with HIV. Arthritis can be a manifestation of infection with mumps (especially in men), influenza, arboviruses, Epstein-

Barr virus (infectious mononucleosis), and varicella. Reviews of viral arthritis have recently been published [8, 38, 39].

2. **Mycobacterial and fungal infections** of joints and bones are **characterized by slow evolution** of physical and radiographic findings [2a]. Fungal arthritis is seen mainly in patients compromised by primary diseases or by medical therapy. Evidence of disseminated disease is common [11]. Among the fungi, sporotrichotic, candidal, and coccidioidal arthritis are the most common, but arthritis can also occur with blastomycosis, cryptococcosis, and histoplasmosis. Bayer and Guze [40] have reviewed fungal arthritis in detail. See further discussion in Chap. 18. *Coccidioides immitis* monoarticular infection typically occurs in non-white immunosuppressed men from endemic areas. Joint infections in patients with blastomycosis primarily spreads from an osteomyelitic focus. Candidal infections of peripheral joints generally are of acute onset following hematogenous spread of the organism [2a].

   M. tuberculosis and atypical mycobacteria are uncommon but important causes of chronic, indolent infectious arthritis [10, 11]. These have been reviewed by Meier and Hoffman [41].

   Cultures of synovial tissue produce a higher yield than cultures of joint fluid **in cases of mycobacterial and fungal infection** [2a].

3. **Lyme disease** [42–46], caused by the tickborne spirochete *B. burgdorferi,* characteristically occurs in summer. It frequently is characterized by a unique skin lesion, erythema chronicum migrans, and often is accompanied by systemic flulike symptoms. From several days to as long as 2 years later, approximately 60% of untreated patients develop brief, recurring episodes of either an asymmetric oligoarthritis affecting primarily large joints such as the knee or a migratory polyarthritis [42, 44]. Diagnostic issues, problems with serologic testing [42, 45], and therapy [42, 46] are **discussed in detail in Chap. 23.**

IV. **Differential diagnosis**
   A. Conditions that may be associated with joint effusion are listed in Table 15-3. Infectious arthritis (group 3) would more commonly have to be distinguished from the inflammatory joint diseases listed in group 2 than from diseases in the other categories. It must be remembered that **bacterial arthritis may complicate, and in part be obscured by, the inflammatory conditions listed in group 2.** The laboratory approach outlined in sec. II should help sort out such possibilities, including crystal-induced synovitis.
   B. Arthritis in the presence of bacterial endocarditis may be due to bacterial seeding of the joint space or of multiple joint spaces or to associated immune complex disease. The development of arthritis in a site unusual for common causes of inflammatory arthritis might warn of the possibility of endocarditis.
   C. **Acute transient synovitis of the hip,** sometimes called "**toxic synovitis** of the hip" or "acute transient epiphysitis," is the most common cause of a painful hip in children under 10 years of age [46a]. Boys are most frequently affected, especially between 3 and 6 years, but the disorder can occur in infancy and early adolescence. The etiology is unknown. The onset of hip pain with motion and weight-bearing may be acute or gradual. There may be a slight fever, usually not higher than 100°F to 101°F [46a]. There are no changes of the bone on conventional radiographs; scintigraphy with technetium-99m studies are normal or show slight diffuse increase in uptake. The peripheral WBC count and ESR are normal. **Aspiration of the hip joint will yield clear fluid that is sterile on culture.** Antibiotics are not indicated once culture results are available. Corticosteroids are not recommended. Antiinflammatory drugs may be useful. This entity is reviewed in more detail elsewhere [46a].
   D. **Postinfectious (reactive) arthritis,** usually with multiple joints involved, can be seen as an immunologic response during infection with certain agents (e.g., hepatitis B); see sec. **III.C.1.** Postinfectious arthritis also can develop following meningococcal infections, sexually transmitted diseases, or enteric infections due to *Shigella, Salmonella, Campylobacter,* and *Yersinia* spp. The presence of the specific histocompatibility antigen HLA-B27 increases the likelihood 50-fold that postinfectious arthritis will develop and appears to predispose to more severe disease [2a] (see related discussion in sec. **III.B.**) Joint fluid cultures are sterile.

V. **Therapy for bacterial joint infections.** Proper therapy **requires both** removal of purulent material (i.e., **adequate drainage**) from the joint **and** administration of appropriate **antibiotics.** Weight bearing probably should be avoided, but immobilization of the joint need be limited only by the symptomatology [4]. In most cases, medical management is highly successful if improvement is noted within 48 hours.

Table 15-3. Differential diagnosis by joint fluid groups

Group 1 (noninflammatory)	Group 2 (inflammatory)	Group 3 (septic)	Hemorrhagic
Degenerative joint disease	Rheumatoid arthritis	Bacterial infections	Hemophilia or other hemorrhagic diathesis
Trauma[a]	Acute crystal-induced synovitis (gout and pseudogout)		Trauma with or without fracture
Osteochondritis dissecans	Reiter's syndrome		Neuropathic arthropathy
Osteochondromatosis	Ankylosing spondylitis		Pigmented villonodular synovitis
Neuropathic arthropathy[a]	Psoriatic arthritis		Synovioma
Subsiding or early inflammation	Arthritis accompanying ulcerative colitis and regional enteritis		Hemangioma and other benign neoplasm
Hypertrophic osteoarthropathy[b]	Rheumatic fever[b]		
Pigmented villonodular synovitis[a]	Systemic lupus erythematosus[b]		
	Progressive systemic sclerosis (scleroderma)[b]		

[a]May be hemorrhagic.
[b]Group 1 or 2.
Source: From G. P. Rodnan, C. McEwen, and S. L. Wallace (eds.), Primer on the rheumatic diseases. *J.A.M.A.* 224(Suppl.):661, 1973. Copyright 1973, American Medical Association.

A. Drainage of purulent material. Even with the first diagnostic joint fluid aspiration, an attempt should be made to remove as much purulent material as possible without any manipulation of the needle that might damage the synovial membrane. Frequent aspiration (daily or more often), both early in the course and as fluid reaccumulates during therapy, is an important adjunct to antibiotic therapy.
   1. Purposes of joint aspiration
      a. To provide drainage of the enclosed space, which functionally is acting like an abscess
      b. To provide symptomatic relief
      c. To relieve joint pressure and remove the products of the inflammatory response, such as enzymes, that may cause destruction of articular cartilage
      d. To ensure that antibiotic therapy is effective by doing follow-up smears, cultures, and leukocyte counts
      e. In certain settings, such as gram-negative bacterial arthritis treated with aminoglycosides, possibly to improve antibacterial activity by removing cells and cell products that lower the pH and thereby could be adversely affecting antibiotic activity
   2. Frequency and duration. The infected joint fluid must be removed periodically (by aspiration) or drained (by open drainage) if fluid reaccumulates or in certain special settings noted later. Repeated aspirations within the first 48 hours of antibiotic therapy often will provide adequate drainage.
B. Repeated aspirations versus open drainage. This remains a controversial subject, with little experimental evidence to support either viewpoint. Several studies [23, 24, 27, 47] support the concept that early drainage is more important than the method of drainage for all joints except the hip, where an initial surgical approach is required (i.e., open drainage). Forty-five children with septic arthritis of less than 6 days' duration in joints other than the hip underwent initial nonoperative treatment. Thirty-four of 49 joints were managed successfully by aspiration and

antibiotics and the remainder by surgical drainage following a lack of response to nonoperative treatment. After an average follow-up of more than 3 years, all joints were normal to clinical and radiographic examination [27]. In a large, pooled retrospective review, a significantly improved outcome was observed with the initial use of needle aspiration compared with initial surgical therapy, and there was no evidence that delay in surgical drainage changed the outcome for those in whom it eventually was required [47]. However, results of treatment in the elderly are generally much less favorable, with mortality ranging from 9 to 33% and a poor functional outcome in approximately half of patients [47, 48].

Whereas repeated needle aspirations (i.e., daily, or more often if fluid accumulates rapidly) of the infected joint are appropriate for most cases of septic arthritis, surgical drainage is to be considered early in the course in certain situations, as follows:

1. **Lack of response to appropriate antibiotic therapy and repeat needle aspirations.** The precise time one should wait is controversial. Some authorities favor open drainage if adequate response has not occurred within 48–72 hours of antibiotic therapy and serial aspirations [2a]; others allow up to 1 week.

2. **Inability to drain the joint adequately by needle aspiration** due to large amounts of debris, fibrin, or loculations [47].

3. **Infection of a prosthetic joint** (see under Prosthetic Joint Infections).

4. **Relative inaccessibility of the joint** or advanced disease and necrosis, as might be the case in an infected hip [4]. The need for surgical (open) drainage of an infected hip often is stated but has not been established by a controlled prospective study. In the absence of such a study, **most clinicians believe that hip joint infections,** except perhaps gonococcal infections, **require surgical drainage.** The shoulder is also special; suppurative arthritis of the shoulder will require either radiographically guided aspiration or surgical drainage [2a].

5. **Gram-negative bacillary arthritis.** These patients have a poorer prognosis. The great majority of patients with staphylococcal or streptococcal joint infections attain complete recovery of the joint. However, only a minority of patients with gram-negative bacillary arthritis achieve such a result. Some authors advocate early explorative arthrotomy to ensure adequate drainage, to assess and drain perisynovial abscesses, and to debride contiguous osteomyelitis (if present) in patients with gram-negative bacillary septic arthritis [31].

C. **Antibiotic therapy**

1. **Instillation of antibiotics directly into the joint is unnecessary and unwise.** Most antibiotics that might be used diffuse readily into the synovial fluid [49, 50], and intraarticular injections of antibiotics may induce a chemical synovitis and prolong or increase the inflammation.

2. **Parenterally administered antibiotics** usually are indicated in the treatment of septic arthritis.

    a. **Penetration** of antibiotics into synovial fluid. According to studies, the following antibiotics have been reported (with varying numbers of observations) to reach levels in synovial fluid, after systemic administration, that would be adequate in the settings in which they were used: penicillin G, ampicillin, methicillin, nafcillin, carbenicillin, cephalothin, cefazolin, cefuroxime, clindamycin, chloramphenicol, tetracycline, sulfonamides, vancomycin, gentamicin, amikacin, ceftriaxone, ceftazidime, aztreonam, imipenem, and probably cefotaxime. It is likely that, for most antibiotics, penetration into synovial fluid is greater earlier in the course of septic arthritis, when the degree of inflammation is greater. Such a possibility would suggest caution regarding too rapid a change in antibiotic therapy as, for instance, to lower doses of parenteral therapy or to oral therapy in nongonococcal infections. Oral ciprofloxacin is a potential agent for susceptible pathogens (see Chap. 28S).

    b. **Specific recommendations for treatment of nongonococcal arthritis.** Initial antibiotic therapy is determined by the interpretation of the synovial fluid Gram stain, as **shown in Table 15-4.** When the culture and sensitivity results are available, the initial regimens can be modified to include the least toxic effective antibiotic. Antibiotic therapy for bite wound infections, which may involve a contiguous joint, are discussed in detail in Chap. 4.

    c. **Gonococcal arthritis** (see also the discussion in Chap. 13). Treatment of gonococcal infections in the United States is influenced by the spread of

Table 15-4. Antibiotic therapy of bacterial arthritis based on initial Gram stain

Gram stain	Drug of choice	Dosage	Alternatives[a]
Gram-positive cocci	Nafcillin (or oxacillin) or vancomycin (if oxacillin-resistant S. aureus is deemed a significant risk)	9 g/day IV in divided doses q4h in adults; 100–200 mg/kg/day IV in divided doses q4h in children (for vancomycin, 1 g q12h in adults, with modifications based on creatinine clearance; see Chap. 28)	First-generation cephalosporin (e.g., cefazolin or cephalothin), clindamycin
Gram-negative cocci			
Adult	Ceftriaxone[b,c]	1 g IV once daily in adults	Cefotaxime,[b,c] ceftizoxime,[b,c] or spectinomycin[b]
Young child (<6 yr)	Ceftriaxone[b,c,d]	50 mg/kg/day (max. 2 g) IV once daily	Cefotaxime 50 mg/kg/day IV in individual doses q8h
Gram-negative bacilli	Gentamicin[e] plus ticarcillin[f]	4.5–5.0 mg/kg/day IM or IV in divided doses 8qh if renal function is normal; 15–18 g/day IV in divided doses q4h in adults; 200–300 mg/kg/day IV in divided doses q4h in children	Gentamicin[e] and third-generation cephalosporin

No organisms seen			
Young adult, healthy	Ceftriaxone	As above	Cefoxitin
Patient with risk factors (see text)	Nafcillin and gentamicin	As above	Third-generation cephalosporin[g]
Young child (<6 yr)	Ceftriaxone[g]	As above	Cefuroxime or ampicillin[h] and nafcillin
Neonate, infant (<3 mo)	Cefotaxime[g,j] or cefotaxime and gentamicin[k]	See Chaps. 3 and 28.	Oxacillin, cefotaxime,[g] and an aminoglycoside[k]

[a] Specific doses of alternative agents are discussed in Chap. 28. In the penicillin-allergic patient with a delayed reaction, cephalosporins often are used as alternative agents. In patients with an immediate, severe reaction to a penicillin, cephalosporins should not be used without skin testing. (See Chap. 27.)

[b] See discussion in text (sec. **V.C.2.c**) under Infectious Arthritis.

[c] When susceptibility data are not available for gonococcal infections, a third-generation cephalosporin now is preferred [51].

[d] May be coccobacillary forms of *Haemophilus influenzae*, which are susceptible to third-generation cephalosporins (e.g., ceftriaxone, cefotaxime), as are gonococci.

[e] Local aminoglycoside susceptibility patterns must be considered. If gentamicin resistance is common, tobramycin or amikacin is preferred.

[f] Or mezlocillin or piperacillin (see Chap. 28E).

[g] In the past, the third-generation cephalosporins were believed to have significantly less antistaphylococcal activity than the semisynthetic penicillinase-resistant penicillins and first-generation cephalosporins, so some clinicians added an antibiotic (e.g., oxacillin) to ensure **optimal** antistaphylococcal activity while awaiting culture data. However, more recent data suggest that some third-generation cephalosporins (e.g., ceftriaxone and cefotaxime) may have adequate antistaphylococcal activity. See Chap. 28F discussion of cephalosporins. Some experts still favor an antistaphylococcal agent (e.g., oxacillin) added to a third-generation cephalosporin [27a] for enhanced *S. aureus* activity.

[h] If ampicillin-resistant *H. influenzae* is common, a third-generation cephalosporin (e.g. ceftriaxone) or cefuroxime is preferred while awaiting culture and susceptibility data (see footnote **d**).

[i] See Chap. 3 for dosages and other options.

[j] If community-acquired infection. See text.

[k] If hospital-acquired infection. See text.

Source: Modified from D. L. Goldenberg and A. S. Cohen, Acute infectious arthritis: A review of patients with nongonococcal joint infections (with emphasis on therapy and prognosis). *Am. J. Med.* 60:369, 1976.

infections due to antibiotic-resistant *N. gonorrhoeae* and the high frequency of chlamydial infections in persons with gonorrhea; guidelines for therapy have recently been revised [51]. If an organism is isolated from joint fluid cultures, antimicrobial susceptibility testing should be performed. Patients should be initially hospitalized for therapy and examined for evidence of endocarditis or meningitis, both of which are rare. The treatment of gonococcal arthritis is similar to that for disseminated gonococcal infection [51]. **See Chap. 13** for specific antibiotic regimens.

3. Duration of parenteral therapy

   a. Gonococcal arthritis. See Chap. 13.

   b. Nongonococcal arthritis

     (1) Adults. Therapy is typically continued until the arthritis appears to be resolved. The usual duration of therapy is 2 weeks for infections due to *H. influenzae,* streptococci, or gram-negative cocci [2a], especially if there is no underlying joint disease and if the patient does well with initial therapy. Longer courses of therapy (e.g., 3 weeks) may be indicated in patients with gram-negative infections, slowly responding infections (despite adequate drainage), or infections with virulent organisms such as *S. aureus* [2a]. Of course, coexisting osteomyelitis also warrants prolonged therapy (see Chap. 16). Whether additional oral therapy is indicated after full courses of parenteral therapy is controversial, although patients with prosthetic joint infections often receive prolonged courses, as noted under Prosthetic Joint Infections.

       When an effective oral regimen is available (e.g., TMP-SMX or oral quinolone very active against the pathogen), oral therapy often is used to complete a full course of therapy (see sec. **(3)**).

     (2) Initial parenteral therapy followed by oral treatment of children. Relatively short courses of parenteral therapy (i.e., 5–7 days) followed by 10–21 days of oral antibiotics in children appears generally to be successful if the initial clinical response is favorable and adequate serum bactericidal activity is demonstrated (i.e., $\geq 1:8$) [52]. However, some guidelines and precautions should be heeded [52].

       (a) The serum bactericidal titer (peak) on the day after the initiation of oral therapy should be at least 1:8 when the pathogen is a gram-negative bacillus, *S. aureus,* or *H. influenzae,* and at least 1:32 when the organism is a streptococcus. Therefore, the pathogen causing the septic arthritis must be isolated so the laboratory can provide information on bactericidal levels necessary to eliminate it (see Chap. 25).

       (b) If the bactericidal level is suboptimal, the dosage of antibiotic must be increased. Usually, the oral dose is 2–3 times that used for minor infections. These higher doses were well tolerated in children [52].

       (c) Ideally, the entire course of oral agents should be given in the hospital, especially if there is any doubt about patient compliance. If the therapy is given at home, three precautions must be taken:

         (i) There must be an **adequate bactericidal titer** of the antibiotic in the serum before discharge.

         (ii) **Compliance** with the oral regimen at home **must be assured** after careful discussion with the patient and family.

         (iii) The patient should be **followed up weekly** to check on his or her clinical condition and to monitor the serum bactericidal level.

       (d) The **duration of therapy** will depend on the organism and the patient's clinical response. For *H. influenzae,* streptococci, or gram-negative cocci, a minimum of 2 weeks of therapy is suggested. For *S. aureus* or gram-negative bacilli, a minimum of 3 weeks is suggested. If the clinical response is slow or the ESR remains elevated, more prolonged therapy and reevaluation are necessary. Therefore, cases must be individualized, especially when *S. aureus* is involved.

       In gram-negative bacillary infections, if susceptible to trimethoprim-sulfamethoxazole or ciprofloxacin, an oral agent may be feasible if compliance can be assured (see Chap. 28).

(3) **In adults, there is far less experience with parenteral short-course therapy followed by oral therapy.** One group [53] suggests the bactericidal level be a trough measurement and be at least a 1:8 level against the isolated pathogen. These investigators acknowledge that whether a peak or trough bactericidal level is necessary is unclear. (See Chap. 25 for additional discussion of bactericidal levels.)

(4) For additional discussion of oral therapy for skeletal infections, see Chap. 16.

D. **Prosthetic joint infections.** See the section Prosthetic Joint Infections later in this chapter.

E. **Repeated aspirations to monitor therapy.** Repeated joint aspirations, within the first 5–7 days of therapy [2a], serve to monitor effectiveness of the antimicrobial therapy as well as to remove debris that may be destructive to the joint. Within a few days of adequate therapy, the joint fluid should become sterile; e.g., serial cultures of joint fluid that become negative within 5 days of the initiation of therapy have been considered to be indicative of a good clinical response [2a]. Within 1 week, the leukocyte count should be substantially lowered if a good outcome is to be expected with the therapeutic regimen in use. In addition, fluid reaccumulation should be markedly decreasing. **In the absence of such indications of response,** despite appropriate antibiotic therapy as determined by cultures and sensitivity testing, **open surgical drainage is to be considered,** as discussed in sec. **B.**

F. **Therapy for nonbacterial joint infections.** Infectious disease consultation is advised for treatment of mycobacterial and fungal infections. See Chaps. 9 and 18 for therapeutic options for fungal and mycobacterial infections, respectively.

VI. **Prognosis.** The prognosis in infectious (septic) arthritis varies greatly. In older children and adults without other comorbidities and for whom a large single joint is infected, the overall prognosis for survival and full return of joint function is excellent. In contrast, infants and neonates in whom the hip joint is involved may have permanent sequelae, including leg length discrepancy [54]. Similarly, in the elderly, permanent sequelae and accompanying osteomyelitis are more common, and death rates approaching 20% have been reported [55]. In a recent review, characteristics of patients with bacterial arthritis associated with a poor outcome included: age of at least 60 years, preexisting (rheumatoid) arthritis, infection of the hip or shoulder, duration of symptoms of more than 1 week before treatment, involvement of more than four joints, and persistently positive cultures after a 7-day course of appropriate antibiotics [2a].

Prosthetic Joint Infections

Under optimal conditions, the overall rate of total joint replacement infections has decreased in recent years to 1–2% [56], although precise rates of infection may be difficult to obtain, and depend on the joint replaced and the extent of time after the operation [56a]. **Risk factors that appear to be associated with the development of infection in prosthetic joints include** advanced age, malnutrition, rheumatoid arthritis, diabetes mellitus, use of corticosteroids, and preexisting infection at another site. Additional risks include prior surgery in the affected joint, location and design of the implanted prosthesis (with knee arthroplasties having a higher incidence of infection than hips), and occurrence of a local hematoma or superficial wound infection in the postoperative period [56, 57]. In a recent review, prior joint surgery, perioperative wound complications, and underlying rheumatoid arthritis were the most well established risk factors [56a].

Prosthetic joint infections have been recently reviewed elsewhere [56a, 57a].

I. **Initiation of infection.** Bacterial contamination of the joint may be initiated either during or after implantation. Despite aseptic surgical techniques, intraoperative contamination can occur via air contamination, generally caused by dispersion of desquamated skin scales from individuals in the operating room; it may also occur from the patient's own skin or contact with the surgeon's hand through a punctured glove [58]. Significantly fewer infections have been found in operating rooms using ultraclean as opposed to conventional air circulation systems [59]. In contrast, deep infection initiated after surgery is caused by hematogenous spread of bacteria from distant sites. Most of these are believed to originate from cutaneous lesions, the respiratory tract, urinary tract, and oral cavity [3, 6].

Most series have demonstrated that 80–90% of prosthetic joint infections, evident in the first 2 years after operation, originate in the operating room, with later, hematogenously acquired infections accounting for the remainder [58].

II. **Biopathogenesis.** Within hours of implantation, the surface of the prosthesis is covered by a layer of glycoproteins, some of which act as receptors that facilitate the adherence of both tissue cells and bacteria. After adherence has taken place, many bacteria produce a slime, the glycocalyx, which renders adherence irreversible, permits optimal concentration of nutrients, and provides protection against both phagocytosis by leukocytes and antibiotics. After the initial invasion of bacteria into tissue, host defenses react within 2–5 hours to localize the infection and prevent spread to adjacent tissues. During this decisive period, antibiotics are successful in reducing the total number of bacteria and tilting the balance in favor of host defenses, but after this time their effect is very limited [58].

III. **Microbiologic features.** More than 50% of prosthesis-related infections are caused by gram-positive organisms. Most of these appear to be due to staphylococci, with coagulase-negative staphylococcal species outnumbering S. *aureus* in some series. Streptococci, including the anaerobic *Peptococcus* species, cause most of the rest of such infections. Enteric gram-negative bacteria account for 10–28% of infections in various series [58]. Many of these agents are skin commensals or transient skin contaminants (Table 15-5).

IV. **Diagnosis**

   A. **Clinical presentation. A high degree of clinical suspicion** is required because the presentation is generally indolent and the degree of pain and systemic symptoms often are considerably less pronounced than in septic arthritis of a native joint. In addition, pain due to mechanical loosening (not due to infection) and that due to sepsis can present with a similar clinical picture. In joint sepsis, **pain is a prominent feature,** usually is constant, is exacerbated by weight bearing, and increases over time. It occurs in 90% of patients, although such hallmarks of infection as fever, localized edema and erythema, and sinus tract drainage each occur in only 30–40% of patients. An acute or fulminant presentation is more common with virulent organisms such as S. *aureus* or pyogenic beta-hemolytic streptococci, while a chronic indolent course is more typical of infection with less virulent organisms, e.g., coagulase-negative staphylococci [56a].

   B. **Radiographic studies**

      1. **Serial x-ray findings.** Loosening or dislocation of the prosthesis in association with cortical bone resorption or periosteal reaction are suggestive of infection but may also be seen with mechanical loosening alone [60].

Table 15-5. Microbiology of 1,033 prosthetic joint infections[a] seen at Mayo Clinic from 1969 to 1991

Microorganism(s)	No. (%) of PJI
Coagulase-negative staphylococci	254 (25)
S. *aureus*	240 (23)
Polymicrobial	147 (14)
Gram-negative bacilli	114 (11)
Streptococci[b]	79 (8)
Unknown[c]	83 (8)
Anaerobes	62 (6)
Enterococci	29 (3)
Other microorganisms	25 (2)
Total	1,033 (100)

PJI = prosthetic joint infections.
[a]All cases met case definition of definite infection. See text for discussion, sec. **IV.D.**
[b]Includes beta-hemolytic streptococci and viridans group streptococci.
[c]Includes cases in which there was no growth on routine bacterial cultures, routine bacterial cultures were not obtained, or microbiological information was not available.
Source: J. M. Steckelberg and D. R. Osman, Prosthetic Joint Infections. In A. L. Bisno and F. A. Waldvogel (eds.): *Infections Associated with Indwelling Medical Devices* (2nd ed.). Washington, D.C.: American Society for Microbiology, 1994. P. 266.

2. **Bone scans.** Recent studies of traditional three-phase ^{99m}Tc bone imaging concluded that this test was "limited in its ability to discern between infection and aseptic loosening as the incidence of false negative results is unacceptably high" [61; also quoted in ref. 56].

3. A summary of seven studies employing ^{111}**In-labeled autologous leukocytes** reported somewhat better results, with an average sensitivity of 79% and a specificity of 81% [62]. ^{111}In-labeled nonspecific IgG scintigraphy may be slightly better still (i.e., overall sensitivity of 97% and specificity of 85%), but both false positive and false negative results occur.

4. **Conclusion. Although useful, none of these tests is entirely satisfactory in defining whether joint sepsis is present in all cases.** Therefore, technetium bone scanning alone cannot usefully distinguish septic and aseptic loose prostheses [57a]. However, a positive scan may be highly suggestive of infection, which can then be confirmed by aspiration and/or biopsy. Gallium scanning has a high reported specificity, indicating that a positive result correlates well with confirmation of infection at aspiration or biopsy, but has a low sensitivity [57a].

C. **Laboratory studies**

1. **Aspiration of joint fluid and subsequent histologic and microbiologic examination of tissue samples obtained at surgery remain the tests of choice for a definitive diagnosis of prosthetic joint infection.** In one recent study, the sensitivity of fine-needle aspiration for detecting the infecting microorganism was 87% and its specificy was 95%, compared to biopsy cultures obtained at the time of surgery [63].

a. **Cultures should be obtained without recent antibiotic therapy.** Because of the critical importance of making a microbiologic diagnosis, in most nonacute cases, antimicrobial therapy should be withheld until all aspirate and/or intraoperative specimens have been obtained. If antimicrobial therapy has already been started, it should be stopped when possible for 10–14 days before any diagnostic procedure to avoid false negative culture results [56a].

b. **Good aerobic and anaerobic cultures** should be routinely processed. As much fluid for culture as possible should be obtained at the time of a diagnostic joint aspiration [56a]. For chronic, indolent infections, fungal and mycobacterial cultures are advised.

c. When prosthesis debridement or removal is performed, the surgeon should obtain multiple tissue samples for culture and histopathology. Intraoperative cultures should include **tissue** from the bone-cement interface, if possible, as well as samples of any purulence [56a]. In chronic infections, mycobacterial and fungal cultures are also advised.

d. **Histopathogic examination** for inflammation, granulomas, and tissue stains for organisms can be very useful.

e. Careful susceptibility studies should be performed on any bacterial pathogens isolated.

f. The predictive value of a single positive surveillance culture at the time of a revision arthroplasty for a failed prosthesis is unknown; such a result requires careful correlation with the clinical context [56a].

g. Cultures of drainage from sinus tracts do not reliably identify the etiologic microorganisms [56a, 57a].

2. **Blood cultures** should routinely be obtained (e.g., two or three samples drawn 30–60 minutes apart).

3. Nonspecific tests such as the ESR and C-reactive protein may be of limited value in raising the clinician's level of suspicion and diagnosing the initial infection or in monitoring the response to therapy.

D. In the recent Mayo Clinic summary **a definite prosthetic joint infection** was defined by at least one of the following criteria: (1) two or more cultures from sterile joint aspirates or intraoperative cultures were positive for the same organism; (2) purulence was observed at the time of surgical inspection; (3) acute inflammation consistent with infection was present on histopathologic examination of intracapsular tissue; or (4) a sinus tract that communicates with the joint spaces was present [56a].

V. **Therapy.** The **optimal approach** to treatment of the infected arthroplasty **remains unclear.** There are few randomized prospective studies reported, and virtually none compare different treatment arms within a single well-controlled study.

A detailed discussion of the infectious disease considerations of the different surgical approaches appears elsewhere [56a, 57a]. In order to consistently achieve microbiology cure, it is necessary to remove the prosthesis and all associated cement and completely debride devitalized tissue and bone. Issues about reimplantation that remain controversial include the optimal time to reimplantation, the role of antibiotic impregnated cement, the need for antibiotic-impregnated polymethylmethacrylate spacers (e.g., in two-stage reimplantation for total knee prosthetic infections), and the optimal type and duration of administration of intravenous and oral antimicrobials [56a]. **Therefore, we suggest close cooperation of the orthopedic surgeon and the infectious disease consultant in managing these patients.**

A. Nonetheless, **two-stage replacement,** involving removal of the hip or knee prosthesis and a 6- to 8-week course of intravenous antibiotic therapy followed by reimplantation, has been widely recommended [56, 60, 64]. Antibiotic-impregnated cement spacers commonly are used as adjunctive therapy in arthroplasty for replacement of the infected knee, in preparation for reimplantation. Success rates for microbiologic cure with this technique vary but average approximately 80–90%.

B. A growing number of reports have suggested that **implant salvage,** employing either antibiotic therapy alone or antibiotics plus surgical debridement, may be feasible in selected patients. This approach has evolved out of multiple concerns, not the least of which are the potential surgical and medical complications attending joint removal and reimplantation in the generally elderly patients, many of whom have other underlying medical illnesses as well as the risk factors outlined earlier.

   1. In addition, new antimicrobial regimens may cure infections that previously were believed to be untreatable without removal of the device [65]. Data from both animal models [65, 66] and human clinical trials now are available to support consideration of this approach. Treatment regimens combining rifampin with either quinolone or beta-lactam antibiotics can be particularly effective, with reported success rates of more than 80% in some studies [65, 66], although such success also has been reported in some series not employing such combinations [56, 67–70]. Treatment durations have generally been prolonged (e.g., ≥ 6–12 months).

   2. **As encouraging as these recent studies may be, enthusiasm must be tempered by numerous other studies demonstrating poorer outcomes (success rates only in the 20–40% range)** [56, 68, 69, 71–73]. The treatment of these infections is clearly evolving.

   3. **In our opinion, patients who might be considered for an attempt at implant salvage must meet at least the following criteria:** (1) A loosened prosthesis is not present. (2) The microorganism is susceptible to antibiotics, including oral antibiotics, that the patient can tolerate. (3) The patient is not septic, requiring immediate removal of the infected prosthesis. It should be recognized that cure rates using this approach appear to be higher with acute (generally defined as symptoms of less than 2–4 weeks' duration) as opposed to chronic infections. (4) Finally, the patient must understand that failure may necessitate, but does not preclude, standard therapy, including prosthesis removal and subsequent reimplantation, arthrodesis, resection arthroplasty, or other treatment options. In contradistinction to others [60, 69], we do not believe that infection with *S. aureus* represents a contraindication to this approach. Experience with gram-negative organisms is more limited.

C. **Debridement with retention of the prosthesis** procedures usually have been unsuccessful for chronic, well-established infections [56a]. For early acute infections (i.e., within less than 3 months of the primary surgery) in the presence of a draining, infected hematoma without cellulitis, thorough open surgical debridement, irrigation, and antibiotics may salvage up to 70% of prosthetic hip or knee replacements [57a]. Recently, delivery of high concentrations of antibiotic via implantable pumps has been used with promising success in acute prosthetic infections [57a]. Further evaluation and experience with this technique is needed.

D. **Suppressive antimicrobial therapy** without concomitant surgical intervention **is not considered standard therapy** for prosthetic joint infection since satisfactory functional outcomes are so low [57a]. In some situations, antibiotic suppression (long-term) is combined with initial surgical debridement with the goal of suppression of symptoms and maintenance of a functioning joint. This may be rational, and often the only option, in some carefully selected patients when (1) removal of the prosthesis is not feasible; (2) the organism is of low virulence and highly susceptible to oral antimicrobial agents; (3) the patient is not systemically ill; (4) the patient is compliant; and (5) the prosthesis is not loose [56a].

VI. **Postoperative superficial wound infection, a major risk for subsequent prosthesis infection.** Aggressive early local care and intravenous antibiotic therapy of these infections have been highly successful in preventing the involvement and removal of the prosthesis [72]. In view of the rapid evolution of treatment options in infections of prosthetic joints, infectious disease consultation is advised.

VII. **Prophylaxis** [74]. Antibiotic prophylaxis reduces the frequency of deep wound infection following total joint replacement, and short courses of cefazolin commonly are recommended (see Chap. 28). The use of operating rooms with ultraclean air has a similar effect. Antibiotic-impregnated cement may be equally as effective, but these data are more preliminary. **See related discussion in Chap. 28B.**

Infectious Bursitis

I. **Clinical presentation.** Septic bursitis usually involves the prepatellar or olecranon bursa of young to middle-aged men [75, 76].

A. **History.** The common background of most patients is **recent trauma** to the site or sustained or intermittent pressure or minor trauma associated with particular occupations (e.g., gardener, plumber, carpet layer, carpenter). Some individuals have a past history of such bursal diseases as gout, rheumatoid involvement, or bursitis of unknown etiology. Some cases of infection have developed after bursal corticosteroid injection for treatment of noninfectious bursitis [77].

1. **Pain** (in >90%) and **swelling** (in 100%) of the involved bursa may occur abruptly over a few hours or may be subacute in onset, often following minor local trauma by a few days [75]. Approximately 10% of patients deny pain or tenderness at initial presentation.

2. **Fever** occurs in approximately one-half of cases, and chills occur occasionally [75, 77].

3. **Prior intrabursal corticosteroid administration** is not uncommon in misdiagnosed cases. This can suppress the inflammatory process, delaying accurate diagnosis and therapy.

B. **Physical examination**

1. **Inflammatory changes occur.** The involved bursa usually is red, warm, tender, and locally distended. **These signs of inflammation are nonspecific and also can be seen in gout and traumatic bursitis.** Associated cellulitis with erythema is common in olecranon bursitis (74%), together with regional adenopathy [75]. Overall, local or distal skin disruption or infection is noted in more than 50% of patients with septic bursitis, although it is less common in cases of abrupt onset.

2. **Joint range of motion,** including rotation, usually is painless, except with full flexion and extension [76]. (This helps to exclude an associated septic arthritis, which would be associated with a marked decrease in range of motion.)

3. In some cases, a laceration or abrasion directly over the involved bursa can be identified.

4. Although the vast majority of cases of septic bursitis occur in the olecranon and prepatellar bursae, infection at other sites including the subdeltoid, iliopsoas, ischial, and trochanteric bursae may occur and require more aggressive imaging and drainage (i.e., CT-guided catheter or open surgical drainage) [78].

II. **Diagnostic aids. The definitive step in establishing the diagnosis is aspiration of the bursal fluid.**

A. **Bursal fluid aspiration.** On gross examination, the fluid can vary from thin, serous material to thick, bloody pus in variable amounts (from a few drops to 40 ml). Analysis reveals findings similar to those seen in septic joint fluids [75].

1. **Leukocyte counts** range from 1,500 to more than 400,000 cells/mm^3 (mean, approximately 75,000) with 52–97% polymorphonuclear leukocytes.

2. **Glucose levels** are variable, ranging from very low to normal.

3. **Gram staining** of the fluid will provide a presumptive etiologic diagnosis in approximately 65% of cases. The Gram stain is particularly important in patients who have received partial antibiotic therapy. In such cases, the smear may be positive and the culture negative.

4. **Urate crystal examination** of the fluid should be undertaken as both gout and infection can appear simultaneously, and gout alone may mimic a septic bursitis.

5. **Cultures** are important in tailoring antibiotic therapy. Few data are available on anaerobically caused septic bursitis, but routine aerobic cultures are essential.

B. **Blood cell count.** The peripheral WBC count and ESR range from normal to markedly elevated, and a leukocytosis greater than 10,000 cells/mm^3 is seen in approximately 60% of cases.

C. **Radiography.** Radiologic examination usually shows only soft-tissue swelling around the infected bursa; adjacent joints usually appear normal but can show evidence of rheumatoid arthritis, gout, or osteoarthritis.

D. **Blood cultures.** These rarely are positive when a single bursa is infected. Cultures should be obtained as an aid in defining concurrent infections elsewhere. It is speculated that in the bacteremic patient, distant bursae may be secondarily infected.

III. **Bacteriology of septic bursitis. *S. aureus* is involved in as many as 90% of cases** [75–77, 79], and the great majority of staphylococci are penicillin-resistant. ORSA or MRSA may be the pathogen in hospital-acquired infections. Streptococci are the next most common organism, especially group A beta-hemolytic strains. In two recent series, infections with gram-negative organisms also were reported [79]. Other, rarer causes of bursitis have been reported and include *M. tuberculosis* as well as atypical mycobacteria, *P. multocida* (after a cat scratch or bite), and certain fungi such as *Cryptococcus neoformans* or *Aspergillus* spp.

IV. **Differential diagnosis.** The bursae usually are closed spaces, and so infection does not imply involvement of the associated joint [75]. However, the suprapatellar bursa commonly communicates with the knee joint. Therefore, if the suprapatellar pouch is adequately drained, so is the knee joint.

A. **Septic arthritis.** The entire joint is usually swollen and inflamed. **The patient will complain of pain** either **with minimal motion of the joint** or throughout the range of motion, rather than solely at full flexion and extension, as is often seen in septic bursitis. Signs of joint effusion will be noted on the roentgenogram in septic arthritis.

B. **Gout and trauma.** The signs associated with septic bursitis are nonspecific and can be seen with gout, especially when the presentation is acute. With nonseptic traumatic bursitis, the fluid leukocyte count usually is less than 1,000 cells/mm^3, whereas it is always higher in septic bursitis. Regional lymphadenopathy and fever are both present in a minority of patients with septic bursitis and will help in distinguishing infection from cases of gout or trauma. **Examination of the fluid for crystals is essential to exclude gout.**

C. **Hemorrhagic olecranon bursitis. In uremic patients** on hemodialysis, this may mimic septic bursitis. In these patients, the bursitis is due to the trauma of local pressure or anticoagulation. It must be noted, however, that several patients reported to have septic bursitis also had renal insufficiency; aspiration and examination of the fluid, including culture, are therefore indicated.

V. **Therapy.** Appropriate therapy includes administration of antibiotics and provision of adequate drainage, which generally can be accomplished by repeated needle aspirations, although some patients will require surgical drainage.

A. **Antibiotics.** Because *S. aureus* (with occasional streptococcal cases) accounts for most cases, antibiotics must be active against *S. aureus*.

Whether therapy should be oral or routinely parenteral has not been fully established, and therapy must be individualized [76, 77]. Parenteral antibiotics and hospitalization generally are indicated to ensure a complete response to therapy in those with underlying host defects (e.g., diabetes mellitus, malignancy, rheumatic disease, renal disease), those undergoing corticosteroid therapy, and those with underlying bursal disease. **The clinical course in patients with underlying HIV infection may also prove refractory to conservative management, and initial parenteral therapy should be considered.** Those with associated cellulitis with systemic symptoms (e.g., fever) and those with radiographic evidence of contiguous joint abnormalities also should receive parenteral antibiotics and should be hospitalized for treatment.

In patients without underlying host defects and with mild disease (i.e., no cellulitis, no fever, and only localized bursal inflammation), oral antibiotics may be sufficient if adequate drainage is provided [80]. However, response to oral antimicrobial therapy alone may be protracted, even in such patients, and a large number of patients fail to respond [77, 80].

   1. **For therapy of known or highly suspected methacillin- (oxacillin-) susceptible S. aureus**

      a. **Parenteral therapy.** A semisynthetic penicillinase-resistant penicillin such as nafcillin or oxacillin, 1.0–1.5 g q4–6h, can be given to adults. In children, 100–150 mg/kg/day is given in divided doses q4–6h.

         In the patient with a delayed penicillin reaction, a cephalosporin commonly is used. Because the first-generation cephalosporins are more active against *S. aureus* than are the second- and third-generation cephalosporins, the first-generation agents are preferred (e.g., cefazolin, 1 g q8h in adults). Ideally, if the patient has a history of an acute, immediate reaction to a penicillin, the cephalosporins should be avoided unless skin testing can be performed (see Chap. 27). Alternative agents in this setting include vancomycin and clindamycin.

      b. **Oral therapy.** Antistaphylococcal agents such as dicloxacillin or cloxacillin, 500 mg qid, can be given to adults. In the adult patient with a delayed penicillin allergy, an oral cephalosporin such as cephalexin or cephradine, 500 mg–1 g qid, can be used and are often better tolerated than oral dicloxacillin or cloxacillin (see Chap. 28F). Oral clindamycin is another alternative agent that is especially useful in the patient with a mild infection and a history of an acute, immediate reaction to penicillin.

      c. **Intrabursal injection of antibiotics. This is not indicated.** Adverse local reactions have been noted when this route was used [75].

   2. **For ORSA or MRSA.** If these organisms are highly likely (e.g., hospital-acquired infection in dialysis patients colonized with MRSA) or are known to be the pathogen by culture, **vancomycin** is the parenteral agent of choice (see Chap. 28O for dosages). If the organism is susceptible to sulfonamides and these drugs are not contraindicated, trimethoprim-sulfamethoxazole is a possible oral agent, potentially combined with rifampin.

   3. **Duration of antibiotic therapy.** The optimal duration of therapy has not been clearly established. In general, antibiotics have often been administered for 14–21 days. Oral antibiotics usually have been used after initial therapy with, and response to, parenteral therapy.

   B. **Adequate drainage is essential** in all patients [75–77, 80]. If adequate drainage cannot be achieved rapidly by serial aspiration (daily or every other day), surgical drainage is indicated.

   C. Warm, moist **soaks** and **analgesics** are important ancillary measures.

VI. **Response to therapy.** With appropriate antibiotic therapy and adequate drainage, many patients respond rapidly, but others have a protracted resolution. Laboratory measurements useful in substantiating clinical and bacteriologic response are the peripheral leukocyte count and ESR (if initially elevated) and, more specifically, repeat analyses of the bursal fluid, with demonstration of conversion of cultures from positive to negative. Bursal fluid leukocyte counts usually decrease with therapy, but the percentage of cells that are polymorphonuclear leukocytes can remain high.

Intervertebral Disc Space Infections

Intervertebral disc space infections (IVDSIs) usually involve lower thoracic and lumbar spaces and appear to arise in two ways. **In children, a hematogenous seeding** of the space is most likely. However, by the third decade, vascularization of the disc space is no longer demonstrable [81]. Most cases of IVDSI **in adults** occur in the **postoperative setting,** with a variable period prior to onset of clinical disease [82], or **after discography** [83]. Spontaneous infections do occur and have recently been reviewed [83a].

It must be noted that there is substantial controversy in the pediatric literature concerning **inflammation (diskitis) versus infection (IVDSI) of vertebral discs in children** [81, 84]. Although some careful studies have found positive blood or disc biopsy cultures (usually isolating *S. aureus*) in half of the patients from whom culture material has been obtained, other studies have found few positive cultures and have reported resolution of illness without antimicrobial therapy. Studies both advocating and questioning a bacterial etiology of diskitis have noted a significant percentage of cases with no bacterial etiology established but with evidence of viral infection either prodromally or early in the disease course. Some reports have described the presence of antecedent trauma in up to one-third of cases, but its role in causation of diskitis has not been adequately assessed. It may be that diskitis represents a broad spectrum ranging from inflammatory or viral involvement to IVDSI to pyogenic vertebral osteomyelitis. **However, at this time, prevailing opinion holds that diskitis is a low-grade bacterial infection** and that failure to obtain positive cultures may be due to sterilization of the area by host defenses between the onset of symptoms and biopsy [85, 85a].

I. **Presentation.** Fever and other systemic signs of infection may be absent in as many as 50% of the patients, both children and adults. Children may be more likely than adults to develop fever unexplained by other intercurrent childhood illnesses. When present, fever can vary from low-grade elevation to high-spiking temperatures.

   A. **Children.** In the child, the **onset** of diskitis is **gradual and subtle.** The presenting symptom is most commonly **back pain,** occasionally with associated difficulties in ambulation. In very young children, however, irritability or refusal to ambulate may be as specific a presentation as can be expected. Children may complain of pain referred to the hip or leg or may show signs suggesting meningeal irritation or an abdominal pathology severe enough to prompt laparotomy [84].

   B. **Adults.** The adult patient most commonly presents with **back pain** that often recurs **after** initial relief of back and leg pain by the **surgical procedure for disc protrusion.** Muscle spasm may be a prominent feature. **It is important to recognize that, by the time of onset of symptoms due to IVDSI, the operative site most often is healed and presents no visible sign of infection** [86]. One retrospective study found histopathologic and clinical evidence of diskitis in 7 of 432 patients who had undergone diskography. Bacteria were isolated from the discs of three of the four patients biopsied less than 6 weeks after diskography [83].

II. **Diagnosis.** There are two laboratory investigations that are of substantial aid in determining the likelihood of IVDSI: the ESR and roentgenographic examination. Needle aspiration can establish the diagnosis.

   A. **ESR and CBC**
      1. **Elevation of the ESR occurs in 90–100% of cases** in both children and adults and is commonly the earliest, and sometimes the only, laboratory abnormality seen [84, 86]. **Any postdiskectomy patient with increasing back pain and an ESR greater than 50 at 2 or more weeks after surgery should be considered to have diskitis until proven otherwise** [87]. The ESR generally may be used as an indicator of therapeutic response, but occasionally it remains elevated for months.
      2. The total leukocyte and differential blood cell counts are normal in 50% or more of patients. These counts, if appreciably elevated or shifted to the left, may suggest extension of infection to structures contiguous to the disc space.

   B. **Roentgenography.** The **hallmark** of IVDSI **is** the roentgenographic finding of **disc space narrowing.** This change may not be present until 2–3 weeks after onset of infection [81] and, if roentgenograms are negative in a potential case, the examination should be repeated after an additional 2–3 weeks. Displacement of vertebrae may occur, and oblique views as well as routine views of the spine should be obtained. Tomography may be helpful.

      Erosion of the vertebral end plates usually follows the narrowing, occurring by 3–5 weeks after onset. This process may give a sawtooth appearance and may progress to destruction of the entire plate and vertebral body. Alternatively, pronounced narrowing of the disc space, with sclerosis, may be the final result.

   C. **Scans**
      1. Experience suggests that ^{99m}**Tc** bone scans may be very useful in establishing an early and accurate diagnosis; such scans are positive in many cases within 7 days of onset [84] and in nearly all cases after 2 weeks of back pain. In one study, false negative results primarily were seen after less than 2 weeks of back pain, but all cases were identified correctly by ^{67}**Ga** bone scanning [88].
      2. There are conflicting reports as to the usefulness of **CT scanning** in making an early diagnosis of diskitis [89, 90]. Disc space narrowing and adjacent bone involvement may appear prior to changes on plain roentgenograms. CT scanning offers greater accuracy than radionuclide scanning in depicting adjacent soft-tissue pathologic processes.

3. Diskitis also gives rise to characteristic changes apparent by **MRI,** with an accuracy of diagnosis similar to radionuclide scans. MRI also provides anatomic information about the adjacent thecal sac and spinal cord not shown by radionuclide scans. A recent prospective, blinded study employing gadolinium-enhanced MRI found that changes in signal intensity in the intervertebral disc space and adjacent marrow are uncommon after routine diskectomy; all seven biopsy and culture-proven diskitis patients had a triad of MRI findings consisting of gadolinium enhancement of the adjacent vertebral bone marrow, disc space, and posterior annulus fibrosus; none of 15 asymptomatic postdiskectomy patients exhibited these changes [90]. **MRI may also be superior to CT scanning** in providing finer resolution of the interface between the disc and adjacent bone [91, 92].

D. **Blood cultures** should be routinely obtained. They are more likely to be positive if the patient is seen early in the course. If they are positive, especially in a child with *S. aureus* infection, a diagnostic needle aspiration may be avoided.

E. **Needle aspiration** of the disc space is the ideal way to obtain material for culture (aerobic, anaerobic, and mycobacterial), **particularly in postoperative diskitis,** so that a specific etiologic diagnosis can be made. In some studies, this procedure has provided culture data on the etiologic agent for as many as 85% of cases in which it was performed. Aspirations should be performed before antibiotic therapy is started. However, it has now become common practice to treat children with uncomplicated diskitis without first performing a culture [85]. A skin test for tuberculosis is recommended.

F. **Operative site wound cultures** are merely superficial cultures in most cases and may reflect colonizing organisms rather than true pathogens. Such cultures can be misleading.

III. **Microbiologic features.** *S. aureus* is the most common pathogen involved, particularly in young patients [81]. In the postoperative setting, a wide spectrum of bacterial etiologies can be found.

A. **Children (with hematogenous seeding).** In those cases in which a bacterial etiology is established, more than 90% are due to *S. aureus* [81, 84]. Streptococci are implicated occasionally.

B. **Adults (with postoperative IVDSI)** [86]

1. *S. aureus* is the most common organism isolated.

2. *S. epidermidis* **and enteric gram-negative bacteria** have been found on needle aspiration cultures [83]. Because the presence of these organisms would directly affect the choice of antibiotic therapy, the importance of a needle aspiration and cultures prior to antibiotic therapy is emphasized.

IV. **Differential diagnosis**

A. **Children**

1. **Acute pyogenic osteomyelitis.** The clinical presentation of this illness may be very similar to that of IVDSI. Osteomyelitis is discussed in Chap. 16 under Special Forms of Osteomyelitis.

2. **Traumatic changes.** Trauma preceding IVDSI appeared to be relatively uncommon. In cases where it has preceded onset, it may merely have served to bring the child to medical attention. A battered child may present with disc space narrowing.

3. **Tuberculous vertebral osteomyelitis.** Changes in this disease occur at a slower rate than in bacterial infections. In general, by the time roentgenographic evidence of IVDSI is present, a negative chest roentgenogram and a negative reaction to intermediate purified protein derivative of tuberculosis (PPD) in the nonanergic patient are helpful in excluding the diagnosis of tuberculosis. A positive skin test does not establish the diagnosis, and a diagnostic aspiration and biopsy are indicated in this setting. (See discussion in Chap. 16 under Special Forms of Osteomyelitis.)

4. **Paraspinal abscess and spinal cord tumor.** These occur less commonly but should be considered, particularly if there are associated neurologic deficits.

B. **Adults.** IVDSI most often has to be differentiated from failure of disc surgery and recurrent herniation, and consideration of such possibilities often leads to a delay in establishing the diagnosis. The diagnostic possibilities discussed in sec. **A** should be considered in the adult patient when there is no prior history of surgery.

V. **Therapy**

A. **Children.** Although diskitis is presumed to be of bacterial etiology in most cases, outcome has generally been reported to be the same whether or not the patient receives antibiotics [93]. **Because no controlled, prospective studies have been done, recommendations for treatment remain controversial.**

1. Many authorities now recommend **a trial of immobilization of the spine,** generally with a body cast, as the key to providing relief of pain [84, 85]. The duration of immobilization may be guided primarily by response of the pain and, secondarily, by changes in the ESR and roentgenograms but is generally in the range of 4 weeks.

2. A reasonable recommendation is that **a child who fails to respond to immobilization should receive intravenous antibiotic therapy,** usually with a first-generation cephalosporin or semisynthetic penicillinase-resistant penicillin for 5–7 days, followed by 7–14 days of an analogous oral antistaphylococcal antibiotic [85]. Generally, 3–4 weeks of antibiotic therapy have been successful. Studies in adults undergoing diskectomy have demonstrated therapeutic levels of cefazolin in the disc within 15–80 minutes after IV drug administration [94].

   a. **Dosages.** Oxacillin or nafcillin, 100–200 mg/kg/day IV, divided and given at 4- to 6-hour intervals, is recommended.

   b. In the **penicillin-allergic patient,** if not contraindicated (see Chap. 28F), a first-generation cephalosporin can be used (e.g., cefazolin, 60–100 mg/kg/day [or its equivalent] IV at 6- to 8-hour intervals).

B. **Adults**

1. **Antibiotic therapy** in adults is more difficult to define because of the wide spectrum of organisms involved in postoperative IVDSI. **Ideally, therapy is guided by results of the Gram stains and by eventual culture information from the diagnostic needle aspiration.**

   a. **For infections with gram-positive cocci, antistaphylococcal therapy** is indicated initially. If methicillin resistance is not likely, a semisynthetic penicillin (oxacillin or nafcillin), 6–12 g/day IV, will treat *S. aureus.* A first-generation cephalosporin or clindamycin can be used in the penicillin-allergic patient.

      For hospitals with a significant incidence of MRSA, intravenous vancomycin can be used at least until susceptibility data are available.

   b. **If gram-negative bacteria are involved,** a cephalosporin or a penicillinase-resistant penicillin (or vancomycin if MRSA is a concern) plus an aminoglycoside should be used while one is awaiting culture results. If *S. aureus* is not found on culture, antibiotics can be adjusted according to the sensitivities of the isolated gram-negative organism. See Chap. 28 for a discussion of the potential roles of new agents such as aztreonam, imipenem-cilastatin, and ciprofloxacin.

   c. **The importance of diagnostic aspirations cannot be overemphasized as gram-negative organisms can be involved.** If the patient refuses such a procedure, or if technically it cannot be performed, a broad-spectrum antibiotic (e.g., a cephalosporin such as ceftriaxone) or a penicillinase-resistant penicillin plus an aminoglycoside (gentamicin, tobramycin, amikacin) are possible options. The role of fluoroquinolones in this setting is unclear. Infectious disease consultation is suggested in these difficult cases.

      If the patient on an empiric regimen fails to show some evidence of clinical improvement by 2–3 weeks, aspiration to obtain tissue for culture will be required to exclude infection with a drug-resistant organism.

   d. If cultures (aspiration) are negative, therapy directed at *S. aureus* should be continued.

2. **The appropriate duration of antibiotic therapy is ill-defined.** Antibiotics probably should be continued at least 4–6 weeks. Any associated wounds should be healed. The ESR may be monitored [81]. If initially elevated, the ESR usually will decrease with appropriate therapy, but at times this is delayed. Antibiotics are continued until there is roentgenographic evidence of bone healing.

3. **Associated surgical wounds need adequate drainage and debridement as indicated.** Some advocate treatment for several days with appropriate antibiotic therapy after initial cultures (aspiration) and before repeat surgical intervention.

4. **Immobilization** often is accomplished using a plaster cast or Stryker frame. The duration of immobilization is determined partially by the response of the pain to therapy and by the tolerance of the patient. Ordinarily, immobilization is used during the initial part of therapy (i.e., the first 2–3 weeks).

5. Repeat surgery

    a. For those not responding to the regimen of antibiotics as just outlined and to immobilization (as measured by diminished pain, roentgenographic improvement, and declining ESR), surgery will be necessary to obtain tissue for cultures to exclude resistant organisms as well as to provide adequate drainage. It is important to obtain cultures on exploration, even if overt pus is not evident.

    b. Early operation is controversial. Some experts believe that infection is slow to subside with the preceding conservative approach and that early surgical drainage of the intervertebral disc space shortens disability and hastens recovery [86].

VI. Prognosis

    A. Children. It appears that in children the disease is fairly short-lived and carries a good prognosis. Extension of the infection to contiguous tissue or metastatic sites is relatively uncommon.

    B. Adults. Recovery can be prolonged in postoperative IVDSI patients who do not have an additional surgical procedure.

References

1. Garcia-Kutzbach, A., and Masi, A.T. Acute infectious agent arthritis (IAA): A detailed comparison of proved gonococcal and other blood-borne bacterial arthritis. *J. Rheumatol.* 1:93, 1974.

2. Goldenberg, D.L., and Reed, J.L. Bacterial arthritis. *N. Engl. J. Med.* 312:764, 1988.

2a. Smith, J.W., and Piercy, E.A. Infectious arthritis. *Clin. Infect. Dis.* 20:225, 1995.
   Recent article from "state-of-the-art" series. For a recent textbook chapter review, see C. Norden, W.J. Gillespie, and S. Nade, Infectious Arthritis. In Infections in Bones and Joints. Boston: Blackwell, 1994. Chap. 18.

3. Kraft, S.M., Panush, R.S., and Longley, S. Unrecognized staphylococcal pyarthrosis with rheumatoid arthritis. *Semin. Arthritis Rheum.* 14:196, 1985.

4. Ward, J.R., and Atcheson, S.G. Infectious arthritis. *Med. Clin. North Am.* 61:313, 1977.

5. Epstein, J.H., Zimmermann, B., and Ho, G. Polyarticular septic arthritis. *J. Rheumatol.* 13:1105, 1986.
   The subset of patients with polyarticular infection superimposed on underlying rheumatoid arthritis may have a higher mortality.

6. Fink, C.W., and Nelson, J.D. Septic arthritis and osteomyelitis in children. *Clin. Rheum. Dis.* 12:423, 1986.

7. Delbarre, F., et al. Pyogenic infection of the sacroiliac joint: Report of thirteen cases. *J. Bone Joint Surg. [Am.]* 57:819, 1975.

8. Saag, K.G., and Naides, S.J. Practical management for suspected viral arthritis. *Contemp. Intern. Med.* 5:35, 1993.
   Succinct reference with useful case presentations, photographs, and tables outlining the diagnosis and management of the various viral arthritides.

9. Naides, S.J. Parvovirus B19 infection. *Rheum. Dis. Clin. North Am.* 19:457, 1993.

10. Enarson, D.A., et al. Bone and joint tuberculosis: A continuing problem. *Can. Med. Assoc. J.* 120:139, 1979.

11. Messner, R.P. Arthritis due to Mycobacteria, Fungi, and Parasites. In D.C. McCarty and W.J. Koopman (Eds.). *Arthritis and Allied Conditions: A Textbook of Rheumatology* (12th ed.). Philadelphia: Lea & Febiger, 1993. Chap. 118.

12. Granfors, K., et al. *Yersinia* antigens in synovial fluid cells from patients with reactive arthritis. *N. Engl. J. Med.* 320:216, 1989.
   See editorial comment, "Do bacteria cause chronic polyarthritis?" by John A. Mills, in the same issue. Approximately 2% of patients who have Yersinia enterocolitica infection, especially those positive for HLA-B27, develop a persistent polyarthritis.

13. Shmerling, R.H., et al. Synovial fluid tests: What should be ordered? *J.A.M.A.* 264: 1009, 1990.

14. Merritt, K., et al. Counterimmunoelectrophoresis in the diagnosis of septic arthritis caused by *Haemophilus influenzae*. *J. Bone Joint Surg. [Am.]* 58:414, 1976.

15. Nocton, J.J., et al. Detection of *Borrelia burgdorferi* DNA by polymerase chain reaction in synovial fluid from patients with Lyme arthritis. *N. Engl. J. Med.* 330:229, 1994.

16. Hendrix, R.W., and Fisher, M.R. Imaging of septic arthritis. *Clin. Rheum. Dis.* 12: 459, 1986.

17. Horgan, J.G., et al. Scintigraphy in the diagnosis and management of septic sacroili-itis. *Clin. Radiol.* 34:337, 1983.
    Report of five cases. The value of scanning in pyogenic sacroiliitis.
18. Guyot, D.R., Manoli, A., and Kling, G.A. Pyogenic sacroiliitis in IV drug abusers. *A.J.R.* 149:1209, 1987.
    Sensitivity of technetium 99 bone scans was 100%, whereas plain radiographs were normal in half the patients in this small series.
19. Ouzounian, T.J., et al. Evaluation of musculoskeletal sepsis with indium 111 white blood cell imaging. *Clin. Orthop.* 221:304, 1987.
20. Wukich, D.K., et al. Diagnosis of infection by preoperative scintigraphy with indium-labeled white blood cells. *J. Bone Joint Surg. [Am.]* 69:1353, 1987.
21. Goldenberg, D.L., and Cohen, A.S. Synovial membrane histopathology in the differential diagnosis of rheumatoid arthritis, gout, pseudogout, systemic lupus erythematosus, infectious arthritis, and degenerative joint disease. *Medicine* 57:239, 1978.
22. Dan, M. Septic arthritis in young infants: Clinical and microbiologic correlations and therapeutic implications. *Rev. Infect. Dis.* 6:147, 1984.
23. Welkon, C.J., et al. Pyogenic arthritis in infants and children: A review of 95 cases. *Pediatr. Infect. Dis.* 5:669, 1986.
24. Wilson, N.I.L., and DiPaola, M. Acute septic arthritis in infancy and childhood. *J. Bone Joint Surg. [Br.]* 68:584, 1986.
25. Nade, S. Acute septic arthritis in infancy and childhood. *J. Bone Joint Surg. [Br.]* 65:234, 1983.
26. Green, N.E., and Edwards, K. Bone and joint infections in children. *Orthop. Clin. North Am.* 18:555, 1987.
27. Herndon, W.A., et al. Management of septic arthritis in children. *J. Pediatr. Orthop.* 6:576, 1986.
27a. Jackson, M.A., et al. The changing face of childhood pyogenic arthritis: Implications for therapy. *Infectious Disease Society of America 33rd Annual Meeting.* San Francisco, CA: Sept. 1995 (abstract 433).
    In the pre H. influenzae b vaccine era (1980–1985), 42% of cases were due to H. influenzae. In recent years, with the increasing use of this vaccine, the incidence of disease due to this pathogen has fallen dramatically: 1986–1988 (29% incidence), 1989–1991 (21%), and 1992–1994 (0%)!
28. Baker, D.G., and Schumacher, H.R., Jr. Acute monoarthritis. *N. Engl. J. Med.* 329: 1013, 1993.
    Comprehensive review emphasizing the extensive differential diagnosis but also reviewing antibiotic therapy and issues of surgical versus medical drainage.
28a. Jackson, L.A., et al. Risk factors for group B streptococcal disease in adults. *Ann. Intern. Med.* 123:415, 1995.
    For a related paper, see M.M. Farley et al., A population-based assessment of invasive disease due to group B streptococcus in nonpregnant adults. N. Engl. J. Med. 328: 1807, 1993.
29. Lam, K., and Bayer, A.S. Serious infections due to group G streptococci. Report of 15 cases with in vitro–in vivo correlations. *Am. J. Med.* 75:561, 1983.
30. Small, C.B., et al. Group B streptococcal arthritis in adults. *Am. J. Med.* 76:367, 1984.
30a. Raymond, N.J., Henry, J., and Workowski, K.A. Enterococcal arthritis: Case report and review. *Clin. Infect. Dis.* 21:516, 1995.
    Enterococci can cause infections in native as well as prosthetic joints. Careful susceptibility studies should be performed.
31. Bayer, A.S., et al. Gram-negative bacillary septic arthritis: Clinical, radiographic, therapeutic, and prognostic features. *Semin. Arthritis Rheum.* 7:123, 1977.
32. Brook, I., and Frazier, E.H. Anaerobic osteomyelitis and arthritis in a military hospital: A 10-year experience. *Am. J. Med.* 94:21, 1993.
33. Dubost, J.-J., et al. Polyarticular septic arthritis. *Medicine* 72:296, 1993.
    Large review detailing the microbiology, underlying host risk factors, and generally poorer prognosis when compared to monoarticular septic arthritis.
34. Deighton, C. β haemolytic streptococci and reactive arthritis in adults. *Ann. Rheum. Dis.* 52:475, 1993.
35. Kingsley, G.H. Reactive arthritis: A paradigm for inflammatory arthritis. *Clin. Exp. Rheumatol.* 11(Suppl. 8):S29, 1993.
36. Rahman, M.U., Schumacher, H.R., and Hudson, A.P. Recurrent arthritis in Reiter's syndrome: A function of inapparent chlamydial infection of the synovium? *Semin. Arthritis Rheum.* 21:259, 1992.

37. Silveira, L.H., et al. Chlamydia-induced reactive arthritis. *Rheum. Dis. Clin. North Am.* 19:351, 1993.
38. Calabrese, L.H. Human immunodeficiency virus (HIV) infection and arthritis. *Rheum. Dis. Clin. North Am.* 19:477, 1993.
38a. Gran, J.T., et al. The variable clinical picture of arthritis induced by human parvovirus B19: Report of seven adult cases and review of the literature. *Scand. J. Rheumatol.* 24:174, 1995.
39. Rynes, R.I. Painful rheumatic syndromes associated with human immunodeficiency virus infection. *Rheum. Dis. Clin. North Am.* 17:79, 1991.
40. Bayer, A.S., and Guze, L.B. Fungal arthritis. *Semin. Arthritis Rheum.* 8:142, 200, 1978–1979, and 9:66, 145, 218, 1979–1980.
    Detailed review of candidal, coccidioidal, sporotrichal, blastomycetic, cryptococcal, and histoplasmal arthritis.
41. Meier, J.L., and Hoffman, G.S. Mycobacterial and Fungal Infections. In W.N. Kelley et al. (eds.), *Textbook of Rheumatology* (4th ed.). Philadelphia: Saunders, 1993. Pp. 1467–1483.
    A recent review of this topic.
42. Kalish, R. Lyme disease. *Rheum. Dis. Clin. North Am.* 19:399, 1993.
43. Rahn, D.W. Lyme disease—where's the bug? [editorial]. *N. Engl. J. Med.* 330:282, 1994.
44. Shrestha, M., Grodzicki, R.L., and Steere, A.C. Diagnosing early Lyme disease. *Am. J. Med.* 78:235, 1985.
45. Lyme disease—Connecticut. *M.M.W.R.* 37:1, 1988.
46. Dattwyler, R.J., et al. Treatment of late Lyme borreliosis—randomized comparison of ceftriaxone and penicillin. *Lancet* 1:1191, 1988.
    Ceftriaxone may be superior to high-dose penicillin in patients with Lyme disease–associated neurologic and rheumatologic disease.
46a. Tachdjian, M.O. Acute Transient Synovitis of the Hip. In *Pediatric Orthopedics* (2nd ed.). Philadelphia: Saunders, 1990. Pp. 1461–1465.
47. Broy, S.B., and Schmid, F.R. A comparison of medical drainage (needle aspiration) and surgical drainage (arthrotomy or arthroscopy) in the initial treatment of infected joints. *Clin. Rheum. Dis.* 12:501, 1986.
    Excellent review of this controversial topic that supports the initial use of medical therapy to manage the acutely infected joint, with surgical drainage reserved for failure of medical management or for initial drainage of hip infections in which needle aspiration is difficult.
48. Cooper, C. Bacterial arthritis in the elderly. *Gerontology* 32:222, 1986.
49. Nelson, J.D. Antibiotic concentrations in septic joint effusions. *N. Engl. J. Med.* 284:349, 1971.
50. Parker, R.H., and Schmid, F.R. Antibacterial activity of synovial fluid during therapy of septic arthritis. *Arthritis Rheum.* 14:96, 1971.
51. Centers for Disease Control. 1993 Sexually transmitted diseases treatment guidelines. *M.M.W.R.* 42 (RR-14):1–102, 1993.
    In these treatment guidelines, gonococcal arthritis is treated similarly to disseminated gonococcal infection. These guidelines are also sumarized in Drugs for sexually transmitted diseases. Med. Lett. Drugs Ther. 37:117, 1995.
52. Syrogiannopoulos, G.A., and Nelson, J.D. Duration of antimicrobial therapy for acute suppurative osteoarticular infections. *Lancet* 1:37, 1988.
    See related discussion by V.Ph. Syriopoulou and A.L. Smith, Osteomyelitis and Septic Arthritis. In R.D. Feigin and J.D. Cherry (eds.), Textbook of Pediatric Infectious Diseases (3rd ed.). Philadelphia: Saunders, 1992. P. 733.
53. Black, J., et al. Oral antimicrobial therapy for adults with osteomyelitis or septic arthritis. *J. Infect. Dis.* 155:968, 1987.
54. Mikhail, I.S., and Alarcon, G.S. Nongonococcal bacterial arthritis. *Rheum. Dis. Clin. North Am.* 19:311, 1993.
55. Vincent, G.M., and Amirault, J.D. Septic arthritis in the elderly. *Clin. Orthop.* 251:241, 1990.
56. Wilde, A.H. Management of infected knee and hip prostheses. *Curr. Opin. Rheum.* 5:317, 1993.
    One of the best recent reviews of this topic.
56a. Steckelberg, J.M., and Osman, D.R. Prosthetic Joint Infection. In A.L. Bisno and F.A. Waldvogel (eds.), *Infections Associated with Indwelling Medical Devices* (2nd ed.).

Washington, D.C.: American Society of Microbiology, 1994. Chap. 11.
This is an excellent discussion.

57. Wymenga, A.B., et al. Perioperative factors associated with septic arthritis after arthroplasty: Prospective multicenter study of 362 knee and 2,651 hip operations. *Acta Orthop. Scand.* 63:665, 1992.
    One of the largest studies available on this topic.

57a. Norden, C., Gillespie, W.J., and Nade, S. Infections in Total Joint Replacement. In *Infections in Bones and Joints.* Boston: Blackwell, 1994. Chap. 17.

58. Wymenga, A.B., et al. Prosthesis-related infection: Etiology, prophylaxis and diagnosis (a review). *Acta Orthop. Belg.* 56:463, 1990.
    One of the most comprehensive reviews available on this topic.

59. Lidwell, O.M., et al. Effect of ultraclean air in operating rooms on deep sepsis in the joint after total hip or knee replacement: A randomised study. *Br. Med. J.* 285:10, 1982.

60. Paya, C.V., Wilson, W.R., and Fitzgerald, R.H., Jr. Management of infection in total knee replacement. *Cur. Clin. Top. Infect. Dis.* 9:222–240, 1988.
    Concise review of this difficult problem.

61. Levitsky, K.A., et al. Evaluation of the painful prosthetic joint. *J. Arthroplasty* 6: 237, 1991.

62. Cuckler, J.M., et al. Diagnosis and management of the infected total joint arthroplasty. *Orthop. Clin. North Am.* 22:523, 1991.

63. Ross, A.C. Infections complicating joint replacement and other orthopedic conditions. *Curr. Opin. Rheum.* 5:461, 1993.

64. Fitzgerald, R.H., Jr. Infections of hip prostheses and artificial joints. *Infect. Dis. Clin. North Am.* 3:329, 1989.

65. Widmer, A.F., et al. Antimicrobial treatment of orthopedic implant–related infections with rifampin combinations. *Clin. Infect. Dis.* 14:1251, 1992.
    Early results of an ongoing prospective study showing excellent outcomes in selected patients with orthopedic implant–related infections treated with the implant left in situ.

66. Drancourt, M., et al. Oral rifampin plus ofloxacin for treatment of *Staphylococcus*-infected orthopedic implants. *Antimicrob. Agents Chemother.* 37:1214, 1993.
    Satisfactory rates of cure demonstrated in this large series of patients with orthopedic device–related infections treated with oral ofloxacin and rifampin with the device left in situ.

67. Davenport, K., Traina, S., and Perry, C. Treatment of acutely infected arthroplasty with local antibiotiocs. *J. Arthroplasty* 6:179, 1991.

68. Hartman, M.B., et al. Periprosthetic knee sepsis: The role of irrigation and debridement. *Clin. Orthop.* 273:113, 1991.

69. Rand, J.A. Alternatives to reimplantation for salvage of the total knee arthroplasty complicated by infection. *J. Bone Joint Surg.* 75-A:282, 1993.

70. Goulet, J.A., et al. Prolonged suppression of infection in total hip arthroplasty. *J. Arthroplasty* 3:109, 1988.

71. Schoifet, S.D., and Morrey, B.F. Treatment of infection after total knee arthroplasty by debridement with retention of the components. *J. Bone Joint Surg.* 72-A:1383, 1990.

72. Rasul, A.T., Jr., Tsukayama, D., and Gustilo, R.B. Effect of time of onset and depth of infection on the outcome of total knee arthroplasty infections. *Clin. Orthop.* 273: 98, 1991.
    In total knee arthroplasty patients, superficial infections, not extending to the joint, were treated successfully with antibiotics without joint removal.

73. Burger, R.R., Basch, T., and Hopson, C.N. Implant salvage in infected total knee arthroplasty. *Clin. Orthop.* 273:105, 1991.

74. Norden, C.W. Antibiotic prophylaxis in orthopedic surgery. *Rev. Infect. Dis.* 13(Suppl. 10):S842, 1991.
    Detailed review of the use of antibiotic prophylaxis in orthopedic procedures either involving or not involving prosthetic devices. Relevant data are presented summarizing antibiotic use during dental procedures in individuals with implantable devices.

75. Ho, G., Jr., Tice, A.D., and Kaplan, S.R. Septic bursitis in the prepatellar and olecranon bursae: An analysis of 25 cases. *Ann. Intern. Med.* 89:21, 1978.

76. Ho, G., Jr., and Mikolich, D.J. Bacterial infection of the superficial subcutaneous bursae. *Clin. Rheum. Dis.* 12:437, 1986.
    Excellent review that emphasizes 89–90% of these infections are due to Staphylococcus aureus. *The olecranon and prepatellar bursae were the most common sites of infection.*

77. Raddatz, D.A., Hoffman, G.S., and Franck, W.A. Septic bursitis: Presentation, treatment and prognosis. *J. Rheumatol.* 14:1160, 1987.

78. Chartash, E.K., et al. Septic subdeltoid bursitis. *Semin. Arthritis Rheum.* 22:25, 1992.
79. Pien, F.D., Ching, D., and Kim, E. Septic bursitis: Experience in a community practice. *Orthopedics* 14:981, 1991.
80. Ho, G., Jr., and Su, E.Y. Antibiotic therapy of septic bursitis. *Arthritis Rheum.* 24: 905, 1981.
81. Boston, H.C., Jr., Bianco, A.J., Jr., and Rhodes, K.H. Disc space infections in children. *Orthop. Clin. North Am.* 6:953, 1975.
82. Dall, B.E., et al. Postoperative discitis. Diagnosis and management. *Clin. Orthop.* 224:138, 1987.
83. Fraser, R.D., Osti, O.L., and Vernon-Roberts, B. Discitis after discography. *J. Bone Joint Surg. [Br.]* 69:26, 1987.
83a. Honan, M., et al. Spontaneous infectious discitis in adults. *Am. J. Med.* 100:85, 1996.
Spontaneous infectious discitis (i.e., no prior surgery or instrumentation) is an uncommon cause of low back pain in adults. If blood cultures are negative, percutaneous disc aspiration for culture is advised. MRI was the most sensitive imaging technique.
84. Wenger, D.R., Bobechko, W.P., and Gilday, D.L. The spectrum of intervertebral disc-space infection in children. *J. Bone Joint Surg. [Am.]* 60:100, 1978.
Diskitis as an infectious process.
85. Cushing, A.H. Diskitis in children. *Clin. Infect. Dis.* 17:1, 1993
Superb review of the many controversies surrounding the etiology and management of this condition, including guidelines for immobilization and antibiotic therapy.
85a. Norden, C., Gillespie, W.J., and Nade, S. Vertebral osteomyelitis and disk space infections. In *Infections in Bones and Joints.* Boston: Blackwell, 1994. Chap. 14.
Authors hypothesize that the same sequence of events may account for both vertebral osteomyelitis and diskitis; therefore, they represent different points in the balance between infecting organisms and host defenses.
86. El-Gindi, S., et al. Infection of intervertebral discs after operation. *J. Bone Joint Surg. [Br.]* 58:114, 1976.
87. Bircher, M.D., et al. Discitis following lumbar surgery. *Spine* 13:98, 1988.
88. Nolla-Sole, J.M., et al. Role of technetium-99m diphosphonate and gallium-67 citrate bone scanning in the early diagnosis of infectious spondylodiscitis. A comparative study. *Ann. Rheum. Dis.* 51:665, 1992.
89. Price, A.C., et al. Intervertebral disk-space infection: CT changes. *Radiology* 149: 725, 1983.
90. Boden, S.D., et al. Postoperative diskitis: Distinguishing early MR imaging findings from normal postoperative disk space changes. *Radiology* 184:765, 1992.
Provides useful guidance in discriminating between routine postoperative changes and those related to diskitis as delineated by MRI.
91. Modic, M.T., Masaryk, T., and Paushter, D. Magnetic resonance imaging of the spine. *Radiol. Clin. North Am.* 24:229, 1986.
92. Hyman, R.A., and Gorey, M.T. Imaging strategies for MR of the spine. *Radiol. Clin. North Am.* 26:505, 1988.
93. Jansen, B.R.H., Hart, W., and Schreuder, O. Discitis in childhood: 12–35-year follow-up of 35 patients. *Acta Orthop. Scand.* 64:33, 1993.
94. Boscardin, J.B., et al. Human intradiscal levels with cefazolin. *Spine* 17(Suppl. 6): S145, 1992.

16

Osteomyelitis and Diabetic Foot Infections

Rathel L. Nolan
and Stanley W. Chapman

Osteomyelitis

Osteomyelitis is an inflammatory process in bone and bone marrow. This condition is most often caused by pyogenic bacteria but may also be due to other microorganisms, including mycobacteria and fungi. Multiple classification schemes have been devised.

I. **Acute versus chronic osteomyelitis.** This clinical distinction sometimes is difficult to make. The following definitions provide a useful separation with implications in therapy and prognosis [1]:

A. **Acute** cases are those in their **first presentation.** The history may be short (days for hematogenous osteomyelitis) or long (weeks to months for contiguous osteomyelitis).

B. **Chronic** osteomyelitis cases are those that have relapsed in a site of previously identified disease. Chronic osteomyelitis is more difficult to treat successfully and carries a poorer prognosis. Surgical intervention usually is required.

II. **Pathogenic classification.** The most useful clinical classification is based on pathogenesis, as outlined by Waldvogel and coworkers [1].

A. **Hematogenous osteomyelitis** results from bacteremia seeding bone.

B. **Contiguous-focus osteomyelitis** is caused by spread from an adjacent area of infection, as in postoperative infections; direct inoculation from trauma; or extension from an area of soft-tissue infection.

C. **Peripheral vascular disease–associated osteomyelitis** usually occurs in patients with diabetes with or without large-vessel insufficiency.

III. **Other classifications.** Other classification systems are based on special circumstances such as (1) a unique age group (neonatal osteomyelitis), (2) a unique clinical setting (e.g., intravenous drug use or sickle cell disease), (3) the microbiologic cause (gram-negative, anaerobic, etc.), or (4) an unusual anatomic location (e.g., vertebral osteomyelitis). A clinicopathologic classification proposed by Cierny and colleagues [2] facilitates comparison of therapeutic outcomes in human case studies and experimental infections. Some of these special areas are discussed separately in this chapter.

IV. **The changing spectrum of osteomyelitis.** Previously, osteomyelitis usually was hematogenous and was most common in children. *Staphylococcus aureus* caused 80–90% of cases. Reviews emphasize a change in the disease presentation [1, 3–6]. Hematogenous osteomyelitis is decreasing in frequency and more commonly involves older patients, often in association with prosthetic devices. There has also been an increase in unusual bacterial causes, including gram-negative bacilli, anaerobes, and mixed infections.

Hematogenous Osteomyelitis

Hematogenous osteomyelitis occurs most often in rapidly growing bone, which explains the increased frequency among children. Recent series note an increasing frequency in older patients, so that the age distribution is bimodal [4–6]. Hematogenous osteomyelitis may occur in any bone, but the long bones—femur, tibia, and humerus—are most frequently involved in children. Older patients tend to have more vertebral involvement.

I. **Pathophysiology and patient age.** The pathophysiology and clinical presentation are age-related [7].

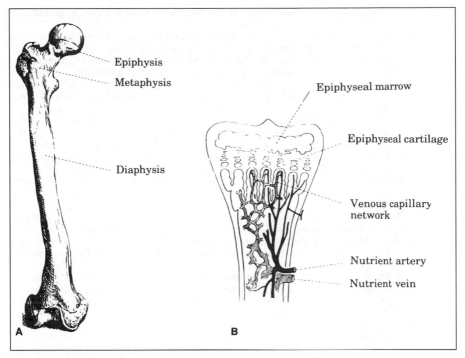

Fig. 16-1. A. Femur, showing diaphysis, metaphysis, and epiphysis. B. Vascular supply of a long bone in the area of the metaphysis and epiphysis. (From F. A. Waldvogel et al., Osteomyelitis: A review of clinical features, therapeutic considerations, and unusual aspects. *N. Engl. J. Med.* 282:198. Copyright 1970, Massachusetts Medical Society.)

A. **Children.** In children 1–16 years of age, disease is most frequent in the metaphysis of long bones (Fig. 16-1). This is believed to result from sluggish blood flow through a sinusoidal venous system, a deficiency of phagocytic cells in this region, and poor collateral circulation. The susceptibility of this region to trauma may also play a role. A history of antecedent trauma may be obtained in 30% of patients with hematogenous osteomyelitis. It is unclear whether this is a true cause-and-effect relationship [8].

  1. **Anatomic considerations.** In childhood, there are no anastomotic vascular channels between the metaphyseal and epiphyseal circulation (see Fig. 16-1). The epiphyseal growth plate acts as a barrier, resulting in the spread of infection laterally and rupture of the cortex into the subperiosteal space, with subsequent subperiosteal abscess formation.

     When infection has reached the subperiosteal space, it may spread longitudinally along the shaft of the bone or rupture through the periosteum. Separation of the bone from the periosteum is accompanied by exuberant periosteal growth and new bone formation. This circumferential new bone covering is referred to as an **involucrum.**

  2. **Sequestrum.** In the course of the infection, segments of bone may lose vascular supply owing to such factors as increased pressure, acidic pH, and effects of leukocytic enzymes. Such an area of **devitalized bone** is referred to as a *sequestrum.* These areas must be surgically removed because they **act as foreign bodies** and will prevent effective antibiotic therapy.

  3. **Associated septic arthritis.** As previously noted, the epiphyseal growth plate serves as a barrier to the spread of infection. In children, osteomyelitis complicated by septic arthritis occurs only in joints in which the metaphysis is intracapsular, such as the proximal femur and proximal humerus.

B. **Neonates and infants younger than 1 year**

  1. **Septic arthritis is common.** In contrast to older children, at this age anastomotic channels exist between the metaphyseal and epiphyseal circulations.

> **Infection may spread rapidly to the epiphysis and joint space, resulting in septic arthritis** (see Fig. 16-1).

2. Involvement of the epiphyseal growth plate may result in growth deformities.
3. The metaphyseal cortex is immature. Spreading exudate rapidly reaches the periosteum and ruptures it, infecting the surrounding periosteal tissues. This accounts for the frequent soft-tissue abscesses found in this age group.

C. **Adults.** Hematogenous osteomyelitis is less common in adults. Initial localization is to the subchondral region of bone, and the vertebrae are most commonly involved.

1. **Anatomic considerations.** In adults, vascular connections between metaphyseal and epiphyseal vessels result after resorption of the growth cartilage. Spread of infection to the joint space by this route can occur. The periosteum is bound tightly to bone and has less osteoblastic activity than that in children, so that subperiosteal abscess and involucrum formation are unusual.
2. **Vertebral osteomyelitis.** This is most common in adults 50 years of age and older and accounts for the bimodal age distribution of hematogenous osteomyelitis.

D. **Special considerations**

1. **Sickle cell disease.** The bone infarcts and marrow thrombosis that complicate this hemoglobinopathy predispose to bacterial localization in bone. Osteomyelitis at multiple sites is common. *Salmonella* spp. are the most common pathogens [8, 9].
2. **Intravenous drug users and hemodialysis patients.** Repeated intravascular injections in intravenous drug users and vascular access infections in hemodialysis patients result in an increased frequency of hematogenous osteomyelitis [10–12].

II. **Microbiologic features**

A. **Staphylococci**

1. *S. aureus* remains the most common pathogen, but the percentage of hematogenous osteomyelitis due to *S. aureus* has declined from 80–90% of cases in the past to 40–60% in recent years [4–6]. In a recent report in children, *S. aureus* was isolated in 64% of patients [12a].
2. *Staphylococcus epidermidis* reportedly causes approximately 5% or fewer cases of disease. It should be considered a pathogen when recovered from a reliable source, such as bone biopsy.

B. **Streptococci**

1. **Group A** streptococcal isolates cause disease in children and occasionally in adults.
2. **Group B** streptococci are common in neonates and may be a more common pathogen in this age group than are staphylococci [13]. Group B streptococci also occur in diabetic patients.

C. *Haemophilus influenzae* causes age-related disease. It incites osteomyelitis in infants and children, particularly those younger than 6–8 years. Passive maternal antibody affords some protection in infants younger than 6 months. Universal vaccination of children in the United States against this pathogen has diminished its importance as a cause of osteomyelitis as invasive infections (e.g., bacteremia) decline in vaccinated populations. In a recent report, there was a dramatic decline in septic arthritis due to *H. influenzae* b in recipients of the conjugated vaccine [13a] (see Chap. 22).

D. **Gram-negative enteric bacilli** (e.g., *Escherichia coli, Salmonella* and *Klebsiella* spp.) most often occur in adults and account for 10–15% of cases of hematogenous osteomyelitis. **Certain patient groups are predisposed** to hematogenous osteomyelitis caused by gram-negative organisms: neonates (Enterobacteriaceae), patients with sickle cell disease (*Salmonella*), and intravenous drug users (*Pseudomonas*). Patients with underlying chronic illness—including chronic renal disease, alcoholism, diabetes, and malignancy—also have an increased risk of gram-negative infections [14].

E. **Anaerobes** are uncommon causes of hematogenous osteomyelitis [15].

F. **Polymicrobial infections** can occur [16].

G. **Mycobacteria,** particularly tuberculosis, can cause vertebral osteomyelitis. This entity is discussed in sec. **IV** under Special Forms of Osteomyelitis.

H. **Fungi** can cause an indolent form of osteomyelitis and may have a propensity to involve bones of the feet or hands and the vertebrae. For further discussion, see sec. **V** under Special Forms of Osteomyelitis. Individual fungal infections are also discussed in Chap. 18. Osteomyelitis due to *Candida* is the subject of a report by Gathe and colleagues [17].

III. **Clinical manifestations.** The classic presentation of sudden onset of bone pain and toxicity with high fever, rigors, and diaphoresis is reported less commonly now than in past reviews of osteomyelitis [4–6, 17a]. Several factors are responsible for this change: (1) the increasing incidence of osteomyelitis due to spread from a contiguous focus of infection or associated with vascular disease; (2) the inclusion in many series of patients with chronic disease; (3) the increasing frequency of vertebral osteomyelitis, which is usually an insidious disease in adults; and (4) the early antibiotic management of extraosseous bacterial infections and extensive perioperative antibiotic therapy, which may modify the clinical course of bone infection. Even in cases of childhood hematogenous osteomyelitis, atypical presentations are becoming more common, and uncommon sites are noted more frequently [18].

A. **Acute symptoms.** Most patients with acute hematogenous osteomyelitis present with symptoms of less than 3 weeks' duration. Children and infants may be symptomatic for less than 1 week. In a recent report, the median duration of symptoms in children prior to presentation was 3 days [12a].

1. **Localized signs and symptoms** include pain, limitation of motion of the involved extremity, soft-tissue swelling, erythema, warmth, and point tenderness over the involved area.

2. **Systemic manifestations** are seen in 50% or fewer patients. They may include fever, chills, night sweats, malaise, anorexia, and weight loss.

3. **Minimal, vague symptoms** may be reported by as many as 40% of patients for 1–2 months. This indolent course is likely in the following situations:

a. **Primary subacute pyogenic osteomyelitis (Brodie's abscess).** This is characterized by the indolent formation of abscess, most frequently occurring at the metaphysis of long bones. Local pain is the most common presenting symptom [19].

b. **Vertebral osteomyelitis** in the adult. See sec. **II** under Special Forms of Osteomyelitis.

c. **Pelvic osteomyelitis.** The presenting symptoms for this condition may be unusual, including abdominal pain, gait disturbance, and sciatica [20, 21].

B. **Neonatal osteomyelitis.** This often poses a difficult diagnostic problem. Soft-tissue swelling, localized tenderness, and decreased motion of an extremity (pseudoparalysis) are the most common findings. See Chap. 3, sec. **VI.A** under Selected Specific Infections in the Newborn, for further discussion.

C. **Sickle cell disease.** The **diagnosis** of osteomyelitis in these patients is **challenging,** because the clinical signs and symptoms mimic those associated with an acute pain crisis. For this reason, **blood cultures should always be obtained in patients presenting with an apparent acute sickle pain crisis.**

IV. **Diagnosis.** Various cultural, hematologic, serologic, and radiographic procedures are helpful in making a clinical diagnosis and substantiating the etiology of disease. It is no longer reasonable to assume that most cases of hematogenous osteomyelitis are due to *S. aureus* and so to direct therapy to this pathogen only. **Vigorous attempts at isolating the etiologic agent are required** to optimize therapy and minimize potential antibiotic toxicity. The diagnostic aids available are applicable to all forms of osteomyelitis.

A. **Blood cultures** should be drawn in all patients with suspected osteomyelitis. Approximately 50% of patients with acute hematogenous osteomyelitis have positive blood cultures. Neonatal osteomyelitis very often is associated with bacteremia. Blood cultures are less likely to be positive in other forms of osteomyelitis, such as contiguous-focus disease, chronic osteomyelitis, and osteomyelitis associated with peripheral vascular disease. In general, two to four separate sets of blood cultures should be drawn.

B. **Leukocytosis** can occur, but normal or minimally elevated leukocyte counts are common and cannot be used as evidence against the diagnosis of osteomyelitis.

C. **The erythrocyte sedimentation rate** (ESR) may be normal early in the disease but usually will rise as the disease progresses. A normal ESR does not exclude the diagnosis. An elevated ESR provides an excellent parameter by which to monitor therapeutic response, as the ESR progressively declines with successful therapy.

D. **Radiographic evaluation** is very helpful, but the radiologic changes may lag days to weeks behind the clinical presentation. Magnification views and tomograms may be of value. Correct radiologic interpretation requires correlation with the clinical time course. The usual sequence of radiologic changes is as follows:
   1. **Roentgenograms are normal** early in the disease course. Bone scans may detect abnormalities at this stage. However, if bone destruction is present, no further imaging may be necessary [21a].
   2. **Soft-tissue swelling and subperiosteal elevation** are the earliest abnormalities. These findings may be subtle and may not appear until 10–14 days after onset of symptoms. Serial radiographic examinations may be required.
   3. **Lytic changes** on roentgenography do not appear until 30–50% of bone has been removed and usually are not detectable until approximately 2–6 weeks after the onset of disease.
   4. **Sclerotic changes** appear weeks after onset of illness owing to delay in mineralization after new matrix formation. Sclerotic changes associated with periosteal new bone formation (involucrum) denote a more chronic process.
   5. **Other diseases** may involve bone primarily or secondarily and result in osteomyelitis-like changes on radiographs. These include (1) chronic venous stasis of the lower extremities, with periosteal reaction involving the tibia; (2) osteoid osteoma; and (3) neoplasms involving bone.
E. **Radionuclide scanning** is most helpful early in the course of acute disease, prior to the development of roentgenographic changes. Positive scans may be seen as early as 24 hours after the onset of symptoms [22].
   1. Scanning with **technetium** radiophosphates is most commonly employed, especially the **three-phase scans.** Radiation exposure approximates that of a standard roentgenogram and is not contraindicated in pediatric patients. Because of the possibility of referred pain or multicentric disease, whole-body images should be obtained in patients with suspected osteomyelitis. More detailed radiographic examination of suspicious areas may then be obtained. Other processes, such as primary and metastatic tumor, osteonecrosis, arthritis, cellulitis, and abscess, may cause false positive examinations. Radionuclide scans remain highly sensitive but are of low specificity. Their use in children has recently been reviewed [21a], and scintigraphy is preferred to magnetic resonance imaging for the initial evaluation of a child with suspected osteomyelitis.
   2. Gallium citrate scans, and indium-labeled leukocyte scans may be helpful in complicated cases [23]. Scans employing an indium-labeled monoclonal antibody against neutrophils provide comparable information to scans with indium-labeled leukocytes but without the labor-intensive leukocyte harvesting and labeling. Radionuclide scans with indium-labeled nonspecific immunoglobulin have been successful in defining focal inflammation in a variety of clinical conditions, including osteomyelitis. Serial immunoglobulin scans have proven helpful in confirming persistence or recurrence of infection in some patients [23–25].
F. **CT scanning** provides excellent images of bone cortex and is used for biopsy localization. The recent trend is to use **MRI,** which is considered the best modality to identify soft-tissue infection, distinguish between cellulitis and abscess, and differentiate bone marrow and soft-tissue involvement. **MRI is particularly useful in the diagnosis of vertebral osteomyelitis** [26], complications from vertebral or pelvic bone osteomyelitis, and/or infections that fail to respond to appropriate antibiotic therapy and may need some type of surgical intervention [21a]. See sec. **II.E.6** under Special Forms of Osteomyelitis.
G. **Needle aspirations** of soft-tissue collections, subperiosteal abscesses, and intraosseous lesions to obtain culture material often are diagnostic. Many authors consider such procedures routine in evaluating patients with osteomyelitis.

   In hematogenous osteomyelitis, the blood cultures may provide the identity of the etiologic agent in many cases. Needle aspiration should be strongly considered in patients who do not respond to initial therapy within 72 hours and in whom gram-negative organisms are suspected.

   In vertebral osteomyelitis, needle aspiration is performed prior to any antibiotic therapy. See sec. **II.E** under Special Forms of Osteomyelitis.
H. **Joint fluid analysis** should be undertaken if there is an associated joint effusion. The aspirated effusion should be analyzed for cellular content, chemistries, Gram stain, and culture. (See Chap. 15, sec. **II.A** under Infectious Arthritis.)

I. **Open biopsy** is indicated in patients in whom response to therapy is unusually slow or incomplete or in situations in which tuberculosis, fungi, metastatic tumor, or Ewing's tumor (which may clinically and radiographically mimic osteomyelitis) is suspected. Biopsy material should be submitted for histopathologic examination with special stains for bacteria, acid-fast bacilli, and fungi. Aerobic, anaerobic, mycobacterial, and fungal cultures should be done.

V. **Initial therapy.** Initial therapy should be aggressive. Inadequate therapy of acute osteomyelitis may result in relapse and development of chronic disease.

A. **Principles of antibiotic use** [27–35]. Antibiotics are the mainstay of therapy. Special aspects of their use in this disease are discussed here.

1. **Parenteral agents** usually are preferred initially to ensure compliance and optimal bone levels. They are given in high doses so that high blood levels are attained, thereby ensuring adequate penetration of bone [27]. Although it is difficult to compare the results of the many studies regarding antibiotic penetration of bone, certain generalizations can be made (see sec. **2**).

a. Antibiotic levels in bone are higher than the minimal inhibitory concentration of most susceptible organisms likely to be encountered with the penicillins (including antistaphylococcal penicillins), the cephalosporins, gentamicin, vancomycin, and clindamycin [27].

(1) Antibiotic levels in diseased bone are higher than in normal bone.

(2) Antibiotic penetration is related to the vascularity of the bone. Cancellous bone levels are higher than cortical bone levels.

(3) In relation to serum levels, clindamycin penetrates bone best. Ciprofloxacin penetrates bone well also.

b. Despite these data, **it should be emphasized that the level of antibiotic penetration into bone is low.** Therefore, when penicillins are used, high-dose therapy (i.e., > 10 million units of penicillin, or nafcillin, 9 g/day in adult patients) is recommended.

2. **Oral antibiotic therapy**

a. **Children.** It is now common practice to treat selected cases of acute hematogenous osteomyelitis in children with oral antibiotics after an initial short course of parenteral therapy. Oral therapy is appealing from the standpoint of patient comfort, economy, and decreased risk of intravenous catheter-related thrombophlebitis and bacteremia. Patients are treated with an initial course of parenteral therapy, usually 5–10 days. After a favorable clinical response is noted, the patient is switched to high-dose oral therapy, which is continued, on average, for 3 weeks. Published studies have demonstrated therapeutic results comparable to those seen with intensive parenteral therapy [30–35]. **Several aspects of oral therapy deserve special emphasis.**

(1) The **causative organism** must be available for study. Pathogens obtained from blood culture or surgical specimens must be saved by the microbiology laboratory for bactericidal testing.

(2) Appropriate surgical debridement or drainage must be performed.

(3) **Compliance must be ensured.** In many studies, the entire course of therapy was administered in an inpatient setting [31, 32]. If therapy is on an outpatient basis, counseling of the patient and family, written instructions, and frequent follow-up are advised. If there is any doubt as to the patient's strict compliance with therapy, outpatient treatment must be abandoned [30].

(4) **Serum bactericidal levels** must be monitored to ensure adequate GI absorption and adequate serum concentrations. **If this monitoring cannot be done, conventional parenteral regimens are necessary.** Higher than usual doses of oral antibiotics are necessary to achieve adequate serum levels [32–35].

(5) **Published studies report success in treating patients without significant underlying diseases** [32–35]. The causative agents were generally susceptible *S. aureus* or streptococci. Oral therapy should not be attempted in a compromised host or a patient with a pathogen that is more difficult to eradicate, such as a gram-negative bacterium. However, there is an increasing body of data to support the use of **oral quinolones as therapy for gram-negative osteomyelitis in adults** [36, 37], as discussed later.

(6) Prolonged follow-up is needed as disease may recur years after an apparent cure.

b. **Adults.** Oral therapy is used in selected cases in adults, applying the same principles as outlined for children. Clindamycin has been very useful in a compliant patient with susceptible *S. aureus* osteomyelitis.

For patients with susceptible gram-negative pathogens, oral ciprofloxacin may allow one to shorten the course of intravenous antibiotics once a clinical response has been achieved with intravenous therapy and any surgical debridement performed. For example, in a patient with a susceptible *E. coli* osteomyelitis, after initial therapy with intravenous antibiotics and in the presence of susceptible strains, oral ciprofloxacin can be used to complete a 6-week total course of antibiotics and dramatically shorten the patient's hospital stay and need for intravenous therapy.

3. **Bactericidal agents** are preferred because fewer effective host defense mechanisms exist in bacterial infections. The exception to this generalization is clindamycin. Although it is usually considered bacteriostatic, it penetrates bone well and in high concentrations may function as a bactericidal agent against susceptible gram-positive cocci.

4. **Synergistic combinations** of antibiotics may be required for some gram-negative organisms, especially *Pseudomonas aeruginosa* or other *Pseudomonas* spp., and particularly for pathogens not susceptible to the fluoroquinolones.

5. **In vitro susceptibility** studies performed against the causative organism aid in the selection of appropriate therapy. **Careful susceptibility studies are particularly important in this disease owing to the prolonged therapy required.** Antibiotic combinations, which may have additive toxicities, are best avoided unless clearly indicated based on susceptibility data. This again emphasizes the need to obtain the etiologic pathogen for susceptibility studies.

6. **Use of serum bactericidal levels to monitor** therapeutic efficacy is a controversial issue. In this technique the patient's serum is obtained immediately prior to and after antibiotic administration. Serial dilutions of the serum then are tested for bactericidal activity against the offending pathogen. It was hoped that this test might predict therapeutic success or failure early in the course of treatment. The real value of the test is unknown, owing to lack of a standardized protocol and absence of large clinical studies to support its use. In one prospective multicenter study using a standardized protocol, the test was able to predict clinical outcome. Trough titers of 1:2 or greater were predictive of cure, whereas lower levels were associated with failure. Peak titers had no predictive value [28] (see Chap. 25).

7. **Prolonged therapy** for acute hematogenous osteomyelitis is important. Antibiotics must be administered for a minimum of 3–4 weeks. Whether longer courses of therapy add any benefit has not been determined.

a. Cure rates of greater than 90% are expected in patients who are given intravenous antibiotics for longer than 3 weeks. Relapse rates of 15–20% occur in patients who receive parenteral therapy for less than 3 weeks [1, 29] (see sec. **VI**).

b. Administration of oral antibiotics does not improve outcome when given as follow-up therapy in patients receiving adequate courses of parenteral therapy for acute osteomyelitis.

8. **Evaluation of initial therapeutic response.** Failure of the patient to show clinical improvement within 48–72 hours should prompt reevaluation. Diagnostic and therapeutic surgery may be necessary.

B. **Initial therapy while awaiting cultures**

1. **Adults**

a. After appropriate cultures are obtained, antistaphylococcal therapy, usually with a penicillinase-resistant semisynthetic penicillin, is recommended for cases of uncomplicated hematogenous osteomyelitis (Table 16-1). In patients with histories of delayed penicillin reactions, a cephalosporin may be used. In patients with histories of immediate penicillin reactions, either clindamycin or vancomycin may be used.

In settings in which methicillin-resistant *S. aureus* (MRSA) is a serious consideration (e.g., after or during a protracted hospitalization, after a documented MRSA bacteremia), intravenous vancomycin would be appropriate while awaiting cultures and susceptibility data. Community-acquired MRSA infection is unusual.

Table 16-1. Empiric initial therapy of the seriously ill patient with acute osteomyelitis

Patient age	Likely pathogens	Therapy[a]
Neonates and infants <2 months old	*Staphylococcus aureus,* enteric gram-negative bacilli, group B streptococci	Penicillinase-resistant semisynthetic penicillin (PRSP) (e.g., oxacillin, nafcillin, or methicillin)[b,c] and an aminoglycoside
Children		
Without associated hemoglobinopathy	*S. aureus* (also *Haemophilus influenzae* in children <6 years old)	PRSP in children >6 years. In those <6 years, cefuroxime or PRSP and ampicillin; a third-generation cephalosporin with or without PRSP[c,d]
With associated hemoglobinopathy	*S. aureus, Salmonella* spp., and *H. influenzae* in children <6 years old	PRSP and ampicillin; cefuroxime; a third-generation cephalosporin with or without PRSP[c]
Adults	*S. aureus* and enteric gram-negative bacilli in high-risk patients[e]	PRSP. In high-risk patients, PRSP and an aminoglycoside; or a third-generation cephalosporin with or without PRSP[e,f]

[a]Dosages are discussed in Table 16-2 and in Chaps. 3 and 28.
[b]Nafcillin should be avoided in the premature and in the very young infant, as the child's hepatic excretion may be deficient. If on Gram staining (of a needle aspiration of the involved bone) gram-negative organisms are seen, ampicillin and an aminoglycoside are initially suggested. See Chap. 3.
[c]In the patient with a history of delayed penicillin allergy, a first-generation cephalosporin is substituted for a PRSP. In a patient with immediate allergy to penicillin, vancomycin or clindamycin may be substituted.
[d]The best initial approach while awaiting culture results has not yet been determined. If *H. influenzae* is highly suspected and ampicillin-resistant strains are prevalent, these organisms must be adequately treated while awaiting cultures. (See sec. **V.B.2** under Hematogenous Osteomyelitis.) Cefuroxime alone or a third-generation cephalosporin (e.g., ceftriaxone), alone or with a PRSP (to ensure optimal *S. aureus* therapy), are suggested. Presumably, young children who are recipients of the *H. influenzae* b conjugate vaccine are less likely to have had invasive bacteremic disease due to this pathogen and therefore are less likely to have osteomyelitis due to this pathogen. See text discussion.
[e]High-risk patients include intravenous drug users, hemodialysis patients, diabetics, and patients with underlying debilitating diseases.
[f]A third-generation cephalosporin (e.g., ceftriaxone), with or without a PRSP (to ensure optimal *S. aureus* therapy), may be used in patients in whom an aminoglycoside is contraindicated or undesirable and in whom *Pseudomonas* spp. are not suspected. If MRSA is a concern, intravenous vancomycin can be used while awaiting susceptibility data.

    b. **When gram-negative organisms are suspected** (see sec. **II.D**), **biopsies for culture** should be performed **prior to administration of antibiotics.** If urgent empiric therapy is required, an aminoglycoside plus an antistaphylococcal agent may be used. A third-generation cephalosporin may also be used as single-agent therapy (see Table 16-1) [38, 39].

  2. **Children.** *S. aureus* remains the most common pathogen in children. *H. influenzae* occasionally causes infections in young children, especially in those between 3 months and 6 years of age who have not received the *Haemophilus* type b conjugate vaccine. In younger children, empiric therapy should be directed at

both *S. aureus* and *H. influenzae*. In children older than 6 years, antistaphylo-coccal therapy is used (see Table 16-1).

The optimal empiric antibiotic regimen in the child younger than 6 years has not yet been determined. A penicillinase-resistant penicillin (e.g., oxacillin or nafcillin) with ampicillin can be used. The cephalosporins also are used in this setting. Cefuroxime, a second-generation cephalosporin, appears to have consistent activity against *H. influenzae* and maintains good activity against *S. aureus*. The third-generation cephalosporins, including cefotaxime, ceftizoxime, and ceftriaxone, are very active against ampicillin-susceptible and ampicillin-resistant *H. influenzae* but are less active against *S. aureus* (see Chap. 28F).

In patients with sickle cell disease, ampicillin has often been used together with a semisynthetic penicillin, owing to these patients' predilection for *Salmonella* infections.

C. **Specific antibiotics and alternatives for commonly used agents** (Table 16-2). The potential roles for new agents, such as aztreonam, imipenem-cilastatin, or the oral fluorinated quinolones, are reviewed in Chap. 28.

Table 16-2. Therapy of osteomyelitis directed at specific pathogens

Pathogen	Antibiotic of choice[a,b]	Alternative antibiotics[c]
Staphylococcus aureus		
Penicillin-susceptible	Aqueous penicillin G (adults: 16–20 million units/day; children: 200,000–300,000 units/kg/day)	Cephalosporin (e.g., cefazolin) (adults: 4 g/day; children: 100 mg/kg/day); or cephalothin (adults: 9–12 g/day; children: 75–100 mg/kg/day)[d] Clindamycin (adults: 1.8–2.4 g/day; children: 20–40 mg/kg/day)
Penicillin-resistant	Penicillinase-resistant semisynthetic penicillin (e.g., nafcillin or oxacillin) (adults: 9–12 g/day; children: 200 mg/kg/day)	First-generation cephalosporin or clindamycin[e] or vancomycin[f]
Methicillin-resistant	Vancomycin (adults: 2 g/day; children: 40 mg/kg/day)	
Streptococcus pyogenes (group A streptococci)	Aqueous penicillin G (adults: 12–18 million units/day; children: 200,000–300,000 units/kg/day)	First-generation cephalosporin or clindamycin[e] or vancomycin[f]
S. agalactiae (group B streptococci)	Aqueous penicillin G (as for group A streptococci)[g]	First-generation cephalosporin[e] or vancomycin[f]
S. pneumoniae[h]		
Penicillin-susceptible	Aqueous penicillin G (as for group A streptococci)	First-generation cephalosporin[e]
Penicillin-resistant	Ceftriaxone or cefotaxime; vancomycin[f]	
Haemophilus influenzae		
Beta-lactamase-negative	Ampicillin (adults: 8–12 g/day; children: 100–200 mg/kg/day)	Cefuroxime, a third-generation cephalosporin[i]; trimethoprim-sulfamethoxazole[j]

Table 16-2 (continued)

Pathogen	Antibiotic of choice[a,b]	Alternative antibiotics[c]
Haemophilus influenzae (cont.)		
Beta-lactamase-positive	Ceftriaxone[i] or cefotaxime[i] or cefuroxime[i]	Trimethoprim-sulfamethoxazole[j]
Salmonella spp.	Ceftriaxone[j] or cefotaxime[j]	Trimethoprim-sulfamethoxazole[j]; ampicillin; fluoroquinolone[c]
Pseudomonas aeruginosa	Aminoglycoside (e.g., tobramycin or gentamicin) with ticarcillin or piperacillin or similar agent[k]	Ciprofloxacin[l]
Escherichia coli	Ampicillin (as for *H. influenzae*) for susceptible strains; cephalosporin for ampicillin-resistant but cephalosporin-susceptible strains[m]	Cephalosporin,[m] fluoroquinolone[c]
Klebsiella pneumoniae	A cephalosporin[m,n]	Fluoroquinolone[c]; aminoglycoside
Bacteroides fragilis	Metronidazole or clindamycin[e]	Ampicillin-sulbactam,[c] imipenem,[c] or cefoxitin[c]
Anaerobic and microaerophilic streptococci	Aqueous penicillin G (as for streptococci)	First-generation cephalosporin[e] or cefoxitin

[a]The daily intravenous dosage recommendations listed are for patients with normal renal function, adults and children older than 4 weeks. See Chap. 3 for dosage recommendations in neonates and infants younger than 4 weeks. See Chap. 28 for a further discussion of antibiotics.

[b]In general, high-dose therapy administered intravenously is recommended for patients with acute osteomyelitis. See text for length of therapy and the role of oral antibiotics in the different categories of disease.

[c]The potential roles of new agents—ciprofloxacin or aztreonam for gram-negative aerobic infections and imipenem-cilastatin, ampicillin with sulbactam, and piperacillin-tazobactam, or ticarcillin with clavulanate for mixed infections—are discussed in Chap. 28.

[d]The first-generation cephalosporins are more active against *S. aureus* than are the second- and third-generation cephalosporins.

[e]In dosages shown for penicillin-susceptible *S. aureus*.

[f]In dosages shown for methicillin-resistant *S. aureus*.

[g]Many experts favor synergistic antibiotic killing of group B streptococci, using penicillin (or ampicillin) plus an aminoglycoside. The higher dosage of penicillin is advised.

[h]Penicillin-resistant isolates are becoming more frequent. Susceptibility studies should be performed on blood or bone isolates. For a detailed discussion of this topic, see Chap. 28C.

[i]Although the second-generation cephalosporin, cefamandole, is active in vitro against *H. influenzae*, its activity is variable and therefore not advised. Cefuroxime is active against *H. influenzae* without an inoculum effect. The third-generation cephalosporins are exquisitely active against both ampicillin-susceptible and ampicillin-resistant *H. influenzae*. Dose regimens are discussed in Chap. 28F.

[j]For dosages, an infectious disease consultation is suggested. See Chap. 28.

[k]An aminoglycoside and a penicillin derivative active against *P. aeruginosa* are used together for synergy. Amikacin may be necessary for more resistant strains. Dosages and monitoring of aminoglycosides are discussed in Chap. 28H. Dosages and possible advantages of one penicillin derivative over another are discussed in Chap. 28E.

[l]Ciprofloxacin may be useful and prevent extended hospitalization in puncture wound osteomyelitis in adults. This drug should not be used in children, teenagers, and pregnant women. Infectious disease consultation is recommended. See discussion in Chap. 28S.

[m]Further study is needed to determine the best cephalosporin in this setting. Because of the excellent activity of the third-generation cephalosporins against these bacteria, the third-generation agents may be preferred in osteomyelitis even if the causative organism is susceptible to a first- or second-generation cephalosporin. The third-generation cephalosporins are discussed in detail in Chap. 28F.

[n]It is unclear whether an aminoglycoside is necessary for synergy. Infectious disease consultation is suggested.

D. Surgery. There is controversy with regard to the importance of early surgical intervention in the treatment of acute hematogenous osteomyelitis [40]. The differences of opinion result from the variability of the cases cited in the literature and center around the adequacy of antibiotic treatment, duration of symptomatic disease prior to therapy, age of the patient, bones involved, and causative organism.

1. **Most cases of hematogenous osteomyelitis, when treated with appropriate and adequate doses of antibiotics, are cured without surgery.** Outcomes are better if therapy is begun within 3–5 days of the onset of symptoms. It is, nonetheless, important for an orthopedic surgeon to follow these patients to help assess the future need for surgery.

2. **Indications for surgery** include the following:

   a. **Diagnosis.** In patients with possible gram-negative osteomyelitis, unusual presentation, or poor clinical response, surgery can substantiate the diagnosis of osteomyelitis, and appropriate cultures can be obtained. Diagnostic aspiration should be routinely performed in vertebral osteomyelitis unless blood cultures provide the pathogen.

   b. **Hip joint involvement** (osteomyelitis of the femoral metaphysis). Drainage needs to be done early in these cases because of the likelihood of rupture of the cortex and spread of infection into the hip joint.

   c. **Neurologic complications** of vertebral or cranial osteomyelitis. See sec. II.D.3 under Special Forms of Osteomyelitis.

   d. **Poor or no response to therapy.** When patients fail to respond clinically after 48–72 hours of therapy, a drainage procedure may be necessary. Surgical drainage most often is needed in patients with disease caused by gram-negative enteric bacilli. A subperiosteal collection of pus that does not respond to therapy also requires drainage. Cultures should be obtained on any surgical specimens because poor response may be due to inappropriate selection of antibiotic.

   e. **Sequestra. This should be removed surgically.**

E. Adjunctive measures. Bed rest or immobilization of the affected area, particularly of weight-bearing joints, often is indicated. The degree of and duration of immobilization are not standard. Strict immobilization for prolonged periods does not appear to be necessary for a successful outcome. Return to mobility should be dictated by improvement of local symptoms. The level of activity should be increased when pain, swelling, and erythema resolve. If surgical intervention is necessary, duration of postoperative immobilization is determined by the orthopedic surgeon and is related to the site involved and the surgical procedure performed.

F. Monitoring therapeutic response

1. **Signs and symptoms.** Successful therapy is indicated by resolution of fever, local tenderness, and erythema.

2. **ESR.** If the ESR was elevated initially, it should decline with appropriate therapy, but it may not return to normal on completion of successful therapy.

3. **Radiography.** Radiographic improvement may lag behind clinical improvement. Serial roentgenograms must be interpreted cautiously. We usually repeat a roentgenogram 2–3 weeks into the course of therapy and at the end of therapy in uncomplicated cases. A radiograph obtained 2–3 months after completion of antibiotic therapy provides a useful baseline should disease recur.

4. **Serial bone scans.** These should not be used to monitor response to therapy. Bone scans may remain positive months after clinical cure owing to the fact that healing bones absorb radiotracers. This healing may be indistinguishable from active infection.

VI. Prognosis. The prognosis for cure in patients with uncomplicated acute hematogenous osteomyelitis is good. Prognosis is, however, related to a variety of factors, including the causative organism, the duration of symptoms prior to therapy, and the length of antibiotic treatment.

A. Adequate antibiotic therapy is essential. There is a 10–20% recurrence rate in patients treated for acute hematogenous osteomyelitis. Recurrences are more common in patients who have received less than optimal therapy. For example, Dich and coworkers [29] noted only a 2% recurrence rate in those receiving more than 3 weeks of parenteral antibiotics compared with a 19% rate in those treated for less than 3 weeks. Waldvogel and coworkers [1] noted recurrent disease in only 1 of 27 patients receiving more than 4 weeks of intravenous antibiotics; in 5 of 6 patients treated with less intensive therapy, disease was not controlled.

B. Although it is not well documented, patients with hematogenous osteomyelitis due to gram-negative organisms appear to have a higher rate of recurrence [14].

C. **The best opportunity for cure is with initial therapy.** Of patients with recurrent disease, only 50% were cured after complete surgical debridement and 4–6 weeks of intravenous antibiotics [1]. **Acute osteomyelitis must be vigorously and adequately treated to prevent the development of chronic infection.**

Contiguous-Focus Osteomyelitis

Contiguous-focus osteomyelitis, due to spread from an adjacent focus of infection, has some special characteristics that require emphasis.

I. **Clinical setting.** Contiguous-focus osteomyelitis is seen primarily in patients older than 50 years.

A. **Postoperative infections** constitute **most cases** of contiguous-focus osteomyelitis.

1. **Open reduction of fractures** is the most common predisposing surgical procedure.

2. **Less common predisposing surgeries** include craniotomies, prosthetic hip and other reconstructive joint surgery, disc surgery, tumor resections, and sternotomy for open heart surgery. These infections can be complicated by the use of foreign materials, including metal, plastic, and bone cement, which serve as a nidus of infection that is resistant to antibiotic therapy. (See Chap. 15 for discussion of prosthetic joint infections.)

B. **Contiguous soft-tissue infections,** with spread to the bone, can involve any site.

1. The bones of the **toes** often are involved. Neonates and infants may develop osteomyelitis of the **os calcis.** These cases presumably occur as a result of blood sampling via multiple heel punctures, which may cause a soft-tissue infection in the heel pad followed by extension to the os calcis [41].

2. Osteomyelitis also may occur by spread from an infected tooth socket or sinuses, skin ulcerations, wounds, or decubitus ulcers, and from infections introduced by foreign bodies (e.g., puncture wounds). Osteomyelitis under pressure sores is especially difficult to diagnose [42, 43].

3. **After head and neck radiation therapy for cancer, mandibular osteomyelitis** can occur [1, 44]. Clinically and radiologically, this is difficult to distinguish from osteoradionecrosis. (**Osteoradionecrosis** refers to bone necrosis after radiation therapy. It most probably results from injury to the bone vasculature with subsequent ischemia.) Surgical biopsy is indicated in such cases for diagnostic histologic workup and cultures.

C. **Puncture wounds** uncommonly cause osteomyelitis, particularly of the small bones of the feet [45, 46]. (See Chap. 4 for initial management of puncture wounds.)

II. **Microbiologic features.** These infections **often are mixed,** because the adjacent wound infections are commonly due to mixed pathogens.

A. **Staphylococci**

1. **S. aureus** is the most common isolate. Approximately 50–60% of cases involve *S. aureus,* especially when disease involves the long bones, hip, and vertebrae. However, *S. aureus* may not be the only pathogen present.

2. **S. epidermidis** must also be considered a pathogen, especially when associated with prosthetic joints. These infections frequently have an indolent course, manifested primarily as constant pain postimplantation [47–50]. (See further discussion in Chap. 15.)

B. **Gram-negative bacteria** often are involved in mixed infections. Waldvogel and associates [1] noted that gram-negative bacteria were found in many or most cases of osteomyelitis of the **mandible, pelvis,** and **small bones.** *Pseudomonas* and other gram-negative bacteria are associated with the osteomyelitis secondary to puncture wounds [46]. *Pasteurella multocida* infection may occur after cat or dog bites [51].

C. **Anaerobic infections** have been underestimated in the past because of poor culture techniques. Anaerobes may be involved in osteomyelitis of the long bones subsequent to trauma and fracture, osteomyelitis related to peripheral vascular disease, pelvic osteomyelitis due to spread from decubitus ulcers, or osteomyelitis of cranial and facial bones due to spread from a contiguous soft-tissue source [15].

III. Clinical manifestations. Although some patients present with acute febrile illnesses, most patients with contiguous-focus osteomyelitis follow an **indolent course.** Most cases are diagnosed within 1–2 months of the onset of disease. Delay in diagnosis often occurs in postoperative infections. This is related in part to the use of prophylactic or postoperative antibiotics, disease due to atypical organisms of low pathogenicity, and the presence of foreign material.

A. **Presenting symptoms** include fever, regional soft-tissue swelling, erythema, and warmth. Purulent drainage from wounds and sinus tracts is common in both the acute and chronic forms.

B. **Site of involvement** may affect the presentation. Osteomyelitis of cranial bones often lacks signs or symptoms of disease, whereas infection of the long bones and pelvis often presents with fever and pain.

IV. Diagnosis

A. **Blood cultures** are less frequently positive in this form of osteomyelitis than in the hematogenous form. Nevertheless, two or three blood cultures should be obtained.

B. **Leukocyte counts** commonly may be normal or exhibit minimal elevations and should not be used to disprove osteomyelitis.

C. The **ESR** may be elevated, but a normal level does not exclude the diagnosis.

D. **Radiographic evaluation** may be useful. In patients with osteomyelitis secondary to a contiguous focus of infection, the diagnosis often is delayed, and roentgenographic changes are likely to be detectable at the time of presentation. Such findings may be difficult to interpret due to radiographic changes associated with the precipitating event (e.g., healing fracture, prosthetic devices). Serial examinations by a radiologist usually are most helpful in these cases. In patients with draining sinuses, **sinograms** may document more extensive involvement of bone than do conventional radiographic examinations.

E. **Technetium radiophosphate bone scans** may be difficult or impossible to interpret in this setting because of adjacent inflammation and infection or postoperative changes. Other techniques, such as MRI (if a metal prosthesis is not present) or indium-labeled leukocyte scanning, may be helpful [25].

F. **Wounds and draining sinus cultures are not as helpful as bone cultures.** In patients with draining sinuses or wounds, the interpretation of cultures is complicated because there may be multiple isolates or isolates of low pathogenicity or cultures may be sterile. A definitive bacteriologic diagnosis often requires careful cultures of bone either by needle aspiration or by open biopsy [52]. Needle biopsy for histopathologic and culture confirmation of osteomyelitis under pressure sores is preferred prior to instituting antibiotic therapy [42, 43].

G. **Open biopsy** may be necessary in those patients who have had an unacceptable response to therapy or in whom needle aspiration is indicated but cannot be performed.

V. Therapy. Treatment of contiguous osteomyelitis is **less successful** than treatment of the acute hematogenous forms. Relapse may occur in 40–50% of cases [1, 4–6]. **Surgery is an essential aspect of therapy in this disease.**

A. **Poor therapeutic response.** This probably is a result of a number of factors including (1) the longer duration of infection prior to the initiation of treatment; (2) the presence of foreign bodies after reconstructive orthopedic procedures; (3) the presence of devitalized bone in postfracture cases; and (4) the increased frequency of mixed infections, which may not be adequately diagnosed or treated.

B. **Antibiotic therapy**

1. **The basic principles** of antibiotic use discussed under Hematogenous Osteomyelitis are true also for contiguous-focus osteomyelitis. Because of the high frequency of mixed infections, **it is critical to obtain good specimens for culture** so that antibiotics can be directed against true pathogens and not wound colonizers.

2. Selection of **specific antibiotics** depends on the results of susceptibility studies. Common dosage schedules are shown in Table 16-2.

3. The ideal **duration of therapy** for this form of osteomyelitis is unknown. Each case is affected by many variables, such as the site of involvement, the adequacy of surgical debridement, underlying chronic illness of the patient, and the presence of a foreign body and whether it can reasonably be removed. Some generalizations can be made.

a. **Prosthetic device–related infections.** (See Chap. 15.)
b. **Wound-associated infection (without prosthetic devices).** In general, we treat these patients for at least 4 weeks, usually with parenteral therapy. Because of the poorer prognosis of this form of osteomyelitis, we may treat with a longer course of parenteral therapy, which sometimes is followed by oral therapy when a suitable agent is available. It must be stressed, however, that there is no proof that these longer courses of therapy improve outcome.

C. **Surgery.** Wounds or abscesses must be adequately debrided or drained. Sequestra must be removed, because they act as foreign bodies and decrease the likelihood of cure. Surgery usually is necessary early in these cases to obtain diagnostic material. Further debridement may be necessary if clinical response is slow.
   1. Whether prosthetic devices should be surgically removed is discussed in Chap. 15.
   2. **Distal lower-extremity osteomyelitis** due to wound infections associated with extensive compound fractures is common. Although treatment outcomes have traditionally been poor in such cases, encouraging results are now being reported in both acute and chronic cases with the use of radical wound debridement, intravenous antibiotics, and microvascular transfer of a muscle or musculocutaneous flap for wound closure [53–55].

D. **Adjunctive measures.** See sec. **V.E** under Hematogenous Osteomyelitis.
E. **Monitoring response.** See sec. **V.F** under Hematogenous Osteomyelitis.

Osteomyelitis Associated with Peripheral Vascular Disease

Most patients with osteomyelitis associated with peripheral vascular disease are diabetic. Osteomyelitis does occur, however, in patients with severe atherosclerosis or vasculitis in the absence of diabetes. Most patients are older than 50 years, and the bones of the toes and feet are most often involved. **For a separate discussion of soft-tissue infections without obvious osteomyelitis in the diabetic foot, see later in this chapter.**

I. **Pathophysiology.** There is **tissue ischemia. Neuropathy** may be present and may predispose to traumatic injury. These factors also explain certain clinical observations: (1) There is poor wound healing with resultant chronic ulcerations; (2) chronic skin ulcerations and tissue ischemia increase the frequency of mixed infections and the likelihood of anaerobic bacterial isolates; and (3) **antibiotics alone are inadequate therapy because of poor penetration to the site of infection. Surgical debridement is often necessary.**

II. **Microbiologic features.** Most wound or sinus drainage cultures and most surgical bone specimens reveal a mixed flora of gram-positive organisms, gram-negative organisms, and anaerobes [56, 57].
   A. **Common mixed infections.** Most infections are due to staphylococci and streptococci or a combination of staphylococci, streptococci, and Enterobacteriaceae.
   B. **Anaerobes.** Ischemia from vascular disease and tissue necrosis in chronic ulcerations provide optimal conditions in which anaerobic organisms flourish. Anaerobic bacteria were present in approximately one-third of isolates in two reports involving diabetic patients [56, 57].

III. **Clinical manifestations.** Few patients have systemic symptoms, and sepsis is rare.
   A. **Local signs and symptoms predominate,** including pain, swelling, and erythema. Most patients have associated cellulitis or long-standing ulceration. Crepitus of the soft tissues may be present, because of either anaerobes or aerobes. A foul odor of anaerobic infection may be present but is often difficult to distinguish from the odor of necrotic tissue [57].
   B. **Long-standing diabetic complications** often are the predominant findings. These include neuropathy, diminished or absent arterial pulses, skin and nail changes, retinopathy, and nephropathy. The presence or absence of such complications may affect disease outcome. For example, in the review by Waldvogel and associates [1], the only patients who were cured with conservative management were those without clinical findings of nephropathy, neuropathy, or retinopathy. Another more recent study, however, noted equivalent clinical outcomes in patients with and without these complications [57].

IV. **Diagnosis**
A. **Blood cultures** seldom are positive. Fever occurs most often in bacteremic patients.
B. **Leukocyte counts** usually are normal.
C. **ESRs** may be elevated but often are normal. A normal ESR in a diabetic patient with a toe or foot ulcer does not rule out osteomyelitis.
D. On **radiographic evaluation,** diagnosis of osteomyelitis is **often difficult.** Diabetics may have bony changes on routine roentgenography as a result of peripheral vascular disease and neuropathy [57]. These changes may be difficult to differentiate from true osteomyelitis. Consultation is indicated in these settings.
E. **Bone scans** [57a]
   1. **Technetium bone scans** are sensitive but expensive and lack adequate specificity.
   2. **Indium-111-labeled** leukocyte scanning is considered the most accurate study [58, 59], but it too is expensive and may be difficult to interpret in the presence of local soft-tissue inflammation.
   3. The usefulness of CT scans and MRI requires further study [57a] but may help identify soft-tissue abscesses.
F. The choice between **wound cultures and bone cultures** is controversial. Although bone biopsy specimens may more accurately detect pathogens in patients with diabetic foot infections, the procedure involves the risk of introducing infection to noninfected bone, causing bone necrosis, or introducing contamination from pathogens from adjacent soft-tissue infections. Percutaneous needle biopsy has, however, been used successfully by some investigators [60]. Bone biopsy specimens should be submitted for both aerobic and anaerobic cultures as well as histopathologic evaluation. (See related discussion in sec. **IV.F** under Contiguous Focus Osteomyelitis.)
G. **Combining plain radiography with a probe for bone** is a reasonable initial approach to the diagnosis of osteomyelitis. The ability to reach bone at the base of an ulcer by gently advancing a sterile probe (prior to any debridement) has a high specificity and positive predictive value in diagnosing osteomyelitis, but the sensitivity of this test is low [57a]. **If bone is detected by probing, treatment for osteomyelitis is recommended.** If bone cannot be detected by probing and the plain radiograph does not suggest osteomyelitis, then some experts suggest treatment can be aimed at a soft-tissue infection [57a]. We concur that this seems to be a useful practical approach to identifying underlying osteomyelitis.
H. **Doppler or angiographic evaluations** are necessary to determine whether there are focal vascular lesions, the correction of which could improve macrocirculation to the involved extremity. Consultation with a vascular surgeon is advised in these cases.
V. **Therapy.** Response to antibiotics alone often is unsatisfactory. Many patients are hospitalized on multiple occasions for treatment of recurrent disease. Initial therapy usually is conservative, with prevention of major amputations the primary goal. Prolonged courses of antibiotics may improve outcomes [57], but surgical debridement is usually essential [57a].
A. **Conservative approach.** To avoid more radical surgery, the following conservative measures are undertaken, though they are time-consuming and may be unsuccessful.
   1. **Limited local incision and drainage** is done to remove necrotic debris.
   2. **Antibiotic therapy** for acute osteomyelitis is outlined in sec. **V.A** under Hematogenous Osteomyelitis. Ideally, aspiration of deep wound or bone biopsy specimens provides the true pathogens, against which therapy is directed.
      a. In one article, high-dose parenteral antibiotics for at least 4 weeks or a combined intravenous and oral regimen for at least 10 weeks was associated with a good outcome (defined as no ablative surgical procedure) in 29 of 51 patients [57].
      b. A poor outcome after limited surgical drainage and antibiotics was noted in patients with abscess, necrosis, or gangrene [57]. Diabetic neuropathy, retinopathy, and arteriopathy were no more common in this group of patients than in those with a good outcome.
      c. Others favor more aggressive surgery [57a].
   3. **Vascular surgery** may improve the macrocirculation to the involved extremity in patients with correctable focal arterial lesions.
   4. **Limited amputations** of digits or parts of digits may prevent more radical future amputations. Adjacent areas of cellulitis should be treated with antibiotics preoperatively [61].

B. **Ablative surgery.** Patients who have done poorly with the conservative approach or who have evidence of abscess or gangrene need ablative surgical therapy. The conservative approach may not be in the best interest of these patients owing to cost, increased time of hospitalization, and risk of antibiotic toxicity.

1. Before amputation, it is important to perform arteriography or Doppler techniques to rule out a surgically correctable arterial lesion and to assess the probability of healing of the proposed surgical wound.

2. Osteomyelitis of the toes may require below-the-knee amputation if a conservative therapeutic approach fails. The conservative approach ranges from minor debridement to digital and transmetatarsal amputations.

Special Forms
of Osteomyelitis

I. **Chronic osteomyelitis** is defined as a **recurrent** problem: The patient has been previously treated for osteomyelitis at the same site [1]. The initial episode may have been due to hematogenous, contiguous, or peripheral vascular disease–associated osteomyelitis. Chronic osteomyelitis occurs most often following contiguous-focus osteomyelitis and peripheral vascular disease–associated osteomyelitis [62].

A. **Special considerations.** Chronic osteomyelitis carries a worse prognosis than acute osteomyelitis. Treatment failure rates in chronic osteomyelitis are higher than in the acute form, and the therapy is different.

B. **Clinical manifestations.** Patients only occasionally have acute symptoms. Systemic manifestations such as fever are uncommon. Localized signs and symptoms are also less common, with the exception of sinus tract or wound drainage, which is very common.

C. **Microbiologic features. *S. aureus* is a common pathogen.** Staphylococcal infections may recur years after the initial episode. Gram-negative bacteria also may be involved. Ideally, specific therapy should be guided by cultures obtained from biopsy.

D. **Diagnosis.** Determining the extent of disease activity and identifying a causative pathogen may be difficult.

1. **Blood cultures** are not often helpful, because bacteremia is rare.

2. **WBC counts** are normal in the majority of patients.

3. The **ESR** may be elevated, but this is a nonspecific finding.

4. **Radiographic evaluation** is complicated by the presence of prior bony abnormalities. It may not be possible to detect new or progressive abnormalities unless older radiographs are available for comparison.

5. **Technetium radiophosphate scans** are less helpful than in cases of acute osteomyelitis. Because scans may remain positive for years in the absence of active infection, a negative scan usually excludes active disease. **Gallium scans and indium-labeled leukocyte scans** are more useful in assessing active infection in areas of old disease [23].

6. **CT scans and MRI** are useful in defining sequestra, directing needle aspiration, and planning the operative approach in chronic osteomyelitis [26].

7. When deciding whether to perform **wound or sinus cultures**, it is important to remember that organisms cultured from draining sinus tracts may not represent the true bacteriology of the underlying bone infection when compared to bone biopsy cultures [62]. **Definitive bacteriologic diagnosis requires culture of bone biopsy specimens.**

8. **Needle aspiration and surgical biopsy** should be performed before any antibiotic is administered [62]. Aerobic, anaerobic, mycobacterial, and fungal cultures should be performed. Most chronic cases eventually require surgery. A diagnostic and therapeutic procedure is preferred prior to initiation of antibiotic therapy. Preoperative antibiotics may decrease the yield of cultures obtained at the time of surgery. Gram stains of the surgical specimens may help in the initial empiric choice of antibiotics.

E. **Therapy** is neither well established nor particularly effective. In addition to surgery and appropriate systemic antibiotics, several adjunctive measures have been advocated. Experience with many of these procedures is limited, and adequate controlled, prospective trials are lacking.

1. **Surgical intervention usually is required** to remove sequestra, to debride necrotic and devitalized material, and to obtain culture material. At times, exten-

sive debridement is done, with attempts at autogenous grafting with pulverized bone to fill in all defects [63]. Protocols using combined extensive debridement, antibiotic therapy, and vascularized muscle flaps to cover the wound have shown promising results [53–55].

2. **Antibiotics** are used, but the best regimen is debatable. In contrast to the basic principles that guide therapy in acute osteomyelitis (see sec. **V.A** under Hematogenous Osteomyelitis), the **optimal approach** to antibiotic therapy in chronic cases **is unknown.**

   a. **Parenteral agents** often are used initially, but the duration of therapy is poorly defined.

   b. **Combination therapy** with an antistaphylococcal penicillin and rifampin has been successful in some patients with chronic staphylococcal osteomyelitis [64].

   c. **The long-term** ($\geq$6 months) **use of oral agents** has been found by several authors to be successful in treating chronic osteomyelitis [65, 66]. Careful monitoring of serum levels was essential to ensure adequate therapy. Although most patients had disease attributable to gram-positive cocci, the quinolone antibiotics may prove useful in treating chronic osteomyelitis caused by aerobic gram-negative bacilli, especially *P. aeruginosa,* which previously required parenteral antibiotics [67]. See Chap. 28 for a detailed discussion of these agents.

      At times, patients with recurrent chronic osteomyelitis flares have been placed on lifetime suppressive oral regimens. Infectious disease consultation is advised.

   d. Closed irrigation with antibiotics or antibiotic and detergent mixtures has been reported [68]. There is a significant risk of superinfection with this approach.

   e. Intraarterial injection of antibiotics for regional perfusion [69] and the implantation of antibiotic beads have also been reported [70].

3. **Hyperbaric oxygen** is advocated by some clinicians in the treatment of particularly difficult cases of chronic osteomyelitis. Large-scale clinical trials using control groups matched for severity of osteomyelitis and severity of chronic underlying diseases are needed to help predict which cases may benefit [71].

4. **Consultation is advised in these difficult cases.** Adequate surgical debridement is essential. A regimen of 3–6 weeks of parenteral antibiotics is often used initially, followed by prolonged oral or ambulatory parenteral therapy.

F. **Complications** of long-standing chronic osteomyelitis

1. **Secondary amyloidosis,** although reported in some reviews, is very rare.

2. **Carcinoma,** primarily epidermoid carcinoma, occurs in the sinus tract of fewer than 1% of cases of chronic osteomyelitis. It usually is heralded by increased pain and drainage from the sinus tract. If cancer is suspected, the entire sinus tract is resected, because the carcinoma may lie deep within the tract.

II. **Vertebral osteomyelitis** is a form of hematogenous osteomyelitis that occurs in older patients [1, 4, 12, 72–73]. (Infection with *Mycobacterium tuberculosis,* which commonly involves the vertebrae, is discussed in sec. **IV.**) Although vertebral osteomyelitis is said to be uncommon, the incidence of this disease is increasing and it accounts for about 2–4% of all cases of pyogenic osteomyelitis [72a].

A. **Special considerations.** Cases often have indolent presentations. The differential diagnosis includes bacterial infection, tuberculosis, and tumor. Because roentgenography cannot always distinguish these entities, **early diagnostic aspiration or biopsy for histopathology and culture is essential.**

B. **Pathogenesis and clinical setting**

1. Vertebral osteomyelitis occurs most often from hematogenous seeding. In addition to arterial spread of infection, retrograde spread of infection is purported to occur from a urinary tract or pelvic source via Batson's plexus, a venous plexus that forms a direct connection between the vasculature of the pelvis and the spinal column. The extensive anastomoses and lack of valves in the veins of Batson's plexus are believed to facilitate spread of infection to adjacent vertebrae.

2. Other cases may occur by spread from a contiguous focus of infection, especially after disc surgery.

3. **The incidence of vertebral osteomyelitis is highest in adults 50 years of age and older.** This increased incidence is considered to be a result of subchondral

vascular changes in vertebrae from the axial stress and osteoarthritis that accompany aging. The relatively higher content of active marrow found in vertebrae compared to other sites may also be a predisposing factor.

4. When associated with intravenous drug use, vertebral osteomyelitis occurs in younger adults, with peak incidence between 20 and 50 years of age. The duration of symptoms is shorter, usually less than 3 months [12]. Pyogenic **vertebral osteomyelitis in children is uncommon** and has been reviewed elsewhere [73a].

5. The lumbar vertebrae are most commonly involved, followed by thoracic and then cervical vertebrae. In drug addicts, there is a high incidence of cervical spinal involvement, whereas only a few cases involve thoracic vertebrae [12, 72, 73].

6. Nosocomial infection, usually due to intravenous cannula-related sepsis with staphylococci, has become an increasingly important problem and occurred in 40% of cases in a recent series, with only 15% of cases in this series secondary to a focus in the genitourinary tract [72a].

C. **Microbiologic features.** S. *aureus* is the most common pathogen. *Salmonella* and gram-negative organisms associated with prior urinary tract infection also are common. *Pseudomonas* spp. are common in drug addicts. Tuberculosis can mimic bacterial infections (this is discussed further in sec. **IV**).

MRSA has been reported, usually with nosocomial infections associated with catheter- or wound-related sepsis [72a].

D. **Clinical manifestations.** In the adult, these may be minimal. Commonly there may be an inordinate delay between symptom onset and diagnosis (e.g., an average inhospital diagnostic delay of up to 11 days) [72a].

1. **Back pain,** described as dull and continuous, is the most common symptom. In a recent series, 85% of patients presented with back pain [72a]. It is present at rest and exacerbated by movement or straining but only slightly relieved by analgesics. Regional paraspinal muscle spasm, percussion tenderness of the spinal column, and point tenderness of the involved spinous processes frequently are present.

2. **Referred pain** due to nerve root irritation may mislead the examiner and direct attention from vertebral involvement. Lumbar disease can, for example, present as pain in the hip or leg.

3. **Neurologic complications** can occur. Owing to the indolent nature of the illness, patients may present with late neurologic sequelae such as paraplegia and meningitis [72, 73]. Limb weakness was noted in about one-half of patients in a recent series [72a].

4. **Fever** is often absent and was reported in only 30% of patients in a recent series and has overall been noted in 20–50% of patients [72a].

E. **Diagnosis**

1. **Blood cultures** should be obtained but often are negative. Blood cultures have been reported positive in 24–50% of patients and when positive (for a pathogen) are assumed to be the etiologic agent [72a].

2. The **WBC** count is elevated in the majority of patients [72a].

3. The **ESR** is usually elevated (80–90 mm/hr) and is considered a useful test supporting the diagnosis of vertebral osteomyelitis. In a recent series [72a], 95% of patients had an elevated ESR (over 80 mm/hr). The ESR is the most consistent laboratory abnormality in vertebral osteomyelitis; a normal ESR makes the diagnosis of vertebral osteomyelitis open to question. The test should be repeated if persistent symptoms continue to be clinically suspicious and if the initial ESR is not elevated [73b].

4. **Radiographic evaluation** (i.e., spinal films) is essential. Intervertebral disc involvement favors the diagnosis of pyogenic infection or tuberculosis. Findings are often nonspecific [72a].

5. **Bone scans** are helpful but have the limitations previously discussed.

6. **MRI scans** are highly sensitive and specific in the diagnosis of spinal infection, and they **provide more accurate anatomic information than bone scans.** Where available, **they have largely supplanted CT scans** in the evaluation of vertebral osteomyelitis [26].

7. **Needle biopsy or open biopsy** is essential to substantiate the diagnosis and provide culture material [72a, 74, 75] if blood cultures are negative. Unfortunately, bone biopsy cultures may be negative in up to 25% of cases for various

reasons, including sampling error and prior antibiotic therapy [72a]. (When this occurs, histologic examination of the biopsy may confirm inflammatory changes compatible with osteomyelitis.) A second needle biopsy is suggested if the first sample is culture negative [73b]. If the second needle biopsy is culture negative, an open surgical biopsy should be considered [73b].

F. **Therapy**

1. **Antibiotics**

   a. The principles of **antibiotic therapy** are as outlined in sec. **V** under Hematogenous Osteomyelitis.

   b. When infection due to MRSA is documented, because intravenous vancomycin may not penetrate bone adequately, combination therapy with rifampin and intravenous vancomycin for MRSA osteomyelitis is indicated. This recommendation is based on studies of animal models that have shown the combination of vancomycin plus rifampin sterilizes bone better than does vancomycin alone [72a].

   c. **Duration.** Antibiotics usually are given for at least 4 weeks [73b] and often for 6 weeks. Often, prolonged IV antibiotics are given at home (see Chap. 28A). If the patient is very compliant and reliable and susceptibility data allow for an oral agent (e.g., oral quinolones for susceptible gram-negative bacteria), a combination of initial intravenous antibiotics followed by oral antibiotics is used.

   The contribution of oral antibiotics after the initial 4–6 weeks of therapy is controversial. Some reviewers recommend them for 3 months after 1 month of IV therapy; other investigators believe that if parenteral therapy is given for 6 weeks, subsequent oral therapy is not required [72a].

   d. Because of the importance of eradicating this infection with the initial regimen and lack of clear-cut guidelines, infectious disease consultation is advised to help select intravenous and oral antibiotic regimens for these difficult problems.

   e. The ESR is a good tool to monitor the success of therapy; with proper antibiotic therapy, it should be expected to decrease to at least half to two-thirds of the pretherapy level [73b].

2. The role of **surgery** is debated. Definite indications include (1) neurologic complications such as cord compression (e.g., with progressive paraplegia), (2) definite paravertebral abscess, (3) failure to make a bacteriologic diagnosis after repeated needle biopsies, (4) poor clinical response [72a, 76], and (5) the presence of gross bone destruction leading to significant deformity or instability [73b].

3. **Adjunctive therapy** includes bed rest and a half-shell cast or body brace if the spine is unstable.

4. Tuberculosis is discussed separately in sec. **IV.** Diskitis is discussed in Chap. 15.

G. **Prognosis.** When early diagnosis is combined with adequate antibiotic therapy, prognosis is generally good. Reviews cite a mortality of less than 5–7%, with residual neurologic deficits occurring in 7–12% [72, 73, 73b]. Between 82% and 91% of patients recovered uneventfully with appropriate antibiotic therapy alone or with antibiotics combined with surgery [72, 73]. If, while on antibiotic therapy for vertebral osteomyelitis, the patient develops symptoms of a compressive neuropathy, MRI can be performed to determine whether there is a collection of pus that may require neurosurgical drainage. Spinal epidural abscesses have been reported in 5–18% of patients [73b].

Relapses can occur. In a recent series, 15% of patients (3 patients) had relapses, and in two of three patients the infecting organism was MRSA [72a].

III. **Infection associated with prosthetic devices** occurs in 1–4% of cases [47–50]. These infections are particularly difficult to manage, but prosthesis removal is not necessary in all cases. Some infections respond to antibiotic management alone.

A. **Special considerations.** Prosthetic devices act as foreign bodies. The question routinely arises as to whether the prosthesis must be removed or whether prolonged antibiotic therapy alone will be adequate.

B. **The approach to these infections** is discussed in Chap. 15 under Prosthetic Joint Infections.

C. **Intramedullary fixation nails.** These nails represent a unique situation, as their premature removal, even when they are infected, often will result in an unstable fracture, nonunion, and persistent infection. The device must usually be left in place and the infection treated with parenteral antibiotics and careful local surgery for debridement and drainage. The nail is removed when union is achieved [77, 78].

IV. **Tuberculous osteomyelitis** should be suspected in any case of vertebral osteomyelitis or osteomyelitis at any site that has not responded to antibiotic therapy. The incidence of tuberculosis in the United States has risen in recent years for a number of reasons. The incidence of tuberculous disease is increased in patients infected with the human immunodeficiency virus (HIV). Tuberculosis often is the first manifestation of HIV; any individual diagnosed with tuberculosis should be offered testing for HIV [79]. Of HIV-seronegative individuals, 15% will have extrapulmonary disease, with osteomyelitis reported in approximately 1% of all cases [80, 81]. The incidence of extrapulmonary disease in HIV-seropositive individuals is 70% [79]. The incidence of osteomyelitis in this group is unknown but can be presumed to be higher than in HIV-seronegative individuals. See related discussions in Chap. 9.

   A. **Pathogenesis.** Bone involvement results primarily from hematogenous spread, most commonly from the lung. Extension from a caseating lymph node or lymphatic drainage also may occur. There is a predilection for renal and skeletal tuberculosis to coexist. In almost all cases, the organism is *M. tuberculosis,* although rare cases of atypical mycobacteria have been reported [82]. *Mycobacterium bovis* was common prior to the pasteurization of milk and still must be considered in countries where unprocessed milk is consumed. *Mycobacterium avium* complex is a common opportunistic pathogen in the late stages of AIDS. Disease typically disseminates to multiple organs, with bone marrow invasion occurring in up to 52%. Localized cases of osteomyelitis have been reported rarely [83].

   B. **Clinical manifestations.** Tuberculous osteomyelitis is seen primarily in adults. Skeletal tuberculosis, like pulmonary tuberculosis, is less common in children.

   1. **Signs and symptoms.** These cases usually have a long, involved course.
      a. **Asymptomatic** bone lesions may be discovered on roentgenograms taken for other reasons. As with pyogenic organisms, patients with tuberculosis of the spine may have a paucity of symptoms and may not present until development of paravertebral abscess or neurologic complications including paraplegia and meningitis (see sec. II).
      b. **Fever** may or may not be present. Tuberculous osteomyelitis should always be considered, however, in the patient with fever of unknown origin and an asymptomatic bone lesion.
      c. **Pain** is the most common complaint and may be accompanied by local swelling and tenderness.
      d. **Chronic draining sinuses** may be present.

   2. **Bones involved.** Although any bone may be involved, 50% of cases in adults involve the spine (especially T11 or T12), 15% the hip, and 15% the knee; in the remaining 20%, the wrist, ankle, elbow, or shoulder may be involved. In children, vertebral involvement is also common.

   C. **Diagnosis.** In addition to the usual methods of diagnosing bacterial osteomyelitis, the following diagnostic tests are important in patients with suspected tuberculous bone disease.

   1. **Chest roentgenography** is necessary to look for evidence of pulmonary tuberculosis. Because only approximately 50% of patients with skeletal tuberculosis have roentgenographic evidence of pulmonary tuberculosis, a negative chest radiograph cannot disprove the diagnosis [80]. Sputum cultures (or gastric cultures if sputum is not available) are necessary if active pulmonary infection is suspected.

   2. A **tuberculin skin test** is part of the workup of any destructive bone or joint lesion, especially when it is monarthric or involves the spine. A negative skin test must never be used to rule out disease (see Chap. 9).

   3. **Needle or open biopsy** is important. In chronic infections in which tuberculosis is suspected and in all cases of vertebral osteomyelitis of unknown etiology, **tissue for histopathologic analysis and culture is crucial.** Special stains as well as cultures for bacteria, mycobacteria, and fungi should be performed.

   D. **Treatment**
   1. Recommendations for **chemotherapy** take into account the increasing incidence of multidrug-resistant tuberculosis and the more prolonged courses of therapy sometimes employed to effect a cure in patients coinfected with HIV. For a detailed discussion, see Chap. 9. In general, empiric therapy should include four drugs: isoniazid, rifampin, pyrazinamide, and usually ethambutol. This

initial regimen is used because there is concern over the presence of drug-resistant organisms [79]. In HIV-seronegative individuals, therapy may continue for as long as 2 years although good outcomes have been documented with shorter courses of 9–12 months. Few data exist regarding the appropriate duration of chemotherapy in HIV-seropositive patients. Usual dose regimens for pulmonary tuberculosis are used (see Chap. 9 under Tuberculosis: Basic Concepts). Infectious diseases consultation is advised.

2. **Surgery**
   a. **Nonvertebral disease.** Except in far-advanced disease, surgery seldom is necessary. Surgery is indicated to prevent deformity, to improve joint function, and to control disease that has not responded to chemotherapy. Surgery usually is delayed until after 2–3 months of chemotherapy [81].
   b. **Vertebral disease.** In the past, spinal tuberculosis (Pott's disease) commonly required surgical fusion. More recent studies show successful treatment in uncomplicated cases by chemotherapy alone. Spinal fusion usually occurs spontaneously with the healing process. Medical therapy may include bed rest or immobilization with plaster jackets. Indications for surgery include severe loss of neurologic function below the level of the vertebral lesion at presentation or progressive loss of neurologic function while on adequate chemotherapy. Surgery may also be indicated for drainage of symptomatic paravertebral abscesses.

E. **Prognosis.** With appropriate chemotherapy, the prognosis in HIV-seronegative patients with skeletal tuberculosis is good. HIV-seropositive patients can often be cured of pulmonary tuberculosis. There are few published data regarding cure rates of osteomyelitis in these patients.
   1. **Nonvertebral disease.** Coexistent joint involvement is frequent. Residual sequelae are often the result of deformity and functional impairment of the involved joint. Most patients, however, do recover normal function following chemotherapy alone. This emphasizes the importance of obtaining a specific etiologic diagnosis in patients with chronic destructive bone and joint lesions.
   2. **Vertebral disease.** Central nervous system involvement, including meningitis or paraplegia, is the most serious complication of tuberculous infection of the spine. Spinal deformities—kyphosis and scoliosis—also occur as a result of destruction of vertebrae. In children, these deformities may be progressive.

V. **Fungal osteomyelitis,** in most cases, is caused by hematogenous spread and are associated with disseminated disease. In some cases, direct inoculation may be involved; this is the pathogenesis for osteoarticular sporotrichosis. See Chap. 18 for more detailed discussions.
A. **Special considerations.** Fungal osteomyelitis should be considered in any indolent osteomyelitis that has not responded to routine measures. In addition, any patient with disseminated fungal disease is at increased risk of localized bone involvement.
B. **Fungal infections.** Bone lesions have been seen in cases of disseminated candidiasis (*C. albicans* is the most common organism), histoplasmosis, blastomycosis, coccidioidomycosis, cryptococcosis, sporotrichosis, and aspergillosis. These fungal infections are discussed in Chap. 18. *Candida* osteomyelitis has been reviewed by Gathe and colleagues [17].
C. **Diagnosis.** Diagnosis of the disease is primarily by culture or histopathologic demonstration of the organism in bone. Joint fluid analysis and culture are indicated when arthritis is present.
D. **Therapy.** The mainstay antifungal agent is amphotericin B, which is discussed in Chap. 18. Ketoconazole and itraconazole have proven successful in selected cases, especially blastomycosis. The role of fluconazole in the treatment of fungal osteomyelitis has not yet been defined. (See Chap. 18 for further discussion.) Surgical intervention for debridement of bone lesions often is necessary. This is especially true with chronic lesions. Infectious diseases consultation is advised.

Diabetic Foot Infections

Treatment of diabetic foot infections requires more days of hospitalization than any other complication of diabetes. Diabetic patients are 17 times more likely to develop gangrene than are nondiabetics. Two-thirds of the major amputations performed in the United States occur as a complication of diabetes. This topic has recently been reviewed [57a, 83a].

I. Pathophysiology

 A. Systemic factors. Whether diabetics are more susceptible to infections is not known, but most authors agree that once an infection is established in a diabetic, it generally is more severe and more refractory to therapy [84–87].

  1. Diabetics are known to have in vitro functional defects in immune defenses. Whether these defects render diabetics more susceptible to infection is unclear. The abnormalities include decreased lymphocyte blastogenic response and decreased lymphocyte glucose metabolism. Polymorphonuclear leukocytes demonstrate defective phagocytosis, intracellular killing, chemotaxis, and adherence [88, 89].

  2. Poor glycemic control is associated with increased incidence of infections in diabetics [89].

  3. Other factors are purported to contribute to the formation of diabetic foot lesions. These include the hypercoagulability of blood due to platelet or RBC changes and connective tissue abnormalities related to glycosylation of glycogen [90].

 B. Ischemia. Patients with diabetic foot infections usually are elderly and obese and have a long history of type 2 diabetes mellitus [57, 91].

  1. A significantly higher proportion of patients with foot lesions smoke than do diabetics without foot lesions [90].

  2. Presence of hypertension and hyperlipidemia may also promote vascular disease. Diabetics with ischemic foot disease have more severe coronary and cerebrovascular disease, which may adversely affect therapy and outcome [92].

  3. Depending on the degree of vascular insufficiency, the poor blood supply may produce (1) trophic skin changes [85]; (2) poor wound healing [93, 94]; (3) decreased tissue oxygenation predisposing to infections, particularly with anaerobes [86]; and (4) poor delivery of antibiotics to the site of infection [91, 95, 96].

 C. Peripheral neuropathy. The protective pain sensation is ablated by peripheral neuropathy, resulting in repetitive injuries to an insensitive extremity [93, 94]. Peripheral neuropathy is present in more than 80% of diabetic patients with foot lesions [57a].

  1. Charcot's joints and diabetic osteopathy. Gait changes and maldistributed weight bearing result in bony resorption, prominences, and joint subluxation. Even in the absence of infection, the extremity may be warm, swollen, and red, with destructive changes on the roentgenogram that are indistinguishable from osteomyelitis [93, 94].

  2. Neuropathic ulcerations (mal perforans). Ulceration is a consequence of the loss of protective sensation, that is a loss of awareness of trauma that can cause the breakdown of skin [57a]. The initial lesion usually occurs at weight-bearing points on the plantar surface, typically under the first or fifth metatarsal heads or on the heel [97]. Blisters or corns from poorly fitting shoes also commonly lead to ulceration and infection [93]. These ulcers may go unnoticed for days to weeks in the painless neuropathic diabetic foot. Bacteria may invade the base of these neglected ulcers and either spread along fascial planes or penetrate fascia and soft tissue to reach the periosteum [86].

  3. Other sources of infection include a break in the skin due to a **superficial fungal infection or improper trimming of nails** [97].

  4. A detailed review of faulty foot mechanics in conjunction with peripheral polyneuropathy in diabetics has recently been published [83a].

II. Microbiologic features. The organisms frequently isolated are related in part to the severity of underlying disease, which has commonly been subdivided into mild, non-limb-threatening infections and more severe limb-threatening infections [57a, 97a] (see discussion in sec. **III**). Whenever possible, deep-tissue aspiration or tissue/bone biopsy provides more reliable specimens in ulcerated lesions; both aerobic and anaerobic cultures should be obtained (see sec. **IV.D**). Recent antibiotic therapy may influence the spectrum of pathogens isolated [97a].

 A. Mild, non-limb-threatening infections are caused primarily by *S. aureus* (more than 50% of patients) and aerobic streptococci. Facultative gram-negative bacilli and anaerobic organisms are infrequent isolates. **In half** of these patients, the infections are **monomicrobial** [57a].

B. Severe, limb-threatening infections, associated typically with far-advanced vascular disease, **usually are polymicrobial.** Deep-tissue cultures that avoid surface contamination usually yield a mixed culture of aerobes and anaerobes. One study demonstrated a mean of 4.8 species per patient [96]. The organisms isolated depend on the severity and chronicity of illness, the methods used to obtain the culture, and the capabilities of the microbiology laboratory.

1. **Aerobes**

a. ***S. aureus* and coagulase-negative staphylococci** are the most common aerobic isolates [57, 96]. Furthermore, staphylococci are found in approximately two-thirds of patients in whom only a single organism is isolated [56].

b. Approximately 20% of isolates are **streptococci** (including group B) **and enterococci** [56, 96]. The pathogenic role of coagulase-negative staphylococci, enterococci, and corynebacteria often is difficult to discern, particularly when these organisms are cultured along with typical virulent organisms. Recent reviewers suggest these organisms can be viewed as skin contaminants and not pathogens (unless they are isolated in pure culture or the patient is not responding to therapy that is not aimed at these organisms) [57a]. Therefore, enterococci can usually be viewed as nonpathogenic, similar to the role of enterococci in intraabdominal infection (see Chap. 11). However, in Bamberger's study [57], enterococci were responsible for one of five relapses. This emphasizes that antibiotics active against enterococci are indicated in patients with enterococci isolated from deep cultures who are not responding to initial empiric antimicrobial therapy.

c. **Enterobacteriaceae** account for 24–27% of organisms isolated. Common isolates include *Proteus, Klebsiella,* and *Enterobacter* spp., *Morganella morganii,* and *E. coli* [56, 96]. *Pseudomonas* and *Acinetobacter* spp. are common contaminants in specimens from ulcers or open draining lesions but are infrequently isolated from deep-tissue cultures [56].

d. ***Corynebacterium* spp.** have been isolated from patients with necrotizing infections, as discussed earlier. Usually these organisms are contaminants, but at times they may be pathogens [56].

2. **Anaerobes** are isolated from 40–80% of patients with severe or advanced disease, depending on the study method. They usually are present in cultures yielding at least four organisms, and the density of growth is higher than that of aerobes [56, 96, 97b].

a. The presence of anaerobes is associated with a higher frequency of fever, foul-smelling lesions, and the presence of a foot ulcer [96].

b. Common anaerobic isolates include anaerobic streptococci (14–17%), *Bacteroides* spp. (9–14%), and *Clostridium* spp. (2–7%). *Bacteroides* spp. are more frequently found in necrotizing infections and osteomyelitis than in abscesses [56]. Although rare, infection due to *Clostridium* spp. may be rapidly progressive. Lack of an inflammatory response on Gram stain in the presence of gram-positive organisms should raise suspicion that *Clostridium* is present [86].

III. **Clinical manifestations.** Meaningful comparison of the many different studies on diabetic foot infections is hindered by the lack of a uniform grading system that includes both the degree of vascular compromise and the extent of infection. Such a system would help the clinician manage patients with various degrees of vascular insufficiency and various extents of soft tissue and/or bone infection. The clinical grading system used at the Rancho Los Amigos Hospital may provide the basis for such a system [94].

A. **Non-limb-threatening versus limb-threatening infections.** Recent reviewers have suggested a practical clinical classification of infections [57a] that appears to be a useful approach.

1. **Non-limb-threatening infections.** Patients have superficial infection, lack systemic toxicity, and have minimal cellulitis (<2 cm of extension from portal of entry). If an ulcer is present, it does not penetrate fully through the skin. These patients do not have bone or joint involvement or significant underlying ischemia.

2. **Limb-threatening infections.** Patients have more extensive cellulitis (>2 cm of extension from the portal of entry) and lymphangitis. Full-thickness ulcers often are present. Infection of contiguous bones or joints occurs frequently.

Significant ischemia with or without gangrene may be present. Fever may be seen in only a minority of these patients and is more common in those with extensive soft-tissue involvement, deep plantar abscesses, bacteremia, or hematogenously seeded remote sites of infection.

B. **Local signs and symptoms** predominate and include those related to infection, vasculopathy, and neuropathy.

    1. **Infection.** The anatomic location of the infection affects prognosis. Proximal infections (along metatarsals, at the heel, or above the ankle) are associated with lower-limb salvage and higher mortality [98].

        a. Most cases of lower-extremity infection in diabetics begin as chronic perforating ulcers [86].

        b. Infection is heralded by warmth, redness, swelling, and purulent exudate. **Tenderness is often minimal or absent owing to neuropathy** [57, 92, 97].

        c. Gas in the soft tissues may be visualized by roentgenography or detected as crepitus on physical examination. Gas usually is from mixed infection with gram-negative bacilli and anaerobes rather than *Clostridium* spp. infection. A foul odor may be present due to necrosis or anaerobic infection [96]. Gangrene owing to infection or ischemia may be seen.

        d. It is important to determine the extent of deep-tissue destruction and possible bone and joint involvement by unroofing all encrusted areas and inspecting the wound carefully [84]. **Surgical consultation should be obtained routinely. Osteomyelitis underlying diabetic ulcers is common.** One study cites an incidence of clinically silent osteomyelitis as high as 68% when sought with bone biopsy and cultures [99].

    2. **Vascular disease.** Patients may complain of intermittent claudication or resting pain relieved by dependency. Pulses may be decreased or absent. Bruits, shiny cold skin, decreased hair and nail growth, atrophy of subcutaneous fat, and a rapid decrease of Doppler pressures may also be present [85, 100]. Other findings include delayed capillary filling time, ischemic rubor, and collapsed veins [87].

    3. **Neuropathy.** This is most prominent in the lower extremities. Commonly, the forefoot may have significant neuropathy while the hind foot and lower leg have relatively normal sensation. A simple method of identifying patients who have lost protective sensation is to press a nylon monofilament (designated 5.07, NC 12750 #14, North Coast Medical, San Jose, CA) against the skin of the foot; the inability of the patient to feel the force of the monofilament correlates with an increased risk of neuropathic foot injury [57a].

        Later findings include decreased sensation of pain, temperature, and touch; impaired proprioception; and sluggish or absent deep-tendon reflexes. Loss of deep-tendon reflexes is a late finding [85, 87].

C. **Systemic signs and symptoms** often occur late and indicate severe infection.

    1. Uncontrolled hyperglycemia is the only reliable sign [84].

    2. Fever occurs when pus is contained (i.e., trapped pus), when a virulent organism is involved, or when bacteremia is present. Otherwise, fever is relatively uncommon. Even in patients with limb-threatening sepsis, only 36% had fever higher than 100°F (37.8°C) during the first day of admission [97a] except in bacteremia and in cases in which anaerobes are recovered from deep cultures [57, 96] (see sec. **A.2**).

IV. **Diagnosis**

A. **Leukocytosis** may be minimal or absent even with severe infection. Even with limb-threatening sepsis, leukocytosis (WBC count > $10,000/mm^3$) was noted in only 53% of patients at admission [97a].

B. The **ESR** usually is elevated [91].

C. **Blood cultures** are positive in approximately 10–15% of patients but should be obtained in all patients. The highest rates of positive cultures are seen in febrile patients [57].

D. The **best method for** obtaining **wound or tissue cultures** from diabetic foot infections **is unknown.** These wounds are chronic and often are colonized superficially with organisms that are not causative (e.g., staphylococci or enterococci). Deep-tissue cultures that avoid contact with the ulcer surface or other draining lesions are preferred [56]. In one study, curettage of the ulcer base correlated better (75%) with results of deep-tissue culture obtained at amputation than did specimens obtained by needle aspiration (69%) or swab of the ulcer (62%) [96].

Various approaches have been suggested. Aerobic and anaerobic cultures should be performed before antibiotics are started.

1. **With debridement.** When debriding is done at the time of presentation, cultures of deep tissue or necrotic tissue, including bone, can be performed. Routine aspirate or biopsy of unexposed bone is not advised [57a].

2. **Direct ulcer culture.** The open ulcer can be cleaned carefully (usually with betadine, which is allowed to dry and then removed with alcohol sponges) and any overlying eschar debrided, and then a swab can be inserted through the opening of the ulcer deeply into the wound to obtain a deep culture. The swab then can be plunged into anaerobic transport media and brought quickly to the laboratory for processing.

3. **Indirect culture of ulcer base.** The skin adjacent to the ulcer can be prepared with betadine and a needle inserted through the intact skin, aiming at the base of the ulcer. (Because of the frequent presence of diabetic neuropathy [i.e., the patient's extremity is anesthetic], this usually can be done without discomfort.) Material is aspirated from the base of the ulcer, or sterile nonbacteriostatic saline is instilled and aspirated, and the aspirate is cultured for aerobes and anaerobes.

4. Bullae or fluctuant collections can be aspirated and cultured [57a].

E. Although **Gram stains** usually reveal mixed flora and may not be especially helpful, the lack of an inflammatory response and the presence of gram-positive rods may indicate a clostridial infection, which may be rapidly progressive [98].

F. **Radiographs**

1. Radiolucent areas within the soft tissues may occur due to dissection of air into open ulcers or as a result of debridement. **Presence of air** in the soft tissue also occurs as a result of gas-forming bacterial infection [100]. Gas formation usually is due to other anaerobes, coliforms, streptococci and, rarely, *Clostridia* spp. [85, 86, 95]. Because air in the soft tissues can occur secondary to a number of benign causes, its presence alone should not be used as justification for amputation.

2. **Sinograms** may detect subfascial plantar extension and involvement of the joint space [87].

3. The differentiation of osteomyelitis from diabetic osteopathy may be difficult [100]. Sequential radiographs may help [86]. Radiographs may be normal in early osteomyelitis [57]. (See sec. **IV.D** under Osteomyelitis Associated with Peripheral Vascular Disease.)

G. **Indium-labeled leukocyte scans are the most sensitive method to detect occult osteomyelitis.** In one study, these scans proved more sensitive than either roentgenograms or bone scans [99] (see sec. **IV.E** under Osteomyelitis Associated with Peripheral Vascular Disease).

H. **CT scanning and MRI** are used mainly to detect soft-tissue abscesses, usually in the plantar spaces, and to identify bone involvement [100].

I. **Probing the base of the ulcer** to detect bone is a useful technique to identify osteomyelitis, as discussed in sec. **IV.G** under Osteomyelitis Associated with Peripheral Vascular Disease (see p. 620). Because necrotic debris frequently masks the ulcer floor, this technique may be the only way to accurately assess ulcer depth and to identify its involvement with contiguous bone [57a].

V. **Therapy.** Early surgical and infectious disease consultation is recommended.

A. **Medical therapy.** Most patients do not require ablative procedures [57]. Furthermore, clinical, radiographic, or radionuclide evaluations cannot distinguish consistently between osteomyelitis and diabetic osteopathy [86].

1. **Antibiotics** are the mainstay of treatment and are recommended in the presence of surrounding cellulitis, a foul-smelling lesion, fever, and deep-tissue infection [95]. No single antibiotic regimen is known to be superior when therapy is based on adequate cultures [57, 57a, 97a].

   a. **Empiric antibiotic therapy is necessary until culture results are available.** Antibiotics are given in full doses because of the potential for poor penetration into the site of infection, especially in patients with advanced vascular disease. Nephrotoxic antibiotics should be avoided when possible. Possible antibiotic options are summarized in Table 16-3.

      (1) **For non-limb-threatening infection,** therapy is aimed at staphylococci and streptococci. Outpatient regimens of 2 weeks of oral cephalexin or clindamycin are quite effective. In patients with superficial ulcers but

Table 16-3. Selected empiric antimicrobial regimens for foot infections
in patients with diabetes mellitus

Non–limb-threatening infection
Oral regimen
  Cephalexin*
  Clindamycin
  Dicloxacillin
  Amoxicillin-clavulanate
Parenteral regimen
  Cefazolin
  Oxacillin or nafcillin
  Clindamycin

Limb-threatening infection
Oral regimen
  Fluoroquinolone and clindamycin
Parenteral regimen
  Ampicillin-sulbactam
  Ticarcillin-clavulanate
  Piperacillin-tazobactam
  Cefoxitin or cefotetan
  Fluoroquinolone and clindamycin

Life-threatening infection
Parenteral regimen
  Imipenem-cilastatin
  Vancomycin, metronidazole, and aztreonam
  Ampicillin-sulbactam and an aminoglycoside
  Piperacillin-tazobactam and an aminoglycoside

Note: These regimens may require adjustment if the patient has a history of allergies or if there are clinical or epidemiologic factors suggesting unusual pathogens. Doses should be commensurate with the severity of infection, with adjustment for renal dysfunction when indicated
*Editors' note: We favor full doses of cephalexin, e.g., 750–1000 mg qid, in the adult. In severe renal failure, doses must be adjusted as described in Chap. 28F (p. 1196).
Source: Modified from G. M. Caputo et al., Assessment and management of foot disease in patients with diabetes. *N. Engl. J. Med.* 331:854, 1994.

with cellulitis that warrants hospitalization and parenteral antibiotics, some reviewers favor cefazolin [57a] rather than the broader regimens typically used for more severe limb-threatening infection (such as cefoxitin or ampicillin-sulbactam). Others have favored monotherapy with cefoxitin, cefotetan, ceftizoxime, ticarcillin-clavulanic acid, ampicillin-sulbactam, and piperacillin-tazobactam [56, 86, 95, 97]. Therapy can be modified as needed after deep-tissue culture results return. **The optimal agent in this setting has not been determined** [57a, 97a].

(2) **For more severe limb-threatening infections,** broad-spectrum antibiotics commonly are used to treat anticipated polymicrobial infection. Although in the past, triple therapy with ampicillin, clindamycin (or metronidazole), and an aminoglycoside was used [56, 86, 95, 97], recent reviewers tend to avoid the aminoglycosides, except in a patient with known or potentially resistant pathogens (see Table 16-3). The new agent piperacillin-tazobactam and the combination of ceftriaxone and clindamycin (or metronidazole) are other options. The role of enterococci remains unclear [57a, 97a] (see related discussion under sec. **II.B.1.a**). The optimal antibiotic regimen has not been defined [57a, 97a].

(3) **For life-threatening infections,** imipenem or combination regimens have been suggested (see Table 16-3). Some experts will include an antibiotic regimen active against enterococci in this setting, at least until culture data are back [97a]. In addition, given the proven efficacy of aminoglycosides in the setting of gram-negative sepsis, these drugs can be used in combination with broad-spectrum agents, at least until

culture data are available; short-term use will minimize their potential for nephrotoxicity [97a]. In nosocomial sepsis, if MRSA is a concern, vancomycin should be included until susceptibility data are available (see Table 16-3).

Once culture data are available, antibiotic therapy can be modified whenever possible.

b. The results of deep-tissue cultures are used to direct continued antibiotic choices.

   (1) If the patient is doing well clinically and is improving on an empiric antibiotic regimen not active against a particular isolate from a deep ulcer culture, the clinical response suggests the organism may just be a colonizer and therefore, this organism(s) needs no directed antibiotic therapy.

   (2) By contrast, if bacteria are isolated that are resistant to the current antibiotic regimen, but the patient is not doing well clinically, it is reasonable to expand antibiotic coverage to include these pathogens. At times, unnecessarily broad antibiotic coverage may be used [56], but this seems unavoidable in this clinical problem.

c. The optimal **duration of antibiotic therapy** for soft-tissue diabetic infections **has not been well established** [57a].

   (1) For osteomyelitis, potential courses are needed as discussed earlier in this chapter. In patients with pedal osteomyelitis, if all infected bone has not been removed, prolonged antibiotics (e.g., 6–12 weeks) may be reasonable [97a].

   (2) For infections limited to soft tissue, intravenous therapy often has been given for 10–14 days. In patients who do well, oral therapy can be used to complete a 2-week course.

   (3) For non-limb-threatening infections, although ulcers may persist beyond a 2-week course of oral therapy aimed at the acute cellulitis, further antibiotics may not be necessary because continued ulcer care depends primarily on local wound care.

   (4) Foot infections with a secondary bacteremia, commonly *S. aureus* or *Bacteroides* spp., requires protracted therapy (see Chap. 2).

   (5) Although prolonged courses of antibiotics along with local incision and drainage may, at times, obviate the need for amputation [57], this approach has been questioned [57a] and early, more definite surgical intervention usually is preferred.

2. Glycemic control should be strict. Insulin should be used for immediate glycemic control even in non-insulin-dependent patients [84]. An excellent monitor of the adequacy of debridement is blood sugar control, which improves as the infection is controlled [83a].

3. Weight bearing of neuropathic ulcers must be eliminated to allow for healing of the ulcers. Various devices are available, among them felted foam inserts and a total-contact cast [57a, 83a]. These are useful after the acute infection has been controlled.

B. In severe infection, urgent surgical intervention may be required to control sepsis. Debridement of necrotic tissue and drainage of pus should not be delayed while awaiting medical stabilization [83a]. Surgery should be postponed only if the patient has had a recent myocardial infarction, especially within the past 2 weeks [85].

1. Nonablative procedures

   a. Surgical considerations include the following:

      (1) Deep infections do not respond to small stab wounds and drains.

      (2) The procedure should ensure later reconstruction, conserving as much healthy tissue as possible.

      (3) Simple dressings are preferred. The use of full-strength solutions, enzymatic debriding agents or other astringents, and hot compresses or soaks leads to more complications.

      (4) The initial surgical debridement and drainage is rarely the definitive procedure. Follow-up procedures usually are required.

   b. Casts, crutches, or braces may be required to immobilize the inflamed part and allow healing [93, 94].

2. Amputations. If at all possible, the limb should be preserved. Prior studies have demonstrated that there is no cost benefit to performing a primary major amputation rather than pursuing an aggressive approach to limb salvage [83a]. Even with conservative treatment, the contralateral foot will be infected within 18 months in 49% of cases [101]. Unfortunately, one-third of all diabetics who have a major amputation of one extremity will have the other extremity amputated within 3 years [94]. Major amputations may be reduced by (1) substituting reconstructive for destructive surgery (muscle and skin flaps may be used to close the lesions); (2) performing radical local debridement; (3) diagnosing early the spread of infections from foot to leg; (4) improving the blood supply; and (5) providing a continuum of care by experienced personnel [60, 92].

3. **Revascularization.** Presence of small-vessel disease elsewhere should not preclude vascular reconstruction in diabetics [93]. **These patients deserve vascular surgical consultation early in therapy once sepsis is controlled, especially prior to any amputation.** There is a predilection in diabetic patients for macrovascular arterial occlusive disease to involve the distal tibial and peroneal vessels between the knee and the foot, but there is no occlusive microvascular disease affecting the diabetic foot [83a]. Arterial reconstructive procedures should be considered in the presence of ulcers, infection, or gangrene. Prior studies have shown that critical ischemia was associated with 62% of cases of nonhealing ulceration and was a causal factor in 46% of amputations [83a]. Such reconstruction may lead to healing of an ulcer, success in a local surgical procedure, lowering of the amputation level, and improved antibiotic delivery [60, 84, 92–94]. Advances in noninvasive vascular testing, vascular surgery, arteriography, angiodilatation techniques, digital techniques, and the use of less nephrotoxic contrast media have improved the outlook for managing diabetics with peripheral vascular disease [93].

VI. Prevention. Diabetic foot infections are better prevented than treated. Success in saving the foot depends on prevention or correction of risk factors, removal of vascular obstruction when possible, early and vigorous treatment of diabetic foot lesions, and patient education in foot care [83a, 102, 103]. **Prophylactic care for diabetics should include the following:**

A. **Periodic examination of the feet** is necessary in all new diabetic patients. In addition, patients with peripheral vascular disease, neuropathy, foot deformities, a history of foot ulcers, or a 10-year or longer history of diabetes, or who are older than 40 years of age should have a foot examination at each visit [102].

1. Examining light touch, position sense of the toes, and tuning-fork sensation can detect early **neuropathy** [93]. The monofilament line test is described in sec. **III.B.3.**

2. The physical examination should also be geared toward the detection of worsening **vasculopathy** and **abnormal foot lesions** such as corns, calluses, ulcers, and nail lesions [85, 93].

B. **Patient education** [90]

1. Smoking should be discouraged [85, 90, 94].

2. The patient should be instructed on proper daily self-examination of the foot. If the patient's vision is poor, other family members should be taught.

3. The patient should avoid extremes of temperature.

4. The patient should seek medical attention early rather than late [85, 93, 94].

5. The patient should also be taught how to file calluses, cut toenails (straight across), wash feet, use lanolin, and care for lesions. The inclusion of a podiatrist on the medical team may be very helpful in this aspect of the patient's care.

6. The patient should not go barefoot [85, 102].

7. Proper footwear and foot care are mandatory.

8. The overweight patient should be counseled regarding weight reduction, which will help lessen the burden on the feet.

9. The diabetic's foot is usually dry and scaly. Application of a skin lubricant is particularly important in these patients [85, 94].

C. **Specific interventions**

1. Absent dorsalis pedis and posterior tibial pulses should lead to further noninvasive vascular studies.

2. In patients with maldistribution of weight on the foot, corns should be debrided periodically by trained personnel [93]. In addition, the podiatrist, orthopedic surgeon, or diabetologist should be consulted for care of calluses, foot deformities, and neuropathic or vascular ulcers [102].

3. Footwear should be examined; shoes should not be too tight [83a, 93, 94]. Selected patients may benefit from static and dynamic measurements of foot pressure, in centers where it is available, to identify areas of the foot at higher risk for ulceration and to aid in the design of appropriate footwear [104].
4. Superficial infections, such as nail infections and paronychia, should be treated early [86].

References

1. Waldvogel, F.A., Medoff, G., and Swartz, M.N. Osteomyelitis: A review of clinical features, therapeutic considerations, and unusual aspects. *N. Engl. J. Med.* 282: 198, 1970.
   A classic.
2. Cierny, G., Mader, J.T., and Pennick, J.J. A clinical staging system for adult osteomyelitis. *Contemp. Orthop.* 10:17, 1985.
   A pathologic classification is included, which may be helpful in comparing therapeutic outcomes in clinical disease and experimental infections.
3. Nelson, J.D. Acute osteomyelitis in children. *Infect. Dis. Clin. North Am.* 4:513, 1990.
4. Waldvogel, F.A., and Vasey, H. Osteomyelitis: The past decade. *N. Engl. J. Med.* 303: 360, 1980.
   An update. Also see excellent recent symposium, C.W. Norden et al. Osteomyelitis. Infect. Dis. Clin. North Am. *4:361, 1990.*
5. Weinstein, A.J. Osteomyelitis: Microbiologic, clinical and therapeutic considerations. *Prim. Care* 8:557, 1981.
   This review emphasizes the difficulty in clinically distinguishing acute and chronic disease. Classification based on pathogenesis of disease is supported.
6. Gentry, L.O. Overview of osteomyelitis. *Orthop. Rev.* 16:255, 1987.
   The incidence of osteomyelitis after orthopedic procedures and bone trauma is increasing. As a result, gram-negative and polymicrobial infections are more common.
7. Kahn, D.S., and Pritzker, K.P.H. The pathophysiology of bone infection. *Clin. Orthop.* 96:12, 1973.
   Discusses the interplay between bacteria and host in determining localization, spread of infection, and factors resulting in chronic infection.
8. Wald, E.R. Risk factors for osteomyelitis. *Am. J. Med.* 78(Suppl. 6B):206, 1985.
   Preceding infection, local trauma, and underlying diseases are major risk factors for hematogenous osteomyelitis. The hemoglobinopathies predispose to Salmonella *osteomyelitis. Chronic granulomatous disease patients are prone to infections by* Serratia marcescens, Aspergillus fumigatus, *and other catalase-positive species.*
9. Piehl, F.C., Davis, R.J., and Prugh, S.I. Osteomyelitis in sickle cell disease. *J. Pediatr. Orthop.* 13:225, 1993.
   Eighty-one percent of cases were due to Salmonella *spp. in this series. Annual incidence of osteomyelitis was 0.36% in sickle cell disease.*
10. Holzman, R.S., and Bishko, F. Osteomyelitis in heroin addicts. *Ann. Intern. Med.* 75:693, 1971.
    Four patients are presented. The clinical course in each case was indolent, and the pathogens included Staphylococcus aureus, *yeast, and* Pseudomonas *spp.*
11. Leonard, A., et al. Osteomyelitis in hemodialysis patients. *Ann. Intern. Med.* 78: 651, 1973.
    Osteomyelitis in five patients mimicked other disease entities, thereby delaying diagnosis and treatment.
12. Sapico, F.L., and Montgomerie, J.Z. Vertebral osteomyelitis in intravenous drug abusers: Report of three cases and review of the literature. *Rev. Infect. Dis.* 2:196, 1980.
    A total of 67 cases are reviewed. Gram-negative aerobic bacilli caused 82% of infections, Pseudomonas *spp. 66%. A high incidence of cervical spinal involvement (27%) was noted.*
12a. Kanwowska, A., et al. Clinical features and outcome of childhood osteomyelitis at a pediatric hospital. Infectious Disease Society of America, 33rd Annual Meeting. San Francisco, CA. September 1995. Abstract #264.
    Review from Alberta, Canada, of 103 cases of osteomyelitis in children with a mean age of 7 years.
13. Edwards, M.S., et al. An etiologic shift in infantile osteomyelitis: The emergence of the Group B streptococcus. *J. Pediatr.* 93:578, 1978.
    Of 21 infants with osteomyelitis, group B streptococcus was the cause in 38%.

13a. Jackson, M.A., et al. The changing face of childhood pyogenic arthritis: Implications for therapy. Infectious Disease Society of America, 33rd Annual Meeting. San Francisco, CA. September 1995. Abstract #433.
In the pre H. influenzae b vaccine era (1980–1985), 42% of cases of infectious arthritis were due to H. influenzae. In recent years, the incidence of disease due to the pathogen has dramatically fallen: from 1986–1988 (by 29%), 1989–1991 (21%), and 1992–1994 (0%)! Presumably the incidence of hematogenous-borne osteomyelitis will show a similar decline of H. influenzae in children who have been vaccinated.

14. Meyers, B.R., et al. Clinical patterns of osteomyelitis due to gram-negative bacteria. *Arch. Intern. Med.* 131:228, 1973.
A good review of the pathogenesis and clinical course of patients with osteomyelitis due to gram-negative bacteria.

15. Brook, I., and Frazier, E.H. Anaerobic osteomyelitis and arthritis in a military hospital: A 10-year experience. *Am. J. Med.* 94:21, 1993.
Retrospective study of 73 cases of anaerobic osteomyelitis using recently developed culture techniques and newer bacterial identification criteria.

16. Pichichero, M.E., and Friesen, H.A. Polymicrobial osteomyelitis: Report of three cases and a review of the literature. *Rev. Infect. Dis.* 4:86, 1982.
Polymicrobial osteomyelitis was associated with contiguous foci in 59% of cases and peripheral vascular insufficiency or neuropathy in 17% of cases and was hematogenous in 13% of cases. Anaerobes were commonly isolated.

17. Gathe, J.C., et al. *Candida* osteomyelitis: Report of five cases and review of the literature. *Am. J. Med.* 82:927, 1987.

17a. Norden, C., Gillespie, W.J., and Nade, S. Hematogenous Osteomyelitis. In *Infections in Bones and Joints.* Boston: Blackwell, 1994.
Nice discussion by experts in the field.

18. Craigen, M.A.C., Watters, J., and Hackett, J.S. The changing epidemiology of osteomyelitis in children. *J. Bone Joint Surg.* 74-B:541, 1992.
The occurrence of osteomyelitis at unusual sites may result in delayed diagnosis.

19. Miller, W.B., Jr., Murphy, W.A., and Gilula, L.A. Brodie abscess: Reappraisal. *Radiology* 132:15, 1979.
A diverse radiologic picture is noted in 25 patients. The average duration of symptoms in these patients was 7 months.

20. Edwards, M.S., et al. Pelvic osteomyelitis in children. *Pediatrics* 61:62, 1978.
Referred pain to the hip, leg, or buttock, often with a gait disturbance, was common.

21. Sequeria, W., et al. Pyogenic infections of the pubic symphysis. *Ann. Intern. Med.* 96:604, 1982.
Infection of this fibrocartilaginous joint is more common in intravenous drug users. Suprapubic and groin pain occurred with walking. For a related paper, see U.B. Hoyme et al., Osteomyelitis pubis after radical gynecologic operations. Obstet. Gynecol. 63:475, 1984.

21a. Jaramillo, D., et al. Osteomyelitis and septic arthritis in children: Appropriate use of imaging to guide treatment. *A.J.R.* 165:399, 1995.

22. Treves, S., et al. Osteomyelitis: Early scintigraphic detection in children. *Pediatrics* 57:173, 1976.
Emphasizes sensitivity of scanning in making a diagnosis of osteomyelitis prior to roentgenographic changes.

23. Shauwecker, D.S., et al. Evaluation of complicating osteomyelitis with Tc-99m MDP, In-111 granulocytes and Ga-67 citrate. *J. Nucl. Med.* 25:849, 1984.
Gallium scanning was excellent in ruling out osteomyelitis when the study was normal. Indium-labeled leukocyte scans were highly sensitive and specific.

24. Oyen, W.J.G., et al. Diagnosis of bone, joint and joint prosthesis infections with In-111-labeled non-specific human immunoglobulin and scintigraphy. *Radiology* 182:195, 1992.
This method avoids the labor-intensive isolation and labeling of the patient's leukocytes.

25. Rosenthall, L. Radionuclide investigation of osteomyelitis. *Curr. Opin. Radiol.* 4:62, 1992.

26. Tehranzadeh, J., Wang, F., and Mesgarzadeh, M. Magnetic resonance imaging of osteomyelitis. *Crit. Rev. Diagn. Imaging* 33:495, 1992.
Extensive review of the role of MRI in all forms of osteomyelitis.

27. Pancoast, S.J., and Neu, H.C. Antibiotic levels in human bone and synovial fluid used in the evaluation of antimicrobial therapy of joint and skeletal infections. *Orthop. Rev.* 9:49, 1980.

This article points out the major problems involved in the bioassay for bone levels of antibiotics. For an update, see L.O. Gentry, Antibiotic therapy osteomyelitis. Infect. Dis. Clin. North Am. 4:485, 1990.

28. Weinstein, M.P., et al. Multicenter collaborative evaluation of a standardized serum bactericidal test as a predictor of therapeutic efficacy in acute and chronic osteomyelitis. *Am. J. Med.* 83:218, 1987.
    Trough serum levels of 1:2 or greater predicted cure in acute osteomyelitis. In patients with chronic osteomyelitis, peak levels of 1:16 or higher and trough titers of 1:4 or greater accurately predicted cure. Also see Chap. 25.

29. Dich, V.Q., Nelson, J.D., and Haltalin, K.C. Osteomyelitis in infants and children. *Am. J. Dis. Child.* 129:1273, 1975.
    An excellent summary of the clinical course, bacteriology, and treatment of 163 cases.

30. Bryson, Y.J., et al. High-dose oral dicloxacillin treatment of acute staphylococcal osteomyelitis in children. *J. Pediatr.* 94:673, 1979.
    Oral therapy was continued on an outpatient basis after initial intravenous therapy in hospital.

31. Tetzlaff, T.R., McCracken, G.H., Jr., and Nelson, J.D. Oral antibiotic therapy for skeletal infections of children: II. Therapy of osteomyelitis and suppurative arthritis. *J. Pediatr.* 92:485, 1978.
    Oral therapy with either cephalexin or penicillin V was used following a short course of parenteral antibiotics.

32. Nelson, J.D. Oral antibiotic therapy for serious infections in hospitalized patients. *J. Pediatr.* 92:175, 1978.
    Editorial comment on the potential advantages and disadvantages of oral therapy in osteomyelitis. One must be able to ensure compliance and monitor serum levels if oral therapy is used.

33. Proher, C.G. Oral therapy for bone and joint infections. *Pediatr. Infect. Dis.* 1:8, 1982.
    An overview. The importance of compliance and careful monitoring is stressed.

34. Syriopoulou, V.P., and Smith, A.L. Osteomyelitis and Septic Arthritis. In R.D. Feigin and J.D. Cherry (eds.), *Textbook of Pediatric Infectious Diseases* (3rd ed.). Philadelphia: Saunders, 1992. Pp. 727–740.
    Concise discussion of oral therapy uses and limitations. Contains a table of suggested oral dosages.

35. Syrogiannopoulous, G.A., and Nelson, J.D. Duration of antimicrobial therapy for acute suppurative osteoarticular infections. *Lancet* 1:37, 1988.
    A minimum of 3 weeks of combined parenteral and oral antibiotic therapy is recommended for acute osteomyelitis due to staphylococci and gram-negative bacilli. Oral therapy should be used only in patients with a prompt clinical response, and bactericidal levels in serum should be monitored.

36. Gentry, L.O., and Rodriguez, G.G. Oral ciprofloxacin compared with parenteral antibiotics in the treatment of osteomyelitis. *Antimicrob. Agents Chemother.* 34:40, 1990.
    Oral ciprofloxacin (750 mg bid) was compared to a parenteral regimen of a broad-spectrum cephalosporin or nafcillin-aminoglycoside in combination. Success rate was 77% for ciprofloxacin and 79% for parenteral therapy.

37. Desplaces, N., and Acar, J.F. New quinolones in the treatment of joint and bone infections. *Rev. Infect. Dis.* 10(S1):79, 1988.
    Cure rates of 73% for ciprofloxacin are cited in the literature reviewed. Development of resistant organisms while on therapy was seen. Thus, careful clinical and microbiologic follow-up are required (see Chap. 28).

38. Sheftel, T.G., and Mader, J.T. Randomized evaluation of ceftazidime or ticarcillin and tobramycin for the treatment of osteomyelitis caused by gram-negative bacilli. *Antimicrob. Agents Chemother.* 29:112, 1986.
    Three treatment failures occurred in nine patients treated with ceftazidime. There were no failures in the nine patients treated with the combination of tobramycin and ticarcillin.

39. Bach, M.C., and Cocchetto, D.M. Ceftazidime as a single-agent therapy for gram-negative aerobic bacillary osteomyelitis. *Antimicrob. Agents Chemother.* 31:1605, 1987.
    In the treatment of 28 patients, a regimen of ceftazidime twice daily was associated with a cure rate of 77% in acute disease and 60% in chronic disease.

40. Gillespie, W.J., and Mayo, K.M. The management of acute hematogenous osteomyelitis in the antibiotic era. *J. Bone Joint Surg.* 63B:126, 1981.
    In this series, surgical intervention was associated with a higher failure rate.

41. Canale, S.T., and Manugian, A.H. Neonatal osteomyelitis of the os calcis: A complication of repeated heel punctures. *Clin. Orthop.* 156:178, 1981.
    Sheds light on the possible association of this relatively common procedure and infection at this unusual anatomic site.
42. Sugarman, B. Pressure sores and underlying bone infection. *Arch. Intern. Med.* 147: 553, 1987.
    A systematic approach to this difficult clinical situation. Osteomyelitis of underlying bone should be considered in patients with nonhealing pressure sores. Those with positive bone scans should undergo bone biopsy after aggressive care of the ulcer.
43. Deloach, E.D., et al. The treatment of osteomyelitis underlying pressure ulcers. *Decubitus* 5:32, 1992.
    Comprehensive review of medical and surgical management as well as diagnostic modalities of this common and refractory problem. See also R.V. Darouiche et al., Osteomyelitis associated with pressure sores. Arch. Intern. Med. 154:753, 1994.
44. Mainous, E.G., and Boyne, P.J. Hyperbaric oxygen in total rehabilitation of patients with mandibular osteoradionecrosis. *Int. J. Oral Surg.* 3:297, 1974.
    Osteoradionecrosis benefits from this therapy.
45. Fitzgerald, R.H., Jr., and Cowan, J.D.E. Puncture wounds of the foot. *Orthop. Clin. North Am.* 6:965, 1975.
    See interesting related article by R.F. Jacobs et al., Pseudomonas of the foot in children. J. Infect. Dis. 160:657, 1989.
46. Fisher, M.C., Goldsmith, J.F., and Gilligan, P.H. Sneakers as a source of *Pseudomonas aeruginosa* in children with osteomyelitis following puncture wounds. *J. Pediatr.* 106: 607, 1985.
    P. aeruginosa was isolated inside the sole of sneakers in seven of eight children with puncture wound osteomyelitis.
47. Fitzgerald, R.H., Jr., et al. Deep wound sepsis following total hip arthroplasty. *J. Bone Joint Surg.* 59A:847, 1977.
    This is an excellent early series describing three stages of clinical infection. See also T.J. Grogan et al., Deep sepsis following total knee arthroplasty. J. Bone Joint Surg. 68A:226, 1986. Of 821 total knee arthroplasties, 1.7% were complicated by deep infection. The constrained type of prosthesis was at greatest risk.
48. Fitzgerald, R.H., Jr. Infections of hip prostheses and artificial joints. *Infect. Dis. Clin. North Am.* 3:329, 1989.
49. Steckelberg, J.M., and Osman, D.R. Prosthetic Joint Infections. In A.L. Bisno and F.A. Waldvogel (eds.). *Infections Associated with Indwelling Medical Devices* (2nd ed.). Washington, D.C.: American Society of Microbiology, 1994. Chap. 11.
    This is an excellent summary of mechanisms, risk factors, pathogenesis, microbiology, diagnosis, and therapy.
50. Norden, C., Gillespie, W.J., and Nade, S. Infection in Total Joint Replacement. In *Infections in Bones and Joints.* Boston: Blackwell, 1994. Chap. 17.
51. Bell, D.B., Marks, M.I., and Eickhoff, T.C. *Pasteurella multocida* arthritis and osteomyelitis. *J.A.M.A.* 210:343, 1969.
    Disease following cat bite or scratch wound may occur acutely or after an extended latent period. Penicillin is the antibiotic of choice. See detailed discussion of animal bite wounds in Chap. 4.
52. Mackowiak, P.A., Jones, S.R., and Smith, J.W. Diagnostic value of sinus-tract cultures in chronic osteomyelitis. *J.A.M.A.* 239:2772, 1978.
    An important paper citing high false positive and false negative rates when sinus tract cultures are compared with operative cultures. (See Letter to the editor, N. Engl. J. Med. 303:1532, 1980.)
53. Irons, G.B., Fisher, J., and Schmitt, E.H., III. Vascularized muscular and musculocutaneous flaps for management of osteomyelitis. *Orthop. Clin. North Am.* 15:473, 1984.
    Although the immediate success rate was 76%, there was a 12% recurrence rate at 1 year of follow-up.
54. Moore, J.R., and Weiland, A.J. Free vascularized bone and muscle flaps for osteomyelitis. *Orthopedics* 9:819, 1986.
    Thorough debridement of infected and nonviable tissue prior to grafting is essential.
55. Hansel, D.P. Vascularized tissue transfer: An adjunct to the treatment of osteomyelitis. *Orthop. Rev.* 18:595, 1989.
    The use of local muscle pedicle flaps, fasciocutaneous flaps, and free tissue transfer is reviewed.

56. Wheat, L.J., et al. Diabetic foot infections: Bacteriologic analysis. *Arch. Intern. Med.* 146:1935, 1986.
Polymicrobial infection was seen in 70% of cases. Different sources of culture are compared.

57. Bamberger, D.M., Daus, G.P., and Gerding, D.N. Osteomyelitis in the feet of diabetic patients. Long-term results, prognostic factors, and the role of antimicrobial and surgical therapy. *Am. J. Med.* 83:653, 1987.
Aggressive treatment with antibiotics was associated with a good outcome in 29 of the 51 patients, even in those with the complications of long-standing diabetes. However, histopathologic evidence of osteomyelitis was documented in only a minority of patients in this study.

57a. Caputo, G.M., et al. Assessment and management of foot disease in patients with diabetes. *N. Engl. J. Med.* 331:834, 1994.
Recent review of this topic. See related, more detailed discussion by A.W. Karchmer and G.W. Gibbons, Foot infections in diabetes: Evaluation and management.. Curr. Clin. Top. Infect. Dis. 14:1, 1994. Authors note that it has been their practice to accept the diagnosis of osteomyelitis when bone can be probed at the base of a foot ulcer, and they have not relied on other costly diagnostic modalities for confirmation. For additional reading, also see L.A. Gavin et al., Prevention and treatment of foot problems in diabetes mellitus: A comprehensive program. West. J. Med. 158:47, 1993, and accompanying editorial comment in the same issue.

58. Maurer, A.H., et al. Infection in diabetic osteoarthropathy: Use of indium-labeled leukocytes in diagnosis. *Radiology* 161:221, 1986.
Indium-labeled leukocytes and technetium scanning had similar sensitivity. However, specificity with leukocyte scanning was greater (89% versus 56%).

59. Newman, L.G., et al. Leukocyte scanning with ^{111}In is superior to magnetic resonance imaging in diagnosis of clinically unsuspected osteomyelitis in diabetic foot ulcers. *Diabetes Care* 15:1527, 1992.
Indium scans were 100% sensitive and 67% specific in diagnosis of osteomyelitis, whereas MRI scans were 29% sensitive and 67% specific.

60. Caprioli, R., et al. Prompt diagnosis of suspected osteomyelitis by utilizing percutaneous bone culture. *J. Foot Surg.* 25:263, 1986.
Percutaneous Jamshidi needle biopsy of suspected osteomyelitis was performed without complications in 13 patients. Poor correlation between ulcer cultures and bone cultures was noted. An algorithm for roentgenograms, scans, and percutaneous biopsy is presented.

61. Ger, R. Prevention of major amputation in the diabetic patient. *Arch. Surg.* 120: 1317, 1985.
A single surgeon's results in treating 48 serious diabetic foot infections over a 7-year period. Major amputation was avoided by reconstructive surgery, debridement, and vascular reconstruction.

62. Gentry, L.O. Approach to the patient with chronic osteomyelitis. *Curr. Clin. Top. Infect. Dis.* 8:62, 1987.
A review by an author with extensive experience in this difficult disease. The poor correlation between sinus tract cultures and bone cultures is especially important in chronic osteomyelitis. The author outlines his experience with percutaneous Craig needle biopsy of bone and his therapeutic approach.

63. Overton, L.M., and Tully, W.P. Surgical treatment of chronic osteomyelitis in long bones. *Am. J. Surg.* 26:736, 1973.
Excellent therapeutic response using autogenous bone grafting.

64. Norden, C.W., et al. Chronic osteomyelitis caused by *Staphylococcus aureus*: Controlled clinical trial of nafcillin therapy and nafcillin-rifampin therapy. *South. Med. J.* 79:947, 1986.
Eight of 10 patients treated with combination therapy had good clinical outcomes versus 4 of 8 in the nafcillin group.

65. Bell, S.M. Oral penicillins in the treatment of chronic staphylococcal osteomyelitis. *Lancet* 2:295, 1968.
Long-term (6 months or longer) oral therapy, with careful attention to serum levels attained, resulted in clinical improvement in patients previously refractory to therapy.

66. Hodgin, U.G. Antibiotics in the treatment of chronic staphylococcal osteomyelitis. *South. Med. J.* 68:817, 1975.
Although good therapeutic results were obtained, significant hepatotoxicity was noted in two patients. The possibility of hematopoietic side effects is also noted.

67. Gentry, L.O., and Rodriguez-Gomez, G. Ofloxacin versus parenteral therapy for chronic osteomyelitis. *Antimicrob. Agents Chemother.* 35:538, 1991.
68. Bansel, P., and Harmit, S. Management of chronic osteomyelitis using an irrigation suction technique. *Int. Orthop.* 12:265, 1988.
    Fifty patients with chronic osteomyelitis were treated with this technique with an overall success rate of 80%.
69. Jones, R.F., Barnett, J.A., and Gregory, C.F. Regional perfusion with antibiotics for chronic bone infections. *Arch. Surg.* 106:142, 1973.
    A small, uncontrolled series showing good clinical response in two-thirds of the patients so treated.
70. Calhoun, J.H., and Mader, J.T. Antibiotic beads in the management of surgical infections. *Am. J. Surg.* 157:443, 1989.
    An excellent review discussing the proposed mechanism of action, clinical use, and complications of antibiotic beads.
71. Mader, J.T., et al. Hyperbaric oxygen as adjunctive therapy for osteomyelitis. *Infect. Dis. Clin. North Am.* 4:433, 1990.
72. Osenbach, R.K., Hitchon, P.W., and Menezes, A.H. Diagnosis and management of pyogenic vertebral osteomyelitis. *Surg. Neurol.* 33:266, 1990.
    The authors review their experience with 40 patients. Disease was insidious in onset; pain was the most common symptom. An association between vertebral osteomyelitis and diabetes was noted.
72a. Torda, A.J., Gottlieb, T., and Bradbury, R. Pyogenic vertebral osteomyelitis: Analysis of 20 cases and review. *Clin. Infect. Dis.* 20:320, 1995.
73. Silverthorn, K.G., and Gillespie, W.J. Pyogenic spinal osteomyelitis: A review of 61 cases. *N.Z. Med. J.* 99:62, 1986.
    The clinical presentation and outcome of 61 cases of pyogenic vertebral osteomyelitis are reviewed. Staphylococcus aureus was cultured in 85% of cases.
73a. Correa, A.G., Edwards, M.S., and Baker, C.J. Vertebral osteomyelitis in children. *Pediatr. Infect. Dis. J.* 12:228, 1993.
    Review of eight cases and literature review; cases of diskitis or tuberculous spondylitis were excluded.
73b. Norden, C., Gillespie, W.J., and Nade, S. Vertebral Osteomyelitis and Disk Space Infections. In *Infections in Bones and Joints.* Boston: Blackwell, 1994. Chap. 14.
74. Cotty, P., et al. Vertebral osteomyelitis: Value of percutaneous biopsy, 30 cases. *J. Neuroradiol.* 15:13, 1988.
    Biopsy was valuable in confirming both the diagnosis and the microbiology of the infection.
75. Hoffer, F.A., Strand, R.D., and Gebbardt, M.C. Percutaneous biopsy of pyogenic infection of the spine of children. *J. Pediatr. Orthop.* 8:442, 1988.
    CT-directed needle biopsy allowed a microbiologic diagnosis without a surgical procedure.
76. Abramovitz, J.N., Batson, R.A., and Yablon, J.S. Vertebral osteomyelitis. The surgical management of neurologic complications. *Spine* 11:418, 1986.
    It is important in planning surgery to determine whether the cord compression is due to intraspinal abscess or spinal deformity or both. Myelography and CT scans are essential procedures in this determination.
77. MacAusland, W.R., Jr. Treatment of sepsis after intramedullary nailing of fractures of femur. *Clin. Orthop.* 60:87, 1968.
    Discusses the combined surgical and antibiotic therapy of this complicated problem.
78. Patzakis, M.J., Wilkins, J., and Wiss, D.A. Infection following intramedullary nailing of long bones. Diagnosis and management. *Clin. Orthop.* 212:182, 1986.
    If fracture stability is dependent on the nail, it should be left in place. Infection should be controlled with adequate debridement and appropriate antibiotics.
79. Banes, P.F., and Barrons, S.A. Tuberculosis in the 1990's. *Ann. Intern. Med.* 119:400, 1993.
80. Davidson, P.T., and Horowitz, I. Skeletal tuberculosis: A review with patient presentations and discussion. *Am. J. Med.* 48:77, 1970.
    The salient features of tuberculous bone disease are presented using a case-oriented discussion.
81. Martini, M., Ajrad, A., and Boudjemaa, A. Tuberculous osteomyelitis. A review of 125 cases. *Int. Orthop.* 10:201, 1986.
    Although any bone can be involved, the tibia and femur were the most common. A favorable outcome with chemotherapy was seen in 92% of cases. Immobilization was not necessary, and surgery was limited to the draining of large abscesses.

82. Wolinsky, E. Nontuberculous mycobacteria and associated diseases. *Am. Rev. Respir. Dis.* 119:107, 1979.
    An extensive review of the spectrum of disease caused by "atypical" mycobacteria.
83. Benson, C.A., and Ellner, J.J., *Mycobacterium avium* complex infection and AIDS: Advances in theory and practice. *Clin. Infect. Dis.* 17:7, 1993.
83a. Gibbons, G.W., and Habershaw, G.M. Diabetic foot infections: Anatomy and surgery. *Infect. Dis. Clin. North Am.* 9:131, 1995.
    Article reviews the mechanical dysfunction leading to ulceration of the foot in patients with diabetes and the nonsurgical and surgical approaches to such ulcers. Contains a good discussion of local measures to prevent or treat neuropathic ulcers.
84. Gibbons, G.W. The diabetic foot: Amputations and drainage of infection. *J. Vasc. Surg.* 5:791, 1987.
    Gives a very helpful description of surgical treatment preceding amputation.
85. Bessman, A. Foot problems in the diabetic. *Compr. Ther.* 8:32, 1982.
    This article presents a very effective discussion of prophylactic foot care.
86. Little, J.R., and Kobayashi, G.S. Infection of the Diabetic Foot. In M.E. Levin and L.W. O'Neal (eds.), *The Diabetic Foot* (4th ed.). St. Louis: Mosby, 1988.
    Also see B.A. Lipsky, et al., The diabetic foot: Soft tissue and bone infection. Infect. Dis. Clin. North Am. 4:409, 1990.
87. Towne, J.B. Management of Foot Lesions in the Diabetic Patient. In R.B. Rutherford (ed.), *Vascular Surgery* (2nd ed.). Philadelphia: Saunders, 1984.
    An excellent description of surgical treatment, with some discussion of vascular reconstruction.
88. Handwerger, B.S., Fernandes, G., and Brown, D.M. Immune and autoimmune aspects of diabetes mellitus. *Hum. Pathol.* 11:338, 1980.
    An extensive review of this vast and controversial subject.
89. Rayfield, E.J., et al. Infection and diabetes: The case for glucose control. *Am. J. Med.* 72:439, 1982.
    Outlines the theoretic basis for glucose control. In the authors' retrospective chart review, urinary tract, respiratory tract, and skin infections were more frequent in patients with poorly controlled diabetes, suggesting that glucose control may benefit patients.
90. Delbridge, L., Appleberg, M., and Reeve, T.S. Factors associated with development of foot lesions in the diabetic. *Surgery* 93:78, 1983.
    Comparing groups of diabetics older than 50 years of age, this study found vascular disease, cigarette smoking, and patient understanding to be significantly associated with the development of foot lesions. Diabetes control and neuropathy were important parameters, although not as important as the aforementioned factors.
91. Leichter, S.B., et al. Clinical characteristics of diabetic patients with serious pedal infections. *Metabolism* 37(Suppl. 1):22, 1988.
    Clinical description of the diabetic with foot infection. Patients are usually obese, type II diabetics.
92. Taylor, L.M., and Porter, J.M. The clinical course of diabetics who require emergent foot surgery because of infection or ischemia. *J. Vasc. Surg.* 6:454, 1987.
    Aggressive surgical treatment and liberal use of lower-extremity revascularization resulted in long-term salvage of 73% of limbs.
93. Corson, J.D., et al. The diabetic foot. *Curr. Probl. Surg.* 23:721, 1986.
    A review of surgical treatment of diabetic foot infections, with emphasis on vascular reconstruction.
94. Wagner, F.W. Treatment of the diabetic foot. *Compr. Ther.* 10:29, 1984.
    In this outline, the author utilizes roentgenographic changes, degree of infection, neuropathy, and gangrene to describe five patterns of diabetic neuropathic bone and joint disease and six grades of the diabetic foot.
95. Jeffcoate, W.J., et al. The Significance of Infection in Diabetic Foot Lesions. In H. Connor, A.J.M. Boulton, and J.D. Ward (eds.), *The Foot in Diabetes.* Chichester, NY: Wiley, 1987.
    A concise review of the topic. Microbiologic results from different studies are summarized.
96. Sapico, F.L., et al. The infected foot of the diabetic patient: Quantitative microbiology and analysis of clinical features. *Rev. Infect. Dis.* 6(Suppl. 1):S171, 1984.
    The authors obtained deep-tissue cultures from 32 patients scheduled for lower-limb amputation and compared them with the results from ulcer curettage and swabs.
97. Goldberg, D., and Neu, H.C. Infectious Diseases of the Diabetic Foot. In M.A. Brenner (ed.), *Management of the Diabetic Foot.* Baltimore: Williams & Wilkins, 1987.

The specific types of nonulcerative diabetic foot infections and the possible antibiotic choices are reviewed in detail.

97a. Grayson, M.L. Diabetic foot infections. *Infect. Dis. Clin. North Am.* 9:143, 1995.

97b. Gerding, D. Foot infections in diabetic patients: The role of anaerobes. *Clin. Infect. Dis.* 20(Suppl. 2):S283, 1995.
The prevalence of anaerobes is dependent on the method of obtaining specimens, the care with which specimens are transported anaerobically, and the sophistication of the laboratory. See related paper by S. Johnson et al., Use of an anaerobic collection and transport swab device to recover anaerobic bacteria from infected foot ulcers in diabetics. Clin. Infect. Dis. 20(Suppl. 2):S289, 1995. The paper concludes that although anaerobes are commonly isolated, their role in infected ulcers remains to be elucidated.

98. Kaufman, J., Breeding, L., and Rosenberg, N. Anatomic location of acute diabetic foot infection: Its influence on the outcome of treatment. *Am. Surg.* 53:109, 1987.
Limb salvage was lower and mortality higher in diabetic patients with infections located at and above the metatarsal level compared with those with distal infections.

99. Newman, L.G., et al. Unsuspected osteomyelitis in diabetic foot ulcers. *J.A.M.A.* 266:1246, 1991.
Osteomyelitis was found to complicate 28 (68%) of 41 diabetic foot infections. Only nine cases of osteomyelitis were diagnosed clinically. Leukocyte scan was 89% sensitive.

100. Zlatkin, M.B., et al. The diabetic foot. *Radiol. Clin. North Am.* 25:1095, 1987.
An excellent review of diagnostic imaging of the diabetic foot.

101. Kucan, J.O., and Robson, M.C. Diabetic foot infections: Fate of the contralateral foot. *Plast. Reconstr. Surg.* 77:439, 1986.
Even with conservative therapy of the initially infected foot, the contralateral foot was infected within 18 months in 49% of patients.

102. National Diabetes Advisory Board. The prevention and treatment of five complications of diabetes: A guide for primary care physicians. *Metabolism* 33:15, 1984.
A short synopsis of recommendations for physicians treating patients with diabetes mellitus.

103. Bild, D.E., et al. Lower extremity amputation in people with diabetes. Epidemiology and prevention. *Diabetes Care* 12:24, 1989.
Reviews prevention programs. The rates of amputation in diabetics have been reduced by 44–85% after the implementation of good foot-care programs.

104. Duckworth, T., et al. Plantar pressure measurements and the prevention of ulceration in the diabetic foot. *J. Bone Joint Surg.* 67B:79, 1985.
In an attempt to prevent pressure ulcerations in patients with neuropathy, static and dynamic pedobarographic screening was helpful in guiding footwear design.

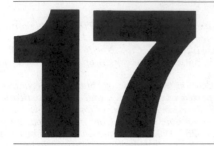

Infectious Mononucleosis and Mononucleosis-like Syndromes

C. Richard Magnussen
and Raphael Dolin

Infectious mononucleosis (IM) is an acute, self-limited infectious disease of children and young adults identified by its characteristic clinical, hematologic, and serologic manifestations. The hallmarks are fever, sore throat, lymphadenopathy, splenomegaly, and lymphocytosis with "atypical" changes in the mononuclear elements of the peripheral blood. Serologic studies reveal the presence of a positive heterophil antibody titer or a positive Monospot slide test. A fourfold rise in antibody titer specific for Epstein-Barr virus (EBV) or the presence of IgM antibody to EBV is indicative of recent infection. A variety of other infectious agents can cause an infectious mononucleosis–like syndrome the unifying characteristic of which is peripheral lymphocytosis with circulating atypical lymphocytes. It is important to distinguish classic infectious mononucleosis caused by EBV infection from infectious mononucleosis–like syndromes caused by other agents, particularly cytomegalovirus (CMV) and *Toxoplasma gondii*.

Classic Infectious Mononucleosis

The term **infectious mononucleosis** was first introduced in 1921 to describe a syndrome characterized by fever, lymphadenopathy, prostration, and a mononuclear lymphocytosis in six previously healthy young adults. Two years later, a more detailed description of the atypical lymphocyte appeared and, in the early 1930s the findings of Paul and Bunnell and others led to the specific heterophil antibody tests now used in the diagnosis of IM. In 1968, Henle and coworkers [1] presented evidence from seroepidemiologic data that EBV was the etiologic agent of heterophil antibody–positive IM.

I. **Etiology.** IM is caused by a double-stranded DNA virus of the herpesvirus group called *EBV*. There is evidence that EBV is the etiologic agent in heterophil-positive IM.

    A. Seroepidemiologic studies revealed that only individuals lacking anti-EBV antibodies developed IM, and the presence of antibody to EBV confers immunity to heterophil-positive IM.

    B. EBV could be demonstrated in cultured B lymphocytes of patients with IM.

II. **Clinical features** [2]

    A. **Age.** Classic IM occurs most commonly in the 15- to 25-year age group. In very young children, the primary infection is either asymptomatic or insidious, producing mild tonsillitis that often is indistinguishable from that caused by other viral agents or group A streptococci. Clinical IM is uncommon in young children. IM also can occur in the elderly, with a clinical presentation different from classic IM [3]. EBV infection in older adults can be severe, with debilitating fever, malaise, and fatigue, but pharyngitis, cervical adenopathy, and splenomegaly may be minimal.

    B. **The incubation period** for primary EBV infection is approximately 30–45 days. The onset usually is accompanied by a prodromal period that may last 7–14 days; it is characterized by fatigue, generalized malaise, myalgias, and headache. In some cases, the onset may be acute, and the first sign is high fever.

    C. **Signs and symptoms.** Common symptoms include fever, sore throat, malaise, headache, myalgias, sweats, anorexia, abdominal pain (due to splenic enlargement or associated hepatitis), chest pain, and cough. The onset of symptoms may be insidious. **Clinical diagnostic clues** that are helpful in distinguishing classic IM at the bedside include:

1. **Tonsillar enlargement, exudative tonsillitis, and pharyngeal inflammation,** which may be indistinguishable from acute pharyngitis caused by group A streptococci or other viruses.
2. **Lymphadenopathy** that primarily involves the posterior cervical area, although generalized adenopathy may occur. The lymph nodes are symmetric, discrete, and tender, but are not fixed.
3. **Hepatomegaly,** seen in 50% of cases. Abnormal liver function tests are obtained in 80% of cases. Compared with classic viral hepatitis, alkaline phosphatase is elevated and is disproportionately higher than transaminase enzymes. Bilirubin usually is only minimally elevated, and **clinical jaundice is rare.**
4. **Splenomegaly,** seen in approximately 75% of cases. If it is present, care should be taken to **avoid traumatic palpation,** which may increase the risk of splenic rupture.
5. **Maculopapular rashes,** which are present in fewer than 5% of cases. However, if ampicillin is given inadvertently to patients with IM, almost all will develop a drug eruption (see Chap. 27).
6. **Petechial enanthema** on the soft palate, which is common but not specific for IM.

D. **Hematologic abnormalities**
   1. **Lymphocytes.** An important feature of IM is an absolute ($>$4,500/mm^3) and relative ($>$50% of the total WBC count) increase in peripheral mononuclear cells, of which 10–20% are atypical lymphocytes. The **atypical lymphocyte (Downey cell)** is a large lymphocyte with an abundant cytoplasm, cytoplasmic vacuoles, loose nuclear chromatin, and indentation of the cell membrane by adjacent erythrocytes. **Atypical lymphocytes in the peripheral blood are not pathognomonic for IM and can be associated with infection by** CMV, adenovirus, rubella, herpes simplex virus, *T. gondii,* and other viral infections. Studies have shown that the atypical lymphocytes are of thymic origin (T lymphocytes), whereas EBV infects bone marrow–derived lymphocytes (B lymphocytes).
   2. **Total WBC count** usually numbers between 10,000 and 20,000 leukocytes per cubic millimeter by the second or third week of illness. On occasion, the total count may rise to as high as 50,000/mm^3, suggesting a leukemoid reaction. Neutropenia with increased immature cells frequently can be present in the early stages of the illness.

E. **Heterophil antibodies** develop in response to primary infection with EBV. They are reactive with antigens of other species, can be present in normal human sera, and are associated with a variety of lymphoproliferative states as well. The heterophil antibody that develops in response to EBV infection is an IgM antibody that reacts with surface antigens of sheep and horse RBCs but not guinea pig kidney cells. Heterophil antibodies unrelated to EBV infection react with guinea pig kidney cells. The differential absorption of heterophil antibodies to guinea pig kidney is the basis of the Paul-Bunnell-Davidsohn test, used to detect heterophil antibodies specific for EBV infectious mononucleosis (see sec. **III.B.1**).

F. **Nonspecific antibody responses** observed during various stages of classic IM include rheumatoid factors, antinuclear factors, antiplatelet antibodies, *Salmonella* agglutinins, *Proteus* OX 19 antibodies, cryoglobulins, and cold-reactive antibodies to the i antigen on RBCs.

III. **Diagnosis**
A. **Differential diagnosis.** A variety of conditions that closely mimic classic EBV-induced IM are now recognized [2]. These IM-like syndromes have as a unifying feature peripheral lymphocytosis with the presence of circulating atypical lymphocytes. In addition, the IM syndromes are characterized by some or all of the following: fever, malaise, pharyngitis, adenopathy, hepatomegaly, and splenomegaly. Unlike classic IM, there is no associated heterophil antibody response. Therefore, these syndromes are also called *heterophil-negative IM.* Proper differentiation of these conditions is necessary to avoid misdiagnosis of serious illnesses (e.g., lymphoma, leukemia, or viral hepatitis) and to prevent patient anxiety and invasive diagnostic procedures for more benign, self-limited illnesses (e.g., CMV or *T. gondii* infections). The following is a list of causes of **heterophil-negative IM,** with some important differentiating features (see discussion under Infectious Mononucleosis–like Syndromes later in the chapter).

1. **Cytomegalovirus IM** uncommonly is accompanied by pharyngitis or adenopathy. Splenomegaly is less prominent than in EBV-induced illness.
2. **T. gondii IM** commonly presents with posterior cervical adenopathy only and no pharyngitis; liver function tests can be completely normal even in the presence of hepatomegaly.
3. **Viral hepatitis** may be associated with atypical lymphocytes, but the percentage is lower than in classic IM. The transaminase enzymes are elevated and are disproportionately higher than levels of alkaline phosphatase, whereas the reverse is true of EBV and CMV hepatitis.
4. **Leptospirosis** has modest pharyngeal symptoms and either a normal differential WBC count or a predominance of polymorphonuclear leukocytes.
5. **Rubella** is associated with postauricular and suboccipital adenopathy, a characteristic exanthem, and a shorter course than classic IM.
6. **Lymphoma** is associated with nontender, fixed adenopathy.
7. **Leukemia** has a characteristic peripheral WBC morphology.
8. **Infectious lymphocytosis** is not accompanied by lymphadenopathy or splenomegaly.
9. **Diphenylhydantoin, para-aminosalicylic acid (PAS), and isoniazid** drug reactions can be associated with fever and generalized lymphadenopathy.
10. **Acute human immunodeficiency virus (HIV) infection** can mimic IM. See Chap. 19 (p. 724).
11. **Miscellaneous** causes include adenovirus infections, herpes simplex virus infections, and brucellosis. A severe infectious mononucleosis–like syndrome caused by human herpesvirus 6 infection has recently been reported in one patient [4].
    The two most common causes of heterophil-negative IM are CMV and *T. gondii*. Except for EBV-induced illness, an IM syndrome is not the most common clinical presentation for any of the diseases just listed. However, IM syndromes do occur frequently enough to cause diagnostic confusion. CMV and *T. gondii* are discussed in more detail under Infectious Mononucleosis–like Syndromes.
B. **Serologic diagnosis.** Clinical suspicion of EBV-induced IM can be confirmed serologically in the majority of cases.
   1. **Heterophil antibody** that agglutinates sheep or horse RBCs develops as a **nonspecific** serologic response to EBV infection. After the onset of IM, heterophil antibodies are detectable at variable levels, depending on the duration of illness: 40% by week 1, 60% by week 2, and 80–90% by week 3. Titers remain elevated for 3–6 months, and this elevation usually implies acute disease; however, a titer occasionally can remain elevated for as long as 1 year. Common laboratory tests used to detect heterophil antibodies include the following:
      a. Tests designed to measure heterophil antibodies have been adapted for purposes of rapid diagnosis. These so-called slide or spot tests have virtually replaced the more traditional tests due to their ease of use. They are highly sensitive for the detection of EBV-induced IM. However, **repeat testing (e.g., at weekly intervals) may be necessary** in some patients because only 60% of individuals will have heterophil antibodies by the second week of the illness. See sec. I.
      b. The spot tests are available from more than 25 different manufacturers. An early prototype test was the Monospot. Some of the more widely used tests now are **Mono-Test** and **Mono-Latex** (Wampole Diagnostics, Cranbury, NJ), **Access Color Slide II** (Seradyn, Inc., Indianapolis, IN), **Monosticon** (Organon Teknika Corp., Durham, NC), and **ImmunoCard Mono** (Meridian Diagnostics, Inc., Cincinnati, OH). As initially formulated, spot tests detected agglutinins to formalized horse RBCs after an absorption step with guinea pig or horse kidney to eliminate cross-reactions with Forssman and serum sickness antibodies (Monosticon). Newer tests use bovine red cell membranes attached to latex particles (Mono-Latex), specially treated horse RBCs (Mono-Test), or solid-phase enzyme-linked immunosorbent assay (ELISA; ImmunoCard Mono) to eliminate the absorption step while maintaining a high degree of specificity.
      c. **The false negative rate of these rapid tests is 10–15%, and false negative results are more frequent among children (the test is usually negative in**

children younger than 5 years). For these patients, EBV-specific serologic testing is needed [5].

   d. False positive spot tests generally are considered uncommon but have been described with rubella, hepatitis, other viral infections, and lymphoma.

   e. The duration of a positive spot test after acute IM is not well described but appears to be in the range of 3–6 months, although the test may occasionally be positive for up to 1 year.

2. **EBV antibody** seroconversion for diagnosis of classic IM is most useful in those adults (approximately 10%) with EBV-induced IM who do not develop heterophil antibodies or who do not have a positive Monospot test. EBV antibody titers may also be necessary for confirming infection in young children, who rarely have a positive heterophil response, or in a patient of any age with an atypical mononucleosis-like illness.

   a. Infected B lymphocytes produce several virus-specific antigens: viral capsid antigen (VCA), early antigen (EA), and Epstein-Barr nuclear antigen (EBNA). Assay of the antibody response to these antigens can be used to differentiate recent from remote EBV infection and to diagnose classic IM in the absence of a heterophil response [2].

      (1) **IgG antibody to viral capsid antigen (VCA-IgG)** is present in active, recent, and past infections and persists for life. A single elevated titer of VCA-IgG does not, by itself, confirm a diagnosis of acute EBV illness but indicates only that infection with EBV has occurred sometime in the past.

      (2) **IgM antibody to viral capsid antigen (VCA-IgM)** is present in primary EBV infection and usually disappears within 1–2 months.

      (3) **Antibody to early antigen** may be detected in up to 70% of patients with acute IM. This antibody resolves after the patient recovers from the infection.

      (4) **Antibody to Epstein-Barr nuclear antigen** appears within 3–4 weeks of the onset of IM and persists for life. The appearance of EBNA in persons who previously had antibody to VCA (see sec. **B.2.a.(1)**) is strong evidence for recent EBV infection.

   b. **EBV-specific antibody studies should be reserved** for the diagnosis of heterophil-negative or atypical primary EBV infection. Acute or recent infection is probable if all four of the following serologic criteria are present: (1) VCA-IgM; (2) high titers ($\geq$ 1:320) of VCA-IgG; (3) anti-EA ($\geq$ 1:10); and (4) absence of antibody to EBNA. Serum should be obtained during convalescence (e.g., at 6–8 weeks) to demonstrate disappearance of VCA-IgM and appearance of anti-EBNA as further confirmation of recent EBV infection.

IV. **Complications.** Although most patients have a benign clinical course with EBV-induced IM, complications occasionally occur.

   A. **Hematologic complications**

   1. **Hemolytic anemia** of the Coombs'-positive type occurs in 1–3% of cases and is mediated by IgM cold-agglutinin antibodies directed at the RBC i antigen.

   2. **Thrombocytopenia** is not uncommon, but associated purpura is rare.

   3. **Granulocytopenia** occasionally progresses to agranulocytosis.

   B. **Hepatitis with clinical jaundice** is uncommon.

   C. **Splenic rupture** occurs in approximately 0.2% of cases. This may be the initial complaint, or it may occur after multiple palpations (which should be avoided).

   D. **Neurologic syndromes** reported in association with classic IM are Landry-Guillain-Barré syndrome, meningitis, encephalitis, mononeuritis, cerebellar dysfunction, and transverse myelitis. Cerebrospinal fluid (CSF) pleocytosis may be more common than has been recognized clinically.

   E. **Miscellaneous complications** include myositis, myopericarditis, pneumonitis [5a], pancreatitis, and postanginal sepsis resulting from phlebitis of the jugular veins [6].

V. **Therapy. No therapy is indicated for the vast majority of cases of classic IM,** but several antiviral agents currently show promise (see sec. **D**). Antibiotics have no effect on uncomplicated cases, and the indiscriminate use of ampicillin may lead to the unnecessary complication of a maculopapular rash.

   A. **Throat cultures** for group A beta-hemolytic streptococci should be obtained (positive in approximately 25% of patients with IM in some series). If they are positive, appropriate treatment is indicated.

B. **Salicylates or other analgesics** usually are adequate to control fever, headaches, and sore throat in the acute phase.

C. **Corticosteroids** are employed **in the management of certain complications,** but their value is uncertain. A short course of prednisone, starting with 40–60 mg/day, can be administered for 7–10 days. Once there is a good clinical response, the dose can be rapidly tapered. Corticosteroids are indicated in:

1. **Severe** toxic exudative **tonsillitis,** pharyngeal edema, or laryngeal edema **when there is impending or early airway obstruction.**

2. **Acute hemolytic anemia and severe thrombocytopenia.**

3. **Neurologic complications.**

4. **Myocarditis and pericarditis.**

Occasionally, in a patient with marked toxicity and a prolonged course, steroids will be employed to abbreviate the course of the disease. In these situations, the diagnosis must be clear so that the corticosteroids do not mask some other disease presenting like IM (e.g., leukemia or lymphoma). The authors generally try to avoid corticosteroids in this setting and try to use analgesics and salicylates unless one of the listed purported indications for steroids also exists.

D. **Specific antiviral chemotherapy** for EBV infection is not currently available. Although phosphonoacetic acid, acyclovir, and interferons all inhibit EBV in vitro, none of these agents has shown consistent clinical benefit to date [7, 8]. (See Chap. 26 for a more detailed discussion of antiviral agents.)

E. **Transmission and implications for isolation.** Since EBV is found in oropharyngeal secretions, kissing is one of the presumed mechanisms of transmission. In the hospital or home, no specific isolation precautions are required other than careful handling of oral secretions. The demonstration of cell-free virus shedding from the human uterine cervix may indicate that sexual transmission of EBV infection is possible [9].

VI. **Prognosis**

A. **Duration** of EBV-induced IM symptoms usually is 2–4 weeks, but 3% of patients may have disease lasting longer than 1 month.

B. **Long-term sequelae** are **unusual** in uncomplicated illness, but neurologic complications may persist with varying degrees of severity.

C. **Reinfection does not occur** because the primary EBV infection confers lifelong immunity.

VII. **Chronic EBV infection.** After acute primary EBV infection, the virus persists in a latent state in B lymphocytes and salivary glands. Reactivation of EBV can result in a **rare, severe illness,** characterized by both cellular and humoral immune defects and histologic evidence of major organ involvement: lymphadenopathy, splenomegaly, hypoplasia of bone marrow presenting as cytopenia (anemia, thrombocytopenia, or leukopenia), chronic persistent hepatitis, interstitial pneumonitis, malabsorption due to lymphocyte infiltration of the small intestine, and uveitis [10, 11]. **Patients with this illness have a unique serologic response to EBV,** with very high titers of VCA-IgG (> 1:5,120), high titers of early antigen (> 1:640), and low titers of EBNA (< 1:2).

Infectious Mononucleosis–like Syndromes

A number of diseases have many clinical signs and symptoms in common with EBV-induced IM [2]. Pharyngitis, adenopathy, hepatosplenomegaly, and lymphocytosis are common to each of these disease entities, although they are not universally present. Careful attention to distinguishing clinical and serologic characteristics of these diseases should enable a proper diagnosis.

I. **CMV mononucleosis** is the **leading cause of heterophil-negative IM-like syndromes.** CMV is a member of the herpesvirus group and is closely related to EBV. Most CMV infection in adults is subclinical, but infection occasionally manifests itself as an IM-like syndrome.

As many as 5–10% of all cases of mononucleosis-like syndrome may be due to CMV infection [12]. The syndrome can occur with naturally acquired infection or may follow extracorporeal circulation in cardiac surgery ("postperfusion syndrome"). CMV infection manifested as an IM-like syndrome also has been associated with multiple blood transfusions, and CMV has been shown to be transmitted through renal allograft or bone marrow transplantation (see Chap. 20). Active homosexual men appear to be at a greater risk of CMV infection than are heterosexual men. Also, CMV frequently causes serious infections in patients with AIDS (see Chap. 19).

A. **Clinical features** of the CMV mononucleosis syndrome in normal hosts vary in certain respects from those of classic EBV-induced IM. In prior retrospective studies, a slightly older patient group (25- to 35-year-olds) are affected. Patients may have fever, malaise, hepatitis, splenomegaly, and lymphocytosis with atypical lymphocytes, as in classic IM. However, CMV is distinguished clinically from classic IM by the **low incidence of pharyngitis and cervical adenopathy.** The splenomegaly also may not be as prominent as in EBV-induced disease. However, in a recent prospective study in children, CMV mononucleosis was significantly more frequent in children younger than 4 years of age and, although symptoms of EBV-IM and CMV mononucleosis were similar, only cervical adenopathy was more frequent in EBV infection (83%) than it was in CMV infection (75%). There was no significant difference in the rates of exudative pharyngitis or splenomegaly in EBV- versus CMV-mononucleosis [12]. CMV lung infections are discussed in Chap. 9.

B. **Transmission** of CMV occurs mainly through close personal contact. CMV shedding has been detected in saliva, urine, cervical secretions, semen, stool, tears, breast milk, and blood. However, the two principal routes of acquisition of primary infection appear to be oral and sexual transmission. Also, CMV infection can be acquired from massive blood transfusions or can follow renal or bone marrow transplantation through transmission in donor leukocytes.

C. **Diagnosis** of CMV is often difficult to establish clearly. Certain laboratory confirmation is necessary.

1. **Viral isolation from saliva or urine** can detect CMV shedding during acute infection. However, shedding may be prolonged and does not unequivocally indicate a direct causal relationship between CMV and an IM-like syndrome. Also, viral culture techniques often may not be available.

2. **Serologic workup.** The heterophil and Monospot tests will be negative. **The most efficient way to make a serologic diagnosis of CMV infection is to screen for the presence of IgG antibody to CMV using an ELISA test. If positive, acute infection can be diagnosed by testing for the presence of IgM antibody to CMV.** Most laboratories use ELISA methodology for the IgM test; rheumatoid factor must be removed to avoid false positive results. A diagnosis of acute CMV infection can also be made by detecting a fourfold or greater rise in antibody using an IgG indirect immunofluorescent antibody test (IgG-IFA), but this requires acute and convalescent blood samples and is recommended only if the IgM ELISA test is not readily available. Most laboratories no longer perform CMV complement fixation antibody testing.

D. **Complications** are infrequent in normal hosts, and in healthy adults the illness usually pursues a benign course. However, the following complications have been associated with CMV infection:

1. **Ampicillin-induced rash.**

2. **Hepatitis** with clinical **jaundice** occasionally.

3. **Hemolytic anemia,** which can result from an IgM cold agglutinin directed against the RBC i antigen.

4. **Thrombocytopenia.**

5. **Neurologic syndromes,** including Landry-Guillain-Barré syndrome, aseptic meningitis, encephalitis, and polyneuritis.

6. **Interstitial pneumonitis.** (See Chaps. 9 and 19 for discussion of CMV infections in the compromised host, including AIDS.)

7. **Chorioretinitis,** which is seen rarely in acute infection of immunocompetent patients but is more common in the immunocompromised host (see Chap. 19).

E. **Therapy** usually is not indicated in most cases of CMV mononucleosis. (The role of ganciclovir in CMV infections in patients with AIDS and other immunocompromised patients is discussed in Chaps. 19 and 26.)

1. **General supportive measures** will allow most normal individuals to recover uneventfully.

2. **Corticosteroids** may be used for the same conditions described for EBV infection. CMV infection does not usually cause pharyngeal inflammation, and upper airway obstruction therefore should not be a problem.

   3. Universal precaution procedures for hospitalized patients shedding CMV is
      sufficient.
   F. Prophylaxis may eventually be possible with a live attenuated CMV vaccine that
      is now undergoing clinical trials. However, indications for future use of this vaccine
      remain controversial.
II. *Toxoplasma gondii* **mononucleosis** is probably the second leading cause of heterophil-negative IM syndromes. *T. gondii* is a protozoan found in many species of warm-
   blooded animals throughout the world. Infection with the protozoan in healthy adults
   is usually subclinical, but it can manifest as an IM syndrome. In the immunocompromised host, *T. gondii* is an opportunistic pathogen and may cause lethal infection.
   CNS toxoplasmosis has been an increasingly recognized opportunistic infection in
   patients with AIDS (see Chap. 19).
   A. Clinical features of *T. gondii* infection in normal hosts can be grouped into three
      distinct syndromes [13, 14]. **See Chap. 19 for a discussion of toxoplasmosis in
      AIDS patients and Chap. 20 for a discussion of toxoplasmosis in transplant
      patients.**
      1. Acute acquired toxoplasmosis in the immunocompetent host may produce
         a syndrome indistinguishable from classic IM, with fever, malaise, adenopathy,
         palpable liver, splenomegaly, maculopapular rash, and a peripheral lymphocy-
         tosis with atypical lymphocytes. The adenopathy may be generalized or, more
         commonly, may involve the posterior cervical nodes alone. In contrast to EBV-
         induced IM, pharyngitis is not prominent, and the spleen is not enlarged to
         the same degree. Also, a rash can occur without ampicillin therapy, and liver
         function tests may be normal in the presence of hepatomegaly. Infections can
         occur in patients with AIDS. Toxoplasmosis in the compromised host is re-
         viewed elsewhere [15]. Neurologic syndromes may occur in these hosts in
         particular and in patients with AIDS (see discussion in Chap. 19).
      2. Ocular toxoplasmosis results from the activation of cysts previously deposited
         in or near the retina during congenital infection or from a subclinical infection
         acquired later in life.
      3. Congenital toxoplasmosis. See Chap. 3, sec. I under Disseminated Uterine
         Infections.
   B. Life cycle. *T. gondii* is a protozoan parasite whose definitive hosts are members
      of the feline family, in particular the domestic cat. The sexual phase of the life
      cycle takes place in the intestine of the cat, where oocysts are produced; these
      are shed in cat feces and deposited in the soil. The oocysts are ingested by interme-
      diate hosts including wild animals, mice, cattle, swine, sheep, and humans. In
      the intermediate host, the oocysts pass into the intestine, where development
      into the trophozoite form takes place; during this phase, the trophozoites encyst
      in the tissue. The tissue cysts persist in a viable latent form in the host for life,
      retaining the potential for reactivation at any time.
   C. Epidemiology and transmission. Humans can acquire the infection by three
      routes.
      1. Ingestion of raw or undercooked meat of another intermediate host (chicken,
         mutton, pork, beef) that contains cysts.
      2. Ingestion of oocysts from cat feces (e.g., while handling cat litter boxes).
      3. Maternal-fetal transmission (congenital toxoplasmosis) during acute parasitic
         infection in the pregnant woman.
   D. Diagnosis. Because there are no pathognomonic clinical features of toxoplasmosis,
      serologic diagnosis is particularly useful and important.
      1. Serologic tests are important and useful in distinguishing individuals with
         recently acquired infection from a large group of individuals who have acquired
         the infection months or years ago. As 30–40% of adults in the United States
         have serologic evidence of prior subclinical infection with *T. gondii*, it is crucial
         to distinguish those with acute serologic changes.
         a. The **Sabin-Feldman dye test** is a neutralization test based on the observa-
            tion that toxoplasma trophozoites exposed to specific immune serum in
            vitro fail to stain with methylene blue dye. It is a sensitive and specific
            test, but titers peak in 6–8 weeks, then slowly decline over 1–2 years, and
            usually remain positive for life. Therefore, it may aid as a screening tool,
            but it has **limited usefulness** in detecting acute infections unless very early
            serum samples are available. Also, because live organisms are required,
            this test is not routinely available.

b. The **IgM immunofluorescent antibody test** (IgM-IFA) is very useful for **detecting early disease** (i.e., within the first 2–4 months of illness). The IgM-IFA detects the early brief IgM antibody response, and a titer of 1:160 or greater is considered diagnostic of active, recently acquired disease.

IgM antibodies to *T. gondii* appear in the first week after onset of acute infection, peak within 1 month, and usually revert to negative within several months. Therefore, if the sample is drawn very early or late in the course of an acute illness, the titer may be negative. For diagnosis of congenital toxoplasmosis, see Chap. 3, sec. I under Disseminated Intrauterine Infections.

c. The **IgG-IFA** uses slide preparations of killed *T. gondii* incubated with serial dilutions of the patient's serum. Reaction between the patient's antibody and the toxoplasma organisms is detected by application of a fluorescein-conjugated antihuman antibody. In virtually all laboratories, the **IgG-IFA test has replaced the Sabin-Feldman dye test.** IgG antibody to *T. gondii* peaks 1–2 months after onset of infection. A serial fourfold titer rise between acute and convalescent sera with the IgG-IFA test is indicative of acute infection. A single elevated titer does not establish a diagnosis of acute infection, because elevated titers may persist in chronic latent infection.

d. **Indirect hemagglutination antibody** (IHA) **and complement fixation antibody** (CFA) titers tend to peak later than antibody measured by the dye test or IgG-IFA. Therefore IHA or CFA testing may be helpful in diagnosis if serum is tested later in the course of the illness. However, a positive test does not prove acute infection and a negative test does not exclude recent infection.

2. **Lymph node biopsy** may reveal a specific histology that is believed to be diagnostic for toxoplasmosis. However, histologic tissue biopsy interpretation requires considerable expertise. There is reactive follicular hyperplasia with irregular clusters of epithelioid histiocytes encroaching on the margins of germinal centers. The organisms usually are not observed.

3. **Identification of *T. gondii*** in muscle, lung, liver, heart, brain, and so on is possible if a biopsy specimen can be obtained. The protozoan rarely is observed in lymph nodes. *T. gondii* can be isolated from body fluids or tissue after intraperitoneal inoculation into mice, but this technique is not available routinely.

E. **Therapy is not necessary for the majority of toxoplasmosis mononucleosis syndromes.**

1. **Indications for treatment** are the following:
   a. **Severe and persistent constitutional symptoms.**
   b. **Vital organ damage,** as in pneumonia, myocarditis, or encephalitis.
   c. **Active chorioretinitis.**
   d. **Infection in the immunocompromised host and patients with AIDS** (see Chap. 19).
   e. **Congenital toxoplasmosis** (see Chap. 3).

2. **Therapeutic regimens** using a combination of sulfadiazine (or triple sulfonamides) with pyrimethamine comprise the only treatment proven effective against acute toxoplasmosis in immunocompetent adults. Various dose regimens have been suggested, and infectious disease consultation is advised. Both drugs are continued for a total of 3–4 weeks. Pyrimethamine has potential bone marrow toxicity, and so WBC and platelet counts may be checked frequently. Folinic acid (leucovorin), 5–15 mg/day PO, may help prevent bone marrow toxicity. See Chaps. 28K and 28U for further discussion of these agents.

F. **Prevention** of toxoplasmosis is of special concern in pregnancy. **Pregnant women should wash their hands after working in garden soil (or wear gloves) and should avoid cat feces.**

III. **Infectious lymphocytosis** is a benign disease of infancy and childhood that may resemble IM.

A. **Clinical features** include fever, malaise, and CNS symptoms, together with headache and slight nuchal rigidity. A generalized morbilliform rash may occur, in addition to GI symptoms such as abdominal pain, nausea, vomiting, and diarrhea. In contrast to classic IM, there is no lymphadenopathy or splenomegaly. Leukocytosis greater than 50,000/mm^3 is common, with a predominance of small lymphocytes that can persist for several weeks to months. The CSF may have increased numbers of lymphocytes.

    B. Diagnosis cannot be made serologically. No infectious agent has been identified, and the heterophil antibody and Monospot tests are negative. Differentiation from lymphoblastic leukemia is based on the presence of a normal hematocrit, normal platelets, and mature lymphocytes in infectious lymphocytosis.

    C. Treatment is symptomatic, and the illness usually pursues a mild, self-limited course.

IV. Rubella (German measles) may closely mimic IM because of the frequent occurrence of fever, sore throat, malaise, myalgia, and posterior cervical adenopathy accompanied by an evanescent exanthem. Differentiation from IM is based on the following observations: (1) The postauricular and suboccipital adenopathy associated with rubella is less common in IM; (2) the brief clinical course of rubella contrasts with the more protracted course of IM; (3) splenomegaly is infrequent in rubella; and (4) specific laboratory diagnosis of rubella can be made either by viral isolation from throat washings or nasopharyngeal secretions or by hemagglutination inhibition antibody response to rubella infection in paired sera.

V. Hematologic neoplasms may be confused with IM. It is essential to be able to differentiate lymphomas and leukemias from IM to prevent unnecessary patient anxiety and performance of invasive diagnostic procedures. Differentiating features can be categorized as follows: (1) Nontender, immobile lymph nodes are associated with lymphomatous conditions, and biopsy may establish the diagnosis; (2) careful examination of the peripheral smear will reveal characteristic, nonmalignant, lymphocytic changes in IM; and (3) nonhemolytic anemia is not characteristic of IM.

VI. Acute HIV infection can mimic IM. This is discussed in Chap. 19 (p. 724).

VII. Cat-scratch disease (CSD) is a frequently overlooked cause of regional adenopathy that may be misinterpreted as IM [16–20]. Unlike IM, however, CSD is a bacterial infection transmitted by cats, and the disease is most frequently detected in children and adolescents who have contact with kittens. CSD occurs in immunocompetent patients of all ages with 60–80% of cases being younger than 21 years of age [21, 22]. CSD is considered the most common cause of chronic, benign adenopathy in children and young adults, with an estimated 24,000 cases recognized each year [21]. CSD may occur in patients without known animal contact [22].

    A. The **etiologic agent** is a delicate, pleomorphic **gram-negative bacillus**, which has been detected in lymph nodes, skin nodules, and ocular granulomas of CSD patients. This organism is best visualized in tissue sections that have been treated with the Warthin-Starry silver impregnation stain.

    Two completely distinct gram-negative bacilli have been touted as the etiologic agents for CSD. *Rochalimaea henselae* (recently reclassified as *Bartonella henselae*) and *Afipia felis* have both been cultured from tissue specimens of patients with CSD [18]. ***B. henselae* appears to be more frequently present, and antibody titers are detectable in up to 88% of CSD patients [19]. Therefore, *B. henselae* currently is considered to be the cause of CSD.** The current evidence suggests that *A. felis* causes few, if any, cases of CSD. However, because CSD is a syndrome, it is possible that more than one agent could produce the clinical findings [17].

    B. Clinical features of the disease include the following:

        1. Single-node or regional **adenopathy** is the **dominant clinical feature** of CSD. The adenopathy usually appears within 2 weeks of the cat scratch or cat contact. More than 80% of the nodes are in the head, neck, and upper extremity proximal to the site of the scratch. In a recent prospective study, lymphadenopathy was seen most commonly in the neck (43%), axilla (38%), and groin (20%); 37% of patients had lymphadenopathy at more than one site [22]. The nodes are usually 1–5 cm in diameter with overlying erythema and tenderness. Although 10–20% may progress to suppuration, most enlarged nodes spontaneously regress over 2–6 months but may take up to 1 year [20].

        2. A **primary inoculation lesion** is commonly present and usually appears as a 2- to 5-mm macule, papule, or vesicle on the skin where the scratch occurred.

        3. Low-grade fever, malaise, headache, anorexia, sore throat, and arthralgias occurring in approximately 50–70% of cases of CSD may cause further confusion in distinguishing this disease from IM.

        4. Severe cases of CSD occur in up to 2% of patients with encephalopathy (which is seen in about 1% of patients [22]); transverse myelitis; facial nerve palsy; involvement of the spleen, lung, liver, or skin; hematologic abnormalities; arthritis; and erythema nodosum.

    C. Diagnosis is primarily clinical and depends on some or all of the following:

        1. Typical single-node or **regional adenopathy in the setting of recent contact with cats** should be present.

2. A **primary inoculation lesion** on the extremity, neck, or head should be carefully sought.
3. **Lymph node biopsy** may occasionally be necessary for diagnosis if the course of the disease is atypical or if a lymphoproliferative disease cannot be excluded. Cultures can be done to isolate *B. henselae* [17].
4. **Other causes of adenitis,** such as other bacteria, HIV, EBV, toxoplasmosis, tuberculosis, malignancy, cystic hygromas, and bronchial cleft cysts, must be differentiated from CSD.
5. A **skin test** reagent prepared from suppurative material of a CSD lymph node is sensitive and specific for CSD. However, **this reagent is not available commercially and is not standardized.** Also, there is the potential risk of transmission of viral hepatitis and HIV because human-derived material is used as the test antigen. Therefore this antigen is seldom used anymore.
6. **Serologic methods** are now **commonly employed to help with epidemiologic studies and diagnosis** [21, 22]. An indirect fluorescent antibody (IFA) is available from the Centers for Disease Control [23]. Also an enzyme immunoassay for the detection of IgG antibody to *B. henselae* is commercially available (Specialty Laboratories, Santa Monica, CA) and is reportedly 5–10 times more sensitive than the IFA test [21]. In a recent report, 67% of patients had positive IFA serology ($\geq 1:64$) [22].

   One attack of CSD appears to confer lifelong immunity in children and adolescents [20].
7. **Polymerase chain reaction** (PCR) assay has been performed on purulent material from lymph nodes and has demonstrated *B. henselae* DNA with great sensitivity and specificity [24].

D. **Treatment is primarily symptomatic** because CSD usually resolves spontaneously over 2–6 months. Patients should be reassured that the prognosis is generally very favorable. Fatal complications and irreversible sequelae have not been documented. Patients with encephalopathy and/or encephalitis have recovered completely [20]. Additional treatment may be necessary for more severe or protracted disease.
1. The involved node should be aspirated if suppuration occurs. Surgical incision and drainage should be performed only if the diagnosis is unclear or for symptomatic relief, because open drainage often will result in a chronic draining fistula.
2. **Antibiotic therapy.** The exact role of antibiotic therapy is unclear [21]. There are no good randomized controlled studies of therapy. Several agents appear to be efficacious, including rifampin, ciprofloxacin, trimethoprim-sulfamethoxazole, and gentamicin [20]. The *Medical Letter* suggests that in adults ciprofloxacin is the preferred agent [25] if therapy is used. Until more information is available, antibiotic therapy seems indicated only in severe cases of CSD or in those patients with severe underlying disease. Conservative, symptomatic therapy is recommended for most patients with mild to moderate CSD [20]. Infectious disease consultation is advised if antibiotic therapy is to be used.
3. Oral corticosteroids are not recommended [20].

Chronic Fatigue Syndrome

Patients with a syndrome of fatigue and malaise have been recognized by clinicians and reported in the medical literature for more than two centuries [26]. In the past decade, a group of patients have had a clinical syndrome consisting primarily of fatigue and cognitive dysfunction, designated as the **chronic fatigue syndrome** (CFS), in whom the **diagnosis is made by exclusion** [26]. It is estimated that there are roughly 6 million office visits per year in the United States for CFS [26].

I. The **etiology** of CFS is unknown. Theories have at various times focused on viral, immunologic, and psychiatric causes. EBV originally was believed to be the etiologic agent, but neither EBV nor other viruses (e.g., human herpesvirus-6) now appear to be responsible. Other agents postulated to be etiologically involved include *Candida albicans* and a number of metabolic or environmental factors whose involvement has not been proven [26]. Although ongoing viral infection is not evident, it is possible that an initial viral infection acts as a trigger for a chronic noninfectious disease process. Immunologic abnormalities have been detected in CFS patients, the two most consistent abnormalities being mild immunoglobulin subclass deficiency and a reduction in the number and activity of a subset of natural killer cells. However, neither of these immunologic defects is pathognomonic for CFS, and there is no definitive evidence that this syndrome is an immune-mediated illness. Depression, conversion reaction, and other psychiatric conditions have been touted as etiologies for CFS, but definitive proof is lacking. Recently, a group at Johns Hopkins Hospital reported that at least in some patients, CFS appears to be related to neurally mediated hypotension and that symptoms may be improved in this subset of patients by therapy directed at this abnormal cardiovascular reflex [27].

II. **History.** About half of the patients with CFS note a discrete flulike illness as the initiating event. Details of travel history, occupational history, and HIV risks should be carefully ascertained to help with the differential diagnosis. Usually the past medical history is unremarkable, although preexisting or concurrent affective disorders should be sought. Patients are primarily 20 to 45 years of age and are more frequently women [26].

III. **Symptoms** include easy fatigability, difficulty concentrating, loss of reasoning (dyslogia), difficulty sleeping, headache, sore throat, feverishness, myalgias, arthralgias, chest pain, and night sweats. These symptoms often wax and wane over weeks to months.

IV. **Physical examination** is usually **normal.** Significant weight loss is not part of this syndrome. In fact, an abnormal physical finding (e.g., generalized adenopathy or significant localized adenopathy) or temperatures over 38.6°C suggests another diagnosis [26].

V. **Laboratory studies** are usually normal. **There are no specific laboratory tests that establish or support the diagnosis of CFS,** and the laboratory should be used sparingly in the evaluation of individuals presenting with fatigue [26].

In his review, Schooley suggests [26] routinely obtaining a complete blood count with differential, sedimentation rate, hepatic enzymes, PPD skin test, and thyroid function tests. If the history or exam suggests possible human immunodeficiency virus (HIV), an ELISA for HIV-1 is recommended. If there is atypical lymphocytosis or hepatic transaminase enzymes are elevated, serologic evaluation for acute or active EBV and/or CMV is suggested. Also, if hepatic transaminase enzymes are elevated, studies for hepatitis A, B, and C are suggested (see Chap. 11).

Schooley emphasizes that it is usually not necessary to perform additional laboratory studies, especially EBV and CMV serology (when the CBC and liver enzymes are normal), *Borrelia burgdorferi* serology, and unfocused serologic studies for other infectious diseases. In addition, skin testing for hypersensitivity to common environmental agents and extensive studies of cellular and hormonal immunologic function are rarely warranted outside the context of clinical research studies [26].

VI. **Differential diagnosis.** If any risk factors for HIV infection are present, HIV infection should be excluded. Other illnesses that must be differentiated from CFS are hypothyroidism, malignancy, immunodeficiency states, collagen vascular disease, endocrinopathies, anxiety, depression, and a primary sleep disorder.

VII. **A working case definition** has been developed that acknowledges the uncertain etiology of this syndrome and emphasizes an evaluation for other causes of fatigue, including careful neuropsychiatric examination [28]. **The case definition of CFS has its greatest utility in epidemiologic studies** or in studies of the etiology or therapy of the syndrome and is much less useful in attempting to make a diagnosis in individual patients or in making disability determinations because it lacks a severity scale [26].

To meet the case definition for CFS, a case must fulfill both major and minor criteria. The original case definition continues to undergo study and revision [28a].

A. **The two major criteria** are as follows [28]:
   1. **New onset** of persistent or relapsing, debilitating **fatigue** in a person without a previous history of such symptoms that does not resolve with bedrest and that is severe enough to reduce or impair average daily activity to less than 50% of the patient's premorbid activity level **for at least 6 months.**
   2. Fatigue that is not explained by the presence of other evident medical or psychiatric illness after a thorough evaluation by history, physical examination, and appropriate laboratory testing.

B. **The minor criteria are at least six symptoms plus at least two signs, or at least eight symptoms from the following list:**
   1. **Symptoms**
      a. Mild fever (oral temperature between 37.5° and 38.6°C if measured by the patient) or chills

   b. Sore throat

   c. Painful adenopathy (posterior or anterior, cervical or axillary)

   d. Unexplained generalized muscle weakness

   e. Myalgias or muscle discomfort

   f. Prolonged generalized fatigue after previously tolerated levels of physical activity

   g. Generalized headaches

   h. Migratory arthralgia without joint swelling or redness

   i. Neuropsychological complaints, including photophobia, transient visual scotomata, forgetfulness, excessive irritability, confusion, difficulty thinking, inability to concentrate, and depression

   j. Sleep disturbance (hypersomnia or insomnia)

   k. Main symptom complex developing over a few hours to a few days

  2. Physical signs

   a. Low-grade fever (oral temperature between 37.6° and 38.6°C, or a rectal temperature between 37.8° and 38.8°C)

   b. Nonexudative pharyngitis

   c. Palpable or tender anterior or posterior, cervical or axillary lymph nodes. However, lymph nodes greater than 2 cm in diameter suggest other diagnoses [26].

VIII. Management is empiric and supportive.

 A. Support. Schooley emphasizes that it is important to reassure the patient about the following issues.

  1. Other serious problems have been excluded.

  2. Even though the etiology and pathogenesis (and treatment) have not been clarified, the fatigue and malaise experienced by the patient are real.

  3. In most cases the illness follows a waxing and waning course but usually subsides [26].

  Also, because it is not infrequent that patients with CFS have a history of concurrent or preexisting affective disorders, psychiatric consultation is often helpful [26]. Serial medical follow-up examinations are important to provide reassurance and rule out evolving organic disease.

 B. Activity. Patients should be encouraged to function at activity levels which are tolerable and within the limits of their fatigue, recognizing that fatigue may wax and wane. There is little objective evidence that enforced rest or gentle exercise exacerbates or ameliorates the illness [26]. Life-style and employment modifications are often necessary. Disability should be used only as a last resort; disability insurers find CFS an extremely challenging syndrome in that there are no diagnostic tests or severity scales with which to classify the syndrome [26]. Schooley has stressed that the CDC case definition should not be used to make disability determinations; a narrative report, coupled with a psychiatric evaluation is much more useful [26].

 C. Pharmacologic therapy. Many agents have been tried. Acyclovir has failed to show efficacy in a controlled trial [29]. Intravenous gammaglobulin is not recommended [26, 30].

  1. Nonsteroidal antiinflammatory agents may help the myalgias and arthralgias of some patients.

  2. Antidepressants (e.g., doxepin, amitriptyline) have been useful in some patients, but no single agent is clearly superior. Management is often facilitated by the involvement of a psychiatrist. Schooley emphasizes that the acceptance by patients of this approach may be better if patients understand these medications are being used to treat symptoms of a physiologic process rather than to treat a primary mental illness [26].

  3. Therapy aimed at neurally mediated hypotension, demonstrated in selected patients, is undergoing clinical evaluation [27].

IX. Because of the many nonspecific symptoms associated with CFS and the lack of a diagnostic test, serious early doubts have been raised about the existence of this syndrome as a single entity [31]. It is probable that CFS eventually will prove to have both somatic and psychosomatic causes. A multifactorial process may occur with predisposing factors (e.g., prior depression, anxiety), precipitating events (e.g., viral infection), and maintaining factors (e.g., immune response to viral process). A symposium on the epidemiology, clinical characteristics, and unsuccessful treatment of CFS has recently been published [32]. In the summary of this symposium, Komaroff and Klimas [33] emphasize that CFS probably is a heterogenous illness or a group of illnesses that share certain symptoms. In addition, despite the active research in the area of CFS, the authors remark that "fundamental questions about the etiology, pathogenesis, diagnosis and treatment of CFS remain unanswered."

References

1. Henle, G., Henle, W., and Diehl, V. Relation of Burkitt's tumor-associated herpes type virus to infectious mononucleosis. *Proc. Natl. Acad. Sci. U.S.A.* 59:94–101, 1968. *Epstein-Barr virus is established as the cause of infectious mononucleosis.*

2. Schooley, R.T. Epstein-Barr Virus (Infectious Mononucleosis). In G.L. Mandell, J.E. Bennett, and R. Dolin (eds.), *Principles and Practice of Infectious Diseases* (4th ed.). New York: Churchill Livingstone, 1995. Pp. 1364–1377.

3. Schmader, K.E., van der Horst, C.M., and Klotman, M.E. Epstein-Barr virus and the elderly host. *Rev. Infect. Dis.* 11:64–73, 1989. *EBV infection in the elderly may be underdiagnosed because not all features typical of infectious mononucleosis are present.*

4. Akashi, K., et al. Brief report: Severe infectious mononucleosis–like syndrome and primary human herpesvirus 6 infection in an adult. *N. Engl. J. Med.* 329:168–171, 1993. *A 43-year-old man developed fever, cervical lymphadenopathy, splenomegaly, tonsillar pharyngitis, skin rash, liver dysfunction, and atypical lymphocytosis associated with seroconversion of antibody to HHV-6 and detection of HHV-6 DNA in peripheral blood mononuclear cells.*

5. Lennette, E.T. Epstein-Barr Virus. In P.R. Murray et al. (eds.), *Manual of Clinical Microbiology* (6th ed.). Washington, DC: American Society for Microbiology, 1995. Pp. 905–910.

5a. Striskandan, S., et al. Diffuse pneumonia associated with infectious mononucleosis: Detection of Epstein-Barr virus in lung tissue by in situ hybridization. *Clin. Infect. Dis.* 22:578, 1996.

6. Dagan, R., and Powell, K.R. Post-anginal sepsis following infectious mononucleosis. *Arch. Intern. Med.* 147:1581–1583, 1987. *Postanginal sepsis is a serious illness in adolescents or young adults due to septic thrombophlebitis of neck veins following an oropharyngeal infection such as infectious mononucleosis. See related discussions in Chap. 4.*

7. Van der Horst, C.M., et al. Lack of effect of peroral acyclovir for the treatment of acute infectious mononucleosis. *J. Infect. Dis.* 164:788–792, 1991. *A 10-day course of oral acyclovir started within 1 week of the first symptoms of infectious mononucleosis had no effect on the resolution of symptoms and signs.*

8. Andersson, J., et al. Effect of acyclovir on infectious mononucleosis: A double-blind, placebo-controlled study. *J. Infect. Dis.* 153:283–290, 1986. *A 7-day course of intravenous acyclovir resulted in modest improvement of pharyngeal symptoms in patients with infectious mononucleosis.*

9. Sixbey, J.W., Lemon, S.M., and Pagano, J.S. A second site for Epstein-Barr virus shedding: The uterine cervix. *Lancet* 2:1122–1124, 1986. *EBV infection of the cervix was detected in 5 of 28 women who either had suspected infectious mononucleosis or had presented to a clinic for sexually transmitted diseases.*

10. Jones, J.F., and Strauss, S.E. Chronic Epstein-Barr virus infection. *Annu. Rev. Med.* 38:195–209, 1987. *Comprehensive review of the spectrum of diseases possibly associated with EBV.*

11. Schooley, R.T., et al. Chronic Epstein-Barr virus infection associated with fever and interstitial pneumonitis. *Ann. Intern. Med.* 104:636–643, 1986. *Report of two patients with fever, interstitial pneumonitis, pancytopenia, and high antibody titers to replicative antigens of the Epstein-Barr virus.*

12. Lajo, A., et al. Mononucleosis caused by Epstein-Barr virus and cytomegalovirus in children: A comparative study of 124 cases. *Pediatr. Infect. Dis. J.* 13:56, 1994. *Prospective study of 104 cases of EBV-IM and 20 cases of CMV mononucleosis in this series from Spain.*

13. Remington, J.S. Toxoplasmosis in the adult. *Bull. N.Y. Acad. Med.* 50:211–227, 1974. *A classic article.*

14. Beaman, M.H., et al. *Toxoplasma gondii.* In G.L. Mandell, J.E. Bennett, and R. Dolin (eds.), *Principles and Practice of Infectious Diseases* (4th ed.). New York: Churchill Livingstone, 1995. Pp. 2455–2475.

In addition to an excellent clinical discussion, this chapter contains a concise review of serologic tests, with their limitations and uses. Coauthored by Dr. Jack Remington who has a long interest and expertise in this disease.

15. Israelski, D.M., and Remington, J.C. Toxoplasmosis in the non-AIDS immunocompromised host. *Curr. Clin. Top. Infect. Dis.* 13:322, 1993.
    Again emphasizes that immunologically normal individuals with acute acquired Toxoplasma *infection usually have a self-limited clinical course and do not require specific treatment directed at the parasite. A related article is that by D.M. Israelski and J.C. Remington, Toxoplasmosis in patients with cancer.* Clin. Infect. Dis. *17(Suppl. 2):S423–S435, 1993.*

16. Moriarty, R.A., and Margileth, A.M. Cat scratch disease. *Infect. Dis. Clin. North Am.* 1:575–590, 1987.
    Excellent review. See also H.A. Carithers, Cat-scratch disease. An overview based on a study of 1,200 patients. Am. J. Dis. Child. *139:1124, 1985; and A.M. Margileth, Cat scratch disease.* Adv. Pediatr. Infect. Dis. *8:1, 1993.*

17. Fischer, G.W. Cat Scratch Disease. In G.L. Mandell, J.E. Bennett, and R. Dolin (eds.), *Principles and Practice of Infectious Diseases* (4th ed.). New York: Churchill Livingstone, 1995. Pp. 1310–1312.

18. Margileth, A.M., and Hayden, G.F. Cat scratch disease. From feline affection to human infection [editorial]. *N. Engl. J. Med.* 329:53–54, 1993.

19. Tompkins, D.C., and Steigbigel, R.T. *Rochalimaea*'s role in cat scratch disease and bacillary angiomatosis [editorial]. *Ann. Intern. Med.* 118:388–390, 1993.
    Reviews the variable clinical manifestations of infection by Rochalimaea *species and develops evidence for a more dominant role of* Rochalimaea henselae *compared to* Afipia felis *in the etiology of cat-scratch disease.*

20. Margileth, A.M. Antibiotic therapy for cat-scratch disease: Clinical study of therapeutic outcomes in 268 patients and a review of the literature. *Pediatr. Infect. Dis. J.* 11:474, 1992.

21. Adai, K.A., et al. Cat scratch disease, bacillary angiomatosis, and other infections due to Rochalimaea. *N. Engl. J. Med.* 330:1509, 1994.
    For a more detailed review, see D.A. Relman, Bacillary angiomatosis and Rochalimaea *species.* Curr. Clin. Top. Infect. Dis. *14:205, 1994.*

22. Hamilton, D.H., et al. Cat scratch disease—Connecticut, 1992–1993. *J. Infect. Dis.* 172:570, 1995.

23. Dalton, M.J., et al. Use of *Bartonella* antigens for serologic diagnosis of cat-scratch disease at a national referral center. *Arch. Intern. Med.* 155:1670, 1995.
    Review of CDC experience with indirect fluorescent antibody serology for cat-scratch disease (CSD). Study concluded that the IFA for Bartonella-*specific antibody is sensitive for the diagnosis of CSD. Redefinition of CSD on the basis of cause and use of this assay as a diagnostic criterion is recommended.*

24. Goral, S., et al. Detection of *Rochalimaea henselae* DNA by polymerase chain reaction from suppurative nodes of children with cat-scratch disease. *Pediatr. J. Infect. Dis.* 11:994, 1994.
    From extraction of DNA to final gel results, it took approximately 12 hours. The authors conclude that the test can eliminate the need for more extensive diagnostic and therapeutic procedures.

25. Medical Letter. The choice of antimicrobial drugs. *Med. Lett Drugs Ther.* 38:25, 1996.
    For Rochalimaea henselae *(cat-scratch bacillus), ciprofloxacin is the drug of first choice for adults. Alternative agents include trimethoprim-sulfamethoxazole, gentamicin, and rifampin.*

26. Schooley, R.T. Chronic Fatigue Syndrome. In G.L. Mandell, J.E. Bennett, and R. Dolin (eds.), *Principles and Practice of Infectious Diseases* (4th ed.). New York: Churchill Livingstone, 1995.
    This chapter is written by an excellent clinician, virologist, and highly regarded infectious disease subspecialist. His chapter is a concise and fair overview of a difficult topic. For a related review, see R. McKenzie and S.E. Straus, Chronic fatigue syndrome. Adv. Intern. Med. *40:119, 1995. This is an extensive review from the National Institute of Allergy and Infectious Diseases, National Institutes of Health, Bethesda, Maryland.*
      See related paper examining viral etiologies and without evidence of such: A.C. Mawle et al., Seroepidemiology of chronic fatigue syndrome: A case-control study. Clin. Infect. Dis. *21:1386, 1995.*

27. Bou-Holaigah, I., et al. The relationship between neurally mediated hypotension and the chronic fatigue syndrome. *J.A.M.A.* 274:961, 1995.
    Patients underwent three-stage upright tilt-table test; 90% of patients with CFS had

an abnormal test. Study suggests that tricyclic antidepressants should be used with caution in this group since neurally mediated hypotension could be exacerbated. Also, 9 of 22 patients reported completed or near complete resolution of their fatigue with an increase in their dietary salt and use of fludrocortisone every day, measures known to help neurally mediated hypotension. Further studies are needed to confirm or refute these preliminary findings (published September 1995).

28. Schluederberg, A., et al. Chronic fatigue syndrome research. Definition and medical outcome assessment. *Ann. Intern. Med.* 117:325–331, 1992.
    Updates the case definition for chronic fatigue syndrome, which was originally published by G.P. Holmes et al., Chronic fatigue syndrome: A working definition. Ann. Intern. Med. 108:387, 1988. For a related paper discussing a set of research guidelines for use in studies of chronic fatigue syndrome, see K. Fukuda et al. and the International Chronic Fatigue Syndrome Study Group, The chronic fatigue syndrome: A comprehensive approach to its definition and study. Ann. Intern. Med. 121:953, 1994. Offers recommendations for initial laboratory evaluation, and advocates careful screening for psychiatric disorders.

28a. Komaroff, A.L., et al. An examination of the working case definition of chronic fatigue syndrome. *Am. J. Med.* 100:56, 1996.
    The revised CDC case definition (see annotation to reference [28], Fukuda et al.) eliminates physical examination criteria and minor criteria symptoms of fever/chills, muscle weakness, and acute onset.

    In Komaroff, the Boston group concludes that patients meeting the major criteria of the current CDC working case definition of CFS reported symptoms that were clearly distinguishable from the experience of healthy control subjects and from the disease comparison groups with depression and multiple sclerosis. Authors further conclude that by eliminating three symptoms (i.e., arthralgias, muscle weakness, and sleep disturbance) and adding others (i.e., anorexia and nausea), the 1994 CDC case definition of CFS appeared to be strengthened.

29. Straus, S.E., et al. Acyclovir treatment of the chronic fatigue syndrome. Lack of efficacy in a placebo-controlled trial. *N. Engl. J. Med.* 319:1692–1698, 1988.
    High, and sometimes toxic, intravenous and oral courses of acyclovir failed to produce significant clinical improvement in 27 adults with chronic fatigue syndrome.

30. Peterson, P.K., et al. A controlled trial of intravenous immunoglobulin G in chronic fatigue syndrome. *Am. J. Med.* 89:554–560, 1990.
    Intravenous immunoglobulin G administered every 30 days for 6 months to 28 adults with chronic fatigue syndrome failed to improve symptoms despite restoration of IgG$_1$ levels to the normal range.

31. Swartz, M.N. The chronic fatigue syndrome—one entity or many? [editorial]. *N. Engl. J. Med.* 319:1726–1728, 1988.

32. Levine, P.H. (ed.). Chronic fatigue syndrome: Current concepts [symposium]. *Clin. Infect. Dis.* 18(Suppl. 1):S1–S167, 1994.
    Recent comprehensive symposium on current concepts, epidemiology, clinical and multidisciplinary research, viral and immunologic studies, and public policy issues.

33. Komaroff, A.L., and Klimas, N. Chronic fatigue syndrome: What have we learned and what do we need to know? *Clin. Infect. Dis.* 18(Suppl. 1):S166, 1994.
    Closing remarks of symposium cited in Levine reference [32].

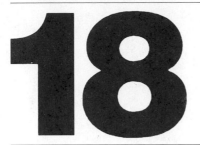

Infections Due to Fungi, *Actinomyces,* and *Nocardia*

Harold M. Henderson
and Stanley W. Chapman

An organized approach to fungal infections is outlined in this chapter, which is divided into sections that describe each mycosis. The epidemiologic settings, host status, skin tests, and serologic information associated with the major fungal diseases are listed in Table 18-1 and should assist the reader in narrowing down the diagnostic possibilities in a given patient. The decision to initiate systemic antifungal chemotherapy may be difficult, and infectious disease consultation is strongly recommended to help determine the indications for the potentially toxic antifungal agents and to assist in their administration.

Actinomycosis and nocardiosis are caused by organisms that are no longer classified as fungi. They are discussed separately at the end of this chapter.

Candidiasis

Candida **species are normal inhabitants of mucocutaneous body surfaces** and commonly cause superficial skin disease and vaginitis. Under certain circumstances, they may overgrow and **cause invasive disease if alterations in host defenses occur.** The incidence of *Candida* infections has increased markedly with the widespread use of antibiotics, immunosuppressive therapy, and intensive care modalities [1].

I. **Growth and identification characteristics. Many** *Candida* **species cause infection in humans,** including *C. tropicalis, C. krusei, C. parapsilosis,* and *C. glabrata* (*Torulopsis glabrata*), **but the most common cause of clinical infection is** *C. albicans. Candida* species are yeasts and can be cultured easily on blood agar and Sabouraud's dextrose agar in 24–48 hours. Presumptive identification of *C. albicans* can be made in 2–3 hours by a positive germ tube test (i.e., characteristic morphologic change seen on incubation of the yeast colony in serum). Definite species identification requires an additional 2–8 days.

II. **Epidemiologic and host factors.** *Candida* species are found worldwide, and are normal commensals of humans.

   A. **Colonization.** *Candida* is commonly cultured from the female genital tract, GI tract, and diseased skin, and from the urine of patients with indwelling Foley catheters. Colonization is more prevalent in hospitalized patients than in healthy individuals and is promoted by antibiotics that suppress normal bacterial growth and allow the overgrowth of yeasts.

   B. **Host defense.** Intact skin, phagocytic cells such as neutrophils and monocytes, and the cell-mediated immune system are all important components of the host's resistance to infection by *Candida* species. **Alterations in host defenses** may lead to a change in the organism's normal commensal status, with subsequent tissue invasion and clinical disease [2]. These alterations may be naturally occurring as in the cases of **diabetes mellitus** and **AIDS.** More often, **iatrogenic factors** predispose to invasive candidiasis. The use of broad-spectrum antibiotics and corticosteroids, mucosal damage from instrumentation or chemotherapeutic agents, or a breach in the integrity of the skin by intravenous catheters or pressure-monitoring devices increases the risk of invasive disease.

Revised from J.W.M. Gold, Infections due to Fungi, *Actinomyces,* and *Nocardia.* In R.E. Reese and R.F. Betts (eds.), *A Practical Approach to Infectious Diseases* (3rd ed.). Boston: Little, Brown, 1991.

Table 18-1. Summary of major fungal infections

Fungus	Epidemiologic features	Major clinical entities	Host/setting	Skin test	Immunologic test	Value of serologic studies
Candida	Worldwide	Cervical; vaginal Oropharyngeal	Normal; antibiotic use Normal; antibiotic use; steroid inhalers; immunocompromised	Not helpful	Precipitating antibody Agglutinating antibody Antigens	Not helpful (false positive and false negative results)
		Gastrointestinal; disseminated; isolated fungemia	Antibiotic use; IV catheters; immuno-compromised; diabetes mellitus; extensive burns			
		Endocarditis	Recent cardiac surgery; IV catheters; heroin addicts			
Histoplasma	Midwestern and south-eastern US[a] Avian feces exposure	Acute pulmonary	Normal	Usually positive in endemic area; can cause false positive *Histoplasma* serologic result	Complement fixation	More than 90% positive; some falsely positive
					Immunodiffusion M band H band	70–80% positive 10–20% positive in active infection
		Progressive disseminated	Immunocompromised; elderly; probably infants	Not useful	Complement fixation	Majority positive[b]
		Chronic cavitary	Chronic obstructive pulmonary disease	Not useful	Complement fixation	Majority positive

Organism	Distribution	Clinical form	Host	Skin test	Serologic test	Result
Cryptococcus	Worldwide	Pulmonary	Normal; immunocompromised	Not useful	Latex agglutination (antigen)	Some positive; false positive results with rheumatoid factor
		CNS	Normal; immunocompromised		Latex agglutination	Sensitive and specific
Coccidioides	Southwestern US	Acute pneumonitis	Normal	95% positive[c]; can cause false positive *Histoplasma* serologic results	Precipitins	75% positive; disappears after 4–6 weeks
					Complement fixation	> 50% positive; develops after 4–12 weeks
		Chronic cavitary	Normal	Minority positive[c]	Precipitins	Usually negative
					Complement fixation	50–60% positive
		Pulmonary nodule	Normal	Not useful[d]	Precipitins	Usually negative
					Complement fixation	Minority positive
		Disseminated	Immunocompromised; Filipinos, Mexicans, blacks, pregnant women	Not useful	Precipitins	Usually negative
					Complement fixation	80–95% positive; 75–95% positive in CSF if meningeal infection

Table 18-1 (*continued*)

Fungus	Epidemiologic features	Major clinical entities	Host/setting	Skin test	Immunologic test	Value of serologic studies
Aspergillus	Worldwide	Allergic broncho-pulmonary asper-gillosis	Asthma	99% positive; false positive results occur	Precipitating antibody (precipitins)	70% or more positive; false positive results occur
		Aspergilloma	Prior pulmonary cavity	Minority positive	Serum IgE Precipitins antibody	Markedly elevated 90–100% positive
		Invasive asper-gillosis	Immunocompromised; rare in normal host	Insufficient data	Precipitins antibody	Not helpful
Blastomyces	Southeastern and mid-western US soil contact	Acute pneumonitis; chronic (lungs, 75%; skin, bone, genitourinary tract)	Normal	Not available	Complement fixation	Not helpful
Mucorales (*Zygomycetes*)	Worldwide	Rhinocerebral; pulmonary Disseminated	Diabetes in poor control; immunocompromised Immunocompromised; extensive burns	Not available	Immunodiffusion	Variable; up to 70–80% in cases of disseminated disease
		Gastrointestinal	Young children with malnutrition or colitis		Not available	

Sporothrix	Worldwide: soil; sphagnum moss; rose and barberry bushes	Cutaneous-lymphatic	Normal	Not available	90% positive
		Pneumonitis	Normal; alcoholics	Agglutinating antibody	
		Disseminated	Normal; immunocompromised; alcoholics	Agglutinating antibody	

[a]May also occur in many cities in the United States. See text.
[b]Tissue histopathologic examination or cultures necessary for diagnosis.
[c]Helpful diagnostically if recent conversion from negative to positive reactivity is shown.
[d]Does not differentiate between active disease and past infection.

III. **Clinical aspects**
A. **Cutaneous infections**
1. **Intertriginous candidiasis** [1]. *Candida* commonly causes infection in warm, moist areas of the skin such as the axillary, inguinal, and intergluteal regions. The spaces between the fingers or toes may be involved with an erythematous, macerated lesion known as *erosio interdigitalis blastomycetica*. Perineal infection with involvement of the perianal area, thighs, scrotum, and penis (balanitis) is common. Diaper rash in infants often is caused by *Candida,* and angular cheilitis at the corners of the mouth may be caused by the organism as well. Each of these conditions is characterized by **erythematous papules or macules that may be confluent and are very pruritic.** Infection tends to be more extensive in the presence of immunosuppression. The diagnosis can be made by wet-mount examination of scrapings from the infected area with 10–20% KOH.
2. **Nail infection.** *Candida* may cause both paronychia and onychomycosis. Persons who frequently immerse their hands in water or wear occlusive gloves are particularly susceptible, and diabetics have a higher incidence of paronychia than does the general population.
3. **Folliculitis.** Inflammation of hair follicles sometimes is caused by *Candida,* especially if maceration or occlusive dressings are present.
4. **Therapy.** Topical agents such as **nystatin** or **miconazole** creams are usually very effective for mild intertriginous infection or folliculitis. More extensive folliculitis or nail involvement that does not resolve with topical therapy may require systemic treatment with an oral azole. Immunocompromised patients with severe cutaneous disease may also require systemic therapy. Ketoconazole, itraconazole, and fluconazole all are effective in these settings.
B. **Mucosal infections**
1. **Oral candidiasis.** Thrush may occasionally occur in normal hosts such as neonates and denture wearers but is **most common in persons with the following predisposing factors:** recent antibiotic treatment, inhaled or systemic steroid use, other immunosuppressive therapy, cancer, and AIDS [3]. The lesions most often appear as raised, white plaques on the tongue and other oral mucosal surfaces. Thrush may also present with an atrophic appearance or as angular cheilitis. The diagnosis may be made by examining scrapings under light microscopy, which reveals masses of yeasts and pseudohyphae.
2. **Esophageal candidiasis.** Esophagitis generally **occurs in immunocompromised patients,** particularly patients with hematologic malignancy or AIDS. **Dysphagia and retrosternal pain with swallowing** are the most common symptoms. Oral candidiasis is often but not always present. Barium studies of the esophagus may suggest the diagnosis, but confirmation requires endoscopy [4]. Many clinicians initiate empiric therapy for esophageal candidiasis in high-risk patients who have typical symptoms in the presence of thrush.
3. **Nonesophageal involvement of the GI tract** by *Candida* is diagnosed most commonly in cancer patients [5]. Antibiotic usage also is associated occasionally with invasive candidiasis of the GI tract. By suppressing the normal endogenous bacterial flora, antibiotics promote increased titers of colonizing *Candida* species, and invasive disease may ultimately result. After the esophagus, the stomach is the organ most often involved. *Candida* may cause significant gastritis, invade ulcer beds, and cause superficial ulcerations in the small and large intestine. Disseminated candidiasis frequently is present in these settings.
4. **Vulvovaginal candidiasis.** See Chap. 13.
5. **Therapy**
a. **Oral candidiasis** may be treated effectively with either **nystatin** oral suspension (5 ml qid) or **clotrimazole** troches (qid for 7–10 days) [1]. Most patients find the clotrimazole troches to be more palatable. The oral azoles (ketoconazole, itraconazole, and fluconazole) are also very effective but are more expensive than clotrimazole or nystatin and can be reserved for patients who do not respond to the more cost-effective regimens.
b. **Esophagitis.** Systemic therapy generally is required for esophageal candidiasis. **Fluconazole** may be given orally or intravenously, is well tolerated, and is highly effective [6]; it is a reasonable first choice for the treatment of esophagitis. A commonly used regimen is 100 mg/day for 10–14 days. Ketoconazole and itraconazole are alternatives. Cases refractory to azole therapy may be treated with amphotericin B.

Relapse of oral or esophageal candidiasis is common in patients whose underlying immunosuppression cannot be reversed, such as patients with AIDS. Maintenance therapy (e.g., weekly fluconazole) may be needed to manage or prevent frequently recurring episodes [7].

C. **Chronic mucocutaneous candidiasis (CMC).** This group of disorders is typified by persistent and recurrent *Candida* infections of the skin, nails, and mucous membranes [8]. CMC may occur in young children or adults and is associated with large, disfiguring cutaneous lesions. Disseminated candidiasis usually is not seen, but other infections with bacteria or dermatophytes may occur. Endocrinopathies, such as Addison's disease, hypothyroidism, or hypoparathyroidism, are present in some patients. Various immune defects have been documented in patients with CMC, but the most consistent finding is that of abnormal T-lymphocyte function, as shown by anergy to delayed hypersensitivity testing. Treatment of CMC centers around therapy for the individual *Candida* infections. The oral azoles are the drugs of choice, and chronic suppressive therapy for many years has proven safe and successful. Therapies to correct the underlying immune defect, such as bone marrow transplantation or transfer factor, have produced inconsistent results.

D. **Disseminated candidiasis.** Once a rare disease, **disseminated candidiasis has become a very important nosocomial infection** because of the increased numbers of susceptible hosts. Disseminated infection affects at least 120,000 patients annually in the United States, accounts for 15% of hospital-acquired infections, and has an overall mortality approaching 50% [1, 9]. In a recent report, from 1980 to 1989 the rates of disseminated candidiasis increased elevenfold [9a]. The clinical spectrum ranges from widespread involvement of multiple organs in a severely ill patient to isolated candidemia that may not be accompanied by tissue invasion. Most cases are caused by *C. albicans,* with *C. tropicalis* the second most common causative agent.

1. **Risk factors.** Disseminated candidiasis is a relatively common infection in patients with neutropenia, transplant recipients, postsurgical patients with complex and protracted hospitalizations, burn victims, low-birth-weight neonates, patients with central intravenous lines, and those receiving hyperalimentation [10, 11]. Several predisposing factors may exist simultaneously in a single patient.

    a. **Broad-spectrum antibiotics** are a well-known risk factor for disseminated disease, allowing overgrowth of *Candida* within the GI tract, with subsequent hematogenous dissemination [11a].

    b. **Central venous and arterial catheters** may provide a conduit by which yeasts move from the skin to the intravascular space. *Candida* species are capable of adhering to plastic catheters, which may also serve as a focus for aggregation of the organism prior to dissemination.

    c. **Functioning neutrophils** are an important defense against *Candida,* and **neutropenia or neutrophil dysfunction** often is present in patients with disseminated *Candida* infection.

    d. **Hyperalimentation** may promote yeast growth due to hyperglycemia and may be a risk factor independent of the intravenous catheter.

    e. **Abdominal surgery,** by decreasing bowel motility, may contribute to *Candida* overgrowth within the GI tract. Also, surgery may compromise the integrity of the bowel wall and predispose to intravascular fungal invasion.

2. **Manifestations.** Dissemination may present as **fever of unclear etiology or as the sepsis syndrome** with chills, spiking fevers, hypotension, and prostration. Multiple organs are usually involved with the formation of diffuse microabscesses. Renal involvement is very common, having been reported in 20 of 22 patients in one series [12]. Myocarditis also occurs frequently, but premortem diagnosis is uncommon.

    Dissemination to brain, lungs, liver, and spleen reflects a major and often preterminal breakdown in host defense. Spread to any organ may occur in this setting, but **infections of the eye and skin** are particularly important, as they may **provide** important **diagnostic clues.**

    a. **Macronodular skin lesions** represent embolic foci [13] but are seen in only a minority of patients. They are 0.5–1.0 cm in diameter, pink or red, and single or multiple and generalized (see Plate III A).

        Punch biopsy may reveal the fungi on histopathologic study and culture. *Candida* may also produce lesions that resemble ecthyma gangrenosum or purpura fulminans.

   b. **Endophthalmitis** [14, 14a] occurs in approximately 20–50% or more of
      disseminated candidiasis patients and correlates closely with multiple vis-
      ceral organ involvement [14a]. Endophthalmitis may cause blurry vision,
      scotomas, or ocular pain, but extensive disease may be present without
      symptoms. Endophthalmitis is a clinical diagnosis made in the proper
      setting and at times requires serial funduscopic examinations [14a]. Fun-
      duscopic examination reveals white, cottonlike, circumscribed exudates
      with filamentous borders in the chorioretina **extending into** the vitreous
      (see Plate III C). Endophthalmitis has become more common as the inci-
      dence of candidemia has increased, and it is highly suggestive of dissemin-
      ated candidiasis. A **good ophthalmologic examination is thus an important
      part of the evaluation** of a patient with risk factors for disseminated disease.
      C. albicans is the candidal species that has the greatest propensity to
      involve the eye [14a].
3. **Diagnosis is problematic.** The definitive diagnosis of disseminated candidiasis
   can be made only by histopathologic demonstration of the organism invading
   tissue or by the isolation of *Candida* from normally sterile body sites. The rate
   of premortem diagnosis is only 10–40%. Thus, a **presumptive clinical diagnosis
   is often the basis for initiating antifungal therapy,** because time is of the
   essence if the underlying disease is severe. The most important diagnostic
   technique in a high-risk patient is a thorough daily physical examination.
   Additional considerations include the following:
   a. **Skin** tests for *Candida* are not useful.
   b. **Serologic tests** are **not yet reliable** enough to use in the diagnosis of
      invasive candidiasis.
      (1) Tests for **antibodies** to *Candida* are **not helpful** because there is a high
          frequency of false positive and false negative results.
      (2) **Antigen testing is more promising.** A variety of antigens have been
          studied, including a cell wall polysaccharide (mannan), cytoplasmic
          antigens, and carbohydrate metabolites such as *d*-arabinatol. Unfortu-
          nately, antigenemia may be transient in systemic infection, and the
          tests have only moderate sensitivity. Antigen tests do not differentiate
          reliably between colonization and invasive disease, and **most of the
          tests developed to date are not simple enough to be commercially
          viable** [15]. Tests for *Candida* antigens thus remain primarily investi-
          gational tools.
   c. **Blood cultures** are negative in more than 50% of patients with disseminated
      candidiasis. The lysis-centrifugation technique may be more sensitive than
      routine methods for detecting candidemia [16]. In addition, isolation of
      Candida from the blood may not always be indicative of disseminated
      disease (see sec. **5**).
   d. **Polymerase chain reaction** (PCR) studies on serum of patients suspected
      of having candidemia are undergoing clinical evaluation [16a].
   e. **Colonization often precedes dissemination.** Positive cultures of urine,
      sputum, or stool are thus common in patients with disseminated disease.
      Isolation of *Candida* species from these specimens has some predictive
      value but is not diagnostic. Only a small proportion of patients who are
      colonized by *C. albicans* develop invasive disease due to this organism
      [17]. The **isolation of *C. tropicalis* from an immunocompromised patient,
      however, has been shown to be more predictive of disseminated disease**
      [18, 19].
4. **Therapy.** Systemic candidal infection mandates systemic antifungal chemotherapy [19a].
   a. **Amphotericin B** has broad activity against various *Candida* species and has
      traditionally been the agent of choice in treating patients with disseminated
      disease [20, 21]. Drug doses and duration of therapy vary considerably and
      depend on the clinical course of the infection, the underlying illness, and the
      toxicity of amphotericin B. For patients with extensive disease, a prolonged
      course with a 2- to 3-g total dose may be required.
         In a recent review, amphotericin B (0.7 mg/kg/day) is suggested in leuko-
      penic patients and in patients with a sepsislike illness. Duration of therapy
      is empiric, but a reasonable approach is to treat for 2 weeks after signs
      and symptoms linked to the *Candida* infection have resolved [19a], and

also when hepatosplenic candidiasis is not involved (see sec. **F.1**) because this complication requires more protracted therapy.

  b. **Oral azoles.** Many patients with disseminated candidiasis are severely ill and tolerate amphotericin B poorly. The search for a less toxic, effective alternative has focused in recent years on **fluconazole.** Two randomized trials comparing fluconazole, 400 mg/day, with amphotericin B **in nonneu-tropenic patients** with disseminated candidiasis have revealed similar outcomes for each drug [22, 23]. Fluconazole, whether used orally or intravenously, has thus been suggested as a **reasonable initial choice for the treatment of disseminated disease in patients without neutropenia** [19a, 22, 23]. Some species, such as *C. krusei,* are resistant to fluconazole, and amphotericin B should be used for fluconazole-resistant strains.

  A comparative study of fluconazole and amphotericin B in neutropenic patients has not been completed. In their review, Filler and Edwards favor using fluconazole as primary therapy only in neutropenic patients who meet the following criteria: (1) clinically stable; (2) no evidence of hematogenous dissemination; (3) the candidemia has occurred in association with an intravascular catheter; (4) not receiving an azole on a prophylactic basis; and (5) infections with *Aspergillus* species are uncommon at that medical center [19a]. Data on itraconazole is limited, and use of ketoconazole is not advised [19a].

  c. **Flucytosine is not used as a single agent** because of the relatively high incidence of primary and secondary drug resistance. Flucytosine is synergistic against *Candida,* however, when used in combination with amphotericin B. Bone marrow suppression may be a complication of combination therapy, particularly if renal insufficiency caused by amphotericin B leads to toxic serum flucytosine levels [21].

  d. Therapy directed at the underlying illness is basic to any approach, especially if in the neutropenic patient the WBC count can be restored to a normal range.

  e. In patients in the intensive care unit (ICU), changing of all lines in the candidemic patient is appropriate. In cancer patients, changing of central venous catheters is advised whenever feasible [19a].

  f. Infectious disease consultation is advised.

 5. **Isolated catheter-related candidemia.** Candidemia frequently occurs in patients with indwelling catheters but in whom signs of disseminated disease are minimal or absent. Removal of the catheter and observation of the patient have been common therapeutic strategies in the past. Several reports have documented late complications of disseminated candidiasis in such patients who did not receive antifungal chemotherapy, particularly immunocompromised patients [24, 25] but also normal hosts [19a, 26]. Most authorities recommend **removal of the catheter and a course of antifungal chemotherapy** in patients in this setting. The principles of therapy are as outlined in sec. **4.** Infectious disease consultation is advised.

E. **Empiric therapy** is raised most commonly in two situations:
 1. **Neutropenic patients,** after chemotherapy, with persisting fever despite treatment with antibiotics. The approach to these patients is discussed in sec. **I.C** under Antifungal Chemotherapy.
 2. **Complex ICU patients who have undergone major surgery.** In those patients without an obvious focal infection, who have *Candida* isolated from superficial cultures (e.g., wound, sputum, urine), and who remain febrile despite broad spectrum antibiotics, empiric therapy is warranted. Because the incidence of disseminated candidiasis diagnosed only at autopsy is unacceptably high and negative blood cultures are common, empiric therapy of disseminated candidiasis is a reasonable approach. Patients who are clinically unstable should receive amphotericin B, those who are febrile but stable may be treated with fluconazole as described in sec. **D.4** [19a].

F. **Specific deep organ infections**
 1. **Hepatosplenic candidiasis** is seen typically in patients with acute leukemia and prolonged leukopenia that has resolved [27]. Recently this condition has been termed **chronic hematogenously disseminated candidiasis** and is characterized by widespread micro- and macroscopic abscesses in the liver, spleen, kidney, and lungs.

    a. Manifestations include persistent fevers, abdominal pain, hepatospleno-megaly, increased alkaline phosphatase levels, and leukocytosis.

    b. Diagnosis. CT scanning, MRI, and ultrasonography reveal multiple hepatosplenic (and occasionally renal) filling defects and/or abscesses. The **CT scan** is the **most specific** diagnostic tool. The lesions are hypodense, and ring enhancement often is seen. Definitive diagnosis requires biopsy with culture and histopathologic examination or, if possible, aspiration of one or more of these abscesses in an attempt to identify the infecting organism. Although *Candida* species frequently can be identified by histopathology, cultures from these lesions are often sterile [19a].

    c. Therapy. Treatment requires long-term antifungal therapy. This syndrome is relatively rare, and thus no randomized trials on its treatment have been performed [19a]. Survival rates with amphotericin B have been no better than 50–60%. Fluconazole was reportedly very effective in one series [28]. In a recent summary of this topic, Filler and Edwards suggest that it is prudent to treat patients with an initial course of amphotericin B and 5-fluorocytosine and then to consider switching to fluconazole oral therapy [19a]. The efficacy of therapy should be monitored by relatively frequent CT scans to assess the size of the lesion(s) [19a]. Infectious disease consultation is advised.

2. Candidal endocarditis is particularly **common in heroin addicts,** in patients with prolonged intravenous catheterization, and after recent cardiac surgery [29]. Most cases are caused by *C. albicans.* Addicts have a predilection for tricuspid involvement (see Chap. 10).

    a. Manifestations are similar to those of bacterial endocarditis, except for a propensity toward large valvular vegetations. Many patients suffer **major embolic episodes** with occlusion of medium-size arteries (brain, extremities, lungs, mesentery). Invasion of the myocardium may occur and generally is irreversible.

    b. Diagnosis. Although early diagnosis is crucial in preventing significant morbidity or death, **only 50% of patients have positive blood cultures** (up to 75% are positive in prosthetic valve endocarditis), and fever and leukocytosis may be absent. **Clinical clues strongly suggestive of the diagnosis** include the presence of endophthalmitis, major embolic episodes, or large vegetations demonstrated by echocardiography. Biopsy of skin lesions may be diagnostic.

    c. Therapy combines early surgical intervention with amphotericin B (0.5–0.8 mg/kg/day). Prolonged intravenous therapy and careful follow-up are vital because relapse is common. (See Chap. 10 under Infective Endocarditis for further details.)

    d. Prognosis has been poor, especially in patients treated with medical therapy alone. Successful therapy is being described with increasing frequency, however, due mostly to earlier diagnosis and surgical intervention. With amphotericin B and surgical therapy, 50% of patients may survive.

3. Genitourinary infection. *Candida* **frequently colonizes the urine,** especially (1) after antibiotic use, (2) in diabetics, and (3) in association with indwelling Foley catheters [30, 31]. For example, approximately 12% of all urine cultures sent to the Barnes Hospital Diagnostic Laboratory in 1990 grew 10^4 or 10^5 colony-forming units (CFU) of *Candida* species per milliliter [31].

    a. Colonization versus infection. Unfortunately, **there are no established criteria that distinguish urinary colonization with *Candida* species from infection** [31, 31a]. Urinary colonization is asymptomatic and does not require antifungal therapy.

    b. True infection is uncommon compared with colonization. The clinical condition of the patient is important [31a]: Is the patient healthy or at risk for disseminated candidiasis? Invasive disease in the form of cystitis or pyelonephritis may occur. The clinical diagnosis of *Candida* cystitis is best confirmed by cystoscopy, which may reveal a nonspecific cystitis, multiple areas of small ulcers, or granulations covered with white membranes. Pyelonephritis may cause fever, flank pain, nausea, vomiting, and dysuria. It is usually acquired hematogenously. Renal involvement is very common in patients with disseminated candidiasis and therefore, when *Candida* is isolated from the urine of patients at risk for disseminated candidiasis (see sec. **D**) these patients require careful assessment.

(1) The **presence of risk factors** such as urinary catheters, anatomic abnormalities of the urinary tract, exposure to multiple antibacterial agents, immunosuppression and/or leukopenia, diabetes, two or more urine cultures showing more than 10^5 CFU/ml of *Candida* species, and *Candida* cultures positive from other sites all **lend support to** the clinical diagnosis of a candidal urinary tract infection [31].

(2) Symptoms of a urinary tract infection and positive serial urine cultures for *Candida* also only suggest underlying infection [31].

(3) Urine should be examined carefully for the presence of white blood cell casts, which suggest renal involvement; the presence of pyuria makes it less likely that the bladder is merely colonized [19a].

c. **Therapy is not well established** [31] except when there is obvious renal involvement in disseminated candidemia. A large study to determine the significance and optimal treatment of candiduria is currently being conducted by the Mycoses Study Group of the National Institute of Allergy and Infectious Diseases (NIAID) [19a].

(1) There is no clear evidence that any therapy in the asymptomatic patient is either necessary or beneficial [31].

(2) **A practical approach** is offered by Medoff [31] and others [31a, 31b].

(a) **If a Foley catheter is in place, it should be removed if possible,** at least for a short trial. Cultures can then be repeated; these often turn negative. If candiduria persists, especially in the settings described in sec. **b.(1)**, fluconazole, 50–100 mg/day for 10 days, can be given; others have used 200 mg/day for 7 days [31b]. If, despite this therapy, candiduria persists, Medoff [31] takes the patient off therapy and monitors him or her, assuming the patient remains asymptomatic.

(b) **If the Foley catheter cannot be removed,** especially in the setting of the risk factors previously outlined, Medoff [31] uses amphotericin B continuous bladder irrigation for 3 days (e.g., 50 mg/liter in sterile water). If follow-up urine cultures remain positive for *Candida* species, patients are monitored until the Foley catheter can be removed. If, after removal, *Candida* species persist in the urine, fluconazole can be used (see sec. **a**).

(c) If no Foley catheter is in place, *Candida* species are shown on serial cultures, and risk factors are present, oral fluconazole can be tried.

(d) If the patient is immunosuppressed, is symptomatic, or has indications of invasive disease, Medoff [31] uses amphotericin B or fluconazole in regimens similar to those for candidemia.

(3) Other reviewers have emphasized that virtually all cases of candiduria should be treated in patients who are neutropenic or have undergone renal transplantation, irrespective of their symptoms [19a].

(4) In a recent study, amphotericin B bladder irrigation and oral fluconazole therapy appeared to be equally efficacious [31b].

d. **In the usual hospitalized patient without multiple special risk factors** (sec. **b.(1)**), we believe serial observation is a reasonable compromise.

4. **CNS infection.** Chronic involvement of the brain generally results in headache, nuchal rigidity, papilledema, or focal neurologic abnormalities. The organism can usually be isolated from the cerebrospinal fluid (CSF). CNS infection in patients with disseminated candidiasis occurs more frequently than was previously appreciated [32]. Other risk factors for CNS infection are trauma and neurosurgical procedures. Therapy with amphotericin B is often effective. Because of its CNS penetration, fluconazole may also be a useful agent. Infectious disease consultation is advised. See related discussion in Chap. 5.

5. **Pulmonary infection** is usually secondary to hematogenous dissemination and results in fever and cough [33]. Although positive sputum cultures are common in hospitalized patients, this usually represents colonization. Definitive diagnosis relies on biopsy, with demonstration of tissue invasion. Primary *Candida* pneumonia is rare except in the compromised host, and even in this setting it is uncommon.

6. **Peritonitis** caused by *Candida* species is generally a complication of peritoneal dialysis or GI surgery [34, 35]. Dissemination is uncommon in infected patients undergoing chronic ambulatory peritoneal dialysis but may occur in association

with bowel surgery. Patients with dissemination should be treated with systemic therapy, usually amphotericin B. See Chap. 11 for a more detailed discussion of this topic.

7. **Musculoskeletal infections** with *Candida* species are uncommon and generally occur in hospitalized patients with disseminated candidiasis or in intravenous drug users [36, 37]. Arthritis is often acute and presents in a fashion similar to bacterial arthritis. Bone disease is usually in the vertebral spine in adults or the long bones in children. Diagnosis requires aspiration of the infected area.

8. **Ocular infection** due to hematogenous dissemination of *Candida* was discussed in sec. **D.2.b.** Exogenous infection following trauma or surgery may also occur. Systemic therapy with amphotericin B with or without flucytosine is indicated [1].

   Recently, in disseminated infection with eye involvement Edwards favored the combination of amphotericin B and flucytosine for therapy, especially for lesions near the macula; ocular penetration of the drug (e.g., amphotericin B) may not correlate with clinical efficacy [14a]. Patients should be followed serially by an ophthalmologist because partial vitrectomy may be very beneficial. After initial therapy with amphotericin B, with or without flucytosine, additional oral therapy with fluconazole is probably reasonable, but Edwards does not advocate primary therapy with fluconazole alone [14a]. Optimal duration of therapy is poorly defined and is in part dependent on serial eye examinations revealing improvement of eye findings; this must be individualized. Both ophthalmology and infectious disease consultations are advised for these patients.

9. **Septic thrombophlebitis** of the peripheral or great vessels may occur in association with intravenous catheters [38, 39]. Fever, signs of sepsis, and persistent candidemia are characteristic of peripheral thrombophlebitis caused by *Candida* species. If suppuration is found with a peripheral phlebitis, the vein should be excised and amphotericin B initiated. Septic thrombophlebitis of the great vessels is uncommon but should be suspected when candidemia persists after removal of a central venous catheter and endocarditis is not believed to be present. A venogram or MRI may be helpful diagnostically. Treatment with amphotericin B is indicated.

Histoplasmosis

Histoplasma capsulatum is a dimorphous fungus that causes histoplasmosis, the most common systemic fungal infection in the United States. Inhalation of the infectious spores of *H. capsulatum* usually results in asymptomatic infection. Symptomatic pulmonary disease may occur in the normal host, and the organism may occasionally produce chronic, progressive pulmonary infection or disseminated disease in some patients. *H. capsulatum* **is an important opportunistic pathogen in the immunocompromised host, especially persons infected with HIV** [40].

I. **Growth and identification characteristics.** *H. capsulatum* can be grown on routine fungal culture media, although growth is augmented on enriched agar such as brain-heart infusion. The mycelial phase requires 10–21 days to grow at room temperature and can be identified in the laboratory by characteristic large tuberculate spores (macroconidia). Conversion to the yeast phase at 37°C requires another 7–14 days. Biopsied tissue specimens should be stained as well as cultured; Gomori's methenamine silver and periodic acid–Schiff preparations may reveal characteristic small, intracellular yeasts. The organism may also be detected by Wright's stain of sputum or blood.

II. **Epidemiologic features**

A. **Endemic areas.** Although histoplasmosis occurs throughout the world, **the disease is endemic in the central United States, particularly in the Ohio and Mississippi River valleys.** In areas of Tennessee and Kentucky, more than 90% of the adult population has been infected with *H. capsulatum,* as manifested by positive skin-test reactions. As far east as Maryland and Virginia, 85% of those tested have been exposed.

B. **Sources of infection.** *H. capsulatum* is found in nature in the soil. The organism grows particularly well in soil contaminated with excreta of birds (e.g., starlings, chickens, and blackbirds) and bats. Persons involved in cleaning chicken houses or blackbird roosts and in exploring caves are at risk for heavy exposures, and these conditions provide the setting for epidemic outbreaks [41]. Histoplasmosis may also be seen in urban residents. Foci of *H. capsulatum* spores may be present in open fields, parks, or old buildings, and an outbreak of acute pulmonary histoplasmosis may result if these foci are disturbed by construction or demolition [42].

III. **Pathogenesis**
  A. **Agent. Infection occurs via inhalation of airborne spores.** The spores are deposited in pulmonary alveoli, where conversion to the yeast form and phagocytosis by macrophages occur. Infected macrophages spread through lymphatic channels to regional lymph nodes, followed by hematogenous spread to organs of the reticuloendothelial system (liver, spleen, and bone marrow).
  B. **In the normal host,** cell-mediated immunity develops within 7–21 days of primary exposure [40]. T lymphocytes secrete cytokines that activate macrophages to kill intracellular yeasts, eventually resulting in caseating or noncaseating granulomas at infected sites. This response controls the infection. The granulomas become calcified over a period of months in children and years in adults, resulting in the characteristic Gohn complex and splenic calcifications commonly seen on roentgenography.
  C. **In some persons, effective cellular immunity never develops.** The infection is not contained, and **disseminated histoplasmosis occurs.** Persons at greatest risk for disseminated disease include the elderly and very young children and immunosuppressed patients such as those with leukemia or lymphoma, transplant recipients, and patients receiving corticosteroids. **AIDS patients are at very high risk for developing disseminated histoplasmosis.**
IV. **Clinical presentation, diagnosis, and therapy**
  A. **Acute pulmonary histoplasmosis**
    1. **Manifestations**
      a. **In the normal host, infection following a mild inhalational exposure is usually subclinical and asymptomatic.** Uncommonly, mild exposure results in symptomatic illness, usually in children or infants. On occasion, massively enlarged nodes may cause tracheal, bronchial, or vena caval obstruction. Caseous nodes may rupture into a bronchus, producing a segmental pneumonitis. Rarely, pulmonary infection may result in disseminated disease, described in sec. **B.**
      b. **Infection following a heavy inhalational exposure** to spores may cause symptomatic disease, referred to as **acute pulmonary histoplasmosis** [41].
        (1) **Acute illness in those without prior exposure** often presents with an **influenzalike picture** (chills, fever, malaise, headache, myalgias, nonproductive cough, and chest pain) after an incubation period of 10–18 days. Erythema nodosum, erythema multiforme, and migrating polyarthritis have been described in this setting. The **chest roentgenogram** generally reveals bilateral patchy, nodular infiltrates with hilar or mediastinal adenopathy. Pleural effusion is uncommon. Symptoms in most patients resolve within 2–3 weeks.
        (2) **Acute disease in a previously exposed individual** follows a slightly different pattern. Symptoms are similar but milder in degree and occur after a shorter incubation period (3–7 days). The chest roentgenogram may be different, in that nodules are fine and miliary and there is no adenopathy, pleural involvement, or late calcification.
    2. **Diagnosis**
      a. **Subclinical infections** are diagnosed retrospectively by skin test conversion or by characteristic x-ray patterns of calcification.
      b. **Acute symptomatic pulmonary histoplasmosis** can be diagnosed by culture and examination of sputum in no more than 10% of patients. Additional diagnostic aids include the following:
        (1) **The chest roentgenogram** may be suggestive, as noted previously.
        (2) **Skin tests** generally are **not useful** because most individuals in endemic areas will react due to prior exposure. Also, the use of skin tests may result in false positive complement fixation titers.
        (3) **Complement fixation tests** detect antibodies to either yeast or mycelial antigens. If either or both tests are performed, more than 90% of patients with acute disease will have titers of 1:8 or greater, and 70% will have titers of at least 1:32 [43]. Titers of 1:8 to 1:16 are suspect because false positive results in healthy persons often fall into this range, particularly in endemic regions. False positive results, generally titers of 1:8 or 1:16, are also seen in 20–40% of persons with other

fungal or granulomatous diseases. A complement fixation titer of at least 1:32, or a fourfold rise in titer, in conjunction with a compatible clinical syndrome is strongly suggestive of acute pulmonary histoplasmosis.

The **immunodiffusion test** for precipitins to the H and M antigens is more specific than complement fixation but is not very sensitive. Antibodies may be undetectable for more than 3 weeks after exposure, and the immunodiffusion and complement fixation tests often are negative if performed early in the course of infection.

   (4) Antigen test. A newly developed radioimmunoassay is able to detect a polysaccharide antigen of *H. capsulatum,* particularly in disseminated disease [44]. In acute pulmonary disease, however, antigen usually is not detectable.

 3. **Therapy.** The vast majority of normal hosts have benign, self-limited infection and require no therapy. A short course of amphotericin B (3–7 mg/kg) has been suggested for severe infection in infants and young children, in patients with the adult respiratory distress syndrome, and in adults with prolonged symptomatic illness of more than 10 days' duration [40]. The use of amphotericin or the oral agents ketoconazole and itraconazole in the treatment of acute disease has not been evaluated in controlled studies. Infectious disease consultation is advised.

B. **Progressive disseminated histoplasmosis** [45, 46] is uncommon, occurring in approximately 1 of 2,000–5,000 acute infections and generally in an immunocompromised host (e.g., an AIDS patient), as noted earlier. On occasion, it has been reported in an otherwise healthy adult. Disseminated disease may occur soon after an acute exposure or years later, after the patient has left an endemic region and subsequently developed immunosuppression. **Infection with HIV should be excluded in patients with disseminated disease** who have no other predisposing conditions.

 1. **Clinical manifestations** may vary from very severe illness (usually seen in infants and patients with AIDS) to more chronic disease, extending over months to years [45].
    a. **Systemic symptoms** of fever, chills, malaise, anorexia, and weight loss are common. Symptoms that follow an acute inhalational exposure and last more than 3 weeks may indicate systemic involvement, as most cases of acute pulmonary histoplasmosis resolve in less than 3 weeks.
    b. **Hepatosplenomegaly** and abnormal liver function tests are common and may be striking in infants.
    c. **Mucosal ulcerations** occur in 35–40% of patients throughout the GI tract, especially the ileum, causing anorexia, nausea, abdominal pain, diarrhea, frank bleeding, or perforation.
       Oropharyngeal, nasal, labial, gingival, and laryngeal ulcers provide **excellent biopsy sites** for diagnostic purposes.
    d. **The adrenal glands** are frequently infected and adrenal insufficiency definitely occurs, but the incidence of clinically significant adrenal insufficiency is unclear.
    e. **Chest roentgenograms** may be normal or show interstitial or nodular infiltrates.
    f. **Anemia and leukopenia** are common, especially in patients with severe disease.
    g. **Uncommon manifestations** include CNS disease (meningitis or focal cerebritis), skin lesions (papules, nodules, or ulcers), endocarditis, and lytic bone lesions.
    h. **Patients with AIDS and disseminated histoplasmosis** frequently have severe disease and may present with shock, adult respiratory distress syndrome, disseminated intravascular coagulopathy (DIC), and CNS involvement [47].

 2. **Diagnosis**
    a. **Complement fixation tests** are positive in 50–70% of patients but should be interpreted with caution, as previously discussed (see sec. **A.2.b.(3)**). Serial testing may be useful.
    b. **Antigen detection.** The polysaccharide antigen of *H. capsulatum* may be detected in the blood of more than 50% and in the urine of more than 90% of patients with disseminated histoplasmosis [44]. **Serial antigen measure-**

ments are helpful in following treatment response because the antigen disappears with treatment and reappears with relapse. The antigen test is commercially available in a single reference laboratory (Histoplasmosis Reference Laboratory, Indianapolis, IN).

  c. **Cultures of bone marrow** are positive in more than 75% of patients with disseminated disease, and **blood cultures** are positive in 40–70% of cases [45–47]. The lysis-centrifugation technique improves the yield from blood cultures and is particularly useful in AIDS patients. The organism can be isolated from **sputum and urine** cultures in more than half of the patients. Growth and identification of *H. capsulatum* in culture generally requires 4–6 weeks.

  d. **Special stains.** Demonstration of organisms by methenamine silver stain provides a diagnosis within 24–48 hours in many patients (e.g., buffy-coat preparations of peripheral blood, bone marrow, and sputum will be positive in >50% of patients). A Wright's stain of the peripheral blood may reveal organisms with leukocytes in patients with severe disease. Biopsy specimens may also be obtained from oral lesions, the liver, and lymph nodes.

3. **Therapy. Antifungal therapy is clearly indicated in all cases of progressive disseminated histoplasmosis.**

  a. **In the immunocompromised HIV-negative patient,** amphotericin B is standard therapy [45]. The usual total dose for adults is 30 mg/kg, whereas infants receive 1 mg/kg/day for at least 6 weeks. Itraconazole, 200 mg/day for a minimum of 6 months, is also effective in adult patients who do not have meningeal involvement or life-threatening disease [48].

  b. **Patients with AIDS** who have CNS involvement or immediately life-threatening disease should receive an **induction course of amphotericin B,** 15–30 mg/kg [47]. AIDS patients with mild to moderate disease may be treated with **itraconazole,** 300 mg bid for 3 days, then 200 mg bid for 12 weeks, as induction therapy [49]. To prevent relapse, all AIDS patients should be placed on **lifelong maintenance** therapy with itraconazole (200–400 mg/day) following resolution of the acute illness [50]. Amphotericin B, 50 mg every 1–2 weeks, is an alternative.

  c. **In nonimmunocompromised HIV-negative patients,** itraconazole, 200 mg/day for 6 months, is well tolerated and very effective [48]. Ketoconazole, 400 mg/day for 6 months, is also effective [51]. Patients with severe disease or involvement of the CNS should be treated with amphotericin B. Infectious disease consultation is advised.

4. **Prognosis.** Without treatment, the mortality is approximately 90%. In HIV-negative patients, treatment with amphotericin B decreases the mortality to 7–15%. The prognosis in AIDS patients is related to the underlying illness and the severity of the infection on presentation. Most relapses occur within 1 year of treatment.

C. **Chronic pulmonary histoplasmosis** [52] occurs in the setting of preexisting chronic lung disease. It manifests initially as a lingering segmental interstitial pneumonitis. Approximately 10–20% of cases progress to chronic cavitary disease.

1. **Early noncavitary pneumonitis**

  a. **Manifestations.** Malaise, fever, cough, and pleuritic pain are common, but some patients may be asymptomatic. Chest roentgenogram shows an interstitial infiltrate occurring typically in the apical-posterior area of the lung. The infiltrate disappears in 2–3 months, and the infarctlike necrotic areas become larger, leading to contraction and volume loss.

  b. **Diagnosis.** Sputum cultures are positive in approximately one-third of cases, and the chest roentgenogram may be suggestive.

  c. **Therapy.** The early pneumonitis episodes usually are self-limited.

  d. **Prognosis.** Although it generally follows a benign course, early pneumonitis may result in the destruction of significant amounts of lung tissue, thereby exacerbating any existing respiratory insufficiency. In many patients, large air spaces, or bullae, become infected, and this progresses to chronic cavitary disease.

2. **Cavitary infection**

  a. **Manifestations.** Cough and sputum production are prominent and are usually accompanied by weight loss, low-grade fever, and easy fatigability. Hemoptysis is common and, in general, there is an acceleration of the manifestations of the underlying chronic lung disease. **Chest roentgen-**

ography reveals cavitation, usually immediately adjacent to a pneumonic lesion and at the extreme apex. If inflammation subsides, cavitary walls remain thin, but active infection leads to wall thickening. As described by Goodwin and coworkers [52], wall thickness of less than 1 mm rarely suggests active infection; most cases with 1- to 2-mm walls heal spontaneously; and established and continuing infection is probable if wall thickness exceeds 2 mm.

   b. **Diagnosis**
   (1) **Definitive bacteriologic diagnosis** by culture or Wright's stain of sputum is not always possible (recovery ranges from 35 to 60%), and positive cultures do not necessarily indicate active disease or threat of relapse.
   (2) **The radiologic picture** affords a better index of disease activity than do microbiologic data.
   (3) **Complement fixation tests** are positive in 75% of patients but should be interpreted with caution.

   c. **Therapy.** Many cases, especially those with thin-walled lesions (<2 mm), may regress spontaneously. Such cases can therefore be managed with an initial period of observation. Without treatment, 30–40% of thin-walled cavities persist and enlarge, and progressive pulmonary insufficiency results. If cavitation progresses and clinical improvement does not occur, antifungal therapy is indicated [40, 52]. Oral therapy with itraconazole (200–400 mg/day) or ketoconazole (400 mg/day) for 6 months or more yields response rates of 65–80% [48, 51], which compare favorably to results seen with amphotericin B. Treatment with one of the oral agents is favored owing to their better side-effect profiles. The indications for surgical resection are not well defined. Underlying lung disease often precludes a surgical approach. Infectious disease consultation is advised.

D. **Uncommon manifestations of histoplasmosis**
   1. **Histoplasmomas** may form during the healing phase of a primary lung infection. These asymptomatic lesions may appear as solitary pulmonary nodules (1–4 cm in diameter) that have central calcification. **No therapy is indicated.** If calcifications are not obvious, comparison with prior x-rays, CT scanning, needle biopsy, or surgical exploration may be indicated to rule out a neoplasm.
   2. **Mediastinal fibrosis** is the term used to describe a very thick (>1 cm), fibrotic capsule in the mediastinal perihilar region, with actual invasion or compression of adjacent structures [53]. The process tends to be slowly but relentlessly progressive, and no therapeutic approach has proven to be reliably effective.
   3. The term **mediastinal granuloma** refers to large caseous lymph nodes that mat together and become encapsulated after primary infection. These rarely cause problems but may occasionally result in symptoms due to compression of adjacent structures in the mediastinum [54]. In selected patients, surgical excision may be beneficial.

Cryptococcosis

Cryptococcus neoformans is a saprophytic fungus that may cause disease in normal hosts as well as in the immunosuppressed. Meningitis and pulmonary infection are the most common manifestations, and *C. neoformans* is a common cause of meningoencephalitis in AIDS patients in the United States [55].

I. **Growth and identification characteristics.** Clinical cryptococcal isolates are encapsulated yeast and often are identifiable on India ink and Wright's stain. Visualization in clinical specimens may yield an early presumptive diagnosis. Standard culture techniques are utilized, but the bacteriology laboratory should be alerted if *Cryptococcus* is a diagnostic possibility. Media used for isolation should not contain cycloheximide because it inhibits growth of the organism. Growth generally occurs in 3–7 days, with identification in 3–4 days. Occasionally growth is slower, however, and incubation should be continued for 4–6 weeks before the culture is discarded as negative.

II. **Epidemiologic features and host factors.** *C. neoformans* is a ubiquitous fungus that is found worldwide in avian feces, particularly pigeon droppings. It has also been found in soil, certain fruits, contaminated milk, and food products [56]. Disease generally occurs following inhalation of the organism. Unlike other airborne mycoses, however, focal outbreaks of cryptococcosis are quite rare. **Many patients have no demonstrable underlying immune defect.** Patients who are immunocompromised, however, especially those with defective cell-mediated immunity, are prone to more serious infections, with rapid progression and dissemination. **Patients at highest risk for severe disease** include those with AIDS, lymphoma or leukemia, transplant recipients, and those receiving corticosteroids [55, 57].

III. **Pulmonary involvement** [58, 59]. The respiratory tract is presumed to be the primary portal of entry of *C. neoformans.* Pulmonary cryptococcosis is probably the **most common form of the disease,** although it is diagnosed less often than meningoencephalitis because it is **usually transient and often subclinical.**

A. **Clinical presentation.** Pulmonary infection usually results in few sequelae, and **many patients are asymptomatic.** If a patient inhales a large inoculum of organisms, or if host defenses are compromised systemically or locally (because of a chronic respiratory disorder), the occurrence of symptomatic pulmonary disease is more likely. Clinically significant illness typically manifests as a subacute or chronic process with minimal constitutional signs and symptoms. The most common symptoms are cough with scant sputum production, dull chest pain, and dyspnea. Low-grade fever and weight loss may occur with illness of longer duration.

B. **Diagnosis.** The manifestations of cryptococcal infection are nonspecific, and diagnosis depends on a high index of suspicion. **Patients who are immunocompromised are especially at risk.** Because of the lack of a vigorous inflammatory response, the routine indices of infection, such as leukocytosis and sedimentation rate elevations, may be absent.

   1. **Sputum cultures** will isolate the organism in only 10–30% of patients with invasive disease. Because saprophytic colonization of the respiratory tract may result in a positive sputum culture, definitive diagnosis often requires open lung or bronchoscopic biopsy and **demonstration of tissue invasion.** Characteristic yeasts are readily seen with methenamine silver, periodic acid–Schiff, or Mayer's mucicarmine stains.

   2. **Chest roentgenographic findings are variable** and may range from solitary nodules in asymptomatic individuals to focal or lobar infiltrates with symptomatic infection. Patients may present with diffuse interstitial infiltrates and the adult respiratory distress syndrome. Cavitation and pleural effusion are uncommon.

   3. **In all patients suspected or proven to have pulmonary cryptococcosis, the spinal fluid, urine, and blood should also be cultured** for *C. neoformans,* and the cryptococcal antigen test should be performed on CSF and serum to rule out disseminated disease [55].

C. **Therapy.** Pulmonary cryptococcosis need not be treated in every patient.

   1. **A 2- to 4-month period of observation without therapy is acceptable in a normal host if** the following conditions are met: (1) There are no extrapulmonary lesions; (2) cultures of blood, CSF, and urine are negative; (3) cryptococcal antigen is negative in the CSF and the serum titer is absent, low, stable, or falling; and (4) pulmonary lesions are small, few, stable, or regressing.

      The ease of giving oral fluconazole makes it tempting to treat pulmonary cryptococcosis. However, this not only may be an unnecessary expense, but also it is unclear whether premature and possibly inadequate therapy may interfere with the host immune response, potentially exposing the host to other consequences of cryptococcal infections (e.g., eventual meningitis). However, this remains a controversial area. Medoff [31] will use oral itraconazole for 6–12 weeks even if there is no meningitis on CSF examination and the patient is not immunosuppressed. Infectious disease consultation is suggested.

   2. **Antifungal therapy.** Therapy **should be instituted if** (1) the radiographic picture worsens; (2) there is evidence of increasing ventilatory impairment; (3) there is any evidence of dissemination; or (4) the patient is immunocompromised. **Patients who are immunosuppressed need antifungal therapy because the risk of dissemination is high** [58, 60]. Particularly troubling are those patients with reticuloendothelial malignancy, severe diabetes, organ transplantation, or AIDS, or those receiving chronic steroids or other immunosuppressive therapy. Antifungal chemotherapy for pulmonary cryptococcosis is not well studied. Many investigators recommend a full course of amphotericin B (total dose,

2–2.5 g) with or without flucytosine. The efficacy of fluconazole in the treatment of cryptococcal pneumonia is unknown at present. Decisions regarding therapy should be individualized based on the immune status of the host, the severity of infection, and the side-effect profiles of the antifungal agents. Infectious disease consultation is recommended.

IV. **Disseminated disease.** Bloodborne cryptococcal yeast may disseminate from the lung to any organ but has an **unexplained preference for the CNS.** Skin and bone involvement may also occur. All patients with disseminated disease should be treated as outlined for meningitis in this section.

A. **Central nervous system.** Meningoencephalitis is the most common clinical manifestation of infection with *C. neoformans* [55, 61]. Due primarily to the prevalence of cryptococcal meningitis in AIDS patients, the majority of persons with cryptococcal CNS infection have compromised immune systems. **See related discussion in Chap. 5.**

1. **The clinical manifestations** of cryptococcal meningitis are highly variable. Patients may present with acute symptoms of only a few days' duration, particularly if they are very immunosuppressed (e.g., HIV-infected persons). Conversely, others may have subtle symptoms for weeks or months before the diagnosis is made. The most common signs and symptoms include headache, fever, nuchal rigidity (often absent), cranial nerve palsies, impaired memory and judgment, lethargy, obtundation, and coma.

2. **Diagnosis**

   a. **Cerebrospinal fluid**

      (1) **Standard tests.** Of symptomatic patients, 90% demonstrate some abnormality of the CSF: increased opening pressure, elevated protein, decreased glucose, or a lymphocytic pleocytosis. On occasion, however, the CSF may be normal. A low CSF inflammatory response (<20 WBCs/μl) is a poor prognostic sign and often is seen in AIDS patients. Normal or only slightly abnormal CSF parameters are common in AIDS patients, and so greater reliance should be placed on more specific tests [62].

      (2) **India ink stains.** Cryptococcal yeast may be demonstrated on India ink stain in at least 50% of non-AIDS patients with CNS involvement and in more than 70% of AIDS patients. False positive results may occur, however, if yeasts are confused with artifact or lymphocytes. Only experienced personnel should interpret India ink preparations. Organisms may also be seen on Gram stain of the CSF.

      (3) **Definitive diagnosis** generally requires isolation of the organism in culture of the CSF. Centrifuged sediments from large volumes of CSF (4–8 ml) should be used.

   b. **The latex agglutination slide test** for detection of the cryptococcal polysaccharide antigen **is the most useful fungal serologic test in clinical practice. The antigen test is particularly useful for making a presumptive diagnosis of cryptococcal meningitis,** with virtually all patients demonstrating titers of 1:8 or higher in the CSF. The test is more than 90% sensitive and specific for cryptococcal infection when performed properly. Rarely, false positive results may occur in the presence of rheumatoid factor or the opportunistic fungus *Trichosporon beigelii* [55]. Cryptococcal antigen may also be detected in serum and urine. **The serum antigen test is usually positive in persons with AIDS and cryptococcal meningitis and is therefore a useful screening test in this cohort of patients.**

   c. **Additional diagnostic tests.** A cryptococcoma or ventricular dilation in a patient with suspected hydrocephalus may occasionally be demonstrated by CT scan or MRI.

3. **Therapy. Cryptococcal meningoencephalitis is an absolute indication for systemic antifungal chemotherapy.** Because of the tendency of this disease to remit and relapse, long-term follow-up is necessary to ensure a cure. Therapeutic outcomes and goals are significantly different in HIV-positive patients compared to those not infected with HIV. Therefore, these two patient populations will be considered separately.

   a. **In non-AIDS patients, amphotericin B** (0.4 mg/kg/day) alone for approximately 10 weeks is a standard therapeutic regimen, with cure rates in excess of 50%. Most authorities, however, now recommend **combination therapy** with amphotericin (0.3 mg/kg/day IV) and flucytosine (25–37.5 mg PO q6h) for 6 weeks, which results in cures of 60–70% of patients. In a

trial comparing combination therapy to amphotericin alone, combination therapy yielded fewer relapses, sterilized the CSF more rapidly, and was less nephrotoxic [63]. **Fluconazole,** a new oral agent highly active against *C. neoformans,* **has been used with success in AIDS patients** with cryptococcal meningitis (see sec. **c**), **but its role in the treatment of non-AIDS patients with CNS cryptococcal infection remains to be defined.**
  b. **Relapses** in HIV-negative individuals after treatment generally occur within 1 year, usually in the first 1–4 months [64]. Posttreatment lumbar punctures should thus be performed every 2–4 months for 1 year following the conclusion of therapy.
  c. **Patients with AIDS** and cryptococcal meningitis cannot be cured. The goal of treatment, therefore, is to **gain control of the acute illness** and then continue therapy with an easily tolerated agent that will **suppress continuing cryptococcal infection** and allow patients to maintain their functional status.
    (1) An aggressive **induction course** of **amphotericin B** (0.7 mg/kg/day) with or without **flucytosine** for the initial 2–3 weeks is used by many experts during the acute phase of the illness. Amphotericin effects more rapid sterilization of the CSF than does fluconazole [65]. **The hematologic toxicity of flucytosine may be magnified in AIDS patients,** and so this drug should be used with caution and probably at slightly reduced doses (e.g., 75–100 mg/kg/day). Combination therapy for approximately 2 weeks still is favored by many clinicians [31], especially in the very ill patient (see related discussion in Chap. 5). Infectious disease consultation is suggested. However, a recent multicenter randomized trial demonstrated no difference in mortality or sterilization of the CSF in patients treated with combination therapy with flucytosine (25 mg/kg q6h) and amphotericin as compared to patients treated with amphotericin B alone [66].
    (2) If clinical and microbiologic improvement is seen with amphotericin B, **consolidation therapy** with **fluconazole,** 400 mg/day for another 8 weeks, is reasonable.
    (3) Selected patients with normal mental status who are at low risk for treatment failure might be treated with fluconazole alone [65]. Consultation with an infectious disease specialist is advised.
  d. **Maintenance therapy** in AIDS patients is critical to prevent the otherwise inevitable relapse. When primary therapy has been completed, patients should receive **fluconazole,** 200 mg/day, indefinitely. This is both a highly effective and well-tolerated maintenance regimen [67, 68]. Fluconazole is preferred over itraconazole for maintenance [66].
  e. **See additional discussion in Chap. 5.**
B. **Skin.** Nearly 10–15% of patients with disseminated disease have skin involvement, which occurs most frequently on the face and scalp. Although rare reports suggest the occurrence of primary skin cryptococcosis, essentially **all patients with cryptococcal skin lesions should be considered to have disseminated disease** and evaluated as such [55].
  1. **Manifestations.** Cryptococcal skin involvement should be suspected in any immunosuppressed patient with erythematous papules, pustules, warts with a molluscum–like appearance, subcutaneous nodules, or ulceration. Mucosal lesions are uncommon.
  2. **Diagnosis.** Skin biopsy with fungal stains and fungal cultures may be diagnostic.
C. **Bone.** Approximately 5% of patients with disseminated disease manifest slow-growing osseous lesions. The prominences of long bones, cranial bones, and vertebrae are involved most commonly. Roentgenograms reveal round lytic areas without sclerosis. **Biopsy with culture is necessary** for diagnosis.
D. Spread to most organs has been documented at postmortem examination in patients with disseminated disease. **Detection of cryptococcal organisms in any organ always mandates a search for the presence of cryptococcal infection elsewhere in the body.** Patients infected with HIV may have a syndrome of disseminated cryptococcal infection without specific organ localization. These patients have fever, chills, myalgias, lethargy, and a positive serum cryptococcal antigen. They require therapy and respond quickly. To prevent CNS localization, chronic suppression is needed.

Coccidioidomycosis

Coccidioides immitis is a highly infectious fungus that frequently causes pulmonary infection in endemic areas of the United States. **Although most disease caused by this organism is benign and self-limited, infection may occasionally result in chronic pulmonary or skin disease, meningitis, or disseminated illness.**

I. **Growth and identification characteristics.** Routine culture methods are employed, with presumptive identification in 2–5 days. The fungus grows readily on most culture media [69, 70]. **All culture plates should be handled with extreme care, for they are highly infectious to laboratory personnel.** Therefore, the laboratory should be alerted about any clinical specimens when coccidioidomycosis is suspected. **Direct human-to-human transmission is not known to occur, however.** The clinician may identify the *Coccidioides* spherule in sputum, drainage material, or infected tissue. It is doubly refractile and thick-walled, measures 20–80 mm, and is typically seen in several stages of development. Several preparations may be utilized to identify spherules, including potassium hydroxide, hematoxylin and eosin, methenamine silver, and periodic acid–Schiff stain.

II. **Epidemiologic features.** Coccidioidomycosis is endemic in the southwestern United States, Mexico, and parts of Central and South America. Cases may be seen outside endemic areas in persons who have traveled through these regions or as reactivation of infection acquired years earlier by a former resident of an endemic area. Because **infection is caused by inhalation of airborne arthrospores,** outbreaks may occur in dry weather in association with fresh diggings, newly plowed ground, and dust storms.

III. **Clinical aspects**

A. **Acute pulmonary coccidioidomycosis.** Most persons with primary infection by *C. immitis* **have an acute, self-limited infection in the lungs** [70, 71].

1. **Subclinical or asymptomatic illness** occurs in approximately 60% of patients. Prior infection in these persons can be detected only by skin testing.

2. **Symptomatic illness.** Forty percent of patients develop flulike symptoms after an incubation period of 7–28 days (average, 10–16 days).

a. **Signs and symptoms.** Fever, malaise, dry cough, shortness of breath, night sweats, anorexia, and pleuritic chest pain are common. Within the first few days of the onset of symptoms, a fine, generalized, erythematous maculopapular rash, sometimes urticarial in appearance, develops in 10–40% of patients. Peripheral eosinophilia may be present. The development of cutaneous hypersensitivity may be manifest as erythema nodosum or erythema multiforme, which occurs in fewer than 25% of infected individuals. This finding often is accompanied by arthralgias and, in association with pneumonitis, constitutes the classic picture of so-called valley fever.

b. **Roentgenographic findings.** The most common radiologic manifestation of acute coccidioidal pneumonitis is a segmental pneumonia, seen in approximately 50% of cases. Minimal infiltrates occur in nearly 30%, whereas hilar adenopathy and pleural effusion, sometimes massive, are seen in approximately 20%. In addition, solitary or multiple nodules, thin- or thick-walled cavities, and mediastinal lymphadenopathy may occur. Roentgenographic abnormalities usually resolve in 1–3 weeks.

3. **Diagnosis**

a. **Sputum.** Approximately 40–70% of primary infections will yield positive cultures [71]. A positive sputum culture is virtually diagnostic of pulmonary coccidioidomycosis, as this organism rarely colonizes the oropharynx.

b. **Skin tests** cannot differentiate between acute and remote infection and often are negative in persons with disseminated disease. They are, therefore, primarily useful only in epidemiologic evaluations.

c. **Serologic tests often are diagnostic** in primary coccidioidomycosis. **Serum precipitins,** as detected by tube precipitin, immunodiffusion, or latex agglutination testing, are IgM antibodies that are demonstrable in more than 75% of patients within 3 weeks of the onset of symptoms. Precipitins usually cannot be detected after 4 weeks. **Complement fixation detects IgG antibodies,** which appear more slowly but persist longer than IgM precipitins. More than 50% of patients will have a positive complement fixation titer, usually less than 1:32, by 3 months after the occurrence of clinical disease. More than 90% of patients with symptomatic acute pulmonary disease will have detectable antibodies by either precipitin testing or complement fixation [69]. Rising or persistently high complement fixation titers are a poor prognostic sign, whereas decreasing titers indicate improvement.

4. **Treatment. In the majority of patients with acute coccidioidomycosis, the disease resolves within 6–8 weeks without specific therapy.** However, systemic **antifungal therapy should be considered in the following settings:** infancy; debilitation; pregnancy; immunosuppression; racial groups predisposed to disseminated disease (see sec. **C**); rising or persistently high (> 1:16) complement fixation titers; progressive pulmonary disease; and persistent symptoms for more than 6 weeks [69, 70]. Amphotericin B has been used most commonly in the past, at a total dose of 0.5–1.5 g depending on clinical response. The activity of itraconazole and ketoconazole in other forms of coccidioidomycosis suggest that they too would be useful in severe primary disease.

B. **Other pulmonary manifestations** may occur.

1. **Chronic pulmonary coccidioidomycosis.** In some patients, symptoms of the acute pneumonia may persist for months or years. These patients have low-grade fever, weight loss, and cough. Serum complement fixation titers are positive, and sputum cultures often grow *C. immitis*. Antifungal therapy is indicated. The efficacy and low toxicity of **itraconazole** at 200 mg bid make this drug a reasonable first choice [72, 73]. Ketoconazole and amphotericin B are alternatives for patients who do not respond to therapy or who relapse after a course of itraconazole.

2. **Solitary pulmonary nodules** (coccidioidomas) may be seen in the asymptomatic patient. In endemic areas, 50% of pulmonary coin lesions may be due to *C. immitis*. Earlier chest roentgenograms should be obtained for comparison, and neoplasm must be excluded.

3. **Cavitary disease** may be seen after acute primary infection but usually resolves spontaneously. Persistent cavitation sometimes occurs. Patients may be asymptomatic or have hemoptysis and low-grade fever. Sputum cultures often are positive. The course of persistent coccidioidal cavities is unpredictable, but the majority will resolve spontaneously over a period of 1–2 years. In a few patients, complications such as hemoptysis or rapid expansion with involvement of the adjacent lung may require some combination of drug therapy and surgery [70].

C. **Disseminated coccidioidomycosis.** Fewer than 1% of infected individuals will develop disseminated (extrapulmonary) infection. This complication **most often occurs in immunocompromised hosts such as transplant recipients, patients with hematologic malignancies, or those receiving immunosuppressive chemotherapy** [69]. **AIDS patients are at increased risk for disseminated disease,** although focal pulmonary disease may also be seen [74, 75]. Dissemination appears to be more common during **pregnancy,** particularly in the third trimester. In addition, **dark-skinned races** (e.g., Filipino, Hispanic, African-American) more commonly have disseminated disease than do whites. Dissemination may occur within a few weeks of the primary infection or years later, following reactivation of quiescent disease. Any organ of the body may be affected, but the major sites of dissemination are discussed next.

1. **Osteoarticular disease.** More than one-third of patients with disseminated disease have **involvement of the bones or joints** [69]. The bones most commonly affected are the skull and vertebrae and the bones of the hands and feet [76]. **Lytic lesions** are typical and frequently involve the overlying soft tissue, producing abscesses or draining sinuses. Articular lesions usually are limited to a single joint, generally the knee or ankle.

2. **Cutaneous disease.** The skin is commonly involved in patients with disseminated coccidioidomycosis. The lesions may vary in appearance from pustules or plaques to verrucous, wartlike growths. Rarely, skin lesions may result from the direct inoculation of *C. immitis*.

3. **Meningitis.** CNS involvement by *C. immitis* usually is subtle and nonspecific and generally occurs within several months of the primary infection. Headache, fever, and weight loss are common symptoms [77]. Examination of the CSF typically reveals a mononuclear pleocytosis with an elevated protein. Peripheral blood eosinophilia has been noted. See Chap. 5 for further discussion.

4. **Other less common manifestations** of dissemination include involvement of the genitourinary tract in the form of prostatitis or epididymitis. Coccidioidal peritonitis and lymphadenitis have been described and, rarely, the eyes may

be involved. **Miliary disease,** as manifested by diffuse, reticular infiltrates on the chest roentgenogram, is a common presentation of disease **in AIDS patients** [75].

5. **Diagnosis.** Definitive diagnosis requires **histopathologic evidence and/or culture of the organism** from infected tissue or fluid (e.g., skin, synovial fluid, or lymph nodes). Positive blood or urine cultures are uncommon. CSF cultures are positive in approximately one-third of patients with meningitis. **Elevated complement fixation titers** are the rule in disseminated coccidioidomycosis. Most patients have serum titers of 1:32 or higher [69]. The exception to this generalization is meningitis, in which serum titers tend to be much lower. Complement-fixing antibodies are **detectable in the spinal fluid** in more than 75% of patients with meningitis. Complement fixation titers show considerable variation between laboratories. The reporting laboratory's experience with these assays should thus be borne in mind when assessing the significance of a particular result.

6. **Therapy. Systemic antifungal therapy is indicated in all forms of disseminated disease.**
   a. **Nonmeningeal** forms of dissemination have traditionally been treated with intravenous **amphotericin B** to a total dose of 1.5–3.0 g, depending on the clinical response [69, 70]. The onset of action with amphotericin B appears to be more rapid than with the oral azoles. **Amphotericin B is therefore indicated for patients with severe, life-threatening disease.**
      Ketoconazole, 400 mg/day, is also effective, but relapse is common even with prolonged therapy [78]. Therapy with **itraconazole,** 400 mg/day for 12 months or longer, has yielded sustained remissions in more than 50% of patients, and relapse appears to be less common than with ketoconazole [72, 73]. Experience with fluconazole is more limited than with the other two azoles. Based on its ease of administration, reduced toxicity, and efficacy compared to amphotericin B, **itraconazole can be recommended as the initial drug of choice for patients without acutely life-threatening disease.** Some clinicians experienced in the treatment of chronic nonmeningeal forms of coccidioidomycosis advocate an initial period of amphotericin B for patients with serious infection, followed by therapy with an oral azole [79]. A combined medical-surgical approach may be beneficial for selected patients with osteoarticular disease [76].
   b. **Treatment of coccidioidal meningitis** in the past has relied on intrathecal amphotericin B. However, prolonged therapy is required, toxicity is considerable, and treatment may not be curative [69, 77]. A recent trial of **fluconazole,** 400 mg/day for 2–4 years, yielded a response rate of 79%, with minimal toxicity [80]. Fluconazole therapy represents a major advance in the treatment of coccidioidal meningitis. However, fluconazole may not be curative, and treatment often needs to be continued indefinitely [80a]. Itraconazole has also been reported to be effective in some patients with meningitis [80a, 81]. Infectious disease consultation is recommended. **See further discussion in Chap. 5.**

Aspergillosis

Aspergillus species are common contaminants in the bacteriology laboratory, and the relationship of a positive culture to clinical disease must always be questioned. However, *Aspergillus* may cause a variety of illnesses, from **hypersensitivity pneumonitis to disseminated, overwhelming infection in immunosuppressed patients** [82].

I. **Growth and identification characteristics.** *Aspergillus* species are easily grown on routine fungal culture media, with identification possible within 48–72 hours. The species most frequently associated with human infections are *A. fumigatus* and *A. flavus.* Although a positive culture may suggest a causative relationship in the setting of a typical clinical syndrome, it may also represent benign colonization. **Definitive diagnosis of *Aspergillus* infection depends on demonstration of the organism invading tissue.** Staining with periodic acid–Schiff and methenamine silver permits ready identification of *Aspergillus* organisms in clinical specimens by visualization of their acutely branching septate hyphae.

II. **Epidemiologic features.** *Aspergillus* species are ubiquitous soil saprophytes that are found in all parts of the world. *Aspergillus* frequently is cultured in hospital wards from unfiltered outside air circulating through open windows. Aspergillosis usually is acquired through the inhalation of airborne conidia by a susceptible host.

III. Clinical aspects. Infection with *Aspergillus* species may result in one of several forms of a broad range of illnesses known as *aspergillosis.*

A. Tracheobronchial colonization. *Aspergillus* may colonize ectatic bronchi or cavities in the lungs of patients with chronic pulmonary disease without invasion of the surrounding pulmonary parenchyma, and occasionally the organism is isolated from sputum specimens in the absence of associated clinical illness. In these instances, allergic or invasive aspergillosis is not present, and no specific therapy is required.

B. Allergic aspergillosis may involve either the alveoli (extrinsic allergic alveolitis) or the airways (allergic bronchopulmonary aspergillosis).

   1. Extrinsic allergic alveolitis is a hypersensitivity pneumonitis that occurs in nonatopic individuals who are repeatedly exposed to conidia of *Aspergillus,* as in farmers who work in close proximity to moldy grain [82]. Cough, dyspnea, fever, chills, and malaise typically develop 4–8 hours after exposure. Repeated attacks can lead to granulomatous disease and pulmonary fibrosis.

   2. Allergic bronchopulmonary aspergillosis (ABPA) results from a **hypersensitivity reaction of the airways** to *Aspergillus* fungal antigens present in the bronchial tree [83]. The pathophysiology of this disorder is complex and only partially understood. The immediate hypersensitivity (type I) reaction is believed to be IgE-mediated, probably accounting for the bronchospastic symptoms that are so characteristic of this disorder. A type III reaction (mediated by immune complexes) is most likely responsible for the roentgenographic features and more destructive changes of the bronchi [84]. A role for the cell-mediated immune system in ABPA has been postulated but is unclear [82, 84].

      a. Manifestations. ABPA is characterized by symptoms of bronchospasm, particularly episodic wheezing and dyspnea. Cough that produces mucopurulent sputum, low-grade fever, peripheral eosinophilia, and pulmonary infiltrates are common. Pleuritic chest pain and hemoptysis may also be seen. The illness may be mild and without sequelae, but recurrent episodes frequently result in progression to bronchiectasis and pulmonary fibrosis. Most patients manifest clinically evident disease when younger than 35 years [83].

      b. Diagnosis. ABPA is highly likely in a patient if several diagnostic criteria are present [84].

         (1) Patients will have a history of episodic asthma.

         (2) Peripheral blood **eosinophilia** is a nearly universal feature.

         (3) The **skin test** with *Aspergillus* antigenic extract usually is positive but is nonspecific, as it may be positive in patients who do not have ABPA.

         (4) Serum precipitating antibodies to *Aspergillus* antigens, measured by immunodiffusion or counterimmunoelectrophoresis (CIE), are present in 70–100% of cases.

         (5) Total serum IgE levels are markedly elevated. Both total IgE and IgE specific for *Aspergillus* antigens are increased in active ABPA and decrease with remissions.

         (6) Chest roentgenograms show a wide variety of abnormalities, from small, patchy, **fleeting infiltrates** (commonly in the upper lobes) to lobar consolidation, atelectasis, or cavitation. A majority of patients eventually develop central bronchiectasis.

         (7) Sputum cultures often are positive for *A. fumigatus* and are suggestive but not diagnostic.

      c. Differential diagnosis. Tuberculosis may be suggested by the upper-lobe infiltrates or cavitation. **Cystic fibrosis** patients often have features in common with ABPA patients, and this disorder must be excluded before treatment with steroids is begun. **Carcinoma of the lung and eosinophilic pneumonia or bronchiectasis** of other etiologies are additional considerations [83].

      d. Therapy is determined by the severity and frequency of attacks. Mild disease may not require specific treatment. Results with inhaled agents such as cromolyn or beclomethasone have been disappointing, perhaps owing to poor penetration into areas obstructed by mucous plugs.

         (1) Corticosteroids are the treatment of choice for ABPA. During acute exacerbations, large daily doses of prednisone (0.5–1.0 mg/kg) have been recommended until the chest roentgenogram has cleared, followed by alternate-day therapy at 0.5 mg/kg. This is continued for 3–6 months and then gradually tapered [82, 83]. Aggressive treatment of early episodes may halt or delay progression to the final fibrotic stage. Unfortunately, prevention of recurrent episodes may require long-term corticosteroid therapy, with its attendant side effects.

(2) **Bronchodilators** and **physiotherapy** with postural drainage may help prevent mucous plugging.

(3) **Serial chest roentgenography and monitoring of IgE levels** are helpful in guiding corticosteroid therapy and detecting exacerbations.

(4) **Preventive aspects.** Patients should avoid locations (e.g., compost heaps and grain silos) and activities (e.g., smoking marijuana) in which exposure to *Aspergillus* spores is likely.

(5) Treatment of ABPA with inhaled aerosolized antifungal agents or inhaled drugs such as cromolyn or beclomethasone has not been successful. The oral antifungal drug **itraconazole,** however, is quite active in vitro against *Aspergillus* and can be expected to achieve much greater levels in affected bronchi than do inhaled agents [85]. The exact role of itraconazole in the treatment of ABPA awaits the completion of clinical trials.

C. **Aspergillomas** ("fungus balls") generally represent **secondary saprophytic colonization of preexisting pulmonary cavities,** most commonly in patients with a history of chronic lung disease such as tuberculosis, sarcoidosis, or emphysema. Primary aspergillomas may occur as a late consequence of invasive aspergillosis and have been described, on occasion, in patients with ABPA. Aspergillomas are masses of tangled hyphal elements, fibrin, and mucus [82].

1. **Manifestations. Hemoptysis** is the most common symptom associated with aspergilloma, occurring in 55–85% of cases. Hemoptysis may vary from blood-streaked sputum to active bleeding that requires urgent surgical resection. Chronic cough is not uncommon. **Many patients are asymptomatic.**

2. **Diagnosis** can be established by a typical radiologic picture, sputum culture, and serologic tests.

   a. **Chest roentgenograms or CT scans usually** show the characteristic intracavitary mass partially surrounded by a crescent of air.

   b. **Sputum cultures** are positive in one-half to two-thirds of patients and are suggestive but not diagnostic.

   c. **Serum precipitins** are present in more than 90% of cases and are suggestive of the diagnosis when accompanied by the characteristic x-ray appearance.

3. **Therapy and prognosis.** The natural history of aspergilloma is variable, and therapy must be individualized based on symptoms and underlying pulmonary status. A conservative approach is prudent, with observation alone indicated for asymptomatic patients and those with mild, infrequent hemoptysis [82, 86]. Spontaneous disappearance or lysis of aspergillomas has been reported in 7–10% of cases. Surgical resection is clearly indicated for patients with severe hemoptysis.

D. **Invasive aspergillosis.** *Aspergillus* **is a common opportunistic pathogen in the compromised host** [82]. Cancer patients with prolonged neutropenia from cytotoxic chemotherapy are particularly prone to infection [87]. Patients receiving high-dose corticosteroids or other immunosuppressive agents or those with chronic granulomatous disease of childhood are also at increased risk. Invasive aspergillosis is being diagnosed increasingly in AIDS patients as well [88, 89]. Usually, this complication occurs in advanced AIDS.

1. **Manifestations**

   a. **Pulmonary involvement** is by far the most common manifestation of invasive aspergillosis [90–92]. The lungs typically manifest a necrotizing bronchopneumonia, ranging from small areas of infiltrate to intensive bilateral hemorrhagic infarction [93]. The most common presentation is that of **unremitting fever and a new pulmonary infiltrate despite broad-spectrum antibiotic therapy in an immunosuppressed patient.** Dyspnea and nonproductive cough are common. Sudden pleuritic pain and tachycardia, sometimes with a pleural rub, may mimic pulmonary embolism. **Hemoptysis is uncommon.** Roentgenograms may reveal patchy bronchopneumonia, nodular densities, consolidation, or cavitation. In immunocompromised patients, invasive pulmonary aspergillosis (IPA) generally is acute and evolves over days to weeks. Less commonly, patients with normal or only mild abnormalities of their immune systems may develop a more chronic, slowly progressive form of IPA [90].

b. **Extrapulmonary dissemination** is found at autopsy in approximately 10–25% of patients with invasive pulmonary aspergillosis [82, 93].

   (1) **Involvement of the CNS** may occur following either hematogenous dissemination or direct extension of invasive disease in the sinuses and usually results in infarction or abscess. The CSF may show a pleocytosis and increased protein content, but **cultures of CSF usually are negative.**

   (2) **Gastrointestinal** involvement has been noted in 10–20% of patients. The esophagus is the most frequently involved area, but ulcers may occur anywhere in the oropharynx, stomach, or intestine, and may cause bleeding or perforation.

   (3) **Necrotizing skin ulcers,** usually on the extremities, may occur secondary to hematogenous dissemination or after direct inoculation from an environmental source.

   (4) **Osteomyelitis** due to *Aspergillus* typically involves a rib or the vertebral column and is most common in the immunosuppressed patient.

   (5) **Myocarditis and pericarditis** have been reported on occasion. Less frequently, *Aspergillus* may involve the thyroid, diaphragm, liver, adrenal gland, spleen, peritoneum, or bladder.

c. **Rapidly invasive infections of the paranasal sinuses** may occur in immunocompromised hosts [82] and may extend into the orbit or cranial vault. *Aspergillus* may also be a cause of sinusitis in normal hosts.

2. **Diagnosis of invasive aspergillosis. Definitive diagnosis requires the demonstration of tissue invasion** as seen on a biopsy specimen (i.e., septate, acute branching hyphae) or a positive culture from tissue obtained by an invasive procedure such as transbronchial biopsy [94]. These patients often are severely ill, however, and invasive procedures may be associated with a high morbidity. **Noninvasive tests in the presence of an appropriate clinical syndrome may suggest the diagnosis.** For example, **pulmonary invasive disease is probable** in (1) patients with chest radiographs that show new nodules or new cavities in the context of neutropenia, (2) those receiving a cytotoxic agent for malignant or immunologic disease, (3) patients on a corticosteroid dosage of more than 10-mg prednisone or its equivalent daily, or (4) those with congenital or acquired immunodeficiency **and** two sputum cultures or one bronchoalveolar lavage (BAL) washing or brush culture for *Aspergillus* species or cytologic examination on BAL that reveals characteristic septate hyphae [94].

a. **Sputum and nasal cultures** are positive in a minority of patients with invasive aspergillosis, and the organisms can sometimes be isolated from these sites in the absence of invasive disease [82]. **In the high-risk patient, isolation of *Aspergillus* from sputum [94a], BAL fluid, or bronchial washings is strongly suggestive of invasive aspergillosis.**

b. **Serologic studies.** The standard *Aspergillus* precipitin assay, usually elevated in ABPA, rarely is elevated in patients with invasive disease and, in general, is **not helpful.** New techniques to detect circulating *Aspergillus* antigen are being developed but are as yet experimental.

c. **Blood cultures** usually are negative. *Aspergillus* fungemia can occur infrequently [94b].

d. **Lung biopsy usually is necessary for definitive diagnosis of IPA,** because parenchymal invasion of lung tissue must be demonstrated to confirm the diagnosis. Most investigators recommend open lung biopsy to ensure adequate tissue for histopathologic evaluation. The transbronchial biopsy approach has also been used. Unfortunately, lung biopsy cannot be performed safely in many patients at high risk for invasive aspergillosis. Therefore, **if the suspicion for IPA is very high, based on the clinical syndrome and positive sputum or nasal cultures, empiric antifungal therapy may be indicated.** Infectious disease consultation is advised.

   Nosocomial *Legionella* pulmonary infection also can occur in these patients and may, at times, be associated with cavity formation on CT or chest roentgenograms. Affected patients will not respond to the usual antibiotics used in febrile leukopenic patients (e.g., piperacillin and an aminoglycoside, imipenem or ceftazidime). Therefore, this diagnosis should be considered and excluded (see Chap. 9). Empiric therapy for *Legionella* may be prudent.

  e. **Biopsy and culture of extrapulmonary lesions** will provide the diagnosis in patients with invasive disease outside the lungs.

  f. **PCR** studies of BAL samples are undergoing clinical evaluation. This technique may merely help identify early colonization.

3. **Therapy.** Invasive aspergillosis is often a fulminating illness that results in death. With early therapy, many patients have survived [91, 92]. Prognosis is highly dependent on the course of the underlying disease.

  a. **Amphotericin B** usually **is** viewed as **the drug of choice.** Most clinicians prescribe high daily doses (0.8–1.0 mg/kg/day). Doses as high as 1.5 mg/kg/day have been given to patients who respond poorly. It is unclear whether combination therapy with flucytosine or rifampin offers any important advantage over amphotericin alone. The optimal duration of therapy has not been defined and should be individualized based on the severity of illness and the degree of immunosuppression.

  b. **Itraconazole.** In mid-1994, the U.S. Food and Drug Administration approved the use of itraconazole for the treatment of pulmonary and extrapulmonary aspergillosis in patients who are intolerant of or refractory to amphotericin B therapy.

    (1) **Primary therapy.** Treatment of invasive aspergillosis infections (with a loading dose of 600 mg/day for 4 days and then 200 mg bid) has been studied in an open trial of patients with various forms of invasive aspergillosis and yielded encouraging results, particularly in patients with IPA [94]. Some of these patients had received a few days of amphotericin B therapy before itraconazole was started. A controlled trial comparing itraconazole directly with amphotericin will be necessary to assess fully the role of itraconazole in the treatment of invasive disease.

    (2) While awaiting recommendations regarding the best therapy for invasive aspergillosis infections, we have tended to initiate therapy with intravenous amphotericin B in patients with severe illness and, if these patients can be stabilized and improve, after an initial course of intravenous amphotericin B and reduction of immunosuppression if appropriate, we sometimes switch to oral itraconazole therapy, which is usually continued until clinical and radiologic resolution.

    (3) Infectious disease consultation is advised for these difficult cases.

    (4) Itraconazole is discussed in more detail in sec. **III** under Antifungal Chemotherapy.

  c. **Reduction of corticosteroids or cytotoxic chemotherapy,** if possible, appears to improve prognosis.

  d. **Surgical resection** may be useful in selected patients with focal lesions.

4. **Prognosis** is improved with early diagnosis and aggressive therapy, remission of the underlying disease, and reversal of chemotherapy-induced bone marrow suppression. **Resolution of neutropenia is particularly important** if a favorable response to therapy is to be seen.

5. **Future chemotherapy if the patient survives.** Patients who have survived a prior episode of invasive aspergillosis are at risk for reactivation of invasive disease during subsequent myelosuppression with repeat courses of chemotherapy. Some studies suggest at least a 50% rate of reactivation during chemotherapy in patients who have recovered from prior invasive aspergillosis. **Many experts advise prophylactic amphotericin B (1 mg/kg/day), beginning at least 48 hours before chemotherapy** and continuing until the time of granulocyte recovery to prevent relapse of invasive disease in patients undergoing repeat chemotherapy [95]. The role of itraconazole in this setting is unknown.

E. **Rare manifestations of aspergillosis**

1. ***Aspergillus* endocarditis** mimics *Candida* endocarditis in that it occurs most commonly on prosthetic heart valves and is associated with large vegetations that embolize to medium-sized vessels [96]. **Diagnosis is difficult because blood cultures are rarely positive.** Early valve replacement is essential if cure is to be achieved.

2. **Allergic *Aspergillus* sinusitis** is a recently recognized form of sinusitis that occurs primarily in young, atopic persons [97]. Nasal polyps and mucoid mate-

rial containing eosinophils and fungal hyphae are found commonly. Optimal therapy requires corticosteroids and surgical debridement. Itraconazole might have some efficacy in the treatment of this disease, but there is no published experience with the drug as yet.

3. **Endophthalmitis** due to *Aspergillus* infection may occur 2–3 weeks after ophthalmic surgery or injury. Manifestations include cloudy vision, redness of the conjunctivae, and pain. Hypopyon may develop, with severe exudation into the anterior and posterior chambers.

Blastomycosis

Blastomyces dermatitidis is a dimorphous fungus that causes the acute and chronic illness blastomycosis. Infection with *B. dermatitidis* occurs via the lungs and may be followed by hematogenous dissemination. Pulmonary disease is most common, followed by disease of skin, bone, and genitourinary tract. **Widely disseminated disease is most common in immunocompromised hosts, especially those with AIDS** [98].

I. **Growth and identification characteristics.** *B. dermatitidis* grows as a mycelial form when specimens are incubated at 30°C, and colonies usually are evident in 1–2 weeks. Conversion to the yeast phase at 37°C is necessary for definitive diagnosis and usually occurs within another 10 days of culture. Microscopic examination of sputum, pus, or drainage from skin lesions is a rapid method for presumptive diagnosis of blastomycosis. When seen in a wet preparation or after digestion with KOH, the **characteristic yeast forms** are apparent as spherical cells with a diameter of 8–15 μm. They have a highly refractile thick cell wall, are multinucleate, and reproduce by a single broad-based bud. These same characteristics allow identification of the organism in histopathologic specimens with the use of special stains such as periodic acid–Schiff, Gomori's methenamine silver, Papanicolaou's, and Giemsa stains.

II. **Epidemiologic and host characteristics.** Infection caused by *B. dermatitidis* has been reported only occasionally outside of North America. Most patients reside in the southeastern and south central states, especially those bordering the Mississippi and Ohio River valleys, and the midwestern states and Canadian provinces that border the Great Lakes [99, 100]. Recent isolates from the environment indicate that *B. dermatitidis* **exists in nature in warm, moist soil that is rich in organic material,** usually decaying vegetation [101, 102]. When these microfoci are disturbed, either during work or recreational activities, the aerosolized spores (conidia) are inhaled into the lungs. Disease at other body sites is the result of dissemination from this initial pulmonary infection. Primary cutaneous disease, however, has been reported after dog bite and after accidental inoculation injury. A rare case of vaginal infection transmitted sexually from a man with genitourinary blastomycosis has been described [100].

B. dermatitidis is a primary pathogen that causes disease primarily in normal hosts. However, recent reports indicate that the organism can also act as an opportunistic pathogen, causing infection in patients with AIDS and other immunosuppressed patients [103, 104].

III. **Clinical manifestations.** Blastomycosis is a systemic disease with both pulmonary and extrapulmonary manifestations. Pulmonary disease may be acute or chronic. Extrapulmonary disease occurs most commonly during the chronic form of illness.

A. **Acute blastomycosis** often is unrecognized and is characterized by **pneumonitis** that occurs after a median incubation time of 30–45 days. Analysis of point source outbreaks indicate that only 50% or so of infected individuals become symptomatic [101, 102].

1. **Symptomatic patients** usually have an influenzalike syndrome with fever, chills, arthralgias, myalgias, cough, fatigue, and pleuritic chest pain. The symptoms may be mild or severe. Spontaneous resolution of disease is well recognized, and the duration of illness in these cases is generally less than 4 weeks [105].

2. **Chest roentgenograms** usually show lobar or segmental consolidation. Small pleural effusions are seen occasionally. Hilar adenopathy usually does not occur [106].

B. **Chronic blastomycosis** is indolent in onset and follows a widely variable course. Recent clinical experience indicates that extrapulmonary disease occurs in only approximately one-fourth of patients with blastomycosis [107]. Infection has been documented in almost every body organ, but skin, bone, and genitourinary sites of disease are most common [99, 100].

1. **Pulmonary manifestations.** Most patients have signs and symptoms of a **chronic pneumonia that mimics tuberculosis.** The most frequent symptoms are cough, sputum production, hemoptysis, pleuritic chest pain, and weight loss. Fever tends to be low-grade. The chest roentgenogram is nonspecific, with a wide variety of findings [106]. Lobar or segmental alveolar infiltrates, especially of the upper lobes, are most common. These infiltrates may progress to cavitation. Masslike infiltrates that mimic lung cancer occur nearly as often as alveolar infiltrates. Other radiologic findings include solitary cavities, lung nodules, and fibronodular infiltrates, with or without cavities. Pleural thickening and small pleural effusions occur, whereas large pleural effusions are uncommon. Miliary disease and diffuse pneumonitis, often associated with respiratory failure, are occasionally reported and are associated with a high mortality.

2. **Skin lesions are the most common form of extrapulmonary blastomycosis.** Skin disease usually occurs in conjunction with pulmonary disease but may occur alone. Skin lesions tend to occur on exposed parts of the body, notably the face and distal extremities. The characteristic lesion begins as a small papule or pustule that gradually enlarges over a period of weeks or months, becoming elevated, verrucous, and crusted. Outer borders are well demarcated and indurated. Older lesions commonly exhibit central healing and scarring at the same time that the outer border of the lesion is active and advancing. Removal of the crust reveals a granulomatous base with numerous small abscesses exuding purulent material. Less frequently, the lesion may begin as a small pustule that ulcerates. These ulcerative lesions bleed easily. Subcutaneous abscesses that sometimes drain spontaneously are seen in a minority of patients. **The organism easily is seen and is cultured from pus aspirated from these abscesses.**

3. **Bone infection** has been reported in 10–50% of patients. Lesions are osteolytic and often painless. The long bones, vertebrae, and ribs are most commonly involved. Some patients present with a contiguous soft-tissue abscess or draining sinus. Contiguous spread to joints may cause a pyarthrosis. **Diagnosis is made by biopsy** of the involved bone or aspiration of the contiguous soft-tissue abscess.

4. **Genitourinary disease** has been noted in 10–30% of patients. The prostate and epididymis are most commonly involved. The kidney usually is spared. Patients may note a painful swelling of the testis or epididymis, a perineal ache, or symptoms of urinary obstruction. The prostate may be tender and enlarged. Cultures of urine or prostatic secretions obtained after massage frequently are positive.

5. **CNS** disease is reported in fewer than 5% of cases. However, recent reports indicate that CNS complications of blastomycosis are more common in AIDS patients, being noted in 40% of patients with blastomycosis and AIDS in one series [103]. Abscesses are most common and present as mass lesions. Meningitis is usually a late complication and is frequently associated with multiorgan disease.

6. **Other sites** of disease are reported less frequently and include the lymph nodes, spleen, larynx, esophagus, thyroid, pituitary, and heart.

C. **Infections in the compromised host.** Blastomycosis in the immunocompromised host is more severe and more often disseminated and is associated with greater mortality than in immunocompetent patients [103, 104]. As noted in the preceding section, CNS infection is especially common in AIDS patients. Death rates of 30–40% are reported despite treatment with amphotericin B.

IV. **Diagnosis.** Definitive diagnosis is **established by culture.** A presumptive diagnosis can be made by visualizing the distinctive yeast forms in clinical specimens and is often sufficient to initiate antifungal therapy. Serologic studies must be interpreted with caution because of their high false positive and false negative rates.

A. **Culture.** Clinical specimens should be cultured on Sabouraud's or more enriched agar. Sputum, pus from soft-tissue abscesses, scrapings from skin lesions, and prostatic secretions may all be cultured successfully.

B. **Direct examination of clinical specimens**
   1. **Wet preparation.** Sputum, scrapings from skin lesions, pus, or pleural fluid

should be examined microscopically as a fresh wet preparation. The use of 10% KOH to digest cellular debris may facilitate seeing the organism. Occasionally, multiple specimens must be collected before the organism can be seen on smear. Bronchoscopy is helpful in patients who are unable to produce sputum.

    2. **Histopathology.** The typical inflammatory response is characterized by pyogranulomas. Yeast forms usually are not seen with hematoxylin and eosin stains but may be demonstrated with special stains, as noted earlier in sec. I.

C. Skin tests. No skin test reagent is currently available for the diagnosis of blastomycosis in patients with suspected disease.

D. Serologic tests for the diagnosis of blastomycosis are complicated by their **lack of sensitivity and specificity** [108]. Thus, negative tests should never be used to rule out disease. Neither should an isolated positive test prompt antifungal therapy. Rather, **a positive result should stimulate the clinician to search diligently for evidence of disease.**

    1. **Complement fixation** tests are neither sensitive nor specific. Fewer than 50% of patients with blastomycosis will develop a positive test, and cross-reactions with *H. capsulatum* and *C. immitis* are common.

    2. **Immunodiffusion tests.** The detection of precipitating antibodies is highly specific for blastomycosis, but sensitivity is variable. Positive results have been reported in up to 80% of patients with blastomycosis. However, lower rates of positivity (33%) have been reported in patients with localized disease [109]. Positive results are most frequently noted in patients with symptoms lasting 50 days or longer. Thus, immunodiffusion is **not helpful in acute disease.**

    3. **Radioimmunoassays and enzyme immunoassays** that are highly sensitive have been developed [109]. False positive results, however, are well documented. An enzyme immunoassay is now commercially available and may prove useful for initial screening of specimens. Positive results should be confirmed with the more specific immunodiffusion test.

    4. **Recent advances** in the characterization of the yeast antigens of *B. dermatitidis* may facilitate the development of more reliable serologic tests. A novel 120-kd surface protein, designated as *WI-1*, has been described by Klein and Jones [110]. Preliminary results using this antigen in a radioimmunoassay appear promising but, currently, this test is investigational.

V. Therapy. Although amphotericin B was previously considered the primary drug for treating all clinical forms of blastomycosis, recent studies have proven that either ketoconazole or itraconazole is an effective alternative for the treatment of immunocompetent patients with mild to moderate disease. Neither azole is indicated for patients with CNS disease.

A. Acute blastomycosis. Some patients may not require therapy. Because the acute form may be a benign, self-limited illness, it has been suggested that patients with acute blastomycosis be followed without specific chemotherapy but with prolonged observation [105]. However, illness progresses in some patients to chronic infection with significant morbidity. Because there are no known clinical characteristics that predict which patients are susceptible to chronic involvement, some authorities recommend that all patients with acute blastomycosis receive chemotherapy. **The indication for antifungal therapy in this group remains controversial,** and infectious disease consultation is advised.

B. Chronic blastomycosis

    1. **Ketoconazole.** Two clinical trials have documented cure rates of approximately 80% for patients treated with a daily dose of 400-mg ketoconazole [51, 111]. For patients who do not respond satisfactorily, the dose may be increased in 200-mg increments to a maximum of 800 mg/day. At least 6 months of treatment is recommended.

    2. **Itraconazole** is highly effective against *B. dermatitidis* both in vivo and in vitro. At doses of 200–400 mg/day, itraconazole was effective in 90–95% of patients with blastomycosis [48]. Because efficacy rates were similar at both doses, the initial recommended daily dose of itraconazole is 200 mg. For patients who fail this initial therapy, the dose may be increased in 100-mg increments to a maximum daily dose of 400 mg. Itraconazole generally has fewer side effects than ketoconazole and is the preferred agent for the treatment of blastomycosis at the authors' medical center.

    3. **Amphotericin B** is the **drug of choice for patients with life-threatening disease,** patients who are **immunocompromised, and** patients **with CNS disease.** A total dose of at least 1.5 g is recommended. For selected patients treated initially

with amphotericin B who are immunocompetent and who do not have CNS disease, an azole may be substituted for amphotericin B after clinical improvement is noted. Cure rates of greater than 90% are reported in immunocompetent patients who complete a full treatment course of amphotericin B, and relapse rates are less than 5%. Relapse is more frequently reported in immunocompromised patients, especially those with AIDS. Maintenance therapy with an oral azole has thus been advocated after successful primary therapy of blastomycosis in AIDS patients.

4. The potential role of **fluconazole** is still under investigation.

5. **Surgery** has a limited role in the treatment of blastomycosis.

6. **Prognosis.** Most patients ($\geq$ 90%) with chronic blastomycosis are cured with therapy. Mortality is greatest in patients with AIDS and those with respiratory failure or CNS disease.

Mucormycosis

Mucormycosis (or *zygomycosis*) is the term for infection caused by fungi of the order Mucorales [112]. A number of families of this order are associated with disease, but the Mucoraceae (which include the genera *Absidia, Mucor, Rhizomucor,* and *Rhizopus*) are the most common. **Mucoraceae may produce severe disease in susceptible individuals, notably patients with diabetes and leukemia.** Mixed infections with other fungi and with bacteria are common.

I. **Growth and identification characteristics.** The Mucorales are cultured on routine fungal media, and growth is abundant in 24–72 hours. A saline preparation will reveal broad (6–20 mm), nonseptate hyphae with right-angle branching. **The laboratory should be alerted when mucormycosis is a diagnostic possibility.** Occasionally, culture media are discarded because the Mucorales may be considered contaminants. Microscopic examination of smears and histopathologic evaluation of scrapings and biopsy material often reveal the diagnosis when cultures are negative. The organisms stain readily with periodic acid–Schiff, methenamine silver, and routine hematoxylin and eosin stains.

II. **Epidemiologic and host characteristics.** The **organisms that cause mucormycosis are ubiquitous** molds commonly found in the soil and on decaying organic debris, as well as on fruit or bread. They are infrequent contaminants in the laboratory. Occasionally, Mucorales species have been isolated from sputum or sinus specimens in the absence of invasive disease. There is **no evidence for person-to-person transmission. Certain conditions predispose** to tissue invasion by these normally saprophytic fungi, including **diabetes mellitus (especially with ketoacidosis), leukemia, lymphoma, corticosteroid therapy, severe malnutrition, organ transplantation, extensive burns, and uremia** [112, 113]. In recent years, several cases of mucormycosis have been reported in dialysis patients who were being treated with the chelating agent **deferoxamine** [114]. Individual predisposing factors are associated with specific patterns of invasive illness.

III. **Clinical aspects.** Mucormycosis is usually an acute, fulminant infection characterized pathologically by the **invasion of major blood vessels, with resultant ischemia and infarction of adjacent tissue.**

A. **Rhinocerebral mucormycosis** most commonly manifests in the setting of **poorly controlled diabetes, especially with ketoacidosis.** The causative organism in most cases is *Rhizopus arrhizus.* The organisms invade through the palate or the mucous membranes of the nose or paranasal sinuses. Subsequently, invasion through the ethmoids may occur, with direct extension into the orbital region and the frontal lobes of the brain. Progression of disease is usually rapid, although it may become indolent if ketoacidosis resolves.

1. **Clinical manifestations.** Local symptoms of sinusitis and palatal or orbital cellulitis may be present. **The nasal septum may be ulcerated, necrotic, or even perforated, and dark, bloody nasal discharge commonly results** [112]. The nasal turbinate bones often are black and necrotic. Soft periorbital or perinasal swelling may progress to induration and discoloration. **Neurologic sequelae** evolve after a few days and usually are rapidly progressive. Ptosis, proptosis, and dilatation or fixation of the pupil may occur. Drainage of **black pus** from the eyes sometimes is seen. Progressive neurologic deficits ensue,

with ophthalmoplegia, blindness, cranial nerve involvement and, finally, contralateral hemiplegia due to thrombosis of the internal carotid artery. Progressive lethargy develops despite control of the diabetes, and coma follows.

2. **Diagnosis** requires a **high degree of suspicion** to permit early and effective therapy.

   a. **A tissue biopsy or wet preparation** of the necrotic areas may demonstrate the characteristic nonseptate hyphae. This is the **best rapid diagnostic procedure** because positive cultures require 1–3 days or are often negative.

   b. **The CSF** usually shows nonspecific findings with a modest mononuclear pleocytosis and slight elevation of protein. CSF cultures typically are negative.

   c. **Radiologic examination** may demonstrate sinusitis or findings suggestive of osteomyelitis. CT scanning or MRI may be useful to demonstrate tissue or bone destruction, cerebritis, or retroorbital disease. Arteriograms may reveal filling defects, narrowing, occlusions, and infarction.

3. **Therapy. Because of the rapidity with which this disease progresses, prompt and aggressive therapy is essential** [113, 115]. Surgical and infectious disease consultations are advised.

   a. **Treatment directed toward reversing the underlying condition** (e.g., diabetic ketoacidosis) or decreasing immunosuppressive therapy is necessary but inadequate.

   b. **Amphotericin B is the only truly effective agent.** The dosage should be rapidly advanced to 1–1.5 mg/kg/day. If there is a favorable clinical response, an alternate-day regimen can be adopted. A total dosage of 2–3 g given over 2–3 months usually is required, depending on the clinical course and control of the underlying disease.

   c. **Surgical debridement.** Extensive surgical extirpation or debridement of devitalized tissue and adequate drainage of sinuses and abscesses are essential elements in controlling infection.

4. **Prognosis.** With aggressive combined chemotherapy and surgery, the mortality is approximately 50%. Survivors often have significant neurologic deficits. Rapid diagnosis and treatment may improve prognosis.

B. **Pulmonary mucormycosis** may occur following inhalation of fungal spores or from hematogenous or lymphatic spread during dissemination. Most patients have leukemia, lymphoma, or severe neutropenia, and most have received glucocorticoid therapy [112].

1. **Manifestations.** The most common picture is one of fever with **pulmonary infiltration or cavitation that progresses despite antibiotic therapy.** Occasionally, subacute cases occur in diabetics, with progression over weeks to months [116].

2. **Diagnosis.** The diagnosis of pulmonary mucormycosis requires **histopathologic evidence of pulmonary invasion.** Cultures of respiratory secretions are usually negative. The chest roentgenogram is nonspecific.

3. **Therapy.** Most patients in whom pulmonary mucormycosis is diagnosed have had advanced disease with extensive tissue destruction, and results of treatment have been disappointing. Early diagnosis, reversal of the underlying disease, and high-dose amphotericin B may improve the prognosis. Surgical resection of pulmonary lesions may be beneficial in selected patients.

C. **Gastrointestinal mucormycosis** has been diagnosed primarily in patients with **severe malnutrition** [112]. Any part of the GI tract may be involved, but the stomach and large bowel are the most common sites of infection. Abdominal pain and bloody diarrhea are typical, and signs of peritonitis may ensue if the intestinal wall is perforated. The disease is usually acute and rapidly fatal. **Diagnosis requires biopsy of involved tissue.** A combination of surgical resection and antifungal chemotherapy with amphotericin B is indicated as treatment.

D. **Cutaneous mucormycosis.** Involvement of the skin with the Mucorales may be primary (following direct inoculation of organisms during minor trauma) or secondary (following dissemination from another site). Cutaneous disease has been associated with the use of elastic bandages [117]. Extensive involvement of burn wounds may result in disseminated disease. **Diagnosis depends on** the demonstration of **tissue invasion in biopsy specimens.** For patients with primary, localized cutaneous disease, surgical debridement may be adequate for cure. However, in patients with evidence of disease distant to the cutaneous site of infection or invasion of hyphal forms into the subcutaneous tissue, systemic therapy with amphotericin B is required.

E. **Disseminated mucormycosis** usually occurs in debilitated patients with hematologic malignancies [118]. Dissemination is most often from the lungs or GI tract and may involve any part of the body, including the CNS. Multiple areas of infarction and abscess formation are common. Cutaneous lesions that resemble ecthyma gangrenosum have been described. The clinical course is acute and rapidly progressive. A high index of suspicion and biopsy of involved tissue are required to make the diagnosis. Intensive therapy with amphotericin B is indicated, but the outcome is generally poor.

F. **Other manifestations** of mucormycosis that have occurred rarely include endocarditis and focal encephalitis or cerebral abscesses (without dissemination) from head trauma, craniotomy, or intravenous narcotic abuse [113].

Sporotrichosis

Sporothrix schenckii is a saprophytic fungus found widely in nature. Infection due to *S. schenckii* generally is limited to the skin and regional lymphatics, although systemic and disseminated disease occasionally occur.

I. **Growth and identification characteristics.** *S. schenckii* is a dimorphous fungus. The mycelial phase can be grown and identified on routine culture media in 3–5 days. Conversion to the yeast phase is desirable for definitive diagnosis. Histopathologic identification requires multiple sectioning and is very difficult. **Isolation of *S. schenckii* in the laboratory usually indicates infection,** as it is not a normal commensal of humans.

II. **Epidemiologic features.** *S. schenckii* is found worldwide. In the United States, the majority of cases have been found in the midwestern river valleys, especially those of the Missouri and Mississippi rivers [119]. This fungus is common in Mexico and Central America. The organism is found in the soil and on rose and barberry bushes, sphagnum moss, tree bark, and other vegetation. **Infection usually occurs following inoculation injury after contact with thorny plants.**

III. **Clinical aspects.** Sporotrichosis can be divided into cutaneous and extracutaneous infection.

A. **Cutaneous disease** accounts for 75–80% of cases of sporotrichosis [119]. Transmission to humans typically occurs through a break in the skin, often after minor or unrecognized injuries. Cutaneous sporotrichosis is therefore an **occupational disease** of gardeners, farmers, horticulturists, nursery workers, and florists.

1. **Manifestations.** The fungus usually gains entry in the fingers or hands, where a **small papule or raised, erythematous, subcutaneous nodule develops.** The lesion may be evident at any time from 1 week to 6 months after inoculation. Spread to regional lymphatics results in **progression of secondary nodules** up the arm, which often ulcerate and drain but do not produce significant pain or disability. Localized cutaneous infection without lymphatic spread is less common; these lesions may be nodular, crusted, weeping, or fungating, and may occur anywhere at a site of trauma. Lesions may wax and wane for months or years. Hematogenous dissemination of cutaneous infection is extremely uncommon.

2. **Diagnosis.** Although the clinical appearance may be very suggestive of sporotrichosis, other infectious entities may cause identical lesions, including nontuberculous *Mycobacteria*, cutaneous nocardiosis, syphilis, pyoderma gangrenosum, and leishmaniasis [119]. **Culture of drainage or aspirated material** should reveal the causative organism and **is diagnostic.** Histopathologic examination of punch biopsy specimens reveals granulomatous lesions with fungal cells confined to the dermis. The fungal cells may be surrounded by an aggregation of material that stains with periodic acid–Schiff, the so-called asteroid body. Serologic tests for antibodies may be positive [120] but contribute little to culture or biopsy results in the setting of cutaneous disease.

3. **Therapy**

a. **Oral potassium iodide** is an effective, inexpensive treatment for cutaneous and lymphatic sporotrichosis and has been the standard regimen for years. Its antifungal effect is not well understood, and it has no direct effect on *S. schenckii* [119]. However, it is associated with frequent allergic reactions and gastrointestinal intolerance.

(1) **Mode of administration.** Saturated potassium iodide solution is given orally in doses of 3–4 ml (maximum) q8h, beginning with 1 ml per dose and gradually increasing the dose while monitoring for toxicity. Some advise putting the drug in root beer to disguise the taste. Treatment is continued until 1 month after the skin lesions disappear.

(2) **Toxicity.** Nausea, vomiting, parotid swelling, iodism (acne) or other skin lesions, coryza, sneezing, eyelid swelling, and depression generally respond to discontinuing the drug for a few days and restarting it at a lower dosage. A brassy or otherwise unpleasant taste in the mouth may be the first symptom of toxicity.

(3) Application of local heat to the lesions may also be helpful.

b. **Itraconazole.** Recent studies have shown that treatment with **itraconazole** results in response rates of greater than 90% [121, 122]. Itraconazole is well tolerated and is thus a reasonable alternative to potassium iodide. Because itraconazole appears to be equally effective and better tolerated than potassium iodide, it should eventually replace iodides for the treatment of sporotrichosis. **This agent is discussed in detail** in sec. III.D under Antifungal Chemotherapy.

B. **Extracutaneous disease** represents approximately 20% of cases of sporotrichosis. Therapy with potassium iodide is ineffective in all forms of extracutaneous disease. Treatment with itraconazole or amphotericin B is required.

1. **Pulmonary sporotrichosis is uncommon.** It may be a primary infection following inhalation of *S. schenckii* spores or may occur secondary to dissemination [123]. Many patients have a history of chronic obstructive pulmonary disease, diabetes, alcohol abuse, or some other chronic medical condition. Symptoms include the insidious onset of cough, sputum production, malaise, weight loss, and fever. **Chest roentgenograms** generally reveal parenchymal infiltration progressing to cavitation, and hilar adenopathy may be marked. Infection is usually indolent but progressive. **Diagnosis depends on isolation of the fungus from sputum, bronchial washings, or lung tissue.** Cure rates of more than 70% have been achieved with amphotericin B in combination with surgical resection, but many patients cannot tolerate this regimen [119]. Itraconazole has been used in a few cases with some success [122, 124].

2. **Osteoarticular sporotrichosis** is an extremely indolent infection that primarily involves the joints and bones. Involvement of a single joint, particularly the knee, is typical [125]. Cutaneous disease usually is absent. Most patients have pain, effusion, and decreased mobility of the affected joint. Cultures of joint fluid are frequently negative, and synovial biopsy may be required for diagnosis. **Amphotericin B** has been the treatment of choice for many years, but prolonged treatment is needed and relapse is common. In a recent study, therapy with **itraconazole** yielded results comparable to those seen with amphotericin and was less toxic [122].

3. **Disseminated sporotrichosis is rare.** Involvement of multiple sites including the skin, lungs, joints, bones, and CNS has been reported [119, 126]. The illness occurs more frequently in the setting of lymphoreticular disease, alcoholism, or chronic corticosteroid therapy. Disseminated disease has also been diagnosed in patients with AIDS [127]. Clinical manifestations depend primarily on the organ systems involved. **Skin lesions**, often ulcerative, are found in most patients. Lymphatic spread generally is not seen due to hematogenous dissemination. **Multifocal joint involvement** is common, in contrast to the normally unifocal osteoarticular disease. Nodular pulmonary lesions are present in 10–20% of patients. **Meningitis** is a rare manifestation of infection with *S. schenckii* and usually presents as a chronic, indolent process.

a. The **diagnosis** may be suspected on the basis of the characteristic skin and joint lesions. **Culture of the fungus** from an infected lesion generally is not difficult, although multiple cultures occasionally are required. Recovery of the organism from blood cultures has been reported. Repeated culture of the CSF often is necessary to isolate the organism in patients with meningitis, and serologic tests of serum and CSF may be useful [128].

b. **Amphotericin B** is the preferred therapeutic agent for disseminated sporotrichosis, including meningitis, with total doses of more than 2 g needed for cure. Itraconazole has been used in only a few patients [124], and firm recommendations regarding its use cannot be given as yet. Infectious disease consultation is advised in these unusual cases.

Miscellaneous Fungal Infections

I. **Paracoccidioidomycosis** is a systemic infection caused by the dimorphous fungus *Paracoccidioides brasiliensis* [129]. The **disease is endemic in Latin America, particularly Brazil,** and is diagnosed only rarely in North America. Pulmonary infection is the most common manifestation, but involvement of the mucous membranes, skin, and lymph nodes following dissemination occurs frequently. **Itraconazole** is the drug of choice for treatment.

II. **Mycetoma** (Madura foot) is a localized, noncontagious infection involving cutaneous tissue, fascia, and bone [130]. The disease is reported most frequently in patients who live in tropical or temperate zones. Mycetoma may be caused by either aerobic actinomycetes or various species of fungi and generally occurs following the traumatic implantation of the organisms into the subcutaneous tissue of a healthy host. Most cases involve the foot or hand and progress very slowly over months to years. Combined surgical-medical treatment is the best therapeutic approach for mycetoma caused by fungi.

III. **Dematiaceous fungi** are a group of darkly pigmented organisms that cause infections termed *phaeohyphomycoses.* These infections occur most frequently in immunocompromised hosts and manifest clinically as subcutaneous, sinus, or cerebral infection [131]. Surgical resection of localized lesions is crucial for diagnosis and treatment, but the prognosis is usually poor.

IV. **Emerging opportunistic fungal infections.** Many fungal species that formerly were considered nonpathogenic or only rarely were associated with invasive disease are now causing increasingly common infections in immunosuppressed hosts. *Trichosporon* and *Malassezia* species are common causes of superficial dermatologic infections but may cause disseminated disease in immunocompromised or debilitated patients [132, 133]. *Fusarium* species cause disseminated infection primarily in patients with hematologic malignancies or severe burns [134]. *Pseudoallescheria boydii* is an agent of mycetoma and may cause more deep-seated infections such as pneumonia or disseminated disease in the immunocompromised host [135]. *Penicillium marneffei* is a dimorphous fungus endemic in Southeast Asia that causes disseminated infection with papular skin lesions in AIDS patients [136]. There is no standard treatment for most of these infections, although infections with *P. marneffei* generally respond to treatment with amphotericin or itraconazole.

Antifungal Chemotherapy

The decision regarding whether to initiate systemic antifungal chemotherapy must be based in part on consideration of the toxicity of these drugs (Table 18-2). **Infectious disease consultation is recommended** to help determine the indications for therapy and to assist in administration of the drugs. The following general guidelines provide an introduction to systemic antifungal chemotherapy.

I. **Amphotericin B (Fungizone)** remains the most reliable agent against most of the fungal pathogens that cause invasive infections [137–138].

A. **Mode of action.** Amphotericin binds to ergosterol, the primary sterol in the membrane of susceptible fungi, which results in the opening of pores in the membrane and leakage of cellular constituents and, ultimately, cell death [139].

B. **The pharmacokinetics** of amphotericin B **are poorly understood.** Amphotericin B is poorly absorbed from the GI tract, and systemic infections must be treated by intravenous administration of the agent. No metabolism of the drug has been identified, and elimination occurs slowly via the biliary tract.

C. **Distribution.** The highest concentrations of amphotericin B are achieved in the liver, spleen, lung, and kidneys [140]. Distribution into spinal fluid, parotid gland fluid, aqueous humor, urine, and hemodialysis solutions is poor. **Outcome of treatment does not appear to be correlated with drug levels in plasma.**

D. **Dosage and administration. The method of calculating the dose of amphotericin B remains a somewhat controversial issue.** Many experts maintain that total duration is the determinant of effective therapy and advocate, for example, low doses daily for 6–12 weeks. Other experts advocate administration of high daily doses, if tolerated, until a specific total dose is achieved. **There is no consensus**

Table 18-2. Principal adverse effects of antifungal agents

Amphotericin B	Flucytosine	Ketoconazole	Fluconazole	Itraconazole
Fever, chills, nausea, vomiting Nephrotoxicity Thrombophlebitis at site of intravenous administration Anemia Electrolyte imbalance (K^+, Mg^{2+}) Pulmonary deterioration (rare)	Suppression of bone marrow Nausea, vomiting Diarrhea Increased hepatic enzymes Rash	Gastrointestinal distress Rash, pruritus Transiently increased hepatic enzymes Severe hepatotoxicity (rare) Alopecia Decreased synthesis of testosterone leading to diminished libido, impotence, gynecomastia Menstrual irregularities Decreased synthesis of cortisol Possible syndrome of mineralocorticoid excess	Gastrointestinal distress (less than with ketoconazole) Rash Headache Transiently increased hepatic enzymes Severe hepatotoxicity (?)	Gastrointestinal distress (less than with ketoconazole) Pruritus Headache Dizziness Transiently increased hepatic enzymes Impotence (?) Possible syndrome of mineralocorticoid excess

Source: From C. L. Terrell and C. E. Hughes, Antifungal agents used for deep-seated mycotic infections. *Mayo Clin. Proc.* 67:69, 1992.

as to the optimal regimen, total dose, or total duration of therapy. General guidelines are available, however, and a total dose of 1–4 g depends on the clinical response, site of infection, identity of the fungus, and the patient's tolerance of the drug [137].

1. **Some authorities suggest an initial test dose** of 1 mg IV over 30 minutes to 1 hour because occasional patients have an idiosyncratic reaction of severe hypotension or an anaphylaxislike reaction. The necessity of this test dose has been questioned [137a] because it may delay therapeutic doses.

2. **Several dosage regimens** are available [137, 138]. The dose may be gradually increased daily (by increments of 5–10 mg/day), or full-dose intravenous administration (e.g., 0.5 mg/kg/day) may begin immediately after a test dose, and **we prefer this latter approach.** The dose may be increased to as much as 0.7–1.0 mg/kg/day, although some prefer to administer a maximum daily dose of 50 mg.

3. **The daily dose has typically been infused over 4–6 hours;** we prefer 4-hour infusion. Some authors believe that a more rapid infusion of 1–2 hours actually may decrease the incidence or intensity of the side effects (e.g., fever, chills, nausea, and vomiting). Preliminary studies suggest that more rapid infusions in patients with normal renal function are as well tolerated as are the more conventional 6-hour infusion rates [141]. Amphotericin B does bind, to some degree, to the cholesterol of mammalian cells, and this may cause the release of intracellular potassium, which can potentially result in severe hyperkalemia, especially in patients with renal failure. Therefore **rapid infusion rates should not be used in patients with renal insufficiency** [142]. In addition, arrhythmias have been reported during amphotericin B administration, and rapid infusion rates should thus not be used in patients with cardiovascular disease [142]. In general, **we favor a 4-hour infusion for most patients.**

4. **Alternate-day or thrice-weekly regimens** often are employed to minimize side effects. Thrice-weekly therapy also facilitates outpatient or home administration. The usual maximum individual dose in these regimens is 50–80 mg.

5. If serum creatinine exceeds 2.5–3.0 mg/dl or BUN exceeds 40 mg/ml, many experts suggest lowering the dose, discontinuing the drug until renal function improves, or switching to alternate-day therapy if the patient is currently on a daily regimen. However, diminishing renal function does not affect the rate of elimination. Although amphotericin B is nephrotoxic, it does not accumulate in renal failure. Dosage adjustments are made to minimize toxicity, but hemodialysis patients usually receive full doses [143].

6. **Intrathecal** or intraventricular amphotericin B may be indicated for coccidioidal meningitis and in some refractory cases of cryptococcal meningitis [77, 144]. Administration is technically complicated, and neurosurgical and infectious disease consultations are suggested.

7. **New formulations** in liposomes, lipid complexes, and colloidal dispersion are being developed [137]. See sec. **J.**

E. **Toxicity**

1. **Fever and rigors** during infusion are common in the first week of therapy and usually diminish thereafter. Recent studies indicate that fever and chills may be the result of amphotericin B–induced release of interleukin 1 (IL-1) and tumor necrosis factor (TNF) from mononuclear cells [137a, 145], which leads to a secondary release of prostaglandin E2. Because they alter the hypothalamic setpoint of the brain, prostaglandins have been implicated as a cause of fever and rigors [137a]. **Some physicians premedicate patients with** a standard dose of acetaminophen (e.g., 650 mg PO for adults), diphenhydramine hydrochloride (Benadryl) (e.g., 25–50 mg IV/PO for adults), and meperidine (e.g., 25–50 mg IV in adults) approximately 30 minutes before the infusion of amphotericin B. Because about 25% of patients receiving amphotericin B with pretreatment do not have any adverse reaction, the authors of a recently published, nationwide prospective surveillance program do not advocate routine pretreatment regimens; but if adverse reactions occur, use of pretreatment regimens in subsequent infusions of amphotericin B is advised [137a]. If the patient has additional chills during the infusion, the dose of meperidine may be repeated at 3-hour intervals. This premedication routine appears to decrease the incidence of fever and rigors in many patients. **Ibuprofen** (a single dose of 10 mg/kg up to a maximum dose of 600 mg) **has also been useful as premedication** [146]. Because protracted use of this agent may be associated with nephrotoxicity,

ibuprofen may be helpful for the initial 1–2 weeks of therapy while tolerance is developing. Simultaneous administration of hydrocortisone, 25–50 mg IV, may be effective when fever is particularly troublesome, but we seldom use it. Corticosteroid alone for pretreatment is not advised [137a].

2. **Anorexia, nausea, and vomiting** are common but usually diminish as therapy progresses. Pretreatment with antiemetics may be helpful.

3. **Nephrotoxicity is the major limiting factor** in amphotericin administration [147]. Early toxicity is dose-dependent, whereas later toxicity is related to the total dose. There is great individual variation in tolerance: Renal function returns to nearly normal levels in most patients several months after therapy is stopped, but irreversible renal failure may result. Renal function should be monitored at least every other day during the early stages of therapy. In the stable patient who is receiving intravenous amphotericin B at home or in an outpatient setting, serum creatinine (and potassium levels) should be monitored at least 2–3 times per week. Other renal abnormalities such as cylindruria and mild renal tubular acidosis are not used as guides to dosage but may be harbingers of renal dysfunction.

   The incidence of renal failure may be reduced if a saline infusion is given prior to each dose or if a high salt intake is maintained [148]. In patients who can tolerate the sodium load, we will often give 500 ml–1 liter of normal saline over 1–2 hours before infusing amphotericin B.

4. **Anemia** develops in more than 75% of patients, secondary to the inhibition of erythropoietin production and also by direct bone marrow suppression [149]. Transfusion therapy may be of temporary benefit but usually is not warranted. Leukopenia and thrombocytopenia are rare.

5. **Hypokalemia** from a renal tubular defect develops in 25% of patients and often requires potassium supplementation. Therefore, **serum potassium levels should be monitored serially. Hypomagnesemia** may also occur.

6. **Phlebitis** resulting from intravenous administration is common. Limiting the concentration of amphotericin to no more than 0.1 mg/ml reduces the incidence of phlebitis. The simultaneous infusion of heparin may also help to ameliorate phlebitis [147].

7. **Serious pulmonary reactions** with acute dyspnea, hypoxemia, and interstitial infiltrates on chest films have been described in patients receiving combined amphotericin B and leukocyte transfusions [150]. Therefore, it is advised that the interval between the infusion of amphotericin B and the leukocyte infusion be as long as possible.

8. **A preprinted order sheet,** including the saline load and premedications described in sec. **1, and preprinted flow sheet** are used by some institutions to monitor the daily and cumulative doses of amphotericin B, serum creatinine, and other therapies.

F. **Pregnancy.** Amphotericin B has been used during pregnancy for the treatment of systemic fungal infections, without any adverse effects on fetal development.

G. **Combination chemotherapy.** Synergistic therapy with flucytosine sometimes is used, especially for cryptococcal infection in non-AIDS patients [63, 64]. Preliminary studies reporting the enhanced efficacy of amphotericin B in combination with other agents, particularly rifampin, are encouraging but have been studied in animal models of infection.

   The combination of fluconazole and amphotericin B is at times antagonistic against *C. albicans* in vitro but not in vivo in the animal model [150a]. However the role of this combination awaits further clinical study.

H. **Empiric amphotericin B therapy in the persistently febrile granulocytopenic patient.** Despite careful serial physical and laboratory examinations (including multiple cultures), no obvious bacterial infection is identified in many febrile neutropenic patients, and fever persists despite broad-spectrum antibiotic therapy. Because the early diagnosis of disseminated fungal infection (e.g., candidemia) is very difficult, the empiric addition of a systemic antifungal agent is a consideration. Typically, if fever persists beyond 5–7 days despite negative blood cultures and broad-spectrum antibiotic therapy, empiric amphotericin B (commonly 0.5 mg/kg/day) often is started and continued until the leukopenia resolves [151]. Empiric amphotericin B sometimes is initiated even more rapidly (within hours) in the hospitalized leukopenic patient who has been stable for several days on broad-spectrum antibiotics and then becomes febrile and acutely ill. In addition to reculturing and broadening antibiotic therapy if indicated, empiric amphotericin B may be added for a possible disseminated fungal infection. The role of fluconazole as a substitute for amphotericin B in such patients is currently being investigated. See discussion under Candidiasis, sec. **III.D.4.b** (p. 665). **Infectious disease consultation is advisable in this setting.** This topic is discussed further in Chap. 2.

I. **Cost.** See Table 18-3.

J. **New formulations under investigation.** With conventional amphotericin B, fungicidal titers are seldom achieved in tissues, and dosages are often limited by adverse effects. Targeted drug delivery systems, such as liposomes, make it possible to give more amphotericin B and to attain a much higher drug concentration in some organs, without any increase in systemic toxic effects [151a]. Liposomal amphotericin B (AmBisome) is undergoing clinical investigation, and the experience of compassionate use of this agent in the United Kingdom was recently reported [151a]. **Amphotericin B lipid complex (Abelcet),** formerly called ABLC, was approved in November 1995 for treatment of patients with invasive aspergillosis who are refractory to or intolerant of conventional amphotericin B therapy. ABLC also has been studied in other fungal infections [151b]. Infectious disease consultation is advised to clarify the potential role and/or availability of these new agents.

II. **Flucytosine (5-fluorocytosine, Ancobon,** 5-FC) is an effective antifungal drug but, because drug resistance develops, it rarely is used alone. It is active against *C. neoformans, Candida* species, and *Torulopsis* species in particular.

A. **Mode of action.** Flucytosine is converted within susceptible fungal cells to 5-fluorouracil and 5-fluor-2-deoxyuredylic acid, which inhibit the function of RNA and DNA, respectively, and result in subsequent cell death [152].

B. **Distribution** is excellent into all body-water spaces, **particularly the CSF, where 60–80% of the serum drug level is achieved.**

C. **Elimination.** Approximately 90% of the drug is excreted unchanged in the urine, and so **reduced renal function will lead to accumulation of the drug.** In contrast, reduced hepatic function does not alter drug excretion. Protein binding is negligible, and flucytosine is removed by hemodialysis and peritoneal dialysis.

D. **Mode of administration and dosage.** This oral agent is well absorbed (> 90%) from the GI tract. Only oral capsules (250 mg and 500 mg) are available.

1. Patients with normal renal function usually receive 12.5–37.5 mg/kg PO q6h (i.e., 50–150 mg/kg/day).

2. **Dosage is reduced in the presence of renal impairment. The dose should be regulated by monitoring serum levels,** which should be maintained at less than 100 µg/ml (preferably 40–60 µg/ml) [152]. Stamm et al. [153] have published a nomogram to guide therapy. Also see dose reductions in Table 18-4.

E. **Toxicity** is noted most often in patients with blood concentrations exceeding 100 µg/ml [152, 153] (see Table 18-2).

1. **Hepatic abnormalities** are seen in approximately 5–7% of patients and are generally asymptomatic and reversible. Fatal hepatic necrosis has been reported, and so weekly liver function panels are suggested.

2. **Leukopenia and thrombocytopenia are potentially lethal complications** [153] and occur more commonly in those with previously damaged marrows. In initial reports, many **AIDS patients** who receive flucytosine along with amphotericin B

Table 18-3. Comparative cost of common antifungal agents

Agent	Route	Typical daily dose	Approximate daily cost[a]
Amphotericin B	IV	50 mg	$30.88
Flucytosine	PO	125 mg/kg/day[b]	31.50[b]
Ketoconazole	PO	200 mg	2.70
Fluconazole	PO	100 mg	6.45
	IV	100 mg	40.62
Itraconazole	PO	200 mg	10.79

[a]Actual wholesale price from *American Druggist Blue Book* 1995.
[b]For example, for a 64-kg adult with normal renal function, if 125 mg/kg/day were given, a total daily dose of 8,000 mg would be given per day or 2,000 mg q6h (four 500-mg capsules q6h).
Source: *American Druggist Blue Book.* New York: Hearst, 1995.

Table 18-4. Recommended dosages of flucytosine in patients with renal insufficiency

Creatinine clearance (ml/min)	Dosage (mg/kg)	Interval (hr)	Total daily dose (mg/kg)
>50	37.5	6	150
26–50	37.5	12	75
13–25	37.5	24	37.5
<13	*	*	*
Hemodialysis	37.5	After each hemodialysis	—

*Avoid or adjust use to maintain peak serum level between 50 and 100 μg/ml.
Source: C. L. Terrell and C. E. Hughes, Antifungal agents used for deep-seated mycotic infections. *Mayo Clin. Proc.* 67:69, 1992. See text discussion.

for the treatment of cryptococcal meningitis were reported to develop significant bone marrow suppression. Therefore, flucytosine use was advised with caution in AIDS patients; amphotericin B is often used alone in the treatment of HIV-related cryptococcal meningitis [61]. Additional clinical studies have determined that together flucytosine and amphotericin B in therapy of cryptococcal meningitis in AIDS patients does not significantly improve results compared to amphotericin B alone [66] (see sec. **IV.A.3** under Cryptococcosis, p. 674).

3. **Gastrointestinal intolerance** usually is limited to mild diarrhea but, in severe cases, patients have had copious diarrhea, anorexia, nausea, vomiting, and abdominal pain.

4. **Teratogenic effects.** Flucytosine has been shown to be teratogenic in animals and, therefore, should be avoided during pregnancy unless the potential benefit is greater than the potential risk to the fetus.

5. **Nursing mothers.** It is not known whether flucytosine is excreted in breast milk. Mothers should be advised to discontinue nursing if flucytosine is administered.

F. **Combination chemotherapy.** Although many initial isolates of *Candida* and most initial isolates of *Cryptococcus* and *Torulopsis* are sensitive to flucytosine, **the rapid emergence of secondary drug resistance precludes the use of the drug as a single agent in serious infections.** The combination of flucytosine with amphotericin B has demonstrated an additive or synergistic effect, both in vitro and in vivo, against *Candida* and *Cryptococcus*. The additive effects may not only offer increased efficacy but may also allow amphotericin B to be given in lower doses, thus decreasing the toxicity of this agent. **Unfortunately, amphotericin B may increase the toxicity of flucytosine by impairing its renal excretion. Therefore, serum concentrations of flucytosine should ideally be monitored in patients who are taking this combination,** and the dosage should be lowered or the drug stopped if flucytosine accumulates. The combination of flucytosine and amphotericin B frequently is recommended for cryptococcal meningitis in the non-AIDS patient [63, 64] and, occasionally, for systemic candidiasis.

G. **Cost.** See Table 18-3.

III. **Azoles.** The azoles have proven to be safe and effective alternatives to amphotericin B for the treatment of many of the systemic mycoses [154]. In addition, they have also proven useful in the management of superficial mycoses that are recalcitrant to topical therapy. The azoles are synthetic and are chemically classified by the number of nitrogen atoms in their five-membered azole rings as either imidazoles (miconazole and ketoconazole) or triazoles (itraconazole or fluconazole). **All the azoles exert their fungistatic activity by the same mechanism:** inhibition of the biosynthesis of ergosterol, the main sterol in the fungal cell membrane, via interference with the cytochrome P450–dependent fungal enzyme C-14 lanosterol demethylase [154]. This results in altered membrane permeability with inhibition of cell growth and replication. **Unfortunately, the azoles may also interact with mammalian enzymes that are dependent on the cytochrome P450 system, and this interaction mediates some of their major toxicities and drug interactions.** The triazoles, as compared to the imidazoles, have much greater affinity for fungal rather than mammalian cytochrome P450 enzymes and, in general, have less toxicity and fewer drug interactions.

A. **Miconazole (Monistat)** is an imidazole that is available as either an intravenous or a topical preparation. See Chap. 13 for its topical uses. Its **usage as a systemic antifungal agent has been supplanted by the availability of more effective and less toxic systemic azoles.**

B. **Ketoconazole (Nizoral),** an oral imidazole, was the first azole to prove clinically useful as a systemic antifungal drug.
   1. **Antifungal activity.** Ketoconazole is active against clinical isolates of *Candida, C. immitis, H. capsulatum, B. dermatitidis,* and *Paracoccidioides brasiliensis.*
   2. **Pharmacokinetics.** Only an **oral** preparation is available. Ketoconazole is well absorbed if there is enough gastric acidity to solubilize the tablet. The administration of antacids or H_2-blocking agents reduces absorption. Other situations that reduce gastric acid secretion (and that may reduce absorption) include aging, gastric surgery, and AIDS gastropathy. **Because of the uncertainty of absorption in these settings, many clinicians may prefer to use fluconazole** when appropriate. Sucralfate does not affect absorption.
      The drug is extensively degraded in vivo, and very little active drug is excreted by either the renal or biliary pathway. Therefore, **the dose does not have to be changed in renal failure.** Whether dosage should be adjusted in hepatic failure is unclear. Isoniazid, phenytoin, and rifampin increase the metabolism of ketoconazole, and concurrent use of these drugs may result in treatment failure. Ketoconazole does not penetrate well into the CSF.
   3. **Clinical uses** [155, 156]
      a. **Chronic mucocutaneous candidiasis.** Ketoconazole has been very effective in treating this uncommon disease [156]. Chronic maintenance therapy over many years has been effective and well tolerated.
      b. **Dermatophyte infections.** Ketoconazole is indicated for the treatment of severe or recalcitrant cutaneous dermatophyte infections that have not responded to topical therapy or oral griseofulvin, or for patients who are unable to take griseofulvin. It has also been used with success in onychomycosis due to *Trichophyton* species, *Microsporum* species, and *Epidermophyton floccosum.*
      c. **Oral thrush and candidal esophagitis.** These conditions in AIDS patients and others often respond well to ketoconazole. Treatment failure may result from the concomitant use of antacids or H_2-receptor antagonists, because an acid gastric pH is necessary for adequate absorption. Patients with AIDS frequently have gastric hypochlorhydria, which impairs ketoconazole absorption and may result in clinical failure. (Fluconazole is another effective agent.)
      d. **Systemic fungal infections.** Ketoconazole may be used for the treatment of a variety of systemic fungal infections in immunocompetent patients who do not have life-threatening or CNS disease. These include **histoplasmosis, blastomycosis, coccidioidomycosis,** and **paracoccidioidomycosis.** Infectious disease consultation is recommended.
      e. **Miscellaneous**
         (1) **Vaginal candidiasis.** The therapy of vaginal candidiasis is discussed elsewhere (see Chap. 13). Ketoconazole is not indicated in the routine management of this problem.
         (2) **Prophylaxis of fungal infections in neutropenic patients with ketoconazole is not advised.**
         (3) *Candida balanitis* often responds well to a 7- to 10-day course of ketoconazole.
   4. **Dosage.** Ketoconazole is available in a scored 200-mg tablet.
      a. **Adults.** The usual starting dose for superficial candidal or dermatophyte infections is 200 mg/day. Higher doses (400–800 mg/day) are used in the treatment of histoplasmosis, blastomycosis, and coccidioidomycosis [51, 79]. In a patient with candidal esophagitis and AIDS, 400 mg/day may be necessary. **Achlorhydria or concurrent administration of agents that decrease gastric acidity** (e.g., antacids, anticholinergics, or H_2-blockers) **decreases the absorption of ketoconazole.** If such agents are being used, they should be given at least 2 hours after ketoconazole administration. Administering ketoconazole with Coca-Cola or another liquid with an acid pH (e.g., orange juice) may improve its absorption. In such circumstances, however, fluconazole, which does not require an acid pH for absorption, is preferable.
      b. **Children.** In small numbers of children older than 2 years, ketoconazole in a single daily dose of 3.3–6.6 mg/kg has been used (see the package insert). The potential benefits should outweigh the risks before using ketoconazole in children.

  c. **The duration of treatment** must be individualized depending on the presence of associated diseases and response to therapy. Usually only 1 or 2 weeks of treatment are necessary for the management of superficial *Candida* infections. A minimum treatment period of 6 months is recommended for the systemic mycoses [51, 78].

  d. **In renal failure,** dose modification is not necessary. Ketoconazole is not substantially removed by hemodialysis or peritoneal dialysis.

  e. **In hepatic insufficiency,** no dose adjustment is necessary for mild to moderate hepatic insufficiency. In patients with severe liver failure, ketoconazole should be avoided or the dose reduced and serum levels monitored if no alternative agent is available.

  f. **Cost.** See Table 18-3.

5. **Contraindications or drug interactions**

  a. **Pregnancy. Ketoconazole** is teratogenic in the rat model and should be avoided in pregnancy.

  b. **Nursing mothers** who must receive ketoconazole should not breast-feed for the duration of treatment.

  c. **Drug interactions**

  (1) Ketoconazole increases the blood levels of **cyclosporine, digoxin, and phenytoin** when administered concurrently. Therefore, serum levels of these drugs should be carefully monitored.

  (2) **The coadministration of ketoconazole with terfenadine or astemizole is contraindicated.** When ketoconazole is administered with either of these agents, it may prolong the QT interval, sometimes causing life-threatening ventricular arrhythmias [157]. Recently, a similar interaction has been described in patients receiving **cisapride (Propulsid)** for upper gastrointestinal motility problems [157a].

  (3) **Isoniazid, rifampin, and phenytoin** increase the metabolism of ketoconazole. Ideally these drugs should not be used concomitantly. Monitoring serum ketoconazole levels may be helpful.

  (4) **The anticoagulant effect of coumadin** may be enhanced by ketoconazole, and so the patient's prothrombin time should be followed closely.

  (5) Ketoconazole may potentiate the hypoglycemic effect of some oral **hypoglycemic agents.**

6. **Adverse effects.** In general, ketoconazole is well tolerated (see Table 18-2) [156, 157].

  a. **Nausea** is the most common side effect. It can be reduced when ketoconazole is taken with food or at bedtime. Abdominal pain may occur.

  b. **Pruritus and skin rashes** are not uncommon. **Anaphylaxis** after the first dose has been reported rarely.

  c. **Hepatotoxicity** due to hepatocellular damage **may occur,** and rare fatalities with progressive hepatic damage have been reported. Liver damage usually is reversible when the drug is discontinued. **Liver function tests should be obtained before starting therapy and at frequent intervals during drug administration,** especially in patients on prolonged therapy or those receiving other potentially hepatotoxic agents. Transient minor liver function test elevations often occur during ketoconazole therapy. The drug should be discontinued if elevated levels persist or are 3–5 times greater than normal.

  d. **Miscellaneous.** Gynecomastia in men, rashes, dizziness, constipation, and diarrhea have been reported. Temporary suppression of serum testosterone levels and of adrenal cortisol production in response to adrenocorticotropic hormone has been described. Rarely, adrenal crisis has been reported in the setting of high-dose ketoconazole therapy [158]. Oligospermia may occur at high daily doses, especially if the dosage exceeds 400 mg/day. Loss of libido and loss of potency also have been reported [159].

C. **Fluconazole (Diflucan)** is a *bis*-triazole antifungal that was released in 1990. Similar to the imidazoles, the triazole antifungals inhibit ergosterol biosynthesis and result in a leaky cell membrane. Fluconazole currently is indicated for the treatment of candidal infections and for initial treatment (of selected patients) and prevention of cryptococcal meningitis in AIDS patients. It is available in both an intravenous and an oral preparation.

1. **Pharmacokinetics**

  a. **Absorption** from the GI tract is **reliable** and complete, with oral bioavailability exceeding 90% [160, 161]. Serum levels are similar following oral and intravenous administration. **Gastric acid is not required for absorption.** Absorption is not reduced by concomitant use of H_2-blockers on antacids.

b. There is little metabolism of fluconazole, and renal excretion accounts for approximately 80% of its elimination as unchanged drug. Therefore, **dosage reduction is necessary in patients with renal failure.**

c. **Urine concentrations of fluconazole are high** as it is minimally metabolized by the liver and excreted largely unchanged in the urine. Thus, it may be an effective agent in urinary tract candidiasis [161].

d. Fluconazole has **excellent penetration into the CSF,** with levels reaching 60–80% of serum levels.

e. In addition to providing good concentrations in the CSF and urine, fluconazole diffuses well into sputum, saliva, skin, and the vitreous and aqueous humor of the eye. Pharmacokinetics are similar in healthy young adults and in the elderly [161].

2. **Clinical uses**

   a. Fluconazole has proven useful for **cryptococcal meningitis in AIDS patients** as both initial therapy and maintenance therapy. Amphotericin B, however, is preferred as initial therapy in those patients who are seriously ill or confused or who have other poor prognostic findings. In these patients, fluconazole may be substituted for amphotericin B once the patient has clinically stabilized and the CSF parameters have improved [65, 66]. (See sec. **IV.A** under Cryptococcosis and Chap. 5.)

   For maintenance therapy of AIDS patients, oral fluconazole is the treatment of choice.

   b. Fluconazole is effective in the treatment of **oropharyngeal and esophageal** candidiasis, primarily in immunocompromised hosts [6, 160].

   c. Fluconazole is not recommended for the routine management of **vaginal candidiasis.** However, it may be helpful in selected patients who fail topical therapy or who have frequent recurrences. (See Chap. 13.)

   d. The use of fluconazole for patients with **candidemia and systemic candidiasis** has been controversial. However, recent studies indicate that fluconazole has equivalent efficacy to amphotericin B for treating these syndromes in patients without neutropenia [22, 23]. See sec. **III.D** under Candidiasis.

   e. Fluconazole has also been used successfully to prevent candidiasis in patients undergoing bone marrow transplantation. Unfortunately, an increased rate of infections due to fluconazole-resistant *C. krusei* was noted in these studies [162, 163]. Many AIDS patients receive fluconazole either continuously or intermittently over long periods of time (see Chap. 19). Concomitant with its widespread use (over 15 million patients since 1988), there have been **increasing reports of fluconazole resistance.** This topic has recently been reviewed elsewhere [163a].

   f. The role of fluconazole in the treatment of coccidioidomycosis, histoplasmosis, blastomycosis, and sporotrichosis is currently under investigation. Initial studies indicate that fluconazole will be a useful agent in treating coccidioidal meningitis [80].

   g. **Hepatosplenic candidiasis** has responded to fluconazole (see sec. **III.F.1** under Candidiasis).

3. **Dosages.** Because fluconazole is well-absorbed after oral therapy, **the daily doses for oral and intravenous therapy are the same.** Intravenous administration is preferred when GI motility is impaired or nasogastric suction is employed. Tablets are available in 50-mg, 100-mg, or 200-mg sizes.

   a. **For oropharyngeal candidiasis,** 200 mg on the first day followed by 100 mg once daily is continued until infection has subsided. Most patients respond in a few days, and treatment for longer than 1 week usually is not necessary. Frequent relapses of disease are noted in AIDS patients, and maintenance therapy has proven helpful in these instances. The authors have found a dose of 100 mg once weekly is effective in preventing relapse in the majority of their patients [7].

   b. **For esophageal candidiasis,** 200 mg on the first day followed by 100 mg once daily is routinely suggested. Higher doses (up to 400 mg/day) may be necessary. Patients should be treated for a minimum of 2 weeks.

   c. **Systemic candidiasis or candidemia.** Two recent randomized trials indicate that nonneutropenic patients treated with fluconazole, 400 mg/day, had an outcome similar to those treated with amphotericin B [22, 23].

However, some non-*albicans* species, such as *C. krusei,* are resistant to fluconazole, and amphotericin B should not be used in individuals infected with these organisms.

  d. **For cryptococcal meningitis**
    (1) **For suppression of relapse** in patients with AIDS, 200 mg once daily is suggested [67, 68].
    (2) **For primary therapy of cryptococcal meningitis** in patients with AIDS, after an initial 400 mg on the first day, 200–400 mg once daily may be effective in selected low-risk patients [65]. However, most experts recommend an initial course of amphotericin, followed by fluconazole once the patient has clinically stabilized and the CSF parameters have improved. Infectious disease consultation is advised in this setting. See sec. **IV.A.3.c** under Cryptococcosis.
    (3) The role of fluconazole in the treatment of cryptococcal meningitis in HIV-negative individuals is yet to be defined.
  e. **Dosage needs to be reduced in patients with renal failure.** After the initial loading dose, the following dose reductions are suggested: For a creatinine clearance in excess of 50 ml/min, give the normal dose; if the clearance is 21–50 ml/min, give 50% of the usual dose; if the clearance is 11–20 ml/min, give 25% of the usual dose. In patients on regular hemodialysis, give the usual dose once after each dialysis treatment.
  f. **Intravenous fluconazole** is used in patients who cannot take the oral, less expensive, route, as in patients who have nausea and vomiting, are NPO, and so on. Otherwise, there is no advantage of the intravenous preparation, which provides serum concentrations similar to the oral preparation. For dosages see sec. 3.
  g. **Pregnancy.** The package insert notes that there are no adequate and well-controlled studies in pregnant women; this agent should be used in pregnancy only if the potential benefit justifies the possible risk to the fetus.
  h. **Nursing.** The package insert notes that fluconazole is excreted in human milk at concentrations similar to plasma. Therefore, the use of fluconazole in nursing mothers is not recommended.
4. **Side effects.** Fluconazole has been well tolerated, with reports of toxicity most frequent in AIDS patients (see Table 18-2) [159, 160].
  a. **Rash** occurs in fewer than 5% of recipients.
  b. **Nausea and vomiting** occur in 2–10% of recipients or fewer. Nausea occurs less frequently with fluconazole than with ketoconazole.
  c. **Stevens-Johnson syndrome** and **hepatotoxicity** have been reported rarely. Transient elevations of liver function tests are relatively common in AIDS patients.
  d. Fluconazole affects adrenal steroid synthesis much less than does ketoconazole. Endocrine side effects including impotence, gynecomastia, and menstrual disturbances are reported less frequently with fluconazole.
5. **Drug interactions.** Drug interactions are less frequent and less pronounced as compared to ketoconazole. When another agent is administered with fluconazole, the following drug interactions may occur.
  a. **Rifampin** decreases serum concentrations of fluconazole.
  b. The hypoglycemic effects of oral agents, especially **tolbutamide,** may be enhanced.
  c. **Warfarin, phenytoin, rifabutin** [163b], **and cyclosporine** levels are variably increased, especially with higher doses of fluconazole. Monitoring the prothrombin time or serum levels is important in patients receiving fluconazole.
  d. **The potential interaction between fluconazole and terfenadine or astemizole has not been adequately studied. Until these data are available, it seems prudent to avoid these combinations.** Recently, data suggest fluconazole may interact with **cisapride** (Propulsid), and these two agents should not be used together [157a].
6. **Cost.** Fluconazole is expensive. See Table 18-3.
D. **Itraconazole (Sporanox),** an oral triazole, is the most recently released agent (1992) for the systemic treatment of fungal infections. Currently, it is approved only for the treatment of histoplasmosis and blastomycosis.
  1. **Pharmacokinetics** [164]
    a. **Absorption** while fasting is only 30–40%. **Bioavailability** is significantly **enhanced by food,** and it is recommended the drug be taken with meals.

Absorption is also enhanced by the presence of gastric acid and is reduced by antacids.

  b. Itraconazole is **highly protein-bound** (99.8%), and there is little or no CSF penetration.

  c. The drug is lipophilic, and **tissue levels exceed serum concentrations.** The drug can be detected in tissue, including the skin and nails, for longer periods of time than in serum after the drug has been discontinued.

  d. Extensive hepatic metabolism occurs, but one of the major metabolites has antifungal activity. Less than 1% of active drug is excreted in the urine.

  e. Renal failure, hemodialysis, and peritoneal dialysis do not alter serum levels or metabolism.

2. Clinical uses [159]

  a. Itraconazole currently is approved for the treatment of **histoplasmosis** and **blastomycosis** and as an alternative agent in aspergillosis. See individual discussions of these topics earlier in this chapter.

  b. Itraconazole has a broad range of in vitro antifungal activity, including *Candida* species, *C. immitis, S. schenckii, C. neoformans,* and *Aspergillus* species. Clinical trials are ongoing to establish the role of itraconazole for treating infections due to these fungi.

  c. Itraconazole may prove helpful in the management of selected patients with chronic skin and nail infections due to dermatophyte fungi. The role of itraconazole for onychomycosis was recently reviewed [164a]; (doses of 200 mg once a day, with a meal, for 3 months are suggested [164a]).

3. Dosage. Itraconazole is available in 100-mg capsules, which **should be taken with meals.** Doses above 200 mg/day should be given in two divided doses.

  a. Histoplasmosis and blastomycosis. In a recent prospective trial, patients treated with 200 mg/day had a similar outcome to those treated with 400 mg/day [48]. Thus, the initial recommended daily dose of itraconazole is 200 mg. Patients whose disease progresses on therapy should have their dose increased in 100-mg increments to a maximum daily dose of 400 mg. A minimum of 6 months' therapy is recommended, but the successful treatment of histoplasmosis frequently requires treatment for 1 year or longer.

  b. Aspergillosis. In mid-1994, itraconazole was approved for use in the treatment of pulmonary and extrapulmonary aspergillosis in patients who are intolerant of or refractory to amphotericin B therapy. A loading dose of 200 mg tid should be given for the first 3 days (in severe infection) and then 200–400 mg/day is suggested by the package insert.

  c. Although not yet approved for **sporotrichosis,** initial studies indicate that itraconazole is an effective alternative to potassium iodide in this setting [121, 122]. For cutaneous or lymphocutaneous disease, the usual dose is 200 mg/day for 3–6 months. Higher doses (200 mg bid) are used for osseous or articular disease and pulmonary disease [122, 124]. Therapy for 1 or 2 years may be required in extracutaneous disease. Infectious disease consultation is recommended.

  d. Pediatric use. The safety and efficacy of itraconazole in children has not been established.

  e. Renal failure. Dosage adjustments are not necessary in renal failure. Neither hemodialysis nor peritoneal dialysis alters serum levels of itraconazole.

  f. Hepatic dysfunction. Whether dosage adjustment is necessary in patients with hepatic dysfunction is unclear. Plasma concentrations should be monitored in patients with severe hepatic insufficiency.

4. Toxicity. Itraconazole is generally well tolerated in the currently recommended doses of 200–400 mg/day. Toxicity is reported more frequently at doses of 600 mg or higher.

  a. Nausea and **vomiting** are seen in approximately 10% of patients but usually do not necessitate discontinuation of therapy. Giving the dose with the evening meal or dividing the daily dosage into two equal doses may be helpful.

  b. Liver function abnormalities are mild and transient; symptomatic hepatitis is rare.

  c. Less common side effects include **pruritus, skin rash, headache, hypertension, hypokalemia, and pedal edema.**

  d. Impotence, usually reversible, has been reported despite normal testosterone levels in these patients.

e. At doses of less than 600 mg/d, itraconazole has little or no effect on adrenal cortisol production.

5. **Drug interactions.** Itraconazole has shown no significant inducing or inhibiting effects on liver enzymes. Compared to ketoconazole, it is a very weak inhibitor of liver microsomal enzymes.

   a. **Antacids, and possibly H₂-receptor antagonists,** will decrease peak serum levels and so should be avoided if possible.

   b. **Rifampin and phenytoin** will induce the metabolism of itraconazole and **result in decreased serum levels.** The dosage of itraconazole may need to be increased in patients failing therapy when these agents are used concurrently. Some suggest that concurrent use of rifampin, phenytoin, carbamazine, and phenobarbital should be avoided in patients receiving itraconazole for life-threatening infection (e.g., invasive aspergillosis) [94].

   c. **The coadministration of itraconazole and terfenadine, or astemizole, is contraindicated. A prolonged QT interval and life-threatening ventricular arrhythmias have been reported** [165]. Recently, a similar potential interaction has been noted for **cisapride** (Propulsid) [157a].

   d. Itraconazole will raise the levels of **cyclosporine, digoxin, and phenytoin** when coadministered with these agents. Monitor levels.

   e. The anticoagulant effect of **warfarin** may be increased by itraconazole.

   f. The hypoglycemic effect of **oral sulfonylurea drugs,** especially tolbutamide, may be enhanced when coadministered with itraconazole.

6. **Pregnancy.** Itraconazole is teratogenic in rats and should not be given during pregnancy unless benefits outweigh potential risks. The drug is secreted in breast milk and should not be administered to nursing mothers.

7. **Cost.** Itraconazole is an expensive agent. See Table 18-3.

IV. **Other agents**

A. **Potassium iodide** has long been an effective agent for the treatment of the cutayneous-lymphatic form of sporotrichosis. See the discussion in sec. III under Sporotrichosis.

B. **Griseofulvin** is produced by a species of *Penicillium.* It exerts its fungicidal activity by inhibiting fungal mitosis, most likely due to the polymerization of cell microtubules and disruption of the mitotic spindle [166]. Griseofulvin is active against the dermatophytes (*Trichophyton, Epidermophyton,* and *Microsporum* species) that cause ringworm of the skin, hair, and nails. It has no clinically significant activity against *Candida* species or any other pathogenic fungi.

   1. **Mode of administration.** Griseofulvin is sold in a microsize form in capsules (125 mg and 250 mg), in an ultramicrosize form in tablets (165 mg and 330 mg), and as a pediatric suspension (125 mg/5 ml).

      a. The **usual adult dose** is 500 mg/day of the microsize preparation or 330 mg of the ultramicrosize preparation given as a single daily dose. In severe or more recalcitrant cases of disease, these doses may be doubled.

      b. The duration of therapy varies depending on the site of infection and clinical response. For skin infections, treatment courses of 4–8 weeks usually are curative. Nail infections are more difficult to treat and usually require a minimum of 4 months for fingernails and 6 months for toenails.

   2. **Toxicity and drug interactions.** Griseofulvin is **generally well tolerated.** Headache is common but usually resolves during the first week of therapy. A variety of skin reactions have been reported and may necessitate stopping the drug. Occasionally nausea, vomiting, a bad taste in the mouth, paresthesias of the hands and feet, insomnia, confusion, or dizziness may occur. Reversible granulocytopenia and hepatotoxicity have been reported. Patients on high-dose or prolonged therapy should have their CBC count and liver tests followed on a routine basis.

Actinomycosis

Actinomyces species are gram-positive, **filamentous bacteria** that once were classified as fungi. The ability of these organisms to cause subacute and chronic granulomatous inflammation perhaps more closely resembles the characteristics of fungal infections than those of most bacterial infections.

I. **Growth and identification characteristics.** Clinical actinomycosis is almost always caused by *Actinomyces israelii* [167]. *Actinomyces* can be grown on routine culture media with augmentation using brain-heart infusion. The **primarily anaerobic character of *Actinomyces* requires rapid transport of abscess material to the laboratory or direct inoculation into an anaerobic container** to maximize the ability to isolate this pathogen. Mature colonies are present after 3–7 days of incubation, and the organism can be identified definitively after an additional 48 hours. *A. israelii* is seen on Gram stains of exudates or tissue sections as pleomorphic, beaded, branching gram-positive rods. Infection with *Actinomyces* may result in the formation of yellow, white, gray, or brown macroscopic particles called **sulfur granules,** which represent conglomerate masses of organisms.

II. **Epidemiologic features.** *Actinomyces* is worldwide in distribution and is a common saprophyte of the oral cavity, pharynx, and intestines. Therefore, **simple recovery of the organism from culture does not necessarily establish the presence of infection.**

III. **Pathogenesis.** The normal commensal status of *Actinomyces* is altered when the organism gains entrance to deeper tissues through a break in intact mucous membranes. Once it enters a microaerophilic or anaerobic atmosphere, *Actinomyces* produces a subacute or chronic granulomatous infection with a tendency to cause externally draining sinuses.

IV. **Clinical syndromes.** Actinomycosis results in three main clinical syndromes depending on the site of involvement: cervicofacial, thoracic, or abdominal.

A. **Cervicofacial actinomycosis** [167] commonly occurs one to several weeks after dental extraction or minor trauma to the oral mucous membrane or in association with poor oral hygiene.

1. **Manifestations.** The patient usually has a bluish, swollen lesion at the angle of the mandible or in the neck. The lesion may enlarge slowly and be painless or may progress rapidly and cause considerable pain. A visible sinus tract or fistula may be present. Sulfur granules may be seen in the exudate. Nonspecific symptoms of fever, weight loss, chills, and trismus may occur. Infection spreads without regard to fascial tissue planes and may involve the salivary and lacrimal glands, mandible, orbit, or paranasal sinuses.

2. **Diagnosis.** Definitive diagnosis is made by culture of the organism from biopsy specimens or exudate. Pus should be collected by aspiration from closed lesions and should be transferred to an anaerobic environment as quickly as possible. Pus should also be examined for the presence of sulfur granules. Roentgenograms may reveal bony changes ranging from a minor subperiosteal reaction to overt lytic destruction, usually involving the mandible.

B. **Thoracic actinomycosis** [168] may result from oropharyngeal aspiration of the organism, direct extension from the neck into the mediastinum, or spread from the abdominal cavity. Severe periodontal disease is commonly present.

1. **Manifestations.** Symptoms often occur relatively late in the course of the illness. Nonproductive cough, low-grade fever, and weight loss gradually progress to mucopurulent sputum production, occasional hemoptysis, and pleuritic chest pain. **Local chest wall spread may involve pleura and ribs and may produce draining sinuses.** Dysphagia may result from mediastinal invasion. Infection may extend to the pericardium, heart, and thoracic vertebrae, or through the diaphragm, producing subphrenic or subhepatic abscesses. Hematogenous dissemination may result in spread to other organs, particularly the skin. Chest roentgenograms may show mass lesions, dense infiltrates, cavities, or pleural disease (effusion or thickening). **Chest wall involvement is particularly suggestive of actinomycosis.** Extension of a pulmonary lesion through the thoracic wall or periostitis or frank destruction of ribs contiguous to an area of lung involvement may occur.

2. **Diagnosis.** Because *A. israelii* may colonize the upper respiratory tract, **definitive diagnosis requires isolation of the organism from a resected specimen,** growth in culture from an **empyema** cavity, **or recovery from a draining sinus.** Identification of sulfur granules is strongly suggestive of the diagnosis.

C. **Abdominal infection** occurs most frequently after appendectomy, appendiceal abscess, or traumatic perforation of the bowel, and represents 20–50% of all cases of actinomycosis [167].

1. **Manifestations.** Infection occurs most commonly in the ileocecal area and produces abdominal discomfort, fever, and a palpable mass. The process may localize or spread directly into the peritoneal cavity, abdominal wall, subphrenic space, or pelvis. The course is usually subacute to chronic. Sinuses may appear in the abdominal wall. Spread through the portal veins may result in jaundice and an enlarged, tender liver. Extension to the urinary tract, pelvic organs, or

vertebral bodies may occur. Anorectal involvement may result from secondary extension or may arise primarily through a break in an anal crypt. Pelvic actinomycosis occurring in association with an intrauterine device in women is well described [169].

2. **Diagnosis** generally is by culture of specimens at the time of exploratory laparotomy, unless draining sinuses are present in the abdominal wall.

V. **Therapy. Penicillin** remains the drug of choice for actinomycosis [169a]. Prolonged treatment with large doses is required to ensure adequate penetration into areas of fibrosis. Intravenous aqueous penicillin G (10–20 million units/day) for 4–6 weeks, followed by oral penicillin for 6–12 months, is suggested. Tetracyclines may be used in the nonpregnant penicillin-allergic patient. Other alternative agents include erythromycin and clindamycin [169a]. Surgical drainage of abscesses and excision of sinus tracts are important aspects of treatment. Infectious disease consultation is advised.

Nocardiosis

Nocardiosis is the localized or disseminated disease most commonly caused by *Nocardia asteroides* and less often by *Nocardia brasiliensis* and *Nocardia caviae*. *Nocardia* species are gaining increased recognition as **opportunistic pathogens, although they also cause illness in normal hosts.** Although originally believed to be fungi, *Nocardia* are now classified as higher-order **bacteria** and are closely related to the genus *Actinomyces*.

I. **Growth and identification characteristics.** *Nocardia* species are gram-positive, aerobic, **weakly acid-fast bacilli,** and are readily isolated on routine bacterial, fungal, and mycobacterial media. Colonies usually appear within 4 days, but in some instances may require 2–4 weeks of culture. *Nocardia* can be difficult to isolate by culture, particularly because of overgrowth by nonpathogenic colonizers. **If nocardiosis is suspected clinically, the bacteriology laboratory should be informed and cultures should be kept longer than usual.** Gram-stained preparations reveal delicately branching, gram-positive, beaded filaments. With a modified Ziehl-Neelsen or Kinyoun stain, *Nocardia* organisms are weakly acid-fast, a characteristic that helps to distinguish them from *Actinomyces*. **However, the histologic appearance of *Nocardia* is not unique, and culture is necessary for definitive diagnosis.**

II. **Epidemiologic and host factors.** *Nocardia* species are found worldwide and maintain a saprophytic existence in the soil. *N. brasiliensis* most often causes primary cutaneous disease and, in the United States, is most frequently reported in the South. Infection with *N. asteroides* most frequently occurs following inhalation of the organism into the lungs of predisposed individuals. The organism is an **opportunistic invader** in the setting of compromised host defenses: Patients with leukemia, lymphoma, solid tumors, AIDS, dysgammaglobulinemia, collagen vascular disease, chronic granulomatous disease, and individuals on steroids or immunosuppression for organ transplantation are especially susceptible. In addition, prior pulmonary disease, including chronic obstructive lung disease and pulmonary alveolar proteinosis, are risk factors. Nevertheless, **approximately 15% of patients with nocardiosis have no underlying disorder** [170–172].

III. **Cinical aspects.** Although a few cases of skin or subcutaneous disease may occur by primary inoculation, clinical infection usually begins in the lungs, with 75% of patients exhibiting a primary pneumonitis. Secondary dissemination occurs by hematogenous spread and is almost always due to *N. asteroides*.

A. **Pulmonary and systemic nocardiosis** usually follows a subacute to chronic course, spanning weeks to months. Acute, fulminating disease may occur in severely immunosuppressed patients.

1. **Manifestations.** Occasional patients may be asymptomatic, but constitutional symptoms of fever, night sweats, malaise, anorexia, and weight loss are reported in most cases. Leukocytosis is not consistently present.

a. **Pulmonary findings.** Cough may be dry but usually is productive of thick, mucopurulent sputum. Hemoptysis and pleuritic chest pain also are reported. **Chest roentgenograms** are variable and **nonspecific.** Localized infiltrates, often in the upper lobes, are common. Single or multiple nodules, cavities, diffuse infiltrates, consolidations, abscesses, large masses, and pleural effusions have all been reported.

b. **CNS** involvement has been noted in approximately 25% of patients. This is usually in the form of a **brain abscess,** and the diagnosis may be suspected on the basis of CT scanning or MRI. Meningitis has been reported. Decreased mental status, unsteadiness, headaches, nausea and vomiting, seizures, or focal neurologic deficits may occur. (CSF does not reveal *Nocardia* on smear or culture, and brain biopsy may be necessary.)

   c. **Skin and subcutaneous abscesses** are present in approximately 10% of patients.

   d. **Pleural and chest wall invasion** from a contiguous pneumonic infection occurs in nearly 10% of cases. Patients may complain of pleuritic pain or may manifest sinus tracts. Intrapleural effusions may become infected, with the development of empyema.

   e. **Metastatic infection** to virtually every organ has been documented.

2. **Diagnosis. Nocardiosis should be considered in any chronic pneumonia that persists despite conventional antimicrobial therapy. The combination of pulmonary and CNS or skin infection in a compromised host is particularly suggestive.**

   a. **Sputum or pulmonary specimens.** Positive sputum cultures are diagnostic, but false negative results are common. Invasive procedures such as thoracentesis, transtracheal aspiration, lung aspiration, or lung biopsy may be necessary.

   b. **Blood cultures** are rarely positive.

   c. **Smears and culture material** obtained from skin lesions, sinus tracts, and tissue biopsy specimens are important sources. Histologic examination is suggestive but not diagnostic.

   d. **Skin and serologic tests are not available.**

3. **Therapy.** Sulfonamide-based regimens have proven to be the most effective treatment for nocardiosis. Infectious disease consultation is advised.

   a. **Trimethoprim-sulfamethoxazole** is considered by most authorities to be the treatment of choice for nocardiosis [169a, 173]. This rationale is supported by the synergy of these two drugs, which has been demonstrated in vitro against *Nocardia,* the excellent tissue levels achieved with both drugs (including the CNS), and their excellent bioavailability when given orally. Sulfa levels in serum should be monitored to achieve concentrations of 12–15 mg/dl [171].

   b. **Sulfonamides** as single agents are also very effective against *Nocardia.* For example, sulfadiazine, 8–12 g/day, can be used (see Chap. 28K). The dosage should be monitored to achieve peak serum concentrations of approximately 15 mg/dl.

   c. **Other regimens** may be necessary if the organisms are resistant or if patients are intolerant to sulfa drugs. Susceptibility testing is difficult and ideally should be performed at reference laboratories. **Minocycline, doxycycline, and amoxicillin-clavulanate** have been effective. Many *Nocardia* strains are susceptible to **amikacin,** and this drug may be added to a sulfa regimen or an alternative regimen [174]. **Imipenem** may be another alternative agent.

   d. The duration of therapy is not well defined, but **most authorities recommend a prolonged course of treatment.** For minor infections and in immunocompetent hosts, therapy is given for at least 2–3 months. For severe infections, or in immunosuppressed individuals, therapy for up to 1 year is recommended. Some experts suggest maintenance therapy to prevent relapse in transplant recipients or in patients continuing on immunosuppressive therapy [171, 172].

   e. **Surgical drainage and excision** should be performed on abscesses, if possible.

4. **Prognosis.** Mortality varies with the site of disease and the severity of the patient's underlying immunosuppression. Survival definitely is improved if therapy is initiated early and before hematogenous seeding occurs. Individuals with CNS infection have the highest mortality, approximately 40%. Mortality in patients with isolated pulmonary disease ranges between 10% and 29%, the higher rate being reported in transplant recipients and other immunocompromised patients [171, 172].

B. *N. asteroides* **is a rare laboratory contaminant, and isolation from sputum usually indicates active disease.** However, positive sputum cultures have been found in asymptomatic patients, individuals with mild upper respiratory tract infections, and some persons with bronchitis. In patients with malignancies or immunosuppressive disorders, the isolation of *Nocardia* from clinical specimens should prompt the initiation of therapy. On the other hand, in immunocompetent individuals a positive culture for *Nocardia* should stimulate further investigation but may not mandate therapy if solid evidence of invasive disease cannot be found. Infectious disease consultation is advised.

References

1. Crislip, M.A., and Edwards, J.E., Jr. Candidiasis. *Infect. Dis. Clin. North Am.* 3:103, 1989.
   Excellent, concise review.
2. Vartivarian, S., and Smith, C.B. Pathogenesis, Host Resistance, and Predisposing Factors. In G.P. Bodey (ed.), *Candidiasis: Pathogenesis, Diagnosis, and Treatment* (2nd ed.). New York: Raven, 1993. P. 59.
3. Epstein, J.B., Truelove, E.L., and Izutzu, K.T. Oral candidiasis: Pathogenesis and host defense. *Rev. Infect. Dis.* 6:96, 1984.
   Good discussion of the host factors important in resistance to oral candidiasis.
4. Wheeler, R.R., et al. Esophagitis in the immunocompromised host: Role of esophagoscopy in diagnosis. *Rev. Infect. Dis.* 9:88, 1987.
5. Eras, P., Goldstein, M.J., and Sherlock, P. *Candida* infection of the gastrointestinal tract. *Medicine* 51:367, 1972.
6. Lopez-Dupla, M., et al. Clinical, endoscopic, immunologic, and therapeutic aspects of oropharyngeal and esophageal candidiasis in HIV infected patients. A survey of 114 cases. *Am. J. Gastroenterol.* 87:1771, 1992.
   The esophagitis was often asymptomatic. Fluconazole therapy was very effective.
7. Marriott, D.J.E., et al. Fluconazole once a week as secondary prophylaxis against oropharyngeal candidiasis in HIV-infected patients. *Med. J. Aust.* 158:312, 1993.
8. Kirkpatrick, C.H. Chronic Mucocutaneous Candidiasis. In G.P. Bodey (ed.), *Candidiasis: Pathogenesis, Diagnosis, and Treatment* (2nd ed.). New York: Raven, 1993. P. 167.
   Excellent discussion of an unusual disorder.
9. Banerjee, S.N., et al. Secular trends in nosocomial primary bloodstream infections in the United States, 1980–1989. *Am. J. Med.* 91:86S, 1991.
   Candidemia is now one of the most common nosocomial bloodstream infections.
9a. Fisher-Hoch, S.P., and Hutwagner, L. Opportunistic candidiasis: An epidemic of the 1980s. *Clin. Infect. Dis.* 21:897, 1995.
   Reviews hospital discharge data from 1980–1989. The rate of debilitating and life-threatening candidiasis among hospitalized patients increased considerably, especially among patients infected with HIV and patients undergoing transplantation or immunosuppression for malignancy. See related papers by J.K. Stamos and A.H. Rowley, Candidemia in a pediatric population. Clin. Infect. Dis. 30:571, 1995; and M.H. Nguyen et al., Candida prosthetic endocarditis. Clin. Infect. Dis. 22:262, 1996.
10. Komshian, S.V, et al. Fungemia caused by *Candida* species and *Torulopsis glabrata* in the hospitalized patient: Frequency, characteristics, and evaluation of factors affecting outcome. *Rev. Infect. Dis.* 11:379, 1989.
    Risk factors and elements affecting prognosis in candidemia are discussed. See related discussion by R.P. Wenzel, Epidemiology of nosocomial Candida infections. Infect. Dis. Clin. Pract. 3(Suppl. 2):56, 1994.
11. Fraser, V.J., et al. Candidemia in a tertiary care hospital: Epidemiology, risk factors, and predictors of mortality. *Clin. Infect. Dis.* 15:414, 1992.
    Large series of patients with candidemia, documenting the associated high mortality.
11a. Rex, J.H. Editorial response: Catheters and candidemia. *Clin. Infect. Dis.* 22:467, 1996.
12. Louria, D.B., Stiff, D.P., and Bennett, B. Disseminated moniliasis in the adult. *Medicine* 41:307, 1962.
13. Bodey, G.P., and Luna, M. Skin lesions associated with disseminated candidiasis. *J.A.M.A.* 229:1466, 1974.
    Color photographs of the skin lesions that, if biopsied, reveal Candida organisms.
14. Edwards, J.E., Jr., et al. Ocular manifestations of *Candida* septicemia: Review of 76 cases of hematogenous *Candida* endophthalmitis. *Medicine* 53:47, 1974.
14a. Edwards, J.E. Candida endophthalmitis, presented in the symposium: In the eye of the beholder: diagnosis and therapy of deep eye infections. 35th Interscience Conference on Antimicrobial Agents and Chemotherapy, San Francisco, CA, September 1995.

15. Jones, J.M. Laboratory diagnosis of invasive candidiasis. *Clin. Microbiol. Rev.* 3: 32, 1990.
    Excellent review of the various tests used to diagnose invasive candidiasis, including a good discussion of the promise and limitations of serologic tests. See a related review by E. Reiss and C.J. Morrison, Nonculture methods for diagnosis of disseminated candidiasis. Clin. Microbiol. Rev. 6:311, 1993. *In a recent review (see reference [19a]), the authors emphasize there is currently no available commercial test to serologically diagnose and/or follow patients with disseminated candidiasis.*

16. Bille, J., et al. Evaluation of a lysis-centrifugation system for recovery of yeasts and filamentous fungi from the blood. *J. Clin. Microbiol.* 18:469, 1983.

16a. Kan, V.I. Polymerase chain reaction for the diagnosis of candidemia. *J. Infect. Dis.* 168:779, 1993.

17. Sandford, G.R., et al. The value of fungal surveillance cultures as predictors of systemic fungal infections. *J. Infect. Dis.* 142:503, 1980.

18. Winegard, J.R., Merz W.G., and Saral, R. *Candida tropicalis:* A major pathogen in immunocompromised patients. *Ann. Intern. Med.* 91:539, 1979.

19. Marina, N.W., et al. *Candida tropicalis* and *Candida albicans* fungemia in children with leukemia. *Cancer* 68:594, 1991.
    This and the preceding study indicate a much higher likelihood of disseminated candidiasis occurring in immunocompromised patients who are colonized with C. tropicalis *compared with those colonized with* C. albicans.

19a. Filler, S.G., and Edwards, J.E., Jr. When and how to treat serious *Candida* infections: Concepts and controversies. *Curr. Clin. Top. Infect.* 15:1, 1995.
    For a related discussion, see L.G. Donowitz and J.O. Hendley, Short-course amphotericin B therapy for candidemia in pediatric patients. Pediatrics 95:888, 1995. *In this paper the authors conclude that once the bloodstream is sterilized and there is no other evidence of invasive fungal disease, 7 to 14 additional days of amphotericin B at 0.5mg/kg/d seems adequate for treatment of candidemia in children. See also J.N. van Der Anker et al., Antifungal agents in neonatal systemic candidiasis.* Antimicrob. Agents Chemother. 39:1391, 1995.

20. Edwards, J.E., Jr., and Filler, S.G. Current strategies for treating invasive candidiasis: Emphasis on infections in nonneutropenic patients. *Clin. Infect. Dis.* 14:S106, 1992.

21. Bodey, G.P. Antifungal Agents. In G.P. Bodey (ed.), *Candidiasis: Pathogenesis, Diagnosis, and Treatment* (2nd ed.). New York: Raven, 1993. P. 371.

22. Anaissie, E.J., et al. A prospective, randomized, multicenter study comparing fluconazole to amphotericin B for nosocomial candidiasis [abstr. 808]. Presented at the 33rd Interscience Conference on Antimicrobial Agents and Chemotherapy, New Orleans, LA, October 1993.

23. Rex, J.H., et al. A randomized trial of fluconazole vs. amphotericin B for the treatment of candidemia in patients without neutropenia. *N. Engl. J. Med.* 331:1325, 1994.
    See editorial comment in this same issue. This randomized study and the preceding one each documented similar outcomes in candidemic patients, whether treated with fluconazole or amphotericin B, with less toxicity in the fluconazole group. (Patients do not have leukopenia.)

24. Havens, P.L., et al. Risk of late infection following transient candidemia [abstr. 69]. Presented at the 29th International Conference on Antimicrobial Agents and Chemotherapy, Houston, TX, September 1989.

25. Young, R.C., et al. Fungemia with compromised host resistance. A study of 70 cases. *Ann. Intern. Med.* 80:605, 1974.

26. Edwards, J.E., Jr. Editorial response: Should all patients with candidemia be treated with antifungal agents? *Clin. Infect. Dis.* 15:422, 1992.
    Good discussion of the rationale for treating all patients with candidemia, regardless of their clinical status or underlying illness.

27. Thaler, M., et al. Hepatic candidiasis in cancer patients: The evolving picture of the syndrome. *Ann. Intern. Med.* 108:88, 1988.
    Excellent description of the manifestations and response to treatment of hepatosplenic candidiasis.

28. Kauffman, C.A., et al. Hepatosplenic candidiasis: Successful treatment with fluconazole. *Am. J. Med.* 91:137, 1991.
    Also see E. Anaissie et al., Fluconazole therapy for chronic disseminated candidiasis in patients with leukemia and prior amphotericin B therapy. Am. J. Med. 91:142, 1991.

29. Rubinstein, E., et al. Fungal endocarditis: Analysis of 24 cases and review of the literature. *Medicine* 54:331, 1975.

Good description of an uncommon disease, emphasizing the crucial role of valve replacement in therapy.

30. Fisher, J.F., et al. Urinary tract infections due to *Candida albicans. Rev. Infect. Dis.* 4:1107, 1982.
    Good discussion of the incidence, predisposing factors, and therapeutic options in candiduria. For a related paper, see B.H. Hamory and R.P. Wenzel, Hospital-associated candiduria: Predisposing factors and review of the literature. J. Urol. 120:444, 1978.

31. Medoff, G. The 10 most common questions about fungal infections. *Infect. Dis. Clin. Pract.* 2:129, 1993.
    Concise summary of one expert's approach to common issues including candidemia, candiduria, cryptococcal pneumonia, and meningitis therapy. Also see A. Voss et al., Fluconazole in the management of fungal urinary tract infections. Infection 22:247, 1994.

31a. Fisher, J.F., Newman, C.L., and Sobel, J.D. Yeast in the urine: Solutions for a budding problem. *Clin. Infect. Dis.* 20:183, 1995.
    A detailed discussion of a rational clinical approach to this difficult topic.

31b. Fan-Havard, P., et al. Oral fluconazole versus amphotericin B bladder irrigation for treatment of candidal funguria. *Clin. Infect. Dis.* 21:960, 1995.
    Patients received either amphotericin B bladder irrigation (50 mg/L over 24 hr or 50 mg/L for 7 days) or fluconazole 200 mg/day for 7 days; urinary catheters were changed at the start and after therapy.

32. Lipton, S.A., et al. Candidal infection in the central nervous system. *Am. J. Med.* 76:101, 1984.

33. Masur, H., Rosen, P.P., and Armstrong, D. Pulmonary disease caused by *Candida* species. *Am. J. Med.* 63:914, 1977.
    Most cases of pulmonary candidiasis are due to hematogenous dissemination.

34. Kerr, C.M., et al. Fungal peritonitis in patients on continuous ambulatory peritoneal dialysis. *Ann. Intern. Med.* 99:334, 1983.

35. Solomkin, J.S., et al. The role of *Candida* in intraperitoneal infections. *Surgery* 88:524, 1980.

36. Bayer, A.S., and Guze, L.B. Fungal arthritis: I. *Candida* arthritis: Diagnosis and prognostic implications and therapeutic considerations. *Semin. Arthritis Rheum.* 8:142, 1978.

37. Gathe, J.C., et al. *Candida* osteomyelitis. Report of five cases and review of the literature. *Am. J. Med.* 82:927, 1987.
    Osteomyelitis may occur as a late complication of inadequately treated disseminated disease.

38. Torres-Rojas, J.R., et al. Candidal suppurative peripheral thrombophlebitis. *Ann. Intern. Med.* 96:431, 1982.

39. Strinden, W.D., Helgerson, R.B., and Maki, D.G. *Candida* septic thrombosis of the great central veins associated with central catheters. *Ann. Surg.* 202:653, 1985.
    The increased use of intravenous catheters has resulted in a greater occurrence of Candida septic thrombophlebitis.

40. Wheat, L.J. Histoplasmosis. *Infect. Dis. Clin. North Am.* 2:841, 1988.
    Excellent review of epidemiology, clinical manifestations, and therapy. For an update by this expert, see J. Wheat, Histoplasmosis: Recognition and treatment. Clin. Infect. Dis. (Suppl. 1):S19, 1994.

41. Goodwin, R.A., Jr., Loyd, J.E., and Des Prez, R.M. Histoplasmosis in normal hosts. *Medicine* 60:231, 1981.
    Detailed discussion of the various forms that histoplasmosis may take in normal hosts.

42. Wheat, L.J., et al. A large urban outbreak of histoplasmosis: Clinical features. *Ann. Intern. Med.* 94:331, 1981.
    Important description of a very large outbreak of histoplasmosis in Indianapolis.

43. Wheat, L.J., et al. The diagnostic laboratory tests for histoplasmosis. Analysis of experience in a large urban outbreak. *Ann. Intern. Med.* 97:680, 1982.

44. Wheat, L.J., Kohler, R.B., and Tewari, R.P. Diagnosis of disseminated histoplasmosis by detection of *Histoplasma capsulatum* antigen in serum and urine specimens. *N. Engl. J. Med.* 314:83, 1986.
    A polysaccharide antigen of H. capsulatum may be detected frequently in serum and urine specimens of patients with disseminated disease and correlates with disease activity.

45. Goodwin, R.A., Jr., et al. Disseminated histoplasmosis: Clinical and pathologic correlations. *Medicine* 59:1, 1980.
    In-depth discussion of disseminated histoplasmosis.

46. Sathapatayavongs, B., et al. Clinical and laboratory features of disseminated histo-plasmosis during two large urban outbreaks. *Medicine* 62:263, 1983.
47. Wheat, L.J., et al. Disseminated histoplasmosis in the acquired immunodeficiency syndrome: Clinical findings, diagnosis, treatment and review of the literature. *Medicine* 69:361, 1990.
   Thorough discussion of disseminated histoplasmosis in AIDS. A fulminant disease presentation is more common, and relapse is inevitable without effective mainte-nance therapy.
48. Dismukes, W.E., et al. Itraconazole therapy for blastomycosis and histoplasmosis. *Am. J. Med.* 93:489–497, 1993.
   Among patients treated for blastomycosis, the success rate was 95% for those treated with more than 2 months of itraconazole. Itraconazole was also very effective as therapy for disseminated histoplasmosis in patients without life-threatening disease.
49. Wheat, L.J., et al. Itraconazole treatment of disseminated histoplasmosis in patients with acquired immunodeficiency syndrome. *Am. J. Med.* 98:336, 1995.
   Itraconazole was very effective for non-severe forms of disseminated histoplasmosis in AIDS patients in this trial.
50. Wheat, L.J., et al. Prevention of relapse of histoplasmosis with itraconazole in patients with the acquired immunodeficiency syndrome. *Ann. Intern. Med.* 118:610, 1993.
   Itraconazole maintenance therapy is well-tolerated and highly effective in preventing relapse in HIV-infected patients who have been treated for disseminated histo-plasmosis.
51. National Institutes of Allergy and Infectious Diseases Mycoses Study Group. Treat-ment of blastomycosis and histoplasmosis with ketoconazole. *Ann. Intern. Med.* 103:861, 1985.
   Ketoconazole was the first azole shown to be effective in the treatment of various forms of blastomycosis and histoplasmosis. It remains a reasonable therapeutic option, particularly in nonimmunocompromised hosts where cost is a concern.
52. Goodwin, R.A., et al. Chronic pulmonary histoplasmosis. *Medicine* 55:413, 1976.
   Exhaustive review, with excellent discussions of pathogenesis and therapy.
53. Loyd, J.L., et al. Mediastinal fibrosis complicating histoplasmosis. *Medicine* 67:295, 1988.
54. Goodwin, R.A., Nickell, J.A., and Des Prez, R.M. Mediastinal fibrosis complicating healed primary histoplasmosis and tuberculosis. *Medicine* 51:227, 1972.
55. Perfect, J.R. Cryptococcosis. *Infect. Dis. Clin. North Am.* 3:77, 1989.
   Very good review of infection with C. neoformans.
56. Levitz, S.M. The ecology of *Cryptococcus neoformans* and the epidemiology of crypto-coccosis. *Rev. Infect. Dis.* 13:1163, 1991.
57. Sugar, A., et al. Cryptococcal disease in patients with the acquired immunodeficiency syndrome. *Ann. Intern. Med.* 104:234, 1986.
   Manifestations and therapeutic outcomes of cryptococcosis in AIDS patients are re-viewed. Disseminated disease with a high mortality is common.
58. Kerkering, T.M., Duma, R.J., and Shadomy, S. The evolution of pulmonary cryptococ-cosis. *Ann. Intern. Med.* 94:611, 1981.
   Manifestations of pulmonary cryptococcosis are presented. Immunocompromised hosts are at risk for extrapulmonary disease, especially meningitis.
59. Hammerman, K.J., et al. Pulmonary *Cryptococcus*: clinical forms and treatment. *Am. Rev. Respir. Dis.* 108:1116, 1973.
60. Cameron, M.L., et al. Manifestations of pulmonary cryptococcosis in patients with acquired immunodeficiency syndrome. *Rev. Infect. Dis.* 13:64, 1991.
61. Chuck, S.L., and Sande, M.A. Infections with *Cryptococcus neoformans* in the acquired immunodeficiency syndrome. *N. Engl. J. Med.* 321:794, 1989.
62. Dismukes, W.E. Cryptococcal meningitis in patients with AIDS. *J. Infect. Dis.* 157:624, 1988.
   Cryptococcal meningitis in AIDS patients may present quite subtly, and therapy is complicated by a high frequency of drug toxicity and relapse.
63. Bennett, J.E., et al. A comparison of amphotericin B alone and combined with flucyto-sine in the treatment of cryptococcal meningitis. *N. Engl. J. Med.* 301:126, 1979.
   The combination of amphotericin B with flucytosine resulted in more rapid sterilization of the CSF in this study of non-AIDS patients with cryptococcal meningitis.
64. Dismukes, W.E., et al. Treatment of cryptococcal meningitis with combination ampho-tericin B and flucytosine for four as compared with six weeks. *N. Engl. J. Med.* 317:334, 1987.

65. Saag, M.S., et al. Comparison of amphotericin B with fluconazole in the treatment of acute AIDS-associated cryptococcal meningitis. *N. Engl. J. Med.* 326:83, 1992.
    Although the difference in overall mortality between the two treatment groups was not statistically significant, amphotericin B effected more rapid sterilization of the CSF than did fluconazole in this randomized trial. Higher doses of amphotericin B than were used in this trial are now used by many infectious diseases clinicians as induction therapy in AIDS patients, followed by fluconazole consolidation therapy.
    See related paper by R.A. Larsen et al., Fluconazole compared with amphotericin B plus flucytosine for cryptococcal meningitis in AIDS. Ann. Intern. Med. *113:183, 1990.*
66. Van der Horst, C., et al. A randomized, double-blind comparison of amphotericin B plus flucytosine to amphotericin B alone (step 1) followed by a comparison of fluconazole to itraconazole (step 2) in the treatment of acute cryptococcal meningitis in patients with AIDS [abstr. I216, I217]. Presented at the 35th Interscience Conference on Antimicrobial Agents and Chemotherapy, San Francisco, CA, September 1995.
67. Bozzette, S.A., et al. A placebo-controlled trial of maintenance therapy with fluconazole after treatment of cryptococcal meningitis in the acquired immunodeficiency syndrome. *N. Engl. J. Med.* 324:580, 1991.
68. Powderly, W.G., et al. A controlled trial of fluconazole or amphotericin B to prevent relapse of cryptococcal meningitis in patients with the acquired immunodeficiency syndrome. *N. Engl. J. Med.* 326:793, 1992.
    Fluconazole was well tolerated and highly effective in preventing relapse of cryptococcal meningitis in AIDS patients in this comparative trial.
69. Stevens, D.A. *Coccidioides immitis.* In G.L. Mandell, and R. Dolin (eds.), *Principles and Practice of Infectious Diseases* (4th ed.). New York: Churchill Livingstone, 1995. P. 2365.
    Excellent, comprehensive review.
70. Ampel, N.M., Wieden, M.A., and Galgiani, J.N. Coccidioidomycosis: clinical update. *Rev. Infect. Dis.* 11:897, 1989.
    See related review by J.N. Galgiani, Coccidioidomycosis. West. J. Med. *159:153, 1993.*
71. Bayer, A.S. Fungal pneumonias: Pulmonary coccidioidal syndromes. I. Primary and progressive coccidioidal pneumonias—diagnostic, therapeutic, and prognostic considerations. *Chest* 79:575, 1981.
72. Tucker, R.M., et al. Itraconazole therapy for nonmeningeal coccidioidomycosis: Clinical and laboratory observations. *J. Am. Acad. Dermatol.* 23:593, 1990.
73. Graybill, J.R., et al. Itraconazole treatment of coccidioidomycosis. *Am. J. Med.* 89:282, 1990.
    This study and the preceding one document the efficacy and tolerability of itraconazole in various forms of nonmeningeal coccidioidomycosis.
74. Bronnimann, A.A., et al. Coccidioidomycosis in the acquired immunodeficiency syndrome. *Ann. Intern. Med.* 106:372, 1987.
75. Fish, D.G., et al. Coccidioidomycosis during human immunodeficiency virus infection. A review of 77 patients. *Medicine* 69:384, 1990.
    AIDS patients infected with C. immitis may present with a variety of manifestations, both pulmonary and extrapulmonary. The optimal treatment is unknown at present.
76. Bried, J.M., and Galgiani, J.N. *Coccidioides immitis* infections in bones and joints. *Clin. Orthop.* 211:235, 1986.
    Good discussion of osteoarticular disease in coccidioidomycosis.
77. Bouza, E., et al. Coccidioidal meningitis. *Medicine* 60:139, 1981.
    Extensive review of manifestations and therapeutic outcomes with amphotericin B.
78. Galgiani, J.N., et al. Ketoconazole therapy of progressive coccidioidomycosis. *Am. J. Med.* 84:603, 1988.
79. Galgiani, J.N. Coccidioidomycosis. *Infect. Dis. Clin. Pract.* 1:357, 1992.
80. Galgiani, J.N., et al. Fluconazole therapy for coccidioidal meningitis. *Ann. Intern. Med.* 119:28, 1993.
80a. Dewsnup, D.H., et al. Is it ever safe to stop azole therapy for *Coccidioides immitis* meningitis? *Ann. Intern. Med.* 124:305, 1996.
81. Tucker, R.M., et al. Itraconazole therapy for chronic coccidioidal meningitis. *Ann. Intern. Med.* 112:108, 1990.
82. Levitz, S.M. Aspergillosis. *Infect. Dis. Clin. North Am.* 3:1, 1989.
83. Glimp, R.A. Fungal pneumonias: III. Allergic bronchopulmonary aspergillosis. *Chest* 80:85, 1981.
    Good discussion of the clinical aspects of ABPA.
84. Rosenberg, M., et al. Clinical and immunologic criteria for the diagnosis of allergic bronchopulmonary aspergillosis. *Ann. Intern. Med.* 86:405, 1977.

Still a relevant article. For recent reviews of this topic, see L.M. Vaughan, Allergic bronchopulmonary aspergillosis. Clin. Pharm. *12:24, 1993; and S.M. Levitz, Aspergillosis.* Infect. Dis. Clin. North Am. *3:1, 1989.*

85. Denning, D.W., et al. Adjunctive therapy of allergic bronchopulmonary aspergillosis with itraconazole. *Chest* 100:813, 1991.
    Adjunctive therapy of ABPA with itraconazole showed promise in this small series of patients.

86. Faulkner, S.L., et al. Hemoptysis and pulmonary aspergilloma: Operative versus nonoperative treatment. *Ann. Thorac. Surg.* 25:389, 1978.

87. Gerson, S.L., et al. Prolonged granulocytopenia: The major risk factor for invasive pulmonary aspergillosis in patients with acute leukemia. *Ann. Intern. Med.* 100: 345, 1984.
    Prolonged granulocytopenia was strongly associated with the development of IPA.

88. Denning, D.W., et al. Pulmonary aspergillosis in the acquired immunodeficiency syndrome. *N. Engl. J. Med.* 324:654, 1991.

89. Pursell, K.J., Telzak, E.E., and Armstrong, D. *Aspergillus* species colonization and invasive disease in patients with AIDS. *Clin. Infect. Dis.* 14:141, 1992.
    The two preceding articles document the occurrence and manifestations of invasive aspergillosis in HIV-infected patients. For a related discussion, see S.H. Khoo and D.W. Denning, Invasive aspergillosis in patients with AIDS. Clin. Infect. Dis. *(Suppl. 1):S41, 1994.*

90. Binder, R.E., et al. Chronic necrotizing aspergillosis: A discrete clinical entity. *Medicine* 61:109, 1982.
    Good review of a rare infectious disease.

91. Aisner, J., Schimpff, S.C., and Wiernik, P.H. Treatment of invasive aspergillosis: Relation of early diagnosis and treatment to response. *Ann. Intern. Med.* 86:539, 1977.
    Early diagnosis and treatment of invasive disease are associated with improved outcome.

92. Denning, D.W., and Stevens, D.A. Antifungal and surgical treatment of invasive aspergillosis: Review of 2,121 published cases. *Rev. Infect. Dis.* 12:1147, 1990.

93. Young, R.C., et al. Aspergillosis: The spectrum of the disease in 98 patients. *Medicine* 49:147, 1970.
    Extensive, classic review of the common sites of infection, predisposing factors, and response to therapy.

94. Denning, D.W., et al. NIAID Mycoses Study Group multicenter trial of oral itraconazole therapy of invasive aspergillosis. *Am. J. Med.* 97:135, 1994.
    In this study of 76 patients, 39% of patients had a complete or partial response to oral itraconazole. This response rate is similar to the overall response rate with amphotericin B, which is in the 30–35% range. Median duration of therapy with oral itraconazole in this study was 46 weeks. Because of side effects from itraconazole, 7% of patients withdrew from the study. The authors conclude that oral itraconazole is a useful alternative therapy for invasive aspergillosis, with response rates apparently comparable to amphotericin B.

94a. Horvatch, J.A., and Dummer, S. The use of respiratory-tract cultures in the diagnosis of invasive pulmonary aspergillosis. *Am. J. Med.* 100:171, 1996.

94b. Duthie, R., and Denning, D.W. Aspergillus fungemia: Report of two cases and review. *Clin. Infect. Dis.* 20:598, 1995.
    Media contamination can cause false-positive blood cultures which may cause problems in the interpretation of the significance of the blood cultures.

95. Karp, J.E., Burch, P.A., and Merz, W.G. An approach to intensive antileukemia therapy in patients with previous invasive aspergillosis. *Am. J. Med.* 85:203, 1988.
    These investigators favor prophylactic use of amphotericin B so that repeat courses of chemotherapy can be given without the occurrence of reactivation of disease.

96. Kammer, R.B., and Utz, J.P. *Aspergillus* species endocarditis. The new face of a not so rare disease. *Am. J. Med.* 56:506, 1974.

97. Spector, J.G., et al. Allergic *Aspergillus* sinusitis: Concepts in diagnosis and treatment of a new clinical entity. *Laryngoscope* 97:261, 1987.

98. Al-Dorry, Y., and DiSalvo, A.F. (eds.). *Blastomycosis.* New York: Plenum Medical Book, 1992.
    A comprehensive, multiauthored text.

99. Bradsher, R.W. Blastomycosis. *Infect. Dis. Clin. North Am.* 2:877–898, 1988.
    Concise review of this topic with discussion of therapeutic options. Colored photographs of skin lesions are shown.

100. Chapman, S.W. *Blastomyces dermatitidis.* In G.L. Mandell, R.G. Douglas, Jr., and

R. Dolin (eds.), *Principles and Practice of Infectious Diseases* (4th ed.). New York: Churchill Livingstone, 1995. P. 2353.

101. Klein, B.S., et al. Isolation of *Blastomyces dermatitidis* in soil associated with a large outbreak of blastomycosis in Wisconsin. *N. Engl. J. Med.* 314:529, 1986.
   An important study in defining the ecologic niche of B. dermatitidis. Additionally, this study also helps to define the clinical spectrum of acute infection. Only 50% or so of infected individuals developed symptomatic disease.

102. Klein, B.S., et al. Two outbreaks of blastomycosis along river banks in Wisconsin are described. Isolation of *B. dermatitidis* from river bank soil and evidence of transmission along waterways is obtained. *Am. Rev. Respir. Dis.* 136:1333, 1987.

103. Pappas, P.G., et al. Blastomycosis in patients with acquired immunodeficiency syndrome. *Ann. Intern. Med.* 116:847, 1992.
   Blastomycosis was a late complicating infection in a few patients with AIDS. Most patients had CD4 counts of fewer than 200 / mm³. Disease was frequently disseminated, CNS disease was common, and mortality was high despite therapy.

104. Pappas, P.G., et al. Blastomycosis in immunocompromised patients. *Medicine* 72: 311, 1993.
   Blastomycosis has been reported in patients treated with corticosteroids, patients with hematologic malignancies, transplant recipients, and patients with a variety of other immunosuppressive disorders.

105. Sarosi, G.A., Davies, S.F., and Phillips, J.R. Self-limited blastomycosis: A report of 39 cases. *Semin. Respir. Infect.* 1:40, 1986.

106. Brown, L.R., et al. Roentgenologic features of pulmonary blastomycosis. *Mayo Clin. Proc.* 66:29, 1991.
   Mass lesions suggestive of bronchogenic carcinoma were the most common roentgenologic finding.

107. Baumgardner, D.J., et al. Epidemiology of blastomycosis in a region of high endemnicity in North Central Wisconsin. *Clin. Infect. Dis.* 15:720, 1992.
   Isolated pulmonary disease was noted in 77% of the 73 patients reported in this series.

108. Turner, S., and Kaufman, L. Immunodiagnosis of blastomycosis. *Semin. Respir. Infect.* 1:22, 1986.

109. Klein, B.S., et al. Comparison of enzyme immunoassay, immunodiffusion and complement fixation tests in detecting antibody in human serum to the A antigen of *B. dermatitidis. Am. Rev. Respir. Dis.* 133:144, 1986.
   A positive immunodiffusion serology was more common in patients with disseminated disease (88%) than in patients with localized disease (33%) in this study.

110. Klein, B.S., and Jones, J.M. Isolation, purification, and radiolabeling of a novel 120-KD surface protein on *Blastomyces dermatitidis* yeasts to detect antibody in infected patients. *J. Clin. Invest.* 85:152, 1990.

111. Bradsher, R.W., Rice, D.C., and Abernathy, R.S. Ketoconazole therapy for endemic blastomycosis. *Ann. Intern. Med.* 103:872, 1985.
   Ketoconazole therapy was successful in 35 of 44 patients (80%) with blastomycosis in this trial.

112. Rinaldi, M.G. Zygomycosis. *Infect. Dis. Clin. North Am.* 3:19, 1989.

113. Sugar, A.M. Mucormycosis. *Clin. Infect. Dis.* 14:S126, 1992.

114. Boelaert, J.R., Fenves, A.Z., and Coburn, J.W. Deferoxamine therapy and mucormycosis in dialysis patients: Report of an international registry. *Am. J. Kidney Dis.* 18:660, 1991.
   Mucormycosis has been diagnosed in a substantial number of dialysis patients receiving treatment with the chelating agent deferoxamine.

115. Parfrey, N.A. Improved diagnosis and prognosis of mucormycosis. *Medicine* 65:113, 1986.

116. Rothstein, R.D., and Simon, G.L. Subacute pulmonary mucormycosis. *J. Med. Vet. Mycol.* 24:391, 1986.

117. Gartenberg, G., and Bottone, E. Hospital-acquired mucormycosis (*Rhizopus rhizopodiformis*) of skin and subcutaneous tissue. *N. Engl. J. Med.* 299:1115, 1978.
   Cutaneous mucormycosis in association with the use of an occlusive bandage was identified in several patients.

118. Ingram, C.W., et al. Disseminated zygomycosis: Report of four cases and review. *Rev. Infect. Dis.* 11:741, 1989.

119. Winn, R.E. Sporotrichosis. *Infect. Dis. Clin. North Am.* 2:899, 1988.
   Excellent review.

120. Blumer, S.D., et al. Comparative evaluation of five serological methods for the diagnosis of sporotrichosis. *Appl. Microbiol.* 26:4, 1973.

121. Restrepo, A., et al. Itraconazole therapy in lymphangitic and cutaneous sporotrichosis. *Arch. Dermatol.* 122:413, 1986.
122. Sharkey-Mathis, P.K., et al. Treatment of sporotrichosis with itraconazole. *Am. J. Med.* 95:279, 1993.
    This and the preceding study provide impressive evidence of the efficacy and favorable side effect profile of itraconazole in the treatment of sporotrichosis.
123. Pluss, J.L., and Opal, S.M. Pulmonary sporotrichosis: Review of treatment and outcome. *Medicine* 65:143, 1986.
124. Winn, R.E., et al. Systemic sporotrichosis treated with itraconazole. *Clin. Infect. Dis.* 17:210, 1993.
125. Crout, J.E., Brewer, N.S., and Tompkins, R.B. Sporotrichosis arthritis. Clinical features in seven patients. *Ann. Intern. Med.* 86:294, 1977.
    Good description of the manifestations of articular disease due to sporotrichosis.
126. Lynch, P.J., Voorhees, J.J., and Harrell, E.R. Systemic sporotrichosis. *Ann. Intern. Med.* 73:23, 1970.
    Description of a rare disease, occurring usually in the immunosuppressed host.
127. Heller, H.M., and Fuhrer, J. Disseminated sporotrichosis in patients with AIDS: Case report and review of the literature. *AIDS* 5:1243, 1991.
    Disseminated sporotrichosis has been identified as another manifestation of infection with HIV.
128. Scott, E.N., et al. Serologic studies in the diagnosis and management of meningitis due to *Sporothrix schenckii. N. Engl. J. Med.* 317:935, 1987.
    Serologic studies performed on the CSF were valuable aids in the diagnosis of meningitis due to S. schenckii.
129. Brummer, E., Castaneda, E., and Restrepo, A. Paracoccidioidomycosis: An update. *Clin. Microbiol. Rev.* 6:89, 1993.
    Detailed, comprehensive review.
130. McGinnis, M.R., and Fader, R.C. Mycetoma: A contemporary concept. *Infect. Dis. Clin. North Am.* 2:939, 1988.
131. Vartivarian, S.E., Anaissie, E.J., and Bodey, G.P. Emerging fungal pathogens in immunocompromised patients: Classification, diagnosis, and management. *Clin. Infect. Dis.* 17:S487, 1993.
    Several fungal organisms, formerly only rarely associated with invasive disease, are now being identified with increasing frequency as a cause of clinical disease in immunosuppressed patients.
132. Walling, D.M., et al. Disseminated infection with *Trichosporon beigelii. Rev. Infect. Dis.* 9:1013, 1987.
    Most patients with trichosporonosis have had hematologic malignancies and neutropenia.
133. Barber, G.R., et al. Catheter-related *Malassezia furfur* fungemia in immunocompromised patients. *Am. J. Med.* 95:365, 1993.
    M. furfur fungemia related to indwelling catheters usually occurs in the setting of a compromised immune system. Intravenous lipids are not a necessary predisposing factor.
134. Gamis, A.S., et al. Disseminated infection with *Fusarium* in recipients of bone marrow transplants. *Rev. Infect. Dis.* 13:1077, 1991.
    Disseminated infection with Fusarium is associated with a particularly poor prognosis.
135. Travis, L.B., Roberts, G.D., and Wilson, W.R. Clinical significance of *Pseudallescheria boydii:* A review of ten years' experience. *Mayo Clin. Proc.* 60:531, 1985.
    Good description of a large series of patients with various manifestations of infection with P. boydii.
136. Hilmarsdottir, I., et al. Disseminated *Penicillium marneffei* infection associated with the human immunodeficiency virus: A report of two cases and a review of 35 published cases. *J. Acquir. Immune Defic. Syndr.* 6:466, 1993.
    Disseminated infection with P. marneffei is being diagnosed with greater frequency in AIDS patients in Southeast Asia.
137. Gallis, H.A., Drew, R.H., and Pickard, W.W. Amphotericin B: 30 years of clinical experience. *Rev. Infect. Dis.* 12:308, 1990.
    A comprehensive review with a bibliography of 190 references.
137a. Goodwin, S.D., et al. Pretreatment regimens for adverse events related to infusion of amphotericin B. *Clin. Infect. Dis.* 20:755, 1995.
    Review of nationwide prospective surveillance of adverse reactions and the role of pretreatment regimens. Although published in 1995, much of the original data was collected in 1988.

138. Peacock, J.E., Jr., Herrington, D.A., and Cruz, J.M. Amphotericin B: Past, present, and future. *Infect. Dis. Clin. Pract.* 2:81, 1993.
139. Brajtburg, J., et al. Amphotericin B: Current understanding of mechanisms of action. *Antimicrob. Agents Chemother.* 34:183, 1990.
140. Christiansen, K.J., et al. Distribution and activity of amphotericin B in humans. *J. Infect. Dis.* 152:1037, 1985.
141. Cruz, J.M., et al. Rapid intravenous infusion of amphotericin B: A pilot study. *Am. J. Med.* 93:123, 1992.
    Similar toxicity was noted with rapid infusions (1–2 hours) vs. standard (4 hours).
142. Drutz, D.J. Rapid infusion of amphotericin B: Is it safe, effective and wise? *Am. J. Med.* 93:119, 1992.
    See related recent discussion by U. Schuler et al., Rapid infusion of amphotericin B: Is it safe, effective and wise? Am. J. Med. *99:104, 1995. The authors discuss the pros and cons of 1- to 2-hour vs. 4-hour infusions.*
143. Graybill, J.R. Therapeutic agents. *Infect. Dis. Clin. North Am.* 2:805, 1988.
144. Polsky, B., et al. Intraventricular therapy of cryptococcal meningitis via a subcutaneous reservoir. *Am. J. Med.* 81:24, 1986.
145. Cleary, J.D., Chapman, S.W., and Nolan, R.L. Pharmacologic modulation of interleukin-1 expression by amphotericin B–stimulated human mononuclear cells. *Antimicrob. Agents Chemother.* 36:977, 1992.
146. Gigliotti, F., et al. Induction of prostaglandin synthesis as the mechanism for the chills and fever produced by infusing amphotericin B. *J. Infect. Dis.* 156:784, 1987.
147. Clements, J.S., Jr., and Peacock, J.E., Jr. Amphotericin B revisited: Reassessment of toxicity. *Am. J. Med.* 88:22–27, 1990.
    A concise review of the major toxicities of amphotericin B and their management.
148. Branch, R.A. Prevention of amphotericin B–induced renal impairment: A review on the use of sodium supplementation. *Arch. Intern. Med.* 148:2389–2394, 1988.
    Oral or intravenous sodium supplementation may prevent or delay the development of renal toxicity associated with the use of amphotericin B. See related paper by A. Llanos et al., Effect of salt supplementation on amphotericin B nephrotoxicity. Kidney Int. *40:302, 1991. The authors used 1 liter of normal saline before infusions.*
149. Lin, A.C., et al. Amphotericin B blunts erythropoietin response to anemia. *J. Infect. Dis.* 161:348, 1990.
150. Wright, D.A., et al. Lethal pulmonary reactions associated with combined use of amphotericin B and leukocyte transfusions. *N. Engl. J. Med.* 304:1185, 1981.
    Amphotericin B and leukocytes should not be infused simultaneously or within a short time interval of one another.
150a. Sugar, A.M., et al. Combination therapy of murine invasive candidiasis with fluconazole and amphotericin B. *Antimicrob. Agents Chemother.* 39:598, 1995.
151. Hughes, W.T., et al. Guidelines for the use of antimicrobial agents in neutropenic patients with unexplained fever. *J. Infect. Dis.* 161:381, 1990.
    A consensus statement by an expert panel of the Infectious Diseases Society of America.
151a. Ng, T.T.C., and Denning, D.W. Liposomal amphotericin B (AmBisome) therapy in invasive fungal infections: Evaluation of United Kingdom compassionate use data. *Arch. Intern. Med.* 155:1093, 1995.
151b. Hiemenz, J.W., et al. Emergency use amphotericin B lipid complex (ABLC) in the treatment of patients with aspergillosis: Historical-control comparison with amphotericin B (abstract 3383) *Blood* 86: 1995.
    For dosage and side effects, see package insert of Abelcet (The Liposome Co., Princeton, NJ). See related references by P.K. Sharkey et al., Amphotericin B lipid complex compared with amphotericin B in the treatment of cryptococcal meningitis in patients with AIDS. Clin. Infect. Dis. *22:315, 1996, with editorial comment by Dr. W. Powderly in the same issue; E.J. Anaissie et al., Amphotericin B lipid complex versus amphotericin B for treatment of hematogenous and invasive candidiasis (abstract LM21). 35th Interscience Conference on Antimicrobial Agents and Chemotherapy. San Francisco, September 18, 1995; and S. Kline et al., Limited toxicity of prolonged therapy with high doses of amphotericin B lipid complex.* Clin. Infect. Dis. *21:1154, 1995.*
152. Francis, P., and Walsh, T.J. Evolving role of flucytosine in immunocompromised patients: New insights into safety, pharmacokinetics, and antifungal therapy. *Clin. Infect. Dis.* 15:1003, 1992.
153. Stamm, A.M., et al. Toxicity of amphotericin B plus flucytosine in 194 patients with cryptococcal meningitis. *Am. J. Med.* 83:236, 1987.
    Hematologic toxicity was noted in 22% of patients.
154. Como, J.A., and Dismukes, W.E. Oral azole drugs as systemic antifungal therapy. *N. Engl. J. Med.* 330:263, 1994.

Good review of the role of azoles in the treatment of the systemic mycoses.

155. Medical Letter. Ketoconazole (Nizoral), a new antifungal agent. *Med. Lett. Drugs Ther.* 23:85, 1981.
156. Symoens, J., et al. An evaluation of two years of clinical experience with ketoconazole. *Rev. Infect. Dis.* 2:674, 1980.
157. Honig, P.K., et al. Terfenadine-ketoconazole interaction: Pharmacokinetic and electro-cardiographic consequences. *J.A.M.A.* 269:1513, 1993.
      Life-threatening arrhythmias may occur as a result of QT prolongation associated with an interaction between ketoconazole and the antihistamine terfenadine.
157a. Klausner, M.A. Letter to Physicians. Janssen Pharmaceutica, Inc. (Titusville, NJ). October 14, 1995.
      Letter to physicians warning them of the potential of serious cardiac arrhythmias (e.g., QT prolongation, ventricular tachycardia) that have been reported in patients taking cisapride (Propulside) with other drugs that inhibit cytochrome P450, such as ketoconazole, fluconazole, itraconazole, miconazole, and erythromycin. Therefore, cisapride is contraindicated in patients taking any of these drugs.
158. Khosia, S., et al. Adrenal crisis in the setting of high-dose ketoconazole therapy. *Arch. Intern. Med.* 149:802, 1989.
159. Medical Letter. Drugs for treatment of deep fungal infections. *Med. Lett. Drugs Ther.* 36:16, 1994.
      For a related discussion, see C.L. Terrell and C.E. Hughes, Antifungal agents used for deep-seated mycotic infections. Mayo Clin. Proc. 67:69, 1992; and G.A. Sarosi and S.F. Davies, Therapy for fungal infections. Mayo Clin. Proc. 69:111, 1994. Also see Medical Letter. Drugs for AIDS and associated infections. Med. Lett. Drugs Ther. 37:87, 1995. Provides a summary of antifungal therapy for AIDS patients.
160. Bennett, J.G. Overview of the symposium on fluconazole: A novel advance in the therapy for systemic fungal infections. *Rev. Infect. Dis.* (Suppl. 3):S263, 1990.
161. Brammer, K.W., Farrow, P.R., and Faulkner, J.K. Pharmacokinetics and tissue penetration of fluconazole in humans. *Rev. Infect. Dis.* 12(Suppl. 3):S318, 1990.
162. Wingard, J.R., et al. Increase in *Candida krusei* infection among patients with bone marrow transplantation and neutropenia treated prophylactically with fluconazole. *N. Engl. J. Med.* 325:1274, 1991.
163. Goodman, J.L., et al. A controlled trial of fluconazole to prevent fungal infections in patients undergoing bone marrow transplantation. *N. Engl. J. Med.* 376:845, 1992.
      Prophylactic use of fluconazole in bone marrow transplant recipients was associated with a decrease in fungal infections in these two trials. However, an increased incidence of infection with C. krusei was noted, and there was no overall impact on mortality.
163a. Rex, J.H., et al. Minireview: Resistance of *Candida* species to fluconazole. *Antimicrob. Agents Chemother.* 39:1, 1995.
      Resistance may be due either to the acquisition of inherently resistant species of Candida (e.g., C. glabrata and C. krusei) or to the acquisition of resistance in a previously susceptible strain. For related papers, see D.W. Denning, Can we prevent azole resistance in fungi? Lancet 346:454, 1995; and J.R. Maenza et al., Risk factors for fluconazole-resistant candidiasis in HIV-infected patients. J. Infect. Dis. 173:219, 1996.
163b. Trapnell, C.B., et al. Increased plasma rifabutin levels with concomitant fluconazole therapy in HIV-infected patients. *Ann. Intern. Med.* 124:573, 1996.
164. Grant, S.M., and Clissold, S.P. Itraconazole: A review of its pharmacodynamic and pharmacokinetic properties, and therapeutic use in superficial and systemic mycoses. *Drugs* 37:310, 1989.
      Also see Medical Letter, Itraconazole. Med. Lett. Drugs Ther. 35:7, 1993.
164a. Medical Letter. Itraconazole for onychomycosis. *Med. Lett. Drug. Ther.* 38:5, 1996.
165. Crane, J.K., and Shih, H. Syncope and cardiac arrhythmia due to an interaction between itraconazole and terfenadine. *Am. J. Med.* 95:445, 1993.
      Also see United States Food and Drug Administration, New box warning added for Seldane, Hismanal. F.D.A. Med. Bull. 22:2, 1992, and 23:2, 1993.
166. Araujo, O.E., Flowers, F.P., and King, M.M. Griseofulvin: A new look at an old drug. *DICP* 24:851, 1990.
      Good review of therapeutic uses and side effects of griseofulvin.
167. Weese, W.C., and Smith, I.M. A study of 57 cases of actinomycosis over a 36-year period. *Arch. Intern. Med.* 135:1562, 1975.
168. Tomm, K.E., Raleigh, J.W., and Guinn, G.A. Thoracic actinomycosis. *Am. J. Surg.* 124:465, 1972.
169. Burkman, R., et al. The relationship of genital tract actinomycetes and the development of pelvic inflammatory disease. *Am. J. Obstet. Gynecol.* 143:585, 1982.

169a. Medical Letter. The choice of antibacterial drugs. *Med. Lett. Drugs Ther.* 38:25, 1996.
   Penicillin remains the drug of choice for actinomycosis, whereas trimethoprim-sulfa-methoxazole is the agent of choice for Nocardia *infections.*
170. Berkey, P., and Bodey, G.P. Nocardial infection in patients with neoplastic disease. *Rev. Infect. Dis.* 11:407, 1989.
   Good review of nocardiosis in cancer patients. For a very recent "state-of-the-art" review, see P.I. Lerner, Nocardiosis. Clin. Infect. Dis. *22:891, 1996.*
171. Wilson, J.P., et al. Nocardial infection in renal transplant patients. *Medicine* 68:38, 1989.
   Extensive review of nocardiosis in kidney transplant recipients.
172. Chapman, S.W., and Wilson, J.P. Nocardiosis in transplant recipients. *Semin. Respir. Med.* 5:74, 1990.
173. Wallace, R.J., et al. Use of trimethoprim-sulfamethoxazole for treatment of infections due to *Nocardia. Rev. Infect. Dis.* 4:315, 1982.
174. Gombert, M.E. Susceptibility of *Nocardia asteroides* to various antibiotics, including newer beta-lactams, trimethoprim-sulfamethoxazole, amikacin and *N*-formidoyl thienamycin. *Antimicrob. Agents Chemother.* 21:1101, 1982.

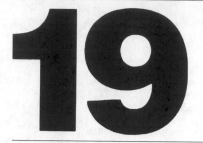

Acquired Immunodeficiency Syndrome

Alice C. Furman,
Kent A. Sepkowitz,
and Rosemary Soave

In 1981, **AIDS** was first reported in previously healthy men [1]. Since then, the catastrophic nature of this epidemic has been recognized and more fully characterized. As of **June 1995**, the Centers for Disease Control (CDC), Atlanta, has received reports of **476,899 cases of AIDS** in the United States, including more than 6,611 children; more than 60% of adults and more than 55% of children with the disease have died [2]. Only 1.4% of cases are in children less than 13 years old [2]. Whites account for 50% of cases, blacks 32%, and Hispanics 17% [2]. Although the overall picture remains grim, significant advances have been made in establishing the epidemiologic features, characterizing the immunopathology, and delineating the clinical manifestations of this infection. A retrovirus, the **human immunodeficiency virus** (HIV), was identified and described as the causative agent in 1983–1984 [3–5]. In addition, in 1987 the first drug, **azidothymidine** (AZT, zidovudine), was approved for antiviral therapy for the disease [6]. The impact of the epidemic, initially felt throughout the medical community, has now come to bear on the entire world. Unraveling the medical and scientific mysteries of HIV infection as well as dealing with the social, political, and economic upheaval precipitated by AIDS will challenge us for years to come.

It is beyond the scope of this chapter to provide a comprehensive list of the rapidly proliferating AIDS literature. Furthermore, due to the tremendous activity in this field, the key articles of today quickly become either classics or obsolete. It is hoped that the references provided in this chapter will serve as stepping stones for the reader who wants to delve further into selected aspects of this disease. **The reader also is directed to various sources that are both practical and useful for keeping up with progress in this disease.** They include: (1) the *Proceedings of the International AIDS Conference,* held in summer each year (e.g., Berlin, 1993; Yokohama, 1994); (2) the *AIDS Commentary Series,* a monthly review article provided in the periodical *Clinical Infectious Diseases;* (3) the monthly *HIV/AIDS Surveillance Report* [7] and frequent *Morbidity and Mortality Weekly Reports;* and (4) *The AIDS Reader,* published six times yearly. In addition, there are a number of recently published reviews and books that deal with the topic [9–16].

The epidemiology, transmission and pathophysiology, and clinical aspects of HIV infection are discussed in this chapter. More detailed discussions of related topics appear in separate chapters (e.g., CNS infections such as cryptococcal meningitis and neurosyphilis in Chap. 5, *Mycobacterium tuberculosis* in Chap. 9, fungal infections in Chap. 18, and the prevention and treatment of *Pneumocystis carinii* pneumonia in Chap. 24). **The indications for and agents used in antiviral therapy for HIV disease are reviewed in detail in Chap. 26.**

I. Epidemiologic features
A. Scope of the epidemic
1. United States
a. **AIDS.** As of June 1995, there have been 476,899 cases reported to the CDC [2]. Eighty-eight percent of patients are between 20 and 49 years of age; of these, 86% are males. Twenty-six percent of the patients are residents of New York City, Los Angeles, or San Francisco [2]. Since 1981,

---

Editors' Note: Because many textbooks cover exclusively the rapidly expanding topic of AIDS and because each week multiple journal articles are published on the evolving therapy of HIV infection and its complications, it would be inappropriate to attempt to cover HIV infection comprehensively in a single chapter in this text. Instead, as indicated in the introduction, this chapter is intended to offer an overview of the broad spectrum of HIV infection. It should help to orient the student and practitioner who occasionally see patients with HIV-related problems.

more than 295,373 patients with AIDS in the United States have died [2, 7, 17].

b. **Seropositive persons (asymptomatic HIV carriers).** The CDC estimates that currently more than 1 million people in the United States are infected with HIV [18]. HIV serosurveys based on blood specimens from newborn infants indicate that 1,500–2,000 HIV-infected infants (0.5 per 1,000 births) were born in 1989 [18]; in a recent report, from 1978–1993, approximately 14,290 HIV-infected infants were born in the United States [18a]. Data from the US Department of Defense indicate that approximately 0.6–0.8 per 1,000 active-duty personnel acquired HIV infection each year since 1986 [19, 20].

c. The **estimated cost** of AIDS in the United States will exceed billions of dollars in the coming years [21, 22].

2. **The world**

a. **AIDS** has been reported throughout the world [23]. The World Health Organization (WHO) estimates there are 11 million seropositive persons worldwide and more than 13 million infected since the beginning of the epidemic [24]. More than 1 million cases are in children. The rate of new infection is rapid: Approximately 1 million new persons become infected every 6 months [24]. Between 600,000 and 2.5 million cases of AIDS have occurred worldwide.

b. **Geographically,** Africa (6.5 million), Asia (2 million), and Latin America (1.5 million) have the highest incidences of infection [25]. The number of cases in Africa is staggering: **Sub-Saharan Africa** currently accounts for nearly 60% of the 11 million infections worldwide [25]. Recently, alarmingly sharp increases in infection rates have been reported from **Thailand** and **India.** In Thailand in 1992, 23.8% of commercial sex workers were seropositive in one survey [25]. Serosurveys of male military recruits revealed that 3.5% were seropositive countrywide; in some areas, more than 10% were seropositive [26, 27]. Reporting is less well developed in India, where WHO estimates that more than 1 million persons are seropositive. In Bombay, WHO estimates that 20% of commercial sex workers are infected. High rates of infection among intravenous drug users in India also are suspected. This explosive increase has led to concern that the number of new infections in Asia may surpass that in Africa by the end of the decade [25].

c. Estimates place the number of **asymptomatic HIV carriers** at more than 10 million worldwide, with a continued exponential increase anticipated.

B. **Transmission.** There are three recognized ways to become infected.

1. **Sexual contact** with an infected person **is the predominant mode of transmission worldwide.**

a. **Homosexual and bisexual men** account for 54% of US cases, with an additional 6% having both intravenous drug use and homosexual activity as risk factors. Multiple sexual partners and receptive anal intercourse appear to be major risk factors [28–30]. Homosexual activity is the main mode of transmission in North America, Europe, and Australia [25, 29]. In 1987, a decline in the incidence of new HIV infections attributable to homosexual transmission was noted [18].

b. **Heterosexual contact** with an infected person **as a risk factor for acquiring HIV has dramatically increased in the United States** from 1.9% to 9.0% from 1985 through 1993. In 1993, the number of AIDS cases attributed to heterosexual contact increased 130% over that in 1992, and it is estimated that this trend will continue [31]. **In the rest of the world, this is the dominant mode of transmission.** The **presence of coincident genital ulcers,** especially chancroid, in either the male or the female partner and lack of male circumcision have been suggested as possible risk factors [32–34]. In a study of infected hemophiliac men and their female sexual partners, HIV transmission occurred more readily as HIV infection progressed [35]. Recently, it has been shown that antiretroviral treatment of men infected with HIV reduced the incidence of heterosexual transmission [36].

2. **Parenteral exposure** to infected blood or blood products

a. **Intravenous drug use** accounts for 24% of US cases, with an additional

6% of cases having both intravenous drug use and homosexuality as risk factors. Transmission occurs when needles or other paraphernalia is shared. **The proportion of AIDS cases attributable to intravenous drug use continues to increase** [2, 37].

b. **Transfusion of infected blood or blood components** [38–40] as a risk factor for acquiring HIV has **dramatically decreased** in incidence **secondary to the availability of a screening blood test and the mandatory screening of all blood products since 1987.** New cases reported are usually secondary to transfusions received prior to 1987, as the risk of acquiring HIV from blood products today is exceedingly low. A study published in December 1995 demonstrated that, in the United States, the estimated risk of transmitting HIV by transfusion of screened blood is very small: one case of transmission for every 450,000–600,000 donations of screened blood [41]. However, the likelihood of becoming infected with HIV after receiving an HIV-positive, single-donor blood product approaches 100% [42, 43].

   (1) **Hemophiliacs** (1% of US cases). The risk of infection has been significantly decreased with implementation of blood-screening procedures and heat treatment of clotting factors [44].

   (2) **Recipients of transfusions,** including whole blood, blood cellular components, plasma, and clotting factors (2% of US cases). However, it has become clear that **recipients of other prepared blood or plasma products, including immunoglobulin, the prior plasma-derived hepatitis B vaccine, and hyperimmune serum, are not at any risk of seroconversion** [45–47]. In Africa, transfusions given for treatment of the anemia associated with malaria and sickle cell disease account for an undetermined but substantial number of cases [17].

   (3) **Recipients of tissue,** including organ transplants and semen (see Chap. 20) [48].

   (4) **Health care workers.** Health care workers have uncommonly become infected following exposure to infected blood via needlestick or through disrupted skin or mucous membranes [49–51]. **The probability of HIV infection after skin puncture with infected materials is estimated to be 0.3–0.5%** [52, 53]. The risk of infection following exposure of nonintact skin and mucous membranes is far lower. The size of the inoculum appears to play a role [52–55]. Health care workers who have sustained needlesticks but have not seroconverted do show increased HIV-specific helper T-cell activity [56]. (See Chap. 26.)

3. **Perinatal transmission** may occur in utero, during birth, or via breast-feeding [17, 57–60]. There is an inherent problem documenting seropositivity in infants because of their **immature immune systems** and due to the **presence of passively acquired maternal antibody.** Prospective studies suggest that perinatal transmission rates range from 22 to 46% [61]. In a recent report, vertical (mother-to-infant) transmission occurred in 15–30% of children born to HIV infected women in the United States [18a]. Mothers with more advanced disease are more likely to give birth to infected children. Maternal infection does not appear to increase the risk of adverse outcomes in pregnancy [62]. **Maternal and neonatal therapy with zidovudine** (see Chap. 26) has recently been shown to **decrease vertical transmission dramatically** to approximately 10% of all newborns [63]. This important finding has raised a difficult ethical issue about requiring HIV testing of pregnant women. Seronegative children of HIV-infected mothers appear to be at higher risk for diarrhea, and perhaps other infections, than do children of HIV-negative mothers [64].

4. Transmission by an **undetermined** route accounts for 3% of US cases. Many of these patients, when reexamined, do have a known risk factor [65, 66]: Up to 40% have a history of sexually transmitted diseases (STDs) and at least one-third of the men have had contact with prostitutes, suggesting that transmission may have occurred by established high-risk behaviors [65].

5. **HIV is not spread by casual contact.** Although HIV has been isolated from saliva, tears, urine, and cerebrospinal fluid (CSF) [17], these bodily fluids have not been implicated in the transmission of HIV [66–68]. The CDC has reported transmission in exceptional circumstances, including between siblings and from a dentist to his patients [69, 70]. It is important to realize that these rare transmissions are the exception and not the rule [71–73].

> a. **Household contacts not sexually involved** with infected persons **are not at risk** for acquiring AIDS. In seroprevalence studies, family members who shared bathrooms and eating utensils with AIDS patients did not become infected [74, 75].
> b. **Mosquitoes do not transmit AIDS** [76].
> c. One of 1,800 surveyed **dental care workers** has become infected from an infected patient [77].
> d. **No cases of transmission from human bites** have been reported. Saliva contains HIV but may also contain neutralizing factors [78, 79].
> e. The risk of contracting HIV by being treated by a seropositive health care worker is small [71–73]. Routine screening of all health care workers does not appear to be cost-effective [80].

II. Etiologic features

A. Background.
In 1984, a **retrovirus** was identified as the causative agent of AIDS in three different laboratories. The virus was named *human T-lymphotropic virus type III* (HTLV-III) at the National Cancer Institute in Bethesda, Maryland [4], lymphadenopathy-associated virus (LAV) at the Pasteur Institute [3], and AIDS-related virus (ARV) at the University of California, San Francisco [5]. After much debate, an international committee adopted the name **human immunodeficiency virus (HIV)** [81]. It has been speculated that this retrovirus has been implicated as an etiologic agent of sporadic, unexplained cases of immunodeficiency that occurred in the 1950s and 1960s [82, 83].

B. Structure and function
1. HIV is an RNA virus that belongs to the lentivirus subfamily of human retroviruses. As a retrovirus, HIV codes for an enzyme, RNA-dependent DNA polymerase or reverse transcriptase, and is thus able to produce DNA from its native RNA. Other properties that HIV shares with lentiviruses include a long genome, highly variable envelope genes, and cytopathic properties in cell culture [3–5, 84, 85].
2. **The mature virion** is composed of a central core surrounded by a spherical lipid envelope that it acquires by budding from the surface of an infected cell. The core contains the reverse transcriptase enzyme in intimate association with two strands of RNA that are structurally similar although sequentially different copies of one another [3–5, 85, 86].

C. HIV life cycle (Fig. 19-1)
1. **Free virus** and possibly virus-infected cells enter the blood during initial infection.
2. **Virus envelope glycoprotein (gp120)** attaches avidly to **CD4 receptors,** although entry occurs into cells without CD4 receptors.
3. The virus **envelope** fuses with the native cell plasma membrane.
4. The **inner core** is removed, freeing the retroviral RNA.
5. Using its **retroviral reverse transcriptase,** the HIV initiates viral DNA synthesis, using its own RNA as a template.
6. Once synthesized, the **proviral DNA** enters the nuclear cytoplasm and is integrated into the native cell's DNA.
7. **Retroviral synthesis** is begun, directed by the cell's infected DNA.
8. New viral particles are produced by budding at the cell plasma membrane.
9. Mature viral cores are produced through action on viral protease *after* budding.
10. **The complete virus** is extruded into the bloodstream.

D. Pathogenesis [86, 87].
HIV infects many different types of cells. The viral gp120 envelope has an affinity for cells expressing the CD4 receptor. Cells that do not express CD4 can also be infected, but the mechanisms currently are unknown.
1. **CD4 T lymphocytes** (helper cells) are depleted progressively by HIV infection, leading to decreased **cell-mediated immunity,** the arm of the immune system that is primarily responsible for containing intracellular pathogens (e.g., viruses, *M. tuberculosis,* and *Toxoplasma gondii*) and humoral immunity; CD4 cell depletion results in an overall lessening of immune function. Thus, HIV infection of CD4 cells destroys the very cells required to control the retrovirus [87]. There is evidence that HIV infection of CD4 cells results in **qualitative impairment** as well [87–89]. As a person's CD4 cell count falls below 200/mm^3, the likelihood of developing opportunistic infections increases. **Depression of T-cell function appears to be most pronounced in AIDS patients with opportunistic infections** [87].
2. **Monocytes and macrophages** are the scavengers of the immune system. HIV infection of these cells occurs either by attachment to the CD4 receptor or by

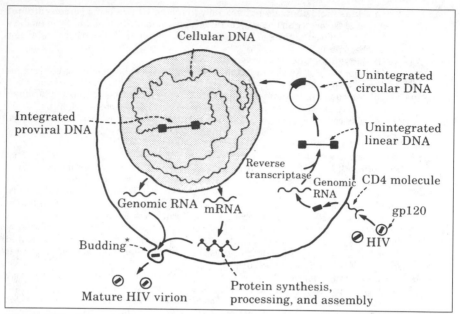

Fig. 19-1. The life cycle of human immunodeficiency virus (*HIV*). (From A. S. Fauci, The human immunodeficiency virus: Infectivity and mechanisms of pathogenesis. *Science* 239:619. Copyright © 1988, American Association for the Advancement of Science.) *Immature viral particles bud.

macrophage phagocytosis of whole HIV [90–95]. The monocyte-macrophage is relatively resistant to the cytopathic effects of the virus. **Once within the macrophage, HIV remains undetected by the body's immune surveillance system and may replicate freely. Thus, the macrophage may serve as both a haven and a reservoir for HIV.** Infected macrophages appear to have impaired chemotaxis, but the implications of this defect are unclear [96].

3. Macrophages may introduce HIV to the **brain** and contribute to the AIDS dementia complex [97, 98]. The infected macrophages may induce an inflammatory response or may activate or infect glial cells. Activated glial cells in turn may harbor HIV [99].

4. Many other cells including **bone marrow cells, B cells, myocardial cells, and cells lining the GI tract** all have been described to harbor HIV. Thus, primary infection by HIV into many cells in the body occurs, and may contribute greatly to various clinical syndromes, such as pancytopenia and diarrhea.

E. **Factors favoring transmission.** Despite our understanding much about transmission, the failure of some high-risk persons to become infected and, conversely, the infection of persons after a single sexual contact, demonstrates that crucial aspects determining transmission are not fully understood. In general, **three factors** must be considered: the status of the **host,** the infectious **inoculum size,** and the relative **virulence of the organism.**

1. **Preconditioning host factors** have long been suspected to play a role, and numerous cofactors have been suggested, including human herpesvirus 6, mycoplasma infection, Epstein-Barr virus, cytomegalovirus, hepatitis B, syphilis, or other STDs [32, 100]. Although no specific cofactor has been found, this remains an area of active research.

2. **The size of infecting HIV inoculum** probably plays a role. This is suggested by studies demonstrating that transmission rates are increased according to the immune status of the host. Immunocompromised hemophiliacs [35, 101] are more likely to transmit infection, presumably due to a high viral load.

3. **Variation exists among HIV strains** [102], and apparent differences in virulence have been noted, including the ability to induce syncytium formation in one laboratory test. However, the association between many virulence factors detected in vitro and actual viral virulence in the human host is poorly understood.

III. The clinical spectrum of HIV infection. The spectrum of HIV infection **is a continuum** from **asymptomatic carriage** to **advanced AIDS,** with a number of intermediate stages. These have been referred to as **AIDS prodrome, pre-AIDS,** or the **AIDS-related complex** (ARC), though the latter term now is used less often. Improved definition of the various stages of HIV infection and identification of HIV-related infections and neoplastic and idiopathic complications became possible with the availability of serologic testing for the retrovirus. As a result of early identification and longitudinal monitoring of HIV-positive individuals, knowledge of the **natural history** of this infection continues to evolve, thus providing greater uniformity in the care of patients and in assessing response to therapeutic strategies [100].

- **A. Classification of HIV infection. Several systems have been proposed.**
  - **1. CDC definition: evolution over time**
    - **a.** In 1982, soon after AIDS was first described, the CDC developed a **case definition,** based on **clinical, immunologic,** and **epidemiologic** features of the first cases. The diagnosis of AIDS was based on the presence of a reliably diagnosed disease at least moderately indicative of underlying cellular immunodeficiency in a person without recognized cause (e.g., neoplastic disease, immunosuppressive therapy) for such a susceptibility [103].
    - **b.** In 1984, the term **ARC** was coined to describe the symptoms of immunodeficiency that were being recognized with increased frequency in persons at risk for AIDS [104]. The symptoms included **unexplained generalized lymphadenopathy, idiopathic thrombocytopenia, oral candidiasis, herpes zoster infection, and a constitutional wasting syndrome. This is now more commonly referred to as** *symptomatic HIV infection.*
    - **c.** In 1984–1985, development of **serologic testing** to identify HIV-infected persons led to further delineation of the spectrum of HIV-associated disease.
    - **d. In 1986, the CDC defined a classification system for the spectrum of HIV infection** to accommodate the increased number of clinical manifestations that had become associated with chronic HIV infection [105]. The new system classified the manifestations of HIV infection into acute infection, asymptomatic infection, persistent generalized lymphadenopathy, and certain other categories.
    - **e. In 1987, the CDC expanded its definition of AIDS** in order to track more effectively the morbidity associated with HIV infection [106].
    - **f. More recently, in 1993, the CDC issued a revised classification system for HIV** infection and expanded the AIDS surveillance case definition. In addition to the original 23 clinical conditions outlined in 1987, the new case definition includes all patients who have fewer than 200 CD4 T lymphocytes or a CD4 T-lymphocyte percentage of total lymphocytes of fewer than 14. In addition, patients with pulmonary tuberculosis, recurrent bacterial pneumonia, and invasive cervical cancer now are included in the AIDS case definition [107]. **The expanded definition for AIDS is summarized in Tables 19-1 and 19-2.**

      The new definition is most useful for surveillance and administrative purposes. It has also fostered the concept that some of the diseases originally considered part of symptomatic HIV infection are now accepted as representing AIDS (i.e., an HIV-infected person can be considered to have AIDS even in the absence of life-threatening opportunistic infections).
      - **(1) Criteria for HIV infection for persons age 13 years or older** include (1) repeatedly reactive screening tests for HIV antibody (e.g., enzyme immunoassay) with specific antibody identified by the use of supplemental tests (e.g., Western blot, immunofluorescence assay); (2) direct identification of virus in host tissues by virus isolation; (3) HIV antigen detection; or (4) a positive result on any other highly specific licensed test for HIV [107].
      - **(2) Table 19-1** demonstrates the three categories corresponding to CD4 T-lymphocyte counts. The percentage of CD4 cells also can be used, with 29% or higher similar to CD4 counts of 500 or more, 14–28% similar to CD4 counts of 200–499, and less than 14% similar to CD4 counts of less than 200.
      - **(3) Table 19-2** summarizes the clinical categories.

Table 19-1. 1993 revised classification system for HIV infection and expanded AIDS surveillance case definition for adolescents and adults*

CD4+ T-cell categories	Clinical categories		
	(A) Asymptomatic, acute (primary) HIV or PGL	(B) Symptomatic, not (A) or (C) conditions	(C) AIDS-indicator conditions
(1) ≥500/mm³	A1	B1	C1
(2) 200–499/mm³	A2	B2	C2
(3) <200/mm³ AIDS-indicator T-cell count	A3	B3	C3

PGL = persistent generalized lymphadenopathy.
*Categories A3, B3, C1, C2, and C3 comprise the expanded AIDS surveillance case definition. Persons with AIDS-indicator conditions (category C) as well as those with CD4+ T-lymphocyte counts of fewer than 200/mm³ (category A3 or B3) will be reportable as AIDS cases in the United States and Territories, effective January 1, 1993.
Source: From Centers for Disease Control, 1993 Revised classification system for HIV infection and expanded surveillance case definition for AIDS among adolescents and adults. *M.M.W.R.* 41(RR-17): 1–19, 1992.

Table 19-2. Clinical categories

Category A
Category A consists of one or more of the following conditions in an adolescent or adult (≥13 years) with documented HIV infection. Conditions listed in categories B and C must not have occurred.
  Asymptomatic HIV infection
  Persistent generalized lymphadenopathy
  Acute (primary) HIV infection with accompanying illness or history of acute HIV infection

Category B
Category B consists of symptomatic conditions in an HIV-infected adolescent or adult that are not included among conditions listed in clinical category C and that meet at least one of the following criteria: (1) the conditions are attributed to HIV infection or are indicative of a defect in cell-mediated immunity; or (2) the conditions are considered by physicians to have a clinical course or to require management that is complicated by HIV infection. **Examples** of conditions in clinical category B include **but are not limited to:**
  Bacillary angiomatosis
  Candidiasis, oropharyngeal (thrush)
  Candidiasis, vulvovaginal; persistent, frequent, or poorly responsive to therapy
  Cervical dysplasia (moderate or severe); cervical carcinoma in situ
  Constitutional symptoms, such as fever (38.5°C) or diarrhea lasting >1 month
  Hairy leukoplakia, oral
  Herpes zoster (shingles), involving at least two distinct episodes of more than one dermatome
  Idiopathic thrombocytopenic purpura
  Listeriosis
  Pelvic inflammatory disease, particularly if complicated by tuboovarian abscess
  Peripheral neuropathy
For classification purposes, category B conditions take precedence over those in category A. For example, someone previously treated for oral or persistent vaginal candidiasis (and who has not developed a category C disease) but who is now asymptomatic should be classified in clinical category B.

Category C
Category C includes the following clinical conditions as listed in the AIDS surveillance case definition. For classification purposes, once a category C condition has occurred, the person will remain in category C.

Table 19-2 (continued)

Category C (cont.)
Candidiasis of bronchi, trachea, or lungs
Candidiasis, esophageal
Cervical cancer, invasive*
Coccidioidomycosis, disseminated or extrapulmonary
Cryptococcosis, extrapulmonary
Cryptosporidiosis, chronic intestinal (>1 month's duration)
Cytomegalovirus disease (other than liver, spleen, or nodes)
Cytomegalovirus retinitis (with loss of vision)
Encephalopathy, HIV-related
Herpes simplex: chronic ulcer(s) (>1 month's duration); or bronchitis, pneumonitis,
    or esophagitis
Histoplasmosis, disseminated or extrapulmonary
Isosporiasis, chronic intestinal (>1 month's duration)
Kaposi's sarcoma
Lymphoma, Burkitt's (or equivalent term)
Lymphoma, immunoblastic (or equivalent term)
Lymphoma, primary, of brain
Mycobacterium avium complex or *M. kansasii,* disseminated or extrapulmonary
Mycobacterium tuberculosis, any site (pulmonary* or extrapulmonary)
Mycobacterium, other species or unidentified species, disseminated or
    extrapulmonary
Pneumocystis carinii pneumonia
Pneumonia, recurrent*
Progressive multifocal leukoencephalopathy
Salmonella septicemia, recurrent
Toxoplasmosis of brain
Wasting syndrome due to HIV

*Added in the 1993 expansion of the AIDS surveillance case definition.
Source: From Centers for Disease Control, 1993 Revised classification system for HIV infection
and expanded surveillance case definition for AIDS among adolescents and adults. *M.M.W.R.*
41(RR-17):1–19, 1992.

2. **The Walter Reed (WR) staging system** for HIV infection classifies patients
   on the basis of CD4 lymphocyte counts, skin-test responsiveness, and the
   presence of lymphadenopathy, oral candidiasis, and opportunistic infections
   [108, 109]. It too has limitations with respect to predictive value and needs
   prospective evaluation before its role in the management of HIV-infected
   individuals can be defined.
3. **WHO** has developed a case definition for AIDS that can be used in developing
   countries where sophisticated diagnostic technologies are lacking [109, 110].
4. **Other classification systems** based primarily on clinical and prognostic parameters have also been proposed [109].

B. **Clinical manifestations of HIV infection.** HIV infection should be considered an
   evolving process. Prototypically, a patient may progress from acute infection to
   an asymptomatic state, through progressive generalized lymphadenopathy and
   symptomatic infection to frank AIDS. In the meantime, there may be progressive
   impairment of immune function as manifested by a decrease in the CD4 cell count.
   Although it has not been determined that all HIV-infected patients will develop
   AIDS, studies show that the rate of progression is high [111] and increases as
   the length of time from initial infection increases [109, 111, 112]. **The time it
   takes to develop AIDS varies considerably and, in many patients, the intermediate stages are not identified.** Recently, attention has focused on **long-term survivors** of HIV infection.
     Although the average time from HIV infection to death is 10 years, clinical and
   immunologic decline is generally evident much earlier. Fewer than 5% of infected
   people are characterized as having nonprogressive infection because they remain
   healthy and do not have the declining CD4 lymphocyte counts that are evident
   in people with progressive disease [112a]. These patients have low levels of circulating viral particles as well as low levels of viral DNA and RNA in their peripheral-
   blood mononuclear cells [112a] and are clinically stable for 10–15 years.

1. **Acute primary HIV infection.** This is defined by the CDC as a **mononucleo-sislike syndrome,** with or without aseptic meningitis, associated with development of HIV antibody [105]. The syndrome was first recognized in 1984 [113, 114] and was further characterized subsequently [115–118].

   a. **The incubation period** is estimated to be between 1 and 12 weeks but most commonly has been reported to be between 2 and 4 weeks [113–117].

   b. **Onset** is sudden and the duration of illness is approximately 3–14 days (range, 3–49 days).

   c. **A variety of nonspecific signs and symptoms** have been associated with the acute retroviral syndrome [117, 118].

      (1) **Fever,** sweats, lethargy, **malaise,** headache, photophobia, arthralgias, myalgias, sore throat, and diarrhea are common symptoms and therefore may mimic classic infectious mononucleosis (see Chap. 17).

      (2) Although approximately one-fourth of patients have a characteristic **truncal maculopapular rash,** other patients have been reported to have a roseolalike or urticarial rash that can be localized or diffuse and last for up to 2 weeks [117–119a]. The rash has also been described as an exanthem much like that seen with other acute viral infections. Asymptomatic, oval, erythematous macules or urticarial plaques, usually 0.5–2.0 cm in diameter, may be generalized, involving the palms and soles, or affect the trunk and upper body only. The lesions may be centrally hemorrhagic, and desquamation may occur. The differential diagnosis of the rash includes viral infections (e.g., Epstein-Barr virus), *Mycoplasma* infection, and secondary syphilis [119a].

      (3) There may also be **oral aphthous ulcers** or **diffuse enanthema** of the oral cavity.

      (4) **Lymphadenopathy** commonly involves the axillary, occipital, and cervical nodes but may be generalized. It may persist for weeks to months after the primary infection.

      (5) **Neurologic manifestations** including meningoencephalitis, myelopathy, peripheral neuropathy, and Guillain-Barré syndrome have also been associated with acute HIV infection [116, 119].

      (6) **Acute opportunistic infections,** including *Candida* esophagitis, *Pneumocystis carinii* pneumonia (PCP), and toxoplasmosis, occurring at the time of acute HIV infection have also been reported.

   d. **Laboratory examination** may reveal lymphopenia, an elevated erythrocyte sedimentation rate, and elevated alkaline phosphatase and serum transaminase levels. After resolution of the infection, some patients are found to have an atypical lymphocytosis and an **inversion of the helper-suppressor T-cell ratio** (CD4/CD8). The inverted ratio (<1.0) is due to an **increase in CD8 lymphocytes** rather than a decrease in CD4 lymphocytes [115, 117]. In contrast, for patients with frank AIDS, the inverted ratio is due to decreased CD4 lymphocytes.

   e. The precise **incidence** of symptomatic acute HIV infection has not been determined. The illness has been reported in all major groups at risk for HIV infection [117].

   f. The **differential diagnosis** of the acute retroviral syndrome should include infectious mononucleosis (due to Epstein-Barr virus or cytomegalovirus), influenza, measles, rubella, herpes simplex infection, disseminated gonococcal infection, secondary syphilis, viral hepatitis, toxoplasmosis, and drug reactions. **Acute HIV infection should be considered in all patients who present with an acute febrile mononucleosislike illness, especially if they are in a high-risk group or have a rash or neurologic symptoms.**

   g. Antibodies to HIV usually are detected within **2 months after HIV exposure.** Seroconversion as early as 2 weeks as well as prolonged antigen-positive antibody-negative states have also been documented. HIV core (p24) antigen may be detected in serum and CSF within 2 weeks of exposure to HIV and may persist for weeks or months. (See the detailed discussion of HIV serologic workup in sec. IV.)

2. **Asymptomatic HIV infection.** The US Public Health Service estimates that approximately 1 million Americans are infected with HIV but are asymptomatic [120]. **Evidence suggests that this period of latency is, in fact, a time of intense viral replication and immune response.**

3. **Persistent generalized lymphadenopathy.** In the early 1980s, generalized lymphadenopathy was suggested as a prodromal state to the development of AIDS in otherwise healthy homosexual men. However, not all homosexuals with persistent generalized lymphadenopathy are infected with HIV.
   a. **The syndrome** of persistent generalized lymphadenopathy is defined as the presence of two or more extrainguinal sites of lymphadenopathy (nodes > 1 cm in diameter) for a minimum of 3–6 months not attributable to other causes and not associated with substantial constitutional symptoms [121, 122].
   b. The prevalence varies widely, ranging from 5 to 70%.
   c. The nodes usually are 0.5–2.0 cm in diameter, symmetric, mobile, and rubbery, and involve the cervical, submandibular, occipital, and axillary chains. Pain and tenderness are uncommon. Mediastinal and hilar adenopathy are not characteristic, whereas mesenteric and retroperitoneal adenopathy are seen often.
   d. Pathologic evaluation of these nodes usually reveals **nonspecific findings of hyperplastic lymphadenopathy with follicular hyperplasia.** Patients with more severe disease (frank AIDS) generally have follicular depletion [123]. Studies of the subclasses of lymphocytes in nodes from HIV-infected patients reveal a proliferation of CD8 ⁣ T cells early in the disease, with a progressive depletion of all lymphoid elements, particularly CD4+ (helper) T cells later [123]. In addition, studies using available techniques, including in situ hybridization, indicate that **lymphadenopathy in HIV-infected patients is a reactive process, with tremendous ongoing antiviral activity** [124].
   e. **The differential diagnosis of persistent generalized lymphadenopathy** includes HIV infection as well as other causes, among them infectious (tuberculosis, secondary syphilis, histoplasmosis), neoplastic (lymphoma, Kaposi's sarcoma), and other processes (sarcoid). **Most asymptomatic patients with persistent generalized lymphadenopathy do not require lymph node biopsy** and can be monitored for occurrence of other AIDS-related manifestations. **A lymph node biopsy (by an experienced individual) is indicated for HIV-infected patients with** (1) localized, rapidly enlarging lymphadenopathy; (2) constitutional symptoms such as fever and weight loss; or (3) an increased risk of tuberculosis (i.e., intravenous drug users, patients from an endemic area or with a previous history of tuberculosis, or those who have a positive purified protein derivative of tuberculin [PPD] test).

4. **AIDS-related complex or symptomatic infection.** The term ARC was coined in 1983 by an extramural AIDS working group of the National Institutes of Health to identify those patients with symptoms indicative of acquired immunodeficiency but without the opportunistic infections or malignancies diagnostic of AIDS [104]. **This stage is now more commonly referred to as symptomatic HIV infection** (category B of the CDC revised classification system for HIV infection; Table 19-2)
   a. Clinical conditions include thrush, persistent or recurrent vulvovaginal candidiasis, cervical dysplasia, oral hairy leukoplakia, idiopathic thrombocytopenic purpura, and herpes zoster involving at least two distinct episodes or more than one dermatome.
   b. Bacterial infections including listeriosis, bacillary angiomatosis, and pelvic inflammatory disease are now classified in this category.
   c. Constitutional symptoms such as fever, diarrhea of greater than 1 month's duration, lymphadenopathy, and weight loss, which previously were included in the definition of ARC, now are included in category B as well [107].

5. **Hematologic abnormalities** are common in HIV-infected patients at any stage of the disease, from asymptomatic infection to frank AIDS [125].
   a. **Depression of one or more blood elements** (e.g., **normochromic, normocytic anemia, neutropenia, lymphopenia, and thrombocytopenia) is common,** and severity can range from mild to extreme. The pathogenesis of these abnormalities has not been delineated and is likely to be multifactorial. (**Erythropoietin** and **granulocyte-monocyte colony-stimulating factors** for pancytopenia in HIV-infected patients are used in selected patients.)

b. Immune thrombocytopenia

(1) This complication usually occurs early in the course of HIV infection. It is usually asymptomatic if the platelet count remains above 50,000, but it may be associated with easy bruising, petechiae, or prolonged bleeding, particularly with counts of less than 10,000.

(2) Immune thrombocytopenia in HIV-infected patients is similar to classic idiopathic thrombocytopenic purpura (ITP) in that there is no splenomegaly and the bone marrow is packed with megakaryocytes, suggesting increased peripheral destruction.

(3) More than half of patients do not require treatment. Active bleeding may be treated with intravenous gamma globulin or platelet transfusions. As with classic ITP, a number of therapeutic options are available (if the HIV-infected patient has severe thrombocytopenia), including corticosteroids, splenectomy, vincristine, danazol, and intravenous gamma globulin. Evaluation and treatment are best guided by a hematologist.

(4) **Although AZT is associated with anemia and leukopenia, it is not usually a cause of thrombocytopenia; in fact, AZT therapy appears to increase platelet counts in most patients** [126, 127].

(5) In the differential diagnosis of thrombocytopenia, one should consider whether the thrombocytopenia might be drug-induced or caused by splenic sequestration, opportunistic infection (*Mycobacterium avium-intracellulare,* histoplasmosis), or neoplasm (lymphoma). Patients with constitutional symptoms and pancytopenia should have a bone marrow aspirate and biopsy with special stains for acid-fast bacilli and fungi. Furthermore, **patients should be instructed to avoid antiplatelet agents** (e.g., aspirin).

c. Thrombotic thrombocytopenic purpura (TTP) has been described in patients with frank AIDS and has an ominous prognosis [128].

6. **AIDS.** AIDS is the **end stage** of long-standing, chronic infection with HIV. The vast majority of individuals infected with HIV are asymptomatic, and this asymptomatic state may be prolonged. Once AIDS develops, this phase of the illness often is relatively brief. **Only a small proportion of individuals infected with HIV have AIDS.** The syndrome is **defined by the various opportunistic infections,** malignancies, and other conditions summarized in the CDC definition **(see Table 19-2, category C)** and discussed in more detail in secs. V–VII. It should be noted that not all HIV-infected patients who die develop opportunistic infections and neoplasms characteristic of AIDS. The rate at which infected patients progress to AIDS and death also varies [109, 111, 112].

7. **Predictors of HIV disease progression.** A most pressing issue facing clinicians is that of **determining when progression from asymptomatic HIV infection to symptomatic disease is beginning** [109, 129–131]. Accurate markers of disease progression would be most useful in identifying those subsets of HIV-infected individuals who would benefit from early therapeutic intervention. The prognostic significance of a number of clinical and laboratory **surrogate markers** has been extensively studied.

a. **Clinical predictors.** Dermatomal or disseminated herpes zoster outbreaks appear to be associated with HIV infection but not with progression to AIDS.

(1) **Oral candidiasis** may herald the development of AIDS [132].

(2) **Involution of persistent generalized lymphadenopathy** appears to correlate with clinical progression.

(3) **Constitutional symptoms,** including fevers, night sweats, and weight loss, are also predictive of progression.

b. **Laboratory markers of HIV disease progression**

(1) **CD4 lymphocyte counts** are a specific test for HIV-induced immunopathology. Some studies of HIV-infected persons show that **the rate of disease progression increases sharply as the CD4 counts drop below 400/mm³** [133]. CD4/CD8 cell ratios of less than 0.6 also show a similar association with disease progression, but the association is not an independent one when CD4 counts are controlled.

(2) **Serum beta₂-microglobulin levels** appear to increase as disease pro-

gresses and, together with CD4 counts, have been used as predictors in heralding the onset of AIDS [134].

(3) The finding of **p24 antigen in serum** is believed to correlate with active HIV replication in vivo, but studies to date have not consistently shown correlation between rising p24 levels and clinical progression.

IV. Methods for serologic testing

A. **Detection of antibody.** Serum antibody appears most commonly 1–3 months after infection. The standard means of testing patients is to use the sensitive but nonspecific **screening enzyme-linked immunosorbent assay (ELISA)** test [135]. In persons with a positive ELISA, a confirmatory **Western blot** must be performed [136]. The Western blot is **more time-consuming and labor-intensive but is extremely sensitive and specific for detection of HIV infection.** Combining these two tests, the false positive rate has been recorded as 1 in 135,187 [137–139].

B. Additional tests to detect antibody include **immunofluorescent antibody** (IFA) test, **radioimmunoprecipitation assay** (RIPA), and other tests [140–142]. The need for highly skilled technicians makes many of these tests impractical for general use.

C. **Detection of virus,** or a marker of virus, is clinically important, especially in three situations: diagnosis of a patient during the "window period" prior to development of antibody (and therefore a positive ELISA–Western blot); diagnosis of infants of HIV-infected mothers, who will continue to have maternal antibody (and therefore a positive ELISA–Western blot) for up to 6–12 months and longer after birth; and for monitoring disease progression and effect of therapy on viral burden (viral load). The following tests can be used [143–145].

1. **Plasma HIV-1 RNA is the most sensitive marker of infectious virus.** RNA is extracted from plasma and then measured by a competitive and noncompetitive reverse transcriptase–based amplification system (i.e., by polymerase chain reaction [PCR]) [143–144a]. **Measurement of plasma HIV RNA viral load (plasma HIV RNA copy number) is also frequently used to assess disease progression and response to therapeutic regimens. See Chap. 26.**

2. Hybridization with DNA extracted from patients' cells and blotted onto nitrocellulose paper has been supplanted by PCR of proviral DNA. Nested primers and PCR have provided increased sensitivity [144b].

3. Infectious virus can be cultured by co-cultivating lymphocytes with target cells. However, the usefulness of this falls mainly in the realm of research studies to monitor sensitivity to the various antiretroviral agents. This is a laborious and expensive procedure.

4. Detection of a core protein, p24, is widely available. This antigen may appear immediately after infection and thus may be detected in the window period; in addition, it does not cross the placenta, and so its presence in an infant's blood is diagnostic of infection with HIV. Usually, acutely infected persons will initially have detectable p24 but, as an immune response is mounted, p24 antigen levels become undetectable. Later, as infection progresses and the patient becomes more ill, free p24 antigen may again appear. Recently, measurement of immune-complex dissociated (ICD) p24 has become available. This method may offer some advantages over routine p24 testing.

V. Routine initial evaluation of the patient with HIV infection has been summarized [145a].

A. A **complete medical history,** with emphasis on specific infections or syndromes suggestive of opportunistic infections is important. Identify current and past high-risk behaviors and exposures that may have resulted in HIV infection [145a] (Table 19-3).

B. Perform a **complete physical examination,** with special attention to signs of mucosal candidiasis, retinal disease, lymphadenopathy, pulmonary abnormalities, hepatosplenomegaly, skin disease, sexually transmitted diseases; a complete gynecological examination should be performed in women.

C. **Obtain initial laboratory studies** as summarized in Table 19-3.

D. **CD4 lymphocyte testing** is an integral part of continued care because it **indicates the need for antiretroviral therapy** and for **chemoprophylaxis of opportunistic infections.**

1. Antiretroviral therapy: see sec. **X** and Chap. 26.

2. See CD4+ lymphocyte considerations in Fig. 19-2 (p. 729).

3. When the CD4 count is $\geq 500/mm^3$, determinations should be repeated every

Table 19-3. Initial evaluation of and measures to prevent opportunistic infections in HIV-infected adults and adolescents[a]

---

1. Obtain a complete medical history, with emphasis on opportunistic infections
    Constitutional symptoms, fever, weight loss
    Mucocutaneous candidiasis
    Pneumonia, gastrointestinal symptoms
    Positive TST result, date and results of last TST, history of treatment with
       antituberculosis drugs
    STDs
    Abnormal cervical Pap smear, date and results of last Pap smear
2. Identify HIV risk behavior and assess ongoing high-risk behavior as well as other
    behaviors, activities, and interests that place patient at risk for opportunistic
    infections[b]
3. Perform physical examination directed by history but including genital and rectal
    examination for signs of STDs and (for women) routine gynecologic examination
4. Conduct laboratory and other tests
    Complete blood count
    CD4+ lymphocyte count
    Blood chemistry profile
    IgG antibody to *Toxoplasma gondii*
    Antibody to CMV (if patient is not at such high risk for CMV that seropositivity
       can be assumed)
    Screening for STDs (RPR or VDRL, HBsAg, and anti-HBc), with possible testing
       for gonorrhea and (in women) for genital chlamydial infection
    Cervical Pap smear
    TST (if result is not already known to be positive)
    Chest radiograph
5. Initiate chemoprophylaxis for PCP if patient has reliable history of PCP or thrush
6. Consider administration of pneumococcal vaccine if it has not already been given
7. Discuss need for future visits
    Emphasis on the importance of opportunistic infections and the fact that many
       can be prevented
    Emphasis on the importance of obtaining CD4+ lymphocyte counts at
       appropriate intervals to determine timing/need for prophylactic interventions
       and antiretroviral therapy

---

anti-HBc = antibody to hepatitis B core antigen; CMV = cytomegalovirus; HBsAg = hepatitis B
surface antigen; PCP = *Pneumocystis carinii* pneumonia; RPR = rapid plasma reagin; STDs =
sexually transmitted diseases; TST = tuberculin skin test; VDRL = Venereal Disease
Research Laboratory.
[a]For initial evaluation suggestions in infants and children see source.
[b]For additional information, see Table 19-10.
Source: J. E. Kaplan et al. and the USPHS/IDSA Prevention of Opportunistic Infections Working
Group, USPHS/IDSA guidelines for the prevention of opportunistic infections in persons infected
with human immunodeficiency virus: An overview. *Clin. Infect. Dis.* 21(Suppl. 1):S12, 1995.
Published by The University of Chicago Press.

6 months. Once the CD4 count is <500/mm^3, determinations should be repeated at least every 6 months and possibly more frequently (e.g., 3–4 times
per year) if there is evidence of rapid decline or if the patient has HIV-related
symptoms [145a].
   4. Follow-up. Asymptomatic persons can be seen 3–4 times per year while symp-
      tomatic patients often require evaluation every 1–2 months.
      a. A tuberculin skin test (TST) can be repeated every 6–12 months in areas
         of high risk for tuberculosis and every 12 months otherwise.
      b. Cervical Papanicolaou smears are suggested every 6–12 months.
E. Immunizations, including pneumococcus and hepatitis B (if a patient is not already
   surface-antibody positive), should be given. The utility of vaccination for *H. influenzae* has not been assessed for this population. Although recent evidence
   suggests that vaccine produces an adverse effect on HIV replication, this effect
   is short lived and of uncertain significance [145b]. Because it is likely that natural
   infection would have an even greater adverse effect, it is prudent to vaccinate
   against diseases where vaccine should be helpful (e.g., influenza).

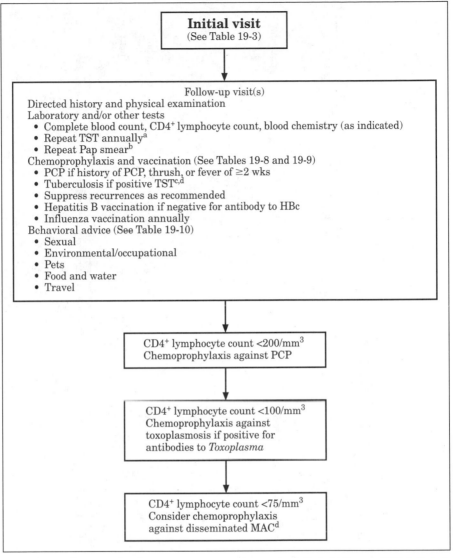

Fig. 19-2. Evaluation of and measures to prevent opportunistic infections in HIV-infected adults and adolescents. HBc = hepatitis B core antigen; MAC = *Mycobacterium avium complex*; PCP = *Pneumocystis carinii* pneumonia; and TST = tuberculin skin test. [a]Although reliability of the TST may diminish as the CD4+ lymphocyte count decreases, repeat the TST at least annually, depending on the risk of exposure to tuberculosis. [b]After an initially negative Pap smear, repeat the Pap smear within 6 months. Thereafter, repeat the Pap smear annually. [c]Patients exposed to an active case of tuberculosis should also receive prophylaxis; those from populations at high risk for tuberculosis (i.e., a prevalence of >10%) may also be candidates for prophylaxis. [d]Exclude active mycobacterial disease before initiating prophylaxis. (From J. E. Kaplan et al. and the USPHS/IDSA Prevention of Opportunistic Infections Working Group. USPHS/IDSA guidelines for the prevention of opportunistic infections in persons infected with human immunodeficiency virus: An overview. *Clin. Infect. Dis.* 21(Suppl. 1):S15, 1995. Published by the University of Chicago Press.)

Table 19-4. Etiologies for common clinical syndromes in patients with HIV infection

	Viral	Bacterial	Fungal	Protozoal	Other
Pneumonia		S. pneumoniae H. influenzae P. aeruginosa M. tuberculosis	H. capsulatum C. neoformans	P. carinii	KS
Change in mental status	JC virus (PML) CMV HIV	Listeria monocytogenes	C. neoformans	T. gondii	Lymphoma
Diarrhea	CMV HIV	Salmonella Shigella Campylobacter spp. C. difficile M. tuberculosis MAI Adherent E. coli	H. capsulatum	E. histolytica G. lamblia Cryptosporidium Microsporidium Isospora Cyclosporeae	
FUO	CMV	M. tuberculosis MAI	H. capsulatum	P. carinii	Lymphoma Drug fever
Esophagitis	Herpes simplex CMV		Candida spp.		Aphthous ulcers KS

CMV = cytomegalovirus; KS = Kaposi's sarcoma; PML = progressive multifocal leukoencephalopathy; FUO = fever of unknown origin; MAI = *Mycobacterium avium-intracellulare.*

F. A baseline ophthalmologic examination is suggested if the CD4 count is less than 200/mm³.

G. Prevention of opportunistic infections is an important part of early and serial follow-up visits. This is discussed in detail in sec. **VIII** on pages 760–765.

VI. Common clinical syndromes in patients with HIV infection. Several **clinical syndromes** occur **frequently** in patients with HIV infection. We will briefly consider the differential diagnosis and clinical approach to seven such common syndromes: **respiratory complaints; diarrhea; fever; oral manifestations; dermatologic manifestations; change in mental status; and esophagitis and biliary tract problems. The pathogens that have been associated with each clinical syndrome are discussed in detail in sec. VII.**

A. Respiratory complaints include cough, dyspnea, chest pain, and sputum production. **Pneumonia** commonly is diagnosed, although **bronchitis, pulmonary embolus,** and **cancer** may cause similar symptoms.

1. **Etiologic agents** include both infectious and noninfectious causes. *P. carinii* continues to cause more than 42% of all AIDS indicator diseases [7] and remains a common pulmonary pathogen, although widespread prophylaxis has changed the frequency and clinical presentation of the disease [146]. See Table 19-4 and discussions in Chap. 24.

    a. In patients with **CD4 counts in excess of 200 mm³,** *Streptococcus pneumoniae* and *M. tuberculosis* are seen.

    b. In patients with **advanced HIV disease,** many additional pathogens must be considered: *P. carinii,* bacteria (*Pseudomonas aeruginosa, Staphylococcus aureus*), fungi (*Aspergillus* spp., *Histoplasma capsulatum, Cryptococcus neoformans*), parasites (*Strongyloides stercoralis*), and atypical mycobacteria. These pathogens may occur in the setting of disseminated disease. *S. pneumoniae* and tuberculosis continue to cause significant morbidity in this population. *P. aeruginosa* can occur as a community-acquired pathogen (see sec. **VII.C;** pp. 747–748).

    c. **Neoplasms,** including non-Hodgkin's lymphoma, Kaposi's sarcoma, and primary or metastatic carcinoma, can also cause lung disease with clinical presentations mimicking pneumonia. In addition, **chemotherapy** for neoplastic disease, such as bleomycin, may cause respiratory symptoms.

2. **Clinical presentation** varies. Classic symptoms such as fever, cough, and sputum production are common, but pneumonia may manifest only by a subtle change in mental status, secondary to hypoxia.

    a. Knowing a patient's CD4 count, PCP prophylaxis history, and history of tuberculosis exposure is essential to a full evaluation.

    b. **Duration of symptoms** may be helpful in distinguishing among various possible etiologies. **PCP** often has an insidious onset with a dry cough and slowly increasing dyspnea on exertion, whereas **bacterial pneumonia** often is more abrupt in onset and is associated with a productive cough and pleuritic chest pain. Symptoms of **tuberculosis** may be indolent or abrupt [147].

3. **Diagnosis** usually is made by **chest roentgenography and sputum exam** [146].

    a. On **chest roentgenography,** the presence of diffuse interstitial infiltrates favors the diagnosis of PCP or tuberculosis, whereas a lobar infiltrate is more common in bacterial pneumonia. Kaposi's sarcoma may have a multicentric stellate appearance on the chest x-ray film. Chest roentgenography, however, is **notoriously nonspecific** and should not be relied on for a diagnosis without supporting microbiologic evidence [148]. Cavitary lesions have been reviewed recently [147a].

    b. **Sputum evaluation,** including Gram stain, Gram-Weigert staining for PCP, acid-fast staining for tuberculosis, and culture for bacteria and mycobacteria, is essential for all patients. **Induced sputum** samples may increase the diagnostic yield in patients with PCP and, possibly, tuberculosis. In selected patients (e.g., those with more chronic symptoms or cavitary changes, or those with a history of travel to or living in endemic areas), fungal cultures are indicated.

    c. **Invasive tests,** including **bronchoscopy** and **lung biopsy,** may be necessary in patients with unrevealing routine evaluations [148]. Overall, the combination of both bronchoalveolar lavage (BAL) and transbronchial biopsy has a diagnostic yield of more than 95% for detecting pulmonary pathogens [149]. **Often a transbronchial biopsy can be avoided when a**

BAL provides the pathogen. In patients in whom an initial BAL study is nondiagnostic, or in whom the presentation or chest roentgenogram is atypical, a BAL and transbronchial biopsy may be done as a single procedure. In general, we try to avoid a diagnostic open lung biopsy.

Noninfectious pulmonary disease can occur and may be identified by biopsy.

(1) **Kaposi's sarcoma** often involves the lung, although not all patients have respiratory complaints. Symptoms include a persistent dry cough and dyspnea. The chest roentgenogram often reveals pleural effusion (up to 50%) and patchy nodularity. Single-breath diffusion capacity is reduced. Superinfection with bacteria, especially *S. aureus,* occurs frequently and usually responds to antibacterial therapy. Treatment consists of chemotherapy directed at the Kaposi's sarcoma.

(2) **Lymphocytic interstitial pneumonia** (LIP) is common in children with AIDS and may also be seen rarely in adults. The etiology involves Epstein-Barr virus–directed transformation of T cells. LIP in non-AIDS patients arises from B cells. Clinical presentation resembles that of other interstitial pneumonias, especially PCP. Diagnosis depends on biopsy, which shows small, noncleaved mature lymphocytes and plasma cells crowding the interstitium but sparing the airways. Treatment with steroids is effective in some patients.

(3) **Nonspecific pneumonitis,** consisting of unexplained interstitial fibrosis, may also occur in AIDS patients with pulmonary complaints. Presentation resembles that of patients with PCP. Diagnosis is made by biopsy and excluding all other potential pathogens. Prognosis and treatment are not known.

d. **Nonspecific tests,** such as gallium scan, CT scan of the chest, lactate dehydrogenase determinations, and ventilation-perfusion (VQ) scans may be required to better elucidate certain aspects of a patient's illness, particularly a patient with a negative routine workup who also has a coagulopathy that precludes biopsy.

4. **Management** is directed at the underlying cause. Patients who are severely ill should be empirically treated for PCP and bacterial pneumonia, with consideration for antituberculous therapy, pending evaluation (see separate discussions later). While awaiting sputum and blood cultures, we often will use cefuroxime for bacteria therapy. In a young to middle-aged patient, we may add erythromycin pending culture data. If *P. aeruginosa* is a concern (see sec. **VII.C**), we will add an aminoglycoside pending culture data (see p. 747). Empiric outpatient management of pneumonia has recently been discussed [149a].

B. **Diarrhea** is a common cause of morbidity in the HIV-infected patient. It occurs in 30–50% of AIDS patients in the United States and in more than 95% of patients from Africa and Haiti. With an aggressive approach, etiologic agents can be identified in 50–85% of patients with enteritis, and more than 50% of identifiable pathogens are treatable [150–152a].

1. **Etiologic agents** for enteritis in HIV-infected patients are listed in Table 19-4. There are two leading explanations for persistent diarrhea and, if chronic, wasting: (1) opportunistic enteric infection and (2) HIV enteropathy [152a]. Neoplasms such as Kaposi's sarcoma and non-Hodgkin's lymphoma also are associated with enteritis in AIDS.

a. **Multiple pathogens,** often occurring concomitantly, **are common.** Systemic infection with *Mycobacterium avium* complex, *M. tuberculosis,* and *Histoplasma* may also involve the intestinal tract and cause diarrhea, but these organisms rarely cause enteritis in the absence of multiorgan disease. The role of *Escherichia coli,* adenovirus, and HIV in causing diarrhea has not been established, and these organisms are not routinely sought. However, in a recent report of patients with chronic diarrhea, adherent bacteria (*E. coli*) demonstrated on histopathology and culture of endoscopic biopsies of the right colon were seen in 17% of AIDS patients [151a]. CMV can infect any level of the gastrointestinal tract [152a].

Parasites such as *Entamoeba coli, Entamoeba hartmanni, Endolimax nana,*and *Blastocystis hominis* are found frequently in stool of HIV-infected patients as well as in nonimmunocompromised hosts. The pathogenic potential of these organisms has not been established. They usually disappear without treatment even in the compromised host.

b. **HIV enteropathy** is suggested by the inability to isolate or demonstrate a known gastrointestinal pathogen. The mechanisms of this entity are complex and are reviewed elsewhere [152a], but an important part is played by dysfunctional immunity, particularly as it relates to the mucosal immune system [152a].

2. Diarrheal episodes may be **acute** or **chronic.** The **severity** of diarrhea ranges from mild and self-limited to fulminant, requiring frequent hospitalizations or intravenous hydration. Duration and severity of diarrhea increase as CD4 cell counts decrease.

3. **Diagnosis and initial approach.** History and physical examination infrequently point to a specific etiology because of the overlap in clinical manifestations of different infections and the presence of multiple concomitant pathogens.

   a. Initial stool studies should include two freshly passed stool samples for **culture for bacterial pathogens, examination for ova and parasites, and** *Clostridium difficile* **toxin assay.** A specific request to look for *Cryptosporidium* and *Microsporidium* must be included in the laboratory request form, because most laboratories do not routinely seek these organisms when performing the ova and parasite examination. (*Microsporidium* stool examination may necessitate sending a sample to a reference laboratory.) The number of negative stool samples needed to document a true negative is unknown; therefore, **at least two samples,** obtained on different days, are examined.

   b. **A blood culture** for bacteria and mycobacterium is suggested [152a].

   c. **If no agent is identified** with the above work-up, as part of a cost-effective approach, some experts suggest for adults a 10-day empiric course of **an oral fluoroquinolone** to ensure that treatable bacterial enteropathogens have been excluded [152a].

   d. **If no treatable condition is identified,** and fever is absent and stools do not show gross evidence of blood, **the adult patient can be treated symptomatically,** usually with loperamide (Imodium) (4 mg initially, followed by 2 mg after each stool passed to a maximum of 16 mg daily) or diphenoxylate HCl (Lomotil) (initially 1–2 tablets qid as needed).

   Octreotide has been used successfully in some cases of microsporidiosis and may have value in chronic diarrhea refractory to other symptomatic treatments [152a] (see sec. **4**).

   The role of antihistamine therapy (e.g., diphenhydramine) and prostaglandin inhibitors (e.g., indomethacin) is undergoing evaluation [152a].

   Psychological counseling and stress management may help some patients.

   e. **Endoscopy** should be considered when repeated stool examinations (see sec. **a**) are negative, therapy directed against a specific pathogen is ineffective, pathogens that may require tissue diagnosis are suspected (e.g., mycobacteria, cytomegalovirus, adenovirus, microsporidia) or symptomatic therapy (see sec. **d**) is not effective. Often, both upper gastroduodenoscopy with small-bowel biopsy and colonoscopy with colonic biopsy are warranted. Biopsy material should be examined for CMV, MAI, adenovirus, fungi, HSV, and parasites [152a].

4. **Miscellaneous.** Maintenance of **optimal hydration** with **glucose- and sodium-enriched fluids** is of paramount importance. **Opiates** are often effective but may have unacceptable side effects. **Octreotide (Sandostatin)** is a subcutaneously administered, synthetic somatostatin analogue that sometimes is useful in controlling severe, dehydrating diarrhea [153]. Cholestyramine has also been tried. Nonspecific antidiarrheal therapy must be individualized for each patient, and this usually is best accomplished by trial and error. **Adequate nutrition** also is important, and supplements containing **medium-chain triglycerides** are better absorbed than those with long-chain triglycerides. The role of **total parenteral nutrition, anabolic steroids,** and other **appetite enhancers** is uncertain. **Dietary guidelines** should include **avoidance of fats, milk and milk-containing products, and caffeine.** Recommendations concerning diet should also be individualized.

5. **Pathogen-specific therapy.** Treatment of specific pathogens is discussed in the sections that describe the pathogens and in Chap. 11. *Shigella, Campylobacter,* **and** *Giardia* **spp., and** *E. histolytica* **can be eradicated with appropriate therapy.** Some infections that do not require treatment (nontyphoid

Salmonella) in the immunocompetent host require **aggressive therapy** and **long-term suppression** in the HIV-infected patient [154].

C. **Fever** is a common symptom among persons with HIV infection. In one prospective study, **46% of a cohort** of patients with advanced HIV infection developed fever within a 9-month period [155]. Most patients with advanced HIV and fever have a recognizable and usually treatable cause [155]. See also related discussion of prolonged fever in HIV patients in Chap. 1, under Fever of Unknown Etiology.

1. **Evaluation** of patients with fever and nonspecific symptoms should include a **chest roentgenogram, routine blood cultures, and a CBC.** Persons with a CD4 count of less than 100/mm^3 should have blood cultures for acid-fast bacilli (e.g., using Dupont Isolator), as well as studies for serum cryptococcal antigen. Viral cultures or serologic tests for cytomegalovirus are not useful in the evaluation of the acutely febrile AIDS patient.

   In one recent report, about 15% of hospitalized patients with fever and neutropenia had documented bacteremia, similar to the incidence of bacteremia documented in febrile leukopenic patients without underlying HIV infection [155a].

   a. The yield from **bone marrow biopsy** and culture and from **liver biopsy** is low in patients without specific signs such as anemia or liver function abnormalities [156, 156a]. When tuberculosis or histoplasmosis is suspected, these tests may be very useful. The indications for a node biopsy include the setting in which lymphoma is a concern (e.g., unexplained fevers despite a routine workup; adequate CD4 cell counts, which indicate that disseminated *Mycobacterium avium-intracellulare* (MAI) is less likely).

   b. **Repeated blood cultures,** particularly for acid-fast bacilli, are suggested.

   c. **Extensive CT scanning generally is not informative** but may be important in patients in whom a superimposed lymphoma is a concern (e.g., see sec. **a**).

2. The majority of fevers have an **identifiable source.** In one study, fever in 83% of outpatients could be explained [155]. Of fevers that take more than 2 weeks to diagnosis, **MAI, PCP** (in persons on aerosol pentamidine prophylaxis), and **lymphoma** are the most likely diagnoses [155]. Empiric therapy for **tuberculosis** should be strongly considered for any patient with an identified risk factor for acute or latent tuberculosis, including persons born in countries endemic for tuberculosis, persons recently imprisoned or hospitalized in facilities with tuberculosis outbreaks, and people with a history of tuberculosis infection or disease. Underlying cancer, including Kaposi's sarcoma [157], should always be considered. The pursuit of the cause of fever must be methodical and thorough. Fevers in patients with advanced HIV infection should not be ascribed to HIV alone [155].

3. **Management** of febrile patients is aimed at antipyretics once the pattern of fever has been established. In patients with high fevers, this may include alternating acetaminophen with nonsteroidal antiinflammatory agents. The concern that such therapy will "mask" the fever and thus obscure the results of empiric trials of therapy probably is unfounded, as few patients will become consistently afebrile on antipyretics.

D. **Oral manifestations** may be identified in 40% of all HIV-infected patients and in more than 90% of AIDS patients [157a] (Table 19-5).

1. **Hairy leukoplakia** is believed to be caused by the Epstein-Barr virus (see Chap. 17) and, although common in HIV-positive patients, has been well described in transplant recipients. Patients may present with painless white plaques anywhere on their tongue or posterior oropharynx, but typically the leukoplakia involves the lateral borders of the tongue. Hairlike projections may be present. This is usually a **clinical diagnosis** based on appearance. The condition is asymptomatic and benign and generally requires no specific therapy [157a].

2. **Human papillomavirus** can cause skin and mucosal warts. Lesions often are multiple and are located throughout the oral cavity. Diagnosis is made by recognition of the typical sessile or cauliflower-appearing papular lesions [157a].

3. **Cytomegalovirus** (CMV) usually is associated with retinitis or systemic CMV disease; mucosal involvement is uncommon. Nonspecific mucositis can occur, as can shallow ulcers that require biopsy for diagnosis.

Table 19-5. Oral manifestations of HIV infection

Fungal diseases
  Candidiasis
Viral diseases
  Herpes simplex virus
  Varicella-zoster virus
  Hairy leukoplakia
  Human papillomavirus
  Cytomegalovirus
Bacterial diseases
  Gingivitis
  Periodontitis
  Syphilis
  Gram-negative infection
  Mycobacterium avium complex infection
Neoplastic diseases
  Kaposi's sarcoma
  Lymphoma
  Squamous cell carcinoma
Miscellaneous conditions
  Aphthous ulcerations
  Xerostomia
  Salivary gland enlargement

Source: From D. L. Battinelli and E. S. Peters, Oral Manifestations. In H. Libman and R. A. Witzburg (eds.), *HIV Infection: A Primary Care Manual* (3rd ed.). Boston: Little, Brown, 1996. P. 88.

4. **Kaposi's sarcoma** (KS) is the most common neoplasm in AIDS. More than half of patients with KS have oral involvement. KS oral lesions are red or purple, nonblanching macules, papules, or nodules. Lesions are especially common on the hard palate and gingival margins and often are asymptomatic. Diagnosis is confirmed by biopsy. Therapy involves surgical excision or radiation therapy [157a]. See related discussion in sec. **E.5.**

5. **Non-Hodgkin's lymphoma** occasionally presents as a firm, painless swelling, with or without ulceration, anywhere in the mouth but especially affecting the gingiva or palate. Any oral nodule or mass should be biopsied to rule out lymphoma [157a]. Squamous carcinoma of the tongue has also been described.

6. **Gingivitis and periodontal disease** can be more severe and rapidly can progress in the HIV-positive patient.

7. **Aphthous ulcerations** are seen often in patients with HIV infection, and they are frequently recurrent. Their etiology is unclear, but systemic illness, trauma, and viruses may play a contributing role. Symptomatic ulcers that do not heal spontaneously can be treated with topical steroids (e.g., fluocinonide ointment, 0.05% mixed with Orabase and applied 3–6 times per day). The differential diagnosis in HIV patients with mouth ulcers includes HSV, syphilis, CMV, zalcitabine (ddC) therapy, and lymphoma. Refractory lesions should be biopsied [157a]. Thalidomide has been used for therapy [157b].

E. **Dermatologic manifestations** of HIV infection are reviewed in detail elsewhere [9, 12–16]. A summary is provided in Table 19-6. Several points deserve emphasis.

1. In **acute primary HIV infection,** a rash can be seen.

2. **Herpes simplex virus and herpes zoster virus** are discussed in Chaps. 4, 13, and 26. In patients with advanced HIV disease, nonhealing herpes simplex virus erosions may enlarge into severe, painful ulcers that can reach up to 20 cm in diameter. Any ulcerative lesion in an HIV-infected patient should be considered herpetic until proven otherwise [119a].

3. **Molluscum contagiosum** develops in approximately 20% of symptomatic HIV-infected patients. These poxvirus-associated lesions classically are pearly, dome-shaped 2- to 4-mm papules with central umbilication. In HIV-infected patients, lesions may disseminate widely, including to the face, and they may enlarge to 1 cm or more. Pathognomonic "molluscum bodies" (large viral inclusion formations) can be demonstrated by KOH touch preparations and

Table 19-6. Dermatologic manifestations of HIV infection

Disease	Clinical manifestations	Diagnosis	Comment
Viral infections			
Acute HIV exanthem (primary HIV infection)	Fever, myalgias, urticaria Truncal, palmar, plantar, maculopapular eruption	HIV antibodies usually within 12 wk of infection Low WBC count, thrombocytopenia, hypergammaglobulinemia	See text
Herpes simplex virus (HSV)	May be widely disseminated, persistent erosions and perirectal ulcers	HSV culture Tzanck smear for multinucleate giant cells	See Chaps. 4, 13, 26
Varicella-zoster virus	May be severe, persistent, dermatomal, disseminated, or deeply scarring Intractable herpetic pain	Herpesvirus culture Tzanck smear for multinucleate giant cells	See Chaps. 4, 13, 26
Molluscum contagiosum	Clusters of white umbilicated papules	Biopsy or KOH preparations of soft central material show large viral inclusions	See sec. **VI.E.3**
Oral hairy leukoplakia	Whitish, nonremovable verrucous plaques on sides of tongue	Biopsy	See sec. **VI.D.1**
Warts (human papilloma-virus)	Increased number, size of verrucous lesions	Biopsy or clinical appearance	See sec. **VI.D.2**

	Clinical features	Diagnosis	Reference
Fungal infections			
Candida albicans	Oral mucosal white plaques, sore throat, dysphagia, deep tongue erosions; Intractable vaginal infection; Nail infection	Culture; KOH slide preparation	See Chap. 18
Tinea versicolor	Thick, scaly hypopigmented or light-brown plaques on trunk	KOH slide shows numerous short hyphae and spores; Wood's light accentuates lesions	See Chap. 13
Dermatophytes (tinea corporis, pedis, cruris)	Extensive involvement, especially groin and feet	KOH slide preparation shows branched, septate hyphae	
Bacterial infections			
Staphylococcal infection	Superficial and subcutaneous infections; Impetigo	Culture	See Chap. 4
Bacillary angiomatosis	Dome-shaped or pedunculated solitary or multiple papules and nodules (4 mm–2 cm); Visceral angiomatosis	Biopsy	See sec. **VII.C.5**
Spirochetal infection			
Syphilis	Painless chancre (primary); Generalized plaques and papulosquamous lesions (secondary); Incubation period for neurosyphilis may be very short (mos)	VDRL or RPR *and* FTA-ABS or MHA-TP; Skin biopsy	See Chap. 13
Neoplastic disorders			
Kaposi's sarcoma	Pale to deep violaceous, oval plaques and papules; Oral lesions (usually palate); Visceral lesions	Biopsy	See sec. **VI.E.5**

Table 19-6 (continued)

Disease	Clinical manifestations	Diagnosis	Comment
Miscellaneous disorders			
Seborrheic dermatitis	Red scaling plaques with yellow greasy scales and distinct margins, on the face and scalp	Biopsy KOH to rule out tinea	
Psoriasis	Activation of previous disease or no previous history	Biopsy	
Xeroderma	Severe dry skin, possible erythroderma	Clinical presentation	
Papular eruption	2- to 5-mm skin-colored papules on head, neck, upper trunk Pruritic, chronic	Biopsy shows lymphocytic perivascular infiltrate	
Eosinophilic (EF) and bacterial folliculitis	Groups of small vesicles and pustules that can become confluent EF: Polycyclic plaques with central hypopigmentation Severe, intractable pruritus	Biopsy Negative culture for atypical organisms	See text

Source: From H. K. Koh and B. E. Davis, Dermatologic Manifestations. In H. Libman and R. A. Witzburg (eds.), *HIV Infection: A Primary Care Manual* (3rd ed.). Boston: Little, Brown, 1996. Pp. 108–111.

skin biopsy. The most common differential diagnosis is warts caused by human papillomavirus (see sec. **D.2**). The diagnosis usually is made clinically, but atypical lesions warrant biopsy. Patients can prevent spread of the lesions by discontinuing blade shaving. Liquid nitrogen applications every 1–2 weeks may be helpful if therapy is needed [119a].

4. *S. aureus* is a common cutaneous pathogen in HIV-infected patients. **Folliculitis** (hair-centered inflammation) is very common. **Follicular pustules** may affect the trunk, face, or groin, especially. Early treatment of folliculitis—for example, with topical agents such as mupirocin or clindamycin (see Chap. 28) and antibacterial soap (chlorhexidine)—may prevent progression to furuncles, carbuncles, abscess, or cellulitis, any of which may require incision and drainage and oral antistaphylococcal agents (e.g., dicloxacillin or a first-generation cephalosporin). See Chap. 4.

   Other types of folliculitis include *Pityrosporum* **disease** (a fungal process confirmed by KOH scraping) and **eosinophilic pustular folliculitis,** which is culture-negative, of unknown etiology, and diagnosed by biopsy, and an acneiform, pruritic, papular, or pustular eruption that can evolve to keratic, lichenified, or indurated plaques. Remissions have occurred with the use of ultraviolet B light treatments [119a].

   In warmer weather, **bullous impetigo** can occur. See Chap. 4.

5. **Kaposi's sarcoma** is reviewed in detail elsewhere [9, 12–16] but is summarized here. HIV-infected patients have a 20,000-fold increased rate of KS [119a].
   a. **Background.** Kaposi's sarcoma is believed to arise from either vascular or lymphatic endothelium. This tumor was previously considered a rare, indolent dermal tumor usually found on the lower extremities of elderly white men of Mediterranean or Eastern European origin. Kaposi's sarcoma also was known to occur in immunosuppressed renal transplant patients in whom lesions often regressed when immunosuppressive agents were discontinued. Recently, an association with a herpes-like virus has been made [157c].
   b. **Presentation.** In AIDS patients, KS is usually aggressive. It is a multicentric tumor that **initially presents as purplish nodules on the skin or mucous membranes.** Patients with high CD4 cell counts (>300–400/ mm³) may develop limited cutaneous lesions. In the early stage, lesions are irregular, reddish-blue or purple to violaceous macules [119a]. The macules may become papular or nodular or coalesce to form large patches, plaques, and fusiform or ovoid tumors. Individual lesions are usually asymptomatic, although pain, itching, and burning can be noted [119a]. Lesions commonly are less than 1 cm in diameter. It frequently spreads to lymph nodes and visceral organs and can be seen in any organ in the body.
   c. **Epidemiologic features. Kaposi's sarcoma is epidemiologically almost entirely confined to the homosexual male population; the reasons remain unclear,** although an infectious agent transmitted sexually but distinct from HIV would explain the observations. Also, in recent years, the incidence of homosexual men developing KS has decreased dramatically.
   d. **Diagnosis.** Kaposi's sarcoma is diagnosed by biopsy, which shows vascular proliferation.
   e. **Therapy.** Treatment often is problematic and palliative unless there is pulmonary or GI involvement. Local therapies, radiation therapy, interferon therapy, and chemotherapy are reviewed elsewhere [9, 12–16].

6. **Seborrheic dermatitis** (SD) may occur as a severe skin problem in HIV-infected patients, affecting up to 50–80% of this population. The etiology of SD is unknown. In contrast to normal hosts, in HIV-infected patients there often is sudden production of markedly erythematous, inflammatory, papular or even psoriasiform lesions. More severe forms may resemble psoriasis. Diagnosis generally is made by clinical appearance. Low-potency topical steroids are useful in mild SD. For resistant cases, topical ketoconazole cream or oral ketoconazole in doses of 200–400 mg/day may be useful [119a].

7. **Skin cancers** (e.g., basal cell carcinoma, squamous cell carcinoma, malignant melanoma). There is an association between cutaneous neoplasms and AIDS. The morbidity and mortality rates of skin cancer are higher in patients with HIV infection than in the general population. This topic has recently been reviewed and the authors encourage that biopsy specimens be obtained from

all suspicious lesions and histopathologic assessment be done. Early and complete excision of the skin neoplasm should be done [119b].

F. Change in mental status may be seen with a number of infections and other conditions, including systemic illnesses outside the CNS.

    1. Common clinical syndromes include meningitis [158], seizures [159], stroke syndromes [160, 161], and cognitive or behavioral changes. Overlap among these syndromes is common.

    2. Anticipated etiologic agents vary according to the presenting syndrome.

        a. *C. neoformans* **is the most common cause of meningitis** [7], although bacterial causes such as *S. pneumoniae* must be excluded.

        b. Seizures often are caused by mass lesions, HIV encephalopathy, and meningitis [159]. Etiologies seldom are found in persons with normal interictal examinations [159].

        c. Stroke syndromes may have infectious (*T. gondii*) or noninfectious etiologies [160, 161]. Syphilis should always be considered in this setting [162].

        d. Progressive dementia is seen relatively frequently among patients with advanced HIV infection. Common causes include **progressive multifocal leukoencephalopathy (PML) and HIV itself.** Persons with progressive dementia in the setting of a new stroke syndrome should be suspected of having PML.

        e. Central nervous system lymphoma may present with altered sensorium with or without a concurrent stroke syndrome.

    3. Diagnosis depends on a thorough physical examination with attention to **concurrent medications. Routine blood work** may disclose a **metabolic cause** for a change in mental status. **Serologic studies** for toxoplasmosis (if not done within the previous 6 months) and serum and CSF cryptococcal antigen studies should be done promptly. Negative serology for toxoplasmosis argues against this infection. Spinal tap and CT or MRI scans generally are obtained. MRI is preferred if available.

        a. In patients with **meningitis** who are suspected of having bacterial meningitis, antibiotics should be begun as discussed in Chap. 5.

        b. Spinal fluid cytology should be obtained on all patients with brain lesions.

        c. Brain biopsy may be necessary in persons with a mass lesion that does not respond to 2 weeks of therapy for toxoplasmosis [163].

    4. The specific CNS infections are discussed later in this chapter and in Chap. 5.

G. Esophagitis. Up to 40% of HIV-infected persons develop esophagitis [163a]. Several different pathogens may cause esophagitis, but the **clinical syndromes are identical,** making empiric therapy or endoscopic diagnosis necessary.

    1. Etiologic agents

        a. *Candida albicans* **causes 50–80% of clinical cases.** In addition, patients may have asymptomatic candidiasis of the esophagus. Other *Candida* spp. may also cause esophagitis. The presence of oral thrush suggests *Candida* as a cause; conversely, **the absence of thrush does not exclude** *Candida* **as a cause.**

        b. Herpes simplex virus (HSV) and **CMV** each account for 5–15% of cases. Empiric treatment with oral acyclovir may identify persons with HSV esophagitis. In proven cases, acyclovir can be given orally or, in severe cases, intravenously. Intravenous ganciclovir or foscarnet is required for CMV esophagitis or CMV ulcers [163b, 163c].

        c. Idiopathic ulcers account for a growing number of cases and may be difficult to treat. In a recent review of esophageal ulcers in HIV-infected patients, **idiopathic ulcers** were diagnosed in 40 of 100 patients. Endoscopic biopsies of these patients' lesions revealed granulation tissue with necrosis of the overlying epithelium and inflammation consistent with ulceration; no viral cytopathic effect or etiologic agent was identified with special stains and neither reflux esophagitis nor drug-induced esophagitis were present [163c]. This is an important diagnosis to confirm since many patients with idiopathic ulcers respond to therapy with either prednisone 40 mg/day PO (tapering 10 mg per week) or prednisone 40 mg/day for 2 weeks [163c]. Among nonresponders, thalidomide has shown benefit.

        d. Other causes include KS, mycobacterial infections, and classic reflux esophagitis. In many series, 8–20% of patients have a normal-appearing mucosa and normal biopsies.

2. **Clinical syndromes are identical** regardless of the etiology. Common symptoms include odynophagia, dysphagia, and retrosternal chest pain.
3. **Diagnosis** usually is made by giving a 1- to 2-week **empiric course of antifungal therapy** for presumed candidiasis (see Chap. 18 for dosages). Esophageal **endoscopy** with biopsy is reserved for those who do not respond to antifungal treatment. (We do not routinely treat empirically for both *Candida* and HSV.) Endoscopy will be necessary to diagnose CMV. **Esophagography** may miss a high percentage of cases of candidiasis and seldom is useful [163a].
4. **Management** includes treatment of pain, nutritional support, and antimicrobials as indicated (e.g., fluconazole for *Candida*). Many patients develop recurrent esophageal symptoms and may require chronic suppressive therapy.

H. **AIDS-related biliary tract disease** [152a].
1. These patients characteristically present with low-grade fever and abdominal pain.
2. Acalculous cholecystitis, sclerosing cholangitis, dilation of bile ducts, and papillary stenosis are recognized complications of HIV infection and characteristically these complications are caused by *Cryptosporidium parvum,* CMV, or a member of the order Microsporidia [152a].
3. The diagnosis is made by examining bile, gallbladder, ductal mucosa, or ampullary tissue [152a].

I. **Miscellaneous syndromes** are discussed in detail elsewhere [9, 12–16], but related topics include the following:
1. **Malignancy.** There is an unusually high incidence of rare neoplasms in AIDS. Opportunistic infections often occur concomitantly. The tumors all are linked to DNA viruses, suggesting that the immunologic lesion in AIDS allows latent viruses to produce neoplasms.
   Non-Hodgkin's lymphoma of B-cell origin is seen with increased frequency in AIDS patients. Extralymphatic involvement is found in more than 90% of patients. Brain and bone marrow are the most common extralymphatic sites, but heart, lung, soft tissue, bile duct, and other areas have been described. Therapy tends to be much less effective in AIDS patients with lymphoma than in immunocompetent patients suffering from the same high-grade lymphoma. Survival tends to be best in those patients without past opportunistic infections.
2. **Renal manifestations.** A variety of renal lesions, including focal and segmental glomerulosclerosis with proteinuria, mesangial proliferation, and acute tubular necrosis, have been described. AIDS patients with AIDS-related nephropathy and renal failure have a poor prognosis and may not benefit from hemodialysis.
3. **Rheumatologic manifestations.** Musculoskeletal complications are common in patients with advanced AIDS. Signs and symptoms include Reiter's syndrome, other forms of arthritis, and myositis. The possible etiologies include a direct effect of HIV or one of its components or a response to the circulating immune complexes generated in the course of infection.
4. **Endocrinologic manifestations.** CMV frequently is found in adrenal glands at autopsy. Clinical Addison's disease may occur rarely.

VII. **Opportunistic infections in AIDS.** With progressive dysfunction of the immune system, patients with HIV infection are at increasingly higher risk for development of opportunistic infections. Although more than 100 microorganisms have been associated with opportunistic infections, the most common opportunistic infections are shown in Table 19-7; they are summarized below and are reviewed elsewhere [9–16].
   In general, most infections, with the exception of tuberculosis, do not occur until the CD4 cell count is less than 200/mm³, and many are not encountered until the counts have dropped below 50/mm³. The probability of developing any AIDS-defining opportunistic infection after the first observation of a CD4 count of <200/mm³ was 33% at 1 year and 58% at 2 years [164] (Fig. 19-3). Because of the continual introduction of new therapies, the specific treatment for many opportunistic infections is a rapidly changing field. In addition, because of the increasing numbers of diseases for which effective prophylaxis now exists, the clinical spectrum of opportunistic infections in AIDS continues to change. **Recently, excellent summaries** of **prophylaxis** [164a] and **therapy** [164b] have been published.
   Recent concepts in the prevention of opportunistic infections are discussed in detail in sec. VIII.

Table 19-7. AIDS-indicator opportunistic infections diagnosed in patients reported to have AIDS in 1993, by age group, in the United States

Opportunistic infection	No. of cases in indicated group	
	Adults/ adolescents	Children (<13 yr)
Bacterial infections, recurrent	NA	165
Candidiasis of bronchi, trachea, or lungs	968	30
Candidiasis of esophagus	8,170	128
Coccidioidomycosis	225	0
Cryptococcosis	2,508	12
Cryptosporidiosis	1,273	34
Cytomegalovirus disease other than retinitis	2,520	57
Cytomegalovirus retinitis	2,623	20
Herpes simplex virus disease	2,883	46
Histoplasmosis	544	1
Isosporiasis	76	1
Mycobacterium avium, M. intracellulare, or *M. kansasii* disease	4,132	62
Mycobacterium tuberculosis infection, disseminated	1,575	5
M. tuberculosis infection, pulmonary	6,288*	NA
Mycobacterial disease, other	774	6
Pneumocystitis carinii pneumonia	20,235	284
Pneumonia, recurrent	2,390	NA
Progressive multifocal leukoencephalopathy	499	2
Salmonella septicemia, recurrent	135	NA
Toxoplasmosis of brain	2,695	9

NA = not applicable.
*Pulmonary tuberculosis was added to the AIDS case definition in 1993 and can be reported retrospectively. Of the 6,288 cases, only 1,937 were diagnosed in 1993.
Note: A total of 105,990 cases of AIDS in adults and adolescents and 959 cases in children were reported. The table includes 61,375 cases (60,513 in adults and adolescents and 862 in children). Excluded are cases with AIDS-indicator conditions of noninfectious or unproven infectious etiology, such as HIV encephalopathy, HIV wasting syndrome, Kaposi's sarcoma, lymphoma, and lymphoid interstitial pneumonia; also excluded are cases in adults and adolescents reported on the basis of CD4+ lymphopenia.
Source: J. E. Kaplan et al. and the USPHS/IDSA Prevention of Opportunistic Infections Working Group, USPHS/IDSA guidelines for the prevention of opportunistic infections in persons infected with human immunodeficiency virus: Introduction. *Clin. Infect. Dis.* 21(Suppl. 1):S1, 1995. Published by The University of Chicago Press.

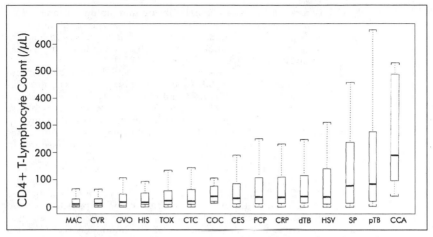

Fig. 19-3. Distribution of CD4+ lymphocyte counts at diagnosis of opportunistic infections. Horizontal line in the interior of each box indicates the median count. The height of the box indicates the interquartile range, representing the 25th and 75th percentiles of the CD4+ distribution. Dotted lines extend to the extreme values of the data. Data are from the CDC Adult and Adolescent Spectrum of Disease Study and cover the period from January 1990 through April 1994. MAC = disseminated infection with *Mycobacterium avium* complex; CVR = cytomegalovirus retinitis; CVO = cytomegalovirus disease other than retinitis; HIS = histoplasmosis; TOX = toxoplasmosis; CTC = cryptococcosis; COC = coccidioidomycosis; CES = *Candida* esophagitis, PCP = *Pneumocystis carinii* pneumonia; CRP = cryptosporidiosis; dTB = disseminated tuberculosis; HSV = chronic mucocutaneous disease due to herpes simplex virus; SP = pneumococcal pneumonia; pTB = pulmonary tuberculosis; and CCA = cervical cancer. (From J. E. Kaplan et al. and the USPHS/IDSA Prevention of Opportunistic Infections Working Group, USPHS/IDSA guidelines for the prevention of opportunistic infections in persons infected with human immunodeficiency virus: Introduction. *Clin. Infect. Dis.* 21(Suppl. 1):S1, 1995. Published by The University of Chicago Press.) Note: μL = mm³.

A. **Viral infections**
   1. **Cytomegalovirus** disease occurs in 40% of AIDS patients [165] and, at autopsy, more than 90% of AIDS patients have documented CMV infection [166]. **Virtually all patients with disease due to CMV have CD4 counts of less than 100/mm³ [167].** As patients with AIDS live longer with severely impaired immune systems, the incidence of CMV disease will increase, with a widening array of clinical syndromes.
      a. **Linking detection of CMV to disease may be difficult** because the presence of CMV in culture does not necessarily indicate invasive disease. Therefore, clinical presentation, physical examination, histopathologic findings, and viral culture all must be considered. **Different criteria are used for diagnosis depending on the affected organ system** (see individual sections). Routinely, CMV is cultured in blood and urine specimens as well as detected histopathologically at autopsy. However, the positive predictive value of CMV viremia (35%) and viruria (28%) for the development of end-organ disease was poor in a recent study [168]. Similarly, positive cultures do not correlate with symptoms of disseminated disease, such as fever and weight loss, but instead correlate with the degree of immunosuppression [168].
      b. **Clinical syndromes**
         (1) **Chorioretinitis** develops in at least 20% of patients with AIDS. It is seldom the presenting manifestation but **occurs when the CD4 count is less than 50/mm³ [169].** Symptoms include decreasing visual acuity, the presence of so-called floaters, or visual field cut defects. Blindness will result if CMV is left untreated [170].

(a) **Diagnosis is made clinically by ophthalmologic examination.** Typical findings include creamy or yellow-white granular areas with perivascular exudates and hemorrhages. These lesions are found initially in the periphery of the fundus but can progress to involve the macula and optic disc [170].

(b) For **therapy,** two drugs currently are available: **ganciclovir** and **foscarnet. These agents,** including oral ganciclovir, **are discussed in detail in Chap. 26.** Induction therapy includes 2 weeks or more of high-dose drug. When retinitis is stable, patients are placed on lifelong maintenance therapy. Ganciclovir therapy (induction dose, 10 mg/kg/day in two divided doses; maintenance dose, 5 mg/kg/day) is associated with an initial response rate of 80–90%; however, 30% of patients relapse within 1 year [171, 172]. Side effects include myelosuppression, particularly neutropenia. Foscarnet (induction dose, 60 mg/kg q8h; maintenance dose, 90–120 mg/kg/day) is similarly effective. Side effects include renal impairment, local periurethral ulceration, paresthesias, seizures, and other CNS symptoms. A trial in 1992 comparing ganciclovir to foscarnet for new retinitis found that there was no difference between the two in the frequency and rate of progression of the retinitis. However, although therapy with foscarnet was not as well tolerated as ganciclovir, it offered a survival advantage, perhaps secondary to its direct antiviral activity [173].

(2) **CMV colitis** develops in 5–10% of patients. **Symptoms are nonspecific** and may include diarrhea, weight loss, abdominal pain and cramping, anorexia, and fever [174].

(a) **Diagnosis is made by endoscopic biopsy** [174a]. Endoscopy reveals mucosal ulceration and submucosal hemorrhage.

(b) **Therapy** with ganciclovir and foscarnet is variably effective. Some studies show improvement of symptoms and the gross and pathologic appearance of the colon, as well as decreased incidence of extracolonic CMV infection [174–175]. However, not all patients respond, and the optimal dose and length of treatment are not well defined. One approach is to treat patients for 2 weeks and follow them clinically. Nonresponders need not receive more therapy, whereas responders may be candidates for chronic suppressive therapy.

(3) **CMV pneumonitis** is a major cause of morbidity and mortality in bone marrow transplantation patients, but invasive pneumonitis very uncommonly occurs in AIDS. **CMV often is isolated in respiratory specimens, along with other pathogens, yet treatment of other pathogens usually results in clinical improvement though CMV infection is not treated** [176]. However, true CMV pneumonitis is seen and may be increasing in incidence as patients are living longer. Clinical symptoms include worsening shortness of breath, dyspnea on exertion, and dry cough. Chest radiograph may show diffuse infiltrates similar to what is seen with PCP.

(a) **Diagnosis** is made by demonstrating pathognomonic intranuclear inclusion bodies ("owl's eyes") on biopsy specimens. The diagnosis may be suggested in patients with positive CMV cultures, no other recovered pathogens, and response to ganciclovir treatment.

(b) **Therapy** is with ganciclovir at routine doses (see Chap. 26). Unlike bone marrow transplant patients, there is no proven benefit to concurrent intravenous immunoglobulin. Maintenance therapy should be considered for responders.

(4) **CMV esophagitis** is less common than that caused by *Candida albicans*. Symptoms include odynophagia, dysphagia, or vague dyspepsia. **Diagnosis is made by endoscopic biopsy.** Ganciclovir is effective for treatment. Maintenance therapy is not used unless symptoms recur.

(5) **CMV encephalitis** usually is diagnosed postmortem [177–178a]. Symptoms are varied and include cognitive deficits, personality changes, and increased somnolence [179, 180]. Diagnosis often is confused with progressive AIDS dementia. Antiviral treatment has not been shown to be effective.

(6) **CMV ventriculitis** has recently been described [178, 178a, 181, 182]. Although the syndrome is still being defined, patients may have headache, diffuse cognitive defects including dementia, and cranial nerve palsies [183]. Patients may either have no history of CMV disease [183] or already be on therapy for CMV [184]. Spinal fluid analysis shows a pleocytosis, usually with lymphocytes but sometimes with polymorphonuclear leukocytes (PMNs), marked increase in protein, and low glucose [183]. MRI may reveal a characteristic periventricular ringlike enhancement [184]. Viral culture of CSF is not always positive; recent studies have suggested a diagnostic role for PCR [185]. Therapy with ganciclovir or foscarnet may ameliorate symptoms if given early, but response is unpredictable and most cases progress [186].

(7) **CMV polyradiculitis** may cause radicular pain, progressive ascending paralysis, and urinary retention [178a, 187]. The CSF may have a pleocytosis with a predominance of PMNs (which is unusual for viral infection), elevated protein, and low glucose [188]. Diagnosis is made by viral culture of CSF; PCR may also be useful [185]. Therapy with ganciclovir has resulted in improvement of symptoms in some patients [189, 190]. Some experts give ganciclovir concurrently with foscarnet.

(8) **CMV involvement of the adrenal glands** is seen at autopsy in up to 50% of patients [191]. However, clinical adrenal insufficiency is less common, and the correlation between adrenal infection and clinical adrenal dysfunction is incomplete. Adrenal insufficiency should be considered in all patients with CMV elsewhere and clinical symptoms consistent with Addison's disease, including electrolyte abnormalities, unexplained hypotension, fever, and fatigue. **Diagnosis is confirmed by the cosyntropin stimulation test.** Dramatic improvement may be seen with steroid replacement therapy.

2. **Herpes simplex virus** (HSV) types 1 and 2 commonly cause disease in HIV-infected persons; 95% of homosexual men with AIDS have positive serology for HSV [192].
   a. **Diagnosis** of HSV infection is made **by clinical presentation or by viral culture.** HSV should be considered as a cause of any chronic nonhealing ulcer.
   b. **Clinical syndromes** of HSV infection include orolabial infection, genital and anorectal infection (see Chap. 13), esophagitis, herpetic whitlow and, rarely, encephalitis [171].
   c. For **therapy,** oral acyclovir (200–400 mg 5 times daily) is the treatment of choice for most routine lesions. Topical acyclovir is not effective.
      (1) **Suppressive acyclovir** therapy is recommended for patients with recurrent infections or relapses after the discontinuation of therapy [193]. Many patients can be controlled with 400–800 mg/day in divided doses. Doses should be individualized, as different patients require different doses.
      (2) **Acyclovir-resistant** HSV infection is increasingly common. Patients at risk usually have had a prior history of acyclovir use. Foscarnet (40 mg/kg/day) is effective at standard doses and should be continued for 7–10 days. Lesions usually recur with sensitive herpesvirus [194], although the second recurrence often is resistant.
      (3) Acyclovir and foscarnet are discussed in more detail in Chap. 26.

3. **Varicella-zoster virus** (VZV) is a common pathogen that causes an array of clinical syndromes, ranging from shingles or disseminated skin involvement to postinfectious vasculitis or visceral disease. **Shingles may be the first clinical evidence of HIV infection and for this reason, many experts recommend HIV testing for any young to middle-aged individual presenting with shingles,** especially if there are any risk factors for HIV infection (see Chap. 4).
   a. The unique unilateral dermatomal distribution of clustered vesicles allows **clinical diagnosis of most cases of shingles.** Early cases with few vesicles or multidermatomal cases may be more difficult to diagnose clinically. In such cases, confirmatory viral culture is recommended.
      HIV-positive patients (regardless of the CD4 cell count) have a higher incidence of dermatomal zoster and are at increased risk for disseminated disease compared to age-matched immunocompetent hosts [195].

    b. Varicella-zoster virus has been recovered from **retinal tissue** in patients with sudden blindness due to **acute retinal necrosis** [196, 197]. **Varicella encephalitis** [198], a subacute encephalitis characterized by slowly progressive dementia and confusion that involves the white matter preferentially, may also be seen.

    c. **Treatment** of VZV requires higher doses of acyclovir than that used for HSV. Some experts treat all patients with dermatomal zoster with intravenous acyclovir (30 mg/kg/day in three divided doses), but it probably is acceptable to treat simple cases in individuals with CD4 cell counts in excess of 200/mm^3 with oral medication (800 mg 5 times daily). All patients with disseminated disease, multidermatomal zoster, or involvement of the ophthalmic division of the trigeminal nerve should receive intravenous acyclovir. See related discussions in Chap. 26.

    As with HSV, **acyclovir-resistant VZV** infection has been reported. The vesicles in this syndrome often are atypical, with a more necrotic base and larger, more leathery appearance. Foscarnet is effective [199].

    The best therapy for retinal necrosis is not known. There is no apparent response to either steroids or antiviral therapy, although antiviral therapy often is tried.

4. JC virus is a papovavirus that infects the oligodendrocytes to cause **progressive multifocal leukoencephalopathy.** Approximately 4% of AIDS patients develop PML, which is caused by reactivation of prior infection [200].

    a. Diagnosis must be **made by brain biopsy,** which shows focal myelin loss with bizarre astrocytes and other changes. Suggestive CT findings include multiple nonenhancing lesions scattered throughout the white matter without mass effect. MRI may also be suggestive: Lesions are hypodense on T_1 images and hyperdense on T_2 lesions [201, 202]. PCR analysis of CSF has been developed but is not yet reliable [203].

    b. Clinical presentation varies depending on the area involved and **ranges from diffuse encephalopathy to focal deficits** such as ataxia, hemiparesis, or speech difficulties. Symptoms tend to progress rapidly over several months, although rare patients have a waxing and waning clinical course extending for years. Unlike global dementia of AIDS, the cognitive deficit of PML often progresses rapidly and can occur with other focal neurologic deficits.

    c. There is **no known treatment** of PML. Some preliminary studies have shown some benefit with cytosine arabinoside (ara-C) given either intravenously or intrathecally [204, 205]; current protocols continue this evaluation. In addition, some patients improve with institution of zidovudine therapy.

5. Hepatitis viruses A, B, and C are prevalent among the HIV-infected, and the course of hepatitis B and C is modified by HIV coinfection. In patients with both HIV and hepatitis B virus (HBV), increased carriage rates and increased viral replication are seen. As CD4 cell counts drop, surface antibody titers decrease and patients can have reactivation of latent HBV [206]. With hepatitis C, small studies have shown increased rates of viremia [207] **(see Chap. 11)**.

B. Spirochetes

1. Syphilis and HIV infection are uniquely associated. Epidemiologic studies have shown that a history of STDs such as syphilis is associated with increased risk of HIV infection, and the genital ulcerations caused by *T. pallidum* may be important in the transmission of the virus [208, 209]. Further, coexistent HIV infection may alter the clinical course of syphilis, especially latent and tertiary disease [210]. **See related discussions of neurosyphilis in Chap. 5 and syphilis in Chap. 13.**

    a. Diagnosis of syphilis remains confusing [210a]. Serologic tests, patient history, clinical examination, and dark-field examination of tissue are all used. The last is the only means of practical, direct diagnosis. **In HIV-infected individuals, serologic tests can have falsely high or false negative results** in patients with low CD4 cell counts [211]. Microhemagglutinating antibody to *T. pallidum* (MHA-TP) may be lost with progression of HIV disease. Therefore, a negative test does not always rule out current or previous infection. Current recommendations for evaluation of latent syphilis **(a positive VDRL greater than 1:2 with no symptoms or history**

of treatment) in an HIV-infected person (regardless of CD4 cell counts) include a CSF examination to rule out neurosyphilis, as 35% of persons with secondary syphilis have asymptomatic CSF involvement [212]. Diagnosis of neurosyphilis is made by a positive CSF serology, high protein, or pleocytosis; however, there are many false negative tests [213].

b. **Clinical presentation is nonspecific** and varies depending on the stage of HIV infection. Symptoms are similar to normal hosts in early infection (see Chap. 13), yet there is a higher incidence of neurosyphilis, which may develop rapidly or years after therapy [210, 214].

c. **Treatment** with benzathine penicillin (2.4 million units) is recommended for **primary or secondary syphilis** in patients who have no evidence of neurosyphilis in CSF. For patients with syphilis of less than 1 year's duration, a single dose is adequate, but in patients with unknown incubation, three doses are needed. In both cases, follow-up serologies should be obtained and, in HIV-positive patients, a slower decrease in serologic response may be seen [215]. **Treatment of neurosyphilis is with high-dose penicillin G** (12–24 million units/day) for 2 weeks.

Even with proper therapy, some HIV-infected patients may have serologic relapse. Therefore, careful long-term follow-up is essential, and repeated courses of therapy may be needed for some patients [215a]. Consequently, the optimal therapy of syphilis in this setting is not entirely clear, and some experts advocate higher doses of penicillin for primary and secondary syphilis in the HIV-positive patient. This topic is discussed further in Chap. 13. Infectious disease consultation is suggested.

The CDC has recently issued **specific guidelines for treatment** of all STDs. This is a valuable and up-to-date resource [216].

d. **Other STDs** that cause ulcerating genital ulcers, including chancroid (*Haemophilus ducreyi*) and HSV may be seen in HIV-infected persons. **Diagnosis** and **treatment** are similar to that for normal hosts. However, the role of these genital ulcer diseases in the transmission of HIV has been well demonstrated. Persons with chancroid, which characteristically causes larger, more friable ulcers, particularly have been found to have higher rates of HIV seroconversion. See Chap. 13.

2. *Borrelia burgdorferi* (Lyme disease) does not appear to be more prevalent or more severe in HIV-positive patients.

C. **Bacterial infections.** Bacterial infections continue to cause significant morbidity and mortality in patients with AIDS [216a]. **Humoral dysfunction** is one of the first clinically evident immunologic sequelae of HIV infection, resulting in bacterial infections caused by *S. pneumoniae, S. aureus* (in intravenous drug users especially, or in those with a central line), other streptococci, *H. influenzae, P. aeruginosa,* and other bacteria **even in patients with high CD4 cell counts.** In addition, antibody responses to vaccines against many bacteria are blunted, limiting their usefulness [217, 218]. Other bacteria, including the mycobacteria, *Salmonella* spp., and *Listeria monocytogenes* are **intracellular pathogens and exploit defects in cell-mediated immunity.**

In a recent report, the incidence of bacterial pneumonia was again emphasized; the rate of bacterial pneumonia increased with decreasing CD4 counts [218a].

1. *S. pneumoniae* is the **most common respiratory pathogen** with associated bacteremia in HIV-positive patients. The **incidence of pneumococcal pneumonia is 5–10 times higher than in the general population** and precedes the diagnosis of AIDS in more than 55% of patients. Overall, 10% of all pneumonias in AIDS patients are bacterial, and *S. pneumoniae* is the most common organism seen [219].

a. **Diagnosis** is made by sputum or blood culture. There is a **higher incidence of bacteremia** in HIV-positive patients with pneumonia than in normal hosts. Some studies found the incidence of bacteremia to be as high as 46% among the HIV-infected versus 10–15% in normal hosts. This suggests higher bacterial loads among the HIV-infected [220].

b. **Clinical presentation** and mortality are similar to that in normal hosts (see Chap. 9), but relapse rates are higher in HIV-positive patients [221]. Symptoms often have an abrupt onset and include fever, productive cough, dyspnea, and acute pleuritic chest pain. The syndrome is usually distinct from PCP, which typically is indolent and associated with dry cough and infrequent chest pain.

   c. **Treatment** is with **penicillin;** however penicillin-resistant pneumococci have recently become more common [222]. In locations in which a high incidence of penicillin resistance to *S. pneumoniae* is present, an alternative antibiotic may be necessary (see Chap. 9 and Chap. 28C for antibiotic therapy).

   d. **Prevention** is best achieved with the 23-valent pneumococcal vaccine, which covers more than 80% of isolates. However, efficacy is blunted by diminished antibody responses seen in HIV-infected patients with decreasing CD4 cell counts. Trimethoprim-sulfamethoxazole used for PCP prophylaxis has protective effect [218a], although disease due to trimethoprim-sulfamethoxazole-resistant *S. pneumoniae* may occur. Some individuals may develop recurrent infections as often as 4–6 times per year. An option we use in such persons is to give chronic suppressive therapy with daily penicillin G, 500 mg PO bid, similar to that given to splenectomized individuals.

  2. *Salmonella* infections, particularly bacteremia, are seen in higher frequency in HIV-positive patients. Non-*typhi* spp., especially *S. enteritidis* and *S. typhimurium,* are isolated most often.

   a. **Diagnosis** is made by culture of blood, stool, or urine.

   b. The **clinical course** in patients with AIDS is more severe than in normal hosts. Rates of bacteremia are increased, fever may persist for 1–2 weeks, and higher relapses are seen as well [154, 223].

   c. **Treatment** with ampicillin, ciprofloxacin, or trimethoprim-sulfamethoxazole is effective. Therapy should extend for at least 7–10 days after defervescence. Some experts place all patients with salmonellosis onto chronic suppressive therapy; others give suppressive therapy only to those with recurrent disease. Oral amoxicillin, ciprofloxacin, and trimethoprim-sulfamethoxazole are equally effective for chronic suppression.

   d. **See related discussion in Chap. 11.**

  3. *Listeria monocytogenes* is seen more often in HIV-positive patients than in age-matched controls; it usually occurs in patients with low CD4 cell counts. Clinical manifestations are similar to those in normal hosts, with a high incidence of bacteremia [224]. Atypical presentations, including brain abscesses and pericarditis, have also been seen.

  4. *P. aeruginosa* is not a common pathogen outside the hospital. Nonetheless, **serious *P. aeruginosa* infections, including community-acquired pneumonia and bacteremia, are occurring more frequently** in children and adults with AIDS [224a]. Recent hospitalization, end-stage disease, and prior antibiotic therapy (possibly including prophylactic or therapeutic regimens with trimethoprim-sulfamethoxazole or multidrug regimens for mycobacterial disease) may be predisposing conditions, although these have not been well defined.

    Until culture data are available in a very ill patient with bacteremia or pneumonia in the setting just described, antibiotic therapy aimed at *P. aeruginosa* (e.g., an aminoglycoside) seems prudent.

  5. **Bacillary angiomatosis** (BA) is a disease caused by small gram-negative organisms of the genus *Rochalimaea* (more recently called *Bartonella*), specifically *R. henselae* and *R. quintana*. This agent was discussed briefly in Chap. 17 under Cat-Scratch Disease [225].

   a. **Clinical presentation** depends on the organ system involved.

     (1) **Cutaneous lesions are raised erythematous areas that bleed when traumatized.** They also can appear as a **cellulitic plaque,** which often overlies osteolytic lesions. They can occur singly or multiply and can occur in any location. Most often they are confused with KS.

     (2) **Osseous BA,** often seen with cutaneous lesions, causes bone pain. Bones most affected include tibia, fibula, and radius.

     (3) **Hepatic BA (peliosis hepatitis)** is characterized by vascular lesions within hepatocytes. Patients present with abdominal pain and fever with high alkaline phosphatase. CT scan demonstrates heterogeneity in the liver. Lesions are seen also in the spleen [226, 227].

     (4) Other systems involved include the **GI tract, respiratory tract, bone marrow, and lymph nodes** [219, 227].

   b. Diagnosis is made by **tissue biopsy and demonstration of the organisms** by modified silver staining (Warthin-Starry). Histopathologic evaluation demonstrates vascular proliferation that can be mistaken for KS, angiosarcoma, or pyogenic granuloma. The organism has also been cultured from the blood but the plates need to be incubated at 35°C for 3 weeks. Use of the Isolator lysis-centrifugation system (Wampole Laboratories, Cranbury, NJ) for blood cultures may also increase the yield of cultures, which should be incubated at least 14 days. Recently, the CDC has developed an indirect immunofluorescent antibody test to detect antibodies to *R. henselae,* which has been useful for diagnosis of both acute disease and relapse [225]. See Chap. 17.
   c. Treatment. Erythromycin is first-line therapy, although cures have also been reported with doxycycline and azithromycin [228]. Despite in vitro susceptibilities, penicillins and first-generation cephalosporins have no activity against *Rochalimaea.* The optimal duration of therapy is unknown, but current recommendations for cutaneous lesions are for 8–12 weeks of therapy (erythromycin, 500 mg qid); for osseous and liver lesions, therapy should probably be continued for at least 3 months [227]. The widespread use of the macrolides in patients with low CD4 cell counts, as prophylaxis against *M. avium* complex disease, may result in a decrease in the incidence of this disease.
 6. Catheter sepsis is increasingly a problem in HIV-positive patients as long-term indwelling catheters are being used more often. The incidence of infection is higher than in other patient populations with catheters. Gram-positive cocci, especially *Staphylococcus* spp., gram-negative bacilli including *P. aeruginosa,* and polymicrobial infection may be encountered [229]. Fungemia due to *C. albicans, C. parapsilosis, Torulopsis glabrata,* and other organisms also is seen. **See related discussion in Chap. 2.**
   a. Diagnosis generally is made by blood culture. However, patients with infusion-associated fever and rigors should be suspected of having catheter-related bacteremia and admitted for intravenous antibiotics.
   b. Treatment should be directed at the most likely bacteria, which vary from medical center to medical center. Generally, empiric therapy to treat both gram-positive and gram-negative bacteria should be given, regardless of the underlying WBC count. Vancomycin and gentamicin is a commonly used regimen pending culture results. Ceftazidime is used by some if an aminoglycoside is contraindicated. Catheters should be **removed** in patients who present with sustained hemodynamic compromise, who have tunnel infections [230], or who are persistently bacteremic despite days of appropriate antibiotic therapy. See related discussion in Chap. 2.
D. Mycobacteria
 1. *Mycobacterium tuberculosis* has emerged in recent years as a **major health threat** to the HIV-infected patient. Beginning in 1984, the decades-long decrease in the annual incidence of tuberculosis ended and, by 1988, annual case rates began to increase [231]. Intensive control efforts led to a decrease in cases in 1993 [232]. The age and race groups with the **greatest increases in** rates of tuberculosis, specifically **black and Hispanic men aged 25–40, are also the groups with the highest rates of HIV infection, demonstrating how closely intertwined these two epidemics have become** [231]. Anonymous HIV testing of serum from tuberculosis clinics demonstrated that as many as 40% of all tuberculosis patients are HIV-infected [233]. This number may be even higher in certain urban areas. In addition, **tuberculosis is unusual among AIDS-related opportunistic infections because it is contagious to nonimmunocompromised persons** as well. This, combined with several well-documented **nosocomial outbreaks** of tuberculosis affecting both patients and staff [234], has led to extensive reconsideration of hospital infection control efforts [235]. Finally, **resistant tuberculosis** has been seen with increasing frequency, especially in urban areas [235–238]. This disease is particularly difficult to treat in the HIV-infected patient.
   A detailed discussion of *M. tuberculosis,* including its pathogenesis, diagnosis, and therapy, is presented in Chap. 9.
   a. Clinical presentation depends largely on the overall immune status of the patient [238]. Patients with high CD4 cell counts (> 200–300/mm^3)

generally will have classic tuberculosis, with apical cavitary lung disease, respiratory symptoms, fevers, and weight loss. **As immunity wanes, presentations become less specific,** and higher rates of extrapulmonary tuberculosis are encountered. Hilar or mediastinal adenopathy may be the primary chest roentgenogram abnormality. Fever, weight loss, and fatigue may be the only symptoms of persons with disseminated tuberculosis, a symptom complex similar to lymphoma, CMV disease, AIDS wasting syndrome, MAC, and other illnesses [155]. In addition, patients with pulmonary tuberculosis may have chest roentgenograms like those of primary tuberculosis, with lobar and interstitial infiltrates; **10–20% may have normal radiographs** [239].

b. **Concurrent HIV and tuberculosis infection alters the natural history of tuberculosis** in several ways:

(1) HIV-infected persons latently infected with tuberculosis will develop **reactivation tuberculosis** at a rate of 8–10% per year, rather than 5–10% per lifetime [240].

(2) **HIV-infected persons exposed to an infectious index case will develop acute tuberculosis at a rate as high as 40% over 6–12 months** rather than 2–5% over 2 years, as is seen in normal hosts [241].

(3) **Tuberculosis may accelerate the progression of HIV infection** by activating expression of HIV from macrophages [242].

c. **Diagnosis** requires culturing *M. tuberculosis* from appropriate specimens. The mainstay of empiric diagnosis, the sputum smear for acid-fast bacilli, is approximately 50% sensitive in HIV-infected persons, a rate similar to that seen in HIV-negative persons [243]. Cultures using a radiometric system (BACTEC) may speed the diagnosis, so that results may be available within 1–2 weeks rather than the 6–8 weeks customary for solid agar media. Because the initial acid-fast bacilli sputum smear cannot distinguish *M. tuberculosis* from *M. avium* complex, mycobacterium cultures with identification and susceptibility data of *M. tuberculosis* isolates should be routinely performed. Newer techniques, including PCR, remain investigational and cannot be relied on in routine care of patients [244].

d. **Treatment** recommendations for tuberculosis have recently been summarized by the American Thoracic Society [245] and are reviewed further in Chap. 9.

(1) The society suggests that HIV-infected persons **with known drug-susceptible tuberculosis** should receive regimens identical to those given HIV-negative persons (four drugs—isoniazid, rifampin, ethambutol, and pyrazinamide—for 2 months, then isoniazid and rifampin for 4 months more). However, because of concern that this regimen may be inadequate in duration [246, 247], clinical trials comparing rates of cure and relapse in 6- versus 9-month courses are currently under way.

(2) The optimal treatment of **resistant and multidrug-resistant** tuberculosis in HIV-infected patients must be individualized, depending on the susceptibility pattern, other underlying diseases, and the severity of the illness [248]. HIV-infected persons with tuberculosis resistant to both isoniazid and rifampin require at least 18–24 months of treatment with a multidrug regimen. If regimens are modified, two or more active agents should be added simultaneously to minimize further selection of resistant organisms (see Chap. 9). Infectious disease or pulmonary consultation is advised to help design optimal treatment regimens.

e. **Prophylaxis** for latent infection among HIV-infected persons includes **12 months of daily isoniazid, 300 mg.** Prophylaxis for tuberculosis may slow progression to AIDS [249]. The recommended prophylaxis for **persons exposed to tuberculosis resistant to both isoniazid and rifampin is unknown** but should include at least two agents to which the index case is sensitive [250]. See Table 19-8 and Chap. 9.

f. *M. tuberculosis* is discussed in detail in Chap. 9.

2. *Mycobacterium avium* **complex (MAC)** is the **most common systemic bacterial infection in AIDS** and is responsible for significant morbidity. The prevalence of diagnosed disseminated MAC (dMAC) for patients with CD4 cell counts of fewer than 100/mm^3 is approximately 10% [251]; at autopsy, prior

to routine use of prophylaxis, the rate was approximately 50% [252–254]. A recent increase in incidence can be attributed to greater surveillance and longer survival of patients with AIDS with low CD4 cell counts [251].

   a. **Clinical presentation** of dMAC includes **fevers, night sweats, weight loss and, less often, diarrhea. Hepatosplenomegaly** may be present but the examination often is quite nonspecific and unrevealing. Common laboratory abnormalities include **anemia** and **elevated alkaline phosphatase.**

   b. **Diagnosis depends on aggressively culturing** possible sites, including rectal swab, blood, lymph nodes, liver, and bone marrow, for mycobacteria. **Blood cultures using special culture media** (e.g., Isolator lysis-centrifugation system) **yield the highest results.** Whereas a single blood culture is diagnostic for dMAC infection, a negative culture does not rule out disseminated infection as patients can have low levels of mycobacteremia [251, 255, 256]. An acid-fast bacilli stain of a rectal swab may be helpful.

   c. **Treatment of MAC continues to improve.** Many drugs have activity, including the macrolides (clarithromycin and azithromycin), the rifamycins (rifabutin and rifampin), clofazimine, ciprofloxacin, ethambutol, and amikacin. **Therapy initially should include a macrolide and ethambutol.** A third agent, such as a rifamycin or ciprofloxacin, can either be included in the initial regimen or added if there is a slow response. The addition of amikacin or a fourth agent may be needed in some patients who fail to respond or who relapse [251, 257–258a]. In patients who are very ill with MAC, we have sometimes used a multidrug regimen initially (e.g., clarithromycin, ethambutol, ciprofloxacin, and amikacin) to try to diminish rapidly the bacteremic load of organisms. Once the patient clinically responds, we then will use at least two oral agents (e.g., ethambutol and clarithromycin) to simplify an outpatient regimen.

   d. **Prophylaxis for MAC infection with rifabutin initially for patients with CD4 cell counts of fewer than 100/mm³ has been approved by the US Food and Drug Administration.** Rifabutin (300 mg/day) did not prevent the development of bacteremia, but the incidence was reduced by 50% and symptoms were less severe in those taking the medication [259, 260]. (The 1995 recommendations suggest consideration of prophylaxis when the CD4 count is $< 75/mm^3$; see sec. **VIII**). Preliminary, nonrandomized studies indicate that clarithromycin (500 mg bid) also is effective in reducing the incidence of MAC bacteremia [261, 262]; see related information in sec. **VIII**.

3. *Mycobacterium kansasii* is the second most common nontuberculous mycobacterial infection in patients with AIDS [263]. Most often, the disease is localized to the lungs, but the organism can cause extrapulmonary infection as well.

   a. **Clinical presentation** resembles tuberculosis and includes fever, cough, and dyspnea. Chest radiograph appearances include either upper-lobe or diffuse infiltrates.

   b. **Diagnosis** is made by culture. *M. kansasii,* similar to *M. tuberculosis,* is always considered to be pathogenic.

   c. **Treatment** recommendations include antituberculous therapy with high-dose isoniazid (600 mg/day), rifampin, and ethambutol. However, other antimycobacterial therapy including clarithromycin has been used with some success [264, 265]. Infectious disease or pulmonary consultation is advised.

4. *Mycobacterium haemophilum* is a rare mycobacterium that causes disease in immunosuppressed patients with and without HIV [266–268].

   a. **Clinical presentation** most often includes involvement of skin lesions, bone, or joints. Lung involvement has also been described [266].

   b. **Diagnosis** is made by special culture of specimens plated on chocolate heme-enriched agar and incubated at 30°C.

   c. **Treatment** has not been standardized but should include a macrolide, rifampin, or rifabutin, and probably one or two more agents from among ciprofloxacin, ethambutol, and amikacin [266]. Duration of therapy is not known, but lifetime suppression probably is required. Infectious disease consultation is advised.

5. **Other mycobacteria,** including *M. malmoense, M. genavense,* and *M. gordonae,* are being recovered more frequently in patients with AIDS [269]. This is due both to improvements in mycobacteriology laboratories and to prolonged survival with severe immunocompromise. Distinguishing colonization from

invasive disease often is difficult, and most infections do not have well-stan-
dardized treatments.

E. **Fungi.** These infections are **discussed briefly here. See Chap. 18 for a more
detailed discussion of these infections and their therapy.** Also see reference
[269a] for a recent summary.

   1. **Candidiasis** is the most common fungal condition seen in HIV-positive persons. Progression of HIV infection to AIDS is associated with the development
   of oral candidiasis [270]. *C. albicans* causes most disease; recently, however,
   other species, including *C. tropicalis* and *C. krusei,* have been seen with
   greater frequency. Chronic courses of azole therapy (e.g., in prophylaxis) may
   result in the selecting out of more resistant species (see Chap. 18).

      a. **Presentation** generally is limited to **oral, vaginal,** or **esophageal** mucosa.
      Systemic disease is rare.

         (1) Symptoms of **oropharyngeal candidiasis** include burning, pain, and
         altered taste sensation, although many patients are asymptomatic.

         (2) **Vaginal candidiasis** presents as a creamy white vaginal discharge
         and often is the first evidence of immune dysfunction in women as it
         can precede the development of oral infection [271]. Recurrent infec-
         tion is common, and chronic suppressive therapy may be necessary.
         See related discussion in Chap. 13.

         (3) **Esophageal candidiasis** may present with severe dysphagia or odyno-
         phagia in patients with or without evidence of oral infection. At endos-
         copy, ulcers and deep erosions are seen lining the esophagus [272].

      b. **Diagnosis** of oral or vaginal disease often is made on clinical appearance
      alone. In patients who fail to respond to standard therapy, KOH prepara-
      tion and fungal cultures are indicated. Esophageal disease is diagnosed
      by endoscopic examination and culture, although response to empiric
      antifungal therapy is increasingly used as an indirect means of establish-
      ing the diagnosis.

      c. Patients with localized candidiasis respond well to topical **therapy,** includ-
      ing oral troches and vaginal creams. For patients who do not respond to
      standard therapy or who have esophageal disease, the antifungal azole
      compounds (ketoconazole, fluconazole, itraconazole) are effective. Azoles
      are begun at 100 mg/day and can be increased if there is no clinical
      response. Although ketoconazole is significantly less expensive, absorption
      is more erratic, sometimes limiting its effectiveness. Fluconazole has been
      shown to be superior in direct comparative trials with ketoconazole [273].

      d. **Drug resistance,** particularly **azole-resistant** candidiasis, is increasingly
      common. Some patients respond to increased doses of the drug, and some
      respond to a switch from one azole to another (e.g., fluconazole to itracona-
      zole). However, low-dose therapy with intravenous amphotericin B (0.3–
      0.5 mg/kg/day for 1–2 weeks or until response is noted) is required for
      many. Maintenance with oral azoles often can be resumed after intrave-
      nous amphotericin B therapy, although some patients must be maintained
      on once- or twice-weekly intravenous amphotericin B.

      e. **Prevention.** See sec. **VIII.**

   2. **Aspergillosis.** Although invasive aspergillosis initially was included as an
   AIDS-defining opportunistic infection [274], it later was deleted from that
   list as it was thought that the disease was related to neutropenia and not
   lymphocyte depletion. However, **recently there have been increasing reports
   of invasive aspergillosis in AIDS.** In some series, fewer than 50% of the
   patients exhibited previously defined risk factors, suggesting that the **immune
   defects of AIDS may be sufficient to allow disease** [275]. Common conditions
   in HIV-infected persons that might be additional risks include chronic lung
   disease from recurrent pneumonias, frequent broad-spectrum antibiotic and
   corticosteroid use, and frequent use of myelosuppressive agents such as zidovudine and ganciclovir.

      a. **Presentation.** With invasive disease, organs most frequently involved in-
      clude lung (76%), CNS (32%), and heart (15%), as well as kidney, sinuses,
      and skin [276]. **AIDS patients appear to have a higher rate of CNS involve-
      ment** compared to patients with other types of immunosuppression [276].
      Most patients have CD4 cell counts of fewer than 50/mm^3 and have had
      numerous previous opportunistic infections. The chest radiograph may

show diffuse or cavitary infiltrates or may be normal, even in advanced disease. Symptoms include cough and fever and, rarely, dyspnea.

  b. **Diagnosis. Biopsy is the best means** of diagnosis. Sputum cultures are inadequate for diagnosis, as *Aspergillus* spp. may colonize the airways and may not correlate with invasive disease [277]. However, recent studies have suggested that BAL cultures often do correlate with invasive disease [275].

  c. **Therapy.** Amphotericin B remains the treatment of choice. Prognosis is still poor for invasive disease, possibly owing to delays in diagnosis. Combinations of amphotericin with flucytosine or rifampin have been used but have not been shown to increase survival. Given the poor prognosis of this rapidly progressive disease, **combination therapy** can be considered for those patients who are able to tolerate it. Itraconazole is active in vitro and may be useful in certain select cases [278]. The use of itraconazole is reviewed in Chap. 18.

3. **Histoplasmosis** occurs in at least 5% of HIV-infected patients residing within endemic regions of the United States. For these HIV-infected patients, it often is their first opportunistic infection (> 70%), and nearly all cases are disseminated at the time of diagnosis. Disseminated infection results either from direct contact with the fungus *H. capsulatum* or from reactivation of latent foci [279].

  a. **Presentation.** More than 95% of patients present with **fever** and **weight loss,** and more than 50% have **pulmonary complaints.** Physical examination is often notable for hepatosplenomegaly, lymphadenopathy and, rarely, skin lesions [279, 280]. The chest roentgenogram may show **streaky infiltrates** but can be normal in half of the cases. An elevated lactate dehydrogenase level, often higher than 1,000 U/L, may be another clue to the diagnosis. With disseminated disease, HIV-infected patients can present with a **sepsislike syndrome** characterized by hypotension, respiratory and liver failure, and disseminated intravascular coagulopathy [279].

  b. **Diagnosis** of active disease is made by **culture of appropriate sites,** including blood, bone marrow, lung tissue, or lymph node. **Sensitivity is approximately 90% for cultures** from blood or bone marrow and slightly less for respiratory specimens. In addition, an antibody-based serologic test is available, although it is less sensitive in HIV-infected patients. A test for *H. capsulatum* polysaccharide antigen from urine and blood has recently been developed and is now widely available. In one series, it had a sensitivity exceeding 90% in urine and approximately 75% in blood in HIV-positive patients [281]. Antigen levels can also be used to detect early relapse [282]. Following the lactate dehydrogenase level is also a sensitive means of following patients and detecting early relapse.

  c. **Therapy** with amphotericin B is effective in most patients. Failures were seen in patients who were severely ill at diagnosis [279]. Lifetime maintenance therapy is required to prevent relapse [283]. Although weekly or biweekly amphotericin B is effective and decreases relapse rates from 80% to 10–15%, itraconazole is equally effective, more convenient, and better tolerated [284].

  d. **Prevention.** See sec. **VIII.**

4. *Cryptococcus neoformans* most often causes meningitis or disseminated disease. Six to ten percent of patients with AIDS will develop cryptococcal infection. Some experts have suggested this may be decreasing because of oral azole use, but cryptococcus continues to account for 5% of 1992 AIDS-indicator diseases. **This topic is reviewed in detail in Chaps. 5 and 18.**

  a. **Presentation.** Cryptococcal meningitis is an **indolent disease,** with symptoms usually present for weeks prior to diagnosis. **Symptoms** include headache, fever, and malaise [285]. The headache often is worse with sneezing or coughing. Classic meningismus and focal neurologic signs are uncommon, occurring less than 10% of the time. Lethargy, mental status changes, and forgetfulness are common. Pulmonary symptoms with an abnormal chest radiograph may be seen. Prostatitis occurs frequently, and the prostate may serve as a nidus for subsequent recurrence [286]. **CSF analysis** reveals a poor inflammatory response. Protein and glucose may be normal, with little pleocytosis. **Poor prognostic factors include** impaired mental status at presentation [287], fewer than 20 WBCs in CSF, raised opening pressure, and a CSF cryptococcal antigen titer of greater than 1:1,054 [286].

b. **Diagnosis.** The latex agglutination test for the cryptococcal polysaccharide antigen is highly sensitive and specific. **In one large study, 98% of patients with culture-proven meningitis had a positive serum antigen titer** [288]. Results vary according to the laboratory and the kit used but, in general, any serum titer in excess of 1:4 should be repeated and consideration given to a full evaluation; any titer in excess of 1:32 should be considered diagnostic. **All patients with a positive serum cryptococcal antigen titer should undergo a spinal tap.** Cerebrospinal fluid India ink stains are positive approximately 75% of the time [288]. Culture of blood and CSF should be obtained.

c. **Therapy** for cryptococcosis in AIDS patients is lifelong and is discussed in detail in Chaps. 5 and 18.

d. **Prevention.** See sec. VIII.

5. **Coccidioidomycosis** is a systemic fungal disease **endemic to areas of the southwestern United States.** Rates and severity of illness are higher in HIV-infected persons [289].

a. **Presentation depends on the immunologic status of patients.** In patients with relatively normal immune function, symptoms are similar to those in immunocompetent hosts—either subclinical illness or lower respiratory symptoms [290]. For patients with CD4 cell counts of less than 250/mm³, **pneumonia** and **meningitis** are more common. The clinical picture may resemble PCP, with fever, dyspnea, nonproductive cough, and a chest radiograph with diffuse nodular infiltrates [289–291]. Coccidioidal meningitis presents with headache, fever, and lethargy. The CSF has more than 50 WBCs (predominantly lymphocytes) with low glucose and high protein. Although it is difficult to culture the organism from the CSF, the presence of complement-fixing antibodies suggests the diagnosis. (See related discussions in Chap. 5.)

b. **Diagnosis.** Coccidioidal **serologic tests** are positive in approximately 90% of HIV-positive patients. Titers reflect the activity of infection and therefore can be used to monitor response to therapy. Definitive diagnosis is made by **culture of the organism** from clinical specimens or identification of coccidioidal spherules on histopathologic examination, using stains that routinely detect *P. carinii* also [292].

c. **Treatment** of systemic disease is with amphotericin B (1 mg/kg/day) for a total dose of as much as 2.5 g. Recently, itraconazole (200 mg bid) and fluconazole (400 mg/day) have also been used with success as initial therapy [293]. Patients have survived for 1 year and longer [294]. All patients with meningitis should receive amphotericin B; intrathecal amphotericin B should be considered for nonresponders. Maintenance therapy with either intermittent amphotericin or oral azoles is recommended because relapse rates are high [295]. Studies are now under way to evaluate optimal therapeutic regimens for both induction and maintenance therapy. For related discussion, see Chaps. 5 and 18.

d. **Prevention.** See sec. VIII.

6. **Blastomycosis** is a systemic fungal disease endemic to areas of the midwestern and south-central United States. It rarely causes disease in HIV-infected persons.

a. **Presentation.** Most patients have had prior opportunistic infections and CD4 cell counts are lower than 200/mm³. Pulmonary or disseminated disease may be seen. Unlike normal hosts, in whom skin, bone, and prostate involvement is common, HIV-positive persons with disseminated disease frequently have infection in the CNS (meningitis or blastomycoma), liver, spleen, and bone marrow.

b. **Diagnosis** is made with **culture;** however, because growth requires 2 to 4 weeks, histopathologic examination of sputum, BAL fluid, and other tissue specimens should be used. Serologic tests lack sensitivity and specificity.

c. **Treatment.** HIV-infected patients should receive amphotericin B until they are stable (usually 10–20 mg/kg total dose) followed by lifelong maintenance therapy with itraconazole [296, 297].

F. Parasitic infections
   1. *Pneumocystis carinii* **pneumocystitis.** See Chap. 24.
   2. *Toxoplasma gondii* **is the most common cause of focal encephalitis in AIDS patients** [298]. Disease usually is due to recrudescence of latent infection, and therefore **all patients with antibodies to** *T. gondii* **are at risk.** Approximately 25–40% of patients with evidence of previous infection will develop disease [299]. Seroprevalence varies between geographic locations: In the United States, 20–40% of adults are latently infected, whereas in France and Germany up to 80% of the general population has evidence of past infection [300, 301].
      a. **Clinical presentation ranges from focal neurologic findings to generalized symptoms,** including weakness, confusion, seizures, and coma. Constitutional symptoms such as fever and malaise are variable, but meningismus is rare. The CSF may show a mononuclear pleocytosis and elevated protein or may be normal.
      b. **Disseminated toxoplasmosis,** involving heart, lung, colon, skeletal muscles, and other organs, has been described with increasing frequency [302–304]. Septic shock has also been seen, with presentation of prolonged fever, dyspnea, thrombocytopenia, and high lactate dehydrogenase levels [305]. Patients may appear to have tuberculosis or pneumocystosis. Diagnosis requires evaluation of appropriate biopsy specimens and serologic data.
      c. **Diagnosis is made definitively by demonstration of the tachyzoite form of** *T. gondii* **in brain biopsy specimens;** however, histologic diagnosis can be difficult because changes can resemble other infectious processes and the organism may be difficult to find [300]. **Most often, diagnosis is made presumptively based on positive serology, radiographic findings, and response to specific therapy.**
         (1) **Radiographic evaluation** of the CNS reveals single or multiple lesions with ring or nodular enhancement. Lesions are most frequently found in the basal ganglia or corticomedullary junction [306]. The **MRI scan is considered the best diagnostic imaging technique** and may detect lesions not seen on CT scanning [306].
         (2) **Serologic diagnosis** is highly reliable. Almost all patients with toxoplasmosis have IgG antibody. From a practical standpoint, if a given patient has a history of a recent negative toxoplasmosis, IgG antibody, and CNS symptoms, he or she is unlikely to have toxoplasmic encephalitis. **Seronegative toxoplasmosis is considered rare** and has been described in 0–3% of cases [298, 307–309]; however, one study did report a seronegative rate of 22% [310]. The level of antibody is not predictive of likelihood of reactivation or severity of disease.
         (3) Recently, other techniques including PCR and direct isolation of the organism have been used for the **diagnosis** of toxoplasmosis. *T. gondii* DNA by PCR has been detected in brain tissue, CSF, sputum, and blood in patients with AIDS [311–313]. *T. gondii* has also been successfully isolated from clinical samples including blood, brain BAL fluid, and muscle [314, 315].
         (4) **Response to empiric treatment is the most practical means of making the diagnosis.** In some series, 50% of patients with toxoplasmosis will respond to therapy by day 3 and 90% by day 14 [316].
         (5) **The main diagnosis of exclusion is CNS lymphoma.** All patients with characteristic lesions on CT scan or MRI and positive serology for *T. gondii* should be treated empirically for toxoplasmosis. In patients with single lesions, the predictive value is less. CNS lymphoma is 4 times more likely to present with single rather than multiple lesions [317]. However, antibody-positive patients with a single lesion should also receive empiric treatment. **For those patients who do not demonstrate a clinical response by day 14 or do not have positive serology, brain biopsy should be considered.** For those who respond, a repeat scan in 1 month may be reasonable.
      d. **The mainstay of treatment is combination chemotherapy.** Most agents act synergistically to block folic acid metabolism. For a detailed discussion of these agents and their side effects, see Chap. 28; sulfadiazine (see Chap. 28K) is commonly used with pyrimethamine (see Chap. 28U). An

Table 19-8. Prophylaxis for first episode of opportunistic disease in HIV-infected adults and adolescents

Pathogen	Indication	Preventive regimens	
		First choice	Alternatives
Strongly recommended as standard of care			
Pneumocystic carinii[a]	CD4+ count or <200/mm^3 or unexplained fever for ≥2 wk or oropharyngeal candidiasis	TMP-SMX, 1 DS tab PO qd (AI)	TMP-SMX, 1 SS tab PO qd (AI) *or* 1 DS tab PO 3×/wk (AII); dapsone, 50 mg PO bid *or* 100 mg/d PO (AI); dapsone, 50 mg/d PO, *plus* pyrimethamine, 50 mg/wk PO, *plus* leucovorin, 25 mg/wk PO (AI); dapsone, 200 mg/wk PO, *plus* pyrimethamine, 75 mg/wk PO, *plus* leucovorin, 25 mg/wk PO (AI); aerosolized pentamidine, 300 mg/mo via Respirgard II nebulizer (Marquest, Englewood, CO) (AI)
Mycobacterium tuberculosis[b]			
Isoniazid-sensitive	TST reaction of ≥5 mm *or* prior positive TST result without treatment *or* contact with case of active tuberculosis	Isoniazid, 300 mg PO, *plus* pyridoxine, 50 mg/d PO × 12 mo (AI); *or* isoniazid, 900 mg PO, *plus* pyridoxine, 50 mg PO 2×/wk for 12 mo (BIII)	Rifampin, 600 mg/d PO × 12 mo (BII)
Isoniazid-resistant	Same as above; high probability of exposure to isoniazid-resistant tuberculosis	Rifampin, 600 mg/d PO × 12 mo (BII)	Rifabutin, 300 mg/d PO × 12 mo (CIII)
Multidrug-resistant (isoniazid and rifampin)	Same as above; high probability of exposure to multidrug-resistant tuberculosis	Choice of drugs requires consultation with public health authorities	None

Pathogen	Indication	First choice	Alternatives
Toxoplasma gondii[c]	IgG antibody to *Toxoplasma* and CD4+ count of <100/mm³	TMP-SMX, 1 DS tab PO qd (AII)	TMP-SMX, 1 SS tab PO qd *or* 1 DS tab PO 3×/wk (AII); dapsone, 50 mg/d PO, *plus* pyrimethamine, 50 mg/wk PO, *plus* leucovorin, 25 mg/wk PO (AI)

Recommended for consideration in all patients

Pathogen	Indication	First choice	Alternatives
Streptococcus pneumoniae[d]	All patients	Pneumococcal vaccine, 0.5 ml IM × 1 (BIII)	None
Mycobacterium avium complex[e]	CD4- count of <75/mm³	Rifabutin, 300 mg/d PO (BII)	Clarithromycin, 500 mg PO bid (CIII); azithromycin, 500 mg PO 3×/wk (CIII)

Not recommended for most patients; indicated for consideration *only* in selected populations or patients

Pathogen	Indication	First choice	Alternatives
Bacteria	Neutropenia	Granulocyte colony-stimulating factor, 5–10 μg/kg/d SC × 2–4 wk; *or* granulcyte-macrophage colony-stimulating factor, 250 μg/m²/d IV over 2 hr × 2–4 wk (CIII)	None
Candida species	CD4+ count of <50/mm³	Fluconazole, 100–200 mg/d PO (CI)	Ketoconazole, 200 mg/d PO (CIII)
Cryptococcus neoformans[f]	CD4+ count of <50/mm³	Fluconazole, 200 mg/d PO (BI)	Itraconazole, 200 mg/d PO (CIII)
Histoplasma capsulatum[f]	CD4+ count of <50/mm³, endemic geographic area	Itraconazole, 200 mg/d PO (CIII)	Fluconazole, 200 mg/d PO (CIII)
Coccidioides immitis[f]	CD4+ count of <50/mm³, endemic geographic region	Fluconazole, 200 mg/d PO (CIII)	Itraconazole, 200 mg/d PO (CIII)
CMV[g]	CD4+ count of <50/mm³ and CMV antibody positivity	Oral ganciclovir, 1 g PO tid (CIII; only preliminary data available)	None
Unknown (herpesviruses?)[h]	CD4+ count of <200/mm³	Acyclovir, 800 mg PO qid (CIII)	Acyclovir, 200 mg PO tid-qid (CIII)

Recommended for consideration[i]

Pathogen	Indication	First choice	Alternatives
Hepatitis B virus[d]	All susceptible (anti-HBc-negative) patients	Energix-B (SmithKline Beecham, Rixensart, Belgium), 20 μg IM × 3 (BII); *or* Recombivax HB (Merck, West Point, PA) 10 μg IM × 3 (BII)	None

Table 19-8 (continued)

Pathogen	Indication	Preventive regimens	
		First choice	Alternatives
Influenza virus[d]	All patients (annually, before influenza season)	Whole or split virus, 0.5 ml/yr IM (BIII)	Rimantadine, 100 mg PO bid (CIII); or amantadine, 100 mg PO bid[j] (CIII)

Anti-HBc = antibody to hepatitis B core antigen; CMV = cytomegalovirus; DS = double-strength; SS = single-strength; TMP-SMX = trimethoprim-sulfamethoxazole; and TST = tuberculin skin test; d = day.

[a]Patients receiving dapsone should be tested for glucose-6-phosphate dehydrogenase deficiency. A dosage of 50 mg/d is probably less effective than a dosage of 100 mg/d. The efficacy of parenteral pentamidine (e.g., 4 mg/kg/mo) is uncertain. Inadequate data are available on the efficacy and safety of atovaquone or clindamycin/primaquine. Sulfadoxine/pyrimethamine (Fansidar) is rarely used because it can elicit severe hypersensitivity reactions. TMP-SMX and dapsone/pyrimethamine (and possibly dapsone alone) appear to be protective against toxoplasmosis. Patients receiving therapy for toxoplasmosis with sulfadiazine/pyrimethamine are protected against P. carinii pneumonia and do not need TMP-SMX. For additional discussion, see Chap. 24.

[b]Directly observed therapy is required for 900 mg of isoniazid 2×/wk; isoniazid regimens should include pyridoxine to prevent peripheral neuropathy. Exposure to multidrug-resistant tuberculosis may require prophylaxis with two drugs; consult public health authorities. Possible regimens include pyrazinamide plus either ethambutol or a fluoroquinolone.

[c]Protection against T. gondii is provided by the preferred antipneumocystis regimens. Pyrimethamine alone probably provides little, if any, protection. Dapsone alone cannot be recommended on the basis of currently available data.

[d]Data are inadequate concerning the clinical benefit of vaccines against S. pneumoniae, influenza virus, and hepatitis B virus in HIV-infected persons, although it is logical to assume that those patients who develop antibody responses will derive some protection. Some authorities are concerned that immunizations may stimulate the replication of HIV. Prophylaxis with TMP-SMX may provide some clinical benefit by reducing the frequency of bacterial infections, but the prevalence of S. pneumoniae resistant to TMP-SMX is increasing. Hepatitis B vaccine has been recommended for all children and adolescents and for all adults with risk factors for hepatitis B infection.

[e]Data on clarithromycin 500 mg PO bid have been presented but have not yet been thoroughly analyzed. Data on the efficacy and safety of azithromycin prophylaxis are not yet available.

[f]There may be a few unusual occupational or other circumstances under which prophylaxis should be considered; consult a specialist.

[g]Data on oral ganciclovir are still being evaluated; the durability of its effect is unclear. Acyclovir is not protective against CMV.

[h]Data regarding the efficacy of acyclovir for prolonging survival are controversial; if acyclovir is beneficial, the biologic basis for the effect and the optimal dose and timing of therapy are uncertain.

[i]These immunizations or chemoprophylactic regimens are not targeted against pathogens traditionally classified as opportunistic but should be considered for use in HIV-infected patients. While the use of those products is logical, their clinical efficacy has not been validated in this population.

[j]During outbreaks of influenza A.

Note: Not all of the recommended regimens reflect current FDA-approved labeling. Letters and Roman numerals in parentheses indicate the strength of the recommendation and the quality of the evidence supporting it. These are summarized on p. 760.

Source: J. E. Kaplan et al. and the USPHS/IDSA Prevention of Opportunistic Infections Working Group, USPHS/IDSA guidelines for the prevention of opportunistic infections in persons infected with human immunodeficiency virus: An overview. Clin. Infect. Dis. 21(Suppl. 1):S12, 1995. Published by The University of Chicago Press.

alternative regimen is clindamycin (see Chap. 28I) [318] and pyrimethamine.

  e. **Primary prophylaxis.** Retrospective studies have found that low-dose trimethoprim-sulfamethoxazole, used for PCP prophylaxis, is effective for toxoplasmosis prophylaxis as well [319]. A prospective study of pyrimethamine for prophylaxis found an unexplained increase in mortality in the treatment arm compared to the placebo-treated patients [320]. As discussed in sec. **VIII** and shown in Table 19-8, chemoprophylaxis is now advised for patients with positive serology for toxoplasmosis and CD4 counts $< 100/mm^3$.

3. **Cryptosporidia** cause diarrhea in 10–20% of AIDS patients in the United States [321] and up to 30–50% of patients in Haiti and Africa [151]. Numerous waterborne outbreaks of cryptosporidiosis in normal hosts in the United States have heightened awareness of this parasite's threat to public health (see Chap. 11).

  a. **Clinical presentation** varies depending on the host. Whereas immunocompetent patients have a self-limited illness, patients with AIDS have a spectrum of disease ranging from asymptomatic carriage to fulminant, persistent choleralike diarrhea [322, 323]. *Cryptosporidium* causes diarrhea, nausea, vomiting, abdominal pain, and weight loss. Biliary tract involvement occurs in at least 15% of AIDS patients and results in severe right upper-quadrant pain and protracted nausea and vomiting. Laboratory studies reveal an elevated alkaline phosphatase, and ultrasonography demonstrates gallbladder wall thickening and dilated bile ducts [324]. Cytomegalovirus and microsporidia cause similar signs and symptoms and often are concomitant pathogens.

  b. **Diagnosis** is made by identifying the red-staining organisms on an **acid-fast-stained stool smear.** Recently developed diagnostic methods that are more sensitive than the acid-fast stain include a **direct immunofluorescence assay** using a monoclonal antibody directed at the oocyst wall (Merifluor, Meridien, Cincinnati, OH) and an **ELISA antigen capture microtiter assay** (ProSpecT, Alexon, Sunnyvale, CA). Biopsy of the small intestine may be less sensitive than stool examinations owing to focal involvement of the intestine and no inflammatory changes to guide the endoscopist.

  c. **Treatment** has been uniformly **dismal.** There are numerous anecdotes of limited success with the nonabsorbable aminoglycoside **paromomycin,** but its limitations in preventing extraintestinal spread have dampened enthusiasm [322, 323]. A placebo-controlled trial is currently in progress. (See Chap. 28H for a discussion of paromomycin.) Lactose-free azithromycin was found to have some promise in a placebo-controlled trial, but further studies are needed to confirm the results. Novel immunomodulatory therapies including bovine colostral immunoglobulins and hyperimmune egg yolks are currently in clinical trials.

4. **Microsporidium spp.** have been widely recognized as a pathogen of animals, but only since 1985 have they been detected in AIDS patients [325, 326]. As diagnostic tests have been simplified, more cases are being diagnosed, but the true prevalence of this infection is not known.

  a. **Clinical presentation.** Three species have been exclusively identified in AIDS patients. **Enterocytozoon bieneusi** is associated with enteritis and cholangitis. **Encephalitozoon hellem** appears to disseminate to lungs and kidneys and often spares the intestine. **Septata intestinalis** involves the intestine but also causes disseminated disease.

  b. **Diagnosis.** Diagnosis **by stool examination** using Weber's chromotrope **stain** [327] or the fluorochrome Uvitex B is rapidly gaining popularity as more technicians are becoming skilled in the use of these agents. Such tests may be available only at reference laboratories or hospitals with a special interest in this diagnosis. Transmission electron-microscopic examination of a small-bowel biopsy specimen commonly is used to confirm the diagnosis of microsporidiosis and to determine genus and species.

  c. **Treatment.** There is **no known effective therapy** for this infection, but numerous anecdotal reports suggest that albendazole may be useful in treating certain microsporidial species. Placebo-controlled trials are currently in progress.

5. ***Isospora belli*** is also an acid-fast coccidian protozoan that causes a clinical syndrome indistinguishable from that of *Cryptosporidium*. *Isospora* can be eradicated with trimethoprim-sulfamethoxazole therapy (one double-strength [DS] tablet qid for 10 days). Because of a high relapse rate, chronic suppression with trimethoprim-sulfamethoxazole (one DS tablet 3 times weekly) or sulfadoxine-pyrimethamine (Fansidar) once weekly is necessary [328].

6. ***Cyclospora*** is a newly recognized acid-fast coccidian that closely resembles *Cryptosporidium* both morphologically and in the disease that it causes [329]. The two coccidians are differentiated by size, *Cyclospora* (8 μm) being twice the size of *Cryptosporidium* (4 μm). Preliminary reports suggest strongly that *Cyclospora* responds to treatment with trimethoprim-sulfamethoxazole (one DS tablet bid) [330].

7. ***Strongyloides stercoralis*** is an intestinal nematode that is endemic in Brazil, Africa, and other tropical areas, but rarely is seen in temperate climates.
   a. **Clinical presentation** varies depending on the host. Most often, intestinal *Strongyloides* is asymptomatic, although some patients develop abdominal pain, nausea, vomiting, and diarrhea [331]. For immunodeficient patients, such as those with AIDS, **hyperinfection** can occur rarely, which is a result of autoinfection leading to extremely high parasite loads [332–335]. The lung is the most frequently involved extraintestinal organ, with symptoms including focal or diffuse infiltrates or asthma. Bacteremic infection with GI pathogens has been reported to occur in up to 45% of patients, with a high incidence of meningitis (30% of bacteremic patients) as well [334]. **Eosinophilia, often present with intestinal disease, is frequently absent in disseminated disease.** Mortality remains high despite treatment.
   b. **Diagnosis** is made by stool or duodenal aspirate, but these tests can be negative in disseminated disease. A skin test and complement fixation test have been developed but are not readily available [334].
   c. **Thiabendazole** is the **treatment** of choice. All patients with infection should be treated for 2–3 days, but patients with hyperinfection should receive longer courses of therapy [332, 333, 335, 335a]. Ivermectin has also been used with good results for patients with refractory disease and is available for compassionate use [336].

VIII. **Guidelines for the prevention of opportunistic infections** in persons infected with HIV were published in the summer of 1995 after a year-long effort by federal authorities, professional societies, researchers, clinicians, community groups, and HIV-infected persons, with comments invited from the general public [164]. This is the first such comprehensive summary of this material. The guidelines are intended to be both patient- and pathogen-oriented. They provide background information and recommendations for clinicians and patients on those behavioral changes, drug regimens, and immunizations that are most likely to be beneficial, safe, feasible, and cost-effective [336a]. A total of 17 opportunistic infections or groups of opportunistic infections are addressed. Although a summary of this material is provided here, the health care provider actively involved in the care of HIV-infected patients is encouraged to review this excellent source material [145a, 164, 164a].

A. **Recommendation ratings**
   1. **Recommendations** designated "**A**" are supported by evidence that is both statistically and clinically persuasive: the measures designated are **strongly recommended,** should **always be offered,** and are considered **standard care;** those designated "**B**" are recommended for consideration; such measures should be generally offered, but their use should involve some discussion of the "pros and cons" between the provider and patient; those designated "**C**" are considered optional; those designated "**D**" generally should not be offered, while those designated "**E**" are contraindicated [164].
   2. **Recommendations are further rated as I** (evidence from at least one properly reported controlled trial), **II** (e.g., evidence from at least one well-designed clinical trial without randomization, or case-controlled studies), or **III** (evidence from opinions of respected authorities based on clinical experience, or descriptive studies, or expert committees) [164].

B. **For prophylaxis for adults and adolescents,** see **Tables 19-8** and **19-9.** (See reference [145a] for similar dosage tables for children and infants or comparable pediatric doses in Chap. 28.)

Table 19-9. Prophylaxis for recurrence of opportunistic disease (after chemotherapy for acute disease) in HIV-infected adults and adolescents

Pathogen	Indication	Preventive regimens	
		First choice	Alternatives
Recommended for life as standard of care			
Pneumocystis carinii	Prior *P. carinii* pneumonia	TMP-SMX, 1 DS tab PO qd (AI)	TMP-SMX, 1 SS tab PO qd (AI) *or* 1 DS tab PO 3×/wk (AII); dapsone, 50 mg PO bid *or* 100 mg/day PO (AI); dapsone, 50 mg/day PO, *plus* pyrimethamine, 50 mg/wk PO, *plus* leucovorin, 25 mg/wk PO (AI); dapsone, 200 mg/wk PO, *plus* pyrimethamine, 75 mg/wk PO, *plus* leucovorin, 25 mg/wk PO (AI); aerosolized pentamidine, 300 mg/mo via Respirgard II nebulizer (Marquest, Englewood, CO) (AI)
Toxoplasma gondii[a]	Prior toxoplasmic encephalitis	Sulfadiazine, 1.0–1.5 g PO q6h, *plus* pyrimethamine, 25–75 mg/day PO, *plus* leucovorin, 10–25 mg/day PO or up to 4×/day	Clindamycin, 300–450 mg PO q6-8h, *plus* pyrimethamine, 25–75 mg/day PO, *plus* leucovorin, 10–25 mg PO qd-qid (AII)
Mycobacterium avium complex[b]	Documented disseminated disease	Clarithromycin, 500 mg PO bid, *plus* one or more of the following: ethambutol, 15 mg/kg/day PO; clofazimine, 100 mg/day PO; rifabutin, 300 mg/day PO; ciprofloxacin, 500–750 mg PO bid (BIII)	Azithromycin, 500 mg/d PO, *plus* one or more of the following: ethambutol, 15 mg/kg/day PO; clofazimine, 100 mg/day PO; rifabutin, 300 mg/day PO; ciprofloxacin, 500–750 mg PO bid (BIII)
Cytomegalovirus[c]	Prior end-organ disease	Ganciclovir, 5–6 mg/kg IV 5–7 days per wk or 1000 mg PO tid (AI); *or* foscarnet, 90–120 mg/kg/day IV (AI)	Sustained-release implants used investigationally
Cryptococcus neoformans	Documented disease	Fluconazole, 200 mg/day PO (AI)	Itraconazole, 200 mg/day PO (BIII); amphotericin B, 0.6–1.0 mg/kg/wk IV or up to 3×/wk

Table 19-9 (continued)

Pathogen	Indication	Preventive regimens	
		First choice	Alternatives
Histoplasma capsulatum	Documented disease	Itraconazole, 200 mg PO bid (AII)	Amphotericin B, 1.0 mg/kg/wk IV (AI); fluconazole, 200–400 mg/day PO (BIII)
Coccidioides immitis	Documented disease	Fluconazole, 200 mg/day PO (AII)	Amphotericin B, 1.0 mg/kg/wk IV (AI); itraconazole, 200 mg PO bid (AII); ketoconazole, 400–800 mg/day PO (BII)
Salmonella species (non-*typhi*)[d]	Bacteremia	Ciprofloxacin, 500 mg PO bid for several months (BII)	
Recommended only if subsequent episodes are frequent or severe			
Herpes simplex virus	Frequent/severe recurrences	Acyclovir, 200 mg PO tid *or* 400 mg PO bid (AI)	
Candida species (oral, vaginal, or esophageal)	Frequent/severe recurrences	Fluconazole, 100–200 mg/day PO (AI)	Ketoconazole, 200 mg/day PO (BII); itraconazole, 100 mg/day PO (BII); clotrimazole troche, 10 mg PO 5×/day (BII); nystatin, 5 × 10⁵ U PO 5×/day (CIII)

DS = double-strength; SS = single-strength; and TMP-SMX = trimethoprim-sulfamethoxazole.

[a]Only pyrimethamine/sulfadiazine confers protection against *P. carinii* pneumonia.

[b]The long-term efficacy of any regimen is not well established. Many multiple drug regimens are poorly tolerated. Drug interactions (e.g., those seen with clarithromycin/rifabutin) can be problematic. Rifabutin has been associated with uveitis, especially when given at daily doses of >300 mg or along with fluconazole or clarithromycin.

[c]Ganciclovir and foscarnet delay relapses by only modest intervals (often only 4–8 weeks). Ocular implants with sustained-release ganciclovir appear promising.

[d]Efficacious eradication of *Salmonella* has been demonstrated only for ciprofloxacin.

Note: Not all of the recommended regimens reflect current FDA-approved labeling. Letters and Roman numerals in parentheses indicate the strength of the recommendation and the quality of the evidence supporting it. These are summarized at the bottom of p. 760.

Source: J. E. Kaplan et al. and the USPHS/IDSA Prevention of Opportunistic Infections Working Group, USPHS/IDSA guidelines for the prevention of opportunistic infections in persons infected with human immunodeficiency virus: An overview. *Clin. Infect. Dis.* 21(Suppl. 1)S12, 1995. Published by The University of Chicago Press.

C. For a summary of suggestions for promoting **behavioral changes,** see **Table 19-10** and source material [145a].
D. For **international travel-related** suggestions for the HIV-infected patient, see Chap. 21.
E. For potential risks of various agents in pregnancy, see related discussions of individual agents in Chaps. 9 and 28 or source material [145a].
F. For **drug interactions,** see source material [145a] and individual agent discussions (Chaps. 9 and 28).
G. For a summary of the **costs** of various prophylactic regimens, see **Table 19-11.**
H. For a detailed discussion of prevention of *P. carinii* pneumonia, see Chap. 24.

Table 19-10. Advising patients about the avoidance of exposure to oppportunistic pathogens

Sexual exposures
1. Patients should use male latex condoms during every act of sexual intercourse to reduce the risk of exposure to cytomegalovirus, herpes simplex virus, and human papillomavirus as well as to other sexually transmitted pathogens (AII). Use of latex condoms will also prevent the transmission of HIV to others.
2. Patients should avoid sexual practices that may result in oral exposure to feces (e.g., oral-anal contact) to reduce the risk of intestinal infections such as cryptosporidiosis, shigellosis, campylobacteriosis, amebiasis, giardiasis, and hepatitis A and B (BIII).

Environmental and occupational exposures
1. Certain activities or types of employment may increase the risk of exposure to tuberculosis (BIII). These include volunteer work or employment in health care facilities, correctional institutions, and shelters for the homeless as well as in other settings identified as high risk by local health authorities. Decisions about whether to continue with such activities should be made in conjunction with the health care provider and should take into account such factors as the patient's specific duties in the workplace, the prevalence of tuberculosis in the community, and the degree to which precautions designed to prevent the transmission of tuberculosis are taken in the workplace (BIII). These decisions will affect the frequency with which the patient should be screened for tuberculosis.
2. Child-care providers and parents of children in child-care facilities are at increased risk of acquiring CMV infection, cryptosporidiosis, and other infections (e.g., hepatitis A and giardiasis) from children. The risk of acquiring infection can be diminished by good hygienic practices, such as hand washing after fecal contact (e.g., during diaper changing) and after contact with urine or saliva (AII). All children in child-care facilities are also at increased risk of acquiring these same infections; parents and other caretakers of HIV-infected children should be advised of this risk (BIII).
3. Occupations involving contact with animals (e.g., veterinary work and employment in pet stores, farms, or slaughterhouses) may pose a risk of cryptosporidiosis, toxoplasmosis, salmonellosis, campylobacteriosis, or bartonella infection. However, the available data are insufficient to justify a recommendation against work in such settings.
4. Contact with young farm animals, especially animals with diarrhea, should be avoided to reduce the risk of cryptosporidiosis (BII).
5. Hand washing after gardening or other contact with soil may reduce the risk of cryptosporidiosis and toxoplasmosis (BIII).
6. In histoplasmosis-endemic areas, patients should avoid activities known to be associated with increased risk, including cleaning chicken coops, disturbing soil beneath bird-roosting sites, and exploring caves (CIII).
7. In coccidioidomycosis-endemic areas, when possible, patients should avoid activities associated with increased risk, including those involving extensive exposure to disturbed soil (e.g., at excavation sites, on farms, or during dust storms) (CIII).

Pet-related exposures
Health care providers should advise HIV-infected persons of the potential risk posed by pet ownership. However, they should be sensitive to the possible psychological benefits of pet ownership and should not routinely advise HIV-infected persons to part with their pets (DIII). Specifically, providers should advise HIV-infected patients of the following:

General
1. Veterinary care should be sought when a pet develops diarrheal illness. If possible, HIV-infected persons should avoid contact with animals that have diarrhea (BIII).

Table 19-10 (continued)

A fecal sample should be obtained from animals with diarrhea and examined for *Cryptosporidium, Salmonella,* and *Campylobacter.*

2. When obtaining a new pet, HIV-infected patients should avoid animals <6 months of age, especially those with diarrhea (BIII). Because the hygienic and sanitary conditions in pet breeding facilities, pet stores, and animal shelters are highly variable, the patient should exercise caution when obtaining a pet from these sources. Stray animals should be avoided. Animals <6 months of age, especially those with diarrhea, should be examined by a veterinarian for *Cryptosporidium, Salmonella,* and *Campylobacter* (BIII).

3. Patients should wash their hands after handling pets (especially before eating) and avoid contact with pets' feces to reduce the risk of cryptosporidiosis, salmonellosis, and campylobacteriosis (BIII). Hand washing by HIV-infected children should be supervised.

Cats

4. Patients should consider the potential risks of cat ownership such as the risk of toxoplasmosis and bartonella infection, as well as enteric infections (CIII). Those who elect to obtain a cat should adopt or purchase an animal that is >1 year of age and in good health to reduce the risk of cryptosporidiosis, bartonella infection, salmonellosis, and campylobacteriosis (BII).

5. Litter boxes should be cleaned daily, preferably by an HIV-negative, nonpregnant person; if the HIV-infected patient performs this task, he or she should wash hands thoroughly afterward to reduce the risk of toxoplasmosis (BIII).

6. Also to reduce the risk of toxoplasmosis, cats should be kept indoors, should not be allowed to hunt, and should not be fed raw or undercooked meat (BIII).

7. Although declawing is not generally advised, patients should avoid activities that may result in cat scratches or bites to reduce the risk of bartonella infection (BII). Patients should also promptly wash sites of cat scratches or bites (CIII) and should not allow cats to lick open cuts or wounds (BIII).

8. Care of cats should include flea control to reduce the risk of bartonella infection (CIII).

9. Testing of cats for toxoplasmosis (EII) or bartonella infection (DII) is not recommended.

Birds

10. Screening of healthy birds for *Cryptococcus neoformans, Mycobacterium avium,* or *Histoplasma capsulatum* is not recommended (DIII).

Other

11. Contact with reptiles (such as snakes, lizards, and turtles) should be avoided to reduce the risk of salmonellosis (BIII).

12. Gloves should be used during the cleaning of aquariums to reduce the risk of infection with *Mycobacterium marinum* (BIII).

13. Contact with exotic pets, such as nonhuman primates, should be avoided (CIII).

Food- and water-related exposures

1. Raw or undercooked eggs (including foods that may contain raw eggs, such as some preparations of hollandaise sauce, Caesar and certain other salad dressings, and mayonnaise); raw or undercooked poultry, meat, or seafood; and unpasteurized dairy products may contain enteric pathogens. Poultry and meat should be cooked until no longer pink in the middle (internal temperature, >165°F). Produce should be washed thoroughly before being eaten (BIII).

2. Cross-contamination of foods should be avoided. Uncooked meats should not be allowed to come into contact with other foods; hands, cutting boards, counters, and knives and other utensils should be washed thoroughly after contact with uncooked foods (BIII).

3. Although the incidence of listeriosis is low, it is a serious disease that occurs unusually frequently among HIV-infected persons who are severely immunosuppressed. Some soft cheeses and some ready-to-eat foods (e.g., hot dogs and cold cuts from delicatessen counters) have been known to cause listeriosis. An HIV-infected person who is severely immunosuppressed and who wishes to reduce the risk of food borne disease can prevent listeriosis by reheating these foods until they are steaming hot before eating them (CIII).

4. Patients should not drink water directly from lakes or rivers because of the risk of cryptosporidiosis and giardiasis. Even accidental ingestion of lake or river water while swimming or engaging in other types of recreational activities carries this risk (BII).

Table 19-10 (continued)

5. During outbreaks or in other situations in which a community "boil-water" advisory is issued, boiling of water for 1 minute will eliminate the risk of cryptosporidiosis (AI). Use of submicron personal-use water filters (home/office types) and/or bottled water* may reduce the risk (CIII). Current data are inadequate to recommend that all HIV-infected persons boil or otherwise avoid drinking tap water in nonoutbreak settings. However, persons who wish to take independent action to reduce the risk of waterborne cryptosporidiosis may choose to take precautions similar to those recommended during outbreaks. Such decisions are best made in conjunction with the health care provider. Persons who opt for a personal-use filter or bottled water should be aware of the complexities involved in selecting the appropriate products, the lack of enforceable standards for the destruction or removal of oocysts, the cost of the products, and the difficulty of using these products consistently.

*See details of personal-use filters and bottled water under cryptosporidiosis discussion in USPHS/IDSA guidelines for the prevention of opportunistic infections in persons infected with human immunodeficiency virus: Disease-specific recommendations. *Clin. Infect. Dis.* 21(Suppl. 1):S32, 1995.
Note: Letters and Roman numerals in parentheses indicate the strength of the recommendation and the quality of the evidence supporting it. These are summarized at the bottom of p. 760.
Source: J. E. Kaplan et al. and the USPHS/IDSA Prevention of Opportunistic Infections Working Group, USPHS/IDSA guidelines for the prevention of opportunistic infections in persons infected with human immunodeficiency virus: An overview. *Clin. Infect. Dis.* 21(Suppl. 1):S12, 1995. Published by The University of Chicago Press.

Table 19-11. Cost of agents used to prevent initial and recurrent disease due to opportunistic pathogens in HIV-infected persons

Opportunistic pathogen	Agent	Dose	Cost[a]
Pneumocystis carinii	Trimethoprim-sulfamethoxazole	160/800 mg/d	$60
	Dapsone	100 mg/d	$60
	Aerosolized pentamidine	300 mg/mo	$1,185
Mycobacterium avium complex	Rifabutin	300 mg/d	$2,387
	Clarithromycin	500 mg bid	$2,088
	Azithromycin	250 mg/d	$2,966
Cytomegalovirus	Ganciclovir (IV)	5 mg/kg/d	$10,800
	Foscarnet (IV)	90–120 mg/d	$27,600
	Ganciclovir (PO)	1000 mg tid	$14,454
Mycobacterium tuberculosis	Isoniazid	300 mg/d	$22
	Rifampin	600 mg/d	$1,542
	Pyrazinamide	1500 mg/d	$957
	Ethambutol	900 mg/d	$1,140
Fungi	Fluconazole	200 mg/d	$5,018
	Itraconazole	200 mg/d	$3,540
	Ketoconazole	200 mg/d	$899
Herpes simplex virus	Acyclovir	400 mg tid	$1,820
Toxoplasma gondii	Pyrimethamine	50 mg/wk	$38
	Leucovorin	25 mg/wk	$1,248
Streptococcus pneumoniae	Pneumovax 23 (Merck, West Point, PA)	0.5 ml IM	$10[b]
Haemophilus influenzae	H. influenzae type b vaccine	0.5 ml IM	$19[b]
Influenza virus	Influenza vaccine	0.5 ml IM	$19[b]
Hepatitis B virus	Recombivax HB (Merck, West Point, PA)	10 μg IM × 3	$167[c]

d = day
[a]Figure, based on average wholesale price as of 1994, is yearly cost except when otherwise indicated.
[b]Cost per dose.
[c]Cost for all three doses. See Chap. 22 for dose schedule.
Source: J. E. Kaplan et al. and the USPHS/IDSA Prevention of Opportunistic Infections Working Group, USPHS/IDSA guidelines for the prevention of opportunistic infections in persons infected with human immunodeficiency virus: An overview. *Clin. Infect. Dis.* 21(Suppl. 1):S12,1995. Published by The University of Chicago Press.

IX. Other retroviruses

A. Human immunodeficiency virus type 2 (HIV-2) is similar to HIV-1. Both are transmitted by the same routes, infect the same cells, and cause similar immune dysfunction and disease. HIV-2 may be less virulent [337]. Genetically, it closely resembles certain variants of the simian immunodeficiency virus (SIV).

1. **Epidemiology.** West Africa has the highest rates of HIV-2 infection. Cases reported in the United States have generally been in persons from endemic areas or their sexual partners. It is believed that HIV-2 may be less easily transmitted than HIV-1 [338].

2. **Diagnosis** is made by specific HIV-2 serologic tests. Routine test results for HIV-1 may also be abnormal: Up to 80% of HIV-2-infected persons have "indeterminate" ELISA determinations for HIV-1 testing. As of June 1992, US blood banks began screening for HIV-2. Culture and PCR testing may also be useful.

3. **Clinical manifestations** of HIV-2 infection resemble those of HIV-1 infection, including dementia, PCP, and other opportunistic infections. However, immune function declines more slowly, with a subsequently slower progression to AIDS.

4. **Treatment** of HIV-2 is aimed at treating specific infections. Zidovudine and other nucleoside analogue retroviral agents are effective against HIV-2 [338].

B. Human T-lymphotropic virus type I (HTLV-I) is endemic in Japan, the Caribbean, and Brazil, and among intravenous drug users in the United States. In the United States, seroprevalence has been reported to be between 0.016% and 0.025% [339–341]. Modes of transmission are identical to HIV-1, and incubation may extend for 20 years or longer. This retrovirus is implicated in two distinct disease entities.

1. **Adult T-cell lymphoma** is an aggressive non-Hodgkin's lymphoma arising from mature T_4 lymphocytes [342, 343]. It is characterized by infiltration of lymph nodes, viscera, and skin, resulting in clinical syndromes including leukemia, generalized lymphadenopathy, hepatosplenomegaly, skin lesions, and bone lesions with hypercalcemia. It occurs in 2–4% of patients infected with HTLV-I. Conventional chemotherapy is not effective, and median survival is 11 months [341].

2. **Tropical spastic paraparesis** is a neurologic disorder characterized by progressive lower-extremity weakness, spasticity, hyperreflexia, sensory disturbances, and urinary incontinence. It is similar to multiple sclerosis without waxing and waning symptoms. Fewer than 1% of patients infected with HTLV-I develop tropical spastic paraparesis [341, 344–346].

C. Human T-lymphotropic virus type 2 (HTLV-II) is seen among intravenous drug users in the United States and Europe and in native populations in North and Central America. Transmission is similar to HTLV-I but, because diagnostic tests only recently were developed to differentiate the two lymphotropic viruses, less is known about the epidemiology and clinical implications of HTLV-II infection. Although initially believed to be associated with hairy-cell leukemia, this association has recently been discounted [341].

X. Overview of an approach to antiretroviral therapy. "Best therapy" for a person infected with HIV continues to be the subject of numerous studies, debates, and reviews. Large, well-conducted trials designed to determine optimal therapy in certain populations defined by CD4 cell counts have yielded conflicting and complicated results. In addition, continued concern about the long-term toxicity of the currently available antiretroviral drugs has become increasingly germaine as long-term survival becomes a reality for many.

A. Chap. 26 discusses the indications for antiretroviral use and the studies on which the current recommendations are based. In addition, an NIH task force has issued guidelines for therapy as discussed in Chap. 26. Even with recommendations, guidelines, and expert opinions, it is important to remember that HIV infection, like hypertension, is a chronic disease and, as with blood pressure medications, therapy for the HIV-infected individual—regardless of CD4 cell count—must be individualized. Working with the patient to determine the best tolerated, most effective regimen requires patience from both physician and patient, as well as an appreciation of the rapidly changing nature of antiretroviral therapy.

B. Several recent reviews emphasize the many unanswered questions related to the therapy of HIV-infected patients [346a–346f]. Underlying many of these questions is the growing recognition of the heterogenicity of HIV-infected patients

and the likelihood that not all patients will benefit equally from antiretroviral therapy [346b].

   None of the drugs currently available to treat HIV-infected patients **can eradicate infection,** but they can decrease the viral load and delay immunologic decline [346d]. The reverse transcriptase inhibition associated with nucleoside analogues (e.g., zidovudine) protects uninfected cells, primarily CD4 lymphocytes, from infection. However, they have no antiviral effect on cells already infected [346c].

1. As of early 1996, monotherapy, particularly with ZDV alone, is no longer the treatment of choice for patients with HIV infection [346f].

   a. Because of the increasing recognition of a large viral load with rapid turnover (i.e., a large pool of virus with the potential for many mutations), it is not surprising that monotherapy, even in early infection, will not be predictably effective over time.

   b. Multiple drug combinations may be needed to effectively reduce the viral load.

2. As reviewed in the *Medical Letter* in April 1996 [346f] and in Chap. 26 (pp. 1019–1020), until more data become available, triple therapy with two nucleosides plus a protease inhibitor (choosing from saquinavir, ritonavir, or indinavir) appears to be the most potent antiretroviral regimen available [346f].

   a. A two-drug regimen with two nucleosides (e.g., ZDV and lamivudine or ZDV and ddI) or one nucleoside plus a protease inhibitor may also be effective in maintaining CD4 cell counts and decreasing HIV RNA [346f]. Furthermore, in some patients, at least initially, a two-drug regimen may be associated with better compliance and patient acceptance.

   b. Which two nucleosides are best together is unknown. ZDV is the best tested. Lamivudine appears to be the best tolerated [346f]. At this point, we favor combining ZDV and lamivudine or ZDV and ddI.

   c. Among the three protease inhibitors now available, saquinavir appears to be well tolerated but the least effective. The use of ritonavir may be limited by its adverse effects and numerous drug interactions [346f]. Therefore, at this point, indinavir is our favored agent.

3. **Quantifying viral load** [144a] (e.g., measurement of plasma HIV RNA copy number) to help understand and/or assess disease progression and response to therapeutic regimens is becoming an important tool.

4. Do standard recommended drug doses actually achieve therapeutic blood levels in a given patient? Preliminary studies suggest a startling variation in blood levels in response to fixed doses of ZDV, ddI, and other agents [346a]. As with aminoglycoside individualized dosing (see Chap. 28H), individualized dosing with pharmacokinetic monitoring of serum levels is anticipated to be an intense area of clinical study during the next few years. Further, can drug toxicity be reduced?

5. Will combination antiviral therapy, early on and/or later on in the course of HIV infection, reduce the likelihood of the development of resistant viral isolates [346a]?

XI. **Prospects for vaccine development.** Once the cause of AIDS was identified, researchers began to hope that containment of this epidemic could be achieved by developing and administering an effective vaccine. Although this remains a central goal of containment efforts, as of early 1996, larger studies are under way. **Efforts to date have been thwarted by several factors,** including (1) incomplete understanding of the determinants of immunity against the establishment and progression of infection, (2) the broad antigenic variation of HIV strains, (3) lack of a suitable animal model to study both immunity and candidate vaccines, and (4) concern about provoking a deleterious immune response [347]. In addition, development has been slowed by ethical and logistic issues surrounding which populations are most suitable for study.

   In general, there are two types of vaccine being developed: vaccines for prevention of infection (traditional vaccines) and vaccines to enhance the immune response of those already infected. Scientifically, vaccine development has focused on enhancing one of three types of immune response: (1) neutralizing antibodies, including the gp120 envelope "V3" loop, (2) antibody-dependent cellular toxicity, and (3) cell-mediated immunity.

   At least 10 trials have been conducted in humans, with modest results. Candidate vaccines have included whole killed virus vaccines (e.g., Salk vaccine); vaccines directed at envelope proteins (e.g., gp120 and gp160 vaccines); vaccines directed at internal or core proteins; live-vector vaccines (e.g., vaccinia-based); and live attenuated vaccines.

Excellent reviews of this topic have been published [347, 348].

XII. Prevention of HIV infection. Prevention of HIV infection can be accomplished only by well-designed interventions that are based on an understanding of the modes of HIV transmission [349].

   A. Strategies to prevent sexual transmission have included **education about safer sex** practices, especially condom use. Consistent **condom use** has been shown to decrease transmission in serodiscordant couples followed prospectively [350]. More advanced patients appear more infectious, and use of antiretroviral agents may decrease transmission risk between serodiscordant heterosexual couples [351]. Sexual abstinence, especially among teenagers, is receiving more attention.

   B. Needle exchange programs have been proposed to help prevent transmission among intravenous drug users. This concept has been adopted in many communities worldwide but has met resistance in some communities over concerns that free, available needles may increase overall injection drug use.

   C. Effective interruption of HIV transmission requires far-sighted, resolute action on the part of public health experts, with the full support of government agencies. We currently have adequate information to reduce transmission of all types. What has been lacking has been a coordinated and effective effort to reach persons at risk.

References

1. Gottlieb, M.S., et al. *Pneumocystis carinii* pneumonia and mucosal candidiasis in previously healthy homosexual men: Evidence of a new acquired cellular immunodeficiency. *N. Engl. J. Med.* 305:1425, 1981.
   See related companion initial articles appearing in the same journal issue: H. Masur et al., An outbreak of community-acquired Pneumocystis carinii *pneumonia: Initial manifestation of cellular immune dysfunction. N. Engl. J. Med. 305:1431, 1981; and F.P. Siegel et al., Severe acquired immunodeficiency in male homosexuals, manifested by chronic perianal ulcerative herpes simplex lesions. N. Engl. J. Med. 305:1439, 1981.*
2. Centers for Disease Control. *HIV/AIDS Surveillance Report* Vol. 7, No. 1, 1995.
3. Barre-Sinoussi, F., et al. Isolation of a T-lymphotropic retrovirus from a patient at risk for acquired immune deficiency syndrome (AIDS). *Science* 220:868, 1983.
4. Gallo, R.C., et al. Frequent detection and isolation of cytopathic retroviruses (HTLV-III) from patients with AIDS and at risk for AIDS. *Science* 224:500, 1984.
5. Levy, J.A., et al. Isolation of lymphocytopathic retroviruses from San Francisco patients with AIDS. *Science* 225:840, 1984.
   The three classic articles associating infection with a retrovirus, later called HIV, and the development of clinical AIDS.
6. Fischl, M.A., et al. The efficacy of azidothymidine (AZT) in the treatment of patients with AIDS and AIDS-related complex: A double-blind, placebo-controlled trial. *N. Engl. J. Med.* 317:185, 1987.
7. Centers for Disease Control. *HIV/AIDS Surveillance Report.*
   A very useful monthly update of the epidemiology of AIDS in the United States that is provided free of charge by the Centers for Disease Control. For additional information, call 800-458-5231.
8. *The AIDS Reader.* SCP Communications, Inc.
9. Sande, M.A., and Volberding, P.A. (eds.). *The Medical Management of AIDS* (4th ed.). Philadelphia: Saunders, 1995.
   Excellent concise chapters devoted to common issues. Written by experts in the field and edited by two national HIV experts from San Francisco General Hospital.
10. Cohen, P.T., Sande, M.A., and Volberding, P.A. (eds.). *The AIDS Knowledge Base: A Textbook on HIV Disease* (2nd ed.). Boston: Little, Brown, 1994.
11. Boswell, S.L. Outpatient management of HIV infection in the adult: An update. *Curr. Clin. Top. Infect. Dis.* 15:301, 1995.
12. Mandell, G.L., Bennett, J.E., and Dolin, R. (eds.). *Principles and Practice of Infectious Diseases* (4th ed.). New York: Churchill Livingstone, 1995. Pp. 1164–1305.
    This infectious disease text has an excellent section on AIDS.
13. DeVita, V.T., Jr., Hellman, S., and Rosenberg, S.A. (eds.). *AIDS Etiology, Diagnosis, Treatment and Prevention* (3rd ed.). Philadelphia: Lippincott, 1992.

14. Glatt, A.E. (ed.). Management of infection in HIV disease. *Infect. Dis. Clin. North Am.* 8:2, 1994.
    Entire issue devoted to AIDS. Excellent summaries.
15. Broder, S., Merigan, T.C., and Bolognesi, D. *Textbook of AIDS Medicine.* Philadelphia: Williams & Wilkins, 1994.
    A comprehensive textbook with extensive references covering both basic science and clinical aspects of HIV infection.
16. Libman, H., and Witzburg, R.A. (eds.). *HIV Infection: A Primary Care Manual* (3rd ed.). Boston: Little, Brown, 1996.
    A useful multiauthored text reflecting the approaches taken in Boston and aimed especially at the practicing physician, house staff, and students.
17. Chamberland, M.E., Ward, J.W., and Curran, J.W. Epidemiology and Prevention of AIDS. In G.L. Mandell, J.E. Bennett, and R. Dolin (eds.), *Principles and Practice of Infectious Disease* (4th ed.). New York: Churchill Livingstone, 1995. P. 1174.
18. Centers for Disease Control. Estimates of HIV prevalence and projected AIDS cases: Summary of a workshop, October 31–November 1, 1989. *M.M.W.R.* 39:110, 1990.
18a. Davis, S.F., et al. Prevalence and incidence of vertically acquired HIV infection in the United States. *J.A.M.A.* 274:952, 1995.
    Vertical transmission accounted for 92% of all new cases of AIDS reported in children in 1994.
19. Garland, F.C., et al. Incidence of human immunodeficiency virus seroconversion in US Navy and Marine Corps personnel, 1986 through 1988. *J.A.M.A.* 262:3161, 1989.
20. McNeil, J.G., et al. Direct measurement of human immunodeficiency virus seroconversions in a serially tested population of young adults in the United States Army, October 1985 to October 1987. *N. Engl. J. Med.* 320:1581, 1989.
21. Bloom, D.E., and Carliner, G. The economic impact of AIDS in the United States. *Science* 239:604, 1988.
22. Hellinger, F.J. The lifetime cost of treating a person with HIV. *J.A.M.A.* 270:474–478, 1993.
23. Piot, P., et al. AIDS: An international perspective. *Science* 239:573, 1988.
24. World Health Organization Global Programme on AIDS. The HIV/AIDS Pandemic: 1993 Overview (WHO/GPA/CVP/EVA/93.1). Geneva: World Health Organization, 1993.
25. Berkley, S. AIDS in the developing world: An epidemiologic overview. *Clin. Infect. Dis.* 17(Suppl. 2):S329–S336, 1993.
26. Narongrid, S., et al. The temporal trend of HIV seroprevalence among men entering the Royal Thai Army, 1989–1991 [abstr. PoC4084]. In *Abstracts of the Eighth International Conference on AIDS,* Amsterdam, 1992.
27. Nelson, K.E., et al. Risk factors for HIV infection among young adult men in northern Thailand. *J.A.M.A.* 270:955–960, 1993.
28. Winkelstein, W., et al. Sexual practices and risk of infection by the human immunodeficiency virus. The San Francisco Men's Health Study. *J.A.M.A.* 257:321, 1987.
29. Moss, A.R., et al. Risk factors for AIDS and HIV seropositivity in homosexual men. *Am. J. Epidemiol.* 125:1035, 1987.
30. Kingsley, L.A., et al. Risk factors for seroconversion to human immunodeficiency virus among male homosexuals. Results from the Multicenter AIDS Cohort Study. *Lancet* 1:345, 1987.
31. Centers for Disease Control. Heterosexually acquired AIDS—United States, 1993. *M.M.W.R.* 43:155, 1994.
32. Holmberg, S.D., et al. Prior herpes simplex virus type 2 infection as a risk factor for HIV infection. *J.A.M.A.* 259:1048, 1988.
33. Kreiss, J.K., et al. AIDS virus infection in Nairobi prostitutes. Spread of the epidemic to East Africa. *N. Engl. J. Med.* 314:414, 1986.
34. Telzak, E.E., et al. HIV-1 seroconversion in patients with and without genital ulcer disease. *Ann. Intern. Med.* 119:1181–1186, 1993.
    Important article associating genital ulcer disease with increased risk of HIV transmission.
35. Eyster, M.E., et al. Natural history of human immunodeficiency virus infections in hemophiliacs: Effects of T-cell subsets, platelet counts, and age. *Ann. Intern. Med.* 107:1, 1987.
36. Musicco, M., et al. Antiretroviral treatment of men infected with human immunodeficiency virus type 1 reduces the incidence of heterosexual transmission. *Arch. Intern. Med.* 154:1971–1976, 1994.

37. Des Jarlais, D.C., et al. Continuity and change within an HIV epidemic. Injecting drug users in New York City, 1984 through 1992. *J.A.M.A.* 271:121–127, 1994.
38. Curran, J.W., et al. Acquired immunodeficiency syndrome (AIDS) associated with transfusions. *N. Engl. J. Med.* 310:69, 1984.
   The original article that described blood transfusion as a risk for AIDS.
39. Evatt, B.L., et al. The acquired immunodeficiency syndrome in patients with hemophilia. *Ann. Intern. Med.* 100:499, 1984.
40. Centers for Disease Control. Update: Acquired immunodeficiency syndrome—United States, 1981–1990. *M.M.W.R.* 40:358, 1991.
41. Lackritz, E.M., et al. Estimated risk of transmission of the human immunodeficiency virus by screened blood in the United States. *N. Engl. J. Med.* 333:1721, 1995.
42. Ward, J.W., et al. The natural history of transfusion-associated infection with human immunodeficiency virus. Factors influencing the rate of progression to disease. *N. Engl. J. Med.* 321:947, 1989.
43. Ward, J.W., et al. Risk of human immunodeficiency virus infection from blood donors who later developed the acquired immunodeficiency syndrome. *Ann. Intern. Med.* 106:61, 1987.
44. Centers for Disease Control. Survey on non-U.S. hemophilia treatment centers for HIV seroconversions following therapy with heat-treated factor concentrates. *M.M.W.R.* 36:121, 1987.
45. Centers for Disease Control. Safety of therapeutic immune globulin preparations with respect to transmission of human T-lymphotropic virus type III/lymphadenopathy-associated virus infection. *M.M.W.R.* 35:231, 1986.
46. Centers for Disease Control. Lack of transmission of human immunodeficiency virus through $Rh_0(D)$ immune globulin (human). *M.M.W.R.* 36:728, 1987.
47. Centers for Disease Control. Hepatitis B vaccine evidence confirming lack of AIDS transmission. *M.M.W.R.* 33:685, 1984.
48. Simonds, R.J., et al. Transmission of human immunodeficiency virus type 1 from a seronegative organ and tissue donor. *N. Engl. J. Med.* 326:726–732, 1992.
49. Centers for Disease Control. Update: Acquired immunodeficiency syndrome and human immunodeficiency virus infection among health-care workers. *M.M.W.R.* 37:229, 1988.
50. Henderson, D.K., et al. Risk of nosocomial infection with human T-cell lymphotropic virus type III/lymphadenopathy-associated virus in a large cohort of intensively exposed health care workers. *Ann. Intern. Med.* 104:744, 1986.
51. Tokars, J.I., et al. Surveillance of HIV infection and zidovudine use among health care workers after occupational exposure to HIV-infected blood. The CDC Cooperative Needlestick Surveillance Group. *Ann. Intern. Med.* 118:913–919, 1993.
   Recent update on the management of health care workers who sustain needlesticks.
52. Hagen, M.D., et al. Human immunodeficiency virus infection in health care workers. A method for estimating individual occupational risk. *Arch. Intern. Med.* 149:1541, 1989.
53. Gerberding, J.L., and Sande, M.A. Real and Perceived Risks of AIDS in the Health Care and Work Environment. In *Information on AIDS for the Practicing Physician, American Medical News.* Vol. 3. Chicago: American Medical Association, 1987. P. 9.
   The authors summarize a number of occupational exposure studies and suggest a probability of HIV infection of approximately 0.3% in health care workers after skin puncture.
54. Marcus, R., and Centers for Disease Control Cooperative Needlestick Surveillance Group. Surveillance of health care workers exposed to blood from patients infected with the human immunodeficiency virus. *N. Engl. J. Med.* 319:1118, 1988.
   One of many articles from the Centers for Disease Control detailing potential risks to health care workers.
55. Centers for Disease Control. Public Health Service statement on management of occupational exposure to human immunodeficiency virus, including considerations regarding zidovudine postexposure use. *M.M.W.R.* 39(RR-1):1–14, 1990.
56. Clerici, M., et al. HIV-specific T-helper activity in seronegative health care workers exposed to contaminated blood. *J.A.M.A.* 271:42–46, 1994.
57. Jovaisas, E., et al. LAV/HTLV-III in 20-week fetus [letter]. *Lancet* 2:1129, 1985.
58. Lapointe, N., et al. Transplacental transmission of HTLV-III virus [letter]. *N. Engl. J. Med.* 312:1325, 1985.
59. Thiry, L., et al. Isolation of AIDS virus from cell-free breast milk of three healthy virus carriers [letter]. *Lancet* 2:891, 1985.
60. Oleske, J., et al. Immune deficiency syndrome in children. *J.A.M.A.* 249:2345, 1983.

61. Ryder, R.W., et al. Perinatal transmission of the human immunodeficiency virus type 1 to infants of seropositive women in Zaire. *N. Engl. J. Med.* 320:1637, 1989.
62. Selwyn, P.A., et al. Prospective study of human immunodeficiency virus infection and pregnancy outcomes in intravenous drug users. *J.A.M.A.* 261:1289, 1989.
63. Cotton, P. Trial halted after drug cuts maternal HIV transmission rate by two thirds. *J.A.M.A.* 271:807, 1994.
    See *E.M. Connor et al., Reduction of maternal-infant transmission of human immunodeficiency virus type 1 with zidovudine treatment.* N. Engl. J. Med. *331:1173, 1994; see editorial comment in this same issue.*
64. Thea, D.M., et al. A prospective study of diarrhea and HIV-1 infection among 429 Zairian infants. *N. Engl. J. Med.* 329:1696–1702, 1994.
65. Castro, K.G., et al. Investigations of AIDS patients with no previously identified risk factors. *J.A.M.A.* 259:1338, 1988.
66. Friedland, G.H., and Klein, R.S. Transmission of the human immunodeficiency virus. *N. Engl. J. Med.* 317:1125, 1987.
67. Lifson, A.R., et al. Unrecognized modes of transmission of HIV: Acquired immunodeficiency syndrome in children reported without risk factors. *Pediatr. Infect. Dis.* 6:292, 1987.
68. Lifson, A.R. Do alternate modes for transmission of human immunodeficiency virus exist? A review. *J.A.M.A.* 259:1353, 1988.
69. Fitzgibbon, J.E., et al. Transmission from one child to another of human immunodeficiency virus type 1 with a zidovudine-resistance mutation. *N. Engl. J. Med.* 329:1835–1841, 1993.
70. Ciesielski, C., et al. Transmission of human immunodeficiency virus in a dental practice. *Ann. Intern. Med.* 116:798–805, 1992.
71. Rogers, A.S., et al. Investigation of potential HIV transmission to the patients of an HIV-infected surgeon. *J.A.M.A.* 269:1795, 1993.
72. Dickinson, G.M., et al. Absence of HIV transmission from an infected dentist to his patients. An epidemiologic and DNA sequence analysis. *J.A.M.A.* 269:1802, 1993.
73. von Reyn, C.F., et al. Absence of HIV transmission from an infected orthopedic surgeon. A 13-year look-back study. *J.A.M.A.* 269:1807, 1993.
74. Berthier, A., et al. Transmissibility of human immunodeficiency virus in haemophilic and non-haemophilic children living in a private school in France. *Lancet* 2:598, 1986.
75. Mann, J.M., et al. Prevalence of HTLV-III/LAV in household contacts of patients with confirmed AIDS and controls in Kinshasa, Zaire. *J.A.M.A.* 256:721, 1986.
76. Castro, K.G., et al. Transmission of HIV in Belle Glade, Florida: Lessons for other communities in the United States. *Science* 239:193, 1988.
77. Klein, R.S., et al. Low occupational risk of human immunodeficiency virus infection among dental professionals. *N. Engl. J. Med.* 318:86, 1988.
78. Ho, D., et al. Infrequency of isolation of HTLV-III virus from saliva in AIDS [letter]. *N. Engl. J. Med.* 313:1606, 1985.
79. Fultz, P.N. Components of saliva inactivate human immunodeficiency virus [letter]. *Lancet* 2:1215, 1986.
80. Phillips, K.A., et al. The cost-effectiveness of HIV testing of physicians and dentists in the United States. *J.A.M.A.* 271:851–858, 1994.
81. Gallo, R., et al. HIV/HTLV gene nomenclature. *Nature* 333:504, 1988.
82. Nahmias, A.J., et al. Evidence for human infection with an HTLV III/LAV-like virus in central Africa, 1959 [letter]. *Lancet* 1:1279, 1986.
83. Huminer, D., Rosenfeld, J.B., and Pitlik, S.D. AIDS in the pre-AIDS era. *Rev. Infect. Dis.* 9:1102, 1987.
84. Gallo, R.C. HIV—the cause of AIDS: An overview on its biology, mechanisms of disease induction, and our attempts to control it. *J. Acquir. Immune Defic. Syndr.* 1:521, 1988.
85. Levy, J.A. Human immunodeficiency viruses and the pathogenesis of AIDS. *J.A.M.A.* 261:2997, 1989.
86. Fauci, A.S. The human immunodeficiency virus: Infectivity and mechanisms of pathogenesis. *Science* 239:617, 1988.
    An excellent, well-written summary. See recent update by A.S. Fanci et al., Immunopathogenic mechanisms of HIV infection. Ann. Intern. Med. *124:634, 1996.*
87. Stanley, S.K., and Fauci, A.S. Immunology of AIDS and HIV Infection. In G.L. Mandell, J.E. Bennett, and R. Dolin (eds.), *Principles and Practice of Infectious Diseases* (4th ed.). New York: Churchill Livingstone, 1995. P. 1203.
88. Lane, H.C., et al. Qualitative analysis of immune function in patients with the acquired immunodeficiency syndrome. *N. Engl. J. Med.* 313:79, 1985.

89. Ho, D.D., Moudgil, T., and Alam, M. Quantitation of human immunodeficiency virus type 1 in the blood of infected persons. *N. Engl. J. Med.* 321:1621, 1989.

90. Levy, J.A., et al. AIDS-associated retrovirus (ARV) can productively infect other cells besides human T helper cells. *Virology* 147:441, 1985.

91. Ho, D.D., Rota, T.R., and Hirsch, M.S. Infection of monocyte/macrophages by human T lymphotropic virus type III. *J. Clin. Invest.* 77:1712, 1986.

92. Nicholson, J.K.A., et al. In vitro infection of human monocytes with human T-lymphotropic virus type III/lymphadenopathy-associated virus (HTLV-III/LAV). *J. Immunol.* 137:323, 1986.

93. Salahuddin, S.Z., et al. Human T lymphotropic virus type II infection by human alveolar macrophages. *Blood* 68:281, 1986.

94. Gartner, S., et al. The role of mononuclear phagocytes in HTLV-III/LAV infection. *Science* 233:215, 1986.

95. Koenig, S., et al. Detection of AIDS virus in macrophages in brain tissue from AIDS patients with encephalopathy. *Science* 233:1089, 1986.

96. Smith, P.D., et al. Monocyte function in the acquired immune deficiency syndrome. *J. Clin. Invest.* 74:2121, 1984.

97. Price, R.W., et al. The brain in AIDS: Central nervous system HIV-1 infection and AIDS dementia complex. *Science* 239:586, 1988.

98. Gyorkey, J.F., Melnick, J.L., and Gyorkey, P. Human immunodeficiency virus in brain biopsies of patients with AIDS and progressive encephalopathy. *J. Infect. Dis.* 155:870, 1987.

99. Dewhurst, S., et al. Susceptibility of human glial cells to infection with human immunodeficiency virus (HIV). *F.E.B.S. Lett.* 213:138, 1987.

100. Lifson, A.R., Rutherford, G.W., and Jaffee, H.W. The natural history of human immunodeficiency virus infection. *J. Infect. Dis.* 158:1360, 1988.

101. Smiley, M.L., et al. Transmission of human immunodeficiency virus to sexual partners of hemophiliacs. *Am. J. Hematol.* 28:27, 1988.

102. Tersmette, M., et al. Association between biological properties of human immunodeficiency virus variants and risk for AIDS and AIDS mortality. *Lancet* May 6, 1984.

103. Centers for Disease Control. Update on acquired immunodeficiency syndrome (AIDS)—United States. *M.M.W.R.* 31:507, 1982.
    The original definition for the diagnosis of AIDS is detailed.

104. Abrams, D.I. AIDS-related conditions. *Clin. Immunol. Allergy* 6:581, 1986.

105. Centers for Disease Control. Current trends: Classification system for human T lymphotrophic virus type III/lymphadenopathy-associated virus infections. *M.M.W.R.* 35:334, 1986.

106. Centers for Disease Control. Revision of the CDC surveillance case definition for acquired immunodeficiency syndrome. *M.M.W.R.* 36(Suppl.):1, 1987.
    A very lucid summary of the Centers for Disease Control attempt to increase the sensitivity and specificity of defining the spectrum of HIV infection.

107. Centers for Disease Control. 1993 Revised classification system for HIV infection and expanded surveillance case definition for AIDS among adolescents and adults. *M.M.W.R.* 41:1–19, 1992.
    The most current case definitions for AIDS with explanations of expanded categories.

108. Redfield, R.R., Wright, D.C., and Tramont, E.C. The Walter Reed staging classification for HTLV III/LAV infection. *N. Engl. J. Med.* 314:131, 1986.

109. Chaisson, R.E., and Volberding, P.A. Clinical Manifestations of HIV Infection. In G.L. Mandell, J.E. Bennett, and R. Dolin (eds.), *Principles and Practice of Infectious Diseases* (4th ed.). New York: Churchill Livingstone, 1995. P. 1217.
    Chap. 102 discusses in detail the various systems (Walter Reed, Centers for Disease Control, World Health Organization) for classifying HIV infection (including the authors' own).

110. World Health Organization. Acquired immunodeficiency syndrome (AIDS). *W.H.O. Weekly Epidemiol. Rec.* 61:69, 1986.

111. Goedert, J.J., et al. Three year incidence of AIDS in five cohorts of HTLV-III infected risk group members. *Science* 231:992, 1986.

112. Moss, A.R., et al. Seropositivity for HIV and the development of AIDS or ARC: Three-year follow-up of the San Francisco General Hospital cohort. *Br. Med. J.* 296:745, 1988.

112a. Baltimore, D. Lessons from people with nonprogressive HIV infection. *N. Engl. J. Med.* 332:259, 1995.
    Editorial comment on 3 companion articles in this same issue discussing long-term seropositive asymptomatic patients.

113. Anonymous. Needlestick transmission of HTLV-III from a patient infected in Africa [letter]. *Lancet* 2:1376, 1984.
     A flulike illness in a nurse 13 days after a needlestick injury.
114. Feorino, P.M., et al. Lymphadenopathy associated with virus infection of a blood donor-recipient pair with acquired immunodeficiency syndrome. *Science* 225:69, 1984.
     Mononucleosislike illness after blood transfusion from a patient who subsequently developed AIDS.
115. Cooper, D.A., et al. Acute AIDS retrovirus infection. Definitions of a clinical illness associated with seroconversion. *Lancet* 1:537, 1985.
116. Ho, D.D., et al. Primary human T-lymphotropic virus type III infection. *Ann. Intern. Med.* 103:880, 1985.
117. Tindall, B., et al. Primary human immunodeficiency virus infection: Clinical and serologic aspects. *Infect. Dis. Clin. North Am.* 2:329, 1988.
118. Tindall, B., et al. Characteristics of the acute illness associated with human immunodeficiency virus infections. *Arch. Intern. Med.* 148:945, 1988.
119. Rustin, M.H.A., et al. The acute exanthem associated with seroconversion to human T-cell lymphotropic virus III in a homosexual man. *J. Infect. Dis.* 12:161, 1986.
119a. Koh, H.K., and Davis, B.E. Dermatologic Manifestations. In H. Libman and R.A. Witzburg (eds.), *HIV Infection: A Primary Care Manual* (3rd ed.). Boston: Little, Brown, 1996. Pp. 107–122.
119b. Wang, C.Y., et al. Skin cancers associated with acquired immunodeficiency syndrome. *Mayo Clin. Proc.* 70:766, 1995.
120. Coolfont report: A Public Health Service plan for prevention and control of AIDS and the AIDS virus. *Public Health Rep.* 101:341, 1986.
121. Metroka, C.E., et al. Generalized lymphadenopathy in homosexual man. *Ann. Intern. Med.* 99:585, 1983.
122. Abrams, D.I., et al. Persistent diffuse lymphadenopathy in homosexual men: Endpoint or prodrome? *Ann. Intern. Med.* 100:801, 1984.
123. O'Hara, C.J. The Lymphoid and Hematopoietic Systems. In S.J. Harawi and C.J. O'Hara (eds.), *Pathology and Pathophysiology of AIDS and HIV-Related Diseases.* St. Louis: Mosby, 1989.
     This book is an excellent compendium of AIDS pathology and pathophysiology.
124. Graziosi, C., et al. HIV-1 infection in the lymphoid organs. *A.I.D.S.* Suppl. 2:S53–S58, 1993.
125. Zon, L.I., and Groopman, J.E. Hematologic manifestations of the human immunodeficiency virus (HIV). *Semin. Hematol.* 25:208, 1988.
126. The Swiss Group for Clinical Studies on AIDS (R. Luthy, Chairman). Zidovudine for the treatment of thrombocytopenia associated with human immunodeficiency virus (HIV): A prospective study. *Ann. Intern. Med.* 109:718, 1988.
127. Hirschel, B., et al. Zidovudine for the treatment of thrombocytopenia associated with human immunodeficiency virus (HIV). *Ann. Intern. Med.* 109:718, 1988.
128. Oksenhendler, E.O., et al. Zidovudine for thrombocytopenic purpura related to human immunodeficiency virus (HIV) infection. *Ann. Intern. Med.* 110:365, 1989.
129. Polk, B.F., et al. Predictors of the acquired immunodeficiency syndrome developing in a cohort of seropositive homosexual men. *N. Engl. J. Med.* 316:61, 1987.
130. Moss, A.R. Predicting progression to AIDS. *Br. Med. J.* 297:1067, 1988.
131. Murray, H.W., et al. Progression to AIDS in patients with lymphadenopathy or AIDS-related complex: Reappraisal of risk and predictive factors. *Am. J. Med.* 86:533, 1989.
132. Greenspan, D., et al. Relation of oral hairy leukoplakia to infection with the human immunodeficiency virus and the risk of developing AIDS. *J. Infect. Dis.* 155:475, 1987.
133. Masur, H., et al. CD4 counts as predictors of opportunistic pneumonias in human immunodeficiency virus (HIV) infection. *Ann. Intern. Med.* 111:223, 1989.
134. Anderson, R.E., et al. Use of B$_2$-microglobulin level and CD4 lymphocyte count to predict development of acquired immunodeficiency syndrome in persons with human immunodeficiency virus infection. *Arch. Intern. Med.* 150:73, 1990.
135. MacDonald, K.L., et al. Performance characteristics of serologic tests for human immunodeficiency virus type 1 (HIV-1) antibody among Minnesota blood donors. *Ann. Intern. Med.* 110:617, 1989.
136. Phair, J.P., and Wolinsky, S. Diagnosis of infection with the human immunodeficiency virus. *J. Infect. Dis.* 159:320, 1989.
137. Ward, J.W., et al. Transmission of human immunodeficiency virus (HIV) by blood transfusions screened as negative for HIV antibody. *N. Engl. J. Med.* 318:473, 1988.
138. Cohen, N.D., et al. Transmission of retroviruses by transfusion of screened blood in

patients undergoing cardiac surgery. *N. Engl. J. Med.* 320:1172, 1989.

139. Burke, D.S., et al. Measurement of the false positive rate in a screening program for human immunodeficiency virus infections. *N. Engl. J. Med.* 319:961, 1988.

140. Jackson, J.B., and Balfour, H.H., Jr. Practical diagnostic testing for human immunodeficiency virus. *Clin. Microbiol. Rev.* 1:124, 1988.

141. Tersmette, M., et al. Confirmation of HIV seropositivity: Comparison of a novel radioimmunoprecipitation assay to immunoblotting and virus culture. *J. Med. Virol.* 24:109, 1988.

142. Kemp, B.E., et al. Autologous red cell agglutination assay for HIV-1 antibodies: Simplified test with whole blood. *Science* 241:1352, 1988.

143. DeRossi, A., et al. Polymerase chain reaction and in-vitro antibody production for early diagnosis of paediatric HIV infection. *Lancet* 2:278, 1988.

143a. Paul, M.O., et al. Laboratory diagnosis of infection status in infants perinatally exposed to human immunodeficiency virus type 1. *J. Infect. Dis.* 173:68, 1996.

144. Loche, M., and Mach, B. Identification of HIV-infected seronegative individuals by a direct diagnostic test based on hybridization to amplified viral DNA. *Lancet* 2: 418, 1988.

144a. Landesman, S.H. quantifying HIV. *J.A.M.A.* 275:640, 1996.

144b. Zazzi, M., et al. Nested polymerase chain reaction for detection of human immunodeficiency virus type 1 DNA in clinical specimens. *J. Med. Virol.* 38:172–174, 1992.

145. Burgard, M., et al. The use of viral culture and p24 antigen testing to diagnose human immunodeficiency virus infection in neonates. *N. Engl. J. Med.* 327:1192–1197, 1992.

145a. Kaplan, J.E., et al., and the USPHS/IDSA Prevention of Opportunistic Infections Working Group. USPHS/IDSA guidelines for the prevention of opportunistic infections in persons infected with human immunodeficiency virus: An overview. *Clin. Infect. Dis.* 21(Suppl. 1):S12, 1995.
    See annotation to reference [164].

145b. Stanley, S.K., et al. Effect of immunization with a common recall antigen on the viral expression in patients infected with human immunodeficiency virus type 1. *N. Engl. J. Med.* 334:1222–1230, 1996.

146. White, D.A., and Zaman, M.K. "Pulmonary disease" in medical management of AIDS patients. *Med. Clin. North Am.* 76:19–44, 1992.

147. Chaisson, R.E., et al. Tuberculosis in patients with the acquired immunodeficiency syndrome: Clinical features, response to therapy, and survival. *Am. Rev. Respir. Dis.* 136:570–574, 1987.

147a. Gallant, J.E., and Ko, A.H. Cavitary pulmonary lesions in patients infected with human immunodeficiency virus. *Clin. Infect. Dis.* 22:671, 1996.

148. Chaisson, R.E., and Volberding, P.A. Clinical Manifestations of HIV Infection. In G.L. Mandell, J.E. Bennett, and R. Dolin (eds.), *Principles and Practice of Infectious Diseases* (4th ed.). New York: Churchill Livingstone, 1995. P. 1233.

149. Broaddus, V.C., et al. Bronchoalveolar lavage and transbronchial biopsy for the diagnosis of pulmonary infections in patients with the acquired immunodeficiency syndrome. *Ann. Intern. Med.* 102:747, 1985.

149a. Masur, H., and Shelhamer, J. Empiric outpatient management of HIV-related pneumonia: Economical or unwise? *Ann. Intern. Med.* 124:451, 1996.

150. Rene, E., et al. Intestinal infections in patients with acquired immunodeficiency syndrome. A prospective study in 132 patients. *Dig. Dis. Sci.* 29:817, 1989.

151. Colebunders, R., et al. Persistent diarrhea, strongly associated with HIV infection in Kinshasa, Zaire. *Am. J. Gastroenterol.* 82:859, 1987.

151a. Kotler, D.P., et al. Chronic bacterial enteropathy in patients with AIDS. *J. Infect. Dis.* 171:352, 1995.
    Chronic infection with adherent bacteria may help explain idiopathic AIDS-associated wasting, especially when CD4 counts were $< 100/mm^3$.

152. Smith, P.D., et al. Infectious diarrheas in patients with AIDS. *Gastroenterol. Clin. North Am.* 22:535, 1993.

152a. Dupont, H.L., and Marshall, S.D. HIV-associated diarrhoea and wasting. *Lancet* 346:352, 1995.

153. Cello, J.P., et al. Effect of octreotide on refractory AIDS-associated diarrhea: A prospective multicenter clinical trial. *Ann. Intern. Med.* 115:705, 1991.

154. Jacobs, J.L., et al. *Salmonella* infection in patients with the acquired immunodeficiency syndrome. *Ann. Intern. Med.* 102:186, 1985.

155. Sepkowitz, K.A., et al. Fever among outpatients with advanced HIV infection. *Arch. Intern. Med.* 153:1909–1912, 1993.

155a. Hambleton, J., et al. Outcome for hospitalized patients with fever and neutropenia who are infected with the human immunodeficiency virus. *Clin. Infect. Dis.* 20:363, 1995. *Clinical presentation (e.g., sepsis or concomitant illness) affected outcome more than cause of neutropenia.*

156. Prego, V., et al. Comparative yield of blood culture, for fungi and mycobacteria, liver biopsy, and bone marrow biopsy in the diagnosis of fever of undetermined origin in human immunodeficiency virus–infected patients. *Arch. Intern. Med.* 150:333, 1990.

156a. Cappell, M.S., Schwartz, M.S., and Biempica, L. Clinical utility of liver biopsy in patients with serum antibodies to the human immunodeficiency virus. *Am. J. Med.* 88:123–130, 1990.

157. Bach, M.C., Bagwell, S.P., and Fanning, J.P. Primary pulmonary Kaposi's sarcoma in the acquired immunodeficiency syndrome: A cause of persistent pyrexia. *Am. J. Med.* 85:274–275, 1988.

157a. Battinelli, D.L., and Peters, E.S. Oral Manifestations. In H. Libman and R.A. Witzburg (eds.), *HIV Infection: A Primary Care Manual.* Boston: Little, Brown, 1996. Pp. 87–95.

157b. Medical Letter. New uses of thalidomide. *Med. Lett. Drugs Ther.* 38:16, 1996.

157c. Moore, P.S., et al. Detection of herpes virus-like DNA sequences in Kaposi's sarcoma in patients with and without AIDS. *N. Engl. J. Med.* 332:1181, 1995.

158. Hollander, H., and Stringari, S. Human immunodeficiency virus–associated meningitis. Clinical course and correlations. *Am. J. Med.* 83:813–816, 1985.

159. Holtzman, D.M., Kaku, D.A., and So, Y.T. New-onset seizures associated with human immunodeficiency virus infection: Causation and clinical features in 100 cases. *Am. J. Med.* 87:173–177, 1989.

160. Bishberg, E., et al. Brain lesions in patients with acquired immunodeficiency syndrome. *Arch. Intern. Med.* 149:941–943, 1989.

161. Engstrom, J.W., Lowenstein, D.H., and Bredesen, D.E. Cerebral infarctions and transient neurologic deficits associated with acquired immunodeficiency syndrome. *Am. J. Med.* 86:528–532, 1989.

162. Matlow, A.G. Neurosyphilis as a cause of cerebral infarction in AIDS. *Am. J. Med.* 88:700–701, 1990.

163. Cohn, J.A., et al. Evaluation of the policy of empiric treatment of suspected *Toxoplasma* encephalitis in patients with the acquired immunodeficiency syndrome. *Am. J. Med.* 86:521–527, 1989.

163a. Wilcox, C.M. Esophageal disease in the acquired immunodeficiency syndrome: Etiology, diagnosis, and management. *Am. J. Med.* 92:412–421, 1992.

163b. Wilcox, C.M., et al. Cytomegalovirus esophagitis in AIDS: A prospective evaluation of clinical response to ganciclovir therapy, relapse rate, and long-term outcome. *Am. J. Med.* 98:169, 1995. *Induction therapy with IV ganciclovir at 10 mg/kg/day for 2 weeks is usually effective. Maintenance therapy does not seem necessary. Ophthalmological examination at the time of diagnosis of CMV esophagitis and/or ulceration is critical since the presence of CMV retinitis would dictate long-term maintenance therapy. Foscarnet given at 60 mg/kg q8h can be used for nonresponders to ganciclovir.*

163c. Wilcox, C.M., et al. Esophageal ulceration in human immunodeficiency virus infection: Causes, response to therapy, and long-term outcome. *Ann. Intern. Med.* 123:144, 1995. *Patients with esophagitis or ulcers due to Candida were excluded. With endoscopic biopsies, 45% of ulcers were due to CMV, 40% were idiopathic, and 5% had HSV. For patients not responding to empiric antifungal therapy for esophagitis symptoms, endoscopy is important. Empiric antivirals not advised. See also C.M. Wilcox and D.A. Schwartz, A pilot study of oral corticosteroid therapy for idiopathic esophageal ulcerations associated with HIV infection. Am. J. Med. 93:131–134, 1992.*

164. Kaplan, J.E., Masur, H., Holmes, K.K., et al., and the USPHS/IDSA Prevention of Opportunistic Infections Working Group. USPHS/IDSA guidelines for the prevention of opportunistic infections in persons infected with human immunodeficiency virus: Introduction. *Clin. Infect. Dis.* 21(Suppl. 1):S1, 1995. *See related references [145a] and [164a]. These recommendations have been summarized in USPHS/IDSA guidelines for the prevention of opportunistic infections in persons infected with human immunodeficiency virus: A summary. M.M.W.R. 44(RR-8):1–34, 1995; and Ann. Intern. Med. 124:349, 1996 (see editorial comment). See also R.D. Moore et al., Natural history of opportunistic disease in an HIV-infected urban clinical cohort. Ann. Intern. Med. 124:633, 1996.*

164a. USPHS/IDSA Prevention of Opportunistic Infections Working Group. USPHS/IDSA guidelines for the prevention of opportunistic infections in persons infected with human immunodeficiency virus: Disease-specific recommendations. *Clin. Infect. Dis.* 21(Suppl. 1):S32, 1995.

164b. Lane, H.C., et al. Recent advances in the management of AIDS-related opportunistic infections. *Ann. Intern. Med.* 120:945–955, 1994.

165. Jacobsen, M.A., and Mills, J. Serious cytomegalovirus disease in the acquired immuno-deficiency syndrome. *Ann. Intern. Med.* 108:58, 1988.

166. Reichert, C.M., et al. Autopsy pathology in the acquired immune deficiency syndrome. *Am. J. Pathol.* 12:357, 1983.

167. Palestine, A.G., et al. A randomized, controlled trial of foscarnet in the treatment of cytomegalovirus retinitis in patients with AIDS. *Ann. Intern. Med.* 115:665–673, 1991.

168. Zurlo, J.J., et al. Lack of clinical utility of cytomegalovirus blood and urine cultures in patients with HIV infection. *Ann. Intern. Med.* 118:12–17, 1993.

169. Back, M.C., et al. 9-(1,3-Dihydroxy-2-propoxymethyl) guanine for cytomegalovirus infections in patients with the acquired immunodeficiency syndrome. *Ann. Intern. Med.* 103:381–382, 1985.

170. Bloom, J.N., and Palestine, A.G. The diagnosis of cytomegalovirus retinitis. *Ann. Intern. Med.* 109:963, 1988.
Contains some good retinal photographs.

171. Drew, W.L., Buhles, W., and Erlich, K. Medical Management of Herpes Virus Infections. In M.A. Sande and D.A. Volberding (eds.), *The Medical Management of AIDS* (4th ed.). Philadelphia: Saunders, 1995. Pp. 512–514.

172. Foscarnet-ganciclovir cytomegalovirus retinitis trial 4: Visual outcomes. Studies of ocular complications of AIDS research group in collaboration with the AIDS clinical trials group. *Ophthalmology* 101:1250, 1994.
These two drugs appear equivalent in their ability to control CMV retinitis.

173. Studies of Ocular Complications of AIDS Research Group. Mortality in patients with the acquired immunodeficiency syndrome treated with either foscarnet or ganciclovir for cytomegalovirus retinitis. *N. Engl. J. Med.* 326:213, 1992.

174. Dieterich, D.T., and Rahmin, M. Cytomegalovirus colitis in AIDS: Presentation in 44 patients and a review of the literature. *J. Acquir. Immune Defic. Syndr.* 4(Suppl. 1):S29, 1991.

174a. Goodgame, R.W. Gastrointestinal cytomegalovirus disease. *Ann. Intern. Med.* 119:924, 1993.
Good review. Endoscopic biopsies are important with histopathology looking for the characteristic cytopathic effect: a large cell containing a basophilic intranuclear inclusion that sometimes is surrounded by a clear halo ("owl's eye" effect).

175. Nelson, M.R., et al. Foscarnet in the treatment of cytomegalovirus infection of the esophagus and colon in patients with acquired immune deficiency syndrome. *Am. J. Gastroenterol.* 86:876, 1991.

176. Miles, P.R., Baughman, R.P., and Linneman, C.C. Cytomegalovirus in the broncho-alveolar lavage fluid of patients with AIDS. *Chest* 97:1072, 1990.

177. Petito, C.K., et al. Neuropathy of acquired immunodeficiency syndrome (AIDS): An autopsy review. *J. Neuropathol. Exp. Neurol.* 45:635–646, 1986.

178. Morgello, S., et al. Cytomegalovirus encephalitis in patients with acquired immunode-ficiency syndrome. An autopsy study of 30 cases and a review of the literature. *Hum. Pathol.* 18:289–297, 1987.

178a. McCutchan, J.A. Clinical aspects of cytomegalovirus infections of the nervous system in patients with AIDS. *Clin. Infect. Dis.* 21(Suppl. 2):S196, 1995.
Discusses the five neurologic syndromes: retinitis, myelitis/polyradiculopathy, enceph-alitis with dementia, ventriculoencephalitis, and mononeuritis multiplex.

179. Masdeu, J.C., et al. Multifocal cytomegalovirus encephalitis in AIDS. *Ann. Neurol.* 23:97–99, 1988.

180. Vinters, H.V., et al. Cytomegalovirus in the nervous system of patients with the acquired immune deficiency syndrome. *Brain* 112:245–268, 1989.

181. Laskin, O.L., Stahl-Bayiss, C.M., and Morgello, S. Concomitant herpes simplex virus type 1 and CMV ventriculoencephalitis in acquired immunodeficiency syndrome. *Arch. Neurol.* 44:843–847, 1987.

182. Barloon, T.J., et al. Cerebral ventriculitis: MR findings. *J. Comput. Assist. Tomogr.* 14:272–275, 1990.

183. Kalayjian, R.C., et al. Cytomegalovirus ventriculoencephalitis in AIDS. *Medicine* 72:67–77, 1993.

184. Berman, S.M., and Kim, R.C. The development of cytomegalovirus encephalitis in AIDS patients receiving ganciclovir. *Am. J. Med.* 96:415–419, 1994.

185. Wolf, O.G., and Spector, S.A. Diagnosis of human CMV central nervous system disease in AIDS patients by DNA amplification from cerebrospinal fluid. *J. Infect. Dis.* 166: 1412–1415, 1992.
186. Price, T.A., Digioia, R.A., and Simon, G.L. Ganciclovir treatment of cytomegalovirus ventriculitis in a patient infected with human immunodeficiency virus. *Clin. Infect. Dis.* 15:606–608, 1992.
187. Kim, Y.S., and Hollander, H. Polyradiculopathy due to CMV: Report of two cases in which improvement occurred after prolonged therapy and review of the literature. *Clin. Infect. Dis.* 17:32–37, 1993.
188. deGans, J., et al. Predominance of polymorphonuclear leukocytes in cerebrospinal fluid of AIDS patients with cytomegalovirus polyradiculomyelitis. *J. Acquir. Immune Defic. Syndr.* 12:1155–1158, 1990.
189. Fuller, G.N., et al. Ganciclovir for lumbosacral polyradiculopathy in AIDS. *Lancet* 335:48–49, 1990.
190. Cohen, B.A., et al. Neurologic prognosis of cytomegalovirus polyradiculopathy in AIDS. *Neurology* 43:493–499, 1993.
191. Bricaire, F., et al. Adrenal cortical lesions and AIDS. *Lancet* 1:881, 1988.
192. Rogers, M.F., et al. National case control study of Kaposi's sarcoma and *Pneumocystis carinii* pneumonia in homosexual men: Part 2. Laboratory results. *Ann. Intern. Med.* 99:151–158, 1983.
193. Douglas, J.M., et al. Double-blind study of oral acyclovir for suppression of recurrences of genital herpes simplex virus infection. *N. Engl. J. Med.* 310:1551–1556, 1984.
194. Balfour, H.H., et al. Management of acyclovir resistant herpes simplex and varicella zoster infections. *J. Acquir. Immune Defic. Syndr.* 7:254, 1994.
195. Friedman-Kien, A.E., et al. Herpes zoster: A possible early clinical sign for development of acquired immunodeficiency syndrome in high risk individuals. *J. Am. Acad. Dermatol.* 14:1023, 1986.
196. Forster, D.J., et al. Rapidly progressive outer retinal necrosis in the acquired immunodeficiency syndrome (AIDS). *Am. J. Ophthalmol.* 110:341–348, 1990.
197. Margolis, T.P., et al. Varicella-zoster virus retinitis in patients with the acquired immunodeficiency syndrome. *Am. J. Ophthalmol.* 112:119–131, 1991.
198. Gray, F., et al. Varicella-zoster virus encephalitis in acquired immunodeficiency syndrome: Report of four cases. *Neuropathol. Appl. Neurobiol.* 18:502–514, 1992.
199. Safrin, S., et al. Foscarnet therapy in five patients with AIDS and acyclovir-resistant varicella-zoster virus infection. *Ann. Intern. Med.* 115:19–21, 1991.
200. Price, R.W., and Worley, J.M. Neurological complications of HIV-1 infections and AIDS. In S. Broder, T.C. Merigan Jr., and D. Bolognesi (eds.), *Textbook of AIDS Medicine.* Baltimore: Williams & Wilkins, 1994. Pp. 494–495.
201. Dalakas, M., Wichman, A., and Sever, J. AIDS and the nervous system. *J.A.M.A.* 261:2396, 1989.
202. Berger, J.R., et al. Progressive multifocal leukoencephalopathy associated with human immunodeficiency virus infection. A review of the literature with a report of sixteen cases. *Ann. Intern. Med.* 107:78, 1987.
    Early article establishing the clinical spectrum, evaluation, and anticipated outcome of PML in AIDS.
203. Henson, J., et al. Amplification of JC virus DNA from brain and cerebrospinal fluid of patients with progressive multifocal leukoencephalopathy. *Neurology* 41:1967–1971, 1991.
204. Bauer, W.R., Turci, A.P., Jr., and Johnson, K.P. Progressive multifocal leukoencephalopathy: Remission with cytarabine. *J.A.M.A.* 226:174–176, 1973.
205. Portegies, P., et al. Response to cytarabine in progressive multifocal leukoencephalopathy in AIDS. *Lancet* 337:680–681, 1991.
206. Waite, J., et al. Hepatitis B virus reactivation or reinfection with HIV-1 infection. *A.I.D.S.* 2:443–448, 1988.
207. Horvath, J., and Raffanti, S.P. Clinical aspects of the interactions between human immunodeficiency virus and the hepatotropic viruses. *Clin. Infect. Dis.* 18:339–347, 1994.
208. Darrow, W.W., et al. Risk factors for human immunodeficiency virus infections in homosexual men. *Am. J. Public Health* 77:479–483, 1987.
209. Greenblatt, R.M., et al. Genital ulceration as a risk factor for human immunodeficiency virus infection. *A.I.D.S.* 2:47–50, 1988.
210. Johns, D.R., Tierney, M., and Felsenstein, D. Alteration in the natural history of neurosyphilis by concurrent infection with the human immunodeficiency virus. *N. Engl. J. Med.* 316:1569–1572, 1987.

210a. Lukehart, S.A., et al. Invasion of the central nervous system by *Treponema pallidum:* Implications for diagnosis and treatment. *Ann. Intern. Med.* 109:855–886, 1988.
Classic article demonstrating the high frequency of culture-positive syphilis in asymptomatic HIV-infected patients with primary or secondary syphilis.

211. Hicks, C.B., et al. Seronegative secondary syphilis in a patient infected with the human immunodeficiency virus with Kaposi's sarcoma: A diagnostic dilemma. *Ann. Intern. Med.* 107:492–495, 1987.

212. Bolan, G. Management of Syphilis in HIV-Infected Persons. In M.A. Sande and P.A. Volberding (eds.), *The Medical Management of AIDS* (4th ed.). Philadelphia: Saunders, 1995. P. 537.

213. Tomberlin, M.G., et al. Evaluation of neurosyphilis in human immunodeficiency virus–infected individuals. *Clin. Infect. Dis.* 18:288–294, 1994.

214. Berry, C.D., et al. Neurologic relapse after benzathine penicillin therapy for secondary syphilis in a patient with HIV infection. *N. Engl. J. Med.* 316:1587, 1987.

215. Telzak, E.E., et al. Syphilis treatment response in HIV-infected individuals. *A.I.D.S.* 5:591–598, 1991.

215a. Malone, J.L., et al. Syphilis and neurosyphilis in a human immunodeficiency virus type-1 seropositive population: Evidence for frequent serologic relapse after therapy. *Am. J. Med.* 99:55, 1995.
Serologic or clinical relapse occurred in 10 of 56 patients (17.9%); 7 of 10 who relapsed had previously received high-dose IV or procaine penicillin.

216. Centers for Disease Control. 1993 Sexually transmitted diseases treatment guidelines. U.S. Department of Health and Human Services. *M.M.W.R.* 42:RR-1, 1993.
Recently updated guidelines for the treatment of STDs.

216a. Bennett, K., and Witzburg, R.A. Conventional Bacterial Infections. In H. Libman and R.A. Witzburg (eds.), *HIV Infection: A Primary Care Manual* (3rd ed.). Boston: Little, Brown, 1996. Pp. 419–430.

217. Ammann, A.S., et al. B-cell immunodeficiency in acquired immune deficiency syndrome. *J.A.M.A.* 251:1447–1449, 1984.

218. Simberkoff, M.S., et al. *Streptococcus pneumoniae* infections and bacteremia in patients with the acquired immunodeficiency syndrome, with report of pneumococcal vaccine failure. *Am. Rev. Respir. Dis.* 130:1174–1176, 1984.

218a. Hirschtick, R.E., et al. Bacterial pneumonia in persons infected with the human immunodeficiency virus. *N. Engl. J. Med.* 333:845, 1995.
Of interest, smokers with a low CD4 count had a higher rate of pneumonias than nonsmokers. Patients receiving TMP-SMX prophylaxis (to prevent PCP) had a 67% reduction in episodes of bacterial pneumonia. The most common pathogens were S. pneumoniae, S. aureus, H. influenzae, K. pneumoniae, and P. aeruginosa.

219. Polsky, B., et al. Bacterial pneumonia in patients with the acquired immunodeficiency syndrome. *Ann. Intern. Med.* 104:38–41, 1986.

220. Yamaguchi, E., Charache, P., and Chaisson, R.E. Increasing incidence of pneumococcal infections associated with HIV infection in an inner-city hospital, 1985–1989 [abstr.]. 1990 World Conference on Lung Health, May 20–24, Boston, Massachusetts. *Am. Rev. Respir. Dis.* 141:A619, 1990.

221. Janoff, E.N., et al. Pneumococcal disease during HIV infection. Epidemiologic, clinical, and immunologic perspectives. *Ann. Intern. Med.* 117:314–324, 1992.
Excellent review of this important topic.

222. Gellert, G., et al. Penicillin-resistant pneumococcal meningitis in an HIV-infected man. *N. Engl. J. Med.* 325:1047–1048, 1991.

223. Gruenewald, R., Blum, S., and Chan, J. Relationship between human immunodeficiency virus infection and salmonellosis in 20- to 59-year-old residents of New York City. *Clin. Infect. Dis.* 18:358–363, 1994.

224. Jurado, R.L., et al. Increased risk of meningitis and bacteremia due to *Listeria monocytogenes* in patients with human immunodeficiency virus infection. *Clin. Infect. Dis.* 17:224–227, 1993.

224a. Kielhofner, M., et al. Life-threatening *Pseudomonas aeruginosa* infections in patients with human immunodeficiency infection. *Clin. Infect. Dis.* 14:403, 1992.
Appears to be an increasing problem. See related papers by I. Roilides et al., Pseudomonas infections in children with human immunodeficiency virus infection. Pediatr. Infect. Dis. J. 11:547, 1992; and G. Flores et al., Bacteremia due to Pseudomonas aeruginosa in children with AIDS. Clin. Infect. Dis. 16:706, 1993.

225. Regnery, R.L., et al. Serologic response to *Rochalimaea henselae* antigen in suspected cat-scratch disease. *Lancet* 339:1443–1445, 1992.

226. Perkocha, L.A., et al. Clinical and pathological features of bacillary peliosis hepatitis in association with human immunodeficiency virus infection. *N. Engl. J. Med.* 323:1573–1580, 1990.
227. Koehler, J.E., and Tappero, J.W. Bacillary angiomatosis and bacillary peliosis in patients infected with human immunodeficiency virus. *Clin. Infect. Dis.* 17:612–624, 1993.
228. Guerra, L.G., et al. Rapid response of AIDS-related bacillary angiomatosis to azithromycin. *Clin. Infect. Dis.* 17:264–266, 1993.
229. Carey, J., Hart, C., and Stoeckle, M. High incidence of gram-negative catheter-associated bacteremia in HIV positive patients. *Clin. Res.* 41:603A, 1993.
230. Benezra, D., et al. Prospective study of infections in indwelling central venous catheters using quantitative blood cultures. *Am. J. Med.* 85:495–498, 1988.
231. Ellner, J.J., et al. Infectious Disease Society of America Symposium: Tuberculosis—emerging problems and promise. *J. Infect. Dis.* 168:537–551, 1993.
    See related paper by R.W. Shafer and B. Edlin, Tuberculosis in patients infected with human immunodeficiency virus: Perspective on the past decade. Clin. Infect. Dis. 22:683, 1996.
232. Centers for Disease Control. Expanded tuberculosis surveillance and tuberculosis morbidity—United States. *M.M.W.R.* 43:361 366, 1994.
233. Onorato, I.M., McCray, E., and Field Services Branch. Prevalence of human immunodeficiency virus infection among patients attending tuberculosis clinics in the United States. *J. Infect. Dis.* 165:87–92, 1992.
234. Sepkowitz, K.A. Tuberculosis and the health care worker: A historical perspective. *Ann. Intern. Med.* 120:71–79, 1994.
235. Frieden, T.R., et al. The emergence of drug-resistant tuberculosis in New York City. *N. Engl. J. Med.* 328:521–526, 1993.
236. Sepkowitz, K.A., et al. Tuberculosis susceptibility trends in New York City, 1987–1991. *Clin. Infect. Dis.* 18:755–759, 1994.
237. Bloch, A.B., et al. Nationwide survey of drug-resistant tuberculosis in the United States. *J.A.M.A.* 271:665–671, 1994.
238. Jones, B.E., et al. Relationship of the manifestations of tuberculosis to CD4 cell counts in patients with human immunodeficiency virus infection. *Am. Rev. Respir. Dis.* 148:1292–1297, 1993.
239. FitzGerald, J.M., Grzybowski, S., and Allen, E.A. The impact of human immunodeficiency virus infection on tuberculosis and its control. *Chest* 100:191–200, 1991.
240. Selwyn, P., et al. A prospective study of the risk of tuberculosis among intravenous drug users with human immunodeficiency virus infection. *N. Engl. J. Med.* 320:545–550, 1987.
241. Daley, C.L., et al. An outbreak of tuberculosis with accelerated progression among persons infected with the human immunodeficiency virus. An analysis using restriction-fragment length polymorphisms. *N. Engl. J. Med.* 326:231–235, 1992.
    Classic article demonstrating the extreme susceptibility of HIV-infected persons to progress to active disease.
242. Wallis, R.S., et al. Influence of tuberculosis on HIV: Enhanced cytokine expression and elevated beta-2-microglobulin in HIV-1 associated tuberculosis. *J. Infect. Dis.* 167:43–48, 1992.
243. Schluger, N., and Rom, W. Current approaches to the diagnosis of active pulmonary tuberculosis. *Am. J. Respir. Crit. Care Med.* 149:264–267, 1994.
244. Noordhoek, G.T., van Embden, J.D.A., and Kolk, A.H.J. Questionable reliability of the polymerase chain reaction in the detection of *Mycobacterium tuberculosis. N. Engl. J. Med.* 329:2036, 1993.
245. American Thoracic Society. Treatment of tuberculosis and tuberculosis infection in adults and children. *Am. J. Respir. Crit. Care Med.* 149:1359–1374, 1994.
    Up-to-date recommendations on how, how long, and whom to treat.
246. Perriens, J.R., et al. Increased mortality and tuberculosis treatment failure rate among human immunodeficiency virus (HIV) seropositive patients compared with HIV seronegative patients with pulmonary tuberculosis treated with standard therapy in Zaire. *Am. Rev. Respir. Dis.* 144:750–755, 1991.
247. Sunderam, G., et al. Failure of optimal four-drug short-course tuberculosis chemotherapy in a compliant patient with human immunodeficiency virus. *Am. Rev. Respir. Dis.* 136:1475–1478, 1987.
248. Iseman, M.D. Treatment of multidrug-resistant tuberculosis. *N. Engl. J. Med.* 329:784–791, 1993.

249. Pape, J.W., et al. Effect of isoniazid prophylaxis on incidence of active tuberculosis and progression of HIV infection. *Lancet* 342:268–272, 1993.
250. Centers for Disease Control. National Action Plan to Combat Multidrug-Resistant Tuberculosis. *M.M.W.R.* 41(RR-11):1–7, 1992.
251. Benson, C.A., and Ellner, J.J. *Mycobacterium avium* complex infection and AIDS: Advances in theory and practice. *Clin. Infect. Dis.* 17:7–20, 1993.
252. Young, L.S. *Mycobacterium avium* complex infection. *J. Infect. Dis.* 157:863, 1988.
253. Armstrong, D., et al. Treatment of infections in patients with the acquired immunodeficiency syndrome. *Ann. Intern. Med.* 103:738, 1985.
254. Glatt, A.E., Chirgwin, K., and Landesman, S.H. Treatment of infections associated with human immunodeficiency virus. *N. Engl. J. Med.* 318:1439, 1988.
255. Young, L.S., et al. Mycobacterial infections in AIDS patients with an emphasis in the *Mycobacterium avium* complex. *Rev. Infect. Dis.* 8:1024, 1986.
256. Kiehn, T.E., et al. Infections caused by *Mycobacterium avium* complex in immunocompromised patients: Diagnosis by blood culture and fecal examination, antimicrobial susceptibility tests, and morphological and seroglutination characteristics. *J. Clin. Microbiol.* 21:168, 1985.
257. Benson, C.A. Treatment of disseminated disease due to the *Mycobacterium avium* complex in patients with AIDS. *Clin. Infect. Dis.* 18(Suppl. 3):S237–242, 1994.
258. Masur, H., and the Public Health Service Task Force of Prophylaxis and Therapy for *Mycobacterium avium* Complex. Recommendations on prophylaxis and therapy for disseminated *Mycobacterium avium* complex disease in patients infected with the human immunodeficiency virus. *N. Engl. J. Med.* 329:898–904, 1993.
     Recent recommendations on prophylaxis and treatment for MAI.
258a. Chaisson, R.E., et al., and the AIDS Clinical Trials Group Protocol 157 Study Team. Clarithromycin therapy for bacteremic *Mycobacterium avium* complex disease. A randomized, double-blind, dose-ranging study in patients with AIDS. *Ann. Intern. Med.* 121:905, 1994.
     Clarithromycin acutely decreased by more than 99% MAI bacteremia. A dose of 500 mg PO bid was well tolerated and was associated with better survival. See editorial comment in this same issue. See also B. Dantzenberg et al., Rifabutin versus placebo in combination with three drugs in the treatment of nontuberculous mycobacterium infection in patients with AIDS. Clin. Infect. Dis. 22:705, 1996.
259. Nightingale, S.D., et al. Two controlled trials of rifabutin prophylaxis against *Mycobacterium avium* complex infection in AIDS. *N. Engl. J. Med.* 329:828, 1993.
260. Centers for Disease Control. Recommendations on prophylaxis and therapy for disseminated *Mycobacterium avium* complex for adults and adolescents infected with human immunodeficiency virus. *M.M.W.R.* 42:RR-9, 1993.
261. Grossman, H.A., et al. Clarithromycin 500 mg bid as primary prophylaxis for disseminated MAC [abstr.]. Presented at the Thirty-Fourth Interscience Conference on Antimicrobial Agents and Chemotherapy, Orlando, Florida, 1994.
262. Keith, P.E., and Schiller, T.L. Clarithromycin as primary prophylaxis in patients with AIDS [abstr.]. Presented at the Thirty-Fourth Interscience Conference on Antimicrobial Agents and Chemotherapy, Orlando, Florida, 1994.
263. Horsburgh, C.R., Jr., and Selik, R.A. The epidemiology of disseminated nontuberculous mycobacterial infection in the acquired immunodeficiency syndrome (AIDS). *Am. Rev. Respir. Dis.* 139:4–7, 1989.
264. Bamberger, D.M., et al. *Mycobacterium kansasii* among patients infected with human immunodeficiency virus in Kansas City. *Clin. Infect. Dis.* 18:395–400, 1994.
265. Levine, B., and Chaisson, R.E. *Mycobacterium kansasii:* A cause of treatable pulmonary disease associated with advanced human immunodeficiency virus infection. *Ann. Intern. Med.* 114:861–868, 1991.
266. Straus, W.L., et al. Clinical and epidemiologic characteristics of *Mycobacterium haemophilum,* an emerging pathogen in immunocompromised patients. *Ann. Intern. Med.* 120:118–125, 1994.
267. Dever, L.L., et al. Varied presentations and responses to treatment of infections caused by *Mycobacterium haemophilum* in patients with AIDS. *Clin. Infect. Dis.* 14:1195–2000, 1992.
268. Kristjansson, M., Bieluch, V.M., and Byeff, P.H. *Mycobacterium haemophilum* infection in immunocompromised patients: Case report and review of the literature. *Rev. Infect. Dis.* 13:906–910, 1991.
269. Stracher, A., and Sepkowitz, K.A. Atypical mycobacteria infections in patients with HIV infection. *AIDS Reader* (in press).

269a. American Thoracic Society. Fungal infection in HIV-infected patients. *Am. J. Respir. Crit. Care Med.* 152:816, 1995.
270. Kaslow, R.A., et al. Infection with the human immunodeficiency virus: Clinical manifestations and their relationship to immune deficiency. *Ann. Intern. Med.* 107:474–480, 1987.
271. Iman, W., et al. Hierarchical pattern of mucosal *Candida* infections in HIV seropositive women. *Am. J. Med.* 89:142–146, 1990.
272. Tavitan, A., Rautman, J.P., and Rosenthal, L.E. Oral candidiasis as a marker for esophageal candidiasis in the acquired immunodeficiency syndrome. *Ann. Intern. Med.* 104:54–55, 1986.
273. Laine, L., et al. Fluconazole compared with ketoconazole for the treatment of *Candida* esophagitis in AIDS. A randomized trial. *Ann. Intern. Med.* 117:655–660, 1992.
274. Jaffe, H.W., Bregman, D.J., and Selik, R.M. Acquired immune deficiency syndrome in the United States: The first 1000 cases. *J. Infect. Dis.* 148:339–345, 1983.
275. Lortholary, O., et al. Invasive aspergillosis in patients with acquired immunodeficiency syndrome: Report of 33 cases. *Am. J. Med.* 95:177–182, 1993.
276. Minamoto, G.Y., Barlam, T.F., and Vander Els, N.J. Invasive aspergillosis in patients with AIDS. *Clin. Infect. Dis.* 14:66–74, 1992.
277. Pursell, K.J., Telzak, E.E., and Armstrong, D.A. *Aspergillus* species colonization and invasive disease in patients with AIDS. *Clin. Infect. Dis.* 14:141–148, 1992.
278. Denning, D.W., et al. Pulmonary aspergillosis in the acquired immunodeficiency syndrome. *N. Engl. J. Med.* 324:654–662, 1991.
279. Wheat, L.J., et al. Disseminated histoplasmosis in the acquired immune deficiency syndrome: Clinical findings, diagnosis and treatment, and review of the literature. *Medicine* 69:361–373, 1990.
280. Johnson, P.C., et al. Progressive disseminated histoplasmosis in patients with acquired immunodeficiency syndrome. *Am. J. Med.* 89.142–146, 1990.
281. Wheat, L.J., et al. *Histoplasma capsulatum* polysaccharide antigen detection in diagnosis and management of disseminated histoplasmosis in patients with acquired immunodeficiency syndrome. *Am. J. Med.* 87:396–400, 1989.
282. Wheat, L.J., et al. Histoplasmosis relapse in patients with AIDS: Detection using *Histoplasma capsulatum* variety capsulatum antigen levels. *Ann. Intern. Med.* 115:936–941, 1991.
283. McKinsey, D.S., et al. Long-term amphotericin B therapy for disseminated histoplasmosis in patients with the acquired immunodeficiency syndrome (AIDS). *Ann. Intern. Med.* 111:655, 1989.
284. Wheat, J., et al. Prevention of relapse of histoplasmosis with itraconazole in patients with the acquired immunodeficiency syndrome. *Ann. Intern. Med.* 118:610–616, 1993.
285. Dismukes, W.E. Cryptococcal meningitis in patients with AIDS. *J. Infect. Dis.* 157:624, 1988.
286. Powderly, W.G. Cryptococcal meningitis and AIDS. *Clin. Infect. Dis.* 17:837–842, 1993.
    Excellent review of this topic.
287. Saag, M.S., et al. Comparison of amphotericin B with fluconazole in the treatment of acute AIDS-associated cryptococcal meningitis. *N. Engl. J. Med.* 326:83–89, 1992.
288. Chuck, S.L., and Sande, M.A. Infections with *Cryptococcus neoformans* in the acquired immunodeficiency syndrome. *N. Engl. J. Med.* 321:794–799, 1989.
289. Bronnimann, D.A., et al. Coccidioidomycosis in the acquired immunodeficiency syndrome. *Ann. Intern. Med.* 106:372–379, 1987.
290. Fish, D.G., et al. Coccidioidomycosis during HIV infection: A review of 77 patients. *Medicine* 69:384–391, 1990.
291. Galgiana, J.N., and Ampel, N.M. Coccidioidomycosis in the human immunodeficiency virus–infected patients. *J. Infect. Dis.* 162:1165–1169, 1990.
292. Sobonya, R.E., et al. Detection of fungi and other pathogens in immunocompromised patients by bronchoalveolar lavage in an area endemic for coccidioidomycosis. *Chest* 97:1349–1355, 1990.
293. Tucker, R.M., et al. Treatment of coccidioidal meningitis with fluconazole. *Rev. Infect. Dis.* 12(Suppl.):S380–S389, 1990.
294. Diaz, M., et al. Itraconazole in the treatment of coccidioidomycosis. *Chest* 100:682–684, 1991.
295. Powderly, W. Fungi. In S. Broder, T.C. Merigan, Jr., and D. Bolognesi (eds.), *Textbook of AIDS Medicine*. Baltimore: Williams & Wilkins, 1994. P. 352.
296. Pappas, P.G., et al. Blastomycosis in patients with the acquired immunodeficiency syndrome. *Ann. Intern. Med.* 116:847–853, 1992.

297. Tan, G., et al. Disseminated atypical blastomycosis in two patients with AIDS. *Clin. Infect. Dis.* 16:107–111, 1993.

298. Luft, B.J., and Remington, J.S. Toxoplasmic encephalitis. *J. Infect. Dis.* 157:1, 1988.

299. Grant, I.H., et al. *Toxoplasma gondii* serology in HIV-infected patients: The development of central nervous system toxoplasmosis in AIDS. *A.I.D.S.* 4:519–521, 1990.

300. Luft, B.J., and Remington, J.S. Toxoplasmic encephalitis in AIDS. *Clin. Infect. Dis.* 15:211–222, 1992.
   Excellent review of this topic.

301. Elder, G.A., and Sever, J.L. Neurologic disorders associated with AIDS retroviral infection. *Rev. Infect. Dis.* 10:286, 1988.

302. Hofman, P., et al. Extracerebral toxoplasmosis in the acquired immunodeficiency syndrome (AIDS). *Pathol. Res. Pract.* 189:894–901, 1993.

303. Pauwels, A., et al. Toxoplasma colitis in the acquired immunodeficiency syndrome. *Am. J. Gastroenterol.* 87:518–519, 1992.

304. Hofman, P., et al. Prevalence of toxoplasma myocarditis in patients with AIDS. *Br. Heart J.* 70:376–381, 1993.

305. Lucet, J.C., et al. Septic shock due to toxoplasmosis in patients infected with the human immunodeficiency virus. *Chest* 104:1054–1058, 1993.

306. Post, M.J., et al. Cranial CT in the acquired immunodeficiency syndrome; spectrum of diseases and optimal contrast enhancement technique. *A.J.R.* 145:929, 1985.

307. Luft, B.J., et al. Toxoplasmic encephalitis in patients with acquired immune deficiency syndrome. *J.A.M.A.* 252:913, 1984.

308. Derouin, F., Thylliez, P., and Garin, Y.J.F. Value and limitations of toxoplasmosis serology in HIV patients. *Pathol. Biol.* 39:255–259, 1991.

309. Renold, C., et al. Toxoplasma encephalitis in patients with the acquired immunodeficiency syndrome. *Medicine* 71:224–239, 1992.

310. Porter, S.B., and Sande, M.A. Toxoplasmosis of the central nervous system in acquired immunodeficiency syndrome. *N. Engl. J. Med.* 327:1643–1648, 1992.

311. Cristina, N., et al. Detection of *Toxoplasma gondii* in AIDS patients by the polymerase chain reaction. *Infection* 21:150–153, 1993.

312. Holliman, R.E., et al. Diagnosis of cerebral toxoplasmosis in association with AIDS using the polymerase chain reaction. *Scand. J. Infect. Dis.* 22:243–244, 1990.

313. Parmly, S., Goebel, F., and Remington, J. Detection of *Toxoplasma gondii* in cerebrospinal fluid from AIDS patients by polymerase chain reaction. *J. Clin. Microbiol.* 30:3000–3002, 1992.

314. Tirard, V., et al. Diagnosis of toxoplasmosis in patients with AIDS by isolation of the parasite from the blood. *N. Engl. J. Med.* 324:634, 1991.

315. Derouin, F., et al. Laboratory diagnosis of pulmonary toxoplasmosis in patients with acquired immunodeficiency syndrome. *J. Clin. Microbiol.* 27:1661–1663, 1989.

316. Luft, B.J., et al. Toxoplasmic encephalitis in patients with the acquired immunodeficiency syndrome. *N. Engl. J. Med.* 329:995–1000, 1993.

317. Ciricillo, S.F., and Rosenblum, M. Use of CT and MR imaging to distinguish intracranial lesions and to define the need for biopsy in AIDS patients. *J. Neurosurg.* 73:720–724, 1990.

318. Dannemann, B.R., Israelski, D.M., and Remington, J.S. Treatment of toxoplasmic encephalitis with intravenous clindamycin. *Arch. Intern. Med.* 148:2477, 1988.

319. Carr, A., et al. Low-dose trimethoprim-sulfamethoxazole prophylaxis for toxoplasmic encephalitis in patients with AIDS. *Ann. Intern. Med.* 117:106–111, 1992.

320. Jacobson, M.A., et al. Primary prophylaxis for toxoplasmic encephalitis in patients with advanced HIV disease: Results of a randomized trial. *J. Infect. Dis.* 169:384–394, 1994.
   See related report by C. Leport et al., Pyrimethamine for primary prophylaxis of toxoplasmic encephalitis in patients with human immunodeficiency virus infection: A double-blind, randomized trial. J. Infect. Dis. 173:91, 1996. Data still favor TMP-SMX if this agent can be tolerated.

321. Laughon, B.E., et al. Prevalence of enteric pathogens in homosexual men with and without acquired immunodeficiency syndrome. *Gastroenterology* 94:984, 1988.

322. Mannheimer, S.B., et al. Protozoal infections in patients with AIDS. *Infect. Dis. Clin. North Am.* 8:483, 1994.
   This review comprehensively covers cryptosporidiosis, isosporiasis, cyclosporiasis, and microsporidiosis.

323. Petersen, C. Cryptosporidiosis in patients infected with the human immunodeficiency virus. *Clin. Infect. Dis.* 15:903, 1992.

324. Margulis, S.J., et al. Biliary tract obstruction in the acquired immunodeficiency syndrome. *Ann. Intern. Med.* 105:207, 1986.
325. Asmuth, D.M. Clinical features of microsporidiosis in patients with acquired immunodeficiency syndrome. *Clin. Infect. Dis.* 18:819, 1994.
     An up-to-date review of the topic.
326. Orenstein, J.M., et al. Systemic dissemination by a newly recognized microsporidia species in AIDS. *A.I.D.S.* 6:1143, 1992.
327. Weber, R., et al. Improved light-microscopical detection of microsporidiaspores in stool and duodenal aspirates. *N. Engl. J. Med.* 326:161, 1992.
     Details of at least one of the new methods for detecting microsporidia in stool.
328. Pape, J.W., et al. Treatment and prophylaxis of *Isospora belli* in patients with the acquired immunodeficiency syndrome. *N. Engl. J. Med.* 320:1044, 1989.
329. Ortega, Y.R., et al. *Cyclospora* species—a new protozoan pathogen of humans. *N. Engl. J. Med.* 328:1312, 1993.
330. Pape, J.W., et al. *Cyclospora* infection in adults infected with HIV. *Ann. Intern. Med.* 121:654, 1994.
331. Neva, F.A. Biology and immunology of human strongyloidiasis. *J. Infect. Dis.* 153:397–406, 1986.
332. Gompels, M.M., et al. Disseminated strongyloidiasis in AIDS: Uncommon but important. *A.I.D.S.* 5:329–332, 1991.
333. Dutcher, J.P., et al. Disseminated strongyloidiasis with central nervous system involvement diagnosed antemortem in a patient with acquired immunodeficiency syndrome and Burkitt's lymphoma. *Cancer* 66:2417–2419, 1990.
334. Igra-siegman, Y., et al. Syndrome of hyperinfection with *Strongyloides stercoralis.* *Rev. Infect. Dis.* 3:397 405, 1981.
335. Jain, A.K., Agarwal, S.K., and El-Sadr, W. *Streptococcus bovis* bacteremia and meningitis associated with *Strongyloides stercoralis* colitis in a patient infected with human immunodeficiency virus. *Clin. Infect. Dis.* 18:253–254, 1994.
335a. Medical Letter. Drugs for parasitic infections. *Med. Lett. Drug. Ther.* 37:99, 1995.
336. Torres, J.R., et al. Efficacy of invermectin in the treatment of strongyloidiasis complicating AIDS. *Clin. Infect. Dis.* 17:900–902, 1993.
336a. Kaplan, J.E., et al. Reducing the impact of opportunistic infections in patients with HIV infection: New guidelines. *J.A.M.A.* 274:347, 1995.
337. Marlink, R., et al. Reduced rate for disease development after HIV-2 infection as compared to HIV-1 infection. *Science* 265:1587–1590, 1994.
338. Markovitz, D.M. Infection with the human immunodeficiency virus type 2. *Ann. Intern. Med.* 118:211–218, 1993.
     Thorough summary of the clinical and epidemiologic features of HIV-2.
339. Williams, A.E., et al. Seroprevalence and epidemiological correlates of HTLV-1 infection in U.S. blood donors. *Science* 240:643, 1988.
340. Scully, R.E., et al. Case records of the Massachusetts General Hospital: Case 36. *N. Engl. J. Med.* 321:663, 1989.
341. Centers for Disease Control and Prevention and the U.S.P.H.S. Working Group. Guidelines for counseling persons infected with human-T-lymphotropic virus type 1 (HTLV-1) and type II (HTLV-2). *Ann. Intern. Med.* 118:448–454, 1993.
342. Centers for Disease Control. Adult T-cell leukemia/lymphoma associated with human T-lymphotropic virus type 1 (HTLV-1) infection—North Carolina. *M.M.W.R.* 36:804, 1987.
343. Wachsman, W., Globe, D.W., and Chen, I.S.Y. HTLV and human leukemia: Perspectives 1986. *Semin. Hematol.* 23:245, 1986.
344. Jacobsen, S., et al. Isolation of an HTLV-1-like retrovirus from patients with tropical paraparesis. *Nature* 331:540, 1988.
345. Sarin, P.S. HTLV-1, adult T-cell leukemia, and tropical spastic paraparesis. *Ann. Neurol.* 23:S181, 1988.
346. Bhagavati, S.B., et al. Detection of human T-cell lymphoma/leukemia virus type 1 DNA and antigen in spinal fluid and blood of patients with chronic progressive myelopathy. *N. Engl. J. Med.* 318:1141, 1988.
346a. Volberding, P. Introduction: Treatment trends in HIV disease. *J. Infect. Dis.* 171(Suppl. 2):S79, 1995.
346b. Volberding, P. The need for additional options in the treatment of human immunodeficiency virus infection. *J. Infect. Dis.* 171(Suppl. 2):S150, 1995.
346c. Murphy, R. Clinical aspects of human immunodeficiency virus disease: Clinical rationale and treatment. *J. Infect. Dis.* 171(Suppl. 2):S81, 1995.

346d. Medical Letter. Drugs for AIDS and associated infections. *Med. Lett. Drugs Ther.* 37:87, 1995.

346e. Executive summary: Abstract ACTG 175. AIDS Clinical Trials Information Service (ACTIS). Sept. 14, 1995.

346f. Medical Letter. New drugs for HIV infection. *Med. Lett. Drugs Ther.* 38:35, 1996.
   This April 12, 1996 issue summarizes the importance of combination therapy, including the role of the new protease inhibitors. See detailed discussion in Chap. 26.

347. Dolin, R., and Keefer, M.C. Vaccines for HIV-1 Infection. In G.L. Mandell, J.E. Bennett, and R. Dolin (eds.), *Principles and Practice of Infectious Diseases* (4th ed.). New York: Churchill Livingstone, 1995. Pp. 1294–1305.
   For a related discussion, see R. Dolin, Human studies in the development of human immunodeficiency virus vaccines. J. Infect. Dis. 172:1175, 1995.

348. Letvin, N.L. Vaccines against human immunodeficiency virus—progress and prospects. *N. Engl. J. Med.* 329:1400–1405, 1993.

349. Chamberland, M.E., Ward, J.W., and Curran, J.W. Epidemiology and Prevention of AIDS and HIV Infection. In G.L. Mandell, J.E. Bennett, and R. Dolin (eds.), *Principles and Practice of Infectious Diseases* (4th ed.). New York: Churchill Livingstone, 1995. Pp. 1192–1203.

350. de Vincenzi, I. A longitudinal study of human immunodeficiency virus transmission by heterosexual partners. *N. Engl. J. Med.* 331:341–346, 1994.

351. Musicco, M., et al. Antiretroviral treatment of men infected with human immunodeficiency virus type 1 reduces the incidence of heterosexual transmission. *Arch. Intern. Med.* 154:1971–1976, 1994.

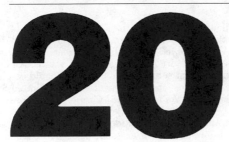

Infections in Transplantation

Sally H. Houston, Robert H. Rubin, and John T. Sinnott

Transplantation, first a reality 40 years ago, dramatically expanded with the addition of cyclosporine to the immunosuppressive regimens of the early 1980s. Improved surgical techniques, innovations in organ procurement, and advances in the diagnosis and treatment of infection have likewise contributed to this remarkable growth. In 1992 alone, there were approximately 10,000 bone marrow transplants, 2,997 liver transplants, 2,161 cardiac transplants, and 9,659 kidney transplants [1]. As lung, heart-lung, and pancreas transplants become accepted therapy, these numbers will increase. Further progress in transplantation currently is hindered by a limited donor pool. As of October 1993, there were 32,603 individuals awaiting organs. Approximately one-third of patients waiting for a heart or liver die before an organ becomes available [2].

All transplant patients require immunosuppression which, while controlling rejection, can produce serious side effects including infection and malignancy. The chronic risk of infection, with its diagnostic challenges and potentially fatal outcome, requires an appreciation of transplant-associated infections. **The following discussion should orient the physician who does not routinely deal with infection in the iatrogenically compromised host.** To avoid repetition, the reader at times is referred to other chapter discussions for the specifics of treatment unless there are transplant-related considerations. **Because these may be complex infections to manage, early infectious disease consultation is advised.** Finally, because of its dramatic impact on the risk and outcome of transplantation, human immunodeficiency virus (HIV) status is a vital consideration in evaluating both donor **and** recipient [3, 4].

Basic Principles

I. **Donor selection** is primarily the responsibility of a trained procurement team. Cadavers are the major source of tissue for all but bone marrow recipients. The scarcity of organs is the major obstacle to the wider use of transplantation as a therapeutic modality. In general, hearts and kidneys are harvested from donors younger than 50 years, and livers are harvested from donors 2 months to 65 years of age [5] with exceptions made on a case-by-case basis. For kidney, heart, and liver transplantation, organ size and ABO compatibility usually are respected, whereas HLA typing plays a limited role. For bone marrow transplantation (BMT), HLA typing is an important factor in success of the therapy [4].
   A. **General contraindications** for organ donation include systemic malignancy and active infections (e.g., pneumonia, upper urinary tract infection, varicella, tuberculosis, or bacteremia) [4]. The possibility of covert bacteremia should be excluded by history and physical examination as well as by scrutiny of blood culture reports.
   B. **Infectious disease considerations are paramount in this setting.** After bacteremia has been excluded, **the donor should be screened for** syphilis, hepatitis B (HBV) and C viruses (HCV), HIV-1, HIV-2, and human T-lymphotropic virus type I (HTLV-I), as well as for toxoplasma and cytomegalovirus (CMV) [4]. The results of these screens are helpful in recognizing infections after transplantation and in selecting appropriate blood products for transfusion [6]. Some centers avoid transplantation of CMV-seropositive tissue into seronegative recipients [7] or, alternatively, initiate prophylactic strategies after transplantation. Studies of cardiac transplant patients demonstrate that primary CMV infection carries a greater risk of mortality than reactivation or secondary CMV infections [6].
II. **Recipient selection.** Recipients should have organ failure refractory to medical therapy and should be free of social and psychiatric problems that may interfere with

the rigid medical regimens entailed by transplantation. Before transplantation, a **laboratory evaluation should include** serologic determinations of varicella-zoster virus (VZV), HIV-1 and -2, HTLV-I, *Legionella,* syphilis, toxoplasma, HBV, HCV, Epstein-Barr virus (EBV), herpes simplex virus (HSV), and CMV status. A purified protein derivative (PPD) test with skin-test controls (see Chap. 9) should be placed. Patients from developing countries and those from the rural southern United States should have their stools screened for *Strongyloides* cysts [8]. Carriers should be treated with thiabendazole.

General contraindications for transplantation include recent hemorrhage, active infection, or malignancy [4]. Active infection must be excluded prior to transplantation because pretransplant bacteremia or pneumonia is associated with a poor outcome. Frustration and disappointment can be avoided by careful attention to intravenous lines and early intubation of the encephalopathic liver transplant candidate to prevent aspiration.

A. **Kidney recipients** should have end-stage renal disease in which recurrence in the transplanted organ is unlikely [4]. Contraindications include coexistent disease that would limit life expectancy to less than 2 years.

B. **Heart recipients** include those with irreversible vascular, valvular, or idiopathic cardiomyopathy. Contraindications include irreversible pulmonary hypertension, recent pulmonary infarction, and severe peripheral vascular disease [4].

C. **Liver recipients** must have end-stage cirrhosis, Budd-Chiari syndrome, or primary hepatocellular carcinoma. Children receive transplants for congenital cirrhosis, primary biliary atresia, and metabolic defects such as alpha$_1$-antitrypsin deficiency, tyrosinemia, and glycogen storage diseases types I and IV. Contraindications include extrahepatic complications such as cholangiocarcinoma or advanced cardiopulmonary disease. Relative contraindications include patient age over 55 years, portal vein thrombosis, HBeAg seropositivity, active alcohol abuse, or prior hepatobiliary or portocaval surgery [9].

D. **Bone marrow recipients.** See later in this chapter, under Bone Marrow Transplantation.

III. **Immunosuppressive therapy.** All patients except those transplanted from an identical twin or those with severe combined immunodeficiency require immunosuppression to prevent graft rejection. The ultimate goal is to induce tolerance after a period of engraftment [4]. Most immunosuppressive regimens employ a combination of cyclosporine, azathioprine, and corticosteroids. Other agents include antilymphocyte antibody preparations or tacrolimus (formerly FK-506); alternative modalities, such as total lymphoid irradiation therapy, may be required. Customarily, a daily maintenance immunosuppressive regimen is established, with pulse therapy (corticosteroids or OKT3–antilymphocyte globulin) employed for managing breakthrough episodes of rejection. These regimens predispose to infection and neoplasia [10]. In cardiac transplantations, approximately 30% of infections develop after pulse therapy for rejection [11]. Immunologic monitoring of T-cell ratios or blastogenesis is experimental.

A. **Antilymphocyte globulins (ALGs), antithymocyte globulins (ATGs), and OKT3 murine monoclonal antibody** are biologic preparations that lyse host immunocytes. OKT3 is effective for both prophylaxis and treatment of rejection. Concurrent administration of corticosteroids, acetaminophen, and diphenhydramine palliates the side effects of fever and rigors [10]. The potential side effects of OKT3 include fever or serum sickness, aseptic meningitis, pulmonary edema, or diarrhea and may be easily confused with infection or ongoing rejection. Furthermore, OKT3 may allow reactivated CMV to become a more severe infection.

B. **Cyclosporine,** a cyclic polypeptide, inhibits interleukin 2 (IL-2) production, thereby suppressing CD4 cell proliferation and activation of cytotoxic T cells. Because interleukin 3 (IL-3) is not inhibited by cyclosporine, the suppressor T-cell population increases, and the ratio of suppressor to cytotoxic cells is increased. Cyclosporine does not lyse effector cells, so it **is more useful for prophylaxis than for treatment of rejection.** The incidence and severity of infections may be reduced with cyclosporine because lower dosages of steroids can be employed. It is metabolized in the liver, and its effects are dose-dependent [10]. Optimum therapeutic levels vary depending on the type of organ transplanted, time interval since transplantation, and level of rejection. Trough levels, determined on plasma, are monitored.

1. **Side effects** include nephrotoxicity, hepatotoxicity, hypertension, hirsutism, tremor, gingival hyperplasia, and tumorigenesis. Nephrotoxicity may be po-

tentiated by aminoglycosides, vancomycin, erythromycin, amphotericin B, acyclovir, ganciclovir, and high-dose trimethoprim-sulfamethoxazole (TMP-SMX) [12]. With long-term cyclosporine use, the transplanted kidney is subject to renal vasoconstriction with the possible induction of hypertension and/or nephrotoxicity. However, most renal-transplant patients tolerate long-term cyclosporine therapy without evidence of progressive toxic nephropathy [12a].

2. **Drug interactions** necessitate frequent monitoring of **cyclosporine** levels. **Ketoconazole and erythromycin increases cyclosporine levels,** with an increase in side effects, whereas rifampin, isoniazid, and TMP-SMX lower levels, increasing the risk of rejection [12]. Drugs stimulating cytochrome P450 activity will result in more rapid metabolism and lower levels of cyclosporine. Idiosyncratic interactions such as renal failure after single doses of aminoglycosides, amphotericin B, or fluoroquinolones may occur.

C. **Corticosteroids** have long been used in the prophylaxis and treatment of transplant rejection. They are believed to interfere with production of interleukins 1, 2, 3, 4, and 5 (and perhaps others) and with immunoglobulin secretion. Additionally, interferon-gamma production is decreased, and acute inflammatory responses are blunted. The immunosuppressive effects of corticosteroids are broad, and their usage predisposes to an array of side effects, especially infection. Leukocytosis frequently is seen, but counts rarely exceed 20,000/mm^3 without an underlying infection. Osteoporosis, aseptic hip necrosis, glucose intolerance, cataracts, and hypercholesterolemia often complicate long-term therapy [10, 12]. **Modern immunosuppressive therapy attempts to minimize the use of corticosteroids.** A maintenance dose is determined empirically by balancing rejection and side effects.

D. **Azathioprine,** a purine analogue, interrupts DNA synthesis, thereby suppressing T-cell proliferation. It is used in rejection prophylaxis. Dose-related side effects include leukopenia, thrombocytopenia, macrocytic anemia, pancreatitis, hepatotoxicity, tumorigenesis, and infection [12]. Azathioprine does not interact with antibiotics but may enhance hematologic toxicity [10]. When administered with allopurinol, the dose should be reduced.

E. **Radiation therapy** is employed routinely for BMT preparation. Total lymphoid irradiation has been used to treat chronic stubborn rejection in heart recipients, and engrafted kidneys have been experimentally irradiated. Total lymphoid irradiation is increasingly used to prepare patients at high risk of rejection for transplantation. The number and nature of infections does not appear to be increased as a result of total lymphoid irradiation [13].

F. **Tacrolimus** (Prograf; **previously called FK506**) was approved for use in 1994 for primary prevention of organ rejection in patients receiving liver transplants. The drug has also been used as rescue therapy for organ-graft rejection unresponsive to cyclosporine and other immunosuppressive drugs [13a]. Tacrolimus is a bacteria-derived macrolide with no chemical resemblance to cyclosporine but with similar activity [13a]. It interferes with cytotoxic T-cell proliferation and production of IL-1 and -2, interferon-gamma, and IL-2 receptors. Tacrolimus is approximately 10 times more active than cyclosporine [14].

G. **Mycophenolate mofetil** (Cell Cept) was approved in 1995 for oral use in preventing organ rejection in patients receiving allogeneic renal transplants [14a].

IV. **Problems resembling infection are myriad**

A. **Allograft rejection** notoriously **mimics infection** in solid-organ transplant recipients. Fever, myalgias or arthralgias, and a leukocytosis may be seen. Alternatively, the patient may feel relatively well, with rejection found only on biopsy. **In all febrile episodes, the clinician must first consider the possibility of rejection, although antibiotics may be initiated empirically after cultures have been obtained.**

B. **Medication side effects** may cause fever, and practically all drugs have been implicated. Azathioprine or cyclosporine hepatotoxicity should be considered in posttransplant hepatitis. Usually OKT3 reactions—fever, chills, or diarrhea—occur early in therapy.

V. **The presentation of infection in patients on immunosuppressive therapy may be vague.** The impaired inflammatory response results in a paucity of physical signs and an atypical presentation of many infectious processes. The insidious onset and possible rapid progression of infection in the transplant patient warrant a prompt, thorough evaluation early in the course of any febrile illness. **The febrile transplant patient should undergo** a complete physical examination, with special attention to the skin and oropharynx. Evaluation with a CBC count, a chest radiograph, urinalysis, and blood cultures is indicated. The initiation of empiric broad-spectrum antibiotics is reasonable in patients in whom the evaluation points to suspected bacteremia or sepsis.

VI. **Cytomegalovirus** is the **most important cause of transplant-associated infection.** Any of three clinical syndromes are commonly encountered during the immunosuppressive period 1–6 months posttransplantation. **Primary infection** may develop in previously uninfected recipients of grafts or blood products from a CMV-seropositive donor. This is usually the most serious syndrome. **Reactivation** can occur when a latently infected patient is unable to contain viral replication because of immunosuppression. **Reinfection** occurs when a different serotype of CMV is transmitted to a CMV-seropositive recipient [15].

   A. **Clinical illness** presents with fever and malaise. Some patients, especially with primary disease, may progress to pneumonitis, encephalitis, hepatitis, and other organ involvement. **Graft dysfunction may ensue** [16].

   B. **Laboratory studies usually show a leukopenia. Viral cultures of blood and urine should be obtained in all patients whose symptoms suggest CMV infection.** Recent studies suggest that antigenemia assays or the polymerase chain reaction (PCR) may be early indicators of CMV disease in transplant patients [7].

   C. Decisions regarding therapy are complex. Because the distinction between CMV infection and CMV disease is important, **infectious disease consultation** is recommended for the appropriate management of CMV syndromes.

   D. **Cytomegalovirus has indirect effects distinct from clinical infectious syndromes** [17].

      1. Cytomegalovirus enhances immunosuppression by depressing neutrophil function and suppressing T-cell activity. This may result in bacterial or opportunistic infections such as with *Pneumocystis, Nocardia,* and *Listeria* spp. [18].

      2. Cytomegalovirus mediates allograft injury, which is probably a form of rejection, in addition to CMV-accelerated atherosclerosis [16, 18].

      3. Malignancy may be induced [19].

VII. **Infection control** in solid-organ transplantation and BMT is complex and subject to frequent change.

   A. **Surgical prophylaxis** varies, but most centers employ a first-generation cephalosporin such as cefazolin prior to renal transplantation. In heart transplantation, cefuroxime often is used for a period of 24–48 hours. Liver transplantation may be preceded by selective bowel decontamination to reduce the carriage of gram-negative organisms and fungi [20]. Prophylaxis with an antipseudomonal cephalosporin and a ureidopenicillin is begun just prior to transplantation and continued for 5 days postoperatively. Concurrent fungal prophylaxis employs clotrimazole or nystatin [17, 21]. Trials with fluconazole prophylaxis in liver transplant recipients are under way.

   B. **Other infection control measures** should be considered.

      1. **A dental evaluation should be undertaken before transplantation** [21]. Due to the presence of a vascular graft, although objective data are not available, **we believe all solid-organ recipients should receive endocarditis prophylaxis for procedures likely to result in bacteremia.** (See Chap. 28B.) The authors would continue this practice for life.

      2. **Environmental exposures** should be minimized by strictly enforcing handwashing on the transplant unit and by isolating transplant recipients from patients and visitors with contagious diseases such as upper respiratory infections, chickenpox, and tuberculosis [17]. Decontaminating hot water supplies and filtering air may be necessary if *Legionella* or *Aspergillus* outbreaks occur. Furthermore, we advise our patients to avoid close contact with zoonotic vectors such as birds (chlamydia) and cats (toxoplasma), and we prohibit fresh floral arrangements in the hospital room or home. For the first 6 months posttransplantation, the patient is advised to wear a mask when exposure to crowds is anticipated. Travel can be fraught with problems for the transplant recipient, particularly if the destination is a developing country. Infectious disease consultation should be obtained well in advance of travel since pathogens, such as salmonella, may pose grave risk to the immunocompromised traveler.

      3. **Vaccination** against pneumococci [22] and, seasonally, influenza is recommended during the pretransplant evaluation. If the spleen is removed, we would also give *Haemophilus influenzae* B vaccine. It is unclear whether immunization offers protection or whether it can trigger rejection if given after transplantation. A live attenuated CMV vaccine shows promise for CMV-nega-

tive recipients of CMV-positive grafts [23]. Because BMT recipients acquire humoral immunity from the donor, vaccination of the donor may be useful [24].

4. **Antimicrobial prophylaxis** of opportunists is problematic. Isoniazid (INH) can be used for tuberculin reactors, but untoward side effects may outweigh benefits. **INH prophylaxis** is particularly indicated in those with a history of active tuberculosis, malnourished individuals, persons with an abnormal chest roentgenogram, converters of nonwhite background, and individuals with other immunocompromising conditions (i.e., diabetes mellitus, achlorhydria). With the increase of INH resistance, consideration may be given to prophylaxis with a fluoroquinolone. The use of prophylactic **TMP-SMX daily for 6 months after renal transplantation has been shown to reduce urinary tract infections** in patients free of anatomic abnormalities. This regimen also protects against *Pneumocystis, Listeria,* and *Nocardia* infections [25, 26]. Many programs use this regimen in heart and liver transplant recipients [27, 28]. Oral acyclovir decreases the frequency of **CMV infection** and disease in CMV-negative recipients of CMV-positive kidneys [29]. Studies looking at ganciclovir prophylaxis and preemptive therapy are promising [18, 30–32] and are discussed further later in this chapter. It is important that CMV-negative recipients of CMV-negative grafts receive CMV-negative blood products. BMT patients often receive oral TMP-SMX and nonabsorbable antibiotics such as vancomycin and neomycin. Additionally, most BMT patients receive oral acyclovir, 400–600 mg/day for 6 months for HSV prophylaxis [33, 34]. Prophylaxis with clotrimazole troche is especially important in liver transplant recipients but is widely used in most transplant patients.

   Antimicrobial prophylaxis in patients undergoing solid organ transplantation has recently been reviewed in detail [34a].

5. **In the transplant unit,** a coordinated effort is required by all health care personnel to minimize postoperative complications and hasten patient recovery. In general, salads and fresh fruits should be avoided to decrease gram-negative colonization. Intravenous lines and Foley catheters should be meticulously cared for and discontinued promptly, and patients should be mobilized as soon as possible. Infections with *Aspergillus* or *Legionella* spp. should prompt an epidemiologic investigation for a source of exposure. Finally, if possible, health care workers with respiratory infections should not care for transplant patients. If this is unavoidable, masks should be worn.

6. **Cytomegalovirus immunoglobulin** reduces the incidence and severity of CMV disease in CMV-negative recipients of CMV-positive renal transplants [35]. Furthermore, CMV-IgG has been shown to be cost-effective in this same patient population [21, 36]. Infectious disease consultation is necessary. **Seronegative patients who are exposed to varicella require prophylaxis with varicella-zoster immunoglobulin (VZIG),** which is available from regional blood banks. See related discussion in Chap. 4.

Infections in Renal Transplantation

It is clear from the analysis of infectious episodes in kidney and heart recipients that the practitioner often can predict the nature of responsible pathogens after considering the time interval from onset of immunosuppression. **During the first month after transplantation, the patient is most likely to experience a nosocomial infection, whereas the second interval (1–6 months) is marked by a predominance of opportunistic infections. After 6 months, if immunosuppression is reduced, community-acquired infections occur primarily [37] (Fig. 20-1). The evaluation of febrile episodes in any of these time periods is hampered by the difficulty encountered in differentiating between infection and rejection. The clinical presentations of these disparate processes are very similar and sometimes can be resolved only by biopsy of the transplanted kidney.** The difficulty in distinguishing infection from rejection requires early and continuous interaction of the infectious disease consultant with the transplant physician. Renal transplant patients differ from other transplant recipients in that immunosuppression may be discontinued in the face of overwhelming infection, thus sacrificing the organ and using dialysis as an alternative therapy. Infectious disease problems of the diabetic renal transplant recipient have recently been reviewed [37a].

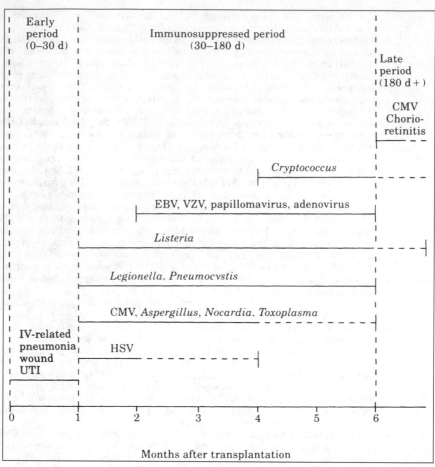

Fig. 20-1. Infection timetable. CMV = cytomegalovirus; EBV = Epstein-Barr virus; VZV = varicella-zoster virus; HSV = herpes simplex virus; UTI = urinary tract infection. (Modified from R. H. Rubin et al., Infection in the renal transplant recipient. *Am. J. Med.* 70:405, 1981.)

I. **Immediate posttransplantation period (first month).** Nosocomial infections must be considered whenever the patient develops a fever during hospitalization, and particularly during the immediate posttransplantation period. Because the net immunosuppression is still low, opportunistic infections occur only rarely in this interval, and their presence should prompt consideration of environmental exposure [38].

   A. **Nosocomial infections** predominate, with intravenous catheters, lung, wound, and urinary tract serving as the most common sites. These infections are frequent sources of fever in the patient with a prolonged postoperative hospitalization or an intensive care unit admission [38]. Other hospital-acquired infections include sinusitis, prostatitis, and disseminated *Candida* infections in patients receiving serial courses of antibiotics.

     1. **Specific syndromes of the early posttransplantation period**

       a. **Intravenous line infections** are common in both central and peripheral sites. Some experts suggest that all intravenous lines discontinued in a febrile transplant patient be quantitatively cultured. See Chap. 2 for a discussion of catheter-related sepsis.

       b. **Pneumonia may be difficult to distinguish from postoperative atelectasis, adult respiratory distress syndrome, hemorrhage, congestive heart failure, or emboli.** Pneumonia in this period is a complex nosocomial process, and the reader is referred to Chap. 9 for further discussion. Empiric therapy should be based on the clinical setting, sputum Gram stain, and local susceptibility patterns. If these studies do not suggest a specific pathogen, the authors would use piperacillin-tazobactam or a third-generation cephalosporin as initial therapy. (Therapy can be modified if cultures reveal a specific pathogen.) Nephrotoxic antibiotics and antibiotics that interact with immunosuppressive agents should be avoided when possible (see sec. **III** under Basic Principles).

c. The reduction of wound infection rates has been a major factor in the overall improvement in transplantation success [39]. **The development of a wound infection** is linked to technical complications that result in urine leaks from ureteral anastomoses, wound hematomas, or lymphoceles [26, 39]. The use of systemic intraoperative antibiotics and improved surgical techniques has decreased the incidence of wound infection to 1% [26]. Wound infections, usually caused by staphylococci or gram-negative organisms, may be difficult to recognize because the presentation is often atypical, the classic findings of incisional pain, erythema, and fever being either mild or absent. **A high index of suspicion and careful scrutiny of all wounds is necessary for early diagnosis.**

(1) When a wound infection is suspected, a Gram stain and culture should be performed on any wound drainage, and blood cultures should be obtained. A CBC count and a urinalysis with culture are indicated.

(2) Routine roentgenography to exclude soft tissue or perirenal gas, and sonography or CT scanning to seek extrarenal fluid should be considered. With most transplanted kidneys, a modest amount of fluid normally is detected by these means. Should no other source of infection be found, an attempt should be made to aspirate existing perirenal fluid collection under CT guidance for Gram stain and culture. Management may include surgical drainage and a 10- to 14-day course of antibiotics. A third-generation cephalosporin or piperacillin-tazobactam should be used empirically until Gram stain or culture results are available. A perinephric infection may involve the vascular anastomosis, and a nephrectomy may be necessary to cure infection or to prevent vascular anastomotic disruption. In early studies, up to 75% of deep infections required a nephrectomy for cure [38].

d. **Urinary tract infections.** Because of surgical manipulation resulting in anatomic alterations, the urinary tract is a prime site of infection and remains so for at least 90 days after transplantation [26]. When infected, an allograft serves as a potential source of life-threatening bacteremia. Infection usually originates with an indwelling catheter, and the organisms are hospital-acquired gram-negative rods.

(1) **Diagnosis.** The clinical presentation may be subtle—a mild febrile episode. In this setting, urinalysis usually will show WBCs and casts. **The importance of obtaining a urine Gram stain cannot be overemphasized as its results can guide therapy.** In the authors' opinion, asymptomatic bacteriuria should be treated for 10 days with oral antibiotics followed by repeat urinalysis and culture.

(2) **Therapy** for these early intrarenal processes should be continued for 4–6 weeks [40]. Intravenous antibiotics often are initiated; completion of therapy with TMP-SMX or a quinolone is reasonable.

Established *Candida* infections infrequently require systemic amphotericin B. Fluconazole is safe and effective for most *Candida* infections of the urinary tract. Significant interactions with cyclosporine are not seen. Search for surgically drainable foci should be undertaken.

(3) **Prophylaxis** of urinary tract infections with TMP-SMX is widely employed [25, 41] and is suggested unless contraindicated.

2. **Nosocomial infections less commonly seen**

a. **Sinusitis** related to nasogastric or nasotracheal tubes is best diagnosed by coronal head CT scans or a bedside Water's view of the sinuses. Oxymetazoline 0.5% and removal of the tube on the affected side may be sufficient therapy. Optimal management may require antral puncture or surgery. Febrile sinusitis should be treated with antibiotics that provide coverage for gram-negative rods as well as anaerobes. We believe piperacillin-tazobactam is a reasonable empiric choice.

b. **Prostatitis** can be precipitated by a Foley catheter, and pus may drain around the indwelling catheter. A rectal examination revealing a boggy, tender prostate is suggestive. Culture of expressed prostatic secretions may identify the involved pathogens. Trimethoprim-sulfamethoxazole is a reasonable empiric choice if cyclosporine levels are followed. Quinolones are an alternative in the sulfa-sensitive patient. In patients receiving quinolones and cyclosporine, we will monitor for nephrotoxicity [41a].

   c. **Disseminated fungal infections** are seen occasionally in patients with line sepsis, intense environmental exposure, or in association with prolonged antibiotic use [38]. Amphotericin B is the drug of choice unless cultures demonstrate that a less toxic alternative may be used.

B. **Reactivated prior infection**

   1. **Cytomegalovirus** often reactivates and usually produces a self-limited febrile illness with malaise and neutropenia. See sec. **VI** under Basic Principles.

   2. **Preexisting tuberculous** disease can disseminate, resulting in miliary disease.

   3. *Strongyloides stercoralis* infestation may evolve into a hyperinfection syndrome with pulmonary infiltrates and polymicrobial bacteremia. Pulmonary manifestations are protean, and mortality approaches 70% [8]. Treatment employs thiabendazole [42]. Screening of stool (five samples), sputum, and duodenal aspirate will identify larvae in 91% of these patients.

C. **Infections may also be transmitted by the allograft,** with pyelonephritis occasionally developing immediately after renal transplantation. The graft may have been seeded hematogenously or by retrograde spread prior to being harvested [43]. Organs from donors who are in the intensive care unit setting for more than 1 week pose the greatest risk. Contamination of the graft during preservation and handling may be more common than donor infection. Culture of the graft and perfusate can identify this potential source of infection. Kidney recipients with a culture-positive perfusate should receive 7–14 days of intravenous antibiotics [44]. Cytomegalovirus and, less commonly, tuberculosis, hepatitis, syphilis, and HIV have also been transmitted by renal allografts [44].

II. **Immunosuppressive period (1–6 months).** This is the interval of maximum immunosuppression. Due to diminished resistance, **infections may present in an unusual fashion and may be caused by exotic and unexpected pathogens.** These infections present the ultimate diagnostic challenge to the clinician and the laboratory. The net immunosuppression is further increased by both primary and reactivated CMV infection [19]. This viral immunomodulation predisposes both to infection and to tumorigenesis [19].

A. **Pulmonary infections mandate a rapid, organized approach** due to the array of potential pathogens. If such infections are diagnosed within 5 days of onset, approximately 80% of patients survive, whereas only 35% survive if diagnosis is delayed [45]. A typical approach is outlined in the following sections. See Chap. 9 for further details. Centers performing invasive pulmonary procedures on immunosuppressed patients should plan their diagnostic approach in an attempt to anticipate the pathogens that may be encountered. A coordinated approach by the pathology, pulmonary, and infectious disease services is necessary to produce a practical protocol. We have developed an "immunocompromised protocol" that encompasses appropriate studies for the diagnosis of pulmonary disease (Table 20-1). Patients with a rapidly deteriorating course should proceed directly to open lung biopsy if the diagnosis is unclear.

   1. **Clinical approach** to pulmonary infections

      a. **A history** should be obtained **and physical examination** shoud be performed, with particular attention to mode of onset, travel, serostatus of the donor and recipient with respect to CMV, EBV, HSV, and VZV, animal contacts, exposure to ill persons, compliance with prophylactic regimens, vaccination history, and receipt of blood products. The type and amount of immunosuppression should be reviewed, with emphasis on courses of pulse immunotherapy for rejection [11]. Recall that CMV infection predisposes to other infectious complications [19].

      b. **Sputum** should be obtained for Gram stain, routine culture, acid-fast stain and culture, *Legionella* culture, and modified acid-fast stain. Specimens may be either expectorated or induced. Expectorated sputum is subject to contamination with oral flora. Atypical pneumonias and opportunistic processes often present with a dry cough. Induced sputum is obtained via inhalation of a 10% saline and 10% glycerin solution for 10 minutes or until productive cough ensues. This technique improves identification of mycobacteria and fungi as well as *Pneumocystis* spp. Cultures should be

Table 20-1. Immunocompromised protocol: Studies done on biopsies of lung tissue

Gram stain and bacterial culture
Fungal culture
Acid-fast bacilli smear and culture
Nocardia smear and culture
Legionella smear and culture
Respiratory viral culture
Cytomegalovirus smear and culture
Smears for herpes simplex virus and adenovirus and, in the proper season, influenza virus, respiratory syncytial virus, and parainfluenza virus
Cytology
Gomori methenamine silver stain for *Pneumocystis carinii* pneumonia

monitored for 2 weeks to detect the delayed growth of *Nocardia*. Additionally, blood cultures, serial arterial blood gases or oximetry, and serial chest films are appropriate. A sputum Papanicolaou smear should be done to search for *Strongyloides*.

c. **Serum cryptococcal antigen and a *Legionella* urinary antigen should be obtained.**

d. **Initial empiric therapy** should be based on clinical setting and Gram stain. In most patients in this interval, the diagnosis will not be readily apparent, and initial therapy should be directed against bacterial pathogens while the laboratory studies are pending. The authors suggest piperacillin-tazobactam or a third-generation cephalosporin with vancomycin as a reasonable choice in this setting. For dosing, see Chap. 28.

e. **Bronchoscopy** can be helpful if a pathogen is not identified within **24–48 hours,** or earlier if the clinical course mandates. Bronchoscopy should include (when available) quantitative cultures obtained by protected catheter, bronchoalveolar lavage, and biopsy. When a protected catheter technique is used, 10^3 bacteria/ml suggests infection. (This approach is used enthusiastically in some centers, whereas others do not routinely employ it.) If these studies are unrevealing, open lung biopsy is indicated [46–48].

f. **Transthoracic needle aspiration** of discrete peripheral lesions or infiltrates can be attempted, especially if the lesions are cavitary. The small amount of tissue is a drawback, compared with an open lung biopsy, when attempting to diagnose a process that may be multifactorial (see Chap. 9).

g. **Immediately after bronchoscopy,** it is our practice to initiate coverage of gram-negative pathogens and staphylococci. For this, we would use a third-generation cephalosporin or piperacillin-tazobactam and vancomycin. Ciprofloxacin provides coverage for *Legionella,* probably without significant interference with cyclosporine levels. Also, although erythromycin use may be associated with elevation of cyclosporine levels, the dose of cyclosporine can be reduced and plasma levels followed (see Chap. 28M). Empiric therapeutic doses of TMP-SMX can be initiated if the patient has not received prophylaxis for *Pneumocystis* (see Chap. 24). Cyclosporine levels should be followed closely when TMP-SMX is used. Sputum for acid-fast bacilli (AFB) smear and culture should be collected postbronchoscopy as there may be an increased yield of mycobacteria after the procedure [49].

2. **The laboratory approach** to pulmonary infections is complex. Our suggestions are not all-inclusive, and the reader is referred to Chap. 9 for further related discussions. The specimens from bronchoscopy and open lung biopsy are valuable aids to diagnosis and must be handled meticulously (see Table 20-1).

a. **Protected brush technique** with quantitative cultures can be used to help differentiate upper airway colonization from lower respiratory infection [48].

b. **Bronchoalveolar lavage** fluid should be stained for *Pneumocystis* spp., fungi, and AFB. The value of direct fluorescent antibody reactive with *Legionella* spp. and viruses such as adenovirus, influenza,* parainfluenza,*

*Seasonal factors dictate testing for these agents. See discussions in Chaps. 7 and 8.

CMV, respiratory syncytial virus,* and HSV is under study and may be useful if available.

   c. **Biopsy tissue** should be stained with hematoxylin and eosin and examined for viral inclusions and granulomas. Tissue should also be cultured for viruses and *Mycobacterium tuberculosis* and stained by the immunoperoxidase technique should toxoplasma be suspected. (See Table 20-1 and Chap. 9.)

   d. **Open lung biopsy** is relatively safe and should not be delayed pending the outcome of noninvasive procedures in the critically ill patient. It is especially useful in the setting of diffuse pulmonary infiltrates. Lung tissue should be comprehensively studied as recommended in sec. **c** and in Chap. 9.

B. **Dermal infections** present a diagnostic challenge, as immunosuppression may modify the appearance of skin lesions. **Biopsy of the lesion is usually necessary for accurate diagnosis.** Lesions should be evaluated promptly because they may be a *forme fruste* of disseminated opportunistic infection at a time when systemic therapy can be successful [40].

   1. **Skin infections** may be similar to those seen in immunocompetent individuals.

      a. **Cellulitis due to staphylococci or streptococci** is frequent because of skin fragility resulting from chronic corticosteroid therapy. Treatment should be initiated with an antistaphylococcal penicillin or a first-generation cephalosporin (e.g., cefazolin). A portal of entry such as dermatophyte infection should be sought and measures to prevent recurrence initiated.

      b. **Cellulitis caused by unusual pathogens may occur.** Gram-negative bacteria, *Candida,* and cryptococci may be clinically indistinguishable from pyogenic cellulitis. **Biopsy with culture is indicated in patients who do not respond to antistaphylococcal therapy within 24–48 hours [38].** See Chap. 4.

   2. **Skin infections producing localized or mild infections in immunocompromised individuals.**

      a. **Herpes simplex viruses.** A major determinant of the incidence and severity of HSV infection is the type and intensity of immunosuppressive therapy. Lympholytic preparations (OKT3, ALG) are major promoters of HSV infection. Approximately one-half of kidney recipients will reactivate cutaneous lesions within 30–60 days after transplantation [38]. With lympholytic therapy, these infections may develop earlier.

         (1) **Herpes labialis** usually is caused by HSV type 1 and is exacerbated by the presence of endotracheal and nasogastric tubes. It may progress to involve the oral and esophageal mucosa and may mimic candidal esophagitis radiographically. The lesions often become superinfected with *Candida* [40]. Acyclovir is effective [21]. (See Chap. 26.)

         (2) **Anogenital lesions due to HSV type 2 are less common.** Lesions after transplantation may be typical vesicles or less characteristic ulcers. A Tzanck preparation is helpful diagnostically, as are viral cultures. There is a potential for secondary infection with GI flora and subsequent bacteremia. Treatment is oral acyclovir (see Chap. 26).

         (3) **Cutaneous dissemination of HSV,** or Kaposi's varicelliform eruption, presents with crops of grouped vesicles arising in separate sites. This is a result of autoinoculation and usually involves areas of prior trauma (burns, abrasions). Treatment is intravenous acyclovir (see Chap. 26).

      b. **Varicella-zoster virus**

         (1) **Reactivation of latent VZV** is dermatomal and occurs in 10% of renal transplant recipients; dissemination is a rare event. Immunosuppression need not be changed. Acyclovir enhances healing, and therapy is particularly indicated for ocular or otic disease and for patients with associated bowel or bladder dysfunction. With normal renal function, acyclovir, 12.5 mg/kg q8h, is indicated. Hospitalized patients should be strictly isolated until the lesions crust [21]. (See Chap. 26.)

         (2) **Primary VZV infection** (chickenpox) is uncommon in renal transplant patients because of prior exposure. When it occurs, hepatitis, pneumonitis, CNS infection, and disseminated intravascular coagulation can result. **Prophylaxis with VZIG is imperative for seronegative transplant patients exposed to VZV.** See Chap. 4 for a discussion of VZIG.

---

*Seasonal factors dictate testing for these agents. See discussions in Chaps. 7 and 8.

If infection occurs, acyclovir, 12.5 mg/kg IV q8h, should be initiated promptly (assuming normal renal function) [38]. Administration of VZIG will prolong the incubation period. (See Chap. 26.)

    c. Papillomavirus, the cause of warts, affects 40% of renal transplant patients and occasionally develops into extensive or disfiguring lesions [38]. Furthermore, malignant transformation of warts can occur in sun-exposed areas. Initial therapy is reduction of immunosuppression followed by cryosurgery. Dermatologic consultation is suggested.

3. Primary skin infections caused by opportunistic organisms usually are diagnosed by biopsy with histologic examination and routine, fungal, and mycobacterial cultures.

    a. Localized infections with atypical mycobacteria, fungi, and even algae can be encountered.

    b. Systemic spread can follow cutaneous infection with *Candida* and the zygomycetes. The lung and GI tract are the usual portals of entry for *Aspergillus* and *Candida* organisms, respectively. The zygomycetes have been introduced by trauma from dressings or intravenous line placement; therefore, care should be taken to protect the skin of the transplant recipient.

4. Disseminated skin Infection may originate from a noncutaneous source, heralding a systemic infection that requires timely systemic therapy. *Nocardia, Cryptococcus,* and *Candida* are noted for this. In 25% of patients with cryptococcosis, dermal lesions appear weeks to months prior to the development of CNS disease. Disseminated candidal infections will present with skin lesions in 15% of patients [38]. *Nocardia* is noted for the concurrence of dermal and lung lesions. Atypical skin lesions should be biopsied (see Chap. 18).

C. Central nervous system infections

1. Meningoencephalitis and brain abscess are the most frequent CNS infections and present in a subacute fashion. Causative organisms include *Aspergillus, Toxoplasma, Nocardia,* and viruses. **See related discussions in Chap. 5.**

    a. *Aspergillus* is most common and usually originates from a pulmonary focus. Patients present with mental status changes that progress to obtundation and death. Occasionally, patients present with focal neurologic findings. **The diagnosis should be suspected in any patient with sinus or pulmonary aspergillosis and changing neurologic status.** Because head CT may be nondiagnostic, **MRI may be preferable.** Cerebrospinal fluid analysis is of minimal utility, but a direct needle aspirate of the lesions evaluated by KOH preparation and culture may be helpful [50]. Amphotericin B is the drug of choice. Most cases end fatally, probably because the infection is widely disseminated by the time CNS involvement is diagnosed and because of the poor penetration of amphotericin B across the blood-brain barrier. There have been anecdotal reports of improved response with the addition of rifampin or itraconazole to amphotericin B [51]. See Chap. 18.

    b. *Toxoplasma gondii* is an uncommon cause of CNS disease in kidney recipients. The initial presentation usually is altered mental status, and CT scanning may demonstrate single or multiple enhancing lesions. A stereotactic biopsy is useful for diagnosis but may not be technically feasible. Sulfisoxazole and pyrimethamine are the agents of choice [50]. Clindamycin may be substituted for the sulfonamide in the sulfa-allergic patient. See Chaps. 5 and 17.

    c. Nocardiosis. See sec. II.A.2 under Infections in Heart Transplantation.

2. Meningitis is another common presentation of CNS infection during this period. Patients may complain of headache, lethargy, or fever, or may demonstrate meningismus. The organism responsible for **acute meningitis usually is *Listeria*, whereas *cryptococcus* and *coccidioides* present in a subacute fashion.** Meningitis often occurs after treatment for rejection, regardless of the time that has elapsed since transplantation [47]. Cerebrospinal fluid analysis is helpful in making the diagnosis, using a cryptococcal antigen assay and India ink to identify cryptococci, and Gram stain and culture to identify *Listeria* and other bacteria [52]. CT scanning often is normal. Treatment includes ampicillin with an aminoglycoside for *Listeria;* the penicillin-allergic patient should receive intravenous TMP-SMX. Fluconazole may prove to be the drug of choice for treatment of cryptococcosis in the transplant recipient in whom interactions with cyclosporine are a primary concern [52, 52a]. It also may have a role in the treatment of coccidioidomycosis; however, amphotericin B administered systemically or, in refractory cases, intrathecally remains the standard of care [53–55]. Most patients respond to therapy. If possible, immunosuppression should be decreased.

   3. **Rhinocerebral phycomycoses** due to *Mucor* and *Rhizopus* are encountered only rarely in renal transplant recipients even during the height of immunosuppression. Physical examination reveals periorbital swelling, cranial nerve palsies, and necrosis of the nasal turbinates. Biopsy with histologic examination demonstrating hyphal elements is diagnostic. Amphotericin B is adjunctive to surgical resection, which must endeavor to remove all infected tissue.

D. **Urinary tract infections** in this period parallel those seen in the immediate post-transplantation period (see sec. **I.A.1.d**).

E. **Gastrointestinal complaints in the renal transplant recipient warrant aggressive diagnostic evaluation, because the severity of illness can be masked by immunosuppression.** See related discussions in Chap. 11.

   1. **Viral infections are common.**
      a. Stomatitis or esophagitis usually is caused by concurrent HSV and *Candida*. In stomatitis, the diagnosis is made clinically, but esophagitis requires endoscopy with biopsy and culture. Treatment of HSV esophagitis is intravenous acyclovir, whereas oral or intravenous fluconazole is used for candidal esophagitis [53].
      b. **Gastrointestinal ulceration** and bleeding may be caused by CMV. Diagnosis requires endoscopy with biopsy and viral culture. Treatment employs ganciclovir [56] (see Chap. 26).

   2. **Bacterial infections are less commonly seen.**
      a. **Acute gastroenteritis** usually is caused by the same pathogens that cause disease in immunocompetent patients.
      b. **Hemorrhagic diarrhea** can be seen with *M. tuberculosis* infection, CMV, pseudomembranous colitis, posttransplantation lymphoproliferative disorder, diverticulitis, or *Campylobacter* or *Salmonella* infection. *Salmonella* is discussed in sec. **III.E.**
      c. **Intraabdominal abscess** can be diagnosed with ultrasonography or CT scanning. Abscesses are associated with chronic steroid therapy, which leads to perforation, abscess formation, and bacteremia. Perforation may occur at any weak area of the bowel.

   3. **Diverticulitis** caused by chronic constipation is seen in patients given long-term phosphate-binding antacids. The physician benefits from awareness of diverticulosis before transplantation as classic signs of peritonitis frequently are absent in the immunosuppressed patient. Diverticulitis should be suspected in any patient with abdominal pain or change in bowel habits. Surgical evaluation, CT scanning, or a water-soluble contrast enema may be helpful (see Chap. 11).

   4. **Cholecystitis** may be calculous or acalculous. In acalculous cholecystitis, dehydration is a contributing factor. **Corticosteroids can mask the manifestations of cholecystitis** [40].

F. **Fever of uncertain origin** in this period often is caused by CMV (see sec. **VI** under Basic Principles). A search for hepatic, neurologic, and GI disease is indicated, and a low threshold for biopsy of the involved organ with routine AFB smear, viral culture, and histology is necessary. Neutropenia, which can accompany CMV infection, may necessitate decreasing the dose of azathioprine. In the authors' experience, CMV infection contributes profoundly to the net immunosuppressive effect. A CMV-infected patient should be observed for the development of other opportunistic infections or malignancies.

III. **The late period (> 6 months) is characterized by community-acquired infections** in patients who are successfully grafted. Patients chronically infected with CMV and hepatitis viruses and those with ongoing rejection remain at risk for opportunistic disease.

A. **Late pulmonary infections**
   1. *M. tuberculosis* **and atypical mycobacterial infections** may exhibit unusual presentations in these patients, and a prior history of exposure or a reactive PPD may be difficult to obtain. Accordingly, a **high index of suspicion** must be maintained when evaluating a patient who develops late pulmonary infiltrates.

Acid-fast stains of sputum can be negative, and bronchoscopy may be necessary to obtain adequate specimens. Optimal treatment for susceptible *M. tuberculosis* infection and atypical mycobacteriosis remains controversial. Though a 9-month course of INH and rifampin may be sufficient, the immunocompromised patient may require an additional 9 months of therapy [21]. See Chap. 9.

Greater controversy surrounds the treatment of multiply resistant tuberculosis. Consideration of this possibility must be made when evaluating individuals exposed to tuberculosis. Resistant and atypical mycobacterial infections require individualized therapy based on the results of susceptibility testing; infectious disease consultation is suggested (see Chap. 9). Lung resection is an alternative in patients with localized pulmonary involvement caused by atypical mycobacteria [21].

2. **Fungal infection** with *Histoplasma, Coccidioides,* and *Cryptococcus* spp. can present without obvious pulmonary involvement. Histoplasmosis and coccidioidomycosis generally are encountered in endemic areas, whereas cryptococcosis occurs throughout the United States. Sputum can be cultured for these fungi (the laboratory will need to be alerted), and growth should be assumed to represent invasive disease. Ideally, tissue should be examined histologically to diagnose invasive disease. For treatment of cryptococcosis, fluconazole is used. Histoplasmosis and blastomycosis respond to itraconazole, which exhibits 90% efficacy [55] (see Chap. 18).

3. **Pneumococcal and *H. influenzae*** pretransplantation vaccination is important. See sec. **VII.B.3** under Basic Principles.

B. **Dermal infections.** See sec. **II.B.**

C. **Central nervous system infection.** If the patient has experienced continued rejection or persistent viral infection, see sec. **II.C.** In the patient requiring low-dose immunosuppression, routine bacterial pathogens and cryptococci should be suspected.

D. **Urinary tract infections.** During this period, urinary tract infections usually are benign, and the incidence of such infections has decreased with the prophylactic use of TMP-SMX. **Low-dose quinolones** are effective and relatively safe in the transplant patient. Bacteremic pyelonephritis during this time frame suggests an anatomic abnormality and warrants urologic evaluation [38].

E. **Gastrointestinal infections**

1. **Chronic hepatitis** caused by HBV, HCV, and hepatitis delta (HDV) viruses is a leading cause of morbidity and mortality in patients with functioning renal allografts who survive 10 years. Hepatocellular injury is cytopathic in HBV and primarily immune-mediated in HCV. Interferon is a difficult drug to use in transplant recipients as it has an immunostimulatory effect [56a]. The long-term effects of posttransplantation HCV infection remain to be seen [57]. A recent study by Pereira et al. demonstrated that the risk of liver disease was increased in recipients of HCV-positive organs. However, they found no difference in the rate of graft loss or mortality during a 3.5 year follow-up period [57a]. Interestingly, HCV exerts an immunomodulating effect in patients during the first year after transplantation, and allograft survival at 1 year is significantly greater in these patients. The infection rate also is greater in the first year. Unfortunately, serum transaminase levels correlate poorly with disease activity in HCV disease. Boletis et al. established that liver biopsy is required to determine the severity of disease, prognosis, and response to treatment [57b]. Cirrhosis may ensue [38].

2. *Salmonella* **infections** may result in metastatic infection or bowel perforation. **Any patient with *Salmonella* gastroenteritis should receive a course of appropriate oral antibiotic therapy** (see Chap. 11).

F. **Visual field defects.** These are a common manifestation of CMV retinitis. The patient may be asymptomatic; a thorough history is helpful. The clinical course evolves over weeks. Ganciclovir, 5 mg/kg q12h for 2 weeks, will halt disease progression, but patients may relapse [52]. See Chaps. 19 and 26 for related discussions. Ophthalmologic consultation is imperative. Toxoplasmosis presents similarly but is very uncommon.

G. **Epstein-Barr virus (EBV)** is associated with a spectrum of B-cell lymphoproliferative diseases that infrequently develop following organ transplantation. These have recently been reviewed [57c].

Infections in Heart Transplantation

There is substantial concordance in the immunosuppression used and resultant problems encountered when comparing cardiac and renal transplantation. Despite many similarities, however, prevention of rejection is the top priority in heart transplant recipients, as retransplantation is risky and expensive. The 1-year survival rate for repeat cardiac transplantation is approximately 55% [58]. The aggressive use of immunosuppression increases the incidence and severity of infection in the heart transplant patient [41]. Other factors that affect the incidence of infection include age, compliance, and the etiology of the underlying heart disease. Patients who receive transplants for ischemic disease tend to experience more infections than those who receive transplants for other reasons, but this may be related to their older mean age [59]. Infection in heart transplant recipients has been recently reviewed [59a].

I. **Immediate posttransplantation period (first month).** The infectious complications encountered during this period are the same as those in renal transplant recipients with the exception of surgical wound infections [60].

   A. **Nosocomial infections** are a common cause of fever in this time period.

      1. **Intravenous catheter** infections should be managed as for renal transplant recipients. The avoidance of bacteremia is paramount because of the vascular anastomoses (see Chap. 2). Lines should be changed every 72 hours, and pacer wires should be removed promptly. No line should be left in place without clear indication.

      2. Refer to sec. **I.A** under Infections in Renal Transplantation and Chap. 9 for the presentation, diagnosis, and treatment of **pneumonia.**

      3. **Surgical wound** infections are uncommon, but potential progression of infection into the mediastinum makes this a grave complication. Responsible organisms include coagulase-positive and -negative staphylococci, and *Enterobacter, Serratia,* and *Pseudomonas* spp. Diagnosis is made by Gram stain and culture of the wound. Sternotomy infections require debridement and systemic antibiotics [38]. When deep infection is suspected, a needle aspirate or bone biopsy is important.

      4. **Urinary tract** infections (UTI) are less common than in renal transplant recipients and are managed as would be any nosocomial urinary tract infection. Prophylaxis with TMP-SMX for *Pneumocystis carinii* pneumonia (PCP) also reduces the incidence of these infections in this group (see Chap. 12).

      5. **Pleural effusions** might occur postoperatively. In an asymptomatic patient, these may be observed, but if infection is suspected, a diagnostic thoracentesis is indicated.

   B. **Reactivation of prior infection can occur.** Refer to sec. **I.B** under Infections in Renal Transplantation.

   C. **Various infections may be transmitted by allograft;** among these are CMV, EBV, HBV, HCV and, rarely, toxoplasmosis. Transplantation of a *Toxoplasma*-seropositive heart into a seronegative patient should prompt consideration of a 6-month course of sulfisoxazole and pyrimethamine prophylaxis. Prevention of CMV transmission by avoiding transplantation of seropositive hearts into seronegative patients is ideal but not always practical. Some programs, extrapolating from renal experience, use CMV hyperimmunoglobulin (CMV-IgG) in an attempt to ameliorate the potentially severe primary infection syndrome [62]. Most centers give high-dose oral acyclovir to both seropositive and seronegative recipients of CMV-positive grafts to reduce the incidence of CMV disease [29, 63]. Prophylaxis regimens combining antiviral drugs and immunoglobulin seem to be more effective than use of either agent alone [63a, 63b]. Hibberd and colleagues recently published their experience administering ganciclovir, 2.5 mg/kg IV daily, during anti-lymphocyte therapy. They found that the incidence of CMV disease was reduced by 52% in patients who received "preemptive" ganciclovir [63c].

II. **Immunosuppressive period (1–6 months).** As in renal transplantation, this is the interval of maximum immunosuppression. Here opportunistic infections surpass hospital-acquired infections as the most common causes of fever. Again, the processes encountered are similar in nature but often more severe than those seen in renal transplant patients. There seems to be an increased number of *Legionella* and *Nocardia* infections in heart transplant recipients. With the use of TMP-SMX prophylaxis, the incidence of *Nocardia* has diminished.

A. Pulmonary infections constitute the most commonly encountered infectious process and are similar to those encountered in renal transplant patients (see sec. II.A under Infections in Renal Transplantation) [64].

   1. Legionellosis occurs with significant environmental and geographic variability in heart recipients. (See related discussion in Chap. 9.)

      a. Legionellosis usually presents as a patchy, interstitial pneumonia that progresses to an alveolar infiltrate. However, any picture may appear, and even cavitation may occur [38].

      b. *Legionella* is difficult to isolate from sputum, and it often is necessary to use bronchoscopy with culture, direct fluorescent antibody (DFA) studies, and histologic examination [65]. An indirect fluorescent antibody (IFA) study is available for serum, but a rise in titer may be delayed. An isolated titer of 1:256 or greater is presumptive evidence of legionellosis [66], whereas paired sera reflecting a fourfold rise are diagnostic. Detection of urinary antigen can be done within 1 day of the onset of symptoms, with good sensitivity and specificity [66]. Histologic examination usually reveals a bronchopneumonia.

      c. Treatment should be started empirically because of the difficulty in confirming the diagnosis. Erythromycin, 4–6 g/day IV, should be given for at least 1 week, though 2 weeks is preferable. Reversible hearing loss may occur at this dosage. Oral erythromycin therapy should then be used at 2 g/day for at least 2 more weeks. Late relapse can occur. Rifampin, 600 mg PO bid may be added in severe or refractory cases [67]. Cyclosporine levels should be followed closely during the treatment course. It appears that the new macrolide agents, azithromycin and clarithromycin, will be useful in the treatment of *Legionella* infections. In particular, clarithromycin, 500 mg bid, is useful in the patient who cannot tolerate oral erythromycin. These drugs demonstrate minimal interaction with cyclosporine.

   2. Nocardiosis is seen in heart transplant recipients.

      a. The incidence of *Nocardia* infections has decreased since the institution of TMP-SMX prophylaxis for PCP. Most patients have symptomatic lung disease. Although x-ray findings are variable, **the concurrence of skin lesions and a pulmonary infiltrate strongly suggests nocardiosis or cryptococcosis.** See related discussion in Chap. 18.

      b. Diagnosis often requires invasive procedures to obtain tissue for culture and histologic examination. Sputum cultures have a yield of only 30% [61]. In sputum or lung tissue, the finding of acid-fast, gram-positive, filamentous bacteria suggests nocardiosis, but culture is necessary for confirmation. All patients with nocardiosis should undergo head CT scanning or MRI to exclude intracranial disease.

      c. The drug of choice is a sulfonamide (e.g., sulfadiazine, 2 g PO q6h) for 3–6 months (see Chaps. 18 and 28K). Serum levels ideally should be monitored, with peak levels adjusted to 12–15 mg/dl. Sulfadiazine at this dose may crystallize in the renal tubules, resulting in acute renal failure. Sodium bicarbonate (or sodium citrate and citric acid [Bicitra]) should be used to maintain the urine pH at greater than 7, which increases the solubility of the sulfonamide.

        In patients allergic to sulfonamides, various combinations of amikacin, minocycline, ceftriaxone, and imipenem have been used with success [68, 69]. Duration of therapy has not been well defined. Infectious disease consultation is advised.

B. Dermal infections. See sec. II.B under Infections in Renal Transplantation.

C. Central nervous system infections. See sec. II.C under Infections in Renal Transplantation.

D. Urinary tract infections. See sec. II.D under Infections in Renal Transplantation.

E. Gastrointestinal infections. See sec. II.E under Infections in Renal Transplantation.

F. Posttransplantation lymphoproliferative disorders (PTLD) are recognized with greater frequency as we gain experience with immunosuppressive agents. **Most** PTLDs are of B-lymphocyte origin and have been shown to be **initiated by EBV infection** [70, 71]. Approximately 90% of the adult population in the United States is seropositive for EBV. This virus may cause primary infection when a seronegative recipient is given a seropositive graft, or reactivation of the host's latent virus may occur [72]. Clinical presentation may mimic CMV with fever, malaise, and leukopenia. Examination may reveal adenopathy or splenomegaly. Involvement of the GI tract, lungs, CNS, or the graft itself are typical presentations [72, 73]. **Early diagnosis is essential as the syndrome may be reversible in the early stages.** If diagnosis is delayed, progression to malignancy occurs. Those at risk for developing PTLD include a seronegative recipient of a seropositive graft, patients receiving antilymphocyte globulin therapy or cyclosporine, recipients of nonrenal grafts [74], and patients with other infections, particularly CMV [73].

Treatment has met with only limited success and initially involves minimizing immunosuppressive regimens and administering antiviral agents—high-dose acyclovir or ganciclovir. Localized symptomatic lesions may be removed surgically; chemotherapy and radiation therapy are reserved for those with systemic involvement who fail to respond to initial treatment. Research into the prevention and treatment of PTLD is a growing field.

G. **Fever of uncertain origin.** See sec. II.F under Infections in Renal Transplantation.

III. **Late period (> 6 months).** The infectious problems encountered in this period are similar to those seen in renal transplant patients. See sec. III under Infections in Renal Transplantation.

Infections in Liver Transplantation

Infection is the most important determinant of morbidity and mortality following orthotopic liver transplantation (OLT) [75, 75a]. Unfortunately, the **diagnosis of infection in the OLT recipient is difficult because of the clinical similarities between infection and rejection** and because of the problem in differentiating between colonization and tissue invasion. Other factors contribute to this confusion. Bacterial infections tend to occur during treatment of rejection episodes, and devitalized liver tissue is a haven for bacteria. Infections or the agents used to treat them may contribute to hepatic dysfunction. Furthermore, liver biopsy results may be altered by infection, making the histologic differentiation between rejection and infection difficult [76].

I. **Noninfectious complications of transplantation that may be confused with infection**
  A. **Rejection** may be acute or chronic.
    1. **Acute rejection** crisis is the most common cause of graft dysfunction and typically occurs on approximately the fifth day after transplantation.
      a. **Symptoms and signs** of malaise, anorexia, abdominal discomfort, fever, increased organ size, or clear bile are present in rejection [75].
      b. **Laboratory abnormalities** (e.g., rapidly rising liver function enzymes, especially bilirubin, and increased prothrombin time) occur [75].
      c. **Radionuclide scans** (HIDA) of the liver will show decreased uptake and excretion not only in rejection but also in ischemic, obstructive, viral, drug, and septic complications. **Liver biopsy remains the most valuable diagnostic tool** to evaluate rejection but may be dangerous because of preexisting coagulopathy or neovascularization of the implanted liver [75]. Ultrasound examination in conjunction with HIDA scan can help distinguish among tumor, biloma, abscess, and hepatic infarction.
      d. **Treatment** of acute rejection requires pulse immunosuppression, which can potentiate infectious complications.
      e. **The prognosis** of rejection is guarded; children fare better than adults. Acute rejection is responsible for 20% of all posttransplantation deaths in OLT [75].
    2. **Chronic rejection** targeting the intrahepatic ducts is an ongoing process and may result in a "vanishing bile duct syndrome" at any time after transplantation [75]. Retransplantation is required in approximately 20% of OLT recipients due to chronic rejection; survival rates average 50% [77, 78].
      a. **Jaundice** is the hallmark of chronic rejection, whereas increasing SGOT and SGPT are less specific. These abnormalities reflect the obliteration of bile ducts during the rejection process.
      b. **The pharmacologic treatment** of this vanishing bile duct syndrome has been disappointing, and retransplantation is often necessary [75].
  B. **Hepatic dysfunction** can occur with viral or bacterial infection. Viral infection with CMV is most common and liver biopsy will establish CMV infection if present; other diagnostic approaches have recently been reviewed [78a]. Less commonly, bacteremia, an intraabdominal abscess, or pneumonia can produce a hyperbilirubi-

nemia, usually in association with an elevated alkaline phosphatase and minimally elevated transaminases [75]. This often is referred to as *cholestatic jaundice*. Hepatotoxic drugs and technical problems such as biliary leak or stricture, bleeding, or hepatic artery thrombosis may simulate infection or rejection [79, 80].

II. **Infection complicates liver transplantation in 80% of recipients.** Many liver transplant recipients will experience infection with more than one organism, and some will experience multiple episodes of infection. Risk factors for infection include postoperative dialysis, age over 20 years, GI or vascular complications, an intensive care unit stay of more than 15 days, and low serum albumin preoperatively [76]. Mortality due to infection runs between 20 and 30% [81]. In OLT, the timing of specific infections is less predictable because the transplanted graft is an "immunologic" organ. Furthermore, the incidence of surgical complications due to the technical difficulty of the procedure is high. **All patients with fever of unclear origin should have a CT scan or ultrasonogram of the liver to rule out abscess formation as well as ductal dilatation. Additionally, because the biliary tree is colonized soon after surgery, antibiotic prophylaxis is essential before biopsy or cholangiogram and should be continued for 48 hours.**

A. **The immediate posttransplantation period (first month)** is marked by rejection with superimposed infection involving the biliary and vascular anastomoses. The difference in infection rates between liver and kidney transplantation can be directly attributed to the technical complexity of the surgery. As a general rule, any procedural problem involving the biliary or vascular anastomoses will result in severe secondary infection.

   1. **Nosocomial infections** are similar to those in renal transplant patients. Differences in the surgical sites and the duration of intubation account for the increased incidence of nosocomial infection in liver transplant patients.

   2. **Procedure-related infections** commonly are encountered due to technical complexity and occur at the sites of vascular and enterobiliary anastomoses. The risk of infection increases with the duration of surgery and the number of prior operations [82].

      a. **Vascular anastomoses can become infected** or undergo thrombosis, especially in children, during the first posttransplantation week. This results in hepatic gangrene with secondary abscess formation. Bacteremias have arisen from hepatic or portal vein thrombosis as well. The clinical onset often is heralded by an isolated episode of fever, although these patients may present with ascites or an increase in liver function tests [75].

      b. **Biliary anastomoses** may leak, become obstructed, or become infected by the adjacent GI flora. The normal flora will not cause clinical infection unless leaks or an obstruction is present. The manifestations are variable and may include cholangitis, liver abscess, or bacteremia [75]. Infection is readily confused with rejection. Postoperative ileus may lead to increased pressure on biliary anastomoses, with subsequent biliary leak and infection [81].

   3. **Invasive candidiasis** arising from the upper small bowel can occur in up to 44% of patients [83]. The donor should undergo decontamination of the small bowel, and the recipient should receive prophylaxis as well. Selective bowel decontamination of recipients seems to lower the incidence of gram-negative and candidal infections in the early postoperative period [84]. Clotrimazole, 10-mg troche 3 times daily dissolved in the mouth, often is given to reduce candidal colonization.

B. **Infection after 30 days** more typically mirrors the processes seen in patients receiving heart or kidney transplants. Mortality is lower than in patients who develop infectious complications during the immediate posttransplantation period [38]. However, the infections are more diverse and reflect prolonged immunosuppression.

   1. **Nosocomial infections** can occur in any hospitalized transplant patient. See sec. **I.A** under Infections in Renal Transplantation.

   2. **Opportunistic infections** are seen in this period and decrease only when immunosuppression is decreased. See sec. **II.A** under Infections in Renal Transplantation.

      a. **Cytomegalovirus infection** may cause mild persistent hepatic dysfunction. In these patients, viral infection can be distinguished from rejection only by biopsy with **histology and viral culture.** Prevention of CMV disease following liver transplantation remains an area of controversy. Singh et al. have found that oral acyclovir is ineffective prophylaxis against CMV in liver transplant recipients and recommend short course preemptive ganciclovir for patients who shed CMV [84a]. Winston's group at the University of California at Los Angeles confirmed the superiority of ganciclovir over acyclovir in liver transplant patients [84b]. See sec. **VI** under Basic Principles and sec. **II** under Infections in Renal Transplantation.

b. **Hepatitis B** can significantly affect graft survival. There is a high rate of recurrence of HBV following OLT, with progression to chronic active hepatitis or fibrosing cholestatic hepatitis. The pathophysiology of fibrosing cholestatic hepatitis is unclear but seems to be related to HBV surface antigen levels; rapid progression to graft failure is the outcome. These patients have more infectious complications and probably a greater risk of hepatic neoplasm if HBV recurs [75].

c. **Hepatitis C.** The implications of HCV infection in the patient who has received a liver transplant are unclear and are undergoing serial assessment. The rate of recurrence of HCV after transplantation is 95–100%. Liver damage is seen in nearly 44% of these patients. However, the long-term consequences of HCV remain to be seen. Interferon-alpha, while demonstrating some success against HCV infection in normal hosts, seems to benefit few OLT patients with HCV [57]. However, a recent study by Thiel et al. revealed that 83% of patients with recurrence of HCV after liver transplantation responded to IFN-gamma therapy and that rejection occurring in the setting of IFN-gamma is no more difficult to treat than rejection in patients who are not receiving IFN-gamma [84c].

C. **In the late period (> 6 months),** opportunistic infections diminish in frequency. The transition from illness caused by opportunistic disease to community-acquired infection is less clear in the liver transplant recipient than in other solid-organ recipients.

Infections in Pancreatic Transplantation

Only a small number of medical centers are performing pancreatic transplantation, and the topic therefore will not be discussed further. A review of infectious complications following pancreatic transplantation has been published recently [84d].

Bone Marrow Transplantation

Bone marrow transplantation differs significantly from solid-organ transplantation. In BMT patients, HLA typing is closely observed; the immunosuppression is profound; and the **possibility of graft-versus-host disease (GVHD) exists.** Furthermore, many marrow recipients have previously undergone therapy for leukemia or have suffered the complications of aplastic anemia, with its attendant infections and blood product requirements. Other differences are the absence of a surgical wound and the presence of an initial period of complete immunosuppression lasting approximately 30 days. The absolute leukopenia as well as the absence of cell-mediated immunity make predictions about putative infectious agents difficult.

I. **Basic principles**

A. **Donor selection**

1. The marrow donor is **ideally an HLA-identical sibling.** The chance of identifying such a donor from among siblings is 25%. The use of partially matched family member donors and closely matched, unrelated donors is becoming more common [85]. It is preferable that the donor and recipient be matched at the HLA–A, -B, and -DR locus of the major histocompatibility complex and necessary that their mixed lymphocyte cultures indicate mutual nonreactivity.

2. **Donors** should be screened for syphilis, CMV, HSV, HIV, HCV, and HBV. Cardiac and pulmonary status must be evaluated if general anesthesia will be used for marrow harvest.

B. **Recipient selection.** Bone marrow transplantation can be employed to treat leukemia, lymphoma, multiple myeloma, aplastic anemia, sickle cell disease, severe combined immunodeficiency, and enzyme deficiencies. Common to all these disorders is an immunologic deficiency that predisposes to infection even prior to marrow irradiation and immunosuppression therapy. Research into BMT treatment of solid-organ tumors is ongoing, with special promise in the management of breast carcinomas.

C. **Immunosuppressive therapy.** Before BMT, patients receive an immunosuppressive regimen that allows donor marrow engraftment and ablates existing disease. Most regimens use chemotherapy, with the addition of total body irradiation for those with malignancy [86–88]. A variety of immunosuppressive agents—including methotrexate (MTX), cyclosporine, ATG, corticosteroids, and pretreatment of donor marrow with monoclonal antibody or lectins to remove T cells—have been employed after BMT in an attempt to prevent GVHD [89]. Patients receiving autologous transplants do not require posttransplantation immunosuppression; neither do those with severe combined immunodeficiency as their underlying illness precludes GVHD.

D. **Fever. Fever is the hallmark of infection** after BMT and almost invariably complicates the early neutropenic period. In BMT as in the leukopenic patient (Chap. 2), fever may be the only sign of infection because the normal inflammatory response is absent [90]. Noninfectious causes of fever—transfusion, embolism, deep hemorrhage, or drugs—may occur.

E. **Infection control**
   1. **Protective environment.** Whereas it is generally accepted that patient hygiene and fastidious hand-washing by staff and visitors is beneficial in infection control, there is controversy regarding the value of laminar air flow (LAF) rooms and nonabsorbable antibiotics. Although LAF decreases the incidence of GVHD and serious bacterial and fungal infections, survival is not necessarily improved, because death resulting from these infections has become less common [91].
   2. **Antibiotic prophylaxis.** Daily prophylaxis with one TMP-SMX double-strength tablet is useful when managing chronic GVHD because of the high incidence of bacterial infections [85]. This also decreases the frequency of PCP [24]. Prophylactic fluconazole, 400 mg/day PO, reduces the incidence of superficial and systemic fungal infections in BMT patients [92].
   3. **Cytomegalovirus prophylaxis** with CMV-IgG should be considered if seropositive tissue is transplanted into a seronegative recipient. However, the risk of CMV disease is greatest in the seropositive recipient: Studies looking at ganciclovir prophylaxis or preemptive therapy are under way and demonstrate a trend toward reduced severity of CMV disease [93–94a].

II. **Infections in BMT** have been recently reviewed [94b].
   A. **The early period (0–21 days after BMT)** is characterized by **neutropenia and lymphopenia.** Chemoradiation therapies leading to mucositis and the use of central venous and Foley catheters contribute to the breakdown of normal anatomic barriers, thereby increasing the chance of infection. Infections of this period are predominantly nosocomial. Herpes simplex virus reactivation occurs at this time [95].
      1. **Bacteremia** with sepsis is the most common infection of this period. The organisms vary but are commonly coagulase-negative staphylococci or gram-negative Enterobacteriaceae. Clinically, patients are febrile and appear septic. Blood cultures, though often negative, should be obtained and a beta-lactam antibiotic (e.g., piperacillin or ceftazidime) and an aminoglycoside should be administered empirically (see Chap. 2). Although the incidence of gram-positive infections in neutropenic patients is rising, most authorities believe that vancomycin can be added if fever persists despite gram-negative coverage [96]. Antibiotics should be continued at least until the patient's neutrophil count rises to 500/mm^3. Treatment may be abbreviated if the patient remains afebrile and clinically stable for more than 1 week and has a neutrophil count of greater than 200/mm^3 and if cultures remain negative. With proven infection, treatment duration after neutrophil recovery should follow standard practice. For indwelling catheter infections, see Chap. 12.
      2. **Fungal infections must be suspected if fever persists despite broad-spectrum antibiotic treatment.** *Candida* is most often implicated [96a], and occasionally molds, such as *Aspergillus,* are encountered. The incidence of these infections is related to the duration of neutropenia following BMT. Patients with suspected fungal infection should have stool, urine, blood, and sputum cultures, biopsy of skin lesions, and retinal examination for fungal endophthalmitis. Radiographic imaging of the chest and sinuses may demonstrate otherwise occult fungal

infections. In neutropenic patients with fever unresponsive to antibacterial therapy, and in patients with positive fungal blood cultures, a course of antifungal therapy is warranted [97]. (See Chaps. 2 and 18.)

3. **Orolabial HSV reactivation** occurs in approximately 75% of seropositive patients and may progress to HSV esophagitis or pneumonia [90, 95, 98–100]. Acyclovir is used orally for prophylaxis and in intravenous preparation for treatment.

B. **The middle period (21–100 days)** is characterized by either continued granulocytopenia from graft failure or rejection, and hence possible bacterial or fungal infection, or successful engraftment with marrow maturation and the gradual return of immune function. In the latter case, viruses and protozoa become important causes of infection. **The main obstacle to survival after marrow engraftment is acute GVHD. This presents with** rash, diarrhea, and hepatic dysfunction, and is believed to result from proliferation of donor T lymphocytes reacting to host tissue antigens. **The second major risk to the patient during this period is interstitial pneumonia** [90].

1. **Interstitial pneumonia** is seen in 40–60% of BMT patients and has an overall mortality that exceeds 50% [101]. The presentation of increased respiratory rate, dry nonproductive cough, and fever occurring approximately 45 days after BMT is suggestive of interstitial pneumonia. Cytomegalovirus is found in one-half of the cases; 30–45% are idiopathic [101]. Pretransplant lung function is a strong predictor of the risk of CMV interstitial pneumonia after BMT. *P. carinii* pneumonia is declining with the use of prophylactic TMP-SMX [90]. Uncommonly, *Aspergillus,* adenovirus, HSV, human herpesvirus 6, parainfluenza, adenovirus, respiratory syncytial virus, or *Chlamydia* are causative agents [102–104].

   a. **Diagnosis.** Hypoxemia and pulmonary infiltrates are hallmarks of interstitial pneumonia. If bronchoscopy with bronchoalveolar lavage and biopsy is nondiagnostic and the patient has not improved after 24–48 hours on a broad-spectrum beta-lactam and aminoglycoside, open lung biopsy should be performed. Open lung biopsy should not be delayed in the critically ill patient.

   b. **Idiopathic interstitial pneumonia** has a similar presentation, but no infectious etiology can be demonstrated. Pulmonary fibrosis may be immune-mediated. Risk factors for idiopathic interstitial pneumonia include preconditioning total body irradiation and chemotherapy, GVHD and the use of MTX to control GVHD, age greater than 20 years, and a low Karnovsky score prior to transplantation [105, 106]. Treatment is supportive. Superinfection is a frequent complication. Overall mortality approaches 60% [101].

   c. **Until biopsy results are known, a broad-spectrum beta-lactam with an aminoglycoside is recommended** [90]. Ganciclovir in combination with CMV immunoglobulin provides the best opportunity for recovery if CMV pneumonitis is confirmed [107].

2. **Dermal infections** of this period are associated primarily with acute GVHD or with indwelling catheters.

   a. **Acute GVHD** with its generalized maculopapular skin rash can evolve into bullae, ulcers, and epidermolysis. The rash of GVHD may mimic the maculopapular rash of a drug eruption. Histologic confirmation may be necessary. Corticosteroids, MTX, ATG, and cyclosporine have been used for treatment [108].

   b. **Skin infections are often associated with an indwelling catheter.** See Chap. 2.

3. **Central nervous system infections can** present as meningitis or as subtle changes in mental status (see Chap. 5).

4. **Urinary tract infections.** See Chap. 12.

5. **Gastrointestinal tract infections.** Complaints of nausea, vomiting, and anorexia during the first 2 weeks after BMT are usually side effects of chemoradiotherapy or side effects of drugs. Between days 15 and 60, acute GVHD, HSV infections, and drug toxicity are diagnostic considerations.

   a. **Diarrhea** is common in this period. Chemoradiotherapy sequelae are diagnosed by biopsy and treated supportively. Drug toxicity is excluded by discontinuation or substitution of medications. Chemotherapeutic agents and antimicrobials may cause *Clostridium difficile* colitis (see Chap. 28A). Patients developing **acute GVHD** present with nausea and vomiting and have hemoccult-positive, watery stools with a high protein content. Barium studies of the small intestine, flat-plate abdominal roentgenography, ultrasonograms showing edematous intestine, or mucosal biopsies of duodenum or colon may aid in the diagnosis [109, 110]. Intestinal infections with viruses—enteroviruses, adenovirus, or rotavirus strains; fungi; parasites; and bacteria may mimic or be associated with GVHD [111]. Stool should be cultured for viruses and enteric pathogens and examined for ova and parasites. Endoscopic biopsy with viral culture should be used if CMV or HSV is suspected or if the diagnosis remains unclear.

b. **Gastrointestinal bleeding** often is caused by mucositis or acute GVHD, but other etiologies include CMV, EBV-induced PTLD, peptic ulcer, and Mallory-Weiss tears [112].

c. **Esophagitis** caused by chemoradiotherapy occurs early in the posttransplantation period and usually is self-limited. Diagnosis of esophagitis generally requires biopsy, as viruses, fungi, or bacteria may cause disease singly or in combination [112]. Stricture formation may be a late sequela.

d. **Abdominal pain**

(1) **Early-onset** abdominal pain may be caused by **chemoradiotherapy or venoocclusive disease.** Right upper quadrant pain, ascites, and fluid retention can be seen with venoocclusive disease. Such disease involves the terminal hepatic venules and sublobular veins, with necrosis of hepatocytes leading to fibrosis and obstruction of sinusoidal blood flow. No intervention has altered the disease course, which carries a mortality of 30% [113].

(2) **Later, acute GVHD and infectious enteritis** are common causes of abdominal pain and may occur simultaneously. Typhlitis, or neutropenic enterocolitis, is characterized by bacterial invasion and inflammation of the bowel wall and also presents with right upper quadrant pain, vomiting, fever, and diarrhea. *Clostridium septicum* may be cultured from blood, though other anaerobes, gram-negative organisms, or yeast may be involved. Sepsis syndrome and edema of the colonic mucosa on CT scanning further suggest this diagnosis. Supportive therapy with appropriate antibiotic treatment is indicated; surgical resection is a consideration while waiting for the neutropenia to resolve [112].

6. **Disseminated infection** often is caused by **CMV,** and GVHD predisposes to symptomatic disease. Approximately 50% of cases are reactivations, but other CMV infections are acquired from the donor or from CMV-seropositive blood products. The nonspecific presentation may include fever, neutropenia, or organ dysfunction. Many patients are asymptomatic [98]. One-fifth or so of CMV infections culminate in pneumonia, with a mortality of 50–60% [94, 95]. Diagnosis requires biopsy of the involved organ and CMV cultures of blood and urine. Alternatively, PCR assays may be helpful. Avoidance of seropositive marrow donors and screening of blood products can prevent most disease. Treatment of visceral disease employs ganciclovir with CMV immunoglobulin [113].

7. **Line-related bacteremias.** The patient's immunosuppressed state, the presence of GVHD, and indwelling venous catheters all contribute to the development of sepsis with fungi such as *Candida* and bacteria such as *Staphylococcus epidermidis* and *Corynebacterium* spp. (see Chap. 2).

C. **The late period (> 100 days)** is associated with fewer infections as most intravenous lines have been removed, fewer immunosuppressive agents are used, and the immune system has progressively recovered. **Chronic GVHD** occurs during this period in 30–50% of patients and may follow acute GVHD or arise de novo [113]. It may be focal and mild, or it may be generalized, resembling autoimmune disease with sclerodermalike skin lesions, hepatitis, malabsorption, and sicca syndrome [112]. Chronic GVHD leads to an increased risk of infection owing to interruption of skin and mucosal barriers, delayed recovery of cell-mediated and humoral immunity, and functional asplenia [113].

1. **Pulmonary infections.** The upper and lower respiratory tracts are common sites of infection because chronic GVHD leads to IgA deficiency and sicca syndrome. *Streptococcus pneumoniae* is a common isolate, whereas fungi, CMV, and *P. carinii* are less common. TMP-SMX is used for bacterial and PCP prophylaxis [98].

2. **Dermal infections.** Varicella-zoster virus is a significant pathogen in the late period, occurring in 30% of all patients and 45% of patients with chronic GVHD.

Both primary and reactivation disease are encountered. Local complications include bacterial superinfection, scarring, postherpetic neuralgia, and trigeminal zoster. Visceral involvement with VZV is a life-threatening complication that can affect pelvic and abdominal organs, the lungs, the oral and genital mucous membranes, and the CNS. Patients with cutaneous or visceral VZV should be treated with intravenous acyclovir and should be strictly isolated. Administration of VZIG is indicated for primary exposures, in the hope of preventing or ameliorating illness. See related discussion in Chaps. 4 and 26.

3. **Disseminated infections.** Pneumococcal sepsis is seen, as are bacteremias with *H. influenzae, Neisseria meningitidis, S. aureus,* and gram-negative aerobes. A beta-lactam and aminoglycoside should be used empirically when these bacteremic syndromes are suspected. TMP-SMX prophylaxis is effective in decreasing the incidence of bacteremia.

References

1. UNOS Scientific Registry, October 15, 1993. *U.N.O.S. Update* 9(9):36, 1993.
2. Youngner, S.J., and Arnold, R.M. Ethical, psychosocial, and public policy implications of procuring organs from non-heart-beating cadaver donors. *J.A.M.A.* 268:2769–2773, 1993.
3. Rubin, R.H., and Tolkoff-Rubin, N.E. The problem of human immunodeficiency virus (HIV) infection and transplantation. *Transpl. Int.* 1:36, 1988.
4. Perlroth, M.G. The Role of Organ Transplantation in Medical Therapy. In E. Rubenstein and D.D. Federman (eds.), *Scientific American Medicine.* New York: Scientific American, 1989. Pp. CTM V, 1–16.
5. Symposium on Liver Transplantation. The Department of Continuing Education in Health Sciences, UCLA Extension, and the Liver Transplantation Program, Department of Surgery, School of Medicine, UCLA, Los Angeles, 1986.
6. Keating, M.R., Wilhelm, M.P., and Walker, R.C. Strategies for prevention of infection after cardiac transplantation. *Mayo Clin. Proc.* 67:676–684, 1992.
7. The, T.H., et al. Monitoring for cytomegalovirus after organ transplantation: A clinical perspective. *Transplant. Proc.* 25(5)(Suppl. 4):5–9, 1993.
8. DeVault, G.A., Jr., et al. Opportunistic infections with *Strongyloides stercoralis* in renal transplantation. *Rev. Infect. Dis.* 12:653–671, 1990.
9. Busuttil, R.W. (Mod.). Liver transplantation today. *Ann. Intern. Med.* 104:377–389, 1986.
10. Council on Scientific Affairs. Introduction to the management of immunosuppression. *J.A.M.A.* 257:1781, 1987.
11. Grossi, P., et al. Infections in heart transplant recipients: The experience of the Italian Heart Transplantation Program. *J. Heart Lung Transplant.* 11:847–866, 1992.
12. McGoon, M.D., and Franz, R.P. Techniques of immunosuppression after cardiac transplantation. *Mayo Clin. Proc.* 67:586–595, 1992.
12a. Burke, J.F., Jr., et al. Long-term efficacy and safety of cyclosporine in renal-transplant recipients. *N. Engl. J. Med.* 331:358, 1994.
  See editorial response, in same issue.
13. Bourge, R.C., et al. Total lymphoid irradiation in cardiac transplantation: Is there a prolonged effect on allograft rejection? *J. Heart Lung Transplant.* 12(1):2(Suppl. 86), 1993.
13a. Medical Letter. Tacrolimus (FK506) for organ transplants. *Med. Lett. Drugs Ther.* 36:82, 1994.
14. Goto, T., et al. FK 506: Historical perspectives. *Transplant. Proc.* 23:2713–2717, 1991.
14a. Medical Letter. Mycophenolate mofetil: A new immunosuppressant for organ transplantation. *Med. Lett. Drugs Ther.* 37:84, 1995.
15. Smyth, R.L., et al. Infection and reactivation with cytomegalovirus strains in lung transplant recipients. *Transplantation* 52:480–481, 1991.
16. Pouteil-Noble, C., et al. Influence of chronic cytomegalovirus and hepatitis B virus infections on the outcome of renal transplantation. *Transplant. Proc.* 22:1820, 1990.
17. Rubin, R.H. Indirect effects of cytomegalovirus infection on the outcome of organ transplantation. *J.A.M.A.* 261:3607, 1989.
18. Abramson, J.S., and Mills, E.L. Depression of neutrophil function induced by viruses and its role in secondary microbial infections. *Rev. Infect. Dis.* 10:326–341, 1988.

19. Tolkoff-Rubin, N.E., and Rubin, R.H. Infection in the Organ Transplant Recipient. In G.J. Cerrill (ed.), *Organ Transplantation and Replacement.* Philadelphia: Lippincott, 1988.

20. Wiesner, R.H., et al. Selective bowel decontamination to prevent gram-negative bacterial and fungal infection following orthotopic liver transplantation. *Transplant. Proc.* 19:2420–2423, 1987.

21. Peterson, P.K., and Anderson, R.C. Infection in renal transplant recipients. *Am. J. Med.* 81(Suppl. 1A):2, 1986.

22. Amber, J.I., et al. Increased risk of pneumococcal infections in cardiac transplant recipients. *Transplantation* 49:122–125, 1990.

23. Brayman, K.L., et al. Prophylaxis of serious cytomegalovirus infection in renal transplant candidates using live human cytomegalovirus vaccine. *Arch. Surg.* 123:1502–1508, 1988.

24. Zaia, J.A., and Forman, S.J. Management of the Bone Marrow Transplant Recipient. In J.E. Parillo and H. Masur (eds.), *The Critically Ill Immunosuppressed Patient.* Rockville, MD: Aspen, 1987. Pp. 381–412.

25. Simmons, R.L., and Migliori, R.J. Infection prophylaxis after successful organ transplantation. *Transplant. Proc.* 20:7–11, 1988.

26. Cuvelier, R., Pirson, Y., and Alexandre, G. Late urinary tract infection after transplantation: Prevalence, predisposition and morbidity. *Nephron* 40:76, 1985.

27. Tolkoff-Rubin, N.E., et al. A controlled study of trimethoprim-sulfamethoxazole prophylaxis of urinary tract infection in renal transplant recipients. *Rev. Infect. Dis.* 4:614, 1982.

28. Evans, R.W., et al. The medical and surgical determinants of heart transplantation outcomes: The results of a consensus survey in the United States. *J. Heart Lung Transplant.* 12:42–45, 1993.

29. Balfour, H.H., Jr., et al. A randomized, placebo-controlled trial of oral acyclovir for the prevention of cytomegalovirus disease in recipients of renal allografts. *N. Engl. J. Med.* 320:1381–1387, 1989.

30. Goodrich, J.M., et al. Early treatment with ganciclovir to prevent cytomegalovirus disease after allogeneic bone marrow transplantation. *N. Engl. J. Med.* 325:1601–1607, 1991.

31. Merigan, T.C., et al. A controlled trial of ganciclovir to prevent cytomegalovirus disease after heart transplantation. *N. Engl. J. Med.* 326:1182–1186, 1992.

32. Schmidt, G.M., et al. A randomized, controlled trial of prophylactic ganciclovir for cytomegalovirus pulmonary infection in recipients of allogeneic bone marrow transplants. *N. Engl. J. Med.* 324:1005–1011, 1991.

33. Kirk, J.L., et al. Analysis of early infectious complications after autologous bone marrow transplantation. *Cancer* 62:2445–2450, 1988.

34. Taylor, C.E., et al. Virus infections in bone marrow transplant recipients: A three-year prospective study. *J. Clin. Pathol.* 43(8):633–637, 1990.

34a. Basgoz, N., and Rubin, R.H. Antimicrobial prophylaxis in patients undergoing solid organ transplantation. *Curr. Clin. Top. Infect. Dis.* 15:344, 1995.

35. Snydman, D.R., et al. Use of cytomegalovirus immune globulin to prevent cytomegalovirus disease in renal-transplant recipients. *N. Engl. J. Med.* 317:1049, 1987.

36. Tsevat, J., et al. Which renal transplant patients should receive cytomegalovirus immune globulin? *Transplantation* 52:259–265, 1991.

37. Migliori, R.J., and Simmons, R.L. Infection prophylaxis after organ transplantation. *Transplant. Proc.* 20(3):395, 1988.

37a. Tolkoff-Rubin, N.E., and Rubin, R.H. The infectious disease problems of the diabetic renal transplant recipient. *Infect. Dis. Clin. North Am.* 9:117, 1995.

38. Rubin, R.H. Infection in the Organ Transplant Recipient. In R.H. Rubin and L.S. Young (eds.), *Clinical Approach to Infection in the Compromised Host* (3rd ed.). New York: Plenum, 1994.

39. Tilney, N.L., et al. Factors contributing to the declining mortality rate in renal transplantation. *N. Engl. J. Med.* 299:1321, 1978.

40. Auchincloss, H., and Rubin, R.H. Clinical Management of the Critically Ill Renal Transplant Patient. In J.E. Parillo and H. Masur (eds.), *The Critically Ill Immunosuppressed Patient.* Rockville, MD: Aspen, 1987. Pp. 347–376.

41. Peters, C., et al. Continuous sulfa prophylaxis for urinary tract infection in renal transplant recipients. *Am. J. Surg.* 146:589, 1983.

41a. American Heart Association Medical/Scientific Statement. Cardiac transplantation: Recipient selection, donor procurement, and medical follow-up. *Circulation* 86(3):1061–1079, 1992.

42. Morgan, J.S., Schaffner, W., and Stone, W.J. Opportunistic strongyloidiasis in renal transplant recipients. *Transplantation* 42:518, 1986.
43. Bijnen, A.B., et al. Infections after transplant of a contaminated kidney. *Scand. J. Urol. Nephrol. Suppl.* 92:49, 1985.
44. Gottesdiener, K.M. Transplanted infections: Donor-to-host transmission with allograft. *Ann. Intern. Med.* 110:1001–1016, 1989.
45. Ramsey, P.G., et al. The renal transplant patient with fever and pulmonary infiltrates: Etiology, clinical manifestations and management. *Medicine* (Baltimore) 59:296, 1980.
46. Toledo-Pereya, L.H., et al. The benefit of open lung biopsy in patients with previous non-diagnostic transbronchial lung biopsy; a guide to appropriate therapy. *Chest* 77:647, 1980.
47. Cockerill, F.R., et al. Open lung biopsy in immunosuppressed patients. *Arch. Intern. Med.* 145:1398–1404, 1985.
48. Winterbauer, R.H., et al. The use of quantitative cultures and antibody coating of bacteria to diagnose bacterial pneumonia by fiberoptic bronchoscopy. *Am. Rev. Respir. Dis.* 128:98, 1983.
49. Bass, J.B., Chairman, Subcommittee of the Scientific Assembly on Microbiology, Tuberculosis and Pulmonary Infections. American Thoracic Society—diagnostic standards and classification of tuberculosis. *Am. Rev. Respir. Dis.* 142:725–735, 1990.
50. Britt, R.H., Enzmann, D.R., and Remington, J.S. Intracranial infection in cardiac transplant recipients. *Ann. Neurol.* 9:107, 1981.
51. Denning, D.W., and Stevens, D.A. New drugs for systemic fungal infections. *Br. Med. J.* 299(6696):407–408, 1989.
52. Paya, C.V. Fungal infections in solid-organ transplantation. *Clin. Infect. Dis.* 16:677–688, 1993.
52a. Dismukes, W.E. Management of cryptococcosis. *Clin. Infect. Dis.* 17(Suppl. 2):S507–S512, 1993.
53. Meyer, R.D. Current role of therapy with amphotericin B. *Clin. Infect. Dis.* 15(Suppl.):S154–S160, 1992.
54. Bodey, G.P. Azole antifungal agents. *Clin. Infect. Dis.* 14(Suppl.):S161–169, 1992.
55. Graybill, J.R. Future directions of antifungal chemotherapy. *Clin. Infect. Dis.* 14 (Suppl.):S170–181, 1992.
56. Sinnott, J.T., Cullison, J.P., and Rogers, K. Treatment of CMV gastrointestinal ulceration in a heart transplant patient. *J. Heart Transplant.* 6:186, 1987.
56a. Rostaing, L., et al. Treatment of chronic hepatitis C with recombinant interferon alpha in kidney transplant recipients. *Transplantation* 59(10):1426, 1995.
57. Wright, T.E. (Lecturer). Hepatitis C and other NANB forms of hepatitis in transplantation. Presented at the North American Transplant Infectious Diseases Symposium, Boston, 1993.
57a. Pereira, B.J., et al. A controlled study of hepatitis C transmission by organ transplantation. *Lancet* 345:484, 1995.
57b. Boletis, J., et al. Liver biopsy is essential in anti-HCV (+) renal transplant patients irrespective of liver function tests and serology for HCV. *Transplant. Proc.* 27(1):945, 1995.
57c. Hanto, D.W. Classification of Epstein-Barr virus–associated posttransplant lymphoproliferative diseases: Implications for understanding their pathogenesis and developing rational treatment strategies. *Annu. Rev. Med.* 46:381, 1995.
58. Ensley, R.D., et al. Predictors of survival after repeat heart transplantation. *J. Heart Lung Transplant.* 11:S142–158, 1992.
59. Cooper, D.K.C., et al. Infectious complications after heart transplantation. *Thorax* 38:822, 1983.
59a. Petri, W.A., Jr. Infections in heart transplant recipients. *Clin. Infect. Dis.* 18:141, 1994. *"State-of-the-art" review article.*
60. Cooper, D.K.C., and Lanza, R.P. (eds.). *Infectious Complications in Heart Transplantation: The Present Status of Orthotopic and Heterotopic Heart Transplantation.* Lancaster, Engl.: Kluwer Academic, 1984. Pp. 195–223.
61. Palmer, D.L., Harvey, R.L., and Wheeler, J.K. Diagnostic and therapeutic considerations in *Nocardia asteroides* infections. *Medicine* (Baltimore) 53:391, 1974.
62. Medical Letter. Cytomegalovirus immune globulin. *Med. Lett. Drugs Ther.* 30:100, 1988.
63. Balfour, H.H. Options for prevention of cytomegalovirus disease. *Ann. Intern. Med.* 114(7):598–599, 1991.
63a. Carrieri, G., et al. Acyclovir/cytomegalovirus immune globulin combination therapy for CMV prophylaxis in high-risk renal allograft recipients. *Transplant. Proc.* 27(1):961, 1995.

63b. Valenza, M., et al. Combined antiviral and immunoglobulin therapy as prophylaxis against cytomegalovirus infection after heart transplantation. *J. Heart Lung Transplant.* 14(4):659, 1995.

63c. Hibberd, P., et al. Preemptive ganciclovir therapy to prevent cytomegalovirus disease in cytomegalovirus antibody-positive renal transplant recipients. *Ann. Intern. Med.* 123:18, 1995.

64. Hofflin, J.M., et al. Infectious complications in heart transplant recipients receiving cyclosporine and corticosteroids. *Ann. Intern. Med.* 106:209, 1987.

65. Rubin, R.H., et al. Infection in the renal transplant recipient. *Am. J. Med.* 70:405, 1981.

66. Peters, J.B. *Use and Interpretation of Tests in Medical Microbiology* (2nd ed.). Santa Monica: Specialty Laboratories, 1990. P. 84.

67. Saravolatz, L.D., et al. The compromised host and Legionnaires' disease. *Ann. Intern. Med.* 90:533–537, 1979.

68. Kim, J., et al. Presumptive cerebral *Nocardia asteroides* infection in AIDS: Treatment with ceftriaxone and minocycline. *Am. J. Med.* 90:656, 1991.

69. Garlando, F., et al. Successful treatment of disseminated nocardiosis complicated by cerebral abscess with ceftriaxone and amikacin: Case report. *Clin. Infect. Dis.* 15(6):1039–1040, 1992.

70. Patton, D.F., et al. Epstein-Barr virus determined clonality in posttransplant lymphoproliferative disease. *Transplantation* 49(6):1080–1084, 1990.

71. Cen, H., et al. Evidence for restricted Epstein-Barr virus latent gene expression and anti-EBNA antibody response in solid organ transplant recipients with posttransplant lymphoproliferative disorders. *Blood* 81(5):1393–1403, 1993.

72. Straus, S.E. (Mod.). Epstein-Barr virus infections: Biology, pathogenesis, and management. *Ann. Intern. Med.* 118(1):45, 1993.

73. Chen, J., et al. Management of lymphoproliferative disorders after cardiac transplantation. *Ann. Thorac. Surg.* 56:527–538, 1993.

74. Penn, I. (Mod.). *Immunosuppression and Lymphoproliferative Disorders Roundtable, Cincinnati, Ohio.* Raritan, NJ: Ortho Biotech, 1992.

75. Busuttil, M.D. Liver transplantation today. *Ann. Intern. Med.* 104:372, 1986.

75a. Winston, D.J., et al. Infections in liver transplant recipients. *Clin. Infect. Dis.* 21:1077, 1995.
     One of the "state-of-the-art" series; published November 1995. Contains good discussion of CMV infections which, without antiviral prophylaxis, may occur in 50–60% of transplant recipients, half of which have symptomatic disease. Liver biopsy typically reveals inclusion bodies. Serological tests are unreliable for immediate diagnosis because they lack sensitivity. Many transplantation centers use the shell-vial culture technique for rapid detection of CMV and supplement the results of cultures with findings from histologic examination of biopsy specimens.

76. Colonna, J.O., et al. Infectious complications in liver transplantation. *Arch. Surg.* 123:360, 1988.

77. Wood, R.P., et al. *A Review of Liver Transplantation for Gastroenterologists.* Omaha: Department of Surgery, University of Nebraska Medical Center. P. 24.

78. Wiesner, R.H., et al. Hepatic allograft rejection: New developments in terminology, diagnosis, prevention, and treatment. *Mayo Clin. Proc.* 68:69–79, 1993.

78a. Kanj, S.S., et al. Cytomegalovirus infection following liver transplantation: Review of the literature. *Clin. Infect. Dis.* 22:537, 1996.
     Includes a discussion of diagnostic approaches including antigenemia assays, serology, PCR, histopathology, etc. Comprehensive review.

79. Goldstein, R.M. *Current Advances in Liver Transplantation: The Role of Candidate Selection.* East Hanover, NJ: Sandoz Pharmaceuticals Corp., 1991.

80. Starzl, T.E., Demetris, A.J., and Thiel, D.V. Liver transplantation medical progress. *N. Engl. J. Med.* 16:1092–1096, 1989.

81. Saint-Vil, D., et al. Infectious complications of pediatric liver transplantation. *J. Pediatr. Surg.* 26:908–913, 1991.

82. Kusne, S., et al. Infections after liver transplantation. *Medicine* (Baltimore) 67:132, 1988.

83. Wajszczuk, C.P., et al. Fungal infections in liver transplant recipients. *Transplantation* 40:347, 1985.

84. Wiesner, R.H. The incidence of gram-negative bacterial and fungal infections in liver transplant patients treated with selective decontamination. *Infection* (Suppl. 1):19–21, 1990.

84a. Singh, N., et al. High-dose acyclovir compared with short-course preemptive ganciclovir therapy to prevent cytomegalovirus disease in liver transplant recipients. *Ann. Intern. Med.* 120:375, 1994.

84b. Winston, D.J., et al. Randomised comparison of ganciclovir and high-dose acyclovir for long-term cytomegalovirus prophylaxis in liver-transplant recipients. *Lancet* 346:69, 1995.

84c. Thiel, D.H., et al. Recurrence of hepatitis C following liver transplantation: Treatment with interferon. *Transplantation Sci.* 4(Suppl. 1):S26, 1994.
   See related paper by E.J. Gane et al., Long-term outcome of hepatitis C infection after liver transplantation. N. Engl. J. Med. *334:815, 1996.*

84d. Lumbreras, C., et al. Infectious complications following pancreatic transplantation: Incidence, microbiological and clinical characteristics, and outcome. *Clin. Infect. Dis.* 20:514, 1995.

85. Meyers, J. Infections in bone marrow transplant recipients. *Am. J. Med.* 81:27, 1986.

86. Thomas, E.D., et al. Bone marrow transplantation. *N. Engl. J. Med.* 292:832, 1975.

87. Storb, R., et al. Marrow transplant for aplastic anemia. *Semin. Hematol.* 21:27, 1984.

88. Thomas, E.D. Current status of bone marrow transplant. *Transplant. Proc.* 17:428, 1985.

89. Martin, P.J., et al. A clinical trial of in-vitro depletion of T-cells in donor marrow for prevention of acute graft-versus-host disease. *Transplant. Proc.* 17:486, 1985.

90. Bowden, R.A., and Myers, J.D. Infection Complicating Bone Marrow Transplantation. In R.H. Rubin and L.S. Young (eds.), *Clinical Approach to Infection in the Compromised Host* (3rd ed.). New York: Plenum, 1994.

91. Saral, R. Infections following bone marrow transplantation. *Transplant. Immunol. Letter* 6(4):9–10, 1990.

92. Goodman, J.L., et al. A controlled trial of fluconazole to prevent fungal infections in patients undergoing bone marrow transplantation. *N. Engl. J. Med.* 326:845–851, 1992.

93. Winston, D.J., et al. Ganciclovir prophylaxis of cytomegalovirus infection and disease in allogeneic bone marrow transplant recipients. *Ann. Intern. Med.* 118:179–184, 1993.

94. Goodrich, J.M., et al. Ganciclovir prophylaxis to prevent cytomegalovirus disease after allogeneic marrow transplant. *Ann. Intern. Med.* 118:173–178, 1993.

94a. Goodrich, J.M., et al. Strategies for the prevention of cytomegalovirus disease after marrow transplantation. *Clin. Infect. Dis.* 19:287, 1994.
   Review concentrates on the role of antiviral chemotherapy. Includes summary of 7 studies showing that ganciclovir reduced the incidence of CMV infection and disease after transplantation. Concludes that ganciclovir is effective to prevent CMV in BMT, but its usefulness is limited by neutropenia.
   Whether all BMT recipients who are CMV positive need antiviral therapy is discussed; ideally weekly centrifugation cultures for CMV can be done with ganciclovir therapy for those who are viremic.

94b. Sable, C.A., and Donowitz, G.R. Infections in bone marrow transplant recipients. *Clin. Infect. Dis.* 18:273, 1994.
   "State-of-the-art" clinical review.

95. Saral, R., et al. Acyclovir prophylaxis of herpes simplex virus infections. A randomized double-blind, controlled trial in bone marrow recipients. *N. Engl. J. Med.* 305:63, 1981.

96. Valteau, D., et al. Streptococcal septicaemia following autologous bone marrow transplantation in children treated with high-dose chemotherapy. *Bone Marrow Transplant.* 7:415–419, 1991.

96a. Rossetti, F., et al. Fungal liver infection in marrow transplant recipients: Prevalence at autopsy, predisposing factors, and clinical features. *Clin. Infect. Dis.* 20:801, 1995.
   The incidence of Candida *infections in BMT recipients is 10–25%. Study revealed that independent predisposing factors for fungal liver infection were multiple positive fungal cultures during life and the presence of underlying veno-occlusive disease of the liver and/or GVDH. Diagnosis of liver involvement is difficult even with imaging studies.*

97. EORTC Cooperative Group. Empiric antifungal therapy in febrile granulocytopenic patients. *Am. J. Med.* 86:668, 1989.

98. Engelhard, D., Marks, M.I., and Good, R.A. Infections in bone marrow transplant recipients. *J. Pediatr.* 108:335, 1986.

99. McDonald, G.B., et al. Esophageal infections in immune suppressed patients after marrow transplantation. *Gastroenterology* 88:1111, 1985.

100. Ramsay, P.G., et al. Herpes simplex pneumonia: Clinical, virological and pathological features in twenty patients. *Ann. Intern. Med.* 100:823, 1984.

101. Crawford, S.W., and Hackman, R.C. Clinical course of idiopathic pneumonia after bone marrow transplantation. *Am. Rev. Respir. Dis.* 147:1393–1400, 1993.

102. Hertz, M.I., et al. Respiratory syncytial virus–induced acute lung injury in adult patients with bone marrow transplants: A clinical approach and review of the literature. *Medicine* (Baltimore) 68:269–281, 1989.
103. Carrigan, D.R., et al. Interstitial pneumonitis associated with human herpesvirus-6 infection after marrow transplantation. *Lancet* 338:147–149, 1991.
104. Yoshikawa, T., et al. Human herpesvirus-6 infection in bone marrow transplantation. *Blood* 78:1381–1384, 1991.
105. Clark, J.G., et al. Idiopathic pneumonia syndrome after bone marrow transplantation. *Am. Rev. Respir. Dis.* 147:1601–1606, 1993.
106. Weiner, R.S., et al. Risk factors for interstitial pneumonia following bone marrow transplantation for severe aplastic anaemia. *Br. J. Haematol.* 71:535–543, 1989.
107. Reed, E.C., et al. Treatment of cytomegalovirus pneumonia with ganciclovir and intravenous cytomegalovirus immunoglobulin in patients with bone marrow transplants. *Ann. Intern. Med.* 109:783, 1988.
108. Meyers, J.D., et al. Biology of Interstitial Pneumonia After Marrow Transplant. In R.P. Gale (ed.), *Recent Advances in Bone Marrow Transplantation.* New York: Alan R. Liss, 1983. Pp. 405–423.
109. Plotkin, S.A. Sensitivity of clinical isolates of human cytomegalovirus to 9-(1,2-dihydroxy-2-propoxymethyl) guanine. *J. Infect. Dis.* 152:833, 1985.
110. Trigs, M.E. Bone marrow transplant for treatment of leukemia in children. *Pediatr. Clin. North Am.* 35:933, 1988.
111. Willoughby, R.E., Wee, S.B., and Yolken, R.H. Non-group A rotavirus infection associated with severe gastroenteritis in a bone marrow transplant patient. *Pediatr. Infect. Dis. J.* 7:133–135, 1988.
112. Wolford, J.L., and McDonald, G.B. A problem-oriented approach to intestinal and liver disease after marrow transplant. *J. Gastroenterol.* 10:419, 1988.
113. Donowitz, G.R. Infections in Bone Marrow Transplant Recipients. In G.L. Mandell, J.E. Bennett, and R. Dolin (eds.), *Principles and Practice of Infectious Diseases* (update 12). New York: Churchill Livingstone, 1992.
See also related update by D.J. Winston, Infections in Bone Marrow Transplant Recipients. In G.L. Mandell, J.E. Bennett, and R. Dolin (eds.), Principles and Practice of Infectious Diseases (4th ed.). New York: Churchill Livingstone, 1995. Pp. 2717–2722.

Bibliography

Dummer, J.S., Ho, M., and Simmons, R.L. Infections in Solid Organ Transplant Recipients. In G.L. Mandell, J.E. Bennett, and R. Dolin (eds.), *Principles and Practice of Infectious Diseases* (4th ed.). New York: Churchill Livingstone, 1995. Pp. 2722–2731.

Ho, M., and Dummer, J.S. Infections in Transplant Recipients. In G.L. Mandell, J.E. Bennett, and R. Dolin (eds.), *Principles and Practice of Infectious Diseases* (4th ed.). New York: Churchill Livingstone, 1995. Pp. 2709–2716.

Rubin, R.H., and Young, L.S. (eds.). *Clinical Approach to Infection in the Compromised Host.* (3rd ed.) New York: Plenum, 1994.
See chapters on infections in transplant recipients.

Rubin, R.H. (ed.). Infection in transplantation. *Infect. Dis. Clin. North Am.* 9:811–1074, 1995.
This December 1995 issue is devoted to transplant-related infections. An excellent resource.

Winston, D.J. Infections in Bone Marrow Transplant Recipients. In G.L. Mandell, J.E. Bennett, and R. Dolin (eds.), *Principles and Practice of Infectious Diseases* (4th ed.). New York: Churchill Livingstone, 1995. Pp. 2717–2721.

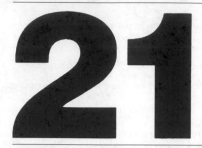

Health Advice for
International Travel

David R. Hill
and Richard D. Pearson

International travel, including visits to the developing world, has become a major pursuit of Americans, with an estimated 8 million Americans traveling to the developing world each year for business, vacation, study, or missionary activities. These travelers often are exposed to bacterial, viral, and parasitic diseases that range from travelers' diarrhea to life-threatening infection with *Plasmodium falciparum*. The changing patterns of disease, changing international health requirements, and complex itineraries make it a challenging task to provide advice on prevention and immunizations for the traveler [1]. Pretravel care should not be taken lightly and, whenever possible, should be provided by an expert in the field. Many hospitals and schools of medicine in the United States have specialized travel clinics or units of tropical medicine that can provide expert advice to the traveler [2].

Vaccinations

I. **General considerations.** To tailor a traveler's vaccines and preventive advice individually, the itinerary (including whether rural areas will be visited), duration of stay, and medical and immunization histories need to be considered [3].
   A. **Types of vaccinations for the traveler.** Vaccinations can be divided into (1) those that are routinely recommended for adults, whether or not they are traveling, (2) those that are required by countries for entry, and (3) those that are recommended because of potential exposure in the country of destination (Table 21-1).
      1. **Routine vaccinations. The pretravel visit is an excellent time to update routinely recommended vaccines** such as tetanus-diphtheria and measles. Immunizations are discussed in the *Guide for Adult Immunization* [4], in *Health Information for International Travel* [5], in Chap. 22, and in sec. II. Recommendations for children have been recently reviewed [5a].
      2. **Required vaccinations—the International Certificate of Vaccination.** The only vaccine now officially required under World Health Organization (WHO) regulations for travel between countries is yellow fever vaccine. Nevertheless, some countries may still ask for evidence of cholera vaccination. This will be discussed in more detail in sec. III. A list of the vaccine requirements by country is published annually by the Centers for Disease Control (CDC) in *Health Information for International Travel* [5]. **According to international health regulations, required vaccinations must be recorded in the document International Certificate of Vaccination [6] and validated** by a stamp issued by state health departments. No vaccinations are required for returning US residents to reenter the United States.
         Smallpox vaccination is no longer required by any country [7]. (See sec. III.)
      3. **Recommended vaccinations.** Travelers and physicians frequently confuse the distinction between **required** and **recommended** vaccines. In reality, only yellow fever may be required. Opinion on which of the other vaccines to administer may differ among health care providers. Some vaccinations are recommended because infection could be acquired in the country of destination or in a particular location within that country. Examples include epidemic meningococcal disease, which is limited to certain areas of the world, and typhoid fever, which is present throughout the developing world but is a risk to travelers only if they encounter poor food and water sanitation. Although vaccines or therapy exist for some diseases transmitted by fecal contamination of the food and water supply (e.g., travelers' diarrhea, typhoid, poliomyelitis, cholera, hepatitis

Table 21-1. Vaccinations to consider for travel to the developing world

Vaccine	Type	Schedule[a]	Indications[a]	Precautions and contraindications[b]	Side effects[b]
Toxoids					
Tetanus-diphtheria (Td)	Adsorbed toxoids	Primary: 2 doses (0.5 ml) IM 4–8 wk apart; third dose 6–12 mo later Booster: every 10 yr	All adults	First trimester of pregnancy Hypersensitivity or neurologic reaction to previous doses Severe local reaction	Local reactions; occasional fever and systemic symptoms Arthuslike reactions in persons with multiple previous boosters Rare, systemic allergy
Inactivated bacteria vaccines					
Cholera	Phenol-killed *Vibrio cholerae* (4×10^9/ml)	Primary: 0.5 ml IM or SC or 0.2 ml ID; give 2 doses 1 wk–1 mo apart at least 6 days before travel Booster: 0.5 ml IM or SC or 0.2 ml ID every 6 mo	No longer required by individual countries May be considered for persons with compromised GI function and high-risk travel (see text)	Safety in pregnancy is unknown Previous severe local or systemic reaction	Local reaction of pain, erythema, and induration lasting 1–2 days Occasional fever, malaise
Haemophilus influenzae type b	Polysaccharide conjugate vaccines	Primary: 2 or 3 doses depending upon vaccine type Booster: usually single dose	Children 2 mo old	Hypersensitivity to any of the vaccine components	Mild local reactions in approximately 10% of patients
Streptococcus pneumoniae	Polysaccharide containing 23 serotypes	Primary: 1 dose (0.5 ml) SC or IM Booster: recommended for high-risk patients after ≥6 yr	Persons ≥2 yr at increased risk of pneumococcal disease and its complications Healthy adults ≥65 years	Safety in pregnancy is unknown	Approximately 50% of patients have erythema and pain at injection site Systemic reaction in <1% of patients Arthuslike reaction with booster doses

Table 21-1 (continued)

Vaccine	Type	Schedule[a]	Indications[a]	Precautions and contraindications[b]	Side effects[b]
Neisseria meningitidis	Polysaccharide containing 4 serotypes (A, C, Y, W-135)	Primary: 1 dose (0.5 ml) SC Booster: not officially recommended; may be given after 5 yr	Travelers to areas with epidemic meningococcal disease Asplenia or certain complement-deficiency states	Safety in pregnancy is unknown	Infrequent, mild local reactions
Typhoid (whole cell)	Acetone and heat-killed *Salmonella typhi* (10^9/ml)	Primary: 2 doses (0.5 ml) SC given 4 or more weeks apart Booster: 0.5 ml SC or 0.1 ml ID every 3 years	Risk for exposure to typhoid fever (see text)	Previous severe local or systemic reaction Acetone-killed vaccines should not be given ID Pregnancy is a relative contraindication	Local reaction of pain, swelling, and induration lasting 1–2 days, can be severe Occasional systemic reaction
Typhoid	Polysaccharide Vi	Primary: 0.5 ml IM in deltoid in adults; in children IM in deltoid or the vastus lateralis Booster: 0.5 ml IM every 2 years	Risk of exposure to typhoid fever in persons ≥2 yr old (see text)	Safety in pregnancy is unknown	Local, mild reactions of pain or tenderness within 48 hr of vaccination
Attenuated live bacterial vaccine					
Typhoid	Attenuated Ty21a mutant of *Salmonella typhi*	Primary: 1 capsule PO given on alternate days for 4 doses Booster: every 5 years	Risk for exposure to typhoid fever (see text)	Safety in pregnancy is unknown Immunocompromised host[b] Children <6 yr Persons with an acute febrile or gastrointestinal illness Persons taking antibiotics Refrigerate capsules	Infrequent gastrointestinal upset or rash

Attenuated live virus vaccines

	Type	Schedule	Indications	Contraindications	Adverse reactions
Measles	Attenuated live virus (available in monovalent form or combined with rubella [MR] ± mumps [MMR])	Primary: 2 doses SC; see text for interval between doses Booster: none	All persons born after 1956 who have not had documented measles infection or received 2 doses of attenuated, live measles vaccine	Pregnancy Immunocompromised host[c] (HIV-infected persons can be considered for vaccination) History of anaphylaxis to eggs or neomycin Recent (<3 mo) administration of immunoglobulin	Temperature of ≥39.4°C, 5–21 days after vaccination in 5–15% Transient rash in 5% Of persons previously immunized with killed vaccine (1963–1967), 4–55% have a local reaction
Mumps	Attenuated live virus	Primary: 1 dose SC (usually given as part of MMR vaccine) Booster: none	Persons born after 1956 who have not had documented mumps or mumps vaccine	Pregnancy Immunocompromised host[c] History of anaphylaxis to eggs or neomycin	Mild allergic reactions uncommon Rare parotitis
Oral poliomyelitis vaccine (OPV)	Attenuated live virus, trivalent	Primary: 3 doses PO, the first two given at a 6- to 8-wk interval, the third 8–12 mo later Booster: 1 dose PO	Children and adolescents <18 yr of age Boost previously immunized persons; complete the series in partially immunized adults; alternative to inactivated poliomyelitis vaccine when there is <1 mo before travel	Immunocompromised host[c] or immuno-compromised contacts of recipients Not used for primary immunization in persons ≥18 yr	Rare paralysis (see text)
Rubella	Attenuated live virus	Primary: 1 dose (0.5 ml) SC (usually given as part of MR or MMR) Booster: none	All persons, particularly women of childbearing age, without documented illness or live vaccine on or after first birthday	Pregnancy Immunocompromised host[c] History of anaphylaxis to neomycin	Up to 40% of postpubertal women have joint pains, transient arthralgias, beginning 3–25 days after vaccination, persisting 1–11 days Frank arthritis in <2%

Table 21-1 (continued)

Vaccine	Type	Schedule[a]	Indications[a]	Precautions and contraindications[b]	Side effects[b]
Yellow fever	Attenuated live virus	Primary: 1 dose (0.5 ml) SC 10 days–10 yr before travel Booster: every 10 yr	As required by individual countries	Avoid in pregnant women, unless high-risk travel Prudent to avoid vaccinating infants <9 mo Immunocompromised host[c] Hypersensitivity to eggs	Mild headache, myalgia, fever 5–10 days after vaccination in 2–5% Rare immediate hypersensitivity
Inactivated virus vaccines					
Hepatitis B	Recombinant-derived hepatitis B surface antigen (Recombivax HB; see Chap. 22 for details)	Primary: 3 doses (1.0 ml) at 0, 1, and 6 mo; IM in deltoid Booster: not routinely recommended	Health care workers in contact with blood Persons residing for >6 mo in areas of high endemicity for hepatitis B surface antigen Others at risk for contact with blood, body fluids, or potentially contaminated medical or dental instruments	Although safety to fetus is unknown, pregnancy not a contraindication in high-risk persons	Mild local reaction in 10–20% Occasional systemic symptoms of fever, headache, fatigue, and nausea
	Energix B (recombinant vaccine)	Primary: 3 doses (1.0 ml) at 0, 1, and 6 mo For expedited pretravel regimen, 1.0 ml at 0, 1, 2, and 12 mo is suggested (see Chap. 22)	As above		

Vaccine	Type	Dose/Schedule	Indications	Contraindications/Precautions	Adverse Reactions
Inactivated poliomyelitis vaccine (eIPV)	Killed poliomyelitis virus, trivalent; enhanced potency	Primary: 2 doses (0.5 ml) SC at a 4- to 8-wk interval; third dose 6–12 mo after second	Preferred for persons ≥18 yr and for immunocompromised hosts	Safety in pregnancy is unknown; Anaphylactic reactions to streptomycin or neomycin	Mild local reaction
Influenza	Inactivated whole and split influenza A and B virus	Annual vaccination with current vaccine	Persons ≥6 mo with high-risk conditions (see text); Healthy persons >65 yr; Medical care personnel	First trimester of pregnancy is a relative contraindication; Anaphylaxis to eggs	Mild local reactions in fewer than one-third; Occasional systemic reaction of malaise, myalgia, beginning 6–12 hr after vaccination and lasting 1–2 days; Rare allergic reaction
Japanese B encephalitis	Inactivated virus	Primary: 3 doses (0.1 ml) SC at days 0, 7, and 30; Booster: 1 dose at 2 yr	Travelers to area of risk with rural exposure or prolonged residence (see text)	Pregnancy; Allergy to mice or rodents; History of anaphylaxis or urticaria	Local mild reactions lasting 1–3 days (20%); Systemic reactions of fever, myalgia, headache or gastrointestinal upset (10%); Allergic reactions with urticaria, rash, angioedema, or respiratory distress (0.1–10/1,000); Rare sudden death or encephalomyelitis
Rabies (human diploid cell vaccine)	Inactivated virus	Preexposure: 1 ml IM in deltoid on days 0, 7, and 21 or 28, or 0.1 ml ID on days 0, 7, and 21 or 28; Booster: depends on risk category and is based on serologic testing; Dose is 1.0 ml IM or 0.1 ml ID[a]	Travel to areas for >1 mo where rabies is a constant threat	Allergy to previous doses; May be given in pregnancy if indicated; Intradermal route should be completed 30 days or more before travel; ID route should not be used with concurrent chloroquine or mefloquine administration	Approximately 30% have local reactions; Approximately 20% have mild systemic reactions of headache, nausea, aches, dizziness; Rare neurologic illness; Occasional (6%) immune reactions with booster doses occurring 2–21 days after vaccination

Table 21-1 (continued)

Vaccine	Type	Schedule[a]	Indications[a]	Precautions and contraindications[b]	Side effects[b]
Hepatitis A (Havrix)	Inactivated virus	Primary: In adults, 1 ml (1440 E.U.) IM in deltoid 14 days before departure; in children 2–18 yr, 0.5 ml (360 E.U.) IM given 1 mo apart To provide long-term protection (≥10 yr?), a second dose in adults and a third dose in children should be given 6–12 mo after original shots	Travel to developing countries (see Chap. 11)	In adults, injection should be given in the deltoid region; the gluteal region should be avoided Data for use in pregnancy are not available	Local reactions with induration, redness
Passive prophylaxis					
Immunoglobulin[d]	Fractionated immunoglobulins (primarily IgG)	Travel of <3 mo duration: 0.02 ml/kg Travel of 4–6 mo duration: 0.06 ml/kg	For prevention of hepatitis A Some travelers may benefit from pretravel hepatitis A antibody testing (see text)		Local discomfort Rare systemic allergy

[a]Manufacturer's full prescribing information should be consulted. Doses given are generally for adults; pediatric doses may vary.
[b]Only major precautions, contraindications, and side effects listed.
[c]Persons immunocompromised because of immunodeficiency diseases, leukemia, lymphoma, generalized malignancy, or AIDS, or immunosuppressed from therapy with corticosteroids, alkylating agents, antimetabolites, or radiation.
[d]Immunoglobulin is now usually given if time before trip does not allow for hepatitis A vaccine antibody response. See text.
Source: Adapted from D. R. Hill and R. D. Pearson, Health advice for international travel. *Ann. Intern. Med.* 108:839–852, 1988.

A, giardiasis, and amebiasis), these may best be prevented by careful monitoring of foods and water. **Exposure in areas of poor food and water sanitation (as may occur in rural areas and small villages) for more than 2–3 weeks may be a reasonable cutoff point for administering vaccines for protection against enteric pathogens (e.g., typhoid).** (See sec. **IV.**) Unfortunately, data are not always available on the precise risk of most infectious diseases by geographic area, and the benefit-to-risk ratio of specific immunizations must be estimated by the physician [5, 8].

B. **Vaccine administration pointers**
 1. **Simultaneous administration** of vaccines is reviewed in detail in Chap. 22. Most viral and bacterial vaccines, whether attenuated, live, or killed, can be administered simultaneously at different sites, although cumulative side effects may preclude this. Attenuated live viral vaccines, which are not given simultaneously, should be separated by 1 month.
 2. **Live viral vaccines generally should not be given to** pregnant women [9], to patients who are immunocompromised, or to persons with a febrile illness.
 3. **Immunoglobulin should not be given for 3 months before or at least 2 weeks after measles, mumps, or rubella vaccine** because the passive transfer of antibodies may interfere with the immune response. These restrictions do not apply to oral poliomyelitis vaccine, yellow fever vaccine, or inactivated viral vaccines.
 4. **A person's risk factors for infection with human immunodeficiency virus (HIV) should be determined before administering vaccines.** Although immunization of healthy, HIV-infected persons is considered safe for most vaccines [10], progressive infection with live attenuated viruses or bacteria remains a theoretic possibility. In addition, there is a general correlation between CD4 cell counts and vaccine immunogenicity, so, in selected cases it may be helpful to check a CD4 count [10–12].
 5. **Documentation.** Prior to the administration of any vaccine, the manufacturer's full prescribing information should be consulted. The date, dose, site, manufacturer, and lot number of each vaccine, as well as any untoward effects should be recorded. (See Chap. 22.)
II. **Routine vaccinations for travelers.** A summary is provided in this section. More detailed discussion may be found in Chap. 22.
 A. **Tetanus-diphtheria toxoids.** Many adults in the United States are not adequately protected against tetanus and diphtheria. This is particularly true for persons older than 50 years in whom most cases of tetanus occur and who may lack protective antibodies against diphtheria [13, 14]. Outbreaks of diphtheria have occurred recently in areas where protection has waned [15]. Each traveler should have completed a primary series of tetanus-diphtheria vaccinations and received boosters with the combined toxoids at 10-year intervals. **Some travelers may benefit from a booster at 5-year intervals,** because a tetanus-prone wound does not require either tetanus immunoglobulin or a booster if a person has been boosted within 5 years [13]. It is easier and safer to be immunized before travel than to obtain a booster in a developing area where sterility of needles and storage conditions are less certain (see Chap. 4).
 B. **Pneumococcal vaccine.** Populations considered for pneumococcal vaccine are generally adults and children older than 2 years who are at increased risk of severe pneumococcal disease. These persons include those with functional impairment of the cardiorespiratory, hepatic, and renal systems, diabetes mellitus, anatomic or functional asplenia, sickle cell disease, chronic alcoholism, or HIV infection, and healthy persons 65 years of age and older [16]. The vaccine consists of 23 polysaccharide serotypes of *Streptococcus pneumoniae* and is given as a one-time dose. High-risk individuals who received the older 14-valent vaccine may be revaccinated. See further discussion in Chap. 9.
 C. **Measles.** Travelers may have substantial exposure to measles overseas. From 1983 to 1988, measles in the United States was epidemiologically linked to international travel in 4–22% of cases, with approximately half of the index cases occurring in returning American travelers [17–19]. Additionally, 8% of all outbreaks of measles in the United States during this time could be traced to imported measles [20]. Many outbreaks occurred on college campuses and in school-age children (5–19 years) who were previously vaccinated.

Because of a marked increase of measles cases in unvaccinated children younger than 5 years and in previously vaccinated individuals, the recommendations for measles immunization recently were changed [21]. Currently, all children should receive two doses of measles vaccine, the first at 15 months and the second at entry to elementary or middle school. Adults born in 1957 or later who have never had measles infection or vaccine should also receive two doses of vaccine separated by an interval of at least 1 month. Travelers born in 1957 or later who have not had two doses of live attenuated vaccine, with the second dose after 1980, should also be given a one-time dose of measles vaccine.

Children traveling to high-risk areas where they are likely to be exposed at a young age can be vaccinated between 6 and 12 months with single-antigen (monovalent) measles vaccine. They should be reimmunized at 15 months with the measles-mumps-rubella vaccine [21]. Vaccination of children younger than 2 years is reviewed elsewhere (see sec. **VIII** under Suggested Readings for the Physician Advising Travelers).

Measles in HIV-infected individuals can be severe, and vaccination with single-antigen vaccine appears to be safe; however, only a limited number of persons have been studied [10, 22]. Asymptomatically infected HIV-positive travelers should be vaccinated; vaccination also should be considered for symptomatic persons after potential risks are explained.

For further discussion of measles vaccinations, see Chap. 22.

D. **Rubella and mumps.** Women of childbearing age who are not immune to rubella should be considered for immunization [23]. Most adults probably were infected naturally with mumps virus and are immune [24]; however, if an adult is susceptible to mumps, vaccination may be considered. If immunity to more than one virus is lacking, combined measles-mumps-rubella vaccine can be given. There are no increased side effects if a person receives a vaccine virus to which he or she is immune (see Chap. 22).

E. **Influenza.** The composition of influenza vaccine is determined annually and includes the viral subtypes projected to cause disease in the United States [25]. Vaccination is recommended for adults with chronic disorders of the cardiovascular or pulmonary system, persons with other chronic medical conditions, nursing home residents, children age 6 months to 18 years who are on chronic aspirin therapy, healthy persons of 65 years and older, and health care workers. Influenza viruses active in the developing world may or may not be included in the vaccine in the United States. Influenza vaccinations should be given to travelers leaving the United States at any time of the year when destined for the tropics, or between April and September when destined for the southern hemisphere. See Chap. 8.

F. *Haemophilus influenzae* **type b.** The *Haemophilus* b conjugate vaccine should be given to children beginning at age 2 months. There are several formulations of this vaccine [26]. Each one conjugates the capsular polysaccharide of type b *Haemophilus* to a different carrier protein to increase immunogenicity at a younger age. None of the conjugate proteins (e.g., diphtheria toxoid) is sufficient to confer immunity against itself, and therefore does not preclude administration of the standard childhood immunizations. Persons with HIV infection should also be immunized. See Chap. 22.

III. **Required vaccinations**

A. **Yellow fever.** Countries that require yellow fever vaccine are listed in *Health Information for International Travel* [5]. Because of its requirement for cold storage and viability for only 60 minutes after reconstitution, **the vaccine is given only in approved yellow fever vaccination centers,** which may be identified by calling state or local health departments. Persons who are traveling or living in areas **infected** with yellow fever and persons who may visit rural areas in countries in the **endemic** zone for yellow fever should receive vaccine [27].

Infected areas are those in which yellow fever cases actually are occurring and lie primarily in equatorial South America and approximately 15 degrees on either side of the equator in Africa. These areas are listed in the *Summary of Health Information for International Travel,* published every 2 weeks by the Centers for Disease Control [28]. Zones **endemic** for yellow fever are areas in Africa and South America where yellow fever could occur. Some countries, particularly those in Asia, that are not in the endemic zones require immunization for persons entering from an area where yellow fever is occurring. These requirements are clearly stated in *Health Information for International Travel* [5].

Travelers infected with HIV generally should not receive yellow fever vaccine and should be advised to avoid infected areas. If they have to travel, such

travelers will need to carry with them a letter of medical exemption to vaccine, and they should adhere meticulously to mosquito avoidance measures. Cholera immunization given within 3 weeks of yellow fever vaccination may reduce antibody responses to both vaccines. Yellow fever vaccine may be given simultaneously with immunoglobulin.

B. **Cholera.** Because of limited vaccine efficacy ($\approx$50%) for only a short duration (3–6 months), uncomfortable side effects, and the low risk of infection in travelers [29–32], **cholera vaccine usually is not recommended for travel.** WHO has removed cholera as a vaccine requirement in international travel. Although no country now requires it for entry, some local authorities may still request documentation. In these circumstances, one dose of vaccine, properly recorded and given at least 6 days before travel, is sufficient. Those who might be considered for vaccination are persons who will work and live in highly endemic areas with poor sanitary conditions and persons with impaired GI defense mechanisms.

Since January 1991, more than 800,000 cases of cholera have occurred throughout Latin America [33]. Although this outbreak has resulted in an increase in cases in Americans, the risk still remains extremely low for those who exercise care in food and water consumption [33, 34]. An outbreak of non-01 *Vibrio cholerae* (0139) in the Indian subcontinent will further complicate cholera prevention [35]. The current vaccine is unlikely to have any protective effect against this strain.

IV. **Recommended vaccinations for travelers**

A. **Typhoid.** Typhoid vaccine is indicated before traveling to areas endemic for typhoid fever where fecally contaminated food and water are likely to be ingested [36]. Travelers to areas where *Salmonella typhi* is resistant to antimicrobial agents should also be considered for vaccination. The risk of typhoid has been estimated to be 0.7 per 1 million travelers to Northern Europe, 20.2 per million travelers to Mexico, and 188 per million travelers to India and Pakistan [37]. Of all cases acquired abroad, 39% of typhoid cases are in travelers to Mexico and 14% in those to India.

1. **Live oral vaccine** (Vivotif Berna, Swiss Serum and Vaccine Institute). This live vaccine utilizing the attenuated Ty21a mutant of *S. typhi* is equally effective and better tolerated by adults and children age 6 years and older than the earlier parenteral, whole-cell killed vaccine. The traveler takes one enteric-coated capsule with a cool to warm drink (<37°C) 1 hour before a meal every other day for a total of four capsules, beginning at least 2 weeks before departure [36]. Capsules should be refrigerated; however, if the vaccine is left at room temperature (20–25°C) for a few days, it usually retains potency. There is no evidence that simultaneous administration of oral poliovirus vaccine interferes with the immune response to either vaccine [38].

   This vaccine should not be given to HIV-positive individuals or persons taking antimicrobials, nor should mefloquine be given simultaneously [32, 38]. Doses of oral typhoid vaccine and mefloquine should be separated by at least 24 hours [5a]. Antibiotic treatment can be commenced as early as 48 hours after completing the vaccine series [38a]. The manufacturer currently recommends revaccination with the four-dose series every 5 years. It is likely that a pediatric formulation for those aged 4 years and older will be released soon.

2. **Parenteral whole-cell vaccine.** Although this vaccine has been available for many years, this killed vaccine is not fully protective (50–70%) and often causes 1–2 days of pain at the site of infection, sometimes accompanied by fever, malaise, and headache [5, 32, 36].

3. **Typhoid Vi polysaccharide vaccine** became available in the United States in early 1995. It consists of purified Vi capsular polysaccharide of *S. typhi*, is given in a single intramuscular dose, and should give approximately 70% protection for 2–3 years [31]. This vaccine can be given to persons 2 years of age or older at least 2 weeks prior to suspected exposure. Local and rare systemic adverse reactions may occur but they are less frequent than with the earlier parenteral vaccine (see sec. **2**) [5a]. Because of the decreased number of adverse reactions and the need for only one dose, the new formulation is preferred for children between 2 and 6 years old [5a]. When compliance is a concern in a patient who is a candidate for the oral vaccine, a single dose of the Vi vaccine intramuscularly may be preferred [38a].

B. **Meningococcal disease.** Most international travelers are at low risk for acquiring meningococcal bacteremia or meningitis [39]. Several areas of the world, however, have had epidemics of meningococcal disease, with consequences severe enough to warrant vaccination. **Trekkers in Nepal, travelers to the New Delhi region of India, religious pilgrims to Saudia Arabia, and long-term visitors to sub-Saharan Africa, Kenya, and Tanzania are at potential risk for meningococcal disease and should be vaccinated** [5, 39–41]. The meningococcal polysaccharide vaccine in the United States is polyvalent for groups A, C, Y, and W-135, and is now available in single-dose vials.

C. **Plague.** Plague vaccine is not required by any country and, because of uncertain efficacy and very low risk of disease, vaccination rarely is recommended for international travel [42]. Adult travelers who will reside in plaque endemic areas with unavoidable exposure to rodents and fleas can take tetracycline (500 mg qid) chemoprophylaxis [5]. The efficacy of this has not been established.

D. **Tuberculosis prevention.** Tuberculosis exposure in the developing world usually occurs as a result of prolonged contact with respiratory droplets from infected persons in a closed setting. For travelers with such exposure, pretravel and posttravel (2 months following return) tuberculin skin testing is indicated and is preferable to administration of the BCG vaccine [43]. For children who will have unavoidable exposure to tuberculosis and for whom other preventive measures such as prophylactic isoniazid cannot be used, BCG vaccine may be considered.

E. **Poliomyelitis.** Worldwide, much progress has been made in the elimination of polio [44, 45]. There have been no documented cases from the Americas since September 1991; however, the disease remains endemic throughout much of Asia and Africa. When vaccine use decreases, outbreaks of poliomyelitis have also occurred in the developed world [46]. The risk to the international traveler is extremely low [47]. In a study of 138 cases of paralytic poliomyelitis in the United States from 1973 to 1984, there were only 13 imported cases [48]. Nevertheless, travelers to endemic areas who are exposed to poor food and water sanitation should be immunized.

Oral poliovirus vaccine (Sabin; live attenuated, trivalent vaccine; OPV) is used for primary vaccination of children in the United States [49]. Because of the rare cases of vaccine-associated paralytic infection, OPV is not recommended as primary immunization of adults. With the first dose of OPV, the risk of paralysis in recipients and contacts of recipients is approximately one case per 1.4 million doses [50]. For all subsequent doses, one case of paralysis occurs per 41.5 million doses. **The risk is actually higher in contacts,** in whom nearly 60% of the cases occurred. Affected contacts usually have been unimmunized or inadequately immunized parents or relatives of a child who has been vaccinated (see Chap. 22).

1. **Primary vaccination with inactivated poliomyelitis vaccine of enhanced potency (eIPV) is recommended for persons 18 years or older** [51]. Although two doses of eIPV should be given before travel, if time is lacking (<4 weeks before departure), a single dose of either eIPV or OPV can be given after risks are explained.

2. If a person has completed or started a primary series with either OPV or eIPV, either vaccine may be used to complete the series or boost the patient.

3. **It is recommended that persons who have completed a primary series receive a one-time booster if traveling to an area of risk.**

4. Oral poliovirus vaccine and eIPV provide long-term immunity. They may be given with immunoglobulin. HIV-infected persons should receive eIPV.

F. **Japanese B encephalitis.** Japanese B encephalitis is a mosquito-borne encephalitis prevalent in many areas of the Indian subcontinent and Asia (Fig. 21-1). It has an unapparent-to-apparent case ratio of 50–500:1 but, among patients with symptomatic disease, the fatality rate is approximately 20%, and there is high morbidity in survivors [52]. The disease occurs primarily in young children and adults older than 65 years, from June through September in temperate zones (China, Japan [little to no risk], Korea, the lowlands of Nepal, Burma, Bangladesh, Cambodia, Laos, northern India and Thailand, and eastern Russia), and throughout the entire year in tropical zones (southern India and Thailand, Taiwan, Indonesia, Philippines, Malaysia, Sri Lanka, and Singapore) [53]. The risk for travelers to the Far East is extremely low. It has been estimated, based on the number of cases in expatriate travelers and the military, to be fewer than one case per 1 million persons. If the risk is based on endemic populations, it could be as high as one case per 5,000 to 20,000.

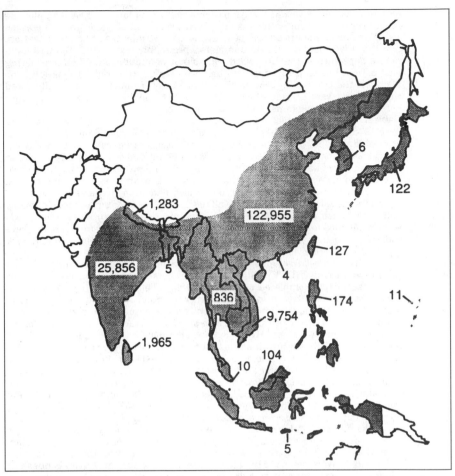

Fig. 21-1. Reported Japanese encephalitis cases by endemic countries and regions of Southeast Asia where viral transmission is proven or suspected, 1986–1990. (From T. F. Tsai and Y. X. Yu, Japanese Encephalitis Vaccines. In S. A. Plotkin and E. Mortimer (eds.), *Vaccines* (2nd ed.). Philadelphia: Saunders, 1994.)

Recently a monovalent inactivated viral vaccine purified from mouse brain (Biken, Osaka University, Japan) was released by Connaught Laboratories for use in the United States [53, 54]. According to the CDC, this vaccine should be considered for travelers spending 4 weeks or more in areas endemic for Japanese encephalitis, especially when there is rural exposure in areas of rice and pig farming [53]. Those planning prolonged residence in endemic countries also should be vaccinated. Therefore, most travelers to endemic countries will not need vaccination because they travel for less than 4 weeks and typically visit only urban and major tourist destinations.

The decision regarding whether to vaccinate the remaining travelers at risk would not be so difficult if the vaccine were completely safe. Although initial studies in the United States indicated that the vaccine was both safe and well tolerated, more recent work has shown that **local (≈20%), systemic (≈10%), and delayed-type hypersensitivity reactions may occur** [53–55]. **The delayed reactions are the most concerning** and have included urticaria, angioedema, anaphylaxis, respiratory distress and, rarely, encephalomyelitis, cardiovascular collapse, and death. Allergic reactions have been estimated to occur in 0.1–10 per 1,000 vaccinees [53]. Reactions can occur after any dose and may be delayed;

88% have occurred within 3 days but some began as late as 2 weeks following immunization. Persons with a history of urticaria or anaphylaxis are at increased risk. **Vaccine recipients should be monitored for 60 minutes after immunization, and the final dose should be completed preferably not sooner than 10 days before departure so that untoward effects may be monitored.** When considering vaccination, the clinician needs to balance carefully the risk of exposure, the ability of the traveler to protect himself or herself against mosquito bites, and the potential vaccine side effects. All travelers should be advised to practice personal protection against the *Culex* mosquito.

G. **Rabies.** The risk of rabies during travel is very low, only 10 cases in travelers from 1975 to 1984 [56]. Although most cases (8 of 10) occurred following the bite of a rabid dog [56, 57], many other animal species are capable of transmitting the rabies virus. Therefore, travelers should be informed about a rabies risk in endemic areas of Latin America, the Far East, the Indian subcontinent, and Africa. Vaccination of dogs in endemic countries is not a guarantee against transmission as some dogs reported to cause rabies cases had been previously vaccinated. Travelers should thoroughly cleanse all animal-bite wounds with soap, if possible, and should seek **postexposure** rabies immunization. **Preexposure** prophylaxis is recommended for persons living in or visiting for 1 month or more areas where rabies is a constant threat [58]. Countries that are rabies-free are listed in *Health Information for International Travel* [5].

The vaccine most frequently used in the United States is the human diploid cell rabies vaccine (HDCV). This vaccine can be administered intradermally or intramuscularly if completed more than 30 days before travel [58]. **If there are fewer than 30 days before departure, intramuscular administration is recommended to ensure development of immunity.** Preexposure immunization consists of three doses of HDCV or rabies vaccine absorbed (RVA), 1.0 ml IM (i.e., deltoid area) (see Table 21-1). Only HDCV may be administered by the intradermal (ID) route (0.1 ml). Preexposure immunization of immunosuppressed persons is not recommended. Routine serologic testing after preexposure immunization is not necessary unless the recipient is believed to be at risk for a diminished immune response. Simultaneous administration of chloroquine (and possibly mefloquine) for malaria prophylaxis should be avoided, because chloroquine may decrease the immunogenicity of intradermally administered vaccine [58]. If the vaccine is given intramuscularly, this interference is overcome. As with all intramuscular vaccines for adults, intramuscular rabies vaccine should be given in the deltoid muscle to ensure adequate absorption. Preexposure prophylaxis may provide protection when there is an inapparent exposure to rabies and when postexposure therapy is delayed. **Travelers should be advised that preexposure prophylaxis does not eliminate the need for prophylaxis after exposure** but simplifies it by eliminating the need for rabies immunoglobulin and decreasing the number of shots (see Chap. 4).

Because the risk of rabies to most travelers is low and the vaccine is expensive, preexposure prophylaxis is sometimes recommended to selected travelers rather than to the general population of long-term travelers [58a].

H. **Hepatitis prophylaxis**
1. **Hepatitis A.** Hepatitis A virus (HAV) is endemic throughout much of the developing world, where the risk increases with duration of travel, rural travel, and exposure to foods and liquids in areas of poor sanitation. Because HAV also occurs in persons on standard tourist itineraries, prevention should be considered for most people who visit the developing world [59]. The risk for HAV in travelers not protected by immunoglobulin varies from 1 to 10 per 1,000 travelers for a 2- to 3-week stay [60, 61]. See related discussion in Chap. 11.
   a. **Immunoglobulin,** a sterile preparation of antibodies (primarily IgG) with high titers against HAV, is available in the United States **for passive immediate protection against infection.** Immunoglobulin provides protection for 2 to 6 months, depending on the dose administered (see Table 21-1). It should be given on a regular basis to persons residing in the developing world for extended periods of time.
   b. **Hepatitis A vaccine.** An inactivated vaccine against hepatitis A was released in the United States in the spring of 1995 [62–63]. After a single intramuscular dose in adults and two doses in children, protective antibodies develop in 14–28 days. A dose at 6–12 months may provide protection for as long as 10–20 years. This vaccine is targeted toward the long-term (≥4 months) or frequent traveler (see Table 21-1).

c. **Pretravel hepatitis A antibody testing may be helpful for frequent visitors to the developing world or those with a higher likelihood of having had infection in the past,** such as persons older than 50, those born in or with prolonged residence in the developing world, and those with a history of hepatitis [64]. In those travelers who are anti–HAV (IgG)–positive, neither immunoglobulin nor hepatitis A vaccine are needed.

2. **Hepatitis B.** Vaccination against hepatitis B virus (HBV) has now been recommended as part of the schedule of routine immunizations in the United States [65]. It may be some time, however, before this is implemented in practice. Travelers at risk are those who will be in contact with blood or body fluid secretions: physicians, nurses, other health care workers and laboratory technicians, and those likely to have sexual exposure [59]. Travelers who will live for more than 6 months in countries with a high prevalence (5–20%) of hepatitis B surface antigenemia (such as parts of Southeast Asia, sub-Saharan Africa, and the interior Amazon basin) should also be vaccinated. Two recombinant vaccines have replaced the original plasma-derived vaccine. Intramuscular injections of hepatitis vaccine should be in the deltoid. **Persons immunized against hepatitis B also will be protected against delta hepatitis** as this incomplete virus requires actively replicating hepatitis B for survival [66] (see Chap. 22).

3. **Hepatitis E** now is recognized as a problem in Africa, the Indian subcontinent, Mexico, Russia, and the Middle East [67]. One outbreak in India affected nearly 80,000 persons [68]. Hepatitis E has also been acquired by US travelers [69]. Water that has been fecally contaminated, often after heavy rains in areas with inadequate sewage disposal, is the most likely source of infection [67, 69]. Pregnant women have a particularly high mortality. There is no evidence that immunoglobulin will prevent hepatitis E [69], and so proper preparation of food and purification of water needs to be emphasized (see Chap. 11).

Advice on Disease Prevention Other than by Vaccination

I. **Travelers' diarrhea**
   A. **Clinical findings.** Travelers' diarrhea affects 30–50% of visitors to developing countries [70–72]. Although illness usually is mild and lasts for only a few days, it can alter a person's plans. Travelers to Latin America, Africa, the Middle East, and portions of Asia are at highest risk. The risk is intermediate in some of the Caribbean islands and eastern Europe. The disease is transmitted through fecally contaminated food or liquids.
      1. **Etiology.** The causative agent is identified in fewer than three-fourths of cases. Enterotoxigenic *Escherichia coli* is the most common cause, accounting for approximately 50% of cases in which the etiology is determined. *Shigella* or *Salmonella* spp. are seen in 10–20% of cases. *Campylobacter* and *Vibrio* spp. and, less commonly, *Aeromonas* and *Plesiomonas* spp. also may cause diarrhea, especially in travelers to the Far East [71, 73]. Norwalk-like agents and rotavirus are implicated in approximately 20% of cases. *Giardia lamblia* is the most common parasite that causes diarrhea (approximately 5% of cases). Symptoms may appear after the traveler has returned to the United States and often persist for more than 2 weeks [74]. *Entamoeba histolytica, Cryptosporidium parvum, Isospora belli, Cyclospora* spp., and other parasites are reported infrequently [71, 75].
      2. **Clinical manifestations.** Travelers' diarrhea usually occurs during the first week after arrival in another country [70, 71, 76]. Diarrhea and abdominal cramps are associated with nausea and malaise. Temperature of more than 38°C occurs in only 10–20% of patients, and vomiting in fewer than 15%. Bloody, dysenteric stools are unusual (2–10%). The duration of travelers' diarrhea, even in persons who are not treated, is 3–4 days, with 60% of patients recovering within 48 hours.
   B. **Prevention**
      1. **Routine precautions. The best precaution against travelers' diarrhea is careful choice of food and drink.** It is particularly important to exercise these precautions when traveling with infants or small children as the consequences of diarrhea at this age may be considerable. A person should ingest only bottled

or carbonated beverages (bottled carbonated water and soda and beer), wine, heated drinks (coffee, tea, boiled water), well-cooked foods and meats (particularly seafood and shellfish), and fruits that can be peeled. Unpasteurized dairy products, tap water, ice cubes, food from street vendors, and fresh, ground-grown leafy greens and salads should be avoided. The most reliable way to purify drinking water is to bring it to a vigorous boil and to continue to boil it for several minutes and longer if at high altitude. If used properly, iodine preparations will kill most viruses, bacteria, and protozoan cysts [77]. *Cryptosporidium* may not be killed by iodine. Chlorine preparations are more sensitive to the effects of water temperature, pH, and turbidity. Small-volume water filters are said to be sufficient for purification of water; however, not all have been rigorously studied against several of the pathogens under field conditions [77].

2. **Antiperistaltic agents.** These should not be used for preventing travelers' diarrhea and should not be ingested when bloody diarrhea or high fever is present.

3. **Prophylactic bismuth subsalicylate.** The prophylactic use of bismuth subsalicylate liquid (Pepto-Bismol) (2 oz qid) or tablets (2 tablets qid) [71, 78] can reduce by approximately 60% the incidence of diarrhea in travelers. Persons taking aspirin-containing compounds may develop salicylate toxicity if bismuth subsalicylate is taken concurrently. **Patients who are allergic to salicylates or are taking salicylates or anticoagulants should not take Pepto-Bismol [79].** Some travelers may want to reserve Pepto-Bismol for use after ingesting food or liquids that they may fear are contaminated.

4. **Preventive antibiotics.** Several antibacterials (trimethoprim, 160 mg, and sulfamethoxazole, 800 mg, 1 tablet daily; trimethoprim, 200 mg/day; doxycycline, 100 mg/day; norfloxacin, 400 mg/day; ciprofloxacin, 500 mg/day) can decrease the incidence of diarrhea to 5–15% for the short-term traveler (<3 weeks) [71, 80], which may be similar to the incidence of diarrhea in persons who take precautions with food and water. **However, prophylactic antibiotics may cause serious allergic reactions in a small number of persons** (e.g., Stevens-Johnson syndrome with sulfonamides) or adverse effects in others (e.g., photosensitivity from doxycycline) and may contribute to the development of resistance to enteric flora. **Therefore, most healthy travelers should not take prophylactic medications to prevent this usually mild illness** [70, 79]. For the short-term traveler on a very important trip or with a medical condition that would be adversely affected by diarrhea, antimicrobial prophylaxis may be considered after potential risks are explained [71].

C. **Treatment**

1. **Fluid replacement and diet.** The most important treatment is to replace fluids and electrolytes lost in diarrheal stools (Table 21-2) [5, 81]. This may be the only treatment necessary for many adults and children because the diarrheal illness will be self-limited and of short duration. Oral rehydration must include glucose, sodium, potassium, chloride, and free water. Except in extreme cases, this may be accomplished in adults and older children by ingesting fruit juices, caffeine-free soft drinks, broths, and bouillons. These may be supplemented with salted crackers, rice, or toast. **Dairy products should be avoided initially** because lactose intolerance may occur.

Breast-fed infants should continue nursing. Bottle-fed children should also continue with lactose-free formulas. For oral rehydration, packets that contain glucose and salts at appropriate concentration after addition of purified water, are available in many developing countries and in the United States (Jianas Brothers Packaging Company, Kansas City, MO). Some formulas may be rice-based. Those who travel with infants and small children should strongly consider taking these packets with them. Children who experience persistent vomiting, bloody diarrhea, or high fever should receive immediate medical attention.

2. **Antimotility agents.** Drugs such as loperamide (Imodium) or diphenoxylate hydrochloride with atropine sulfate (Lomotil) relieve cramping and help to control diarrhea, allowing patients to participate in planned activities, which may be invaluable [82]. Loperamide is now available as an over-the-counter preparation and appears to be better tolerated than diphenoxylate-atropine in many patients, particularly the elderly. It is favored by most physicians advising travelers.

Table 21-2. Treatment of travelers' diarrhea[a]

Agent	Dose
Fluids and electrolytes World Health Organization composition[b]	Sodium chloride, 3.5 g/L Glucose,[c] 20.0 g/L Sodium citrate,[d] 2.9 g/L Potassium chloride, 1.5 g/L
Nonspecific agent Bismuth subsalicylate	1 oz q$\frac{1}{2}$h × 8 doses, or 2 tab q$\frac{1}{2}$h × 8 doses as needed
Antimotility agent[e] Loperamide, 2 mg	2 capsules initially, then 1 with each subsequent loose stool, not to exceed 8/d

Antibacterials[f]
    Ciprofloxacin, 500 mg
    Norfloxacin, 400 mg[g]
    Ofloxacin, 300 mg
    Trimethoprim, 160 mg, and
        sulfamethoxazole, 800 mg[h]
    Doxycycline, 100 mg[h]
	1 tablet bid
	1 tablet bid
	1 tablet bid
	1 tablet bid
	
	1 tablet bid

[a]Travelers who have a temperature of more than 38.5°C, severe cramping, and blood or mucus in their stools should seek prompt medical attention if symptoms do not resolve.
[b]Composition is in grams per liter.
[c]Sucrose (table sugar), 40 g/L, may be substituted.
[d]Sodium bicarbonate, 2.5 g/L, may be substituted.
[e]Antimotility agents should generally not be taken if there is a temperature of more than 38.5°C and blood or mucus in the stools.
[f]Antibacterials may be taken for 3 days.
[g]Treatment of enteric infections is not an approved indication for norfloxacin.
[h]Because in recent years resistance to TMP, TMP-SMX, and doxycycline is more common, the quinolones are often preferred if not contraindicated.
Source: Adapted from D. R. Hill and R. D. Pearson, Health advice for international travel. *Ann. Intern. Med.* 108:839–852, 1988.

Antimotility agents may predispose to complications, particularly in patients with invasive or inflammatory enterocolitis. Therefore, **these agents should not be used when there is a temperature greater than 38.5°C or if blood appears in the stool** [71]. They **should also not be used in children younger than 2 years.**

Liquid bismuth subsalicylate has been effective treatment for mild diarrhea [71]. Experience with it in children is limited [83], and it could potentially lead to salicylate toxicity if not used properly [84].

If symptoms persist beyond 48 hours after any of these agents are initiated, they should be discontinued and medical attention sought.

3. **Antibiotic therapy.** Patients with moderate travelers' diarrhea can be treated with 3 days of trimethoprim-sulfamethoxazole (TMP-SMX), doxycycline, or any of the new quinolone antibiotics such as norfloxacin, ciprofloxacin, or ofloxacin (see Table 21-2) [71, 85–88]. **The quinolones are likely to be more effective in areas with widespread sulfonamide and tetracycline resistance or where** *Campylobacter* **is endemic.** These appear to encompass most areas of the world except interior Mexico [71]. **Combined therapy of mild to moderate diarrhea using an antibiotic plus loperamide has also been shown promptly to improve symptoms** [71, 85, 89].

Patients with high fever or bloody diarrhea should seek medical evaluation. At times, medical attention may not be available, and empiric antibiotic therapy can be initiated by the traveler. This could also be done cautiously for children older than 2 years using TMP-SMX combined with erythromycin until medical help is obtained [71].

II. **Malaria.** Malaria is a febrile, flulike illness caused by one of four species of malaria parasites: *Plasmodium falciparum, P. vivax, P. ovale,* and *P. malariae.* Effective and safe prophylaxis against malaria has become increasingly difficult because the species that causes the most severe illness, *P. falciparum,* has become widely resistant to chloroquine phosphate and, in some areas, to other antimalarials as well (Fig. 21-2). A major goal of malaria prevention in travelers is to prevent *P. falciparum* infection because nearly all cases of fatal malaria are associated with this species [5, 90]. In the decade of the 1980s, most cases of falciparum malaria (82%) imported to the United States by US citizens originated in sub-Saharan Africa [5, 91]. Because many of these countries, especially Kenya and Tanzania, are popular tourist destinations, it is important to give travelers accurate information.

The risk of exposure to malaria depends on the itinerary and duration of a trip, time of year, and prevalence of *Plasmodium* spp. The risk for malaria by country is published both by the CDC in *Health Information for International Travel* [5] and by WHO [92]. A multifaceted approach is needed that emphasizes protection against mosquitoes, safe and effective preventive drugs, and plans for medical care if malaria occurs. **All travelers should be informed that no prophylactic regimen is 100% effective and that malaria can develop several months or longer after returning to the United States.** Travelers must be advised to seek prompt medical attention for any acute illness that might be malaria and to inform their physician of their exposure. **Important aspects of prevention include the following:**

A. **Mosquito avoidance.** The first step in malaria prevention is avoiding the female *Anopheles* mosquito, which typically feeds from dusk until dawn. During these times, travelers should wear long-sleeved protective clothing appropriate to the climate, avoid the use of perfumes, use mosquito repellents, and sleep under netting or in well-screened rooms. Mosquito repellents that contain diethyltoluamide (DEET) in a concentration of 30–35% protect best. Preparations of DEET, however, should be used cautiously in children, because of potential neurologic side effects [93]. DEET should also be used sparingly in pregnant women. The possibility of adverse reactions to DEET will be minimized if repellent is applied sparingly only to exposed skin or clothing; highly concentrated products are not used in children; repellents are not inhaled, ingested, or applied to mucosal membranes, the eyes, or irritated skin; and repellents are washed off after coming indoors [5]. If a suspected reaction to a repellent occurs, treated skin should be washed and medical attention promptly sought. Insect sprays containing pyrethrum can be used in living and sleeping areas. Clothing and netting may be

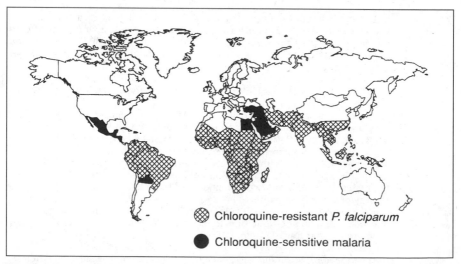

Fig. 21-2. Distribution of malaria and chloroquine-resistant *Plasmodium falciparum,* 1994. (From Centers for Disease Control, *Health Information for International Travel, 1994.* [HHS Publication no. 94-8280]. Atlanta: US Department of Health and Human Services, Public Health Service, 1994.)

sprayed or dipped in permethrin (Permanone), which will confer weeks of protection against mosquitoes [94].

B. **Prophylactic drugs. Current recommendations for antimalarial drugs and their dosing should always be consulted** because they are being reviewed on an ongoing basis as the efficacy and safety of various regimens are evaluated [5, 92, 95]. Table 21-3 lists antimalarial drugs in adult and pediatric doses. A recent report emphasizes that antimalarial chemoprophylaxis is very cost effective [95a].

   1. **For travel to areas with chloroquine-sensitive malaria.** Currently, only the Dominican Republic, Haiti, Central America west of the Panama Canal, Mexico, Egypt, and most countries in the Middle East have *P. falciparum* that still is sensitive to chloroquine. For travel to these areas, chloroquine phosphate, a four-aminoquinoline, remains the drug of choice. It can prevent clinical illness due to the erythrocytic stages of sensitive strains of *P. falciparum* and all other *Plasmodium* spp. No agent, including chloroquine, will prevent mosquito bites or kill sporozoites or hepatic-phase organisms.

      Chloroquine is taken as a single oral dose weekly, beginning 1–2 weeks before travel, each week in the malarious zone, and for 4 weeks after leaving the endemic area. Because of the risk of life-threatening toxicity with accidental ingestion or overdose of chloroquine in children, only the necessary amount of drug should be prescribed and it should be stored in childproof containers [96]. The infrequent side effect of minor GI distress can be reduced by taking the drug after meals. Rare cases of chloroquine-resistant *P. vivax* have been reported from Indonesia and Papua New Guinea [97].

   2. **Travel to areas where chloroquine resistance occurs**
      a. **Mefloquine (Lariam)** is highly effective against both chloroquine-resistant and sulfadoxine-pyrimethamine-resistant *P. falciparum* infections [98, 99]. Mefloquine alone has been recommended as the chemoprophylactic drug of choice for travel to areas where chloroquine resistance occurs [5]. In spite of the recent introduction of mefloquine, however, reports of resistance of *P. falciparum* have been received from West Africa and from Thailand's border regions with Cambodia and Myanmar (formerly Burma) [100, 101]. Thus, while mefloquine has been an important addition, it is not 100% effective.
         (1) **Dosage.** Mefloquine is taken as a single dose weekly (250 mg for adults), 1–2 weeks before travel, which will achieve adequate blood levels and

Table 21-3. Drugs used in the prophylaxis of malaria

Drug	Adult dose	Pediatric dose
Mefloquine (Lariam)	228 mg base (250 mg salt) per wk PO	15–19 kg: $^1/_4$ tab/wk 20–30 kg: $^1/_2$ tab/wk 31–45 kg: $^3/_4$ tab/wk >45 kg: 1 tab/wk
Doxycycline	100 mg/d PO	>8 yr old: 2 mg/kg/d of body weight PO up to adult dose of 100 mg/d
Chloroquine phosphate (Aralen)	300 mg base (500 mg salt) once per wk PO	5 mg/kg base (8.3 mg/kg salt) per wk PO, up to maximum adult dose of 300 mg base
Hydroxychloroquine sulfate (Plaquenil)	310 mg base (400 mg salt) once per wk PO	5 mg/kg base (6.5 mg/kg salt) per wk PO, up to maximum adult dose
Proguanil	200 mg/d PO, in combination with weekly chloroquine	<2 yr: 50 mg/d 2–6 yr: 100 mg/d 7–10 yr: 150 mg/d >10 yr: 200 mg/d
Primaquine	15 mg base (26.3 mg salt) per day PO, for 14 days	0.3 mg/kg base (0.5 mg/kg salt) per day PO for 14 days

day = day
Source: From Centers for Disease Control, *Health Information for International Travel* (HHS publication no. 95-8280). Atlanta: US Department of Health and Human Services, Public Health Service, 1995.

allow potential side effects to be assessed. Mefloquine is continued once weekly during travel in malarious areas and once per week for 4 weeks after a person leaves the malarious areas.

(2) **Side effects.** Mefloquine is well tolerated by most persons. However, because it is still a relatively new agent, serious adverse reactions should be reported to the CDC, Malaria branch.

  (a) Minor side effects with prophylactic doses include GI disturbance and dizziness, which tend to be transient and self-limited.

  (b) Serious adverse reactions (e.g., hallucinations, convulsions) have been reported rarely (one to two cases per 10,000) with prophylactic doses but more frequently with the higher doses used for treatment [102, 103].

(3) **Contraindications to the use of mefloquine**

  (a) Travelers with a known hypersensitivity to mefloquine.

  (b) Children weighing less than 15 kg, although according to CDC information, its use in this group is safe and may be considered when exposure to chloroquine-resistant *P. falciparum* is unavoidable.

  (c) Pregnant women in their second and third trimester can take mefloquine safely when exposure to chloroquine-resistant malaria is unavoidable, according to CDC guidelines [5]. Its use in the first trimester may be safe but should be monitored and reported to the CDC (770-488-7760). Mefloquine in pregnancy is not FDA approved.

  (d) Travelers with underlying cardiac conduction abnormalities but not those on beta-blockers if they have normal underlying rhythms.

  (e) Travelers with a history of epilepsy or psychiatric disorder.

  (f) There is no evidence that travelers involved in tasks requiring fine coordination and spatial discrimination, such as airline pilots, are adversely affected by mefloquine.

b. **Alternatives to mefloquine**

(1) **Doxycycline** alone is an alternative regimen for short-term travelers who are intolerant of mefloquine, for whom mefloquine is contraindicated, and for travelers to areas where mefloquine resistance is well documented as in the rural, border areas of Thailand [5, 95]. Doxycycline is taken daily, beginning 1–2 days before departure and continued daily during travel in the malarious areas and for 4 weeks after the traveler leaves the malarious area (see Table 21-3). Doxycycline is contraindicated in pregnancy and in children younger than 8 years. Potential problems with doxycycline include cost, photosensitivity dermatitis, and vaginal candidiasis (see Chap. 28N). If patients cannot minimize sun exposure, use of a sunscreen with a reasonably high protection factor (e.g., $\geq$ 15) is suggested.

(2) **Proguanil,** a dihydrofolate reductase inhibitor, can be combined with chloroquine. Limited data suggest that it is more effective in Africa than is chloroquine alone but not in Thailand and Papua New Guinea [5, 92, 105]. The lack of effectiveness may be due to drug resistance or lack of compliance. If travelers use proguanil, it should be taken as a daily 200-mg dose (for adults) in combination with weekly chloroquine. Proguanil is not available in the United States but can be obtained in Canada, many European countries, and many African countries.

(3) **Chloroquine alone with a self-treatment dose of sulfadoxine-pyrimethamine (Fansidar) should be carried** by the traveler [5, 95]. This regimen is an option for pregnant women and children weighing less than 15 kg. However, some authorities suggest that pregnant women not travel to malarious areas [5].

  In the event of a febrile, flulike illness that could be malaria, the traveler should first seek medical help. If help is not available, adults should take three sulfadoxine-pyrimethamine tablets at one time and continue to seek medical evaluation. The pediatric dose of sulfadoxine-pyrimethamine is based on weight. For children weighing 5–10 kg: one-half tablet; for 11–20 kg: one tablet; for 21–30 kg: one and one-half tablets; for 31–45 kg: two tablets; and for more than 45 kg, the usual adult dose is given (i.e., three tablets once only). **Sulfadoxine-**

pyrimethamine use is contraindicated in persons with a history of sulfonamide intolerance and in infants younger than 2 months [5]. Weekly chloroquine must be continued. Some experts prefer to use pyrimethamine with a short-acting sulfonamide, such as sulfadiazine, rather than sulfadoxine-pyrimethamine for empiric treatment because of sulfadoxine-pyrimethamine's small but defined risk for a severe cutaneous reaction [104]. This has occurred in 1 in 5,000–8,000 users of weekly prophylactic sulfadoxine-pyrimethamine. (**Note:** In some foreign countries, a fixed combination of mefloquine and sulfadoxine-pyrimethamine is marketed under the name Fansimef. **Fansimef** should not be confused with mefloquine, and it is **not recommended** for prophylaxis of malaria.)

3. **Prolonged exposure to malaria in areas intensely endemic for** *P. vivax* **or** *P. ovale* **may warrant terminal malaria prophylaxis with primaquine phosphate** to eradicate persistent hepatic forms of these species [5]. Missionaries, Peace Corps volunteers, or refugee camp workers with prolonged exposure may be at risk. Because primaquine may cause hemolysis in the presence of glucose-6-phosphate dehydrogenase (G-6-PD) deficiency, a G-6-PD level should be checked before prescribing this drug. Primaquine is **contraindicated during pregnancy** because the G-6-PD status of the fetus cannot be easily ascertained. Most travelers do not need to take primaquine.

4. **Malaria hotline.** Detailed recommendations for the prevention of malaria may be obtained 24 hours per day by calling the CDC Malaria Hotline at 404-332-4555 or by fax: 404-332-4565.

III. **Other diseases**
  A. **Dengue fever.** Dengue fever is a mosquitoborne arboviral illness characterized by the sudden onset of fever, headaches, severe myalgias and arthralgias (break bone fever), abdominal discomfort, rash, and mild liver enzyme abnormalities. The rash appears 3–5 days after onset of fever and may spread from the torso to the extremities and face. It has been a long-standing problem in the Far East, and during the last 10 years, dengue has also spread throughout the Caribbean basin and surrounding countries of Latin America [106, 107]. Several outbreaks have included cases that progressed to fatal dengue hemorrhagic shock syndrome, although most cases in travelers are self-limited and resolve [106]. In recent years, 20–50 cases of confirmed dengue have occurred in US travelers [108]. **Travelers should avoid the mosquito vectors,** *Aedes* **spp., by using the personal protection measures discussed for malaria. No vaccine is available.**
  B. **Schistosomiasis.** Acute schistosomiasis (Katayama fever), sometimes associated with severe neurologic sequelae, may occur in travelers [109]. **Travelers are exposed to the parasite while swimming in fresh water in endemic areas of the Caribbean, South America, Africa, or Asia. Travelers should avoid swimming, wading, or bathing in fresh water unless it is chlorinated.** In some areas, the popular opinion may be that the fresh water is free of risk (such as in Lake Malawi); however, cases of schistosomiasis have occurred in these situations, so the safest course is to avoid fresh-water swimming in endemic areas altogether. Swimming in salt water or bathing in fresh water heated to 50°C for 5 minutes or that has stood more than 48 hours is safe. Praziquantel is effective treatment for schistosomiasis caused by any *Schistosoma* spp. [95].
  C. **Sexually transmitted diseases.** Travelers who engage in sexual activity abroad are at risk for sexually transmitted diseases [60, 60a]. Drug-resistant isolates of *Neisseria gonorrhoeae* are prevalent in many areas, especially Southeast Asia and Africa, and syphilis, herpes simplex, and venereal diseases uncommon in the United States (chancroid, lymphogranuloma venereum, and granuloma inguinale) occur (see Chap. 13).

     The rapid spread of HIV infection throughout the world (particularly in recent years in Southeast Asia; more than 180 countries have reported cases of AIDS), especially in prostitutes, poses a major risk for transmission via the sexual route [110–112]. Despite these risks, many travelers still do not use adequate protection [113, 114]. Seroprevalence of HIV in urban female prostitutes from some Central and East African countries exceeds 50% [111, 115]. **Although the risk of transmission of HIV may be lessened by the use of condoms, diaphragms, and spermicides, the safest course for the traveler is abstinence.** Additionally, condoms manufactured outside the United States may not be reliably protective [116]. Genital lesions enhance the transmission of HIV and should be an absolute indication for abstinence [117].

Other Considerations
for the Traveler

I. **Jet lag.** Many travelers' first days are disrupted because jet lag affects their sleep and wakefulness cycles. While there is interest in dietary measures, these have never been rigorously evaluated [118]. Pharmacologic management of jet lag has been extensively studied [119]. Benzodiazepines may help travelers adapt by helping to maintain sleep when a traveler's body clock tells it to be awake. However, they should not be used during air travel. If these drugs are used, they should be started at the lowest effective dose, their duration of action should be matched with the time available for sleep, and they should be reserved for the first few nights only in the new time zone. Investigations with melatonin are promising [120], but the reliability of currently available preparations has not been rigorously demonstrated.

II. **Motion sickness.** There are several agents for motion sickness. For short-term use, over-the-counter preparations of diphenhydramine (e.g., Benadryl) are usually effective, especially for children, but the sedative effects may cause problems for adults. For longer trips, such as cruises, a sustained-release transdermal preparation of scopolamine (Transderm-Scōp) may be preferred. The package insert instructions for these products should be carefully followed and, after the disc is applied, the traveler should thoroughly wash his or her hands to remove any scopolamine.

III. **Sun protection.** Travelers should avoid excessive exposure to the sun to prevent heat exhaustion and sunburn. Sunburn can be caused by the effects of both ultraviolet B (UVB) and ultraviolet A (UVA) radiation. Most sunscreens offer excellent protection against both types of ultraviolet radiation; those with sun protection factors of 15 or higher protect best [121]. The major protective ingredient is paraaminobenzoic acid (PABA), although some persons may develop photoallergic reactions to PABA and, for them, PABA-free preparations should be used. Water insolubility is another feature that may extend the life of the sunscreen.

IV. **Skin care.** Skin problems are a major health issue for the traveler [121]. Insect bites, sunburn, dermatophyte infections, and cellulitis all can occur. Many dermatophytoses are made worse by warm and humid tropical conditions. Therefore, skin should be kept as clean and dry as possible, especially in skinfold areas. A tropical antifungal preparation can be carried by travelers prone to such infections. Arthropod infections such as scabies and lice can be avoided by carefully washing hands and clothes. Persons should refrain from scratching insect bites to avoid pyoderma and cellulitis. Shoes or sandals should be worn at all times to prevent penetration by various nematodes.

V. **Acute mountain sickness.** Acute mountain sickness, characterized by headache, nausea, vomiting, insomnia, and lassitude, may affect up to 50% of persons who rapidly ascend altitudes of more than 9,000–12,000 feet during mountain treks to Nepal, Africa, the Andes, or areas within the United States [122]. Acute mountain sickness occasionally is associated with the fatal complications of high-altitude pulmonary edema or cerebral edema. Acclimatization—spending a few days at an intermediate altitude of 5,000–7,000 feet—and gradual ascent to higher altitudes [122, 123] are the best prevention against mountain sickness. Acetazolamide (Diamox), a carbonic anhydrase inhibitor, may help travelers who start out at high elevations and gain a rapid ascent. It hastens acclimatization but will not necessarily prevent acute mountain sickness. Acetazolamide, 250 mg bid, may be taken 24–48 hours before and for a few days during the ascent. The drug increases urine output, can have side effects of circumoral and peripheral paresthesias, and is contraindicated in the sulfa-allergic patient. Dexamethasone has also been investigated for the prevention of acute mountain sickness, but its routine use is not recommended [122, 123]. The safest course of action if mountain sickness occurs is to descend.

VI. **Personal safety.** Travelers should be cautioned about personal safety. Although many travelers may feel at higher risk for exotic infections, far more deaths in Americans overseas are attributable to accidents, injuries, and homicides than to infectious diseases [124, 125]. Travelers should take care to avoid accidents and injuries during public and private transportation and to avoid swimming and diving in unfamiliar waters. Travelers may decrease the risk of personal assault by dressing conservatively, traveling in groups, and avoiding areas of potential risk. Avoiding personal injury will also decrease the possibility that a blood transfusion will be necessary. The US State Department (202-647-5225) will provide callers with updated travel advisory or visa information regarding any country, along with safety tips related to foreign travel and the names, addresses, and telephone numbers of foreign service locations.

VII. **Chronic illness and pregnancy.** Many travelers have chronic illnesses. Patients with severe chronic obstructive pulmonary disease should undergo pulmonary function testing with arterial blood gases to determine whether they will need supplemental oxygen during air flight [126]. Insulin-dependent diabetics should discuss with their physician the proper adjustment of insulin and diet schedules for time zone changes [127]. The pregnant traveler should consider the potential health risks to self and fetus by air flight, exposure to chloroquine-resistant *P. falciparum* malaria, and receipt of vaccinations and prophylactic medicines [9]. All travelers need to be cautioned about the effects of changes in diet, jet lag, altitude, and climate, and should carry on their person each of their medications in labeled bottles.

VIII. **Emergency medical help.** Emergency medical aid may be required during travel. Insurance companies may also provide coverage that includes baggage and trip cancellation protection, money for hospitalization, access to an interpreter, names of physicians, and air evacuation if necessary. The availability of medical care in remote areas may be ascertained by inquiring at US consulates or embassies or by visiting mission hospitals, which often are staffed by expatriates.

IX. **Travel and HIV infection.** The rapid spread of HIV infection has threatened the safety of the blood supply in many areas, especially if blood is not screened. There is no evidence that HIV is transmitted by mosquitoes. Blood products, previously used needles or intravenous administration sets, dental equipment, and other skin-piercing instruments should be avoided. Providing travelers with kits containing gloves, alcohol swabs, needles, and syringes in case an injection is needed has been considered. Some have also considered obtaining blood needed for transfusion from fellow travelers or members of the expatriate community who have tested negative for HIV and who have no risk factors for HIV infection.

For the HIV-positive traveler, issues of vaccine safety and efficacy, exposure to unusual or prevalent infectious agents overseas, and health care access all need to be considered and discussed in the pretravel visit [11, 115, 128]. Some countries now require HIV testing before granting entrance visas. **HIV infected travelers** who travel to developing countries appear to be at higher risk for acquiring foodborne and waterborne infections. Special guidelines have recently been suggested for the HIV-positive international traveler; these are summarized in Table 21-4.

For related suggestions on food and water related exposures, see Table 19-10.

X. **Transporting personal items for someone else.** The traveler should be advised to refuse if someone he or she befriends while in a foreign country (e.g., personal guide)

Table 21-4. Travel-related exposures in the HIV-infected patient

1. Travel, particularly to developing countries, may carry significant risks for the exposure of HIV-infected persons to opportunistic pathogens, especially for patients who are severely immunosuppressed. Consultation with health care providers and/or with experts in travel medicine will help patients plan itineraries (BIII).
2. During travel to developing countries, HIV-infected persons are at even higher risk for food- and waterborne infections than they are in the United States. Foods and beverages—in particular, raw fruits and vegetables, raw or undercooked seafood or meat, tap water, ice made with tap water, unpasteurized milk and dairy products, and items purchased from street vendors—may be contaminated (AII). Items that are generally safe include steaming-hot foods, fruits that are peeled by the traveler, bottled (especially carbonated) beverages, hot coffee or tea, beer, wine, and water brought to a rolling boil for 1 minute (AII). Treatment of water with iodine or chlorine may not be as effective as boiling but can be used, perhaps in conjunction with filtration, when boiling is not practical (BIII).
3. Waterborne infections may result from the swallowing of water during recreational activities. To reduce the risk of cryptosporidiosis and giardiasis, patients should avoid swallowing water during swimming and should not swim in water that may be contaminated (e.g., with sewage or animal waste) (BII).
4. Antimicrobial prophylaxis for traveler's diarrhea is not recommended routinely for HIV-infected persons traveling to developing countries (DIII). Such preventive therapy can have adverse effects and can promote the emergence of drug-resistant organisms. Nonetheless, several studies (none involving an HIV-infected population) have shown that prophylaxis can reduce the risk of diarrhea among travelers. Under selected circumstances (e.g., those in which the risk of infection is very high and the period of travel brief), the provider and patient may weigh the potential risks and benefits and

Table 21-4 (continued)

decide that antibiotic prophylaxis is warranted (CIII). For those individuals to whom prophylaxis is offered, fluoroquinolones, such as ciprofloxacin (500 mg qd) can be considered (BIII). Trimethoprim-sulfamethoxazole (TMP-SMX) (1 DS tab daily) has also been shown to be effective, but resistance to this drug is now common in tropical areas. Persons already taking TMP-SMX for prophylaxis against *Pneumocystis carinii* pneumonia (PCP) may gain some protection against traveler's diarrhea. For HIV-infected persons who are not already taking TMP-SMX, the provider should use caution when prescribing this agent for prophylaxis of diarrhea because of the high rates of adverse reactions and the possible need for the agent for other purposes (e.g., PCP prophylaxis) in the future.

5. All HIV-infected travelers to developing countries should carry with them a sufficient supply of an antimicrobial agent to be taken empirically should diarrhea develop (BIII). One appropriate regimen is 500 mg of ciprofloxacin bid for 3–7 days. Alternative antibiotics (e.g., TMP-SMX) should be considered as empirical therapy for use by children and pregnant women (CIII). Travelers should consult a physician if their diarrhea is severe and does not respond to empirical therapy, if their stools contain blood, if fever is accompanied by shaking chills, or if dehydration develops. Antiperistaltic agents such as diphenoxylate and loperamide are used for the treatment of diarrhea; however, they should not be used by patients with high fever or with blood in the stool, and their use should be discontinued if symptoms persist beyond 48 hours (AII). These drugs are not recommended for children (DIII).

6. Travelers should be advised about other preventive measures appropriate for anticipated exposures, such as chemoprophylaxis for malaria, protection against arthropod vectors, treatment with immunoglobulin, and vaccination (AII). They should avoid direct contact of the skin with soil and sand (e.g., by wearing shoes and protective clothing and using towels on beaches) in areas where fecal contamination of soil is likely (BIII).

7. In general, live virus vaccines should be avoided (EII). An exception is measles vaccine, which is recommended for nonimmune persons. Inactivated (killed) poliovirus vaccine should be used instead of oral (live) poliovirus vaccine. Persons at risk for exposure to typhoid fever should be given inactivated parenteral typhoid vaccine instead of the live attenuated oral preparation. Yellow fever vaccine is a live virus vaccine with uncertain safety and efficacy in HIV-infected persons. Travelers with asymptomatic HIV infection who cannot avoid potential exposure to yellow fever should be offered the choice of vaccination. If travel to a zone with yellow fever is necessary and immunization is not performed, patients should be advised of the risk, instructed in methods for avoiding the bites of vector mosquitoes, and provided with a vaccination waiver letter.

8. In general, killed vaccines (e.g., diphtheria-tetanus, rabies, Japanese encephalitis) should be used for HIV-infected persons as they would be for non–HIV-infected persons anticipating travel (BIII). Preparation for travel should include a review and updating of routine vaccinations, including diphtheria-tetanus for adults and all routine immunizations for children. The currently available cholera vaccine is not recommended for persons following the usual tourist itinerary, even if travel includes countries reporting cases of cholera (DII).

9. Travelers should be told about other area-specific risks and instructed in ways to reduce those risks (BIII). Geographically focal infections that pose a high risk to HIV-infected persons include visceral leishmaniasis (a protozoan infection transmitted by the sandfly) and several fungal infections (e.g., *Penicillium marneffei* infection, coccidioidomycosis, and histoplasmosis). Many tropical and developing areas have high rates of tuberculosis.

Note: Letters and Roman numerals in parentheses indicate the strength of the recommendation and the quality of the evidence supporting it. These are summarized in Chap. 19, p. 760.
Source: J. E. Kaplan et al. and the USPHS/IDSA Prevention of Opportunistic Infections Working Group, USPHS/IDSA Guidelines for the prevention of opportunistic infections in persons infected with human immunodeficiency virus: An overview. *Clin. Infect. Dis.* 21(Suppl. 1):S12, 1995.

asks the traveler to carry a package from one country to another (e.g., to another guide in the next country); illicit drugs or other illegal items may be hidden in the "gift" or "package."

The Returned Traveler

Many illnesses may not become manifest until after a person has returned from travel. Diseases with prolonged incubation periods such as giardiasis, amebiasis, viral hepatitis, typhoid fever, malaria, leishmaniasis, and tuberculosis can occur from weeks to months after a traveler's return [8, 60, 129]. Fortunately, for most travelers, serious illness is unusual; however, **diarrhea (11% of all travelers), upper respiratory tract infections (8%), skin rash (3%), and fever (2%)** are not uncommon [129]. Therefore, travelers should be informed that an illness presenting after their return could be related to travel and should be evaluated. Persons who were ill during their trip or who lived for a prolonged period in a developing country should receive posttravel medical follow-up.

When formulating a differential diagnosis, one needs to consider the incubation periods of potential infections, the geographic locations visited and the traveler's activities, the frequency of specific diseases among travelers to these areas, and the prophylactic measures used. **Febrile illness warrants immediate attention because it may be due to malaria or another potentially life-threatening pathogen.**

I. **Traveler's diarrhea.** Traveler's diarrhea may begin abroad or after return [71, 129]. Patients should be carefully examined and stools should be tested for blood and fecal leukocytes and sent for culture and ova and parasite examination, as discussed later. Although traveler's diarrhea in the returned traveler can be managed by hydration alone; prolonged or disabling cases may benefit from antibiotic treatment or loperamide (see Table 21-2 **and related discussions in Chap. 11**).

   A. **Noninflammatory diarrhea.** Most cases of acute traveler's diarrhea are due to toxigenic *E. coli.* Fecal leukocytes and blood are absent, and the temperature is normal or only mildly elevated. Treatment is best accomplished by rapid and appropriate hydration; antibiotics or antimotility agents may not be needed. Hydration, in most cases, can be accomplished orally with fluids, glucose, and electrolytes. Some cases of *V. cholerae* have been imported and may present as rapidly dehydrating diarrhea [33].

   B. **Bacterial dysentery.** The presence of fever higher than 38°C, bloody stools, or tenesmus suggests inflammatory enterocolitis caused by bacterial pathogens such as *Shigella* spp., *Campylobacter jejuni, Salmonella* spp., *Yersinia enterocolitica,* and invasive *E. coli.* **Fecal leukocytes usually will be in the stool.** Hydration is important, and treatment with an antibiotic, such as one of the quinolones in adults, frequently is indicated pending the results of stool culture. Loperamide and other antimotility agents should not be used. See related discussions in Chap. 11.

   C. **Amebic colitis.** Although not common among travelers, amebic colitis is a consideration in persons with dysentery. Gross or occult blood is almost always present in the stool, but fecal leukocytes may be pyknotic or absent. The diagnosis is confirmed by finding cysts or trophozoites in the stool or in biopsies or scrapings of colonic lesions. Metronidazole will eradicate tissue parasites and most cysts but should be followed with a luminal agent such as iodoquinol, paromomycin, or diloxanide furoate. Loperamide and other antimotility agents are contraindicated.

   D. **Prolonged diarrhea.** Noninflammatory diarrhea of more than 10 days' to 2 weeks' duration raises the possibility of giardiasis or other protozoal infection. Stools should be examined for trophozoites and cysts. Three stools properly examined usually will yield the diagnosis. Occasionally, empiric therapy is warranted if other etiologies have been excluded. Metronidazole is currently the drug of choice. Cyclospora and cryptosporidium may also be a cause of prolonged diarrhea. Stool acid-fast stains should be done to detect it. Treatment for cyclospora may be effective with SMX/TMP [129a]. See Chap. 11.

II. **Upper respiratory tract infections.** Upper respiratory tract infections are the second most common illness in travelers. Although not carefully studied, **most are presumed to be viral.** They should be managed symptomatically. Influenza should be considered in returned travelers with fever, myalgia, headache, coryza, and cough. Penicillin-resistant *S. pneumoniae* is common in some countries (e.g., Spain), and it seems prudent to test *S. pneumoniae* isolates for penicillin resistance (see Chaps. 9 and 28C).

III. **Dermatitis.** Travelers may suffer sun-related skin injuries, insect bites, drug reactions, or cutaneous infections due to *Staphylococcus aureus, Streptococcus pyogenes,* fungi, or other pathogens. Recently, several cases of cutaneous leishmaniasis have been described [130]. Systemic diseases can also present with cutaneous manifestations. The differential diagnosis of rash in the returned traveler is extensive and is reviewed in detail elsewhere [121].

Many American travelers and physicians are unfamiliar with **cutaneous leishmaniasis,** which is a potential risk to the traveler in the Americas, the Middle East and northern Africa [130, 130a]. Sandflies are the vectors. Untreated skin lesions typically evolve over weeks to months from **papules to nodules to ulcers** with raised indurated borders [130]. Researchers with extended stays (e.g., ornithologists) and intensive nocturnal exposure are at higher risk. For diagnosis, Giemsa-stained thin smears of dermal scrapings of ulcerative lesions and cultures of lesion aspirates (using a special medium available from the CDC Parasitic Branch [770-488-4050]) is advised. Serologic tests are not useful. Although chemoprophylaxis and vaccines for American cutaneous leishmaniasis are not available, many lesions might be prevented if travelers consistently minimize the amount of exposed skin with protective clothing. Repellents, screening, and bed nets of sufficiently fine mesh to keep out sandflies (which are approximately one-third the size of mosquitoes) will help reduce the risk [130].

IV. **Fever.** The differential diagnosis of fever in returned travelers includes diseases that are common in North America as well as those that are endemic abroad. The following are important considerations.

A. **Malaria. Malaria is the first consideration in a traveler returning from Africa or other malaria-endemic regions who develops fever.** The mortality of *P. falciparum* malaria among nonimmune Americans is 3–4%, primarily because of delayed or missed diagnosis. Symptoms of malaria can begin as early as a week after sporozoites are inoculated by an infected mosquito, but they may be delayed for months to years. Compliance with antimalarial chemoprophylaxis does not exclude the diagnosis.

1. **The symptoms** of malaria often are systemic and nonspecific and can include malaise, myalgia, anorexia, confusion, and headache, or they may be focal with headache, chest pain, abdominal pain, diarrhea, obtundation, or seizures. Although a tertian or quartan pattern points to the diagnosis of malaria, the majority of US travelers have **hectic fever patterns.** Splenomegaly may be present, but there are **no pathognomonic physical findings.**

2. **The diagnosis** of malaria is confirmed by identifying parasites in thick or thin blood smears; however, parasites may sometimes be sparse and therefore missed by inexperienced laboratory workers. **If no other diagnosis is apparent in a toxic-appearing, febrile traveler, empiric treatment for malaria should be initiated.**

3. **Therapy** for persons returning from areas with chloroquine-resistant *P. falciparum* is quinine sulfate plus either sulfamethoxazole-pyrimethamine or tetracycline [95, 131], unless the malarial smear shows another malaria species, not *P. falciparum,* in which case chloroquine alone may be reasonable therapy in the mildly ill patient who can be serially observed. Persons returning from areas with chloroquine-sensitive *P. falciparum* can be treated with chloroquine phosphate. Parenteral quinidine gluconate is administered in patients with severe *P. falciparum* infection who cannot take medications orally [95, 131, 132]. *P. vivax* or *P. ovale* infection is treated with chloroquine followed by primaquine to eradicate hypnozoites in the liver, provided that the traveler is not G-6-PD-deficient (Table 21-5). Infectious disease consultation is advised.

B. **Typhoid fever.** *S. typhi* is endemic throughout developing areas. A progressive increase in fever over a period of days, malaise, headache, abdominal symptoms, a pulse-temperature deficit, Rose spots, and eventually hypotension suggest the diagnosis. The isolation of *S. typhi* from blood, bone marrow, stool, or urine confirms it. See Chap. 11.

C. **Viral infections.** Some of the major viral infections encountered by travelers are discussed here.

1. **Arthropodborne viruses.** Dengue, yellow fever, and other arthropodborne viruses are endemic in tropical areas. Fortunately, cases of yellow fever are extremely rare among travelers owing to the high degree of efficacy of the vaccine. **Dengue,** in contrast, remains a risk, and there is no effective form of immunoprophylaxis. The incubation period is short (5–7 days), so a disease that begins a week or more after a traveler leaves the tropics is not dengue (see sec. **III.A** under Advice on Disease Prevention Other than by Vaccination).

Table 21-5. Treatment of malaria

Drug	Adult dose	Pediatric dose
P. vivax, P. ovale, P. malariae, and chloroquine-susceptible *P. falciparum*		
Chloroquine	600 mg base (1000 mg chloroquine phosphate) PO initially, followed by an additional 300 mg base (500 mg salt) 6 hours later, and again at 24 and 48 hr	10 mg base/kg PO initially, not to exceed 600 mg base, followed by an additional 5 mg base/kg 6 hours later and at 24 and 48 hr (total dose of 25 mg base/kg over 3 days)
Chloroquine-resistant *P. falciparum*		
Oral regimens		
Quinine sulfate plus pyrimethamine-sulfadoxine	650 mg q8h × 3–7 days 3 tab on the last day of quinine treatment	25 mg/kg/day in 3 divided doses 1–3 yr: 0.5 tablet 4–8 yr: 1.0 tablet 9–14 yr: 2.0 tablets
OR		
Quinine followed by tetracycline[a]	250 mg qid × 7 days	20 mg/kg/day in 4 divided doses × 7 days
OR		
Quinine followed by clindamycin[a]	900 mg tid × 3–5 days	20–40 mg/kg/day in 3 divided doses × 3–5 days
Mefloquine[b]	1250 mg single dose	25 mg/kg single dose
Halofantrine[c]		

Table 21-5 (continued)

Drug	Adult dose	Pediatric dose
Parenteral regimens		
Quinidine gluconate[d]	10 mg/kg loading dose (max 600 mg) in normal saline infused slowly over 1–2 hours, followed by continuous infusion of 0.02 mg/kg/min until patient is able to begin oral treatment	Same as adult dose
Quinine dihydrochloride[d,e]	20 mg/kg loading dose in 5% dextrose over 4 hr, followed by 10 mg salt/kg over 2–4 hr q8h (max 1800 mg/day) until patient is able to begin oral treatment	Same as adult dose
Prevention of relapse due to *P. vivax* or *P. ovale*		
Primaquine phosphate	15.3 mg base (26.5 mg phosphaste salt) per day PO × 14 days OR 45 mg base (79 mg salt) per wk × 8 wk	0.3 mg base (0.5 mg salt) per kg/day × 14 days

[a]Tetracycline and clindamycin are typically begun after 2–3 days of treatment with quinine to ensure that side effects from quinine are not confused with those of tetracycline or clindamycin. Tetracycline should not be given to children <8 yr.

[b]At this dosage, severe side effects such as nausea, vomiting, diarrhea, dizziness, psychosis, and seizures may occur. Medical Letter suggests giving adult single dose as 750 mg followed 6–8 hours later by 500 mg.

[c]Halofantrine has not been approved by the FDA for use in the United States for either adults or children. Cardiac toxicity from halofantrine can be fatal. Because of its potential side effects, other agents are preferred.

[d]Continuous cardiac [EKG], blood pressure, and glucose monitoring is recommended.

[e]Quinine dihydrochloride is not available in the United States.

Note: For a related reference see Medical Letter, Drugs for parasitic infections. *Med. Lett Drug Ther.* 37:99, 1995.

Source: Modified from D. J. Krogstad, Plasmodium species (Malaria). In G. L. Mandell, J. E. Bennett, and R. Dolin (eds.), *Principles and Practice of Infectious Diseases* (4th ed.). New York: Churchill Livingstone, 1995. P. 2424.

2. **Hepatitis A, E, B, and D.** Fever, nausea, vomiting, fatigue, and malaise suggest the possibility of viral hepatitis. If the liver enzymes are elevated, serologic studies are indicated to make the specific diagnosis (see Chap. 11).
3. **Measles, rubella, and varicella.** The common childhood viral exanthems must be considered in travelers with fever and rash. Measles has been acquired by young adult US travelers who failed to develop immunity following a single childhood immunization. Rubella and chickenpox may also be acquired abroad.
4. **Viral hemorrhagic fevers.** Fortunately, viral hemorrhagic fevers, such as Lassa fever, Ebola virus infection, and Marburg virus infection, are rare in travelers but must be considered in those with unexplained fever, prostration, multiorgan system involvement and coagulopathies [133]. Barrier nursing techniques are important in preventing the spread of these viruses to health care workers. If a returning patient has a syndrome suggestive of viral hemorrhagic fever, expert help should be sought, including consultation with the CDC.
5. **Other viral diseases.** Many other viruses can produce febrile diseases in returning travelers. Clinicians should consider infections endemic to the United States, such as cytomegalovirus, Epstein-Barr virus, and HIV, as well as viral infections that may have been acquired overseas.

D. **Rickettsial diseases.** Typhus and other rickettsial diseases may be acquired during travel [134]. Many are associated with a rash, but the rash may develop relatively late in the course of infection. If a rickettsial disease is suspected, empiric therapy with a tetracycline or chloramphenicol should be initiated.

E. **Other infectious diseases.** A number of bacterial diseases—such as brucellosis, leptospirosis, relapsing fever, plague, and *Legionella pneumophila* pneumonia— and parasitic disease—such as visceral leishmaniasis, Katayama fever (acute schistosomiasis), and Chagas' disease—must be considered in the differential diagnosis of fever in travelers who have had potential exposure in endemic areas [135].

F. **Noninfectious disease.** Drug fever should be considered in travelers who are taking antibiotics or other medications. Deep venous thrombosis with or without pulmonary emboli can occur in persons who have been seated for long periods of time.

V. **Eosinophilia.** The finding of eosinophilia (>500 total eosinophils) in a returned traveler suggests the possibility of a helminthic infection [136]. However, many persons will have increased eosinophil counts secondary to drug allergy or atopic conditions, so these should be ruled out before extensive investigations are performed for parasites. Although many parasites can cause eosinophilia, those worms that have an extensive tissue phase do so most commonly. *Strongyloides stercoralis,* heavy infestation with hookworms, *Schistosoma* spp., visceral larva migrans (*Toxocara* spp.), *Trichinella spiralis,* and filarial worms are the most common culprits. Appropriate studies are dictated by the clinical impression but may include three stools for ova and parasites, a string test for *Strongyloides,* blood smears for filaria, serology, and skin or tissue biopsies. Testing may need to be repeated after 3–6 months because of the prolonged time it can take for many filarial or intestinal helminth infections to become clinically manifest.

Suggested Readings for the Physician Advising Travelers

I. **Centers for Disease Control.** *Health Information for International Travel* (HHS publication no. [CDC] 95-8280). Atlanta: US Department of Health and Human Services, Public Health Service, 1995.

This publication is for sale by the Superintendent of Documents, US Government Printing Office, Washington, DC 20402; (202) 512-1800. **It is published annually** and lists all the countries with their requirements for yellow fever vaccination and their malaria risk. It provides information on each immunization that should be considered for travel and contains other detailed advice on prevention, focusing on malaria prevention. A section describes the health risks by geographic area. **This is an important and essential reference for any physician advising travelers.**

II. **Centers for Disease Control.** *Summary of Health Information for International Travel* (HHS publication no. 396). Atlanta: U.S. Department of Health and Human Services, Public Health Service.

Known as the **blue sheet,** this biweekly publication lists countries and areas within those countries (for yellow fever) that are reporting yellow fever, cholera, and plague. This publication is used in conjunction with *Health Information for International Travel* to determine whether yellow fever vaccine should be given. To request the biweekly blue sheet, write the US Department of Health and Human Services, Public Health Service, Centers for Disease Control, Center for Prevention Services, Quarantine Division, Atlanta, GA   30333.

III. *Morbidity and Mortality Weekly Report (M.M.W.R.).*

This CDC publication periodically reports official changes in vaccination requirements and disease outbreaks and is another source of information that can be invaluable in advising travelers. It is available in most hospital libraries. Individual subscriptions are available by writing: Massachusetts Medical Society, P.O. Box 9120, Waltham, MA   02254-9120.

IV. American College of Physicians Task Force on Adult Immunization, Infectious Diseases Society of America. *Guide for Adult Immunization* (3rd ed.). Philadelphia: American College of Physicians, 1994.

This publication is available from the American College of Physicians, Independence Mall West, Sixth Street at Race, Philadelphia, PA   19106-1572. It is an excellent review of vaccines for immunization in adults. Each vaccine is discussed thoroughly, giving background, indications, side effects and adverse reactions, and precautions and contraindications. Immunization of special groups, such as the immunocompromised host, are also discussed in detail.

For additional discussions of routine immunizations, see Chap. 22.

V. Superintendent of Documents, US Public Health Service. *International Certificate of Vaccination* (PHS-731). Washington, DC: US Government Printing Office.

This booklet is used to record required immunizations, other immunizations, and some personal medical history. Required immunizations need to be validated by a stamp issued by state health departments.

VI. World Health Organization. *International Travel and Health. Vaccination Requirements and Health Advice.* Geneva: World Health Organization, 1995.

The World Health Organization's version of *Health Information for International Travel.*

VII. Wolfe, M.S. *Health Hints for the Tropics* (11th ed.). Washington: The American Society of Tropical Medicine and Hygiene, 1993.

One of several practical text summaries that help provide travel consult data. Useful.

VIII. *Journal of Travel Medicine.*

A new journal (1994) published by the International Society of Travel Medicine devoted to reviews and primary literature in the field. For subscriptions, contact Decker Periodicals at 1-800-568-7281 or fax to 905-522-7859.

IX. Centers for Disease Control, Voice and Fax Information Service.

This service provides current information on health risks and prevention recommendations on topics such as immunizations, food and water hygiene, and disease outbreak bulletins for 16 regions throughout the world. It can be accessed 24 hours a day. For voice information, (404) 332-4559; for information by fax, (404) 332-4565. CDC internet address on the World Wide Web Server is http://www.cdc.gov.

References

1. Hill, D.R., and Pearson, R.D. Health advice for international travel. *Ann. Intern. Med.* 108:839–852, 1988.
2. Kozarsky, P.E., Lobel, H.O., and Steffen, R. Travel medicine 1991: New frontiers. *Ann. Intern. Med.* 115:574–575, 1991.
3. Hill, D.R. Immunizations. *Infect. Dis. Clin. North Am.* 6:291–312, 1992.
4. American College of Physicians Task Force on Adult Immunization, Infectious Diseases Society of America. *Guide for Adult Immunization* (3rd ed.). Philadelphia: American College of Physicians, 1994.
5. Centers for Disease Control. *Health Information for International Travel* (HHS publication no. [CDC] 95-8280). Atlanta: US Department of Health and Human Services, Public Health Service, 1995.
5a. Barnett, E.D., and Chen, R. Children and international travel: Immunizations. *Pediatr. Infect. Dis. J.* 14:982, 1995.
6. Superintendent of Documents, US Public Health Service. *International Certificates of Vaccination* (PHS-731). Washington, DC: US Government Printing Office.

7. Centers for Disease Control. Vaccinia (smallpox) vaccine. Recommendations of the Immunization Practices Advisory Committee (ACIP). *M.M.W.R.* 40(RR-14):1–10, 1991.
8. Wilson, M.E. *A World Guide to Infections: Disease, Distribution, Diagnosis.* New York: Oxford University Press, 1991.
9. Bia, F. Medical considerations for the pregnant traveler. *Infect. Dis. Clin. North Am.* 6:371–388, 1992.
10. Centers for Disease Control. Recommendations of the Advisory Committee on Immunization Practices (ACIP): Use of vaccines and immune globulins in persons with altered immunocompetence. *M.M.W.R.* 42(RR-5):1–18, 1993.
11. Vardinon, N., et al. Poliovirus vaccination responses in HIV-infected patients: Correlation with T4 cell counts. *J. Infect. Dis.* 162:238–241, 1990.
12. Steinhoff, M.C., et al. Antibody responses to *Haemophilus influenzae* type B vaccines in men with human immunodeficiency virus infection. *N. Engl. J. Med.* 325:1837–1842, 1991.
13. Centers for Disease Control. Diphtheria, tetanus, and pertussis: Recommendations for vaccine use and other preventive measures. Recommendations of the Immunization Practices Advisory Committee (ACIP). *M.M.W.R.* 40(RR-10):1–28, 1991.
14. Karzon, D.T., and Edwards, K.M. Diphtheria outbreaks in immunized populations. *N. Engl. J. Med.* 318:41–43, 1988.
15. Centers for Disease Control. Diphtheria outbreak epidemic—New independent states of the former Soviet Union, 1990–1994. *M.M.W.R.* 44:177–181, 1995.
16. Immunization Practices Advisory Committee (ACIP). Pneumococcal polysaccharide vaccine. *M.M.W.R.* 38:64–68, 73–76, 1989.
17. Centers for Disease Control. Measles—United States, 1988. *M.M.W.R.* 38:601–605, 1989.
18. Markowitz, L.E., et al. International measles importations, 1980–1985. *Int. J. Epidemiol.* 17:187–192, 1988.
19. Hill, D.R., and Pearson, R.D. Measles prophylaxis for international travel [editorial]. *Ann. Intern. Med.* 111:699–701, 1989.
20. Markowitz, L.E., et al. Patterns of transmission in measles outbreaks in the United States, 1985–1986. *N. Engl. J. Med.* 320:75–81, 1989.
21. Centers for Disease Control. Measles prevention; recommendations of the Immunization Practices Advisory Committee (ACIP). *M.M.W.R.* 38(S-9):1–18, 1989.
22. Onorato, I.M., Markowitz, L.E., and Oxtoby, M.J. Childhood immunization, vaccine-preventable diseases and infection with human immunodeficiency virus. *Pediatr. Infect. Dis. J.* 6:588–595, 1988.
23. Centers for Disease Control. Rubella prevention: Recommendations of the Immunization Practices Advisory Committee (ACIP). *M.M.W.R.* 39(RR-15):1–18, 1990.
24. Centers for Disease Control. Mumps vaccine. *M.M.W.R.* 38:388–400, 1989.
25. Centers for Disease Control. Prevention and control of influenza: Recommendations of the Advisory Committee on Immunization Practices (ACIP). *M.M.W.R.* 44(RR-3):1–22, 1995.
26. Centers for Disease Control. *Haemophilus* b conjugate vaccines for the prevention of *Haemophilus influenzae* type b disease among infants and children two months of age and older: Recommendations of the Immunization Practices Advisory Committee (ACIP). *M.M.W.R.* 40(RR-1):1–7, 1991.
27. Centers for Disease Control. Yellow fever vaccine: Recommendations of the Immunization Practices Advisory Committee (ACIP). *M.M.W.R.* 39(RR-6):1–6, 1990.
28. Centers for Disease Control. *Summary of Health Information for International Travel* (HHS publication no. 396). Atlanta: US Department of Health and Human Services, Public Health Service, 1995.
29. Snyder, J.D., and Blake, P.A. Is cholera a problem for US travelers? *J.A.M.A.* 247:2268–2269, 1982.
30. MacPherson, D.W., and Tonkin, W. Cholera vaccination: A decision analysis. *Can. Med. Assoc. J.* 146:1947–1952, 1992.
31. Immunization Practices Advisory Committee (ACIP). Cholera vaccine. *M.M.W.R.* 37:617–618, 623–624, 1988.
32. Skiest, D., and Hill, D.R. Current Vaccines to Prevent Enteric Infections. In M.J. Blaser et al. (eds.), *Infections of the Gastrointestinal Tract.* New York: Raven, 1995.
33. Centers for Disease Control. Update: *Vibrio cholerae* 01—Western hemisphere, 1991–1994, and *V. cholerae* 0139—Asia, 1994. *M.M.W.R.* 44:215–219, 1995.
34. Swerdlow, D.L., and Ries, A.A. Cholera in the Americas. Guidelines for the clinician. *J.A.M.A.* 267:1495–1499, 1992.
35. Cholera Working Group. Large epidemic of cholera-like disease in Bangladesh caused by *Vibrio cholerae* 0139 synonym Bengal. *Lancet* 342:387–390, 1993.

36. Centers for Disease Control. Typhoid immunization—Recommendations of the Advisory Committee on Immunization Practices (ACIP). *M.M.W.R.* 43(RR-14):1–7, 1994.
37. Ryan, C.A., Hargrett-Bean, N.T., and Blake, P.A. *Salmonella typhi* infections in the United States, 1975–1984: Increasing role of foreign travel. *Rev. Infect. Dis.* 11:1–8, 1989.
38. Cryz, S.J. Postmarketing surveillance experience with live oral Ty21a vaccine [letter]. *Lancet* 341:49–50, 1993.
38a. Canadian Communicable Disease Report. Statement on overseas travellers and typhoid fever. *Can. Med. Assoc. J.* 151:989, 1994.
    See related paper by M.S. Wolfe, Typhim Vi: A new typhoid vaccine. Infect. Dis. Clin. Pract. *4:186, 1995.*
39. Immunizations Practices Advisory Committee (ACIP). Meningococcal vaccines. *M.M.W.R.* 34:255–259, 1985.
    For a recent discussion see review in Canada Communicable Disease Report, Statement on meningococcal vaccination for travelers. Can. Med. Assoc. J. *153:303, 1995. This paper suggests that vaccination is not necessary for people making short-term business or holiday trips to areas of heightened meningococcal activity who will have little contact with or exposure to local populations in crowded conditions.*
40. Schwartz, B., Moore, P.S., and Broome, C.V. Global epidemiology of meningococcal disease. *Clin. Microbiol. Rev.* 2(Suppl.):S118–S124, 1989.
41. Centers for Disease Control. Epidemic meningococcal disease—Kenya and Tanzania: Recommendations for travelers, 1990. *M.M.W.R.* 39:13–14, 1990.
42. Centers for Disease Control. Human plague—India, 1994. *M.M.W.R.* 43:689–691, 1994.
43. Immunizations Practices Advisory Committee (ACIP). Use of BCG vaccines in the control of tuberculosis: A joint statement by the ACIP and the advisory committee for elimination of tuberculosis. *M.M.W.R.* 37:663–664, 669–675, 1988.
44. Centers for Disease Control. Progress toward global poliomyelitis eradication, 1985–1994. *M.M.W.R.* 44:273–275, 1995.
45. Hull, H.F., et al. Paralytic poliomyelitis: Seasoned strategies, disappearing disease. *Lancet* 343:1331–1337, 1994.
46. Centers for Disease Control. Update: Poliomyelitis outbreak—Netherlands, 1992. *M.M.W.R.* 41:917–919, 1992.
47. Kubli, D., Steffen, R., and Schär, M. Importation of poliomyelitis to industrialised nations between 1975 and 1984: Evaluation and conclusions for vaccination recommendations. *Br. Med. J.* 295:169–171, 1987.
48. Strebel, P.M. Epidemiology of poliomyelitis in the United States one decade after the last reported case of indigenous wild virus-associated disease. *Clin. Infect. Dis.* 14:568–579, 1992.
49. Centers for Disease Control. Poliomyelitis prevention. *M.M.W.R.* 31:22–26, 31–34, 1982.
50. Centers for Disease Control. General recommendations on immunization: Recommendations of the Advisory Committee on Immunization Practices (ACIP). *M.M.W.R.* 43(RR-1):1–38, 1994.
51. Immunization Practices Advisory Committee (ACIP). Poliomyelitis prevention: Enhanced-potency inactivated poliomyelitis vaccine—supplementary statement. *M.M.W.R.* 36:795–798, 1987.
52. Japanese encephalitis: Report of a World Health Organization working group. *M.M.W.R.* 33:119–120, 125, 1984.
53. Centers for Disease Control. Inactivated Japanese encephalitis virus vaccine. Recommendations of the Advisory Committee on Immunization Practices (ACIP). *M.M.W.R.* 42(RR-1):1–15, 1993.
54. Poland, J.D., et al. Evaluation of the potency and safety of inactivated Japanese encephalitis vaccine in US inhabitants. *J. Infect. Dis.* 161:878–882, 1990.
55. Andersen, M.M., and Rønne, T. Side effects with Japanese encephalitis vaccine [letter]. *Lancet* 337:1044, 1991.
56. Centers for Disease Control. Human rabies acquired outside the United States. *M.M.W.R.* 34:235–236, 1985.
57. Centers for Disease Control. Human rabies—Alabama, Tennessee, and Texas, 1994. *M.M.W.R.* 44:269–272, 1995.
58. Centers for Disease Control. Rabies prevention—United States, 1991: Recommendations of the Immunization Practices Advisory Committee (ACIP). *M.M.W.R.* 40 (RR-3):1–19, 1991.
58a. Canada Communicable Disease Report. Statement on travellers and rabies vaccine. *Can. Med. Assoc. J.* 152:1241, 1995.

59. Centers for Disease Control. Protection against viral hepatitis: Recommendations of the Immunization Practices Advisory Committee (ACIP). *M.M.W.R.* 39(RR-2):1–26, 1990.
60. Steffen, R., et al. Health problems after travel to developing countries. *J. Infect. Dis.* 156:84–91, 1987.
60a. Canadian Communicable Disease Report. Statement on travellers and sexually transmitted diseases. *Can. Med. Assoc. J.* 152:1826, 1995.
    A good summary of this important topic. Hepatitis B, hepatitis C, HIV, N. gonorrhoeae, *and* Haemophilus ducreyi *infections are a significant risk for individuals who engage in unprotected sex, especially with overseas commercial sex workers.*
61. Steffen, R., et al. Epidemiology and prevention of hepatitis A in travelers. *J.A.M.A.* 272:885–889, 1994.
62. Innis, B.L., et al. Protection against hepatitis A by an inactivated vaccine. *J.A.M.A.* 271:1328–1334, 1994.
63. Werzberger, A., et al. A controlled trial of a formalin-inactivated hepatitis A vaccine in healthy children. *N. Engl. J. Med.* 327:453–457, 1992.
64. Parry, J.V., et al. Rational programme for screening travellers for antibodies to hepatitis A virus. *Lancet* 1:1447–1449, 1988.
65. Centers for Disease Control. Hepatitis B virus: A comprehensive strategy for eliminating transmission in the United States through universal childhood vaccination: Recommendations of the Immunization Practices Advisory Committee (ACIP). *M.M.W.R.* 40(RR-13):1–24, 1991.
66. Hadler, S.C., et al. Delta virus infection and severe hepatitis. An epidemic in the Yucpa Indians of Venezuela. *Ann. Intern. Med.* 100:339–344, 1984.
67. Krawczynski, K. Hepatitis E. *Hepatology* 17:932–941, 1993.
68. Waik, S.R., et al. A large waterborne outbreak viral hepatitis E epidemic in Kanpur, India. *Bull. World Health Organ.* 70.597–605, 1992.
69. Centers for Disease Control. Hepatitis E among U.S. travelers, 1989–1992. *M.M.W.R.* 42:1–4, 1993.
70. National Institutes of Health Consensus Conference. Travelers' diarrhea. *J.A.M.A.* 253:2700–2704, 1985.
71. DuPont, H.L., and Ericsson, C.D. Prevention and treatment of traveler's diarrhea. *N. Engl. J. Med.* 328:1821–1827, 1993.
72. Guerrant, R.L., and Bobak, D.A. Bacterial and protozoal gastroenteritis. *N. Engl. J. Med.* 325:327–340, 1991.
73. Taylor, D.N., et al. Etiology of diarrhea among travelers and foreign residents in Nepal. *J.A.M.A.* 260:1245–1248, 1988.
74. Hill, D.R. Giardiasis: Issues in management and treatment. *Infect. Dis. Clin. North Am.* 7:503–525, 1993.
75. Ortega, Y.R., et al. *Cyclospora* species—a new protozoan pathogen of humans. *N. Engl. J. Med.* 328:1308–1312, 1993.
76. Steffen, R., et al. Epidemiology of diarrhea in travelers. *J.A.M.A.* 249:1176–1180, 1983.
77. Ongerth, J.E., et al. Backcountry water treatment to prevent giardiasis. *Am. J. Public Health* 79:1633–1637, 1989.
78. DuPont, H.L., et al. Prevention of travelers' diarrhea by the tablet form of bismuth subsalicylate. *J.A.M.A.* 257:1347–1350, 1987.
79. Medical Letter. Advice for travelers. *Med. Lett. Drugs Ther.* 36:41–44, 1994 and update 38:17, 1996.
80. DuPont, H.L., et al. Prevention of travelers' diarrhea with trimethoprim-sulfamethoxazole and trimethoprim alone. *Gastroenterology* 84:75–80, 1983.
81. Avery, M.E., and Snyder, J.D. Oral therapy for acute diarrhea. The underused simple solution. *N. Engl. J. Med.* 323:891–894, 1990.
82. Johnson, P.C., et al. Comparison of loperamide with bismuth subsalicylate for the treatment of acute travelers' diarrhea. *J.A.M.A.* 255:757–760, 1986.
83. Figueroa-Quintanilla, D., et al. A controlled trial of bismuth subsalicylate in infants with acute watery diarrheal disease. *N. Engl. J. Med.* 328:1653–1658, 1993.
84. Barry, M. Medical considerations for international travel with infants and older children. *Infect. Dis. Clin. North Am.* 6:389–404, 1992.
85. Ericsson, C.D., et al. Treatment of traveller's diarrhea with sulfamethoxazole and trimethoprim and loperamide. *J.A.M.A.* 263:257–261, 1990.
86. Ericsson, C.D., et al. Ciprofloxacin or trimethoprim-sulfamethoxazole as initial therapy for travelers' diarrhea. *Ann. Intern. Med.* 106:216–220, 1987.
87. Wiström, J., et al. Short-term self-treatment of travellers' diarrhea with norfloxacin: A placebo-controlled study *J. Antimicrob. Chemother.* 23:905–913, 1989.

88. DuPont, H.L., et al. Five versus three days of ofloxacin therapy of traveller's diarrhea: A placebo-controlled study. *Antimicrob. Agents Chemother.* 36:87–91, 1992.
89. Taylor, D.N., et al. Treatment of travelers' diarrhea: Ciprofloxacin plus loperamide compared with ciprofloxacin alone. A placebo-controlled, randomized trial. *Ann. Intern. Med.* 114:731–734, 1991.
90. Greenberg, A.E., and Lobel, H.O. Mortality from *Plasmodium falciparum* malaria in travelers from the United States, 1959 to 1987. *Ann. Intern. Med.* 113:326–327, 1990.
91. Lackritz, E.M., et al. Imported *Plasmodium falciparum* malaria in American travelers to Africa. Implications for prevention strategies. *J.A.M.A.* 265:383–385, 1991.
92. World Health Organization. *International Travel and Health. Vaccination Requirements and Health Advice.* Geneva: World Health Organization, 1995. Pp. 67–82.
93. Roland, E.H., Jan, J.E., and Rigg, J.M. Toxic encephalopathy in a child after brief exposure to insect repellents. *Can. Med. Assoc. J.* 132:155–156, 1985.
94. Alonso, P.L., et al. A malaria control trial using insecticide-treated bed nets and targeted chemoprophylaxis in a rural area of The Gambia, West Africa: 6. The impact of the interventions on mortality and morbidity from malaria. *Trans. R. Soc. Trop. Med. Hyg.* 87(Suppl. 2):37–44, 1993.
95. Medical Letter. Drugs for parasitic infections. *Med. Lett. Drugs Ther.* 37:99, 1995.
95a. Behrens, R.H., and Roberts, J.A. Is travel prophylaxis worthwhile? Economic appraisal of prophylactic measures against malaria, hepatitis A, and typhoid in travellers. *Br. Med. J.* 309:918, 1995.
Controversial report suggesting hepatitis A and typhoid prophylaxis may not be cost-effective. See follow-up commentary in Br. Med. J. *310:61, 401, 1995.*
96. Centers for Disease Control. Childhood chloroquine poisonings—Wisconsin and Washington. *M.M.W.R.* 37:437–439, 1988.
97. Baird, J.K., et al. Resistance to chloroquine by *Plasmodium vivax* in Irian Jaya, Indonesia. *Am. J. Trop. Med. Hyg.* 44:547–552, 1991.
98. Lobel, H.O., et al. Long-term malaria prophylaxis with weekly mefloquine. *Lancet* 341:848–851, 1993.
99. Steffen, R., et al. Mefloquine compared with other malaria chemoprophylactic regimens in tourists visiting East Africa. *Lancet* 341:1299–1303, 1993.
100. Fontanet, A.L., et al. High prevalence of mefloquine-resistant falciparum in eastern Thailand. *Bull. World Health Organ.* 71:377–383, 1993.
101. Brasseur, P., et al. Multi-drug resistant falciparum malaria in Cameroon in 1987–1988: II. Mefloquine resistance confirmed in vivo and in vitro and its correlation with quinine resistance. *Am. J. Trop. Med. Hyg.* 46:8–14, 1992.
102. Weinke, T., et al. Neuropsychiatric side effects after the use of mefloquine. *Am. J. Trop. Med. Hyg.* 45:86–91, 1991.
103. Bem, J.L., Kerr, L., and Sturchler, D. Mefloquine prophylaxis: An overview of spontaneous reports of severe psychiatric reactions and convulsions. *J. Trop. Med. Hyg.* 95:167–179, 1992.
104. Miller, K.D., et al. Severe cutaneous reactions among American travelers using pyrimethamine-sulfadoxine (Fansidar) for malaria prophylaxis. *Am. J. Trop. Med. Hyg.* 35:451–458, 1986.
105. Fogh, S., et al. Malaria chemoprophylaxis in travellers to East Africa: A comparative prospective study of chloroquine plus proguanil with chloroquine plus sulfadoxine-pyrimethamine. *Br. Med. J.* 296:820–822, 1988.
106. Dengue and dengue hemorrhagic fever in the Americas, 1986. *M.M.W.R.* 37:129–131, 1988.
107. Malison, M.D., and Waterman, S.H. Dengue fever in the United States. A report of a cluster of imported cases and review of the clinical, epidemiologic, and Public Health aspects of the disease. *J.A.M.A.* 249:496–500, 1983.
108. Centers for Disease Control. Imported dengue—United States, 1993–1994. *M.M.W.R.* 44:353, 1995.
For diagnosis of dengue, acute and convalescent serum samples should be obtained for viral isolation and serodiagnosis through the state health department and/or the CDC's Dengue Branch, San Juan, Puerto Rico (809-766-5181).
Dengue fever recently has been reported to be on the increase in the Caribbean (and Central America), with over 1,500 cases reported in the Caribbean. Outbreaks were reported in Belize, British Virgin Islands, Barbados, Dominica, Grenada, Guadaloupe, Guyana, Jamaica, Martinique, Montserrat, Puerto Rico, St. Vincent, Trinidad, and Tobago. See A. Manning, Caribbean caution: Dengue fever rising. USA Today Nov. 24, 1995.

Plate I. Rashes and Skin Lesions

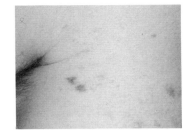

A. Meningococcal rash.

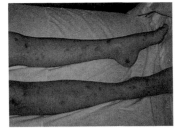

B. Meningococcal rash.

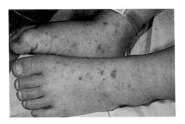

C. Meningococcal rash.

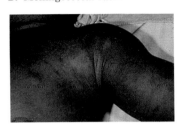

D. Meningococcal rash.

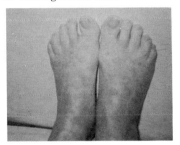

E. Methicillin drug rash.

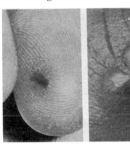

F. Disseminated gonococcal skin lesion.

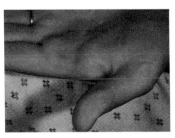

G. Disseminated gonococcal skin lesion.

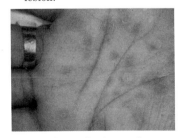

H. Macular rash of secondary syphilis.

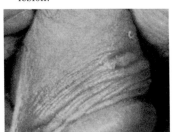

I. Herpes simplex lesion.

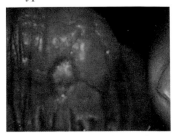

J. Primary syphilis (chancre).

, and **J** courtesy of Dr. D.O. Pollock, Bassett Healthcare, Cooperstown, NY; **F** courtesy of Dr. K.K. Holmes, U.S. Public Health Service Hospital, Seattle, and American College of Physicians, Philadelphia; **G** courtesy of Dr. W.A. Franck, Bassett Healthcare, Cooperstown, NY; **I** courtesy of Dr. J.D.J. Parker and Mosby–Year Book, Chicago.

Plate II. Scabies

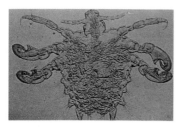

A. Crab louse.

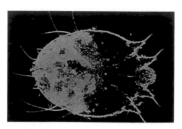

B. Scabie mite.

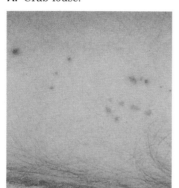

C. Skin rash of scabies.

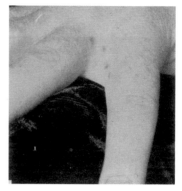

D. Skin rash of scabies.

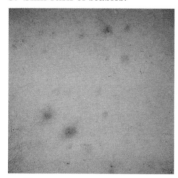

E. Skin rash of scabies.

A and **B** courtesy of Reed and Carnrick Pharmaceutical Co., Jersey City, NJ; **C** courtesy of Dr. A.S. Lurie and Cliggott Publishing Co., Greenwich, CT; **D** courtesy of Dr. L.C. Parish and Cliggott Publishing Co., Greenwich, CT; **E** courtesy of Dr. D.O. Pollock, Bassett Healthcare, Cooperstown, NY.

Plate III. Miscellaneous Disorders

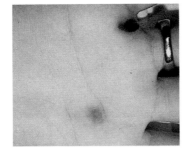

A. *Candida* skin lesions.

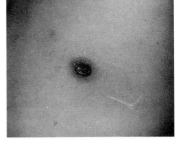

B. Ecthyma gangrenosum.

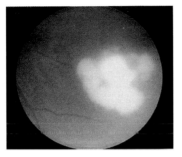

C. *Candida* ophthalmitis.

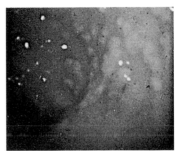

E. Pseudomembranous colitis (sigmoidoscopy view).

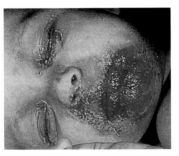

D. Staphylococcal scaled skin syndrome.

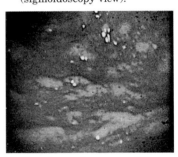

E. Pseudomembranous colitis (sigmoidoscopy view).

A courtesy of Dr. D. Armstrong, Memorial Sloane-Kettering Cancer Institute, New York; **C** courtesy of Dr. T.A. Farrell, Bassett Healthcare, Cooperstown, NY; **E** courtesy of Dr. F.J. Tedesco, Medical College of Georgia, Augusta, GA, and American College of Physicians, Philadelphia.

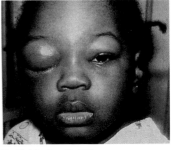

F. Orbital cellulitis.

Plate IV. Lyme Disease

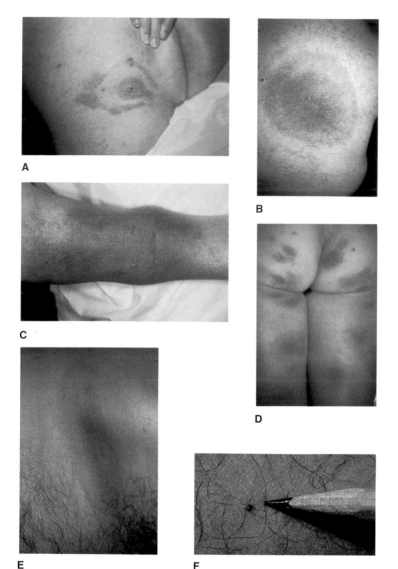

A–E. Skin lesions show examples of erythema migrans (see text discussion).
F. Actual deer tick compared to a pencil point.

A–E courtesy of Dr. B.W. Berger, Department of Dermatology, New York University School of Medicine, New York (**A–C** reprinted from B.W. Berger, Dermatologic manifestations of Lyme Disease. *Rev. Infect. Dis.* 11[Suppl.]:S1475, 1989.); **F** reprinted from M.H. Zaki and D.C. Graham, *Lyme Disease.* Happauge, NY: Suffolk County Department of Health Services, 1990.

109. Centers for Disease Control. Schistosomiasis in U.S. Peace Corps volunteers—Malawi, 1992. *M.M.W.R.* 42:565–570, 1993.
110. World Health Organization. Acquired immunodeficiency syndrome (AIDS)—data as of 30 June 1993. *Weekly Epidemiol. Rec.* 68:193–196, 1993.
111. Mann, J.M., Tarantola, D., and Netter, T. *AIDS in the World.* Boston: Harvard University Press, 1993.
112. Padian, N.S. Heterosexual transmission of acquired immunodeficiency syndrome: International perspectives and national projections. *Rev. Infect. Dis.* 9:947–960, 1987.
113. Gillies, P., et al. HIV-related risk behavior in UK holiday-makers. *AIDS* 6:339–341, 1992.
114. Howeling, H., and Coutinho, R.A. Needlesticks and Sexual Behavior Among Dutch Expatriates in Sub-Saharan Africa. In H.O. Lobel, R. Steffen, and P.E. Kozarsky (eds.), *Travel Medicine 2.* Atlanta: International Society of Travel Medicine. 1992. Pp. 204–206.
115. von Reyn, C.F., Mann, J.M., and Chin, J. International travel and HIV infection. *Bull World Health Organ.* 68:251–259, 1990.
116. Centers for Disease Control. Update: Barrier protection against HIV infection and other sexually transmitted diseases. *M.M.W.R.* 42:589–591, 597, 1993.
117. Telzak, E.E., et al. HIV-1 seroconversion in patients with and without genital ulcer disease. A prospective study. *Ann. Intern. Med.* 119:1181–1186, 1993.
118. Ehert, C.F., and Scanlon, L.W. *Overcoming Jet Lag.* New York: Berkley Books, 1983.
119. Jet lag and its pharmacology [editorial]. *Lancet* 2:493–494, 1986.
120. Petrie, K.J., Dawson, A.G. Recent developments in the treatment of jet lag. *J. Trav. Med.* 1:79–83, 1994.
121. Kelsall, B.L., and Pearson, R.D. Evaluation of skin problems. *Infect. Dis. Clin. North Am.* 6:441–472, 1992.
     See related paper by E. Caumes et al., Dermatoses associated with travel to tropical countries: A prospective study of the diagnosis and management of 269 patients presenting to a tropical disease unit. Clin. Infect. Dis. 20:542, 1995.
122. Johnson, T.S., and Rock, P.B. Current concepts. Acute mountain sickness. *N. Engl. J. Med.* 319:841–845, 1988.
     For related discussions see S. Bezruchka, High-altitude medicine. Med. Clin. North Am. 76:1481, 1992; and C.C.W. Hsia, Southwestern internal medicine conference: Pulmonary complications of high altitude exposure. Am. J. Med. Sci. 307:448, 1994.
123. Medical Letter. High altitude sickness. *Med. Lett. Drugs Ther.* 34:84–86, 1992.
124. Baker, T.D., Hargarten, S.W., and Guptill, K.S. The uncounted dead—American civilians dying overseas. *Public Health Rep.* 107:155–159, 1992.
125. Frame, J.D., Lange, W.R., and Frankenfield, D.L. Mortality trends of American missionaries in Africa, 1945–1985. *Am. J. Trop. Med. Hyg.* 46:686–690, 1992.
126. Gong, H. Advising patients with pulmonary diseases on air travel [editorial]. *Ann. Intern. Med.* 111:349–351, 1989.
127. Benson, E. Management of diabetes during intercontinental travel. *Bull. Mason Clin.* 38:145–151, 1985.
128. Wilson, M.E., von Reyn, C.F., and Fineberg, H.V. Infections in HIV-infected travelers: Risks and preventions. *Ann. Intern. Med.* 114:582–592, 1991.
129. Hill, D.R. Evaluation of the returned traveler. *Yale J. Biol. Med.* 65:343–356, 1992.
129a. Hoge, C.W., et al. Placebo-controlled trial of co-trimoxazole for cyclospora infection among travellers and foreign residents in Nepal. *Lancet* 345:691–693, 1995.
130. Herwaldt, B.L., Stokes, S.L., and Juranek, D.D. American cutaneous leishmaniasis in U.S. travelers. *Ann. Intern. Med.* 118:779–784, 1993.
130a. Melby, P.C., et al. Cutaneous leishmaniasis: Review of 59 cases seen at the National Institutes of Health. *Clin. Infect. Dis.* 15:924–937, 1992.
131. Wyler, D.J. Malaria: Overview and update. *Clin. Infect. Dis.* 16:449–458, 1993.
132. Centers for Disease Control. Treatment of severe *Plasmodium falciparum* malaria with quinidine gluconate: Discontinuation of parenteral quinine from CDC drug service. *M.M.W.R.* 40:239, 1991.
133. Centers for Disease Control. Update: Management of patients with suspected viral hemorrhagic fever—United States. *M.M.W.R.* 44:475–479, 1995.
134. Wilson, M.E., Brush, A.D., and Meany, M.C. Imported rickettsial disease: Clinical and epidemiologic features. *Am. J. Med.* 87:233–234, 1989.
135. Strickland, G.T. (ed.). *Hunter's Tropical Medicine* (7th ed.). Philadelphia: Saunders, 1991.
136. Wolfe, M.S. Eosinophilia in the returning traveler. *Infect. Dis. Clin. North Am.* 6:489–508, 1992.

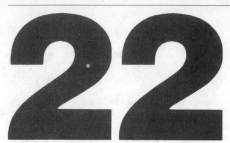

Immunizations

Paul J. Edelson

Immunization has been an effective, cost-efficient tool for preventing a wide range of bacterial, viral, and toxic diseases [1, 2] and has played a major role in controlling or eliminating such diseases as smallpox, poliomyelitis, and congenital rubella. Until recently, in the United States, most vaccination programs were directed primarily at universal childhood immunization, and childhood immunization remains the primary control strategy for diphtheria, pertussis, tetanus, poliomyelitis, measles, mumps, rubella, and life-threatening *Haemophilus influenzae* disease. However, major programs for adult immunization against hepatitis B, pneumococcal sepsis, and influenza have been developed in the past several years [3], making prophylactic immunization an important aspect of primary care at all ages. In addition, the development of new vaccines (e.g., for varicella and hepatitis A), passage of the National Childhood Vaccine Injury Act [4], and changing patterns of epidemic disease have affected our practice responsibilities for immunization of the adult patient [5]. Perhaps most importantly, immunization levels in some children [6] and young adults [7] have been disturbingly low until recently, threatening the resurgence of such nearly controlled diseases as measles and pertussis, and new immunization strategies are actively being developed for programs based in the office, hospital, and emergency room [8].

For example, on October 1, 1994, the US Department of Health and Human Services implemented the Vaccines for Children (VFC) program, which will provide free vaccine to children at participating private and public health care provider sites of their choice. Children who are eligible for free vaccines include those on Medicaid, those without insurance, and Native Americans or Alaskan Natives. In addition, children whose insurance does not cover vaccination (i.e., who are underinsured) can receive vaccines through the VFC at federally qualified health centers and rural health clinics. Other children can receive free vaccines at public clinics under existing programs [6].

Vaccination recommendations have now been formulated to address the special needs of such groups as adolescents, the elderly, the homeless, college students, prisoners, immunocompromised patients, and hospital employees.

Reports of the recommendations of the US Advisory Committee on Immunization Practices (ACIP) of the US Public Health Service are published in **Morbidity and Mortality Weekly Reports,** issued by the Centers for Disease Control and Prevention (CDC), Atlanta. This valuable publication may be obtained through MMS Publications, P.O. Box 9120, Waltham, MA 02254-9120. Similar recommendations of the Canadian expert group are published in the *Canadian Medical Association Journal.* Recommendations of other expert panels are collected in the *Report of the Committee on Infectious Diseases* (the so-called Red Book) [9] for infants and children, in summaries from the CDC [9a], and in the *Guide to Adult Immunization* (the so-called Green Book) [10] for adults. Excellent summaries of current recommendations for immunization of the adult patient have been published [11–12a], and the entire field of vaccines has been authoritatively surveyed in two texts [13, 14]. These recommendations are for use in the United States only because epidemiologic circumstances and vaccines differ in other countries [15]. Advice regarding immunization for travel abroad can be found in Chap. 21.

I. **General principles** [15]
   A. **Active immunization** involves the use of immunogens, such as live attenuated virus, inactivated virus, isolated viral proteins, bacterial components, or inactivated toxins (toxoids), to stimulate a protective antibody or cell-mediated immune response, or both (Table 22-1).
      1. **Live attenuated virus vaccines** generally stimulate greater and more durable immunity than do inactivated virus vaccines. The live attenuated vaccines, however, have greater inherent risks and are not appropriate for use in all individuals.

Table 22-1. Major types of vaccines

Live attenuated virus
  Measles
  Mumps
  Rubella
  Poliovirus (oral)
  Yellow fever
  Varicella
  Respiratory syncytial virus*
  Parainfluenza virus*

Live attenuated bacteria
  Typhoid (oral)
  Bacillus Calmette-Guérin (BCG)
  Tularemia

Inactivated virus
  Hepatitis B
  Influenza
  Poliovirus (subcutaneous)
  Rabies
  Hepatitis A
  Human papillomavirus*

Inactivated bacteria
  Anthrax
  Cholera
  Diphtheria (toxoid)
  Haemophilus influenzae type b (polysaccharide-protein conjugate)
  Meningococcus (polysaccharide)
  Pertussis
  Pneumococcus (polysaccharide)
  Plague
  Tetanus (toxoid)
  Typhoid (subcutaneous)
  Gonococcus*

Inactivated rickettsiae
  Q fever (*Coxiella burnetii*)

Inactivated protozoa
  Malaria*

*Under development.

    a. Live attenuated preparations include measles, mumps, rubella, oral poliovirus, varicella, and yellow fever vaccines.
    b. Limitations. Except under special circumstances, **live attenuated vaccines should not be administered to patients with** congenital or acquired immunodeficiency, leukemia or lymphoma, or generalized malignancy, or to patients receiving immunosuppressive therapy or, in certain cases, to members of their households, as there is the potential for these attenuated agents to be associated with viral replication after administration in immunocompromised individuals and to spread to susceptible hosts. In addition, because these agents could present a theoretic risk to the developing fetus, live attenuated virus vaccines are not generally recommended for use in pregnant women or those likely to become pregnant within 3 months after immunization. For special recommendations concerning the use of live attenuated measles or trivalent measles-mumps-rubella (MMR) vaccine in children with human immunodeficiency virus (HIV) infection, see sec. **III.A.5.h.**
   2. Inactivated virus or synthetic viral components are used to produce **influenza** and **hepatitis B** vaccines. Because an inactivated virus is employed, the limitations in sec. **1.b** may not apply to these vaccines. For example, if poliomyelitis immunization is indicated for immunosuppressed patients, their household contacts, or other close contacts, the (enhanced) inactivated poliovirus vaccine

can safely replace the live attenuated vaccine, as discussed in sec. **III.D.3.** Under certain conditions, some vaccines may also be administered after the first trimester of pregnancy.

3. **Inactivated bacterial vaccines** include the currently available **pertussis, typhoid** (parenteral), and **cholera** vaccines. Bacterial-component immunogens may not produce lifelong immunity and may therefore require booster doses at appropriate intervals to ensure adequate and long-lasting protection.

4. **Toxoids. Diphtheria** and **tetanus** vaccines are inactivated toxins, referred to as *toxoids*.

B. **Passive immunization** is produced by the administration of **immunoglobulin** (IG), which contains specific protective antibodies derived from human blood plasma. This form of immunization **provides immediate protection** but is of very limited duration and is most useful for time-limited prophylaxis. It may be given up to 3 weeks before or up to 72 hours after specific disease exposure.

1. **Immunoglobulin** is prepared from large plasma pools by ethanol fractionation (the Cohn method) and was previously called *immune serum globulin* or *gamma globulin*. It **contains specified amounts of antibody against measles, diphtheria, and poliovirus type 1.** In addition, IG contains **variable amounts of antibody against hepatitis A and B viruses, varicella virus, respiratory syncytial virus,** and possibly some non-A, non-B hepatitis viruses. Immunoglobulin must be further processed to be safe for intravenous administration. It is not specifically designated as safe for intravenous use and should be used only intramuscularly.

   Immunoglobulin has never been associated with the transmission of HIV, although some lots prepared before 1985 have passively transferred transient HIV seropositivity. The Cohn procedure has been shown to inactivate HIV; nonetheless, since 1985 all IG used in the United States must be prepared from HIV-seronegative blood.

2. **Specific human IGs** are obtained from immunized donors, from individuals recovering from recent disease or, in some instances, from units known to contain high-titered antibody to specific infectious agents. Human IGs are much less likely to provoke serious hypersensitivity reactions than are IGs derived from animals, which human IGs have generally replaced. Recommendations for the use of both specific and pooled IGs have been published [16]. Examples of pathogens for which specific IGs are available include the following:

   a. **Varicella-zoster virus.** See Chap. 4 under Mucocutaneous Vesicles.
   b. **Tetanus.** See Chap. 4 under Tetanus.
   c. **Rabies.** See Chap. 4 under Bite Wounds and Rabies Prevention.
   d. **Hepatitis B.** See sec. **IV.A.**

3. **Animal-derived IGs. Except for treatment of snake and spider bites, animal sera are no longer recommended for human use.** In the past, tetanus and rabies antisera were derived from immunized animals. These were far more likely than human products to cause serum sickness or anaphylaxis.

C. **Passive and active immunizations** sometimes are combined to provide both immediate protection (with preformed antibody) and sustained protection (antigenic stimulation of host immune response).

1. For postexposure **rabies** prophylaxis, for example, human rabies IG (passive) is combined with human diploid cell rabies vaccine (active), or HDCV.

2. For postexposure **tetanus** prophylaxis in the previously nonimmunized individual, human tetanus (IG) passive is combined with tetanus toxoid (active). Note, however, that in this situation **only the alum-precipitated or adsorbed toxoid, and not the fluid toxoid, should be used** (see sec. **V.E**).

3. Similar active-passive immunization is used in the prophylaxis of neonates born to mothers who are hepatitis B carriers. (See sec. **IV.A.**)

4. **Immunoglobulin should never be administered to modify the reaction to a live attenuated virus vaccine,** as was previously done with the measles vaccine.

D. **Simultaneous administration of vaccines.** Studies have shown that it is safe and, in most instances, effective to administer multiple vaccines simultaneously [15]. This often is more convenient for individuals who require many different immunizations. When several vaccines are being administered at the same time, the vaccines should not be combined in the same syringe or administered at the same site. **Only prepackaged combination vaccines should be administered at a single site.**

However, the antibody **response of both cholera and yellow fever vaccines may be decreased if given simultaneously** or within a short time of each other. If possible, cholera and yellow fever vaccinations should be separated by at least 3 weeks [15]. (See Chap. 21.)

1. **Live attenuated virus vaccines** were previously administered 1 month apart, but studies have shown that simultaneous administration of some live virus vaccines (e.g., MMR) is just as effective as single injections and does not result in higher rates of adverse reactions [15].

2. **Inactivated vaccines** can be administered simultaneously at separate sites. When vaccines commonly associated with local or systemic side effects (e.g., cholera, parenteral typhoid, or plague) are given simultaneously, side effects could be accentuated. For patients who have a history of a reaction to one or more vaccines, it is prudent to administer each on a separate occasion.

3. **An inactivated and a live attenuated vaccine** can be given simultaneously.

4. **Inactivated bacterial and viral vaccines** can be given simultaneously. An example is the simultaneous administration of influenza and pneumococcal vaccines (at separate sites).

E. **Contraindications and adverse reactions [17].** The manufacturer's guidelines and recommendations, as contained in the US Food and Drug Administration–approved package insert, should be followed carefully.

1. **Hypersensitivity reactions**
   a. **Some vaccine antigens are derived from embryonated chicken eggs or embryonic chick cells.** In general, **if patients can eat a whole egg, these vaccines can be safely administered.** Protocols have been developed for immunization of the highly egg-allergic patient [18].
   b. **Anaphylactic antibiotic reactions.** Some vaccines contain trace amounts of antibiotics. In patients with a history of anaphylactic reactions to specific antibiotics, the current package insert should be carefully reviewed to ascertain whether the antibiotic of concern is in the vaccine. If the vaccine does contain the antibiotic, the vaccine should be avoided. No current vaccines contain penicillin or penicillin derivatives. The history of a minor local contact dermatitis from prior neomycin use is not a contraindication to any vaccine containing neomycin [15].

2. **Altered immunity.** Live attenuated virus vaccines may cause serious disease in some immunocompromised individuals and so, in general, these vaccines should not be used in such patients. Measles vaccine, however, has been recommended for use in certain individuals infected with HIV (see sec. **III.A.5.h**). **Live attenuated poliovirus vaccines should not be administered to any household member of an immunocompromised person** (see sec. **VI.F**).

3. **Severe febrile illness.** Minor illness, such as a mild upper respiratory infection, should not preclude immunization. Vaccination of patients with severe febrile illnesses should be deferred so that side effects of the vaccine do not complicate the existing illness and so that symptoms of the illness are not incorrectly ascribed to the vaccine.

4. **Pregnancy.** Because **live attenuated virus vaccines pose a theoretic risk to the developing fetus,** these vaccines generally should not be given to a pregnant woman or to a woman likely to become pregnant within 3 months of immunization. Concerns and risks of immunization during pregnancy are further addressed in sec. **VI.B.**

5. **Recent administration of IG.** Passively acquired antibody (e.g., IG) **can interfere with the response to live attenuated virus vaccines. Administration of such vaccines should be deferred until approximately 3 months after IG administration** when possible. In addition, **IG should not be administered for at least 2 weeks after vaccine has been given** (when possible) to avoid inhibiting the immune response to the vaccine. This is an important aspect of the timing of IG for travelers (e.g., those who need measles immunization) who may require several vaccines and IG before departure (see Chap. 21, sec. **I**).

Most bacterial or inactivated viral vaccines may be administered with IG for specific postexposure prophylaxis (see sec. **I.C**).

II. **Immunization schedules**
A. **Pediatric immunization schedules.** The details of these schedules are published

in the serial editions of the Red Book [9] and updated reports of the Committee on Infectious Diseases in *Pediatrics,* and in recommendations made by the ACIP as published in *Morbidity and Mortality Weekly Reports.*

In February 1994 a working group, comprising members of the American Academy of Pediatrics (AAP), ACIP, American Academy of Family Physicians, the Food and Drug Administration, National Institutes of Health, CDC, Maternal and Child Health Bureau, vaccine manufacturers, and state immunization programs, met to develop a **single, scientifically valid immunization program** (reviewed elsewhere [9a]), which was revised in 1996 [9b] and is **summarized in Table 22-2.** This meeting was intended in part to help resolve some variations in prior recommendations. Important recommendations of the working group include:

1. The third dose of oral polio vaccine (OPV) should be administered routinely at 6 months of age; vaccination at as late as 18 months remains an acceptable alternative.
2. The first dose of measles, mumps, and rubella (MMR) vaccine is suggested at 12–15 months of age. The second dose of MMR can be administered at either 4–6 years or 11–12 years of age.
3. Universal hepatitis B vaccination of infants was recommended in 1991.
   a. For infants whose mothers are hepatitis B surface antigen (HBsAg) negative, routine hepatitis B vaccination series should begin at birth, with the second dose administered at 2 months of age (see acceptable ranges in Table 22-2). The third dose should be administered at 6–18 months.
   b. For infants of HBsAg-positive mothers, the infant should receive the first dose of vaccine at birth (along with hepatitis B immunoglobulin [HBIG]), the second dose at 1 month of age, and the third dose at 6 months (see related discussion in Chap. 3).
4. The current schedule for diphtheria-tetanus-pertussis (DTP) vaccination is still recommended (see Table 22-2).

B. **Adult immunizations.** The indications for adult immunizations are reviewed in the individual vaccine discussions (see secs. III–V). See also Table 22-3 and related discussion in Chap. 21.

C. **Requirements of the National Childhood Vaccine Injury Act of 1988.** This act, which provides for certain indemnifications for vaccine-related injuries, imposes certain record-keeping and reporting obligations on individuals who administer vaccines. Requirements of most relevance to adult vaccinees apply to the administration of tetanus and diphtheria toxoids, tetanus toxoid, and both oral and inactivated poliovirus vaccines. As of March 21, 1988, **physicians and others providing these vaccines are required to maintain permanent immunization records specifying for each recipient** the date of administration, manufacturer, and lot number of the vaccine, and the name, address, and title of the person administering the vaccine. In addition, the law specifies a list of reportable events occurring within specified times after vaccine administration and names authorities to whom reports must be made. (Additional details are presented in appendices 9 and 10 of the Green Book [10].)

III. **Live attenuated virus vaccines**

A. **Measles (rubeola)** can be a severe disease, with respiratory and neurologic complications. Encephalitis occurs in approximately 1 of every 2,000 cases, and survivors may suffer permanent neurologic impairment or mental retardation. Death occurs in 1 in 3,000 cases [19]. Measles during pregnancy increases the rate of spontaneous abortion, the risk of premature labor and low birth weight and, when infection occurs in the first trimester, the risk of congenital malformation. Subacute sclerosing panencephalitis is also considered to be a rare but devastating complication of natural infection with measles virus.

Before measles vaccine became available in 1963, more than 400,000 measles cases were reported annually in the United States, and it is estimated that only 10% of cases were reported. Since then, reported cases (including imported cases representing overseas exposures) have fallen by 100- to 1,000-fold, and a national goal of measles eradication has been set by the US Public Health Service [19]. There has also been a striking decline in the incidence of subacute sclerosing panencephalitis, a chronic progressive encephalopathy believed to be caused by the measles virus.

The currently available measles vaccine and the measles eradication program are reviewed in detail elsewhere [19]. Recommendations for measles outbreak control are reviewed in that same CDC publication [19].

1. **Measles outbreaks in the United States.** Despite the availability of the measles vaccine, measles outbreaks continue to occur in the United States. The major settings for outbreaks include the following:
    a. **Preschoolers living in densely populated urban areas in which proper vaccination rates are low** (e.g., approximately 50%). These young unvaccinated children in crowded conditions are particularly susceptible to measles [19]. Improved immunization programs aimed at preschoolers are essential to decrease this type of outbreak.
    b. **Youths and young adults** (i.e., school-age children and college students) who have not been vaccinated at all or who received primary vaccination that has failed [20]. Primary vaccine failures (i.e., patients who have been vaccinated but fail to seroconvert) occur in 2–10% of patients. Failure to seroconvert is more likely (1) in patients vaccinated before 15 months of age, (2) with less-than-optimal vaccine storage and handling, or (3) with the use of measles vaccine manufactured before 1980, owing to its greater lability. A new stabilizer was used in 1979, and **vaccines available since 1980 appear to be associated with a better antibody response in vaccine recipients.** To avoid future outbreaks in educational settings, it will be important for educational facilities to require adequate documentation of measles vaccination (see sec. **4**).
2. **Control of measles in the United States.** To reduce the number of cases and outbreaks of measles in the United States, the inadequate vaccination status of preschoolers and young adults must be addressed. When this approach has been pursued aggressively by a country (e.g., Finland), it has been very successful [20a].
    a. **Preschoolers**
        (1) **Improved compliance** with recommended measles vaccination programs for young children is essential.
        (2) **Two-dose measles vaccine schedule.** To reduce the number of primary vaccine failure–related cases, the ACIP has recommended a routine two-dose measles vaccine schedule [9a]. The initial dose is administered at 12–15 months of age. (In an actual outbreak of measles, children can be vaccinated initially at 6–9 months of age, then reimmunized at 12 months, and boosted before beginning school.) The second dose is recommended at school entry (4–6 years of age), or at age 11–12 but may be administered at any visit provided at least 1 month has elapsed since receipt of the first dose. See Table 22-2. MMR is used for both doses.
    b. **Young adults** (high school and college age). Educational institutions need to adopt certain requirements.
        (1) Evidence of measles immunity (i.e., prior diagnosis by a physician or laboratory evidence) must be provided by entering students born in or after 1957.
        (2) Documentation of two doses of live measles vaccine, with the second dose after 1980, must be provided. If this has not been done already, a dose of measles vaccine should be given before school begins to ensure adequate immunity.
        (3) In an outbreak of measles, all persons at risk (e.g., students attending schools where measles has occurred who have not been adequately vaccinated) should be vaccinated. See secs. **(1)** and **(2)**.
        (4) **Although MMR has been considered reasonable for revaccinating college-age students,** because of the increased incidence of arthritic reactions seen in young adults after revaccination with MMR, **it may be prudent to revaccinate with measles vaccine alone [21] if rubella immune status is not a concern** (see sec. **5** and Table 22-4). Arthritis and arthralgias are known adverse effects of rubella vaccine in nonimmune vaccinees. They occur in approximately 12–20% of adults and 0–3% of children and have an intermediate incidence in adolescents. Neither MMR nor measles vaccine is recommended in pregnancy.
        (5) When colleges have state-mandated prematriculation immunization guidelines for measles, measles outbreaks in colleges can be reduced [21a].

Table 22-2. Recommended childhood immunization schedule[a]—United States, January–June 1996

Vaccine		Age									
	Birth	1 Mo	2 Mo	4 Mo	6 Mo	12 Mo	15 Mo	18 Mo	4–6 Yr	11–12 Yr	14–16 Yr
Hepatitis B[b]	Hep B-1	Hep B-2			Hep B-3					Hep B[c]	
Diphtheria and tetanus toxoids and pertussis vaccine[d]			DTP	DTP	DTP	DTP (DTaP at ≥15 mo)			DTP or DTaP	Td	
Haemophilus influenzae type b[e]			Hib	Hib	Hib	Hib					
Poliovirus[f]			OPV	OPV	OPV				OPV		
Measles-mumps-rubella[g]						MMR			MMR or MMR	MMR	
Varicella zoster virus[h]							Var			Var[i]	

Note: Boxed information indicates range of acceptable ages for vaccination.

[a] Vaccines are listed under the routinely recommended ages.

[b] **Infants born to hepatitis B surface antigen (HBsAg)-negative mothers** should receive 2.5 µg of Recombivax HB (Merck) or 10 µg of Engerix-B (SmithKline Beecham). The second dose should be administered ≥1 month after the first dose. **Infants born to HBsAg-positive mothers** should receive 0.5 ml hepatitis B immune globulin (HBIG) within 12 hours of birth, and either 5 µg of Recombivax HB or 10 µg of Engerix-B at a separate site. The second dose is recommended at age 1–2 months and the third dose at age 6 months. **Infants born to mothers whose HBsAg status is unknown** should receive either 5 µg of Recombivax HB or 10 µg of Engerix-B within 12 hours of birth. The second dose of vaccine is recommended at age 1 month and the third dose at age 6 months.

cAdolescents who have not received three doses of hepatitis B vaccine should initiate or complete the series at age 11–12 years. The second dose should be administered at least 1 month after the first dose, and the third dose should be administered at least 4 months after the first dose and at least 2 months after the second dose.

dThe fourth dose of diphtheria and tetanus toxoids and pertussis vaccine (DTP) may be administered at age 12 months, if at least 6 months have elapsed since the third dose of DTP. Diphtheria and tetanus toxoids and acellular pertussis vaccine (DTaP) is licensed for the fourth and/or fifth dose(s) for children aged ≥15 months and may be preferred for these doses in this age group. Tetanus and diphtheria toxoids, adsorbed, for adult use (Td) is recommended at age 11–12 years if at least 5 years have elapsed since the last dose of DTP, DTaP, or diphtheria and tetanus toxoids, absorbed, for pediatric use (DT).

eThree *Haemophilus influenzae* type b (Hib) conjugate vaccines are licensed for infant use. If PedvaxHIB (Merck) *Haemophilus* b conjugate vaccine (meningococcal protein conjugate) (PRP-OMP) is administered at ages 2 and 4 months, a dose at 6 months is not required. After completing the primary series, any Hib conjugate vaccine may be used as a booster.

fOral poliovirus vaccine (OPV) is recommended for routine infant vaccination. Inactivated poliovirus vaccine (IPV) is recommended for persons—or household contacts of persons—with a congenital or acquired immune deficiency disease or an altered immune status resulting from disease or immunosuppressive therapy, and is an acceptable alternative for other persons. The primary three-dose series for IPV should be given with a minimum interval of 4 weeks between the first and second doses and 6 months between the second and third doses.

gThe second dose of measles-mumps-rubella vaccine (MMR) is routinely recommended at age 4–6 years or at age 11–12 years but may be administered at any visit provided at least 1 month has elapsed since receipt of the first dose.

hVaricella zoster virus vaccine (Var) can be administered to susceptible children any time after age 12 months.

i"Catch-up" vaccination (see also footnote c). Unvaccinated children who lack a reliable history of chickenpox should be vaccinated at age 11–12 years.

Source: Modified from Advisory Committee on Immunization Practices, American Academy of Pediatrics, and American Academy of Family Physicians. *M.M.W.R.* 44:942–943, 1996.

Table 22-3. Vaccines to be considered for patient groups[a]

Patient group	Major vaccines[b]	Other considerations[c]
Healthy adults		
Adolescents and young adults	Td, MMR up to date, hepatitis B, completion of childhood immunizations	Varicella (see text)
25–64 years	Td, rubella (women only), polio	
65 years and older	Td, influenza, pneumococcal	Varicella (see text)
Pregnant women	MMR is contraindicated; test for rubella antibody and hepatitis B surface antigen	
Environmental situations		
Nursing home residents	Influenza, pneumococcal	Tuberculin test
Institutionalized mentally retarded	Hepatitis B	Hepatitis A
Prison inmates	Hepatitis B	Hepatitis A
Homeless persons	Review all vaccines; consider pneumococcal vaccine	Tuberculin test
Occupational groups		
College students	MMR; consider hepatitis B, polio, influenza	Varicella
Health care workers	Hepatitis B, influenza, MMR	
Essential community services	Influenza	
Daycare center personnel	MMR, polio, influenza	Hepatitis A, hepatitis B
Laboratory personnel	Hepatitis B	Consider individually
Veterinarians, animal handlers, rural workers, and other field personnel	Rabies	Plague, anthrax
Immigrants and refugees	Review all vaccines, test for hepatitis B surface antigen	Tuberculin test

	Major vaccines[b]	Other considerations[c]
Life-styles		
Homosexual and bisexual men	Hepatitis B, hepatitis A	
Intravenous drug abusers	Hepatitis B, Td, hepatitis A	
Prostitutes, persons with multiple sexual partners or sexually transmitted diseases	Hepatitis B	Hepatitis A (see Chap. 11)
Accidents		
Wounds	Td	TIG
Animal bites	Td	Rabies vaccine, RIG
Snake and spider bites	Td	Specific antivenins
Immunocompromise		
HIV infection and AIDS	Pneumococcal, hepatitis B	IG (measles), VZIG
Splenic disorders	Pneumococcal, influenza	Haemophilus influenzae type b, meningococcal
Diabetes	Pneumococcal, influenza	
Renal failure and dialysis	Pneumococcal, influenza, Hepatitis B	Hepatitis B vaccine, Haemophilus influenzae type b
Alcoholism, cirrhosis	Pneumococcal, influenza	
Organ transplantation, immunosuppressive therapy	Pneumococcal, influenza	
Malignant diseases	Consider individually	
International travel	Review Td, MMR, polio; consider influenza, pneumococcal, hepatitis B	Yellow fever, IG or hepatitis A, meningococcal, typhoid, cholera, rabies, Japanese encephalitis, antimalarial prophylaxis (see Chap. 21)

[a]See text for specific details on indications, administration, adverse reactions, precautions, contraindications, and special considerations for each vaccine, toxoid, and immunoglobulin preparation. Also see reference [10].

[b]Major vaccines include combined tetanus and diphtheria (Td) toxoids; measles-mumps-rubella (MMR) vaccine; oral polio vaccine and enhanced-potency inactivated polio vaccine; influenza vaccine; pneumococcal vaccine; and hepatitis B vaccine.

[c]Other considerations include immunoglobulin (IG), tetanus immunoglobulin (TIG), rabies immunoglobulin (RIG), varicella-zoster immunoglobulin (VZIG), and intravenous immunoglobulin (IVIG).

Source: Modified from ACP Task Force on Adult Immunization and Infectious Diseases Society of America, *Guide to Adult Immunization* (3rd ed.). Philadelphia: American College of Physicians, 1994. See also P. Gardner et al., Adult immunizations. *Ann. Intern. Med.* 124:35, 1996.

3. **Vaccine.** The current live attenuated measles vaccine, prepared in chick embryo cell cultures, is less reactogenic than its predecessor, the Edmonston B strain. The current vaccine produces a mild or inapparent noncommunicable infection, with antibody developing in 95% of susceptible recipients vaccinated at 15 months of age or older. Both monovalent (measles only) and combination (i.e., measles and rubella, and MMR) forms of the vaccine are available.

4. **Persons can be considered immune to measles if one of the following conditions is met:**

   a. **Born before 1957.** These individuals are likely to have been infected naturally and are considered immune.

   b. **Documentation of physician-diagnosed measles.** A clinical case definition includes a generalized maculopapular rash of 3 days' duration or longer (often appearing first at the hairline, forehead, and behind the ears and upper neck, then spreading downward to involve the face and neck and then the trunk and upper extremities), **and** fever of at least 101°F orally **and** one or more of the following: cough, coryza, and conjunctivitis. A confirmed case has seropositivity or meets the preceding definition and is epidemiologically linked to a known case or outbreak of measles. A suspected case meets the preceding definition (but rash can be of less than 3 days' duration) but has no serologic confirmation or epidemiologic link. Serologic confirmation involves either a positive IgM test or a fourfold rise in acute to convalescent specimen in complement fixation testing without a history of recent vaccination.

   c. **Documented laboratory evidence of measles immunity.** The most commonly used test for measles immunity is the hemagglutination inhibition (HI) test. Most, but not all, measles-immune individuals will have measles HI antibody titers of 4 or more. Routine serologic screening to determine measles immunity is not recommended, except possibly for health care workers. See sec. **11** and Appendix B on employee health.

   d. **Adequate immunization with live measles vaccine at or after 15 months of age.** The maximum rate of seroconversion after measles vaccine occurs at 15 months of age or later. An adequate two-dose measles vaccination schedule in children or a booster dose in young adults is necessary (see sec. **2**).

5. **Persons needing measles vaccine** (Table 22-4)

   a. **Susceptible children older than 15 months, adolescents, and adults** should be vaccinated if there are no contraindications. For persons who did not receive the two-dose measles vaccine, see sec. **2**.

   b. **Those vaccinated with live measles virus before 12 months of age** should be identified and revaccinated.

   c. **Those immunized with the inactivated (killed) measles vaccine in use from 1963 to 1967** (or to 1969 in Canada) are at risk for developing **atypical measles** when exposed to natural infection. This is a disease of significant morbidity in young adults and some adolescents. It may present as a diagnostic challenge. It has been reviewed in detail elsewhere [22]. Patients may have conjunctivitis and a characteristic erythematous, maculopapular rash progressing to vesicular, petechial, or purpuric lesions. The rash initially involves the palms and soles, with subsequent spread to the proximal extremities and trunk, sparing the face. Pulmonary involvement, with significant hypoxemia, is common. Although recipients of the killed vaccine may have an increased risk of adverse reaction when revaccinated with the live vaccine, these risks are minor compared to the severity of atypical measles.

   d. **Young adults** (secondary school or college age) **who have not had measles vaccine since 1980** require revaccination. (See sec. **2**.)

   e. **Persons who received IG at the time of measles vaccination** should be revaccinated. Although immunization with the Edmonston B strain vaccine probably was effective even when administered with IG, the use of IG with other vaccines, including the current one, could render the dose ineffective. All individuals in whom IG was used in combination with a vaccine other than the Edmonston B strain, or in whom the vaccine type is not known, should be reimmunized.

   f. **Susceptible persons exposed to a person with measles** may benefit from vaccination if the vaccine is given within 72 hours of measles exposure.

Table 22-4. Current recommendations for measles vaccination

Routine childhood schedule, United States	
Most areas	Two doses[a,b]
	First dose at 12–15 months
	Second dose at 4–6 years (entry to kindergarten or first grade)[d]
High-risk areas[c]	Two doses[a,b]
	First dose at 12 months
	Second dose at 4–6 years (entry to kindergarten or first grade)[d]
Colleges and other educational institutions after high school	Documentation of receipt of two doses of measles vaccine after the first birthday[b] or other evidence of measles immunity[e]
Medical personnel beginning employment	Documentation of receipt of two doses of measles vaccine after the first birthday[b] or other evidence of measles immunity[e]

[a]Both doses should preferably be given as combined measles-mumps-rubella vaccine (MMR).
[b]No less than 1 month apart. If no documentation of any dose of vaccine, vaccine should be given at the time of school entry or employment and no less than 1 month later.
[c]A county with more than five cases among preschool-aged children during each of the last 5 years, a county with a recent outbreak among unvaccinated preschool-aged children, or a county with a large inner-city urban population. These recommendations may be applied to an entire county or to identified risk areas within a county.
[d]Some areas may elect to administer the second dose at an older age or to multiple age groups (see reference [19] and text). Also see Table 22-2.
[e]Prior physician-diagnosed measles disease, laboratory evidence of measles immunity, or birth before 1957.
Source: Centers for Disease Control, Measles prevention: Recommendations of the Immunization Practices Advisory Committee. *M.M.W.R.* 38(Suppl. 9):4, 1989.

   g. **Travelers to high-risk areas** may require vaccination. Measles continues to be endemic throughout many parts of Asia, Africa, and Central and South America. Nonimmune visitors run the risk of acquiring measles and of exposing others on their return. **Travelers born after 1956 who are planning trips to these areas should have their measles immune status reviewed** (see sec. **2**). Although serologic screening is not routinely recommended, it may be useful in evaluating prospective travelers. If the traveler has prior immunity, there is no evidence of enhanced risk from receiving the live attenuated measles vaccine. For infants traveling to measles-endemic areas, vaccination is recommended as early as 6 months of age, with a second measles immunization at age 15 months, and a third dose at school entry. **For further discussion, see Chap. 21.**
   h. **Children with HIV infection** may be at special risk for measles complications. Because of several reports of severe or fatal cases of measles in children with HIV infection [23], it has been recommended that measles vaccine be administered to all such children, regardless of the stage of their HIV disease.
 6. **The dosage** is the same for children and adults, a subcutaneous dose of properly stored vaccine in the 0.5-ml volume recommended by the manufacturer. The trivalent MMR form is the vaccine of choice for routine childhood immunization. **IG should not be administered with the measles vaccine or, ideally, sooner than 3 months before measles vaccine or 2 weeks after it.** (See Chap. 21.)
 7. **Precautions and contraindications**
   a. **Pregnancy.** Live measles vaccine should not be administered to women who are pregnant. Also, women should avoid becoming pregnant for 3 months after vaccination. Although there is no clinical experience of harm to the developing fetus, there is a theoretic risk of such harm.
      Pregnant women exposed to natural measles infection may wish to consider the use of IG within 6 days of the exposure.

b. **Allergies.** Because the live attenuated virus vaccine is prepared in chick embryo cells, patients with a history of **egg allergy** associated with anaphylactic reaction should be vaccinated only with extreme caution. A protocol for immunizing such individuals has been published [18]. There is no evidence that persons with other allergies to chicken or to feathers are at increased risk of reaction to the vaccine.

The vaccine contains trace amounts of **neomycin.** Therefore, persons who have experienced anaphylactic reactions to topical or systemic neomycin also should not receive this vaccine. See related discussion in sec. **I.E.**

c. **Febrile illness, recent use of IG, and states of altered immunity** are discussed in sec. **I.E.**

8. **Side effects.** The currently available measles vaccine has an excellent safety record. Side effects include **fever** (beginning approximately the sixth day after inoculation and lasting up to 5 days) in 5–15% of recipients, **transient rashes** in approximately 5% of recipients, and **encephalitis** occurring approximately once in every million doses administered. It is estimated that severe illness or death is more than 1,000 times more likely to occur in a person who acquires the disease naturally than in one who becomes ill as a result of vaccination [19].

9. **Revaccination.** Two doses of vaccine are recommended for full immunity. No additional doses are recommended for persons already immune. However, there is no evidence that revaccination of an immune individual carries an enhanced risk.

10. **Immunoglobulin is effective in preventing or modifying measles in a susceptible normal host exposed within the preceding 6 days.** The dose used is 0.25 ml/kg IM, with a maximum dose of 15 ml. **The common intramuscular immunoglobulin preparation should never be administered intravenously.** Immunoglobulin may be particularly indicated for susceptible household contacts of measles patients, especially contacts younger than 1 year, or for susceptible pregnant women. If not contraindicated, live attenuated virus vaccine should be administered 3 months later to those more than 12 months old. Whether IG is protective in patients with impaired immunity is unclear. (See reference [23] for the use of IG in exposed patients with HIV infection.)

11. **Nosocomial measles** can occur, and inadequately vaccinated medical personnel are sometimes the vectors [24].

B. **Mumps** is principally a disease of school-age children, but approximately 15% of cases occur in adolescents or adults. It usually is self-limited, but deafness is a rare complication. Although orchitis may occur in up to 20% of cases in postpubertal male patients, sterility is very rare. Naturally acquired mumps infection, including the estimated 30% of cases that occur subclinically, confers durable immunity [25].

There is no evidence that mumps during pregnancy causes congenital malformations [25].

In recent years, there has been an increased occurrence of mumps in susceptible adolescents and young adults, with several outbreaks in high schools, colleges, and occupational settings. This is due to the relative underimmunization of children born between 1967 and 1977, when the mumps vaccine was not used routinely.

1. **Mumps live virus vaccine,** introduced in 1967, produces a subclinical, noncommunicable infection with very few side effects. The live attenuated vaccine is prepared from chick embryo cell cultures and induces antibodies in more than 95% of recipients. Immunity is long-lasting, but the precise duration is unclear.

Mumps vaccine is available both in a monovalent form (mumps only) and in combination (e.g., measles, mumps, and rubella). The MMR vaccine is the vaccine of choice for routine administration and should be used in all situations where there is no contraindication and recipients are also likely to be susceptible to measles or rubella [25]. There is no evidence that persons who have previously had mumps or received mumps vaccine are at any increased risk of local or systemic reactions to live mumps vaccine [25].

2. **Persons can be considered immune to mumps** if one of the following conditions is met:

a. **Born before 1957.** Those born before 1957 are likely to have been infected naturally.

b. **Documentation of physician-diagnosed mumps.**

    c. **Documented laboratory evidence of mumps immunity.** Reliable serologic studies (neutralization, complement fixation, enzyme-linked immunosorbent assay [ELISA], or radial hemolysis antibody tests) are not readily available. The mumps skin test does not predict immunity reliably. Routine susceptibility testing before vaccination is unnecessary. Persons who are immune from prior infection or immunization are not at an increased risk for reaction if they receive live mumps virus vaccine.

    d. **Documentation of adequate immunization** with live mumps virus vaccine when 12 months old or older.

3. **Vaccination is indicated for any susceptible person older than 12 months.** Susceptible children, adolescents, and adults should be vaccinated against mumps unless vaccination is contraindicated. Mumps vaccine is of particular value for children approaching puberty, especially adolescent and young adult men who have not had mumps and who have not previously been immunized. However, it should be recognized that the most serious consequence of mumps infection—deafness—may occur at any age.

4. **Dosage.** A single dose of vaccine in the volume specified by the manufacturer should be administered subcutaneously. It should not be administered to infants younger than 12 months as persisting maternal antibodies may interfere with seroconversion.

5. **Side effects.** The mumps vaccine is very well tolerated. Rarely, parotitis and allergic reactions (transient rashes and pruritus) have been reported. Very infrequently, febrile seizures or encephalitis occurring within 30 days of immunization have been reported, but an etiologic relationship between these events and prior vaccination has not been established.

6. **Precautions and contraindications**

    a. **Pregnancy.** The precautions in pregnancy are the same as for measles (see sec. **A.7.a**).

    b. **Allergies.** The vaccine is produced in chick embryo culture (see discussion in sec. **I.E**). Some vaccines contain traces of **neomycin;** if the patient has a history of anaphylaxis to neomycin, the vaccine should be avoided. A history of contact dermatitis to neomycin is not a contraindication to receiving mumps vaccine.

    c. **Prior IG administration and immunodeficiency** (see sec. **I.E**). An exception to these general recommendations relates to children infected with HIV. All HIV-infected children should receive MMR at 15 months of age (see sec. **III.A.5.h**).

    d. **Febrile illness.** See sec. **I.E.3**.

7. **International travel.** Although mumps vaccine is not a requirement for entry into any country, susceptible children, adolescents, and adults would benefit from a single dose of vaccine, usually as MMR, unless contraindicated. Persons younger than 12 months need not be given the vaccine because of the likelihood of persisting maternal antibodies affecting seroconversion and because the risk of serious disease from mumps is relatively low. See Chap. 21.

8. **Mumps control** measures are reviewed elsewhere [25].

9. **Nosocomial mumps** can occur rarely and is, at least in part, preventable [24].

C. **Rubella** is a common childhood disease with nonspecific signs and symptoms including postauricular and suboccipital adenopathy, low-grade fever, and a transient erythematous rash [26]. **Because of the nonspecific nature of this infection, a history of rubella illness is not a reliable indicator of immunity. Assessment of immune status is based on the presence of demonstrable antibody.**

1. **Background. The goal of rubella immunization is unique: the prevention of the congenital rubella syndrome** rather than prevention of rubella infections per se. The most important consequences of rubella are fetal anomalies resulting from rubella infection early in pregnancy, particularly early in the first trimester (see Chap. 3). School and infant vaccination programs have reduced the overall incidence of rubella in the United States more than 1,000-fold, but cases continue to occur among nonimmunized adolescents and young adults. **Outbreaks have been reported from schools, colleges, the military, office buildings, prisons, hospitals,** and other institutions in which large numbers of young adults live or work. Therefore, a combined approach to vaccinating both infants and susceptible adolescents and young adults has been recommended.

2. **Live rubella vaccine** is prepared in human diploid cell culture. Since 1979, the available vaccine has been based on the RA 27/3 virus strain. With a single dose, approximately 95% of recipients develop antibody that provides lifelong protection.

3. **Susceptibility status** is determined by serologic studies. Hemagglutination inhibition antibody usually is used to screen for rubella immunity. Other screening tests include passive hemagglutination, hemolysis in gel, and ELISA tests. **Any detectable titer,** whether from natural infection or immunization, and no matter how low, **protects against subsequent viremic infection** (i.e., the type of infection that may affect the fetus). The ACIP suggests that revaccination of persons with low levels of rubella HI antibody is unnecessary. Rather, attention should be directed toward vaccinating the truly susceptible population.

   Routinely performing serologic tests in all women of childbearing age to determine susceptibility is expensive and has been ineffective in some areas. Therefore, the ACIP recommends that rubella vaccination be given, without prior serologic testing, to a woman who is not pregnant, who has been counseled to avoid pregnancy for the subsequent 3 months, and who has no history of vaccination [26, 27].

4. **Indications for vaccination**
   a. **All children older than 12 months.** These individuals should be vaccinated to protect against rubella and to prevent spread of the virus to susceptible women.
   b. **Susceptible** prepubertal, adolescent, and adult **women of childbearing age.**
   c. **Susceptible hospital employees. Both male and female employees should be vaccinated because any infected employee may transmit rubella to pregnant patients [26].**
   d. **All susceptible military recruits, applicants to educational and training institutions, and prisoners.**

5. **Risks to the pregnant patient.** Because of the theoretic risk of this live virus vaccine to the fetus, women of childbearing age should receive this vaccine only if they are not pregnant and are counseled to avoid pregnancy for 3 months after vaccination. However, all available data indicate that teratogenicity from live rubella vaccines has not occurred. The CDC has followed more than 200 known rubella-susceptible pregnant women who were vaccinated within 3 months before or 3 months after conception [27]. None of the babies had malformations consistent with congenital rubella infection. Therefore, the ACIP states that inadvertent rubella vaccination just before or in early pregnancy should not be a reason to recommend interruption of pregnancy routinely [26, 27]. Vaccinating susceptible children whose mother or other household member is pregnant poses no risk to the pregnant woman.

6. **Side effects** include occasional rash and lymphadenopathy in children. Arthralgia of the small joints may occur in up to 40% of those vaccinated, but frank arthritis occurs in fewer than 1%. These symptoms are more common in adults and usually occur 7–21 days after immunization and persist for 1–3 days. The risk of these reactions is no greater if persons already immune are vaccinated [26].

7. **Contraindications**
   a. **Pregnancy.** See sec. **5.** As of April 1989, the CDC discontinued accepting new enrollees into the Vaccine in Pregnancy (VIP) registry [27]. However, any suspected case of congenital rubella syndrome, whether presumed to be due to wild-type or vaccine virus infection, should continue to be reported through state and local health departments.
   b. **Immunocompromised hosts.** Because live attenuated vaccine strains may cause disease in immunocompromised patients, such patients **should not receive this live virus vaccine** (see sec. **I.E.2**).
   c. **Severe allergy to neomycin.** This vaccine contains trace amounts of neomycin, so persons who have experienced anaphylactic reactions to neomycin should not receive rubella vaccine.

D. **Poliomyelitis** has been nearly eliminated in the United States since the introduction of poliovirus vaccines in 1955. This has been due primarily to the widespread use of live attenuated OPV, first developed by Sabin. The inactivated poliovirus vaccine (IPV) prepared by Salk is, however, still indicated for use in certain special situations. The licensure of an enhanced-potency inactivated poliovirus vaccine (E-IPV) is likely to encourage further the use of inactivated virus preparations in certain special circumstances. Although routine immunization of persons over the age of 18 years is not recommended, **when polio immunization is appropriate in the adult, E-IPV is recommended.** The status of OPV and IPV has been reviewed [28], and supplements to that statement have been issued containing recommendations on the use of E-IPV [29, 30]. In addition, modification of the number of doses necessary for primary immunization has been recommended (see sec. **2**).

1. **Indications for vaccination.** Routine primary immunization of adults (generally those 18 years old or older) in the United States is not necessary. Most adults are immune because of prior immunization or prior wild-type poliovirus infection. In addition, the small number of cases of poliomyelitis that currently occur in this country make the risk of exposure to wild-type virus very small. **Major emphasis on primary poliovirus vaccinations in the United States is aimed at children.** Certain adults at special risk are also candidates for primary or booster vaccination (see sec. **4**). See footnote below.*

2. **OPV.** Available since 1963, this **live attenuated vaccine,** containing all three poliovirus strains, provides long-lasting immunity in more than 95% of recipients after primary vaccination.

   a. **Indications. For primary immunization of normal infants and young children,** OPV is preferred because it is simple to administer, is well accepted by patients, induces intestinal and systemic immunity, results in immunization of some contacts, and has a record of having essentially eliminated disease associated with wild poliovirus in the United States.

   b. **Risks and contraindications.** Rarely (1 in approximately 3.2 million doses distributed), OPV has been associated with the development of paralytic poliomyelitis in a vaccine recipient or close contact. This risk is increased in immunocompromised individuals (e.g., those with a primary immunodeficiency [sec. **I.E**] or receiving immunosuppressive agents) and in adults.

      (1) **OPV should not be used in immunocompromised hosts or for household contacts of such patients.**

      (2) **Healthy adults requiring primary vaccination may also be at increased risk of vaccine-associated paralysis after OPV. In these situations, the inactivated form of the poliovirus vaccine (E-IPV) should be used.**

      (3) **Pregnancy.** Because there is a theoretic risk to the fetus, vaccination of pregnant women should be avoided. However, in special circumstances, if the risk of exposure to natural infection is substantial and immediate, protection is needed: e.g., for the young pregnant woman traveling to a country with endemic poliomyelitis, the risk of poliovirus exposure outweighs the theoretic risk of the vaccine. In pregnancy, OPV is preferred. (IPV may be considered if the complete vaccination series can be administered before the anticipated exposure [15].)

      (4) Although the risk of vaccine-associated paralysis is extremely rare with OPV (estimated, for healthy adults, to be one case in 5.5 million doses of vaccine), recipients should be informed of this risk.

   c. **Administration.** For primary vaccination, three doses, rather than the previous four-dose regimen, are recommended [15]. The second dose should be administered at least 4 weeks, and preferably 8 weeks, after the first. The third dose should be given at least 6 months, and preferably 12 months, after the second. In infants, immunization may begin as early as 6 weeks of life but preferably closer to 2 months of age. Interrupted primary immunization schedules may be taken up wherever they left off, regardless of the length of time elapsed since the last vaccine dose. For children, a fourth supplemental dose is recommended before they enter school (see Table 22-2). See footnote below.*

3. **The inactivated poliovirus vaccine has been used extensively since 1955 and is given by the subcutaneous route.** The original inactivated vaccine has been superseded by a new enhanced-potency vaccine released in March 1988. Primary vaccination of children with three doses of the **E-IPV** resulted

---

*The ACIP is considering a new sequential dosing schedule for children: two inactivated doses administered subcutaneously at 2 and 4 months, followed by two oral doses at 6–12 months and 12–18 months.

in immunity to all three poliovirus types in more than 99% of recipients [30, 31]. Early studies suggested that the durability of immunity following IPV will be excellent [32].

   a. **Indications.** In the United States, IPV is used commonly **to vaccinate immunodeficient patients and their household contacts and adults requiring primary immunization.** This vaccine can also be used as a booster dose in adults planning international travel to developing countries (see Chap. 21). See footnote, p. 861.

   b. **Risks and side effects.** No paralytic reactions to IPV have occurred with recent preparations. In 1955, a cluster of poliomyelitis cases occurred after use of an IPV preparation containing live poliovirus that had escaped inactivation.

   c. **Allergic history.** Because this preparation contains trace amounts of streptomycin and neomycin, **individuals with a history of anaphylactic reactions to systemic or topical streptomycin or neomycin should not receive this vaccine.**

   d. **Administration.** Primary vaccination consists of three doses given subcutaneously in the volume recommended by the manufacturer. The first two doses are given at a 4- to 8-week interval, and the third dose should follow the second in 6–12 months.

4. Vaccination of adults. Routine vaccination of those older than 18 years is not indicated (see sec. **1**).

   a. **These adults are at special risk and deserve vaccination:**

     (1) **Travelers** to areas of countries where poliomyelitis is endemic or epidemic (see Chap. 21).

     (2) **Laboratory workers** handling specimens that may contain poliovirus.

     (3) **Medical workers** in close contact with patients who may be excreting poliovirus, including those who administer live virus vaccine.

     (4) **Members of communities or specific population groups** with a high prevalence of natural disease.

   b. **Regimens.** In general, for adults without prior primary vaccination, a full series of E-IPV is recommended as adults may be at a slightly increased risk of vaccine-associated paralytic disease caused by OPV. The details of vaccination schedules were described previously (see sec. **2.c**).

     For adults who have completed primary immunization with OPV, a booster OPV dose (or E-IPV) may be given. If adults have completed the primary series with IPV, either E-IPV or OPV may be used for the booster dose. In general, we prefer to use E-IPV in adults.

5. Precautions and contraindications

   a. **Pregnancy.** Although there is no convincing evidence documenting adverse effects of either OPV or IPV in the pregnant woman or developing fetus, it is prudent to avoid vaccinating pregnant women. Exceptions may be made if the risk of exposure to poliovirus outweighs the theoretic risk of vaccine use (see sec. **2.b**).

   b. **Immunodeficient persons should not receive OPV. Likewise, OPV should not be used to immunize their household contacts.** If OPV is inadvertently administered to a household contact of an immunodeficient individual, close contact between the two should be avoided for approximately 1 month after vaccination. The family member and the immunosuppressed individual in particular must be carefully counseled to avoid exposure to fecal-oral contamination, essentially by practicing good personal hygiene (i.e., enteric precautions).

E. Varicella. Live attenuated varicella vaccines have been used routinely in Japan for nearly 20 years now. Studies of these vaccines have been under way in the United States since 1980, first in immunocompromised children [33] and more recently in healthy children [34] and adults [35]. The vaccine has been generally well tolerated in all groups, although mild chickenpox developed in 7% of healthy children and up to one-third of children who had received chemotherapy [36]; in the latter group children with rash may transmit the virus. In immunocompromised children, a significant number of vaccinees subsequently developed natural infection, although no severe cases were reported. The risk of varicella-zoster infection following vaccine appears comparable to [37] or lower than that after natural infection.

In March 1995, the Food and Drug Administration licensed a live-attenuated varicella vaccine (Varivax, Merck, West Point, PA) for use in individuals 12 months of age or older who have not had varicella [37a]. In addition to its routine use in infants, the vaccine has also been recommended for use in adolescents and young adults [37b] to prevent the serious complications of adult varicella [37c] and varicella during pregnancy [37d]. Adult immunization may also be useful in controlling disease in health care workers [37e].

1. **Recommendations for vaccine use** have been reviewed in detail elsewhere [37a, 37f].

   a. **Age 12 to 18 months.** One subcutaneous dose is recommended for universal immunization for all healthy children who lack a reliable history of varicella [37a].

   b. **Age 18 months to 13 years.** One dose is recommended for children who have not been immunized previously and who lack a reliable history of varicella infection [37a].

   c. **Healthy adolescents and young adults.** Healthy adolescents older than 13 years who have not been immunized previously and have no history of varicella infection should be immunized by administration of two doses of vaccine 4–8 weeks apart [37a]. **A two-dose regimen is necessary for adults because of their diminished responsiveness to the vaccine** [37g]. One recent report suggests that higher serum titers of antibody are achieved when the second dose is given at the 8-week interval rather than the 4-week interval [37h].

   d. **Adults.** In healthy individuals older than 18 years who have no history of varicella, **performing serologic tests** and looking for prior infection with VZV before vaccination **is optional** [37a].

   Precise recommendations for adults await an official statement from the ACIP that will probably be available in mid- to late 1996. In the meantime, **for adults with negative serology** for varicella:

   (1) Health care workers and susceptible family and/or close contacts of immunocompromised hosts would seem good potential candidates for the vaccine.

   (2) Those adults whose occupations place them at risk for exposure (e.g., teachers, day care workers) should be considered for vaccination. College students, military personnel, and nonpregnant women of childbearing age should be considered for vaccination.

   (3) Other susceptible adults may be candidates for the vaccine after discussion with their personal physicians. The role of the vaccine in routine international travel (i.e., in non-health care providers) is being evaluated.

2. **Contraindications and cautions** [37a]

   a. Varicella vaccine **should not be given to immunodeficient patients** or to patients who have received **high doses of systemic corticosteroids** in the previous month. The vaccine is probably safe for children using only inhaled steroids [37a] (see sec. **e**).

   b. Varicella should not be administered to **pregnant women** because the possible effects on fetal development are unknown [37a]. When postpubertal females are immunized, pregnancy should be avoided for 1 month after immunization [37a].

   c. Varicella vaccine should not be administered to individuals who have had an **anaphylactoid reaction to neomycin** because trace amounts of neomycin are in the vaccine. A contact dermatitis history to neomycin is not a contraindication of the vaccine [37a].

   d. The vaccine manufacturer recommends that **salicylates not be administered for 6 weeks** after the varicella vaccine has been given because of the association between Reye syndrome, natural varicella, and salicylates [37a].

   e. Under special circumstances, in patients with acute lymphocytic leukemia in remission at least 1 year, vaccine may be reasonable under a special protocol. (See reference [37a] for details.)

   f. **Households with potential immunocompromised contacts.** In their recent recommendations, the Committee on Infectious Diseases emphasized the following.

Transmission of vaccine type VZV from healthy individuals has been infrequently if at all documented. Thus, even in families with immuno-compromised individuals, including those with HIV infection, no pre-cautions need to be taken after vaccination of healthy children (and presumably adults) who do not develop a rash. Vaccinees who develop a rash (up to 7–8% of recipients) should avoid contact with immunocom-promised susceptible hosts for the duration of the rash. If contact inad-vertently occurs, the use of varicella-zoster immunoglobulin is not recommended currently, because transmission is rare and disease, if it develops, is mild [37a].

3. Doses are given subcutaneously. The **cost** of the new varicella vaccine to physicians is $39 per dose; the cost of serum antibody testing to varicella is about $70 [37f] but will vary depending on the laboratory used.

F. **Rabies.** See Chap. 4 under Bite Wounds and Rabies Prevention, and Chap. 21, sec. **IV** under Vaccinations.

G. **Yellow fever.** See Chap. 21.

IV. **Inactivated virus vaccines**
   A. **Hepatitis B**
      1. **Preexposure HBV** vaccine **now is recommended for routine use in all new-born infants in the United States** [38]. **In addition, the ACIP recently rec-ommended vaccination of all 11- to 12-year-old children who have not pre-viously received the hepatitis vaccine and vaccination of all unvaccinated children under 11 years who are Pacific Islanders or who reside in house-holds of first generation immigrants from countries where HBV is of high or intermediate endemicity** [38a].

      Preexposure HBV vaccine **also is recommended for** high-risk health care workers, clients and staff of institutions for the mentally retarded, hemodialy-sis patients, homosexually active men, intravenous drug users, hemophiliacs who receive factor VIII or IX blood products, sex workers, and household and sexual contacts of HBV carriers [39].

      In addition, the HBV vaccine should be considered for others who might be at high risk for contracting HBV. These include inmates of long-term correctional facilities, heterosexually active persons with multiple sexual part-ners, international travelers to areas endemic for HBV (see Chap. 21), and certain high-risk population groups in special settings, including certain health care providers. (The details of these recommendations are reviewed carefully elsewhere [38, 39].)

      All HBV vaccines currently available in the United States are recombinant DNA–derived. Heptavax, a human plasma–derived vaccine, is no longer pro-duced in the United States.
         a. **Recombivax HB** (Merck) is produced by common baker's yeast into which a plasmid containing the gene for hepatitis B surface antigen (HBsAg) has been inserted. Heptavax B and Recombivax are equally effective, and approximately 90% of healthy adults will develop protective antibody.
         b. **Engerix-B** (SmithKline Beecham, Philadelphia) is a recombinant DNA–derived vaccine. Studies show it is as effective as the Recombivax HB vaccine.
      2. **Dosages of vaccines.** Hepatitis B vaccines are packaged to contain 10–40 μg HBsAg protein per milliliter. Table 22-5 shows the currently recommended dosage schedules [39]. **Primary vaccination consists of** three intramuscular doses, with the second and third doses given at 1 and 6 months after the first, respectively. For more rapid protection, **an accelerated regimen** has been effective [40] for certain high-risk groups (e.g., needlestick exposures, certain travelers, infants born of infected mothers) with standard doses of **Engerix-B** given at 0, 1, 2, and 12 months. Other accelerated regimens have undergone preliminary investigation and may be useful in some international travelers [40a]. If routine dose schedules are interrupted, alternative dose regimens are available [39].
         a. **Antibody response.** Antibody response **is higher when the HBV vaccine is given in the arm (deltoid muscle) than in the buttock (gluteal muscle).** Therefore, the arm should be used as the site of injection **in adults** (unless it may jeopardize shunt access in the hemodialysis patient). **For infants born to mothers who are HBV carriers, the preferred site for vaccination**

Table 22-5. Recommended doses and schedules of currently licensed hepatitis B vaccines

Group	Recombivax HB[a] dose (μg)	(ml)	Engerix-B[a,b] dose (μg)	(ml)
Infants of HBV-carrier mothers	5	(0.5)	10	(0.5)
Other infants and children < 11 yr	2.5	(0.25)	10	(0.5)
Children and adolescents 11–19 yr	5	(0.5)	20	(1.0)
Adults > 19 yr	10	(1.0)	20	(1.0)
Dialysis patients and other immunocompromised persons	40	(1.0)[c]	40	(2.0)[d,e]

[a]Usual schedule: three doses at 0, 1, and 6 months.
[b]Alternative schedule: four doses at 0, 1, 2, and 12 months.
[c]Special formulation for dialysis patients.
[d]Two 1.0-ml doses given at different sites.
[e]Four-dose schedule recommended at 0, 1, 2, and 6 months.
Source: Centers for Disease Control, Hepatitis B virus. Recommendations of the Immunization Practices Advisory Committee. *M.M.W.R.* 40(RR-13):5, 1991.

remains the anterolateral thigh. The total hospital cost of the three vaccine adult doses in the United States is approximately $55 to $65.

b. **Booster doses of vaccine are not routinely recommended; nor is routine serologic testing to assess antibody levels. However, previously vaccinated persons who experience percutaneous or needle exposure to HBsAg-positive blood should be tested for antibody level.** If the antibody level is lower than 10 mIU/ml, two booster doses at 1-month intervals may be useful. Hemodialysis patients should be tested semiannually and may require booster doses.

c. **Nonresponders.** Why some adults do not respond to the conventional hepatitis B immunization series is only partially understood. Older age, smoking, and obesity seem to be related to decreased responsiveness to hepatitis B vaccine. Determination of whether real differences exist between antibody response to the two currently available vaccines awaits further prospective studies [40b].

The optimal approach to the nonresponder is unclear [40b]. Giving two booster doses at 1-month intervals appears to result in an adequate response in only a minority of recipients (see sec. **b**). Other preliminary protocols have been suggested for nonresponders [40c].

3. **Postexposure prophylaxis of HBV** infection should be exercised in the following situations: (1) accidental percutaneous or permucosal exposure to HBsAg-positive blood, (2) sexual exposure to an HBsAg-positive person, and (3) perinatal exposure of an infant born to an HBsAg-positive mother (see Chap. 3 for details). Recent recommendations include the use of both HBIG (single dose) and the HBV vaccine in persons known or suspected to be negative for anti-HBs. This affords an immediate passive immunity combined with long-lasting active immunization. The cost of this new combined therapy is lower compared to previous recommendations, which called for two HBIG immunizations at a total hospital cost of approximately $300 to $350 for an average-sized adult. In addition, HBIG alone is only approximately 75% effective.

For details of postexposure prophylaxis, see Table 22-6 and the ACIP recommendations [39]. If HBIG is not immediately available, IG should be used. The latter contains low-level anti-HBs and, although not as good as HBIG, is probably better than no therapy.

4. **Prevaccination serologic screening for susceptibility.** Carriers of HBV and those having antibody from previous infection need not be vaccinated. Sero-

Table 22-6. Recommendations for postexposure prophylaxis for hepatitis B virus

	HBIG		Vaccine	
Exposure	Dose	Recommended timing	Dose	Recommended timing
Perinatal[a]	0.5 ml IM	Within 12 hours of birth	0.5 ml IM[b]	Within 12 hours of birth
Percutaneous	0.06 ml/kg IM	Single dose within 12 hours	1.0 ml IM[b]	Start vaccination series as soon as possible after exposure[b]
	or[c]			
	0.06 ml/kg IM	Within 24 hours; repeat at 1 month		
Sexual	0.06 ml/kg IM	Single dose within 14 days of sexual contact	Vaccine is recommended for sexually active homosexual men and for regular sexual contacts of chronic hepatitis virus carriers	
Household contact Chronic carrier	—	—	Footnote[b]	Start vaccination series as soon as possible[b]
Acute case Known exposure	None, unless known exposure 0.06 ml/kg IM	Single dose within 14 days of exposure	None unless known exposure Vaccine is recommended if household case becomes chronic carrier	
In primary caregiver—infant < 12 months	0.5 ml IM	As soon as possible	0.5 ml[b]	Start vaccination series as soon as possible[b]

HBIG = hepatitis B immunoglobulin.
[a]For further discussion, see Chap. 3.
[b]For vaccine doses and time intervals, see Table 22-5. The first dose can be given the same time as the HBIG dose but at a separate site.
[c]For those who choose not to receive hepatitis B vaccine.
Source: Adapted from Centers for Disease Control, Hepatitis B virus. Recommendations of the Immunization Practices Advisory Committee. *M.M.W.R.* 40(RR-13):6, 1991.

logic screening to detect such individuals before vaccination may or may not be cost-effective in a given setting. This topic and an approach to the variables involved in screening are discussed elsewhere [41]. The vaccine is well tolerated in carriers or those with protective antibody so that these patients are not at excess risk of side effects if they receive the vaccine when screening is not done.

B. Inactivated poliovirus vaccine is discussed in sec. **III.D.**
C. Influenza. See Chap. 8.
D. Rabies. See Chap. 4 under Bite Wounds and Rabies Prevention, and Chap. 21, sec. **IV** under Vaccinations.

V. Bacterial vaccines. Certain of these vaccines are discussed elsewhere. For such cases, only recent developments in vaccines and vaccine regimens are discussed here.

A. Pneumococcal vaccine. (See Chap. 9.) Although the polyvalent pneumococcal vaccine currently available in the United States has been shown to be effective in preventing pneumococcal bacteremia and sepsis in otherwise healthy young adults [42] and children [43], two studies in Veterans Administration patients [44, 45] reported efficacy rates as low as 60–70%. An excellent review of these data [46] concludes that pneumococcal vaccine is effective in healthy individuals of all ages but that these reports must raise serious concerns about its immunogenicity and long-term efficacy in the high-risk elderly patient, the population in greatest need of effective prophylaxis.

One approach to this problem may be to immunize persons routinely at age 55, before most age-related debilities have developed, in order to establish protection later in life. Another approach currently under consideration is to reimmunize high-risk elderly patients 5–6 years after their initial inoculation with pneumococcal vaccine [10, 47]. If these strategies are not effective, it may become important to develop conjugate vaccines, in which the pneumococcal polysaccharide is combined with a more immunologically stimulating protein molecule, as has been done for the *H. influenzae* type b vaccine [48, 49] (see sec. **F**).

B. Meningococcal vaccine. (See Chap. 5 under Prophylaxis of Meningitis, and Chap. 21.) The status of this vaccine has been reviewed [50].

C. Typhoid. See Chap. 21.

D. Plague. See sec. **VII.D** and Chap. 21.

E. Diphtheria, tetanus, and pertussis. The recommendations for DTP immunization in the United States have been comprehensively reviewed [51].

    1. Background

        a. Diphtheria remains a serious, although rare, disease in the United States, with fatalities in approximately 5–10% of respiratory cases. Most cases, both in adults and children, occur in nonimmunized or inadequately immunized individuals. However, waning immunity many years after primary vaccination may also be a contributor to some adult outbreaks [52]. Cutaneous diphtheria occurs primarily in certain groups of Native Americans and among indigent adults. Adequate immunization is believed to protect for at least 10 years. Unfortunately, recent serosurveys in the United States suggest that many adults do not have protective levels of antibodies.

        b. Tetanus incidence in the United States has declined dramatically with the routine use of tetanus toxoid in childhood. Though vaccine-induced immunity may not be lifelong, it is extremely durable. Currently, the fewer than 100 annual cases of tetanus that occur in this country involve elderly people who never received primary immunization [53]. Tetanus control therefore depends most on universal primary vaccination. The control strategy also includes reimmunizations every 10 years and appropriate use of toxoid and human hyperimmune antitetanus globulin in accident and emergency rooms. A significant number of emergency room patients are overtreated or, worse, undertreated for tetanus-prone injuries [54]. See related discussion in Chap. 4 under Tetanus.

        c. Pertussis is caused by toxicogenic strains of the gram-positive rod *Bordetella pertussis*. Its precise incidence is unclear. The disease is highly communicable, with attack rates of more than 90% reported in susceptible household contacts. Most reported illness occurs in children younger than 1 year, with classic lower respiratory symptoms. In older children or adults, however, the disease may be manifest as merely a modest upper respiratory or catarrhal illness, permitting such persons to serve as unrecognized reservoirs and disseminators of infection [55, 56] and increasing the difficulty of providing effective secondary prophylaxis for susceptible contacts. Hence, **in the United States, adults constitute the majority of patients infected with *B. pertussis* [55].**

        Naturally acquired immunity is long-lasting. **The vaccine does not confer either complete or lifelong immunity.** Studies suggest a loss of protection in approximately 20% of vaccine recipients 3 years after vaccination and a lack of protection in more than 90% of individuals 12 years after vaccination. This lack of long-term protection means that even in the absence of recognizable outbreaks of pertussis in the community, it is likely that many infants will be exposed to pertussis while they are still young enough to be at risk for severe or life-threatening disease. This is of particular concern for high-risk hospitalized children, among whom outbreaks have been unwittingly caused by infected hospital personnel [57].

2. Vaccines

  a. **Diphtheria toxoid** is prepared by formaldehyde treatment of purified diphtheria toxin. The concentration of diphtheria toxoid in preparations for adult use (designated **d**) is lower than that in pediatric formulations (designated **D**) to reduce the incidence of adverse reactions, which are considered to be related to both dose and age.

  b. **Tetanus toxoid** is likewise prepared by formaldehyde inactivation of purified tetanus toxin. It is available in fluid and aluminum salt–adsorbed forms. The adsorbed toxoid induces more persistent antitoxin titers and is strongly recommended for routine use.

  c. **Pertussis vaccine** has been comprehensively reviewed [58–61]. **Until recently,** all pertussis vaccine as used in the United States was a suspension of inactivated *B. pertussis* bacteria. The **use of whole, killed organisms in this vaccine probably accounted for its higher rate of adverse side effects. Two acellular vaccines,** in which some of the contaminating bacterial components of the whole-organism vaccine have been removed, **have now been approved for use in the United States for the fourth and fifth vaccine doses only.** Since 1981, such vaccines have been in routine use in Japan and appear to be associated with lower rates of adverse reactions while still being protective. However, the vaccine has primarily been used in children 2 years of age and older and, at this age, rates of reaction to the whole killed vaccine also are considerably lower. The acellular vaccine may be especially suitable for immunization or boosting of adults [60]. Acellular pertussis vaccines have been reviewed recently [61a].

3. Preparations and dosages. Simultaneous immunization against diphtheria, pertussis, and tetanus during infancy and childhood has been routine in the United States since the late 1940s.

  a. **For infants and children younger than 7 years,** diphtheria toxoid, tetanus toxoid, and pertussis vaccine adsorbed (DTP), and diphtheria and tetanus toxoids adsorbed (DT) are most commonly used. Dose schedules are reviewed elsewhere [15].

  b. **For persons 7 years old or older,** tetanus and diphtheria toxoids adsorbed (Td) is recommended. This product contains a smaller amount of diphtheria antigen (as indicated by the lowercase **d**) for use in older children and adults. **Tetanus toxoid should be given with adult-dose diphtheria toxoid every 10 years as part of routine primary medical care.** If a dose is given sooner as part of wound management, the next booster is not needed for 10 years thereafter. The use of tetanus toxoid in wound management is discussed in Chap. 4. **Some travelers may benefit from a booster at 5-year intervals,** because a tetanus-prone wound does not require tetanus IG or a booster if a person has been boosted within 5 years [51]. (See Chap. 21.)

  c. **Single-antigen products** are available (i.e., pertussis vaccine adsorbed [P], tetanus toxoid adsorbed [T], and diphtheria toxoid adsorbed [D]) for use when combined preparations are not appropriate. For example, pertussis vaccine has been used in hospital personnel to help control a pertussis outbreak [62].

4. Side effects and adverse reactions

  a. **DTP** administration commonly is associated with local reactions such as erythema, induration, and tenderness. These usually are self-limited and require no therapy. Fever beginning several hours after administration also is common and may persist for up to 2 days. Mild somnolence, vomiting, irritability, or malaise can occur, especially with pertussis-containing vaccines. Rarely, severe systemic reactions such as generalized urticaria, anaphylaxis, or neurologic complications may occur after DPT administration (see sec. **c**).

  b. **Arthus-type hypersensitivity reactions,** characterized by severe local reactions 2–8 hours after an injection, may be seen in persons receiving many booster injections at too-frequent intervals, as may happen with tetanus.

   c. **Pertussis. Severe reactions can occur** occasionally after pertussis vaccine injection [51], including (1) collapse or a shocklike state, (2) persistent screaming episodes (prolonged episodes of peculiar crying or screaming that cannot be controlled by comforting the infant), (3) high fever (i.e., > 40.5°C or 105°F), (4) isolated convulsions (with or without fever), and (5) possibly encephalopathy with or without convulsions or focal neurologic findings. **However, recent large studies indicate that there is no evidence of a causal relationship between pertussis vaccine and permanent neurologic illness [63–64a].** The incidence of major adverse reactions is low (< 1 in 1,000 for any symptom, and 100–1,000 times less frequent for the most serious reactions); in many cases, the occurrence of major reactions may be merely coincidental with the recent immunization rather than attributable to it. Sudden infant death syndrome (SIDS) is not more likely to occur following a DTP immunization [65, 66].

   d. **Use of multiple reduced-dose regimens.** Some physicians have suggested using reduced doses of pertussis, or other vaccines, in a multidose regimen, to reduce the risk of an adverse reaction. **There is no rationale for doing this as vaccine reactions do not appear to be dose-related.** In addition, efficacy of such idiosyncratic dosing schedules is unknown, and children receiving such vaccines would be considered nonimmune for the purpose of school entrance requirements.

5. **Precautions and contraindications**
   a. **When an infant or child returns for the next dose of DTP injections, the parent should be questioned about severe side effects or adverse reactions after the previous dose.** If any of the severe reactions listed previously has occurred, or if a severe systemic allergic reaction has occurred, the immunizations should be completed with DT. **The presence of an evolving neurologic disorder contraindicates the use of pertussis vaccine until neurologic status stabilizes.** However, a personal or family history of seizures is not an indication to withhold pertussis vaccine. A CDC statement on contraindications to the use of pertussis vaccine has been distributed [67].
   b. The main contraindication to the use of tetanus or diphtheria toxoids is a history of neurologic or systemic hypersensitivity reaction following a previous dose. Local side effects alone do not preclude further use. When an Arthus-like local reaction occurs after frequent tetanus toxoid doses (e.g., with frequent immunizations such as every 2 or 3 years), further routine or emergency booster doses of Td should not be given more frequently than every 10 years.
   c. Immunosuppressive therapies may reduce the efficacy of these vaccines. When possible, routine vaccination should be deferred while patients are receiving such therapy or for 3 months thereafter (see also sec. **VI.F**).

F. *Haemophilus influenzae* **b polysaccharide conjugate vaccine.** Until the licensing of the *H. influenzae* type b (Hib) conjugate vaccines for use in infants [68], Hib was the leading cause of systemic bacterial infection in children in the United States. **Since conjugate vaccine introduction, rates of both meningitic and nonmeningitic childhood Hib disease have decreased by 90% [69].**

Hib vaccines do not affect nonencapsulated (nontypeable) strains, which commonly colonize the respiratory tract and cause otitis media in childhood and pneumonia in the elderly but rarely cause bacteremic disease.

1. **Vaccines.** The purified capsular polysaccharide vaccine (PRP), which was licensed in 1985, has now been superseded by more immunogenic polysaccharide-protein conjugate vaccines. Four such conjugate vaccines have been licensed for use in the United States: a PRP-diphtheria toxoid conjugate (**PRP-D**), a meningococcal protein conjugate (**PRP-OMP**), a mutant diphtheria toxin conjugate (**HbOC**), and a tetanus toxoid conjugate (**PRP-T**). Tetravalent vaccines composed of DPT/HbOC or DPT/PRP-T have also been licensed. The various conjugated vaccines have been reviewed in detail elsewhere [70]. Antibodies to the polyribose-phosphate capsular polysaccharide correlate with protection against invasive disease.

2. **Responses.** Excellent responses in infants have been achieved with multidose regimens of all the conjugate vaccines except PRP-D, which is licensed for

use only at 15 months of age or older. Persons with immunologic impairment may have a substandard response to the usual immunizing regimen but may benefit from additional booster doses.

3. **Efficacy.** Clinical experience in the United States shows the conjugate vaccines to be highly effective in preventing Hib meningitis and septicemia (see Chap. 5, sec. **I.B.1** under Meningitis, page 136). Less clear is whether it will affect the incidence of Hib epiglottitis. It should be appreciated that vaccine failures do occur, particularly in individuals with IgG_2 subclass deficiencies. There is no evidence that immunization with the conjugate vaccines increases the risk for Hib disease in the immediate postimmunization period [70].

4. **Recommendations for use.** Specific recommendations are discussed in detail elsewhere [70] but, briefly, they include the following:

   a. **Routine immunization of all children beginning at 2 months of age is recommended** [9a, 70, 71]. Children receiving HbOC or PRP-T should be given two additional doses at 4 and 6 months and a booster dose at 15 months. Children receiving PRP-OMP should receive one additional dose at 4 months and a booster dose at 12 months.

   b. **Children older than 11 months who have not been vaccinated should be vaccinated.** These children should receive one dose of HbOC, PRP-T, or PRP-OMP, and a booster at 15 months if their initial dose was given before 15 months. Children between 15 and 59 months do not need a booster. Children older than 59 months do not normally need immunization. Injections given at 15 months or later may use any of the four licensed vaccines, including PRP-D.

   c. **Children who received the unconjugated vaccine between ages 18 and 23 months should be revaccinated with the conjugate.** Revaccination should take place at least 2 months after the initial dose of vaccine.

   d. **Children who had invasive Hib disease when they were younger than 24 months** should also receive the conjugate vaccine.

   e. Insufficient data are available on which to base a recommendation concerning vaccine use in older children or adults with conditions associated with an increased risk of Hib disease. (See related discussion in secs. **VI.F–G.**)

   f. Because those who have received their full primary series of immunizations (including booster doses if needed) are considered fully immunized, such children do not require rifampin for secondary prophylaxis of Hib case contacts. However, they may still require rifampin for household prophylaxis if other members of the household younger than 60 months are not fully immunized. Fully immunized immunocompromised children and their household contacts should still receive rifampin prophylaxis as appropriate, because the immunization may have been ineffective.

   g. Conjugate vaccine (other than DPT/HbOC) and routine DPT immunization may be given simultaneously at different sites.

5. **Side effects.** PRP conjugate vaccines are among the safest of all vaccine products. Fever has been reported in 1% of vaccinees and local reactions in up to 25% [70, 71]. DTP/HbOC carries with it all the cautions and potential side effects of the DTP vaccine (see sec. **E.4–5**). For children in whom DTP immunization is contraindicated (see sec. **E.5**), the combined HbOC/DTP vaccine also is contraindicated.

6. **Miscellaneous**

   a. **Because these vaccines will not protect against nontypeable strains of *H. influenzae*, recurrent upper respiratory disease, including otitis media and sinusitis, are not considered indications for vaccination.**

   b. Use of the diphtheria or tetanus toxoid conjugates (PRP-D or PRP-T) is not sufficient to ensure immunity to diphtheria or tetanus, and the conjugates should not be used in place of routine DPT immunization.

VI. **Immunization considerations for special-risk groups.** Special immunization programs have been formulated for certain groups with recognized special risks.

   A. **The elderly.** Immunization recommendations for the elderly are well addressed elsewhere [6, 72], and useful reviews have appeared [73, 74]. Recommendations for pneumococcal and influenza vaccine were discussed previously (see sec. **V.A** and Chap. 8, respectively). Only approximately 22% of the elderly receive influenza vaccine each year, and only 10% have received pneumococcal vaccine [75]. A survey of the attitudes and practices of the elderly concerning pneumococcal and influenza vaccines emphasizes that the most important factor in determining immunization status of the elderly is the recommendation of the individual's physician [75].

B. **Pregnant women.** Immunization of the pregnant woman recently was reviewed [76]. **In general, immunization during pregnancy should be avoided.** Although there is little evidence that currently available live virus vaccines can harm the developing fetus, the theoretic risk exists, making it prudent to avoid such exposures. Inactivated vaccines do not carry this same risk, but it has been suggested that maternal fever may be a risk factor for certain congenital abnormalities, making it prudent to avoid these vaccines as well. When necessary, it is possible to administer OPV to pregnant women, as discussed more fully in sec. **III.D.5.a.** Influenza vaccination during pregnancy is discussed in Chap. 8 under Influenza.

C. **College students.** These young adults are at special risk for epidemic illness spread by the respiratory route; outbreaks of measles, rubella, and influenza have repeatedly been reported on college campuses [77]. Since May 1983, the American College Health Association has encouraged institutions to adopt a recommended preadmission immunization policy [78], but serious gaps in immunization among college students persist [79].

D. **Prison populations.** Rubella outbreaks in prisons in several different parts of the country [80] have emphasized the need for immunization programs for young adults in prison [81]. Such outbreaks also represent occupational risks for prison staff.

E. **Homeless persons.** The fragmentary, episodic, and disorganized medical care that many of the homeless receive leaves a large pool of individuals susceptible to a variety of vaccine-preventable diseases, for whom new immunization strategies may be required [82]. Homeless adults have been targets of a diphtheria epidemic [83] and a cluster outbreak of pneumococcal pneumonia [84]. Homeless adolescents may be at high risk for HBV infection [85].

F. **Immunosuppressed individuals.** Immunization of the immunocompromised individual has recently been reviewed [86–88]. Immunizations in this population is problematic for two reasons. **Live virus vaccines generally are contraindicated** because of their potential for causing disease, whereas many inactivated or component vaccines may not be as effective in this population. However, **certain exceptions** to these general rules should be noted. Because of reports of severe and even fatal measles occurring in children who were HIV-infected, it has been recommended that both **symptomatic and asymptomatic HIV-infected children be immunized with measles vaccine [23].** Children who are HIV-infected and who have a measles exposure should also receive IG prophylaxis. Pneumococcal vaccination appears to be cost-effective in the adult with HIV infection, though routine influenza immunization may be more problematic [89].

The use of bacterial polysaccharide vaccines has been an important issue in Hodgkin's disease patients who have previously undergone staging splenectomy. In these individuals, the risk of pneumococcal or *Haemophilus* sepsis is appreciably elevated. Studies of the responses of such individuals show that, although vaccine immunogenicity and durability of the antibody response may be poorer in such persons, protective levels can be achieved in some [90]. Immunization efficacy is not influenced by the scheduling of splenectomy, but better responses are achieved when chemotherapy can be delayed 3 weeks after vaccine administration [90].

G. **Additional special vaccinee categories.** Special studies and recommendations have been made for alcoholics [91], persons with rheumatologic disease [92], persons receiving hemodialysis [93], patients after splenectomy [94], and patients who have undergone bone marrow transplantation [95]. Recommendations have also been reviewed for health care workers [96, 97]. See Appendix B.

VII. **Vaccines for use in special occupational groups**

A. **Anthrax.** Anthrax vaccine is recommended for persons whose occupations bring them into frequent close contact with imported animal hides or hair and for laboratory workers studying the agent. The vaccine is available through the Biologic Products Program, Michigan Department of Public Health, East Lansing, MI.

B. **Q fever.** An investigational inactivated vaccine is available for use in animal handlers working with sheep and in laboratory workers exposed to *Coxiella burnetii*. It is available through the U.S. Army Medical Research Institute of Infectious Diseases, Fort Detrick, MD.

C. **Tularemia.** A live attenuated vaccine is available from the CDC, Atlanta, GA, for use in individuals whose work regularly brings them into contact with wild mammals or vectors in tularemia-endemic areas.

  D. **Plague.** Plague vaccine is used rarely except in laboratory or field personnel who are working with *Yersinia pestis* or in certain workers (e.g., Peace Corps volunteers and agricultural advisers) who reside in rural areas where enzootic or epidemic plague exists and where avoidance of rodents and fleas is impossible. Detailed indications and recommendations for the use of this vaccine have been reviewed [98].

  E. **Rabies vaccine.** This is discussed in Chap. 4 under Bite Wounds and Rabies Prevention.

VIII. **Vaccines** are currently **being developed** de novo for gonorrhea, malaria, and respiratory syncytial virus, and improved vaccines also are being developed for cholera and typhoid [99].

  IX. **Vaccine use in developing countries.** This topic is beyond the scope of this chapter. However, it has been reviewed in an international symposium [100] and updated [101].

References

1. Williams, J.S., and Saunders, C.R. Cost-effectiveness and cost-benefit analysis of vaccines. *J. Infect. Dis.* 144:486, 1981.
2. LaForce, F.M. Immunizations, immunoprophylaxis, and chemoprophylaxis to prevent selected infections. US Preventive Services Task Force. *J.A.M.A.* 257:2464, 1987.
3. Williams, W.W., et al. Medicine and public issues. Immunization policies and vaccine coverage among adults: The risk for missed opportunities. *Ann. Intern. Med.* 108:616–625, 1988.
4. Current trends. National Childhood Vaccine Injury Act: Requirements for permanent vaccination records and for reporting of selected events after vaccination. *M.M.W.R.* 37:197, 1988.
5. Gardner, P., and Schaffner, W. Immunization of adults. *N. Engl. J. Med.* 328:1252, 1993.
6. Current trends. Vaccination coverage of 2-year old children—United States, 1993. *M.M.W.R.* 43:705, 1994.
   This is a further update of a similar report appearing in M.M.W.R. *42:785, 1994. For related discussions, see H.D. Mustin et al., Adequacy of well-child care and immunizations in U.S. infants born in 1988.* J.A.M.A. *272:1111, 1994. In this survey of more than 7,000 infants, although adequate visits were reported for 82% of white infants and 75% of black infants, adequate immunizations were received by only 46% and 34%, respectively. See editorial response in the same issue, which emphasizes the critical role of providers in ensuring that infants receive proper immunizations.*
7. Kelley, P.W., et al. The susceptibility of young adult Americans to vaccine-preventable infections. A national serosurvey of US Army recruits. *J.A.M.A.* 266:2724, 1991.
8. Successful strategies in adult immunization. *M.M.W.R.* 40:700, 1991.
9. *Report of the Committee on Infectious Diseases* (23rd ed.). Evanston, IL: American Academy of Pediatrics, 1994.
9a. Centers for Disease Control. Recommended childhood immunization schedule—United States, 1995. *M.M.W.R.* 44(RR-5):1–9, 1995.
   Refs 9a and 9b summarize the uniform recommendations from the American Academy of Pediatrics (AAP) and the Advisory Committee on Immunization Practices (ACIP). See related CDC summary in M.M.W.R. *43:959, 1995. See also related commentary by C.B. Hall, The recommended childhood immunization schedule of the United States.* Pediatrics *95:135, 1995.*
9b. Centers for Disease Control. Recommended childhood immunization schedule—United States, January–June 1996. *M.M.W.R.* 44:940, 1996.
10. ACP Task Force on Adult Immunization and Infectious Diseases Society of America. *Guide to Adult Immunization* (3rd ed.). Philadelphia: American College of Physicians, 1994.
   This superb reference can be obtained by writing Subscriber Services, American College of Physicians, Independence Mall West, Sixth Street at Race, Philadelphia, PA 19106-1572 or by calling 1-800-523-1546, X2600.
11. Fedson, D.S. Adult Immunization. In J. Noble (ed.), *Textbook of General Medicine and Primary Care.* Boston: Little, Brown, 1987. Pp. 1681–1695.

See also D.S. Fedson, Adult immunization: Summary on the National Vaccine Advisory Committee Report. J.A.M.A. 272:1188, 1994, which again emphasizes that although effective and safe vaccines are available, they are poorly used. Also see Medical Letter, Routine immunization for adults. Med. Lett. Drugs Ther. 32:54, 1990; and P. Gardner et al., Adult immunizations. Ann. Intern. Med. 124:35, 1996.

12. Orenstein, W.A., et al. Immunization. In G.L. Mandell, J.E. Bennett, and R. Dolin (eds.), *Principles and Practice of Infectious Diseases* (4th ed.). New York: Churchill Livingstone, 1995. Pp. 2270–2790.

12a. Gardner, P., and Eickhoff, T. Immunization in adults in the 1990s. *Curr. Clin. Top. Infect. Dis.* 15:271, 1995.
See related editorial comment from the Task Force on Adult Immunization, Adult Immunization 1994. Ann. Intern. Med. 121:540, 1994.

13. Plotkin, S.A., and Mortimer, E.A., Jr. *Vaccines* (2nd ed.). Philadelphia: Saunders, 1994.

14. Fulginiti, V.A. *Immunization in Clinical Practice*. Philadelphia: Lippincott, 1982.

15. Centers for Disease Control. General recommendations on immunization. *M.M.W.R.* 43(RR-1):1–38, 1994.

16. NIH Consensus Conference. Intravenous immunoglobulin. Prevention and treatment of disease. *J.A.M.A.* 264:3189, 1990.

17. Zimmerman, B., Gold, R., and Lavi, S. Adverse effects of immunization. Is prevention possible? *Postgrad. Med.* 82:225, 1987.

18. Herman, J.J., et al. Allergic reactions to measles (rubeola) vaccine in patients hypersensitive to egg protein. *J. Pediatr.* 102:196, 1983.

19. Centers for Disease Control. Measles prevention: Recommendations of the Immunization Practices Advisory Committee. *M.M.W.R.* 38(Suppl. 9):1, 1989.
See related update: Centers for Disease Control, Measles—United States, 1994. M.M.W.R. 44:496, 1995.

20. Kelley, P.W., et al. The susceptibility of young adult Americans to vaccine-preventable infections. A national serosurvey of US Army recruits. *J.A.M.A.* 266:2724, 1991.

20a. Peltola, H., et al. The elimination of indigenous measles, mumps, and rubella from Finland by a 12-year, two-dose vaccination program. *N. Engl. J. Med.* 331:1397, 1994.
Fascinating report published in late November 1994. MMR vaccine was given to children at 16–18 months of age and again at 6 years and to selected groups of older children and young adults. Vaccination was voluntary and free. In this same issue, see the editorial comment by M.B. Heisler and J.B. Richmond, Lessons learned from Finland's successful immunization program.

21. Medical Letter. Measles revaccination—an additional note. *Med. Lett. Drugs Ther.* 31:85, 1989.

21a. Baughman, A.L., et al. The impact of college prematriculation immunization requirements on risk for measles outbreaks. *J.A.M.A.* 272:1127, 1994.
Of selected schools, 11% of the 796 responding schools reported one or more measles cases from 1988 through 1991. Schools with a state-mandated prematriculation immunization requirement for measles were significantly less likely than other institutions to report measles outbreaks of two or more cases.

22. Martin, D.B. Atypical measles in adolescents and young adults. *Ann. Intern. Med.* 90:877, 1979.
Contains excellent color photos of the characteristic skin lesions.

23. Epidemiologic notes and reports: Measles in HIV-infected children. *M.M.W.R.* 37:183, 1988.
In this same issue of M.M.W.R., a supplementary statement on the immunization of children with HIV appears, including the therapeutic uses of immunoglobulin in HIV patients (vaccinated or unvaccinated) who are exposed to measles. Also see K. Krasinski et al., Measles and measles immunity in children with human immunodeficiency virus. J.A.M.A. 261:2512, 1989.

24. Murray, D.L. Vaccine-preventable diseases and medical personnel. *Arch. Intern. Med.* 150:25, 1990.
This brief editorial reviews the importance of medical personnel being properly protected against measles, mumps, and rubella. See companion articles on nosocomial spread of these infections.

25. Centers for Disease Control. Mumps prevention. *M.M.W.R.* 38:388, 1989.

26. Centers for Disease Control. Rubella prevention. *M.M.W.R.* 33(RR-15):1, 1990.

27. Centers for Disease Control. Rubella vaccination during pregnancy—United States, 1971–1988. *M.M.W.R.* 38:289, 1989.

28. Centers for Disease Control. Poliomyelitis prevention. *M.M.W.R.* 31:22, 1982.
29. Centers for Disease Control. Poliomyelitis prevention: Enhanced-potency inactivated poliomyelitis vaccine—supplementary statement. *M.M.W.R.* 36:795, 1987.
   For a recent discussion of the possible expanded role for E-IPV, see S.A. Plotkin, Inactivated polio vaccine for the United States: A missed vaccination opportunity. Pediatr. Infect. Dis. J. 14:835, 1995.
30. Medical Letter. A more potent inactivated polio vaccine. *Med. Lett. Drugs Ther.* 30:49, 1988.
31. Simoes, E.A., et al. Antibody response of infants to two doses of inactivated poliovirus vaccine of enhanced potency. *Am. J. Dis. Child.* 139:977, 1985.
32. Bernier, R.H. Improved inactivated poliovirus vaccine: An update. *Pediatr. Infect. Dis.* 5:289, 1986.
33. Brunell, P.A., et al. Administration of live varicella vaccine to children with leukemia. *Lancet* 2:1069, 1982.
34. Weibel, R.E., et al. Live attenuated varicella virus vaccine: Efficacy trial in healthy children. *N. Engl. J. Med.* 310:1409, 1984.
   See C.J. White et al., Varicella vaccine (VARIVAX) in healthy children and adolescents: Results from clinical trials, 1987–1989. Pediatrics 87:604, 1991.
35. Gershon, A.A., et al. Immunization of healthy adults with live attenuated varicella vaccine. *J. Infect. Dis.* 158:132, 1988.
   For related discussion, see I.R. Hardy and A.A. Gershon, Prospects for use of a varicella vaccine in adults. Infect. Dis. Clin. North Am. 4:159, 1990. An important topic because 5–10% of people who reach adulthood are susceptible to varicella-zoster virus.
36. Gershon, A.A., et al. Live attenuated varicella vaccine. Efficacy for children with leukemia in remission. *J.A.M.A.* 252:355, 1984.
37. Lawrence, R., et al. The risk of zoster after varicella vaccination in children with leukemia. *N. Engl. J. Med.* 318:543, 1988.
37a. American Academy of Pediatrics Committee on Infectious Diseases. Recommendations for the use of live attenuated varicella vaccine. *Pediatrics* 95:791, 1995 [erratum appears in *Pediatrics* 96(Pt 1):172, 1995].
   For an editorial comment favoring use of this vaccine, see S.A. Plotkin, Varicella vaccine. Pediatrics 97:251, 1996.
37b. Lieu, T.A., et al. Cost-effectiveness of varicella serotesting versus presumptive vaccination of school-age children and adolescents. *Pediatrics* 95:632, 1995.
37c. Gogos, C.A., Bassaris, H.P., Vagenakis, A.G. Varicella pneumonia in adults: A review of pulmonary manifestations, risk factors and treatment. *Respiration* 59:339, 1992.
37d. Enders, G., et al. Consequences of varicella and herpes zoster in pregnancy: Prospective study of 1739 cases. *Lancet* 344:950, 1994.
37e. Lewis, D.A., et al. Varicella-zoster vaccination for health care workers. *Lancet* 343:1362, 1994.
37f. Medical Letter. Varicella vaccine. *Med. Lett. Drugs Ther.* 37:55, 1995.
37g. Gershon, A.A., et al. Varicella vaccine: The American experience. *J. Infect. Dis.* 166(Suppl. 1):S63, 1992.
37h. Kuter, B.J., et al. Safety, tolerability, and immunogenicity of two regimens of Oka/ Merck vaccine (Varivax) in healthy adolescents and adults. *Vaccine* 13:967, 1995.
   Higher titers are achieved using a 2-month dose interval; we favor this interval.
38. Centers for Disease Control. Hepatitis B virus: A comprehensive strategy for eliminating transmission in the United States through universal childhood vaccination. *M.M.W.R.* 40(RR-13):1, 1991.
38a. Centers for Disease Control. Update recommendations to prevent Hepatitis B virus transmission—United States. *M.M.W.R.* 44:574, 1995.
   The editorial note of this reference emphasizes that of the estimated 1 million Asian and Pacific Islander children aged 2–10 years in the United States, less than 10% have received hepatitis B vaccine.
   At a routine adolescent vaccination visit at 11 to 12 years of age, the visit can be used to ensure that all adolescents have received three doses of hepatitis B vaccine, two doses of MMR, a booster dose of tetanus and diphtheria, and to assess whether adolescents are immune to varicella. Compliance in adolescents can be a problem. See N.A. Halsey, Hepatitis B immunization of adolescents. Pediatr. J. Infect. Dis. 14:1124, 1995.
   See related editorial comment by T.G. Ganiats, Hepatitis B immunization for adolescents. West. J. Med. 163:70, 1995; the author emphasizes the importance of vaccinating adolescents because about 25% of cases of hepatitis B occur between the ages of 10 and 20 years, especially since many teenagers are sexually active.

39. Centers for Disease Control. Protection against viral hepatitis. *M.M.W.R.* 39(RR-2):1, 1990.

40. Safary, A., et al. An accelerated dosing schedule of hepatitis B vaccination for those needing rapid protection [abstract 197]. Twenty-Ninth Interscience Conference on Antimicrobial Agents and Chemotherapy, Houston, Sept. 18, 1989.

40a. Marchou, B., et al. A 3-week hepatitis B vaccination schedule provides rapid and persistent protective immunity: A multicenter, randomized trial comparing accelerated and classic vaccination schedules. *J. Infect. Dis.* 172:258, 1995.
   Report from France in which a recombinant vaccine, GenHevac B, was given at days 0, 10, 21, and a booster at 1 year.

40b. Margolis, H.S., and Presson, A.C. Host factors related to poor immunogenicity of hepatitis B vaccine in adults: Another reason to immunize early. *J.A.M.A.* 270: 2971, 1993.
   An editorial on this topic and two related articles in this journal issue.

40c. Bertino, J.S., Jr. et al. Booster doses of hepatitis B vaccine for low/non-responding employees. Submitted for publication, 1996.
   In this preliminary study for hospital employees who failed to respond to the conventional three-dose regimen of Engerix-B (20 μg at 0, 1, and 6 months) with low to no antibody titers 1–2 months after the third dose, the following regimen was used: (1) those with titers of < R = 10 or negative were given a second series of Engerix-B 20 μg on the accelerated dosing schedule of 0, 1, 2 months; (2) anti-HBs titer was obtained 1–2 months after third dose to determine the effectiveness of this second series; (3) if this titer returned ≤ R = 10, a third series of vaccine was begun using Recombivax 40 μg, given on the accelerated dosing schedule of 0, 1, 2 months; (4) anti-HBs titer was obtained 1–2 months after third injection. (5) Regimen stops here regardless of titer results. Using this approach, most employees developed protective antibody levels.

41. Stevens, C.E., and Taylor, P.E. Hepatitis B vaccine: Issues, recommendations, and new developments. *Semin. Liver Dis.* 6:23, 1986.

42. Austrian, R. Some observations on the pneumococcus and on the current status of pneumococcal disease and its prevention. *Rev. Infect. Dis.* 3(Suppl.):S1, 1981.

43. Riley, I.D., et al. Pneumococcal vaccine prevents death from acute lower-respiratory tract infections in Papua, New Guinea children. *Lancet* 2:877, 1986.

44. Simberkoff, M.S., et al. Efficacy of pneumococcal vaccine in high-risk patients. *N. Engl. J. Med.* 315:1316, 1986.

45. Forrester, H.L., et al. Inefficacy of pneumococcal vaccine in a high-risk population. *Am. J. Med.* 83:425, 1987.

46. LaForce, F.M., and Eickhoff, T.C. Pneumococcal vaccine: An emerging consensus [editorial]. *Ann. Intern. Med.* 108:757, 1988.

47. Centers for Disease Control. Pneumococcal polysaccharide vaccine. *M.M.W.R.* 38: 64, 1989.

48. Musher, D.M., Watson, D.A., and Dominguez, E.A. Pneumococcal vaccination: Work to date and future prospects. *Am. J. Med. Sci.* 300:45, 1990.

49. Clancy, C.M., Gelfman, D., and Poses, R.M. A strategy to improve the utilization of pneumococcal vaccine. *J. Gen. Intern. Med.* 7:14, 1992.

50. Lepow, M.L., and Gold, R. Meningococcal A and other polysaccharide vaccines: A five-year progress report [editorial retrospective]. *N. Engl. J. Med.* 308:1158, 1983.

51. Centers for Disease Control. Diphtheria, tetanus, and pertussis: Recommendations for vaccine use and other preventive measures. *M.M.W.R.* 40(RR-10):1, 1991.

52. Karzon, D.T., and Edwards, K.M. Diphtheria outbreaks in immunized populations. *N. Engl. J. Med.* 318:41, 1988.

53. Centers for Disease Control. Tetanus—United States, 1985–1986. *M.M.W.R.* 36: 477, 1987.

54. Brand, D.A., et al. Adequacy of antitetanus prophylaxis in six hospital emergency rooms. *N. Engl. J. Med.* 309:636, 1983.

55. Hewlett, E.L. *Bordetella* Species. In G.L. Mandell, J.E. Bennett, and R. Dolin (eds.), *Principles and Practice of Infectious Diseases* (4th ed.). New York: Churchill Livingstone, 1995. Pp. 2078–2086.
   Also see J.D. Cherry et al., The past, present, and future of pertussis. West. J. Med. 150:319, 1989.

56. Nelson, J.D. The changing epidemiology of pertussis in young infants. *Am. J. Dis. Child.* 132:371, 1978.

57. Linnemann, C.C., Jr., et al. Use of pertussis vaccine in an epidemic involving hospital staff. *Lancet* 2:540, 1975.

58. Report of the Task Force on Pertussis and Pertussis Immunization—1988. *Pediatrics* 81:939, 1988.

59. Centers for Disease Control. Pertussis vaccination: Acellular pertussis vaccine for the fourth and fifth doses of the DTP series. Update to supplementary ACIP Statement. *M.M.W.R.* 41(RR-15):1, 1992.

60. Edwards, K.M., et al. Adult immunization with acellular pertussis vaccine. *J.A.M.A.* 269:53, 1993.

61. Blennow, M., et al. Primary immunization of infants with an acellular pertussis vaccine in a double-blind randomized clinical trial. *Pediatrics* 82:293, 1988.

61a. Edwards, K.M., and Decker, M.D. Acellular vaccines for infants. *N. Engl. J. Med.* 334:391, 1996.
    Excellent editorial comment and summary. Review of this topic and two controlled trials that appear in this issue. Authors favor acellular vaccines and encourage their licensure in the U.S.

62. Linnemann, C.C., Jr., et al. Use of pertussis vaccine in an epidemic involving hospital staff. *Lancet* 2:540, 1975.

63. Cherry, J.D. "Pertussis vaccine encephalopathy": It is time to recognize it as the myth that it is. *J.A.M.A.* 263:1679, 1990.

64. Pertussis immunization and the central nervous system. Ad Hoc Committee for the Child Neurology Society Consensus Statement on Pertussis Immunization and the Central Nervous System. *Ann. Neurol.* 29:458, 1991.

64a. Halsey, N.A., et al. Committee on infectious diseases. *Pediatrics* 97:279, 1996.
    Whole-cell pertussis vaccine has not been proven to be a cause of brain damage.

65. Hoffmann, H.J., et al. Diphtheria-tetanus-pertussis immunization and sudden infant death: Results of the National Institute of Child Health and Human Development Cooperative Epidemiological Study of Sudden Infant Death Syndrome Risk Factors. *Pediatrics* 79:598, 1987.

66. Waler, A.M., et al. Diphtheria-tetanus-pertussis immunization and sudden infant death syndrome. *Am. J. Public Health* 77:945, 1987.

67. Centers for Disease Control. Supplementary statement of contraindications in receipt of pertussis vaccine. *M.M.W.R.* 33:301, 1984, and 36:281, 1987.

68. *Haemophilus* b conjugate vaccines for prevention of *Haemophilus influenzae* type b disease among infants and children two months of age and older. *M.M.W.R.* 40(RR-1):1, 1991.

69. Adams, W.G., et al. Decline of childhood *Haemophilus influenzae* type b (Hib) disease in the Hib vaccine era. *J.A.M.A.* 269:221, 1993.

70. American Academy of Pediatrics. Committee on Infectious Diseases. *Haemophilus influenzae* type b conjugate vaccines: Recommendations for immunization with recently and previously licensed vaccines. *Pediatrics* 92:480, 1993.
    See related report by D.M. Granoff et al., Effect of carrier protein priming on antibody responses to Haemophilus influenzae *type b conjugate vaccines in infants. J.A.M.A. 272:1116, 1994. Vaccination with DT at 1 month of age increases the magnitude of the anti-PRP antibody responses to conjugate vaccination.*

71. Centers for Disease Control. Supplemental statement: Changes in administration schedule for *Haemophilus* b conjugate vaccines. *M.M.W.R.* 39:232, 1990.

72. Fedson, D.S. Clinical practice and public policy for influenza and pneumococcal vaccination of the elderly. *Clin. Geriatr. Med.* 8:183, 1992.

73. Bentley, D.W. Immunizations in the elderly. *Bull. N.Y. Acad. Med.* 63:533, 1987.

74. Harward, M.P. Preventive health for the elderly. Role of vaccination. *J. Fla. Med. Assoc.* 79:687, 1992.

75. Current trends. Adult immunization—knowledge, attitudes, and practices: DeKalb and Fulton counties, Georgia, 1988. *M.M.W.R.* 37:657, 1988.

76. Immunization during pregnancy (ACOG tech. bull. no. 160, October 1991). *Int. J. Gynaecol. Obstet.* 40:69, 1993.

77. Current trends. Immunization practices in colleges—United States. *M.M.W.R.* 36:209, 1987.

78. American College Health Association. Position statement on immunization policy. *J. Am. Coll. Health* 32:7, 1983.

79. Williams, W.W. Immunizations in college health: The remaining tasks. *J. Am. Coll. Health* 37:197, 1989.

80. Rubella outbreaks in prisons—New York City, West Virginia, California. *M.M.W.R.* 34:615, 1985.

81. Krupp, L.B., et al. Prisoners as medical patients. *Am. J. Public Health* 77:859, 1987.

82. Brickner, P.W., et al. Medicine and public issues: Homeless persons and health care. *Ann. Intern. Med.* 104:405, 1986.

83. Pedersen, A.H.B., et al. Diphtheria on Skid Road, Seattle, WA, 1972–75. *Public Health Rep.* 92:336, 1977.

84. Mercat, A., Nguyen, J., and Dautzenberg, B. An outbreak of pneumococcal pneumonia in two men's shelters. *Chest* 99:147, 1991.
85. Wang, E.E., et al. Hepatitis B and human immunodeficiency virus infection in street youths in Toronto, Canada. *Pediatr. Infect. Dis. J.* 10:130, 1991.
86. Hibbard, P.L., and Rubin, R.H. Approach to immunization in the immunosuppressed host. *Infect. Dis. Clin. North Am.* 4:123, 1990.
87. Sixbey, J.W. Routine immunizations and the immunosuppressed child. *Adv. Pediatr. Infect. Dis.* 2:79, 1987.
88. Centers for Disease Control. Use of vaccines and immune globulins in persons with altered immunocompetence. *M.M.W.R.* 42(RR-4):1, 1993.
89. Rose, D.N., Schechter, C.B., and Sacks, H.S. Influenza and pneumococcal vaccination of HIV-infected patients: A policy analysis. *Am. J. Med.* 94:160, 1993.
90. Siber, G.R., et al. Antibody response to pretreatment immunization and posttreatment boosting with bacterial polysaccharide vaccines in patients with Hodgkin's disease. *Ann. Intern. Med.* 194:467, 1986.
91. McMahon, B.J., et al. Response to hepatitis B vaccine in Alaska natives with chronic alcoholism compared with non-alcoholic control subjects. *Am. J. Med.* 88:460, 1990.
92. Turner-Stokes, L., and Isenberg, D.A. Immunisation of patients with rheumatoid arthritis and systemic lupus erythematosus. *Ann. Rheum. Dis.* 47:529, 1988.
93. Schwebke, J., and Mujais, S. Vaccination in hemodialysis patients. *Int. J. Artif. Organs* 12:481, 1989.
94. Konradsen, H.B., et al. Antibody persistence in splenectomized adults after pneumococcal vaccination. *Scand. J. Infect. Dis.* 22:725, 1990.
95. Ljungman, P., Duraj, V., and Magnius, L. Response to immunization against polio after allogeneic marrow transplantation. *Bone Marrow Transplant.* 7:89, 1991.
96. Williams, W.W., et al. Vaccines of importance in the hospital setting. Problems and developments. *Infect. Dis. Clin. North Am.* 3:701, 1989.
97. Valenti, M.M. Infection control and the pregnant health care worker. *Nurs. Clin. North Am.* 28:673, 1993.
98. Centers for Disease Control. Plague vaccine. *M.M.W.R.* 31:302, 1982.
99. Robbins, F.C., and Robbins, J.B. Current status and prospects for some improved and new bacterial vaccines. *Annu. Rev. Public Health* 7:105, 1986.
100. Bart, K.J., Hinman, A.R., and Jordan, W.S., Jr. International symposium on vaccine development and utilization. *Rev. Infect. Dis.* 11(Suppl. 3):S491–S667, 1989.
    Extensive symposium on vaccine development, delivery, and strategies in developing countries.
101. Hall, A.J., Greenwood, B.M., and Whittle, H. Modern vaccines. Practices in developing countries. *Lancet* 335:774, 1990.

23

Lyme Disease (Tickborne Borreliosis)

Henry F.C. Weil, Walter A. Franck, and Daniel W. Rahn

Lyme disease (LD) was newly recognized as an infectious disease within the past two decades. It is an illness that may be compared to tuberculosis or syphilis in terms of its protean findings, delays in development of a clinical syndrome, and its most significant manifestations, which occur in a chronic rather than an acute setting. This chapter is designed for clinicians wishing to obtain an effective working knowledge of and approach to LD. Such an understanding requires acquisition of geographic, epidemiologic, pathophysiologic, clinical, and pharmacologic data bases.

Lyme disease was first described in the United States in 1976, but its occurrence in Europe has been recognized since the early years of the twentieth century [1, 2]. It now is known that this illness is caused by a spirochete, *Borrelia burgdorferi,* which is transmitted to humans by the bite of *Ixodes* ticks [3, 4]. It may cause symptoms in several organ systems days to years after initiation of the infection and **may mimic other illnesses.** Diagnosis of this disease in its early stage is critical, for then it is reversible. Nonetheless, it is responsive to treatment, to varying degrees, in most stages.

Overview

I. **Endemic versus nonendemic areas.** Whether a patient has been present in an endemic area is very important when assessing the possibility of LD. The clinician should study the accompanying map of the United States (Fig. 23-1) **to determine whether a given patient is from (or has traveled to)** (1) an **endemic** area, (2) a **periendemic** area or, (3) a **nonendemic** area.

A. **For persons exposed to endemic or periendemic areas,** a suspicion for LD may be entertained in the presence of a variety of signs and symptoms, but diagnosis of LD must be methodical and well justified.

B. For those clinicians evaluating **patients from nonendemic areas,** detailed knowledge of LD is still of great importance. **The travel history,** with respect to regions endemic for LD, is **crucial** to the workup of any patient presenting symptoms compatible with LD. In addition, whereas areas inhabited by spirochete-bearing ticks expand slowly and usually into contiguous areas, discrete new foci of infected ticks infrequently do occur, possibly as ticks are transported to new areas by birds [5].

C. In the absence of a classic LD presentation, **ruling out geographic exposure to LD vastly reduces the possibility of LD.**

D. The **distribution of LD** in the United States is represented in **Figure 23-1.** Most cases are reported from the northeastern, mid-Atlantic, north central, and Pacific coastal regions.

E. The overall incidence rate for the United States was 3.9 per 100,000 population in 1992 [6]. In parts of California, Connecticut, Massachusetts, New York, and Wisconsin, reported rates exceeded 200 per 100,000 cases. The respective areas were well recognized to harbor established enzootic cycles [6].

II. **Special aspects of LD**

A. **Overdiagnosis. Lyme disease has a confounding variability of signs and symptoms.** Because of its clinical heterogeneity and the consequent ready confusion with many other illnesses, there is a **tendency toward overdiagnosis.**

B. **Underdiagnosis.** Accurate diagnosis is hampered by both the variability of presentation and the **absence of an available reliable serologic test** [7]. **At best,** LD will present with a known tick bite and its hallmark rash (erythema chronicum migrans) and will be easy to diagnose and treat. **At worst,** the tick bite will go

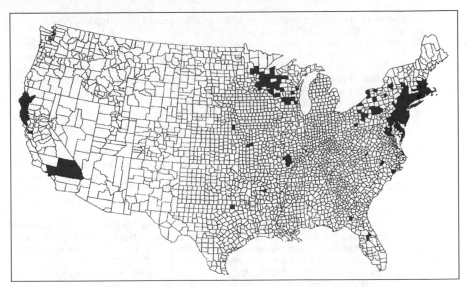

Fig. 23-1. U.S. counties averaging at least five Lyme disease cases during 1991–1993. (From D. Fish, Environmental risk and prevention of Lyme disease. *Am. J. Med.* 98(Suppl. 4A): 2S, 1995.)

   unnoticed, the rash will not appear, and the disease will present as a confusing constellation of complaints and physical findings, making definitive diagnosis difficult. Furthermore, **serologic tests** are not standardized and will be **falsely negative** in some individuals and **falsely positive** in others. Thus, the skill and judgment of the clinician often are challenged.
   C. **Consequences of infection.** Although LD is **potentially debilitating** physically and psychologically, it is almost never fatal and usually resolves spontaneously, though the course in some patients gradually tapers to remission through a series of flares. Only a small minority of patients with infection experience chronic, persistent symptoms.
   D. **Response of the general public.** The public is generally confused about LD, in part due to the occasional difficulties in making a definitive diagnosis and in part due to the media attention this disease has received. **Intense nervousness and paranoia often are present among both populations at risk and populations at no risk.**
   E. **Geographic zones of risk.** The endemic areas of LD are expanding, with the known range enlarging slowly (over four decades) from one small Massachusetts island to current reports of cases in 43 states. However, it must be emphasized that LD can be conveyed only by certain subspecies of *Ixodes* ticks and that these particular ticks are **not** found in most places in the United States.
III. **Lyme disease challenges for the physician and scientific community include the following:**
   A. **To diagnose accurately** and **to avoid overdiagnosis** and treat effectively
   B. **To educate** (i.e., to inform the populations at risk and to reassure the populations at no risk)
   C. **To prevent** (i.e., to ensure that individuals who inhabit or visit areas endemic for LD know where, when, and how they are at risk and how to avoid infection)

Background

I. **History.** The history of LD is well documented elsewhere [8–11]. Some brief highlights are presented.
   A. **1909.** A red, slowly expanding rash, persisting weeks to months, was described in Sweden [1]. Association with tick bite was recognized, but an infectious etiology was not established. The lesion was named **erythema chronicum migrans** (ECM).

   B. 1940s. An infectious etiology for ECM was suspected by European investigators when ECM was found to respond to penicillin.
   C. 1975. Stimulated by observations and concerns of astute parents, researchers at Yale University and the Connecticut State Department of Health investigated an epidemic of oligoarticular arthritis in children living in the town of Lyme and neighboring areas, suspecting an infectious etiology from the outset of their investigation. The association between tick bite, ECM, and later neurologic sequelae was discovered by this group [2, 8, 11].
   D. 1982. Dr. Willie Burgdorfer isolated a spirochete from the midgut of *Ixodes scapularis* ticks and identified this agent as "the long-sought cause of ECM and Lyme disease" [10].
   E. Since 1975, a multinational research effort has resulted in a clearer understanding of the epidemiology, clinical range, pathogenesis, diagnosis, and treatment of LD.
II. **Epidemiologic factors. Knowledge of LD epidemiology**—the spirochete, tick vector, important tick hosts, tick habitat and life cycle, seasonality of infection, and distribution of disease—**is essential to effective diagnosis, prevention, and treatment of LD.**
   A. Spirochete
      1. A newly recognized spirochete, designated **Borrelia burgdorferi,** has been isolated from tissues and body fluids of numerous patients with LD, has been grown in culture, and has been isolated from *Ixodes* ticks [12]. **This spirochete is known to be the causative agent of LD.**
      2. Antigenic variability has been demonstrated in isolates of *B. burgdorferi* obtained from different geographic locations and may play a role in causing differences in the clinical presentation of Lyme disease [13].
      3. *B. burgdorferi* has been isolated from numerous mammalian and avian hosts [14] as well as from domestic animals, including dogs, cats, horses, and cows [15].
      4. Several **subspecies of Ixodes** (or hard-shelled) **ticks have been implicated as the principal vectors of spirochetal transmission to humans** [8, 16].
      5. Other arthropods and insects are suspected to host the spirochete, and LD has apparently been diagnosed abroad in areas not endemic for *Ixodes* ticks, raising the possibility that other ticks or insects may have vector competence [17–20]. At this time, **human infection in the United States other than by Ixodes ticks is virtually unknown.**
   B. Tick
      1. **Four geographically and morphologically distinct subspecies of Ixodes** tick are the principal vectors of transmission of LD to humans: **I. scapularis** (formerly *I. dammini*) on the eastern seaboard and in the midwestern United States; **I. pacificus** on the West Coast; **I. ricinus** in Europe; and **I. persulcatus** in Asia [16, 21]. The northern population of *I. scapularis*, previously believed to be a distinct subspecies and named *I. dammini*, has recently been found to be cospecific with *I. scapularis* and now is subsumed under that name [22]. **Because of their small size, these ticks are not easy to identify by inspection.** Ideally, potentially infected ticks should be identified only by those versed in *Ixodes* tick taxonomy.
      2. **Lyme disease has spread with the spread of ticks** [23, 24]. Prior to 1950, *I. scapularis* ticks were found only on Naushon Island, off the Massachusetts coast. In the 1950s and 1960s, the ticks spread to nearby islands and the mainland, and a clinical entity nicknamed *Nantucket knee* appeared, now recognized to be Lyme arthritis. Similarly, in New York State, *I. scapularis* originally flourished only on Long Island and in the lower Hudson Valley. In New York, the tick appears to have migrated northward, and case reports of LD have burgeoned from 100 prior to 1980 to approximately 50,000 through 1992 [25, 26].
      3. There are two principal determinants of infection rates in humans in a given endemic area:
         a. The density of *Ixodes* ticks in that area
         b. The prevalence of ticks infected with the spirochete
      4. Thus, **the presence of Ixodes ticks alone is not predictive of human infection; it is rather the regional density of ticks and the percentage of ticks parasitized by B. burgdorferi spirochetes that predict human risk.** Up to 60% of *I. scapularis* collected from endemic areas on the East Coast and in the Midwest have been documented to carry spirochetes as opposed to approximately 1% of *I. pacificus* in the San Francisco Bay area of California [3, 27, 28]. Similarly,

a low percentage of *I. scapularis* infection exists in the south. As one might expect, the incidence of LD in endemic areas on the East Coast is far greater than on the West Coast [29–31]. These differences in prevalence of infected ticks apparently result from the tendency of *I. scapularis* in the northeastern and upper midwestern United States to parasitize mammals and birds, whereas *I. pacificus* and *I. scapularis* in the southern states primarily parasitize lizards, less effective reservoirs of spirochetes, yielding lower rates of tick-to-tick transmission.

5. **Endemic areas for LD are expanding as the range of *Ixodes* ticks gradually enlarges. Spread usually is contiguous and gradual, although sporadic non-contiguous foci have been documented** [5]. The typical pattern of expansion of an endemic focus is for uninfected ticks to colonize a new area and to become hosts to spirochetes subsequently.

6. The widening range of *Ixodes* populations may correlate with recent increases in the abundance of deer (*recent* here meaning within the last 30 years) [31].

7. Limitations to expansion of the *Ixodes* tick range are not known, but expansion rates are slow [5]. This may be a consequence of the 2-year life cycle of *Ixodes* ticks, which prohibits rapid colonization of new areas.

8. The *Ixodes* ticks have a broad host range and have been collected from numerous species of mammals, both wild and domestic, as well as from numerous species of birds and reptiles [14, 32].

C. **The life cycle of the tick is very complex. Knowledge of the tick life cycle is a valuable aid to diagnosis and patient education,** second in utility only to knowledge of the geographic distribution of infected ticks and of clinical presentation of LD. Ticks, like other arthropods, pass through three stages: larval, nymphal, and adult. See Fig. 23-2, which summarizes the tick life cycle.

1. *Ixodes* ticks live approximately 2 years. During most of its life, an *Ixodes* tick is not attached to an animal. Rather, it "hibernates," either in the nesting material of its previous host or on the forest floor. The tick feeds only once in each stage of its life (or a total of three times).

2. **Eggs** typically are laid on the ground in the spring. During the summer, the eggs hatch into larvae, which feed once and detach from the host animal thereafter.

3. Transovarial transmission of spirochetes does occur but is rare and ineffective in maintaining infection in the tick population. **A larva must feed on an effective reservoir host (and one that is colonized with spirochetes) to become infectious to humans.** Thus, **only nymphal or adult ticks have the capacity to infect humans.**

4. Larvae spend the winter unattached and molt into nymphs (the second stage) in the second spring. Nymphs then enter the "questing stage," when they search for a host from which to take a blood meal. **Although only 30% of people who contract LD and the ECM rash recall tick bite, most ticks that have been saved and identified have been nymphs** (i.e., not larvae and not adults) [16].

5. Note that nymphs feed during the late spring and early summer months, so that this is the most likely time of transmission from tick to human. **The period when humans are most likely to become infected corresponds to the questing nymph season—namely, June, July, and August.**

6. Nymphs molt after feeding and become adults during the summer of the second year. They then attach to a third host as adults. While feeding on the third host, the adults mate. This occurs in the late summer and fall of the second year. The female ticks are dormant through the winter and lay their eggs in the spring, thus completing the cycle. Adult male ticks die shortly after mating.

D. **Why is LD a successful human zoonosis?**

1. Many larvae and nymphs take their single blood meal on mice; a mouse in an area populous with ticks may harbor many ticks of both stages simultaneously [31]. Mice remain spirochetemic (though asymptomatic) for weeks. Thus, a mouse may be made bacteremic by previously infected nymphs, and **uninfected larvae will take a blood meal on that mouse and become infected.** An infected larva will then winter over and molt into a nymph in the spring and may **either attach to another mouse and complete the cycle by horizontally infecting members of the next generation of larvae or incidentally attach to and infect a human.**

2. **Mice are predominant hosts.** Mice are competent reservoirs of spirochetes, whereas deer may not be [31, 33]. However, deer appear to be important for the biologic success of *I. scapularis*.

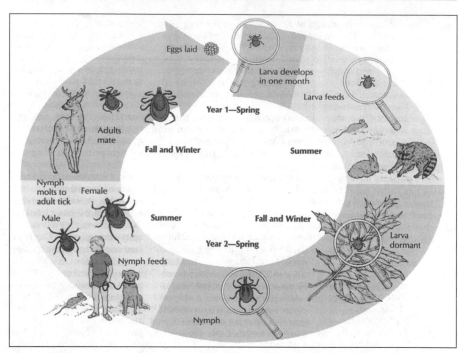

Fig. 23-2. The 2-year life cycle of *B. burgdorferi* in *Ixodes* ticks depends on horizontal transmission between immature ticks and mice. The larval tick is infected in summer when it feeds on a mouse that carries the spirochete. After a dormant period, the larva emerges as a nymph the next spring, when it again feeds on a mouse and infects it with the spirochete. It is the nymphal stage that usually transmits the infection to humans. Nymphs become adults during the summer, feed once in the fall (preferably on a deer), and then produce more larvae, which are spirochete-free until the spring, when the cycle begins again with larvae feeding on mice. (From A. C. Steere, Current understanding of Lyme disease. *Hosp. Pract.* Apr. 15, 1993.)

   3. **A key point is that nymphs quest during the summer months, the season when humans are most likely to enter their habitat. This explains the predominance of the first stage of LD (ECM rash, etc.) presenting in the late spring through early fall.**
   E. **Why is LD appearing now?** Success of *Ixodes* ticks is essential to success of the spirochete. On the East Coast, from whence the **spirochete** probably has spread in the United States, farming as a vocation has declined. Fields have given way to woodlands, the natural habitat of deer. Deer, once uncommon, are now again plentiful. Deer probably are necessary for the ecologic success of *Ixodes* ticks, ergo *B. burgdorferi* spirochetes. Mice are ubiquitous in areas inhabited by deer. Unless there are unknown supervening factors, ***Ixodes* ticks may spread into any area heavily populated with deer.** Because of the long life cycle, spread is slow and can be monitored, a fact of great importance to the clinician when assessing probability of infection in a given patient.
   F. **Humans come in contact with ticks most commonly on the edges of fields in low brush,** where questing larvae and nymphs await host mammals. Neighboring wooded areas are necessary. Lawns are less likely to harbor questing ticks [33a]. Transportation of ticks by pets is not believed to be a common mode of spread but may infrequently play a role in endemic areas. Dogs in two California coastal counties had a prevalence of 26% infection by serologic testing [34].
   G. **Human demographics.** The annual number of reported cases of LD increased sevenfold between 1980 and 1986. **LD is now the most common vectorborne illness in the United States [30]. However, LD remains an uncommon disease** and is misdiagnosed in both endemic and nonendemic areas.

1. **The prevalence of clinical LD is extremely variable within different endemic areas** [25, 35, 36].
2. In one study, the ratio of symptomatic to asymptomatic patients with positive serologic findings was as high as 1:1 [35]. The significance of a positive titer in an asymptomatic individual is, however, unclear. (See sec. **VII.B** under Clinical Manifestations of Lyme Disease.)
3. **Men are slightly more likely to become infected** than women [25], and **children more so than adults** (probably because of more likely exposure). The incidence drops off with increasing age (> 70 years) [25].
4. In the area surrounding Lyme, Connecticut, an overall prevalence rate of 4.3 per 1,000 residents was documented, and 12.2 per 1,000 children [11].

H. **Distribution of LD.** Fig. 23-1 displays the currently known endemic areas for LD in the United States. Fig. 23-1 displays counties in the United States from which more than 5 cases of LD were reported during 1991–1993 [33a]. Lyme disease has now been reported in 43 of the 50 states. Eighty-six percent of the 5,731 provisional cases reported to the Centers for Disease Control (CDC), Atlanta, were acquired in New York, New Jersey, Massachusetts, Rhode Island, Connecticut, Minnesota, and Wisconsin [29]. Pennsylvania, Virginia, Oregon, and California have also had significant numbers of cases [29]. Again, **most of these cases were contracted in well-demarcated endemic regions of these states.**
   1. There are three primary groups of foci: (1) seaboard areas from Massachusetts to Maryland; (2) the upper Midwest, in parts of Minnesota and Wisconsin; and (3) the West Coast, in parts of California and Oregon.
   2. Lyme disease has now been documented in more than 20 countries and on 3 continents [36].
I. **Importance of the travel history.** Clearly, **travel history may play a critical role in triggering suspicion for LD,** particularly for the clinician whose practice lies in a nonendemic area. **A patient who has not had exposure to an area endemic, or at least periendemic, for LD is most unlikely to have LD.**

III. **Pathogenesis. During the 1980s and early 1990s, LD was characterized as having three distinct stages (stages 1, 2, and 3),** correlating with the interval from infection to appearance of findings. **These divisions were arbitrary,** as symptoms and signs of two stages may overlap, and there is no uniform clinical evolution. **What follows is a more detailed view of pathogenesis within the above-named categories of LD. The disease is better understood as evolving from an early localized infection through a period of dissemination (involving early and later features) to a chronic stage.** Thus, the new way of looking at the disease is to categorize the spectrum of presentations according to clinical behaviors. As an overview, the **early localized** manifestation is the hallmark rash, ECM; the **early disseminated** manifestations include fever, arthralgias, myalgias, secondary skin lesions, and possibly Bell's palsy; **late disseminated** manifestations include intermittent frank arthritis, carditis, acute CNS symptoms and signs and radiculoneuropathy; and **chronic** manifestations include arthritis and CNS findings lasting longer than 1 year.

A. **Early localized LD**
   1. An infected questing *Ixodes* tick crawls onto a human and begins to feed. Spirochetes within the tick translocate from the midgut to the salivary glands. The tick **regurgitates** or **salivates** material that contains spirochetes into the bite [37]. Alternatively, spirochetes may be inoculated by fecal contamination of the bite.
   2. The site of the tick bite may become inflamed for two reasons: either **in reaction to the bite itself** (not indicative of infection) **or in response to the presence of the spirochete.**
      a. The tick with which most people are familiar, *Dermacentor variabilis,* or "the dog tick," probably does not transmit LD but frequently incites an immediate local reaction with its bite.
      b. **In experimental studies, ticks must often be attached for 24 hours or more before there is sufficient transfer of spirochetes to cause an infection [38]. The ECM rash typically does not appear until several days after tick bite, as opposed to the local reaction, which is immediate.**
   3. **ECM skin lesion.** The organism moves centrifugally within the skin away from the site of tick bite (associated with the rash enlarging centrifugally); organisms have been isolated by biopsy at the margin of the expanding rash (ECM). (For a clinical description of ECM, see sec. **I.B** under Clinical Manifestations of Lyme Disease.)

B. Early disseminated LD
1. **The organism may enter the bloodstream and widely disseminate to sites throughout the body. It is believed that the flulike manifestations of LD as well as other subsequent manifestations are consequent to bloodborne metastasis shortly after inoculation.**
2. **In the early phase after dissemination, the organism may inhabit new skin sites and cause several to numerous additional ECM lesions in up to 50% of patients.** The appearance of these lesions is similar to the initial one, but they generally are smaller.
3. Myalgias and arthralgias are due either to local reaction to spirochetes or to release of nonspecific factors.
4. **In as many as 50% of infected individuals, no early localized disease (ECM) is noted; nevertheless, these individuals may progress to later stages** [39].
5. Some patients appear to clear infection locally after ECM without antibiotic treatment, whether or not there are signs or symptoms of dissemination.
6. Most individuals who experience the ECM rash and are not treated, do not clear infection and progress to later manifestations of the disease. Others may be incompletely treated with oral antibiotics and progress to late disease.
7. Treatment in the early disseminated phase usually prevents progression to later stages [40]. A Jarisch-Herxheimer reaction may be seen with treatment, possibly due to release of a lipopolysaccharide from dying organisms, which in turn liberates interleukin-1 and tumor necrosis factor [40–42].

C. Late disseminated LD
1. **As noted previously, the late disseminated phase is a delayed consequence of bloodborne spread of organisms. Manifestations are seen most often in joints, neural tissue, and myocardium.**
2. The **arthritis** of late disseminated LD is due, at least in part, to the presence of organisms in the joint space. In some individuals, inflammatory activity may persist in the absence of live organisms.
3. **Meningitic manifestations of late disseminated LD** are probably the consequence of infection within the cerebrospinal fluid (CSF), with clinical manifestations due to local inflammation. Evidence for this includes isolation of spirochetes from CSF and the presence of locally produced antibody to spirochetes in the CSF [12, 43, 44], occasionally in the absence of measurable serum antibodies.
4. Evidence of humoral antineuronal activity and cellular autoimmune activity to neuronal antigen suggests that the **pathogenesis of LD neurologic disease may include autoimmune mechanisms in addition to local damage resulting from infection** [45–47]. Certain spirochetal antigens have been shown to possess homology with human cellular antigens.
5. **Radiculoneuropathy and cranial neuropathy (particularly Bell's palsy)** also occur commonly, with or without accompanying meningitis. Nerve conduction studies and biopsy suggest that axonal injury is the lesion in radiculoneuropathy [48].
   A recent report from Japan emphasizes the importance of herpes simplex virus (HSV) in many cases of so-called idiopathic Bell's palsy in nonendemic areas of LD [48a]. The exact role HSV plays in causing Bell's palsy awaits further study, but this report further complicates the evaluation of patients presenting with this problem.
6. Spirochetes have been recovered from CSF and other tissues early in disease, **suggesting that dissemination shortly after tick bite may eventually cause later manifestations of the disease** [39]. This probably accounts for the occasional meningitic symptoms noted during the first week after inoculation.
7. Myocarditis is a direct consequence of infection and pathologically shows infiltrates of lymphocytes [49]. Spirochetes have been isolated from cardiac tissue [50].
8. Response of late disseminated LD to antibiotics is variable both between and within affected organ systems, highlighting the dual roles of infection and self-perpetuating injury in pathogenesis.

D. Chronic LD
1. *B. burgdorferi* spirochetes have been isolated from foci of infection months to years after inoculation, suggesting that these organisms may participate directly in the chronic phases of disease.

2. The **pathogenesis** of chronic LD is **controversial.** Antibiotics may fail to prevent arthritic relapses and chronic neurologic lesions, raising the question as to whether live organisms are necessary to continue inflammation at these sites [47]. Response to antibiotics in approximately 55% of patients with chronic arthritis (and occasional recovery of organisms) implicates chronic infection in the pathogenesis of chronic joint disease; however, the failure to cure 45% of these suggests other mechanisms [51–53].

E. **Overview of pathogenesis**
   1. *Borrelia burgdorferi* **spirochetes are not aggressive organisms and do not cause fulminant infection. Rather, bacteremia is tolerated well, and infection progresses in an indolent fashion.**
   2. Pathogenesis of some aspects of LD remains controversial. Early phases probably are primarily infectious, but late and chronic manifestations may have components of infectious and parainfectious pathology.

Clinical Manifestations

As with other spirochetal illnesses, the clinical manifestations of LD can appear in many organ systems and at widely variable intervals from the time of infection. Table 23-1 summarizes the clinical manifestations, categorized by the nomenclature of chronicity.

I. **Early localized infection. Early localized LD occurs in the first month after infection and manifests as the definitive skin lesion of LD.**
   A. The first evidence of LD infection might be the finding of an attached tick or the nonspecific swelling and local inflammation that result from any tick bite, whether or not it is a tick parasitized by *B. burgdorferi.* (See sec. **III.A.1–2** under Background.)
   B. **The cardinal lesion of LD—ECM—occurs between 3 and 32 days after the tick bite,** with a median of 7 days. The lesion may be located anywhere, with the thigh, groin, and axilla being common sites [39]. **(See Plate IV.)**

Table 23-1. Clinical manifestations of Lyme disease

Early localized infection
  Erythema migrans
  Erythema migrans with a mild viral illness
Early disseminated infection
  Erythema migrans in areas distant from tick bite
  Mild to severe systemic symptoms or other evidence of systemic spread (e.g.,
    abnormal liver function tests)
  Bell's palsy (may occur early or later)
  Myalgias, arthralgias without frank arthritis
Late disseminated infection
  Cardiac abnormalities
    Atrioventricular block
    Myopericarditis
  Neurologic disorders
    Acute meningitis
    Acute encephalitis
    Cranial neuritis
    Radiculoneuritis (Bannwarth syndrome)
    Peripheral neuropathy
  Arthritis
Chronic infection (lasting > 1 year)
  Neurologic disorders
    Peripheral neuropathy
    Chronic meningoencephalitis
    Chronic encephalitis
  Arthritis
  Acrodermatitis chronica atrophicans

1. The median diameter of the lesion is roughly 15 cm; the range is 3–68 cm. The rash is hot but painless.
2. Most lesions are **flat** (although occasionally they are raised), with **red to bright red outer borders and partial central clearing** and, after they have been present for days to several weeks, may become blue. Lesions usually are **painless** but may be hypersensitive to touch. Uncommon findings include intensely erythematous and indurated, vesicular, or necrotic centers of early lesions [39].
3. Several days or more after the appearance of the original ECM, as few as 1 to as many as 100 additional lesions may develop. These **multiple annular secondary lesions** are similar in appearance to the original one, though usually smaller, with less migration, and lacking an indurated center. These lesions are one **sign of early dissemination of the spirochete.** Secondary lesions have been described anywhere except the palms of the hands and soles of the feet. Individual lesions may appear or disappear at different times, and their borders may become merged [39].
4. **Untreated, the ECM rash and secondary lesions fade within a median of 28 days** and a range of 1 day–14 months. There is occasionally residual scaling or pigmentary change [39]. Some untreated individuals have recurrences of secondary lesions intermittently over periods of years.
5. Among patients given antibiotic agents, the skin lesions usually resolve after several days of therapy.

II. **Early disseminated infection**
   A. **Signs of LD**
      1. In addition to secondary ECM lesions, regional and generalized lymphadenopathy, pain on neck flexion, malar rash, erythematous throat, and conjunctivitis all occurred in from 10 to 41% of patients in one carefully performed study [39].
      2. Right upper quadrant tenderness, frank arthritis, splenomegaly, hepatomegaly, muscle tenderness, periorbital edema, evanescent skin lesions, abdominal tenderness, and testicular swelling occurred less commonly [39]. Fever is an uncommon sign.
   B. **Symptoms of LD**
      1. **Nonspecific complaints.** Malaise, fatigue, and lethargy are the most common systemic symptoms in early disseminated LD.
      2. **Meningeal symptoms.** In some patients, symptoms suggesting meningeal irritation predominate. These patients may have excruciating headache, which is usually intermittent (typically lasting hours) and localized (frontal, temporal, or occipital) but in some cases is generalized and persistent. Neck pain, stiffness, or pressure may also be present. (CSF usually is normal at this point [39, 54].)
      3. **Arthralgias, myalgias,** backache, anorexia, sore throat, nausea, and vomiting occur in 10% or more of patients [39].
      4. Abdominal pain, photophobia, hand stiffness, dizziness, cough, chest pain, ear pain, and diarrhea are uncommon early symptoms of LD [39].

III. **Late disseminated infection.** This phase of LD **occurs weeks to months** after the initial tick bite. **Late disseminated disease includes nervous system, cardiac, musculoskeletal, and ophthalmologic involvement.** Once again, **migratory and intermittent signs and symptoms may be observed. The syndromes listed here are rare sequelae of LD:**
   A. **Neurologic manifestations**
      1. **General considerations.** The neurologic manifestations may mimic other neurologic processes; thus, any patient who resides in or near an area endemic for LD who presents with a disorder ranging from Bell's palsy to a multiple sclerosis–type syndrome should be questioned carefully regarding tick bite or prior ECM rash and should have a serologic test for LD. However, **multiple sclerosis–like presentations occur very rarely in LD and should be attributed to LD only when compelling evidence is present.** Objective testing will discriminate actual multiple sclerosis from LD [55].
         a. A number of patients with documented LD will have abnormalities of nerve conduction studies **without symptoms** [48].
         b. **Aseptic meningitis may be the presenting symptom of LD,** with severe relapsing headache and stiff neck as well as nonspecific CSF abnormalities [56].
         c. **Neuritis** is a common manifestation of late disseminated disease, involving approximately 15% of all patients [54, 57]. **Bell's palsy** is the most common

clinical manifestation of neurologic LD. **Bell's palsy develops in up to 50% of patients with frank meningitis** [56]. It often occurs early in LD, which has prompted some investigators to classify it as an early disseminated finding.

d. As with all manifestations of LD, there is potential for overlap. Thus, some patients who develop clinical manifestations of late disseminated neurologic LD may persist in having primary or secondary ECM lesions or may have already progressed to chronic arthritis [56].

e. It must be emphasized that the neurologic manifestations, or any manifestation of LD for that matter, may appear in the absence of prior LD abnormalities. Bell's palsy, for example, may present without any other symptoms or signs suggestive of LD.

f. **Some patients present with one neurologic finding and subsequently develop another neurologic finding.** For example, patients have initially experienced a right-sided facial palsy, followed weeks later by left-sided facial palsy. Alternatively, some patients have had a painful radiculopathy in a bandlike distribution around the abdomen, as well as meningitis.

g. **CSF findings** range from normal profile to typical aseptic meningitis and are described elsewhere (see sec. **VII**). Spirochetes have only rarely been cultured from CSF. (See also Chap. 5.)

2. **Specific neurologic syndromes associated with LD**

   a. **Headache.** Most patients with Lyme meningitis will have the predominant symptom of headache, which typically fluctuates in intensity. On some days it will be excruciating and on other days mild or absent [56]. In addition to headaches, some patients experience nausea, vomiting, photophobia, and pain on eye motion [56]. Most will have mild stiffness on extreme neck flexion, but Kernig's and Brudzinski's signs will be absent.

   Encephalitis also is recognized in up to 30% of patients with neurologic manifestations of LD. The symptoms usually are subtle. Difficulty concentrating, poor memory, irritability, and emotional lability have been documented in a few patients [56]. **These symptoms do not necessarily correlate with the severity of headache and stiff neck and also vary from day to day.** Seizures and coma have not been observed [56].

   b. **Cranial neuritis** is the second most common neurologic manifestation of LD. **It frequently will overlap with meningitis.** Seventh nerve palsy is common. A small number of patients will have bilateral facial palsies. Often, weakness is accompanied by a sensation of numbness and tingling on the weak side of the face, but a clear sensory abnormality cannot be demonstrated [56]. **Unilateral Bell's palsy should not be assumed to be due to LD, even in a patient residing in an endemic area.** (See under sec. **III.C.5**, p. 884.)

   c. Patients may have pain around the ear or jaw [56]. Localization of the lesion in the facial nerve has usually been distal to the branching of the chorda tympani, similar to classic Bell's palsy. Patients have been observed who have changes in hearing but not hyperacusis or loss of taste, and vice versa, findings atypical for Bell's palsy [56].

   d. **Other cranial neuropathies.** The other most commonly affected cranial nerves are the third, fourth, and sixth nerves. When the fifth cranial nerve is affected, the symptoms are likely to be sensory rather than motor. Eighth cranial nerve involvement has been observed with dizziness, otalgia, and sore throat [58].

   e. Optic atrophy and Argyll Robertson pupils have been noted.

   f. **Radiculopathy, usually painful,** may occur. Findings of dermatomal thoracic sensory radiculitis, motor radiculoneuritis in one or more extremity, or mononeuritis multiplex have been described. In extremity involvement, there often is severe radicular pain, dysesthesias, subtle sensory loss, focal weakness, and loss of reflexes [56]. Significant muscle atrophy has been observed. When extremities are involved bilaterally, one side usually is more severely affected. Onset of symptoms may be separated by weeks or months. **Thoracic radiculitis is usually experienced as intense pain** [56, 59].

   g. Patients have been observed with frank psychoses and auditory hallucinations, sleep disturbances, and personality changes [56].

   h. In addition, pseudotumor cerebri has been described. In these patients, LD serologic studies and lumbar puncture may be helpful in making the diagnosis [56].

        i. Complete or partial recovery is commonplace with most neurologic complications of late disseminated LD. However, that is not invariable. The goal of therapy is to arrest symptoms [60].

        j. Retinitis and panophthalmitis have been seen infrequently.

  3. Some patients previously treated for ECM have gone on to develop facial paralysis and other manifestations of later disease **despite standard treatment.** Treatment with antibiotics seems to shorten the course of late disseminated manifestations and was clearly superior to prednisone for meningitic manifestations, but treatment with prednisone was reported to be equally efficacious for radiculoneuritis [48, 61].

B. Cardiac abnormalities of late disseminated disease. Cardiac manifestations occur in **8–10% of patients with LD** [62], a median of 5 weeks after infection, with a range of 3–21 weeks. **Cardiac manifestations of LD include myopericarditis, pancarditis, and varying degrees of atrioventricular (AV) block, from first-degree to complete heart block. Cardiac valves are never involved.** The injury probably is a consequence of direct invasion of spirochetes. Cardiac disease may appear de novo or with other findings of LD [63, 64].

  1. Syncope, dizziness, palpitations, and exertional dyspnea are common symptoms of cardiac involvement. S3 gallops have been detected on examination [39].

  2. Patients with high-degree AV block or first-degree block with a P-R interval longer than 0.3 seconds should be hospitalized, because they appear to be at marked risk for developing complete heart block [63]. Temporary pacemaker insertion has been necessary in some symptomatic patients with high degrees of AV block.

  3. Treatment is currently not well defined and may include antibiotics and salicylates (see sec. **VIII.D**). Permanent heart damage usually does not occur; however, **antibiotic treatment has not been shown necessarily to alter the natural history of cardiac involvement** [64].

C. Musculoskeletal manifestations of late disseminated disease. Arthritis is a common manifestation of disseminated *B. burgdorferi* infection. There is a broad spectrum of presentation. A deep myositis can occur. The division of early, late, and chronic musculoskeletal conditions is arbitrary and represents a continuum, with differences in presentation that may be attributable to individual host response. (See further discussion in sec. **IV.A.**)

IV. Chronic infection. Chronic LD consists of frank arthritis and late neurologic complications, sometimes defined as having a duration of more than 1 year. Particular class II major histocompatibility genes may determine host immune response to *B. burgdorferi* that results in chronic arthritis and lack of response to antibiotics [65].

A. Arthritis. Because late disseminated and chronic musculoskeletal aspects of LD represent a continuum, they are discussed together.

  1. Musculoskeletal pain may occur in all stages of LD and may be severe. Complaints may include migratory pain in tendons, muscles, and bones. Musculoskeletal symptoms begin an average of 2 weeks after onset of ECM. They may recur intermittently for years without evidence of joint injury [66].

  2. Frank arthritis occurs in 60% of untreated patients who have had ECM [67]. Often a recurrent monoarticular or asymmetric oligoarticular arthritis appears, primarily affecting large joints and reminiscent of the arthritis of Reiter's syndrome [67, 68]. Attacks may persist for 1 week to 3 months, with intervening symptom-free periods ranging from 1 week to several months [67]. Severity, duration, and disease-free interval is unpredictable in the individual patient [68]. The knee is the most commonly afflicted joint, with heat and intense swelling but often little pain. Baker's cyst occurs commonly and may rupture and dissect, especially early in the course of arthritis [67]. Even when swelling is bilateral, it often starts at a different time on each side and frequently is more severe on one side than the other [66]. It is rare that more than five joints are involved [66]. The temporomandibular joint may be affected [66]. Joint fluid is inflammatory and is described elsewhere (see sec. **VII.C.3**).

  3. In some individuals, particularly children, septic arthritis is suggested by high fever and the acuteness and intensity of synovitis [67, 69].

  4. In approximately 10% of cases, the intermittent pattern evolves into chronic arthritis, usually after at least a year of intermittent attacks. **Erosive joint damage may occur, particularly in one or both knees.** Difficulty walking is the primary functional disability [67, 68]. Even in patients who suffer chronic arthritis, inflammation rarely continues for more than several years [54], after which inflammation spontaneously subsides.

B. Neurologic manifestations of chronic disease. There are three major chronic neurologic syndromes, characterized by neuropsychiatric symptoms, focal CNS disease, or severe, incapacitating fatigue [70]. **Many patients will have arthritis accompanying neurologic manifestations of late disease** [70]. Arthritis may precede chronic neurologic manifestations by as many as 5–10 years [70]. **The syndromes listed here are rare sequelae of LD.**

   1. Neuropsychiatric symptoms occur in children and include difficulties with concentration and interaction with peers, wide mood swings, and decline in grades. Most often, these patients will have been infected by the age of 10 [70].

   2. Focal CNS lesions include progressive meningoencephalitis, which may primarily involve the spinal cord and mimic multiple sclerosis; or focal encephalitis, transverse myelitis, vestibular neuronitis, optic neuritis, or other forms of CNS inflammation that have occurred rarely [70–72].

   3. Incapacitating fatigue constitutes the third category of chronic CNS symptoms, if energy depletion may be considered a CNS complaint. Fatigue may be episodic and last days to a few weeks. Subtle neurologic signs may or may not be detected on examination. Patients feel well between attacks [66, 67, 73]. **This diagnosis should not be made without objective evidence of borrelial infection** (e.g., a rising or significant antibody titer, previous ECM). Fatigue alone, without other manifestations of active LD, should not be considered indicative of neurologic infection.

C. European LD. Several syndromes associated with *B. burgdorferi* infection have been described in Europe that have not been seen on the North American continent. These entities involve the nervous system and skin and are well described elsewhere [9, 54].

V. Lyme disease in pregnancy. Lyme disease affects the pregnant woman in a similar manner to the nonpregnant woman. However, **fetal fatalities and other adverse fetal outcomes have been documented in pregnant women with LD** [74, 75].

A. Occurrence in each of the trimesters has been reported, and both early and late LD may be associated with fetal injury or death [76].

B. One case report described a pregnant woman who received a short course of low-dose oral penicillin for LD early in her pregnancy and delivered a baby who survived only 23 hours after birth. Autopsy revealed spirochetes in brain and liver [77].

C. Anomalies observed in the infants of patients with LD during pregnancy include syndactyly, cortical blindness, rash in the newborn, prematurity, and intrauterine fetal death. **It is unclear whether these outcomes are a consequence of spirochetal infection or whether the coexistence of LD was unrelated.** In conclusion, while it is likely that the LD spirochete can cause an adverse fetal outcome, it is thought to be rare [54, 73a, 74].

D. Patients known to have LD or strongly suspected of having LD during pregnancy should be considered for immediate treatment until data clarifying this issue are available. Appropriate antibiotics for the pregnant patient should be used (see Chap. 28A).

VI. Reinfection. Prior infection with *B. burgdorferi* does not uniformly confer immunity. Patients who have been successfully treated for early LD probably resume their prior risk of acquiring LD [74]. Reinfection has not been observed in patients with an expanded antibody response to *B. burgdorferi* [74]. In vaccine trials in mice, an immune response, including reaction to certain outer surface proteins, does confer protection against subsequent infection [78].

VII. Laboratory findings. LD is a clinical diagnosis. Routine laboratory tests are nonspecific. Serologic testing is the only widely available diagnostic test being utilized at this time, there being both immunofluorescent antibody (IFA) and enzyme-linked immunosorbent assay (ELISA) tests. **Serologic tests should not be ordered indiscriminately but rather to confirm a diagnosis based on epidemiologic and clinical evidence** [79]. The serologic tests have limitations. Both false positives and false negatives occur. **Unfortunately, an ideal serologic test is not available.**

A. Laboratory findings in early LD. Routine laboratory tests may be abnormal but are of little diagnostic value. Note that *B. burgdorferi* organisms are almost never successfully cultured from human blood or CSF in any stage of LD [54]. However, skin biopsies cultured on appropriate media are positive 50% of the time [80].

The **nonspecific** laboratory tests in early LD that are most commonly abnormal include the following:

1. **Erythrocyte sedimentation rate,** which is greater than 20 mm/hr in 53% (median level, 35 mm) [11].
2. Serum IgM level, which is elevated in 33% of patients [11].
3. Liver function tests, including serum aspartate aminotransferase (AST, SGOT), alanine aminotransferase (ALT, SGPT), and lactic dehydrogenase (LDH), which are abnormal in 19% of patients [39].
4. Hematocrit, which is lower than 37% in 12% of patients, and WBC count (> 10,000/mm) in 8% of patients [39].
5. Urinalysis, which reveals microscopic hematuria in 6% of patients [39].
6. Lumbar puncture, which should be performed in patients with symptoms suggestive of meningitis, although the CSF in early LD usually is unremarkable (as opposed to the CSF in later stages; see sec. **C.2**).

B. **Serologic testing,** when used in the setting of thoughtful epidemiologic and clinical considerations, is beneficial. For reasons that are unclear, antibodies develop slowly. Both IFA and ELISA are widely available, **ELISA generally being the superior assay.** Western blot assays are also available. They are more difficult to perform but are more specific [81]. Currently, experts advocate a two-step approach. Initially an ELISA serology is performed, in preference to IFA. Then, for those patients with a positive ELISA, or borderline positive ELISA, or false positive ELISA tests, a Western blot test can be performed as a confirmatory serology [81a–81e]. In evaluating neurologic complaints, simultaneous serum and CSF antibody titers may be useful [82]. The results of serologic studies are incorporated in the surveillance case definition for LD by state health departments and the CDC [83].

1. Patients are aware of the existence of serologic tests because of the extensive media attention to LD. Therefore, **serologic testing may be an expectation of patients who do not understand its limitations.**
2. **The readily available serologic tests,** both IFA and ELISA, **have many limitations.** They are reasonably sensitive in late disseminated and chronic stages. However, false positive results render screening of asymptomatic patients useless and misleading, and serologic test results are interpretable only in the presence of a carefully considered clinical suspicion for LD.
3. **In early localized and early disseminated disease, serologic tests will be negative in up to 65% of infected patients** [74]. The specific IgM response to *B. burgdorferi* does not peak until 3–6 weeks after onset of disease; peak titers of IgG are reached only after months to years [12].
4. **Antibiotic treatment of a patient with ECM may truncate or eliminate both IgM and IgG antibody responses.** Antibody usually will diminish in a successfully treated patient, though this is not a useful criterion by which to monitor treatment success or failure [54].
5. Antibody will fluctuate with disease intensity, especially with respect to IgM. Persistence or reappearance of IgM antibody is sometimes a helpful indicator of incipient neurologic and cardiac manifestations of late disseminated disease.
6. **There is no standardization of tests, and great variability exists among results from different laboratories.** Each laboratory uses its own antigen and provides its own quality control. **No standardized antigen or externally evaluated proficiency testing is available at this time** [7, 81d, 84, 85]. In a study in Minnesota, a marked variability in results of IFA testing was found in different laboratories [7, 84]. In addition, **only 34% of patients with diagnosed ECM had a titer greater than or equal to 1:256 between 30 and 60 days after onset of rash** [84]. It is believed that "failure of patients to have an antibody response during the early stages of LD may have contributed to this demonstrated lack of sensitivity" [84].

   There is controversy about cutoff levels of IFA: Some believe 1:128 should be the cutoff, whereas others prefer 1:256. In either case, sensitivity or specificity will be diminished [86].
7. The **Western blot** [86] is a useful supplemental test in selected patients, particularly as a confirmatory test to positive, borderline, and suspected false positive ELISA and IFA tests. Results must be interpreted with caution, due to lack of standardization and variability between laboratories. Antibody to outer surface protein A (OSP-A), protein B (OSP-B), and protein C (OSP-C) is specific for LD; antiflagellar antibody is a less specific finding. Immunoblotting methods

play an important role, and standardized criteria for interpretation are currently under development [81d].

8. **Cross-reactivity and false positive results.** Serum antibodies to *Borrelia hermsii, Borrelia recurrentis*, treponemes, and leptospires cross-react with *B. burgdorferi* in IFA and ELISA tests. Therefore, **patients with syphilis may have** positive LD serologic studies, but patients with LD will not have positive rapid plasma reagin (RPR) or microhemagglutination antibody to *T. pallidum* (MHA/TP) tests [86]. Therefore, in patients with positive serologic tests for LD and with risk factors for syphilis, serologic workup for syphilis should be done to rule out false positive LD study results.

9. **False positive serologic results also occur with polyclonal B-cell activation and in individuals with rheumatoid factors and antinuclear antibodies.** Patients with **active infectious mononucleosis** may have false positive LD titers [86].

10. In patients suspected clinically to have LD but who have negative serologic tests, T-cell functional changes may be demonstrable, such as heightened T-cell blastogenic response to *B. burgdorferi* [74].

11. **Concluding remarks.** The sensitivity varies for both IFA and ELISA tests in early LD, but both tests are specific and sensitive in complicated LD (i.e., late disseminated and chronic stages) [87]. **Serologic tests should be used only to confirm a diagnosis based on epidemiologic and clinical suspicion and should not be relied on as the only criteria to make the diagnosis of LD.** This practice will minimize false positive test results and avoid misdiagnosis.

   The polymerase chain reaction (PCR) test may offer a more specific method to diagnose LD [88, 88a] but is a research tool at this time [81d]. As an example of future application, PCR of joint fluid may provide information critical to identifying those patients likely to respond to antibiotics versus those who have progressed to a postinfectious mechanism [89]. PCR has also been used to identify *B. burgdorferi* in the blood of patients with early disseminated disease [88a]. (See Chap. 25 for a general discussion of PCR testing.)

C. **Other laboratory tests in disseminated LD**
   1. **Cardiac disease**
      a. As cited earlier, varying degrees of AV block may be noted on the electrocardiogram. **Patients with first-degree AV block greater than 0.3 seconds or a higher-grade block should be hospitalized** for observation and intravenous antibiotic therapy [63, 64].
      b. In severe cases of carditis, chest roentgenogram may reveal cardiomegaly, and echocardiogram may show diffuse wall motion abnormalities [63, 64].
   2. **Neurologic disease**
      a. It is currently believed that *B. burgdorferi* causes primarily axonal injury [48]. Neurophysiologic testing may reveal abnormalities in patients with LD who do not have overt neuropathy [48].
      b. Although this issue is debated by some, it would be prudent to examine the CSF by lumbar puncture in the setting of meningitic findings or possibly in patients with Bell's palsy in a situation suspicious for LD [81d, 89a]. Appropriate selection of patients who should undergo lumbar puncture is a difficult area to define. Patients in whom there is low suspicion of LD and who have not had prior antibiotic therapy may first undergo serum testing and follow-up. Those for whom there is strong suspicion of neurologic involvement with LD should have serum determination with ELISA and Western blot but should probably undergo lumbar puncture if therapy for CNS disease is contemplated. The role of lumbar puncture in patients with Bell's palsy is poorly defined [89a] and must be individualized. Cerebrospinal fluid abnormalities in individuals with Lyme meningitis are typical of aseptic meningitis (see Chap. 5). Characteristic features include a mild pleocytosis consisting of predominantly mononuclear cells, a modest elevation of protein, and a normal glucose level [62]. Locally produced antiborrelial antibody may be detected through finding a CSF antibody titer out of proportion to a simultaneous serum antibody titer in a patient in whom LD was previously diagnosed, either with or without prior treatment. An increased CSF–serum antibody ratio may confirm a clinical suspicion of late disseminated neurologic disease, but not all patients with CNS disease will have elevated titers in CSF [62, 82]. **Such a determination should be made by a subspecialist familiar with LD.**

   3. Joint disease
   a. Joint fluid WBC counts range from 500 to more than $100,000/mm^3$, with predominantly polymorphonuclear leukocytes.
   b. Radiography may reveal erosive changes in individuals with chronic arthritis.
VIII. Treatment. Optimal treatment of LD is still being defined. Appropriate antibiotic therapy abbreviates the disease by weeks to months to years, depending on the individual and phase of illness. In all stages, residual (usually milder) symptoms may occur after treatment. In general, best results occur in treating early disease [40].

   At this time, the diagnostic complexity of LD dictates that overtreatment in endemic areas is unavoidable. However, this overtreatment should be minimized by a disciplined and rigorous approach to diagnosis. Media and public expectations conspire to exert pressure for overtreatment in nonendemic areas, but physicians should strenuously attempt to avoid this [90–93a].
A. Endemic areas
   1. Tick bite. The issue of whether to treat tick bite in an endemic area is a difficult one, as scientific data must be balanced against psychological issues for the individual patient [74]. It is the opinion of the authors that **tick bite alone,** no matter what the geographic area, **should be closely observed but not routinely treated.** The following facts pertain:
   a. The risk of LD after tick bite appears to be low (fewer than five cases per 100 bites) [94, 95]. These numbers are now confirmed in two small prospective studies, both in heavily endemic areas for ticks infected with *B. burgdorferi.*
   b. A recent cost-effectiveness analysis supported empiric therapy of tick bites in settings of very high probability, but consultants to the *Medical Letter* found the data "unconvincing" [96, 97].
   c. The site of the tick bite may be closely observed, and patients should be counseled about the signs and symptoms of LD. (See also sec. **D.5.e.**)
   d. The proportion of complications of therapy approximates the proportion of prevented disease [94, 95].
   e. Patients are less likely to fully treat a tick bite than actual disease (i.e., they may not take the full course of prescribed antibiotics).
   f. The authors recognize that a counterargument may be posed.
      (1) Treatment of tick bites in an endemic area, if initiated immediately, **may** prevent dissemination of spirochetes in a subset of patients.
      (2) In rare instances, the failure to treat tick bite may impose an unacceptable psychological burden on the patient.
      (3) For further discussion, see the correspondence section of the *New England Journal of Medicine,* in which several experts debate this difficult issue [98].
   2. Erythema chronicum migrans in any area should be treated.
   3. In a known endemic area, manifestations of early disseminated, late disseminated, or chronic LD accompanied by a positive titer should be treated.
   4. Pregnancy. Suspected or known LD in pregnancy should be treated. The extent of risk to the fetus appears to be low, but the precise risk is unclear [74].
   5. Generalized screening in at-risk populations will yield a number of false positive results. **There are no data to support treatment in the event of a positive LD titer in the absence of findings compatible with LD** [98a; see this important reference and its annotation].
B. Periendemic area. The same recommendations apply in periendemic areas as in endemic areas (see sec. **A**).
C. Nonendemic area
   1. Only those cases in which diagnostic confidence is high should be treated. Diagnosis of LD should be made with extreme rigor. The exception would be history of travel to an endemic area within a clinically plausible time frame and conditions as listed in sec. **A.**
   2. Definite ECM with known tick bite in a nonendemic area should be treated. It is important to differentiate between the immediate local reactions of any tick bite and ECM. Reporting of an index case to the state health department is of utmost importance in this setting (see sec. **4** also).
   3. Patients with symptoms or signs compatible with LD in the absence of ECM and in conjunction with a positive serologic workup from a reliable laboratory fall into a difficult category. Treatment should be reserved for those patients

in whom the highest suspicion of LD is entertained ' y the clinician—for example, when a history of ECM or tick bite is related or a history of travel to an endemic area is reported. In the overwhelming majority, patients who have no exposure to a known endemic area will **not** have LD, and positive serologic results may well be false positive. (See sec. **4** also.)

4. **Although overtreatment is an unfortunate necessity in endemic and periendemic areas, overtreatment should be avoided in cases not clearly LD in areas believed to be nonendemic. A diagnosed case from such an area should be scrutinized with the greatest care, probably in consultation** with a rheumatologist, neurologist, or infectious disease specialist, **and with input from the state health department.**

An index case from such an area has profound implications for all local residents and physicians. Cases should be reported to state health departments (see sec. **XI**). When possible, ticks should be saved, both for species identification and for isolation of spirochetes.

D. **Specific treatment regimens** have been summarized [92, 93, 97] (Table 23-2).
1. **Early localized disease.** Oral antibiotic therapy shortens the duration of the rash and associated symptoms and prevents later illness in most patients. Some patients with severe early disease have progressed to later stages despite recommended courses of oral antibiotics [99]. **The duration of therapy for all regimens is not well established**; it is often based on severity of disease and rapidity of response [99].
    a. **Doxycycline,** 100 mg PO bid for 3 weeks, has been recommended **for men, nonpregnant women, and children older than 8 years** [97]. Patients taking this agent should be cautioned regarding sun exposure. (See Chap. 28N for additional comments on doxycycline.) Tetracycline was once recommended, but doxycycline is considered more effective [100].
    b. Alternatively, **amoxicillin,** 500 mg PO qid in adults or 20–40 mg/kg/day in three divided doses in children, for 3 weeks, is effective and **preferred for children younger than 8 years and for pregnant or lactating women** who are not allergic to amoxicillin. Amoxicillin plus probenecid has been shown recently to be equally efficacious to doxycycline [101]. The addition of probenecid to the amoxicillin regimen may be an advantageous option, although one study showed a high rate of drug rash, and comparisons to amoxicillin alone have not been published [101, 102]. **Probenecid, tetracycline, and doxycycline should not be used during pregnancy.**
    c. In one report, **cefuroxime axetil** has been demonstrated to be equal in efficacy to doxycycline in the treatment of early LD and the prevention of late sequelae [103]. A second recent study supports this finding [103a].
    d. **Macrolides. Erythromycin,** 250 mg PO qid in adults or 30 mg/kg/day for children, can be used but may be less effective [97]. In a small pilot study, **clarithromycin,** 500 mg bid for 21 days, showed promise for therapy of erythema migrans [103b]. In a small, randomized, open study of therapy of erythema migrans, **azithromycin** (500 mg on day 1, and 250 mg daily on days 2–5) was reported to be as effective as a 10–20-day course of doxycycline or amoxicillin with probenecid [101]. However, in a more recent 1996 report, azithromycin (500 mg once daily for 7 days) was not as effective as amoxicillin (500 mg tid for 20 days) [103c]. The macrolides are discussed further in Chap. 28M.
    e. The *Medical Letter* suggests that for Lyme disease, doxycycline or amoxicillin (unless contraindicated) is the drug of choice, whereas cefuroxime, penicillin G, azithromycin, clarithromycin, and ceftriaxone (or cefotaxime) are alternative agents [103d].
2. **Early disseminated disease—neurologic**
    a. **Mild symptoms** (e.g., **Bell's palsy alone**) may be treated with oral doxycycline or amoxicillin with or without probenecid, as described in sec. **1**, but **dosages are generally continued for 1 month** [97].
    b. For cranial or peripheral **neuropathies, meningitis, or encephalitis** due to LD, intravenous therapy is recommended.
        (1) **Penicillin,** 20–24 million units/day IV (in divided doses q4–6h) in adults or 250,000–400,000 units/kg/day IV in children with normal renal function, for 10–21 days, has been used. See Chap. 28C for dose modification in renal failure.
        (2) **Ceftriaxone** at 2 g IV once daily in adults for 14 days was superior to intravenous penicillin for 10 days in one small study [104]. In children,

Table 23-2. Therapy of Lyme disease

Drug	Adult dosage[a]	Pediatric dosage
Early localized or early disseminated disease[b]		
Amoxicillin[c]	500 mg qid × 21 days	20–40 mg/kg/day × 21 days
± probenecid	500 mg qid × 21 days	
or doxycycline	100 mg bid × 21 days	
Cefuroxime axetil	500 mg bid × 21 days	250 mg bid × 21 days
Alternative		
Erythromycin	250 mg qid × 21 days	30 mg/kg/day × 10–21 days
Azithromycin	See text	
Late disseminated and chronic disease[b]		
Seventh nerve palsy with normal lumbar puncture		
Doxycycline	100 mg bid × 21–30 days	
or amoxicillin	500 mg qid × 21–30 days	
± probenecid	500 mg qid × 21–30 days	
Radiculoneuropathy, meningitis, peripheral neuropathy, and encephalopathy		
Ceftriaxone	2 g/day × 21 days[b]	50–80 mg/kg/day IV × 10–21 days
or penicillin	20–24 million units/day, divided doses × 21 days[b]	250,000–400,000 units/kg/day, divided doses × 10–21 days
Arthritis (early and late)		
Amoxicillin	500 mg qid × 30 days	40 mg/kg/day × 21 days
± probenecid	500 mg qid	
or doxycycline	100 mg bid × 30 days	
or ceftriaxone	2 g/day × 14–21 days	50–80 mg/kg/day × 10–21 days
or penicillin	20–24 million units/d, divided doses × 14–21 days	250,000–400,000 units/kg/day, divided doses × 10–21 days

Cardiac disease		
Mild	Doxycycline	100 mg bid–tid × 21 days
	or amoxicillin	500–1,000 mg qid
	± probenecid	500 mg qid × 21 days
More serious	Ceftriaxone	2 g/day × 14 days
	or penicillin	20–24 million units/day, divided doses × 14 days
Chronic neurologic disease (chronic meningitis or encephalitis)[b]	Ceftriaxone	2 g/day × 21–30 days
	or penicillin	20–24 million units/day, divided doses × 21–30 days

50–80 mg/kg/day IV × 10–21 days
250,000–400,000 units/kg/day, divided doses × 10–21 days

50–80 mg/kg/day IV × 14–21 days
250,000–400,000 units/kg/day, divided doses × 14–21 days

[a]See text for comments on these regimens.
[b]Duration of therapy is not well established for any indication.
[c]A range of doses and dosing intervals has been proposed for amoxicillin, from 250 mg to 1,000 mg, tid–qid. The authors of this chapter favor the regimen given in table until there is further clarification; we also favor a qid probenecid regimen.
Source: Adapted from several sources [52, 64, 88, 93, 101–104, 106, 108–110].

50–80 mg/kg IV can be used for a daily dose. Whether this program is superior to penicillin is unclear. However, it has become a popular regimen, in part because of the ease of administration of a once-daily dose (for 10–21 days), which can often be given in the home or outpatient setting. (See Chap. 28F.)

3. **Late disseminated disease—neurologic.** Late complications (e.g., focal CNS disease and fatigue syndromes sometimes associated with LD) have been treated with intravenous penicillin or ceftriaxone, with variable success [104]. Some of these patients probably did not have actual LD.

4. **Early disseminated disease—cardiac**
   a. **Minor conduction system involvement** (first-degree AV block but a P-R interval of < 0.30 seconds) and no other significant symptoms can usually be treated with doxycycline or amoxicillin plus probenecid, as for early localized disease (see sec. 1).
   b. **More severe conduction system disease** (including first-degree AV block with a P-R interval > 0.30 seconds) warrants hospitalization and intravenous antibiotic therapy. Ceftriaxone, 2 g/day for adults (50–80 mg/kg/day for children), or penicillin G, 20–24 million units/day for adults (250,000–400,000 units/kg/day for children), for 10–21 days, depending on the rapidity of the patient's response, has been recommended [97]. The conduction system abnormalities associated with LD are not permanent, but temporary pacemaker insertion may be necessary in some patients [105].

5. **Arthritis (early and late)**
   a. **Arthritis may be treated with oral doxycycline, or amoxicillin with or without probenecid, as described in sec. 1.** Recalcitrant arthritis sometimes resolves after retreatment with the same or an alternative antibiotic regimen. Based on limited data, patients with arthritis who did not respond to oral antibiotics often did not respond to intravenous penicillin or ceftriaxone [99, 106].
   b. Arthritis that fails oral therapy warrants treatment with intravenous antibiotics. Penicillin G in patients with normal renal function, 20–24 million units/day for adults or 250,000–400,000 units/kg/day for children in divided doses q4–6h for 10–21 days, is commonly used.
   c. **Ceftriaxone,** 2 g IV once daily for 2 or 3 weeks, in one small controlled study was more effective than intravenous penicillin G and effective in some patients who had not responded to penicillin [104].
   d. Arthroscopic synovectomy may be an effective treatment of chronic Lyme arthritis in patients who do not respond to antibiotic therapy [107].
   e. **The misdiagnosis of chronic LD in many patients with fibromyalgia has frequently resulted in inappropriate antibiotic therapy.** Empiric antibiotic therapy should be withheld in these vague circumstances, as there are well-documented cases of serious consequences to overzealous antibiotic use [108–110].

IX. **Prevention.** For those residing in or traveling to endemic areas, this information is crucial:
   A. Wear **light-colored clothing,** on which the tiny *Ixodes* ticks will be easy to spot.
   B. Wear **long pants** tucked into socks or boots.
   C. Wear **long-sleeved shirts.**
   D. **Stay on paths** and avoid contact with brush.
   E. **Search exposed skin** every 3–4 hours when outside.
   F. **After being outside, carefully check all areas of the skin,** particularly skin folds in groin, axillae, and thighs.
   G. **Consider the use of insecticides.**
      1. Diethyltoluamide (DEET) is a component of many over-the-counter insect repellents that are applied to the skin. It is a potent acaricide. Overuse should be avoided because of the potential for CNS toxicity. It is probably prudent to use a concentration of 35% or less (see Chap. 21).
      2. Permethrin is an acaricide approved for use on clothes but not on the skin. It is not licensed for use in all states and is potentially oncogenic. Applications of permethrin may survive washing of clothes.
   H. Spraying of yards and other areas to kill ticks has not been shown to be effective.
   I. Damminix, a commercially available product consisting of a tube full of an acaricide-impregnated cotton that mice will use in bedding material, thereby killing ticks, has been demonstrated effectively to reduce the numbers of ticks in yards

and other small areas. It is expensive, however, and one must realize that it will not significantly lower the number of infectious ticks in the first year of its use.
  J. Mouse population control is prohibitively difficult.
  K. Deer population control has been used on some islands but could not be used short of wholesale destruction of deer herds in other areas.
X. **Role of the media**
  A. The media has considerably raised consciousness of LD. Unfortunately, two aspects of media coverage have been problematic.
    1. Though the media has generally described the tick, the symptoms, and the worst scenario of consequences, **geographic limitations of the disease have not been emphasized.** The general public often is not aware that persons not living in or visiting an endemic area need not worry about this illness. Thus, unnecessary anxiety prevails in many individuals, who no longer go in the woods or allow their children to do so; who have disposed of their pets; and who may imagine that their everyday aches and pains are the stirrings of a dread disease.
    2. **Except for ECM,** which does not occur in all patients, **the signs and symptoms of LD are nonspecific.** However, the media often has developed a definite association, in the public eye, between LD and symptoms such as chronic fatigue, malaise, forgetfulness, arthritis, Bell's palsy, and sundry aches and pains. As a result, lay people often come to physicians either wondering whether they have LD or convinced that they do have LD. It becomes difficult for the physician to persuade them otherwise even after a careful negative evaluation. Indeed, many LD clinics have been established in endemic areas but are visited primarily by patients with chronic fatigue, arthritis, and other ailments in no way related to LD.
  B. Furthermore, the media has implied explosive spread of LD, which is, in fact, contrary to the nature of the illness. Rather, the current phenomenon is an explosion of awareness.
XI. **Reporting. All cases of LD should be reported to state departments of health, which in turn report data to the CDC.** Reports should include pertinent laboratory tests and clinical circumstances. In areas not known to be endemic, any suspicious ticks should be saved and transported to state health departments or other designated agencies for definitive identification.
XII. **Future advances.** Much work is currently being done with regard to the clinical diagnosis and treatment of LD. It is hoped that a set of diagnostic criteria will be generally agreed on and widely adopted at some future time. Diagnostic tests with improved sensitivity and specificity are in an experimental stage, but no new diagnostic test with clear advantages over current tests is near marketing stage. Studies intended to clarify treatment decisions with regard to tick bite, pregnancy, and late complicated disease are ongoing. Work on a vaccine that deters ticks as well as an antispirochetal vaccine is in progress [111–113].

References

1. Afzelius, A. Verhandlungen der dermatologischen Gesellschaft zu Stockholm. *Arch. Dermatol. Syph.* 101:405–406, 1910.
2. Steere, A.C., et al. Lyme arthritis: An epidemic of oligoarticular arthritis in children and adults in three Connecticut communities. *Arthritis Rheum.* 20:7–17, 1977.
3. Steere, A.C., Broderick, T.F., and Malawista, S.E. Erythema chronicum migrans and Lyme arthritis: Epidemiologic evidence for a tick vector. *Am. J. Epidemiol.* 108:312–321, 1978.
4. Burgdorfer, W., et al. Lyme disease—a tick-borne spirochetosis? *Science* 216:1317–1319, 1982.
5. Schulze, T.L., et al. Evolution of a Focus of Lyme Disease. In G. Stanek, et al. (eds.), *Proceedings of the Second International Symposium on Lyme Disease and Related Disorders, Vienna, 1985.* New York: Verlag, 1987.
6. Centers for Disease Control. Lyme Disease: United States, 1991–1992. *M.M.W.R.* 42:345, 1993.
    Also see the update: Centers for Disease Control, Lyme disease: United States–1993. M.M.W.R. *43:561, 1994.*
7. Baaken, L.L., et al. Performance of 45 laboratories participating in a proficiency testing program for Lyme disease serology. *J.A.M.A.* 268:891–895, 1992.

8. Burgdorfer, W. The discovery of Lyme disease spirochete and its relation to tick vectors. *Yale J. Biol. Med.* 57:515, 1984.
9. Steere, A.C., et al. Historical Perspectives. In G. Stanek et al. (eds.), *Proceedings of the Second International Symposium on Lyme Disease and Related Disorders, Vienna, 1985.* New York: Verlag, 1987.
10. Burgdorfer, W. The Discovery of the Lyme Disease Spirochete. In G. Stanek et al. (eds.), *Proceedings of the Second International Symposium on Lyme Disease and Related Disorders, Vienna, 1985.* New York: Verlag, 1987.
11. Steere, A.C., et al. The clinical spectrum and treatment of Lyme disease. *Yale J. Biol. Med.* 57:453–460, 1984.
12. Steere, A.C., et al. The spirochete etiology of Lyme disease. *N. Engl. J. Med.* 308:733, 1983.
13. Wilske, B., et al. Antigenic variability of *Borrelia burgdorferi. Ann. N.Y. Acad. Sci.* 539:126–143, 1988.
14. Anderson, J. Mammalian and avian reservoirs for *Borrelia burgdorferi. Ann. N.Y. Acad. Sci.* 539:180–191, 1989.
15. Burgess, E. *Borrelia burgdorferi* infection in Wisconsin horses and cows. *Ann. N.Y. Acad. Sci.* 539:235–243, 1989.
16. Steere, A.C., and Malawista, S.E. Cases of Lyme disease in the United States: Locations correlated with distribution of *Ixodes dammini. Ann. Intern. Med.* 91:730–733, 1979.
17. Anderson, I.F., and Magnarelli, L. Avian and mammalian hosts for spirochete-infected ticks and insects in a Lyme disease focus in Connecticut. *Yale J. Biol. Med.* 57:627–641, 1984.
18. Piesman, J. Vector competence of ticks in the Southeastern United States for *Borrelia burgdorferi. Ann. N.Y. Acad. Sci.* 539:417–418, 1988.
19. Rawlings, J. Lyme Disease in Texas. In G. Stanek et al. (eds.), *Proceedings of the Second International Symposium on Lyme Disease and Related Disorders, Vienna, 1985.* New York: Verlag, 1987. Pp. 483–487.
20. Schulze, T., et al. *Amblyomma americanum:* A potential vector of Lyme disease in New Jersey. *Science* 224:601–603, 1984.
21. Weber, K., et al. European erythema migrans disease and related disorders. *Yale J. Biol. Med.* 57:465–471, 1984.
22. Oliver, J., Jr., et al. Conspecificity of the ticks *Ixodes scapularis* and *I. dammini. J. Med. Entomol.* 30(1):54–63, 1993.
23. Centers for Disease Control. Lyme disease—Connecticut. *M.M.W.R.* 37:1–3, 1988.
24. Main, A.J., et al. *Ixodes dammini (Acarus ixodidae)* on white-tailed deer (*Oedocoileus virginianus*) in Connecticut. *J. Med. Entomol.* 18:487–492, 1981.
25. Zaki, M.H., and Graham, D.C. *Lyme Disease,* vol. 3. Hauppauge, NY: Suffolk County Department of Health Services, March 1988.
26. Lyme Disease Surveillance Spreadsheet. Case totals as reported to the CDC by state health departments, 1992.
   For a related discussion, see Centers for Disease Control, Lyme disease—United States, 1991–1992. M.M.W.R. *42:345, 1993.*
27. Schulze, T.L., et al. Comparison of Rates of Infection by the Lyme Disease Spirochete in Selected Populations of *Ixodes dammini* and *Amblyomma americanum.* In G. Stanek et al. (eds.), *Proceedings of the Second International Symposium on Lyme Disease and Related Disorders, Vienna, 1985.* New York: Verlag, 1987. Pp. 507–513.
28. Lane, R.S., and Lavoie, P.E. Lyme borreliosis in California: Acarological, clinical, and epidemiological studies. *Ann. N.Y. Acad. Sci.* 539:192–203, 1988.
29. Ciesielski, C.A., et al. The geographical distribution of Lyme disease in the United States. *Ann. N.Y. Acad. Sci.* 539:283–288, 1988.
30. Spach, D.H., et al. Tick-borne diseases in the United States. *N. Engl. J. Med.* 329:936–947, 1993.
31. Spielman, A., Levine, J.F., and Wilson, M.L. Vectorial capacity of North American *Ixodes* ticks. *Yale J. Biol. Med.* 57:507–513, 1984.
32. Anderson, J.F. Epizootology of *Borrelia* in *Ixodes* tick vectors and reservoir hosts. *Rev. Infect. Dis.* 11(6):S1451–S1459, 1989.
33. Telford, S.R., et al. Incompetence of deer as reservoirs of *Borrelia burgdorferi. Ann. N.Y. Acad. Sci.* 539:429–430, 1988.
33a. Fish, D. Environmental risk and prevention of Lyme Disease. *Am. J. Med.* 98(Suppl. 4A):2S, 1995.
34. Teitler, J., et al. Prevalence of *Borrelia burgdorferi* antibodies in dogs in northern California. *Ann. N.Y. Acad. Sci.* 539:126–143, 1988.

35. Steere, A., et al. Longitudinal assessment of the clinical and epidemiological features of Lyme disease in a defined population. *J. Infect. Dis.* 154:295–301, 1986.

36. Schmidt, G.P. The global distribution of Lyme disease. *Rev. Infect. Dis.* 7:41–50, 1985.

37. Benach, J.L., et al. Adult *Ixodes dammini* on rabbits: A hypothesis for the development and transmission of *Borrelia burgdorferi*. *J. Infect. Dis.* 155:1300–1306, 1987.

38. Piesman, J., et al. Duration of tick attachment and *Borrelia burgdorferi* transmission. *J. Clin. Microbiol.* 25:557–558, 1987.

39. Steere, A.C., et al. The early clinical manifestations of Lyme disease. *Ann. Intern. Med.* 99:76–82, 1983.

40. Steere, A.C., et al. Treatment of the early manifestations of Lyme disease. *Ann. Intern. Med.* 99:22–26, 1983.

41. Beck, G., et al. A Role for Interleukin I in the Pathogenesis of Lyme Disease. In G. Stanek et al. (eds.), *Proceedings of the Second International Symposium on Lyme Disease and Related Disorders, Vienna, 1985*. New York: Verlag, 1987. Pp. 133–136.

42. Beck, G., et al. *Borrelia burgdorferi* Lipopolysaccharide and Its Role in the Pathogenesis of Lyme Disease. In G. Stanek et al. (eds.), *Proceedings of the Second International Symposium on Lyme Disease and Related Disorders, Vienna, 1985*. New York: Verlag, 1987. Pp. 137–150.

43. Lake, L., et al. Neurologic abnormalities of Lyme disease. *Medicine* (Baltimore) 58:281–294, 1979.

44. Link, H., et al. B-cell response at cellular level in CSF and blood in Lyme disease and controls. *Ann. N.Y. Acad. Sci.* 539:389–392, 1988.

45. Sigal, L.H., and Tatum, A.H. Lyme disease patients' serum contains IgM antibodies to *Borrelia burgdorferi* that cross-react with neuronal antigens. *Neurology* (NY) 38:1439–1442, 1988.

46. Martin, R., et al. *B. burgdorferi* as a trigger for autoimmune T-cell reactions within the CNS. *Ann. N.Y. Acad. Sci.* 539:400–401, 1988.

47. Andriole, V.T. Lyme disease and other spirochetal diseases. *Rev. Infect. Dis.* 11(Suppl. 6):S1433–S1525, 1989.

48. Halperin, J.J., et al. Nervous system abnormalities in Lyme disease. *Ann. N.Y. Acad. Sci.* 539:24–34, 1988.

48a. Murakami, S., et al. Bell palsy and herpes simplex virus: Identification of viral DNA in endoneurial fluid and muscle. *Ann. Intern. Med.* 124:27, 1996.
   Using a polymerase chain reaction technique, 11 of 14 patients with Bell's palsy had demonstrated herpes simplex type 1 as the presumed etiologic agent. See favorable editorial comment in the same issue. The implications of this study argue for the use of acyclovir in the management of acute Bell's Palsy. See J.R. Baringer, Herpes simplex virus and Bell palsy. Ann. Intern. Med. *124:64, 1996.*

49. Duray, P.H. Clinical pathologic correlations of Lyme disease. *Rev. Infect. Dis.* 11(6):S1487–S1493, 1989.

50. Stanek, G., et al. Isolation of *Borrelia burgdorferi* from the myocardium of a patient with longstanding myocardiopathy. *N. Engl. J. Med.* 322:249, 1990.

51. Snydman, D.R., et al. *Borrelia burgdorferi* in joint fluids in chronic Lyme arthritis. *Ann. Intern. Med.* 104:798–800, 1986.

52. Steere, A.C., et al. Successful parenteral penicillin therapy in established Lyme arthritis. *N. Engl. J. Med.* 312:869–874, 1985.

53. Steckenberg, B.W. Lyme disease: The latest great imitator. *Pediatr. Infect. Dis. J.* 7:402–409, 1988.

54. Steere, A.C. Lyme disease. *N. Engl. J. Med.* 321:586–596, 1989.

55. Coyle, P.K. *Borrelia burgdorferi* antibodies in multiple sclerosis patients. *Neurology* (NY) 39:760–761, 1989.

56. Pachner, A.R., and Steere, A.C. The triad of neurologic manifestations of Lyme disease: Meningitis, cranial neuritis, and radiculoneuritis. *Neurology* (NY) 35:47–53, 1985.

57. Steere, A.C., et al. Clinical Manifestations of Lyme Disease. Historical Perspectives. In G. Stanek et al. (eds.), *Proceedings of the Second International Symposium on Lyme Disease and Related Disorders, Vienna, 1985*. New York: Verlag, 1987. Pp. 201–205.

58. Finkel, M. Lyme disease and its neurologic complications. *Arch. Neurol.* 45:99–104, 1988.

59. Reik, L., Burgdorfer, W., and Donaldson, J. Neurologic abnormalities in Lyme disease without ECM. *Am. J. Med.* 81:73–78, 1986.

60. Pachner, A.C. *Borrelia burgdorferi* in the nervous system: The new "great imitator." *Ann. N.Y. Acad. Sci.* 539:56–64, 1988.

61. Steere, A., et al. Neurologic abnormalities of Lyme disease: Successful treatment with high-dose intravenous penicillin. *Ann. Intern. Med.* 99:767–772, 1983.

62. Luft, B.J., and Dattwyler, R.J. Lyme borreliosis. *Curr. Clin. Top. Infect. Dis.* 10:56–81, 1989.

63. Steere, A.C., et al. Lyme carditis: Cardiac abnormalities of Lyme disease. *Ann. Intern. Med.* 93:8–16, 1980.
    For a related discussion, see H.F. McAlister, et al. Lyme carditis: An important cause of reversible heart block. Ann. Intern. Med. *110:339, 1989.*

64. Olssen, L., Okafor, E., and Clements, I. Cardiac involvement in Lyme disease: Manifestations and management. *Mayo Clin. Proc.* 61:745–749, 1986.

65. Steere, A.C., et al. Association of chronic Lyme arthritis with HLA-DR4 and HLA-DR2 alleles. *N. Engl. J. Med.* 323:219–223, 1990.

66. Steere, A.C., Schoen, R.T., and Taylor, E. The clinical evolution of Lyme arthritis. *Ann. Intern. Med.* 107:725–731, 1987.

67. Duffy, J. Lyme disease. *Infect. Dis. Clin. North Am.* 1(3):511, 1987.

68. Steere, A.C., et al. Chronic Lyme arthritis: Clinical and immunogenetic differentiation from rheumatoid arthritis. *Ann. Intern. Med.* 90:896–901, 1979.

69. Eichenfield, A., et al. Childhood Lyme arthritis: Experience in an endemic area. *J. Pediatr.* 109:753–758, 1986.

70. Pachner, A.R., and Steere, A.C. Neurological Manifestations of Third Stage Lyme Disease. In G. Stanek et al. (eds.), *Proceedings of the Second International Symposium on Lyme Disease and Related Disorders, Vienna, 1985.* New York: Verlag, 1987. P. 301.

71. Wokke, J., et al. Chronic forms of *Borrelia burgdorferi* infection of the nervous system. *Neurology* (NY) 37:1031–1034, 1987.

72. Ackerman, R., et al. Chronic neurological manifestations of erythema migrans borreliosis. *Ann. N.Y. Acad. Sci.* 539:16–23, 1988.

73. Pachner, A.R. Spirochetal diseases of the nervous system. *Neurol. Clin.* 4:207–222, 1986.

73a. Sigal, L. A symposium: National Clinical Conference on Lyme Disease. Panel discussion. *Am. J. Med.* 98(Suppl. 4A):79S, 1995.
    An excellent discussion conducted by experts on the topic.

74. Steere, A.C. *Borrelia burgdorferi* (Lyme Disease, Lyme Borreliosis). In G.L. Mandell, J.E. Bennett, and R. Dolin (eds.), *Principles and Practice of Infectious Diseases* (4th ed.). New York: Churchill Livingstone, 1995. Pp. 2143–2155.

75. Markowitz, L.E., et al. Lyme disease during pregnancy. *J.A.M.A.* 255:3394–3396, 1986.

76. Kaplan, K. Lyme disease: An update. *Infect. Dis. Pract.* 10(8):1–8, 1987.

77. Weber, K., et al. *Borrelia burgdorferi* in a newborn despite oral penicillin for Lyme borreliosis during pregnancy. *Pediatr. Infect. Dis. J.* 7:286–289, 1988.

78. Fikrig, E., et al. Long-term protection of mice from Lyme disease by vaccination with OspA. *Infect. Immun.* 60:773–777, 1992.

79. Dattwyler, R., et al. Seronegative Lyme disease. *N. Engl. J. Med.* 319:1441–1446, 1988.

80. Nadelman, R., et al. Failure to isolate *Borrelia burgdorferi* after antimicrobial therapy in culture-documented Lyme borreliosis associated with erythema migrans: Report of a prospective study. *Am. J. Med.* 94:583–588, 1993.

81. Dressler, F., et al. Western blotting in the serodiagnosis of Lyme disease. *J. Infect. Dis.* 167:392–400, 1993.

81a. Aguero-Rosenfeld, M.E., et al. Serodiagnosis in early Lyme disease. *J. Clin. Micro.* 31:3090, 1993.

81b. Engstrom, S.M., Shoop, E., Johnson, R.C. Immunoblot interpretation criteria for serodiagnosis of early Lyme disease. *J. Clin. Micro.* 33:419, 1995.

81c. Sood, S.K., Zemel, L.S., Ilowite, N.T. Interpretation of immunoblot in pediatric Lyme arthritis. *J. Rheum.* 22:758, 1995.

81d. Magnarelly, L.A. Current status of laboratory diagnosis for Lyme disease. *Am. J. Med.* 98(Suppl. 4A):10S, 1995.

81e. Recommendations for test performance and interpretation from the Second National Conference on Serologic Diagnosis of Lyme Disease. *M.M.W.R.* 44:590, 1995.

82. Steere, A.C., et al. Evaluation of the intrathecal antibody response to *Borrelia burgdorferi* as a diagnostic test for Lyme neuroborreliosis. *J. Infect. Dis.* 161:1203–1209, 1990.

83. Lyme Disease National Surveillance Case Definition.

84. Hedberg, C., et al. An interlaboratory study of antibody to *Borrelia burgdorferi*. *J. Infect. Dis.* 155:1325–1327, 1987.

85. Schwartz, B.S., et al. Antibody testing in Lyme disease: A comparison of results in four laboratories. *J.A.M.A.* 262:3431, 1989.

For editorial comments on the difficulties of diagnosing Lyme disease, see L.A. Magnarelli, Quality of Lyme disease test. J.A.M.A. 262:3464, 1989; and A.G. Barbour, The diagnosis of Lyme disease: Rewards and perils. Ann. Intern. Med. 110:501, 1989. Also see related articles: S.W. Luger, Serologic tests for Lyme disease: Interlaboratory variability. J.A.M.A. 150:761, 1990; and the associated editorial comment by E.M. Reiman and M.A. Mintun, Serologic tests for antibody to Borrelia burgdorferi: Another Pandora's box for medicine? J.A.M.A. 150:732, 1990.

86. Grodzicki, R., and Steere, A.C. Comparison of immunoblotting and indirect enzyme-linked immunosorbent assay using different antigen preparations for diagnosing early Lyme disease. *J. Infect. Dis.* 157:790–797, 1988.

87. Russell, H., et al. Enzyme-linked immunosorbent assay and indirect immunofluorescence assay for Lyme disease. *J. Infect. Dis.* 149:465–470, 1984.

88. Nocton, J., et al. Detection of *Borrelia burgdorferi* DNA by polymerase chain reaction in synovial fluid from patients with Lyme arthritis. *N. Engl. J. Med.* 330:229–234, 1994.

88a. Goodman, J.L., et al. Bloodstream invasion in early Lyme disease: Results from a prospective, controlled, blinded study using the polymerase chain reaction. *Am. J. Med.* 99:6, 1995.
PCR detected early spirochetemia and may be useful in rapid diagnosis. PCR positivity correlated with clinical evidence of disease dissemination.

89. Rahn, D. Lyme disease—where's the bug. *N. Engl. J. Med.* 330:282–283, 1994.

89a. Sigal, L. A symposium: National Clinical Conference on Lyme Disease. Panel discussion. *Am. J. Med.* 98(Suppl. 4A):37S, 1995.
An excellent discussion conducted by experts on the topic.

90. Sigal, L.H. Summary of the first 100 patients seen at a Lyme disease referral center. *Am. J. Med.* 88:577, 1990.
Incorrect diagnosis often leads to unnecessary treatment. Only 37 of the 100 referrals was thought to have Lyme disease. On review, 25 had fibromyalgia. Probably 50% of the 91 patients who received antibiotics before referral were "overtreated."

91. Steere, A.C., et al. The overdiagnosis of Lyme disease. *J.A.M.A.* 269:1810–1816, 1993.

92. Rahn, D.W., and Malawista, S.E. Lyme disease: Recommendations for diagnosis and treatment. *Ann. Intern. Med.* 114:472–481, 1991.

93. Dattwyler, R.J., and Luft, B.J. Lyme Borreliosis. In S.L. Gorbach, J.G. Bartlett, and N.R. Blacklow (eds.), *Infectious Diseases.* Philadelphia: Saunders, 1992.

93a. Sigal, L.H. Anxiety and persistence of Lyme disease. *Am. J. Med.* 98(Suppl. 4A):74S, 1995.

94. Costello, C.M., et al. Prospective study of tick bites in an endemic area for Lyme disease. *J. Infect. Dis.* 159:136–139, 1989.

95. Shapiro, E., et al. A controlled trial of antimicrobial prophylaxis for Lyme disease after deer-tick bites. *N. Engl. J. Med.* 327:1769–1773, 1992.

96. Magid, D., et al. Prevention of Lyme disease after tick bites. *N. Engl. J. Med.* 327:534–541, 1992.

97. Medical Letter. Treatment of Lyme disease. *Med. Lett. Drugs Ther.* 34:95–97, 1992.

98. Genter, J., et al. Antimicrobial prophylaxis after tick bites. *N. Engl. J. Med.* 328:1418–1420, 1993.
In the May 13, 1993, issue, see the series of letters to the editor and authors' replies discussing the pros and cons of antimicrobial prophylaxis after tick bites. This remains a controversial issue.

98a. Luft, B.J., et al. Empiric antibiotic treatment of patients who are seropositive for Lyme disease but lack classic features. *Clin. Infect. Dis.* 18:111, 1994.
This is a joint statement and practice policy position paper of the American College of Rheumatology and the Council of the Infectious Diseases Society of America on the treatment of "possible" Lyme disease. *The report again emphasizes that the methods of serological testing used in different laboratories have not been standardized, so that substantial variability exists. Immunoblotting methods have not been systematically assessed yet. Problems arise especially if serology is done in patients with nonspecific symptoms. Because fibromyalgia and other nonspecific rheumatic syndromes are more common than LD, positive LD serology results in patients with nonspecific findings are more likely to represent false positive results rather than proof of LD, with increasing uncertainty as one goes from an area of high to low endemicity of LD. The report emphasizes that a positive serology is not definitive evidence for the diagnosis of LD in the absence of classic clinical symptoms. The paper concludes that "in patients whose only evidence for LD is a positive immunologic test, the risks for empiric antibiotic treatment outweigh the benefits."*

99. Steere, A.C., et al. Treatment of Lyme arthritis. *Arthritis Rheum.* 37:878–888, 1994.
100. Dattwyler, R.J., et al. Failure of tetracycline in early Lyme disease. *Arthritis Rheum.* 30:448–450, 1987.
101. Massorotti, E.M., et al. Treatment of early Lyme disease. *Am. J. Med.* 92:396–403, 1992.
102. Dattwyler, R.J., et al. Amoxicillin plus probenecid versus doxycycline for treatment of erythema migrans borreliosis. *Lancet* 336:1404–1406, 1990.
103. Nadelman, R.B., et al. Comparison of cefuroxime axetil and doxycycline in the treatment of early Lyme disease. *Ann. Intern. Med.* 117:273–280, 1992.
103a. Luger, S.W., et al. Comparison of cefuroxime axetil and doxycycline in patients with early Lyme disease associated with erythema migrans. *Antimicrob. Agents Chemother.* 39:661, 1995.
103b. Dattwyler, R.J., Grunwalt, E., and Luft, B.J. Clarithromycin in treatment of early Lyme disease: A pilot study. *Antimicrob. Agents Chemother.* 40:468, 1996.
    In this study, 41 patients with erythema migrans were enrolled in an open-labeled study. Authors conclude that clarithromycin shows promise as an effective agent for the treatment of early Lyme disease and warrants further study.
103c. Luft, B.L., et al. Azithromycin compared with amoxicillin in the treatment of erythema migrans: A double-blind, randomized, controlled study. *Ann. Intern. Med.* 124:785–791, 1996.
    Interesting study published in May 1996 in which 246 adult patients with erythema migrans lesions at least 5 cm in diameter were studied at 12 centers. Patients who received azithromycin also received a dummy placebo so that the dosing schedules were identical. Of 217 evaluable patients, those treated with amoxicillin were significantly more likely than those treated with azithromycin to achieve complete resolution of disease at day 20 (88% vs 76%; P = 0.024). More azithromycin recipients had relapse. Patients were followed for 180 days.
103d. Medical Letter. The choice of antibacterial drugs. *Med. Lett. Drugs Ther.* 38:25, 1996.
104. Dattwyler, R.J., et al. Treatment of Lyme borreliosis—randomized comparison of ceftriaxone and penicillin. *Lancet* 1:1191–1194, 1988.
105. McAlister, H.F., et al. Lyme carditis: An important cause of reversible heart block. *Ann. Intern. Med.* 110:339–345, 1989.
106. Lin, N.Y., et al. Randomized trial of doxycycline vs. amoxicillin probenecid for the treatment of Lyme arthritis: Treatment of nonresponders with IV penicillin or ceftriaxone [abstract]. *Arthritis Rheum.* 32:546, 1989.
107. Schoen, R.T., et al. Treatment of refractory chronic Lyme arthritis with arthroscopic synovectomy. *Arthritis Rheum.* 34:1054–1062, 1991.
108. Lightfoot, R.W., et al. Empiric parenteral antibiotic treatment of patients with fibromyalgia and fatigue and a positive serologic result for Lyme disease. *Ann. Intern. Med.* 119:503–509, 1993.
109. Appropriateness of parenteral antibiotic treatment for patients with presumed Lyme disease: A joint statement of the American College of Rheumatology and the Council of Infectious Diseases Society of America. *Ann. Intern. Med.* 119:518, 1993.
110. Ceftriaxone-associated biliary complications of treatment of suspected disseminated Lyme disease—New Jersey, 1990–1992. *M.M.W.R.* 42:39–42, 1993.
111. Keller, D., et al. Safety and immunogenicity of a recombinant outer surface protein A Lyme vaccine. *J.A.M.A.* 271:176–179, 1994.
112. Wormser, G.P. Prospects for a vaccine to prevent Lyme disease in humans. *Clin. Infect. Dis.* 21:1267, 1995.
113. Wormser, G.P. A vaccine against Lyme disease? *Ann. Intern. Med.* 123:627, 1995.

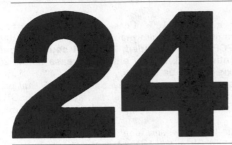

Prevention and Therapy of *Pneumocystis carinii* Pneumonia

Anne M. Traynor,
Richard E. Reese, and
Robert F. Betts

Basic Principles

Pneumocystis carinii pneumonia (PCP) occurs in newborns with agammaglobulinemia, patients with lymphoproliferative disorders, and patients on high-dose corticosteroids (e.g., in patients following organ transplantation and those with systemic lupus erythematosus), but it is most common in patients with the acquired immunodeficiency syndrome (AIDS).

Before antipneumocystic prophylaxis was widely prescribed in the United States, most North American patients with AIDS ultimately developed one or more episodes of PCP, resulting in hospital admission and considerable morbidity, mortality, and cost [1–1b]. During the mid-1980s, considerable progress was made in the early diagnosis and therapy of PCP, yet it continued to be a serious problem. For patients infected with the human immunodeficiency virus (HIV), fatality rates remained in the range of 20–40% for patients with severe hypoxemia at the onset of therapy of PCP [2], and morbidity and cost of PCP were still significant. **Prevention of PCP became an important goal of the late 1980s and 1990s.** General discussion of the pathogenesis, clinical presentation, and diagnosis of PCP appears elsewhere [3–8]. This chapter focuses on **primary prophylaxis** (prevention of the first episode of PCP), **secondary prophylaxis** (prevention of PCP in an individual who has recovered from an episode of PCP), and the **therapy for PCP.**

The rationale, various regimens available, dosages used, and brief overview of side effects for prophylaxis and therapy of PCP will be discussed in the first part of this chapter. Later in this chapter, we review special aspects of the individual agents and provide a more complete discussion of their toxicities. This format, of necessity, involves some repetition, but overall we believe it will expedite the retrieval of useful information for the busy clinician.

For those patients at risk for PCP, preventive therapy significantly reduces the rates of PCP [1, 5–12]. **The initial impact of PCP prophylaxis has been examined** in a large natural-history cohort study [11]. It was demonstrated that effective primary PCP prophylaxis delays the onset of AIDS by approximately 6–12 months, so that patients receiving prophylaxis do not develop AIDS-defining infections until their CD4+ lymphocyte cell counts are substantially lower. Correspondingly, AIDS-defining diagnoses among patients on prophylaxis were infections that occur at a lower level of immune function than does PCP and included disseminated *Mycobacterium avium* complex, CMV disease, and the generalized wasting syndrome [11]. Therefore, it is important to identify patients at risk for PCP and to provide them preventive therapy [1, 5–12].

Even with appropriate prophylaxis, PCP is one of the most common serious opportunistic infections (OI) among persons in the United States (both adults and children) who are infected with HIV [1b,11].

I. **Prevention of PCP in adult and adolescent patients infected with HIV** has been reviewed [1, 5–12].

   A. **Prevention of initial infection (primary prevention).** The following criteria are used to define patients at risk.

      1. **Based on CD4 cell counts.** Retrospective and prospective studies have shown that CD4+ lymphocyte cell counts are excellent predictors of whether PCP infection will develop [1, 9, 13]. Once the CD4 cell count drops below 200/mm³, the risk begins to increase, with further increasing risk as the CD4 T-cell count decreases. The majority of cases of PCP occurs in persons with CD4 cell counts

of less than 50/mm³ [1b]. Only about 10% of cases of PCP occur in patients with CD4 counts in excess of 200 and then mainly in the range of 200–250 [1a, 9, 14, 15]. **So that PCP can be avoided, CD4 cell counts should be monitored every 3–6 months** [1, 9]. **If they either decrease below 200 or decline rapidly, prophylaxis should be started.**

2. **Unexplained prolonged fever.** Patients with a fever above 100°F that persists for more than 2 weeks appear to be at increased risk, even if their CD4 cell counts do not warrant prophylaxis. Therefore, prophylaxis should be initiated in these patients [1, 1a].

3. **Oropharyngeal candidiasis** has also been identified as an independent risk factor for the development of PCP in the HIV-positive patient [1, 1a, 9].

B. **Secondary preventive.** Secondary prevention measures are indicated for any patient who has recovered from an episode of PCP, irrespective of the CD4 cell count, as these patients are at great risk for recurrent PCP—that is, more than 60% recur by 1 year if given no prophylaxis [9].

C. **Regimens effective** in preventing PCP [1–1b, 9, 12, 16–21]

1. **Trimethoprim-sulfamethoxazole (TMP-SMX).** If not contraindicated, TMP-SMX is the **preferred agent.**

   a. **Efficacy.** In primary prophylaxis, a prospective, randomized trial comparing TMP-SMX to placebo revealed that TMP-SMX both reduced the rate of PCP over 2 years of follow-up (0% incidence versus 53%) and lengthened survival (23 months versus 12 months) [15]. Although one study detected that both TMP-SMX and aerosolized pentamidine, when taken consistently, were effective prophylactic agents in disease prevention and survival prolongation [18], direct head-to-head comparisons between the two agents have demonstrated TMP-SMX's superior efficacy [16, 17]. In a prospective trial of primary prophylaxis, no patients randomized to receive TMP-SMX developed PCP, compared to 11% of those who received aerosolized pentamidine. A similar multicenter trial (AIDS Clinical Trials Group Protocol [ACTG] 021) of secondary prophylaxis reported that patients on aerosolized pentamidine were more than 3 times more likely to contract PCP over the study period than were patients receiving TMP-SMX [16, 17]. These findings led the US Public Health Service (USPHS) to recommend TMP-SMX as the drug of choice for PCP prophylaxis [1–1b]. The recent ACTG 081 trial again demonstrates that TMP-SMX is as effective or more effective in preventing PCP than dapsone or inhaled pentamidine [21a].

   b. **Protection against other pathogens.** Oral TMP-SMX provides protection against cerebral toxoplasmosis [16, 17, 20, 22] and protection against respiratory pathogens, e.g., *Streptococcus pneumoniae* or *Haemophilus influenzae* [22a], and possibly gastrointestinal pathogens (e.g., *Salmonella* spp.). Since the recognition of *Bartonella henselae* as the cause of bacillary angiomatoses and this pathogen's known susceptibility to TMP-SMX, there is speculation that this infection might be prevented as well.

   c. **Dosage.** Although a common recommendation is a daily dose of 160 mg TMP and 800 mg SMX orally (one double-strength [DS] tablet), **the minimum dosage of TMP-SMX in PCP prophylaxis is not firmly established** [1b, 19]. *The Medical Letter* recommendations reflect the different dosage options available, with drug administration of one DS tablet suggested every day or 1 DS tablet for 3 days per week [19]. Recent studies have used lower doses, such as one DS tablet 3 times weekly or one single-strength (SS) tablet daily, without loss of efficacy and with improved drug tolerance [17, 20, 21]. However, fewer data are available with regard to intermittent-dosing regimens for HIV-infected persons; one SS dose daily may be as effective as one DS tablet daily for primary prophylaxis [1b]. Pending further data, we recommend following the USPHS guidelines and administering TMP-SMX as one DS tablet daily, 7 days per week, or using one DS tablet twice daily on 3 consecutive days per week, for PCP prophylaxis.

   d. **Adverse effects. These are more common in HIV-infected patients than in uninfected persons** (see Chap. 28K for further discussion of the adverse effects of TMP-SMX). Pruritus, rash, leukopenia, transaminase elevation, and nausea are common. Most side effects are mild and reversible and respond to supportive therapy. In general, drug tolerance is greater with prophylaxis than with treatment regimens and has improved with the lower dosages used in prophylaxis, although rates of drug discontinuation due to adverse effects still approach 25–40% [1b, 15–17, 20, 22]. Initially, experts differed in their opinions about the safety of rechallenging a patient who had a non–life-threatening reaction (e.g., mild to moderate diffuse rash) to TMP-SMX. Such a rechallenge seems reasonable, in part because in ACTG 021 it was demonstrated that adverse reactions to TMP-SMX were no more frequent or severe among patients with a history of mild to moderate adverse reactions to TMP-SMX than among patients without such a history [16]. Furthermore, recent recommendations emphasize that because TMP-SMX is the preferred agent for patients with an adverse reaction that is non–life-threatening, treatment with TMP-SMX should be continued if clinically feasible; for those whose therapy has been discontinued for minor adverse reactions, its reinstitution should be strongly considered [1–1b]. Oral desensitization regimens to TMP-SMX have been described in the literature [22b]; completion of this allows patients to continue TMP-SMX despite a prior history of mild to moderate adverse reactions to TMP-SMX.

For patients with a vague history of sulfonamide intolerance or a history of minor intolerance only, many experts suggest using TMP-SMX prophylaxis initially. TMP-SMX should be avoided in patients with a history of a severe reaction (e.g., rashes with mucosal involvement [Stevens-Johnson syndrome] or desquamation, drug-induced hypotension, or anaphylaxis). See further discussion on page 912.

e. **Cost.** The estimated wholesale monthly cost of generic TMP-SMX, one DS tablet daily, as of 1995 is $5, whereas that for aerosolized pentamidine approaches $100 [23].

f. **Future considerations.** At the conclusion of the ACTG trial 081 summary [21a], the authors raised an important question. Because, overall, TMP-SMX was found to be the most effective agent in the prevention of PCP, and as routine early use of TMP-SMX might prematurely expose patients to adverse side effects that would preclude its use later on, the authors wondered whether the uniform preference for TMP-SMX as the initial preventive therapy in patients at lower risk (i.e., CD4 counts > 100/mm^3) should be reconsidered. Instead, different strategies might limit the intolerance to TMP-SMX or TMP-SMX might be reserved for the most vulnerable patients [21a].

2. **Dapsone.** Dapsone (alone or in combination with pyrimethamine) has emerged as the second-line agent for PCP prophylaxis in patients who are intolerant of TMP-SMX [1–1b, 5, 10, 19]. Because of the frequency of sulfonamide allergies (which preclude the use of TMP-SMX), increasing concerns about the use of aerosolized pentamidine, the low cost and ease of administration of dapsone, and the protective effects against *T. gondii,* when dapsone is combined with pyrimethamine, **dapsone is an appealing alternative for use in PCP prophylaxis.**

a. **Efficacy.** A randomized prospective trial comparing primary PCP prophylaxis with dapsone (100 mg/day) to that with TMP-SMX (one DS tablet daily) yielded similar clinical efficacies and rates of drug intolerance, with prophylaxis being interrupted in most patients in both groups owing to adverse effects (see sec. **d**) [24]. In a subsequent prospective trial of primary PCP prophylaxis, patients randomized to receive either aerosolized pentamidine (300 mg/mo) or the combination of dapsone (50 mg/day) and a second antifolate agent, pyrimethamine (50 mg/wk), revealed that both regimens were equally effective in preventing PCP (approximately 6% incidence for both groups) [24a]. Although the combination of dapsone with pyrimethamine allowed the daily dosage of dapsone to be reduced, discontinuation was still significantly more frequent in patients taking the combination regimen of dapsone-pyrimethamine.

In a recent trial, dapsone (50 mg bid) was as effective as TMP-SMX and inhaled pentamidine in preventing primary PCP; failures to prevent PCP were more common with 50 mg of dapsone daily than with 100 mg daily [21a].

b. **Protection against other agents.** A trial of 100 mg dapsone twice weekly versus inhaled pentamidine revealed equal efficacy in PCP prevention but a reduction of *T. gondii* clinical disease in dapsone recipients [25]. In another study, the use of the dapsone-pyrimethamine combination regimen was associated with a significantly reduced incidence of opportunistic toxoplasmic encephalitis, compared to the aerosolized pentamidine group [24a]. Regimens of dapsone in combination with pyrimethamine provide protection against both PCP and toxoplasmosis, although the magnitude of protection against PCP is about the same as that provided by aerosolized pentamidine [1b].

  c. **Dosage.** The recommended oral dose of dapsone for PCP prophylaxis is 50–100 mg/day (e.g., 50 mg bid) [5, 10, 21, 24–26]. One study used 100 mg twice weekly because of dapsone's long half-life [25]. In combination regimens (which also provide prophylaxis against toxoplasma encephalitis, desirable when CD4 counts are $< 100/mm^3$ in toxoplasmosis antibody-positive patients) 50 mg of dapsone daily plus 50 mg of pyrimethamine per week plus 25 mg of leucovorin per week have been used [1a, 1b, 19]. However, the manufacturer of dapsone prefers a dose of 100 mg of dapsone daily to ensure optimal protection against PCP, especially in patients with CD4 cell counts of less than $100/mm^3$. Another regimen includes 200 mg of dapsone plus 75 mg of pyrimethamine plus 25 mg of leucovorin once a week [1, 1a, 1b, 25a]. See regimen summaries in Tables 19-8 and 19-9.

  Furthermore, when significant concerns about the potential for drug toxicity with dapsone are apparent, we recommend consideration of titrating the dosage upward from an initial daily dose of 12.5–25.0 mg, then to 50 mg/day, and finally to 100 mg/day, as tolerated.

  d. **Adverse effects. A glucose-6-phosphate dehydrogenase (G-6-PD) screen must be done before treatment is begun.** Patients who experience mild to moderate adverse reactions to TMP-SMX often can tolerate dapsone [10, 24]. **See** sec. **III** under Selected Aspects of Antipneumocystic Agents **for a detailed discussion** of the adverse effects of dapsone (pp. 920–923). A mild decrease in hematocrit and a rise in the serum lactate dehydrogenase (LDH) level were the only two side effects unique to dapsone [24]. Most side effects in the dapsone-pyrimethamine combination regimen were mild and transient: anemia, rash, fever, nausea, and headache. Occasionally, methemoglobinemia develops while a patient is on dapsone.

  e. **Cost.** As of 1995 the estimated wholesale monthly cost of dapsone for PCP prophylaxis at a dose of 100 mg/day is $5 [23].

3. **Aerosolized pentamidine**
  a. **Efficacy.** Aerosolized pentamidine has been shown to be effective in primary and secondary prophylaxis of PCP, with annual relapse rates averaging 10–20%, and is recommended **for patients who cannot tolerate oral TMP-SMX or dapsone** [1–1b, 5, 7, 9, 12, 13, 18, 27]. In a recent trial, aerosolized pentamidine was less effective in preventing primary PCP in patients with CD4 counts less than $100/mm^3$ than was TMP-SMX or full doses of dapsone [21a]. Because the aerosolized drug is delivered almost exclusively to the patient's lungs, there is no protection against extrapulmonary pneumocystosis, which can occur (see page 920). Furthermore, the fact that extrapulmonary PCP does occur leads to an investigation of this possibility whenever unexplained fever develops in these patients.

  b. **Protection against other pathogens. Aerosolized pentamidine has no known effect against other opportunistic pathogens** or against bacteria [16, 17, 24a].

  c. **Special issues associated with inhaled pentamidine.** See further discussion, pages 919–920.
    (1) **Potential spread of tuberculosis. Before aerosolized pentamidine is initiated, patients should be evaluated for tuberculosis** and serially reassessed, at future treatments, for signs and symptoms of tuberculosis as aerosol-induced coughing can be associated with the spread of tuberculosis. In persons with known tuberculosis, aerosolized pentamidine should be administered following special precautions [28].
    (2) **Potential for extrapulmonary *P. carinii* infection** (see sec. **a**).
    (3) Aerosolized pentamidine should not be administered, if possible, to patients who have had hypoglycemia, pancreatitis, arrhythmias, or severe hypotension associated with any form of prior pentamidine administration. If no suitable alternative exists, close monitoring of the patient is important.

(4) The diagnostic yield of bronchoalveolar lavage (BAL) is reduced in episodes of PCP breaking through aerosolized pentamidine. See sec. **F.2** and pages 919–920.

d. **Dosages.** A **jet nebulizer (Respirgard II,** Marquest, Englewood, NJ), uses compressed air or oxygen to generate the aerosol. This device generates the aerosol continuously, and patients inhale, at best, for one-third of the time, which results in considerable waste of the drug. The requirements for compressed air and supervision by a respiratory therapist for home use make this method of administration awkward and expensive [3].

   The standard dose is 300 mg once monthly. However, in a recent randomized pilot study, patients receiving higher dosages of either 300 mg biweekly or 600 mg once monthly experienced lower rates of PCP when compared to historical controls receiving 300 mg/mo [29]. Residual lung volumes increased slightly, compared to baseline values, with the high-dose regimen. Overall, the higher-dose regimen was well tolerated, and no cases of extrapulmonary *P. carinii* developed. These investigators have begun a larger trial to examine their hypothesis of a dose-response effect with aerosolized pentamidine [29]. Pending further evaluation of this higher-dose regimen and given its significantly higher cost, we recommend that the standard dosage of 300 mg/mo be employed.

e. **Toxicity.** Several issues of toxicity are raised with the use of aerosolized pentamidine.

   (1) Patients who develop cough, wheezing, or chest pain should receive immediate intervention with an inhaled beta₂-agonist (e.g., albuterol inhaler) and inhaler pretreatment 10 minutes before subsequent pentamidine administration.

   (2) Substantial environmental contamination may result from the aerosol delivery system and coughing by the patient. After the treatment room or booth has been used, adequate time should be allowed for dissipation of residual pentamidine and any infectious organisms from the air before the room or booth is used by another patient. Ideally, all **patients should receive aerosol treatment in individual rooms or booths with negative ventilation.**

   (3) **Health care workers administering aerosol pentamidine should wear particulate respirators** whenever they are in a room or booth during administration of aerosolized pentamidine. Although there is concern about the effects of aerosolized pentamidine on health care workers who might inhale and absorb drug that was released into the environment by the nebulizer or by the patient during exhalation or coughing, there is no evidence for teratogenicity or carcinogenicity [5].

   (4) Patients who have substantial bullous lung disease or obstructive lung disease may not distribute aerosolized drug adequately. In addition, it has been well recognized that these patients have a high incidence of spontaneous pneumothorax. Thus, such patients are likely to be poor candidates for prophylaxis with aerosolized pentamidine [9].

f. **Cost.** Aerosolized pentamidine costs about 20 times that of TMP-SMX or dapsone [23].

D. **Investigational regimens to prevent PCP.** Data using these regimens are only preliminary; thus, these regimens are not routinely recommended [1, 1a, 9]. For patients who have had life-threatening intolerance to TMP-SMX, dapsone, and aerosolized pentamidine or who are intolerant to TMP-SMX and dapsone and have breakthrough episodes despite treatment with aerosolized pentamidine, these investigational regimens are potential alternatives. Infectious disease consultation is advised. Note that sulfadoxine-pyrimethamine (Fansidar) is no longer recommended.

1. Intermittent parenteral pentamidine (e.g., 4 mg/kg IV every 2–4 weeks) [3, 8, 29a].

2. Clindamycin and primaquine.

3. Intramuscular pentamidine once monthly. This is undergoing clinical investigation and may provide an alternative for those patients who cannot tolerate other regimens [30].

4. In preliminary studies, aerosolized pentamidine delivered by metered-dose inhaler was well tolerated [31].

E. **Patients receiving pyrimethamine and sulfadiazine therapy for toxoplasmosis** probably are receiving adequate prophylaxis against PCP and do not need additional therapy with TMP-SMX, dapsone, and the like (see Chap. 28U under Pyrimethamine) [32].

F. **Monitoring patients**

1. **Watch for *Pneumocystis* infection.** Because prophylaxis is not 100% effective, patients should be serially assessed for the development of *Pneumocystis* infection. In particular, physicians should be alert for the unusual radiographic presentation of PCP or extrapulmonary *Pneumocystis* infection seen in aerosolized pentamidine recipients [1, 9].

2. The diagnostic yield of BAL is reduced in episodes of PCP that develop in patients who are receiving aerosolized pentamidine prophylaxis. Bronchoscopy must not be confined only to the middle or lower lobes; upper-lobe or site-directed bronchoscopy is recommended [33–35] (see pp. 919–920).

3. Recent survival data indicate that recurrent episodes of PCP in patients receiving secondary prophylaxis may be less severe and not necessarily associated with diminished survival rates [34, 36].

G. **Breakthrough PCP in patients receiving prophylaxis can occur.** Why this is so is unclear. When TMP-SMX is used, poor compliance or possible inadequate GI absorption may be the explanation for breakthrough. When aerosolized pentamidine is used, poor pulmonary ventilation distribution and the inability to use the aerosol device properly are possible explanations.

1. **Therapy for breakthrough PCP.** Many experts suggest using a different therapeutic agent: For example, if prophylaxis was with TMP-SMX, parenteral pentamidine is used to treat breakthrough PCP. However, there are no data to support this approach [1, 9]. For instance, in cases of breakthrough PCP on inhaled pentamidine, PCP has been treated successfully with therapeutic parenteral doses of pentamidine [1, 9].

2. **Prophylaxis of future PCP after a breakthrough episode of PCP.** Unless contraindicated, TMP-SMX still is preferred [1, 12].

H. **Prevention of exposure.** The sources of *P. carinii* that cause pneumonia in humans are unknown, although transmission is presumed to be through the air [1b]. Consequently, some authorities have suggested that patients with known or suspected PCP should not be placed in the same room with other persons at risk for PCP. However, when reviewing this issue, Simonds et al. conclude that in the absence of specific studies that evaluate the risk of person-to-person transmission, data are insufficient to support isolation of patients with PCP as a standard practice [1b].

II. **Prevention of PCP in children.** This topic has been reviewed elsewhere [12].

A. **Impact of PCP on HIV-infected children.** *Pneumocystis carinii* pneumonia is the most common serious HIV-associated opportunistic infection among children [1b].

1. **Age onset.** Although PCP can occur at any age among children, it is most commonly diagnosed between 3 and 6 months of age. PCP in infants (i.e., children < 12 months of age) is often acute in onset and results in a poor prognosis [12].

2. **Initial manifestation of HIV.** *Pneumocystis carinii* pneumonia is often the initial clinical sign of HIV infection, especially among infants.

3. **Implications.** Effective prevention of PCP among HIV-infected infants requires that exposure to HIV be identified either before or immediately following birth so that prophylaxis can be initiated before 2 months of age—the age at which the risk of PCP begins to increase dramatically. At present, many HIV-exposed children are not identified early enough to be offered prophylaxis before the period of highest risk for PCP. Recent studies show that only 35–55% of HIV-exposed children have been identified by their health care providers [12]. One study of HIV-infected children diagnosed with PCP in the United States during 1991–1993 indicated that 59% of the children who had not received prophylaxis had not been identified as being at risk for HIV infection soon enough for prophylaxis to be initiated [12].

B. **Special problems in defining infants at risk for PCP**

1. **Use of CD4 cell counts.** Since the 1991 CDC guidelines that emphasized using CD4 cell counts to help determine when PCP chemoprophylaxis should be started, further study has indicated that **the usefulness of CD4 counts in determining the need for prophylaxis among infants is limited** [12]. In addition, the formerly used CD4 percentages [37] are no longer suggested as a criterion for PCP prophylaxis [12].

2. **Diagnosis of HIV.** HIV infection can be diagnosed by using the standard HIV immunoglobulin G (IgG) antibody tests in children over 18 months of age [12]. However, because maternal IgG can be present in children less than 18 months of age, standard serologic tests relying on HIV-IgG assays cannot be used to diagnose HIV infection in this age group. However, recent techniques allow for the diagnosis to be made in infants usually by 4–6 months of age [12].

   a. **HIV culture and polymerase chain reaction (PCR)** assays are very useful. The sensitivity of PCR is over 90% by 3 months of age and nearly 100% by 6 months of age [12].

   b. Use of the standard p24 antigen-capture assay has relatively low sensitivity, and use of this assay alone is not recommended [12].

C. **Revised 1995 CDC recommendations for PCP prevention** [12]

   1. **Promptly identify children born to HIV-infected mothers and initiate regular diagnostic and immunologic monitoring** of such children. Diagnosing HIV infection among women before or during pregnancy is the most beneficial way to accomplish this goal [12].

      a. The use of HIV culture or PCR is the preferred method of diagnosing infection among infants, and these assays should be performed at least twice (once at ≥ 1 month of age and once at > 4 months of age). If the result of any test is positive, testing should be repeated to confirm the diagnosis [12].

      b. Serial CD4 counts in infants are not necessary to determine PCP prophylaxis but are useful to measure level of immunosuppression in HIV exposed children (Table 24-1).

   2. **All infants born to HIV-infected mothers should be started on PCP prophylaxis at 4–6 weeks of age, regardless of their CD4 counts** (see Table 24-1).

      a. Infants who are first identified as being HIV exposed after 6 weeks of age should be started on prophylaxis at the time of identification [12].

Table 24-1. Recommendations for PCP prophylaxis and CD4 monitoring for HIV-exposed infants and HIV-infected children, by age and HIV-infection status

Age/HIV-infection status	PCP prophylaxis	CD4 monitoring
Birth to 4–6 wk, HIV exposed	No prophylaxis	1 mo
4–6 wk to 4 mo, HIV exposed	Prophylaxis	3 mo
4–12 mo		
HIV infected or indeterminate	Prophylaxis	6, 9, and 12 mo
HIV infection reasonably excluded[a]	No prophylaxis	None
1–5 yr, HIV infected	Prophylaxis if: CD4 count is <500 cells/mm^3 or CD4 percentage is <15%[c,d]	Every 3–4 mo[b]
6–12 yr, HIV infected	Prophylaxis if: CD4 count is <200 cells/mm^3 or CD4 percentage is <15%[d]	Every 3–4 mo[b]

[a]HIV infection can be reasonably excluded among children who have had two or more negative HIV diagnostic tests (i.e., HIV culture or PCR), both of which are performed at ≥1 mo of age and one of which is performed at ≥4 mo of age, or two or more negative HIV IgG antibody tests performed at >6 mo of age among children who have no clinical evidence of HIV disease.
[b]More frequent monitoring (e.g., monthly) is recommended for children whose CD4 counts or percentages are approaching the threshold at which prophylaxis is recommended.
[c]Children 1–2 yr of age who were receiving PCP prophylaxis and had a CD4 count of <750 cells/mm^3 or percentage of <15% at <12 mo of age should continue prophylaxis.
[d]Prophylaxis should be considered on a case-by-case basis for children who might otherwise be at risk for PCP, such as children with rapidly declining CD4 counts or percentages or children with category C conditions (see revised classification of HIV infection, Table 19-2). Children who have had PCP should receive lifelong PCP prophylaxis.
Source: Centers for Disease Control. 1995 Revised guidelines for prophylaxis against *Pneumocystis carinii* pneumonia for children infected with or perinatally exposed to human immunodeficiency virus. *M.M.W.R.* 44(RR-4):6, 1995.

   b. **Prophylaxis for PCP should not be administered to infants less than 4 weeks of age,** because they are at low risk for PCP and sulfonamide use in neonates is not advised (see Chap. 3). In addition, the concurrent use of sulfa drugs in neonates who are receiving zidovudine during the first 6 weeks of life to prevent perinatal transmission could potentially aggravate the anemia associated with zidovudine [12].

3. **PCP prophylaxis for infants 4–12 months of age**
   a. All HIV-infected infants and infants whose infection status has not yet been determined should continue prophylaxis until 12 months of age [12].
   b. PCP prophylaxis should be discontinued among infants in whom HIV infection has been reasonably excluded on the basis of two or more negative viral tests (see sec. **1**).
   c. For children who do not have access to such testing, prophylaxis should be continued until 12 months of age unless HIV infection has been excluded on the basis of two or more negative HIV IgG antibody tests performed at least 6 months of age [12].

4. **For children over 1 year of age,** see Table 24-1.

5. **Prophylaxis against recurrent PCP. HIV infected children who have had an episode of PCP should receive lifelong PCP prophylaxis to prevent recurrence,** regardless of CD4 measurement or clinical status [12].

D. **Regimens for PCP prophylaxis.** Although no randomized, placebo-controlled trials of PCP chemoprophylactic regimens for PCP among HIV-infected children have been performed, extrapolations may be made from experience with drugs used for PCP prophylaxis for children with other diseases and from PCP prophylaxis data in adults [1b, 12].

1. **TMP-SMX is the drug of choice for PCP prophylaxis in HIV-infected candidates older than 1 month** (Table 24-2).
   a. **TMP-SMX is not recommended for neonates** because of concerns about bilirubin displacement by sulfonamides. Although this potential adverse effect is a realistic concern in the premature neonate and the duration of the risk is not known, infants older than 2 months and probably those between 1 and 2 months of age are not likely to suffer adverse sequelae. However, it also is noteworthy that intravenous TMP-SMX contains benzyl alcohol, which may cause toxicity in the neonate [12, 38].
   b. **Adverse reactions** to TMP-SMX appear to be more frequent and severe in HIV-infected adult patients (40–60% of recipients have reactions) than among HIV-infected children (15% of recipients have reactions) [12]. If life-threatening toxicity (anaphylaxis, Stevens-Johnson syndrome, or hypotension) occurs, TMP-SMX should be permanently discontinued. If other poten-

Table 24-2. Drug regimens for PCP prophylaxis for children ≥4 wk of age

Recommended regimen
   Trimethoprim-sulfamethoxazole (TMP-SMX) 150 mg TMP/m^2/day with 750 mg SMX/m^2/day PO administered in divided doses bid 3×/wk on consecutive days (e.g., Monday, Tuesday, Wednesday)

Acceptable alternative TMP-SMX dosage schedules
   150 mg TMP/m^2/day with 750 mg SMX/m^2/day PO administered **as a single daily dose** 3×/wk on consecutive days (e.g., Monday, Tuesday, Wednesday)
   150 mg TMP/m^2/day with 750 mg SMX/m^2/day PO divided bid and **administered 7 days per week**
   150 mg TMP/m^2/day with 750 mg SMX/m^2/day PO divided bid and administered 3×/wk on **alternate days** (e.g., Monday, Wednesday, Friday)

Alternative regimens if TMP/SMX is not tolerated
   Dapsone*: 2 mg/kg/day PO (not to exceed 100 mg) given once daily
   Aerosolized pentamidine* (children ≥5 yr): 300 mg administered via Respirgard II inhaler monthly

---

*If neither dapsone nor aerosolized pentamidine is tolerated, some clinicians use **intravenous pentamidine** (4 mg/kg) administered every 2 or 4 weeks.
Source: Centers for Disease Control. 1995 Revised guidelines for prophylaxis against *Pneumocystis carinii* pneumonia for children infected with or perinatally exposed to human immunodeficiency virus. *M.M.W.R.* 44(RR-4):8, 1995.

tially related reactions are noted (e.g., rash, neutropenia), the drug may be temporarily discontinued and restarted within 2 weeks [12, 38]. Desensitization is a consideration and, if carried out, TMP-SMX should be given daily because of the potential for serious adverse reactions on reintroduction of the drug after any interruption of dosing [12].

   c. **Dosages. See Table 24-2. In children, TMP-SMX 3 times weekly on consecutive days (e.g., Monday, Tuesday, Wednesday) is recommended.** Doses should be adjusted upward as the child grows, with a maximum dose not to exceed 320 mg TMP plus 1,600 mg SMX daily [12].

   d. **Monitoring.** Complete blood cell counts with differentials and platelet counts should be done at the initiation of TMP-SMX prophylaxis and at monthly intervals to assess for potential hematologic toxicity [12].

2. **Dapsone** may be considered for those older than 1 month who cannot tolerate TMP-SMX. Dosages are reviewed in Table 24-2.

   a. As of early 1996 a liquid formulation is not commercially available but is under study in the ACTG clinical trials. It is anticipated that a liquid preparation will become available in 1996. See related discussion of dapsone in sec. **III** under Selected Aspects of Antipneumocystic Agents. The 25- and 100-mg tablets are crushable so that an appropriate dose can be administered and the drug can be given in or with food.

   b. Monitoring of monthly CBC count is advised as described in sec. **1.d.**

   c. Breakthrough episodes of PCP can occur in children receiving dapsone prophylaxis. The reasons for this are unclear [38a].

3. **Aerosolized pentamidine** is recommended for HIV-infected children 5 years of age or older if TMP-SMX and dapsone cannot be tolerated. Use of aerosolized pentamidine in younger children usually is limited by the child's ability to use the nebulizer [12]. (See Table 24-2.) The dose and method of delivery is extrapolated from adult data, as there are limited data on the use of aerosolized pentamidine in children. Reductions in pediatric dosages of aerosolized pentamidine may be considered in the future, as drug concentrations delivered to the lungs of children—especially to the large, central airways—appear to exceed those in adults [39]. However, in a preliminary report, standard doses of aerosolized pentamidine for prophylaxis were well tolerated in infants [39a].

4. **Intravenous pentamidine** given every 2 or 4 weeks has been used in patients who cannot tolerate any of the aforementioned regimens (see Table 24-2).

E. PCP prophylaxis in non–HIV-positive patients has been discussed [39b].

III. **Therapy for PCP** has been reviewed [2, 3–5, 8, 40].

A. **Severity of illness. This should be assessed at the start of therapy because the severity of illness in PCP has an effect on therapeutic options.**

1. **Mild (to moderate) episodes** are defined by **initial room air PaO$_2$ greater than 70 mm Hg** or an alveolar-arterial oxygen difference (A-a)DO$_2$ of less than 35. Mortality rates of mild to moderate PCP are in the range of 10–20% [2].

2. **Severe PCP** is defined as patients with a room air PaO$_2$ of less than 70 mm Hg or (A-a)DO$_2$ of greater than 35 mm Hg. Mortality rates in these patients are in the 20–40% range despite therapy [2].

3. **Adjunctive corticosteroids** should be given **early** in the course of treatment of severe PCP as they have been shown to improve outcome and reduce mortality. The rationale and dosages are discussed in detail in sec. **IV.**

B. **Agent of choice**

1. **TMP-SMX is considered the initial therapy of choice** for both mild to moderate and severe cases of PCP [2, 5–8, 19, 40]. It is microbiostatic against *P. carinii.* This drug combination interferes with sequential steps of folate synthesis. **Adjunctive therapy with folinic acid (or folic acid) should be avoided [40a].** A prospective, randomized study of AIDS patients with PCP revealed that patient survival without respiratory support was significantly greater (86% versus 61%) for patients treated with TMP-SMX compared to those treated with intravenous pentamidine [41]. Although TMP-SMX has proven efficacious in the treatment of PCP in studies of immunocompromised children since the mid-1970s, it remains far from the ideal antipneumocystic agent in AIDS patients as the majority will experience some type of drug-related toxicity.

   a. **Dosage.** The optimal daily dose of TMP-SMX in PCP is not well established. Although formerly the usual dose recommended was 15–20 mg/kg/day, based on the TMP component, given equally in divided doses q6h, recent recommendations typically prefer 15 mg/kg/day, based on the TMP component, divided into 3 or 4 doses, in both children and adults [19, 40]. Therapy in patients with AIDS usually is given **for** at least **21 days;** other patients may require only 14 days. The intravenous route is preferred for initial therapy in very ill patients. Oral therapy often is used in mild infections or to complete therapy in severe infection.

   (1) Sattler and colleagues [41] determined that some adverse effects of TMP-SMX could be reduced with pharmacokinetic monitoring by maintaining serum trimethoprim concentrations between 5 and 8 µg/ml. Using this method, no loss of efficacy was encountered when patients were treated with TMP-SMX dosages of 10–15 mg/kg/day.

   (2) Because pharmacokinetic monitoring usually is not available, a reasonable approach for patients with normal renal function is to start with the dose of the trimethoprim component at 15 mg/kg/day and after 4–5 days of clinical stability, then consider reducing the daily trimethoprim dose further to 10 mg/kg/day if the patient is responding well.

   (3) In a related report, in patients receiving therapy for PCP pneumonia, the incidence of anemia, neutropenia, and azotemia increased with increasing TMP plasma concentrations, while other adverse effects (gastrointestinal disorders, rash, fever, and liver function abnormalities) were independent of plasma drug concentration [41a]. The authors do not recommend plasma drug concentrations to monitor patients because of the low predictive value of these measurements [41a].

   (4) See dosing of TMP-SMX in renal failure in Chap. 28K.

   b. **Adverse effects. More than 60% of all AIDS patients have experienced adverse reactions to TMP-SMX and 20–50% or more have had to discontinue therapy** (although these data derive largely from trials that used full-dose TMP-SMX for the duration of the treatment period) [5–7]. See related discussions on pages 904–905.

   (1) Much of the toxicity of TMP-SMX is attributed to the cytotoxicity toward lymphocytes of sulfamethoxazole's hydroxylamine metabolite [42]. It is hypothesized that clearance of this active metabolite is impaired in AIDS patients because this population, as compared to non–HIV-infected persons, has significantly reduced concentrations of the antioxidant scavenger glutathione [42]. Greater tolerance to therapy with TMP-SMX is conceivably related to less accumulation of this cytotoxic metabolite [20, 41]. This postulated mechanism of toxicity is substantiated by the finding that development of hypersensitivity to TMP-SMX is less likely to occur with lower CD4 cell counts [43].

   (2) **Most side effects are mild** and reversible and usually appear 7–14 days into therapy. Severe reactions are rare [44]. Commonly encountered adverse reactions to TMP-SMX include rash (seen in 27–37% of AIDS patients), leukopenia (19%), elevation of serum transaminases (20%), nausea and vomiting (7%), fever, and thrombocytopenia [6, 7]. Hyperkalemia (seen in 20% of patients) and hyponatremia are likely related to trimethoprim's blockage of sodium channels in the distal tubule, resulting in impaired potassium secretion and salt wasting [45].

   (3) **Most adverse effects can be treated with supportive care or dosage reduction and should not necessarily prompt discontinuation of the drug** (although this decision must obviously be individualized). Severe rashes with desquamation or mucosal involvement (e.g., Stevens-Johnson type), drug-induced hypotension, or anaphylaxis requires drug discontinuation [44].

   2. Some physicians may prefer to use **trimethoprim-dapsone** therapy rather than TMP-SMX **in first-episode mild to moderate PCP** in patients with AIDS, based on the findings of Medina and coworkers [46], which show both regimens were equally effective. However, it is noteworthy that TMP-dapsone was better tolerated by patients than was TMP-SMX, and it can be used in sulfa-allergic patients. (See sec. **C.2.**) Sattler and Feinburg [2] point out that this trial did not establish whether TMP-dapsone is of comparable efficacy to TMP-SMX because of the relatively small study population (only 60 patients). Likewise, dosage reduction of TMP-SMX and supportive care with antihistamines often permits the uninterrupted continuation of TMP-SMX therapy [2, 41].

C. **Therapy for mild to moderate PCP in adults.**
   1. **TMP-SMX,** if not contraindicated, **is preferred** by many clinicians [19]. The usual initial dose regimen is 15 mg/kg/day of the TMP component, given in

divided doses q6–8h [3, 41] for 14–21 days, although lower doses in the range of 12–15 mg/kg/day of TMP have been effective [41]. See sec. **B.1.a.(2)** for a detailed discussion of TMP-SMX dosing.

2. **TMP-dapsone** may be used [19, 46]. In a double-blind trial reported by Medina and colleagues [46], 60 patients with AIDS and a **mild to moderately severe** first episode of PCP were randomly assigned to 21 days of therapy with either TMP-SMX (at 20 mg/kg/day of the TMP component divided into four doses) or TMP and dapsone (doses follow). The regimens were equally effective, but with the TMP-dapsone regimen, fewer serious adverse effects occurred. **Patients were screened for G-6-PD deficiency and monitored for signs of methemoglobinemia** along with serial blood counts. See pages 920–923 for further discussion of dapsone.

Perhaps if doses had been reduced gradually, as described in sec. **B.1.a.(2)**, adverse effects would have been fewer in TMP-SMX recipients.

   a. **Dosages**
      (1) **Dapsone:** 100 mg/day as a single oral dose.
      (2) **Trimethoprim:** 20 mg/kg/day in four divided oral doses.
   b. **Side effects** reported by Medina [46] included the following:
      (1) **Major** side effects (hepatitis and neutropenia) were seen more frequently in the TMP-SMX recipients. Minor side effects (mild neutropenia or increased aminotransferase levels) were also seen in the TMP-SMX recipients. Overall, because of major adverse reactions, TMP-SMX had to be discontinued in 57% of recipients compared to 30% of recipients of TMP-dapsone.
      (2) Diffuse maculopapular **rashes,** often with fever, occurred in 30% of TMP-dapsone recipients and 37% of TMP-SMX recipients. In most patients, the rash and fever resolved within 48–72 hours, even though therapy continued at full dosages. The drug was stopped if the rash was subjectively intolerable or if there was desquamation or involvement of mucous membranes.
      (3) **Mild hyperkalemia** was observed in 53% of TMP-dapsone recipients, compared with 20% of TMP-SMX recipients and was most likely related to dapsone's inhibition of trimethoprim's clearance or metabolism, thereby exacerbating trimethoprim's reduction of potassium secretion from the distal nephron.
   c. **Conclusion.** Medina's group [46] concluded that "because trimethoprim-sulfamethoxazole induced a higher incidence of major toxic effects (including neutropenia and hepatitis), ... [Medina and colleagues] ... believe that trimethoprim-dapsone is preferable for oral therapy for ambulatory or mildly ill patients and ... [these investigators] ... now use it as initial therapy for outpatients with mild to moderate *P. carinii* pneumonia." They stressed careful serial follow-up and encouraged additional study of dosage regimens that may help reduce further the side effects of TMP-dapsone therapy.

We concur that this study suggests that **in first-episode mild to moderate PCP in patients with AIDS, TMP-dapsone is a reasonable initial choice of therapy.** This is especially appealing for a patient allergic to sulfonamides. For severe PCP infection, hospitalization and conventional therapy (e.g., intravenous TMP-SMX or pentamidine) are indicated initially.

3. **Dapsone alone is not effective for PCP** [2, 47].
4. **Intravenous pentamidine** is an effective alternative therapy when **patients cannot receive TMP-SMX** (e.g., sulfonamide allergy) **or are not candidates for TMP-dapsone therapy** (e.g., severely ill at presentation). Pentamidine usually is effective when used in patients who cannot tolerate TMP-SMX or TMP-dapsone. The **dose** of intravenous pentamidine in the treatment of mild to moderate PCP is 3 mg/kg/day, diluted in 50–250 ml of 5% dextrose in water, infused over 1–2 hours [48, 49]. For more serious cases, a dose of 4 mg/kg/day is used. See pages 918–920 for a further discussion of pentamidine therapy in PCP.
5. **Clindamycin plus primaquine** together have excellent activity against *P. carinii* in a limited culture system and in cortisone-treated rats, although neither is effective alone [2]. Clinical efficacy data using this combination involves small numbers of patients, but this combination appears promising, as published recommendations suggest that clindamycin-primaquine can be considered an

effective alternative therapy for mild to moderate PCP [50]. A pilot study of AIDS patients with mild to moderate PCP yielded similar rates of response (91% for TMP-SMX and 89% for clindamycin-primaquine) and drug tolerance (20% of TMP-SMX patients discontinued treatment due to adverse effects, compared to 18% of clindamycin-primaquine patients), prompting the authors to encourage further evaluation of this regimen [51]. See reference [51a].

   a. Dosages. This regimen is listed as an alternative regimen in *The Medical Letter's* "Drugs for Parasitic Infections" [19], although its use in this setting is **considered investigational** by the FDA. Clindamycin, 600 mg IV q6h for 21 days or 300–450 mg PO q6h for 21 days, plus primaquine, 15 mg base PO once daily for 21 days, is suggested [19].

   b. Side effects

   (1) Generalized rash was the most common side effect in preliminary studies but often was not treatment limiting. The rash probably is related to clindamycin therapy [2]. (See Chap. 28I.)

   (2) There is the **potential for hemolytic anemia.** Hemolysis can be precipitated by primaquine in patients with G-6-PD deficiency. This deficiency is most common in blacks, Asians, and Mediterranean peoples [19].

   c. Precautions

   (1) Patients should be screened for G-6-PD deficiency before primaquine treatment is initiated [19].

   (2) Primaquine should not be used during pregnancy [19].

   (3) The incidence of primaquine-related methemoglobinemia is reduced using doses of 15 mg primaquine base daily; venous methemoglobin levels should be monitored, especially during weeks 2 and 3 of treatment [50, 51].

6. Atovaquone (Mepron, BW566C80) was approved in 1992 for treatment of mild to moderate PCP and is an alternative agent available for use against *P. carinii* [19].

   a. Background. In a multicenter trial, AIDS patients with mild to moderate PCP were randomized to receive oral therapy with either atovaquone (750 mg 3 times daily) or TMP-SMX (320 mg trimethoprim and 1,600 mg sulfamethoxazole 3 times daily) [52]. Atovaquone use was associated with significantly lower rates of clinical efficacy and survival but was better tolerated. Bioavailability of this agent appears to be a major determinant of clinical response, in that the authors were able to correlate therapeutic success with atovaquone plasma concentrations.

   In another report, in patients with known HIV infection and histologically confirmed mild to moderate PCP, 56 patients received atovaquone (750 mg tid with meals) and 53 received intravenous pentamidine (3–4 mg/kg/day). Both agents demonstrated similar rates of success, but atovaquone had significantly fewer treatment-limiting adverse effects [52a].

   b. Dosage. The initial dosage regimen for atovaquone in treating mild to moderate PCP was 750 mg (three 250-mg **tablets**) administered orally 3 times daily for 21 days. Recently, a **suspension** of atovaquone has become available. The recommended oral dose for PCP in the package insert is **750 mg (5 ml) administered with meals twice daily for 21 days.** The package insert emphasizes that the suspension formulation provides an approximately twofold increase in atovaquone bioavailability compared with the tablet form. Therefore, the more convenient twice daily suspension regimen is now preferred [19, 40], and the manufacturer no longer makes the oral tablets. The **absorption of atovaquone is markedly enhanced by the presence of food,** especially foods high in fat, resulting in a two- to threefold increase in plasma drug concentrations [53]. Therefore, atovaquone can be used only in patients who can take oral medications and eat dependably [52a].

   c. Adverse reactions to atovaquone appear to occur less frequently than with TMP-SMX [52, 53]. In the study by Hughes and colleagues [52], 7% of patients receiving atovaquone experienced treatment-limiting adverse effects, compared to 20% of patients taking TMP-SMX. Reported adverse effects included rash, liver function abnormalities, fever, and vomiting, each occurring in fewer than 5% of patients. Diarrhea occurred significantly more often in patients receiving atovaquone (19%) but was not associated with lack of efficacy [52]. In addition, atovaquone has fewer side effects than intravenous pentamidine [52a].

   d. See sec. **V** under Selected Aspects of Antipneumocystic Agents for a further discussion of atovaquone use in PCP.

 7. Aerosolized pentamidine. Although initial data were encouraging about the use of inhaled pentamidine for therapy of PCP [2], additional studies suggested an unacceptably high failure rate seen especially in moderate to severe PCP [54, 55]. However, this observation was not confirmed in a more recent multicenter study [56].

   In their review of the treatment of PCP, Sattler and Feinburg [2] suggest that **aerosolized pentamidine is best suited for patients with mild PCP who cannot tolerate other therapies,** whereas other reviewers have voiced stronger reservations about its use in the treatment of PCP [5, 6]. Interestingly, *The Medical Letter* in 1993 and 1995 did not list aerosolized pentamidine as an alternative regimen in the treatment of PCP [19]. See sec. **II.E.** under Selected Aspects of Antipneumocystic Agents for a further discussion of issues associated with aerosolized pentamidine use in prophylaxis of PCP.

D. Therapy for severe PCP
 1. Conventional therapy
   a. **TMP-SMX** is viewed as the gold standard and **is preferred** unless contraindicated [2, 19, 41].
   b. **Intravenous pentamidine** is an alternative [2, 19]. Comparison trials with TMP-SMX demonstrated inferior survival rates with intravenous pentamidine, but it remains an important therapeutic agent due to the patient's frequent intolerance of TMP-SMX [41]. When this agent is substituted because the patient has not responded to 5–7 days of TMP-SMX, pentamidine often is ineffective [7]. There is no evidence that combining pentamidine with TMP-SMX increases the effectiveness of therapy, although toxicity may increase [7].
     (1) **Slow intravenous infusion over 1–2 hours.** Because pentamidine regularly produces painful sterile abscesses at the site of intramuscular injections, intravenous infusion is advised [7, 8]. Pentamidine is diluted in 50–250 ml of 5% dextrose in water [48, 49].
     (2) **Dose.** The dose of pentamidine for adults and children is 4 mg/kg once daily [3, 19] for 21 days for severe PCP.
     (3) **In renal failure,** see separate discussion on pages 918–919.
     (4) For further discussion of pentamidine, see pages 918–920.
 2. Adjunctive corticosteroids are recommended early in the course of treatment of severe PCP as they have been shown to improve outcome and reduce mortality. The rationale and dosages are **discussed in detail in sec. IV.**
 3. Trimetrexate is an antifolate drug that is concentrated in protozoan cells and binds to the dihydrofolate reductase of *P. carinii* nearly 1,500 times more avidly than does TMP. **Concurrent therapy with leucovorin (folinic acid) protects against trimetrexate-induced hematologic toxicity [2, 57].**
   a. **Background.** The initial trial of trimetrexate in patients intolerant of or who failed on TMP-SMX appeared promising in that 85% of recipients survived [58]. However, a multicenter trial initiated by the ACTG to compare trimetrexate (45 mg/m²/day) with TMP-SMX (20 mg/kg/day of TMP) revealed a significant benefit in favor of those treated with TMP-SMX. In this report of a double-blind study of 215 patients with moderate to severe PCP, failure rates occurred in 20% of those treated with TMP-SMX versus 38% of trimetrexate/leucovorin recipients. By day 49, the mortality rates were significantly different (16% versus 31%, respectively). Trimetrexate-treated patients had fewer severe side effects [58a].
   b. In their review, Sattler and Feinburg [2] suggest that **trimetrexate should be reserved for patients (requiring parenteral therapy) who are intolerant of or have failed TMP-SMX and pentamidine.**
     (1) **Availability** of this agent is discussed in sec. **IV.A** under Selected Aspects of Antipneumocystic Agents.
     (2) Therapy requires frequent hematologic monitoring and leucovorin, which is expensive.
   c. **Dosages.** Trimetrexate, 45 mg/m² IV over 60–90 minutes every day for 21 days, and folinic acid, 20 mg/m² PO or IV q6h for 24 days, which must be

continued for a full 3 days following cessation of trimetrexate therapy according to the package insert.

    d. See further discussion on pages 923–925.

4. Clindamycin-primaquine. Although a single retrospective uncontrolled trial determined that salvage therapy with clindamycin-primaquine in AIDS patients with severe PCP who were previously intolerant of, or refractory to, conventional therapy was successful in 24 of 28 episodes [59], further studies are needed to examine the role of this combination regimen in severe PCP.

5. Eflornithine (DMFO, Ornidyl), which appeared to be useful in preliminary studies for salvage therapy, is **not available,** even on a compassionate basis [2].

6. Experimental therapies

    a. Piritrexin is an oral antifolate drug similar to trimetrexate and is undergoing clinical study. Leucovorin is administered with this agent, which adds to the expense of its clinical use. Studies are planned to determine whether piritrexin plus pulsed doses of dapsone for the initial 5–7 days of therapy will improve outcome [2].

    b. Atovaquone (Mepron, BW566C80) **has been approved for oral therapy in mild to moderate PCP** [52]. See sec. **C.6.** Its role in the treatment of severe PCP or prophylaxis of PCP awaits further clinical study.

E. Therapy in children. The same principles are used in children as in adults except that *The Medical Letter* recommends only standard therapy be employed—that is, TMP-SMX or intravenous pentamidine. Doses per kilogram are the same as for adults [19].

F. Duration of therapy generally is 2–3 weeks.

    1. For mild disease, 2 weeks of therapy may be appropriate. This is followed by lifelong prophylaxis therapy for PCP.

    2. For severe disease, it seems prudent to treat the patient for 3 weeks with conventional therapy. This is followed by lifelong prophylaxis therapy for PCP.

    3. For investigational regimens, a 3-week duration of therapy is typically recommended [19]. Again, this would be followed by lifelong PCP prophylaxis.

G. Intensive care issues. With adjunctive corticosteroids (see sec. **IV**) and appropriate therapy, intubation and consequent transfer to the intensive care unit is less frequent.

    Those individuals who do require transfer are much more severely ill and, hence, the cost-effectiveness of their care has fallen [59a].

IV. Adjunctive corticosteroids in the treatment of selective cases of PCP

A. Clinical studies have demonstrated that adjunctive steroid therapy initiated within 72 hours of the diagnosis of PCP in patients infected with HIV who have moderate to severe hypoxemia from PCP significantly reduces the risk of transfer to the intensive care unit, intubation, and death due to respiratory failure [60–63].

B. Consensus statements

    1. The National Institutes of Health–University of California Expert Panel on the Use of Corticosteroids as Adjunctive Therapy for *Pneumocystis* Pneumonia in AIDS [64], in its November, 1990 report, emphasized the following:

        a. Adults and adolescents (children >13 years) with HIV and PCP should be given corticosteroid therapy for severe PCP (i.e., patients with a room air $PaO_2 < 70$ mm Hg or an $(A-a)DO_2$ of > 35 mm Hg), as corticosteroids clearly can reduce the likelihood of death, respiratory failure, or progressive hypoxemia. Whether patients with mild to moderate PCP will benefit from corticosteroids is unknown, and no recommendation was made for this group.

        b. Adjunctive corticosteroid therapy should be started when specific antipneumocystic therapy is started. A benefit for patients given corticosteroids more than 72 hours after specific antipneumocystic therapy begins has not been consistently demonstrated [65]. The panel [64] believed that it is reasonable to begin treatment with corticosteroids in patients with presumed AIDS-associated PCP, but the diagnosis of HIV and PCP should be confirmed rapidly to minimize the likelihood of missing other treatable diseases (e.g., tuberculosis) and to minimize the adverse effects of unnecessary drugs.

        c. Corticosteroid regimen. The regimen with the largest clinical experience was preferred, although the optimal regimen is unknown. Recent summaries still favor this dose regimen [19].

  (1) Oral regimen: Prednisone
  - **(a)** 40 mg bid on days 1–5
  - **(b)** 20 mg bid on days 6–10
  - **(c)** 20 mg each day on days 11–21

  (2) Intravenous regimen: Methylprednisolone at 75% of the prednisone doses (45–60 mg/day initially and then tapered).

  d. **Children younger than 13 years.** The pathogenesis of PCP in children may differ. Data still are needed to address the role of corticosteroids in children younger than 13, especially in very young children. (See Sleasman and colleagues [66].) Early reports suggest that steroids are beneficial in children [66].

  e. **Corticosteroids in patients with PCP and immunosuppression but without HIV.** No studies have yet evaluated this population, but the panel [64] believed it was reasonable to use adjunctive corticosteroids, as in the HIV population, as described previously.

  f. **Adjunctive corticosteroids in pregnant women with HIV infection and PCP.** Again, although no studies are available, the panel [64] believed that these patients may similarly benefit from corticosteroids.

  g. **Rescue therapy.** The role of adding corticosteroids for those in whom standard antipneumocystic therapy is failing and the role of higher doses of corticosteroids for patients not responding to standard regimens is unclear and awaits further clinical study. As reported in a recent review, five of six patients with severe PCP and refractory hypoxia given rescue steroids at a mean of 12 days after the initiation of specific treatment of PCP were alive at 6 months of follow-up [65]. The authors suggest that, although clinical trials clarifying the role and timing of corticosteroid therapy in PCP now are difficult to perform given the acceptance of the consensus statement [64], consideration should be given to the possible role of rescue corticosteroid therapy for PCP patients who deteriorate while receiving conventional antipneumocystic regimens [65].

2. **Working Group on Steroid Use, Antimicrobial Agents Committee, Infectious Disease Society of America** [67]

  a. This group recommends selective use of corticosteroids in early moderate to severe hypoxemia, similar to the summary in sec. **B.1.a.** The report emphasizes that the published data, reviewed in sec. **A**, provide **good evidence** to support the recommendation of corticosteroid use in this group of patients [67].

  b. This group reports that few data are available for younger patients, but some clinical trial protocols have recommended the same guidelines for children older than 2 years.

  c. The report **emphasizes the importance of confirming the diagnosis of PCP** as steroids may mask the symptoms of untreated infections (e.g., *Mycobacterium tuberculosis*). However, steroid therapy should not be withheld while awaiting confirmation of the diagnosis of PCP (or the delay may prevent steroids from exerting their beneficial effect).

C. **Miscellaneous**

1. Other experts have expressed concern that empiric adjunctive corticosteroids could have detrimental effects if given to patients with other opportunistic infections, especially tuberculosis or fungal infections [2]. In fact, these infections may respond initially to steroids, giving one the false impression that the patient has "improving" PCP. **Therefore, the diagnosis of PCP should be confirmed as early as possible, and consideration should be given also to beginning antituberculous therapy in patients at risk for tuberculosis** (those with evidence for past exposure to tuberculosis, those of certain ethnicity associated with high rates of tuberculosis, and intravenous drug users) and in whom diagnostic tests are not possible [2].

2. **Corticosteroids may aggravate and accelerate the progression of cutaneous and pulmonary Kaposi's sarcoma** [2]. Thus, corticosteroids should be prescribed with caution in patients with cutaneous Kaposi's sarcoma, and consideration should be given to withholding their use in patients with typical radiographic features or documented evidence of pulmonary Kaposi's sarcoma.

3. Overall, with adherence to the precautionary measures outlined in section **C.1**, no evidence exists to implicate adjuvant corticosteroid therapy as a cause of increased risk of serious AIDS-related opportunistic infections or malignancies [7, 68].

4. **Skin rashes** appear to occur less frequently in TMP-SMX recipients who receive corticosteroids. In one report, 18 of 38 patients (47%) who were treated with TMP-SMX alone developed cutaneous side effects; whereas 3 of 23 patients (13%) who received TMP-SMX and corticosteroids developed cutaneous side effects [68a].

D. **Potential mechanisms of action of corticosteroids in PCP.** Although the exact mechanisms of action of corticosteroids in PCP remain unclear, recent in vitro experiments have demonstrated that corticosteroids play a role in inhibiting the release of inflammatory cytokines from the alveolar macrophages of AIDS patients with pathologic pulmonary processes [69].

Selected Aspects of Antipneumocystic Agents

I. **Trimethoprim-sulfamethoxazole** is reviewed in detail in Chap. 28K.

II. **Pentamidine isethionate** (Pentam 300) is an antiprotozoal agent, that, in the United States, has as its main indication **the treatment and prevention of PCP** [19]. Pentamidine interferes with the biosynthesis of DNA, RNA, phospholipids, and proteins; although its precise mechanism of action is unclear, it may interfere with nuclear metabolism [48, 49].

A. **Pharmacokinetic data** are limited [6, 48, 49].

1. **Excretion** is primarily nonrenal. However, after cessation of parenteral therapy, patients continue to excrete decreasing amounts of pentamidine in urine for up to 6–8 weeks.

2. Pentamidine slowly accumulates in **tissue,** with the highest **concentrations** in the liver, spleen, and kidney. The amount of pentamidine that accumulates in the lungs is a small fraction (approximately 10%) of the amount measurable in other visceral organs in humans.

3. **Aerosol administration** delivers pentamidine to the target organ (i.e., the lungs) while limiting potentially toxic concentrations in other visceral organs. Pentamidine is retained in the lungs for many weeks after a single aerosol dose. The therapeutic implications of these observations are discussed in pages 906–907, 911.

B. **Dosage in renal failure.** Some studies suggest that a dose modification is necessary in moderate to severe renal insufficiency [70–72], whereas one study suggested that dose modification in renal failure may not be necessary [73]. The 1996 *Physicians' Desk Reference* does not address dose modification of pentamidine in renal failure [49].

1. **Dose modification.** In 1987, Conte and coworkers [70] reported that in patients with a creatinine clearance of 35 ml/min or more, no dosage adjustments are necessary [70]. Standard published tables on dosages in renal failure for antimicrobial agents [71, 72] suggested dose modifications in renal failure. Using these data, some clinicians have given intravenous pentamidine as follows:

   a. When the creatinine clearance is 35 ml/min or more, the standard dose is given q24h.

   b. When the creatinine clearance is 10–35 ml/min, a standard dose q24–36h is suggested.

   c. When the creatinine clearance is 10 ml/min or less, a standard dose q48h is suggested.

   d. **Dialysis.** No supplemental dose is suggested after hemodialysis or chronic ambulatory dialysis [72].

2. **No dose modification. In a 1991 report,** Conte [73] concludes that **dose reduction for renal impairment is not necessary,** even if the patient is undergoing hemodialysis, because little pentamidine is excreted by the kidney normally. Renal clearance accounts for a small fraction (2.1%) of plasma clearance [73]. In addition, renal excretion increased only marginally with repeated dosing in this study.

The effect of hepatic metabolism on the kinetics of intravenous pentamidine is unknown [73]. The true half-life of pentamidine is difficult to measure accurately, and plasma and tissue concentrations persist long after the last dose is administered. The plasma and tissue concentrations of pentamidine associated with toxicity are unknown [73].

3. **Although a dose modification may not be necessary in terms of plasma concentrations of pentamidine, a prudent approach may be to use the lower dose range of pentamidine (i.e., 3 mg/kg/dose) when the intravenous drug is used in patients with severe renal failure, possibly to reduce the risk of added nephrotoxicity.**

C. **Toxicity.** Toxicity is common **with parenteral pentamidine** therapy [41, 48, 49, 74].

1. **Dysglycemia** can occur. **Hypoglycemia** can be severe (< 25 mg/dl) in 2.0–2.5% of recipients and can be seen to a lesser extent in 20% [41]. This can occur after a single dose, especially if the infusion is too rapid. Hypoglycemia is more common in patients with renal dysfunction or those who receive a higher total dose [6]. **Hyperglycemia,** attributable to a direct cytolytic effect of the drug on pancreatic beta cells, can be irreversible and require insulin [74].

2. **Nephrotoxicity** with serum creatinine elevation in the 2.4- to 6.0-mg/dl range is common (23%), whereas severe acute renal failure (serum creatinine > 6 mg/dl) occurs in fewer than 0.5% of recipients [49]. **Because of the potential added nephrotoxicity if both intravenous pentamidine and intravenous amphotericin B are indicated, an alternative agent for one of these two drugs is indicated.**

3. **Hematologic** effects occur. **Neutropenia** ($< 1,000$ cells/mm^3) requiring discontinuation of therapy has been reported in 7% of recipients. More commonly, leukopenia and **thrombocytopenia** are mild and reversible; anemia, likewise, has been reported [7, 74].

4. **Hypotension** may be severe (systolic blood pressure < 60 mm Hg in 1–5% of patients); mild hypotension is seen in approximately 4%, as noted in the package insert. **If the intravenous infusion is given slowly over 60–120 minutes, hypotension can usually be avoided.**

5. **Sterile abscesses,** pain, or induration at the site of the intramuscular injection is seen in approximately 10% of patients. Intramuscular use is discouraged for therapeutic regimens but has been investigated for prophylaxis [30].

6. **Other side effects** include modest elevation of liver function tests in 8% or so of patients, nausea or anorexia in approximately 6%, rashes (which may respond to antihistamines or epinephrine), and urticaria eruption; rarely, Stevens-Johnson syndrome, facial flushing, dysgeusia, phlebitis, confusion, cardiac arrhythmias, hypocalcemia, and hypomagnesemia may occur [74, 75].

D. **Use in pregnancy.** The package insert indicates that animal reproduction studies have not been conducted with pentamidine and that it is not known whether pentamidine can cause fetal harm when it is administered to a pregnant woman. Therefore, the package insert suggests that pentamidine should be given to a pregnant woman only if clearly needed [48, 49].

E. **Special issues associated with the use of aerosolized pentamidine**

1. See discussion of aerosolized pentamidine in the prevention of PCP in sec. **I.C.3** and therapy for PCP in sec. **III.C.7** under Basic Principles.

2. **Effect on diagnostic tests and presentation of PCP.** With further experience using aerosolized pentamidine, the following observations have been reported:

   a. **Atypical roentgenographic findings** may be present. Usually PCP presents with rather typical diffuse bilateral interstitial infiltrates. In patients who have received prophylactic aerosolized pentamidine, **upper-lobe infiltrates are more common,** often appearing in more than one-third of relapsing patients [33–35, 76]. It is speculated that drug delivery is less efficient to this region, accounting for the disparate radiographic findings. This explanation may be incomplete, however, as higher semiquantitative rates of organism recovery have been detected in the upper lobes of PCP patients who did not receive aerosolized pentamidine prophylaxis or therapy [77].

   b. **Bronchoalveolar lavage for identification of *P. carinii* in recipients of aerosolized pentamidine** remains a sensitive mechanism for diagnosis if site-directed (corresponding to the area of greatest radiographic abnormality) or upper-lobe lavage is conducted [33–35], with the diagnostic yield exceeding 95%. These findings refute those of earlier reports.

     c. Transbronchial biopsies, which expose the PCP patient to a greater risk of pneumothorax and pulmonary hemorrhage, are largely unnecessary to verify the diagnosis [33–35].

   3. Disseminated *P. carinii* infection in patients receiving aerosolized pentamidine. In the past, *P. carinii* infection beyond the lung rarely was described. However, more recently, case reports of disseminated *P. carinii* infection (with liver, lymph node, spleen, bone marrow, heart, pancreas, kidney, and other organ involvement at autopsy) have appeared, especially in patients who have received aerosolized pentamidine. Aerosolized pentamidine provides excellent lung tissue concentration but inadequate tissue concentration levels elsewhere. In these cases, presumably the aerosolized pentamidine suppresses intraalveolar infection but not extrapulmonary infection due to *P. carinii*. **Therefore, clinicians should be aware of the possibility of disseminated *P. carinii* in patients receiving chronic aerosolized pentamidine therapy,** particularly in unusual patient settings such as unexplained worsening liver function abnormalities, hypoalbuminemia, or unexplained embolic disease [1, 78].

   4. Cost issues. For preventive therapy, aerosolized pentamidine is about 20-fold more expensive than daily TMP-SMX or dapsone [23, 79, 80].

III. Dapsone (diaminodiphenylsulfone, DDS) is a synthetic sulfone antiinfective that has been a drug of choice for the treatment of leprosy [81]. In HIV-infected patients, dapsone and trimethoprim have been used in the treatment of PCP [2, 3, 19, 46], and dapsone has been used alone as prophylaxis to prevent PCP [1, 79]. See discussions in secs. I.C.2, II.D.2, and III.B.2, under Basic Principles.

  A. Mechanism of action. Dapsone probably has a mechanism of action similar to that of sulfonamides, which involves inhibition of folic acid synthesis in susceptible organisms. Dapsone is usually **static** in action [81].

  B. Spectrum of activity. Dapsone is active in vitro against *M. leprae, M. tuberculosis,* and other species of *Mycobacterium.* In vivo dapsone is active against *P. carinii, Plasmodium* spp., and *T. gondii* [1, 81].

  C. Pharmacokinetics. Only an oral preparation (tablet) is available currently. (A liquid preparation is undergoing clinical investigation.)

   1. Absorption. After oral administration, dapsone is absorbed slowly, with the maximum concentration in plasma reached at approximately 4 hours [82].

   2. Distribution. Dapsone is distributed into most body tissues, including sputum, liver, bile, and kidneys, but probably has limited penetration into ocular tissue [81]. Dapsone crosses the placenta and is excreted in breast milk [82]. The drug is highly bound to plasma proteins (70–90%) [81].

   3. Metabolism and excretion. The elimination half-life varies in individuals but averages 20–30 hours [6, 81, 82].

    a. In humans, approximately half the dose of dapsone is **acetylated** in the liver to monoacetyldapsone. The remainder undergoes *N*-hydroxylation to hydroxylamine dapsone (NOH-DDS), which appears to be responsible for methemoglobinemia and hemolysis induced by dapsone [6, 81].

    b. An **enterohepatic circulation** occurs. This is supported by the fact that orally administered charcoal substantially enhances the elimination of dapsone. This approach has been used in the treatment of acute overdoses of dapsone [81, 82].

    c. Approximately 20% of each dose of dapsone is excreted in urine as unchanged drug, 70–85% is excreted in urine as water-soluble metabolites, and a small amount is excreted in feces [81].

    d. Hemodialysis also reportedly enhances the elimination of dapsone [81].

  D. Clinical uses

   1. Leprosy. A discussion of dapsone in the treatment of leprosy is beyond the scope of this book. This topic is summarized elsewhere [81].

   2. Therapy for PCP in patients with AIDS. In 1990, Medina and associates [46] reported that **TMP-dapsone therapy for mild to moderate PCP was as effective as conventional TMP-SMX** and was associated with fewer side effects than TMP alone. This study, including dosage regimens, is reviewed on page 913. Monotherapy with dapsone is not effective treatment for PCP [47].

   3. Prevention of recurrent episodes of PCP. Dapsone is being used increasingly in the prevention of PCP in HIV-infected individuals [5, 10, 24, 24a]. Because of the frequency of sulfonamide allergies (which preclude the use of TMP-SMX), the concerns about the use of aerosolized pentamidine, the low cost and ease of administration of dapsone, and the possible protective effects when combined with pyrimethamine against *T. gondii,* **dapsone is an appealing alternative for use in PCP prophylaxis.**

Although there is no package insert indication for this use, daily dapsone is used in the prevention of PCP in HIV-infected patients [1, 19, 79]. This is discussed in detail in sec. I.C.2 under Basic Principles.

    a. **G-6-PD screen.** Before dapsone therapy is initiated, the patient is screened for G-6-PD deficiency and renal function.

    b. **Dosages. The optimal dosage regimen** for PCP prevention **still is being evaluated.**

        (1) **Adults.** Recent data favor 100 mg/day (e.g., 50 mg bid) as discussed on pages 905–906. When lower doses are used (50 mg/day) failure to prevent PCP is more likely to occur [21a]. Some authors suggest initiation of therapy in a stepwise fashion, starting with 25 mg PO once daily and increasing the dose weekly by 25 mg/day to a final dose of 25 mg q6h [83]. In general, the dose of dapsone has been reduced in recent trials when combined with a second antifolate agent [6, 24a].

        (2) **Children.** See Table 24-2 for the dosage used to achieve serum levels similar to those in adults.

    c. If dapsone is used to prevent PCP, the potential side effects (see sec. I) and routine monitoring (see sec. J) should be followed.

E. **Dosage in renal failure.** Guidelines for dose reduction are not available (see sec. C). Hemodialysis will remove dapsone. In moderately severe renal failure, monitoring serum levels would be useful; alternatively, carefully assess the patient serially for hematologic toxicity (see sec. I) as an indirect measurement of accumulating dapsone levels. In mild renal failure, for PCP prophylaxis, it may be prudent to avoid doses in excess of 50 mg/day while awaiting better guidelines.

F. **Contraindications or special precautions**

    1. **Pregnancy.** Although dapsone has been used in pregnant women without producing fetal abnormality, the drug should be used only when clearly indicated. It is a category C agent (see Chap. 28A) [23].

    2. **Dapsone should not be used in nursing women.**

    3. **Hypersensitivity.** Dapsone is contraindicated in patients who are hypersensitive to the drug.

G. **Use in patients with prior reactions to TMP-SMX.** Patients who cannot tolerate TMP-SMX often are able to take dapsone, as illustrated by a clinical trial in which almost half the patients intolerant of TMP-SMX due to toxicity were crossed over successfully and tolerated prophylaxis with dapsone [24]. Furthermore, in a preliminary report, more than 80% of HIV-positive patients intolerant of TMP-SMX were able to tolerate dapsone for PCP prophylaxis [83a].

H. **Drug interactions** (in nonleprosy therapy)

    1. **Rifampin** decreases serum dapsone concentrations by inducing liver enzymes. The exact significance of this interaction is unclear, and generally dosage modification of dapsone is not currently recommended [81, 82] when both drugs are being used.

    2. **Folic acid antagonists** (e.g., **pyrimethamine**) may increase the likelihood of hematologic reactions. If pyrimethamine is used concomitantly with dapsone, the patient should be monitored more frequently than usual for adverse hematologic effects.

    3. **Trimethoprim** and dapsone exhibit a bidirectional drug interaction, resulting in higher concentrations of each in the presence of the other, possibly secondary to an inhibition of or competition with renal secretion of these drugs [74]. This interaction is believed to be responsible for the higher incidence of hyperkalemia seen with TMP-dapsone therapy, as compared to TMP-SMX, due to TMP's inhibition of potassium secretion [45].

    4. **Didanosine** (ddI) may interfere with dapsone's efficacy. Failure of PCP prophylaxis with dapsone has been reported in a significant proportion of patients concurrently taking didanosine [81, 84]. Although pharmacokinetic studies are not yet available, the most likely mechanism for this failure is the presence of the citrate-phosphate buffer system contained in didanosine that is necessary to facilitate the antiretroviral agent's absorption. Dapsone requires an acidic environment for absorption, so it is **recommended that dapsone be administered 2 hours before or after the buffered didanosine.** Similar interference with absorption due to the neutralization of gastric acidity by the didanosine buffer system is seen with ketoconazole [81, 84].

I. **Side effects.** The most frequent adverse side effects of dapsone are dose-related hemolytic anemia and methemoglobinemia [81]. These effects occur in all patients on dapsone but usually are so mild that they go unnoticed. These effects are **dose-dependent,** but some individuals are more susceptible because of enzyme deficiencies or hemoglobinopathies [82]. Unless severe, methemoglobinemia or hemolysis does not generally require treatment or discontinuation of dapsone therapy [46].

1. **Methemoglobinemia** formation is caused by the NOH metabolite of dapsone (see sec. **C**). In normal individuals, methemoglobin is formed continuously under physiologic conditions in very low amounts and is reduced again by NADH-dependent methemoglobin reductase [82]. Methemoglobinemia describes that clinical state in which more than 1% of the hemoglobin of the blood has been oxidized to the ferric form [85]. Methemoglobinemia decreases the oxygen capacity of blood, because the oxidized iron cannot reversibly bind oxygen.

   a. After dapsone administration and subsequent formation of NOH metabolites, more methemoglobin is formed, and its percentage rises.

   b. **Excessive methemoglobinemia may cause cyanosis,** tiredness, dyspnea, tachycardia, headache, dizziness, nausea, mild jaundice [82], or the symptoms of an associated anemia. Methemoglobinemia may be poorly tolerated by patients with severe cardiopulmonary disease, preexisting hypoxemia, or anemia [81].

   c. **Severe cases** of methemoglobinemia (concentrations $\geq 20\%$) can be treated with intravenous methylene blue, 1 mg/kg given by slow intravenous infusion. Alternatively, in nonemergent situations, methylene blue can be given orally at 3–5 mg/kg q4–6h [81]. Methylene blue enhances the reduction of methemoglobin by activating a second, NADPH-dependent methemoglobin reductase [82].

      Methemoglobinemia may be life-threatening when the level of the pigment exceeds half the total hemoglobin [85]. **Methylene blue should not be administered to patients with G-6-PD deficiency,** as methylene blue reductase depends on G-6-PD. **Fortunately, with G-6-PD deficiency subjects are less susceptible to methemoglobin formation.**

      Orally administered charcoal (20 g qid) **has been shown to enhance the elimination of dapsone substantially** (see sec. **C.3.b**), and some clinicians recommend it as the treatment of choice for managing acute dapsone intoxications. Hemodialysis also enhances the elimination of dapsone.

2. **Hemolysis** with Heinz-body formation is the second most important hematologic side effect. The life span of the erythrocytes is reduced in all subjects taking dapsone [82].

   a. **Individuals with G-6-PD deficiency or diminished activity of glutathione reductase are more prone to this adverse effect** [82]. Hemoglobinopathy M patients are also at risk [81]. These are patients who have methemoglobinemias due to the inheritance of an abnormality in the structure of the globin portion of the hemoglobin molecule, known as *hemoglobin M disease* [85].

   b. Short-term studies suggest that **daily dapsone doses of 100 mg or less in normal healthy persons and 50 mg or less in healthy G-6-PD-deficient persons will not produce clinically important hemolysis** [82, 86]. Hemolysis occurs in most patients receiving 200 mg or more of dapsone daily [81, 86]. **Hemolysis appears to be dose-related, and this may explain why patients may tolerate a 4-times-daily dose regimen rather than a higher, single-dose-per-day regimen.**

   c. The A⁻ type of G-6-PD deficiency is the most common variant in the American black population, with an incidence rate among black men of approximately 11% [87]. In this type of G-6-PD deficiency, the drug-induced hemolytic anemia is self-limited because the young red cells produced in response to hemolysis have near-normal G-6-PD levels and are relatively resistant to hemolysis [87]. In contrast, patients with homozygous B⁻ G-6-PD deficiency may have such severe hemolysis if exposed to dapsone that the drug should be avoided in these patients. (See sec. **D.3.b.(1)** regarding careful initiation of drug therapy.)

   d. Primaquine has a greater hemolytic effect in G-6-PD-deficient persons but causes less hemolysis in normal individuals than does dapsone [41].

3. Miscellaneous side effects

a. **"Sulfone syndrome"** is a severe dapsone hypersensitivity reaction that has been reported sporadically in the literature and has been reviewed [88]. In general, this syndrome includes **fever,** maculopapular **rash,** and hepatic injury (hepatomegaly, jaundice, or hyperbilirubinemia), typically occurring within 2 months of the patient's starting dapsone. Hemolysis can occur, and the syndrome can be seen in patients with normal G-6-PD activity [88]. Because dapsone is being used more frequently as alternative therapy to prevent PCP in AIDS patients, this syndrome may become more common [88]. For those patients with fever and rash after dapsone therapy, a desensitization protocol has been proposed [83].

b. Occasionally, **leukopenia** and, rarely, agranulocytosis have been reported.

c. **Gastrointestinal intolerance** occurs with anorexia, with occasional nausea and vomiting [24, 81].

d. Mild **hepatitis and cholestatic jaundice** have been reported.

e. **Hyperkalemia** may occur. Plasma TMP concentrations have been detected to be 49% higher in patients receiving TMP-dapsone, compared to those receiving TMP-SMX, probably because of the positive bidirectional interaction between dapsone and TMP [45, 74]. Trimethoprim increases serum potassium via amiloridelike blockage of sodium channels in the distal nephron, which in turn impairs the transepithelial voltage gradient responsible for maintaining potassium secretion. Furthermore, AIDS patients may be at greater risk for developing hyperkalemia due to coexistent, but clinically asymptomatic, impairment of aldosterone secretion [45, 89].

J. Monitoring patients receiving dapsone

1. **Complete blood cell counts** should be performed weekly during the first month of therapy and then at least monthly. If patients are also receiving folic acid antagonists, even more frequent CBCs may be indicated (see sec. **H.2**).

2. **A screening test for G-6-PD deficiency should be done before initiation of dapsone therapy.** Dapsone should be administered with caution, if at all, to patients with this deficiency, and a reduced dose is suggested—for example, for prevention of PCP, 50 mg/day instead of 100 mg/day. Initially, in PCP prevention, regimens could start with 25 mg/day to ensure that the patient can tolerate the drug, and then the dose could be increased to 25 mg bid (see sec. **D.3**).

3. **A methemoglobin level should be obtained if symptoms of methemoglobinemia occur** (see sec. **I**). Generally, following methemoglobin levels is not suggested in asymptomatic patients who are undergoing routine serial blood counts. In one study [46], asymptomatic mild elevations of methemoglobin commonly occurred, but in only 1 of 30 patients was the level high enough (i.e., > 20%) to merit discontinuation of therapy.

4. **Mild hyperkalemia** can occur in patients on TMP-dapsone therapy [46]. Therefore, in patients who may be at risk for this complication, serial serum potassium levels are a consideration.

5. **Hepatic dysfunction.** Because hepatitis and cholestatic jaundice have been described early in dapsone therapy, **baseline and serial liver function tests are suggested.** Patients should be advised of possible symptoms of hepatitis, and liver function tests should be performed if these symptoms occur.

6. **Rashes.** Usually, therapy with dapsone can be continued in the presence of diffuse maculopapular rash. However, if the rash is subjectively intolerable or if there is desquamation or involvement of the mucous membranes, the drug should be stopped [46]. (See sec. **I.3**.)

K. **Cost.** Dapsone (100 mg/day) costs about the same as TMP-SMX (1 DS tablet per day) which is about $5 per month [23].

L. **Summary.** Dapsone, along with TMP, has emerged as a useful agent in the treatment of mild to moderate PCP and in prevention of PCP. Future dosage recommendations may be modified as we learn more about dose regimens that may reduce side effects but maintain clinical efficacy.

IV. **Trimetrexate (TMTX, NeuTrexin)** was discussed briefly in sec. **III.D.3** under Basic Principles [2, 19]. This drug **recently was approved by the FDA as an alternative agent in the treatment of moderately severe PCP in AIDS patients who are intolerant of, or refractory to, TMP-SMX therapy or in whom TMP-SMX is contraindicated. Trimetrexate must be given with leucovorin to avoid serious toxicity.** See earlier discussion on pages 915–916.

A. **Availability**
   1. **For adults.** Trimetrexate with leucovorin is commercially available for adult use from pharmaceutical wholesalers under the trade name NeuTrexin.
   2. **For infants and children infected with HIV.** The safety and efficacy of trimetrexate for the treatment of PCP in patients younger than 18 years has not been established. The use of trimetrexate in infants has been reviewed [90]. For additional experience and/or information of trimetrexate's use in children, the medical information number of U.S. Bioscience can be consulted (1-800-872-4672).
B. **Pharmacokinetics.** Structurally, trimetrexate resembles methotrexate, but its greater lipid solubility allows for better penetration into pneumocystic cells, which lack the folate membrane transport system necessary to take up classic folate structures such as leucovorin, thereby allowing leucovorin to be used for host cell protection [57, 91]. The terminal half-life is approximately 12 hours [57]. Trimetrexate is cleared hepatically and renally, with up to 41% excreted unchanged in the urine [57].
C. **Standard dose.** The package insert indicates the dosage regimen for trimetrexate is 45 mg/m² once daily by intravenous infusion over 60–90 minutes for 21 days and, for leucovorin (folinic acid), the dose is 20 mg/m² PO or IV (over 5–10 minutes) q6h [19, 92] for 24 days (total daily dose: 80 mg/m²). The leucovorin (5-formyl tetrahydrofolate) protects the mammalian cells from the cytotoxic effects of trimetrexate without compromising the antiprotozoan effect of the drug [92].

   Leucovorin should be given in the proper dosage and schedule for 3 full days after cessation of trimetrexate therapy. **If folinic acid (leucovorin) is not given** in the proper dosage and schedule for the duration of trimetrexate therapy and for 3 days after completion of trimetrexate therapy, **lethal toxicity can occur.** (The oral dose should be rounded up to the next higher 25-mg increment per the package insert.)
D. **Dosage modifications** in different settings (per package insert)
   1. **Hematologic toxicity.** Trimetrexate and leucovorin doses should be modified based on the worst hematologic toxicity, according to Table 24-3. If leucovorin is given orally, doses should be rounded up to the next higher 25-mg increment.
   2. **Hepatic toxicity.** Transient elevations of transaminases and alkaline phosphatase have been observed in patients treated with trimetrexate. Interruption of treatment is advisable if transaminase levels or alkaline phosphatase levels increase to more than 5 times the upper limit of normal range.
   3. **Renal toxicity.** Interruption of trimetrexate therapy is advisable if serum creatinine levels increase to more than 2.5 mg/dl and the elevation is considered to be secondary to trimetrexate.

Table 24-3. Dose modifications of trimetrexate for hematologic toxicity

Toxicity grade	Neutrophils (polys and bands)	Platelets	Recommended dosages	
			NeuTrexin	Leucovorin
1	>1,000/mm³	>75,000/mm³	45 mg/m² once daily	20 mg/m² q6h
2	750–1,000/mm³	50,000–75,000/mm³	45 mg/m² once daily	40 mg/m² q6h
3	500–749/mm³	25,000–49,999/mm³	22 mg/m² once daily	40 mg/m² q6h
4	<500/mm³	<25,000/mm³	Day 1–9: Discontinue Day 10–21: Interrupt up to 96 hours*	40 mg/m² q6h

*If grade 4 hematologic toxicity occurs prior to day 10, NeuTrexin should be discontinued. Leucovorin (40 mg/m² q6h) should be administered for an additional 72 hours. If grade 4 hematologic toxicity occurs at day 10 or later, NeuTrexin may be held up to 96 hours to allow counts to recover. If counts recover to grade 3 within 96 hours, NeuTrexin should be administered at a dose of 22 mg/m² and leucovorin maintained at 40 mg/m² q6h. When counts recover to grade 2 toxicity, the NeuTrexin dose may be increased to 45 mg/m², but the leucovorin dose should be maintained at 40 mg/m² for the duration of treatment. If counts do not improve to ≤ grade 3 toxicity within 96 hours, NeuTrexin should be discontinued. Leucovorin at a dose of 40 mg/m² q6h should be administered for 72 hours following the last dose of NeuTrexin.
Source: *Physicians Desk Reference* (50th ed.) Montvale, NJ: Medical Economics Data, 1996. P. 2575.

4. **Other toxicities.** Interruption of treatment is advisable in patients who experience severe mucosal toxicity that interferes with oral intake. Treatment should be discontinued for fever (oral temperature ≥ 105°F [40.5°C] that cannot be controlled with antipyretics.

5. **Pregnancy.** Trimetrexate can cause fetal harm when administered to a pregnant woman (category D, see Chap. 28A). **Trimetrexate should therefore be avoided in pregnant women,** and women of childbearing age should be advised to avoid becoming pregnant if they receive this drug.

6. **Nursing mothers.** It is not known whether trimetrexate is excreted into human milk. The package insert suggests that breast-feeding be discontinued if the mother is treated with this drug.

E. **Adverse reactions.** Most patients who participated in the clinical trials of trimetrexate had complications of advanced HIV disease, making it difficult to distinguish true adverse reactions to this drug from events secondary to the patients' underlying disease or other medications. In this setting, the package insert emphasizes the following possible adverse outcomes:

1. **Hematologic toxicity** with neutropenia ($< 1,000/mm^3$) in 30.3%, thrombocytopenia ($< 75,000/mm^3$) in 10.1%, and anemia (hemoglobin < 8 g/dl) in 7.3%, per package insert. (**Note:** These percentages are similar to the side effect profile of AIDS patients treated with TMP-SMX.)

   Because myelosuppression can occur, it may be prudent to discontinue other myelosuppressive agents (e.g., zidovudine) [57]. Serial CBC should be monitored.

2. **Hepatotoxicity.** Increases in serum transaminases (> 5 times normal) occur in 11–13%, increase in alkaline phosphatase (> 5 times normal) in 4.6%, and hyperbilirubinemia (≥ 2.5 times normal) in 1.8%, per package insert. (**N.B.:** Again, these % are similar to TMP-SMX recipients in AIDS populations.)

3. **Nephrotoxicity** with a serum creatinine rise in excess of 3 times normal was seen in 0.9% of recipients.

4. **Miscellaneous**
   a. Fever (8.3%), rash or pruritus (5.5%), nausea or vomiting (4.6%), confusion (2.8%), and fatigue (1.8%) have been reported.
   b. Hyponatremia (4.6%) and hypocalcemia (1.8%) have been documented.

V. **Atovaquone** (Mepron, BW566C80) was approved in 1992 for **oral treatment of mild to moderate PCP** in patients who are intolerant of TMP-SMX [52, 53, 93]. (See also sec. **III.C.6** under Basic Principles.)

A. **Mechanism of action.** Atovaquone apparently interferes with mitochondrial electron transfer in *P. carinii,* ultimately interrupting pyrimidine synthesis. It is believed that this novel mechanism of action, in contrast to folate antagonism, may have a microbicidal, rather than microbiostatic, effect on *P. carinii* [93]. This agent also is active against *Plasmodium falciparum* and *T. gondii* [93].

B. **Pharmacokinetics.** As of late 1995, only an oral suspension is available (750 mg/ 5 ml).

1. **Bioavailability is increased** approximately two- to threefold when administered **with meals.** In particular, the package insert emphasizes that fat has been shown to enhance absorption [53]. The package insert indicates that the suspension formulation provides approximately a twofold increase in bioavailability of atovaquone compared with the prior tablets.

2. **Half-life.** Atovaquone has a long half-life (2.2 ± 0.6 days) in AIDS patients, presumably due to its enterohepatic cycling and eventual fecal elimination. No metabolism of atovaquone appears to take place, alleviating the need for dosage adjustments in patients with renal or hepatic impairment [93].

C. **Indications.** Atovaquone is indicated as an alternative agent for treatment of mild to moderate PCP. A recent trial demonstrated that atovaquone is better tolerated but has lesser efficacy when compared to TMP-SMX [52]. In another study, the drug had similar overall efficacy to intravenous pentamidine [52a]. In addition, atovaquone is undergoing clinical evaluation for its role in the prevention of PCP and treatment of severe PCP, as well as its possible use in the treatment of toxoplasmosis in AIDS patients [94].

D. **Dosages**
1. **Adults.** The oral dose used initially was three 250-mg tablets (750 mg) administered **with food** three times daily for 21 days. More recently, the oral suspension is preferred and 750 mg twice daily for 21 days is suggested [19, 40]. The oral tablets are no longer manufactured since the oral suspension is better absorbed

and requires only twice-daily dosing. Failure to administer atovaquone with food may result in lower plasma concentrations and therapeutic failures [52, 53, 93].

   2. Pediatric use. As of early 1996 there are no efficacy studies in children.
   3. Pregnancy. There are no well-controlled studies of atovaquone in pregnant women. Therefore the package insert emphasizes that atovaquone should be used in pregnancy only if the potential benefit justifies the potential risk to the fetus. (It is a category C drug. See Chap. 28A.)
   4. Nursing mothers. Because it is not known whether atovaquone is excreted into human milk, caution should be exercised when atovaquone is administered to nursing women.
E. Adverse reactions. Relatively speaking, this agent has been used in only a small number of patients. Its exact safety profile will be determined by further experience with this agent. The following side effects are summarized in the package insert based on patients receiving atovaquone: rash, nausea and vomiting, diarrhea, headaches, fever, insomnia, asthenia, pruritus, abdominal pain, constipation, dizziness, anemia, neutropenia, elevated liver function tests, and hyponatremia.
F. Cost. The cost of a 3-week therapeutic course of the oral suspension of atovaquone for PCP is about $325 (manufacturer's wholesale price).
G. Summary. Atovaquone offers another oral, nonsulfonamide regimen for mild to moderate PCP in patients who cannot tolerate other regimens. Further clinical experience with this agent will better define its clinical role and safety profile.

References

1. Centers for Disease Control. USPHS/IDSA Guidelines for the prevention of opportunistic infections in persons infected with human immunodeficiency virus: A summary. *M.M.W.R.* 44(RR-8):1–34, 1995.
   For a more detailed discussion of these guidelines, see tables and text in Chap. 19 and reference [1a].
1a. USPHS/IDSA Prevention of Opportunistic Infections Working Group. USPHS/IDSA guidelines for the prevention of opportunistic infections in persons infected with human immunodeficiency virus: Disease-specific recommendations. *Clin. Infect. Dis.* 21(Suppl. 1):S32, 1995.
   See preceding two summary articles in this same symposium supplement and reference [23].
1b. Simonds, R.J., et al. Preventing *Pneumocystis carinii* pneumonia in persons infected with human immunodeficiency virus. *Clin. Infect. Dis.* 21(Suppl. 1):S44, 1995.
2. Sattler, F.R., and Feinburg, J. New developments in the treatment of *Pneumocystis carinii* pneumonia. *Chest* 101:451, 1992.
3. Moe, A.A., and Hardy, W.D. *Pneumocystis carinii* infection in the HIV-seropositive patient. *Infect. Dis. Clin. North Am.* 8:331, 1994.
4. Leoung, G.S., and Hopewell, P.C. In P.T. Cohen, M.A. Sande, and P.A. Volberding (eds.), *The AIDS Knowledge Base: A Textbook on HIV Disease* (2nd ed.). Boston: Little, Brown, 1994.
   Contains a series of chapters on PCP by these authors.
5. Hopewell, P.C., and Masur, H. *Pneumocystis carinii* Pneumonia: Current Concepts. In M.A. Sande and P.A. Volberding (eds.), *The Medical Management of AIDS* (4th ed.). Philadelphia: Saunders, 1995.
   An excellent resource. Serially revised.
6. Voehringer, H.F., and Keikawus, A. Pharmacokinetic optimisation in the treatment of *Pneumocystis carinii* pneumonia. *Clin. Pharmacokinet.* 24:388, 1993.
7. Viner, B.L. Pneumocystis Pneumonia. In H. Libman and R.A. Witzburg (eds.), *HIV Infection: A Primary Care Manual* (3rd ed.). Boston: Little, Brown, 1996.
8. Masur, H. Prevention and treatment of pneumocystis pneumonia. *N. Engl. J. Med.* 327:1853, 1992.
9. Kovacs, J.A., and Masur, H. Prophylaxis for *Pneumocystis carinii* pneumonia in patients infected with human immunodeficiency virus. *Clin. Infect. Dis.* 14:1005, 1992.
   Good discussion from experts from the National Institutes of Health.
10. Hecht, F.M., and Solway, B. Changing approaches to prophylaxis for *Pneumocystis carinii* pneumonia. *AIDS Clin. Care* 4:61, 1992.

11. Hoover, D.R., et al. Clinical manifestations of AIDS in the era of Pneumocystis prophylaxis. *N. Engl. J. Med.* 329:1922, 1993.
    This analysis from the Multicenter AIDS Cohort Study revealed that approximately 28% of HIV-infected patients receiving PCP prophylaxis developed PCP over roughly 5 years. During this time, the percentage of patients presenting with PCP as their AIDS-defining illness dropped from 57% in 1986 to 25% in 1991. Compared to patients not taking PCP prophylaxis, those receiving prophylaxis had significantly lower CD4 cell counts at the time of their AIDS diagnosis, and they presented with four diseases significantly more often: Mycobacterium avium *complex infection, cytomegalovirus, wasting syndrome, and esophageal candidiasis. For related papers further discussing the impact of prophylaxis, see R.M. Selik et al., Trends in infectious diseases and cancers among persons dying of HIV infection in the United States from 1987 to 1992.* Ann. Intern. Med. *123:933, 1995; R.D. Moore, R.E. Chaisson, Natural history of opportunistic disease in an HIV-infected urban clinical cohort.* Ann. Intern. Med. *124:633, 1996.*

12. Centers for Disease Control. 1995 revised guidelines for prophylaxis against *Pneumocystis carinii* pneumonia for children infected with or perinatally exposed to human immunodeficiency virus. *M.M.W.R.* 44(RR-4):1–11, 1995.
    In March 1994, the National Pediatric and Family HIV Resource Center, in collaboration with the CDC, convened to review new information on PCP prevention in children and revise the 1991 guidelines. This report summarizes their recommendations.
    See related papers by S. Grubman and R.J. Simonds, Preventing Pneumocystis carinii *pneumonia in human immunodeficiency virus–infected children: New guidelines for prophylaxis.* Pediatr. Infect. Dis. J. *15:165, 1996; and D.M. Thea et al., Benefit of primary prophylaxis before 18 months of age in reducing the incidence of* Pneumocystis carinii *and early death in a cohort of 112 human immunodeficiency virus infected infants.* Pediatrics *97:59, 1996.*

13. Casale, L., et al. Decreased efficacy of inhaled pentamidine in the prevention of *Pneumocystis carinii* pneumonia among HIV-infected patients with severe immunodeficiency. *Chest* 103:342, 1993.

14. Veugelers, P.J., et al. Recommendations for prophylaxis against *Pneumocystis carinii* pneumonia. *Lancet* 341:758, 1993.

15. Fischl, M.A., et al. Safety and efficacy of sulfamethoxazole and trimethoprim chemoprophylaxis for *Pneumocystis carinii* pneumonia. *J.A.M.A.* 259:1185, 1988.

16. Hardy, W.D., et al. A controlled trial of trimethoprim-sulfamethoxazole or aerosolized pentamidine for secondary prophylaxis of *Pneumocystis carinii* pneumonia in patients with the acquired immunodeficiency syndrome. *N. Engl. J. Med.* 327:1842, 1992.
    TMP-SMX was significantly more effective (11.4% of TMP-SMX recipients had recurrent PCP at 18 months) than pentamidine (27.6% with recurrent PCP).

17. Schneider, M.M.E., et al. A controlled trial of aerosolized pentamidine or trimethoprim-sulfamethoxazole as primary prophylaxis against *Pneumocystis carinii* pneumonia in patients with human immunodeficiency virus infection. *N. Engl. J. Med.* 327:1836, 1992.
    Aerosolized pentamidine (300 mg monthly) or TMP-SMX (either one single-strength or one double-strength tablet daily) for primary PCP prophylaxis was used.

18. Chaisson, R.E., et al. Pneumocystis prophylaxis and survival in patients with advanced human immunodeficiency virus infection treated with zidovudine. *Arch. Intern. Med.* 152:2009, 1992.

19. Medical Letter. Drugs for parasitic infections. *Med. Lett. Drugs Ther.* 37:99, 1995.
    See also related reference [40].

20. Ruskin, J., and LaRiviere, M. Low-dose co-trimoxazole for prevention of *Pneumocystis carinii* pneumonia in human immunodeficiency virus disease. *Lancet* 337:468, 1991.

21. Coker, R.J., et al. Co-trimoxazole versus dapsone-pyrimethamine for prevention of *Pneumocystis carinii* pneumonia. *Lancet* 340:1099, 1992.

21a. Bozzette, S.A., et al. A randomized trial of three antipneumocystis agents in patients with advanced human immunodeficiency virus infection. *N. Engl. J. Med.* 332:693, 1995.
    This is a report of the ACTG 081 trial. When the CD4 count was 100–200/mm³, TMP-SMX (1 DS tablet bid), dapsone (50 mg bid) and aerosolized pentamidine (300 mg q4wk via Respirgard II nebulizer) had similar efficacy in preventing primary PCP. For patients with CD4 counts < 100/mm³, aerosolized pentamidine was less effective in preventing PCP. Also, failures to prevent PCP were more common with 50 mg of dapsone than with 100 mg of dapsone daily. There was no difference in survival in this study. (See editorial comment in the same issue.)

22. Carr, A., et al. Low-dose trimethoprim-sulfamethoxazole prophylaxis for toxoplasmic encephalitis in patients with AIDS. *Ann. Intern. Med.* 117:106, 1992.
    Study concludes that low-dose TMP-SMX (one double-strength tablet bid given 2 days/ wk) appears to be effective prophylaxis against toxoplasmic encephalitis in HIV-infected patients with previous PCP. A prospective, randomized, controlled study is needed to evaluate these findings further. See editorial comment in the same issue.

22a. Hirschtick, R.E., et al. Bacterial pneumonia in persons infected with the human immunodeficiency virus. *N. Engl. J. Med.* 333:845, 1995.
    Prophylaxis with TMP-SMX was associated with a 67% reduction of confirmed episodes of bacterial pneumonia. Risk of pneumonia in HIV positive patients increases as CD4 counts are less than 200/mm³, especially in smokers.

22b. Gluckstein, D., and Ruskin, J. Rapid oral desensitization to trimethoprim-sulfamethoxazole (TMP-SMZ): Use in prophylaxis for *Pneumocystis carinii* pneumonia in patients with AIDS who were previously intolerant to TMP-SMZ. *Clin. Infect. Dis.* 20:849, 1995.
    See related papers: N. Absar et al., Desensitization to trimethoprim-sulfamethoxazole in HIV-infected patients. J. Allergy Clin. Immunol. 93:1001, 1994; A. Carr et al., Efficacy and safety of rechallenge with low-dose trimethoprim-sulfamethoxazole in previously hypersensitive HIV-infected patients. AIDS 7:63, 1993; M.T. Nguyen et al., Two-day oral desensitization to trimethoprim-sulfamethoxazole in HIV-infected patients. AIDS 9:573, 1995.

23. Kaplan, J.E., et al. USPHS/IDSA guidelines for the prevention of opportunistic infections in persons infected with human immunodeficiency virus: An overview. *Clin. Infect. Dis.* 21(Suppl. 1):S12, 1995.
    Contains a good cost table of prophylactic regimens used in AIDS patients, which is reproduced in Chap. 19 (see Table 19-8).

24. Blum, R.N., et al. Comparative trial of dapsone versus trimethoprim-sulfamethoxazole for primary prophylaxis of *Pneumocystis carinii* pneumonia. *J. Acquir. Immune Defic. Syndr.* 5:341, 1992.
    In this single-institution prospective trial of PCP prophylaxis, 47 patients were randomized to receive dapsone (100 mg/day), whereas 39 received TMP-SMX (one double-strength tablet daily). Over 18 months, 1 patient in each group developed PCP. Although most patients stopped therapy due to adverse effects (70% of patients on dapsone and 64% on TMP-SMX), approximately half of these patients successfully crossed over and tolerated their subsequent prophylactic regimen.

24a. Girard, R.M., et al. Dapsone-pyrimethamine compared with aerosolized pentamidine as primary prophylaxis against *Pneumocystis carinii* pneumonia and toxoplasmosis in HIV infection. *N. Engl. J. Med.* 328:1514, 1993.
    This prospective French trial of PCP prophylaxis randomized 176 patients to receive aerosolized pentamidine (300 mg/mo) and 173 to receive the combination regimen of dapsone (50 mg/day) and pyrimethamine (50 mg/wk). Equivalent rates of survival and the development of PCP (approximately 6% in each group) were detected at 539 days of follow-up. The dapsone-pyrimethamine combination was less well tolerated than aerosolized pentamidine, with 24% of patients discontinuing prophylaxis due to adverse effects, but its use was associated with a significantly reduced rate of cerebral toxoplasmosis (11% versus 18%).

25. Torres, R.A., et al. Randomized trial of dapsone and aerosolized pentamidine for the prophylaxis of *Pneumocystis carinii* pneumonia and toxoplasmic encephalitis. *Am. J. Med.* 95:573, 1993.
    Dapsone (100 mg twice weekly) or aerosolized pentamidine (100 mg every 2 weeks) was used. Dapsone was found to be as effective, less expensive, and easier to use, and had a preventive effect against toxoplasmosis.
    See related paper by M.A. Slavin et al., Oral dapsone versus nebulized pentamidine for Pneumocystis *prophylaxis. AIDS 6:1169, 1992. The authors favor dapsone as it had equivalent efficacy and low cost and was easier to administer. Fifty patients received dapsone (100 mg twice weekly) compared to 46 who received nebulized pentamidine (400 mg monthly).*

25a. Opravil, M., et al. Once-weekly administration of dapsone/pyrimethamine vs. aerosolized pentamidine as combined prophylaxis for *Pneumocystis carinii* pneumonia and toxoplasmic encephalitis in human immunodeficiency virus-infected patients. *Clin. Infect. Dis.* 20:531, 1995.
    Dapsone/pyrimethamine (200 mg/75 mg once weekly) was as effective as aerosolized pentamidine as prophylaxis for PCP and significantly reduced the incidence of toxo-

plasmic encephalitis among those participants who tolerated it. The combination was tolerated by 30% of participants.

26. Antinori, A., et al. Failure of low-dose dapsone-pyrimethamine in primary prophylaxis of *Pneumocystis carinii* pneumonia. *Lancet* 340:788, 1992.
    A letter that reports a small open trial, which compares primary PCP prophylaxis with TMP-SMX (one double-strength tablet every other day), aerosolized pentamidine (300 mg monthly), and dapsone (100 mg weekly) plus pyrimethamine (25 mg twice weekly), demonstrated improved efficacy with TMP-SMX.

27. Pretet, S., et al. Long term results of monthly inhaled pentamidine as primary prophylaxis of *Pneumocystis carinii* pneumonia in HIV infected patients. *Am. J. Med.* 94:35, 1993.
    Study from France: 232 patients with CD4 cell counts below 20% of the total lymphocyte count were given aerosolized pentamidine once monthly. The regimen was effective and well tolerated.

28. Centers for Disease Control. Guidelines for preventing the transmission of tuberculosis in health-care-settings with special focus on HIV-related issues. *M.M.W.R.* 39(No. RR-17):1–29, 1990.

29. Golden, J.A., et al. A randomized comparison of once-monthly or twice-monthly high-dose pentamidine prophylaxis. *Chest* 104:743, 1993.

29a. Ena, J., et al. Once-a-month administration of intravenous pentamidine to patients infected with human immunodeficiency virus as prophylaxis for *Pneumocystis carinii* pneumonia. *Clin. Infect. Dis.* 18:901, 1994.
    Fifty-two patients received intravenous pentamidine at a dosage of 4 mg/kg over 60–90 minutes each month for primary (37 patients) and secondary (15 patients) prophylaxis. During 387 months of administration, no cases of PCP were seen in primary prevention; during 200 months of secondary prevention, one case of PCP was seen. Side effects were mild and did not necessitate withdrawal of the drug. The authors concluded that this is a valid approach for patients who cannot tolerate sulfonamides.

30. Cheung, T.W., et al. Intramuscular pentamidine for the prevention of *Pneumocystis carinii* pneumonia in patients infected with human immunodeficiency virus. *Clin. Infect. Dis.* 16:22, 1993.
    Intramuscular pentamidine was given monthly by the Z-track technique in 96 patients at a dose of 300 mg (4 mg/kg if the patient weighed < 50 kg). Sterile abscess formation at the site of injection occurred in three instances (3% of patients or four cases per 1,000 injections). The approach was effective in primary and secondary PCP prophylaxis, with only three cases of PCP occurring in recipients. The authors conclude that monthly intramuscular pentamidine is an alternative for PCP prevention, and a prospective study should be undertaken to provide more data.

31. Phillips, L., et al. Tolerability and Safety Assessment of Pentamidine Delivered by Metered-Dose Inhaler [abstract 1087]. In *Proceedings of the Thirty-third Interscience Conference on Antimicrobial Agents and Chemotherapy*, American Society for Microbiology, New Orleans, 1993.

32. Heald, A., et al. Treatment for cerebral toxoplasmosis protects against *Pneumocystis carinii* pneumonia in patients with AIDS. *Ann. Intern. Med.* 115:760, 1991.

33. Read, C.A., et al. Differential lobe lavage for diagnosis of acute *Pneumocystis carinii* pneumonia in patients receiving prophylactic aerosolized pentamidine therapy. *Chest* 103:1520, 1993.

34. Fahy, J.V., et al. Effect of aerosolized pentamidine prophylaxis on the clinical severity and diagnosis of *Pneumocystis carinii* pneumonia. *Am. Rev. Respir. Dis.* 146:844, 1992.

35. Teuscher, A.U., et al. Predictive value of bronchoalveolar lavage in excluding a diagnosis of *Pneumocystis carinii* pneumonia during prophylaxis with aerosolized pentamidine. *Clin. Infect. Dis.* 16:519, 1993.
    Determined a 94% negative predictive value of bronchoalveolar lavage for patients receiving aerosolized pentamidine prophylaxis who underwent site-directed sampling.

36. Dohn, M.N., et al. Equal survival rates for first, second, and third episodes of *Pneumocystis carinii* pneumonia in patients with acquired immunodeficiency syndrome. *Arch. Intern. Med.* 152:2465, 1992.
    Single-institution prospective cohort study that followed AIDS patients treated for 222 occurrences of PCP over 5 years demonstrated that survival rates after the first, second, and third episodes were similar (86%, 84%, and 88%, respectively). Patients with second and subsequent episodes had lesser degrees of hypoxemia at presentation.

37. Waecker, N.J., et al. Age-adjusted CD4+ lymphocyte parameters in healthy children at risk for infection with human immunodeficiency virus. *Clin. Infect. Dis.* 17:123, 1993.

38. Mueller, B.U., and Pizzo, P.A. Trimethoprim-sulfamethoxazole prophylaxis of *Pneumocystis carinii* pneumonia in infants. *Pediatr. Infect. Dis. J.* 11:1072, 1992.

38a. Barnett, E.D., et al. Dapsone for prevention of *Pneumocystis* pneumonia in children with acquired immunodeficiency syndrome. *Pediatr. Infect. Dis. J.* 13:72, 1994.
Breakthrough infections can occur, and the onset is insidious and mild in nature.

39. O'Doherty, M.J., et al. Lung deposition of nebulised pentamidine in children. *Thorax* 48:220, 1993.
See also T.A. Orcutt et al., Aerosolized pentamidine: A well-tolerated mode of prophylaxis against Pneumocystis carinii *pneumonia in older children with human immunodeficiency virus infection.* Pediatr. Infect. Dis. J. *11:290, 1992.*

39a. Hand, I.V., et al. Aerosolized pentamidine for prophylaxis of *Pneumocystis carinii* pneumonia in infants with human immunodeficiency virus infection. *Pediatr. Infect. Dis. J.* 13:100, 1994.
Seven infants, ages 3.5–11 months, received a total of 45 monthly aerosolized pentamidine treatments of 300–600 mg/mo, adjusted for minute ventilation and weight. Sixty-two percent of treatments were associated with no discernible side effects. Observed toxicity included coughing, mild wheezing, and arterial desaturation. Authors concluded that aerosolized pentamidine appears to be a relatively safe, well-tolerated.

39b. Sepkowitz, K.A. *Pneumocystis carinii* pneumonia without acquired immunodeficiency syndrome: Who should receive prophylaxis? *Mayo Clin. Proc.* 71:102,1996.
Editorial comment. Suggests that any patient with an underlying immunologic disorder (e.g., chemotherapy, transplantation, or an inflammatory disorder) who receives the equivalent of ≥ 20 mg prednisone daily for more than 1 month probably deserves PCP prophylaxis. See article in same journal.

40. Medical Letter. Drugs for AIDS and associated infections. *Med. Lett. Drugs Ther.* 37:87, 1995.

40a. Safrin, S., et al. Adjunctive folinic acid with trimethoprim-sulfamethoxazole for *Pneumocystis carinii* pneumonia in AIDS patients is associated with an increased risk of therapeutic failure and death. *J. Infect. Dis.* 170:912, 1994.

41. Sattler, F.R., et al. Trimethoprim-sulfamethoxazole compared with pentamidine for treatment of *Pneumocystis carinii* pneumonia in the acquired immunodeficiency syndrome: A prospective non-crossover study. *Ann. Intern. Med.* 109:280, 1988.

41a. Hughes, W.T., et al. Adverse events associated with trimethoprim-sulfamethoxazole and atovaquone during the treatment of AIDS-related *Pneumocystis carinii* pneumonia. *J. Infect. Dis.* 171:2295, 1995.
For description of original trial, see reference [52]. Treatment-limiting adverse effects occurred in 9% of the atovaquone-treated patients and 24% of the TMP-SMX patients.

42. van der Ven, A.J.A.M., et al. Adverse reactions to co-trimoxazole in HIV infection. *Lancet* 338:431, 1991.

43. Carr, A., et al. Clinical and laboratory markers of hypersensitivity to trimethoprim-sulfamethoxazole in patients with *Pneumocystis carinii* pneumonia and AIDS. *J. Infect. Dis.* 167:180, 1993.
In this retrospective analysis of PCP patients, 27% developed hypersensitivity (as manifested by a mild rash) after an average of 12 days of therapy with TMP-SMX. Authors conclude hypersensitivity to TMP-SMX is less likely to occur with advanced AIDS.

44. Kelly, J.W., et al. A severe, unusual reaction to trimethoprim-sulfamethoxazole in patients with human immunodeficiency virus. *Clin. Infect. Dis.* 14:1034, 1992.
Report of 3 patients who developed fever and hypotension rapidly after administration of TMP-SMX and who had exhibited minor intolerance to the drug 2–3 weeks earlier.

45. Velazquez, H., et al. Renal mechanisms of trimethoprim-induced hyperkalemia. *Ann. Intern. Med.* 119:296, 1993.
A retrospective analysis of 30 AIDS patients receiving TMP (20 mg/kg/day) that demonstrated reversible increases in serum potassium of an average of 0.6 mmol/liter after 5 days of therapy. Half of these patients had serum potassium levels in excess of 5.0 mmol/liter, whereas 10% had serum potassium levels greater than 6.0 mmol/liter. In the same issue, see also S. Greenberg et al., TMP-SMX induces reversible hyperkalemia, Ann. Intern. Med. *119:291, 1993.*

46. Medina, I., et al. Oral therapy for *Pneumocystis carinii* pneumonia in the acquired immunodeficiency syndrome: A controlled trial of trimethoprim-sulfamethoxazole versus trimethoprim-dapsone. *N. Engl. J. Med.* 323:776, 1990.
Both regimens were equally effective, but there were fewer adverse reactions in the TMP-dapsone group.

47. Mills, J., et al. Dapsone therapy of *Pneumocystis carinii* pneumonia in the acquired immunodeficiency syndrome. *Antimicrob. Agents Chemother.* 32:1057, 1988.
Oral dapsone therapy alone was less effective than conventional therapy or the combination of dapsone-TMP.
48. American Hospital Formulary Service. Pentamidine isethionate. In *Drug Information*. Bethesda, MD: American Society of Hospital Pharmacists, Inc., 1993. P. 510.
49. *Physicians' Desk Reference* (50th ed.). Montvale, NJ: Medical Economics, 1996. P. 1042.
50. Vilde, J.L., and Remington, J.S. Role of clindamycin with or without another agent for treatment of *Pneumocystis* in patients with AIDS. *J. Infect. Dis.* 166:694, 1992.
51. Toma, E., et al. Clindamycin/primaquine versus trimethoprim-sulfamethoxazole as primary therapy for *Pneumocystis carinii* pneumonia in AIDS: A randomized, double-blind pilot trial. *Clin. Infect. Dis.* 17:178, 1993.
See related paper by J.R. Black et al., Clindamycin and primaquine therapy for mild-to-moderate episodes of Pneumocystis carinii *pneumonia in patients with AIDS: AIDS clinical trials group 044. Clin. Infect. Dis. 18:905, 1994, which indicates that this combination is effective and well tolerated. See also related discussions in Chap. 28I.*
51a. Safrin, S., et al. Comparison of three regimens for treatment of mild to moderate *Pneumocystis carinii* pneumonia in patients with AIDS: A double-blind randomized trial of oral trimethoprim-sulfamethoxazole, dapsone-trimethoprim, and clindamycin-primaquine. *Ann. Intern. Med.* 124:793,1996.
In this May 1996 report, no statistical differences were seen among treatment groups; survival during therapy or for 2 months thereafter did not differ. Choice of regimen may ultimately be based on expected toxicity. The authors conclude that evidence of hepatic insufficiency at the time of presentation should prompt clinicians to consider a regimen other than TMP-SMX and that severe myelosuppression at baseline may suggest a regimen other than clindamycin-primaquine be used.
52. Hughes, W.T., et al. Comparison of atovaquone (566C80) with trimethoprim-sulfamethoxazole to treat *Pneumocystis carinii* pneumonia in patients with AIDS. *N. Engl. J. Med.* 328:1521, 1993.
This ACTG trial demonstrated atovaquone's potential for use as an alternative therapy for mild to moderate PCP. Patients treated with atovaquone (750 mg tid), compared to TMP-SMX (two double-strength tablets tid), had significantly higher rates of therapeutic failure (20% versus 7%) and 4-week mortality (11% versus 0.6%). However, atovaquone was better tolerated. See reference [41a].
52a. Dohn, M.N., et al. Oral atovaquone compared with intravenous pentamidine for *Pneumocystis carinii* pneumonia in patients with AIDS. *Ann. Intern. Med.* 121:174, 1994.
Multicenter randomized study. Discontinuation of original therapy because of treatment-limiting adverse events was more frequent in the pentamidine group (36%) than the atovaquone group (4%). For a related review, see L.J. Epstein et al., Clinical experience with atovaquone: A new drug for treating Pneumocystis carinii *pneumonia. Am. J. Med. Sci. 308:5, 1994.*
53. Artymowicz, R.J., and James, V.E. Atovaquone: A new antipneumocystic agent. *Clin. Pharm.* 12:563, 1993.
54. Soo Hoo, G.W., et al. Inhaled or intravenous pentamidine therapy for *Pneumocystis carinii* pneumonia in AIDS: A randomized trial. *Ann. Intern. Med.* 113:195, 1990.
55. Conte, J.E., Jr., et al. Intravenous or inhaled pentamidine for treating *Pneumocystis carinii* pneumonia in AIDS. *Ann. Intern. Med.* 113:203, 1990.
Inhaled pentamidine therapy of PCP was associated with unacceptably high relapse rates.
56. Montgomery, A.B., et al. Aerosolized pentamidine vs. trimethoprim/sulfamethoxazole for acute *Pneumocystis carinii* pneumonia [abstract 395]. In *Proceedings of the Sixth International Conference on AIDS* 6:220, 1990.
57. Amsden, G.W., Kowalsky, S.F., and Morse, G.D. Trimetrexate for *Pneumocystis carinii* pneumonia in patients with AIDS. *Ann. Pharmacother.* 26:218, 1992.
For an update see B. Fulton et al., Trimetrexate: A review of its pharmacokinetic properties and therapeutic potential in the treatment of Pneumocystis carinii *pneumonia. Drugs 49:563, 1995.*
58. Allegra, C.J., et al. Trimetrexate for treatment of *Pneumocystis carinii* pneumonia in patients with acquired immunodeficiency syndrome. *N. Engl. J. Med.* 317:978, 1987.
In this study of 16 patients, 30 mg/m² of trimetrexate was used intravenously once daily.
58a. Sattler, F.R., et al. Trimetrexate with leucovorin versus trimethoprim-sulfamethoxazole for moderate to severe episodes of *Pneumocystis carinii* pneumonia in patients

with AIDS: A prospective, controlled multicenter investigation of the AIDS clinical trials group protocol 029/031. *J. Infect. Dis.* 170:165, 1994.
Trimetrexate plus leucovorin was effective, although inferior to, TMP-SMX for moderate to severe PCP but was better tolerated than TMP-SMX.

59. Noskin, G.A., et al. Salvage therapy with clindamycin/primaquine for *Pneumocystis carinii* pneumonia. *Clin. Infect. Dis.* 14:183, 1992.
Eighty-six percent of 26 patients (who experienced 28 episodes of PCP) in this dual-institution retrospective study who received salvage therapy for PCP responded when treated with clindamycin (900 mg IV q8h, followed by 450 mg PO qid) and primaquine (30 mg/d). Half the patients developed a mild rash, but 25% developed methemoglobinemia, 2 of whom required treatment. The authors advocated a larger, controlled analysis of this regimen (d = day).

59a. Wachter, R.M., et al. Cost and outcome of intensive care for patients with AIDS, *Pneumocystis carinii* pneumonia, and severe respiratory failure. *J.A.M.A.* 273:230, 1995.

60. Montaner, J.S.G., et al. Corticosteroids prevent early deterioration in patients with moderately severe *Pneumocystis carinii* pneumonia and the acquired immunodeficiency syndrome (AIDS). *Ann. Intern. Med.* 113:14, 1990.
Oral prednisone (60 mg/day for 7 days and then tapered over 2 weeks) was beneficial in first-episode PCP. In this prospective, randomized, double-blind placebo-controlled trial, steroids prevented early deterioration of oxygenation and increased exercise tolerance.

61. Bozzette, S.A., et al. A controlled trial of early adjunctive treatment with corticosteroids for *Pneumocystis carinii* pneumonia in the acquired immunodeficiency syndrome. *N. Engl. J. Med.* 323:1451, 1990.
This report from the California Collaborative Treatment Group summarizes the beneficial results from a multicenter, randomized, controlled trial of twice-daily prednisone therapy (initially 40 mg bid × 5 days, then 40 mg/day × 5 days, and then 20 mg/day while being treated for PCP). It showed that steroids reduced by one-half the risk of respiratory failure and death in patients with AIDS and moderate to severe PCP. Clinical benefits could not be demonstrated for patients with mild PCP. The authors emphasize the importance of confirming the diagnosis of PCP so as not to mask another infection (e.g., tuberculosis). This was a large study of 250 patients. In steroid recipients, there was a slightly increased incidence of reactivation of localized herpetic lesions.

62. Gagnon, S., et al. Corticosteroids as adjunctive therapy for severe *Pneumocystis carinii* pneumonia in the acquired immunodeficiency syndrome: A double-blind, placebo-controlled trial. *N. Engl. J. Med.* 323:1444, 1990.
Double-blind, placebo-controlled study showed steroid can improve survival and decrease the occurrence of respiratory failure in severe PCP. Patients were given methylprednisolone, 40 mg IV q6h for 7–10 days, or placebo.

63. Nielsen, T.L., et al. Adjunctive corticosteroid therapy for *Pneumocystis carinii* pneumonia in AIDS: A randomized European multicenter open label trial. *J. Acquir. Immune Defic. Syndr.* 5:726, 1992.

64. National Institutes of Health–University of California Expert Panel for Corticosteroids as Adjunctive Therapy for *Pneumocystis* Pneumonia. Consensus statement on the use of corticosteroids as adjunctive therapy for *Pneumocystis* pneumonia in the acquired immunodeficiency syndrome. *N. Engl. J. Med.* 323:1500, 1990.
Report completed August 15, 1990, and published November 22, 1990. Summarizes published and nonpublished studies and favors use of corticosteroids in patients with moderate to severe PCP.

65. LaRocco, A., et al. Corticosteroids for *Pneumocystis carinii* pneumonia with acute respiratory failure: Experience with rescue therapy. *Chest* 102:892, 1992.

66. Sleasman, J. W., et al. Corticosteroids improve survival of children with AIDS and *Pneumocystis carinii* pneumonia. *Am. J. Dis. Child.* 147:30, 1993.
Steroids were beneficial in infants who have acute respiratory failure due to PCP. Also see G.E. McLaughlin et al., Effect of corticosteroids on survival of children with immunodeficiency syndrome and Pneumocystis carinii–related respiratory failure. J. Pediatr. 126:821, 1995, in which steroids were beneficial.

67. McGowan, J.E., Jr., et al. Guidelines for the use of systemic glucocorticosteroids in management of selected infections. *J. Infect. Dis.* 165:1, 1992.
Report from the Working Group on Steroid Use, Antimicrobial Agents Committee, Infectious Disease Society of America. Good summary, with categorization of the extent to which data are, or are not, supportive of steroid use in a variety of settings: gram-negative sepsis, toxic shock syndrome, tuberculosis complications, herpes zoster, meningitis, and the like. Well-referenced.

68. Lambertus, M.W., et al. Complications of corticosteroid therapy in patients with the acquired immunodeficiency syndrome and *Pneumocystis carinii* pneumonia. *Chest* 98:38, 1990.

68a. Caumes, E., et al. Effect of corticosteroids on the incidence of adverse cutaneous reactions to trimethoprim-sulfamethoxazole during treatment of AIDS-associated *Pneumocystis carinii* pneumonia. *Clin. Infect. Dis.* 18:319, 1994.

69. Huang, Z.B., and Eden, E. Effect of corticosteroid release on IL1-beta release by alveolar macrophages from patients with AIDS and *Pneumocystis carinii* pneumonia. *Chest* 104:751, 1993.

70. Conte, J.E., Jr., et al. Pentamidine pharmacokinetics in patients with AIDS with impaired renal function. *J. Infect. Dis.* 156:885, 1987.

71. Gilbert, D.N., and Bennett, W.M. Use of antimicrobial agents in renal failure. *Infect. Dis. Clin. North Am.* 3:517, 1989.
    See update by L.L. Livornese et al., Antibacterial agents in renal failure. Infect. Dis. Clin. North Am. 9:591, 1995.

72. Bennett, W.M., et al. *Drug Prescribing in Renal Failure: Dosing Guidelines for Adults* (3rd ed.). Philadelphia: American College of Physicians, 1994.
    This is a useful handbook.

73. Conte, J.E., Jr. Pharmacokinetics of intravenous pentamidine in patients with normal renal function or receiving hemodialysis. *J. Infect. Dis.* 163:169, 1991.
    Dose adjustment of intravenous pentamidine does not appear necessary.

74. Lee, B., and Safrin, S. Interactions and toxicities of drugs used in patients with AIDS. *Clin. Infect. Dis.* 14:773, 1992.

75. Gradon, J.D., Fricchione, L., and Sepkowitz, D. Severe hypomagnesemia associated with pentamidine therapy. *Rev. Infect. Dis.* 13:511, 1991.
    Case report. See related report by G.M. Shah, Symptomatic hypocalcemia and hypomagnesemia with renal magnesium wasting associated with pentamidine therapy in a patient with AIDS. Am. J. Med. 89:380, 1990.

76. Jules-Elysee, K.M., et al. Aerosolized pentamidine: Effect on diagnosis and presentation of *Pneumocystis carinii* pneumonia. *Ann. Intern. Med.* 112:750, 1990.
    This type of prophylaxis may make the diagnosis of relapses difficult.

77. Baugham, R.P., et al. Increased *Pneumocystis carinii* recovery from the upper lobes in pneumocystis pneumonia: The effect of aerosolized pentamidine prophylaxis. *Chest* 103:426, 1993.

78. Berman, S.M., et al. Disseminated *Pneumocystis carinii* in a patient receiving aerosolized pentamidine prophylaxis. *West. J. Med.* 153:82, 1990.
    Case report of a patient with hypoalbuminemia and progressive liver function test abnormalities due to disseminated disease. Reviews literature on this topic up to early 1990. See a related brief report by G.A. Noskin and R.L. Murphy, Extrapulmonary infection with Pneumocystis carinii *in patients receiving aerosolized pentamidine. Rev. Infect. Dis. 13:525, 1991.*

79. Kemper, C.A., et al. Low dose dapsone prophylaxis of *Pneumocystis carinii* pneumonia in AIDS and AIDS-related complex. *AIDS* 4:1145, 1990.
    Includes a cost analysis that estimates oral dapsone costs about 5% of what aerosolized pentamidine costs per year.

80. Castellano, A.R., and Nettleman, M.D. Cost and benefit of secondary prophylaxis for *Pneumocystis carinii* pneumonia. *J.A.M.A.* 266:820, 1991.

81. American Hospital Formulary Service. Sulfones. In *Drug Information.* Bethesda, MD: American Society of Hospital Pharmacists, 1993. P. 482.

82. Zuidema, J., et al. Clinical pharmacokinetics of dapsone. *Clin. Pharmacokinet.* 11: 299, 1986.

83. Metroka, C.E., Lewis, N.J., and Jacobus, D.P. Desensitization of dapsone in HIV-positive patients. *J.A.M.A.* 267:512, 1992.
    This brief correspondence described a desensitization protocol that was successful in 13 of 14 patients who had had fever and a diffuse erythematous macular pruritic rash 8–14 days after initiation of dapsone for PCP prophylaxis. The authors speculate whether a gradual increase in the dose of dapsone may actually have desensitized some patients who might otherwise have had an allergic reaction had they been given 100 mg/day from the start.

83a. Beumont, M.G., et al. Safety of dapsone as PCP prophylaxis in HIV-infected patients with TMP-SMX intolerance [abstract I167]. *Proceedings of the Thirty-Fourth Interscience Conference on Antimicrobial Agents and Chemotherapy,* Orlando, FL, Oct. 6, 1994. American Society for Microbiology.
    Of 53 patients with a clinical history of allergy to TMP-SMX, 19% had adverse reactions

to dapsone prophylaxis. Anemia was common (30%) in those with prior PCP compared to those without prior PCP (15%). Dapsone dose and the use of azidothymidine were not obviously associated with adverse experiences.

84. Metroka, C.E., et al. Failure of prophylaxis with dapsone in patients taking dideoxy-inosine. *N. Engl. J. Med.* 325:737, 1991.
85. Beutler, E. Methemoglobinemia and Sulfhemoglobinemia. In W.J. Williams et al. (eds.), *Hematology* (4th ed.). New York: McGraw-Hill, 1990. Pp. 743–746.
86. DeGowin, R.L. A review of therapeutic and hemolytic effects of dapsone. *Arch. Intern. Med.* 120:242, 1967.
    A classic article describing some of the hematologic side effects of dapsone, especially hemolysis.
87. Beutler, E. Glucose-6-phosphate Dehydrogenase Deficiency. In W.J. Williams et al. (eds.), *Hematology* (4th ed.). New York: McGraw-Hill, 1990. Pp. 591–602.
88. Mohle-Boetani, J., et al. The sulfone syndrome in a patient receiving dapsone prophylaxis for *Pneumocystis carinii* pneumonia. *West. J. Med.* 156:303, 1992.
89. Grinspoon, S.K., and Bilezikian, J.P. HIV disease and the endocrine system. *N. Engl. J. Med.* 327:1360, 1992.
90. Smit, M.J.M., et al. Trimetrexate efficacy and pharmacokinetics during treatment of refractory *Pneumocystis carinii* pneumonia in an infant with severe combined immunodeficiency disease. *Pediatr. Infect. Dis.* 9:212, 1990.
    See commentary by B.A. Kamen, which follows this report in the same issue. See also annotation of reference [57].
91. Medical Letter. Trimetrexate for *Pneumocystis carinii* pneumonia. *Med. Lett. Drugs Ther.* 31:51, 1989.
92. Sattler, F.R., et al. Trimetrexate-leucovorin dosage evaluation study for treatment of *Pneumocystis carinii* pneumonia. *J. Infect. Dis.* 161:91, 1990.
93. Medical Letter. Atovaquone for *Pneumocystis carinii* pneumonia. *Med. Lett. Drugs Ther.* 35:28, 1993.
94. Kovacs, J.A. Efficacy of atovaquone in treatment of toxoplasmosis in patients with AIDS. The NIAID–Clinical Center Intramural AIDS Program. *Lancet* 340:637, 1992.
    Preliminary report of eight patients with AIDS and presumed or biopsy-confirmed toxoplasmosis who were intolerant of or had not responded to standard therapy and who were treated with atovaquone, 750 mg qid. Seven patients showed radiologic improvement. The study concluded that atovaquone is a well-tolerated drug that appears to be an effective alternative for patients with toxoplasmosis who are intolerant of standard therapy. Further data are needed.

25

Microbiology Laboratory Tests

Paul S. Graman and
Marilyn A. Menegus

Diagnostic Laboratory Tests

Smear and Stain Techniques

The most direct, rapid, and technically least restricted tests are the microscopic examination of stained and unstained smears of material from the site of infection. Direct microscopic evaluation can provide immediate data in such life-threatening illnesses as pneumonia and meningitis. Isolation of the potential etiologic agent may otherwise take hours to days (bacteria) or weeks (mycobacteria and fungi). Sometimes, as in malaria and other parasitic diseases, culture cannot be done [1].

I. **Gram stain**
   A. Differential staining characteristics are based on cell wall lipid content and the cell wall's decreased permeability to organic solvents of gram-positive organisms compared to gram-negative organisms. Gram-positive organisms stain purple from the retained crystal violet–iodine complex, whereas gram-negative organisms do not retain this complex and stain red owing to a counterstain.
   B. **Uses**
      1. **Diagnostic aid.** Smears of clinical specimens are particularly useful for determining quickly the morphologic features and staining characteristics (gram-positive or gram-negative) of organisms in clinical material. Gram stains can help one make a clinical diagnosis by providing clues to the etiologic agent involved in an infection, which in turn will help one choose the appropriate antibiotic while awaiting culture results. (See Chap. 28A under Principles of Antibiotic Use.)
      2. **Adequacy of specimens.** Gram stains also help one to assess the adequacy of culture material. Sputum samples, in particular, often are contaminated with oral secretions. When large numbers of epithelial cells are present, it is likely that the sample has been collected improperly and that culture results may be misleading. Many laboratories will not culture "sputum" samples that contain more than 10 squamous epithelial cells per low-magnification field ($10\times$ objective).
      3. **Purulence of a specimen.** Many polymorphonuclear cells are more likely to be seen in infected, versus colonized, sputum specimens (see Chap. 9). The absence of polymorphonuclear cells, however, does not exclude an acute bacterial infection (e.g., in leukopenic patients and in asymptomatic bacteriuria).
      4. **Quantitation of bacteria.** When one or more organisms per oil-immersion field are seen on a Gram stain of a drop of fresh, unspun bodily fluid such as urine, the culture usually shows more than 10^5 organisms per milliliter.
   C. **Technique of preparation**
      1. Make a **thin smear** of the clinical specimen on a clean glass slide.
         a. **Body fluids.** Cerebrospinal fluid (CSF) and other normally sterile fluids, such as joint or pleural fluid, can be applied directly to the slide or centrifuged to concentrate the organisms. Either conventional centrifugation or cytocentrifugation may be used. Thicker smears can be made by placing successive loopsful of sediment on the same spot. Allow the spot to dry before applying the next loopful.
         b. **Sputum.** Use purulent-appearing samples and spread the sample on the slide.

2. **Air-dry and gently heat-fix** the smear by passing the slide through a flame 1 or 2 times. Do not make the slide too hot to touch, as this could cause staining artifacts and altered cell morphology. Grossly bloody smears can be cleared by flooding with distilled water for 5 minutes after they have been heat-fixed.

3. **Staining**

   a. **After cooling** the slide, flood it with **crystal or gentian violet** for 10 seconds and then rinse gently with tap water.

   b. **Flood with Gram's iodine** for 10 seconds and then rinse again. The duration of staining in the first two steps is not particularly critical.

   c. **Decolorize** with 95% ethanol or an acetone-ethanol mixture (95% ethyl alcohol, 100 ml; acetone, 100 ml), and repeat the tap-water rinse. **Decolorization is the critical step in the staining procedure.** Decolorization of the smear is complete when the blue stain is no longer visible and when the solvent is colorless as it runs from the slide.

   Thick smears of sputum or purulent exudates resist decolorization, and attempts to clear all portions of the specimen will result in excessive decolorization of the interpretable areas. Such specimens should therefore be decolorized only until the thin parts of the smear are colorless. Solvents that contain acetone will act more rapidly than 95% ethanol, and decolorization may be adequate after only 1 or 2 seconds.

   d. **Counterstain** with safranin for 10 seconds and repeat the rinse.

   e. **Air-dry or blot** gently with clean, absorbent paper.

D. **Factors affecting smear interpretation**

   1. **Incomplete decolorization** will result in excessive gram-positive staining of cells and bacteria. These will appear dark, and gram-negative organisms could thereby be misclassified and read as gram-positive. If the stain is inadequately decolorized, prepare a new smear. If the clinical sample is not available, remove the immersion oil with xylene and repeat the decolorization and counterstaining steps.

   2. **Overdecolorization** can cause gram-positive organisms to appear gram-negative. Only gram-negative cells and bacteria are seen. One's staining technique can be evaluated by parallel staining of a sample known to contain gram-positive flora (e.g., oral secretions). A repeat smear should be made or the immersion oil should be removed with xylene and the entire staining process repeated if further specimens are unavailable.

   3. **Precipitates of crystal violet** may be misinterpreted as gram-positive cocci or fungi. These precipitates usually are irregular in size and shape, more refractile than organisms, and more likely to be seen in under-decolorized smears, especially in thick portions of the smear.

   4. **Variations of morphologic features on Gram staining.** Gram-positive organisms may appear gram-negative or both gram-positive and gram-negative (gram-variable) when the organisms are old, damaged after exposure to an acidic environment, or exposed to antibiotics. Some organisms (e.g., *Acinetobacter* spp. and some *Bacillus* spp.) are naturally gram-variable.

   5. **Background interference.** Look carefully for small, pleomorphic, gram-negative organisms, such as *Haemophilus* spp., which can easily be missed because of the staining of the amorphous background material.

   6. When **gram-positive cocci** are seen, it may not be possible to make a specific etiologic diagnosis. Almost any gram-positive coccus can appear in pairs or short chains. Staphylococci may not appear in clusters but may be seen as a single coccus or in pairs.

II. **Acid-fast stains.** Organisms that stain well with particular dyes (e.g., carbol-fuchsin or auramine) and resist decolorization with acid-alcohol are termed *acid-fast*. Acid-fast bacilli (AFB) include mycobacteria (which stain poorly or not at all with Gram stain) and *Nocardia* spp. The initial step in the laboratory diagnosis of tuberculosis is examination of smears by an acid-fast procedure. Two types of acid-fast stains are commonly used.

A. The basic fuchsin stain (**Kinyoun** or **Ziehl-Neelsen**) combined with conventional light microscopy.

B. **Fluorochrome stains** offer the advantages of speed and ease of observation. The most well-established technique, Truant stain, employs auramine-rhodamine fluorescent dyes. Smears are examined under low power using a fluorescence microscope. Large areas can be easily examined in a short time, making fluorochrome stains **more sensitive than conventional basic fuchsin stains** [2, 3]. See related discussion in Chap. 9 (sec. **IV** under Tuberculosis: Basic Concepts), in which the role of gastric and urine AFB smears also is discussed.

C. **Application and interpretation**

1. The sensitivity of microscopy for the diagnosis of mycobacterial infection is relatively low, requiring approximately 5×10^3 bacilli per milliliter for detection. Therefore, all specimens examined by smear should also be cultured (see related discussion in Chap. 9, sec. **IV** under Tuberculosis: Basic Concepts). **Whenever possible, sputum specimens should be concentrated** for microscopic examination as well as culture. For example, mycobacteria are recovered optimally from clinical specimens when methods both to release them from body fluids and cells (digestion) and to remove or sufficiently reduce competing organisms (decontamination) are used. Using the N-acetyl-L-cysteine–sodium hydroxide method, the N-acetyl-L-cysteine is a mucolytic agent that can digest tenacious sputum. Decontamination is achieved by the addition of sodium hydroxide [3a]. The sample can then be centrifuged and the sediment stained and cultured, with an improved yield of organisms compared with a direct stain of the patient's sputum.

2. The number of tubercle bacilli in respiratory secretions is directly related to the risk of transmission.

3. One cannot, on the basis of smear results, differentiate *Mycobacterium tuberculosis* from the nontuberculous ("atypical") mycobacteria. Culture and identification tests, or special DNA probes, are needed.

4. *Nocardia* spp. are AFB but they retain acid-fast stains less tenaciously than do mycobacteria. Modified acid-fast stains with milder decolorization must be used to detect *Nocardia* reliably.

III. **Wet-mount preparations** of a variety of specimens can be examined microscopically for fungal, bacterial, parasitic, and other pathogens. In general, for the preparations described here, a drop or small portion of specimen (feces, exudate, CSF, urine sediment, sputum, or scrapings) is mixed in a drop of physiologic saline on the surface of a glass slide. Coverslips are applied to prevent evaporation. Slides are scanned under a dim substage light with a $10\times$ or $45\times$ objective, depending on the organism sought. In some cases, dark-field illumination may be helpful.

A. **Wet mounts with physiologic saline** are useful to examine for trichomonads of the genital tract and intestinal parasites. Slides should be examined as soon as possible to avoid drying. A cold environment should also be avoided as it causes organisms to become immobile and therefore more difficult to identify. Appropriate specimens for diagnosis of *Trichomonas* infection include vaginal secretions, urethral discharges, or urine sediment. *Trichomonas vaginalis* will appear as clear, actively motile forms, approximately the size of neutrophils. Cultures for *T. vaginalis* are not widely available, but they are significantly more sensitive (20–30%) than wet mounts [4]. (See the discussion in Chap. 13 under Vulvovaginitis.)

B. **Potassium hydroxide** (KOH) is used primarily for identification of fungal forms.

1. **Specimens.** Cervical discharge, skin scrapings (taken with a no. 11 blade), sputum, and tissue scrapings can be examined with this technique.

2. **Method.** A drop of 10–20% KOH solution is mixed with the clinical specimen and allowed to stand for 10–15 minutes. (Alternatively, the back of the slide can be gently heated.) KOH lyses debris and background material, so fungal forms can be seen more easily.

C. **India ink preparations** are used to visualize the capsule of *Cryptococcus neoformans*.

1. **Technique.** Cerebrospinal fluid, urine, and exudates can be examined. Mix a drop of centrifuged specimen with a small drop of India ink on a clear glass slide. Cover with a coverslip and examine when wet.

2. **Interpretation.** The mucoid capsule will appear as a clear halo that surrounds the yeast cell. In inexperienced hands, mononuclear cells (especially lymphocytes) may be mistaken for *C. neoformans*. Budding forms must be observed before a specimen is interpreted as positive. **The latex test for polysaccharide antigen is now the preferred test for the rapid diagnosis of cryptococcosis because it is more sensitive than direct microscopy** [5]. (See additional discussion in Chaps. 5 and 18.)

D. **Dark-field microscopy** is particularly useful in diagnosing primary syphilis. This is discussed in Chap. 13 under Genital Lesions.

IV. **Other useful staining methods.** A number of different stains can be used to detect and identify infectious agents in blood, impression smears, exfoliated cells, and tissue sections.

A. **Giemsa and Wright's stains** are available in every hematology laboratory.

1. **Malaria and babesiosis smears.** Although textbooks often recommend that thick smears be made of the blood of patients suspected of having malaria or babesiosis, these smears contain numerous artifacts and require significant clinical experience to interpret. Consequently, routinely prepared thin smears of the patient's peripheral blood or a special malarial smear preparation (e.g., smear of platelet-depleted RBCs) are suitable for screening for these intracellular parasites. Platelets overlying RBCs can mimic intracellular parasites to the untrained observer.

2. **Herpes simplex and varicella-zoster viral skin lesions** can be distinguished from pustular pyodermas by a Giemsa or Wright's stain of a scraping of the bottom at the periphery of an unroofed vesicle. Herpetic lesions show the characteristic multinucleate giant cells and, rarely, intranuclear inclusions. Other staining methods (e.g., methylene blue [**Tzanck preparation**]) and routine Papanicolaou smears are better suited for this purpose because nuclear detail is more easily visualized.

3. *Pneumocystis carinii, Toxoplasma gondii, Histoplasma capsulatum,* yeast, and bacteria can be detected in **Giemsa stains of touch preparations of tissue.**

B. **Silver stains** (Gomori's methenamine silver, Warthin-Starry, and Dieterle) are difficult to perform properly and should be used only by skilled individuals. They are most useful for the detection of *Treponema pallidum* fungi, *P. carinii, Legionella* spp., rickettsiae, and the organism associated with cat-scratch disease. Many of these organisms stain poorly or not at all on Gram staining and other methods.

C. **Periodic acid–Schiff (PAS) and calcofluor white stains** are used to demonstrate fungi in clinical specimens. PAS and Gomori's methenamine silver stains often reveal fungi not well visualized by more conventional techniques (e.g., hematoxylin-eosin and Gram stain).

D. **Acridine orange,** a fluorochrome DNA stain, can be used to detect a variety of microorganisms (e.g., bacteria, fungi, and trichomonads). It is more sensitive than Gram stain for bacteria because organisms can be seen under low-power magnification, and organisms partially damaged by antibiotics can still be detected [1].

E. **Methylene blue smears for fecal leukocytes** are discussed in Chap. 11 under Infectious Gastroenteritis (p. 383).

F. **Fluorescent antibody and immunocytochemical stains** are discussed later in this chapter under Direct Detection of Microbial Antigens in Clinical Specimens.

General Principles for Specimen Collection and Handling

This topic has recently been reviewed in detail [5a].

I. **Obtain specimens before initiating or changing antibiotic therapy.**

II. **Collect specimens in a manner that minimizes or avoids contamination by resident bacterial flora.**

A. Many potential pathogens can be transient colonizers of body sites. The mere isolation of these organisms does not necessarily establish the organism's clinical significance. On the other hand, recovery of certain organisms such as *Neisseria gonorrhoeae* or *M. tuberculosis* is significant in any clinical specimen.

B. When possible, **avoid sites of resident flora** in reaching normally sterile tissue areas or body cavities. Procedures such as suprapubic bladder aspiration, transtracheal or percutaneous lung aspiration, and percutaneous aspiration of vesicles, bullae, or abscesses all effectively avoid contamination of the specimen with resident flora.

III. **Use appropriate collection systems.** Specimens should be collected in clean, sterile containers free of inhibitory materials such as residual detergents or disinfectants. Saline or water with antibacterial preservatives should be avoided in the collection of specimens (e.g., tissue aspirates). Lidocaine also has antibacterial activities that can adversely affect recovery of organisms from bronchoscopy samples. Because of problems with inadequate sample size and drying of specimens, **applicator swab collection (especially ordinary cotton swabs) generally is less satisfactory than needle or catheter aspiration with a syringe.** Aspirated samples generally provide sufficient material for both culture and Gram stain.

Some anaerobes are sensitive to atmospheric oxygen and desiccation, and so special care must be taken in specimen collection and handling. Specimens aspirated into a syringe can be transported after one has expelled all residual air. Alternatively, the specimen can be inoculated into special oxygen-free transport systems.

IV. **Transportation to the laboratory**
   A. Although transport media are useful if culturing of specimens must be delayed, **rapid transport to the microbiology laboratory is preferable.** Except in emergencies, specimens should be routinely collected at times when prompt inoculation and handling in the laboratory is possible. Certain aerobes such as *Streptococcus pneumoniae* and *Neisseria* spp. are fastidious and may not survive adverse transport conditions (e.g., temperature extremes or drying). Long delays in transport can also result in the growth of clinically insignificant bacterial contaminants.
   B. **Label all specimens** to avoid errors in later identification.
   C. **Clearly inform the diagnostic laboratory about the information being sought** through the cultures and note their source. Certain culture techniques will minimize the effect of contamination and enhance the yield of useful information. The inoculation of highly selective media will increase the probability of recovering certain organisms such as species of *Salmonella, Shigella, Campylobacter,* and *Yersinia.*

V. **Blood culture collection technique.** Attention to strict aseptic technique is imperative to minimize the risk of contaminating blood cultures with resident skin flora (e.g., coagulase-negative staphylococci, diphtheroids, and *Propionibacterium acnes*). Contaminated cultures are often misleading. Furthermore, some organisms that are usually skin contaminants can, under certain circumstances (e.g., catheter-related sepsis, prosthetic valve endocarditis), be true bloodborne pathogens. (See Chap. 2 under Positive Blood Cultures.) Therefore, adequate preparation of the skin is the most important aspect of this procedure.
   A. Wear gloves when drawing blood, to reduce the risk of infection with bloodborne agents (e.g., hepatitis B and human immunodeficiency virus [HIV]).
   B. Obtain and set up equipment: appropriate media, 2% tincture of iodine or povidone, alcohol swabs, tourniquet, syringe, and needles.
   C. Remove the caps from the culture bottles and, using friction, swab the stopper twice with alcohol.
   D. Select the venipuncture site (usually antecubital) and prepare a circular area with a radius of approximately 2 inches. Starting at the puncture site, scrub the area with povidone-iodine, using a circular motion with overlapping strokes and working toward the periphery. Perform the procedure twice. (If the patient is allergic to povidone-iodine, use 70% isopropyl alcohol, cleansing the area for 1–2 minutes.)
   E. For better visualization of the actual puncture site, clean povidone-iodine off the vein site with one or two alcohol swabs, using the same "clean-to-dirty" circular motion.
   F. With the 10- to 20-ml syringe (for adults), perform the venipuncture carefully. Avoid touching the needle or prepared skin site. (If it is necessary to palpate the site to find a vein, use a sterile glove.)
   G. Remove the needle from the vein (avoid touching the needle to skin outside the prepared area). For adults **transfer 5–10 ml** of blood, **using the maximum amount suggested by the manufacturer,** into each broth bottle or transfer the appropriate volume into the recommended blood culture tube.
   H. Carefully label the blood culture slip as to the **date** and **exact time** the culture was drawn. **Blood drawn through intravascular catheters should be specifically identified.** This information is important in interpreting culture results.

Culture Techniques

I. **Blood cultures.** Blood cultures are indicated whenever there is reason to suspect clinically significant bacteremia or fungemia. In severely ill patients, cultures might be the only source demonstrating the causative agent.
   A. **Blood culture methods.** Recovery of microorganisms can be accomplished by placing the blood into a broth medium or by lysing the RBCs and then inoculating the lysate onto solid media [6–9].
      1. **Broth cultures** are used by most laboratories for the detection of bacteremia. A variety of broth culture media are available, and most laboratories use both an aerobic and an anaerobic broth. Growth of microorganisms can be detected

by visual examination of the bottles for turbidity, by blind subculture to solid media, or by a variety of automated systems that detect microbial metabolism. With older instruments, cultures are read at intervals (1–3 times) during the day. However reading is essentially continuous with newer systems [9].

   a. **Types of bacteremia.** Bacteremias are characterized as continuous, intermittent, or transient. Continuous bacteremias are associated with endocarditis and other intravascular infections. Intermittent bacteremia is by far the most common form and occurs in many different infections. Transient bacteremia is self-limited and often follows the manipulation of nonsterile mucosal surfaces or infected tissues [6–9]. (See Chap. 2.)

   b. **Volume of sample.** The ideal volume of blood to be collected for broth culture is unknown. Because of the low density of most bacteremias, 10- to 20-ml samples (e.g., 5–10 ml per bottle, depending on the manufacturer's recommendation) for adults and 1- to 5-ml samples for children commonly are recommended. When the sample is inoculated into the culture media, a 1:5 to 1:10 dilution of the blood appears to be best to reduce intrinsic serum antibacterial activity and to reduce the concentration of antimicrobials to subinhibitory levels. Some studies suggest improved recovery with higher dilutions of blood [7–9].

   c. **Timing and number of blood cultures.** Blood should be collected as soon as possible after the onset of fever or chills or whenever serious infection is suspected. **Two to three blood cultures, drawn at intervals of at least 20 minutes, are recommended** because of the intermittent nature of most bacteremias. However, the ideal time interval between cultures has not been established. Of course, blood cultures should be drawn before antibiotic therapy is initiated [7–9]. (See further discussions in Chaps. 2 and 10.)

   d. **Media.** Many relatively comparable, conventional broth media are available for use in blood cultures. Hypertonic media (usually prepared by the addition of 10–15% sucrose to a conventional broth media) appear to improve both the speed and overall recovery of certain organisms and are said also to enhance the recovery of organisms from patients being treated with antibiotics. In addition, resin devices and resin-containing media improve the recovery of organisms (staphylococci, in particular) from treated patients, but this general approach is costly, and its usefulness is debated [7].

2. **Blood lysis tubes** are available in two forms—one designed for centrifugation and concentration of organisms and the other, a smaller pediatric tube, from which the contents can be plated directly onto solid media. Blood lysis permits quantitation of organisms in blood, which may be useful in certain clinical situations (e.g., distinguishing intravascular catheter-related sepsis from sepsis originating at another site) (see Chap. 2). In addition, the blood lysis method results in increased recovery and decreased detection time for certain microorganisms (particularly yeast) and increased recognition of polymicrobial bacteremia compared with broth cultures [6–9]. The major disadvantages of the blood lysis technique identified thus far are a high contamination rate and poor recovery of anaerobic organisms.

B. **Fastidious organisms.** Blood cultures for brucellosis, tularemia, leptospirosis, systemic fungal infections, *Bartonella henselae* (formerly *Rochalimaea henselae,* the organism believed to be responsible for cat-scratch disease [see Chap. 17]), and *Mycobacterium avium* require special media and incubation for optimal isolation. For example, the Isolator lysis-centrifugation system (Wampole Laboratories, Cranbury, NJ) has been used to detect *B. henselae* and *M. avium* complex. Individual laboratories should be alerted to these diagnostic possibilities for specific recommendations regarding collection and processing of the specimens [7–9].

II. **Special methods for bacterial culture**

A. **Tissue specimens** can be cultured quantitatively and qualitatively. The former may, at times, be helpful for burn specimens because criteria based on the number of organisms per gram of tissue have been established for the diagnosis of burn wound sepsis. **Touch preparations** and subsequent staining for appropriate microorganisms may be helpful (e.g., rapid diagnosis of *P. carinii* pneumonia by staining of touch preparations of lung biopsy specimens).

B. **Foley catheter tips should not be submitted for bacterial culture** because they are invariably contaminated with resident periurethral flora.

C. **Intravenous catheters** are cultured qualitatively or semiquantitatively, depending on the laboratory. One technique for semiquantitative culture consists of rolling the catheter on a blood agar plate and reporting the total number of colonies of organisms that grow. To interpret these results, blood cultures must be positive. Using this approach, 15 colonies or more correlate with bacteremia caused by catheter infection, whereas fewer than 15 colonies probably represent extraneous contamination [10]. The optimal laboratory diagnostic method to define catheter-related sepsis has not been established. See related discussion in Chap. 2, sec. **III** under Catheter-Related Sepsis.

  D. Genital tract cultures are more likely to yield *N. gonorrhoeae* if they are transported to the laboratory within 6 hours of collection or if inoculated directly onto a selective medium. Special devices containing a layer of agar in a rectangular dish to which a carbon dioxide–generating tablet (Jembec) is added are available.

III. Anaerobic cultures. Most anaerobic bacteria of clinical importance are oxygen-tolerant. Nevertheless, special anaerobic containers often are recommended for specimen collection and transport. Rapid processing of samples also is important in avoiding overgrowth by facultative anaerobes [11, 12].

  A. Whenever possible, specimens should be aspirated and transported to the laboratory in the syringe used for collection or via an oxygen-free transport system.

  B. Swabs are less desirable because of the potential for inadequate sample size, air exposure, and sample desiccation. If swabs must be used, they should be placed in an oxygen-free transport system.

  C. Sites for anaerobic culture. Because many body sites are colonized by anaerobic organisms, only certain sites are appropriate for culture (Table 25-1).

  D. A Gram-stained smear should be performed on all specimens submitted for anaerobic culture. Because anaerobic cultures take considerable time for processing and identification, the Gram stain can provide useful clues regarding the infecting organisms. **Anaerobes should be considered when organisms are seen on smear but do not grow on routine aerobic cultures.** The unique morphologic features of many anaerobes might suggest their presence to the experienced observer. For example, in a Gram-stained smear, pale, unevenly stained, pleomorphic gram-negative rods with rounded ends and bipolar staining suggest *Bacteroides fragilis*. Broad gram-positive rods, generally without visible spores, suggest *Clostridium perfringens*. Other *Clostridium* spp. may be thin and gram-variable, with or without spores.

IV. Viral cultures. The same viral syndrome often can be produced by a variety of viral agents, and clinical differentiation of the specific infecting virus may be difficult, if not impossible (see Chap. 7). The etiology of a viral syndrome can often be established by viral culture, serologic tests, or both. Table 25-2 outlines the appropriate specimens necessary for virus isolation for the different clinical syndromes. Rapid diagnostic tests recommended for viral agents are discussed later under Direct Detection of Microbial Antigens in Clinical Specimens.

  A. General guidelines

  1. Specimens should be obtained from patients early in the course of illness, when virus shedding is greatest, preferably within 3 days after the onset of symptoms.

  2. Because many viruses are labile, samples should be placed in viral transport media and transported promptly to the virology laboratory. Many specimens

Table 25-1. Sites of culture for anaerobic specimens

Appropriate sites	Inappropriate sites
Normally sterile bodily fluids; blood; bile; pleural, peritoneal, joint, and spinal fluid; surgical specimens from normally sterile sites	Specimens contaminated by indigenous anaerobic flora; sputum, throat swabs, fecal specimens, rectal and vaginal swabs
Abscess contents, deep-wound aspirates, surgical biopsy specimens	Superficial-wound swabs, sites obviously contaminated by intestinal contents
Transtracheal or percutaneous lung aspirates	Sputum, bronchoscopy washings, nasopharyngeal or throat swabs
Suprapubic bladder aspirates	Voided or catheterized urine specimens
Culdocentesis fluid	Cervical or vaginal swabs

Table 25-2. Viruses associated with specific syndromes and recommended specimens for viral isolation

Syndrome	Common agents	Less common agents	Source of specimen for viral isolation
Upper respiratory tract infection	Influenza A, B Rhinovirus Parainfluenza 1, 3 Respiratory syncytial virus Adenovirus	Parainfluenza 2 Coxsackievirus A, B Echovirus Coronavirus	Nasal wash Nose or throat swab
Lower respiratory tract infection			
Child	Respiratory syncytial virus Parainfluenza 3, 1, 2 Influenza A, B	Adenovirus Influenza B	Nasal wash
Adult	Coxsackievirus A, B	Adenovirus	Nose or throat swab Sputum
Pleurodynia			Throat swab Stool
Central nervous system infection			
Meningitis	Coxsackievirus A, B Echovirus	Human immunodefi- ciency virus (HIV) type 1 Lymphocytic choriomenin- gitis Mumps	Cerebrospinal fluid Throat swab Stool
Encephalitis and encephalopathy	HIV type 1 Herpes simplex virus type 1	Arboviruses Mumps	Blood, brain biopsy
Myocarditis and pericarditis	Coxsackievirus B	Coxsackievirus A Influenza	Throat swab Stool

Gastroenteritis	Rotavirus Norwalk-like viruses	Adenovirus Calicivirus Astrovirus Coronavirus	Stool
Urinary tract infection: acute hemorrhagic cystitis		Adenovirus 11	Urine
Orchitis and epididymitis	Mumps	Coxsackievirus B(?)	Throat swab Stool
Parotitis	Mumps		Throat swab Stool
Exanthemas (nonspecific, with fever)	Coxsackievirus A9, A16 Echovirus 9, 16, 11	Echovirus 1–6, 14, 18, 19 Coxsackievirus A(2, 4, 23) Coxsackievirus B(1–5) Adenovirus	Skin vesicle fluid Throat swab Stool
Herpangina	Coxsackievirus A(1–6, 8, 10, 16, 22)	Echovirus 9, 17 Coxsackievirus B	Skin vesicle fluid Throat swab Stool
Hand-foot-and-mouth disease	Coxsackievirus A		Skin vesicle fluid Throat swab Stool
Nonspecific febrile illness	HIV type 1 Cytomegalovirus Coxsackievirus A, B Echovirus Influenza A, B	Adenovirus	Urine (for cytomegalovirus) Nose and throat swab Stool Blood

Source: Adapted from M. A. Menegus and R. G. Douglas, Jr., Viruses, Rickettsiae, Chlamydiae, and Mycoplasmas. In G. L. Mandell, R. G. Douglas, Jr., and J. E. Bennett (eds.), *Principles and Practice of Infectious Diseases* (3rd ed.). New York: Churchill Livingstone, 1990.

can be held at 4°C for up to 48 hours (on wet ice or in a refrigerator) without significant decrease in virus recovery. For prolonged storage, specimens should be frozen at −70°C.

3. Samples collected on swabs (conjunctival, pharyngeal, nasopharyngeal, rectal) should be placed quickly in a liquid viral transport medium provided by the laboratory.

4. The type of specimen and clinical syndrome should be clearly recorded, as different processing steps prior to attempted isolation are necessary for different types of samples.

B. Specimen collection and transport guidelines

1. **Blood.** Whole blood (anticoagulated with heparin or ethylenediaminetetra-acetic acid [EDTA]) can be used to isolate viruses from the leukocytes (e.g., cytomegalovirus, HIV). Enteroviruses can be isolated from both serum and leukocyte-rich preparations.

2. **Nasal secretions.** A cotton swab on a fine wire is introduced through the anterior nares into the nasopharynx. Alternatively, a regular cotton swab is inserted into each anterior naris. These are placed in a viral transport medium. **Nasal washings** (e.g., for respiratory syncytial virus) are collected by instilling 4–5 ml of veal infusion broth into each nostril while the patient extends his or her neck slightly and closes the posterior pharynx (by pushing against the *K* sound). The head is tilted forward, and a sample is collected in a clean container held beneath the nose.

3. **Pharynx.** A swabbing of the posterior pharynx should be accomplished by vigorously rubbing the swab over both tonsillar areas and the posterior pharyngeal wall.

4. **Vesicular fluid.** After decontamination of overlying skin, lesion is aspirated with a Pasteur pipette or a small-gauge needle attached to a tuberculin syringe, or the vesicle is opened and fluids and cellular elements collected from the base onto a swab. If a crust is present, the crust should be lifted off; the fluid beneath the crust can then be swabbed.

5. **Cerebrospinal fluid.** Collect 1–3 ml into a sterile container.

6. **Urine.** Collect 5–10 ml of a clean-catch, midstream urine into a sterile container and process immediately or store refrigerated. **Urine should never be frozen.**

7. **Feces.** Place a 2- to 5-g sample into a clean specimen container without transport medium. A rectal swab is less satisfactory but can be obtained by inserting a cotton-tipped swab stick 5 cm into the rectum and gently rotating the swab. In contrast to rectal cultures for the recovery of gonococci, some fecal material **should** be obtained when doing swabs for viral studies.

C. Viral cultures require living cells to support their replication. Most microbiology laboratories now rely on cell cultures rather than eggs or laboratory animals for virus isolation. Patient specimens are inoculated into cell cultures and incubated at 33°–36°C for 2–14 days. Periodically, the inoculated cultures are examined microscopically for evidence of viral growth. Most viruses are detected within 7 days [13].

V. Mycobacterial cultures. The major obstacle in culturing specimens for mycobacteria is the presence of large numbers of contaminating organisms. Prompt processing of individually collected fresh specimens is preferable to pooled samples, in which overgrowth of other microorganisms can occur.

A. Take appropriate specimens. See Table 25-3.

B. If delays in processing are anticipated, specimens should be refrigerated at 4°C. **If gastric specimens cannot be processed promptly, they should be adjusted to pH 7** with sodium bicarbonate so that the gastric acidity will not affect the viability of the organisms.

C. Because mycobacteria may be present in the sample in low numbers, multiple specimens of relatively large volumes should be cultured when possible (sputum, fluid [CSF, in particular]).

D. Sterile, wide-mouth containers with fitted caps should be used. Mycobacteria sometimes adhere to wax-coated surfaces; therefore, **waxed containers should be avoided.**

E. During specimen collection and handling, care should be taken to avoid the production of infectious aerosols, and **specimens should be labeled clearly to indicate a possible biologic hazard.**

F. *M. tuberculosis* usually grows on conventional solid media (e.g., Lowenstein-Jensen) in 2–4 weeks, but cultures routinely are observed for 6–10 weeks before

Table 25-3. Specimens for culture of mycobacteria

Source	Recommended number	Volume	Comments
Respiratory tract			
Sputum	3	5–10 ml	Saliva inappropriate
Bronchoscopy washing (e.g., bronchoalveolar lavage, BAL)	1		See Chap. 9
Gastric washing	2–3	30–50 ml	Useful if respiratory secretions are not available; early-morning specimens required before eating or activity; small volume of sterile water can be used in the tube placement (20–30 ml); requires rapid delivery (within 30–60 min) to microbiology laboratory to prevent inactivation of organism; stains may at times be helpful (saprophytes may cause false positive smears) (see Chap. 9)
Urine	2–3	Maximum volume of single specimen	Use first-voided midstream collections; avoid 24-hr collection (too much bacterial overgrowth); stains may at times be helpful (saprophytes may cause false positive smears) (see Chap. 9)
Cerebrospinal fluid		Maximum volume available	
Other: joint, pleural, and peritoneal fluid		Maximum volume available	
Blood	1–2	10 ml	Useful for the recovery of *Mycobacterium avium* from patients with AIDS (see Chap. 19)

being reported as negative. The introduction of a radiometric system for the cultivation of mycobacteria has significantly shortened the time required for the recovery of *M. tuberculosis* as well as other *Mycobacterium* spp. [2, 3].

G. Most laboratories differentiate between *M. tuberculosis* and atypical mycobacteria or mycobacteria other than tuberculosis (MOTT) with a few simple biochemical tests. This usually is accomplished within 1 or 2 weeks. Complete speciation of MOTT usually is done by larger laboratories; others send such isolates to reference laboratories for speciation [2, 3, 14]. See related discussion in Chap. 9.

H. Nucleic acid probes. In some laboratories, *M. tuberculosis* and *M. avium* are identified specifically through the use of commercially available nucleic acid probes [2]. See related discussion later in this chapter (sec. **II** under Nucleic Acid Techniques for Direct Detection).

I. Susceptibility tests were not routinely performed on *M. tuberculosis* isolates in the past, unless there were epidemiologic reasons to suspect drug resistance, because prior to 1989 resistance was rare. However, owing to the recent emergence of multidrug-resistant *M. tuberculosis* (MDR-TB), past practice has changed. The **Centers for Disease Control** (Atlanta) **now recommends that initial isolates from all patients be tested for susceptibility to first-line antituberculous drugs** [3] (see Antimicrobial Susceptibility Testing, under Laboratory Guidance in Therapy).

VI. Chlamydiae. Because of the importance of chlamydiae as etiologic agents in conjunctivitis, pneumonia in infancy, urethritis, cervicitis, and pelvic inflammatory disease, isolation of this organism is a potentially helpful diagnostic maneuver. Chlamydiae, like viruses, are obligate intracellular parasites and must be cultivated in living cells. Diagnosis may be attempted either by culture or by direct antigen detection in the clinical specimens. See related discussions in Chap. 13.

A. Growth in cell culture is the most sensitive method for detecting *Chlamydia trachomatis*. Patient specimens (e.g., sputum, cervical scrapings, urethral discharge) must be placed in special transport media and delivered promptly to the laboratory. Chlamydial growth can be demonstrated by staining with iodine, Giemsa, or fluorescent antibody 2–3 days after cell culture inoculation.

B. Direct detection of *C. trachomatis* in clinical specimens using immunodiagnostic and nucleic acid probe tests is now more widely available than cell culture. Though not as sensitive as cell culture, such tests are more convenient and generally less expensive [15, 16]. (See Chap. 13.)

VII. Mycoplasma. Despite the clinical importance of *Mycoplasma pneumoniae* in respiratory infections, techniques to culture *M. pneumoniae* from clinical specimens are not widely available. This organism is slow-growing, and positive culture results often are not available for 7–14 days. Therefore, serologic studies (cold-agglutinin titers or complement-fixing antibodies) are still most commonly used for diagnosis (see Chap. 9).

VIII. Tests for bacterial exotoxins

A. Exotoxins are the major virulence determinant for a number of organisms. Well-known exotoxin-induced disease processes include tetanus, diphtheria, toxic shock syndrome, botulism, cholera, and diarrhea caused by *Clostridium difficile* and enterotoxigenic *Escherichia coli* among others. Most laboratory tests for the detection of bacterial toxins are complex and technically difficult. **With the exception of *C. difficile*, tests for bacterial toxin production generally are performed only in reference laboratories** and only in special circumstances.

B. *C. difficile* appears to cause up to 25% of antibiotic-associated diarrhea and is known to play an important role in the development of pseudomembranous colitis. A variety of assays are available for the detection of *C. difficile* in stool specimens, but tests based on demonstration of cytotoxic activity in cell culture are viewed as the gold standard. Such assays are sensitive and correlate well with the presence of disease [17]. (See Chap. 28A.)

Interpretation of Culture Results

I. Contamination, colonization, and infection. Growth of microorganisms in culture does not necessarily represent infection.

A. Contamination refers to the introduction of extraneous organisms into the culture during specimen collection or processing. Contaminating organisms may originate from the skin of the patient, the clinician, or the laboratory technician, or from laboratory materials and the inanimate environment.

B. Colonization of a body site refers to the **presence of organisms,** including potential pathogens, that are **not causing infection** (i.e., without evidence of illness, tissue invasion, or inflammation). Colonizing bacteria, for example, normally inhabit the oropharynx, skin, colon, vagina, and surfaces of wounds.

C. **To determine the clinical significance of culture data, the clinician must interpret all culture results in the context of (1) the clinical condition of the patient, (2) the site cultured, (3) the method of specimen collection, and (4) the identity and quantity of organisms recovered.** See chapters on specific infections for further discussion—for example, wound infections in Chap. 4, and pneumonia in Chap. 9.

II. **Failure to culture or detect a suspected pathogen** can be caused by a number of factors; many are related to improper collection and transport.

  A. **Incorrect diagnosis** can occur. Infection may not be present or may be caused by organisms that are not cultured routinely (e.g., viruses, rickettsiae, or mycoplasmas).

  B. **Misinterpretations of Gram-stained smears** also can occur, and artifacts might be interpreted as organisms.

  C. **Inadequate specimens** that are not representative of material at the true site of infection may be examined.

  D. **Improper technique or delayed transport of specimens** may cause overgrowth by indigenous flora or loss of anaerobes or fastidious organisms.

  E. **Antimicrobial therapy** prior to specimen collection may kill or inhibit the growth of organisms.

  F. **Improper culture methods** may be employed. Special isolation techniques are necessary for anaerobes, mycobacteria, viruses, and certain fungi and bacteria. The physician must inform the microbiology laboratory of clinically suspected pathogens so that appropriate cultures can be performed.

III. **Preliminary identification of bacteria,** though not definitive, may assist the clinician in early diagnosis and choice of empiric antibiotic therapy. Clinical microbiology personnel can provide guidance in the interpretation of preliminary results. In addition to the Gram stain, results of several tests often are available before an organism is finally identified [18, 19].

  A. **Gram-positive cocci**

   1. **Blood agar hemolysis.** Colonies of streptococci may produce various patterns of hemolysis on blood agar plates.

     a. **Beta-hemolysis** is a clear, colorless zone in the agar surrounding colonies of group A streptococci (*S. pyogenes*), group B streptococci (*S. agalactiae*), and other less common streptococcal pathogens.

     b. **Alpha-hemolysis,** or partial hemolysis, refers to a greenish zone surrounding colonies of *S. pneumoniae* and many species of viridans streptococci that commonly inhabit the upper respiratory and GI tracts.

     c. **Gamma-hemolysis** actually denotes **nonhemolysis** and is observed typically with group D streptococci, including enterococcal and nonenterococcal species.

     d. Note that the **Lancefield serogrouping** of streptococci (groups A, B, C, D, etc.), based on antigenic differences in cell wall carbohydrates, is an independent classification system that **should not be confused with the hemolytic patterns** of streptococci.

   2. **Catalase test.** The Gram stain often will help to distinguish between streptococci (chains or pairs) and staphylococci (clusters). If the distinction remains uncertain, a simple catalase test can be helpful. Hydrogen peroxide will bubble on exposure to catalase-positive organisms. Streptococci are catalase-negative, and **staphylococci are catalase-positive.**

   3. **Coagulase test.** Coagulase-positive staphylococci produce an enzyme that coagulates rabbit plasma. A coagulase **slide test** can be performed in minutes but is less sensitive than an overnight coagulase **tube test.** Negative results of a coagulase slide test should be confirmed with a coagulase tube test. *S. aureus* is **coagulase-positive;** *S. epidermidis, S. saprophyticus,* and other staphylococcal species are coagulase-negative. Many laboratories have adopted latex agglutination tests in place of the traditional coagulase test for differentiation between *S. aureus* and other staphylococcal species.

   4. **Nomenclature of gram-positive cocci** is a frequent source of confusion.

     a. **Group A** beta-hemolytic streptococci are *S. pyogenes.*

     b. **Group B** beta-hemolytic streptococci are *S. agalactiae.*

     c. **Group D** streptococci include:

          (1) Enterococcal spp. The majority of clinical isolates of enterococci will be *Enterococcus faecalis* (80–90%) and *E. faecium* (5–10%). Infrequently, *E. avium, E. raffinosus,* and *E. gallinarum* will be found.

          (2) Nonenterococcal species (*S. bovis*). See discussion of this organism in Chap. 2, under Positive Blood Cultures.

      d. Viridans group streptococci, often referred to as *strep viridans,* is not a single species but encompasses many species of alpha-hemolytic streptococci including the *S. milleri* group (*S. anginosus, S. constellatus, S. intermedius*), *S. mitis, S. mutans, S. salivarius,* and *S. sanguis* [20].

   B. Gram-negative bacilli

      1. Lactose fermentation. MacConkey agar plates are used to promote selective growth of gram-negative bacilli. Colonies of **lactose fermenters** (*E. coli* and species of *Klebsiella, Enterobacter,* and *Citrobacter*) appear red on MacConkey plates within 24 hours. **Non–lactose fermenters** (species of *Proteus, Serratia, Salmonella, Shigella, Pseudomonas,* and others) appear colorless or white. **Caution:** Although certain species are typically lactose fermenters (e.g., *E. coli*), some strains of these species are occasionally non–lactose fermenters.

      2. Oxidase test. When oxidase reagent is applied to colonies on a culture plate, oxidase-positive colonies appear purple. *Pseudomonas* spp. are oxidase-positive and Enterobacteriaceae are oxidase-negative.

   C. Gram-positive bacilli often are nonpathogens and viewed as contaminants. At times, they may be true pathogens. These organisms can be spore-forming or non–spore-forming. The most commonly isolated non–spore-forming bacilli are "diphtheroids"—corynebacteria that normally inhabit the skin. However, when repeatedly isolated from normally sterile fluids or sites, they may be pathogenic (e.g., prosthetic device infection) [18]. When isolated from blood or CSF, it is important to distinguish corynebacteria from another non–spore-forming bacillus, *Listeria monocytogenes,* which is motile at room temperature and may cause meningitis in newborn infants, immunocompromised hosts [18], and the elderly.

      The clinical significance of gram-positive bacilli and *Bacillus* spp. is reviewed in detail elsewhere [20a, 20b]. (**Note:** Anaerobic gram-positive bacilli often may be important clostridial spp.)

Direct Detection of Microbial Antigens in Clinical Specimens

A variety of immunodiagnostic tests can be used to detect the presence of microbial antigens in clinical specimens. The basis for all such tests is the reaction of an antibody with the target antigen in the clinical specimen.

  I. Antigen detection methods have successfully been applied to the diagnosis of virtually all classes of microorganism: bacteria, fungi, parasites, and viruses. The target organisms for the most widely used tests are listed in Table 25-4 [21].

  II. There are **advantages and disadvantages specific to** each of the different **types of immunodiagnostic test methods.**

   A. Counterimmunoelectrophoresis (CIE) consists of the application of an electrical current to drive the antigen-antibody precipitin reaction to completion in a gel. Once widely used to detect bacterial antigens in the CSF, urine, and serum of patients with bacterial meningitis and suspected sepsis, **CIE now has been largely replaced by simpler and more sensitive latex agglutination and coagglutination tests.**

   B. Latex agglutination tests generally are rapid (10–15 minutes) and can be performed by individuals with minimal training. However, in some cases, interpretation of the agglutination reactions may pose a problem for the unskilled reader. Latex agglutination tests are used commonly to detect group A beta-hemolytic streptococci in pharyngeal specimens (see Chap. 7) and a variety of bacterial antigens in meningitis (e.g., *H. influenzae* type b, *S. pneumoniae,* and *N. meningitidis*). Kits are also available to test for group B streptococci and cryptococci (see Chap. 5).

   C. Coagglutination testing takes advantage of the fact that protein A in the cell wall of *Staphylococcus aureus* binds the Fc fragment of most IgG immunoglobulins. Heat-inactivated *S. aureus* is coated with specific antibody and, as with the latex agglutination tests, agglutination occurs in the presence of the target antigen.

Table 25-4. Microorganisms commonly detected in clinical specimens
by immunodiagnostic methods

Agent	Name
Bacteria	*Haemophilus influenzae*
	Streptococcus pneumoniae
	Neisseria meningitidis
	Streptococcus, groups A and B
	Legionella pneumophila
	Bordetella pertussis
Fungi	*Cryptococcus neoformans*
Viruses and chlamydiae	Respiratory syncytial virus
	Rotavirus
	Hepatitis B (surface antigen)
	Herpes simplex virus
	Chlamydia trachomatis

    D. **Immunofluorescent** (IF) **and immunocytochemical stains** (e.g., peroxidase, anti-peroxidase) are especially useful for detecting and localizing virus-infected cells in infected organs and tissues. IF stains also are widely used to detect virus-infected cells in specimens from the respiratory tract, *C. trachomatis* elementary bodies in cervical and urethral discharge, and a variety of bacteria (e.g., *T. pallidum, Bordetella pertussis, Legionella* spp.) in clinical specimens.

    E. **ELISA (enzyme-linked immunosorbent assay) tests** have largely replaced their somewhat more difficult to standardize predecessors, **radioimmunoassays,** as tools for antigen detection in clinical laboratories. Although ELISA tests for most agents remain complex and must be performed in the laboratory setting, some are now available in kit form and are so simple that they can be performed in the office or even in the home setting with reasonable accuracy. Simple kits for the detection of group A beta-hemolytic streptococci, *C. trachomatis,* rotavirus, respiratory syncytial virus, and herpes simplex virus are already commercially available and are as reliable as their more complex laboratory counterparts.

III. **Monoclonal and polyclonal antibodies** can be used as both capture and detector antibodies in antigen detection tests. Although monoclonal antibodies are not suitable for all immunodiagnostic tests, they are preferred because they represent a consistent and reliable antibody source. This technique is reviewed in detail elsewhere [22].

IV. The **sensitivity and specificity of antigen detection tests** varies depending both on the test method used and on the target organism. **In general, antigen detection tests are not as sensitive or specific as culture,** but they often do produce results more rapidly and are a less expensive alternative than culture [21].

V. **Clinical applications**

    A. The sensitivity of immunodetection tests (CIE, coagglutination, and latex agglutination) in patients with **meningitis** on initial evaluation of CSF ranges from 82 to 95% for *H. influenzae,* from 40 to 80% for *N. meningitidis,* and from 70 to 80% for *S. pneumoniae.* Unfortunately, immunodetection is less sensitive in cases in which the Gram-stained smear of CSF is negative. In such cases, testing urine and serum for antigen may be of value. Antigen detection tests are most useful in partially treated patients and when CSF indices do not distinguish between bacterial and nonbacterial meningitis [23] (see Chap. 5).

    B. The polysaccharide antigen of **C. neoformans** is readily detected in both the CSF and the serum of patients with active infection. Properly controlled, the **sensitivity of the cryptococcal latex agglutination test approximates that of culture** [5] (see Chaps. 5 and 18).

    C. **The IF test** frequently is used for the rapid diagnosis of infections with *Legionella pneumophila* because cultures may take as long as 3–5 days to become positive. Unfortunately, the sensitivity of IF is low (25–50%) and, although its specificity is high, the generally low prevalence of disease compromises the predictive value of positive results [24] (see Chap. 9).

    D. More than 20 different commercial immunodiagnostic kits are available for the detection of **group A beta-hemolytic streptococci** in pharyngeal specimens. When compared to culture, the sensitivity of such tests ranges from 60 to 90% or more, and the specificity generally is found to be in excess of 95%. Many recommend culture for all antigen-negative specimens because of the reports of low sensitivity [25] (see Chap. 7).

E. Immunodiagnostic tests for **respiratory syncytial virus** now are used widely. Most have very good performance characteristics, with sensitivities and specificities in excess of 90% and 95%, respectively. In large measure, the apparently good performance of such tests is due to intrinsic deficiencies of the gold standard (growth in cell culture) against which they are measured [26].

F. **Legionella urinary antigen.** This test has been discussed in Chap. 9, sec. **VI.F,** under Specific Considerations and Specific Therapy (p. 287) and has been reviewed recently [26a]. Commercially available kits using radioimmunoassay or enzyme immunoassay (EIA) (Binax, Portland, ME) can detect *L. pneumophila,* serogroup 1 in the urine. In a recent report, this was a valuable test to help diagnose legionella pulmonary infection [26a]. Although the urinary assay detects only *L. pneumophila* serogroup 1, this serogroup causes about 80% of cases of legionnaires' disease [26a, 26b]. Because bacterial antigen may persist in urine for days to weeks after initiation of antibiotic therapy, the assay may be positive when other diagnostic tests are negative [26b]; the test could also be positive from a prior and no longer active infection.

G. **Influenza direct antigen tests** were briefly discussed in Chap. 8, sec. **V.B,** under Influenza. For example, the Directigen Flu A antigen detection test (Becton Dickinson, Cockeysville, MD) employs an enzyme immunomembrane filter assay to detect influenza A antigen extracted from suitable patient specimens [26c]. Nasopharyngeal washes or aspirates are preferred as they have more viral particles than do nasal and/or pharyngeal swabs. In patients in whom wash or aspirate techniques are contraindicated, swabs can be used. When positive, this rapid test (which takes less than 1 hour to perform in the laboratory) is very useful in making a rapid diagnosis. The manufacturer reports a specificity of 95%. The sensitivity of the test in multiple laboratories awaits further experience. A negative antigen test therefore should be processed for influenza A viral cultures before the diagnosis of influenza A is excluded. By using a direct antigen test as an adjunct to culture isolation in nursing homes, influenza A often can be identified rapidly so that proper antiviral therapy and infection control measures can be initiated [26d]. A positive test also helps plan isolation and/or therapy in the acute care setting.

Nucleic Acid Techniques for the Direct Detection and Characterization of Microbial Pathogens in Clinical Specimens

In recent years, nucleic acid techniques have been used to address a variety of problems in clinical microbiology. **Although many methods remain research tools, a number are already in use in clinical laboratories.** The general principles of such tests and their applications are summarized in this section.

I. **Molecular epidemiology.** A wide variety of typing methods can be used to determine whether multiple isolates of a species represent a single strain or unrelated strains of the same species. **Phenotypic typing schemes** use characteristics expressed by the organism to determine strain relatedness and include biotyping, antimicrobial susceptibility testing, serotyping, phage typing, and multilocus enzyme electrophoresis. Strain relatedness can also be established with **genotypic typing methods** based on direct analysis of chromosomal and extrachromosomal DNA. Two commonly used techniques, plasmid profile analysis and restriction enzyme analysis, are described in this section; others including pulse field electrophoresis, arbitrarily primed polymerase chain reaction, ribotyping, and Southern blot analysis of chromosomal DNA are described in detail in recent reviews [27–29].

A. **Plasmid fingerprinting** consists of using plasmids (independent circular DNA molecules) as markers for bacterial strains. The plasmids are separated by agarose gel electrophoresis based on their molecular weights. Similar strains of bacteria generally contain the same number of plasmids with the same molecular weight, whereas dissimilar strains have distinct profiles. Plasmid fingerprinting is **useful in epidemiologic studies** and is available through research centers.

1. Plasmid fingerprinting is said to be more accurate than other phenotyping

methods (e.g., biotyping, phage typing, serotyping), but this may be more situational than intrinsic.

2. Plasmid fingerprinting is especially helpful in differentiating species for which no accurate phenotyping schemes have been developed.

3. The application of restriction enzyme analysis (described in **B**) to plasmids increases the sensitivity of the technique in terms of demonstrating differences among strains.

B. Restriction enzyme analysis. Restriction enzymes recognize defined DNA nucleotide sequences and cleave the nucleic acid at specific sites. Once cleaved, the fragmented nucleic acid (plasmid, viral genome, or bacterial genome) is separated by agarose gel electrophoresis based on fragment size. When identical patterns result, regardless of the number of enzymes used, the organisms or plasmids under analysis are considered identical. Identity is more certain if it is established with a number of enzymes with different specificities.

II. **Nucleic acid probe assays** are based on the combination of labeled, single-stranded DNA or RNA molecules (probes) with single-stranded target nucleic acid. Several techniques, including filter, liquid, Southern blot, Northern blot, and in situ hybridization, are in common use, and each exploits the technology in a slightly different way.

Nucleic acid probes are pieces of DNA or RNA labeled with chemiluminescent (light-emitting), affinity (antibody-based), or radioactive reporter molecules that are able to bind to complementary sequences of either DNA or RNA in the target organism. Probe technology exploits the presence of nucleotide sequences that are unique to a given organism or species as a molecular fingerprint for identification [28].

A. Nucleic acid probes have been used to detect directly a wide variety of microorganisms in clinical specimens. Although very useful for specific microorganisms, in many cases, the nucleic acid probe assays appear no more sensitive than antigen detection assays.

The most successful commercial probe systems are those for the direct detection of *N. gonorrhoeae* and *C. trachomatis* in cervical samples [28] (see Chap. 13).

B. Nucleic acid probe–based tests have also been developed to identify rapidly grown organisms in vitro, to detect virulence determinants (e.g., toxins), and to localize antibiotic resistance determinants. For a review of this subject, see Tenover [28].

1. *Mycobacterium* **spp.** The probes that have made the greatest impact on the diagnosis of respiratory disease are the culture confirmation assays designed to identify organisms growing on solid medium or in a liquid medium, such as BACTEC (Becton Dickinson Diagnostic Instrument Systems, Sparks, MD). Probes are available for *M. tuberculosis, M. avium* complex (MAC), *M. kansasii,* and *M. gordonae.* When a combination of the BACTEC and DNA probe is used, *M. tuberculosis* frequently can be identified in less than 2 weeks from the time of specimen collection. Mixed infections (e.g., *M. tuberculosis* and MAC) can likewise be identified [28] (see Chap. 9).

2. *N. gonorrhoeae* culture confirmation probes are available and do not require viable organisms [28].

3. **Other probes** are available for *S. pneumoniae, S. aureus,* group B streptococci, enterococci, *Listeria monocytogenes,* and gram-negative pathogens [28].

III. The **polymerase chain reaction** (PCR) is a nucleic acid amplification method. Within hours, as many as 1 billion copies of DNA can be made from a single target segment of DNA or RNA. The technique has been applied to amplify target microbial nucleic acid in many types of clinical specimens. The amplified product can be detected by any one of a number of methods. The specific advantage of the PCR is its enormous potential for increasing the sensitivity of probe and other nucleic acid–based detection methods. For a recent review of this topic, see Tenover [28] and Eisenstein [30].

Polymerase chain reaction technology is evolving and, at present, many of the tests available through commercial, hospital, and research laboratories cannot be considered standardized. Significant variation in both sensitivity and specificity of such tests has been observed in blinded, interlaboratory comparisons. Until PCR tests are better standardized, the results of such testing for clinical diagnostic purposes must be interpreted with great caution. Woods and Washington [18] emphasize that this **methodology requires extreme care to prevent false-positive reactions due to contamination.** PCR is very useful for the rapid detection of the human immunodeficiency virus [18] (see Chap. 19). Also, in some settings, as in the diagnosis of herpes simplex encephalitis, a carefully performed PCR on the patient's CSF is the optimal way to confirm this diagnosis, short of a brain biopsy (see Chap. 5). The role of PCR is further addressed in individual chapter discussions when relevant.

Serodiagnostic and Immune Status Tests

When attempts to recover an infectious agent are unsuccessful or impractical, or when culture techniques or facilities are not available, **serologic studies** frequently are used to provide a specific diagnosis. Unfortunately, serologic diagnoses often are retrospective, and therapeutic decisions must frequently be made before the serology results are available. Examples of infectious diseases that commonly are diagnosed by serologic methods are syphilis, rubella, *M. pneumoniae,* leptospirosis, toxoplasmosis, Lyme disease, and infectious mononucleosis.

I. **General principles.** The **interpretation of serologic tests** depends on the determination of antibody titers in blood.
   A. **Many different assay techniques exist** for demonstrating antibody titers in various infections. Whether antibody is measured by agglutination, complement fixation, neutralization, ELISA, or other techniques depends on the nature of the antigen, the availability of the assay and, most important, the ability of a given serologic technique to detect antibody. For certain infections such as rubella, the titers obtained with different antibody tests can be used to help assess the likelihood of recent infection.
   B. **Clotted blood specimens** are acceptable for most serologic tests. Blood should be collected in tubes without anticoagulant and can be refrigerated for 2 or 3 days prior to testing. If longer delays are anticipated, the blood should be centrifuged and the serum frozen at $-20°C$.

II. **Clinical applications** of serologic testing are to diagnose acute infection and to determine the immune status of an individual.
   A. **Diagnosis of acute infection** usually is accomplished by comparing acute and convalescent sera pairs. Occasionally, a single acute-phase serum or a single convalescent-phase serum can also be used to diagnose acute infection.
      1. **Paired sera.** Using acute and convalescent sera, a conversion from seronegative to seropositive or a fourfold or greater rise in antibody titer is considered indicative of recent infection. A single blood specimen containing antibody to a specific antigen may indicate that the patient has had prior exposure to that antigen or to a cross-reacting one. **In most cases, single titers are difficult to interpret.**
         a. **Acute-phase serum** should be obtained as early in the course of the illness as possible. In any patient hospitalized with an undiagnosed febrile illness, a 5-ml serum specimen should be frozen for potential use as an acute-phase serum in future serologic studies. It can be discarded if not needed. Blood should be collected aseptically and, to avoid lipemia, preferably during fasting.
         b. **Convalescent-phase serum** should be collected at least 10 days, but preferably 2–4 weeks, after the onset of the illness. **For testing to be valid, both the acute and convalescent sera should be analyzed simultaneously.**
      2. **A single acute-phase serum may be helpful diagnostically in some cases.** IgM antibody typically develops early during primary infection, persists for several weeks, and then becomes undetectable. Therefore, **the presence of IgM** often indicates recent infection, and commercial kits are now available for detecting IgM to hepatitis A virus and to rubella virus.
      3. **A single convalescent-phase serum** can also be used occasionally to diagnose recent infection. For example, a presumptive diagnosis of *Legionella* infection can be made on the basis of a single elevated indirect fluorescent antibody titer (1:256 or greater), because high titers persist only transiently after infection.
   B. **Immune status testing** of an individual may be important in certain situations. For example, rubella vaccine is recommended for seronegative women of childbearing age as a means of preventing congenital rubella syndrome. Because of the complexity and variety of serologic tests now available, communication with the microbiology laboratory or infectious diseases unit prior to ordering a test is often essential to ensure that the maximum amount of useful information is obtained from the test. **Chapters on individual infectious diseases should be consulted for serologic testing specific for that infection.**

Laboratory Guidance
in Therapy

The two general types of laboratory tests used as aids in therapy are in vitro tests that assess the susceptibility of the infecting organism to various antimicrobial agents and the measurement of antimicrobial concentration or activity in serum or other bodily fluids [18, 19, 31, 32].

Antimicrobial Susceptibility Testing

I. **Disc diffusion test (Kirby-Bauer).** Worldwide, the most widely used method for testing the activity of antimicrobials against bacteria is the disc diffusion test (also called the *agar diffusion test*). Although dilution tests are believed to provide more exact determinations of susceptibility, the standardized Kirby-Bauer disc diffusion test is the initial susceptibility test used in most laboratories because of its ease of performance, reproducibility, and proven value as a guide to antimicrobial therapy.

A. **Method.** Paper discs impregnated with a standardized quantity of antimicrobial agent are applied to the surface of an agar plate that has been inoculated with a suspension of the organism to be tested. The antimicrobial agent diffuses from the paper disc through the agar in a continuously decreasing gradient. After 16–20 hours of incubation, a concentric zone of growth inhibition around the paper disc can be measured. In general, large zones of inhibition are associated with susceptibility of the organism to the antibiotic, and small or absent zones with resistance. Standards for interpretation of the zones of inhibition have been based on quantitative determinations of susceptibility or resistance by broth or agar dilution tests. The disc diffusion test is applicable only to rapidly growing organisms such as the Enterobacteriaceae and *Staphylococcus* and *Pseudomonas* spp. Its reproducibility depends on strictly standardized methods.

B. **Clinical application.** Disc diffusion susceptibility testing is indicated for clinically significant isolates that have unpredictable sensitivity patterns, such as the Enterobacteriaceae and *Staphylococcus* and *Pseudomonas* spp. Susceptibility testing also is indicated for any isolate from normally sterile bodily fluids such as blood and CSF. Disc diffusion testing need not be performed routinely for organisms that are uniformly sensitive or resistant to a particular antibiotic; for example, group A streptococci and *N. meningitidis* are uniformly sensitive to penicillin G.

C. **Interpretation.** A three-category system of reporting results of disc diffusion testing often is used.

   1. **Susceptible (sensitive)** implies that an infection due to the tested strain should respond to an appropriate dose of the antibiotic recommended for that type of infection.

   2. **Resistant** indicates that the strain is not completely inhibited by antimicrobial concentrations within the therapeutic range, and it strongly predicts failure when that particular antibiotic is used alone.

   3. **Intermediate** indicates that a clinical response may occur if unusually high concentrations of relatively nontoxic antibiotics can be achieved at the site of the infection. **For most situations, however, a strain classified as intermediate should be considered resistant until proven otherwise.** If clinical circumstances favor the use of that particular antimicrobial, dilution susceptibility testing may be performed to determine the actual sensitivity or resistance of the organism to the drug. **Some laboratories will routinely report all intermediate zones of inhibition as resistant.**

D. **Limitations**

   1. **For some organisms, susceptibility testing by the disc diffusion method is not applicable.**

      a. Organisms that are fastidious, slow-growing, or have special growth requirements (e.g., anaerobes) cannot be tested. Anaerobic susceptibility testing is discussed in sec. **IV.**

      b. Mycobacterial and fungal susceptibility testing requires specialized techniques that are usually available only in reference laboratories.

   c. Organisms that are part of the normal flora of nonsterile body sites are not routinely tested.

2. Special techniques may be required to detect penicillin-resistant *S. pneumoniae,* oxacillin-resistant (or methicillin-resistant) *S. aureus,* and aminoglycoside-resistant or penicillin-resistant enterococci. See related discussions in Chap. 28 and discussion of the E test in sec. **III.B.**

3. Disc diffusion testing may indicate in vitro susceptibility, despite lack of therapeutic efficacy in actual practice. Examples are *Salmonella typhi* susceptibility to aminoglycosides and enterococcus susceptibility to cephalosporins.

4. **Standards for interpreting zones of growth inhibition are based on achievable serum levels of antimicrobials. Disc diffusion testing, therefore, is not always applicable to urinary tract isolates, because the achievable levels of certain antibiotics in urine are much higher than in serum [33].** For example, an enterococcal isolate resistant to ampicillin by disc diffusion testing may nevertheless be successfully treated with ampicillin if the infection is limited to the urinary tract.

5. Certain antibiotics cannot be accurately tested (e.g., methenamine mandelate and the polymyxins).

6. Bactericidal activity cannot be tested because the disc diffusion method yields bacteriostatic data only.

7. **Simple matching of antibiotic to infecting organism susceptibility pattern is a superficial approach to therapy.** The disc diffusion test is only one aid to assessing potential response of the infection. Factors such as host defense mechanisms; site of infection; underlying illnesses; route, dose, and penetration of the antibiotic into the infected site; and duration of antibiotic therapy must always be considered (see Chap. 28).

II. **Dilution susceptibility tests** are used to determine the **minimum inhibitory concentration** (MIC) and the **minimum bactericidal concentration** (MBC) of an antibiotic for an infecting organism. The **MIC of the drug is defined as the lowest concentration that prevents visible growth of the test organism** under a standardized set of conditions (Fig. 25-1). The **MBC of the drug is the lowest concentration that results in complete killing of the test organism** or that permits no more than a 0.1% survival of the initial inoculum under standardized conditions. The MIC and MBC are expressed quantitatively in micrograms, international units, or micromoles of antibiotic per milliliter. Dilution susceptibility testing can be done by a broth dilution or agar dilution method.

A. **Methods**

1. **Broth dilution tests.** Serial, twofold dilutions of an antimicrobial are incorporated into broth-containing tubes, which are then inoculated with a standard number of organisms, usually 10^5–10^6 colony-forming units (CFU) per milliliter. After the culture has been incubated at 35°C for 16–20 hours with traditional technology, the tubes are inspected for visible growth. (Rapid techniques are also available. See sec. **E.**) The MIC of the drug is the lowest concentration that prevents visible growth. If the tubes with no visible growth are subcultured quantitatively to a drug-free medium, the MBC of the antimicrobial can be determined, as indicated in Fig. 25-1. **Microdilution susceptibility** testing employs the same principles but uses wells on a microtiter tray rather than dilution tubes, permitting miniaturization and automation of the MIC determination.

2. **Agar dilution test.** The agar dilution test is very similar to the broth technique except that the antibiotic dilutions are incorporated into a solid medium and the inoculum, usually 10^4 CFU/ml, is applied as a spot to a small portion of the agar plate. The MIC again is recorded as the lowest antibiotic concentration that prevents visible growth. In contrast to the broth dilution technique, an MBC cannot be determined with agar dilution.

B. **Clinical application.** Several commercially manufactured **semiautomated systems are now available that permit routine MIC determinations for all clinically significant bacterial isolates.** Therefore, microbiology laboratories now have the option of using disc diffusion susceptibility testing or semiautomated microdilution susceptibility testing on a routine basis. The dilution susceptibility principles discussed in this chapter are applicable to MIC testing performed on an individual basis or by commercial, semiautomated methods. **If not routinely performed on all isolates, dilution susceptibility testing (MIC and MBC determinations) should be considered when the following conditions apply:**

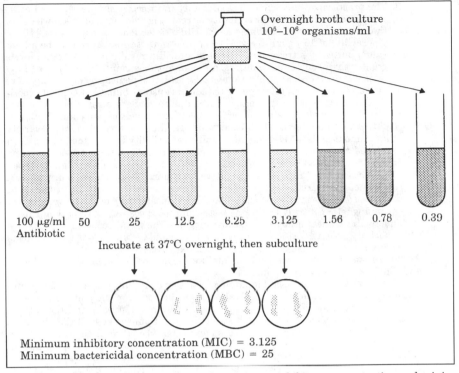

Fig. 25-1. Dilution susceptibility testing for minimum inhibitory concentration and minimum bactericidal concentration determination.

1. Disc diffusion testing has yielded intermediate susceptibility to an antibiotic (e.g., an aminoglycoside) chosen to treat a serious infection.
2. Complicated or life-threatening infections exist owing to organisms with an unpredictable susceptibility pattern.
3. Serious infections caused by organisms susceptible only to relatively toxic agents exist.
4. Determination of a bactericidal end point is desirable, as in endocarditis.
5. Disc diffusion results are unreliable, as with relatively fastidious or slow-growing organisms.
6. An infection has failed to respond to an antibiotic, despite in vitro susceptibility of the infecting organism determined by disc diffusion testing.

C. **Interpretations.** The MIC of an organism may be useful in selecting an antibiotic that will be active against that organism at the site of the infection. Generally, if an antibiotic can be administered so that its serum or tissue level exceeds its MIC for the responsible organism at the site of infection, the infection should respond to therapy. Because it usually is not possible to measure tissue concentrations of the antibiotic, a blood level that exceeds the MIC twofold to eightfold is a commonly accepted guideline. This is an arbitrary definition of acceptable blood levels of antibiotic and does not take into account variable penetration into different tissues or the role of host defense mechanisms. See related discussions of time-dependent and concentration-dependent bactericidal activity in Chap. 28A (pp. 1080–1081).

D. **Limitations**
1. Dilution tests for MIC and MBC values often are more expensive and more technically demanding than is disc diffusion testing.
2. Lack of interlaboratory standardization makes interpretation difficult.

3. The practitioner may experience difficulty in interpreting the MIC and MBC results. Assessment of susceptibility or resistance depends on a knowledge of the antibiotic levels achievable at the site of infection. For example, a MIC of piperacillin of 16 μg/ml to *Pseudomonas aeruginosa* may appear to be a high value, but a 3-g intravenous dose of piperacillin results in peak serum levels greater than 100 μg/ml, and thus, a *Pseudomonas* strain with a MIC of 16 μg/ml is considered susceptible. Conversely, a MIC of penicillin G of 0.5 μg/ml to viridans streptococci may appear to indicate susceptibility, but clinical experience has documented that endocarditis due to viridans streptococci with this MIC is relatively resistant to achievable serum levels of penicillin G.

E. **Rapid versus conventional MIC methods.** In the last several years, a variety of instrument-assisted identification and susceptibility test methods have been developed that permit generation of test results in a period of 6–9 hours, as opposed to the 15–24 hour time frame required with traditional overnight methods [33a]. These newer "rapid" methods have, in general, been shown to provide test results nearly as accurate as those derived from traditional overnight tests, but the newer tests are more expensive [33a]. The clinical impact of this newer technology and whether it truly facilitates faster and more cost-effective patient care is undergoing clinical study. One study suggests the rapid tests have a positive impact on patient care [33a]. The exact role of rapid tests versus traditional tests awaits further clinical experience and comparative studies.

III. **Antimicrobial concentration gradient methods** combine features of disc diffusion and dilution susceptibility testing.

A. The **spiral gradient endpoint method** employs an agar plate containing a continuous gradient of antibiotic concentration from the center of the plate to the edge; the test organism is applied to the plate in a radial streak, and the MIC is determined by measuring the distance of growth from the edge of the plate.

B. **E test** (AB Biodisk, Solna, Sweden) is a method based on the diffusion of a continuous concentration gradient of an antimicrobial agent from a plastic strip into an agar medium. This newly developed (1988) in vitro technique was created to overcome several of the disadvantages of the disc diffusion and dilution techniques and also to retain the principle of the agar dilution method by producing an accurate, reproducible, quantitative MIC result [33b] (Fig. 25-2).

1. **Procedure** [33b]

   a. An inert thin plastic carrier strip with a predefined continuous concentration gradient of dried and stabilized antibiotic on one side and a continuous MIC interpretive scale corresponding to a range of 15 log₂ dilutions on the other side is used.

   b. After an agar plate is inoculated with a broth suspension of the test organism, four to six E strips can be placed on the plate, which is incubated.

2. **MIC result.** After incubation, an ellipse of inhibition is formed around the strip, and the MIC is read at the point where the ellipse intersects the strip edge (see Fig. 25-2). Studies evaluating E test performance compared with routine susceptibility testing methods have demonstrated excellent agreement [33b].

3. **Potential uses.** The role the E test will play in microbiology laboratories awaits further clinical study. However, it appears to be a useful laboratory technique especially for in vitro susceptibility testing of organisms for which there is not a "routine" or "standardized" approach or **for fastidious organisms.** Examples include *S. pneumoniae* [33c], *H. influenzae, Neisseria* spp., anaerobes (see sec. **IV.B**), enterococci, methicillin-resistant *S. aureus,* and testing for the presence and susceptibility of extended-spectrum beta-lactamase–producing organisms.

4. Its major drawback may be its relatively higher cost when compared with currently available susceptibility tests. However, in certain clinical situations **(e.g., in the isolation of *S. pneumoniae* from a normally sterile bodily fluid), this appears to be an easy and useful technique to determine whether the clinical isolate is susceptible, intermediately susceptible, or resistant to penicillin (see Chap. 28C).**

IV. **Susceptibility testing of anaerobic bacteria is not routinely available in most hospitals.** In recent years, however, anaerobic susceptibility testing has assumed greater importance because susceptibility patterns are known to be less predictable than once was believed, susceptibilities vary between institutions, and the clinical significance of anaerobic bacteria is more widely appreciated [34]. Total reliance on published susceptibility patterns may be misleading. For example, 10% or more of *B. fragilis* infections may be resistant to clindamycin in many institutions [35, 36]. These variable

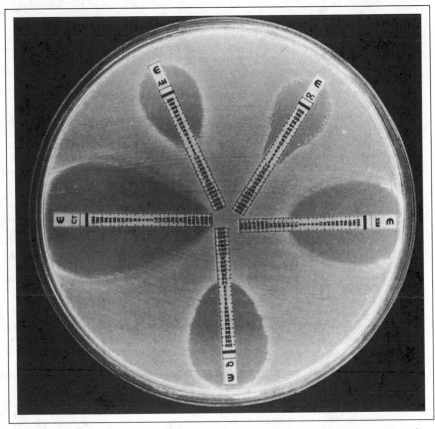

Fig. 25-2. E tests with a beta-lactamase-producing *Haemophilus influenzae* strain performed with HTM agar. Antibiotic abbreviations on the E-test strips and minimum inhibitory concentration interpretations (indexed to base 1) are as follows: *AM* = ampicillin, 8 µg/ml; *DC* – doxycycline, 4 µg/ml; *XM* = cefuroxime, 1 µg/ml; *CF* = cefaclor, 2 µg/ml; *CT* = cefotaxime, 0.015 µg/ml. (From J. H. Jorgensen et al., Quantitative antimicrobial susceptibility testing of *Haemophilus influenzae* and *Streptococcus pneumoniae* by using the E test. *J. Clin. Microbiol.* 29:109, 1991.)

patterns of resistance among institutions must be considered when choosing therapy. Hospitals may elect to monitor anaerobic susceptibility patterns periodically as a general guide to empiric antibiotic selection [18, 36a].

A. **Susceptibility testing of specific anaerobic isolates can assist in the management of patients with selected infections** [34, 37], as follows:

  1. **Serious anaerobic infections** such as endocarditis, brain abscess, empyema, or bone and joint infections, especially when an anaerobic pathogen is isolated in pure culture

  2. **Anaerobic infections that persist or recur** despite presumed appropriate empiric antibiotic therapy directed at anaerobes

B. **Methods** of anaerobic susceptibility testing [18, 19, 31, 34].

  1. **Agar dilution** susceptibility tests are performed in reference laboratories but are time-consuming and impractical for most clinical microbiology laboratories.

  2. **Broth microdilution** tests are manageable for clinical laboratories. Microdilution trays are commercially available.

  3. **Antimicrobial density gradient** methods, such as the E test, are applicable to anaerobic susceptibility testing and are simple to perform (see sec. **II.B**). Although expensive, these simpler tests may play an increasing role in the hospi-

tal laboratory. The E test compared favorably with the reference agar dilution method in a recent study [37a].

4. **Determination of beta-lactamase production.** Laboratories unable to perform susceptibility tests may assay gram-negative anaerobes for beta-lactamase activity, which is indicative of resistance to penicillins and cephalosporins. A commercial disc test is available. However, a negative result must be interpreted with caution, as resistance to beta-lactam antibiotics may also be mediated by mechanisms other than beta-lactamase production.

V. **Susceptibility testing of antibiotic combinations** in vitro attempts to identify antibiotic combinations that are superior to therapy with single agents. (See the discussion of the use of antibiotic combinations in Chap. 28A under Principles of Antibiotic Use.) A combination of antibiotics is considered to be synergistic when the effect of the combination is greater than the sum of the independent effects of each agent and antagonistic when the combined effect of the two antibiotics is less than the effect of each single antibiotic. Testing for synergistic and antagonistic activity can be done by a "checkerboard" technique, a "killing curve" technique, or disc diffusion [31, 38].

Susceptibility testing of antibiotic combinations has been advocated for certain situations such as *P. aeruginosa* sepsis in the immunocompromised patient [39, 40], but **the techniques used to assess antibiotic synergy lack interlaboratory standardization and are cumbersome and often expensive.** Moreover, correlation between in vitro testing and in vivo (clinical) efficacy of combination antibiotic therapy is uncertain. For these reasons, the **usefulness** of susceptibility testing of antibiotic combinations is **debatable,** and consultation with a specialist in infectious diseases is recommended if such testing is contemplated.

VI. **Beta-lactamase test**

A. **Principle and technique.** Resistance of *H. influenzae* and *N. gonorrhoeae* to the penicillin class of antibiotics may be due to the production of plasmid-mediated beta-lactamase enzymes. The development of rapid assays for beta-lactamase permits an assessment of sensitivity to the penicillins before standard disc diffusion or broth dilution susceptibility testing results are available. Rapid acidometric, iodometric, and chromogenic cephalosporin methods currently are used to detect beta-lactamase production. Bacteria can be tested after overnight growth in media, and results usually are available within 30 minutes [19].

B. **Clinical application**

1. *H. influenzae* **infections** will not respond to ampicillin if the strain produces beta-lactamase. Because ampicillin resistance is an increasing problem, **no serious or life-threatening** *H. influenzae* **infection should be treated with ampicillin alone until sensitivity to ampicillin has been established.** Rapid testing of the isolate for beta-lactamase should be performed, and ampicillin should not be used if the test is positive. The absence of beta-lactamase signifies ampicillin sensitivity. However, certain rare strains of *H. influenzae* are negative by beta-lactamase testing but are resistant to ampicillin by disc diffusion testing. Therefore, ideally, a negative beta-lactamase test (implying ampicillin sensitivity) should be confirmed by disc diffusion testing (see Chaps. 5 and 9).

2. *N. gonorrhoeae* **strains** may exhibit plasmid-mediated production of beta-lactamase, resulting in resistance to penicillin and failure to respond to penicillin therapy. Because of the high prevalence of beta-lactamase-positive *N. gonorrhoeae* in the United States, treatment with a regimen (e.g., ceftriaxone) active against resistant strains of gonorrhea is required [41]. **Note:** Absence of beta-lactamase does not guarantee susceptibility of *N. gonorrhoeae* to penicillin, as some strains may possess chromosomally mediated resistance to penicillin (CMRNG), which is independent of beta-lactamase production. (See also Chap. 13, sec. **IV** under Urethritis.)

VII. **Susceptibility testing of** *M. tuberculosis* is essential to the selection of appropriate antibiotic therapy, especially in the setting of increased prevalence of multidrug-resistant tuberculosis. Testing is performed by either a proportion method on solid media or a radiometric method in liquid media (BACTEC system). In the proportion method, which requires 2–3 weeks after isolation of the organism, susceptibility to a drug is defined as growth of the mycobacterial isolate on drug-containing medium that is less than 1% of growth of the same organism on control (drug-free) medium. The radiometric BACTEC system measures and compares growth, by release of carbon 14, of an isolate in a drug-containing vial compared with growth of the same organism in a control vial. Results of radiometric susceptibility testing may be available within 1 week after isolation of the organism. Hospital laboratories that perform susceptibility testing of *M. tuberculosis* routinely test isoniazid, rifampin, ethambutol, and strepto-mycin; reference laboratories perform testing for other agents including pyrazinamide, cycloserine, ethionamide, and fluoroquinolones. Susceptibility testing of mycobacteria other than *M. tuberculosis* is less commonly performed, and correlations between in vitro drug susceptibility of these species and in vivo response to therapy are not well established [42, 42a]. See related discussion in Chap. 9 sec. **IV.A,** under Tuberculosis: Basic Concepts.

VIII. **Fungal and viral susceptibility testing** are not routinely performed in clinical labora-tories. Testing methods and interpretive criteria are not well standardized, and these tests are considered experimental. Infectious disease consultation is advised when questions of antifungal or antiviral susceptibility arise.

Monitoring Antimicrobial Therapy

Two general types of in vitro tests are used to monitor antimicrobial therapy: measure-ment of blood or bodily fluid antibiotic activity against the responsible organism, and assay of actual antibiotic concentrations in blood or other bodily fluids.

I. **The serum bactericidal test** determines the "killing power" **of patient serum** against the infecting organism. The result is expressed as the highest dilution of serum that will produce the desired effect.

A. **Method.** The serum bactericidal test involves a modification of the broth dilution technique. Serum usually is obtained from the patient at times believed to correlate with the maximum or minimum antibacterial activity. Serial, twofold **dilutions of the patient's serum are inoculated with a standard quantity of the infecting organism.** After overnight incubation of the mixtures, the inhibitory and lethal end points are determined as in broth dilution susceptibility testing, shown sche-matically in Fig. 25-3. **The serum inhibitory or bacteriostatic activity** is defined as the highest dilution of serum that demonstrates a visible inhibitory effect. **The serum lethal or bactericidal activity** is similarly expressed as the highest dilution that produces a lethal effect, usually defined as a 99.9% or greater reduction of viable organisms in the initial inoculum. Bactericidal activity of other bodily fluids such as CSF, urine, and synovial fluid also can be measured by a modification of this method.

1. **Variables.** The measurement of serum bactericidal activity is influenced by numerous technical variables. These include the type of serum or broth diluent used, whether serum complement is or is not inactivated, the concentration of magnesium and calcium ions in the media, and the definition of the bacteri-cidal end point. For example, a patient's serum containing highly protein-bound antibiotics may show greater bactericidal activity if diluted in nutrient broth (which has a low protein concentration) rather than in pooled human serum (which has a high protein concentration). **The lack of interlaboratory standardization in the performance of these tests makes it difficult to com-pare results between studies** [43, 43a].

2. **Timing of sample.** Several authors favor collection of the serum sample at peak, whereas others prefer trough levels. The utility of peak versus trough serum bactericidal activity remains controversial [43].

B. **Clinical application.** Many authorities advocate using serum inhibitory or bacteri-cidal activity as the best indicator of potential therapeutic efficacy. The test is the most reliable in vitro correlate of actual in vivo conditions because it accounts for other components of the antibacterial activity of serum in addition to the antibiotic (i.e., serum complement, opsonins, lysozymes). However, clinical appli-cability of the serum bactericidal titer remains to be proven rigorously [43], and its use remains somewhat controversial [18, 44]. **Infectious disease consultation is advised to assist in the appropriate utilization and interpretation of serum bactericidal tests.**

A determination of serum bactericidal activity may prove useful in guiding therapy, particularly in the following situations:

1. **Endocarditis** may be more effectively treated when higher serum bactericidal activity can be achieved. However, the results of serum bactericidal tests are not necessarily predictive of survival or clinical cure, and the peak and trough bactericidal titers that best correlate with outcome are not yet clear [43, 43a, 45]. Although a peak bactericidal titer of at least 1:8 is most frequently recommended, one study concluded that a peak titer of 1:64 or more and a trough titer of 1:32 or more were most predictive of bacteriologic cure

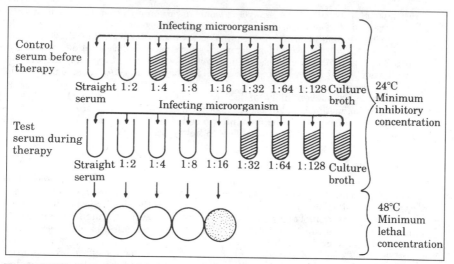

Fig. 25-3. Dilution susceptibility testing for serum inhibitory and serum lethal activity. Serum minimum inhibitory concentration = 1:16; serum bactericidal concentration = 1:8. (Adapted from H. M. Sommers, Drug Susceptibility Testing in Vitro—Monitoring of Antimicrobial Therapy. In G. P. Youmans, P. Y. Paterson, and H. M. Sommers [eds.], *The Biologic and Clinical Basis of Infectious Diseases* [2nd ed.]. Philadelphia: Saunders, 1980.)

of endocarditis; the test was a poor predictor of bacteriologic failure [46]. **The bactericidal titer may be particularly helpful in the following circumstances** [43]:

a. When endocarditis is caused by organisms that are not highly sensitive to the antibiotics being used, and a synergistic combination of antibiotics might be more effective

b. When less well established treatment regimens are employed

c. When the patient fails to improve on standard therapy

d. When the serum bactericidal titer is very high and drug toxicity is a significant risk, in which case the drug dose might be reduced without compromising antibacterial effect

2. In acute and chronic **osteomyelitis,** serum bactericidal titers that exceed certain levels have been correlated with cure [47]. When changing from parenteral to oral therapy of acute hematogenous osteomyelitis in children, bactericidal titers often are monitored to adjust antibiotic dosage to achieve a bactericidal level of 1:8 or more [43a]. The usefulness of serum bactericidal tests in the management of osteomyelitis, particularly in adults, remains uncertain.

3. In the **immunocompromised host,** a serum bactericidal titer of 1:8 or greater has been correlated with successful treatment of bacteremia and soft-tissue infections [48]. Higher bactericidal titers may be desirable in the granulocytopenic patient with gram-negative rod bacteremia [49].

4. In patients with acute pulmonary exacerbations of **cystic fibrosis,** peak serum bactericidal titers of 1:128 or greater against the patients' pulmonary pathogens have been correlated with favorable bacteriologic responses to therapy [50].

II. **Antimicrobial levels** may be obtained to assess the adequacy of the chosen dose and route of administration and to avoid toxicity [19].

A. **Methods**

1. **Correct timing of samples is necessary for accurate interpretation of the significance of antibiotic levels.** The two measurements usually performed are the anticipated peak and trough blood levels of the antimicrobial after a dose has been given.

a. **Peak blood levels** usually are obtained 1 hour after an intramuscular dose, 30 minutes after the completion of an intravenous infusion, or 1–2 hours after an oral dose. In patients with renal insufficiency who receive antimicrobials by the parenteral route, peak levels may be delayed 2–4 hours after an intramuscular antibiotic dose or 1 hour after an intravenous dose.

   b. **Trough blood levels** are obtained immediately before the next dose is due.

   c. The blood should be obtained in tubes free of anticoagulant.

   d. **The sample should be taken promptly to the laboratory** and quickly processed. Some antibiotics rapidly lose activity, and the simultaneous presence of two antibiotics may result in one agent inactivating the other (e.g., carbenicillin can inactivate gentamicin).

   e. The **laboratory requisition** should indicate clearly the antibiotic level desired, time of most recent dose, amount of most recent dose, and any concomitant treatment with other antibiotics.

   2. **Techniques for assay of antibiotic levels.** Prior to 1970, bioassays (agar diffusion and broth dilution) were the most commonly used techniques to assay for levels of antibiotics in bodily fluids. Bioassays have been largely supplanted by a variety of more accurate and reproducible methods (e.g., immunoassays and high-pressure liquid chromatography).

   a. **Bioassays** are performed by parallel dilution of both antibiotic standards and the patient's bodily fluid. The dilutions then are tested for their ability to inhibit the growth of an indicator organism. The quantity of antibiotic in the bodily fluid is derived from the relationship between the degree of inhibition of the indicator organism by the bodily fluid and the inhibition by the antibiotic standards. Because bioassays depend on the inhibitory effects of an antibiotic on an organism, they lack specificity (i.e., they cannot differentiate between the effects of two or more antibiotics present in a bodily fluid). **Therefore, it is essential to submit complete and accurate information about combination antimicrobial therapy with specimens sent for bioassay.** With such information, the laboratory can sometimes circumvent the problem by technical manipulations (e.g., add beta-lactamase to inhibit penicillins, use multidrug-resistant indicator organisms, or remove antibiotics with cation-exchange resins). **Most bioassay systems are not as precise as other types of assays** but, when the tests are performed carefully with adequate controls, the precision generally is adequate for clinical use.

   b. **Immunologic assays** are presently the **most widely used** method for determining antibiotic levels in bodily fluids. They exploit the specificity of the antigen-antibody (antimicrobial-antibody) reaction and use sophisticated instrumentation. More simple latex agglutination tests have also been developed and marketed for the semiquantitative assay of aminoglycoside antibiotics. Immunoassays have gained widespread acceptance because they are rapid, accurate, specific, and easier to perform than bioassays. **Aminoglycoside** and **vancomycin** levels now are routinely available in many laboratories using the immunoassay method.

   c. **High-pressure liquid chromatography** is a method for separating compounds; quantitation is subsequently achieved by analysis of the separated compounds. Liquid chromatographic procedures have been developed to measure almost all antibiotics in clinical specimens but are used most widely for chloramphenicol because no suitable immunoassay has been developed for this drug. Immunoassays generally are favored because they are simpler to perform.

B. **Clinical application.** Determination of antibiotic levels may be considered in the following situations:

   1. When complicated or life-threatening infections exist secondary to organisms with MIC or MBC values near the maximum achievable levels of the antibiotic being used. Pneumonia and bacteremia due to gram-negative organisms may respond more favorably to treatment when therapeutic plasma levels of aminoglycosides are achieved [51, 52]. A high peak concentration of aminoglycoside relative to the MIC for the infecting organism has been correlated with improved clinical response to therapy [53]. For further discussion of the role of aminoglycoside levels, see Chap. 28H.

   2. When one wishes to monitor therapy with an antibiotic that could have toxic side effects, particularly in the presence of altered hepatic or renal function (e.g., aminoglycosides; see Chap. 28H).

   3. When an infection due to a sensitive organism is not responding to antibiotic treatment and all other therapeutic approaches have been optimized.

C. Interpretation. As a general guide, it is anticipated that an infection will respond to therapy if a level of antibiotic greater than the MIC of the infecting organism can be achieved at the site of infection. However, the relationship between achievable serum levels and response at an extravascular site of infection is variable. Also, factors other than an absolute serum level may be important (e.g., magnitude of level in comparison to MIC, duration of level above the MIC, and effect of serum protein binding). **Determination of an antibiotic level is not a substitute for clinical judgment,** and other therapeutic modalities must always be optimized (e.g., draining abscesses, removing foreign bodies, and bolstering host defense mechanisms). See related discussions of **time-dependent and concentration-dependent bactericidal activity** in Chap. 28A (pp 1080–1081).

References

1. Murray, P.R. Microscopy. In B.B. Wentworth (ed.), *Diagnostic Procedures for Bacterial Infections.* Washington, DC: American Public Health Association, 1987. Pp. 681–691.
2. Nolte, F.S., and Metchock, B. Mycobacterium. In P.R. Murray et al. (eds.), *Manual of Clinical Microbiology* (6th ed.). Washington, DC: American Society for Microbiology, 1995. Pp. 400–437.
3. Tenover, F.C., et al. The resurgence of tuberculosis: Is your laboratory ready? *J. Clin. Microbiol.* 31:767–770, 1993.
3a. Isenberg, H.D. *Clinical Microbiology Procedures Handbook,* Vol. 1. Washington, DC: American Society for Microbiology, 1993. P. 3.4.1.
4. Bickley, L.S., et al. Comparison of direct fluorescent antibody, acridine orange, wet mount, and culture for detection of *Trichomonas vaginalis* in women attending a public sexually transmitted disease clinic. *Sex Transm. Dis.* 16:127–131, 1989.
5. Wu, T., and Koo, S.Y. Comparison of three commercial cryptococcal latex kits for detection of cryptococcal antigen. *J. Clin. Microbiol.* 18:1127, 1983.
5a. Wilson, M.I. General principles of specimen collection and transport. *Clin. Infect. Dis.* 22:766, 1996.
   First article in a series of diagnostic microbiology updates that will appear in this journal.
6. Reller, L.B. Recent innovative methods for detection of bacteremia. *Am. J. Med.* (Suppl. 1B):26, 1983.
   Good review of radiometric, acridine orange, and lysis centrifugation culture techniques.
7. Strand, C.L., and Shulman, J.A. *Blood Stream Infections.* Chicago: ASCP Press, 1988.
   A comprehensive resource on blood cultures.
8. Aronson, M.D., and Bor, D.H. Blood cultures. *Ann. Intern. Med.* 106:246–253, 1987.
9. Smith-Elekes, S., and Weinstein, M.P. Blood cultures. *Infect. Dis. Clin. North Am.* 9:221, 1993.
10. Press, O.W., et al. Hickman catheter infections in patients with malignancies. *Medicine* (Baltimore) 63:189:200, 1984.
   For a related discussion and more recent references, see Catheter-Related Sepsis in Chap. 2.
11. Jousimies-Somer, H.R., and Feingold, S.M. Problems encountered in anaerobic bacteriology. *Rev. Infect. Dis.* 6(Suppl 1):45–50, 1984.
12. Citron, D.M. Specimen collection and transport, anaerobic culture techniques, and identification of anaerobes. *Rev. Infect. Dis.* 6(Suppl 1):51, 1984.
13. Menegus, M.A., and Douglas, R.G., Jr. Viruses, Rickettsiae, Chlamydiae, and Mycoplasmas. In G.L. Mandell, R.G. Douglas, Jr., and J.E. Bennett (eds.), *Principles and Practice of Infectious Diseases* (3rd ed.). New York: Churchill Livingstone, 1990. Pp. 193–205.
   An overview of diagnostic methods.
14. Woods, G.L., and Washington, J.A., II. Mycobacteria other than *Mycobacterium tuberculosis:* Review of microbiologic and clinical aspects. *Rev. Infect. Dis.* 9:275–294, 1987.
15. Batteiger, B.E., and Jones, R.B. Chlamydial infections. *Infect. Dis. Clin. North Am.* 1:55, 1987.
16. Tilton, R.C., et al. Multicenter comparative evaluation of two rapid microscopic methods and culture for detection of *Chlamydia trachomatis* in patient specimens. *J. Clin. Microbiol.* 26:167, 1988.
   Published erratum appears in J. Clin. Microbiol. *26:2233, 1988.*

17. Peterson, L.R., and Kelly, P.J. The role of the clinical microbiology laboratory in the management of *Clostridium difficile*–associated diarrhea. *Infect. Dis. Clin. North Am.* 7:277, 1993.
18. Woods, G.L., and Washington, J.A. The Clinician and the Microbiology Laboratory. In G.L. Mandell, J.E. Bennett, and R. Dolin (eds.), *Principles and Practice of Infectious Diseases* (4th ed.). New York: Churchill Livingstone, 1995. Pp. 169–199.
    An overview of specimen collection and processing, identification of organisms, and determinations of antimicrobial activity.
19. Murray, P., et al. (eds.). *Manual of Clinical Microbiology* (6th ed.). Washington, DC: American Society for Microbiology, 1995.
    Excellent in-depth reference on culture techniques, identification, and significance of microorganisms, antimicrobial susceptibility testing, and the like.
20. Finegold, S.M. (ed.). Summary of current nomenclature, taxonomy, and classification of various microbial agents. *Clin. Infect. Dis.* 16:597–615, 1993.
20a. Sliman, R., et al. Serious infections caused by *Bacillus* species. *Medicine* (Baltimore) 66:218, 1987.
20b. Berkowitz, F.E. The gram-positive bacilli: A review of the microbiology, clinical aspects, and antimicrobial susceptibilities of a heterogeneous group of bacteria. *Pediatr. Infect. Dis. J.* 13:1126, 1994.
21. Tilton, R.C. Microbial Antigen Detection. In B.B. Wentworth (ed.), *Diagnostic Procedures for Bacterial Infections*. Washington, DC: American Public Health Association, 1987. Pp. 693–702.
22. Payne, W.J., Jr., et al. Clinical laboratory applications of monoclonal antibodies. *Clin. Microbiol. Rev.* 1:313–329, 1988.
23. Wilson, C.B., and Smith, A.L. Rapid tests for the diagnosis of bacterial meningitis. *Curr. Clin. Top. Infect. Dis.* 7:134–156, 1986.
24. Winn, W.C., Jr. *Legionella* and the clinical microbiologist. *Infect. Dis. Clin. North Am.* 9:377, 1993.
25. Gerber, M.A. Rapid diagnosis of group A beta-hemolytic streptococcal pharyngitis. Use of antigen detection tests. *Diagn. Microbiol. Infect. Dis.* 4(Suppl.):5–15, 1986.
    A comprehensive review. See related discussions in Chap. 7 on page 218 of this book.
26. Welliver, R.C. Detection, pathogenesis, and therapy of respiratory syncytial virus infections. *Clin. Microbiol. Rev.* 1:27–39, 1988.
    See related discussions in Chap. 8, under Bronchiolitis.
26a. Plouffe, J.F., et al. Reevaluation of the definition of legionnaire's disease: Use of the urinary antigen assay. *Clin. Infect. Dis.* 20:1286, 1995.
    The urinary antigen assay gave a positive result in fewer than 1% of non-cases but was positive in 55.9% of all cases. The assay was most sensitive (80%) in cases in which L. pneumophila serogroup 1 was isolated. The commercially available radioimmunoassay kit was used. Study concludes that the urinary antigen assay will be a valuable tool in the prompt diagnosis of legionnaires' disease. The test is currently not in widespread use.
26b. Edelstein, P.H. Legionnaires' disease. *Clin. Infect. Dis.* 16:741, 1995.
    State-of-the-art review. See related references in Chap. 9.
26c. Johnston, S.L., and Bloy, H. Evaluation of a rapid enzyme immunoassay for detection of influenza A virus. *J. Clin. Microbiol.* 31:142, 1993.
26d. Leonardi, G.P., et al. Comparison of rapid detection methods for influenza A virus and their value in health-care management of institutionalized geriatric patients. *J. Clin. Microbiol.* 32:70, 1994.
27. Tompkins, L.S. The use of molecular methods in infectious diseases. *N. Engl. J. Med.* 327:1290–1297, 1992.
    See related update by S.P. Naber, Molecular pathology: Diagnosis of infectious disease, N. Engl. J. Med. 331:1212, 1994, which reviews probes and the polymerase chain reaction.
28. Tenover, F.C. DNA hybridization techniques and their application to the diagnosis of infectious diseases. *Infect. Dis. Clin. North Am.* 7:171, 1993.
    For further discussions of rapid techniques to diagnose M. tuberculosis, see also related update, reference [42a].
29. Maslow, J.N., Mulligan, M.E., and Arbeit, R.D. Molecular epidemiology: Application of contemporary techniques to the typing of microorganisms. *Clin. Infect. Dis.* 17:153–162, 1993.
    See related editorial by J.R. Lupski, Molecular epidemiology and its clinical application, J.A.M.A. 270:1363, 1993, in which the author comments on the molecular epidemiologic methods used to study two nosocomial outbreaks (one due to methicillin-resistant

S. aureus *and the other due to erythromycin-resistant* S. aureus*), which are reported in separate journal articles in this same issue.*
See also L.S. Tompkins et al., New technology in the clinical microbiology laboratory: What you always wanted to know but were afraid to ask. J. Infect. Dis. 170:1068, 1994; this paper briefly discusses molecular epidemiology.

30. Eisenstein, B.I. The polymerase chain reaction. *N. Engl. J. Med.* 322:178, 1990.
A description of the method, its research applications, and its specific applications in the field of medicine. For an additional discussion, see K.B. Mullis, The unusual origin of the polymerase chain reaction. Sci. Am. 262:56, 1990.

31. Lorian, V. (ed.). *Antibiotics in Laboratory Medicine* (4th ed.). Baltimore: Williams & Wilkins, 1996.
Detailed discussion of antimicrobial susceptibility testing, antimicrobial synergism, and measurement of antibiotic levels.

32. Rosenblatt, J.E. Laboratory tests used to guide antimicrobial therapy. *Mayo Clin. Proc.* 66:942–948, 1991.
Excellent, concise summary of testing for antimicrobial susceptibility and serum bactericidal activity. See also G.L. Woods, In vitro testing of antimicrobial agents. Infect. Dis. Clin. North Am. 9:483, 1995.

33. Stamey, T.A., et al. Serum versus urinary antimicrobial concentrations in cure of urinary tract infections. *N. Engl. J. Med.* 291:1159–1163, 1974.
Cure of urinary tract infections is dependent on antimicrobial levels achieved in urine rather than in serum.

33a. Doern, G.V., et al. Clinical impact of rapid in vitro susceptibility testing and bacterial identification. *J. Clin. Microbiol.* 32:1757, 1994.
This study is from the University of Massachusetts, Worcester, MA. The mean lengths of time to provision of susceptibility and identification test results in the rapid test (the Baxter-Microscan WALKAWAY-96 System, Baxter-Microscan, Sacramento, CA) group were 11.3 and 9.6 hours, respectively. In the conventional overnight group, these values were 19.6 and 25.9 hours, respectively. In terms of outcome, mean lengths of hospitalization were the same in both groups, but mortality rates were lower in the rapid test group (8.8% vs. 15.3%). Statistically, significantly fewer laboratory studies, days of intubation, days in an ICU, and imaging studies were observed in the rapid test group. Rapid testing was also associated with significantly shortened lengths of elapsed time prior to alterations in antibiotic therapy and lower patient costs for hospitalization.

33b. Sanchez, M.L., and Jones, R.N. E test, an antimicrobial susceptibility testing method with broad clinical and epidemiologic application. *Antimicrob. News.* 8(1):1, 1992.
Contains a general description of the E test and overview. For related references, see: E.A. Macias et al., Comparison of E test with standard broth microdilution for determining antibiotic susceptibilities of penicillin-resistant strains of S. pneumoniae, J. Clin. Microbiol. 32:430, 1994; J.H. Jorgensen et al., Detection of penicillin and extended-spectrum cephalosporin resistance among S. pneumoniae clinical isolates by use of the E test, J. Clin. Microbiol. 32:159, 1994; J.E. Schulz and D.F. Sahm, Reliability of the E test for detection of ampicillin, vancomycin, and high-level aminoglycoside resistance in Enterococcus spp., J. Clin. Microbiol. 31:3336, 1993.*

33c. Kiska, D.L., et al. Comparison of antimicrobial susceptibility methods for detection of penicillin-resistant *Streptococcus pneumoniae. J. Clin. Microbiol.* 33:229, 1995.
For determining penicillin MICs for S. pneumoniae, *the E test was the most accurate commercial system studied.*

34. Finegold, S.M., Jousimies-Somer, H.R., and Wexler, H.M. Current perspectives on anaerobic infections: Diagnostic approaches. *Infect. Dis. Clin. North Am.* 7:257–275, 1993.

35. Cuchural, G.J., et al. Susceptibility of the *Bacteroides fragilis* group in the United States: Analysis by site of isolation. *Antimicrob. Agents Chemother.* 32:717, 1988.
Antimicrobial susceptibility patterns of anaerobes vary among hospitals.

36. Goldstein, E.J.C., et al. Comparative susceptibility of the *Bacteroides fragilis* group species and other anaerobic bacteria to meropenem, imipenem, piperacillin, cefoxitin, ampicillin/sulbactam, clindamycin and metronidazole. *J. Antimicrob. Chemother.* 31:363–372, 1993.

36a. Wexler, H.M., and Doern, G.V. Susceptibility Testing of Anaerobic Bacteria. In P.R. Murray et al. (eds.), *Manual of Clinical Microbiology* (6th ed.). Washington, DC: American Society for Microbiology, 1995. P. 1350–1355.
Notes that the clinical utility of anaerobic susceptibility testing is frequently considered limited. However, given regional variations in susceptibility patterns, hospitals could

periodically batch-test anaerobes, either in their own facility or by sending them to a reference laboratory.

37. Finegold, S.M., and the National Committee for Clinical Laboratory Standards. Susceptibility testing of anaerobic bacteria. *J. Clin. Microbiol.* 26:1253, 1988.
Clinical indications for susceptibility testing of anaerobes and interpretation of results.

37a. Schieven, B.C., et al. Evaluation of susceptibility of anaerobic organisms by the E test and the reference agar dilution method. *Clin. Infect. Dis.* 20(Suppl. 2):S337, 1995.

38. Moellering, R.C. Antimicrobial synergism—an elusive concept. *J. Infect. Dis.* 140: 639, 1979.
Editorial reviewing the concepts and uncertainties of antimicrobial synergism testing. For an update, see G.M. Eliopolous, Synergism and antagonism, Infect. Dis. Clin. North Am. 3:399, 1989.

39. Anderson, E.T., Young, L.S., and Hewitt, W.L. Antimicrobial synergism in the therapy of gram-negative rod bacteremia. *Chemotherapy* 24:45, 1978.
Antimicrobial synergism correlated with successful outcome of gram-negative rod bacteremia in patients with serious underlying disease, neutropenia, shock, or Pseudomonas infections.

40. Klastersky, J., Meunier-Carpentier, F., and Prevost, J. Significance of antimicrobial synergism for the outcome of gram-negative sepsis. *Am. J. Med. Sci.* 273:157, 1977.
Cancer patients with gram-negative infections responded more favorably to synergistic combinations of antibiotics.

41. Centers for Disease Control. 1993 Sexually transmitted disease treatment guidelines. *M.M.W.R.* 42(no. RR-14):1–102, 1993.

42. Witebsky, F.G., and Conville, P.S. The laboratory diagnosis of mycobacterial diseases. *Infect. Dis. Clin. North Am.* 7:359–376, 1993.

42a. Shinnick, T.M., and Good, R.C. Diagnostic mycobacteriology laboratory practices. *Clin. Infect. Dis.* 21:291, 1995.
In addition to a discussion of conventional procedures, newer diagnostic tests under clinical study, which expedite the identification and susceptibilities of M. tuberculosis, are reviewed.

43. Wolfson, J.S., and Swartz, M.N. Serum bactericidal activity as a monitor of antibiotic therapy. *N. Engl. J. Med.* 312:968, 1985.
Excellent current review of this controversial topic. For additional discussion of this topic, see K. Vosti, Serum bactericidal test: Past, present, future use in the management of patients with infections, Curr. Clin. Top. Infect. Dis. 10:43, 1989.

43a. Reller, L.B. The serum bactericidal test. *Rev. Infect. Dis.* 8:803, 1986.
See related summary by K. Vosti, Serum bactericidal test: Past, present, and future use in the management of patients with infections. Curr. Clin. Top. Infect. Dis. 10:43, 1989.

44. Stratton, C.W. Bactericidal testing. *Infect. Dis. Clin. North Am.* 7:445, 1993.
Reminds reader there is little evidence to support the use of serum bactericidal levels clinically. With standard dose regimens, clinical cure often depends on host factors, not antibiotic levels. Bactericidal testing, especially if it can become more standardized, may prove to be most useful in the research setting as there is need to assess newer classes or agents for bactericidal activity.

45. Coleman, D.L., Horwitz, R.I., and Andriole, V.T. Association between serum inhibitory and bactericidal concentrations and therapeutic outcome in bacterial endocarditis. *Am. J. Med.* 73:260, 1982.
There is insufficient evidence contained in published studies to conclude that serum inhibitory or bactericidal concentrations of 1 : 8 or more predict successful treatment of bacterial endocarditis.

46. Weinstein, M.P., et al. Multicenter collaborative evaluation of a standardized serum bactericidal test as a prognostic indicator in infective endocarditis. *Am. J. Med.* 78:262, 1985.
Bacteriologic cure of endocarditis was correlated with peak serum bactericidal titers of 1 : 64 or more and trough bactericidal titers of 1 : 32 or more. Bactericidal activity was not predictive of treatment failures.

47. Weinstein, M.P., et al. Multicenter collaborative evaluation of a standardized serum bactericidal test as a predictor of therapeutic efficacy in acute and chronic osteomyelitis. *Am. J. Med.* 83:218, 1987.
Serum bactericidal titers correlated with cure of acute and chronic osteomyelitis. In acute osteomyelitis, a trough bactericidal level of 1 : 2 or greater and, in chronic osteomyelitis, a trough bactericidal level of 1 : 4 or greater were associated with im-

proved outcome. Optimal bactericidal levels are unclear; some favor peak levels in excess of 1 : 32.

48. Klastersky, J., et al. Antibacterial activity in serum and urine as a therapeutic guide in bacterial infections. *J. Infect. Dis.* 129:187, 1974.
   Peak serum bacteriostatic titers of 1 : 8 or greater correlated with a favorable outcome in wound and bloodstream infections in cancer patients.

49. Sculier, J.P., and Klastersky, J. Significance of serum bactericidal activity in gram-negative bacillary bacteremia in patients with and without granulocytopenia. *Am. J. Med.* 76:429, 1984.
   Peak serum bactericidal titers of 1 : 8 or more in nongranulocytopenic patients, or 1 : 16 or more in granulocytopenic patients, were predictive of a favorable response to antimicrobials.

50. Cahen, P., et al. Serum bactericidal test as a prognostic indicator in acute pulmonary exacerbations of cystic fibrosis. *Pediatrics* 91:451–455, 1993.

51. Moore, R.D., Smith, C.R., and Lietman, P.S. The association of aminoglycoside plasma levels with mortality in patients with gram-negative bacteremia. *J. Infect. Dis.* 149:443, 1984.
   Aminoglycoside plasma concentrations in the therapeutic range 1 hour after infusion are associated with lower mortality in patients with gram-negative bacteremia.

52. Moore, R.D., Smith, C.R., and Lietman, P.S. Association of aminoglycoside plasma levels with therapeutic outcome in gram-negative pneumonia. *Am. J. Med.* 77:657, 1984.
   Successful outcome of gram-negative pneumonia correlates with therapeutic peak plasma levels of aminoglycosides.

53. Moore, R.D., Leitman, P.S., and Smith, C.R. Clinical response to aminoglycoside therapy: Importance of the ratio of peak concentration to minimal inhibitory concentration. *J. Infect. Dis.* 155:93–99, 1987.

Antiviral Agents

Susan E. Cohn, Taimor Nawaz, and Mala R. Gupta

26

An Introduction to Antiviral Chemotherapy

I. **Overview.** Antiviral drugs with proven therapeutic and prophylactic effectiveness currently are available for a variety of viral infections (Table 26-1). Because viral replication depends primarily on host cell metabolic functions, it has been difficult to identify agents that inhibit virus-specific activities such as attachment to the cell, uncoating of the viral genome, or assembly of progeny virions, without damaging the host cell. Many of the currently approved antivirals selectively inhibit specific events in ongoing viral replication and, hence, have a limited spectrum of antiviral activity and fail to eliminate nonreplicating or latent viruses. Development of viral resistance by some antiviral agents has also limited their usefulness and become an important clinical issue.

II. **Relative activity of antiviral agents**
   A. **Potency.** The potency of antiviral agents is determined by the concentration required to inhibit the growth of a standard inoculum by 50% or **a 50% inhibitory dose (ID$_{50}$).**
   B. **Therapeutic index.** This index is the ratio of the toxic concentration to the therapeutic concentration. The larger the therapeutic index, the greater the potential clinical applicability of the antiviral agent. Therefore, an important concept in antiviral chemotherapy is to compare the cytotoxic concentration of a drug with its viral inhibitory concentration (i.e., an in vitro therapeutic index).
   C. **Application of therapeutic index.** Although cytosine arabinoside (ara-C) and acyclovir each have an ID$_{50}$ of approximately 0.1–0.2 μM, ara-C also inhibits cellular growth at 0.1 μM, whereas acyclovir inhibits cellular growth only at concentrations greater than 300 μM. Therefore, while both agents are equally potent against herpes simplex virus (HSV), ara-C has an in vitro therapeutic index of 1, whereas acyclovir has a therapeutic index of greater than 3,000 [1]. This difference explains why ara-C-treated patients were not benefited in clinical trials and why acyclovir has been effective against infections due to herpesviruses.

III. **Special antiviral agents. Twenty antiviral agents** currently are approved in the United States (as of spring 1996): iododeoxyuridine, vidarabine, trifluorothymidine (trifluridine, TFT), amantadine, rimantadine, acyclovir, famciclovir, valacyclovir, ribavirin, interferon, zidovudine (ZDV), zalcitabine (dideoxycytidine, ddC), didanosine (ddI), stavudine (d4T), ganciclovir, foscarnet, and, most recently, lamivudine (3TC), saquinavir, ritonavir, and indinavir. See Table 26-1 for a brief overview of the antiviral agent of choice for various viral infections.

IV. **Chapter organization.** This chapter is divided into two major sections. The first section focuses on antiviral medications used for non-HIV viral infections. The second section focuses on antiretroviral medications and provides some background on recently completed clinical trials to help readers assess the potential benefit of various antiretroviral regimens.

Revised from O.L. Laskin and R.G. Douglas, Jr., Antiviral Agents. In R.E. Reese and R.F. Betts (eds.), *A Practical Approach to Infectious Diseases* (3rd ed.). Boston: Little, Brown, 1991.

Table 26-1. Drugs for viral infections

Viral infection	Drug of choice
Condyloma acuminatum	Interferon-alfa-2b, interferon-alfa-n3
Cytomegalovirus	Ganciclovir
Retinitis	Foscarnet
Hepatitis B virus	Interferon-alfa-2b
Chronic hepatitis	Lamivudine*
Hepatitis C virus	Interferon-alfa-2b
Chronic hepatitis	
Hepatitis D virus	Interferon-alfa-2b
Chronic hepatitis	
Herpes simplex virus	
Genital herpes	
First episode	Acyclovir
Recurrence	Acyclovir
Frequent recurrences	Acyclovir
Encephalitis	Acyclovir
Mucocutaneous disease in immuno-compromised hosts	Acyclovir
Neonatal herpes	Acyclovir
Acyclovir-resistant herpes	Foscarnet, trifluridine
Keratoconjunctivitis	Trifluridine
Human immunodeficiency virus (see Table 26-15)	Zidovudine, didanosine, zalcitabine, stavudine,* lamivudine,* saquinavir,* ritonavir,* indinavir*
Influenza A virus	Amantadine, rimantadine
Respiratory syncytial virus	Ribavirin
Varicella-zoster virus	
Varicella	Acyclovir
Herpes zoster	Acyclovir, famciclovir,* valacyclovir*
Varicella or zoster in immuno-compromised hosts	Acyclovir
Acyclovir-resistant virus	Foscarnet

*Additional agents added as they were approved for use.
Source: Adapted from Medical Letter. Drugs for non-HIV viral infections. *Med. Lett. Drugs Ther.* 36:30–31, 1994.

Antiviral Agents for Non-HIV Viral Infections

Acyclovir

Acyclovir (9-[2-hydroxyethoxymethyl] guanine, Zovirax) is an acyclic nucleoside analogue of guanosine. The drug has potent antiviral activity against most herpesviruses [2, 3].

I. **Mechanism of action.** The selective activity of acyclovir for herpesvirus replication is due to its selective phosphorylation by the herpes-encoded thymidine kinase to its monophosphate form [4]. Cellular enzymes then are capable of converting acyclovir monophosphate to acyclovir diphosphate and triphosphate. Acyclovir triphosphate is the active antiviral compound and **inhibits viral replication in three ways.** First, it selectively inhibits viral DNA polymerase. Second, the triphosphate competitively inhibits the incorporation of guanosine triphosphate into herpesvirus DNA. Third, the triphosphate also is incorporated into newly formed herpesvirus DNA. Because acyclovir lacks the 3'-hydroxyl group necessary for further elongation, its incorporation results in termination of the viral DNA chain. Additional mechanisms of action may exist.

II. **In vitro activity.** Acyclovir is active against HSV types 1 and 2 (ID_{50}, 0.1–1.6 μM) and varicella-zoster virus (VZV) (ID_{50}, 3–4 μM). Most strains of cytomegalovirus (CMV) appear to be relatively resistant ($ID_{50} > 200$ μM). Because mammalian cell growth is inhibited only at very high concentrations (> 300 μM), the in vitro therapeutic index for acyclovir is very favorable (i.e., with respect to HSV, the therapeutic index $> 3,000$) [1].

III. **Resistance.** Resistance to acyclovir **can be induced in several ways.** The **most common** mechanism seen clinically is the mutation of the herpesvirus to a thymidine kinase deficient (TK-deficient) strain [5, 6]. Because these TK-deficient strains do not produce a virus-specific TK, acyclovir is not phosphorylated to its monophosphate form. A **second,** far less frequent mutation results in a virus-specific TK that does not recognize acyclovir as a substrate. The **final** known mechanism of resistance results from a mutation that alters the sensitivity of the virus-specific DNA polymerase to acyclovir triphosphate [5]. The latter has been observed only in the laboratory setting.

Acyclovir-resistant mutants have been isolated not only from patients who are on therapy with acyclovir [6] but also in a few patients not receiving any antiviral chemotherapy [7]. Patients who shed resistant mutants may improve clinically. Therefore, these resistant mutants may improve without therapy. In addition, experimental data show that acyclovir-resistant mutants are less virulent than the parent strains, and it is more difficult to establish latency with TK-deficient mutant strains of HSV [8]. However, treatment failures in immunocompromised patients due to acyclovir-resistant strains of HSV have occurred [9].

IV. **Pharmacology**
   A. **Absorption**
      1. **Topical.** Plasma acyclovir concentrations are undetectable after topical administration.
      2. **Oral.** Oral absorption of acyclovir is **slow, variable,** and between **15 and 30% of the dose.** After oral administration of multiple doses of 200 or 800 mg acyclovir, the mean steady-state peak plasma concentrations are approximately 0.6 and 1.6 μg/ml, respectively [2].
      3. **Intravenous.** Steady-state peak plasma concentrations after intravenous doses of acyclovir, 5 or 10 mg/kg q8h, are approximately 10 and 20 μg/ml, respectively [2].
   B. **Distribution.** The drug is distributed into all tissues, with highest concentrations in the kidney and lowest in the CNS. Acyclovir enters the cerebrospinal fluid (CSF), saliva, and vesicular and vaginal secretions at concentrations inhibitory to HSV. In patients with herpes zoster, the acyclovir concentration in the vesicle fluid approximates the plasma level.
   C. **Elimination**
      1. **Adults with normal renal function. Renal excretion is the major route of elimination.** After an intravenous infusion of acyclovir, most of the dose is excreted unchanged in the urine, with only a small percentage (8.5–14.0%) of the dose recovered in the urine as the oxidized metabolite, carboxymethoxymethylguanine. Acyclovir is eliminated via the kidney by renal tubular secretion as well as by glomerular filtration [10–12]. Probenecid inhibits the renal clearance of acyclovir, presumably by inhibiting the organic acid tubular transport system [11]. In patients with normal renal function, the elimination half-life of acyclovir is 2–3 hours.
      2. **Renal impairment.** In patients with end-stage renal disease, acyclovir clearance is reduced by 90% [2]. The half-life of acyclovir in patients who are anuric is approximately 20 hours [13]. Therefore, the **dose must be adjusted according to the degree of renal dysfunction** (see sec. **VIII**).
         a. **Hemodialysis.** Acyclovir is removed by hemodialysis, 60% of the drug being removed from the body during a single 6-hour course of hemodialysis. The patient's dosing schedule should be adjusted so that an additional dose is administered after each course of dialysis [13].
         b. **Peritoneal dialysis** does not remove acyclovir and so no supplemental dose is necessary after dialysis [2, 3].
      3. **Children.** The pharmacokinetics in children (> 1 year old) are similar to those seen in adults [10].
      4. **Neonates.** In neonates, the acyclovir total body clearance is approximately one-third of that found in children and adults [10]. Therefore, the dose determined on a per-square-meter basis will result in higher serum levels in neonates as compared with adults and children (> 1 year old).

V. Clinical uses. The efficacy and safety of acyclovir have been demonstrated in numerous clinical trials, with most of these trials being conducted in a prospective, randomized, double-blind controlled fashion [14]. **We do not recommend the use of topical acyclovir.**

A. Immunocompromised patients

1. Herpes simplex infections

a. Prophylaxis or suppression of infections in immunocompromised patients. Acyclovir has been shown to be effective for prophylaxis and therapy of infections caused by HSV. Organ transplant recipients and patients with leukemia who have latent infection (i.e., who have antibodies to HSV) have a high incidence of severe reactivated HSV infections in the weeks after intensive immunosuppressive therapy (see Chap. 20). Acyclovir, when administered either intravenously or orally, prevents reactivation of HSV infections in bone marrow recipients and patients with leukemia [15–17]. However, latency is not eradicated, and the patients develop reactivated infections after the drug is discontinued.

In immunocompromised patients who are successfully treated with acyclovir for established mucocutaneous infections but who have recurrences once therapy is discontinued, acyclovir has been shown to suppress recurrent disease effectively. This is particularly useful in patients in whom the immunocompromised state does not improve (such as in AIDS).

b. Therapy for HSV infections. Immunosuppressed patients treated with acyclovir have a significantly shorter median time to cessation of pain (from 13.1 to 8.9 days), to termination of viral shedding (from 16.8 to 2.8 days), to lesion healing (from 20.1 to 13.7 days), and to lesion crusting (from 13.5 to 9.3 days), and a decreased time to cessation of new lesion formation [18]. Oral acyclovir (2 g/day) appears to be effective and safe for HSV infections in immunocompromised hosts [19].

c. Resistant virus. The development of resistance is indicated by the presence of persistent ulcers on therapy and continued detection of virus. High-dose oral acyclovir (4 g/day) or continuous intravenous infusion of acyclovir may be effective in some instances [20]. Herpes simplex virus resistant to acyclovir may require treatment with intravenous foscarnet.

2. Varicella-zoster virus

a. Herpes zoster. In immunocompromised patients with herpes zoster, acyclovir IV, 500 mg/m^2 q8h for 7 days, when compared with a placebo, halted progression of disease [21]. Acyclovir reduced the period of viral shedding and prevented visceral dissemination. Patients started on therapy within 72 hours of the onset of rash had the greatest benefit from therapy. However, patients did benefit from acyclovir even when therapy was begun later. The most important benefit occurred in patients with severe pain at the outset. Pain reduction occurs more rapidly in the treated group. Acyclovir is superior to vidarabine for this indication [22].

b. Varicella. Acyclovir is beneficial for varicella (chickenpox) in the immunocompromised patient [23–25]. When acyclovir was given at 500 mg/m^2 q8h for 7 days to immunocompromised children with primary varicella, none of the acyclovir recipients developed visceral complications whereas 45% of the placebo group developed pneumonitis, hepatitis, or thrombocytopenia [25].

c. Herpes zoster prophylaxis. Oral acyclovir appears to be effective in preventing herpes zoster for the first 6 months after bone marrow transplantation. However, 6 months after the drug was discontinued, the incidence of herpes zoster was similar to that seen in the placebo group [26].

3. Human CMV infections

a. Therapeutic trials. Acyclovir, even in doses as high as 28 mg/kg q8h, has little or no therapeutic benefit for infections caused by CMV.

b. Prevention of reactivation. Systemic acyclovir prophylaxis appears to reduce the likelihood of CMV disease in renal [27], liver [28], and bone marrow transplant recipients [29] but not in liver transplant recipients receiving OKT 3 [30]. Acyclovir does not appear to be effective in preventing CMV retinitis in patients with AIDS.

4. Epstein-Barr virus

a. Studies of acyclovir in Epstein-Barr virus (EBV) infections are extremely limited. Acyclovir does not appear to have a clinically important effect in the therapy of acute EBV infections (causative agent of mononucleosis) in either the immunosuppressed or the immunocompetent patient [32–34].

b. **Acyclovir** (400 mg 5 times daily) **may be beneficial** in patients infected with human immunodeficiency virus (HIV) who have **oral hairy leukoplakia,** a tongue lesion believed to be caused by EBV. Continuous acyclovir therapy (200 mg 5 times daily) appears to prevent recurrence of lesions [35, 36], although the need to treat this lesion is questionable.

B. Nonimmunocompromised patients

1. Herpes simplex infections

a. **Herpetic keratoconjunctivitis.** Although prior studies have shown that acyclovir is effective in this setting [37], topical trifluorothymidine (TFT) is the treatment of choice [14]. An ophthalmic preparation of acyclovir is available in some countries [14]. The 5% ointment for topical use should not be used in the eye. Oral acyclovir also appears to be effective for this condition.

b. **Herpes simplex encephalitis.** Acyclovir is the treatment of choice for herpes simplex encephalitis (HSE) and is given intravenously 10 mg/kg q8h. The optimal duration of therapy for HSE has not been clearly established. Although patients have often been treated for 10 days, some relapses have occurred after this course of therapy and a 14- to 21-day duration may be preferable [14, 38, 39]. (See related discussion in Chap. 5.)

c. **Neonatal herpes simplex infections.** Newborns with HSV can have localized disease (skin, eyes, and mouth), CNS infections, or disseminated disease. The treatment of choice for neonatal HSV is acyclovir [2]. The recommended dose is 10 mg/kg IV q8h and the duration of therapy is 10–14 days [2].

d. **Herpes genitalis.**

(1) **First episode.** For herpes genitalis, both intravenous and oral acyclovir are beneficial [40, 41]. Although intravenous therapy seems to be superior to oral therapy, when given orally at a dose of 200 mg 5 times daily for 10 days, acyclovir resulted in a decreased duration of viral shedding, time to crusting, time to healing, duration of pain, and new lesion formation, compared to placebo [40, 41].

(2) **Recurrent disease**

(a) **Therapy.** Topical acyclovir provides no clinical benefit [42]. Although oral acyclovir therapy has some effect in recurrent herpes genitalis, the benefit is less than that seen in primary herpes genitalis. It is not known whether intravenous therapy is beneficial for recurrent disease. Even if benefit is derived in patients with recurrent herpes genitalis treated with intravenous acyclovir, the cost and inconvenience of hospitalization and intravenous therapy would probably outweigh any benefit obtained. However, oral acyclovir, 200 mg 5 times daily for 5 days, does have therapeutic benefit with respect to decreasing viral shedding, halting new lesion formation, and decreasing time to complete crusting and healing in patients with recurrent disease [43, 44]. On average, oral acyclovir decreased the duration of disease manifestations by a day.

(b) **Suppressive therapy.** When given orally to patients who have frequent recurrences (more than 6–12 episodes per year) of herpes genitalis, acyclovir is effective in reducing the attack rate [45, 46]. However, once the drug is discontinued, most patients have recurrent HSV genital infections. The doses used in these studies ranged from 400 to 1,000 mg/day. The duration of therapy was 4–6 months. Data from patients treated longer show that acyclovir is safe and effective in suppressing disease for at least 7 years [47, 48].

(c) **Latency.** Acyclovir does not have any effect on latency. In addition, acyclovir therapy for primary infections has not been shown to prevent the establishment of latency.

e. **Herpes labialis (cold sore, fever blister).** Topical acyclovir is of no benefit and is not recommended [2].

(1) Oral therapy, 400 mg 5 times daily, has a slight benefit and only if initiated early after recurrences. It is not recommended for routine treatment of herpes labialis [2, 38].

(2) Short-term prophylactic therapy with oral acyclovir, 200 mg 5 times daily, may benefit some patients with recurrent labialis who anticipate engaging in activity likely to lead to recurrence (e.g., skiers with intense sun exposure) [2].

(3) For immunocompetent adults with frequent recurrences (i.e., ≥ six episodes per year), oral therapy is effective in suppressing recurrences [49].

2. **Herpes zoster.** The role of acyclovir therapy in normal hosts must be individualized. **Ophthalmic herpes zoster virus (HZV) deserves therapy.** Most healthy patients with nonophthalmic zoster need not be treated, especially if the lesions have been present for more than 72 hours and are limited to one dermatome. Healthy patients with cutaneous dissemination (i.e., more than 15 lesions outside the primary and adjacent dermatomes) are candidates for oral therapy [38]. Patients older than 60 years with other underlying disease probably deserve therapy [50]. Human immunodeficiency virus testing should be considered in patients with herpes zoster, especially in patients younger than 60 years (see Chap. 19).

There are now two other antiviral agents licensed for the treatment of herpes zoster in immunocompetent adults, famciclovir and valacyclovir. (See Famciclovir and Valacyclovir sections on pp. 977–980 and summary of agents in sec. **VIII** under Valacyclovir, p. 980.)

   a. **Intravenous acyclovir. In immunocompetent patients,** acyclovir (5 mg/kg q8h for 5 days) enhances the relief of acute severe pain and the rate of healing [51], especially in those who are older than 60 years, who have had their pain for fewer than 4 days, and who are febrile. **Acyclovir has no effect on post-herpetic neuralgia.** Using a dose approximately 2.5 times greater (500 mg/m^2 or approximately 12.4 mg/kg 3 times daily), acyclovir reduces pain, decreases erythema, prevents the formation of new vesicles, decreases viral shedding, and accelerates lesion healing [52]. However, 35% of the patients have persistence of pain after therapy has been stopped.

   b. **Oral acyclovir.** In immunocompetent individuals with either ophthalmic zoster [53, 54], or nonophthalmic zoster [55], 600–800 mg oral acyclovir given 5 times daily leads to more rapid decrease in viral and clinical parameters. Four hundred milligrams per dose appears ineffective. It is important that the drug be initiated within 48 hours of the onset of cutaneous lesions. In view of the usual pattern of zoster, this can be as late as 120 hours after the onset of pain. Although benefit from therapy may be most pronounced when treatment is initiated within 48 hours after the cutaneous manifestations become evident, ocular complications may be diminished when treatment begins as late as 7 days after the onset of rash [38, 53]. The usual duration of therapy is 7–10 days [38, 54]. This high dose was chosen for study based on knowledge of oral acyclovir pharmacokinetics (i.e., relatively poor absorption) and the levels required to inhibit VZV in tissue culture.

3. **Chickenpox**
   a. **In adults.** Chickenpox (primary varicella) can be a more serious disease in adults than in children. Although uncommon, clinical pneumonia can occur in conjunction with the rash. Less commonly, an encephalopathy develops. In one study, oral acyclovir, 800 mg PO 5 times daily for 7 days, reduced the duration of morbidity, including days of fever, if the drug was started within the first 24 hours of the appearance of rash [56]. Studies suggest that acyclovir, IV 500 mg/m^2 for 7 days, reduces mortality in varicella-associated pneumonia in immunocompetent hosts [38]. See Chap. 22 on the role of the varicella vaccine in both immunocompetent and immunosuppressed persons. **In view of the more serious consequences of varicella infection in adults, the expense of oral acyclovir in adults with varicella seems justified** [50].
   b. **In children.** Oral acyclovir reduces the duration and severity of chickenpox in normal children when therapy is initiated within the first 24 hours at a dose of 20 mg/kg body weight (with a maximum of 800 mg/dose) 4 times daily for 5 days [2, 57]. **The need for treatment of normal children must be evaluated on a case-by-case basis** [2]. Whether acyclovir can reduce the rare, serious complications of chickenpox remains unknown [57]. Therapy may help reduce time missed from daycare centers [57, 58]. Secondary cases within the family may warrant therapy [50].

VI. **Adverse effects.** Acyclovir has a very high therapeutic index, and toxicity with this agent has been **minor.** The most frequent adverse events reported with short-term orally administered acyclovir for genital herpes were nausea or vomiting (2.7%) and headache (0.6%). Less frequent side effects (0.3% each) included diarrhea, dizziness, anorexia, fatigue, edema, skin rash, leg pain, inguinal adenopathy, medicinal taste, and sore mouth [3].

   A. **Phlebitis** and local **intravenous site irritation** have been observed. These may be related to the rather high pH of the infusing solution (pH > 9.0) rather than to a direct effect of the drug [59].

   B. **Renal dysfunction.** Acyclovir causes a reversible elevation of serum creatinine level, which may be due to crystallization of acyclovir in the renal tubules or collecting ducts [60]. The development of renal dysfunction is related to the method of administration and the degree of hydration. It is more likely to occur when the drug is given as a bolus injection rather than a 1-hour infusion and is more common in patients with dehydration. This renal dysfunction is completely reversible following hydration and discontinuation of drug therapy and, in most cases, is not clinically important. It rarely occurs after oral acyclovir use except perhaps with very high doses [38].

   C. **Liver enzyme elevation.** Acyclovir has caused elevation in the liver transaminases (SGOT, SGPT), but the clinical importance of this has not been established [61].

   D. **Neurotoxicity.** Acyclovir-induced neurotoxicity has been reported in a number of cases. Renal dysfunction that causes impaired drug clearance and produces elevated acyclovir concentration increases the risk of neurotoxicity. Other risk factors have not been well defined. In a series of 24 patients, the reported CNS effects, in order of decreasing frequency, included tremor, myoclonus, confusion, agitation, lethargy, hallucination, extrapyramidal symptoms, clouding of consciousness, dysarthria, and unilateral focal symptoms [62]. The relation between CNS effects and acyclovir serum concentration remains unclear. Drug toxicity occurs most commonly when serum acyclovir levels exceed 25 μg/ml but may better correlate with the area under the concentration time curve and the elimination half-life than with single (peak) concentration [38, 62]. Neurotoxicity is reversible, and improvement of neurologic symptoms occurs after discontinuation of drug or after its removal by hemodialysis [63, 64].

   E. **Lack of bone marrow toxicity.** Acyclovir has been shown not to have any bone marrow suppressive toxicity at clinically relevant concentrations [15, 61].

   F. **Mutagenicity, carcinogenicity, or teratogenicity.** In preclinical studies, acyclovir was not found to be carcinogenic, mutagenic, or teratogenic [60]. Teratogenic data in humans are not available.

VII. **Drug interactions**

   A. **Probenecid** inhibits the renal clearance of acyclovir, thereby enhancing the plasma concentrations [11].

   B. Presumably, other anionic drugs secreted by the renal tubular organic acid transport system would have an effect similar to probenecid in decreasing acyclovir clearance. These drugs would include penicillins, cephalosporins, methotrexate, and paraaminohippuric acid (PAH). However, the influence of probenecid (and presumably these other agents) on acyclovir kinetics, while statistically significant, is small and probably of limited clinical importance. By contrast, acyclovir may decrease the renal clearance of other drugs that are eliminated by active renal secretion. This could be very significant for a drug such as **methotrexate for which decreased elimination may result in methotrexate toxicity.**

VIII. **Dosing recommendations** (Tables 26-2 and 26-3)

   A. **Topical administration.** Topical administration has questionable efficacy; we do not recommend it.

   B. **Oral administration.** Now 200 mg, 400 mg and 800 mg tablets are available. For recommended doses for treatment of herpesvirus infections, see Table 26-2. See Table 26-3 for adjustment in oral dosage in renal insufficiency.

   C. **Intravenous preparation.**

      1. For recommended doses for treatment of herpesvirus infections, see Table 26-2.

      2. **Adjustments will need to be made in the dosages in renal failure** to prevent accumulation of acyclovir (see Table 26-3). During a 6 hour hemodialysis, approximately 60% of acyclovir in the body will be removed and should be replaced [19]. No supplemental dose appears to be necessary after peritoneal dialysis, other than adjustment of the dose interval per Table 26-3.

Table 26-2. Treatment of herpes simplex and varicella-zoster viral infections

Virus	Regimen[†]	Comments
Herpes simplex		
Genital, primary	*Acyclovir:* Oral—200 mg 5 times/day or 400 mg tid × 7–10 days; IV—5 mg/kg q8h × 5 days	Mild lesions and symptoms usually are not treated
Genital, recurrent	*Acyclovir:* Oral—200 mg PO 5 times/day or 400 mg tid × 5 days	Initiate during prodrome or at first sign of lesions
Genital, prophylaxis	*Acyclovir:* Oral—200 mg PO 2–5 times/day or 400 mg PO bid	Indicated only with ≥ 6 recurrences/yr
		Good efficacy and good safety profile with treatment up to 6 yr; contraindicated in pregnancy
Encephalitis	*Acyclovir:* IV—10 mg/kg q8h × 14–21 days	Pediatric dose is 500 mg/m² IV q8h
Mucocutaneous progressive	*Acyclovir:* IV—5–10 mg/kg q8h × 7–14 days Oral—200–400 mg PO 5 times/day × 7–14 days	AIDS patients often require preventative therapy with acyclovir 200–400 mg PO 3–5 times/day indefinitely
		Pediatric dose is 250 mg/m² IV q8h for 7–14 days
Prophylaxis in high-risk patients	*Acyclovir:* IV—5 mg/kg q8h; oral—200 mg 3–5 times/day or 400 mg PO bid	Organ and bone marrow transplant recipients; treat seropositive patients for 1–3 mo post-transplantation
Keratoconjunctivitis, adult	*Trifluridine:* Topical—(1%) 1 drop q2h, up to 9 drops/day × 10 days	Ophthalmologist should supervise treatment; oral acyclovir also is effective
Keratoconjunctivitis, neonatal	*Acyclovir:* IV—10 mg/kg q8h × 10–21 days	Not FDA-approved for this indication
Acyclovir-resistant strains	*Foscarnet:* IV—40 mg/kg q8h	Thymidine kinase–deficient strains, usually from immunosuppressed patients unresponsive to acyclovir; duration of therapy depends on the clinical response
Varicella-zoster		
Chickenpox, adult	*Acyclovir:* Oral—20 mg/kg (800 mg max) 5 times/day × 7–10 days Varicella vaccine (prophylaxis)*	Must treat within 24 hr of exanthem; efficacy established
Chickenpox, children	*Acyclovir:* Oral—20 mg/kg up to 800 mg PO q6h × 5 days Varicella vaccine (prophylaxis)*	Must treat within 24 hr of exanthem; no reduction in serologic response noted; there is no consensus, though considered cost-effective due to decrease in parent work time lost
Pneumonia	*Acyclovir:* IV—10–12 mg/kg q8h × 7 days; oral—800 mg 5 times/day × 10 days	Efficacy not clearly established, but appears best if treatment is initiated within 36 hr of admission

Table 26-2 (continued)

Virus	Regimen[†]	Comments
Varicella-zoster (*cont.*)		
Dermatomal Immunosuppressed	*Acyclovir:* IV—10–12 mg/kg q8h × 7 days	Indications to treat are greater for severe disease, early disease, or zoster in immunosuppressed host
Normal host	*Acyclovir:* Oral—800 mg 5 times/day × 7–10 days *Famciclovir:* Oral—500 mg q8h × 7 days* *Valacyclovir:* Oral—1 g q8h × 7 days*	Acyclovir and/or corticosteroids (prednisone, 40 mg/day × 7 days, then taper over 3 wk) may reduce post-herpetic neuralgia. Steroids usually reserved for persons > 40 yr. Acyclovir should be started ≤ 4 days and famciclovir and valacyclovir < 72 hr of onset of rash. Post-herpetic neuralgia: amitriptyline
Ophthalmic zoster	*Acyclovir:* Oral—600–800 mg 5 times/day × 10 days	Consult ophthalmologist
Disseminated zoster or varicella (immunosuppressed host)	*Acyclovir:* IV—10–12 mg/kg q8h × 7 days	Foscarnet (40 mg/kg q8h) or vidarabine (10 mg/kg/day IV) × 5–7 days
Acyclovir-resistant strains	*Foscarnet:* IV—40 mg/kg q8h	Consider a trial of topical trifluridine 1% ophthalmic solution (see text)
Exposure (zoster or chickenpox) Immunosuppressed	*Varicella-zoster immunoglobulin*	
Susceptible health care worker	None Varicella vaccine (prophylaxis)*	Must refrain from patient contact on days 10–21
Prophylaxis in transplant recipients	*Acyclovir:* 5 mg/kg IV q8h or 200 mg PO q6h days 8–35	

[†]Regimens assume normal renal function. Adult dosages given unless otherwise indicated.
*Recently approved for this indication.
Source: Adapted from Medical Letter. Drugs for non-HIV viral infections. *Med. Lett. Drugs Ther.* 36:30–31, 1994.

- **D. Miscellaneous**
  - **1. Pregnancy.** All formulations of acyclovir are assigned U.S. Food and Drug Administration (FDA) pregnancy category C status, which indicates that safety in human pregnancies has not been determined. A recent report from the Acyclovir in Pregnancy Registry, however, indicates no increased risk for birth defects among infants born to 425 women exposed to acyclovir during the first trimester [65].

    Untreated varicella pneumonia in pregnant women has a higher mortality than in untreated nonpregnant women. Recent studies suggest that treatment of varicella pneumonia in pregnancy with acyclovir lowers the mortality rate [66, 67].
  - **2. Nursing.** Acyclovir has been documented in breast milk, and so caution should be exercised when acyclovir is administered to nursing women [3].
  - **3. Pediatric use.** Safety and effectiveness in children younger than 2 years have not been adequately studied [3].
- **IX. Cost** (Table 26-4)

Table 26-3. Adjustment of acyclovir regimens in patients with varying degrees of renal function

Usual dosage	Estimated creatinine clearance (ml/min)	Adjustment Dose (mg)	Adjustment Dose interval (hr)
Oral regimens[a]			
200 mg q4h	> 10	200	q4h 5×/day
	0–10	200	q12h
400 mg q12h	> 10	400	q12h
	0–10	200	q12h
800 mg q4h	> 25	800	q4h 5×/day
	11–25	800	q8h
	0–10	800	q12h
Intravenous regimens[b]			
	> 50		q8h
	25–50		q12h
	10–25		q24h
	0–10		q24h

[a]Based on manufacturer's recommendation.
[b]Data from *Physicians' Desk Reference* (49th ed.). Montvale, NJ: Medical Economics, 1995. Pp. 829, 833. Usual dose (mg/kg) given but dose interval adjusted.

Table 26-4. Average wholesale cost of antiviral agents to pharmacy (1995)

Drug	Quantity	Cost (dollars)
Acyclovir (Zovirax)		
Capsules (200 mg)	100 capsules	97.63
Capsules (400 mg)	100 capsules	156.37
Capsules (800 mg)	100 capsules	368.44
Suspension (200 mg/5 ml)	473 ml (1 pint)	84.13
IV infusion	500 mg vial	50.90
Famciclovir		
Famvir (500 mg)	50 tablets	340.07
Valacyclovir		
Valtrex (500 mg)	42 capsules	96.70*
	100 capsules	235.24*
Ganciclovir (Cytovene)		
IV infusion	500 mg vial	34.80
Capsules (250 mg)	180 capsules	702.00
Foscarnet (Foscavir)		
IV infusion (24 mg/ml)	250 ml	73.28
Trifluorothymidine (Trifluridine, Viroptic)		
1% Ophthalmic solution	7.5 ml	48.29
Zidovudine (ZDV, Retrovir)		
Capsules (100 mg)	100 capsules	154.80
Syrup (10 mg/ml)	240 ml	37.15
IV infusion (10 mg/ml)	20 ml	16.74
2'3'-Dideoxyinosine (didanosine, ddI, Videx)		
Chewable tablets		
25 mg	60 tablets	21.61
50 mg	60 tablets	43.21
100 mg	60 tablets	86.42
150 mg	60 tablets	129.63

Table 26-4 (continued)

Drug	Quantity	Cost (dollars)
2'3'-Dideoxyinosine (*cont.*)		
Powder (packet)		
167 mg	30 tablets	72.17
250 mg	30 tablets	108.03
Solution, pediatric	2 gm	28.80
(20 mg/ml)	4 gm	57.60
Zalcitabine (ddC, HIVID)		
Tablets		
0.375 mg	100 tablets	178.07
0.750 mg	100 tablets	223.22
Stavudine (d4T, Zerit)		
15 mg	60 capsules	200.01
20 mg	60 capsules	208.00
30 mg	60 capsules	217.00
40 mg	60 capsules	225.00
Lamivudine (Epivir)		
Liquid (10 mg/5 ml)	240 ml	59.71*
Tablets (150 mg)	60 tablets	223.92*
Amantadine		
Capsules (100 mg)	100 capsules	19.13
Syrup (50 mg/5 ml)	480 ml	47.90
Rimantadine (Flumadine)		
Tablets (100 mg)	100 tablets	127.57
Syrup (50 mg/5 ml)	240 ml	25.80
Ribavirin (Virazole)		
6 g	1 vial	1,319.85
Interferon-alpha (alfa):	3 million units	29.87
Intron A (interferon-alfa-2b)	vial	
Influenza virus vaccine (Flu-immune)	10 dose vial	27.00
Varicella vaccine (Varivax)	10 dose vial	394.50

*Wholesale price per manufacturer.
Note: See also related Table 28-15.
Source: From *Red Book,* Montvale, NJ: Medical Economics, 1995. Copyright *Drug Topics Red Book* 1995. Reprinted by permission. All rights reserved.

Famciclovir

Famciclovir (Famvir) is an oral antiviral agent **approved for use in mid-1994 for the treatment of uncomplicated herpes zoster in the normal host** [68].
I. **Mechanism of action.** Famciclovir is the oral form of penciclovir which, like acyclovir, is a guanosine analogue that inhibits herpes DNA synthesis by interfering with the action of viral DNA polymerase [68].
II. **In vitro activity.** Penciclovir is initially phosphorylated by a virally encoded thymidine kinase and, subsequently, by cellular kinases to penciclovir triphosphate, which inhibits HSV-1, HSV-2, and VZV DNA polymerases. Most acyclovir-resistant HSV and VZV clinical isolates are resistant to penciclovir. Penciclovir also is active in vitro against hepatitis B virus [68].
III. **Pharmacology** [68]
   A. **Absorption**
      1. Famciclovir is well absorbed from the GI tract (systemic bioavailability of 77%) and is rapidly converted by deacetylation and oxidation to penciclovir.
      2. Food slows the absorption of famciclovir and the rate of conversion to penciclovir but has no effect on the ultimate bioavailability of penciclovir.

B. Elimination
1. Penciclovir is excreted in the urine mostly unchanged by both glomerular filtration and tubular secretion.
2. The serum half-life of penciclovir is 2 hours, but the intracellular half-life of penciclovir is 7 to 20 times longer, which is markedly prolonged compared to that of acyclovir triphosphate.

IV. Clinical trials
   A. Herpes zoster. Two multicentered, double-blind controlled trials in **immunocompetent adults with a herpes zoster rash** present no more than 72 hours showed that famciclovir was superior to placebo in resolution of skin lesions, viral shedding, and duration of post-herpetic neuralgia [69].
   1. The first trial compared 7-day therapy with famciclovir, 500 mg tid in 138 patients, versus 750 mg tid in 135 patients, versus placebo in 146 patients. Median time to full crusting in the treated groups was 5 days versus 7 days in the placebo group [70].
      a. There was **no difference** between groups in the duration of acute pain or incidence of post-herpetic neuralgia.
      b. The **median duration** of **post-herpetic neuralgia** was shorter in patients treated with famciclovir 750 mg tid (61 days) and famciclovir 500 mg tid (63 days) compared with placebo (119 days) [69]. In the subgroup of patients 50 years of age or older, post-herpetic neuralgia resolved 2.6 times faster in famciclovir versus placebo recipients. No such benefit was seen for patients younger than 50 years [70].
   2. **A second trial** compared famciclovir, 250 mg, 500 mg, or 750 mg tid, with acyclovir, 800 mg five times daily, in 545 patients with acute herpes zoster [68].
      a. Times to crusting and resolution of acute pain were similar with famciclovir and acyclovir.
      b. The duration of post-herpetic neuralgia was similar with both drugs.
   3. See sec. **VIII** under Valacyclovir (p. 980) for a summary comment on the role of acyclovir versus famciclovir versus valacyclovir for HZV infections.
   B. Investigational uses. Controlled studies of famciclovir in patients with hepatitis B and recurrent herpes simplex infections are underway. Preliminary data suggest that famciclovir, like acyclovir, can be effective in the therapy and prevention of recurrent HSV genital infections [68]. **The role of famciclovir in the immunocompromised host awaits further study.**

V. Adverse effects. Famciclovir is well tolerated, with occasional headache and nausea reported in frequencies similar to those seen in placebo recipients [69].

VI. Drug interactions. The package insert indicates that no clinically significant alterations of single-dose pharmacokinetics of famciclovir were noted with multiple doses of cimetidine, allopurinol, or theophylline. Concurrent use of probenecid and famciclovir may be associated with increased levels of penciclovir.

VII. Dosing recommendations (adults)
   A. For therapy of acute herpes zoster in the nonimmunocompromised host with rash no longer than 72 hours' duration, famciclovir 500 mg tid for 7 days is recommended. The efficiency of famciclovir initiated after 72 hours of rash onset has not been studied.
   B. The recommended dosage interval (q8h) should be adjusted for **renal insufficiency.** There is insufficient data to recommend famciclovir if the creatinine clearance is less than 20 ml/min (Table 26-5).
   C. Pediatric use. The safety and efficacy in children 18 years of age and younger have not been established.
   D. Pregnancy. Famciclovir is classified as a category B drug. There are no well-controlled studies in pregnant women. Famciclovir should be used during pregnancy only if the benefit to the patient clearly exceeds the potential risk to the fetus.
   E. Nursing. The drug's safety during nursing is unknown [68]. High doses of famciclovir given for 2 years were associated with increased incidence of mammary adenocarcinoma in female rats, but the clinical significance of this finding is unknown [69].

VIII. Cost (see Table 26-4)

Valacyclovir

Valacyclovir (Valtrex), the l-valyl ester of acyclovir, is an oral antiviral agent approved

Table 26-5. Adjustment of famciclovir (penciclovir) regimens in patients with varying degrees of renal function

Creatinine clearance (ml/min)	Dose regimen
≥ 60	500 mg q8h
40–59	500 mg q12h
20–39	500 mg q24h
< 20	Insufficient data

Source: *Physicians' Desk Reference* (50th ed.). Montvale, NJ: Medical Economics, 1996. P. 2488. Copyright *Physicians' Desk Reference* 1996. Reprinted by permission. All rights reserved.

in June 1995 **for use in the treatment of uncomplicated herpes zoster in immuno-competent adults** and in December 1995 for recurrent genital HSV.

I. **Mechanism of action.** Because valacyclovir is rapidly absorbed from the GI tract and is nearly completely converted to acyclovir and L-valine by first-pass intestinal and/or hepatic metabolism, its mechanism of action is identical to acyclovir [71, 71a].

II. **Pharmacology**
   A. The **bioavailability** of acyclovir from oral valacyclovir is three to five times that of high-dose oral acyclovir [71].
   B. There was no accumulation of acyclovir after the administration of valacyclovir at the recommended dosage regimen in volunteers with normal renal function. The binding of valacyclovir to plasma proteins ranged from 13.5% to 17.9% [72].
   C. The elimination of valacyclovir and acyclovir is similar. A dosage reduction is recommended in patients with creatinine clearance less than 50 ml/min (Table 26-6).

III. **Clinical trials**
   A. **Herpes zoster.** Two randomized double-blind clinical trials in immunocompetent adults with a herpes zoster rash present for no more than 72 hours were conducted.
      1. Valacyclovir, 1000 mg tid for 7 days or 14 days, was compared with acyclovir, 800 mg five times daily, in 1141 persons **older than 50 years** [71]. In an intent-to-treat analysis, valacyclovir provided up to 34% faster resolution of pain than acyclovir, significantly shortened the duration of post-herpetic neuralgia, and decreased the proportion of patients with pain persisting for 6 months by 26% compared with acyclovir [71].
      2. Valacyclovir, 1000 mg tid for 7 days or 14 days, was compared to placebo in immunocompetent patients less than 50 years of age with localized herpes zoster [72]. In patients **younger than 50 years,** the median time to cessation of new lesion formation was 2 days for those treated with valacyclovir, compared with 3 days for those treated with placebo. **No difference** was found with respect to the duration of pain after rash healing (post-herpetic neuralgia) between recipients of valacyclovir and placebo.
   B. **Cytomegalovirus disease.** To study the effect of valacyclovir in suppressing AIDS-related CMV diseases, 1227 patients with CD4 cell counts below 100 cells/mm^3 (median CD4 cell count, 32 cells/mm^3) who were taking antiretroviral therapy were given valacyclovir, 2000 mg qid, or acyclovir, 800 mg qid or 400 mg bid, and

Table 26-6. Adjustment of valacyclovir regimens in patients with varying degrees of renal function

Creatinine clearance (ml/min)	Dose regimen
≥ 50	1 g q8h
30–49	1 g q12h
10–29	1 g q24h
< 10	500 mg q24h*

*Patients requiring hemodialysis should receive the recommended dose of valacyclovir after hemodialysis. No supplemental doses of valacyclovir are required following chronic ambulatory peritoneal dialysis (CAPD) or continuous arteriovenous hemofiltration/dialysis (CAVHD). Source: Data from Valtrex (Valacyclovir). *Package Insert.* August 1995.

followed for 1 year after the last patient was enrolled. Although valacyclovir at 8 g/day resulted in delayed onset of symptomatic CMV disease, this high dosage resulted in an elevated incidence of gastrointestinal adverse effects and allergic reactions (e.g., rash), and in turn caused a number of persons to withdraw from the valacyclovir group sooner than participants in the acyclovir groups. Although the study was stopped prematurely when a decreased survival was noted in patients in the valacyclovir treatment group, subsequent follow-up data have not found a statistically significant increase in mortality in patients assigned to the valacyclovir group [72a].

C. **Genital herpes.** Preliminary reports suggest that valacyclovir significantly accelerates the resolution of signs and symptoms of recurrent genital herpes in immunocompetent adults compared with placebo, and is comparable in efficacy to acyclovir.

IV. **Adverse effects**

A. **Thrombotic thrombocytopenic purpura/hemolytic uremic syndrome** (TTP/HUS) has been reported in patients with advanced HIV disease and also in bone marrow transplant and renal transplant recipients participating in valacyclovir clinical trials, resulting in death in some cases. This syndrome has not been observed in immunocompetent patients treated with valacyclovir in clinical trials.

B. No other adverse effects have been reported that differ significantly from acyclovir.

V. **Drug interactions.** Cimetidine and probenecid, separately or together, reduced the rate but not the extent of conversion of valacyclovir to acyclovir and reduced the renal clearance, resulting in higher plasma acyclovir concentrations.

VI. **Dosage recommendations (adults)**

A. **For the treatment of acute herpes zoster in immunocompetent adults** with rash no more than 72 hours' duration, the recommended dosage is two 500 mg caplets (1 g) tid for 7 days. The efficacy of valacyclovir started more than 72 hours after onset of rash has not been studied. For recurrent genital herpes, 500 mg bid for 5 days is suggested in adults.

B. The recommended dosage interval should be adjusted **for renal insufficiency** (see Table 26-6). Patients requiring hemodialysis should receive the recommended dose of valacyclovir after hemodialysis.

C. **Pediatric use.** Safety and effectiveness of valacyclovir in pediatric populations have not been established.

VII. **Cost** (see Table 26-4)

VIII. **Summary.** There are currently three drugs approved for the treatment of herpes zoster infections in immunocompetent adults: acyclovir, famciclovir, and the recently approved valacyclovir. Famciclovir has been studied only in immunocompetent adults with nonophthalmic zoster. Valacyclovir and famciclovir appear to offer significant improvement over acyclovir in the treatment of acute herpes zoster in immunocompetent adults in terms of simplicity of dosing, duration of abnormal sensations, and duration of post-herpetic pain, if it were to develop [68]. As of January 1996, there are no published data about the use of valacyclovir or famciclovir in the immunocompromised host or the immunocompetent adult with ophthalmic zoster.

Ganciclovir

Ganciclovir (9-[1,3-dihydroxy-2-propoxymethyl] guanine, DHPG, Cytovene) is an acyclic nucleoside analogue of guanine, approved in 1989 for the treatment and chronic suppression of CMV retinitis in immunocompromised patients.

I. **Mechanism of action.** Ganciclovir is phosphorylated intracellularly to its active triphosphate form. The antiviral activity of ganciclovir triphosphate is believed to be the result of inhibition of viral DNA synthesis by two known modes: competitive inhibition of viral DNA polymerases and direct incorporation into viral DNA that results in slowing and subsequent cessation of viral DNA elongation [73]. In cells infected with HSV and VZV, phosphorylation to ganciclovir triphosphate is similar to that described for acyclovir and involves a herpes-specific thymidine kinase. In cells infected with EBV or CMV, which do not produce herpes-specific thymidine kinase, the phosphorylation of ganciclovir appears to be attributable to a virally induced host cell–encoded enzyme. There is an approximately 10-fold greater concentration of ganciclovir-triphosphate in CMV-infected cells than in uninfected cells, indicating a preferential phosphorylation of ganciclovir in virus-infected cells [74]. **Ganciclovir is virostatic,** and relapse of CMV disease may occur on discontinuation of therapy.

II. **In vitro activity.** The in vitro activity (ID_{50}) of ganciclovir against CMV ranges from 0.5 to 3.0 μM; against HSV type 1, from 0.2 to 2 μM; against HSV type 2, from 0.3

to 10.0 μM; against VZV, from 3 to 10 μM; and against EBV, from 5 to 25 μM [73]. In vitro cytotoxicity ranges from a mean of 1.6 to 250.0 μM, with hematopoietic progenitor cells being particularly more sensitive than cells with low rates of DNA synthesis [75, 76].

III. **Resistance to ganciclovir.** Resistance can develop in CMV after exposure to ganciclovir [77–79]. Mechanisms of resistance are similar to those for acyclovir in HSV. Two mechanisms of resistance in CMV isolates have been identified: reduced intracellular phosphorylation and point mutations in the viral DNA polymerase that lead to partial resistance to ganciclovir [80, 81]. Ganciclovir resistance may be manifested by progressive disease and persistent CMV viremia despite therapy [78]. In one study, 6 of 72 AIDS patients on ganciclovir (8%) had progressive disease and shed resistant CMV after 3 months or more of continuous ganciclovir therapy [82]. Ganciclovir-resistant isolates are usually sensitive to foscarnet (see Foscarnet section).

IV. **Pharmacology**

    A. **Oral administration.** Oral bioavailability of ganciclovir is low (2.6%–9.0%) and, therefore, relatively large doses (1 g tid) need to be administered when oral ganciclovir is prescribed [83, 84]. A dose of oral ganciclovir of 3000 mg daily yielded plasma concentrations of ganciclovir between 0.5 and 1.0 μg/ml [83, 85]. Within this concentration range, ganciclovir exceeds the median in vitro inhibitory concentration (IC_{50}) of most CMV clinical isolates [85].

    B. **Intravenous administration.** Following a 1-hour infusion, doses of 1, 2.5, and 5 mg/kg resulted in mean steady-state peak concentrations of 9.4, 20.3, and 44.5 μM, respectively [86]. Steady-state trough concentrations are 2.7 and 4.4 μM after 2.5 and 5.0 mg/kg q8h, which indicates that plasma concentrations for most of the interval exceed the in vitro ID_{50} for most human strains of CMV [87].

    C. **Distribution.** The concentration of ganciclovir in lung, liver, and testes is approximately equal to that seen in plasma. The ratio of CSF to plasma concentration of ganciclovir was found to range from 0.3 to 0.67 [88, 89]. Concentrations in various tissues compared to corresponding plasma concentrations were as follows: CNS, 38%; aqueous fluid, 40%; and kidney, 300–700% [89].

    D. **Elimination.** Ganciclovir is almost entirely eliminated by renal excretion, probably by both glomerular filtration and renal tubular secretion [86]. The plasma half-life is 2–4 hours in patients with normal renal function and 11.5 hours in renal failure. The half-life in vitreous fluid has been found to be 13.3 hours when injected intravitreally [90]. Approximately half the dose is eliminated during a single 4-hour course of hemodialysis [91, 92], which is similar to acyclovir.

V. **Clinical uses.** Ganciclovir is indicated for the treatment and chronic suppression of **CMV retinitis** in immunocompromised individuals, including patients with AIDS. It is also indicated for the **prevention of CMV disease in transplant patients at risk** for CMV disease.

    A. **Nonimmunocompromised patients.** There currently are **no indications** for ganciclovir therapy in nonimmunocompromised patients with herpesvirus infections because of the drug's inherent toxicity.

    B. **Immunocompromised patients**

        1. **Cytomegalovirus retinitis**

            a. **Intravenous therapy.** Cytomegalovirus retinitis, if untreated, causes progressive retinal disease and blindness [93]. In transplant patients, CMV retinitis may resolve spontaneously with a reduction in immunosuppression. Ganciclovir is given initially as induction therapy for 2–3 weeks, followed by maintenance therapy (Table 26-7). Ganciclovir induced initial improvement in approximately 85% of AIDS patients with CMV retinitis, although reactivation rates were high [94]. Reactivation of CMV retinitis occurred in all patients with AIDS who did not receive maintenance therapy [95]. Intravenous ganciclovir is comparable to foscarnet in the treatment of CMV retinitis and is better tolerated, although the median survival of patients appears to be shorter on ganciclovir (8.5 months versus 12.6 months) [96]. **Recent data also suggest that combination ganciclovir and foscarnet therapy is effective** in stabilizing progressive CMV disease in patients whose disease is refractory to single-agent therapy and is well tolerated [97, 97a]. See related discussions in Chaps. 6 and 19.

            b. **Intravitreal ganciclovir therapy**

                (1) In early studies, ganciclovir was injected intravitreally with successful control of progressive CMV retinitis. However, the injections had to be repeated at least once weekly and were associated with risk of

Table 26-7. Adjustment of ganciclovir regimens in patients with varying degrees of renal function

Parenteral induction treatment*

Creatinine clearance (ml/min)	Ganciclovir intravenous dose (mg/kg)	Ganciclovir dosing interval (hr)
≥ 70	5	12
50–69	2.5	12
25–49	2.5	24
10–24	1.25	24
< 10	1.25	3 ×/wk following hemodialysis

Oral maintenance treatment*

Creatinine clearance (ml/min)	Ganciclovir capsule doses
≥ 70	1,000 mg tid or 500 mg q3h, 6×/day
50–69	1,500 mg qd or 500 mg tid
25–49	1,000 mg qd or 500 mg bid
10–24	500 mg qd
< 10	500 mg 3 ×/wk following hemodialysis

*Data from *Physicians' Desk Reference* (50th ed.). Montvale, NJ: Medical Economics, 1996. P. 2109.

endophthalmitis and retinal detachment; in addition, there was a high relapse rate of 53% in 8 weeks [98].

(2) Ganciclovir intraocular devices (GIOD) were implanted in the vitreous in a phase 1 study involving 22 patients, 17 of whom had progressive CMV retinitis despite intravenous ganciclovir and 5 of whom were previously untreated. There was stabilization of retinitis in 90% of the treated eyes, and the survival analysis revealed a mean time of progression of retinitis of 19 weeks. In a study of 173 patients, GIOD prevented progression of CMV retinitis about three times longer than intravenous ganciclovir, for 220 days versus 72 days, respectively [98a]. The procedure was associated with acceptable risks and toxicities. However, GIODs did not prevent systemic CMV disease (26%) or development of bilateral CMV retinitis when the initial presentation was unilateral. Bilateral GIOD implants have been associated with higher rates of endophthalmitis [99, 100]. Subtherapeutic levels of ganciclovir in the vitreous have been reported with intravenous ganciclovir and may explain, in part, the high rates of CMV retinitis reactivation [101].

(3) Intraocular devices were recommended for approval in December 1995 and, therefore, their use may increase significantly in the future. **Current recommendations continue to support the use of intravenous ganciclovir, foscarnet, or both for CMV retinitis.**

2. **Prevention of CMV disease**

    a. **In transplant recipients,** ganciclovir prophylaxis appears to be effective and reasonably well tolerated for the prevention of CMV disease in bone marrow transplant recipients who are shedding CMV (blood, urine, bronchoalveolar lavage) [102–104], in seropositive but not seronegative cardiac transplant patients [105], and in liver transplant recipients [106]. Short-term prophylaxis is ineffective in seronegative lung transplant recipients experiencing primary infection [31]. See related discussion in Chap. 20.

    b. **In AIDS patients,** the use of oral ganciclovir as prophylaxis against CMV disease is currently under evaluation [107].

3. **Cytomegalovirus pneumonia**

    a. **AIDS patients.** Patients with progressive pulmonary disease in whom biopsy has been carried out and **in whom CMV is demonstrated** in the absence of another cause are assumed to have CMV pneumonitis. Improvement in these patients with ganciclovir therapy has been difficult to evaluate. In patients with documented *Pneumocystis carinii* pneumonia (PCP), patients who are also culture positive for CMV do no worse than those who are culture negative [108]. **Because CMV in these patients may not be clinically important, unlike in those with retinitis or gastritis, there has been a reluctance to initiate therapy** because the risks of the drug are greater than its potential benefit.

    b. **Bone marrow recipients.** In allogeneic bone marrow recipients with pneumonia related to CMV, ganciclovir alone reduces the duration of detection of virus but does not affect the clinical outcome. Ganciclovir combined with CMV immunoglobulin therapy in bone marrow transplant recipients reduces mortality from CMV pneumonitis from 80–90% to 30–50% [81]. See related discussion in Chap. 20.

    4. **Cytomegalovirus gastrointestinal disease.** Ganciclovir therapy appears to be beneficial in the treatment of GI infections caused by CMV [87]. In posttransplantation patients with gastrointestinal CMV disease, ganciclovir causes resolution of symptoms and promotes healing of lesions [109]. In AIDS patients, ganciclovir therapy for CMV esophageal ulcers and CMV colitis results in improved symptoms in most patients [110, 111]. The need for continued secondary prophylaxis with ganciclovir for gastrointestinal CMV disease is being evaluated.

    5. **Cytomegalovirus CNS disease.** Uncontrolled data suggest that therapy with ganciclovir provides benefit in some, but not all, cases. Polyradiculomyelopathy due to CMV in AIDS patients has been treated with intravenous ganciclovir with some success [112]. See Chap. 19 also.

    6. **Cytomegalovirus syndrome** (i.e., fever, abnormal liver function tests, and, occasionally, pulmonary infiltrates in transplant recipients). In a study of cardiac transplant recipients who were CMV seropositive, there were significantly fewer illnesses if ganciclovir was given in the first 28 days after transplantation [105].

    7. **Congenital CMV.** Currently, a protocol is being developed to evaluate ganciclovir in children with congenital CMV. Because the presence of active viral infection is not obviously detrimental or life-threatening to most children with congenital CMV, there is no reason to treat this group of patients until studies demonstrate that the benefit offsets the risk of this drug.

C. **Maintenance therapy.** Although most persons with AIDS respond to an initial 2- to 3-week course of ganciclovir therapy, the disease in most (if not all) patients reactivates 1–2 months after ganciclovir is stopped [87]. Because of these relapses, **long-term suppressive therapy usually is necessary in AIDS patients.** The drug usually is given intravenously once daily for 5–7 days per week, which greatly extends the time to reactivation. However, relapses do still occur, but these generally (80%) respond to reinduction doses of ganciclovir, foscarnet, or both concomitantly [113, 114]. A recent study comparing maintenance therapy with oral versus intravenous ganciclovir in patients with AIDS, following stabilization of acute CMV retinitis, found no difference in survival, changes in visual acuity, or incidence of adverse gastrointestinal events [107].

    Oral ganciclovir was approved in 1995 as an alternative to the intravenous formulation for maintenance treatment of CMV retinitis in immunocompromised patients in whom retinitis is stable (following appropriate induction therapy) and for whom the risk of more rapid progression is balanced by the benefit associated with avoiding daily intravenous infusions [84].

VI. **Adverse effects**

A. **Myelosuppression is** the most frequent adverse effect of ganciclovir [73, 87, 89, 113, 114]. Myelosuppression occurs more frequently with intravenous ganciclovir than with oral ganciclovir [83].

    1. **Neutropenia occurs frequently,** the incidence during induction therapy being approximately 25–40%. This neutropenia is usually reversible when the drug is discontinued. Granulocyte colony stimulating factors (GM-CSF, G-CSF) have been used to treat ganciclovir-induced neutropenia.

    2. **Thrombocytopenia** has been seen in approximately 20% of transplantation patients and in about 9% of patients with AIDS [74].

B. **Gastrointestinal dysfunction.** Nausea, vomiting, and diarrhea have been reported. Mucositis may occur if suppression is severe.

C. **Liver dysfunction.** Abnormal liver function tests may develop.

D. **Neurologic dysfunction.** Confusion, seizure, and abnormal mentation have been infrequently reported.

E. **Renal dysfunction.** Impairment of renal function with a rise in serum creatinine has been reported in cardiac transplant patients.

F. **Other adverse effects.** Decreased sperm synthesis, skin rash, infusion site reaction, and eosinophilia have also been reported [14].

VII. **Drug interactions**

A. **Myelosuppressive agents. When given with other drugs that have a tendency to produce leukopenia (zidovudine** [ZDV], trimethoprim-sulfamethoxazole [TMP-SMX], pyrimethamine), **ganciclovir may produce severe neutropenia** [115]. In these instances, the other drug (e.g., ZDV) may have to be withheld, an agent that stimulates WBC production (e.g., G-CSF) may need to be given, or an alternate agent to treat CMV (e.g., foscarnet) may need to be selected [14, 38].

B. **Probenecid.** Probenecid may interfere with the renal secretions of ganciclovir, resulting in greater-than-expected plasma concentrations.

C. **Imipenem-cilastatin.** Seizures have been reported in patients receiving both ganciclovir and imipenem-cilastatin. However, seizures have been reported with either of these agents when given alone as well. See related discussion of imipenem, Chap. 28G.

VIII. **Dosing recommendations**

A. **Induction therapy**

1. **Dose** (see Table 26-7). Infusions are given over a 1-hour period.

2. **Duration.** The duration of induction therapy is 14–21 days for the treatment of CMV disease and 7–14 days for the prevention of CMV disease in transplant recipients.

B. **Maintenance therapy**

1. After induction therapy, maintenance therapy is given as 5 mg/kg/day IV **or** 6 mg/kg IV 5 days/wk when renal function is normal.

   a. Patients with AIDS and CMV disease are treated indefinitely. The duration of therapy in transplant recipients depends on the degree and duration of immunosuppression. In clinical trials in bone marrow allograft recipients, the treatment was continued 100–120 days posttransplantation; treatment duration was 28 days in heart allograft recipients.

   b. The recommended maintenance dose of oral ganciclovir is 1000 mg tid with food. Alternatively, the dosing regimen of 500 mg 6 times daily, every three hours with food while awake, may be used [84].

   c. Patients who experience progression of retinitis while on maintenance therapy may be retreated with a twice daily regimen or switched to foscarnet or another anti-CMV retinitis regimen.

2. **Dosage adjustments in renal failure** are outlined in Table 26-7.

C. **Hemodialysis.** Dosing for patients undergoing hemodialysis should not exceed 1.25 mg/kg/day [74]. On days when hemodialysis is performed, the dose should be given shortly after completion of the procedure, as hemodialysis removes ganciclovir.

D. **Pregnancy.** Ganciclovir is embryotoxic in animal models. There are no controlled studies in pregnant women. Therefore, ganciclovir should be used in pregnancy only if the potential benefit justifies the potential risk to the fetus.

E. **Nursing.** The package insert suggests that mothers should be instructed to discontinue nursing while receiving ganciclovir [74].

F. **Pediatric use.** The package insert emphasizes that the use of ganciclovir in children warrants extreme caution due to the probability of long-term carcinogenicity and reproductive toxicity. Administration in children should be undertaken only after careful evaluation and only if the potential benefits outweigh the risks.

G. **Monitoring patients.** Neutrophil and platelet counts are suggested every 2–3 days while patients are on induction therapy and weekly while on maintenance therapy. Serum creatinine or creatinine clearance should be monitored at least once every 2 weeks, and ganciclovir dosing should be adjusted accordingly. If significant myelosuppression occurs, the dose may be reduced or the drug temporarily discontinued. Bone marrow suppression is more likely to occur after the first week of ganciclovir therapy, especially in those patients who already have a mild neutropenia. Patients who develop neutropenia may be treated with G-CSF or GM-CSF while continuing ganciclovir. If the **neutrophil count falls below 500 cells/mm^3 or the platelet counts are lower than 25,000/mm^3,** the drug should be temporarily discontinued. Depending on the clinical situation and the previous clinical response, the drug may be restarted (at either the full or reduced dose) after resolution of the abnormality. The decision about whether to restart ganciclovir, and at what dose, should be made after consultation with someone with experience in treating CMV disease.

IX. **Cost** (see Table 26-4)

Foscarnet

Foscarnet (trisodium phosphonoformate, Foscavir) is an antiviral drug approved by the FDA in 1991 for the intravenous treatment of CMV retinitis in AIDS. The antiviral activity of foscarnet includes HSV 1 and 2, VZV, CMV, EBV, and HIV, among others [116]. It also inhibits ganciclovir-resistant CMV and acyclovir-resistant HSV and VZV [116, 117].

I. **Mechanism of action.** Foscarnet is a pyrophosphate analogue that reversibly blocks viral DNA polymerase and inhibits pyrophosphate exchange from deoxynucleotide triphosphates, thus preventing DNA chain elongation [118]. Unlike ganciclovir, acyclovir, and ZDV, foscarnet does not require intracellular phosphorylation by viral (thymidine kinase) or cellular enzymes to be active. Foscarnet is a noncompetitive inhibitor of HIV reverse transcriptase [119] and appears to bind to reverse transcriptase at a site that is distinct from the nucleoside triphosphate binding site. Foscarnet is **virostatic to CMV,** and reactivation of CMV may occur after stopping the drug.

II. **Mechanism of resistance.** The mechanism of resistance is unclear. In vitro studies show that herpesviruses and HIV-1 resistance to foscarnet are associated with mutations in the DNA polymerase genes. The mechanism of resistance is different from ganciclovir resistance. Strains of HSV, VZV and CMV resistant to foscarnet in vitro may emerge during therapy but have not always been associated with decreased clinical response [14].

III. **Pharmacology**
   A. **Absorption.** Foscarnet is poorly absorbed orally and is only administered parenterally [120].
   B. **Distribution.** Foscarnet appears to be widely distributed throughout the body. Cerebrospinal fluid drug levels have been measured at 54–80% (mean, 66%) of simultaneous plasma drug levels at steady state [121]. The relationship between CSF drug levels and brain drug levels has not been established [122]. Sequestration in bone accounts for 10–20% of a dose [83, 120].
   C. **Metabolism.** No metabolism of foscarnet has been detected in animals or humans [123].
   D. **Elimination.** Approximately 80–90% of intravenous foscarnet is excreted unchanged in the urine of patients with normal renal function by both glomerular filtration and tubular secretion [124, 125]. Foscarnet is removed by hemodialysis [126].

IV. **Clinical studies and use.** Foscarnet is approved for treatment of CMV retinitis in patients with AIDS [96, 127]. It also is effective in acyclovir-resistant HSV or VZV infections [128–131] and ganciclovir-resistant CMV retinitis in immunocompromised patients [132]. The safety and efficacy of foscarnet have not been established for the treatment of other CMV infections (e.g., pneumonitis, gastritis, congenital or neonatal CMV disease) or disease in normal hosts. Studies are under way to help assess its role in these settings. **There is no clear consensus on whether foscarnet or ganciclovir should be used for initial treatment of CMV retinitis** [14]. Many practitioners use ganciclovir instead of foscarnet for initial therapy for CMV retinitis in nonneutropenic AIDS patients because ganciclovir has more predictable toxicities, lower cost, and does not require large volumes of fluid.
   A. **Cytomegalovirus retinitis in AIDS**
      1. **Induction.** Prior uncontrolled studies suggested that foscarnet was useful in the treatment of CMV retinitis in AIDS patients [133]. A controlled trial (FOS-03) was conducted with 24 patients with AIDS and peripherally located CMV retinitis. Patients randomized to treatment with foscarnet had a significant delay in progression of CMV retinitis compared to untreated controls [127]. In a clinical trial comparing long-term foscarnet and ganciclovir in 234 AIDS patients with CMV retinitis, there was no difference in the rate of progression of retinitis [96]. Although ganciclovir was better tolerated than foscarnet, there was excess mortality in the ganciclovir group (median survival, 8.5 months

versus 12.6 months), perhaps related to greater ZDV use in the foscarnet group or additive anti-HIV effects of foscarnet [96, 134, 135]. Foscarnet has also been reported to be useful in the treatment of ganciclovir-resistant CMV retinitis in AIDS patients [132].

2. **Maintenance.** A study of 32 patients with CMV retinitis and AIDS documented increased survival and increased time to retinitis progression with a foscarnet maintenance dose of 120 mg/kg (adjusted for renal function) compared with 90 mg/kg/day, without increased toxicity [135]. Based on the study, it might be worth considering a maintenance dose of 120 mg/kg/day, with prompt reduction to a lower dosing regimen for those who experience unacceptable toxicity.

3. **Intravitreal foscarnet therapy.** Although foscarnet has been injected intravitreally with successful control of progressive CMV retinitis, as with intravitreal ganciclovir injection its use has been associated with an increased risk of endophthalmitis and retinal detachment [135a]. Use of intravitreal foscarnet is being studied.

B. **Acyclovir-resistant HSV infections.** AIDS patients treated with foscarnet experience improvement of chronic ulcerative mucocutaneous lesions that fail to heal with acyclovir therapy and from which acyclovir-resistant HSV are isolated [129, 131]. Unfortunately, clinically significant foscarnet-resistant HSV may develop [136].

C. **Investigational uses of foscarnet** [14, 137]
  1. **Cytomegalovirus pneumonia.** Foscarnet has been used successfully for treatment of severe CMV infections in allograft recipients.
  2. **Varicella zoster virus resistant to acyclovir** may respond to foscarnet therapy [130]. AIDS patients who do not respond to acyclovir may benefit from foscarnet.
  3. **Human immunodeficiency virus.** In one study of the effect of foscarnet on p24 antigen of HIV, a reduction was seen in 21 of 22 patients [138]. In a second study, HIV ribonucleic acid (RNA) was quantitated in 17 patients before and during foscarnet therapy. A decrease in HIV RNA was observed in 16 of 17 patients [119]. No data is available on the impact of foscarnet on HIV viremia, but its antiretroviral activity may result in increased survival for patients with CMV retinitis compared with ganciclovir therapy.
  4. **CMV gastrointestinal disease** in AIDS. Uncontrolled studies suggest that foscarnet is an effective therapy for CMV esophageal ulceration and CMV colitis [110, 139]. An open label comparative trial of ganciclovir and foscarnet in patients with symptomatic CMV gastrointestinal disease found both drugs to be effective. No difference in survival or relapse rate despite maintenance therapy was seen [140].

V. **Adverse effects. Foscarnet is less well tolerated than ganciclovir, except that ganciclovir is myelosuppressive, whereas foscarnet usually is not.** The most common dose-limiting adverse effect of foscarnet is nephrotoxicity. In addition, foscarnet binds bivalent metal ions and therefore can produce metabolic abnormalities. In five controlled US clinical trials in which 189 patients with AIDS and CMV retinitis were treated with foscarnet, the most frequently reported events were the following: fever, 65%; nausea, 47%; anemia, 33%; diarrhea, 30%; abnormal renal function, 27%; vomiting, 26%; headache, 26%; and seizure, 10%. Genital ulcerations have also been reported [124, 141].

A. **Renal impairment.** Nephrotoxicity with azotemia and possibly tubular necrosis is the major dose-limiting effect [83]. Renal toxicity may be increased with concurrent use of other nephrotoxic drugs (e.g., amphotericin B, aminoglycosides, pentamidine). **Patients should be pretreated with 0.5–1.0 liter of intravenous normal saline prior to foscarnet therapy [142],** because adequate hydration may decrease the risk of nephrotoxicity. Recovery of renal function usually occurs within 1 week of drug discontinuation.

B. **Mineral and electrolyte imbalance.** Foscarnet chelates divalent ions and has been associated with changes in serum electrolytes, including hypocalcemia and hypercalcemia, hypophosphatemia and hyperphosphatemia, hypomagnesemia, and hypokalemia. Ionized serum calcium levels should be measured when neurologic or cardiac disturbances develop, because **decreases in ionized calcium may occur** and may not be reflected in total serum calcium levels. The risk of severe hypocalcemia, sometimes fatal, is increased by concurrent intravenous pentamidine [14]. Transient changes in electrolytes may contribute to a patient's risk for cardiac disturbance and seizure.

C. **Neurotoxicity and seizures.** Foscarnet has been associated with seizures in 18 of 189 AIDS patients (10%) in five controlled studies [124]. In most cases, the patients had an active CNS condition (e.g., toxoplasmosis, HIV encephalopathy) or a history of CNS disease. Several cases of seizures were associated with death. However, the rate of seizures did not increase with the duration of therapy. Occurrence of seizures did not always necessitate discontinuation of foscarnet therapy; the drug was continued after treatment of underlying diseases or after dose decreases [124].

D. **Hematopoietic system dysfunction.** Anemia has been reported in 33% of patients and granulocytopenia in 17% of patients in controlled studies [124]. However, foscarnet is less myelosuppressive than ganciclovir and can usually be taken with ZDV.

E. **Overdosage.** Adverse events and death produced by overdosage has been reported with foscarnet. There is no specific antidote, but hemodialysis and hydration may be of benefit in reducing drug plasma levels.

F. **Drug interactions.** A possible drug interaction with intravenous pentamidine, producing severe hypocalcemia and death in one patient, has been reported. Foscarnet preferably should be avoided in combination with potentially nephrotoxic drugs such as aminoglycosides, amphotericin B, and pentamidine, unless the benefit outweighs the risk [124].

VI. **Dosing recommendations for CMV retinitis**

A. **Induction therapy**

1. **Normal renal function.** The recommended dose of foscarnet for patients with normal renal function is 60 mg/kg IV (at a constant rate via infusion pump over a minimum of 1 hour) q8h for 2–3 weeks, depending on the clinical response. Although foscarnet may be given peripherally, administration centrally is preferred. Adequate hydration is recommended to establish a diuresis, both prior to and during treatment, to minimize renal toxicity. The standard 24 mg/ml solution may be used without dilution when administered centrally. When a peripheral vein catheter is used, the solution must be diluted to 12 mg/ml with 5% dextrose or normal saline to avoid local irritation of peripheral veins.

2. **With any degree of renal dysfunction, the dose must be modified on an individual basis** so that serum levels of foscarnet do not rise excessively and thereby potentiate renal toxicity. **To individualize doses,** first the patient's creatinine clearance must be known or estimated as discussed in Chap. 28A, in sec **VI.C** under Antibiotic Checklist (p. 1079). Then, the patient's creatinine clearance is divided by the patient's body weight (in kilograms) to determine the number of milliliters per minute per kilogram (ml/min/kg) for that patient. Use Table 26-8 to determine the actual induction dose.

    For example, if the patient's estimated creatinine clearance is 60 ml/min, and his weight is 60 kg, then:

$$\frac{\text{Estimated creatinine clearance}}{\text{Weight (kg)}} = \frac{60 \text{ ml/min}}{60 \text{ kg}} = 1 \text{ ml/min/kg}$$

    Based on Table 26-8, the proper dose would be 39 mg/kg q8h.

    If the patient's creatinine clearance divided by his or her weight is less than 0.4 ml/min/kg, the package insert suggests that foscarnet should be discontinued and the patient monitored (e.g., daily) until resolution of minimal renal function is ensured.

B. **Maintenance therapy.** After induction treatment, the package insert recommends that most patients be started on maintenance treatment with a dose of 90 mg/kg/day (individualized for renal function) given as an intravenous infusion over 2 hours. Adequate hydration is important. Patients who demonstrate escalation of retinitis or who tolerate very well the 90 mg/kg/day dose may benefit from treatment with an escalated maintenance dose of 120 mg/kg/day, especially given the recently reported study of improved outcome on this higher dose [135].

    See Table 26-9 for modification of maintenance doses depending on the patient's renal function. If the patient's renal function is below 0.4 ml/min/kg, foscarnet should not be used.

C. **Progression of retinitis.** Patients receiving foscarnet maintenance therapy in whom retinitis progresses should be retreated with induction followed by maintenance regimens. Combined use of foscarnet and ganciclovir may benefit some patients failing monotherapy [97, 97a].

D. **Pregnancy.** There are no adequate and well-controlled studies in pregnancy; foscarnet should be used during pregnancy only if clearly needed [124].

Table 26-8. Induction doses of foscarnet in patients with varying degrees of renal function

Creatinine clearance (ml/min/kg)	Equivalent to 60 mg/kg dose q8h
≥ 1.6	60
1.5	57
1.4	53
1.3	49
1.2	46
1.1	42
1.0	39
0.9	35
0.8	32
0.7	28
0.6	25
0.5	21
0.4	18

Source: *Physicians' Desk Reference* (49th ed.). Montvale, NJ: Medical Economics Data, 1995. P. 567. Copyright *Physicians' Desk Reference* 1995. Reprinted by permission. All rights reserved.

Table 26-9. Maintenance doses of foscarnet

Creatinine clearance (ml/min/kg)	Equivalent to 90 mg/kg dose q24h	Equivalent to 120 mg/kg dose q24h
> 1.4	90	120
1.2–1.4	78	104
1.0–1.2	75	100
0.8–1.0	71	94
0.6–0.8	63	84
0.4–0.6	57	76

Source: *Physicians' Desk Reference* (49th ed.). Montvale, NJ: Medical Economics Data, 1995. P. 567. Copyright *Physicians' Desk Reference* 1995. Reprinted by permission. All rights reserved.

E. **Nursing.** It is not known whether foscarnet is excreted in human milk. It would therefore seem prudent for mothers to avoid nursing while receiving foscarnet.

F. **Pediatric use.** The strategy and effectiveness of foscarnet in children have not been studied. Administration to children should be undertaken after careful evaluation and only if the potential benefits outweigh the risks [124].

G. **Patient monitoring.** It is recommended that a 24-hour creatinine clearance be determined at baseline and periodically thereafter to ensure correct dosing. Serum creatinine and electrolytes (calcium, magnesium, potassium, and phosphate) should be checked 2–3 times per week during induction and at least once every 1–2 weeks during maintenance therapy.

VII. **Doses in investigational uses.** No dosage recommendations can be made at this time for other investigational uses of foscarnet. Foscarnet, 40 mg/kg IV q8h, has been suggested as an alternative for acyclovir-resistant HSV infections or VZV infection in AIDS patients [14].

VIII. **Cost** (see Table 26-4)

Investigational Drugs for Non-HIV Viral Infections

I. **Sorivudine** (BV-araU). Sorivudine is a nucleoside analogue with in vitro activity against VZV that is more than a thousandfold greater than the activity of acyclovir [143]. In addition, the compound retains activity against HSV-1 and EBV, but not HSV-2 or CMV. Sorivudine triphosphate inhibits viral DNA synthesis and is concentrated in virus-infected cells. It is well absorbed orally, generally well tolerated, and can be given with once-daily dosing. It has had potentially fatal drug interactions with 5 fluorouracil, and has been removed from the market in Japan for this reason. Sorivudine has shown great promise in clinical trials in HZV infections in immunocompromised adults in the United States. Ongoing trials in nonimmunocompromised patients with HZV are also in progress. Use of the compound in progressive ocular retinal necrosis, which has responded poorly to other antiviral agents, has also been reported [144].

II. **Cidofovir** (HPMPC, Vistide). Cidofovir is a nucleotide analogue of cytosine and can therefore bypass the initial phosphorylation step by viral thymidine kinase that is utilized by nucleosides such as acyclovir and ganciclovir [145]. The compound is highly active against CMV, including some ganciclovir- and foscarnet-resistant strains. It is administered intravenously and cleared largely by the kidney with a serum half-life of 2.6 hours. Concomitant administration with probenecid markedly prolongs its half-life and protects against the major dose-limiting side effect, nephrotoxicity. The intracellular half-life of cidofovir diphosphate is 17–30 hours and is the basis for its administration at weekly to biweekly intervals. Results from a randomized, controlled clinical study of cidofovir in patients with AIDS and previously untreated peripheral CMV retinitis suggest that cidofovir markedly delays time to progression of CMV retinitis with infrequent intravenous dosing (one dose each week for 2 weeks as induction therapy, followed by one dose every 2 weeks as maintenance therapy). Cidofovir also has been successful in healing acyclovir- and foscarnet-resistant HSV infections [146]. Cidofovir is now available through a Treatment Investigational New Drug (IND) Program (1-800-445-3235) for the intravenous treatment of CMV retinitis in patients with AIDS who had relapsed on or cannot tolerate existing therapies.

Cidofovir also is currently being evaluated for intravitreal use for the treatment of CMV retinitis in patients with AIDS. Adverse effects from intravitreal injection include an intraocular pressure decrease, mild iritis, and retinal detachment [147].

Vidarabine

Vidarabine (Ara-A, adenine arabinoside) was the first parenterally administered antiviral agent licensed in the United States. Although it is efficacious for a number of herpesvirus infections, including herpetic encephalitis, neonatal infections, and herpes zoster in immunocompromised hosts, vidarabine has largely been replaced by acyclovir in clinical practice.

Iododeoxyuridine

Iododeoxyuridine (IDU, idoxuridine, 5-iodo-2'-deoxyuridine) is an analogue of thymidine. This drug was the first antiviral agent demonstrated to have a therapeutic effect and to be licensed for use in the United States. Iododeoxyuridine has one of the lowest therapeutic indices (< 2) of licensed drugs and an unacceptably high toxicity when administered systemically. The toxicity of IDU is not significant when administered topically, and it currently is approved for topical treatment of herpetic keratitis. Topical IDU use has largely been replaced by the more efficacious topical trifluorothymidine.

Trifluorothymidine (Trifluridine)

Trifluorothymidine (TFT, trifluridine, Viroptic) is a fluorinated pyrimidine in which three fluorine atoms substitute for the three hydrogens of the methyl group in thymidine. Although it was initially investigated as an antineoplastic agent, TFT was found to have antiherpesvirus activity [148].

I. **Mechanism of action.** Trifluridine is phosphorylated by host-cell thymidine kinase to TFT triphosphate and then is incorporated into both cellular and viral DNA, although there is some preferential uptake by viral DNA. Viral replication is believed to be inhibited by TFT in a manner similar to that in IDU. In addition, TFT monophosphate has the potential to inhibit thymidylate synthetase, the enzyme responsible for the conversion of dUMP to dTMP, which is necessary for DNA synthesis. This inhibition in the formation of dTMP probably accounts for the anticellular and antineoplastic properties of TFT. **Trifluridine is not very selective and therefore has significant toxicity when given parenterally to humans.**

II. **Pharmacology.** The plasma terminal half-life of TFT is approximately 18 minutes. **Currently, there is no indication for the use of the parenteral form of the drug because TFT is extremely toxic when given intravenously.**

III. Toxicity. Because TFT inhibits cellular DNA synthesis when given intravenously, rapidly replicating cells are inhibited. This results in unacceptable bone marrow suppression. **The topical ophthalmic solution toxicities are minor and infrequent.**

IV. Clinical uses

A. Herpetic keratoconjunctivitis. Trifluridine is more effective than IDU and is either as effective or more effective than vidarabine for the **treatment of herpetic kerato-conjunctivitis** [14]. Because TFT is never used parenterally, the emergence of resistant strains against TFT is of lesser potential clinical importance than the emergence of vidarabine resistance. For **herpetic keratoconjunctivitis,** the 1% ophthalmic solution is used as follows: one drop is instilled onto the cornea q2h while awake to a maximum of nine drops per day; on reepithelialization, treatment is continued for an additional 7 days at one drop q4h 5 times daily. If there is no improvement after 7 days or if reepithelialization has not occurred after 14 days, other forms of therapy should be considered. Treatment of HSV ocular infections should be supervised by an ophthalmologist.

B. Mucocutaneous acyclovir-resistant HSV infections. Acyclovir-resistant HSV infections are increasingly frequent in patients with advanced HIV disease, and treatment typically requires intravenous foscarnet (preferably through a central venous catheter). Topical TFT has been used successfully both alone [149, 150] and in combination with interferon-alpha [151] in small numbers of AIDS patients with severe cutaneous HSV infection resistant to acyclovir or resistant to both acyclovir and foscarnet. Although generally well tolerated, reported adverse effects of topical TFT have included a mild burning sensation after application and contact dermatitis [149]. For HSV infections, the 1% ophthalmic solution typically is applied three times daily as a thin film to each lesion and is covered with bacitracin-polymyxin ointment and a nonabsorbent dressing [150].

V. Cost (see Table 26-4)

Amantadine

Amantadine (1-adamantanamine hydrochloride) was first licensed in the United States in 1966 for the prevention of influenza A_2 and in 1976 for prophylaxis and therapy for all strains of influenza A. Amantadine is a primary symmetric amine that has a unique cagelike structure. Rimantadine, an amantadine analogue, was licensed in 1993 for prophylaxis and treatment of influenza A virus but has a lower potential for side effects.

I. Mechanism of action. The mechanism of action has **not been completely established.** However, amantadine does not appear to have any effect on virus attachment, and it does not affect the ability of the virus to penetrate into the cell, as it has been shown that both these activities occur normally in the presence of high concentrations of amantadine. The antiviral effect of amantadine is believed to be due to its ability to inhibit uncoating of the virus once it enters the cell.

II. In vitro sensitivity. All strains of influenza A virus are inhibited at concentrations that can readily be achieved clinically, with relatively good tolerance and safety. **Amantadine does not have activity against influenza B and parainfluenza virus** at concentrations that can be tolerated by humans.

III. Resistance. Amantadine-resistant strains of influenza A viruses can be selected in vitro. Studies have found amantadine-resistant and rimantadine-resistant strains of influenza A isolated from patients and children receiving antiviral therapy and in family members receiving postexposure prophylaxis [152–154]. Because rimantadine or amantadine will not prevent or treat infections caused by these resistant strains, one must question the use of these agents in low-risk patients who will have close contact with susceptible high-risk patients.

IV. Pharmacology. Amantadine is 85–95% absorbed after oral administration. Therapeutic concentrations are 0.2–0.6 μg/ml. The drug is not metabolized and is slowly excreted in the urine, with a half-life of approximately 15 hours in those with normal renal function. Amantadine is eliminated by both renal tubular secretion and glomerular filtration. The drug accumulates in patients with impaired renal function, and blood levels from 1 to 5 μg/ml have been associated with severe neuropsychiatric toxicity. In the elderly, the total body clearance of amantadine is reduced, and the half-life of amantadine is approximately twice as long as in the young adult (29 hours versus 15 hours, respectively). Therefore, **doses should be reduced in the elderly and in patients with renal insufficiency** [155, 156].

V. Toxicity

A. **In young adults with normal renal function,** the adverse effects are relatively mild and reversible. When adverse effects occur, they usually appear in the first 2 days of therapy. The incidence of side effects may be reduced by administering the drug as a divided dose twice daily rather than as a single daily dose.

  1. **Central nervous system.** Adverse effects occur in approximately 5–10% of healthy adults and consist of difficulties in thinking, confusion, lightheadedness, anxiety, insomnia and, rarely, hallucinations.

  2. **Anticholinergiclike effects.** In addition, even though amantadine does not block cholinergic receptors, anticholinergiclike side effects may be seen, such as dry mouth and urinary retention.

B. **Elderly** patients are **more likely to have both CNS and anticholinergiclike side effects.** There are several possible reasons for this:

  1. Because renal function declines with age (with renal tubular secretion decreasing even more than glomerular filtration rate), the clearance of amantadine is reduced in the elderly.

  2. On the average, the **elderly tend to weigh less** than the average young adult. Therefore, if one gives the standard dose of 200 mg/day, the elderly patient receives a higher dose (based on mg/kg) than does the young adult.

  3. **Tissue sensitivity.** The elderly may be more sensitive to the CNS effects of amantadine even at the same serum concentrations. This is true with other drugs such as the benzodiazepines.

  4. **Recommendations.** Ideally, the dose of amantadine in elderly patients should be adjusted in proportion to their amantadine clearance. The elderly probably should receive approximately 1.4 mg/kg/day [155]. See Table 26-10 for dose recommendations relative to varying degrees of renal function.

C. **Pregnancy.** Because of amantadine's teratogenic potential, it should be used in pregnancy only when the benefit to the patient outweighs the risk to the fetus.

D. **Drug interactions.** Anticholinergic drugs, when administered with amantadine, may result in an increase in adverse effects due to cholinergic blockade.

VI. Clinical indications

A. **Prophylaxis.** In numerous controlled studies, it has been shown that amantadine (200 mg/day), when given prophylactically during influenza A epidemics, is approximately 70–90% effective in preventing illness, a value similar to the efficacy of the influenza vaccines [157, 158]. This has been documented in normal adults, children, and chronically ill and debilitated patients. Controlled clinical trials are not available in high-risk elderly patients. Amantadine, 100 mg/day, also appears to be effective in some populations [157]. Because the protective effect of amantadine is present only while the patient is taking the drug, the amantadine must be given during the entire epidemic period, usually 5–7 weeks or for at least 2 weeks after the patient is given a vaccine containing the current epidemic strain. Chemoprophylaxis, however, is not a substitute for vaccine [158]. Persons at high risk for influenza A should be vaccinated unless it is contraindicated.

B. **Therapy.** Amantadine has been widely tested as a therapeutic agent in naturally occurring influenza A infections in previously healthy young adults [157, 158]. Amantadine, 200 mg/day for 3–5 days, reduced by 50% the duration of fever and

Table 26-10. Adjustment of amantadine in patients with varying degrees of renal function

Creatinine clearance (ml/min/m^2)	Dose
> 80	200 mg daily
60–80	200 mg; 100 mg on alternate days
40–60	100 mg qd
30–40	200 mg 2 ×/wk
20–30	100 mg 3 ×/wk
10–20	200 mg; 100 mg alternating every 7 days

Source: From V.W. Horadam et al. Pharmacokinetics of amantadine hydrochloride in subjects with normal and impaired renal function. *Ann. Intern. Med.* 94: 454, 1981.

systemic symptoms. Other data suggest that amantadine-treated students with influenza returned to class more rapidly than those receiving a placebo. Also, amantadine has been shown to enhance resolution of abnormalities in peripheral airway function. **To be effective, the drug probably needs to be started within 24–48 hours after onset of disease.** A major problem with the use of amantadine for the treatment of influenza A infections lies in the lack of a rapid diagnostic test for influenza infections. (See discussion of influenza direct antigen testing, Chap. 8, sec. **V.B** under Influenza, p. 241). Until these tests become more readily available, it would seem reasonable to treat those patients, especially the high-risk group, who develop influenzalike symptoms during a documented influenza A outbreak in the community or facility in which the patient lives. Amantadine use in children is undefined [159].

C. **Pneumonic complications.** There are no trials investigating the effectiveness of amantadine in patients with influenza who develop pulmonary complications (such as primary influenza pneumonia). Nevertheless, in this setting it seems reasonable to use amantadine or rimantadine at therapeutic doses for 5 days.

VII. **Dosing guidelines (as a single daily dose or split bid dose)** [158]

A. **Prophylaxis of influenza A** [160] **in high-risk groups (defined as** those with cardiac or pulmonary disease, residents of nursing homes and chronic care facilities, those who provide medical care, the elderly, and those with other chronic diseases) who have not received or cannot receive the vaccine (e.g., those who are allergic to egg products or who have had hypersensitivity reactions to the vaccine). The dose in patients with normal renal function is 100 mg bid for the entire epidemic period except in those older than 65 years, who typically receive 100 mg/day (see secs. **V.B.** and **VIII**). Such lower daily doses (100 mg/day) also protect against influenza A in semiclosed populations of teenage students [157]. As an alternative to giving amantadine for 5–7 weeks, one can give the nonimmunized patient influenza vaccine and then administer amantadine (e.g., 100 mg bid if renal function is normal) for only 10–14 days, to protect against influenza infection until protective antibodies develop. Amantadine does not affect the antibody response to influenza vaccines.

B. **Prophylaxis of high-risk people** during an epidemic with a new subtype of influenza A for which no current vaccine is available. In this case, amantadine (100 mg bid if renal function is normal) must be administered during the entire epidemic, usually 6–8 weeks.

C. **Prophylaxis of profoundly immunocompromised patients.** In patients in whom adequate antibody response to vaccination is not expected (e.g., those with AIDS, chronic renal disease, and other forms of immunosuppression), supplemental administration of amantadine, in addition to vaccination, may enhance the protective effect over vaccine alone.

D. **For the treatment of influenza A** (especially in those patients in the high-risk group). Amantadine therapy (100 mg bid if renal function is normal for 3–5 days) should be started within 24–48 hours [158]. Similar doses are used in complicated cases of influenza (primary influenza pneumonia or mixed viral-bacterial pneumonia), even though efficacy for this indication has not been studied in properly performed trials (see Chap. 8). As previously noted (see sec. **III**), however, one should exercise caution in treating low-risk patients who are likely to have contact with susceptible high-risk patients.

VIII. **Dose modifications for children, the elderly, and patients with renal impairment**

A. **Age-adjusted doses.** In children between the ages of 1 and 9 years, use 5 mg/kg/day up to 150 mg in two divided doses. In children and adults between 10 and 64 years of age, use 100 mg bid if renal function is normal. In the elderly (> 65 years), 100 mg/day is suggested.

B. **Impaired renal function (adult doses).** See Table 26-10. Alternatively, one can reduce the dose in proportion to the patient's renal function. For example,

Daily amantadine dose (mg) = 200 × (patient's Cl_{cr}/120)

where *200* represents the usual daily amantadine dose (in mg); *patient's Cl_{cr}* represents either the measured or the estimated creatinine clearance (in ml/min) of the patient; and *120* represents the average normal creatinine clearance (in ml/min).

IX. **Vaccine versus amantadine.** There are advantages of the influenza vaccine over amantadine chemoprophylaxis.

A. **Advantages of vaccines**

1. **Compliance.** Vaccine requires the patient to be compliant only once, whereas amantadine needs to be taken twice daily for 6 weeks.
2. **Cost.** The average wholesale cost of a dose of influenza vaccine is less than $4.00, whereas the average wholesale cost for a 6-week course of amantadine is approximately $18.00 (see Table 26-4).
3. **Protection against influenza B** often is provided by the multivalent vaccine but not by amantadine.

B. **Advantage of amantadine.** Amantadine protects against all strains of influenza A, even if an antigen shift occurs.

Rimantadine

Rimantadine (alpha-methyl-1-adamantane methylamine, Flumadine) hydrochloride is an analogue of amantadine that was licensed in 1993 for prophylaxis and treatment of illness caused by influenza A virus in adults and for prophylaxis against influenza A virus in children. **Rimantadine has a similar efficacy to but a lower potential for side effects compared with amantadine** [161].

I. **Mechanism of action, in vitro activity, and resistance.** The mechanism of action and in vitro spectrum of activity are similar to those for amantadine, though rimantadine is somewhat more active [157]. Resistance to rimantadine does occur clinically [152–154]. When the drug is administered for prophylaxis to close contacts of patients who develop resistant strains of influenza, rimantadine is ineffective. Like amantadine, rimantadine use in patients with influenza probably should be avoided when there is likely to be close contact with a susceptible high-risk person.

II. **Pharmacology.** Unlike amantadine, which is essentially eliminated entirely by renal excretion, rimantadine is extensively metabolized in the liver, with less than 25% of a dose excreted in urine as unchanged drug [162, 163]. The absolute bioavailability of rimantadine is unknown. The average plasma half-life is approximately 1–1.5 days, twice as long as that of amantadine.

A. **Renal disease.** In patients with end-stage renal disease, the mean half-life increased approximately 60%, with an approximately 40% decrease in total body clearance [164]. Rimantadine, like amantadine, is not removed by hemodialysis. Therefore, **in patients with end-stage renal disease, the ideal dose administered probably should be decreased by approximately 40%.**

B. **Hepatic disease.** No clinically significant alteration was seen in rimantadine kinetics in patients with mild chronic hepatic disease (total bilirubin concentration or prothrombin times of less than 2 times the upper limit of normal) [165]. **In persons with severe liver dysfunction, rimantadine clearance was 50% lower than that reported for persons without liver disease [158]. A dose reduction to 100 mg/day is recommended for persons with severe hepatic dysfunction [158].**

III. **Adverse effects. Rimantadine is well tolerated.** The rate of adverse experiences appears to be similar to that seen in placebo recipients and is less than that seen with amantadine [157, 166]. Rimantadine is contraindicated in patients with known hypersensitivity to amantadine. The incidence of some adverse effects in the elderly, from pooled data from controlled studies, was increased with the recommended dose of rimantadine (100 mg bid) compared to controls: Central and peripheral nervous system dysfunction affected 12.5% versus 8.7%, and GI system dysfunction affected 17% versus 11.3% [167].

IV. **Pregnancy.** Rimantadine should be used during pregnancy only if the potential benefit to the patient outweighs the risk to the fetus.

V. **Drug interactions.** Data are limited, but no significant interactions have been described. Concurrent use of cimetidine (Tagamet) can increase, and aspirin or acetaminophen can decrease, plasma concentrations of rimantadine, but the magnitude of these effects is unlikely to be important clinically [163].

VI. **Clinical indications and dose recommendations.** These are similar to those for amantadine. **Rimantadine may be preferred over amantadine in the elderly and persons in institutions, because of the lower risk of CNS toxicity [157]. Rimantadine may also be the drug of choice in younger persons because of the lower incidence of associated CNS effects. Its potential benefits must be weighed against its increased cost (see Table 26-4).**

A. **Influenza A prophylaxis.** The recommended dose of rimantadine for adults and children older than 10 years is 100 mg bid. In patients with severe hepatic dysfunction, renal failure (creatinine clearance ≤ 10 ml/min) and elderly nursing home patients, a dose reduction to 100 mg/day is recommended. The recommended dose of rimantadine for children 1 to 9 years old is 5 mg/kg/day in two divided doses, not to exceed 150 mg [158].

B. **Treatment of influenza A infections.** Placebo-controlled trials have demonstrated the benefit of rimantadine, 200 or 300 mg/day, in reducing the signs and symptoms of disease in patients with naturally occurring influenza A illness [157]. The recommended adult dose is 100 mg bid. In patients with severe hepatic dysfunction, renal failure (creatinine clearance $\leq$ 10 ml/min) and elderly nursing home patients, a dose reduction to 100 mg/day is recommended. Based on data on disease in close contacts caused by resistant strains of influenza A, **one probably should avoid treatment of otherwise healthy patients who will be in contact with susceptible individuals at high risk of mortality from influenza disease.** The drug has not been approved for treatment of children with influenza A infections.

VII. **Vaccine versus rimantadine.** The advantages and disadvantages of vaccine versus rimantadine are similar to those for amantadine (see sec. **IX** under Amantadine).

VIII. **Cost** (see Table 26-4)

Ribavirin

Ribavirin (1-beta-D-ribofuranosyl-1H-1,2,4-triazole-3-carboxamide, Virazole) is a broad-spectrum antiviral agent that is active against most RNA and DNA viruses. Ribavirin is related structurally to the naturally occurring ribonucleoside guanosine. **Ribavirin is approved for aerosol therapy for respiratory syncytial virus (RSV).** Used as an aerosol, it can decrease morbidity in children hospitalized with RSV bronchiolitis and pneumonia, including those requiring mechanical ventilation [14]. Ribavirin has a broad spectrum of antiviral activity in vitro, where it inhibits replication of RSV, influenza A and B, parainfluenza, adenovirus, measles, Lassa fever, and Hantaan viruses. It has been shown to be effective for influenza A and influenza B by aerosol and for Lassa fever and epidemic hemorrhagic fever when given intravenously, but it is not FDA-approved for these uses [168]. Neither oral nor intravenous ribavirin has been marketed in the United States [14].

I. **Mechanism of action.** The mechanism of action of ribavirin is not well established, and the mechanism of action by which different classes of viruses are inhibited probably varies.

II. **Pharmacology**

A. **Metabolism and elimination.** The drug exhibits a very complex kinetic profile, and the decay of the plasma ribavirin concentrations appears to have three phases of elimination: alpha, or disposition phase; beta, or elimination phase; and gamma, or deep compartment phase. In humans, the elimination of ribavirin appears to be by both renal elimination and metabolism. In addition, the drug accumulates and is concentrated into RBCs, presumably as the phosphorylated nucleotides. This accumulation into RBCs probably accounts for the gamma or terminal-phase half-life. The decay of ribavirin from RBCs is slow (half-life of 40 hours).

B. **Plasma concentrations**

1. **Oral preparation.** Bioavailability is 35–50%, with peak plasma concentrations achieved approximately 2 hours after administration [169]. Mean peak ribavirin plasma concentrations are 1.7–5.3 μM (0.4–1.3 μg/ml) following ribavirin administration, 1,000 mg/day PO given in three divided doses.

2. **Aerosol preparation.** Peak plasma ribavirin concentrations are in the range of 3.3–6.1 μM (0.8–1.5 μg/ml), whereas mean peak ribavirin concentrations in the respiratory secretions are in the range of 1–8 mM (0.25–2.00 mg/ml) [170].

3. **Intravenous preparation.** Mean plasma ribavirin concentrations are 94 μM and 68 μM, respectively, following 1,000 mg q6h and 500 mg q6h [171]. These concentrations do not necessarily represent peak concentrations.

III. **Clinical use**

A. **Small-particle aerosol preparation.** Ribavirin was found to be effective for the treatment of the following infections:

1. **RSV infections in infants and young children** [172, 173]. In addition, infants with RSV infections who were treated with ribavirin were less likely to develop specific IgE-anti-RSV antibodies in their sputum [174]. Because IgE-anti-RSV antibodies are postulated to mediate the postinfectious complication of bronchospastic disease seen following RSV infections in infants, ribavirin may be useful both for the therapy of the acute illness and perhaps in preventing the postinfectious sequelae.

The American Academy of Pediatrics has recommended that infants hospitalized with lower respiratory tract disease caused by RSV **in the following categories may be considered for therapy with ribavirin aerosol** [175–176a].

  a. **Infants at high risk for severe or complicated RSV** (e.g., immunosuppressed infants, infants with congenital heart or lung conditions).

  b. **Infants hospitalized with RSV lower respiratory tract disease who are severely ill** (e.g., those with PaO_2 levels < 65 mm Hg and those with increasing $PaCO_2$ levels).

  c. **Infants mechanically ventilated for RSV infection.**

  d. Infants who may not be severely ill at presentation but who may be at some increased risk of progressing to a more complicated course by virtue of young age (< 6 weeks) or in whom prolonged illness might be particularly detrimental to an underlying condition, such as multiple congenital anomalies or neurologic or metabolic disease.

  2. **Influenza A and B infections** in otherwise healthy adults when therapy was initiated within 24 hours of onset of illness [177–179].

B. **Intravenous preparation.** Infectious disease consultation and consultation with the Centers for Disease Control are advised when using intravenous ribavirin in the following rare situations and for investigational use.

  1. **Lassa fever.** The intravenous form has been used in the therapy of Lassa fever when given intravenously in daily doses of 2–4 g/day (in four divided doses) for 10 days [38, 180]. Ribavirin also is useful in prophylaxis for persons who have been exposed to a patient with Lassa fever [38].

  2. **Hantavirus infection.** Ribavirin has been reported to be of clinical benefit in the treatment of hemorrhagic fever with renal syndrome and hantavirus pulmonary syndrome caused by the Sin Nombre virus [181]. See Chap. 9 (pp. 291–293).

C. **Oral preparation**

  1. Oral ribavirin has been proposed for prophylaxis of Lassa fever and in Congo-Crimean hemorrhagic fever contacts but is not approved for marketing for this use [14].

  2. Oral ribavirin has beneficial effects on serum amino-transaminase and histologic findings in the liver of patients with chronic **hepatitis C** (HCV), but these effects are not accompanied by HCV RNA level changes and are not sustained when therapy is stopped [182]. Therefore, ribavirin alone is unlikely to be beneficial in the treatment of chronic hepatitis C [182].

  3. Oral ribavirin has not been shown to be effective in HIV infection [183].

IV. **Toxicity**

A. When ribavirin is administered by aerosolization, no clinically significant toxicity is seen. When doses greater than 600 mg/day are given orally or when the drug is given intravenously, a reduction in the number of RBCs or a normochromic, normocytic anemia may occur. This is believed to be due to a decrease in RBC production by maturation arrest in the bone marrow. A reticulocytosis may occur after therapy is discontinued.

B. Health care workers exposed to aerosolized ribavirin have experienced minor toxicity, including eye and respiratory tract infections [184].

C. Ribavirin has been shown to produce testicular lesions in rodents and to be teratogenic in all animal species in which studies have been performed [184].

V. **Dosing.** For aerosol use, ribavirin (6 g reconstituted in 300 ml sterile water to a final concentration of 20 mg/ml) usually is given by small-particle aerosol (using a special small-particle aerosol generator), administered 12–20 h/day for approximately 3 days for influenza disease in young adults and for 3–5 or 7 days in the treatment of RSV infections in infants. Preliminary studies in animals and in humans suggest that hour-long inhalation 3 or 4 times per day is as effective as longer durations [175, 185]. Maximal therapeutic responses usually are noted after 2–4 days of treatment [175]. If ribavirin therapy is given to a patient on assisted ventilation, special precautions are necessary, and this should be done in facilities where the personnel have specific training and expertise in the administration of ribavirin to ventilated infants [175, 176].

A. Treatment with ribavirin does not eliminate the need for contact isolation of patients with RSV [175].

B. Earlier concerns of environmental contamination and the potential risk to hospital personnel, especially pregnant health care workers, has largely disappeared as further experience has been gained with this agent. This topic has been reviewed elsewhere; the teratogenicity of ribavirin in humans remains highly questionable [175].

VI. Resistance. The development or selection of resistance to ribavirin has not been observed in clinical isolates or in vitro.

VII. Cost. It is uncertain whether the use of this very expensive drug will reduce the cost of hospitalization of children with RSV infection. The cost of ribavirin, not including administration, is approximately $1,300 a day (see Table 26-4).

Interferons

Interferons are a family of functionally related, species-specific proteins synthesized in eukaryotic cells in response to viruses and a variety of other stimuli. Interferon-alpha (alfa) is available as alfa-2a (Roferon A), alfa-2b (Intron A), and interferon-alfa-n3 (Alferon) [186–188]. Recombinant interferon-alpha has been approved for use both as an anticancer agent and as an antiviral drug. Many of the malignancies for which it is indicated are associated with viral infections (hairy cell leukemia, human T-lymphotropic virus type I, Kaposi's sarcoma in patients with AIDS). Interferon-gamma is indicated for reducing the frequency and severity of serious infections associated by chronic granulomatous disease, primarily of bacterial origin [188, 189]. **This section will address only interferons used for viral infections. The use of interferon gamma has recently been reviewed by Gallin et al. [189].**

I. **Spectrum of antiviral activity and mechanism of action.** A wide range of different RNA and DNA viruses are susceptible in vitro to interferon. Interferon is not directly antiviral but causes a series of biological reactions within the cell that lead to the production of an antiviral substance. Despite its relatively short half-life in plasma, this intracellular antiviral substance persists for several days.

II. **Pharmacology.** Interferon-alpha is not orally bioavailable. After intravenous administration, the decline in plasma concentration is biphasic, with a terminal plasma half-life of 2 hours. After intramuscular or subcutaneous administration, the time to peak concentration is 4–8 hours, and return to baseline occurs by 18–36 hours. However, biochemical effects of interferon persist for days after a single intramuscular injection. The antiviral state, as judged by ex vivo challenge of lymphocytes to vesicular stomatitis virus, peaks at 1 day and decreases to baseline in slightly less than 1 week [190]. Therefore, the antiviral state persists much longer than that of the plasma concentrations.

III. **Clinical uses**

A. **Papillomavirus**

1. **Condylomata acuminata.** Intralesional use of interferon is useful in refractory cases of this disease [191–194]. In a placebo-controlled trial, intralesionally administered natural interferon-alpha, given twice weekly for up to 8 weeks, completely eliminated lesions in 62% of patients compared to only 21% in the control group [192]. Other studies using thrice-weekly intralesional injections for 3 weeks have demonstrated efficacy [191]. Unfortunately, after complete remission, relapses may occur in at least 20–30% of patients. The average time to relapse was 4 months [192]. Retreatment usually is successful. Parenteral therapy has also been advocated for extensive disease [195, 196].

    Less expensive alternatives (e.g., cryotherapy; trichloroacetic acid, 80–90%; podophyllin, 10–25%) are available for therapy of condylomata acuminata [14]. See related discussion in Chap. 13.

2. **Juvenile laryngeal papillomatosis.** Although most children with juvenile laryngeal papillomatosis have some response to interferon-alpha, the recurrence rate is high after treatment is stopped. The long-term response to interferon treatment is highly variable [196, 197]. The role of interferon for this indication awaits further clarification from clinical experience.

B. **Herpesviruses**

1. **Varicella-zoster virus.** Interferon has been demonstrated to be beneficial for the treatment of infections caused by VZV in the immunosuppressed patient when given at relatively high doses, but frequent side effects were observed [198, 199]. **Acyclovir therapy is preferred,** and interferon rarely, if ever, is used for this indication.

2. **Herpes simplex virus.** Topically applied interferon appears to have some activity in recurrent genital herpes and, in combination with TFT, may be beneficial in drug-resistant mucocutaneous HSV infections [151]. **Acyclovir remains the treatment of choice for HSV infections [14].**

C. **Hepatitis B virus** (HBV). Interferon-alpha administration to patients with chronic HBV infections appears to be beneficial [200–206]. Therapy with parenteral interferon-alfa-2b (5 million units daily for 4 months) was associated with loss of HBV DNA, seroconversion to anti-HBe, and biochemical and histologic improvement in approximately 40% of patients with chronic HBV infection [202–204]. In patients with HBV who are positive for hepatitis B e antigen, serum HBV e antigen is eliminated, which may be associated with clinical improvement, normalization of aminotransferase activity, sustained histologic improvement, improved survival, and lower costs [207]. Women may be more likely than men to respond.

D. **Non-A, non-B hepatitis virus including hepatitis C and D viruses**

1. **Hepatitis C virus (HCV).** A placebo-controlled trial has demonstrated that interferon-alpha, 2 million units subcutaneously 3 times weekly for 6 months, was helpful in reducing the disease activity in chronic infections caused by HCV [208]. In more than half the patients, there was a beneficial effect on the serum aminotransferase activity. The degree of hepatic injury, particularly the amount of lobular necrosis and inflammation, was also decreased. However, patients frequently relapsed after treatment was stopped. A related study showed similar results, with 50% of responding patients relapsing after treatment was stopped [209]. Some reviewers suggest therapy for HCV should not be recommended in asymptomatic patients or individuals with slowly progressive disease [210]. See Katkov and Dienstag [211] for a summary of an approach to therapy of HCV.

2. **Hepatitis D virus (HDV).** In a randomized controlled trial comparing high doses (9 million units) or low doses (3 million units) of interferon-alfa for 48 weeks with no treatment in patients with chronic HDV, approximately half the patients on the high dose had normalization of their serum alanine aminotransferase level, HDV RNA became undetectable in serum, and histologic improvement was noted [212]. Unfortunately, most patients had a relapse within 6 months after stopping therapy.

3. **Autoimmune chronic hepatitis.** This form of hepatitis may be exacerbated by treatment with interferon [14, 213]. Therefore, it is important to make an accurate diagnosis of HCV before using interferon treatment. In a small group of patients in whom the HCV cannot be reliably distinguished from autoimmune chronic hepatitis, some experts suggest that a course of corticosteroids should be administered on a trial basis, and then interferon treatment should be instituted in patients unresponsive to corticosteroids [214], as these patients are more likely to have chronic HCV.

4. The optimal dose and duration of therapy for chronic viral hepatitis infections await further clinical study.

E. **Miscellaneous.** In HIV infections, particularly in early-stage infection, interferon treatment has been associated with dose-related antiretroviral effects, although significant adverse effects have occurred [215]. Combination studies with various nucleoside reverse transcriptase inhibitors are under way. In vitro resistance to interferon has been observed in HIV isolates [216]. In addition to clinical investigational studies in AIDS, interferon-alpha is undergoing clinical evaluation in rhinovirus infection and visceral leishmaniasis [217]. Intranasal interferon-alfa-2b, in conjunction with oral naproxen and ipratropium, has been shown to reduce incidence and severity of colds after rhinovirus inoculation [218]. Oral interferon is not effective in HIV infections [219].

IV. **Adverse effects.** Interferon is associated with a high frequency of dose-related toxicity that limits its use. Fortunately, however, reactions are generally well tolerated, mild to moderate, reversible, and, if monitored closely, rarely life threatening [217].

A. **Flulike syndrome.** Fever, headache, chills, nausea, vomiting, myalgias, or diarrhea can be seen within hours of administration of interferon-alpha, given by either intramuscular or subcutaneous injection, especially during the first week of therapy [14]. Even after intralesional administration, flulike symptoms occur in approximately 50% of patients, although they usually resolve during the first week of therapy.

B. **More serious toxicity includes** granulocytopenia, thrombocytopenia, neurotoxicity (including confusional states, depression, and, rarely, seizures), profound fatigue, depression, anorexia, weight loss, alopecia, hypothyroidism or hyperthyroidism, autoantibody formation, and, possibly, cardiotoxicity [14].

V. **Dose regimens.** Our understanding of dosing of interferon-alpha is rapidly evolving, and optimal doses, routes of administration, dose intervals, and duration of therapy are still being assessed, especially for the treatment of hepatitis.

A. **Currently approved interferon dosages** are listed in this section. The package insert recommendations should be carefully followed, and consultation with sub-specialists familiar with the use of interferons is advised.

   1. **Interferon-alfa-2b,** recombinant (Intron A), has been approved for use in selected cases of condylomata acuminata, chronic HCV (chronic non-A, non-B), chronic HBV in patients older than 18 years, selected patients with Kaposi's sarcoma, and hairy cell leukemia [187].

      a. The optimal regimen for **condylomata acuminata** has not been determined, but the manufacturer recommends 1.0 million IU into each lesion thrice weekly on alternate days, for 3 weeks. Patients with more than five lesions may need additional courses of treatment.

      b. The optimal regimen for **chronic non-A, non-B (C) hepatitis** is currently under investigation, but the manufacturer recommends 3 million IU thrice weekly, administered subcutaneously or intramuscularly.

      c. The recommended dosage for the treatment of **chronic HBV** is 30–35 million IU per week, administered subcutaneously or intramuscularly either as 5 million IU daily or 10 million IU thrice weekly for 16 weeks.

   2. **Interferon-alfa-N3** (Alferon N), derived from human leukocytes, has been approved for use in refractory or recurrent **condylomata acuminata** in patients older than 18 years [188]. The recommended dose is 250,000 IU per wart, administered twice weekly for up to 8 weeks, with a maximum dose of 2.5 million IU per treatment session [188].

   3. **Interferon-alfa-2a,** recombinant (Roferan A) is currently approved only for hairy cell leukemia and AIDS-related Kaposi's sarcoma.

   4. **Interferon-gamma-1b** (Actimmune) is currently approved only for reducing the frequency and severity of serious infections associated with chronic granulomatous disease.

B. **Because dosage recommendations are subject to revision and are influenced by ongoing clinical trials, especially in chronic viral hepatitis therapy, consultation with a gastroenterologist or infectious disease expert with a special interest in viral hepatitis is advised before using these expensive agents for chronic hepatitis.** For a discussion of the specifics of therapy for viral hepatitis, see Katkov and Dienstag [211].

VI. **Cost** (see Table 26-4).

Antiretroviral Agents

Much progress has been made in the development of antiretroviral agents for the treatment of HIV infection. Unfortunately, with the approval of each new antiretroviral drug, the therapy of HIV infection becomes more complex. **Combination therapy appears to hold much promise in enhancing our ability to suppress HIV viral load, delay the progression of AIDS, and prolong survival.** In addition, new classes of drugs are being developed, and numerous clinical trials are currently under way to help determine optimal combinations of antiretroviral agents.

As of January 1996, there **currently** is **no consensus** as to when to initiate antiretroviral therapy and with what drugs, when and how to modify antiretroviral regimens, and when, if ever, to discontinue antiretroviral medications. Results from a state-of-the-art conference panel on antiretroviral therapy for adult HIV-infected patients were published in 1993 and are woefully out of date [220]. Plans for updating and revising recommended antiretroviral regimens are under way.

This section reviews the pharmacology of available anti-HIV medications and highlights the results of major monotherapy and combination therapy clinical trials. The section concludes with clinical perspectives on selecting antiretroviral regimens and **guidelines for antiretroviral therapy** based on current knowledge that provide reasonable alternatives for patients, depending on their levels of immunosuppression. **With the field of antiretroviral therapy changing so quickly, any guidelines or options for antiretroviral therapy undoubtedly will need to be revised frequently.** Hence, the guidelines provided should be viewed as just that—guidelines or options—and it must be remembered that the optimal antiretroviral regimen for a particular patient will need to be individualized.

Zidovudine

Zidovudine (ZDV, azidothymidine [AZT], Retrovir) is a nucleoside analogue of thymidine that inhibits HIV reverse transcriptase. **It was the first antiviral agent shown to be of benefit in the treatment of HIV infection** [221]. Zidovudine was approved in 1987 by the FDA and has been shown to decrease transient plasma RNA levels and increase circulating CD4 cell counts, decrease the number of opportunistic infections and progression to AIDS, prolong survival in persons with AIDS, and to decrease progression to AIDS in patients with HIV disease [116, 222, 223].

I. **Mechanism of action.** Zidovudine is a prodrug that is phosphorylated by cellular enzymes to its active 5'-triphosphate form [224]. Zidovudine triphosphate is a competitive inhibitor and a chain terminator of viral DNA synthesis [225]. Because of this, **ZDV inhibits or terminates the reverse transcriptase–mediated production of proviral DNA.**

II. **In vitro activity.** Zidovudine is active against HIV-1 and HIV-2 in vitro.

III. **Resistance.** Resistance to ZDV has been associated with readily inducible point mutations in the reverse transcriptase gene; multiple changes are required to confer high-level resistance [226, 227]. Mutations associated with resistant strains have had amino acid substitutions on multiple loci, including positions 41, 67, 70, 215, and 219 [228]. Of the HIV-1 mutations reported to be associated with ZDV resistance, the mutation at codon 215 of the reverse transcriptase gene is the most commonly occurring and has the greatest impact on susceptibility [229, 230]. Most resistant strains have been isolated from HIV-infected patients treated with ZDV for 6 months or longer [226]. Clones of HIV with four or five mutations have a greater than 100-fold reduction in ZDV sensitivity [228]. **Development of resistance appears to correlate with advanced stage of disease and increased duration of ZDV use** [231, 232].

With continued use of ZDV monotherapy, in vitro resistance develops and has been associated with clinical deterioration [233]. Strains of HIV resistant in vitro to ZDV may be susceptible to didanosine (ddI), zalcitabine (dideoxycytidine, ddC), and other recently approved antiretroviral agents [234]. Recent studies suggest that ZDV-resistant HIV-1 can be transmitted sexually, through blood exposure, and vertically to newborns [235–237]. **Strategies for the use of ZDV in combination therapies are designed, in part, to decrease the emergence of resistant viral strains.**

IV. **Pharmacology** [221]. Although drug levels can be measured by high-performance liquid chromography (HPLC), radioimmunoassay, and bioassay, they are not available clinically.

A. **Absorption.** Zidovudine is well absorbed from the GI tract, with an oral bioavailability of 65–70% and peak concentrations of 1 μg/ml occurring 0.5–1.0 hour following doses.

B. **Half-life.** After oral (or intravenous) administration, ZDV is cleared rapidly from the plasma with a half-life of 1 hour.

C. **Elimination and metabolism.** Zidovudine is eliminated by hepatic metabolism to a glucuronide, which is excreted rapidly into the urine.

   1. **Hepatic disease.** In patients with cirrhosis, oral clearance of the drug is reduced by 70% [221, 238], resulting in two to threefold increases in peak plasma levels and half-life. Although controlled clinical trials have not studied dosage and efficacy **in patients with severe hepatic dysfunction, a reduced dose seems appropriate** [221].

   2. **Renal disease.** In uremic patients, the peak concentration of ZDV is increased by approximately 50%, and studies are under way to determine the effect of renal dysfunction on the half-life of ZDV. Zidovudine doses in patients with impaired renal function have not been established, but preliminary reports suggest **reduction of doses (e.g., 100 mg tid) and more frequent monitoring for potential toxicities (anemia or neutropenia) may be reasonable** [221].

D. **Cerebrospinal fluid penetration.** ZDV crosses the blood-brain barrier, producing therapeutic CSF levels, but penetration can be variable.

V. **Clinical uses.** An excellent reference guide to major clinical trials in patients infected with HIV was published in 1995 [239], and the authors plan to publish an update of their summary tables annually.

A. **Initial antiretroviral therapy**

   1. **Primary HIV infection.** Zidovudine appears to be useful in patients who present with primary HIV infection. A recent study of 77 patients with primary HIV infection were randomly assigned to ZDV, 250 mg bid, versus placebo for 6 months [240]; HIV disease progression was significantly less frequent in the

ZDV group. After adjusting for baseline CD4 count, patients treated with ZDV had an average monthly CD4 cell count gain of 8.9 cells/mm³ during the first 6 months, whereas the placebo group had an average monthly loss of 12 cells/mm³.

2. **Asymptomatic HIV disease**
   a. In 1990, ZDV was shown to slow the clinical progression to AIDS in persons with asymptomatic HIV infection and CD4 cell count < 500 cells/mm³ compared to placebo (AIDS Clinical Trials Group **[ACTG] 019**) [241]. Long-term follow-up of these asymptomatic HIV-infected patients with CD4 counts < 500 cells/mm³ revealed a benefit in ZDV's delaying disease progression, but no differences were seen in overall survival during a 4-year period [242].
   b. The results of several trials of ZDV monotherapy in early stages of HIV disease may appear inconsistent. **The Concorde I trial**, which compared immediate versus deferred ZDV therapy, found no difference in progression of disease or survival during a 3-year study period in the subgroup of asymptomatic patients with < 500 CD4 cells/mm³ [243, 244]. The rate of progression to severe AIDS-related complex (ARC) and AIDS was slower during the initial 55 weeks of study in the immediate ZDV treatment group, which was consistent with ACTG 019 results [241, 243].
   c. **The European-Collaborative Group** compared ZDV (500 mg bid) versus placebo treatment in ZDV-naive patients with CD4 cell counts > 400 cells/mm³ and found a slower progression to AIDS in ZDV-treated patients [245]. This study was not designed to evaluate survival.
   d. In an observational Multicenter AIDS Cohort Study (MACS) of HIV-infected men, patients treated with ZDV had reduced mortality at 6, 12, and 18 months. Survival advantage of ZDV was noted at 24 months, only if PCP prophylaxis was given concomitantly [223].
   e. Although as of early 1996 **studies do not support the use of antiretroviral medication in asymptomatic HIV-infected persons with CD4 cell counts ≥ 500** cells/mm³, studies are under way with various combinations of antiretroviral agents because there is active viral proliferation during all stages of disease [246, 247].

3. **Symptomatic HIV disease**
   a. Symptomatic patients with CD4 cell counts between 200 and 500 cells/mm³ were treated with ZDV, 1,200 mg/day, in divided doses versus placebo. Zidovudine delayed disease progression significantly and with less drug toxicity than in patients with more advanced disease [222].
   b. The Veterans Affairs Cooperative Study Group compared immediate ZDV versus deferred ZDV (1,500 mg/day) in symptomatic patients with CD4 cell counts between 200 and 500/mm³ [248]. In the deferred group, ZDV was initiated when the CD4 cell count fell below 200 cells/mm³ or when AIDS developed. Although immediate therapy significantly delayed disease progression compared with deferred therapy, follow-up of more than 2 years revealed that survival did not lengthen.
   c. A study involving patients who had recovered from *Pneumocystis carinii* pneumonia **(ACTG 002)** demonstrated that a reduced dose of ZDV (1,200 mg/day for 4 weeks, followed by 600 mg/day in divided doses) resulted in better survival and less toxicity than the higher dosage [249].
   d. The lowest effective dose of ZDV has not been established, and doses as low as **300 mg/day** appear to be efficacious [250].
   e. An early open-label study of varying doses of ZDV and ddI suggests that **combination therapy was associated with higher and more sustained improvements in HIV surrogate markers (e.g., CD4 counts, HIV-1 plasma titers) than ZDV alone,** although no clinical endpoint data were presented [251].
   f. Results from **ACTG 175**—a study which compared the safety and efficacy of monotherapy with ZDV or ddI, versus combination therapy with ZDV/ddI or ZDV/ddC, as well as benefits of immediate versus delayed combination therapy in HIV-infected persons without AIDS and CD4 cell counts between 200 and 500 cells/mm³—recently became available [252]. In ZDV-naive patients, ZDV-ddC was superior to ZDV monotherapy. In ZDV-experienced patients, ZDV-ddI was superior to ZDV monotherapy. Overall, **ZDV monotherapy was less effective than ZDV-ddI or giving ddI alone, in slowing**

progression to AIDS and prolonging survival. Little benefit was seen when ddC was added to ZDV monotherapy in patients with prior ZDV experience.

g. The results of the Delta studies have been presented at conferences [253, 254]. The **Delta Study** compared ZDV to ZDV-ddI and ZDV-ddC in ZDV-naive patients **(Delta I)** with ZDV-experienced participants with CD4 cell counts between 50 and 350 cells/mm³ **(Delta II)**. The baseline CD4 cell counts in Delta I were around 200 cells/mm³, lower than those of the ZDV-naive patients in ACTG 175. Delta II participants had lower CD4 cell counts than the ZDV-experienced cohort in ACTG 175 (189 versus 338, respectively). More patients stopped ZDV-ddI than ZDV-ddC due to side effects. **In ZDV-naive patients, either ZDV-ddI or ZDV-ddC was superior to ZDV** alone in slowing the progression to AIDS and prolonging survival. In ZDV-experienced patients, no difference in drug regimens was noted. **Overall, ZDV-ddI and ZDV-ddC were determined to be superior to ZDV monotherapy.**

h. Additional multicenter studies are under way comparing various nucleoside analogues both alone and in combination regimens.

B. **Modification of antiretroviral therapy.** There are no firm guidelines for when initial therapy should be modified. Many consultants would adjust the patient's current antiretroviral regimen to conform to what is currently known about effective antiretroviral regimens. See related discussion at the end of this chapter under Clinical Perspectives on Selecting Antiretroviral Regimens.

1. Patients with more than 8 and less than 16 weeks of prior ZDV therapy **(ACTG 116A)** had fewer AIDS-defining illnesses than patients continued on ZDV if they had been randomized to ddI [255]. Similarly, patients with more than 16 weeks prior ZDV therapy **(ACTG 116B/117)** had fewer new AIDS-defining illnesses if they were randomized to ddI, 500 mg/day, than patients continued on ZDV [256]. No differences in survival were noted among the three treatment groups: (1) ddI, 500 mg/day; (2) ddI, 750 mg/day; and (3) ZDV, 600 mg/day [256].

2. Patients with advanced HIV disease, CD4 cell counts ≤ 300 cells/mm³, and at least 6 months of prior ZDV therapy (ACTG 155) showed no difference in survival when they were continued on ZDV, when they were switched to ddC alone, or when they received ZDV-ddC combination therapy [257]. A later analysis revealed that a subset of **patients with CD4 cell counts > 150 cells/mm³ appeared to benefit from switching to ZDV-ddC combination therapy** [257].

3. In a small study of patients with advanced HIV disease who had tolerated ZDV for at least 6 months, open-label ddC (2.25 mg/day) was no more effective than ZDV (500–1,200 mg/day) in improving survival or decreasing disease progression [258].

C. **Other potential uses of ZDV**

1. **Prevention of vertical transmission of HIV.** Results from a randomized, controlled trial found that **the rate of HIV transmission from mothers to infants was reduced from 25.5% in pregnant women and their infants who received placebo to 8.3% in women and infants treated with ZDV [259]**. In the study **(ACTG 076)**, HIV-infected pregnant women with CD4 cell counts higher than 200 cells/mm³ were randomized between the fourteenth and thirty-fourth week of gestation to ZDV, 100 mg, or placebo five times daily until the onset of labor. Zidovudine or placebo was administered intravenously during labor, with a loading dose of 2 mg/kg over 1 hour, followed by continuous infusion of 1 mg/kg/hr until delivery. Infants also received 2 mg/kg of ZDV or placebo in syrup q6h within 24 hours after birth and for 6 weeks thereafter. Fifty-three of 364 infants had positive cultures for HIV, and of these, 40 were in the placebo group and 13 in the ZDV group. Zidovudine is well tolerated in pregnancy, although studies of long-term toxicity are under way [259, 260]. **Until the potential risk for teratogenicity and other complications from ZDV therapy given in the first trimester can be assessed, ZDV therapy only for the purpose of reducing the risk for perinatal transmission is not recommended before the fourteenth week of gestation.**

2. **HIV-induced thrombocytopenia.** Zidovudine is currently the preferred treatment for HIV-related thrombocytopenia [221].

3. **Central nervous system involvement.** Zidovudine has been found to be effective in the treatment of HIV-associated neurologic disease, with improvement in

attention, memory, and visual motor skills noted [261, 262]. The optimal dosage regimen is unclear.

4. **Postexposure prophylaxis for needlesticks and mucosal splashes.** While trials are in progress, demonstration of the benefit of ZDV therapy will be difficult in view of the low incidence of infection after such an exposure (estimated risk is 1:250) [263]. **Animal and human data are inadequate to support a definite role of ZDV for this use [263].** Failures of ZDV prophylaxis after exposure to HIV-1 have been reported [264, 265]. As of early 1990, the exposed individual and his or her physician have had to decide jointly whether to use postexposure prophylaxis with ZDV [263]. Doses and duration of therapy used have varied. Some use ZDV doses of 200 mg q4h (5 or 6 times/day) for 4–6 weeks (see sec. **VIII.H**). Because as many as 10% of new infections may be ZDV resistant, some clinicians favor using a combination of antiretroviral agents such as ZDV-ddI. This remains a controversial area. In a June 1996 report from the CDC, ZDV appeared to have a beneficial effect when used in this setting, typically in combination therapy [266]. **Infectious disease consultation is advised for the optimal approach** to this evolving issue (see p. 1004).

5. **Pediatric patients.** In children, the benefits of ZDV appear to be similar to those in adults [267]. Those with neurologic involvement seem to have benefited most. Recent data suggest that ddI may be preferable to ZDV in pediatric populations [268, 269].

6. ZDV has a beneficial effect on **HIV-induced psoriasis** [221].

7. **Racial differences.** Prior studies have failed to detect any racial differences in response to ZDV therapy [270]. **Access to care and late initiation of ZDV therapy appear to be more important factors** in the differential survival of minority patients than does a different response to ZDV therapy [221].

VI. **Adverse effects.** Low-dose regimens of ZDV (600 mg/day) are much less toxic and better tolerated than the initial higher-dose regimens (1,200–1,500 mg/day).

A. **Hematologic dysfunction** [271]. The incidence and severity of hematologic toxic effects appear related to the dose of ZDV and the stage of HIV disease when treatment is begun. More toxicity is likely in advanced disease [116].

1. **Anemia** with high-dose regimens in patients with AIDS is very common (15–30%) but, with low-dose regimens, especially in asymptomatic HIV-infected patients, anemia is seen in only 2% of recipients compared to 9.7% of asymptomatic recipients of high-dose ZDV [271]. The risk for the development of severe anemia in asymptomatic HIV-infected patients is greatest in months 3–8 of treatment and more likely to occur if the patient is mildly anemic or thrombocytopenic at the onset of ZDV therapy. Recombinant erythropoietin may decrease transfusion requirements in severely anemic patients receiving ZDV, but only in patients with low erythropoietin levels (< 500 IU/liter)[271–273].

2. **Neutropenia** is more likely to be seen in more advanced cases of AIDS. Although severe neutropenia may occur in high-dose ZDV recipients, mild neutropenia can also occur with low-dose ZDV. Granulocyte-stimulating factors (e.g., G-CSF and GM-CSF) may increase the number of neutrophils in ZDV-induced neutropenia, but the treatment is expensive and the results transient. Many clinicians would switch antiretroviral agents rather than supplement ZDV with growth factors or transfusions [272].

3. **Macrocytosis** occurs in 90% of ZDV recipients but does not correlate with the development of anemia [221].

4. The mechanism of ZDV myelosuppression is unclear [221]. Thrombocytopenia is not a significant side effect of ZDV.

B. **Myopathy.** Although myopathies can be seen with HIV-1 infection, ZDV can cause an insidious onset of proximal muscle weakness and exercise-induced myalgias, occurring in approximately 6–18% of patients after 6–12 months of ZDV therapy [221].

1. **Laboratory findings.** Creatine kinase levels are often elevated. With electro-myelographic evaluation, a myopathic pattern with fibrillations and positive sharp wave activity is seen in proximal muscles. Light microscopy shows mild-to-moderate myonecrosis, and electron microscopy shows mitochondrial abnormalities of enlargement and increased number [221, 274].

2. In symptomatic patients, discontinuation of ZDV has resulted in gradual resolution of symptoms over 6–8 weeks in 70–100% of patients [221].

C. **Less serious but more frequent adverse reactions.** These tend to occur early, and many subside with continued therapy. Undoubtedly, in some instances, the adverse events are caused by the underlying disease. Frequent adverse reactions include (1) **CNS effects** (especially headache and insomnia); (2) **gastrointestinal effects** (nausea, vomiting, diarrhea, and abdominal discomfort, which typically diminish with continued use and seldom require lowering the dose or stopping ZDV [14]); (3) **systemic effects** (rash, fever, malaise, and myalgias); and (4) **dermatologic effects** (hyperpigmentation of the skin and nails). Melanonychia occurs in 40% of patients on therapy, with a much higher incidence occurring in blacks than in whites or Hispanics [221].

D. **More serious but less frequent adverse events.** Severe hepatitis with fatty infiltration and increased lactate levels has been associated with several nucleoside reverse transcriptase inhibitors (NRTIs) including zidovudine [271, 275]. This complication has been noted more commonly in women but, fortunately, it occurs rarely.

VII. Drug interactions

A. **Probenecid** inhibits both glucuronidation of ZDV and renal secretion, resulting in increased serum levels and an increased half-life [221]. Preliminary studies with combination therapy of **ZDV and probenecid resulted in a surprisingly high frequency of rash, suggesting that these two drugs should not be used concomitantly [276].**

B. **Myelosuppressive drugs (e.g., ganciclovir) may have added bone marrow toxicity** when coadministered with ZDV. The use of ganciclovir and ZDV is associated with a very high incidence of neutropenia, and very few patients tolerate full doses of both drugs [277]. As newer agents for HIV and CMV become available, the need for ganciclovir and ZDV coadministration will diminish.

C. **Acetaminophen** was believed initially to increase the incidence of anemia with ZDV use. Further studies have shown that acetaminophen has no effect on the metabolism of ZDV [221] and therefore **can be given to patients receiving ZDV.**

VIII. Dosage regimens

A. **Forms available.** A 100-mg capsule, strawberry-flavored syrup (50 mg/5 ml), and an intravenous infusion preparation with 10 mg/ml are available [278].

B. **Adults (oral therapy)**

1. Zidovudine, 200 mg q8h, is considered the standard daily dose; however, the ideal dose and interval are not known. Some physicians elect to treat with 100 mg PO 3–5 times daily [116]. Although the package insert recommends a dosage of 200 mg q4h for the first month of therapy, most clinicians believe this is unnecessary or necessary only in suspected HIV encephalopathy. Lower doses are generally better tolerated and appear to have clinical and virologic effects similar to higher doses [250, 272].

2. **For asymptomatically infected patients with CD4 cell counts of > 500 cells/ mm³,** antiretroviral therapy is not currently recommended.

3. For **neurologic HIV involvement,** the optimal dose regimen is unclear. Because prior studies typically used high doses of ZDV, most clinicians would favor higher doses (800–1,200 mg/day) as tolerated.

4. For **HIV-related thrombocytopenia,** ZDV is the treatment of choice, but the optimal dose regimen remains unsettled. The mechanism of action of ZDV on HIV-related thrombocytopenia remains unknown [221]. The standard dose (500–600 mg/day) for HIV-associated thrombocytopenia has not been carefully evaluated and some prefer a higher dose (1,000–2,000 mg/day) as this dose was used in prior trials demonstrating efficacy.

C. **Children.** In children 3 months to 12 years of age the package insert suggests a starting dose of 180 mg/m² q6h (720 mg/m²/day) not to exceed 200 mg q6h. Doses in infants are being studied [279].

D. **In patients with renal and hepatic insufficiency,** dosage reductions have not been fully established. Preliminary guidelines are given in sec. **IV.C.2** (e.g., 100 mg tid).

E. **Pregnancy.** Taken after the first trimester, ZDV is generally well tolerated and has not been associated with malformations of the fetus. Zidovudine remains the treatment of choice for preventing vertical transmission of HIV [259, 260].

F. **Nursing.** The package insert indicates that it is unknown whether ZDV is excreted in human milk. Because HIV might be spread to infants through breast milk, women with HIV in the United States are advised not to breast-feed, regardless of whether they are receiving antiretroviral agents.

G. **Intravenous formulation.** The intravenous dose is 1–2 mg/kg infused q4h (6 times daily). The intravenous dosing regimen equivalent to the oral administration of

100 mg q4h is approximately 1 mg/kg IV q4h, per the package insert [278]. (See the package insert for a detailed discussion of dosing with this formulation.)

H. **Postexposure prophylaxis.** Many physicians and institutions have developed guidelines with respect to the management of the health care worker who is exposed to HIV-infected material [263]. Recent data suggest ZDV has a beneficial effect in postexposure prophylaxis [266] with or without other antiretroviral agents; **the CDC has reviewed this topic through June 1996** [266]. Because this is an evolving important issue, the hospital infection control physician and/or an infectious disease specialist with expertise in this area should be consulted for their current recommendations. See sec. **V.C.4** and Chap. 19.

IX. **Monitoring of chemistries and hematologic parameters.** With the introduction of the lower dose of ZDV, the hematologic system and liver function are much less subject to effect even in more advanced cases of HIV. However, it is reasonable to monitor therapy at the outset, as some subjects will have more significant toxicity than others. Furthermore, in patients receiving other agents (e.g., ganciclovir) that may be myelosuppressive, serial monitoring is important.

A. **If the hemoglobin exceeds 10 g/dl,** those individuals are not likely to have significant problems. For them, monitoring of the CBC count and hepatic transaminases, monthly at first and then bimonthly thereafter, is reasonable.

B. **If the initial hemoglobin is less than 10 g/dl;** weekly monitoring initially and then, if stable, monthly monitoring is a reasonable approach. Transaminase monitoring can be undertaken as discussed previously.

C. **Patients with renal insufficiency** who are treated with ZDV should be closely monitored as the risk of developing toxicity is increased.

X. **Dose adjustments.** If the patient develops anemia or granulocytopenia while receiving ZDV, the decision regarding whether to stop or reduce the ZDV dose or change to another agent (e.g., ddI) or use erythropoietin or G-CSF must be individualized. Severe anemia (e.g., hemoglobin < 7.5 g/dl) or granulocytopenia (e.g., granulocytic counts < 750/mm²) may require dose interruption of ZDV until evidence of marrow recovery is observed. For less severe anemia or granulocytopenia, a dose reduction of ZDV may be adequate.

XI. **Combination therapy** with **ZDV** and other agents is an area of **intense clinical investigation.** See secs. **III** and **IV** under Clinical Perspectives on Selecting Antiretroviral Regimens (p. 1019).

A. **ZDV and/or another reverse transcriptase inhibitor** (see sections on ddI, ddC, lamivudine) and/or **protease inhibitors** in combination are under clinical study. In a recent pilot study of **alternating or simultaneous ZDV and ddI** therapy in patients with symptomatic HIV infection, simultaneous therapy provided more sustained rises in CD4 counts than alternating therapy, without increased toxicities [280].

B. **Acyclovir**

1. Acyclovir has been studied intensively to determine its role in the treatment of HIV. Although it has no activity against HIV, synergistic inhibition of HIV was reported in vitro with a combination of acyclovir and ZDV [281]. Early clinical studies of the combination of ZDV and acyclovir failed to find any additional benefit regarding immunologic markers or on measures of viral replication [281]. Two randomized clinical trials found the combination of high-dose acyclovir (3.2 g/day) with ZDV was associated with improved survival compared with ZDV alone [282, 283].

2. A recent report from the Multicenter AIDS Cohort Study found that acyclovir 600–800 mg/day was associated with prolonged survival after an AIDS diagnosis in ZDV-treated homosexual men [284]. Data from an observational cohort of patients with AIDS or ARC treated with ZDV recently found no survival benefit for the third of patients that used concomitant acyclovir [281].

C. **Ribavirin** and ZDV have antagonistic effects.

D. Zidovudine combined with either **foscarnet or interferon-alpha** are currently being studied.

XII. **Cost** (see Table 26-4)

Didanosine

Didanosine (ddI, 2′,3′-dideoxyinosine, Videx) is a derivative of inosine that inhibits viral reverse transcriptase and functions as a chain terminator, thus inhibiting viral DNA synthesis. Didanosine was approved in the fall of 1991 for use in treating advanced HIV infection in adult and pediatric patients older than 6 months who were unresponsive to or intolerant of ZDV [272, 285]. **Recent studies provide data supporting the use of ddI as the initial antiretroviral agent of choice,** either alone or in combination with ZDV [252, 286].

I. **Mechanism of action.** Like ZDV, ddI is a product that is converted intracellularly to an active triphosphate with antiretroviral activity.

II. **In vitro.** Didanosine has excellent in vitro activity against HIV, including ZDV-resistant strains [287]. The concentration of ddI that inhibits HIV is well below that which is achievable in the serum. Didanosine possesses a higher therapeutic ratio than ZDV [288].

III. **Resistance of HIV to ddI.** Although there are five nucleoside reverse transcriptase inhibitors currently available to treat HIV infection (e.g., ZDV, ddI, zalcitabine [ddC], stavudine [d4T], and lamivudine [3TC]), HIV-1 resistance to one compound does not necessarily confer resistance to another [289]. Resistance to ddI has been observed in patients treated with ddI. Some HIV isolates from patients switched from ZDV to ddI became less sensitive to ddI but regained susceptibility to ZDV [116, 290, 291]. Resistance of HIV-1 to ddI is primarily associated with a mutation in viral reverse transcriptase at codon 74 [287]. Mutations in reverse transcriptase codons 65, 70, 72, and 184 have also been associated with ddI resistance [289]. Prolonged ddI monotherapy has been associated with mutations that may decrease the efficacy of subsequent ZDV therapy in some patients [289]. Strains resistant to ddI may also be resistant to ddC. The clinical significance of ddI resistance is unknown.

IV. **Pharmacology.** The active metabolite of ddI, ddATP, has a prolonged intracellular half-life of 8–24 hours.

   A. **Phase I** dose escalation studies, using doses between 0.4 and 66 mg/kg, revealed that 12–20 mg/kg were the highest tolerated doses.

   B. **The drug is much better absorbed on an empty stomach.** The bioavailability after oral administration varies widely and depends on the drug formulation, the patient's gastric acidity, and whether there is food in the stomach. **Didanosine is very acid labile, and food reduces absorption by 50% or more** [292]. **It should be taken 1 hour before or 2 hours after a meal** (i.e., 1 hour before breakfast and at bedtime). The chewable (dispersible) tablet has 20–25% greater bioavailability than does the powder. Because ddI is rapidly degraded in an acidic pH, oral formulations contain buffering agents designed to increase the pH of the gastric environment (see sec. **IV.E**).

   C. Didanosine penetrates CSF and the CSF-to-plasma ratio at 1 hour after administration is approximately 20% [293].

   D. After oral administration of ddI, the average **elimination** half-life is 1.6 hours but, in uremic patients, this is prolonged to 4.5 hours; thus doses must be adjusted in renal failure. Approximately 20% of the dose is cleared by a 4- to 6-hour hemodialysis; an additional dose is given after dialysis [294].

   E. **Drug interactions. Didanosine can decrease the absorption of tetracyclines, fluoroquinolones, itraconazole, ketoconazole, and possibly dapsone** [272].

V. **Clinical uses.** Didanosine was licensed originally for use in patients who were intolerant to or failing ZDV treatment in terms of favorable effects on surrogate markers of HIV (e.g., CD4 cell counts and p24 antigen levels) [295].

   A. **Phase III trials of ddI monotherapy**

      1. **A multicenter, double-blind study compared ddI to ZDV in 913 patients who had been treated with ZDV for 16 weeks or more.** Changing treatment from ZDV to ddI, 500 mg/day, was superior to continued ZDV in reducing new AIDS-defining events and deaths, but not in prolonging survival (ACTG 116B/117) [256]. Therapeutic benefit was observed in patients with asymptomatic infection and CD4 cell counts $\leq$ 200 cells/mm^3 and in those with symptomatic HIV infection, but not in patients with AIDS [256]. There were more increases in the CD4 cell count and decreases in p24 antigen levels in ddI-treated versus ZDV-treated participants. Patients with a high-level of HIV-1 resistance to ZDV predicted more rapid clinical progression and death when adjusted for other factors [233]. Because patients with advanced AIDS benefited after switching from ZDV to ddI, regardless of their level of HIV-1 resistance, the authors conclude that assessment of ZDV resistance is not necessary when deciding to switch monotherapy from ZDV to ddI [233].

      2. In a similar study of 312 patients with progressive HIV disease who had received at least 6 months of ZDV, patients switched to ddI had fewer clinical

endpoints than patients continued on ZDV [296]. Patients with CD4 cell counts of 100 to 300 cells/mm³ benefited more than patients with lower CD4 counts [296].

3. Didanosine was compared with continuous ZDV therapy in HIV-infected patients with CD4 cell counts between 200 and 500 cells/mm³ who had tolerated ZDV for more than 6 months [297]. Changing to ddI led to a decrease in the rate of disease progression, a sustained increase in CD4 cell counts, and a decrease in the chances of developing high-level resistance to ZDV [297].

B. **Comparison of ddI to ZDV as primary therapy**

1. **ACTG 175** found ZDV to be inferior to ddI, ZDV-ddI, and ZDV-ddC when given as primary therapy (see detailed discussion on ACTG 175 study results under zidovudine, sec. **V.A.3.f**) [253].

2. In **ACTG 116A,** ddI and ZDV were compared in a randomized, blinded fashion in 617 HIV-infected patients who had AIDS or advanced HIV disease and fewer than 16 weeks of prior ZDV therapy [255]. Generally, ZDV appeared more efficacious than ddI among patients who were ZDV-naive on entering the study, while ddI appeared more efficacious than ZDV among those who were ZDV-experienced, particularly in those who had 8–16 weeks of prior ZDV therapy. Measures of efficacy included both the time to new AIDS-defining events and survival [255].

3. In **ACTG 152,** long-term safety and efficacy of treatment with ZDV versus ddI versus a combination of ZDV-ddI were compared in children age 3 months to 18 years. Patients receiving either ddI or ddI-ZDV fared better than those taking ZDV alone, according to preliminary analyses [268]. Because ddI was relatively well tolerated [298], it may become the antiretroviral agent of choice in this population [268].

VI. **Adverse effects**

A. **Pancreatitis.** Pancreatitis, which has been fatal in some cases, is the major clinical toxic event occurring with ddI therapy and **must be considered whenever a patient receiving ddI therapy develops abdominal pain, nausea, or vomiting** [298a]. Didanosine use should be suspended until the diagnosis of pancreatitis is excluded. In the recent trial comparing ZDV to low-dose ddI (500 mg/day), pancreatitis was relatively uncommon (7%) among ddI recipients and similar in frequency to that occurrence in recipients of ZDV [256], although increases in amylase (> 1.3 times the upper limit of normal) were more common among those receiving ddI, 500 mg/day, than ZDV, 600 mg/day (20% versus 6%, $p = 0.001$, respectively) [256]. The risk of pancreatitis increases with increasing doses, a history of pancreatitis, alcohol abuse, advanced HIV disease, or exposure to intravenous pentamidine [14].

B. **Peripheral neuropathy** [299, 300, 301]. Peripheral neuropathy was seen frequently in phase 1 studies of ddI and was more common in patients taking higher doses of ddI [300, 301]. The sensory symptoms usually improve in patients who discontinue ddI, and some patients have tolerated reintroduction of ddI at lower doses [299]. Subsequent studies showed that the incidence of peripheral neuropathy on low-dose ddI was similar to that on ZDV (600 mg/day) [256].

C. **Hematologic dysfunction.** There is an improvement in the number of WBCs and neutrophils among treated subjects compared to recipients of ZDV [256]. Thrombocytopenia, possibly due to HIV, also improves in some instances.

D. **Hepatitis.** Fulminant hepatitis with severe lactate acidosis has been reported [302] in patients taking ddI as well as ZDV. Liver biopsies have shown diffuse microvesicular steatosis, and the outcome is often fatal.

E. **Miscellaneous effects** [14]

1. Diarrhea is relatively common with ddI therapy but appears to be less frequent with tablets than with the powder form of ddI.

2. **Other** reported **adverse effects** include headache, insomnia, nausea, emesis, abdominal pain, myelosuppression, increased aminotransferase activity, and hyperuricemia. Retinal toxicity (depigmentation) has been reported in pediatric patients [303].

VII. **Doses of ddI** [295]

A. **Availability.** Didanosine is available **only for oral use. All formulations should be administered on an empty stomach.**

1. **Chewable (dispersible) buffered tablets** are available in 25-, 50-, 100-, and 150-mg sizes.

Table 26-11. Adult dosages of didanosine (ddI, Videx)

Patient weight	Videx tablets*	Videx buffered powder
≥ 60 kg	200 mg bid	250 mg bid
< 60 kg	125 mg bid	167 mg bid

*Use two tablets to provide dose (i.e., for 200 mg bid, use two 100-mg tablets bid to provide adequate buffering). See text.
Source: *Physicians' Desk Reference* (50th ed.). Montvale, NJ: Medical Economics Data, 1996. P. 726. Copyright *Physicians' Desk Reference* 1996. Reprinted by permission. All rights reserved.

2. **Buffered powder** is supplied in single-dose, child-resistant foil packages (sachets) in 100-, 167-, and 250-mg strengths.
3. **Pediatric powder for oral solution** is supplied in 4- and 8-ounce glass bottles containing 2 or 4 g of ddI, respectively. This preparation may be the best tolerated; some adults who do not tolerate ddI tablets and powder well can successfully tolerate the pediatric suspension. When mixed by the pharmacist with purified water and antacid, the final concentration is 10 mg/ml.
B. **In adults. Adult dosages** of ddI are shown in Table 26-11. **Two tablets should be taken at each dose so that adequate buffering is provided to prevent gastric acid degradation of ddI (see sec. IV.B).**
C. **In children.** To prevent gastric degradation, children older than 1 year should receive a two-tablet dose; children younger than 1 year should receive a one-tablet dose (Table 26-12). The optimal dose for children has not been established. Some investigators suggest doses up to 300 mg/m²/day divided into three doses [295].
D. **Dose adjustment**
1. **Clinical signs of pancreatitis should prompt dose discontinuation and careful evaluation** of the possibility of pancreatitis.
2. Many patients who develop symptoms of **peripheral neuropathy** will tolerate a reduced dose of ddI after resolution of these symptoms on drug discontinuation.
3. Dose reduction should be considered in patients with **renal insufficiency or hepatic impairment** [295], although insufficient data exist to recommend specific dose adjustments.
E. **Pregnancy.** There are no adequate and well-controlled studies on the use of ddI in pregnant women. The drug should be used during pregnancy only if clearly indicated [295].
F. **Nursing.** It is not known whether ddI is excreted in breast milk. Because HIV potentially may be spread to infants through breast milk, women with HIV in the United States are advised not to nurse, regardless of whether they are receiving antiretroviral agents.
G. **Combination therapy.** Coadministration of ddI and ZDV is not thought to alter significantly the pharmacokinetics of ZDV [304]. ZDV and ddI can be given concomitantly.

Table 26-12. Pediatric doses of didanosine (ddI, Videx) (based on 200 mg/m²/day average recommended dose)*

Body surface area (m²)	Videx tablets	Videx pediatric powder Dose	Vol/10 mg/ml admixture
1.1–1.4	100 mg bid	125 mg bid	12.5 ml bid
0.8–1.0	75 mg bid	94 mg bid	9.5 ml bid
0.5–0.7	50 mg bid	62 mg bid	6 ml bid
≤ 0.4	25 mg bid	31 mg bid	3 ml bid

*Based on Videx pediatric powder. See text.
Source: *Physicians' Desk Reference* (50th ed.). Montvale, NJ: Medical Economics Data, 1996. P. 726. Copyright *Physicians' Desk Reference* 1996. Reprinted by permission. All rights reserved.

VIII. Serial monitoring

A. **Serial blood counts** and **liver function tests** are indicated. Amylase levels should be monitored in patients with a history of elevated amylase, pancreatitis, or alcohol abuse, and in patients who are on parenteral nutrition or who are otherwise at high risk for pancreatitis.

B. Serial **clinical assessment for signs and symptoms of pancreatitis** and peripheral neuropathy is indicated.

C. Dose reduction or elimination should be carried out if either severe pancreatitis or peripheral neuropathy occurs (see sec. **VII.D.1–2**).

IX. Cost (see Table 26-4)

Zalcitabine

Zalcitabine (ddC [dideoxycytidine], HIVID) is a dideoxynucleoside analogue of cytidine that inhibits the in vitro replication of HIV by inhibiting reverse transcriptase and improves certain surrogate measures of HIV infection, including CD4 cell count [258, 305].

Zalcitabine was approved for use in mid-1992 only in combination therapy with ZDV to treat adult patients with advanced HIV infection (with CD4 cell counts of < 300 cells/mm^2) who have demonstrated significant clinical or immunologic deterioration (typically after prolonged ZDV therapy). Recent studies suggest ddC may also have a role as single-agent therapy in patients intolerant of ZDV [306].

I. **In vitro activity.** Like ZDV and ddI, ddC requires intracellular conversion to an active triphosphate to exercise antiretroviral activity [232, 307]. It is active against HIV-1 and HIV-2 and inhibits replication in vitro at a concentration of 0.01–0.50 μM. Zalcitabine also is active against most ZDV-resistant strains of HIV [307].

II. **Resistance.** Resistance occurs, but its clinical significance is uncertain [308]. The use of ddC in combination with ZDV does not prevent the emergence of ZDV-resistant HIV isolates [307, 309, 310]. A mutation at residue 69 produced a fivefold reduction in ddC susceptibility, and mutations in the reverse transcriptase gene at residues 135 and 184 also have been associated with diminished susceptibility to ddC after prolonged therapy [228]. The codon 74 mutation that confers ddI resistance also produces cross-resistance with ddC [287]. The clinical significance of in vitro resistance to all dideoxynucleosides among strains of HIV is unclear at present [307].

III. **Pharmacology** [305]

A. **Absorption.** Zalcitabine is rapidly absorbed from the GI tract.

B. **Penetration.** Low levels of ddC can be detected in CSF.

C. **Half-life.** The half-life of ddC ranges from 1 to 3 hours [307]. Zalcitabine is largely cleared by the kidney [307].

D. **Pediatric populations.** The pharmacology of ddC in pediatric populations appears to be similar to that in adults [307].

IV. **Clinical studies**

A. **Phase 1 trials.** In phase 1 studies in adults with advanced HIV disease, treatment with ddC, 2–4 mg q8h, resulted in weight gain, a decrease in serum p24 antigen, and transient increases in CD4 cell counts [232, 305]. Early studies using doses of 0.06–5.40 mg/kg/day were limited by the frequent occurrence of painful, peripheral neuropathy. Lower doses (0.375–0.750 mg tid) are associated with less neuropathy. In a few patients, pancreatitis has developed [232].

B. **Zalcitabine as primary therapy.** Patients who have received ZDV for only a limited period of time (< 3 months) or not at all had poorer survival when randomized to receive ddC as compared with continuing on ZDV (ACTG 114); hence, this study was interrupted [311]. Zidovudine also had substantial advantages over ddC in initial monotherapy of AIDS in terms of functional and health status [312].

When patients had already been receiving ZDV for 1 year or more before randomization, patients, when continued on ZDV compared to switching to ddC, appeared to do equally well in overall survival and in time to death or AIDS-defining events (ACTG 119) [258]. In another trial, the efficacy of ddC was equivalent to that of ddI in patients in whom ZDV therapy had been unsuccessful or who could no longer tolerate ZDV [306].

C. **Combined therapy with ddC and ZDV**

1. A small phase I/II open-label study evaluated the safety and immunologic and antiviral effects of combination therapy with ZDV and ddC in **patients with advanced HIV infection** [310]. Six different dose regimens were used: ZDV, 50-, 100-, or 200-mg doses tid combined with either 0.005 mg/kg or 0.01 mg/kg of ddC or no ddC. **Combination therapy with ddC and the higher doses of**

ZDV (100 or 200 mg tid) produced greater and more persistent effects (rising CD4 cell counts and a decline of p24 antigenemia) in patients with advanced HIV infection compared with other study regimens and with the results of previous trials of ZDV monotherapy. Patients had CD4 cell counts of < 200 cells/mm³ and had not previously been exposed to ZDV. Neither drug affected the pharmacokinetic profile of the other [310], nor were the drugs' toxicities increased.

2. Another study compared continuous ZDV treatment with a switch to ddC or to ZDV-ddC combination therapy in patients with symptomatic HIV disease and CD4 cell counts < 300 cells/mm³, or asymptomatic HIV disease and CD4 cell counts < 200 cells/mm³ (ACTG 155) [257]. Overall analysis revealed no differences in survival or in progression to AIDS and death among the treatment groups. Further post hoc analysis by entry CD4 cell count subgroups suggested a possible advantage of the ZDV-ddC combination in patients with an entry-level count > 150 cells/mm³ [257]. However, this subgroup was small, and the results should be interpreted with caution. Further studies are under way to assess the efficacy and role of this combination.

3. Results from ACTG 175, a study designed to compare the safety and efficacy of monotherapy with ZDV or ddI versus combination therapy with ZDV-ddI or ZDV-ddC, and of immediate versus delayed combination therapy in HIV-infected persons without AIDS and CD4 cell counts between 200–500 cells/mm³, recently became available [252] (see Zidovudine, sec. **V.A.3.f**). In ZDV-naive patients, ZDV-ddC was superior to ZDV monotherapy. In ZDV-experienced patients, ZDV-ddI was superior to ZDV monotherapy. Overall, ZDV monotherapy was less effective than ZDV-ddI or ddI alone, in slowing progression to AIDS and prolonging survival. Little benefit was seen when ddC was added to ZDV monotherapy in patients with prior ZDV experience.

4. Because HIV potentially may be spread to infants through breast milk, **women with HIV in the United States are advised not to nurse,** regardless of whether they are receiving antiretroviral agents.

5. In the Delta study, either ZDV-ddC or ZDV-ddI was superior to ZDV alone in ZDV-naive patients in slowing the progression to AIDS and prolonging survival [254]. Additional benefit was not seen when adding ddC or ddI to ZDV monotherapy in ZDV-experienced patients. See Zidovudine, sec. **V.A.3.g.**

D. **Ongoing studies**

1. **Zalcitabine has been tested in children** with symptomatic HIV infection and, after 8-week courses, seemed to be safe and have antiviral activity [313]. Further studies are pending.

2. Although **alternating regimens** of ZDV and ddC have been studied, most favor concomitant use [314].

V. **Adverse effects**

A. **Peripheral neuropathy** can occur and may be severe, especially when higher doses are used (0.03–0.06 mg/kg) [315]. The risk of neuropathy increases with increased dose, duration of continuous therapy, and perhaps in patients with CD4 cell counts < 50 cells/mm³ [258].

B. **Other side effects** include oral and esophageal ulceration, nausea, abdominal discomfort, hepatic dysfunction, pancreatitis, diarrhea, pruritus, rash, headache, myalgias, cardiomyopathy, fatigue, fever, and leukopenia [116, 258, 272, 316].

C. Rare cases of lactic acidosis and severe hepatomegaly with steatosis have been reported with ddC as well as other nucleoside analogues (e.g., ZDV, ddI). Rare cases of hepatic failure and death have been reported in patients with underlying hepatitis B and ddC (monotherapy) [317].

D. In a **preliminary study, ddC and concurrent ZDV** were well tolerated without unusual toxicity associated with this combination therapy. The toxicities seen had been described when each drug was administered alone [310].

VI. **Dosing recommendations**

A. **Availability.** Oral tablets of ddC containing 0.375 mg per tablet or 0.750 mg per tablet are available. There is no intravenous form.

B. **For combination therapy,** one 0.750-mg tablet of ddC PO q8h, administered concomitantly with 200 mg ZDV q8h. There is no need to reduce the dose for body weight of 30 kg or more. **For monotherapy,** doses of ddC are similar to those used in combination therapy regimens.

C. **Pregnancy.** There are no adequate and well-controlled studies on the use of ddC in pregnant women. The drug should be used during pregnancy only if clearly indicated [317].

D. **Nursing.** It is not known whether ddC is excreted in breast milk. Because HIV potentially may be spread to infants through breast milk, women with HIV in the United States are advised not to nurse, regardless of whether they are receiving antiretroviral agents.

E. **In renal failure.** The package insert suggests that if the estimated creatinine clearance is 10–40 ml/min, the usual dose interval should be prolonged to q12h; if the creatinine clearance is < 10 ml/min, the ddC dose should be reduced to 0.750 mg q24h.

F. **In preexisting hepatic disease,** dose reduction guidelines are not yet available. Serial monitoring is especially important in these patients.

VII. **Serial monitoring**

A. Serial blood counts and liver function tests are indicated. Amylase levels should be monitored in patients with a history of elevated amylase, pancreatitis, or alcohol abuse, and in patients who are on parenteral nutrition or who are otherwise at high risk for pancreatitis [317].

B. Serial clinical assessment for signs and symptoms of a peripheral neuropathy is indicated, especially in patients with low CD4 cell counts who may be at increased risk for the development of peripheral neuropathy.

C. Dose reduction or elimination should be carried out if either severe peripheral neuropathy or oral ulcers occur.

VIII. **Cost** (see Table 26-4)

Stavudine

Stavudine (d4T, Zerit) is a thymidine nucleoside analogue approved in mid-1994 for the treatment of adults with advanced HIV infection who are intolerant of or are failing approved therapies [116, 318].

I. **Mechanism of action.** Stavudine is phosphorylated by cellular kinases to the active triphosphate form, which has an intracellular half-life of 3.5 hours in cells. Stavudine triphosphate inhibits HIV-1 replication by inhibiting viral reverse transcriptase by competing with thymidine triphosphate and causing DNA chain termination [319]. It has relatively little inhibition of cellular thymidine mechanism, which may account for its relative lack of bone marrow suppression.

II. **In vitro activity.** Stavudine is active in vitro against both HIV-1 and HIV-2. In vitro selection studies have yielded HIV-1 strains with reverse transcriptase mutations at codons 75 and 50, resulting in 7- and 30-fold reduced sensitivity, respectively [319, 320]. The risk of developing resistance to stavudine awaits further clinical trials and experience with this drug [319]. Stavudine and didanoside are synergistic in vitro. However, ZDV inhibits the phosphorylation of stavudine, which may result in antiviral antagonism. Currently, stavudine is approved only as monotherapy. However, studies of stavudine in various combination regimens with nucleoside and nonnucleoside reverse transcriptase inhibitors as well as protease inhibitors are under way.

III. **Pharmacology**

A. **Absorption.** Stavudine is well absorbed after oral administration, with the maximum plasma concentration reached by 0.5 to 1.5 hours [321]. Its bioavailability is more than 85%. The volume of distribution is 0.7 liter/kg, and it is not protein bound.

B. **Elimination.** Stavudine undergoes both tubular secretion in addition to glomerular filtration. The drug appears largely unchanged in urine, but approximately 60% of the drug's clearance is by nonrenal mechanisms.

C. **Cerebrospinal fluid.** Because the levels of stavudine in CSF are relatively high (25–75% of serum level), stavudine may be a reasonable alternative to ZDV in patients with advanced HIV disease and AIDS dementia complex [228].

IV. **Clinical use.** Stavudine was licensed based on studies in which administration of stavudine was associated with improvement in CD4 cell counts and p24 antigen level—surrogate markers and not clinical endpoints.

A. At present, there are no results from controlled trials evaluating the effect of stavudine therapy on the clinical progression of HIV infection, such as the incidence opportunistic infection or survival.

B. Data supporting FDA approval for stavudine were obtained from an ongoing multicenter randomized double-blind trial of stavudine versus continued ZDV in HIV-infected adults with CD4 cell counts of 50–500 cells/mm³ and at least 6 months of prior ZDV treatment. An interim analysis of 359 patients with a mean baseline CD4 cell count of 250 cells/mm³ revealed that at 12 weeks, patients switched to stavudine had a mean increase in CD4 cell count of 22 cells/mm^3, while patients who continued on ZDV had a mean decrease in CD4 cell count of 22 cells/mm^3 [322].

  C. An interim analysis of 10,438 patients randomized to receive either stavudine or placebo failed to demonstrate a survival advantage with stavudine. No CD4 cell count data are available to date [322].

  D. Currently, stavudine is being studied as part of various combination therapies.

V. **Adverse effects**

  A. **Peripheral neuropathy** is the major dose-limiting toxicity and occurred in 15–21% of recipients. Patients with a history of peripheral neuropathy and more advanced HIV disease are at increased risk, and careful monitoring is essential if they receive stavudine [323]. Peripheral neuropathy may be a consequence of the fact that mitochondrial DNA gamma-polymerase is very sensitive to stavudine triphosphate. The neuropathy seen resembles that which occurs in recipients of ddI and ddC [324].

  B. **Pancreatitis** seems to be infrequent and may reflect the background incidence of pancreatitis in HIV disease [324].

  C. **Other side effects** occur at rates similar to ZDV and include headache, asthenia, insomnia, anxiety, myalgias, diarrhea, rash, nausea and/or vomiting. Stavudine has much less bone marrow toxicity than ZDV [320].

VI. **Dosing recommendations** [318]

  A. **Availability.** Stavudine is only available for oral use in capsules of 15-, 20-, 30-, and 40-mg strengths.

  B. **Adult dosages.** Adults can receive this drug without regard to meals. The recommended dose of stavudine is as follows:

   1. For patients weighing 60 kg or more, 40 mg bid.

   2. For patients weighing less than 60 kg, 30 mg bid.

  C. **Monitoring patients and dose adjustments.** Patients should be **serially assessed for the development of peripheral neuropathy,** which usually is suggested by complaints of numbness, tingling, or pain in the feet or hands. If these symptoms develop, the package insert suggests therapy be stopped.

   1. In some patients, symptoms may worsen temporarily following discontinuation of therapy.

   2. If symptoms resolve completely, resumption of therapy at half doses can be considered.

  D. **In renal failure,** dose reduction is suggested for a creatinine clearance of ≤ 50 ml/min as shown in Table 26-13.

  E. **Pregnancy.** There are no adequate and well-controlled studies in pregnant women; use in pregnancy only if clearly indicated.

  F. **Pediatric use.** The safety and efficacy of stavudine in children have not been established. Clinical trials of stavudine in children are under way.

VII. **Cost** (see Table 26-4)

Lamivudine

Lamivudine (3TC, Epivir) is a synthetic **nucleoside approved in November 1995 for use only in combination with zidovudine** [325]. To date, improvements in surrogate

Table 26-13. Adjustment of stavudine (Zerit) in patients with varying degrees of renal function

Creatinine clearance (ml/min)	Recommended stavudine dose by patient weight	
	> 60 kg	< 60 kg
> 50	40 mg q12h	30 mg q12h
26–50	20 mg q12h	15 mg q12h
10–25	20 mg q24h	15 mg q24h

Note: There are insufficient data to recommend a dose for patients with creatinine clearance < 10 ml/min or for patients undergoing dialysis.
Source: *Physicians' Desk Reference* (50th ed.). Montvale, NJ: Medical Economics Data, 1996. P. 732. Copyright *Physicians' Desk Reference* 1996. Reprinted by permission. All rights reserved.

markers were seen in antiretroviral-naive and antiretroviral-experienced patients, and these provided the basis for approval. Ongoing trials are in place to evaluate its clinical and survival benefits. **Lamivudine should not be used as monotherapy** as high-level resistance uniformly develops in 4–8 weeks of monotherapy [228]. This resistance (mutation codon 184 of HIV reverse transcriptase) [326] to lamivudine appears to decrease phenotypic development of ZDV resistance. Further data are needed to explain this phenomenon. Lamivudine has a lower toxicity profile than the other four nucleoside reverse transcriptase inhibitors.

I. **Mechanism of action.** Lamivudine is a synthetic $(-)$ enantiomer of the dideoxy analogue of cytidine, which is phosphorylated intracellularly to its active 5′ triphosphate (TP) metabolite. This 5-TP moiety inhibits HIV reverse transcriptase and acts as a chain terminator. Lamivudine is a weak inhibitor of mammalian DNA polymerases, and hence may have less potential to cause bone marrow suppression or peripheral neuropathy than other nucleoside reverse transcriptase inhibitors [228, 325].

II. **In vitro activity.** Lamivudine is active against HIV-1 and HIV-2, including ZDV-resistant strains [228]. It also is a potent inhibitor of HBV [327]. Its actions are synergistic with those of ZDV, and additive with those of ddC and ddI [228].

III. **Resistance**

A. **Monotherapy with lamivudine leads to development of high-level resistance** (100- to 1000-fold increases in phenotypic resistance), characterized primarily by a mutation at reverse transcriptase **codon 184** with a methionine, which is replaced by either a valine or isoleucine [328, 329]. A mutation at **codon 65** may also confer various degrees of resistance to lamivudine as well as to ddI and ddC [228].

B. A marked decline in HIV-1 RNA levels (95% below baseline) and p24 antigen was observed within 2 weeks of treatment with lamivudine, followed by a rise that corresponded with the appearance of lamivudine-resistant viruses in serum [329]. After 12 weeks, a partial antiretroviral effect persisted despite the presence of codon 184 mutant viruses [329]. Antiviral effects, despite evidence of in vitro lamivudine resistance, may be attributable to in vivo phenotypic sensitivity, altered HIV mutant replication, and/or improvement of sensitivity to a second drug [329]. Improvements in surrogate markers have been most significant in patients given a combination of lamivudine and ZDV [330]. The **mutation at codon 184 may also lead to suppression of ZDV resistance** and may partially account for maintenance of improved surrogate markers [330].

IV. **Pharmacology**

A. **Absorption.** Lamivudine is rapidly absorbed after oral administration with an oral bioavailability of 86%. If given with food, the time to peak level is prolonged. This, however, has no effect on systemic exposure, and lamivudine can be given with or without food.

B. **Elimination.** The elimination half-life of lamivudine ranges from 5–7 hours [325]. Lamivudine metabolism is the minor route of elimination; it is primarily excreted unchanged in urine. Dose modification of lamivudine is required in patients with renal dysfunction (Table 26-14).

C. **Cerebrospinal fluid.** Cerebrospinal fluid concentrations of lamivudine are low and equal that of ddC and ddI, but are much less than that of ZDV [331]. The CSF to serum ratio ranges from 0.04 to 0.08 [331].

Table 26-14. Adjustment of lamivudine (Epivir) in patients with varying degrees of renal function

Creatinine clearance (ml/min)	Dosage of lamivudine
≥ 50	150 mg bid
30–49	150 mg qd
15–29	150 mg first dose, then 100 mg/day
5–14	150 mg first dose, then 50 mg/day
< 5	50 mg first dose, then 25 mg/day

Note: There are insufficient data to recommend a dosage of lamivudine in patients undergoing hemodialysis.
Source: From Epivir (Lamivudine). *Package Insert*. November 1995.

V. Clinical uses in HIV disease
A. Phase I/II studies
1. A phase I/II trial of lamivudine in asymptomatic and mildly symptomatic HIV-infected patients observed sustained reductions in HIV RNA load and immune complex–dissociated p24 antigen levels, which were maintained over 12 weeks [332].
2. Another phase I/II study evaluated lamivudine in patients with asymptomatic and mildly symptomatic HIV-1 infection and CD4 cell counts $\le$ 400 cells/mm^3 [331]. Small and transient increases in CD4 cell counts were seen during the first 4 weeks of treatment, followed by progressive declines during extended monotherapy. Sustained decreases in HIV p24 antigen levels and other immunologic measures were observed during the 52-week study [331].

B. Phase II/III studies
1. **Study NUCB 3001** compared combination therapy with lamivudine and ZDV to ZDV alone in 129 ZDV-naive patients with CD4 cell counts of 100–400 cells/mm^3 [333]. The mean baseline CD4 cell count was 271 cells/mm^3, which rose by 34 cells/mm^3 after 4 weeks on ZDV monotherapy but fell 7 below baseline at 24 weeks (i.e., 264 cells/mm^3). With combination therapy, on the other hand, the CD4 cell count rose by 85 cells/mm^3 at 8 weeks, with increases of 80 cells/mm^3 that were sustained at 24 weeks. The decline in immune complex–dissociated p24 antigen and HIV RNA also was less in combination therapy.

   All HIV isolates in combination-arm patients were found to have codon 184 mutation by week 24. This improvement in the combination arm may be due to a lack of ZDV resistance. At 24 weeks, monotherapy patients were offered an open-label combination ZDV-lamivudine regimen. At 48 weeks, the original combination group had sustained improvements in surrogate markers. Patients who switched to combination therapy also demonstrated significant improvements in viral load and surrogate markers. In patients receiving ZDV monotherapy, 75% of viral isolates had developed ZDV resistance at codon 70 of reverse transcriptase by week 24, while less than 30% of viral isolates in patients on combination therapy were found to have ZDV resistance. The maximum mean change in viral RNA level was a -1.8 log in the combination-therapy group and -0.7 log in the monotherapy group [228].
2. **In NUCB 3002,** the comparison of ZDV monotherapy and lamivudine-ZDV combination therapy with both high dose (300 mg bid) and low dose (150 mg bid) was evaluated in 223 ZDV-experienced patients (mean 24 months) with a CD4 cell count range of 100–400 cells/mm^3 (median 251 cells/mm^3) [334]. In patients who continued with ZDV monotherapy, CD4 cell counts declined from baseline by 21 cells at week 24, while in the combination arm CD4 cell counts increased from baseline by 33 cells at week 24. There were no significant differences in the two lamivudine doses.
3. In **NUCA 3001,** 366 patients with CD4 cell counts of 200–500 cells/mm^3 and less than 4 weeks of prior ZDV treatment were randomized to receive lamivudine monotherapy (300 mg bid versus 150 mg bid), ZDV monotherapy, or combination therapy [335]. Mean initial HIV RNA levels were well balanced between the three groups (median 31,600 copies/ml), and 23% of the patients overall were p24 antigen-positive at entry [228]. The mean CD4 cell count was lower in the monotherapy arms (322 cells/mm^3) than in the combination regimen (370 cells/mm^3). At week 24, the best response of surrogate markers was found in the combination group, with high-dose lamivudine. At week 24, in ZDV monotherapy CD4 cell counts were 8 cells above baseline; in lamivudine monotherapy, 15 cells above baseline; in the low-dose combination group, 36 cells above baseline; and in the high-dose combination group, 58 cells above baseline. By week 24, the median changes in HIV RNA levels were -0.3 log with ZDV monotherapy, -0.5 log with lamivudine monotherapy, -0.8 log with low-dose combination therapy, and -1.0 log with high-dose combination therapy [228]. The frequency of adverse events was similar across the four groups [335].
4. In **NUCA 3002,** ZDV-experienced patients were randomized to receive ZDV with either ddC or lamivudine (300 mg bid versus 150 mg bid) [336]. Patients had CD4 cell counts of 100–400 cells/mm^3 with a mean of 211 cells/mm^3. At 24 weeks, patients in the ddC group had a decrease in CD4 cell count of 15 cells from baseline. In contrast, the lamivudine-ZDV groups had increases in CD4 cell counts of 32 cells in the low-dose lamivudine group and 15 cells in

the high-dose group. Differences in HIV RNA levels were not observed between groups [336].

VI. Clinical uses in HBV. In a preliminary trial, 32 patients with chronic HBV (17 of whom had no response to prior interferon treatment) received 25-, 100-, or 300-mg daily of lamivudine for 12 weeks [327]. Levels of HBV DNA became undetectable in 70% of patients receiving 25-mg daily and in 100% of patients receiving 100- or 300-mg daily of lamivudine [327]. HBV DNA reappeared, however, in most patients after lamivudine was stopped; suppression was sustained in 6 of 32 patients (19%), 5 of whom had failed previous interferon treatment. Larger controlled trials of lamivudine alone or in combination with interferon are under way.

VII. Adverse effects [325]

    A. Side effects of lamivudine include headache, nausea, malaise, fatigue, diarrhea, and abdominal pain. **Peripheral neuropathy** also has been associated with lamivudine but less so than with other antiretroviral agents. **Pancreatitis** has been reported in 15% of pediatric patients in an open trial and in less than 0.5% in adult patients. Hematologic side effects include **anemia, neutropenia, and thrombocytopenia.**

    B. Lamivudine has been associated with **elevated transaminase, amylase,** and **lipase levels.** It is unclear what effects medications used in combination with lamivudine (e.g., ZDV) have on the side-effect profile of lamivudine.

VIII. Dosing recommendations [325]

    A. Lamivudine is available in 150-mg tablets. It also is supplied as an oral solution that is pale yellow and fruit flavored. The solution comes in a 10-mg/ml concentration in 240-ml bottles. No intravenous preparation is available.

    B. Adults and adolescents (12–16 years). Lamivudine, 150 mg PO bid **in combination with ZDV.**

    C. Pediatric dosing. For patients age 3 months to 12 years, lamivudine, 4 mg/kg bid (maximum 150 mg bid), **in combination with ZDV.** No data are available on the use of lamivudine in combination with ZDV in pediatric patients [325]. An open trial of lamivudine in pediatric patients revealed similar pharmacokinetics to adults but a **higher incidence of pancreatitis.**

    D. Monitoring patients for lamivudine toxicity should include evaluation for symptoms of pancreatitis, peripheral neuropathy, and gastrointestinal symptoms. Laboratory monitoring should include hematologic parameters and chemistry profiles. In pediatric patients, amylase should be monitored.

    E. Lamivudine **dosing must be adjusted in patients with renal insufficiency** (see Table 26-14). No data are available to recommend a dosage of lamivudine in patients on hemodialysis.

    F. Pregnancy. Lamivudine is classified as category C and should be used in pregnancy only if the benefit to the patient outweighs the risk to the fetus. No human data on the teratogenic potential of lamivudine are available. In animal models, lamivudine does cross the placenta into the fetus.

    G. Nursing. It is not known whether lamivudine is excreted in breast milk. Because HIV potentially may be spread to infants through breast milk, in the United States women with HIV are advised not to nurse, regardless of whether they are receiving antiretroviral agents.

IX. Cost (see Table 26-4)

Protease Inhibitors

HIV-1 protease is a critical component in the development of the HIV particle. It cleaves protein precursors into enzymes and structural proteins during the last phase of viral assembly and during budding. If assembly is blocked, the viral particles become noninfectious (see Fig. 19-1). Because the structure of HIV-1 protease is well established as a homodimer with an active site [337], the enzyme is an ideal target for rationally designed inhibitors. A number of pharmaceutical companies have specifically designed and developed molecules that fit into and bind to the cleavage site of the protease enzyme, thus rendering it inactive. To date, more than 300 HIV protease inhibitors have been designed with about ten currently in clinical development [338]. **From December 1995 through spring 1996, three protease inhibitors were approved for treatment of HIV infection: saquinavir, ritonavir, and indinavir** [338a].

HIV protease inhibitors in vitro are active against HIV-1 and HIV-2 at nanomolar concentrations, do not need intracellular processing as with nucleoside reverse transcriptase inhibitors, are active in both acutely and chronically infected cells, and appear to have antiviral activity in macrophages (where nucleoside reverse transcriptase inhibitors are not active). Problems with HIV protease inhibitors include poor bioavailability, high plasma protein binding leading to decreased intracellular levels, and a laborious and expensive production process. Lastly, development of resistance and cross-resistance of protease inhibitors also may be a limiting factor in their use as monotherapy.

SAQUINAVIR (INVIRASE)

The approval of saquinavir for use in the United States was based on studies demonstrating surrogate marker improvements, although studies with clinical endpoint outcomes are ongoing [339]. Saquinavir is approved for use in combination with nucleoside analogues.

I. **Mechanism of action.** Saquinavir is a synthetic peptide analogue that specifically inhibits HIV protease, thus preventing the development of infectious virions.

II. **In vitro activity.** Saquinavir, in vitro, inhibits HIV-1 and HIV-2 in acutely infected and chronically infected cells. It is synergistic to additive in cell cultures in combination with nucleoside reverse transcriptase inhibitors.

III. **Resistance.** Resistance to saquinavir has been found in vitro and in vivo at codons 48 and 90 of HIV protease. In phase I/II studies, 45% of patients on monotherapy had developed genotypic and phenotypic resistance, with a median time of 52 weeks. In contrast, patients on combination therapy with nucleosides had 31% genotypic resistance and 38% phenotypic resistance [340]. The development of resistance mutations at codons 48 and 90 appears to correlate with higher viral loads, but the relationship between dosage and mutation rate remains unclear [228].

IV. **Pharmacology**
   A. **Absorption and bioavailability** are poor, with an average bioavailability of 4% due to incomplete absorption and first-pass metabolism. Saquinavir's absorption rate is improved by high-fat meal intake.
   B. **Metabolism** of saquinavir occurs in the liver using the cytochrome p450 system. Saquinavir undergoes extensive first-pass metabolism and is rapidly metabolized to inactive compounds. Its metabolites are excreted primarily by the GI tract, with minimal metabolites recovered in the urine. Data is not available on saquinavir's CSF penetration, but presumably it is low due to its poor bioavailability
   C. A new oral formulation of saquinavir, which is expected to have five times the bioavailability of the parent compound, may enter trials soon [338].

V. **Clinical uses**
   A. In ZDV-naive patients, saquinavir monotherapy, 600 mg tid, was tolerated well and resulted in a 0.6 log reduction in plasma HIV RNA level [341]. The combination of saquinavir (1800 mg/day) and ZDV (600 mg/day) in antiretroviral-naive patients resulted in a median increase in CD4 cell count of 99 cells from baseline, along with a median decrease of plasma RNA of 1.5 log, which persisted through week 20 [338].
   B. In ACTG 229 [342], 300 patients with advanced HIV disease and previous ZDV experience were randomized to receive saquinavir-ZDV-ddC, saquinavir-ZDV, or ZDV-ddC. At 24 weeks, the triple drug regimen had the best laboratory response with CD4 cell count increases of at least 50 cells in 39%, and a decrease in viral RNA of 0.3 logs in 50% patients, with the two drug combinations having less of a response. Although at 48 weeks, the triple combination was superior to the double-drug combinations, viral load and CD4 cell count tended to return to the pretreatment level over time [338]. Viral resistance studies are under way in this patient group.
   C. As of December 1995, saquinavir should be used only in combination with other nucleoside analogues. Additional trials to evaluate saquinavir combination therapy are ongoing and include clinical endpoints.

VI. **Adverse effects**
   A. Saquinavir has been associated with diarrhea, abdominal discomfort, nausea, and rash. Overall, it is well tolerated [338a].
   B. No consistent alterations in laboratory tests have been associated with saquinavir.

VII. **Drug interactions**
   A. Saquinavir coadministered with **rifampin** decreases saquinavir concentration by 80%. Similarly, **rifabutin** decreases saquinavir concentration by 40%.
   B. Other drugs that may decrease saquinavir levels include **phenobarbital, phenytoin, carbamazepine, and dexamethasone.**
   C. Coadministration of **terfenadine-astemizole**—potent inhibitors of the cytochrome

p450 pathway—with saquinavir is a concern: high concentrations of these antihistamines may cause fatal cardiac arrhythmias [338a]. Alternative antihistamines are advised.

   D. Coadministration of saquinavir with **calcium channel blockers, clindamycin, dapsone, triazolam, and quinidine** may elevate their plasma levels [340].

VIII. **Dosing recommendations**

   A. Saquinavir is available in capsules of 200 mg (light brown and green opaque). The daily recommended dose for adults is 600 mg tid taken within 2 hours after a full meal. Saquinavir should be prescribed in combination with ZDV, 200 mg tid, and/or ddC, 0.75 mg tid. Lower than recommended doses of saquinavir do not have significant antiviral efficacy.

   B. Safety and efficacy of saquinavir in patients younger than 16 years have not been established [340].

   C. **Pregnancy.** Saquinavir is classified as category B drug. No human data are available on saquinavir teratogenicity.

   D. **Nursing.** It is unknown if saquinavir is excreted in human milk. Because HIV potentially may be spread to infants through breast milk, in the United States women with HIV are advised not to nurse, regardless of whether they are receiving antiretroviral agents.

   E. Data on use of saquinavir in renal insufficiency are not available.

IX. **Cost** (see Table 26-4)

RITONAVIR (NORVIR)

Ritonavir (Norvir, ABT-538) is a HIV protease inhibitor with good oral bioavailability, potent antiretroviral activity, and favorable safety profile [338a].

I. **Phase I/II trials**

   A. Phase I/II trials of ritonavir as monotherapy found statistically significant decreases in plasma HIV RNA levels by 0.86–1.70 log, which were partly sustained at week 12, with a mean reduction of approximately 1.1 log. The patients' CD4 cell count rose by a median of 83 cells/mm^3, from baseline to week 12 [337, 343]. The durability of the partial loss of activity beyond 12 weeks of therapy may be due to decreased trough levels of drug or emergence of drug resistant HIV-1 variants. Viral resistance has been observed in vitro, but the clinical implications remain uncertain [228].

   B. In the European-Australian collaborative ritonavir study, each of four ritonavir regimens initially yielded similar increases in CD4 cell count and declines in HIV RNA load [343]. Only the group receiving the highest dose (600 mg bid) showed a sustained effect on surrogate markers at 32 weeks. In this group, there was an increase in CD4 cell count of 230 cells above baseline and a decline of viral RNA by 0.81 log.

II. **Adverse effects.** Adverse effects of ritonavir are common and include diarrhea, nausea, perioral paresthesias, alteration in taste, and headaches. Transient elevations of triglyceride and aminotransferase concentrations have also been noted. No hematologic toxicity attributable to ritonavir has been detected [337]. **Ritonavir significantly affects the metabolism of many drugs** that are contraindicated or must have doses adjusted or closely monitored when ritonavir is used [338a]. **See package insert.**

III. **Dosing.** Ritonavir is available in capsules and oral solution. The recommended dosage is 600 mg PO bid in adults, beginning with 300 mg bid and increasing over 5 days to 600 mg bid (i.e., 300 mg bid for 1 day, then 400 mg bid for 2 days, 500 mg bid for 1 day, and then 600 mg bid). Ritonavir should be taken with food. The oral solution may have an unpleasant taste; the manufacturer suggests that it be taken with chocolate milk or a liquid nutritional supplement [338a].

IV. **Indications.** Ritonavir is indicated in combination with nucleoside analogs [338a] or as monotherapy for the treatment of HIV infection when therapy is warranted. See sec. III under Clinical Perspectives on Selecting Antiretroviral Regimens (p. 1019).

INDINAVIR (CRIXIVAN)

Indinavir (Crixivan, MK 639) is a potent inhibitor of HIV protease that is being evaluated in monotherapy and combination trials. It is well tolerated, has good bioavailability, and exerts significant antiviral effect. Indinavir, in combination therapy (see pp. 1019–1020), has been associated with decreases in plasma viral RNA of up to 2 logs for up to 24 weeks.

I. **Phase I studies.** In an open-label phase I trial, five subjects with mean CD4 cell counts of 66 cells/mm^3 and CD4 percentages of 4.4 received 600 mg of indinavir qid for 24 weeks. The mean increase in CD4 cell count was 143 cells/mm^3, and the mean change in CD4 percentage points was 5.2 points [228]. The mean decrease in the number of HIV RNA copies/ml was 1.52 log and was maximal at week 4.

II. **Phase II/III studies.** Indinavir has been evaluated in comparison with ZDV. In a 24-week blinded study, 73 patients were randomized to one of three groups: low-dose indinavir (200 mg q6h), high-dose indinavir (400 mg q6h), or ZDV (200 mg tid) with an optional change to ddC [344]. All subjects were p24 antigenemic, with a median baseline CD4 cell count of 118 cells/mm^3. Although most patients had had prior ZDV exposure, the median change in CD4 cell count was 80 cells/mm^3 above baseline in the high-dose group, 60 cells/mm^3 above baseline in the low-dose group, and 17 cells/mm^3 below baseline in the ZDV-ddC group. At 24 weeks, these results were largely sustained, the changes being +65 cells/mm^3, +43 cells/mm^3, and −11 cells/mm^3, respectively [228]. Higher doses of indinavir (600 mg q6h) appear to have the most sustainable antiviral effect. Other studies have been summarized [338a].

III. **Resistance.** Resistant strains appear after a few weeks of monotherapy in most patients [338], especially with suboptimal dosing. Combination therapy with appropriate dosing is less likely to be associated with the rapid development of resistance.

IV. **Adverse effects.** Indinavir is generally well tolerated. Mild **hyperbilirubinemia** (indirect) occurs in about 10% of patients and usually resolves without intervention [338a]. **Kidney stones** occurred in 2–3% of recipients: patients taking indinavir should drink at least 48 ounces of water daily [338a]. Indinavir interacts with many other drugs (see package insert), but with fewer than ritonavir [338a].

V. **Dosages.** Indinavir is available in a 200- and 400-mg capsule. For adults, 800 mg q8h has been used. The drug should be taken with water, 1 hour before or 2 hours after a meal. Indinavir lowers gastric pH and may interfere with absorption of ddI; if used concurrently, the two drugs should be taken at least 1 hour apart [338a]. The pharmacokinetics in renal failure have not been studied as of early 1996.

VI. **Indications.** Indinavir is indicated for the treatment of adults with HIV-1 infection. Combination therapy is advised [338a] as discussed in sec. **IV.B**, pp. 1019–1020.

Investigational Drugs for HIV Infection

The goal of this summary is not to detail all drugs now under consideration for trials against HIV. However, a few comments may help the reader become aware of some of the alternative agents now undergoing clinical investigation.

I. **Nonnucleoside reverse transcriptase inhibitors.** A number of structurally unrelated compounds (**nevaripine, delavirdine**) specifically inhibit reverse transcriptase of HIV-1, but not HIV-2, and are being studied in clinical trials. Unfortunately, although these compounds are relatively nontoxic, resistant mutants appear rapidly in vitro and in vivo, thus limiting the usefulness of these agents in monotherapy [233]. The most common adverse reaction associated with nevaripine and delavirdine has been rash that usually is relatively mild but which, at times, has progressed to Stevens-Johnson reaction [228].

In a recent phase II trial comparing a triple combination of ZDV-ddI-nevaripine to a two-drug combination of ZDV-ddI, the addition of nevaripine was associated with improvements in CD4 cell counts and lowered viral infectivity, which were sustained over 48 weeks [345]. Although no clinical benefit was noted, the study was not designed to detect clinical differences between the two regimens. Additional analyses are planned to define virologic and/or pharmacologic factors associated with sustained antiviral response to triple therapy with ZDV-ddI-nevaripine. Several of these agents (nevaripine, delavirdine) are currently under study in combination regimens at various stages of HIV infection.

II. **Pentoxifylline.** Pentoxifylline (Trental) is a trisubstituted xanthine used for intermittent claudication that has been shown to decrease tumor necrosis factor (TNF). Tumor necrosis factor increases the expression of HIV, reverses the therapeutic efficacy of ZDV, and may contribute to the wasting syndrome [346, 347]. In a phase I trial, pentoxifylline was well tolerated by patients with advanced HIV disease and was associated with decreased levels of TNF, mRNA, and triglycerides but was not associated with significant changes in HIV viral burden or CD4 lymphocyte counts. Although pentoxifylline is unlikely to be effective as a single agent, its role in combination with other nucleoside analogues is currently being evaluated [347].

III. **Interleukin-2.** Decreased intrinsic production of interleukin-2 (IL-2) is seen in HIV-1 infection, and replacement of this cytokine has been viewed as a possible form of immunotherapy [348, 349]. Because IL-2 is known to upregulate the production of HIV-1 in vitro, IL-2 therapy may actually increase the viral load, the rate of CD4 destruction, and theoretically worsen clinical progression. For this reason, this recombination therapy is almost always given in the setting of concurrent antiretroviral therapy [350, 351]. In clinical trials of high-dose intermittent intravenous IL-2 therapy, impressive increases in peripheral CD4 cell counts have been seen with small increases in viral burden [351]. The impact of these changes on long-term clinical outcome is unknown. In addition, **lower doses** of IL-2 are associated with a sustained increase in natural killer (NK) cell function and interferon-gamma production, both of which could be beneficial [352, 353]. Ongoing protocol ACTG 248, which examines the effects of low-dose subcutaneous IL-2 therapy, takes a rational approach by carefully evaluating the full range of effects of IL-2 therapy on immune function. Until further results are published, IL-2 use in HIV should be restricted to experimental protocols.

IV. **Hydroxyurea.** Because HIV is known to be present in large amounts at early stages of HIV infection, antiretroviral regimens are being designed to suppress HIV in both activated and resting cells [247]. The combination of ddI and hydroxyurea, known to suppress viral production in vitro in both of these cell types, was given to 12 patients with asymptomatic HIV infection [354]. The treatment was well tolerated and a large reduction of viral load was noted in all 12 patients, becoming nonquantifiable in 7 of 12 patients, as measured by infectious virus titer, and in 6 of 12, as measured by plasma HIV RNA. The reduction in viral load was accompanied by a median increase in CD4 cell count of 120 cells/mm^3 at day 90, with a median increase of 244 cells/mm^3 among the six patients with nonquantifiable viral RNA [354]. A randomized multicenter European trial designed to validate these results is being planned.

V. **Vaccines.** Several HIV candidate vaccines (MN-rgp120, HIV-1, MN-rgp160) are under investigation as potential therapeutic agents to slow the progression of HIV and prevent vertical transmission [355]. Most trials involve patients with early HIV infection in the hope of strengthening the host response to HIV. Unfortunately, preliminary results from a large multicenter study of patients with CD4 cell counts > 500 cells/mm^3 who received MN-rgp120 vaccinations failed to show a significant antiretroviral effect [356].

Clinical Perspectives on Selecting Antiretroviral Regimens

I. **HIV pathogenesis.** A full discussion of HIV pathogenesis is beyond the scope of this chapter. However, as our understanding of the dynamics of viral load improves, so will our ability to manage antiretroviral therapy for individual patients with HIV disease. The burden of HIV can be assessed by measuring: (1) **viral proteins** (e.g., p24 antigen); (2) **plasma RNA levels** (e.g., branched-chain DNA, reverse transcriptase-polymerase chain reaction [RT-PCR] assays); (3) **viral DNA** (e.g., quantitative measurements of proviral DNA in active or latently infected cells); and (4) **viral culture** (e.g., HIV in plasma or peripheral blood mononuclear cells). Our understanding of HIV burden is also affected by **viral phenotype** (e.g., syncytium cell–inducing (SI) associated with poorer outcome than non-SI strains) and **drug resistance** (e.g., depressed sensitivity to antiretroviral agents).

II. **Timing of intervention. Recent studies have found that the level of viral replication is very high during early HIV infection,** when HIV appears to be latent and persons with HIV have no clinical symptoms. Quantitative plasma RNA assays indicate that viral burden is very high during acute HIV infection with about 10^6 to 10^7 RNA copies/ml. During the so-called latency period of HIV infection, the viral burden is downregulated to approximately 10^3 to 10^4 copies/ml [228, 357]. In addition, lymph nodes of persons with early asymptomatic HIV infection show replicating viruses and intense immunologic reactions in lymphoid tissue. **Thus, theoretical considerations support early treatment of HIV-1 infection.**

Early treatment of asymptomatic HIV infection, however, remains controversial. Several studies have failed to detect a survival advantage to early therapy with ZDV [241–244, 358]. One recent study has shown that early use of ZDV during primary infection and 6 months thereafter results in improved clinical course and increased CD4 cell counts [240]. The currently available nucleoside reverse transcriptase inhibitors are relatively weak antiretroviral agents that lower the viral load by 0.5–1.0 log at best [359]. Some protease inhibitors may lower plasma load by about 2.0 log [247, 359]. Certain nonnucleoside reverse transcriptase inhibitors, such as nevaripine, have an inhibitory effect of 1.0–1.5 log, whereas the combination of ZDV and lamivudine is reported to lower plasma viremia by 1.7 log [359]. Some recently released data on nonnucleoside reverse transcriptase inhibitors in combination with protease inhibitors (e.g., indinavir) have reported reductions in plasma load in excess of 3.0 that have persisted over several months. Equally large reductions in viral burden are noted early on in therapy but, unfortunately, rarely are sustained. As safe and more effective treatment regimens are defined, our ability to detect whether early intervention is effective in prolonging survival and quality of life will improve.

III. **Monotherapy versus combination therapy.** HIV-1 replication is a dynamic process where half the virus in plasma is cleared and replenished every 2 days or less, with about 1 billion virus particles produced daily [246, 247, 359]. Given the known mutation rate of HIV-1 reverse transcriptase of about 1 in 1000 to 1 in 10,000 per base occurring in the setting of a high HIV viral replication rate, numerous viral variants are presumably generated. Hence, **monotherapy is theoretically less likely than combination therapy to be effective in the long run,** especially since substitution of a single base can result in HIV-1 becoming resistant [359].

Combination therapy has been shown to be superior to monotherapy in clinical trials [228, 252, 360]. The use of combination therapy has resulted in greater suppression of HIV replication, increased CD4 cell counts, delayed clinical progression, and delayed emergence of resistance [228]. However, it is difficult to make specific treatment recommendations from the results of the many clinical trials. Most studies are analyzed on an intent-to-treat basis using the regimen to which the participant was assigned. Some studies, for example, have large dropout rates that may favor the combination group, given the potential for additional side effects with additional medications. If the participants who remain in the study do well, the results may be distorted somewhat. In addition, some of the more successful combination therapies have never been compared in a head-to-head comparison.

At this time, we can only provide **options** for reasonable regimens based on the results of clinical trials. Even more effective regimens may exist, but as yet no data exist to support their use.

IV. **Individualizing therapy**

   A. Many experts believe that the purpose of clinical trials is to define the safety and efficacy of an agent or a combination of medications rather than to define one standard treatment regimen. The results offer information on potential therapeutic options [228]. For individual patients, the goals are to increase CD4 cell counts, reduce viral load, and prolong quality of life. In current practice, treatment regimens are determined on an individual basis, based on results of clinical trials, availability of medications, side-effect profiles, cost considerations, quality-of-life issues, and provider and patient preferences [228]. Because patients may be infected and living with HIV for well over a decade, providers should consider the need for long-term antiretroviral therapy. Some clinicians prefer to start with regimens that are simpler and better tolerated while building a rapport with their patients. Then, as patients adapt to taking medications on a regular basis, their regimens may be expanded to include more potent agents or combinations of agents that may have additional side effects. While some providers prefer to reserve the most effective combinations of medications for later stages of the disease process, when more aggressive therapy is warranted, others prefer to hit "early and hard" with combinations of potent agents when the overall viral burden may be less, thus resembling an oncologic model [359]. Providers also should consider the role of resistance when selecting the optimal antiretroviral treatment regimen. **Clearly, there are no right answers, but the best decisions are ones that are made when both patients and providers work together as a team.**

   B. **Options for antiretroviral therapy.** The optimal antiretroviral regimens for HIV infection continue to evolve. As of early May 1996, several points deserve emphasis and have recently been reviewed [338a].

      1. Monotherapy, particularly with ZDV alone, is no longer the treatment of choice for patients with HIV infection.

      2. Until more data become available, **triple therapy with two nucleosides plus a protease inhibitor** (choosing from saquinavir, ritonavir, or indinavir) appears to be the most potent antiretroviral regimen available [338a].

         a. A two-drug regimen with two nucleosides (e.g., ZDV and lamivudine or ZDV and ddI) or one nucleoside plus a protease inhibitor may also be effective in maintaining CD4 cell counts and decreasing HIV RNA [338a].

            Furthermore, in some patients, at least initially, a two-drug regimen may be associated with better compliance and patient acceptance.

Table 26-15. Cost of drugs for HIV infection

Drug	Usual dosage	Cost[a]
Nucleoside analogs		
Zidovudine (Retrovir, Glaxo Wellcome)	200 mg tid	$278.64
Didanosine (Videx, Bristol-Myers Squibb)	200 mg bid	186.04
Zalcitabine (HIVID, Roche)	0.75 mg tid	206.93
Stavudine (Zerit, Bristol-Myers Squibb)	40 mg bid	242.74
Lamivudine (Epivir, Glaxo Wellcome)	150 mg bid	223.92
Protease inhibitors		
Saquinavir (Invirase, Roche)	600 mg tid	572.06
Ritonavir (Norvir, Abbott)	600 mg bid	667.82
Indinavir (Crixivan, Merck)	800 mg tid	360.00[b]

[a]Cost to the pharmacist for 30 days' treatment with the usual recommended dosage based on wholesale price (AWP) listings in *First DataBank PriceAlert,* March 15, 1996.
[b]Direct price. Currently available only from Stadtlander Pharmacy (1-800-238-1548).
Source: Medical Letter. New drugs for HIV infection. *Med. Lett. Drugs Ther.* 38:35, 1996.

      b. Which two nucleosides are best together is unknown. ZDV is the best tested. Lamivudine appears to be the best tolerated [338a]. At this point, we favor combining ZDV and lamivudine or ZDV and ddI.

      c. Among the three protease inhibitors now available, saquinavir appears to be well tolerated but the least effective. The use of ritonavir may be limited by its adverse effects and numerous drug interactions [338a]. Therefore, at this point, indinavir is our favored agent.

   3. The **costs** of these antiretroviral agents as of spring 1996 are shown in Table 26-15.

   4. How early these drugs should be started remains to be determined. At this point, for asymptomatic patients with CD4 counts $\geq$ 500 cells/mm^3, no antiretroviral therapy has been recommended; this too is being reassessed.

   5. Quantifying viral load [361] (e.g., measurement of plasma HIV RNA copy number) to help understand and/or assess disease progression and response to therapeutic regimens is becoming an important tool. (See Chap. 19)

References

1. De Clerq, E., et al. Comparative efficacy of antiherpes drugs against different strains of herpes simplex virus. *J. Infect. Dis.* 141:563, 1980.
   Compares the activity of many antiviral agents against numerous strains of herpes simplex virus and host cell growth. Determines not only potency but also the in vitro therapeutic indexes.
2. Whitley, R.J., and Gnann, J.W., Jr. Acyclovir: A decade later. *N. Engl. J. Med.* 327:782, 1992.
   An excellent review.
3. Zovirax (acyclovir). *Physicians' Desk Reference* (49th ed.). Montvale, NJ: Medical Economics, 1995. Pp. 827–834.
4. Elion, G.B. Mechanism of action and selectivity of acyclovir. *Am. J. Med.* 73(1A):7, 1982.

5. Coen, D.M., et al. Mutations in the herpes simplex virus DNA polymerase gene can confer resistance to 9-beta-D-arabinofuranosyladenine. *J. Virol.* 41:909, 1982.
6. Crumpacker, C.S., et al. Resistance to antiviral drugs of herpes simplex virus isolated from a patient treated with acyclovir. *N. Engl. J. Med.* 306:343, 1982.
   Describes acyclovir resistance occurring in a patient receiving acyclovir.
7. Parris, D.S., and Harrington, J.E. Herpes simplex virus variants resistant to high concentrations of acyclovir exist in clinical isolates. *Antimicrob. Agents Chemother.* 22:71, 1982.
   Found that thymidine kinase–deficient mutants that are resistant to acyclovir can be isolated from patients if they had not previously been exposed to acyclovir.
8. Sibrack, C.D., et al. Pathogenicity of acyclovir-resistant herpes simplex virus type 1 from an immunodeficient child. *J. Infect. Dis.* 146:673, 1982.
   Describes how acyclovir-resistant mutants of HSV are also less pathogenic than the parent strain.
9. Englund, J.A., et al. Herpes simplex virus resistant to acyclovir. *Ann. Intern. Med.* 112:416, 1990.
10. Blum M.R., and de Miranda, P. Overview of acyclovir pharmacokinetic disposition in adults and children. *Am. J. Med.* 73(1A):186, 1982.
11. Laskin, O.L., et al. Effects of probenecid on the pharmacokinetics and elimination of acyclovir in humans. *Antimicrob. Agents Chemother.* 21:804, 1982.
    Found that probenecid inhibits the elimination of acyclovir.
12. Laskin, O.L. Clinical pharmacokinetics of acyclovir. *Clin. Pharmacokinet.* 8:187, 1983.
    A detailed review describing the pharmacokinetics, metabolism, elimination, absorption, and distribution of acyclovir in humans.
13. Laskin, O.L., et al. Effect of renal failure on the pharmacokinetics of acyclovir. *Am. J. Med.* 73(1A):197, 1982.
    Compares the pharmacokinetics of acyclovir in patients with normal renal function with those who were anuric.
14. Medical Letter. Drugs for non-HIV viral infections. *Med. Lett. Drugs Ther.* 36:27–32, 1994.
    Nice, concise, recent clinical summary.
15. Saral, R., et al. Acyclovir prophylaxis of herpes simplex virus infections: A randomized, double-blind, control trial in bone marrow transplant recipients. *N. Engl. J. Med.* 305:63, 1981.
    A trial showing that intravenous acyclovir can suppress reactivation of HSV infections in bone marrow transplant patients while they are receiving drug. Acyclovir was unable to eradicate latency.
16. Saral, R., et al. Acyclovir prophylaxis against herpes simplex virus infection in patients with leukemia. *Ann. Intern. Med.* 99:773, 1983.
17. Wade, J.C., et al. Oral acyclovir for prevention of herpes simplex virus reactivation after marrow transplantation. *Ann. Intern. Med.* 100:823, 1984.
18. Meyers, J.D., et al. Multicenter collaborative trial of intravenous acyclovir for treatment of mucocutaneous herpes simplex virus infection in the immunocompromised host. *Am. J. Med.* 73(1A):229, 1982.
    A prospective double-blind, randomized, placebo-controlled trial of intravenous acyclovir involving 97 immunosuppressed patients. Demonstrated that acyclovir had a therapeutic benefit with respect to reducing viral shedding, decreasing lesion pain, and enhancing lesion healing. No serious adverse effects were seen.
19. Shepp, D.H., et al. Oral acyclovir therapy for mucocutaneous herpes simplex virus infection in immunocompromised recipients. *Ann. Intern. Med.* 102:783, 1985.
20. Engel, J.P., et al. Treatment of resistant herpes simplex virus with continuous infusion acyclovir. *J.A.M.A.* 263:1662, 1990.
21. Balfour, H.H., Jr., et al., and the Burroughs-Wellcome Collaborative Acyclovir Study Group. Acyclovir halts progression of herpes zoster in immunocompromised patients. *N. Engl. J. Med.* 308:1448, 1983.
    A prospective double-blind, randomized, placebo-controlled trial demonstrating that acyclovir was able to halt progression of herpes zoster virus in immunosuppressed patients.
22. Shepp, D.H., Dandliker, P.S., and Meyers, J.D. Treatment of varicella-zoster virus infection in severely immunocompromised patients. *N. Engl. J. Med.* 314:208, 1986.
23. Balfour, H.H., Jr. Intravenous acyclovir therapy for varicella in immunocompromised children. *J. Pediatr.* 104:134, 1984.
    A series of eight immunosuppressed patients with varicella that demonstrates the

importance for early administration of acyclovir. In four children who were treated with acyclovir within 2 days of onset of rash, disease resolved quickly, whereas the other four who were treated after 5 days of onset of rash had progressive disease.

24. Novelli, V.M., et al. Acyclovir administered perorally in immunocompromised children with varicella-zoster infections. *J. Infect. Dis.* 149:478, 1984.
    Series of ten immunocompromised children with varicella who received oral acyclovir; all appeared to do well.

25. Prober, C.G., Kirk, L.E., and Keeney, R.E. Acyclovir therapy of chickenpox in immuno-suppressed children: A collaborative study. *J. Pediatr.* 101:622, 1982.
    A placebo-controlled trial that looks at the therapeutic response of intravenous acyclovir.

26. Perren, T.J., et al. Prevention of herpes zoster in patients by long-term oral acyclovir after allogenic bone marrow transplantation. *Am. J. Med.* 85(2A):99, 1988.

27. Balfour, H.H., et al. A randomized placebo-controlled trial of oral acyclovir for the prevention of cytomegalovirus disease in recipients of renal allografts. *N. Engl. J. Med.* 320:1381, 1989.

28. Stratta, R.J., Shaefer, M.S., Cushing, K.A., et al. Successful prophylaxis of CMV disease after primary CMV exposure in liver transplant recipients. *Transplantation.* 51:90–97, 1991.

29. Meyers, J.D., et al. Acyclovir for prevention of cytomegalovirus infection and disease after allogeneic marrow transplantation. *N. Engl. J. Med.* 318:70, 1988.
    Acyclovir prevented or lengthened the time of CMV infection after transplant.

30. Stratta, R.J., et al. A randomized prospective trial of acyclovir and immune globulin prophylaxis in liver transplant recipients receiving OKT 3 therapy. *Arch. Surg.* 127:55–64, 1992.

31. Bailey, T.C., et al. Failure of prophylactic ganciclovir to prevent CMV disease in recipients of lung transplants. *J. Infect. Dis.* 165:548–552, 1992.

32. Andersson, J., et al. Effect of acyclovir on infectious mononucleosis: A double-blind, placebo-controlled study. *J. Infect. Dis.* 153:283, 1986.

33. Andersson, J., and Ernberg, I. Management of Epstein-Barr virus infections. *Am. J. Med.* 85(2A):107, 1988.

34. Straus, S.E., et al. Acyclovir treatment of the chronic fatigue syndrome: Lack of efficacy in a placebo-controlled trial. *N. Engl. J. Med.* 319:1692, 1988.

35. Resnick, L., et al. Regression of oral hairy leukoplakia after orally administered acyclovir therapy. *J.A.M.A.* 259:384, 1988.

36. Schofer, H., et al. Treatment of oral "hairy" leukoplakia in AIDS patients with vitamin A acid (topically) or acyclovir (systemically). *Dermatologica* 174:150, 1987.

37. La Lau, C., et al. Multicenter trial of acyclovir and trifluorothymidine in herpetic keratitis. *Am. J. Med.* 73(1A):305, 1982.
    Comparative trial of acyclovir and trifluorothymidine showing that acyclovir 3% ointment healed 90% of patients in 14 days compared with 75% in the trifluorothymidine 2% ointment-treated group. Commercially, trifluorothymidine is available only in the 1% solution.

38. Keating, M.R. Antiviral agents. *Mayo Clin. Proc.* 67:160, 1992.

39. Van Landingham, K.E., et al. Relapse of herpes simplex encephalitis after conventional acyclovir therapy. *J.A.M.A.* 259:1051, 1988.
    See article in same issue favoring 21-day course of therapy.

40. Bryson, Y.J., et al. Treatment of the first episodes of genital herpes simplex virus infection with oral acyclovir: A randomized double-blind controlled trial in normal subjects. *N. Engl. J. Med.* 308:916, 1983.
    A placebo-controlled trial showing that oral acyclovir had a marked therapeutic effect in primary HSV genitalis.

41. Corey, L., et al. Intravenous acyclovir for the treatment of primary genital herpes. *Ann. Intern. Med.* 98:914, 1983.
    A placebo-controlled trial showing that intravenous acyclovir is effective in treating primary herpes genitalis.

42. Corey, L., et al. A trial of topical acyclovir in genital herpes simplex virus infections. *N. Engl. J. Med.* 306:1313, 1982.
    Placebo-controlled trial showing that topical acyclovir 5% ointment resulted in a statistically significant therapeutic response and antiviral effect in patients with first-episode herpes genitalis, but only an antiviral effect was seen in patients with recurrent herpes genitalis.

43. Reichman, R.C., et al. Topically administered acyclovir in the treatment of recurrent

herpes simplex genitalis: A controlled trial. *J. Infect. Dis.* 147:336, 1983.
Describes trial of topical acyclovir for recurrent herpes genitalis.

44. Reichman, R.C., et al. Treatment of recurrent genital herpes simplex infections with oral acyclovir. *J.A.M.A.* 251:2103, 1984.
A trial of oral acyclovir versus placebo where drug therapy was patient initiated.

45. Douglas, J.M., et al. A double-blind study of oral acyclovir for suppression of recurrences of genital herpes simplex virus infection. *N. Engl. J. Med.* 310:1551, 1984.
Acyclovir was able to prevent herpes simplex reactivation in 71% of patients during therapy.

46. Straus, S., et al. Suppression of frequently recurring genital herpes. *N. Engl. J. Med.* 310:1545, 1984.
Oral acyclovir prevented recurrences in 75% of patients on therapy.

47. Goldberg, L.H., et al. Long-term suppression of recurrent genital herpes with acyclovir: A 5-year benchmark. *Arch. Dermatol.* 129:582–587, 1993.

48. Fife, K.H., et al. Recurrence and resistance patterns of herpes simplex virus following cessation of ≥ 6 years of chronic suppression with acyclovir. *J. Infect. Dis.* 169:1338–1341, 1994.

49. Rooney, J.F., et al. Oral acyclovir to suppress frequently recurrent herpes labialis: A double-blind, placebo-controlled trial. *Ann. Intern. Med.* 118:268, 1993.

50. Whitley, R., and Straus, S. Therapy for varicella-zoster virus infections: Where do we stand? *Infect. Dis. Clin. Pract.* 2:100, 1993.
Adolescents and adults with chickenpox deserve therapy, which should be instituted within 24 hours of disease onset. Secondary family cases of chickenpox in children 2–12 years of age deserve therapy if within 24 hours of onset of rash. Most immunocompetent children do not need acyclovir for chickenpox.

51. Peterslund, N.A., et al. Acyclovir in herpes zoster. *Lancet* 2:827, 1981.
A trial demonstrating that acyclovir enhanced pain relief and shortened time to healing in nonimmunocompromised patients with herpes zoster.

52. Bean, B., Braun, C., and Balfour, H.H., Jr. Acyclovir therapy for acute herpes zoster. *Lancet* 2:118, 1982.
There was some benefit of intravenous acyclovir for herpes zoster in otherwise healthy adults.

53. Cobo, L.M., et al. Oral acyclovir in the therapy of acute herpes zoster ophthalmicus. *Ophthalmology* 92:157, 1985.
See related article: M. Cobo, Reduction of the ocular complications of herpes zoster ophthalmicus by oral acyclovir. Am. J. Med. 85(Suppl. 2A):90, 1988.

54. Hoang-Xuan, T., et al. Oral acyclovir for herpes zoster ophthalmicus. *Ophthalmology* 99:1062, 1992.
Authors suggest 800 mg of oral acyclovir 5 times daily for 7 days.

55. McKendrick, W.M., et al. Oral acyclovir in acute herpes zoster. *Br. Med. J.* 293:1529, 1986.

56. Wallace, M.R., et al. Treatment of adult varicella with oral acyclovir: A randomized placebo-controlled trial. *Ann. Intern. Med.* 117:358, 1992.

57. Dunkle, L.M., et al. A controlled trial of acyclovir for chickenpox in normal children. *N. Engl. J. Med.* 325:1539, 1991.
See editorial comment, reference [58], and related comment by A.A. Gershon in West. J. Med. 158:180, 1993, indicating exactly who should receive acyclovir is controversial because it is expensive and of modest clinical benefit.

58. Brunell, P.A. Chickenpox: Examining our options. *N. Engl. J. Med.* 325:1577, 1991.

59. Keeney, R.E., Kirk, L.E., and Bridgen, D. Acyclovir tolerance in humans. *Am. J. Med.* 73(1A):176, 1982.
Reviews the tolerance of acyclovir in humans.

60. Tucker, W.E. Preclinical toxicology profile of acyclovir: An overview. *Am. J. Med.* 73(1A):27, 1982.
Looks at preclinical toxicity of acyclovir.

61. Laskin, O.L., et al. Acyclovir concentrations and tolerance during repetitive administration for 18 days. *Am. J. Med.* 73(1A):221, 1982.
Looks at toxicity and levels of acyclovir in bone marrow transplant recipients on prolonged acyclovir therapy.

62. Haefeli, W.E., et al. Acyclovir-induced neurotoxicity. *Am. J. Med.* 94:212, 1993.

63. Spiegal, D.M., and Lau, K. Acute renal failure and coma secondary to acyclovir therapy (letter). *J.A.M.A.* 255:1882–1883, 1986.

64. Swan, S.K., and Bennett, W.M. Oral acyclovir and neurotoxicity (letter). *Ann. Intern. Med.* 111:188, 1989.

65. Centers for Disease Control. Pregnancy outcomes following systemic prenatal acyclovir exposure—June 1, 1984–June 30, 1993. *M.M.W.R.* 42:806–809, 1993.
66. Mego, R.A., et al. Use of acyclovir for varicella pneumonia during pregnancy. *Obstet. Gynecol.* 78(6):1112–1116, 1991.
67. Broussard, R.C., et al. Treatment with acyclovir of varicella pneumonia in pregnancy. *Chest* 99(4):1045–1047, 1991.
68. Medical Letter. Famciclovir for herpes zoster. *Med. Lett. Drugs Ther.* 36:97, 1994.
69. Famvir (famciclovir). *Physicians' Desk Reference* (49th ed.). Montvale, NJ: Medical Economics, 1995. Pp. 2374–2376.
70. Tyring, S., et al. Famciclovir for the treatment of acute herpes zoster: Effects on acute disease and postherpetic neuralgia. *Ann. Intern. Med.* 123:89–96, 1995.
71. Beutner, K.R., et al. Valacyclovir compared with acyclovir for improved therapy for herpes zoster in immunocompetent adults. *Antimicrob. Agents Chemother.* 39:1546–1553, 1995.
71a. Medical Letter. Valalcyclovir. *Med. Lett. Drugs Ther.* 38:3, 1996.
72. Valtrex (valacyclovir). *Product Insert,* August 1995.
72a. National Institutes of Allergy and Infectious Disease, ACTG 204. Executive Summary. February 1995.
73. Faulds, D., and Heel, R.C. Ganciclovir: A review of its antiviral activity, pharmacokinetic properties, and therapeutic efficacy in cytomegalovirus infections. *Drugs* 39: 597, 1990.
74. Cytovene (ganciclovir). *Physicians' Desk Reference* (49th ed.). Montvale, NJ: Medical Economics, 1995. Pp. 2471–2475.
75. Bowden, R.A., et al. Immunosuppressive effects of ganciclovir on in vitro lymphocyte responses. *J. Infect. Dis.* 156:899, 1987.
76. Sommadossi, J-P., and Carlisle, R. Toxicity of 3'-azido-3'-deoxythymidine and 9-(1,3-dihydroxy-2-propoxymethyl)guanine for normal human hematopoietic progenitor cells in vitro. *Antimicrob. Agents Chemother.* 31:452, 1987.
77. Biron, K.K., et al. A human cytomegalovirus mutant resistant to the nucleoside analog, 9-[(2-hydroxy-1-(hydroxymethyl)ethoxy)methyl]guanine (BW B759U), induces reduced levels of BW B759U-triphosphate. *Proc. Natl. Acad. Sci. U.S.A.* 83: 8769, 1986.
78. Erice, A., et al. Progressive disease due to ganciclovir-resistant cytomegalovirus in immunocompromised patients. *N. Engl. J. Med.* 320:289, 1989.
79. Plotkin, S.A., et al. Sensitivity of clinical isolates of human cytomegalovirus to 9-(1,3-dihydroxy-2-propoxymethyl)guanine *J. Infect. Dis.* 152:833, 1985.
80. Sullivan, V., et al. A protein kinase homologue controls phosphorylation of ganciclovir in human CMV-infected cells. *Nature* 358:162–164, 1992.
81. Hayden, F.G., Douglas, R.G. Antiviral Agents. In G.L. Mandell, R.G. Douglas, J.E. Bennett (eds.), *Principles and Practice of Infectious Diseases* (3rd ed.). New York: Churchill Livingstone, 1990. Pp. 370–393.
82. Drew, W.L., et al. Prevalence of resistance in patients receiving ganciclovir for serious cytomegalovirus infection. *J. Infect. Dis.* 163:716–719, 1991.
83. Spector, S.A., et al. Pharmacokinetic, safety, and antiviral profiles of oral ganciclovir in persons infected with human immunodeficiency virus: A Phase I/II study. *J. Infect. Dis.* 171:1431–1437, 1995.
84. Cytovene (ganciclovir capsules). *Package Insert.* October 1995.
85. The Oral Ganciclovir European and Australian Cooperative Study Group. Intravenous versus oral ganciclovir: European/Australian comparative study of efficacy and safety in the prevention of cytomegalovirus retinitis recurrence in patients with AIDS. *AIDS.* 9:471–477, 1995.
86. Weller, S., et al. The pharmacokinetics of ganciclovir in patients with cytomegalovirus (CMV) infections. *J. Pharm. Sci.* 76:S120, 1987.
87. Laskin, O.L., et al. Ganciclovir for the treatment and suppression of serious infection caused by cytomegalovirus. *Am. J. Med.* 83:201, 1987.
88. Fletcher, C., et al. Human pharmacokinetics of the antiviral drug DHPG. *Clin. Pharmacol. Ther.* 40:281, 1986.
89. Shepp, D.H., et al. Activity of 9-[(2-hydroxy-1-(hydroxymethyl)ethoxymethyl)]guanine in the treatment of cytomegalovirus pneumonia. *Ann. Intern. Med.* 103:368, 1984.
90. Henry, K., et al. Use of intravitreal ganciclovir (dihydroxy propoxy methyl guanine) for cytomegalovirus retinitis in a patient with AIDS. *Am. J. Ophthalmol.* 103:17, 1987.
91. Lake, K.D., et al. Ganciclovir pharmacokinetics during renal impairment. *Antimicrob. Agents Chemother.* 32:1899, 1988.
92. Sommadossi, J-P., et al. Clinical pharmacokinetics of ganciclovir in patients with normal and impaired renal function. *Rev. Infect. Dis.* 10(suppl. 3):S507–S514, 1988.

93. Spector, S.A., et al. A randomized controlled study of intravenous ganciclovir therapy for cytomegalovirus peripheral retinitis in patients with AIDS. *J. Infect. Dis.* 168:557–563, 1993.
    This study indicates that ganciclovir delays the progression of CMV peripheral retinitis in patients with AIDS.

94. Jabs, D.A., Enger, C., Bartlett, J.G. CMV retinitis and acquired immunodeficiency syndrome. *Arch. Ophthalmol.* 107:75–80, 1989.

95. Holland, G.N., Sakamoto, M.J., Hardy D. Treatment of CMV retinopathy in patients with AIDS. *Arch. Ophthalmol.* 104:1794–1800, 1986.

96. Studies of the Ocular Complications of AIDS Research Group in collaboration with the AIDS Clinical Trial Group. Mortality in patients with the acquired immunodeficiency syndrome treated with either foscarnet or ganciclovir for cytomegalovirus retinitis. *N. Engl. J. Med.* 326:213–220, 1992.
    Multicenter, randomized, unblinded clinical trial of 234 patients. The median survival was 8.5 months in the ganciclovir group and 12.6 months in the foscarnet group. Although the patients assigned to ganciclovir received less antiretroviral therapy on average than those assigned to foscarnet, the excess mortality could not be explained entirely by the differences in exposure to antiviral drugs. There was no difference in the two groups in the rate of progression in retinitis. Although patients may not tolerate foscarnet as well as ganciclovir, treatment with foscarnet seemed to have a survival advantage. For a related paper, see M.A. Polis, et al. Am. J. Med. 94:175, 1993. Study from National Institutes of Health; data suggest foscarnet may prolong the survival of persons with AIDS and CMV retinitis. Authors suggest, therefore, that foscarnet should be the initial treatment of choice in these patients.

97. Dieterich, D.T., Poles, M.A., Lew, E.A. Concurrent use of ganciclovir and foscarnet to treat CMV infections in AIDS patients. *J. Infect. Dis.* 167:1184–1188, 1993.

97a. The Studies of Ocular Complications of AIDS Research Group in Collaboration with the AIDS Clinical Trials Group. Combination foscarnet and ganciclovir therapy vs. monotherapy for the treatment of relapsed cytomegalovirus retinitis in patients with AIDS: The cytomegalovirus retreatment trial. *Arch. Ophthalmol.* 114:23, 1996.
    Combination therapy, if tolerated, is more effective.

98. Cocherau-Massin, I., Lehoang, P., Lautier-Frau, M. Efficacy and tolerance of intra-vitreal ganciclovir in CMV retinitis in AIDS. *Ophthalmology* 98:1348–1355, 1991.

98a. Advance on AIDS Eye Disease. *New York Times.* December 10, 1995. P. 28.

99. Anand, R., Nightingale, S.D., Fish, R.H. Control of CMV retinitis using sustained release of intraocular ganciclovir. *Arch. Ophthalmol.* 111:223–227, 1993.

100. Anand, R., et al. Pathology of CMV retinitis treated with sustained release intravitreal ganciclovir. *Ophthalmology* 100:1032–1039, 1993.

101. Kuppermann, B.D., et al. Intravitreal ganciclovir concentration after intravenous administration in AIDS patients with cytomegalovirus retinitis: Implications for therapy. *J. Infect. Dis.* 168:1506–1509, 1993.

102. Goodrich, J.M., et al. Early treatment with ganciclovir to prevent cytomegalovirus disease after allogeneic bone marrow transplantation. *N. Engl. J. Med.* 325:1601–1607, 1991.

103. Goodrich, J.M., et al. Ganciclovir prophylaxis to prevent CMV disease after allogenic marrow transplant. *Ann. Intern. Med.* 118:173–178, 1993.

104. Schmidt, G.M., et al. A randomized controlled trial of prophylactic ganciclovir for cytomegalovirus pulmonary infection in recipients of allogeneic bone marrow transplants. *N. Engl. J. Med.* 324:1005, 1991.

105. Merigan, T.C., et al. A controlled trial of ganciclovir to prevent cytomegalovirus disease after heart transplantation. *N. Engl. J. Med.* 326:1182, 1992.

106. Winston D.J., et al. Randomised comparison of ganciclovir and high-dose acyclovir for long term cytomegalovirus prophylaxis in liver-transplant recipients. *Lancet* 346:69–74, 1995.

107. Drew W.L., et al. Oral ganciclovir as maintenance treatment for cytomegalovirus retinitis in patients with AIDS. *N. Engl. J. Med.* 333:615–620, 1995.

108. Bozzette, S.A., et al. Impact of Pneumocystis carinii and cytomegalovirus on the course and outcome of atypical pneumonia in advanced human immunodeficiency virus disease. *J. Infect. Dis.* 165:93–98, 1992.

109. Mayoral, J.L., et al. Diagnosis and treatment of CMV disease in transplant patients based on gastrointestinal tract manifestations. *Arch. Surg.* 126:202–206, 1991.

110. Goodgame, R.W. Gastrointestinal cytomegalovirus disease. *Ann. Intern. Med.* 119:924–935, 1993.

111. Dieterich, D.T., et al. Ganciclovir treatment of CMV colitis in AIDS: A randomized, double blind, placebo-controlled multicenter study. *J. Infect. Dis.* 167:278–282, 1993.

112. Cohen, B.A., McArthur, J.C., Grohman, S. Neurologic prognosis of CMV polyradiculo-myelopathy in AIDS. *Neurology* 43:493–499, 1993.
113. Collaborative DHPG Treatment Study Group. Treatment of serious cytomegalovirus infections with 9-(1,3-dihydroxy-2-propoxymethyl)guanine in patients with AIDS and other immunodeficiencies. *N. Engl. J. Med.* 314:801, 1986.
114. Laskin, O.L., et al. Use of ganciclovir to treat serious cytomegalovirus infections in patients with AIDS. *J. Infect. Dis.* 155:323, 1987.
115. Balfour, H.H., Jr. Management of cytomegalovirus disease with antiviral drugs. *Rev. Infect. Dis.* 12(S7):S849, 1990.
116. Medical Letter. Drugs for AIDS and associated infections. *Med. Lett. Drugs Ther.* 37:87–94, 1995.
117. Balfour H.H., Jr., et al. Management of acyclovir-resistant herpes simplex and vari-cella-zoster virus infections. *J. Acquir. Immune Defic. Syndr.* 7:254–260, 1994.
118. Crumpacker, C.S. Mechanism of action of foscarnet against viral polymerases. *Am. J. Med.* 92(Suppl 2A):3S–7S, 1992.
119. Kaiser, L., et al. Foscarnet decreases human immunodeficiency virus RNA. *J. Infect. Dis.* 172:225–227, 1995.
120. Sjovall, J., et al. Oral absorption and pharmacokinetics after intravenous administra-tion of foscarnet to patients with HIV infection. *Clin. Pharmacol. Ther.* 44:65–73, 1988.
121. Hengee, U.R., et al. Foscarnet penetrates the blood-brain barrier: Rationale for ther-apy of cytomegalovirus encephalitis. *Antimicrob. Agents Chemother.* 37:1010–1014, 1993.
122. Sjovall, J., et al. Pharmacokinetics of foscarnet and distribution to cerebrospinal fluid after intravenous infusion in patients with HIV infection. *Antimicrob. Agents Chemother.* 33:1023–1031, 1989.
123. Oberg, B. Antiviral effects of phosphonoformate (PFA, foscarnet sodium). *Pharmacol. Ther.* 44:65–73, 1988.
124. Foscavir (foscarnet). *Physicians' Desk Reference* (49th ed.). Montvale, NJ: Medical Economics, 1995. Pp. 564–567.
125. Lietman, P.S. Clinical pharmacology: Foscarnet. *Am. J. Med.* 92(suppl 2A):8S–11S, 1992.
126. Aweeka, F.T., et al. Pharmacokinetics of concomitantly administered foscarnet and zidovudine for treatment of human immunodeficiency virus infection (AIDS Clinical Trials Group Protocol 053). *Antimicrob. Agents Chemother.* 36:1773, 1990.
127. Palestine, A.G., et al. A randomized, controlled trial of foscarnet in the treatment of cytomegalovirus retinitis in patients with AIDS. *Ann. Intern. Med.* 115:665, 1991.
128. Chatis, P.A., et al. Successful treatment with foscarnet of an acyclovir-resistant muco-cutaneous infections with herpes simplex virus infection in a patient with acquired immunodeficiency syndrome. *N. Engl. J. Med.* 320:297–300, 1989.
129. Safrin, S., et al. Foscarnet therapy for acyclovir-resistant mucocutaneous herpes simplex virus infection in 26 patients, preliminary data. *J. Infect. Dis.* 161:1078–1084, 1990.
130. Safrin, S., et al. Foscarnet therapy in five patients with AIDS and acyclovir-resistant varicella zoster virus infection. *Ann. Intern. Med.* 115:19, 1991.
131. Safrin, S., et al. A controlled trial comparing foscarnet with vidarabine for acyclovir-resistant mucocutaneous herpes simplex in the acquired immunodeficiency syndrome. *N. Engl. J. Med.* 325:551, 1991.
132. Jacobson, M.A., et al. Foscarnet therapy for ganciclovir-resistant cytomegalovirus retinitis in patients with AIDS. *J. Infect. Dis.* 163:1348–1351, 1991.
133. Jacobson, M.A., O'Donnell, J.J., Mills, J. Foscarnet treatment of CMV retinitis in patients with the acquired immunodeficiency syndrome. *Antimicrob. Agents Chemo-ther.* 33:736–741, 1989.
134. Harb, G.E., Bacchetti, P., Jacobson, M.A. Survival of patients with AIDS and cytomeg-alovirus disease treated with ganciclovir or foscarnet. *AIDS* 5:959–965, 1991.
135. Jacobson, M.A., Causey, D., Polsky, B. A dose-ranging study of daily maintenance intravenous foscarnet therapy for CMV retinitis in AIDS. *J. Infect. Dis.* 168:448, 1993.
135a. Diaz-Llopis, M., et al. High-dose intravitreal foscarnet in the treatment of cytomegalo-virus retinitis in AIDS. *Br. J. Ophthalmol.* 78:120–124, 1994.
136. Safrin, S., et al. Foscarnet-resistant herpes simplex virus infection in patients with AIDS. *J. Infect. Dis.* 169:193–196, 1994.
137. Medical Letter. Foscarnet. *Med. Lett. Drugs Ther.* 34:1, 1992.
138. Reddy, M.M., et al. Effect of foscarnet therapy on human immunodeficiency virus p24 antigen levels in AIDS patients with cytomegalovirus retinitis. *J. Infect. Dis.* 166:607–610, 1992.

139. Nelson, M.R., et al. Foscarnet in the treatment of cytomegalovirus infection of the esophagus and colon in patients with the acquired immune deficiency syndrome. *Am. J. Gastroenterol.* 86:876–881, 1991.

140. Blanshard, C., et al. Treatment of AIDS-associated gastrointestinal cytomegalovirus infection with foscarnet and ganciclovir: A randomized comparison. *J. Infect. Dis.* 172:622–628, 1995.

141. Gross, A.S., Dretler, R.H. Foscarnet-induced penis ulcer in an uncircumcised patients with AIDS. *Clin. Infect. Dis.* 17:1076–1077, 1993.

142. Deray, G., et al. Foscarnet nephrotoxicity: Mechanism, incidence, and prevention. *Am. J. Nephrol.* 9:316, 1989.

143. Andrei, G., et al. Comparative activity of selected antiviral compounds against clinical isolates of varicella-zoster virus. *Eur. J. Clin. Micro. Infect. Dis.* 14:318–329, 1995.

144. Pinnolis, M.K., Foxworthy, D., Kemp, B. Treatment of progressive ocular retinal necrosis with sorivudine. *Am. J. Ophthalmol.* 119:516–517, 1995.

145. Lalezari, J.P., et al. (S)-1-[3-Hydroxy-(Phosphonylmethoxy) propyl]-cytosine (Cidofovir): Results of a phase I/II study of a novel antiviral nucleotide analogue. *J. Infect. Dis.* 171:788–796, 1995.

146. Snoeck, R., et al. Successful treatment of progressive mucocutaneous infection due to acyclovir- and foscarnet-resistant herpes simplex virus with (S)-1-[3-hydroxy-2-(phosphonylmethoxy)propyl] cytosine (HMPMC). *Clin. Infect. Dis.* 18:570–578, 1994.

147. Kirsch, L.S., et al. Intravitreal cidofovir (HPMPC) treatment of cytomegalovirus retinitis in patients with acquired immune deficiency syndrome. *Ophthalmology* 102:533–542, 1995.

148. Heidelberger, C., and King, D.H. Trifluorothymidine. *Pharmacol. Ther.* 6:427, 1979. *Good general review of trifluorothymidine.*

149. Murphy, M., et al. Topical trifluridine for mucocutaneous acyclovir-resistant herpes simplex II in AIDS patient. *Lancet* 340:1040, 1992.

150. Kessler, H., et al. ACTG 172: Treatment of acyclovir-resistant (ACV-R) mucocutaneous herpes simplex virus (HSV) infection in patients with AIDS: Open label pilot study of topical trifluridine (TFT) (WeB 1056). *Antimicrob. Agents Chemother.* Final Program, July 19–24, 1992.

151. Birch, C.J., et al. Clinical effects and in vitro studies of trifluorothymidine combined with interferon-alpha for treatment of drug-resistant and -sensitive herpes simplex virus infection. *J. Infect. Dis.* 166:108–112, 1992.

152. Belshe, R.B., et al. Genetic basis of resistance to rimantadine emerging during treatment of influenza virus infection. *J. Virol.* 62:1508, 1988.

153. Hayden, F.G., et al. Emergence and apparent transmission of rimantadine-resistant influenza A virus in families. *N. Engl. J. Med.* 321:1696, 1989.

154. Hall, C.B., et al. Children with influenza A infection: Treatment with rimantadine. *Pediatrics* 80:275, 1987.

155. Aoki, F.Y., and Sitar, D.S. Amantadine kinetics in healthy elderly men: Implications for influenza prevention. *Clin. Pharmacol. Ther.* 37:137, 1985. *Determines the pharmacokinetics in the elderly and suggests dose modification for this group.*

156. Horadam, V.W., et al. Pharmacokinetics of amantadine hydrochloride in subjects with normal and impaired renal function. *Ann. Intern. Med.* 94:454, 1981.

157. Douglas, R.G., Jr. Drug therapy: Prophylaxis and treatment of influenza. *N. Engl. J. Med.* 322:443, 1990.

158. Centers for Disease Control. Prevention and control of influenza: Recommendations of the advisory committee on immunization practices (ACIP). *MMWR.* 44:10–18, 1995.

159. Glezen, W.P. Indications for amantadine in otherwise healthy children. *Pediatr. Infect. Dis. J.* 12:106, 1993.

160. Betts, R.F. Amantadine and rimantadine for the prevention of influenza A. *Semin. Respir. Infect.* 4:304, 1989.

161. Monto, A.S., Arden, N.H. Implications of viral resistance to amantadine in control of influenza A. *Clin. Infect. Dis.* 15:362–367, 1992.

162. Hayden, F.G., et al. Comparative single-dose pharmacokinetics of amantadine hydrochloride and rimantadine hydrochloride in young and elderly adults. *Antimicrob. Agents Chemother.* 28:216, 1985.

163. Medical Letter. Rimantadine for prevention and treatment of influenza. *Med. Lett. Drugs Ther.* 35:109–110, 1993.

164. Capparelli, E.V., et al. Rimantadine pharmacokinetics in healthy subjects and patients with end-stage renal failure. *Clin. Pharmacol. Ther.* 43:536, 1988.

165. Wills, R.J., et al. Pharmacokinetics of rimantadine hydrochloride in patients with chronic liver disease. *Clin. Pharmacol. Ther.* 42:449–454, 1987.
166. Dolin, R., et al. A controlled trial of amantadine and rimantadine in the prophylaxis of influenza A infection. *N. Engl. J. Med.* 307:580, 1982.
167. Flumadine (rimantadine). *Physicians' Desk Reference* (49th ed.). Montvale, NJ: Medical Economics, 1995. Pp. 1028–1030.
168. Huggins, J.W., et al. Prospective, double-blind, concurrent, placebo-controlled clinical trial of intravenous ribavirin therapy of hemorrhagic fever with renal syndrome. *J. Infect. Dis.* 164:1119–1127, 1991.
169. Laskin, O.L., et al. Ribavirin disposition in high-risk patients for acquired immunodeficiency syndrome. *Clin. Pharmacol. Ther.* 41:546, 1987.
170. Connor, J.D., et al. Ribavirin Pharmacokinetics in Children and Adults During Therapeutic Trials. In R.A. Smith, V. Knight, and J.A.D. Smith (eds.), *Clinical Applications of Ribavirin*. New York: Academic, 1984. Pp. 107–123.
171. Austin, R.K., et al. Sensitive radioimmunoassay for the broad-spectrum antiviral agent ribavirin. *Antimicrob. Agents Chemother.* 24:696, 1983.
172. Hall, C.B., and McBride, J.T. Respiratory syncytial virus: From chimps with colds to conundrums and cures. *N. Engl. J. Med.* 325:57, 1991.
     Editorial that contains a nice summary of the clinical impact of RSV in children. Concludes that further studies are needed to define more clearly the pathophysiology of progressive disease as the basis for unambiguous guidelines for antiviral therapy in infants with RSV infection.
173. Hall, C.B., et al. Aerosolized ribavirin treatment of respiratory syncytial virus by ribavirin. *N. Engl. J. Med.* 308:1443, 1983.
     Placebo-controlled trial describing efficacy of ribavirin in infants with infections due to RSV.
174. Ciardullo-Geraci, K., et al. IgE anti-RSV secretory immune response in infants treated with ribavirin aerosol. *Pediatr. Res.* 19:290A, 1985.
     Study describing the effect that ribavirin treatment has on the IgE immune response in infants with RSV infections.
175. American Academy of Pediatrics, Committee on Infectious Diseases. Use of ribavirin in the treatment of respiratory syncytial virus infection. *Pediatrics* 92:501–504, 1993.
     See related discussion of the use of ribavirin in the therapy for RSV in G. Peter et al. (eds.), 1994 Red Book: Report of the Committee on Infectious Diseases (23rd ed.). Elk Grove Village, IL: American Academy of Pediatrics, 1994. P. 571.
176. Smith, D.W., et al. A controlled trial of aerosolized ribavirin in infants receiving ventilation for severe respiratory syncytial virus infection. *N. Engl. J. Med.* 325:24, 1991.
     Concludes that in infants who require mechanical ventilation because of severe RSV infection, treatment with aerosolized ribavirin decreases the duration of mechanical ventilation, oxygen treatment, and hospital stay. Therefore, ribavirin therapy in the ICU setting is not only clinically effective but also cost-effective.
176a. Committee on Infectious Diseases. Reassessment of the indications for ribavirin therapy in respiratory syncytial virus infections. *Pediatrics* 97:137, 1996.
     The clinical effectiveness of ribavirin is unclear.
177. Knight, V., et al. Ribavirin small particle aerosol treatment of influenza. *Lancet* 2:945, 1981.
     Trial showing the efficacy of ribavirin for influenza A.
178. Knight, V., and Gilbert, B.E. Chemotherapy of respiratory viruses. *Adv. Intern. Med.* 31:95, 1986.
179. McClung, H.W., et al. Ribavirin aerosol treatment of influenza B virus infection. *J.A.M.A.* 249:2671, 1983.
     Describes trial of ribavirin for the therapy of influenza B viral infections.
180. McCormick, J.B., et al. Lassa fever. Effective therapy with ribavirin. *N. Engl. J. Med.* 314:20, 1986.
181. Morrison, Y.Y., Rathbun, R.C. Hantavirus pulmonary syndrome: The Four Corners disease. *Ann. Pharmacotherapy.* 29:57–65, 1995.
182. Bisceglie, A.D., et al. Ribavirin as therapy for chronic hepatitis C. *Ann. Intern. Med.* 123:897–903, 1995.
183. The Ribavirin ARC Study Group. Multicenter clinical trial of oral ribavirin symptomatic HIV-infected patients. *J. Acquir. Immune Defic. Syndr.* 6:32–41, 1993.
184. Virazole (ribavirin). *Physicians' Desk Reference* (49th ed.) Montvale, NJ: Medical Economics, 1995. Pp. 1154–1156.

185. Englund, J.A., et al. High-dose short duration ribavirin aerosol therapy in children with suspected respiratory syncytial virus infection. *J. Pediatr.* 117:313, 1990.
186. Roferon-A (interferon alfa-2A). *Physicians' Desk Reference* (49th ed.). Montvale, NJ: Medical Economics, 1995. Pp. 2055–2058.
187. Intron A (interferon alfa-2B). *Physicians' Desk Reference* (49th ed.). Montvale, NJ: Medical Economics, 1995. Pp. 2263–2271.
188. Alferon N (interferon alfa N3). *Physicians' Desk Reference* (49th ed.) Montvale, NJ: Medical Economics, 1995. Pp. 1926–1929.
189. Gallin, J.I., et al. Interferon-gamma in the management of infectious diseases. *Ann. Intern. Med.* 123:216–224, 1995.
190. Barouki, F.M., et al. Time course of interferon levels, antiviral state, 2',5'-oligoadenylate synthetase and side effects in healthy men. *J. Interferon Res.* 7:29, 1987.
191. Eron, L.J., et al. Interferon therapy for condylomata acuminata. *N. Engl. J. Med.* 315:1059, 1986.
192. Friedman-Kien, A.E., et al. Natural interferon alfa for treatment of condylomata acuminata. *J.A.M.A.* 259:533, 1988.
193. Reichman, R.C., et al. Treatment of condyloma acuminatum with three different interferons administered intralesionally. *Ann. Intern. Med.* 108:675, 1988.
194. Vance, J.C., et al. Intralesional recombinant alpha-2 interferon for the treatment of patients with condyloma acuminatum or verruca plantaris. *Arch. Dermatol.* 122: 272, 1986.
195. Trofatter, K.F., Jr. Interferon. *Obstet. Gynecol. Clin. North Am.* 14:569, 1987.
196. Weck, P.K., Brandsma, J.L., and Whisnant, J.K. Interferons in the treatment of human papillomavirus diseases. *Cancer Metastasis Rev.* 5:139, 1986.
197. Lusk, R.P., McCabe, B.F., and Mixon, J.H. Three-year experience of treating recurrent respiratory papilloma with interferon. *Ann. Otol. Rhinol. Laryngol.* 19:158, 1987.
198. Ho, M. Interferon for the treatment of infections. *Annu. Rev. Med.* 38:51, 1987.
199. Winston, D.J., et al. Recombinant interferon alpha-2a for treatment of herpes zoster in immunosuppressed patients with cancer. *Am. J. Med.* 85:147, 1988.
200. Davis, G.L., and Hoffnagle, J.H. Interferon in viral hepatitis: Role in pathogenesis and treatment. *Hepatology* 6:1038, 1986.
201. Alexander, G.J.M., et al. Loss of HB$_s$Ag with interferon therapy in chronic hepatitis B virus infection. *Lancet* 2:66, 1987.
202. Perrillo, R.P., et al. A randomized, controlled trial of interferon alfa-2b alone and after prednisone withdrawal for the treatment of chronic hepatitis B. *N. Engl. J. Med.* 323:295, 1990.
    In chronic hepatitis B, treatment with interferon-alfa-2b (5 million units per day for 16 weeks) was effective in inducing a sustained loss of viral replication and achieving remission, assessed biochemically and histologically, in more than one-third of patients. In about 10% of treated patients, hepatitis B surface antigen disappeared.
203. Perrillo, R.P. Antiviral therapy of chronic hepatitis B: Past, present and future (review). *J. Hepatol.* 17(Suppl 3):S56–S63, 1993.
204. Korenman, J., et al. Long-term remission of chronic hepatitis B after alpha-interferon therapy. *Ann. Intern. Med.* 114:629, 1991.
    Remissions in chronic hepatitis B induced by alpha-interferon are of long duration and are usually followed by the loss of HBsAG and all evidence of viral replication.
205. Perrillo, R.P., and Brunt, E.M. Hepatic histologic and immunohistochemical changes in chronic hepatitis B after prolonged clearance of hepatitis B antigen and hepatitis B surface antigen. *Ann. Intern. Med.* 115:113, 1991.
206. Wong, D.K., et al. Effect of alpha-interferon treatment in patients with hepatitis B e antigen-positive chronic hepatitis B: A meta-analysis. *Ann. Intern. Med.* 119:312–323, 1993.
207. Wong, J.B., et al. Cost-effectiveness of interferon-α2b treatment for hepatitis B e antigen-positive chronic hepatitis B. *Ann. Intern. Med.* 122:664–675, 1995.
208. DiBisceglie, A. M., et al. Recombinant interferon alfa therapy for chronic hepatitis C. A randomized, double-blind, placebo-controlled trial. *N. Engl. J. Med.* 321:1506, 1989.
    Interferon alpha therapy was beneficial in reducing disease activity in chronic hepatitis C, but in the great majority of patients (90%), the response was only transient. See editorial comment in this same issue.
209. Davis, G.L., et al. Treatment of chronic hepatitis C with recombinant interferon alfa: A multicenter randomized, controlled trial. *N. Engl. J. Med.* 321:1501, 1989.
    A 6-month course of interferon was effective in controlling disease activity after 3

million or 1 million units of recombinant interferon alfa 3 times weekly, although relapse was seen in 44–51% of recipients once therapy was stopped.

210. Hess, G. Treatment of chronic hepatitis C. *J. Hepatol.* 13(Suppl. 1):S17, 1991.
   A review article.

211. Katkov, W.N., and Dienstag, J.L. Prevention and therapy of viral hepatitis. *Semin. Liver Dis.* 11:187, 1991.
   Has a good discussion of the role of interferon in the therapy of chronic hepatitis B, C, and D.

212. Farci, P., et al. Treatment of chronic hepatitis D with interferon alfa-2a. *N. Engl. J. Med.* 330:88–94, 1994.
   See editorial comments in this same issue.

213. Papo, T., et al. Autoimmune chronic hepatitis exacerbated by interferon. *Ann. Intern. Med.* 116:51, 1992.

214. Black, M., and Peters, M. Alpha-interferon treatment of chronic hepatitis C: Need for accurate diagnosis in selecting patients. *Ann. Intern. Med.* 116:86, 1992.
   Discusses some of the therapeutic implications of the difficulties in making a precise diagnosis of hepatitis C.

215. Lane, H.C., et al. Interferon-alpha in patients with asymptomatic human immunodeficiency virus (HIV) infection. *Ann. Intern. Med.* 112:805–811, 1990.

216. Edlin, B.R., et al. In vitro resistance to zidovudine and alpha interferon in HIV1 isolates for patients: Correlation with treatment duration and response. *Ann. Intern. Med.* 117:457–460, 1992.

217. Volz, M.A., and Kirkpatrick, C.H. Interferons 1992: How much of the promise has been realized? *Drugs* 43:285, 1992.

218. Gwaltney, J.M. Combined antiviral and antimediator treatment of rhinovirus colds. *J. Infect. Dis.* 166:776–782, 1992.

219. Hulton, M.R., Levin, D.L., Freedman, L.S. Randomized, placebo-controlled, double-blind study of low-dose oral interferon-alpha in HIV-1 antibody positive patients. *J. Acquir. Immune Defic. Syndr.* 5:1084–1090, 1992.

220. Sande, M.A., et al. Antiretroviral therapy for adult HIV-infected patients: Recommendations from a state-of-the-art conference. *J.A.M.A.* 270:2583, 1993.

221. McLeod, G.X., and Hammer, S.M. Zidovudine: Five years later. *Ann. Intern. Med.* 117:487, 1992.
   An excellent review.

222. Fischl, M.A., et al. The safety and efficacy of zidovudine (AZT) in the treatment of subjects with mildly symptomatic human immunodeficiency virus type 1 (HIV) infections. *Ann. Intern. Med.* 112:727, 1990.

223. Graham, N.M.H., et al. The effects on survival of early treatment of human immunodeficiency virus infection. *N. Engl. J. Med.* 326:1037, 1992.

224. Furman, P.A., et al. Phosphorylation of 3'-azido-3'-deoxythymidine and selective interaction of the 5'-triphosphate with human immunodeficiency virus reverse transcriptase. *Proc. Natl. Acad. Sci. U.S.A.* 83:8333, 1986.

225. St. Clair, M.H., et al. 3'-azido-3'-deoxythymidine triphosphate as an inhibitor and substrate of purified human immunodeficiency virus reverse transcriptase. *Antimicrob. Agents Chemother.* 31:1972, 1987.

226. Larder, B.A., Darby, G., and Richman, D.D. HIV with reduced sensitivity to zidovudine (AZT) isolated during prolonged therapy. *Science* 243:1731, 1989.

227. Larder, B.A., Kemp, S.D. Multiple mutations in HIV-1 reverse transcriptase confer high-level resistance to zidovudine (AZT). *Science* 246:1155–1158, 1989.

228. Richman, D., Volberding, P.A., Co-chairs. The biology of antiretroviral treatment: New findings. Proceedings of a roundtable held in Denver, CO, June 26–27, 1995.

229. Richman, D.D., et al. Detection of mutations associated with zidovudine resistance in human immunodeficiency virus by use of polymerase chain reaction. *J. Infect. Dis.* 164:1075–1081, 1991.

230. Boucher, C.A., et al. Ordered appearance of zidovudine resistance mutations during treatment of 18 human immunodeficiency virus positive subjects. *J. Infect. Dis.* 165:105–110, 1992.

231. Erice, A., Balfour, H.H. Resistance of human immunodeficiency virus type 1 to antiretroviral agents: A review. *Clin. Infect. Dis.* 18:149–156, 1994.

232. Hirsch, M.S., D'Aquila, R.T. Therapy for human immunodeficiency virus infection. *N. Engl. J. Med.* 328:1686–1695, 1993.

233. D'Aquila, R.T., et al. Zidovudine resistance and HIV-1 disease progression during antiretroviral therapy. AIDS Clinical Trials Group protocol 1167B/117 team and the virology committee resistance working group. *Ann. Intern. Med.* 122:401–408. 1995.

234. Larder, B.A., Chesebro, B., Richman, D.D. Susceptibilities of zidovudine-susceptible and -resistant human immunodeficiency virus isolates to antiviral agents determined by using a quantitative plaque reduction assay. *Antimicrob. Agents Chemother.* 34:436–441, 1990.

235. Erice, A., et al. Primary infection with zidovudine-resistant human immunodeficiency virus type 1. *N. Engl. J. Med.* 328:1163–1165, 1993.

236. Fitzgibbon, J.E., et al. Transmission from one child to another of human immunodeficiency virus type 1 with a zidovudine-resistant mutation. *N. Engl. J. Med.* 329:1835–1841, 1993.

237. Frenkel, L.M., et al. Effects of zidovudine use during pregnancy on resistance and vertical transmission of human immunodeficiency virus type 1. *Clin. Infect. Dis.* 20:1321–1326, 1995.

238. Taburet, A.M., et al. Pharmacokinetics of zidovudine in patients with liver cirrhosis. *Clin. Pharmacol. Ther.* 47:731, 1990.

239. Spooner, K.M., Lane, H.C., Masur, H. Antiretroviral therapy: Reference guide to major clinical trials in patients infected with human immunodeficiency virus. *J. Infect. Dis.* 20:1145–1151, 1995.

240. Kinloch-De Loes, S., et al. A controlled trial of zidovudine in primary human immunodeficiency virus infection. *N. Engl. J. Med.* 333:408–413, 1995.

241. Volberding, P.A., et al. Zidovudine in asymptomatic human immunodeficiency virus infection: A controlled trial in persons with fewer than 500 CD4 positive cells per cubic millimeter. *N. Engl. J. Med.* 322:941–949, 1990.

242. Volberding, P.A., et al. A comparison of immediate with deferred zidovudine therapy for asymptomatic HIV-infected adults with CD4 cell counts of 500 or more cubic millimeter. *N. Engl. J. Med.* 333:401–407, 1995.

243. Aboulker, J.R., Swart, A.M. Preliminary analysis of the Concorde trial [Letter]. *Lancet.* 341:889–890, 1993.

244. Concorde Coordinating Committee. Concorde MRC/ANRS randomized double-blind controlled trial of immediate and deferred zidovudine in symptom-free HIV infection. *Lancet* 343:871–881, 1994.

245. Cooper, D.A., et al. Zidovudine in persons with asymptomatic HIV infection and CD4 + cell counts greater than 400 per cubic millimeter. *N. Engl. J. Med.* 329:297–303, 1993.

246. Ho, D.D., et al. Rapid turnover of plasma virions and CD4 lymphocytes in HIV-1 infection. *Nature* 373:123–126, 1995.

247. Wei, X., et al. Viral dynamics in human immunodeficiency virus type 1 infection. *Nature* 373:117–122, 1995.

248. Hamilton, J.D., et al. A controlled trial of early versus late treatment with zidovudine in symptomatic human immunodeficiency virus infection: Results of a Veterans Affairs Cooperative Study. *N. Engl. J. Med.* 326:437–443, 1992.

249. Fischl, M.A., et al. A randomized controlled trial of a reduced daily dose of zidovudine in patients with the acquired immunodeficiency syndrome. *N. Engl. J. Med.* 323:1009–1041, 1990.

250. Collier, A.C., et al. A pilot study of low-dose zidovudine in human immunodeficiency virus infection. *N. Engl. J. Med.* 323:1015–1021, 1990.

251. Collier, A.C., et al. Combination therapy with zidovudine and didanosine compared with zidovudine alone in HIV-1 infection. *Ann. Intern. Med.* 119:786–793, 1993.

252. National Institutes of Allergy and Infectious Disease, ACTG 175. Executive Summary. September 1995.

253. Torres, G. ACTG 175 and Delta. *Treatment Issues* 9:3–4, 1995.

254. Choo, V. Combination superior to zidovudine in Delta trial. *Lancet* 342:895, 1995.

255. Dolin, R., et al. Zidovudine compared with didanosine in patients with advanced HIV type 1 infection and little or no previous experience with zidovudine. AIDS Clinical Trials Group. *Arch. Intern. Med.* 155:961–974, 1995.

256. Kahn, J.O., et al. A controlled trial comparing continued zidovudine with didanosine in human immunodeficiency virus infection. *N. Engl. J. Med.* 327:581–587, 1992.
In this multicenter, double-blind study of 913 patients, changing treatment from ZDV to 500 mg qd of ddI appeared to slow the progression of HIV disease, especially in asymptomatic HIV infection or AIDS-related complex. Also, ddI was better tolerated than ZDV.

257. Fischl, M.A., et al. Combination and monotherapy with zidovudine and zalcitabine in patients with advanced HIV disease. *Ann. Intern. Med.* 122:24–32, 1995.

258. Fischl, M.A., et al. Zalcitabine compared with zidovudine in patients with advanced HIV-1 infection who received previous zidovudine therapy. *Ann. Intern. Med.* 118:762–769, 1993.

259. Connor, E.M., et al. for the Pediatric AIDS Clinical Trials Group Protocol 076 Study Group. Reduction of maternal-infant transmission of human immunodeficiency virus type 1 with zidovudine treatment. *N. Engl. J. Med.* 331:1173, 1994.
   ZDV therapy reduced the risk of maternal-infant HIV transmission by approximately two thirds. See editorial comment, M.F. Rogers and H.W. Jaffe, Reducing the risk of maternal-infant transmission of HIV: A door is opened. N. Engl. J. Med. 331:1222, 1994. See also Centers for Disease Control, Recommendations of the U.S. Public Health Service Task Force on the use of zidovudine to reduce perinatal transmission of human immunodeficiency virus. M.M.W.R. 43(RR-11):1–20, 1994.
260. Sperling, R.S., et al. A survey of zidovudine use in pregnant woman with human immunodeficiency virus infection. *N. Engl. J. Med.* 326:857–861, 1992.
261. Schmitt, F.A., et al. Neuropsychological outcome of zidovudine (AZT) treatment of patients with AIDS and AIDS-related complex. *N. Engl. J. Med.* 319:1573, 1988.
262. Sidtis, J.J., et al. Zidovudine treatment of the AIDS dementia complex: Results of a placebo-controlled trial. AIDS Clinic Trials Group. *Ann. Neurol.* 33:343–349, 1993.
263. Centers for Disease Control. Public Health Service statement on management of occupational exposure to human immunodeficiency virus, including considerations regarding zidovudine postexposure use. *M.M.W.R.* 39:1–14, 1990.
264. Lange, J.M.A., et al. Failure of zidovudine prophylaxis after accidental exposure to HIV-1. *N. Engl. J. Med.* 322:1375–1377, 1990.
265. Miller, R.A. Failure of zidovudine prophylaxis after exposure to HIV-1. (Letter) *N. Engl. J. Med.* 323:915–916, 1990.
266. CDC. Update: Provisional Public Health Service Recommendations for chemoprophylaxis after occupational exposure to HIV. *M.M.W.R.* 45:468, 1996.
267. Pizzo, P.A., et al. Effect of continuous intravenous infusion of zidovudine (AZT) in children with symptomatic HIV infection. *N. Engl. J. Med.* 319:889, 1988.
268. National Institutes of Allergy and Infectious Disease, ACTG 152. Executive Summary. February 1995.
269. Gibb, D.M., et al. Treatment of children with HIV infection. *Lancet* 345:1115, 1995.
270. Lagakos, S., et al. Effects of zidovudine therapy in minority and other subpopulations with early HIV infection. *J.A.M.A.* 266:2709–2712, 1991.
271. Koch, M.A., et al. Toxic effects of zidovudine asymptomatic patients with HIV infection and with CD4 cell count 0.5×10^9/L or less. *Arch. Intern. Med.* 152:2286–2292, 1992.
272. Medical Letter. Drugs for AIDS and associated infections. *Med. Lett. Drugs Ther.* 35:79–86, 1993; with update 37:87, 1995.
273. Fischl, M., et al. Recombinant human erythropoietin for patients with AIDS treated with zidovudine. *N. Engl. J. Med.* 322:1488–1493, 1990.
274. Dalakas, M.C., et al. Mitochondrial myopathy caused by long-term zidovudine therapy. *N. Engl. J. Med.* 322:1098–1105, 1990.
275. Stein, D. A new syndrome of hepatomegaly with severe steatosis in HIV seropositive patients. *AIDS Clin. Care* 6:17–20,26, 1994.
276. Petty, B.G., Kornhauser, D.M., Leitman, P.S. Zidovudine with probenecid: A warning. *Lancet* 335:1044–1045, 1990.
277. Jacobson, M.A., et al. Prolonged pancytopenia due to combined ganciclovir and zidovudine therapy. *J. Infect. Dis.* 158:489, 1988.
278. Retrovir(zidovudine). *Physicians' Desk Reference* (49th ed.). Montvale, NJ: Medical Economics, 1995. Pp. 802–809.
279. Boucher, F.D., et al. Phase I evaluation of zidovudine administered to infants exposed at birth to HIV. *J. Pediatr.* 122:137, 1993.
280. Yarchoan, R., et al. A randomized pilot study of alternating or simultaneous zidovudine and didanosine therapy in patients with symptomatic human immunodeficiency virus infection. *J. Infect. Dis.* 169:9–17, 1994.
281. Gallant, J.E., et al. Lack of association between acyclovir use and survival in patients with advanced human immunodeficiency virus disease treated with zidovudine. Zidovudine Epidemiology Study Group. *J. Infect. Dis.* 172:346–352, 1995.
282. Cooper, D.A., et al. The efficacy and safety of zidovudine alone or as co-therapy with acyclovir for the treatment of patients with AIDS and AIDS-related complex: A double blind, randomized trial. *AIDS* 7:197–207, 1993.
283. Youle, M.S., et al. Effects of high-dose oral acyclovir on herpes virus disease and survival in patients with advanced HIV disease: A double-blind, placebo-controlled study. *AIDS* 8:641–649, 1994.
284. Stein, D.S., et al. The effect of the interaction of acyclovir with zidovudine on progression to AIDS and survival. Analysis of data in the Multicenter AIDS Cohort Study. *Ann. Intern. Med.* 121:100–108, 1994.

285. Corey, L., et al. Clinical perspectives in the treatment of HIV disease: The role of didanosine. *Clin. Infect. Dis.* 16(Suppl. 1):S1–S73, 1993.
286. Dolin, R., Fischl, M.A., Pettinelli, C. Executive summary for the final analysis of ACTG 116A, 1992.
287. St. Clair, M.H., et al. Resistance to ddI and sensitivity to AZT induced by a mutation in HIV-1 reverse transcriptase. *Science* 253:1557–1559, 1991.
288. Yarchoan, R., et al. In vitro activity against HIV and favorable toxicity profile of 2'3' dideoxyinosine. *Science* 245:412, 1989.
289. Demeter, L.M., et al. Development of zidovudine resistance mutations in patients receiving prolonged didanosine monotherapy. *J. Infect. Dis.* 172:1480–1485, 1995.
290. Reichman, R.C., et al. ddI and ZDV susceptibilities of HIV isolates from long term recipients of ddI. *Antiviral Research* 20:267–277, 1993.
291. McLeod, G.X., et al. Didanosine and zidovudine resistance patterns in clinical isolates of human immunodeficiency virus type 1 as determined by a replication endpoint concentration assay. *Antimicrob. Agents Chemother.* 36:920–925, 1992.
292. Hartman, N.R., et al. Pharmacokinetics of 2',3' dideoxyinosine in patients with severe immunodeficiency infection II: The effects of different oral formulations and the presence of other medications. *Clin. Pharmacol. Ther.* 50:278–285, 1991.
293. Hartman, N.R., et al. Pharmacokinetics of 2',3'-dideoxyadenosine and 2',3'-dideoxy-inosine in patients with severe human immunodeficiency virus infection. *Clin. Pharmacol. Ther.* 47:647–654, 1990.
294. Singlas, E., et al. Didanosine pharmacokinetics in patients with normal and impaired renal function: Influence of hemodialysis. *Antimicrob. Agents Chemother.* 36:1519–1524, 1992.
295. Videx (didanosine). *Physicians' Desk Reference* (49th ed.) Montvale, NJ: Medical Economics, 1995. Pp. 688–694.
296. Spruance, S.L., Pavia, A.T., Peterson, D., et al. Didanosine compared with continuation of zidovudine in HIV-infected patients with signs of clinical deterioration while receiving zidovudine. *Ann. Intern. Med.* 120:360–368, 1994.
297. Montaner, J.S.G., et al. Didanosine compared with continued zidovudine therapy for HIV-infected patients with 200 to 500 CD4 cells/mm³. *Ann. Intern. Med.* 123:561–571, 1995.
298. Butler, K.M., et al. Dideoxyinosine in children with symptomatic human immunodeficiency virus infection. *N. Engl. J. Med.* 324:137, 1991.
298a. Seidlin, M., et al. Pancreatitis and pancreatic dysfunction in patients taking dideoxy-inosine. *AIDS* 6:831–835, 1992.
299. Kieburtz, K.D., et al. Extended follow-up of peripheral neuropathy in patients with AIDS and AIDS-related complex treated with dideoxyinosine. *J. Acquir. Immune Defic. Syndr.* 5:60–64, 1992.
300. Lambert, J.S., et al. 2',3' dideoxyinosine (ddI) in patients with acquired immunodeficiency syndrome or AIDS-related complex: A phase I trial. *N. Engl. J. Med.* 322:1333, 1990.
301. Cooley, T.P., et al. Once daily administration of 2'3' dideoxyinosine (ddI) in patients with acquired immunodeficiency syndrome or AIDS related complex: Results of a phase I trial. *N. Engl. J. Med.* 322:1340, 1990.
302. Bossuel, F., et al. Fulminant hepatitis with severe lactate acidosis in HIV-infected patients on didanosine therapy. *J. Intern. Med.* 235:367–371, 1994.
303. Whitcup, S.M., et al. Retinal toxicity in human immunodeficiency virus-infected children treated with 2',3'-dideoxyinosine. *Am. J. Ophthalmol.* 113:1–7, 1992.
304. Sahai, J., et al. Pharmacokinetics of simultaneously administered zidovudine and didanosine in HIV-seropositive male patients. *J. Acquir. Immune Defic. Syndr.* 10:54–60, 1995.
305. Gustavson, L.E., et al. A pilot study of the bioavailability and pharmacokinetics of 2,3 dideoxycytidine in patients with AIDS or AIDS-related complex. *J. Acquir. Immune Defic. Syndr.* 3:28, 1990.
306. Abrams, D.I., et al. A comparative trial of didanosine and zalcitabine in patients with human immunodeficiency virus infection who are intolerant or have failed zidovudine therapy. *N. Engl. J. Med.* 330:657–662, 1994.
307. Shelton, M.J., O'Donnell, A.M., Morse, G.D. Zalcitabine. *Ann. Pharmacother.* 27:480–489, 1993.
308. Fitzgibbon, J.E., et al. Human immunodeficiency virus type 1 pol: Gene mutations which cause decreased susceptibility to 2,3-dideoxycytidine. *Antimicrob. Agents Chemother.* 36:157, 1992.

309. Richman, D.D., et al. Resistance to AZT and ddC during long-term combination therapy in patients with advanced infection with human immunodeficiency virus. *J. Acquir. Immune Defic. Syndr.* 7:135–138, 1994.

310. Meng, T., et al. Combination therapy with zidovudine and dideoxycytidine in patients with advanced human immunodeficiency virus infection: A phase I/II study. *Ann. Intern. Med.* 116:13–20, 1992.

311. Dear Doctor Letter. January 13, 1992. ddC information amendment: Closure of N330 (ACTG 114). Nutley, NJ: Hoffman LaRoche, Inc.

312. Bozzette, S.A., et al. Health status and function with zidovudine or zalcitabine as initial therapy for AIDS: A randomized controlled trial. Roche 3300/ACTG 114 Study Group. *J.A.M.A.* 273:295–301, 1995.

313. Pizzo, P.A., et al. Dideoxycytidine alone and in an alternating schedule with zidovudine in children with symptomatic human immunodeficiency virus infection. *J. Pediatr.* 117:799, 1990.
    A small study in which four different dosage levels of ddC were given for 8 consecutive weeks, then stopped. After a 30-day rest, a schedule of ddC for 1 week was followed by 3 weeks of ZDV; this schedule was alternated as tolerated. Longer courses of ddC and optimal dosing studies need to be undertaken.

314. Skowron, G., et al. Alternating and intermittent regimens of zidovudine and dideoxycytidine in patients with AIDS or AIDS-related complex. *Ann. Intern. Med.* 118:321–330, 1993.
    Unblinded, randomized, phase II multicenter study. Data suggest alternating therapy with ZDV and ddC reduces toxicity while maintaining antiviral activity. (The ZDV dose used was 200 mg q4h.)

315. Berger, A.R., et al. 2',3'-dideoxycytidine (ddC) toxic neuropathy: A study of 52 patients. *Neurology.* 43:358–362, 1993.

316. Indorf, A.S., and Pegram, P.S. Esophageal ulceration related to Zalcitabine (ddC). *Ann. Intern. Med.* 117:133, 1992.

317. HIVID (zalcitabine). *Physicians' Desk Reference* (49th ed.) Montvale, NJ: Medical Economics, 1995. Pp. 2040–2044.

318. Zerit (stavudine). *Physicians' Desk Reference* (49th ed.). Montvale, NJ: Medical Economics, 1995. Pp. 697–700.

319. Lin, P.F., et al. Genotypic and phenotypic analysis of human immunodeficiency virus type 1 isolates from patients on prolonged stavudine therapy. *J. Infect. Dis.* 170:1157–1164, 1994.

320. Browne, M.J., et al. 2',3'-didehydro-3'-deoxythymidine (d4T) in patients with AIDS or AIDS-related complex: A phase I trial. *J. Infect. Dis.* 167:21–29, 1993.

321. Dudley, M.N., et al. Pharmacokinetics of stavudine in patients with AIDS or AIDS-related complex. *J. Infect. Dis.* 166:480–485, 1992.

322. Bristol Myers Squibb. Review of stavudine (Zerit) clinical trials. Evansville. Indiana: B202, 1994.

323. Food and Drug Administration. Stavudine approved for certain patients with advanced HIV. *J.A.M.A.* 272:582, 1994.

324. Volberding, P.A. Perspectives on the use of antiretroviral drugs in the treatment of HIV infection. *Infect. Dis. Clin. North Am.* 8:303, 1994.

325. Epivir (Lamivudine). *Package Insert.* November 1995.

326. Boucher, C.A.B., et al. High level resistance to ($-$) enantiomeric 2'-deoxy-3'-thiacytidine in vitro is due to one amino acid substitution in catalytic site of HIV-1 reverse transcriptase. *Antimicrob. Agents Chemother.* 37:2231–2234, 1993.

327. Dienstag, J.L., et al. Preliminary trial of lamivudine for chronic hepatitis B infection. *N. Engl. J. Med.* 333:1657–1661, 1995.

328. Wainberg, M.A., et al. Development HIV-1 resistance to($-$)2'-deoxy 3'-thiacytidine in patients with AIDS or advanced AIDS related complex. *AIDS* 9:351–357, 1995.

329. Schuurman, R., et al. Rapid changes in HIV-1 RNA load and appearance of drug resistant virus population in persons treated with lamivudine (3TC). *J. Infect. Dis.* 171:141–149, 1995.

330. Larder, B., Kemp, S.D., Harrigan, R. Potential mechanism for sustained antiretroviral efficacy of AZT-3TC combination therapy. *Science* 269:696–699, 1995.

331. VanLeeuwen, R., et al. Evaluation of safety and efficacy of 3TC (lamivudine) in patients with asymptomatic or mildly symptomatic HIV infection: A phase I/II study. *J. Infect. Dis.* 171:1166–1171, 1995.

332. Ingrand, D., et al. Phase I/II study of lamivudine in HIV positive, asymptomatic or mild AIDS related complex patients: Sustained in reduction in viral mother. *AIDS* 9:1323–1329, 1995.

333. Katlama, C. European Lamivudine HIV working group combination 3TC/ZDV vs ZDV monotherapy in ZDV naive HIV-1 positive patients with a CD4 of 100–400 cells/mm³ (Abstract LB31). Presented at Second National Conference on Human Retroviruses and Related Infections, Washington DC: January 29–February 2, 1995.

334. Staszewski, S. European Lamivudine HIV Working Group Combination 3TC/ZDV vs ZDV monotherapy in ZDV experienced HIV-1 positive patients with a CD4 of 100–400 cells/mm³ (Abstract LB32). Presented at Second National Conference on Human Retrovirus and Related Infections. Washinton DC: January 29–February 2, 1995.

335. Eron, J.J., et al. Treatment with lamivudine, zidovudine, or both in in HIV-positive patients with 200 to 500 CD4+ cells per cubic millimeter. *N. Engl. J. Med.* 333:1662–1669, 1995.

336. Bartlett, J., et al. A randomized double blind multicenter comparative trial of lamivudine (3TC)/zidovudine (ZDV) combination therapy vs ZDV/dideoxycytidine (ddC) combination in ZDV experienced patients CD4 100–300 mm³ (Abstract LB35). Second National Conference on Human Retroviruses and Related Infections. Washington DC: January 29–February 2, 1995.

337. Markowitz, M., et al. A preliminary study of ritonavir, an inhibitor of HIV-1 protease, to treat HIV infection. *N. Engl. J. Med.* 333:1534–1539, 1995.

338. Vella, S. Update on HIV Protease Inhibitors. *AIDS Clin. Care.* 7:79, 1995.

338a. Medical Letter. New drugs for HIV infection. *Med. Lett. Drugs Ther.* 38:35, 1996.
This April 1996 issue briefly summarizes the new protease inhibitors. A placebo-controlled trial in over 1000 patients with advanced HIV disease and extensive previous treatment found that the addition of ritonavir to the therapeutic regimen decreased the incidence of clinical progression or death after 6 months' treatment: among patients treated with ritonavir, 5% died compared with 8% among patients given placebo. In another trial, the triple combination of ritonavir plus ZDV and zalcitabine for 6 months lowered plasma HIV counts below detectable levels in 5 of 21 patients with advanced, previously untreated HIV infection.
Includes a brief summary of combination therapy of indinavir with ZDV and indinavir with ZDV plus lamivudine: These combinations were effective in reducing HIV levels during the study period.
For a related paper, see S.A. Churchill, Protease inhibitors: Implications for HIV research and treatment. J. Internat. Assoc. of Physicians in AIDS Care 2:13, 1996, with a summary from the Fifth European Conference on Clinical Aspects and Treatment of HIV Infection.

339. Soo, W., et al. Inter-Company Collaboration Combination Trials. *J. Acquir. Immune Defic. Syndr.* 10(Suppl. 2):592, 1995.

340. Invirase (Saquinavir mesylate). *Product Insert.* December 1995.

341. Kitchen, V.S., et al. Safety and activity of saquinavir in HIV Infection. *Lancet.* 345:952, 1995.

342. Bassett, R., Schoenfeld, D., Collier, A. ACTG 229 Extension Phase. Executive Summary. December 7, 1995.
See recent report of ACTG 229 by A.C. Collier et al., Treatment of human immunodeficiency virus infection with saquinavir, zidovudine, and zalcitabine. N. Engl. J. Med. 334:1011, 1996. Study concludes that further studies are warranted to evaluate whether the three-drug combination will reduce morbidity and mortality.

343. Danner, S.A., et al. A short term study of the safety, pharmacokinetics and efficacy of ritonavir, an inhibitor of HIV-1 protease. *N. Engl. J. Med.* 333:1528–1533, 1995.

344. Mellors, J., et al. A randomized, double blind study of the oral HIV protease inhibitor, L-735,524 vs zidovudine in p24 antigenemic, HIV-1 infected patients with < 500cells/mm³ (Abstract 183). Presented at Second National Conference on Human Retroviruses and Related Infections. Washington DC: January 29–February 2, 1995.

345. National Institutes of Allergy and Infectious Disease, ACTG 241. Executive summary. November 16, 1994.

346. Dezube, B.J., et al. Pentoxifylline decreases tumor necrosis factor expression and serum triglycerides in people with AIDS. *J. Acquir. Immune Defic. Syndr.* 6:787–794, 1993.

347. Dezube, B.J., et al. High-dose pentoxifylline in patients with AIDS: Inhibition of tumor necrosis factor production. *J. Infect. Dis.* 171:1628–1632, 1995.

348. Nokta, M.A., Pollard, R.B. Differential reconstitution of zidovudine-induced inhibition of mitogenic responses by interleukin-2 in peripheral blood mononuclear cells from patients with human immunodeficiency virus infection. *Antiviral Research* 11:191–202, 1989.

349. Ebert, E.C., et al. Diminished interleukin 2 production and receptor generation characterize the acquired immunodeficiency syndrome. *Clin. Immunol.* 37:283–297, 1985.
350. McMahon, D.K., et al. A phase I study of subcutaneous recombinant interleukin-2 in patients with advanced HIV disease while on zidovudine. *AIDS* 8:59–66, 1994.
351. Teppler, H., et al. Efficacy of low doses of the polyethylene glycol derivative of interleukin-2 in modulating the immune response of patients with human immunodeficiency virus type 1 infection. *J. Infect. Dis.* 167:291–298, 1993.
352. Kovacs, J.A., et al. Increases in CD4 T lymphocytes with intermittent courses of interleukin-2 in patients with human immunodeficiency virus infection. *N. Engl. J. Med.* 332:567–575, 1995.
353. Schnittman, S.M., et al. A Phase I study of interferon-alpha 2b in combination with interleukin-2 in patients with human immunodeficiency virus infection. *J. Infect. Dis.* 169:981–989, 1994.
354. Biron, F., et al. Anti-HIV activity of the combination of didanosine and hydroxyurea in HIV-1-infected individuals. *J. Acquir. Immune Defic. Syndr.* 10:36–40, 1995.
355. Graham, B.S., and Wright, P.F. Drug therapy: Candidate AIDS vaccines. *N. Engl. J. Med.* 333:1331–1337, 1995.
356. Allan, J., et al. Safety and immunogenicity of MN and IIIB rgp 120/HIV-1 vaccines in HIV-1 infected subjects with CD4 counts > 500 cells per cubic millimeter. *Ninth International Conference on AIDS.* Berlin: June 1993.
357. Piatak, M., Jr., et al. High levels of HIV-1 in plasma during all stages of infection determined by competitive PCR. *Science* 259:1749–1754, 1993.
358. Volberding, P.A., et al. The duration of zidovudine benefit in persons with asymptomatic HIV infection. *J.A.M.A.* 272:437–442, 1994.
359. Ho, D.D. Time to hit HIV, early and hard. *N. Engl. J. Med.* 333:450–451, 1995.
360. *Centers for Disease Control.* Case-Control Study of HIV Seroconversion in Health-Care Workers After Percutaneous Exposure to HIV-Infected Blood—France, United Kingdom, and United States, January 1988–August 1994. *M.M.W.R.* 44:929–935, 1995.
361. Landesman, S.H. Quantifying HIV. *J.A.M.A.* 275:640, 1996.

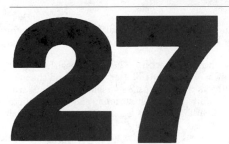

Allergy to Penicillin and Other Antibiotics

John J. Condemi
and Michael G. Sheehan

It should not be surprising that adverse reactions to drugs are an important medical problem: They contribute significantly to iatrogenic disease and limit the pharmacologic agents available to treat patients. Adverse drug reactions are, however, more of a problem than most realize. Prior studies have estimated that up to 3–5% of medical hospital admissions are attributable to this cause and that 6–30% of hospitalized patients experience at least one adverse drug reaction, which often prolongs their hospitalization [1–4]. Allergic reactions to drugs contribute to 1% of admissions and 2% of prolonged hospitalizations. Antibiotics contribute significantly to these statistics in that they are one of the three classes of drugs most frequently associated with adverse reactions [3, 5]. This chapter deals predominantly with penicillin allergy, because penicillins G and V, semisynthetic penicillins, and the cephalosporins continue to be the most widely used antibiotics in the United States. Our understanding of the mechanism of allergic reactions to penicillin should allow us to reduce their frequency in patients who are to receive penicillin.

I. **Reactions to penicillin.** Adverse reactions are estimated to occur in 1–10% of patients receiving penicillin. The frequency varies depending on the type of reaction. Immediate systemic reactions or anaphylaxis occurs in approximately 0.01–0.05% (1 to 5/10,000 courses of treatment) [1a], death in 0.002% [6], and urticaria in 4.5%; the 10% incidence figure includes those patients experiencing a morbilliform rash after receiving penicillin.

   A. **Allergic nature of reactions.** The evidence, besides positive skin tests, that some of the penicillin reactions are allergic in nature and treatable with antiallergic medications, is inferred on clinical grounds by applying the following criteria.

   1. The observed manifestation does **not** resemble the known **pharmacologic** actions of the drug.

   2. There is a **latent period** during which the drug has been taken with no ill effects. This latent period may vary from a few days to many years but is commonly 7–10 days after initiation of drug administration.

   3. Once a reaction has occurred, it generally **recurs on readministration** of the same, or a closely related, drug, either immediately or faster after reexposure than was the case for the initial reaction.

   4. On **reexposure** to the drug, there is an **increase in severity** of symptoms, even when small doses have been administered.

   5. The **reaction occurs only in a minority of persons** receiving the drug.

   6. The reaction **resembles** those that have been associated with **known allergic manifestations,** such as anaphylaxis, serum sickness, urticaria, angioedema, asthma, and contact dermatitis.

   7. The reaction is accompanied by **eosinophilia,** or histologic studies reveal eosinophilic infiltrates within the tissues, or they reveal a **vasculitis.** Antibiotic-induced vasculitides are uncommon but have occurred when an agent is continued despite the presence of a progressive maculopapular rash and/or in the presence of a rash with so called "palpable purpura." This topic has been reviewed recently [6a].

   B. **Pathogenesis of reaction.** Although these criteria would suggest that immunologic phenomena are causing the reaction, proof that a drug causes an allergic reaction requires the demonstration of either an antibody or cell-mediated hypersensitivity to the drug. These types of observations have been made in patients experiencing some of the reactions to penicillin and have allowed a more rational classification of penicillin-allergic reactions. Such findings have rarely been observed with other drug reactions.

C. Classification of reactions. The classification of the different types of penicillin-allergic reactions **based on the time of onset** as suggested by Levine [1a] is given in Table 27-1.

1. **Immediate reactions are the most dangerous.** These occur within 30–60 minutes after initiation of penicillin or other antibiotic therapy, and the symptoms are related to the release of histamine and other vasoactive amines from IgE-sensitized mast cells and basophils. The most serious reaction is hypotension, which may progress to shock and be fatal. Urticaria (hives), wheezing, or rhinitis can also occur.

2. **Accelerated allergic reactions** occur 1–72 hours after initiating the penicillin therapy. These usually are not life-threatening, except for laryngeal edema, which can cause death by asphyxia. As with the immediate allergic reaction, these reactions appear to be IgE-mediated, but they differ in that they have been modified by IgG.

3. **Late reactions** are the most frequent type with penicillin use, accounting for approximately 80–90% of all reactions. They begin days to weeks after initiation of penicillin therapy, and the **most common is that of a morbilliform eruption.** Although this reaction is included in Table 27-1, **no definite allergic mechanism has been demonstrated.** The major distinction between urticaria arthralgic syndrome and serum sickness is the absence of fever, adenopathy, splenomegaly, and renal or cardiac involvement in urticaria arthralgic syndrome.

4. The **less common (late) reactions** occur rarely. In many of them, the immunologic basis has not been established; nonetheless, they are included because they fulfill many of the previously mentioned criteria. Drug fever is discussed in Chap. 1. If this is the sole manifestation of a penicillin reaction, penicillin or its derivatives can probably be readministered in the future at no additional risk to the patient. However, fever may accompany other more severe manifestations, such as vasculitis, but the fever may precede the development of skin involvement. Because there may be a risk of their developing vasculitis on subsequent administration of penicillin (in the patient with a history of drug fever due to penicillin), these patients need careful observation.

Table 27-1. Allergic reactions to penicillin and semisynthetic penicillins

Immediate allergic reactions (2–30 min after penicillin)
  Erythema or pruritus
  Urticaria
  Angioedema
  Wheezing, rhinitis
  Hypotension or shock
Accelerated allergic reactions (1–72 hr)
  Erythema or pruritus
  Urticaria
  Angioedema
  Laryngeal edema
  Wheezing, rhinitis
Late allergic reactions (more than 72 hr)
  Morbilliform eruptions
  Urticaria—angioedema
  Urticaria—arthralgia
  Serum sickness
Less common reactions
  Immune hemolytic anemia
  Pulmonary infiltrates with eosinophilia
  Interstitial nephritis
  Granulocytopenia
  Thrombocytopenia
  Drug fever
  Hypersensitivity vasculitis
  Erythema multiforme
  Drug-induced systemic lupus erythematosus

D. Immunologic response. To understand how individuals become allergic to penicillin, it is important to appreciate how a simple chemical of low molecular weight can elicit an immune response. It has been clearly established that low-molecular-weight substances capable of producing an allergic reaction are **haptens.** These are substances that can react specifically with antibodies but that are unable to induce antibody formation unless attached to carrier molecules, usually proteins, by a strong covalent bond. In the case of penicillin, it has been determined that the **patients do not exhibit an immune response to penicillin itself but rather to those breakdown, or metabolic, products of penicillin** that are capable of forming the necessary strong covalent linkage with tissue and serum proteins. **Some, if not all, of the degradation products responsible for the immunologic stimulus occur in the vial, tablet, or powder prior to its being administered to the patient.**

These degradation products form covalent bonds with proteins that result in antigens. They have been divided into two groups, designated as **major** and **minor** (Fig. 27-1).

1. **The major antigenic determinant** is the breakdown product produced in the largest amount, benzylpenicilloyl (BPO), which accounts for approximately 95% of the breakdown products. A commercially available reagent is available for skin testing with this breakdown product (see sec. **II.A**).

2. **The minor antigenic determinants** are produced in lesser amounts (approximately 5% of breakdown products) and, in the literature, minor-determinant mixtures (MDMs) of penicillin are prepared containing benzylpenicilloate and

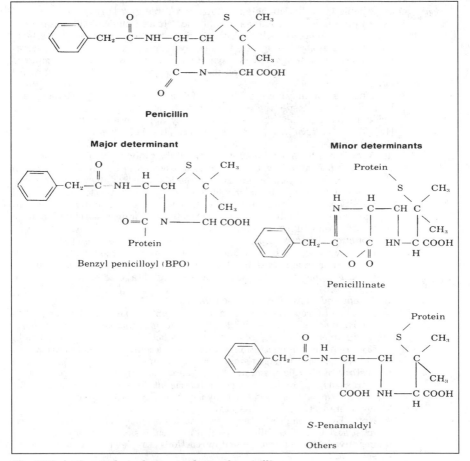

Fig. 27-1. Antigenic degradation products of penicillin.

benzylpenicilloate haptens. These form antigens by disulfide binding with cysteine-containing proteins, producing benzylpenicillinate, benzylpenamaldyl, and others [7, 8]. Other MDMs used for skin testing are alkaline hydrolysis products of ampicillin, methicillin [9, 10], or penicillin itself [5, 11].

E. **Clinical significance of immune response to major versus minor determinants. The terms** major **and** minor **refer only to the quantity of hapten available for covalent protein binding and not to the relative immunologic or clinical importance of each hapten.** On receiving penicillin, an individual therefore is exposed to a number of antigens and may develop an immune response, with the production of IgM, IgG, IgE, and sensitized lymphocytes capable of mediating cellular immunity to each or some of the antigens.

   1. **The minor determinants appear to be very important in causing the immediate IgE-mediated reactions,** and more than 90–95% of such immediate reactions seem to be due to minor determinants.

   2. **The major determinants** therefore are related only occasionally to immediate reactions. They are, however, the **predominant antigens responsible for the accelerated allergic IgE-mediated reactions.** These reactions are more frequent than the immediate reactions but less severe. The major concern is the development of laryngeal edema.

   3. **The IgG and IgM responses** to the major determinant are responsible for hemolytic anemia and immune complex–mediated diseases.

F. **A more detailed discussion of the mechanisms of hypersensitivity** reactions has recently been reviewed [1a]. **Hypersensitivity reactions** are the result of the interaction between drugs or their metabolites and components of the immune system [1a]. **Drug hypersensitivity reactions can occur via one of several immunopathogenic mechanisms as summarized in Table 27-2** [1a].

   1. **Type I IgE mediated reactions are the most feared clinically** because of the risk of death from anaphylaxis. This risk is increased significantly in patients receiving beta-blocking agents, because systemic beta blockade complicates the management of anaphylactic symptoms [1a]. The onset of IgE symptoms may occur immediately after parenteral therapy or up several hours after oral administration [1a].

   2. **Risk factors** that may increase the risk of drug hypersensitivity reactions have been identified. Most of these risk factors are derived from studies of allergic reactions to penicillin, but presumably they apply to antibiotics in general [1a]. They are reviewed in data elsewhere [1a], but several points deserve special emphasis.

      a. **Age. Those between 20–49 years are at the highest risk** for allergic reactions to penicillin. Faster declines in antipenicillin IgE antibody titers in children than in adults may explain the lower risk of allergic reactions in children. Although the elderly have fewer penicillin reactions, the risk of fatality caused by penicillin-induced anaphylaxis, if it occurs, is higher in the elderly, probably because of age-related and/or disease-related compromised cardiopulmonary function [1a].

      b. **Concurrent disease.** Epstein-Barr virus infection, acute lymphocytic leukemia, or cytomegalovirus infection increases the risk for ampicillin-amoxicillin macular papular rash to 60–100% [1a]. The reason for this is unknown, but it does not appear to be mediated by IgE [1a] (see related discussion in sec. **V.B**).

      c. **Extent and route of drug exposure** [1a]
         (1) The oral route is less immunogenic than the parenteral route.
         (2) High doses with sustained serum levels may increase risk. (Therefore, in an early, delayed reaction, dose reduction is sometimes beneficial.)
         (3) Frequent administration of intermittent courses seems to have an increased risk versus a single prolonged course.

      d. **History of allergic reaction to penicillin.** Not only are these patients at increased risk for allergic reactions if accidentally exposed to penicillin, but also they are at increased risk of hypersensitivity reactions when exposed to non–beta-lactam antibiotics [1a].

      e. **Note:** Even though a patient gives no history of prior penicillin allergy, most serious or fatal allergic penicillin reactions occur in patients with a negative history of prior penicillin reactions [1a] (see related discussion in sec. **II.A.2**).

G. **For late allergic reactions, morbilliform rashes,** etc., see discussion under sec. **V.**

Table 27-2. Classification of immunopathologic reactions to penicillin

Type of Reactions*	Description	Primary effector mechanism(s)			Clinical Reactions
		Antibody	Cells	Other	
I	Immediate hypersensitivity	IgE	Basophils, mast cells		Anaphylaxis, urticaria
II	Cytotoxic or cytolytic damage	IgG, IgM	Any cell with isoantigen	C', RES	Coombs-positive hemolytic anemia; cytopenias; drug-induced nephritis
III	Immune complex disease	Soluble immune complexes (Ag-Ab)	None directly	C'	Serum sickness; drug fever
IV	"Delayed" or cell-mediated hypersensitivity	None known	Sensitized T lymphocytes		Contact dermatitis
V	Idiopathic	?	?	?	Maculopapular eruptions; Stevens-Johnson syndrome; exfoliative dermatitis; eosinophilia

C' = complement; RES = reticuloendothelial system; Ag-Ab = antigen-antibody; (?) = immunopathologic mechanisms unknown.
*According to the scheme of Gell and Coombs. (Gell, P. G. H., and Coombs, R. R. A., Classification of Allergic Reactions Responsible for Clinical Hypersensitivity and Disease. In P. G. H. Gell, R. R. A. Coombs, and P. J. Lachmann (eds.), *Clinical Concepts of Immunology*. Oxford: Blackwell, 1975. P. 761–781.)
Source: Modified from Boguniewicz, M., and Leung, D. Y. M., Hypersensitivity reactions to antibiotics commonly used in children. *Pediatr. Infect. Dis J.* 14:221, 1995; and Weiss, M. E., and Adkinson, N. F. Jr., β-Lactam Allergy. In G. L. Mandell, J. E. Bennett, and R. Dolin (eds.), *Principles and Practice of Infectious Diseases* (4th ed.). New York: Churchill Livingstone, 1995. P. 273.

II. **Immunologic tests**
   A. **Skin tests for detection of IgE. The most important test for the evaluation of patients with penicillin allergy is the skin test for detecting the presence of penicillin IgE–sensitized mast cells.**

   Reagents available are penicilloyl polylysine (**PPL,** available commercially as **Pre-pen,** Kremers-Urban Co, a division of Schwarz-Pharma, Milwaukee, WI) and penicillin G. Penicilloyl polylysine is prepared by replacing the amino group of lysine with benzylpenicilloyl residues and substituting the protein with polylysine (see Fig. 27-1). It, therefore, has multiple penicilloyl determinants and is able to elicit an allergic response by direct skin testing without having to conjugate with cutaneous proteins. **By direct skin testing, it will detect IgE antibody to the major determinant BPO.**

   At the present time, there is no commercial MDM available [1a, 5]. But, by skin testing with potassium penicillin G (KPG), which does contain degradation products, one can expect to identify 90–95% of patients who have the potential to react to the minor determinant antigens [12]. A stable MDM preparation has been developed and is awaiting clinical evaluation [12a].

   Antihistamines, tricyclic antidepressants, and adrenergic drugs, all of which may inhibit skin test results, should be discontinued 48–96 hours prior to skin testing. Antihistamines with long half-lives need to be discontinued for appropriate durations [4], and astemizole (Hismanal) ideally should be discontinued for 6–8 weeks before skin testing [1a].

   1. **Skin test procedure for history-positive patients.** Skin tests are performed by using PPL at a concentration (supplied by manufacturer) of 6×10^{-5} M (M = moles per liter) and KPG at a concentration of 1,000 and 10,000 units/ml. The tests are performed first by applying the test solutions to **scratches or shallow punctures of skin;** only after this are the solutions injected intradermally. The **former** procedure is **safer** because less antigen is introduced: It is **performed to identify materials that could cause a systemic reaction if injected intradermally.**

      a. **Scratch or prick test.** A scratch test is performed by breaking the skin in a 1-cm-long scratch with the side of the beveled portion of a sterile needle and placing a drop of test material on the scratch. Alternatively, the skin may be punctured through a drop of testing material with commercially available scarifiers or with a darning needle prick technique. In both techniques, production of bleeding should be avoided. In testing for the presence of penicillin allergy, **scratch or prick tests are performed prior to proceeding with the intradermal skin testing.** A scratch or prick test therefore is performed with PPL, 6×10^{-5} M, and penicillin G, 10,000 units/ml. A positive response is a wheal-and-flare reaction that usually is obvious within 15–20 minutes after the test solution is applied; if scratch testing is **positive, an intradermal test should not be performed.**

      b. **Intradermal test.** A tuberculin syringe and short beveled no. 26 needle are used to inject 0.02 ml of test solution into the skin. If the patient is scratch test– or prick test–negative, then testing is performed with PPL and penicillin G at 1,000 units/ml and, if this is negative, at 10,000 units/ml. A wheal that is more than 0.3 cm (with erythema) larger than the diluent control that appears in 15–20 minutes is considered a positive reaction.

      c. **Conservative approach.** A more conservative approach is that of using penicillin G in concentrations of 5 units/ml and 10,000 units/ml. Scratch testing is performed first with 5 units/ml; if this is negative, it is followed by 10,000 units/ml. If the scratch tests are negative, intradermal skin testing is performed with penicillin G, 10,000 units/ml.

      d. **Control tests.** These are performed simultaneously using a **diluent** (e.g., normal saline), **histamine** (0.01 mg histamine base per milliliter), and **morphine sulfate** (0.1 mg/ml), which is a mast cell degranulator. The **diluent** should result in a **negative test,** and the **latter two substances** should **produce a wheal measuring 0.8–1.2 cm.**

      The histamine and morphine tests determine the reactivity of the capillaries in the skin and the presence of mast cells capable of releasing histamine. They are especially important as controls when patients are extremely ill or on medications such as antihistamines, hydroxyzine, and tricyclic antidepressants, which are known to inhibit skin tests by binding to the histamine receptor sites. (These agents ideally should be held at least 48 hours before skin testing.) While a patient is on these drugs, both the histamine control and morphine sulfate skin tests may be negative. In patients who are on drugs such as codeine or morphine, which are known to be mast cell degranulators, the morphine control may be negative and the histamine control positive. **When the normal positive controls (i.e., morphine and histamine) are negative, or the negative control is positive (e.g., in people with dermatographia), further skin tests are not predictive, and the risk of penicillin therapy cannot be determined.**

2. **Skin testing of history-negative patients.** The role of **skin testing in history-negative patients is not defined.** It would appear on the surface that with a 3–7% positive skin test frequency in a history-negative patient, it would be useful to screen by skin testing for the occasional immediate reaction that will occur in such patients.

   The risk to these history-negative patients, should they receive penicillin, however, has not been determined, as no challenge studies have been performed. The time and cost of routine skin testing prior to penicillin administration need to be balanced against the benefits of detecting those patients with a negative history but a positive skin test. One would assume, however, that a history-negative patient with a positive skin test is at risk for experiencing an allergic reaction. **Weiss** [4] **concluded that skin testing in history-negative patients is not indicated.**

3. **Timing of skin tests.** Although the probability of inducing an IgE antibody with PPL is extremely small, the probability of inducing an anamnestic response with penicillin does exist. Therefore, we have **limited skin tests to patients who are to receive penicillin (if skin tests allow) or to those patients who have had a reaction to penicillin in the previous 3 months.** These are usually patients who were on multiple drugs at the time of the adverse reaction in whom one wants to confirm the diagnosis of penicillin allergy. Because of the anamnestic response to penicillin skin tests that may occur, the information gained from such tests can be used only for a short time (24 hours); therefore, antibiotic therapy should be initiated within 24 hours. Beyond this time, if the patient is to receive penicillin, skin tests should be repeated [8].

   In children and adolescents, however, one study [13] evaluated the resensitization that could result from skin tests and challenge: 240 patients with a history of penicillin allergy were skin-tested when well and in no immediate need of penicillin. Of these patients, 219 were negative and were given a 10-day course of oral penicillin; they were skin-tested again 4 weeks or more after completion of the oral challenge. Only 2 patients (fewer than 1%) had a positive skin test on retesting. This study forces us to consider this procedure or the role of routine skin testing in individuals not in immediate need of penicillin [13].

B. **Skin test for delayed sensitivity.** In addition to immediate skin-test responses, penicillin may produce a tuberculin-type delayed reaction in the skin. Such reactions are observed in approximately 15% of patients. They occur in 7% of patients who have had recent penicillin therapy and 21% of patients who have had no recent penicillin therapy [14]. This type of cellular immunity is important in the pathogenesis of allergic eczematoid dermatitis and may play a part in organ-directed allergic reactions [15]. It is evident, however, that the great majority of patients with positive delayed skin tests to penicillin tolerate penicillin therapy with no untoward reactions.

C. **Serologic test for detection of IgE**
   1. The **radioallergosorbent test (RAST)** may be applicable in detecting specific circulating IgE antibody to penicillin [4, 16]. In this test, the antigen is conjugated to insoluble materials such as paper discs or beads. This insoluble polymer-antigen conjugate is mixed with the serum to be tested: Any IgE in the serum that is specific for the penicillin antigen will attach to the surface. By adding radiolabeled anti-IgE antibody and measuring the amount of radioactivity taken up by the polymer-antigen conjugate, one can determine the quantity of antigen-specific IgE that is present in the patient's serum.
      a. **Problems with RAST.** In recent years, **RAST** has come to be **considered less sensitive than direct skin testing** for the detection of IgE-specific antibody because it detects antibody in the circulation after all the IgE-specific sites on mast cells have been saturated and usually only those IgE antibodies to the major determinant BPO. Recently, testing for two minor determinants has been studied [1a]. Studies comparing RAST with skin testing in terms of ability to predict allergic reactions to penicillin are insufficient.

Another major disadvantage of RAST is the time necessary to perform the test. The advantage of direct skin testing is that, in most situations, the results of the tests will be noted immediately and clinical decisions can be made at the bedside.

   b. **Advantages of RAST. The role of RAST may therefore be in following a patient who is both skin test–positive and RAST-positive.** Disappearance of RAST positivity and therefore specific IgE antibody can be determined. In addition, because skin testing can induce an IgE response, RAST may be useful in determining whether a patient has penicillin IgE when the patient is not to receive penicillin.

   c. **Summary.** Because it is more time-consuming, more expensive, less sensitive for detection of IgE antibodies than skin testing, **RAST has limited clinical utility at this time** [4]. It may be useful for patients who cannot be skin tested [1a].

  2. **Hemagglutination. Antibodies** of the **IgG** or **IgM class** specific for **BPO can be detected through hemagglutination** by using RBCs coated with penicillin.

   a. **Antibodies of the IgG class are responsible for penicillin-induced hemolytic anemia.** This is an unusual, but not a rare, reaction in patients receiving high-dose penicillin therapy; it can occur particularly when renal function is compromised. At high blood penicillin levels, circulating RBCs become extensively coated by BPO and, if antibody is present, the patient will develop a positive Coombs' test and may develop hemolytic anemia. **The reaction occurs in the absence of other manifestations of penicillin allergy.** Therefore, one would predict that skin testing would be of little or no value in detecting persons who are prone to this complication, or in making a diagnosis. **Early detection is possible** by performing **Coombs' tests** in all patients on high-dose penicillin therapy [17].

   b. **High serum antibody titers due to IgM** commonly are associated with symptoms of **serum sickness** and the **morbilliform eruption** but also are observed in the **absence of any known allergic reaction.** The absence of demonstrable antibody therefore can be used to exclude the diagnosis of penicillin allergy, and its presence can be used to support a diagnosis of exposure to penicillin. However, this does not establish a diagnosis of allergy to penicillin. This conclusion is based on the fact that these antibodies can be detected in all patients who have recently received penicillin and in 97% of individuals who have a recent history of penicillin therapy [18].

   c. **Blocking antibodies.** Although it is difficult to assign a pathogenic role (except in penicillin-induced hemolytic anemia) to BPO-specific IgG or IgM, there are data to suggest that IgG antibodies may function in a protective, blocking role in those patients who have immediate, positive skin tests to PPL.

 D. **Duration of beta-lactam IgE antibodies.**
  1. The half-life of beta-lactam IgE antibodies has been shown to range from as short as 10 days to an indeterminantly long interval (>1000 days) [4].
  2. In general, the likelihood of sustaining IgE-specific beta-lactam antibodies declines with increasing time from the previous reaction. Prior studies have shown that skin tests performed within 1–2 months after an acute allergic reaction are positive 80–90% of the time. Therefore, there is a time-dependent decline in the rate of positive skin tests to fewer than 20% by 10 years [4].

   Patients who have serum sickness–like reactions to beta-lactam antibiotics often persist with an intense antibody reaction and for many years may remain at high risk for allergic reactions [4].

III. **Significance of KPG, PPL, and MDM skin tests**
 A. **Frequency of positive skin tests.** By performing **skin tests** with major and minor determinants, it has been possible to confirm which patients have **had an IgE-mediated reaction to penicillin.**
  1. In patients with a **positive history of penicillin allergy,** the frequency of positive skin tests varies from 9 to 63% [8, 9, 11, 13, 19]. The reasons for this wide variation include the different reagents used for skin testing, the time the skin tests were performed following the reaction to penicillin, the nature of the penicillin reaction, and different criteria for positive skin tests. The frequency of positive skin tests is highest when the skin tests are performed within 1 year of the allergic reaction [8]. Patients with anaphylaxis, asthma, and urticaria are

more likely to have positive skin tests than are those with a history of a morbilliform eruption [8, 11].

2. In patients with a **negative history of penicillin allergy,** Levine and Zolov [19] obtained positive, immediate skin tests in 3%, Greene and colleagues [11] in 7%, and Sogn and coworkers [20] in 4%, to one or both reagents used. This figure is no higher than in those with a history of a morbilliform eruption.

In Sogn's study [20], 1,227 patients were skin test–negative and received either penicillin or a semisynthetic derivative. There were seven (0.6%) reactions of either an immediate or accelerated nature. Five of seven were urticarial. None were fatal or life-threatening. One skin test–negative patient who experienced urticaria at 2 hours was found to be skin test–positive when tested after the reaction. All these patients had positive histories. No suspected IgE-mediated reactions were noted in any of 568 history-negative, skin test–negative patients.

B. **Significance of negative skin tests.** When patients are given penicillin after skin tests, it is obvious that those **with positive tests are at a higher risk of reactions than are those with negative skin tests** [9, 19]. Levine and Zolov [19] determined that in 185 patients who were skin test–negative to PPL and MDM, only one patient developed a mild accelerated urticarial reaction and six developed morbilliform reactions when given penicillin. In the study by Greene and associates [11], of the 346 who were skin test–negative to PPL and penicillin G, 12 (3%) developed some type of reaction. Only three (1%) of these reactions, however, were believed to be mediated by IgE and therefore likely to be predicted by the skin tests. The potentially predictive adverse reactions not detected using PPL and penicillin were hypotension and urticaria within 10 minutes of receiving penicillin in one patient and, in the other two, hives and generalized pruritus 24 hours after receiving penicillin. The remainder of the reactions not expected to be predicted included five morbilliform eruptions; one case of petechiae, fever, and arthralgia; one case of fever and leukopenia; one case of fever alone; and one case of Coombs'-positive hemolytic anemia. As can be seen from this study **using PPL and KPG** without an MDM, **99% of patients who were skin test–negative were able to receive penicillin therapy without an IgE-mediated reaction.** This is higher than the figure estimated by Parker [12].

To determine the frequency of resensitization in hospitalized adults with a history of penicillin allergy who are receiving beta-lactam antibiotics, we skin-tested patients prior to and following treatment. Three of 17 patients converted from negative to positive. This **emphasized the importance of informing patients who have a history of penicillin allergy, have undergone skin testing, and have received beta-lactam antibiotics that skin testing should be carried out in the future prior to receiving another course of penicillin or a penicillin derivative** [21].

C. **Significance of positive skin test**

1. **PPL-positive skin test.** In patients who were **skin test–positive** to PPL, Levine and Zolov [19] noted an **accelerated urticarial reaction** in four of six. Two patients did not experience any reactions. Greene and coworkers [11] noted that three of four patients who were PPL-positive experienced an accelerated urticarial reaction and the other an immediate reaction. Further studies on those who were skin test–positive to PPL revealed that patients who did not experience a reaction were noted to have BPO-specific IgG antibody at the beginning of therapy, the level of which rose during penicillin administration. Patients with no BPO-specific IgG experienced immediate reactions. Patients who experienced accelerated reactions when given penicillin were noted to have BPO-specific IgG antibody at the beginning of therapy, which decreased prior to the reaction. One can conclude, therefore, that the severity of the reaction and whether a reaction occurs at all during penicillin therapy in a PPL-positive individual depends on the presence and amount of BPO-specific IgG. Patients with preceding PPL-positive skin tests who tolerated penicillin continued to be skin test–positive to PPL while being treated with penicillin; this indicates that desensitization or utilization of mast cell–fixed IgE had not occurred as a result of therapy. These data have suggested that the IgG antibody present in the circulation may serve a protective function and act as a blocking antibody by binding the BPO determinant of penicillin in the circulation and thereby preventing this antigen from diffusing into the tissue and combining with the IgE present on mast cells.

2. **Penicillin- or MDM-positive skin test.** In the studies of Levine [19] and Greene

[11] and coworkers, all **patients with positive skin tests to penicillin or MDM experienced an immediate allergic reaction. Patients who are skin test–positive to penicillin G are therefore at great risk for immediate reactions to penicillin, and only in unusual circumstances is the risk of desensitization warranted.** When desensitization is attempted, the patients must be converted from skin test–positive to skin test–negative; this indicates utilization of the IgE-coated mast cells.

D. **Conclusions.** It is obvious from the studies cited above that the ideal situation would be to skin test with an MDM and PPL, or alternatively penicillin G alkaline hydrolysis products and PPL to predict immediate and accelerated allergic reactions. Because MDM is not yet commercially available, PPL and a solution of penicillin that is easily prepared are used. It is anticipated that by using these two reagents, a small number of patients at risk for reactions to penicillin may remain undetected by skin testing. It is hoped that MDM reagents will be available soon to detect almost all the patients at risk of developing IgE-mediated reactions when given penicillin. In the clinical situation, using PPL and penicillin without an MDM, one must balance the risk of giving penicillin against its therapeutic advantage when compared to other antibiotics.

IV. **Reactions to other antibiotics**
  A. **General comments**
    1. **Patients allergic to one penicillin should generally be considered allergic to all other semisynthetic penicillins, but the risk of cross-reaction with other beta-lactam antibiotics is less clear** [5]. Penicillin-allergic individuals given cephalosporins occasionally have reactions, but the percentage who do probably is less than the 10% commonly quoted. The true incidence awaits prospective studies. See related discussion under Cephalosporins, Chap. 28F.
      a. The semisynthetic penicillins all contain the six-amino penicillinic acid nucleus, which is responsible for their ability to react with body proteins to produce antigenic conjugates (Fig. 27-2).
      b. The cephalosporins contain the seven-amino cephalosporinic acid nucleus and hence chemically are not penicillin, but they do share the common, highly reactive beta-lactam ring structure (see Fig. 27-2, p. 1048).
    2. Based on structure, there is reason to believe that the **fourth-generation penicillins** (e.g., piperacillin) **and the third-generation cephalosporins may not be as cross-reactive as the earlier generation agents in these classes.** These newer antibiotics have stable beta-lactam rings that are cleaved poorly and therefore react poorly with tissue proteins. In addition, the large structural modifications of these newer antibiotics may change their antigenicity and contribute to a decrease in cross-reactivity [4].
    3. **Two other beta-lactam antibiotics**—carbapenems (e.g., imipenem) and monobactams (e.g., aztreonam)—have been studied for their ability to produce positive skin tests in penicillin-allergic subjects who are skin test–positive.
      a. **Imipenem** is the first of a new class of beta-lactam antibiotics. The carbapenem nucleus is characterized by a beta-lactam ring with an associated unsaturated five-member ring containing a carbon atom at the position analogous to sulfur in penicillin (see Fig. 27-2, p. 1048).
      b. Monobactams (e.g., **aztreonam**) are clinically unique, consisting of a monocyclic beta-lactam ring (see Fig. 27-2, p. 1048).
  B. **Immunologic studies** in humans and animals have demonstrated cross-reaction with penicillin G, semisynthetic penicillins, and the cephalosporins, but rarely with aztreonam [8, 10, 22–27]. **Of the semisynthetic penicillins and cephalosporins, one would predict from their structure that the cephalosporins would be the least cross-reactive with penicillin.** The frequency is not determined.
     Saxon and colleagues [27–29], by performing skin tests with imipenem and aztreonam in **penicillin-allergic,** skin test–positive subjects, have data indicating that **imipenem cross-reacts frequently** [28] **and aztreonam not at all** [27, 29] or uncommonly after multiple exposures to aztreonam [30].
    1. **Imipenem**, therefore, **should not be used in a patient known or suspected by history to be penicillin allergic** [1a].
    2. **Aztreonam** can usually be administered to the penicillin-allergic patient, but caution should be exercised in patients who receive repeated courses of this drug (see sec. **C.2**).
    3. See Chap. 28G for more discussion of these agents.
  C. **Clinical studies**

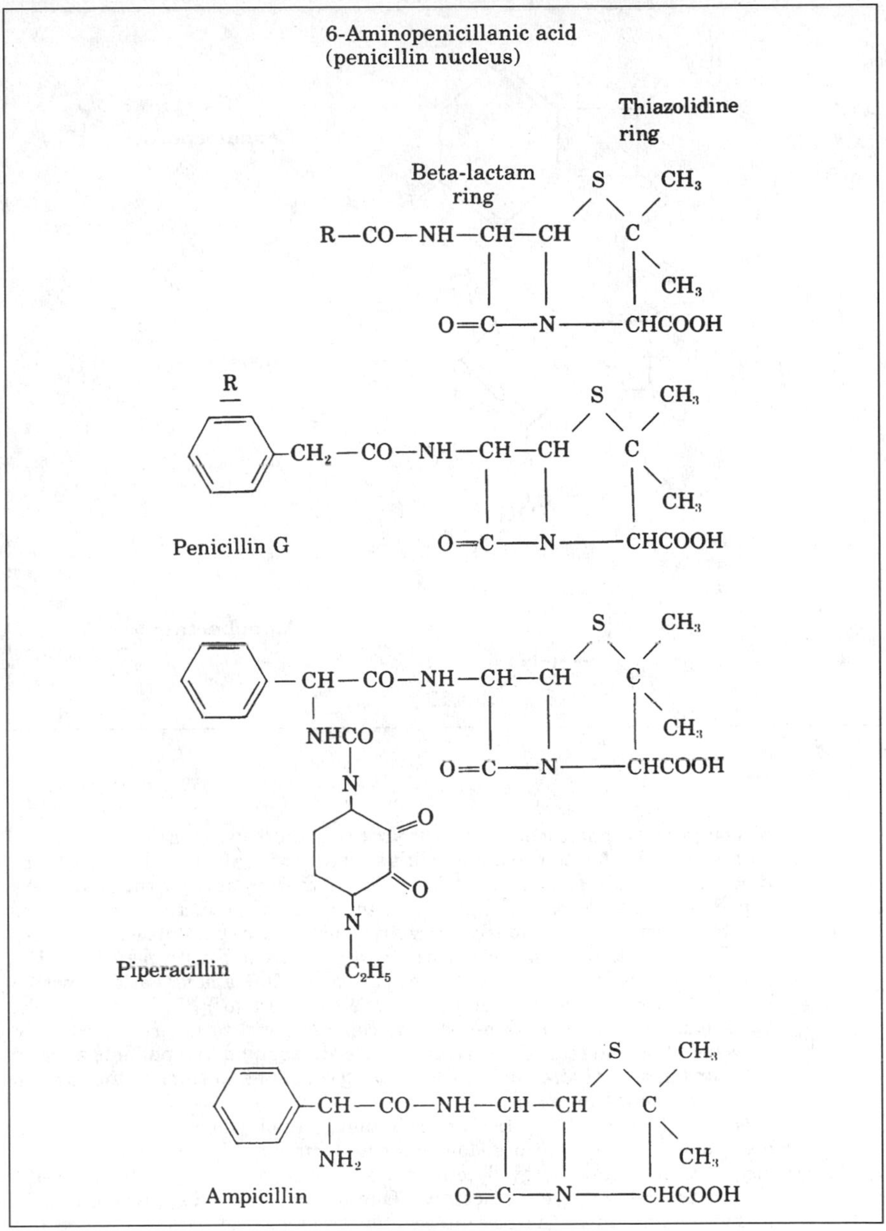

6-Aminopenicillanic acid
(penicillin nucleus)

Thiazolidine
ring

Beta-lactam
ring

$$R{-}CO{-}NH{-}CH{-}CH \quad \overset{S}{\diagup} \overset{}{\diagdown} \overset{CH_3}{\diagup} C$$

$$CH_3$$

$$O{=}C{-}N{-}{-}{-}CHCOOH$$

R

$$\text{(phenyl)}{-}CH_2{-}CO{-}NH{-}CH{-}CH \quad \overset{S}{\diagup}\overset{}{\diagdown}\overset{CH_3}{\diagup} C$$

$$CH_3$$

$$O{=}C{-}N{-}{-}{-}CHCOOH$$

Penicillin G

$$\text{(phenyl)}{-}CH{-}CO{-}NH{-}CH{-}CH \quad \overset{S}{\diagup}\overset{}{\diagdown}\overset{CH_3}{\diagup} C$$

$$NHCO$$

$$CH_3$$

$$O{=}C{-}N{-}{-}{-}CHCOOH$$

$$N$$

$$=O$$

$$=O$$

$$N$$

Piperacillin $\quad C_2H_5$

$$\text{(phenyl)}{-}CH{-}CO{-}NH{-}CH{-}CH \quad \overset{S}{\diagup}\overset{}{\diagdown}\overset{CH_3}{\diagup} C$$

$$NH_2$$

$$CH_3$$

Ampicillin $\quad O{=}C{-}N{-}{-}{-}CHCOOH$

Fig. 27-2. Structures of the beta-lactam antibiotics. (Figure continues.)

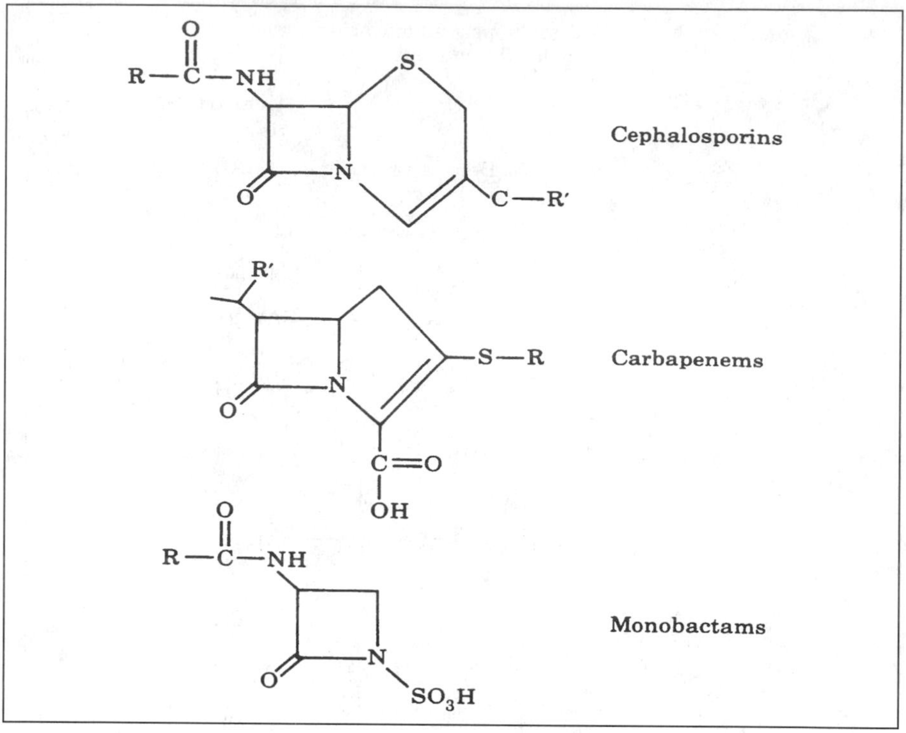

Fig. 27-2 (continued)

1. Although the cephalosporins do appear to be the least cross-reactive, prior data have indicated that patients with a history of penicillin allergy had four times as many allergic reactions to cephalothin therapy as those with no history of penicillin allergy. This is slightly less than the sixfold increase in reactions that have been found previously in bacterial endocarditis patients with a history of allergic reactions to penicillin who had been treated with penicillin. The reaction frequency to cephalosporins approached 50% among patients with a history of penicillin allergy and a positive skin test to PPL. Unfortunately, these patients were not skin-tested to cephalosporin to determine whether they were likely to react. It therefore is **safer to assume that patients allergic to penicillin are at increased risk for having reactions to semisynthetic penicillins and cephalosporins.**

2. Moss [30] described 21 cystic fibrosis patients, all of whom had high levels of previous exposure to antipseudomonal beta-lactam antibiotics and a previous history of penicillin allergy. Twenty patients were given aztreonam if specific skin tests were found to be negative. One patient's skin test proved positive to aztreonam and so the patient was not treated. One patient developed a systemic reaction on initial exposure, and three additional patients developed systemic reactions on reexposure to the drug. Repeat skin tests showed positive conversion in all four of these patients. Hence, a 20% sensitization rate to aztreonam was noted in this study, with one patient being sensitized from previous beta-lactam exposure by skin testing [30]. Therefore, aztreonam can be given to patients with cystic fibrosis who are allergic to other beta-lactam antibiotics, but it should be administered cautiously, especially with repeated use.

D. **Skin testing.** Although not extensively studied, it would appear that many of the semisynthetic penicillins can be used for skin testing. In studies using penicillin G, ampicillin, methicillin, and the cephalosporins, a marked variability in the patterns of positive skin tests is noted [9, 10, 24, 25]. Therefore, one cannot predict by history the form of penicillin that a patient might tolerate. The skin test materials in these studies have included the plain drug, minor-determinant preparations, and polylysine conjugates. In some patients who were skin test–positive to one penicillin or cephalosporin but negative to others, treatment with the antibiotic to which they were negative resulted in no unusual reactions. It should be emphasized, however, that patients with positive skin tests to semisynthetic penicillins, cephalosporins, or carbapenems have not been treated with the drug to which they were positive in order to determine whether they were at increased risk of experiencing a reaction.

One study looking at specific side-chain determinants in patients with a history of penicillin allergy was able to identify 10 of 21 patients who did not respond to conventional major and minor determinants [31]. The clinical implications of this observation need to be evaluated further by challenges, because in all previous studies patients who are skin test–negative to the major and minor determinants had a very low frequency of reactions when given penicillin.

E. **Materials. The concentrations of antibiotic used in these studies** were **0.25 mg/ml** and **2.5 mg/ml** for cephalothin, cefazolin, ampicillin, and methicillin. Ampicillin and the cephalosporins should be freshly prepared (at least monthly) because ampicillin loses reactivity, which results in false negative reactions, and because the cephalosporins become more reactive and cause false positive reactions in time. For carbenicillin, ticarcillin, and presumably piperacillin, the researchers used freshly prepared solutions at a concentration of 1.0 mg/ml. The concentration of imipenem is 5×10^{-3} M and, for aztreonam, 6×10^{-3} M in L-arginine buffer. It is assumed, however, that information available for predicting allergic reactions to penicillin G itself is applicable to the semisynthetic penicillins and cephalosporins and that individuals who are skin test–positive to these antibiotics probably are at high risk for a reaction. **There is insufficient experience with the predictive value of a negative skin test to the semisynthetic penicillins and cephalosporins to recommend testing with these agents without simultaneous penicillin skin testing.** In a patient who has an allergic reaction to penicillin, it is not likely that the IgE antibody to penicillin would be lost and the IgE to the reacting semisynthetic be maintained. If the patient is skin test–positive to penicillin, PPL, or MDM, and negative to the semisynthetic drug or to cephalosporin, the reason for the negative reaction may be the lack of an MDM or major-determinant antigen to this antibiotic. As the use of semisynthetic penicillins and cephalosporins has increased, patients have been seen who are skin test–positive to these materials and not to penicillin. It is important, therefore, to determine the antibiotics to which a patient is exposed in order to interpret the skin test pattern [8, 9].

V. **Other allergic reactions**

A. **Late allergic reactions.** Until now, we have been discussing the ability of **skin tests** to predict IgE-mediated reactions that result in immediate and accelerated allergic reactions. It should be emphasized that these tests **do not predict either the late or less common allergic reactions.** However, **the skin tests are of value in determining whether a patient is having a serum sickness [32], urticarial, angioedematous, or arthralgic reaction to penicillin.** These patients will develop a positive reaction to PPL, penicillin, or MDM, so skin testing with these reagents can be diagnostic. There is no information available as to the value of semisynthetic penicillins in the diagnosis of these syndromes.

B. **Morbilliform eruption.** Of all the reactions to penicillins, the **morbilliform eruption is the most common** (see Plate I.E). At present, it is clear that it is not an IgE-mediated reaction and therefore cannot be predicted by skin tests, nor can skin tests be used in the diagnosis of this rash. Because of its frequency, morbilliform eruption presents a major problem to the clinician: Many patients with this reaction are labeled *penicillin-allergic* with the implication that they are at risk for a more severe reaction if they were to receive penicillin again.

1. **Frequency.** The eruption is estimated to occur in 3% of patients treated with penicillin and 3–9% of patients treated with ampicillin. Of patients who also have infectious mononucleosis, 70–90% treated with ampicillin will develop this complication. It also is seen more frequently in patients with lymphatic leukemia or cytomegalovirus infection and in those using allopurinol [4, 33].

2. **The reason** ampicillin or amoxicillin has a higher rate of rashes compared with penicillin is unclear [1a]. It has been postulated that the diamino acyl side chain contained in ampicillin or amoxicillin allows more readily for the formation of linear polymers of varying lengths, which may explain the higher cutaneous reaction rates seen with ampicillin or amoxicillin [4].

3. **Treatment.** If the rash develops while a patient is on the antibiotic treatment, the agent often can be continued without worsening the rash; that is, the rash will progress and improve whether or not the drug is continued. Whether one continues or discontinues the drug should depend on the severity of the infection being treated, the discomfort of the eruption, and the possibility that the morbilliform eruption is actually the onset of a desquamative dermatitis or vasculitis. For symptomatic treatment, one may use an antipruritic agent such as hydroxyzine or diphenhydramine.

4. **Skin testing.** Although patients who have experienced morbilliform eruptions are at no more risk for an IgE-mediated reaction than individuals who have not experienced an eruption, in the present medicolegal climate, good judgment dictates that these patients be skin-tested prior to receiving penicillin therapy. It should be emphasized that the skin test is of no value in predicting a possible eruption of a morbilliform rash. In addition, after the onset of a morbilliform rash, skin testing will not help establish that the rash is due to a penicillin reaction.

   There are, however, studies [8, 13] that report increased frequency of positive skin tests in patients with morbilliform eruptions. In one, the authors comment that the presence of pruritus had a significant correlation with positive skin tests [8].

C. **Less common reactions.** Information on the other manifestations of penicillin allergy listed in Table 27-1, except for hemolytic anemia, is inadequate to demonstrate that such events are immunologically mediated. The evidence we do have is as follows:

1. Some patients with pulmonary infiltrates with eosinophilia have been noted to be skin test–positive, but no repeat exposures have been performed.

2. Thrombocytopenia, drug fever, and granulocytopenia are well-described adverse reactions to penicillin that have been reproduced by repeat exposure, but no immunologic studies have been performed that might support the notion that these are allergic reactions.

3. Hypersensitivity vasculitis [6a], erythema multiforme, and the systemic lupus erythematosus syndrome occurring during the course of penicillin therapy have pathologic findings similar to those described in persons not receiving penicillin. In many situations, it is difficult to decide whether the symptoms are due to the condition being treated or to an adverse reaction to penicillin. The major evidence suggesting a relationship with penicillin is that the patients improve on discontinuation of the drug.

VI. **Clinical situations.** It is obvious from the previous discussion that in a patient with a history of an adverse reaction to penicillin, the type of reaction and the advantage of penicillin over other antibiotics should determine whether skin tests should be performed. The skin-test results themselves should then be considered in making a therapeutic decision (Table 27-3).

A. **Interpretation of skin tests and desensitization**

1. **Positive PPL skin test.** In a patient who has a positive skin test to PPL, a decision concerning penicillin therapy must be made even though the presence of blocking antibody has not been, or cannot be, determined. In many situations, a positive skin test to PPL is sufficient to warrant serious consideration of alternate therapy. If it is believed that penicillin therapy is **strongly indicated,** the patient and the family should be made aware of the risks. In this situation, one should avoid a large initial dose in case the patient does not have any blocking antibody, and one should **administer further doses cautiously** to avoid any severe, accelerated reaction. **The schedule we have found useful** begins with 2,000 units of penicillin, followed by 20,000 units SC, and then 200,000 units IM (in an extremity) at 15- to 30-minute intervals. If no reaction occurs, therapeutic doses can be given. The initial dose of 2,000 units/ml was selected because the skin test itself has introduced 200 units of penicillin into the skin with no reaction. The injections should be administered in an extremity so that a tourniquet can be applied above the injection site. Epinephrine (adrenalin) should be drawn and available for rapid administration against the possibility of a reaction. In general, it is recommended that no premedication be given but, in patients who are PPL-positive, one should more strongly consider the use of antihistamines to prevent accelerated reactions. The reason for this is not the potential severity of reaction anticipated but that a reaction may occur while a physician is not in attendance—hours or days after penicillin

therapy has been started. Others in this situation have performed routine desensitization (see sec. **2**).

   2. **Positive penicillin G skin test.** Despite the risk of a severe immediate reaction to penicillin, penicillin therapy may still be desirable if the infection is serious and no alternative antibiotic can be used. Before **penicillin** is administered, **desensitization is necessary.**

      a. **Precautions.** Because at least one death has occurred in conjunction with attempted desensitization, the nature and potential risks of the procedure must be explained to the patient and the family. A physician should be in attendance throughout desensitization, and an emergency cart should be

Table 27-3. Immediate skin-test responses in penicillin allergy

PPL (major)	Penicillin G or MDM	Semisynthetic penicillin, cephalosporin	Allergic reaction expected	Treatment
+	+	0	Immediate reaction to penicillin G	Alternative nonpenicillin antibiotic; desensitization to penicillin G
0	+	0	Immediate reaction to penicillin G	Alternative nonpenicillin antibiotic; desensitization to penicillin G; test dose of semisynthetic penicillin or cephalosporin prior to therapeutic dose
+	0	0	Accelerated reaction to penicillin G	Alternative nonpenicillin antibiotic; cautious administration of penicillin G; test dose of semisynthetic penicillin or cephalosporin prior to therapeutic dose
0	0	+	Immediate reaction to skin test–positive antibiotic	Test dose or cautious administration of skin test–negative antibiotic
0	0	0	None	Test dose or therapeutic dose, depending on type of initial penicillin reaction

PPL = penicilloyl polylysine; MDM = minor-determinant mixture; + = positive; 0 = negative.

available so that immediate treatment can be instituted should a severe reaction occur. At present, there is no uniform procedure that is followed by everyone, but **the basic principle is to start at a dose that is low enough not to produce a reaction and then to increase the dose at short intervals.**

b. **Approach.** Tables 27-4 and 27-5 outline the dilutions and suggest a schedule. Initial doses of less than 100 units/ml should be considered if the patient is scratch test– or prick test–positive to weaker concentrations of penicillin G. Parker [12] has used an alternate schedule of desensitization in patients with a high degree of sensitivity. He suggests that desensitization should begin with very small quantities of the drug, such as 100 units or less, given by mouth, and gradually this oral dose should be increased over 4–24 hours until therapeutic levels are reached. Parker [12] prefers the oral route initially because of the infrequency of fatal anaphylaxis due to oral penicillin. When the oral dose of penicillin has reached approximately 50,000 units, one begins parenteral penicillin injections, starting with 1,000 units or less, intradermally or subcutaneously, while continuing oral penicillin administration. The amount of injected penicillin is doubled every 20–30 minutes until comparable parenteral and oral doses of penicillin have been reached and allergic skin reactivity has markedly diminished. At that point, full therapeutic doses of penicillin are administered and oral therapy is discontinued. It should be emphasized that desensitization in

Table 27-4. Preparation of solutions, using aqueous crystalline penicillin G

Dilute 20,000,000-unit vial to 20 ml = 1,000,000 units/ml (solution 1)
Dilute 1 ml of solution 1 to 10 ml = 100,000 units/ml (solution 2)
Dilute 1 ml of solution 2 to 10 ml = 10,000 units/ml (solution 3)
Dilute 1 ml of solution 3 to 10 ml = 1,000 units/ml (solution 4)
Dilute 1 ml of solution 4 to 10 ml = 100 units/ml (solution 5)

Source: G. R. Greene, G. A. Peters, and J. E. Geraci, Treatment of bacterial endocarditis in patients with penicillin hypersensitivity. *Ann. Intern. Med.* 67:235, 1967.

Table 27-5. Penicillin hyposensitization: Administration of solutions

Solution no.	Concentration (units/ml)	Amount of solution injected SC (ml/15 min)	Amount of penicillin per SC dose (units)
5	100	0.05	5
		0.1	10
		0.2	20
		0.4	40
		0.8	80
4	1,000	0.15	150
		0.3	300
		0.6	600
		1.0	1,000
3	10,000	0.2	2,000
		0.4	4,000
		0.8	8,000
2	100,000	0.15	15,000
		0.3	30,000
		0.6	60,000
		1.0	100,000
1	1,000,000	0.2	200,000
		0.4	400,000
		0.8	800,000

Source: G. R. Greene, G. A. Peters, and J. E. Geraci, Treatment of bacterial endocarditis in patients with penicillin hypersensitivity. *Ann. Intern. Med.* 67:235, 1967.

patients with positive skin tests to penicillin attempts to convert a positive skin test to negative. It should come as no surprise that there are some patients who will experience systemic reactions even with small doses of penicillin and in whom it will not be possible to administer therapeutic doses. As a rule, no premedication is given; if marked skin reactivity is present, however, repeated subcutaneous injection of epinephrine during the early stages of desensitization is worth considering.

3. **Future precautions.** Caution patients who are skin test–negative and have been given penicillin (and their families) that **although one may have received penicillin without an adverse reaction, this should not be taken as an indication that one can receive penicillin without prior testing at some future date. Such patients should consider themselves allergic to penicillin** and should carry identification, such as medical alert tags, indicating the allergy.

In view of the report by Mendelson and colleagues [13], we have again skin-tested hospitalized adult patients 1 month or more after receiving beta-lactam antibiotics to determine the actual conversion rate. To date, we have observed conversion of skin tests from negative to positive in 3 of 17 patients tested [21].

4. **Use of semisynthetic penicillins.** In patients who are skin test–positive to PPL or penicillin G but skin test–negative to a semisynthetic or cephalosporin, the latter antibiotics may be given cautiously. The reason for cautious administration is that neither a major-determinant antigen nor an MDM of the semisynthetic penicillin is available for testing. Patients who are to be treated with semisynthetic penicillins therefore should be skin-tested with penicillin G, PPL, and the semisynthetic penicillin. **The method of administration** that we have found helpful is to start with approximately 5 mg and increase every 15–20 minutes to 50–100 mg, followed by 1 g. This **cautious** administration is necessary even if cephalosporins are to be used, as there are data to suggest an increased reaction rate in patients who receive cephalosporins and who are PPL-positive.

If a patient with a positive history of a morbilliform eruption due to penicillin is skin test–negative to all reagents, the semisynthetic penicillin or cephalosporin can be given in therapeutic amounts, or **a test dose (5–10 mg) can be given prior to the therapeutic amount.** When the patient has a history of an immediate reaction and negative skin tests, a test dose is recommended. In a patient who is skin test–negative to penicillin G, PPL, and cephalosporin, and who is positive to one semisynthetic penicillin, the penicillin, the cephalosporin, or a skin test–negative semisynthetic can be given after a test dose. The **test dose of penicillin is 1,000 units.**

5. **Cephalosporin use in patients with a penicillin-allergic history. If a patient had a prior immediate reaction to a penicillin, penicillin and cephalosporin skin testing should be performed before a cephalosporin is used.** If the patient had a delayed, nonpruritic morbilliform rash with prior penicillin use, cephalosporins can be administered without skin testing (see clinical example in sec. **B.1**). A recent report emphasizes the safety of giving cephalosporins (especially second- and third-generation agents) in patients with histories of penicillin allergy [33a]. Imipenem, however, should be avoided in the penicillin-allergic patient, whereas aztreonam should be safe. See related discussions in sec. **IV.A.3** and Chap. 28G.

B. **Clinical examples.** As a guide, a few clinical examples using the algorithm in Fig. 27-3 will demonstrate how the information discussed can help one to make clinical decisions.

1. An elderly patient is hospitalized with a pneumococcal pneumonia. The chart is labeled *penicillin-allergic*. On review of the chart, one notes that the patient was reported 3 years previously to have had a diffuse morbilliform rash beginning on the seventh day of penicillin therapy.

Following the algorithm, one can determine that this patient had a late allergic reaction. The current infection—pneumonia in an elderly patient requiring hospitalization—is serious. **In this situation, the cephalosporins can be administered without special skin testing.** The possibility of a more severe IgE-mediated reaction is no greater than in a history-negative patient and, because the cephalosporins are the least cross-reactive, there is not much likelihood of inducing another morbilliform eruption. **If this same patient had the history of an immediate allergic reaction to penicillin, then, because of the risk of cross-reactivity, the cephalosporins could not be used safely**

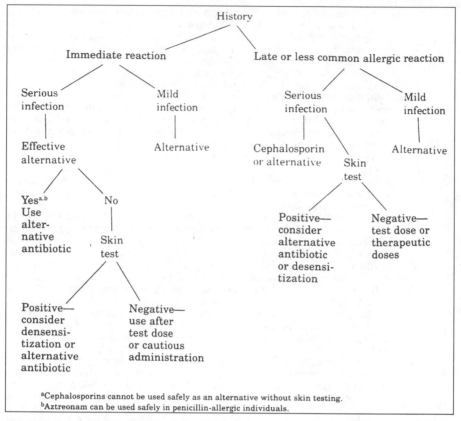

History

Immediate reaction | Late or less common allergic reaction

Serious infection | Mild infection | Serious infection | Mild infection

Effective alternative | Alternative | Cephalosporin or alternative | Skin test | Alternative

Yes[a,b] Use alternative antibiotic | No | Positive— consider alternative antibiotic or desensitization | Negative— test dose or therapeutic doses

Skin test

Positive— consider densensitization or alternative antibiotic | Negative— use after test dose or cautious administration

[a]Cephalosporins cannot be used safely as an alternative without skin testing.
[b]Aztreonam can be used safely in penicillin-allergic individuals.

Fig. 27-3. Approach to penicillin skin testing. (Courtesy of William Mitchell, M.D., Bassett Healthcare, Cooperstown, NY.)

without prior skin testing. Alternative antibiotics (erythromycin, vancomycin) are available, so these should be used (see Chap. 9 under **Special Considerations and Specific Therapy**).

2. A teenager is seen in the office with a documented streptococcal group A pharyngitis. Five years previously, the patient had developed a **morbilliform rash** after taking ampicillin for otitis media. This can be considered **a mild infection** with the possibility of using **alternate antibiotics** (erythromycin or a cephalosporin).

3. A 60-year-old patient with an aortic valve prosthesis and mild renal failure is about to undergo cystoscopy. He says he is penicillin-allergic because of a **urticarial reaction** that had occurred 3 days after prior penicillin therapy.

   This is a **late allergic reaction.** There is no strong indication for penicillin therapy in this case because the patient does not have an infection, and **prophylactic antibiotics** are to be used only for 6–12 hours. Because an acceptable **alternative to penicillin or ampicillin is available** (i.e., vancomycin), it should be used. The dose can be adjusted to provide adequate levels for 12–24 hours, without excessive toxicity.

   If a more prolonged course of vancomycin therapy were needed in a patient with a hearing deficit and an active infection (e.g., enterococcal endocarditis), then penicillin skin testing could be considered. (See next example.)

4. A 50-year-old man develops **enterococcal endocarditis.** He has known chronic renal failure with a baseline serum creatinine of 3.0. He was told 5 years previously that he was allergic to penicillin when he developed **angioedema 5 days after intravenous penicillin.**

In this case, the patient had a **late allergic reaction.** The cephalosporins currently available are not effective against enterococci. If susceptibility data reveal a vancomycin-susceptible organism, vancomycin, in combination with low-dose gentamicin (see Chap. 10), is an acceptable alternative, but this patient has renal failure and, if vancomycin is used, doses must be carefully adjusted (see Chap. 28O) to avoid toxicity. In view of the high probability of a negative penicillin skin test, skin testing may be performed with penicillin (KPG, PPL, and MDM) and ampicillin. If these tests are negative, the patient can be given either drug and an aminoglycoside. If the patient reacts positively to either PPL or penicillin G and is skin test–negative to ampicillin, then ampicillin should first be given in a test dose prior to being given in therapeutic amounts. The **test dose is very important** because there is significant cross-reaction between penicillin and ampicillin and because the reason for the negative skin test to ampicillin may be inadequacy of testing reagents.

If the patient is skin test–positive to both penicillin and ampicillin, one has to decide whether to attempt desensitization or to use vancomycin. This decision would be based on skin-test reactivity. A skin test that is positive to PPL only would indicate a high probability of successful desensitization, in which case desensitization can be seriously considered. If the scratch or prick test were positive to penicillin (KPG or, in particular, MDM) or ampicillin, the patient is likely to react even with careful desensitization, thus an alternate agent (vancomycin with low-dose gentamicin) may be the best compromise. (See Chap. 10.)

5. A 70-year-old woman develops a postoperative *Pseudomonas aeruginosa* pneumonia. She is intubated and is unable to give a history. Her chart indicates she is *penicillin-allergic,* but there are no details of the type of allergy. Ideally, one would like to use a synergistic antibiotic combination of piperacillin or a similar agent with an aminoglycoside to achieve synergy. Skin testing should be performed using PPL, KPG, MDM, and the desired penicillin derivative. Table 27-2 summarizes the possible results from skin testing. Even if all the skin tests are negative, we would probably begin with a test dose of piperacillin in this patient because there is no available history of the type of presumed prior penicillin allergy.

VII. **Reactions to other antibacterial agents**

A. **Sulfonamides** have been implicated in the development of such reactions as drug fever, pruritus, and rashes; the worst of these is Stevens-Johnson syndrome, developing between days 7 and 10 of treatment. In addition, these agents frequently have been implicated in the development of hypersensitivity vasculitis.

The mechanism is believed to be both toxic and immunologic in nature. Sulfonamides normally are metabolized in the liver either by N-acetylation or via the cytochrome P450 catalyzed oxidation pathway. The latter pathway produces toxic multivalent metabolites of the N4-sulfonamidoyl group. These compounds are highly reactive with protein, forming hapten-carrier complexes against which immunologic reactions may be directed. IgE-mediated responses to these metabolites have been demonstrated both by skin testing and in vitro [34, 35]. The risk of **cross-sensitization among sulfonamides** and related compounds such as sulfonylurea, oral hypoglycemic agents, thiazide diuretics, and carbonic anhydrase inhibitors has been raised and, although such sensitization is rare, it should be considered in prescribing these drugs to patients who are known to be sensitive to sulfonamides. Some patients who are allergic to sulfanilamide also may react to other compounds containing the *p*-aminophenyl group, such as local anesthetics of the procaine type. The combination of trimethoprim and sulfamethoxazole does not appear to alter the incidence of allergic reactions to sulfonamide. (See Chap. 28K.)

1. **AIDS patients** who receive sulfonamides (e.g., TMP-SMX for *Pneumocystis carinii* prophylaxis or treatment) have a high incidence of cutaneous reactions to sulfonamides. In the absence of severe cutaneous reactions and in those without mucosal involvement, many of these patients have been desensitized to sulfonamides and can continue sulfonamides [36]. See detailed discussion of this topic and related references with specific protocols in Chaps. 24 and 28K.

2. In patients with inflammatory bowel disease who must receive sulfasalazine, desensitization has been undertaken [37, 38]. In this setting, desensitization should be supervised by an allergist or a physician experienced in reexposing patients to sulfonamides.

B. Aminoglycosides. Streptomycin, kanamycin, gentamicin, tobramycin and amikacin have similar structures, pharmacology, and toxicology. Allergic reactions to streptomycin have followed injections and skin contact. The contact dermatitis is documented by patch testing. Although skin testing has been performed with streptomycin, study results are inconclusive regarding the test's significance in predicting anaphylactic reactions. Delayed skin-test reactions to streptomycin are associated with contact dermatitis.

C. General concepts. It is safe to assume that **allergic reactions have been described for most antibiotics.** At present, however, there are no in vitro tests to support the existence of immunologic reactions to such drugs. Clearly, it would be desirable to have appropriate antigens for testing patients with antibiotics other than penicillin but, at the present time, such reagents are not available, and physicians must use probabilities and drug removal as the major diagnostic tool, with provocative challenge being considered in unusual situations.

1. Provocative challenge. In certain situations, such as drug fever, accelerated allergic reactions, and pulmonary infiltrates with eosinophilia, when skin-test antigenic material is not available (e.g., sulfonamides, aminoglycosides), the clinician may have to decide whether a provocative challenge is appropriate. In those situations where alternative drugs are available and the possibility of requiring a repeat course of the drug is small, it is not appropriate to perform a provocative challenge in most patients.

In patients with presumed antibiotic-related drug fever, the suspect antibiotic usually can be discontinued and the drug fever typically resolves in 72–96 hours. In the great majority of patients, it is not necessary nor recommended to rechallenge the patient with the same antibiotic because alternative agents are typically available (see related discussion in Chap. 1, under Drug Fever).

In general, we try to avoid rechallenging patients. If a specific agent is essential for a patient, and without an obvious alternative agent, then rechallenge may be considered on an individualized basis and, ideally, with the input of an allergist. The risk of rechallenge should be fully explained to both the patient and the family.

2. Common antibiotic reactions. See separate discussions in Chap. 28.

References

1. Jick, H. Adverse drug reactions: The magnitude of the problem. *J. Allergy Clin. Immunol.* 74:555, 1984.
   Data from the Boston Collaborative Drug Surveillance Program indicate that the average medical inpatient in the United States receives approximately nine different drugs per hospitalization and 30% develop an adverse reaction. On average in the United States, adults take two drugs regularly.
1a. Boguniewicz, M., and Leung, Y.M. Hypersensitivity reactions to antibiotics commonly used in children. *Pediatr. Infect. Dis. J.* 14:221, 1995.
2. Hurwitz, N. Admissions to hospital due to drugs. *Br. Med. J.* 1:539, 1969.
   For related reviews, see M.C. Lakshmanan et al., Hospital admissions caused by iatrogenic disease. Arch. Intern. Med. *146:1931, 1986; and L.G. Seidel et al., Studies on the epidemiology of adverse drug reactions.* Bull. Johns Hopkins Hosp. *119:299, 1966.*
3. Report of the International Conference on Adverse Reactions Reporting Systems. Washington, DC: National Academy of Science, 1971.
   Information concerning specific reactions.
3a. Segretig, J., Trenholme, G.M., and Levin, S. Antibiotic allergy in the allergic patient. *Med. Clin. North Am.* 79:935, 1995.
   Review emphasizes alternative agents for various pathogens and/or settings.
4. Weiss, M.E. Evaluation and treatment of patients with prior reactions to B-lactam antibiotics. *Curr. Clin. Top. Infect. Dis.* 13:131, 1993.
   For a related discussion, see M.E. Weiss and N.F. Adkinson, Jr., β-Lactam Allergy. In G.L. Mandell, J.E. Bennett, and R. Dolin (eds.), Principles and Practice of Infectious Diseases (4th ed.). New York: Churchill Livingstone, 1995. Pp. 272–278.
5. Medical Letter. Penicillin allergy. *Med. Lett. Drugs Ther.* 30:79, 1988.
6. Idsol, O., et al. Nature and extent of penicillin side reactions with particular reference to fatalities from anaphylactic shock. *Bull. World Health Organ.* 38:159, 1968.

6a. Somer, T., and Finegold, S.M. Vasculitides associated with infections, immunization, and antimicrobial drugs. *Clin. Infect. Dis.* 30:1010, 1995.
Comprehensive literature review. Most antibiotic-induced vasculitis is a small-vessel vasculitis (usually leukocytoclastic vasculitis) and is thought to be caused by immune-complex deposition, a process in which the drug is believed to act as a hapten / antigen.

7. Levine, B.B., and Redmond, A.P. Minor haptenic determinant specific reagents of penicillin hypersensitivity in man. *Int. Arch. Allergy Appl. Immunol.* 35:445, 1969.
Details the preparation of the minor determinant mixture used by Dr. Bernard Levine.

8. Sullivan, T.J., et al. Skin testing to detect penicillin allergy. *J. Allergy Clin. Immunol.* 68:171, 1981.
Authors review their experience with skin testing, emphasizing the importance of skin testing to detect patients at risk of having a reaction.

9. Solley, G.O., Gleich, G.J., and Van Dellen, R.G. Penicillin allergy: Clinical experience with a battery of skin test reagents. *J. Allergy Clin. Immunol.* 69:238, 1982.
Summarizes the experience at Mayo Clinic in skin testing more than 700 patients.

10. VanDellen, R.G., et al. Differing patterns of wheal and flare skin reactivity in patients allergic to penicillins. *J. Allergy* 47:230, 1971.

11. Greene, G.R., Rosenblum, A.H., and Sweet, L.C. Evaluation of penicillin hypersensitivity. Value of clinical history and skin testing with PPL and penicillin G. *J. Clin. Immunol.* 60:339, 1977.

12. Parker, C.W. Drug allergy. *N. Engl. J. Med.* 292:511, 732, 957, 1975.
This is a classic review of pathogenesis, clinical manifestations, occurrence, diagnosis, prevention, and treatment of drug allergies. See also R.M. Ten et al., Allergy skin testing. Mayo Clin. Proc. *70:783, 1995, for a recent review of methods and interpretation.*

12a. Personal communication. Kremers-Urban, a division of Schwarz-Pharma, Milwaukee, WI. Dec. 14, 1995.

13. Mendelson, L.M., et al. Routine elective penicillin allergy skin testing in children and adolescents: Study of sensitization. *J. Allergy Clin. Immunol.* 73:76, 1984.

14. Redmond, A.P., and Levine, B.B. Delayed skin reactions to benzyl-penicillin in man. *Int. Arch. Allergy Appl. Immunol.* 33:193, 1968.

15. Baldwin, D.S., et al. Renal failure and interstitial nephritis due to penicillin and methicillin. *N. Engl. J. Med.* 279:1245, 1968.
This paper concerns itself with seven patients who developed renal failure, rash, fever, and eosinophilia while on penicillin or methicillin. Also see Chap. 28D.

16. Wide, L., and Jublin, L. Detection of penicillin allergy of the immediate type by radioimmunoassay of reagins (IgE) to penicilloyl conjugates. *Clin. Allergy* 4:161, 1974.

17. Petz, L.D., and Fudenberg, H.H. Coombs positive hemolytic anemia caused by penicillin administration. *N. Engl. J. Med.* 274:171, 1966.

18. Levine, B.B., et al. Penicillin allergy and the heterogeneous immune responses of man to benzylpenicillin. *J. Clin. Invest.* 45:1895, 1966.
Describes preparation of RBCs with penicillin for hemagglutination assay.

19. Levine, B.B., and Zolov, D.M. Prediction of penicillin allergy by immunological tests. *J. Allergy* 43:4, 1969.

20. Sogn, D.D., et al. Results of National Institute of Allergy and Infectious Diseases Collaborative Clinical Trial to test the predictive value of skin testing with major and minor penicillin derivatives in hospitalized patients. *Arch. Intern. Med.* 152:1025, 1992.
See related article in same journal issue by R.Y. Lin, A perspective on penicillin allergy. Arch. Intern. Med. *152:930, 1992. See also summary and overview of these two articles and penicillin allergy by S. Levin, Ask the Expert.* Infect. Dis. Clin. Pract. *2:70, 1993.*

21. Parker, P.J., et al. Penicillin resensitization in hospitalized patients. *J. Allergy Clin. Immunol.* 88:213, 1991.

22. Brandriss, M.W., Smith, J.M., and Steinmen, H.H. Common antigenic determinants of penicillin G, cephalothin and 6 amino penicillin acid in rabbits. *J. Immunol.* 94:696, 1965.

23. Gerard, J.P. Common antigenic determinants of penicillin G, ampicillin, and the cephalosporins demonstrated in man. *Int. Arch. Allergy Appl. Immunol.* 33:428, 1968.
Demonstrated that patients who were skin test–positive to penicillin frequently were positive also to ampicillin and occasionally positive to cephalosporins.

24. Levine, B.B. Antigenicity and cross reactivity of penicillin and cephalosporins. *J. Infect. Dis.* [Suppl.] 128:364, 1973.

25. Thoburn, R., Johnson, J.E., III, and Cluff, L.E. Studies on the epidemiology of adverse

drug reactions: IV. The relationship of cephalothin and penicillin allergy. *J.A.M.A.* 193:345, 1966.

26. Petz, L.D. Immunologic cross-reactivity between penicillins and cephalosporins: A review. *J. Infect. Dis.* 137(Suppl.):74, 1978.

27. Saxon, A., et al. Immediate hypersensitivity reactions to beta-lactam antibiotics. *Ann. Intern. Med.* 107:204, 1987.
This UCLA conference report is an excellent review of this topic.

28. Saxon, A., et al. Imipenem cross-reactivity with penicillin in humans. *J. Allergy Clin. Immunol.* 82:213, 1988.
Patients allergic to penicillin were skin-tested with imipenem, and a significant proportion had positive skin tests to imipenem, suggesting cross-reactivity.

29. Saxon, A., et al. Lack of cross reactivity between aztreonam, a monobactam antibiotic, and penicillin in penicillin-allergic individuals. *J. Infect. Dis.* 149:16, 1984.
Patients allergic to penicillin can receive aztreonam safely.

30. Moss, R.B. Sensitivity to aztreonam and cross-reactivity with other beta-lactam antibiotics in high-risk patients with cystic fibrosis. *J. Allergy Clin. Immunol.* 87:78, 1991.
See related paper by R.B. Moss et al., Evaluation of immunologic cross-reaction of aztreonam in patients with cystic fibrosis who are allergic to penicillins or cephalosporin antibiotics, or both. Rev. Infect. Dis. *13(Suppl. 7):S598, 1991.*

31. Silviu-Dan, F., McPhillips, S., and Warrington, R.J. The frequency of skin test reactions to side chain penicillin determinants. *J. Allergy Clin. Immunol.* 91:694, 1993.

32. Fellner, M.J., and Baer, R.L. Immunologic studies in patients with serum sickness–like reactions following penicillin therapy. *J. Invest. Dermatol.* 48:384, 1967.

33. Kagan, B.M. Ampicillin rash. *West. J. Med.* 126:333, 1977.
Discusses the natural history of the morbilliform eruption due to ampicillin when the medication is continued or administered a second time.

33a. Anne, S., and Reisman, R.E. Risk of administering cephalosporin antibiotics to patients with histories of penicillin allergy. *Ann. Allergy Asthma Immunol.* 74:167, 1995.
Literature and review of post-marketing pharmaceutical data suggest that in patients with a history of penicillin allergy, the incidence of cephalosporin reactions is minimally if at all increased; post-marketing studies of second- and third-generation cephalosporins showed no increase in allergic reactions in patients with histories of penicillin allergy. Penicillin skin tests do not predict the likelihood of allergic reactions to cephalosporins in patients with histories of penicillin allergy. The authors conclude that on review of these data, it is safe to administer cephalosporin antibiotics to penicillin-allergic patients and that penicillin skin tests do not identify potential reactors.

34. Gruchalla, R.S., and Sullivan, T. Detection of IgE to sulfamethoxazole by skin testing with sulfamethoxazoyl-poly-L-tyrosine. *J. Allergy Clin. Immunol.* 88:784, 1991.

35. Carrington, D.M., Earl, H.S., and Sullivan, T.J. Studies of human IgE to a sulfonamide determinant. *J. Allergy Clin. Immunol.* 79:442, 1987.

36. Finegold, I. Oral desensitization to trimethoprim-sulfamethoxazole in a patient with AIDS. *J. Allergy Clin. Immunol.* 78:905, 1986.
See related discussion and references in Chaps. 24 and 28K.

37. Taffet, S.L., and Das, K.M. Desensitization of patients with inflammatory bowel disease to sulfasalazine. *Am. J. Med.* 73:520, 1982.

38. Purdy, B.H., Philips, D.M., and Summers, W. Desensitization for sulfasalazine skin rash. *Ann. Intern. Med.* 100:512, 1984.

28

Antibiotic Use

Richard E. Reese and
Robert F. Betts

A. Principles of Antibiotic Use

The clinician facing an ill febrile patient has the task of deciding whether an antibiotic is indicated and then choosing a clinically effective, safe, and cost-effective antibiotic. There are now more than 15 penicillin derivatives and more than 15 cephalosporins from which to choose. New agents continue to be released, such as the fluoroquinolones, clarithromycin, and azithromycin. To assist the beginning clinician in particular, **this discussion emphasizes** general concepts of antibiotic use and **a logical, stepwise approach to the selection of a specific antibiotic for a given patient.** It is hoped that these general principles still will apply when new agents are introduced. Prophylactic antibiotics are discussed in Chap. 28B.

After a careful history and physical and clinical assessment, a series of 10 important questions can and should be routinely addressed before selecting a specific antibiotic (Table 28A-1).

Antibiotic Checklist

I. **Question 1. Is an antibiotic indicated on the basis of clinical findings?**
   A. **Obvious bacterial infections** require antibiotic therapy.
      1. **Localized infection.** Patients with pneumonia, urinary tract infection, wound infection, or cellulitis require therapy.
      2. **Urgent "probable" infections** deserve therapy, as discussed in sec. **B.3.**
   B. **Probable bacterial infection.** The patient with fever and systemic symptoms but no focal findings is more problematic. The severity of symptoms, patient's age, and underlying illnesses must be considered before one chooses an antibiotic for such patients. Travel history, exposure to community infections (e.g., influenza) and, in hospitalized patients, the presence of an implantable device used for prolonged venous access or prolonged antibiotic therapy affect the decision about antibiotic treatment.
      1. **Nonspecific nature of symptoms, signs, and laboratory test results.** Many of the clinical manifestations that suggest bacterial infection (fever; leukocytosis; chills; rapid onset of symptoms; acute, tender adenopathy; myalgias; and localizing symptoms such as pharyngitis, dysuria, and cough) are not diagnostic and may be due to noninfectious causes or nonbacterial agents. **Fever** may be due to drugs, tumor, or connective tissue diseases as well as infection. Shaking chills may be the first sign. By contrast, some patients, especially elderly patients, may have bacteremia with little or no fever. The peripheral WBC count can be normal even in patients with bacteremia.
      2. **Viral infections.** Viruses may produce symptoms and signs similar to those of bacterial infection. In early viral infections, leukocytosis with a predominance of polymorphonuclear leukocytes may be seen, causing further confusion. Antibiotics are ineffective against viruses and may be associated with adverse side effects. In addition to false expectations, the risks inherent in antibiotic exposure (i.e., potential allergies, side effects, superinfection, and added cost)

Revised from Richard E. Reese and Robert F. Betts, *Handbook of Antibiotics* (2nd ed.). Boston: Little, Brown, 1993. Chaps. 1–20, pp. 1–434.

Table 28A-1. Important questions to answer routinely before selecting an antibiotic

1. Is an antibiotic **indicated**?
2. Have appropriate **specimens** been obtained, examined, and cultured?
3. **What organisms** are most likely?
4. If several antibiotics are available, **which is best**? (This question involves such factors as drugs of choice, pharmacokinetics, toxicology, cost, narrowness of spectrum, and bactericidal compared with bacteriostatic agents.)
5. Is an antibiotic **combination** appropriate?
6. What are the important **host factors**?
7. What is the best **route of administration**?
8. What is the appropriate **dose**?
9. Will initial therapy require **modification** after culture data are returned?
10. What is the optimal **duration** of treatment, **and** is development of **resistance** during prolonged therapy likely to occur?

are real. **Unnecessary treatment of viral infections is a major source of excess antibiotic use.**

   a. **Upper respiratory tract infections,** including pharyngitis, are commonly caused by viruses. Characteristically, exudates are not present in most viral infections. Only by throat culture or properly performed positive rapid streptococcal screening can one reliably differentiate between the bacterial causes that require treatment.

   b. **Influenza** is a viral syndrome in which antibiotics play no role unless there is bacterial superinfection. Because influenza occurs in epidemics, the presence of this virus in the community should affect one's thinking about empiric antibiotic therapy. In an influenza epidemic, patients presenting with fever, myalgias, sore throat, and cough most probably will have infection with influenza virus. Antibiotics are not indicated unless there is secondary bacterial pneumonia, bronchitis, or sinusitis (see Chap. 8). Furthermore, some viruses—for example, influenza and respiratory syncytial virus—can cause nosocomial infections. Viral infection must be considered in fever workups in hospitalized patients (children and adults) during community epidemics.

3. **Urgency of the situation.** A very important factor in the decision to use antibiotics is the **urgency** of the problem.

   a. **Nonurgent situation.** The otherwise healthy patient with mild illness and no focal findings does not require treatment until a diagnosis has been reached. Furthermore, unnecessary antibiotic therapy may confuse the clinical picture. Even a single dose of parenteral antibiotic may suppress follow-up cultures for several days, especially urine and blood cultures.

   b. **Urgent situation.** In contrast, a patient with **presumed infection who is severely ill,** with or without focal findings, **needs immediate therapy.** Because cultures may require 24–48 hours to become positive, the patient should be treated presumptively. A careful history, physical examination, and laboratory assessment provide the information for a rational choice of antibiotics that should be active against the organisms most likely to be involved. Once cultures have revealed the offending pathogen, the therapeutic regimen can be altered to be more specific. In fact, initiation of antibiotic therapy is carried out most commonly on the basis of clinical judgment. The laboratory results help one refine and adjust therapy.

   The following are **examples of patients who require presumptive therapy.**

   (1) **Patients with** signs or symptoms of a **focal infection** such as pneumonia, urinary tract infection (UTI), or biliary tract infections. These patients should be treated even if they are only moderately ill but especially if they are severely ill. In elderly patients, even those mildly ill with focal symptoms, therapy must be initiated early.

   (2) **Septic patients.** Any patient with sepsis from an obvious or unclear source (see Chap. 2).

(3) **Febrile leukopenic patients.** In these high-risk patients, empiric antibiotics are used for unexplained fever even if the patient is not septic in appearance (see Chap. 2).

(4) **Possible acute endocarditis.** The patient with valvular heart disease or the narcotic addict who presents with fever and chills may have endocarditis with a virulent organism that quickly could lead to destructive changes in the heart valve if empiric therapy is not initiated (see Chap. 10).

(5) **Bacterial meningitis** (known or suspected). See Chap. 5.

(6) **Acute necrotizing cellulitis** is a rapidly progressive infection and deserves empiric antibiotic therapy and often surgical debridement. See Chap. 4.

II. **Question 2. Before antibiotics are initiated, have appropriate clinical specimens been obtained, examined, and cultured?** This is extremely important. Even in the most urgent situations, blood and appropriate cultures (e.g., sputum and urine) must be obtained prior to initiation of antibiotics.

A. A **Gram stain** of any exudate or bodily fluid **may help one to recognize the major organism** or organisms (Table 28A-2) and thus help guide selection of specific agents. Specific identification of an organism from the Gram stain may not be possible. For example, gram-positive cocci in pairs or short chains may represent aerobic streptococci (including *Streptococcus pneumoniae* or enterococci), anaerobic streptococci, or even staphylococci. The classic grapelike clusters of staphylococci are quite helpful if detected but may not be present. Nevertheless, the Gram stain indicates that antibiotic therapy in these instances must be directed against gram-positive organisms. The technique and interpretation of Gram stains are discussed in Chap. 25.

B. **It is important to obtain appropriate cultures** (aerobic, anaerobic) of bodily fluids, exudates, and blood **before starting antibiotic treatment.**

1. **When the pretreatment cultures become available, the initial antibiotic regimen often can be altered** (see sec. **IX**). If cultures are not obtained, it is difficult to determine which drugs to continue or discontinue in the patient who responds clinically to multiple antibiotics.

2. **Follow-up cultures** are much less reliable than pretreatment cultures. Because antibiotics may rapidly sterilize blood and urine cultures and alter surface bacterial flora (e.g., sputum or wound swabs) quickly after their initiation, subsequent cultures usually do not reflect the initial causative organisms.

3. **Anaerobic cultures.** It is important to obtain anaerobic cultures when anaerobic infections are considered (e.g., abscesses that are incised and drained or aspirated). See Chap. 25.

III. **Question 3. What organisms are most likely to be causing the infection?** Often the clinician must start antibiotics empirically. Based on clinical information and Gram stains, an educated guess about the likely pathogens is desirable in order to select an antibiotic with good activity against the most likely pathogen(s).

A. **Focal findings** (i.e., genitourinary, pulmonary, skin, or biliary) will strongly influence the decision about whether coverage will be directed against gram-positive, gram-negative, or anaerobic organisms.

1. **Table 28A-2 lists the common organisms seen in focal infections.** Presumptive antibiotic therapy must cover these organisms.

2. **Gram stains** of clinical specimens **may provide additional clues** that certain organisms among those listed in Table 28A-2 are more likely to be causative agents.

3. **Table 28A-3 lists the antibiotics of choice for common organisms.** Using focal findings, Gram stains, and the information obtained in Tables 28A-2 and 28A-3, a rational choice can be made.

4. **Examples using Tables 28A-2 and 28A-3**

a. A patient develops a fever and shaking chills on the third postoperative day following a hernia repair. Clinical evaluation reveals a postoperative incision with erythema, tenderness, and induration at the margins of the incision site. No other focus of infection can be found, and there is some purulent drainage from the wound. The Gram stain of the wound drainage reveals gram-positive cocci. Although hospital-acquired infections after this surgery can occasionally be caused by gram-negative bacilli, it is quite uncommon, and the Gram stain indicates otherwise. Table 28A-2 indicates

Table 28A-2. Common pathogens in focal infections

Presumed location of infection	Common pathogens	Gram stain characteristics of exudate—if available
Urinary tract infections	Community-acquired: *Escherichia coli*	GNB
	Recurrent or nosocomial: *E. coli; Klebsiella, Proteus, Pseudomonas* spp.	GNB
	Enterococci	GPC
Intravenous catheter phlebitis or sepsis		
Peripheral catheter	*Staphylococcus aureus* or *S. epidermidis*	GPC
	Klebsiella, Enterobacter, Pseudomonas spp.	GNB
Hyperalimentation line	*Candida* spp., *S. aureus,*	Budding yeast; GPC
	S. epidermidis, enterococci	
	Klebsiella, Enterobacter spp., etc.	GNB
Arteriovenous fistula	*S. aureus, S. epidermidis*	GPC
Septic bursitis	*S. aureus*	GPC
Biliary tract	*E. coli, Klebsiella* spp., and enterococci; *Bacteroides fragilis* (in elderly patients), *Clostridium* spp.	
Intraabdominal abscess, peritonitis, or large bowel perforation; diverticulitis[a]	*E. coli*	GNB
	B. fragilis	GNB (thin, irregularly stained)
	Klebsiella spp.	GNB
	(Enterococci)	GPC

Condition	Organisms	
Burn wounds	Early: S. aureus, streptococci	
	Later: gram-negative bacilli, fungi	
Cellulitis, wound and soft-tissue infections	S. aureus	GPC
	Streptococci	GPC
	Clostridium spp.	GPB
Meningitis	See Chap. 5	
Pneumonia	See Chap. 9	
Pelvic abscess, postabortal or postpartal	Anaerobic streptococci	GPC
	B. fragilis	GNB (thin, irregularly stained)
	Clostridium spp.	GPB
	E. coli	GNB
	Enterococci	GPC
Septic arthritis	S. aureus	GPC
	Group B streptococci (in neonates)	GPC
	Gram-negative organisms[b]	GNB
Acute osteomyelitis	S. aureus	GPC
	Group B streptococci (in neonates)	GPC
	Gram-negative organisms[b]	GNB

GNB = gram-negative bacilli; GPC = gram-positive cocci; GPB = gram-positive bacilli

[a]The precise role of enterococci in intraabdominal infections is unclear. In mild to moderate infections, it may not be necessary to provide antibiotic activity against enterococci.

[b]In high-risk patients (e.g., immunocompromised, elderly, intravenous drug abusers, diabetics, debilitated patients).

Table 28A-3. Antibiotics of choice for common pathogens

Pathogen	Antibiotic of first choice[a]	Alternative agents[a]
Gram-positive cocci		
Staphylococcus aureus or *S. epidermidis**		
Non-penicillinase-producing	Penicillin	A first-generation cephalosporin preferred, vancomycin, imipenem, or clindamycin; a fluoroquinolone[b]
Penicillinase-producing	Penicillinase-resistant penicillin (e.g., oxacillin or nafcillin)	A first-generation cephalosporin, vancomycin, clindamycin, imipenem, amoxicillin–clavulanic acid, ticarcillin–clavulanic acid, ampicillin–sulbactam, piperacillin-tazobactam; a fluoroquinolone[b]
Methicillin-resistant	Vancomycin with or without gentamicin with or without rifampin	TMP-SMX, minocycline; a fluoroquinolone
Streptococci		
Group A, C, G	Penicillin	A cephalosporin[a], vancomycin, erythromycin; clarithromycin; azithromycin; clindamycin
Group B	Penicillin (or ampicillin)	A cephalosporin[a], vancomycin, or erythromycin
Enterococcus*		
Endocarditis or other serious infection	Penicillin (or ampicillin) with gentamicin	Vancomycin with gentamicin (see text; Chap. 28O)
Uncomplicated urinary tract infection	Ampicillin or amoxicillin	A fluoroquinolone, nitrofurantoin
Viridans group*	Penicillin G (with or without gentamicin)	A cephalosporin[a], vancomycin
S. bovis	Penicillin G	A cephalosporin[a], vancomycin
S. pneumoniae*	See text (Chap. 28C)	
Gram-negative cocci		
Neisseria gonorrhoeae*	Ceftriaxone, see text (Chap. 13)	Spectinomycin, a fluoroquinolone, cefoxitin, cefixime, cefotaxime (see Chap. 13)
N. meningitidis	Penicillin G	Third-generation cephalosporin, chloramphenicol
Moraxella (Branhamella) catarrhalis	TMP-SMX	Amoxicillin–clavulanic acid; an erythromycin; clarithromycin, azithromycin, cefuroxime, cefixime, third-generation cephalosporin, tetracycline

Gram-positive bacilli

Organism	First Choice	Alternative
Clostridium perfringens (and *Clostridium* spp.)	Penicillin G	Metronidazole, clindamycin, imipenem, chloramphenicol
Listeria monocytogenes	Ampicillin with or without gentamicin	TMP-SMX

Gram-negative bacilli

Organism	First Choice	Alternative
*Acinetobacter**	Imipenem	Tobramycin, gentamicin, or amikacin, usually with ticarcillin or piperacillin (or similar agent); TMP-SMX; a fluoroquinolone
Aeromonas hydrophila	TMP-SMX	Gentamicin, tobramycin; imipenem; a fluoroquinolone
*Bacteroides**		
Bacteroides spp. (oropharyngeal)	Penicillin G or clindamycin	Cefoxitin, metronidazole, cefotetan, ampicillin-sulbactam, piperacillin-tazobactam, chloramphenicol
B. fragilis strains (gastrointestinal strains)	Metronidazole	Clindamycin; imipenem; ampicillin-sulbactam; piperacillin-tazobactam; ticarcillin–clavulanic acid; cefoxitin^c; cefotetan^c; piperacillin^c; chloramphenicol; cefmetazole^c
*Campylobacter fetus**	Imipenem	Gentamicin
*Campylobacter jejuni**	A fluoroquinolone or an erythromycin	A tetracycline, gentamicin
Enterobacter spp.*	Imipenem	An aminoglycoside and piperacillin or ticarcillin or mezlocillin; a third-generation cephalosporin^d; TMP-SMX; aztreonam; a fluoroquinolone
*Escherichia coli**		
Uncomplicated urinary tract infection	TMP-SMX	A cephalosporin or a fluoroquinolone
Recurrent or systemic infection	A cephalosporin^e	Ampicillin with or without an aminoglycoside, TMP-SMX, oral fluoroquinolones useful in recurrent infections, ampicillin-sulbactam, ticarcillin–clavulanic acid, piperacillin-tazobactam, aztreonam
Haemophilus influenzae (coccobacillary)*		
Life-threatening infections	Cefotaxime or ceftriaxone	Chloramphenicol; cefuroxime (for pneumonia but not meningitis)
Upper respiratory infections and bronchitis	TMP-SMX	Cefuroxime; cefuroxime-axetil; third-generation cephalosporin, amoxicillin–clavulanic acid, cefaclor, tetracycline; ampicillin or amoxicillin; clarithromycin; azithromycin; cefixime
Helicobacter pylori	See Chap. 11	See Chap. 11

Table 28A-3 (continued)

Pathogen	Antibiotic of first choice[a]	Alternative agents[a]
Gram-negative bacilli (*cont.*)*		
*Klebsiella pneumoniae**	A cephalosporin[e]	An aminoglycoside, imipenem, TMP-SMX, ticarcillin–clavulanic acid, ampicillin–sulbactam, piperacillin-tazobactam; aztreonam; a fluoroquinolone; amoxicillin–clavulanic acid
Legionella spp.	Erythromycin with rifampin	TMP-SMX; clarithromycin; azithromycin; ciprofloxacin
Pasteurella multocida	Penicillin G	Tetracycline, cefuroxime, cefuroxime-axetil; amoxicillin–clavulanic acid, ampicillin–sulbactam, piperacillin-tazobactam
Proteus spp., indole-positive*	Cefotaxime, ceftizoxime, or ceftriaxone[f]	An aminoglycoside; ticarcillin or piperacillin or mezlocillin; TMP-SMX; amoxicillin–clavulanic acid; ticarcillin–clavulanic acid, ampicillin-sulbactam, piperacillin-tazobactam; a fluoroquinolone; aztreonam; imipenem
*Providencia stuartii**	Cefotaxime, ceftizoxime, or ceftriaxone[f]	Imipenem; an aminoglycoside often combined with ticarcillin or piperacillin or similar agent; ticarcillin–clavulanic acid; piperacillin-tazobactam; TMP-SMX; a fluoroquinolone; aztreonam
*Pseudomonas aeruginosa** Non-urinary tract infection	Gentamicin or tobramycin or amikacin (combined with ticarcillin, piperacillin, etc., for serious infections)	An aminoglycoside and ceftazidime; imipenem, or aztreonam plus an aminoglycoside; ciprofloxacin
Urinary tract infections	A fluoroquinolone (e.g., ciprofloxacin)	Carbenicillin; ticarcillin, piperacillin, or mezlocillin; ceftazidime; imipenem; aztreonam; an aminoglycoside
*Pseudomonas (Burkholderia) cepacia**	TMP-SMX	Ceftazidime, chloramphenicol
*Salmonella typhi**	Ceftriaxone or a fluoroquinolone	TMP-SMX, chloramphenicol; ampicillin, amoxicillin
Other species	Cefotaxime or ceftriaxone or a fluoroquinolone	TMP-SMX, chloramphenicol; ampicillin or amoxicillin
*Serratia**	Cefotaxime, ceftizoxime, or ceftriaxone[f]	Gentamicin or amikacin; imipenem; TMP-SMX; ticarcillin, piperacillin, or mezlocillin, which can be combined with an aminoglycoside; aztreonam; a fluoroquinolone

Shigella*	A fluoroquinolone	TMP-SMX; ceftriaxone: ampicillin
Vibrio cholerae (cholera)	A tetracycline	TMP-SMX; a fluoroquinolone
Vibrio vulnificus	A tetracycline	Cefotaxime
Xanthomonas (Pseudomonas) maltophilia[g]	TMP-SMX	Minocycline, ceftazidime; a fluoroquinolone
Yersinia enterocolitica*	TMP-SMX	A fluoroquinolone; an aminoglycoside; cefotaxime or ceftizoxime
Yersinia pestis (plague)	Streptomycin	A tetracycline; chloramphenicol; gentamicin

TMP-SMX = trimethoprim-sulfamethoxazole.

[a]**See later individual discussions of agents for details of agent use and contraindications of use.** Choice presumes susceptibility studies indicate that the pathogen is susceptible to the agent.

[b]The experience with fluoroquinolone use in staphylococcal infections is relatively limited. Resistance during therapy may occur. See Chap. 28S.

[c]Up to 15–20% of strains may be resistant.

[d]Enterobacter spp. may develop resistance to the cephalosporins. See discussions in Chaps. 28A and 28F.

[e]Specific choice will depend on susceptibility studies. Third-generation cephalosporins may be exquisitely active against many gram-negative bacilli (e.g., E. coli, Klebsiella spp.). In some geographic areas, 20–25% of community-acquired E. coli infections may be resistant to ampicillin (amoxicillin).

[f]In severely ill patients, this often is combined with an aminoglycoside while awaiting susceptibility data.

[g]Renamed Stenotrophomonas maltophilia.

Note: The fluoroquinolones should be used only in adults. See Chap. 28S.

*****Resistance may be a problem;** susceptibility tests should be performed.

Source: Adapted from Medical Letter. The choice of antibacterial drugs. Med. Lett. Drugs Ther. 36:53, 1994; and update of the same article 38:25, 1996.

that wound infections commonly involve *Staphylococcus aureus* and streptococci. Because the infection was hospital-acquired, the *S. aureus* is presumed to be a penicillinase producer. To provide adequate antibiotic therapy
while awaiting cultures, Table 28A-3 suggests a penicillinase-resistant
penicillin both for the *S. aureus* (e.g., oxacillin) as well as for most streptococci. It is unlikely that methicillin-resistant *S. aureus* (MRSA) would be a
factor in this clinical situation but, if a particular hospital had a nosocomial
outbreak of MRSA, vancomycin could be used while awaiting cultures and
therapy modified after culture data became available.

   b. A 55-year-old woman with a prior history of gallstones presents with right-
upper-quadrant abdominal pain, fever, chills, leukocytosis, and hyperbilirubinemia. Her presentation is consistent with **acute cholecystitis** and
possibly an early cholangitis. Table 28A-2 indicates that *Escherichia coli*,
Klebsiella spp. and, much less commonly, *Enterobacter* spp. are the major
pathogens. Enterococci can usually be ignored unless culture is proven.

   Several antibiotic options are possible to use in this setting; this topic
is reviewed in detail in Chap. 11. For the mildly ill patient, cefazolin alone
would be reasonable for community-acquired infection, although cefoxitin
is preferred by some in this setting. For the sicker patient, ceftriaxone
would provide excellent gram-negative bacterial activity (with or without
metronidazole for anaerobic activity, which is more of a concern in the
elderly patient with biliary infection).

   c. A 70-year-old patient has a tender abdomen, with mild rebound left-lower-
quadrant abdominal tenderness, fever, and leukocytosis. He has a past
history of diverticulitis. After surgical evaluation, he is believed to have
acute diverticulitis. Table 28A-2 indicates that the major potential pathogens are *E. coli, Bacteroides fragilis,* and *Klebsiella* spp. From Table 28A-
3 one can see that a cephalosporin is listed as the antibiotic of choice against
E. coli (in non-UTI) and *Klebsiella* spp. For serious *B. fragilis* infections,
metronidazole is preferred, but for mild to moderate infections, as in our
example, cefoxitin is an alternative. This cephalosporin is active against
community-acquired *E. coli* and *Klebsiella* spp. and could be used as monotherapy. Ampicillin-sulbactam or piperacillin-tazobactam would be other
alternatives for monotherapy.

   In a very ill patient with diverticulitis with a protracted course and with
possible perforation, focal peritonitis, and possible intraabdominal abscess,
several options are available. A cephalosporin very active against *E. coli*
and *Klebsiella* spp. (e.g., ceftriaxone) can be combined with metronidazole.
Although triple antibiotics, ampicillin, metronidazole or clindamycin, and
an aminoglycoside have often been used in this setting, some clinicians are
concerned that aminoglycosides do not provide adequate tissue concentrations in severe intraabdominal infections, especially when early abscess
formation is present. See related discussions in Chap. 11.

   d. See the example of an **arteriovenous shunt infection** discussed later under
Using the Antibiotic Checklist.

B. The **age** of the patient at times may provide important additional **clues to the
likely organisms** or may affect the choice of agent.

   1. **In meningitis,** neonates usually are infected with group B streptococci or enteric
organisms. In children younger than 2 years, *Haemophilus influenzae* in the
unvaccinated child is common but *S. pneumoniae* and *Neisseria meningitidis*
also occur. The latter two organisms are the most common pathogens in adults.
Recipients of the conjugated *H. influenzae* b vaccine are less likely to have
invasive disease due to this pathogen. See Chap. 22.

   2. **The choice and dosage of an antibiotic** are also affected by age. For example,
tetracycline should be avoided in children younger than 8 years because of its
effect on teeth. If chloramphenicol must be used in the neonate, serum levels
must be monitored to avoid the development of the gray-baby syndrome. The
fluoroquinolones are avoided generally in children and prepubertal teenagers
because they may affect cartilage and bone formation. See sec. **3.**

   3. **The elderly patient poses special problems.** These topics have been reviewed
elsewhere in detail [1, 2, 2a].

      a. **Infections occur more frequently** in the elderly, in part because mechanical
barriers such as skin and mucosa undergo structural and functional decline
with age. Immune dysregulation and immunodeficiency are well-described

phenomena accompanying aging. Age-related chronic diseases (e.g., diabetes, chronic pulmonary disease) may compromise host defenses. The elderly are hospitalized more often than young adults, and the incidence of nosocomial infections, often with resistant pathogens, is threefold higher in elderly patients [1].

b. The **mortality** for specific infections **is higher** in older patients versus younger. There is a threefold increase in death rates with pneumonia, sepsis, meningitis, and endocarditis; a two- to eightfold increase with cholecystitis; a five- to tenfold increase with kidney infection; and a fifteen- to twentyfold increase with appendicitis [1].

In addition to the compromised host defenses and underlying chronic diseases, other factors help explain these higher death rates, including the atypical presentation of infections (see sec. **d**), delays in seeking help, and poorer tolerance to invasive diagnostic procedures and therapeutic interventions, among them surgery [1].

c. **Morbidity rates are higher** in the elderly with infections. Pneumonias are more apt to be associated with bacteremia and slow resolution; UTI is associated with bacteremias commonly; intraabdominal infection is more commonly associated with perforation, bacteremia, or abscess formation than in younger patients [1].

d. **Infection** in elderly persons **may present atypically** with minimal or subtle findings, often without signs pointing to a specifically involved organ system. This is particularly common in the so-called frail elderly (often older than 80 years, typically nursing home residents, with underlying debilitating illnesses as well as cognitive impairment). In these patients, **any unexplained change in functional status** (e.g., lethargy or agitation, anorexia, falls, confusion) should lead the clinician to consider and evaluate for infection [2].

Fever may be blunted or absent in up to one-third of infected elderly patients. Elderly patients may have lower baseline temperatures so that with an infection, their temperature may not elevate above 101°F (38°C). **Therefore, in nursing home patients, in the setting of changes of functional status, an increase from baseline temperature of more than 1.4°F or an absolute oral temperature of greater than 100°F is highly suggestive of an underlying infection** [2].

e. **Clinical implications.** Because of these special problems in the elderly and the higher death and morbidity rates, some experts emphasize [1]:

(1) **Early empiric antibiotics.**

(2) **Initial broad-spectrum antibiotics.** Focal infections may not be defined, hospital-acquired infections are common, and gram-negative infections in nursing home patients are common. (Antibiotics can be modified once culture data are back).

(3) **Careful selection and dosing of antibiotics. All elderly patients have some degree of renal impairment** (see sec. **VI.C**) and may be on other drugs that may interact with antibiotics. Aminoglycosides should be used cautiously in these patients. See Chap. 28H.

(4) **Compliance** with oral antibiotics is a concern in the elderly [2a]. **Reasons for noncompliance** in the elderly **include:** forgetfulness, poor understanding of the drug regimen, impaired hearing or vision, polypharmacy, fear of side effects, disappearance of symptoms, complexity of the drug regimen, concerns regarding expense, inability to open child-resistant containers, and intentional nonadherence [2a].

Studies indicate that antimicrobial **compliance is enhanced with once-per-day and twice-per-day dosing;** some of the newer antibiotics with these easier dosing schedules may be more useful in the elderly because their use improves compliance, even though the newer agents may be more expensive than traditional agents [2a].

(5) **Drug-drug interactions** are a potential concern in the elderly patient on multiple medications [2a]. Similarly, **adverse drug reactions** also are a concern in these older patients with decreased renal function, problems with compliance, and often malnourished status [2a].

C. **Severity of illness** dictates not only whether antibiotic therapy should be initiated but also, at times, whether multiple agents should be used. In sepsis of unclear etiology, combinations of antibiotics often are indicated (see Chap. 2). In pelvic and other severe abdominal infections, multiple agents may be necessary to ensure sufficiently broad-spectrum coverage.

  D. Epidemiologic features

    1. Hospital-acquired infections often are caused by gram-negative bacteria that are resistant to penicillin, ampicillin, erythromycin, and other antibiotics commonly used in the outpatient setting. The incidence of hospital-associated gram-negative bacteria resistant to cephalosporins and aminoglycosides varies among institutions, and local resistance patterns will affect the initial antibiotic choice. Because approximately 10–20% of these organisms may be sensitive only to an aminoglycoside, the latter is used often in the therapy of presumptive severe gram-negative infections in the hospital setting. This is even more likely if the patient has previously received antibiotics. Patients who develop infections in the intensive care or burn unit are especially likely to be infected with resistant gram-negative organisms. See also sec. **4.**

    2. As noted, **prior antibiotic use** in a given patient may predispose to infections with more resistant organisms. Thus, a patient with one or more recent infections requiring gentamicin may, in a subsequent infection, be infected with an organism resistant to gentamicin.

    3. All suspected **staphylococcal infections,** whether **hospital-acquired or community-acquired, should be presumed to be penicillin-resistant** for initial antibiotic therapy. When susceptibility studies are available, penicillin should be substituted if the staphylococcus is shown to be susceptible. If methicillin resistance to *S. aureus* or *S. epidermidis* organisms is shown or is highly suspected, vancomycin is used (see Chap. 28D). **Therefore, susceptibility data for staphylococci should be carefully examined.**

    4. Is the patient at risk for recently emerging resistant bacteria, which may be community-acquired or hospital-acquired? In some geographic areas or special settings, in addition to high rates of ampicillin-resistant *H. influenzae* and MRSA, an increasing incidence of **penicillin-resistant *S. pneumoniae*** (see Chap. 28C), **vancomycin-resistant enterococci** (see Chap. 28O), **and multidrug-resistant gram-negative bacilli** are seen. See related discussion in sec. **II** under Miscellaneous Aspects of Antibiotic Use.

  E. Prior culture data often provide helpful clues. For example, an elderly man who recently had a positive culture for enterococci prior to removal of an indwelling catheter and who develops a UTI and sepsis associated with gram-positive cocci in an unspun urine Gram stain should have an antibiotic directed against enterococci (e.g., ampicillin) included in his empiric antibiotic regimen. Similarly, if prior cultures showed that the most recent gram-negative bacteria colonizing the urine was gentamicin-resistant, the clinician should be concerned about a resistant gram-negative infection and should choose amikacin.

IV. Question 4. If several antibiotics are available to treat the likely or known pathogen, which agent is best for a particular patient? This question involves many variables.

  A. Is there an obvious **drug of choice** [3] (see Table 28A-3) and, if so, can this agent be used?

  B. Are there antibiotic allergies? For example, if a patient is allergic to a penicillin, the patient must be presumed to be allergic to all the penicillin derivatives unless appropriate skin tests can be done to test specifically for cross-reactivity. It is important to consider both trade and generic names of antibiotics when evaluating a patient's allergic history. **See discussion of penicillin and other drug allergies in Chap. 27.**

  C. Antibiotic penetration and pH. Will the antibiotic under consideration **penetrate** the infected area? This may be particularly important in infections involving the CNS, into which clindamycin, aminoglycosides, and first- and some second-generation cephalosporins penetrate poorly. Two other sites of poor penetration are the prostate and the obstructed biliary tree. The **pH of the site of infection may affect antibiotic activity;** for example, aminoglycosides are much more effective in a physiologic medium (pH 7.4) than in an acid environment (e.g., abscess). In pus or sputum, an acid pH may alter the activity of these antibiotics.

  D. Because of potential side effects, some agents may be contraindicated in certain settings. Examples include the following:

    1. Chloramphenicol use is tempered by the rare occurrence of aplasia (probably 1/25,000–1/50,000 courses of therapy).

    2. The dental effects of tetracycline limit its use in children younger than 8 years and during pregnancy.

3. The fluoroquinolones may affect cartilage formation and therefore are not recommended for use in prepubertal children [4] and pregnant women.

4. **Certain antibiotics** (e.g., the second- and third-generation cephalosporins, clindamycin) **may pose a greater risk for the development of *Clostridium difficile* diarrhea** than other antibiotics (e.g., aminoglycosides, aztreonam). In certain patients, this may be a consideration in the selection of one antibiotic over another. This topic is discussed in detail at the end of this chapter.

E. **Bactericidal versus bacteriostatic agents.** The laboratory definitions and determination of bactericidal and bacteriostatic antibiotics are discussed in Chap. 25.

1. **Bacteriostatic agents** primarily **inhibit** bacterial growth. Killing of the organism depends on host defense mechanisms. One of the disadvantages of bacteriostatic agents is that, in the setting of inadequate host mechanisms, any partially inhibited organisms may survive, replicate, and produce recurrent disease when the antibiotic is discontinued.

2. **Bactericidal agents** depend less on host factors. These agents are preferable if the host is compromised (e.g., neutropenic or immunosuppressed patients) or when host defense mechanisms do not operate well (e.g., in patients with bacterial endocarditis or meningitis).

3. **Clinical implications.** In minor infections of the healthy host, bacteriostatic or bactericidal agents are probably of equal efficacy. However, **in severe, life-threatening infections (particularly bacteremias in leukopenic patients or patients with endocarditis or meningitis), bactericidal agents are necessary.** A brief summary of antibiotics falling into these different categories is given in Table 28A-4.

F. **Cost of antibiotics.** From the 1950s through the 1970s, the cost of an antibiotic and its administration seemed to have had little impact on the prescribing habits of house officers and most physicians. Now, with the spiraling costs of these agents and, in particular, the expense of hospitalization, the cost of administering antibiotics is an important consideration.

This is a complex issue, and only a brief summary follows. A hospital's pharmacy and therapeutic committee (or formulary committee) will consider all these factors when evaluating new versus old agents.

1. **The cost of the antibiotic itself** is the easiest component to sort out. See Tables 28A-5, 28A-6, and 28F-5. **Generic preparations** should be ordered whenever possible (e.g., generic oral trimethoprim-sulfamethoxazole [TMP-SMX]; see Table 28A-5). It is **essential that the clinician recognize that the cost per day of the antibiotic is only one component of the cost of antibiotic administration in hospitalized patients.** Other factors include the following:

2. **Frequency of administration** per day. The more frequently the antibiotic is given (q4h versus q8h versus q24h), the more expensive it is to administer in

Table 28A-4. Bactericidal and bacteriostatic agents

Bactericidal	Bacteriostatic[a]
Penicillins	Erythromycin
Cephalosporins	Clindamycin
Aminoglycosides	Tetracycline
Vancomycin	Sulfonamides
Aztreonam	Chloramphenicol[c]
Imipenem[b]	
Fluoroquinolones	
Metronidazole	

[a]At high concentration, these agents may be bactericidal against some susceptible organisms. In general, however, they are still classified as bacteriostatic antibiotics.
[b]Some strains of *Listeria monocytogenes* and enterococci may show tolerance (see Chap. 28G).
[c]Generally, chloramphenicol has been considered a bacteriostatic antibiotic. However, data indicate that chloramphenicol is bactericidal against some bacteria (e.g., *S. pneumoniae, H. influenzae, N. meningitidis*) and bacteriostatic against other bacteria (e.g., *S. aureus* and Enterobacteriaceae). See J.J. Rahal, Jr., and M.S. Simberkoff. Bactericidal and bacteriostatic action of chloramphenicol against meningeal pathogens. *Antimicrob. Agents Chemother.* 16:13, 1979.

Table 28A-5. Cost of common oral regimens

Drug	Dosage	Cost (dollars) for 10 days[a]
Penicillin V	250 mg qid	
Rugby (generic)		2.31
V-cillin K		8.58
Dicloxacillin	250 mg qid	
Schein (generic)		15.00
Dynapen		37.58
Cloxacillin (generic)	250 mg qid	13.96
Amoxicillin	250 mg tid	
Rugby (generic)		3.76
Polymox (Trimox)		7.17
Ampicillin	250 mg qid	
Moore (generic)		4.40
Principen		4.50
Augmentin	tid	
250-mg Tablets		55.95
Chewables (250 mg)		50.00
125-mg Suspension		26.25
Chewables (125 mg)		26.25
Carbenicillin (Geocillin)	382 mg qid (1 tab)	72.06
	2 tab qid	144.11
Cephalexin	250 mg qid	
Rugby (generic)		22.74
Keflex		51.51
Rugby (generic)	500 mg qid	44.28
Keflex		101.24
Cefadroxil	1 g bid	
Generic		39.77
Duricef		121.45
Cephradine	250 mg qid	
Rugby (generic)		21.99
Velosef		33.02
Rugby (generic)	500 mg qid	43.44
Velosef		64.85
Cefaclor (Ceclor)	250 mg tid	62.18
Mylan (generic)		55.66
Cefuroxime axetil (Ceftin)	125 mg bid	34.86
	250 mg bid	65.35
	500 mg bid	123.98
Cefixime (Suprax)	400 mg q24h	61.96
Cefprozil (Cefzil)	250 mg q12h	55.30
Loracarbef (Lorabid)	200 mg bid	62.90
Cefpodoxime proxetil (Vantin)	200 mg bid	66.14
Ceftibuten (Cedax)	400 mg qd	61.80
Clindamycin (Cleocin)	300 mg q8h	66.38
TMP/SMX	1 double-strength bid	
Bactrim		23.82
Septra (generic)		22.98
Rugby (generic)		2.10
Trimethoprim	100 mg bid	
Rugby (generic)		3.83
Proloprim		15.05
Erythromycin (base)	250 mg qid	
Abbott		5.59
E-mycin (delayed release)		9.45

Table 28A-5 (continued)

Drug	Dosage	Cost (dollars) for 10 days[a]
Erythromycin sterate Rugby (generic)	250 mg qid	6.07
Azithromycin (Zithromax)	1 g once only[b]	24.15
	500 mg, day 1, plus 250 mg, days 2–5 (Z-pak)[b]	36.23
Clarithromycin (Biaxin)	250 mg bid	59.77
	500 mg bid	59.77
	Pediatric suspension 7.5 mg/ kg given bid (for 17kg patient, 125 mg bid)	26.59
Tetracycline hydrochloride	250 mg qid	
Mylan		1.62
Sumycin 250		2.16
Doxycycline	100 mg/day (with 200-mg initial load)	
Lederle (generic)		6.57
Vibramycin		38.86
Vancomycin (Vancocin HCl [oral solution powder])	Capsules: 125 mg q6h PO	189.00
Metronidazole	250 mg qid	
Rugby (generic)		3.28
Flagyl		53.23
Norfloxacin (Noroxin)	400 mg bid	51.63
Ciprofloxacin (Cipro)	250 mg bid	54.10
	500 mg bid	62.61
	750 mg bid	108.60
Ofloxacin (Floxin)	200 mg bid	58.29
	300 mg bid	64.37
	400 mg bid	73.16
Lomefloxacin (Maxaquin)	400 mg once daily	61.07

[a]Actual wholesale prices (rounded off) to pharmacist from *American Druggist Blue Book,* 1994–1995. **Retail and patient prices would be higher based on local mark-up and bidding practices.**
[b]See text discussion in Chap. 28M on single-dose and once-daily dosing × 5 for azithromycin.
Source: Courtesy of Joseph S. Bertino, Jr., Pharm.D., Bassett Healthcare, Cooperstown, NY.

terms of personnel time, intravenous materials used, and so on. In one study, the estimated average nonantibiotic cost associated with the mixing and administration of a single intravenous antibiotic dose was $3.35 [5]. Agents with longer half-lives may be more cost-effective. For example, if a third-generation cephalosporin is indicated, ceftriaxone may be a good choice because it can often be given once daily (see Chap. 28F).

3. **Number of antibiotics.** The use of multiple antibiotics often increases costs. In some situations, instead of using triple antibiotics for intraabdominal sepsis (e.g., ampicillin, gentamicin, clindamycin, or metronidazole), it may be appropriate and cost-effective to use an expensive single agent (e.g., cefoxitin, cefotetan, ampicillin-sulbactam, or imipenem-cilastatin), which is less toxic than an aminoglycoside and does not require antibiotic serum monitoring.

4. **Intravenous administration costs.** In addition to the **nursing time** involved in giving the agent, the **tubing,** plastic **bags,** and infusion **pumps** all add to the costs of intravenous administration.

5. **Intravenous versus intramuscular versus oral administration.** Because less nursing time and materials are required, intramuscular administration is less expensive, and oral therapy (if appropriate) saves even more. The new oral fluoroquinolones (see Chap. 28S) are very exciting agents that often are cost-effective if they are used appropriately instead of using a parenteral agent. However, the absorption of intramuscularly administered antibiotics may be impaired in diabetic patients [4].

Table 28A-6. Costs of common parenteral regimens (moderately severe infection)

Drug	Dose/day	Cost (dollars) per day[a]
Penicillin G	2,400,000 units	3.04
Pfizerpen G (Pfizer)	12 million units	6.05
Oxacillin	12 g	128.28
Prostaphlin (Bristol) Apothecon		
Nafcillin	12 g	96.12
Nafcil (Bristol)		
Ampicillin	6 g	23.22
Omnipen (Wyeth)		
Ticarcillin	18 g	51.43
Ticar (Beecham)		
Piperacillin	18 g	99.13
Pipracil (Lederle)	16 g	88.12
Mezlocillin	18 g	73.48
Mezlin (Miles)	16 g	65.31
Ticarcillin-clavulanate	18 g/0.6 g	80.10
Timentin (Beecham)	12 g/0.4 g	53.40
Ampicillin-sulbactam	6 g	37.42
Unasyn (Roerig)	12 g	74.83
Piperacillin-tazobactam	3.375 g q6h	60.75
Zosyn (Lederle)	4.5 g q6h	81.00
Cephalothin	9 g (1.5 g q4h)	30.79
Keflin (Lilly)		
Cefazolin	4 g (1 g q6h)	12.00
Ancef (SKF)	3 g (1 g q8h)	9.00
Cefuroxime	2.25 g (750 mg q8h)	21.33
Zinacef (Glaxo)	4.5 g (1.5 g q8h)	42.65
Cefamandole	9 g (1.5 g q4h)	87.59
Mandol (Lilly)		
Cefoxitin	8 g (2 g q6h)	73.54
Mefoxin (MSD)	6 g (2 g q8h)	55.16
Cefonicid	1 g q12h	52.20
Monocid (SKF)		
Cefotetan	2 g q12h	43.80
Cefotan (Stuart)		
Cefmetazole		
Zefazone (Upjohn)	2 g q8h	51.41
Ceftriaxone	2 g (2.0 g q24h)	70.57
Rocephin (Roche)	1 g (1.0 g q24h)	40.18
Ceftazidime	6 g (2 g q8h)	
Fortaz (Glaxo)		85.36
Tazicef (SKF)		88.92
Tazidime (Lilly)		86.44
Cefotaxime	2 g q6h	83.98
Claforan (Hoechst)	2 g q8h	62.99
Cefoperazone	8 g (2 g q6h)	131.35
Cefobid (Pfizer)	6 g (2 g q8h)	98.51
Ceftizoxime	(2 g q8h)	63.42
Ceftizox (SKF)		
Aztreonam	2 g q8h	85.98
Azactam (Squibb)	1 g q8h	43.05
Imipenem	2,000 mg (500 mg q6h)	101.65
Primaxin (MSD)		

Table 28A-6 (continued)

Drug	Dose/day	Cost (dollars) per day[a]
Gentamicin		
Garamycin (Schering)	360 mg (1.5 mg/kg q8h for an	18.09
(generic) (Elkins-Sinn)	80-kg patient)	4.69
Tobramycin	360 mg (1.5 mg/kg q8h for an	32.76
Nebcin (Dista)	80-kg patient)	
(Lederle)		30.33
Amikacin	1,200 mg (7.5 mg/kg q12h for	140.98
Amikin (Bristol)	an 80-kg patient)	
Clindamycin	2,400 mg (600 mg q6h)	23.20
Cleocin (Upjohn)	2,700 mg (900 mg q8h)	18.18
	1,800 mg (600 mg q8h)	17.40
Chloramphenicol	4 g (1 g q6h)	16.60
Chloromycetin (P/D)		
TMP/SMX	1,400 mg TMP (5 mg TMP/kg	62.06
Septra (Burroughs	q6h for a 70-kg patient[b])	
Wellcome)	700 mg TMP (5 mg TMP/kg	31.02
	q12h for a 70-kg patient)	
Erythromycin	2,000 mg (500 mg q6h)	23.20
Erythromycin (Elkins-Sinn)		
Doxycycline	200 mg (100 mg q12h)	42.14
Vibramycin (Pfizer)		
Vancomycin	2,000 mg (500 mg q6h)	31.20
Vancocin (Lilly)		
Metronidazole	2,000 mg (500 mg q6h)	35.40
(generic) (Elkins-Sinn)		
Ciprofloxacin	200 mg q12h	31.21
Cipro	400 mg q12h	60.02
Ofloxacin	400 mg q12h	52.80
Floxin		
Pentamidine	280 mg (4 mg/kg q24h for a	92.17
Pentam (LyphoMed)	70-kg patient)	
Spectinomycin	2 g (IM)	18.81

[a]Actual wholesale prices (rounded off) to pharmacist from *American Druggist Blue Book,* 1994–1995. **Retail (patient) prices would be higher based on local mark-up and bidding practices.**
[b]Maximum initial dose for *P. carinii* pneumonia; usual dose is lower than this. See Chap. 24. Lower doses used in other settings. See Chap. 28K.
Note: The daily cost of an antibiotic itself represents only a portion of the total administration cost per day. See text.
Source: Courtesy of Joseph S. Bertino, Jr., Pharm.D., Bassett Healthcare, Cooperstown, NY.

6. **Monitoring of serum levels and toxicity.** The potential for toxicity with certain agents (e.g., aminoglycosides, chloramphenicol) is real, and the toxicity, if it occurs, may prolong the patient's hospitalization, increase the level of care of the patient (e.g., dialysis), or be associated with increased morbidity and even mortality. Monitoring for potential toxicities is expensive. Therefore, if an alternative choice of a "safer" agent is available, it often is wise as well as cost-effective to use the alternative. (See individual agent discussions.)

7. **Outpatient oral therapy.** Cost factors are less complex than in hospitalized patients but are still very important to control. For example, if a 55-year-old woman presents with an uncomplicated cystitis and no drug allergies, 10 days of generic TMP-SMX therapy will be approximately 10% of the cost of an unnecessarily broad-spectrum agent such as ciprofloxacin (250 mg bid) (see Table 25A-6).

G. **Narrow versus broad spectrum of activity.** For empiric therapy, antibiotics with a broad spectrum of activity are used initially. Once susceptibility data are known, it is preferable to use as narrow-spectrum an agent as possible.

A precise definition of the term **broad-spectrum agent** is one active against more than one of the major groups of infectious agents (i.e., bacteria, rickettsias, chlamydiae, mycoplasmas, viruses, fungi, protozoa, or spirochetes). **Narrow-spectrum** antibiotics are effective against only one or two varieties of microorganisms. For example, penicillin is active against bacteria and spirochetes. In routine clinical use, the term **broad-spectrum** agent or **wide-spectrum** agent is used to refer to those antibiotics that are active against many gram-positive and gram-negative bacteria (e.g., the newer cephalosporins). A **narrow-spectrum** agent such as penicillin is active against fewer organisms (e.g., primarily gram-positive bacteria).

V. **Question 5. Is an antibiotic combination appropriate?**

A. **Current indications for antibiotic combinations.** Although in vitro and animal studies support the use of antibiotic combinations, documentation of increased efficacy for human infections is difficult to obtain. Synergistic combinations in bacteremic leukopenic patients do seem to be associated with improved outcome when compared with single-agent therapy [4, 6].

1. In the **febrile leukopenic patient,** two or sometimes three antibiotics often are used to provide activity against gram-positive and gram-negative organisms and, it is hoped, to provide synergy against gram-negative bacilli [7] and cover, at times, gram-positive cocci. However, the optimal antibiotic regimen in this setting is unclear [4], and monotherapy often is useful. See Chap. 2.

2. **In infections in which multiple organisms are likely or proved** (e.g., intraabdominal sepsis or pelvic abscess), more than one antibiotic may be required for adequate treatment. For example, therapy for an intraabdominal abscess and peritonitis often includes an aminoglycoside or cephalosporin (to treat the gram-negative aerobes) and clindamycin or metronidazole (to treat *B. fragilis* and other anaerobes). Although in the past a third agent (e.g., ampicillin) was added synergistically with gentamicin against enterococci, recently reviewers have suggested that therapy aimed at enterococci usually is not necessary. See Chap. 11 for a discussion of this topic. With the increased spectrum of activity of the newer cephalosporins (e.g., cefoxitin and cefotetan) and agents such as piperacillin-tazobactam, a single antibiotic may be useful in community-acquired mixed infections, saving the broader-acting imipenem-cilastatin for hospital-acquired infections. (See individual agent discussions.)

3. **Synergism.** When one antibiotic greatly enhances the activity of another, with more than an additive effect, this interaction is called **synergy.** Synergy can be measured in the laboratory by timed killing curves and checkerboard methods, but these tests are time-consuming and can be difficult to interpret. Examples of mechanisms of synergy include the following:

   a. **Serial inhibition of microbial growth.** Fixed combinations of trimethoprim (80 mg) and sulfamethoxazole (400 mg) will block successive steps in the synthesis of folic acid (see Chap. 28K).

   b. **One antibiotic enhances the penetration of another.** The synergistic interaction between penicillin and aminoglycosides may be mediated by this mechanism. It is believed that enterococci are impermeable to aminoglycosides. The penicillin alters the cell wall, allowing the aminoglycoside to penetrate the bacteria and thereby act effectively at the ribosomal level.

4. **Limiting or preventing the emergence of resistance.** This principle applies primarily to the treatment of tuberculosis. More than one agent is used routinely in an attempt to prevent the replication of preexisting resistant organisms (see Chap. 9). Whether or not two agents minimize the occurrence of resistance with gram-negative bacilli is unclear [6], but available data suggest that it does not.

B. **Antibiotic combinations commonly used** are briefly outlined here:

1. Penicillin and gentamicin are synergistic against many enterococci.

2. Ticarcillin or piperacillin (and related penicillins) and aminoglycosides are synergistic against *Pseudomonas aeruginosa* and other gram-negative organisms (see Chap. 28E).

3. Cephalosporins and aminoglycosides may be synergistic against *Klebsiella pneumoniae.*

4. **The drug combinations clavulanic acid–amoxicillin, clavulanic acid–ticarcillin, sulbactam-ampicillin,** and **tazobactam-piperacillin** are discussed under the penicillins (see Chap. 28E). In these combinations, the clavulanic acid, sulbactam, and tazobactam are inhibitors of beta-lactamase enzymes. They extend the activity of the antibiotic combined with these agents.

C. **Unique drug combination. Imipenem-cilastatin** is another type of combination. The enzyme inhibitor (cilastatin) prevents metabolic breakdown of imipenem by the kidney (see Chap. 28G for a detailed discussion).

D. **Disadvantages of multiple antibiotics**
   1. **An increased risk of drug sensitivities or toxicity** is more likely when more agents are used.
   2. **An increased risk of colonization with a resistant bacterial organism** may occur. If superinfection develops, such resistant organisms are more difficult to treat.
   3. **Possibility of antagonism**
      a. Antagonism is present when the combined effect of two drugs is less than the effect of either drug alone; one of the drugs appears to interfere with the action of the second. How often this occurs clinically is unknown [6]. However, prior data suggest that the combination of tetracycline and penicillin for treatment of meningitis resulted in a poorer outcome than when penicillin was used alone, presumably due to the inhibition of growth by tetracycline, which interferes with the bactericidal action of penicillin.
      b. There has been recent interest in using the newer broad-spectrum beta-lactams in combination with one another to obtain broad-spectrum coverage without exposing the patient to the possible toxicity of aminoglycosides, for example. Although this seems reasonable, there is in vitro and in vivo evidence that some beta-lactam–beta-lactam combinations may be antagonistic against certain organisms such as *Enterobacter, Serratia,* or *Pseudomonas* spp. This antagonism seems to be the result of the induction or derepression of chromosomally mediated beta-lactamases by one of the agents, leading to inactivation of the second antibiotic [4]. For example, antagonism has also been described when cefoxitin, cefamandole, or imipenem cilastatin is combined with another cephalosporin or expanded penicillin. Apparently the cefoxitin or imipenem can induce a chromosomal beta-lactamase, which in turn may decrease the effectiveness of the cephalosporin or expanded penicillins [6].
         (1) Moellering [4] concludes that the exact clinical significance of this phenomenon is not presently clear, but it must be kept in mind when one considers the clinical use of such drug combinations.
         (2) We tend to minimize the use of such combinations.
   4. **Higher costs.** Combination antibiotics often are more expensive than single agents.
   5. **False sense of security.** Although appealing at times, the use of multiple agents to treat all possible organisms often is not possible, practical, or necessary and may be associated with significant complications.

VI. **Question 6. What are the important host factors?** There may be special characteristics of the host that must be considered in choosing an antibiotic for use in individual patients. Some examples are given here.
   A. **Genetic factors.** Patients with glucose-6-phosphate dehydrogenase (G-6-PD) deficiency may develop hemolysis from sulfonamides, nitrofurantoin, and chloramphenicol [4].
   B. **Pregnancy and lactation.** Certain drugs may pose special problems (e.g., the tetracyclines, which may cause hepatotoxicity in the mother and dentition problems in the infant). Because of the physiologic changes that occur in the mother during pregnancy (e.g., increases in total body water, with an increase in the apparent volume of distribution, increases in glomerular filtration rates and renal excretion of many antibiotics), overall serum drug levels of antibiotics are lower during gestation [7a]. Therefore, in critical infections, serum levels of antibiotics may need to be monitored and compensatory dosage adjustments may be necessary [7a].
      1. **Placental transfer of antibiotics.** Whenever possible, pregnant women should avoid all drugs because of the risk of fetal toxicity. Table 3-3 (on p. 71) shows the infant and maternal serum concentrations of selected antibiotics. This topic

has been reviewed in detail [7a, 8, 9] and is summarized as follows:

   a. Antibiotics considered safe in pregnancy include the penicillins (with the possible exception of ticarcillin) [4], the cephalosporins, erythromycin base, and probably aztreonam.

   b. Antibiotics to be used with caution include the aminoglycosides, vancomycin, clindamycin, imipenem-cilastatin, trimethoprim, and nitrofurantoin.

   c. Antibiotics contraindicated in pregnancy include chloramphenicol, erythromycin estolate, tetracycline, fluoroquinolones, and TMP-SMX (Bactrim, Septra). Although controversial, we would avoid metronidazole because of its carcinogenic potential (see Chap. 28P). Sulfonamides should be avoided in the last trimester of pregnancy. Some experts suggest avoiding ticarcillin as it has been shown to be teratogenic in rodents [4]. See Chap. 28E.

  2. Antibiotics in breast milk. Limited information is available regarding adverse effects in nursing neonates from antibiotics administered to their mothers. If possible, nursing mothers should avoid all drugs. As in pregnancy, chloramphenicol, tetracycline, sulfonamides, and metronidazole should be avoided. Until further data are available, we suggest avoiding the use of fluoroquinolones. Table 3-4 (on p. 72) shows the concentrations of selected antibiotics in breast milk and milk-plasma ratios. The total daily dose a nursing baby receives often probably is not toxicologically significant.

  3. The US Food and Drug Administration's (FDA's) use-in-pregnancy drug-rating system is shown in Table 28A-7. These pregnancy categories are based on the degree to which available information has ruled out risk to the fetus balanced against the drug's potential benefits to the patient. This topic has recently been reviewed [7a].

    The human embryo is most vulnerable to teratogenic insult during the first trimester (days 1–70 of gestation). During the second trimester (days 70–154 of gestation), the fetal organs have been developed and growth continues; agents with antimetabolic activity, such as the folate antagonists, have the most theoretical potential for adverse effects. The third trimester (day 154 to delivery) is characterized by an impaired fetal ability to metabolize toxic agents and competition of the drugs with endogenous substances (e.g., bilirubin) for plasma protein-binding sites [7a].

C. Renal function. Renal failure may affect not only the choice of antibiotic but also its dosages [10, 10a] (see discussions of individual agents). Consequently, renal function should be monitored in patients treated with antibiotics that are potentially nephrotoxic and primarily excreted by the kidney. These are summarized in Table 28A-8. Serum antibiotic levels, especially when aminoglycosides are used, should be monitored, as should serum creatinine, every 2–4 days.

  1. Dosages of antibiotics excreted by the kidney are modified based on the patient's creatinine clearance.

Table 28A-7. US Food and Drug Administration use-in-pregnancy ratings

Category	Interpretation
A	**Controlled studies show no risk.** Adequate, well-controlled studies in pregnant women have failed to demonstrate risk to the fetus.
B	**No evidence of risk in humans.** Either animal findings show risk but human findings do not; or, if no adequate human studies have been done, animal findings are negative.
C	**Risk cannot be ruled out.** Human studies are lacking, and animal studies are either positive for fetal risk or lacking as well. However, potential benefits may justify the potential risk.
D	**Positive evidence of risk.** Investigational or postmarketing data show risk to the fetus. Nevertheless, potential benefits may outweigh the potential risk.
X	**Contraindicated in pregnancy.** Studies in animals or humans, or investigational or postmarketing reports have shown fetal risk that clearly outweighs any possible benefit to the patient.

Source: *Physicians' Desk Reference* (49th ed.). Montvale, NJ. Medical Economics, 1995. P. 2797.

Table 28A-8. Major pathways of antibiotic excretion

Antibiotics primarily excreted by the liver[a]	Antibiotics primarily excreted by the kidneys
Cefoperazone	Aminoglycosides
Chloramphenicol	Aztreonam
Clindamycin	Cephalosporins (other than cefoperazone)
Doxycycline	Imipenem
Erythromycin	Fluoroquinolones[b]
Metronidazole	Penicillin and penicillin derivatives
Nafcillin	Trimethoprim
Rifampin	Tetracycline
Sulfamethoxazole	Vancomycin

[a]In renal failure, dosages usually do not need modifications. See individual chapter discussions.
[b]The fluoroquinolones are excreted by the kidneys to a variable degree depending on the specific agent (see Chap. 28S).

2. **The serum creatinine may not accurately reflect the patient's renal function, especially in the elderly,** who may have decreased creatinine production. The **creatinine clearance is a better measure** of renal function. By modifying the equation of Cockcroft and Gault [11], it is possible to estimate the patient's creatinine clearance from the patient's age, gender, body weight (in kilograms), and serum creatinine [10] as follows:
   a. **Male estimated creatinine clearance =**

   $$\frac{(140 - \text{age}) \times (\text{weight})}{72 \times \text{serum creatinine}}$$

   (1) **Female estimated creatinine clearance = 85% of male value**
   (2) Some prefer to use ideal body weight (IBW), which can be calculated as:
       (a) Male = 50 kg + 2.3 kg per each inch over 5 feet (in height)
       (b) Female = 45.5 kg + 2.3 kg per each inch over 5 feet
   (3) **In the obese patient,** we use IBW to estimate the creatinine clearance.
   b. **If the patient is oliguric,** the creatinine clearance is estimated at < 10 ml/min [10].
   c. **Example:** A 70-year-old man has a weight of 70 kg and a serum creatinine of 2.2. His estimated creatinine clearance is:

   $$\text{Cl}_{cr} \, (\text{ml/min}) = \frac{(140 - 70) \times 70}{72 \times 2.2}$$
   $$= \frac{4,900}{158.4}$$
   $$= 31 \, \text{ml/min}$$

   d. **In patients with severe hepatic insufficiency,** this formula may overestimate the creatinine clearance. See sec. **D.4.**
D. **Liver function.** The half-life of an antibiotic excreted by the liver may be prolonged if there is relative hepatic insufficiency [12] (see individual agent discussions of chloramphenicol, nafcillin, clindamycin, and erythromycin). Unfortunately, there is no easily performed laboratory test to assess for hepatic insufficiency (except possibly a prolonged prothrombin time) comparable to the serum creatinine test in renal failure. Table 28A-8 summarizes agents excreted primarily by the liver. Our understanding of modifying dosages in hepatic insufficiency is not as sophisticated as it is for renal insufficiency [12]. However, **four issues deserve special emphasis** in patients with hepatic insufficiency.
   1. **Aminoglycoside use may be associated with an increased risk of nephrotoxicity,** as reviewed in Chap. 28H.
   2. **Beta-lactam antibiotic use** in one study was **associated with an increased risk of leukopenia** when standard doses of beta-lactam antibiotics were used in patients with underlying liver disease [13]. The probable mechanism is

impaired hepatic metabolism of the beta-lactam antibiotics, resulting in bone marrow suppression of white cell precursors from excessive antibiotic concentrations. The authors proposed a reduction in dosages of beta-lactam antibiotic when used in patients with significant hepatic dysfunction [13].

3. **Drugs primarily excreted or detoxified by the liver** (e.g., chloramphenicol, clindamycin) **need dose adjustments.** Other drugs that should be used with caution or for which serum levels should be monitored include fluconazole, itraconazole, nitrofurantoin, and pyrazinamide [4, 14]. See Table 28A-8 and individual chapter discussions.

4. When selecting a dose for a potentially nephrotoxic drug, creatinine clearance (glomerular filtration rate [GFR]) should be estimated (just as in the elderly) even when the serum creatinine is normal [14].

   a. Normal GFR values are reliable in this setting.

   b. Low GFR may overestimate the true GFR (by two- to threefold) as measured by an inulin clearance. This may be accounted for by underproduction of creatinine resulting from diminished muscle mass or by a decreased rate of hepatic production of creatine, the substrate for the production of creatinine in muscle [14]. To provide a better estimate of GFR in this setting, determination of a creatinine index sometimes is suggested [14].

   In practice for those with an estimated low GFR and severe hepatic disease, we assume their estimated creatinine clearance may be approximately 50% of the calculated estimate using the formula in sec. C.2.

E. **Humoral and cellular host defense mechanisms.** Patients receiving corticosteroid therapy, chemotherapy, or radiation therapy, especially if they are leukopenic, are at risk for bacterial infections. Bactericidal antibiotics usually are preferred in such patients for previously stated reasons.

F. **Prosthetic devices** predispose the host to infections that may be highly subacute at times [15]. See individual chapter topics (e.g., prosthetic valve endocarditis, Chap. 10). It often is necessary to remove the foreign body to cure an infection in the vicinity of a prosthetic heart valve or joint implant [4].

VII. **Question 7. What is the best route of administration?**

A. **Parenteral antibiotics** are almost always used in **serious infections** to ensure adequate blood levels.

1. **Intravenous therapy** is mandatory if **hypotension** is present or in a patient with a **bleeding diathesis** or thrombocytopenia and is preferred when high blood levels are important (e.g., in sepsis, meningitis, at least initial therapy of endocarditis, and gram-negative pneumonias). The absorption of intramuscularly administered antibiotics may be impaired in **diabetic patients** [4]. Therefore, intravenous therapy is preferred in diabetic patients with presumed or known bacteremia [4] or serious illness.

2. **Intramuscular therapy.** Many drugs cannot be tolerated by this route for more than a few doses. Some of the cephalosporins (e.g., cefazolin and ceftriaxone) provide excellent levels after intramuscular injection. Both procaine penicillin and aminoglycosides are well tolerated by intramuscular injection, although absorption of the latter can be unpredictable. Imipenem can be given IM.

3. **Continuous versus intermittent bolus intravenous infusion.** Whether intravenously administered antibiotics should be given by continuous infusion or by intermittent bolus remains controversial [4]. This is reviewed elsewhere [16, 16a].

   a. **Continuous** infusions may result in less vein irritation and phlebitis. Prior animal model studies suggested that concentrations of penicillins and cephalosporins in fibrin clots were related to peak serum levels achieved; therefore, intermittent bolus therapy seemed appropriate for endocarditis and tissue infections [4].

      Recent data suggest that the clinical effectiveness of beta-lactam antibiotics is optimal when the concentration at the site of infection exceeds the minimum inhibitory concentration (MIC) of the infecting organism for a prolonged time (i.e., animal model data favors continuous infusion for serious systemic infections) [4]. This is called **time-dependent bactericidal activity,** which has little relationship to the magnitude of drug concentrations as long as the concentrations are above the MIC or really the minimal bactericidal concentration (MBC, see related discussion in Chap. 25) and includes the **beta-lactam antibiotics and vancomycin** [16a].

Multiple, small, frequent doses or continuous infusions produce similar or superior bactericidal effects compared with infrequently administered larger doses. The exception would be a beta-lactam with a prolonged half-life (e.g., ceftriaxone) that provides persistence of effective levels with infrequent dosing. At this point, while awaiting other clinical data, **we do not advocate using continuous infusions** of time-dependent antibiotics (e.g., beta-lactams).

   b. **Intermittent infusions** may be preferred for antibiotics that exhibit **concentration-dependent bactericidal activity** over a wide range of drug concentrations; i.e., the rate and extent of bactericidal action increase with increasing concentrations above the MBC up to a point of maximum effect, usually 5–10 times the MBC [16a]. The **aminoglycosides and fluoroquinolones** demonstrate this type of activity [4, 16a]; the higher the drug level, the greater the rate of bacterial clearance, which slows as the drug level falls [16a].

   (1) **Potential implications.** Large, infrequently administered doses of concentration-dependent agents (e.g., aminoglycosides) that achieve maximal concentrations at peak at the site of infection should produce optimal bactericidal effect [16a]. This is in large part the **basis for once-daily regimens of aminoglycoside** dosing, which is discussed in detail in Chap. 28H.

   (2) However, clinical studies that clearly prove this approach (e.g., once-daily aminoglycoside dosing) superior to other dosing regimens are still not available.

   Moellering emphasizes that "definitive clinical studies providing unequivocal support for these concepts remain to be carried out" [4]. In his 1995 review, Levison concludes: "The optimal dosing interval of concentration-dependent antimicrobial agents remains an unanswered question for any individual patient and type of infection, and is under study for aminoglycosides" [16a]. Therefore, the long-term clinical implications of this dosing approach await further study.

B. **Oral absorption** of an antibiotic, in general, is often too unpredictable to trust in serious infections.

   1. **Completion of antibiotic therapy.** Well-absorbed oral agents may be used to complete a full course of therapy in uncomplicated infections. For example, in the patient with pyelonephritis, initially with dehydration, who is responding well after 1–4 days of intravenous therapy, one may elect to complete the course of therapy with oral therapy. A patient with a wound infection that required intravenous clindamycin may complete the course with oral clindamycin, as this is well absorbed. See specific discussions of oral cefuroxime (Chap. 28F), clindamycin (Chap. 28I), TMP-SMX (Chap. 28K), metronidazole (Chap. 28P), and the fluoroquinolones (Chap. 28S).

   The new erythromycinlike oral antibiotics (e.g., azithromycin and clarithromycin) are discussed in Chap. 28M.

   2. **Common outpatient infections.** Many common minor infections respond to oral medications: pharyngitis, skin infections, UTIs, mycoplasmal pneumonia, and bronchitis.

   3. **Special situations.** In special circumstances, well-absorbed oral agents may be used in serious infections; for example, TMP-SMX is available as an oral agent and has been used either initially or following intravenous therapy (e.g., in patients with AIDS and *Pneumocystis carinii* pneumonia). See Chap. 24. The new **fluoroquinolones** may allow oral therapy in certain settings (see Chap. 28S).

C. **Home intravenous antibiotics.** In the mid-1970s, various groups began to report their experiences with self-administration of intravenous antibiotics at home. This approach is cost-effective but also has many difficult-to-measure variables in terms of the patient's being at his or her own home and often able to return to school, work, or social functions.

   1. **Types of infections.** Patients with stable infections requiring prolonged intravenous therapy—for example, bone and joint infections, subacute endocarditis, and pulmonary infections in cystic fibrosis patients—are potential candidates.

   2. **Typical criteria for home intravenous therapy** have been reviewed elsewhere and usually include the following [17–22]:

a. **Evidence that infection is controlled.** This includes patients who are afebrile and ready for discharge except for intravenous antibiotics. The patient's course is anticipated to be stable.

b. **Cooperative, motivated patient or family.**

c. **Adequate patient and family education.** The family and patient need to understand the rationale, risks, and necessity for prolonged intravenous therapy. The intravenous team and nursing staff provide this education. **Currently, several intravenous administration approaches are available** [22–25].

(1) **Intravenous minibag administration** of the antibiotic allows the premixed medication to be infused by a **gravity flow system.** This technique has been used since the late 1970s. The patient or designated caregiver administers the antibiotic intermittently, and therefore he or she must understand aseptic technique and demonstrate proficiency at this. Compliance must not be a concern. The patency of these systems is maintained by flushing the intravenous device with heparin and saline [24, 25].

Clinicians have used this approach successfully when a caregiver or patient is able to self-administer the intravenous agent and care for the intravenous access site. Clinicians have tended to prefer simple antibiotic regimens (e.g., monotherapy with dosing q24h, q12h, or possibly q8h) whenever possible.

(2) **Fixed-rate infusion pumps** can infuse a specified volume at a specified rate. For example the elastomeric infusion pump uses a disposable, single-use elastomeric balloon. When filled, the distended balloon forces the medication through a capillary tube with a fixed resistance, thereby allowing fixed-rate drug infusion with no risk of air embolism. Patients can attach the pump to their belts with no impairment of motion [23].

(3) **Computerized ambulatory infusion devices** became available for clinical use in the early 1990s. This device has programmable features that allow a variety of antibiotics to be administered over a wide range of infusion schedules including q4h infusions. In addition, patients who are not candidates for minibag administration of antibiotic, because of age, physical handicaps, lack of family support, or inappropriate home environment, often are candidates for this technique [24].

(4) **Infectious disease consultation is advised** to help determine the optimal antibiotic, dose regimen, and mode of administration as this must be individualized. At times, an oral regimen may be appropriate in some compliant patients. Reimbursement issues may limit options.

d. **Adequate venous access.** Peripheral vein intravenous catheters (changed every 3 days), peripheral inserted central catheter lines, or a Hickman catheter have been used; the best method must be individualized [23].

e. **Backup plan for problems.** A sequential plan (e.g., nurse, doctor, emergency room) must be known to the patient and family. A summary, given to the patient, of the patient's problem, plan, dosage, and supervising physicians will be helpful in case an emergency arises.

f. **Inpatient trial of all medications before home use.** This is important to exclude any obvious immediate side effects or potential drug interactions. Consultation with an individual with a special interest in infectious diseases and with the pharmacy will help ensure the proper choice of drug and the most convenient dose interval.

g. **Proper refrigeration.** The patient must have access to a refrigerator (or freezer) at home to store the medications (usually a 3- to 7-day supply is provided at a time).

3. **Periodic follow-up,** either by a visiting nurse or by return for outpatient visits, is essential.

4. **Serial blood work** (e.g., blood counts, urinalysis, hepatic or renal function tests, aminoglycoside levels when indicated) can be obtained at the home or by periodic clinic visits.

5. **Side effects and problems.** These do not seem to occur any more frequently than in hospitalized patients and usually occur less often.

6. **Miscellaneous**
   a. **Patient satisfaction** usually is very high with this approach.

   b. **A team approach** is necessary for selection of patients, patient education, selection of proper agent, and follow-up [17–22].
   c. **Cost-effectiveness.** Home parenteral antibiotic therapy has been shown to save between 68 and 78% of the costs required for in-hospital care [21]. Third-party reimbursement schedules may vary and need to be considered in planning home programs.

VIII. **Question 8. What is the appropriate dose?** To reduce the risk of side effects, the potential of superinfection, and the cost of therapy, generally the lowest dose of antibiotic that will be efficacious is used.
   A. **Dosage in neonates.** See Chap. 3.
   B. **Dosage in children and adults.** See discussions under individual agents.

IX. **Question 9. Will initial therapy need modification after culture data are available?** Once the results of cultures and antibiotic susceptibility data are available, the antibiotic regimen should be modified when possible. Some general guidelines follow:
   A. **Narrow- versus broad-spectrum agent.** A narrow-spectrum agent should be used whenever possible to decrease the risk of colonization and possible superinfection with resistant organisms. (See sec. **X.B.**)
   B. ***S. aureus* susceptible to penicillin.** If *S. aureus* organisms are susceptible to penicillin, this narrow-spectrum agent should be used rather than a semisynthetic penicillin because it is the most active agent against that organism.
   C. **Gram-negative infections.** In known or suspected gram-negative infections, an aminoglycoside often is used in initial presumptive therapy. If the identified pathogen is susceptible to an agent with narrow spectrum (e.g., ampicillin or a cephalosporin), a change is made to these agents as long as the patient has no contraindication to their use [3].
   D. **Multiple negative initial cultures.** If appropriate cultures were obtained and handled properly, negative cultures raise the question of other diagnostic possibilities. For example, in the patient with pneumonia doing poorly on ampicillin yet in whom the routine cultures yield only normal flora, other infectious agents (mycoplasma, *Mycobacterium tuberculosis, Legionella* spp.) or even noninfectious possibilities (e.g., pulmonary infarct, pulmonary vasculitis) must be considered.
   E. **Assessment after antibiotics are initiated.** It is important for the clinician to assess the clinical course of the patient as well as the culture data. For example, colonization with new organisms is expected with antibiotic use. New colonization must be differentiated from new infection. If the patient is improving and then an organism resistant to the antibiotic in use is isolated on follow-up cultures, it can usually be ignored. This is particularly important in wound and sputum culture interpretation. (See Chaps. 4 and 9.)

X. **Question 10. What is the optimal duration of therapy, and is the development of resistance during prolonged therapy likely to occur?**
   A. **Duration.** The optimal duration of antibiotic therapy may be well established (e.g., a minimum of 4 weeks in osteomyelitis) or relatively empiric (10–14 days of therapy for peritonitis). This must be individualized. Typical durations of therapy for common problems are shown in Table 28A-9.
      With the increasing concerns of bacterial resistance, it will become even more important for the clinician to treat the patient for an adequate, but not an unnecessarily prolonged, period to reduce the likelihood of selecting out resistant pathogens.
   B. **Development of resistance.** A detailed discussion of bacterial resistance is beyond the scope of this discussion but is reviewed elsewhere [26–32]. Bacteria have several mechanisms of acquired antimicrobial resistance, including a change in the drug target, the production of a detoxifying enzyme, or decreased antibiotic uptake (see Table 28A-10).
      1. **See related discussion of increasing bacterial resistance** in sec. II under Miscellaneous Aspects of Antibiotic Use, later in this chapter (p. 1089).
      2. **Broad versus narrow antibiotic therapy.** What has become increasingly clear is that **using a broader-spectrum agent than is necessary** (e.g., a third-generation cephalosporin rather than a first-generation cephalosporin) **appears to be associated with an increased likelihood of the development of multiresistant bacteria** [29–31]. Patients infected with antibiotic-resistant organisms are more likely to require hospitalization, have a longer hospital stay, and be at an increased risk of death [26, 29, 30].

Table 28A-9. Duration of antibiotic therapy for common infections

Diagnosis	Duration of therapy (days)
Meningococcal meningitis	7–10
Pneumococcal meningitis	10–14
Haemophilus influenzae type b meningitis	10–14
Streptococcal group A pharyngitis	10
Otitis media	7–10
Bacterial sinusitis	10–14
Pneumococcal pneumonia	? optimal[a]
Gram-negative pneumonias (*Klebsiella, Enterobacter, Pseudomonas*)	? 21[b]
Mycoplasma pneumonia	14[c]
Legionella pneumonia	21[c]
Endocarditis (nonprosthetic)	
Viridans streptococci	28[d]
Staphylococcal	28–42
Peritonitis	10–14
Septic arthritis (nongonococcal)	14–21[e]
Osteomyelitis	28[f]

[a]Most experts agree that therapy should be continued at least 3 days after the temperature returns to normal. Elderly patients probably deserve 7 days of parenteral therapy.
[b]Difficult to eradicate; patients may require even longer courses.
[c]To prevent relapse, a full therapeutic course should be given.
[d]Some patients may be candidates for 2 weeks of penicillin combined with an aminoglycoside. Infectious disease consultation is advised.
[e]Four weeks of therapy may be indicated in patients with gram-negative infections, slowly responding infections (despite adequate drainage), or infections with virulent organisms such as *S. aureus*.
[f]In vertebral osteomyelitis, patients often are treated for 6 weeks.

Table 28A-10. General mechanisms of resistance to antimicrobial agents

Resistance mechanism	Specific examples
Diminished intracellular drug concentration	
Increased efflux	Tetracyclines
	Quinolones
Decreased outer membrane permeability	Beta-lactams
	Quinolones
Decreased cytoplasmic membrane transport	Aminoglycosides (decreased energy)
Drug inactivation (reversible or irreversible)	Beta-lactams (beta-lactamases)
	Aminoglycosides (modifying enzymes)
	Fosfomycin (glutathione binding)
	Choramphenicol (inactivating enzymes)
Target modification	Quinolones (gyrase modifications)
	Rifampin (DNA polymerase binding)
	Beta lactams (PBP changes)
	Macrolides (rRNA methylation)
Target bypass	Glycopeptides
	Trimethoprim (thymine-deficient strains)

PBP = penicillin-binding proteins.
Source: From H.S. Fralmow and E. Abrutyn, Pathogens resistant to antimicrobial agents: Epidemiology, molecular mechanisms, and clinical management. *Infect. Dis. Clin. North Am.* 9:497, 1995.

Therefore, it is particularly important for the clinician to use the new broad-spectrum agents carefully to help minimize the development of bacterial resistance [26, 29–31]. This usually involves some type of hospitalwide antibiotic control program [32] and rational use of antibiotics [33, 34]. Cautious conservation is advocated in the use of new antimicrobial agents [34]. See related discussions in Chaps. 28F and 28H, and later in this chapter in sec. **II,** under Miscellaneous Aspects of Antibiotic Use.

Using the Antibiotic Checklist

The stepwise approach to antibiotic therapy is emphasized in the following complex clinical problem.

I. **Using the checklist (see Table 28A-1)**
  A. **Illustrative case.** A 45-year-old woman on chronic hemodialysis comes to the emergency room with shaking chills, malaise, and fever of 2 days' duration. She has no localizing symptoms or signs except for a wound infection around her arteriovenous (AV) fistula site. A Gram stain of the wound drainage reveals gram-positive cocci, and the exudate is submitted for culture. The patient has a mild leukocytosis. She has been taking no antibiotics recently but claims she had an immediate anaphylactic reaction after intravenous penicillin 1 year ago. Two blood cultures are obtained over a 45- to 60-minute period. The series of questions given in Table 28A-1 is applied as follows.
    1. **Is an antibiotic indicated on the basis of the clinical findings?** Yes. The patient has chills and leukocytosis and probably is bacteremic.
    2. **Have appropriate specimens been obtained, examined, and sent for culture?** Because the patient has chills, two blood cultures separated in time (by at least 20–30 minutes) are drawn to help identify the organism involved and determine the duration of the bacteremia. The duration of bacteremia may, in turn, help determine duration of the antibiotic therapy. A swab of the exudate from the AV fistula site is submitted for culture, and a Gram stain of this material reveals many polymorphonuclear leukocytes and clumps of gram-positive cocci.
    3. **What organisms are most likely to be causing the infection?** The Gram stain reveals gram-positive cocci. In the absence of other findings, antibiotics must be directed against a presumed gram-positive cocci infection, particularly staphylococci (*S. aureus* and *S. epidermidis*) (see Table 28A-2).
    4. **If several antibiotics are available to treat this likely or known organism, which agent is the best for this patient?** (See Table 28A-3.) While awaiting susceptibility results for presumed *S. aureus* or streptococcal infection, the drug of choice would usually be a penicillinase-resistant penicillin. However, because MRSA are potential pathogens, vancomycin is preferred, especially in institutions that have high rates of MRSA infections.
        Is there something about the pharmacology, toxicology, or cost of the agent that affects the initial choice? Yes; because this patient is penicillin-allergic, an alternative agent must be used. A cephalosporin is a common alternative agent for *S. aureus,* but because the patient had immediate anaphylaxis to penicillin a year ago, she requires skin testing and an allergy consultation before using these agents (see Chap. 27). Clindamycin is an alternative choice but is not a bactericidal agent nor is it active against *S. epidermidis*. In the septic patient in whom a secondary endocarditis is possible, one would prefer a bactericidal drug. The third choice listed in Table 28A-3 is vancomycin. This is a bactericidal agent, safe in penicillin-allergic patients, and effective against gram-positive cocci, including *S. aureus* and coagulase-negative staphylococci, including methicillin-resistant strains.
    5. **Is an antibiotic combination appropriate?** Because the patient is penicillin-allergic, a semisynthetic penicillin and an aminoglycoside cannot be used for a possible *S. aureus* bacteremia (see Chap. 2). Vancomycin is typically used as a single agent against staphylococcal and nonenterococcal streptococcal infections.
    6. **Are there special considerations related specifically to host factors** involving the use of vancomycin in this particular patient? Yes, the patient's renal failure must be considered. Vancomycin is primarily excreted by the kidneys,

and it is poorly dialyzed; therefore, the interval between doses must be prolonged and levels ideally should be monitored. See Chap. 28O.

7. **What is the best route of administration?** Oral vancomycin is poorly absorbed, and intramuscular vancomycin is painful. Therefore, vancomycin should be given intravenously.

8. **What is the appropriate dose and dose interval?** See Chap. 28O, in which vancomycin dosages are discussed.

9. **Will initial therapy need modification after culture data are returned?** If the cultures yield methicillin-resistant *S. aureus,* vancomycin will be continued. If methicillin-susceptible *S. aureus* is isolated, skin testing to see whether a first-generation cephalosporin can be used is a consideration, although in a patient with renal failure, periodic doses of vancomycin probably are more practical. (When oxacillin is contraindicated but a first-generation cephalosporin is not, some experts prefer a first-generation cephalosporin rather than vancomycin as an antistaphylococcal agent. See Chap. 28O).

10. **What is the optimal duration of treatment, and is the development of resistance during prolonged therapy likely to occur?** This must be individualized. If the patient continued to have fever and chills and further blood cultures were drawn and were positive for *S. aureus,* endocarditis or endothelial infection of the vascular access site is likely. Resistance to vancomycin does not develop during therapy.

B. **Conclusion.** Going through the checklist of questions is helpful for achieving a rational choice and recognizing obvious potential problems (drug allergies, dose adjustments in renal failure, choice of route of administration, and so on). Because of all the variables, a **stepwise approach helps one to reach a rational decision.** The important clinical, pharmacokinetic, toxic, and special characteristics of the major antibiotic agents are discussed in the chapters that review specific antibiotics.

Miscellaneous Aspects of Antibiotic Use

I. **Important side effects** of each agent are discussed in the individual chapters that follow. Some side effects warrant special attention.

A. **Morbilliform rash and other antibiotic allergic reactions** with penicillin or penicillin derivatives are discussed in Chap. 27.

B. *Clostridium difficile* diarrhea associated with antibiotic use has been reviewed elsewhere [35–40].

1. **Pathophysiology.** Bartlett [35] emphasized the four critical components for *C. difficile*–induced disease.

a. There must be a **disturbance** in the mechanisms responsible for the **balance of bacteria** in the colon. Alterations of the intestinal flora permit overgrowth by *C. difficile* and production of its toxins. **Antibiotics usually are implicated;** occasionally, only chemotherapeutic agents are involved, and these agents have been associated with alteration of bowel flora and growth of *C. difficile* [41]. The diarrhea can develop while the patient is receiving antibiotics or up to 4–6 weeks after a course of antibiotics. Clindamycin, ampicillin, and the cephalosporins have particularly been implicated [35], whereas metronidazole, vancomycin, the fluoroquinolones, TMP-SMX, or the aminoglycosides have less frequently been associated with it [38].

b. There must be a **source of *C. difficile* in the colon, either from endogenous flora (e.g., *C. difficile* is located in the stool of approximately 3% of healthy, nonhospitalized patients) or from an exogenous source. After a few days in the hospital, stool cultures of 10–30% of patients become colonized with this organism** [35, 36]. Although *C. difficile* has been isolated from a variety of healthy animals, animals are not considered important in the transmission of the organism to humans [36].

c. The *C. difficile* must have the potential for producing **toxin. Nearly 25% of isolates** from humans lack genes for production of toxins A and B and are **nontoxicogenic;** these never cause diarrhea or colitis [36]. Toxin-producing strains produce both toxin A and toxin B. Presumably, toxin A is associated with producing the clinical findings, whereas toxin B is responsible for the cytopathic changes detected in the standard cell culture assay. Epidemiologic studies have shown that patients colonized with *C. difficile* non-toxin-producing strains are asymptomatic. In contrast, patients colonized with a toxin-producing strain often develop clinical symptoms.

   d. **Age** of the host is important. For unexplained reasons, patients older than 50 years are most susceptible to *C. difficile* diarrhea. In contrast, neonates can often be colonized (60–70%) with this organism yet have no symptoms [36]. Patients undergoing surgery (especially abdominal surgery) and patients in intensive care units may also be at higher risk [36].

2. **Clinical manifestations.** *C. difficile* **causes a spectrum** of disease ranging from asymptomatic carriage, to mild or severe diarrhea, to life-threatening colitis [35–38].

   a. **Diarrhea** is watery and profuse and foul-smelling and, usually, more than six episodes occur per 24 hours. Typically, diarrhea begins 4–9 days after starting antibiotics but may begin as soon as 24 hours after administration. Diarrhea can occur after single doses of prophylactic antibiotics. In as many as 20% of patients, diarrhea does not begin until up to 6 weeks after antibiotics have been stopped [36]. Sometimes the stool is bloody. Approximately 50% of the patients will have leukocytes in smears of the stool [36].

   b. **Crampy abdominal pain** is common, and abdominal tenderness may be present on examination.

   c. **Fever** (39–40°C or more) can occur [36].

   d. **Laboratory studies.** Leukocytosis is common, and even a leukemoid reaction can occur. **Hypoalbuminemia** is frequent.

   e. **Course of untreated disease.** This is variable. Some patients have trivial diarrhea that stops when the antibiotic is discontinued. Others may have chronic diarrhea for weeks or even months [35]. **Probably the majority develop fever, abdominal tenderness, leukocytosis, and hypoalbuminemia.**

   f. **Complications** of severe disease (pseudomembranous colitis) include toxic megacolon, colonic perforation, severe electrolyte imbalance, dehydration, hypoalbuminemia, and anasarca. Some patients may have little or no diarrhea but present with toxic megacolon, colonic perforation, or peritonitis. (The diagnosis of *C. difficile* may be suggested on abdominal CT scanning; see sec. **3.e**). Rare cases of polyarthritis have occurred [39].

3. **Diagnosis.** *C. difficile* **diarrhea is a common cause of diarrhea of hospitalized patients, especially in those patients with onset of diarrhea more than 3 days after admission** [39].

   a. **Cell culture toxin assay,** originally used to identify this entity, still is the **most sensitive diagnostic test** [35]. Because the cell lines are difficult to maintain in the laboratory, this assay often is not available.

   b. **Stool cultures** for *C. difficile* are facilitated by special selective culture media (containing cycloserine, cefoxitin, and fructose in agar [CCFA media]), but precise identification of this clostridial species may be difficult, particularly for small microbiology laboratories.

   c. **Rapid tests**

      (1) **Latex-particle agglutination assay.** Though this assay was originally thought to detect toxin A, subsequent work indicates that the capturing antibody is not antibody to toxin A but antibody to another protein of no clear biologic significance [35]. Although experience with this assay is variable, overall **the positive predictive value of this test is** a **disappointing** 60–80% [35]. **We are not in favor of using this test** as the sole method of diagnosing *C. difficile* diarrhea, if at all.

      (2) **Counterimmunoelectrophoresis (CIE)** has been used to detect toxin B in stool, but because this test uses nonspecific antisera, the results have been nonspecific [36].

      (3) **Enzyme immunoassay (EIA)** for toxin A is available and **is a useful** technique, especially for hospital laboratories that are unable to perform the tissue culture assay and *C. difficile* stool cultures.

      (4) **Investigational tests.** Hybridization probe or polymerase chain reaction (PCR) for toxin A and toxin B are undergoing evaluation.

   d. **Endoscopy.** Although useful, endoscopy seldom is used for diagnosis because of its cost, inconvenience, and the availability of the toxin assay [35]. It is a **useful procedure if an immediate answer is needed or in patients with relapsing diarrhea in whom another diagnosis may be confirmed**

      with endoscopy. Routine flexible sigmoidoscopy may miss 10–30% of the characteristic mucosal lesions; therefore, colonoscopy is the most definitive procedure [35].

    e. Computerized tomography (CT) of the abdomen may be helpful if colonoscopy is contraindicated [36], but specific CT features of *C. difficile* are uncommon [42]. Positive scans may show a characteristic thickening of the colon, with contrast medium trapped in the folds (i.e., the so-called accordion sign) [38].

    f. In severe colitis, **barium studies** may precipitate toxic megacolon, perforation, or other complications and are **not recommended** [36].

  4. Therapy in adults. The offending antibiotic should be discontinued if possible. This alone may be adequate therapy for mild cases. If patients improve in 48 hours, supportive therapy can be continued and the diarrhea usually will subside over the next several days. For moderate to severe cases or prolonged symptoms, specific therapy is indicated. **Oral antibiotic therapy is required** to ensure high stool concentrations of the antibiotic used. If systemic antibiotics are important to continue for other sites of infection, therapy for *C. difficile* is added to the patient's regimen as follows [35, 36]:

    a. Mild to moderate cases are treated with oral metronidazole, 250 mg qid, usually for 10–14 days [38]. **Oral vancomycin is much more expensive** than metronidazole (see Table 28A-5), **and widespread use of oral vancomycin may be contributing to the increasing noted problems with vancomycin-resistant enterococci** (see Chap. 28O). Therefore, in mild to moderate disease, **metronidazole is preferred** [3].

    b. Severe disease. Many experts prefer oral vancomycin in very severe or life-threatening disease [35–38]. The dose of oral vancomycin in adults is 125 mg qid for 10–14 days. **Because of increasing concerns with vancomycin-resistant enterococci (see Chap. 28O), we try to limit the use of oral vancomycin.**

    c. Oral bacitracin (25,000 units or 500 mg qid) has been used for 10–14 days instead of metronidazole or vancomycin. Clinical response is slower and less reliable; further data are needed [36].

    d. If oral therapy is not possible, the best approach is unclear. Preliminary data suggest that intravenous metronidazole is preferred over intravenous vancomycin [43]. Fekety [36] suggests that when parenteral therapy is essential (as in patients with adynamic ileus), treatment with both intravenous vancomycin and intravenous metronidazole (500 mg q6h) is reasonable. This is supplemented with vancomycin given by nasogastric tube at higher-than-usual dosages (500 mg PO q6h) or into ileostomies or colostomies or by enema. Serum vancomycin levels should be monitored in this setting [36].

    e. Cholestyramine resin (4 g PO q6h) **may be used alone in mild disease** (or relapses). It binds toxin B, and probably toxin A [36], and firms up the stool due to its naturally desiccating side effects. It may also bind vancomycin, so their simultaneous use should be avoided [36].

    f. The role of lactobacilli replacement is unclear. See sec. **7.**

    g. Opiates and antiperistaltic agents should be avoided. They are especially dangerous in infants. These agents may provide symptomatic relief (because of pooling of fluid within the lumen of the intestines) but, because of toxin retention in the colon, more severe damage to the colon may occur [36].

  5. Therapy in children [44]. Whenever feasible, antibiotic therapy should be discontinued.

    a. Vancomycin. In patients with severe toxicity or in whom diarrhea persists after antimicrobial therapy is discontinued, oral vancomycin is the **drug of choice** at a dose of 40 mg/kg/day in four divided doses, usually for 10 days.

    b. Metronidazole, orally and intravenously, at 35 mg/kg/day in four divided doses, also is effective and less expensive. However, its **safety has not been established in children,** and the drug is not currently approved by the FDA for this indication [44].

    c. Cholestyramine has not been evaluated in children in this setting [44].

  6. Infection control aspects. *C. difficile* diarrhea has been recognized as a common nosocomial pathogen capable of causing epidemics [45, 46]. The **hands of caregivers are important in nosocomial spread** [45–47]. Routine handwashing with chlorhexidine helps reduce hand colonization with *C. difficile* organisms and, presumably, subsequent spread [45]. However, many caregivers develop a dermatitis if this agent is used routinely. One study suggests that the **use of vinyl gloves by hospital personnel** during patient care is beneficial in controlling this nosocomial problem [47]. DNA fingerprinting techniques have shown that a toxin-producing strain of *C. difficile* may spread rapidly from patient to patient if proper infection control methods are not used.

7. **Relapses after a therapeutic course.** The exact role environmental contamination with *C. difficile* plays in nosocomial transmission remains unclear [48]. **Approximately 10–20% of patients have recurrent diarrhea after a course of oral vancomycin or metronidazole** [35–37]. Some of these cases probably represent a new infection, with a new strain of *C. difficile*, usually in a debilitated host, rather than true relapse. **The best approach** in these patients **is unclear.** Repeat 7- to 14-day courses of oral metronidazole or vancomycin therapy usually are used. Longer courses of therapy do not eradicate the carrier state and do not appear to be more efficacious in preventing recurrences. In fact, shorter courses of antibiotics may permit more rapid restoration of normal fecal flora, which in some way inhibits *C. difficile* [36].

Approximately 3% of *C. difficile* isolates may be metronidazole-resistant; vancomycin resistance has not been identified. For mild to moderate recurrent illness, we often use another course of oral metronidazole. For patients with severe disease, we would favor oral vancomycin. Treatment options for refractory cases with several relapses is unclear [35–38]. See references [36] and [38] for options.

The role of colonizing the colon with oral lactobacilli is unclear. We have anecdotally tried lactobacilli (Bacid capsules, one capsule = 500,000 organisms) with a dose of one to two capsules tid in adults.

Saccharomyces boulardii is a novel living nonpathogenic biotherapeutic agent that has been used in France since the 1950s for the treatment of diarrhea. It is undergoing clinical study in the United States, and preliminary studies suggest it may be beneficial in *C. difficile* diarrhea. Further studies with this agent are under way [36].

C. **Nephrotoxicity** is of concern especially with the aminoglycosides (see Chap. 28H). Interstitial nephritis is discussed in Chap. 28D and under individual agents.

D. **Neurotoxicity** manifested as seizure disorders, encephalopathy, neuropsychiatric symptoms, cranial nerve dysfunction, or peripheral neuropathies may occasionally occur with antimicrobial agents [49]. Imipenem-associated seizures are reviewed in Chap. 28G.

E. **Bone marrow suppression** occurs fairly commonly with some agents (e.g., chloramphenicol) and infrequently with other agents (e.g., nafcillin, vancomycin, TMP-SMX). Patients on prolonged antibiotic therapy need serial complete blood cell counts to help monitor for this side effect. See related discussion of leukopenia seen in patients with underlying hepatic disease and beta-lactam antibiotic use in sec. **VI.D.2.**

F. **Hypoprothrombinemia** is discussed in Chap. 28F under Individual Agents, sec. **V.D.** (p. 1209).

G. **Hepatotoxicity** occurs more commonly with antituberculous agents but can be seen at times with antibacterials such as oxacillin and TMP-SMX (the latter especially in AIDS patients). (See individual agent discussions.) Patients on prolonged antibiotic therapy should probably have liver function tests weekly.

H. **Drug interactions** can occur at times and may be clinically relevant (e.g., erythromycin and ciprofloxacin may elevate theophylline levels; erythromycin and the newer macrolides may elevate serum terfenadine [Seldane] or astemizole [Hismanol] levels). Potentially important drug interactions are discussed in the chapters on individual antibiotics and are summarized elsewhere [50, 51].

II. **Increasing bacterial resistance** has been emphasized in recent reviews [52–56] as well as in the media. Although an extensive discussion of this topic is beyond the scope of this text, several issues deserve special emphasis.

A. **Background.** After the introduction of sulfonamides in the middle to late 1930s and penicillin in the early 1940s, pharmaceutical companies have introduced antibiotics to combat resistant bacteria. These agents included, in the late 1950s, the semisynthetic penicillins to treat penicillin-resistant *S. aureus* and, in the 1960s–1980s, cephalosporins and aminoglycosides for hospital-acquired organisms, especially gram-negative bacilli. Vancomycin (available 1958) has been useful to treat increasing problems associated with MRSA. The concept of an untreatable bacterial disease is foreign to most physicians in the developing world [52] but, if recent bacterial-resistant trends continue, it may become a reality.

B. **Current dilemma.** In the past decade, there has been a **worrisome rise in resistant,** often multidrug-resistant, **bacteria**—not only in hospital-acquired bacteria but also community-acquired bacteria and *M. tuberculosis*—in the United States and worldwide [52–56]. Many of these topics are discussed elsewhere in this book.

1. **Nosocomial infections.** In the past decade, gram-positive bacteria have emerged as the most frequent causes of nosocomial infection [56].

   a. **Coagulase-negative staphylococci** commonly cause prosthetic device and catheter-related infections, and 60–90% of strains are methicillin-resistant [56].

   b. Methicillin-resistant *S. aureus* can account for 5–40% of *S. aureus* infections, depending on the size and type of hospital. See Chap. 28D.

   c. **Enterococci** are the third most common nosocomial pathogen (after *S. aureus* and *E. coli*) and in 1993 vancomycin-resistant enterococci were reported in up to 14% of intensive care unit enterococcal isolates, a 20-fold increase since 1987 [56]. See Chap. 28O.

   d. Multidrug-resistant *P. aeruginosa* and *P. cepacia* have become common in patients with cystic fibrosis. Multidrug-resistant *Acinetobacter* spp. can occur in intensive care units [56].

   e. When broad-spectrum cephalosporins are used, cephalosporin-resistant *Enterobacter* spp. emerge. Fortunately, they usually remain susceptible to aminoglycosides (see Chap. 28F).

      Multidrug-resistant outbreaks of *Klebsiella* spp. have been reported [57], presumably related to selection pressure from widespread use of late-generation cephalosporins; they usually are susceptible to imipenem.

2. **Community-acquired infections**

   a. In recent years, *Neisseria gonorrhoeae* (see Chap. 13), *Salmonella,* and *Shigella* spp. (see Chap. 11) have shown increasing resistance.

   b. **Multidrug-resistant *M. tuberculosis*** is a serious and increasing problem in the United States and worldwide (see Chap. 9). Case fatality rates of 40–60% occur in patients with normal immunity, and 80% mortality occurs in the immunocompromised population [56].

   c. The increasing and ominous problem of *S. pneumoniae* resistant to penicillin and other antibiotics is discussed in detail in Chap. 28C.

   d. Ampicillin-resistant *H. influenzae* and *Branhamella (Moraxella) catarrhalis* are reviewed in Chaps. 5, 7, and 28E.

C. **Risk factors** for emergence of resistant bacteria are partially understood and reviewed in detail elsewhere [52–58]. Several points should be emphasized.

1. **Antibiotic use, and abuse** helps to select out resistant bacteria [52–57].

   a. Enterococci are intrinsically resistant to cephalosporins. With the increased popularity of cephalosporins in recent years, enterococcus as a colonizer and as a cause of nosocomial infections has increased. Furthermore, intravenous vancomycin used for staphylococcal infections and oral vancomycin used for *C. difficile* may help select vancomycin-resistant enterococci. See Chap. 28O.

   b. **Often, new antibiotics are used excessively** so that resistance develops more rapidly than anticipated and, in time, the agent has lost its effectiveness. Kunin [55] emphasizes "the pattern of discovery, exuberant use, and predictable obsolescence has been repeated after the introduction of each new antimicrobial drug." See related discussion of the fluoroquinolones' use and abuse in Chap. 28S. A recent report notes the increased use of broad-spectrum antibiotics in office practices [59]. Not only is resistance an increasing problem with aerobic cocci and gram-negative bacilli, but also excess antibiotic use may be selecting out resistant anaerobes (e.g., *Bacteroides* spp.). See Chap. 28I.

   c. **Long-term use** of antibiotics may pose a greater risk for antimicrobial resistance than short-term use or prophylaxis [52].

   d. **Widespread use of antibiotics in animals**—both short-term therapeutic use and subtherapeutic doses to prevent infection and promote growth—promotes resistance in animals and humans [52, 60].

2. **Microbial characteristics** [52] may facilitate the development of resistance.

   a. The **propensity to exchange genetic material easily or mutate** and adapt to a changing environment are important properties of bacteria [58].

   b. **Reservoirs** or "niches" may be important to allow the organism to prolifer-
      ate. Patients who harbor resistant organisms may be reservoirs and spread-
      ers of resistant pathogens.
   c. The **intrinsic resistance** of an organism may help facilitate resistance. See
      sec. **1.a.**
   d. The ability of an organism to survive on inanimate surfaces (e.g., *C. difficile*)
      may allow it to spread and survive.
3. **Society and environmental aspects**
   a. **Daycare centers** allow for "sharing" of many bacteria, with secondary
      spread to family members and other attendees.
   b. **Crowding, homelessness, poor nutrition,** and **inadequate care** are condu-
      cive to the transmission of infectious diseases and therefore promote multi-
      drug-resistant organisms (e.g., *M. tuberculosis*).
   c. **Poor sanitation and crowding** facilitate the spread of bacteria in devel-
      oping countries.
   d. **Behavioral aspects** of a society can affect the spread of bacteria, as in the
      sexual transmission of gonococci and disease associated with intravenous
      drug use.
   e. **Erosion of the public health infrastructure in the United States** due to
      cost-containing policies or complacency has decreased public health activi-
      ties such as supervised therapy for tuberculosis and surveillance of im-
      portant infectious diseases [52, 58, 61]. For example, national surveillance
      of drug-resistant *M. tuberculosis* was discontinued in 1984 and was only
      reinstituted in 1993. Surveillance of foodborne disease is inadequate in
      most areas of the United States, and many outbreaks go undetected [58].
   f. **Changes in food production, processing, and distribution** may compro-
      mise food safety and increase foodborne illnesses [58]. See Chap. 11.
4. **Other contributing factors**
   a. **International travel** exposes the traveler to resistant pathogens in both
      developing and developed countries and allows the traveler to spread infec-
      tion from one country to another.
   b. As **patients live longer and undergo more immunosuppression,** a larger
      population is at risk for infection, invasive procedures, and antibiotic
      therapy.
   c. **Invasive procedures** (including central venous catheters) **and foreign bod-
      ies** as a consequence of these procedures expose patients to nosocomial
      infectious complications.
   d. **Resistant bacteria are as virulent as susceptible bacteria.** Because of
      the disproportionately high incidence of multidrug-resistant bacteria in
      hospitals, the argument has been made that resistant pathogens are dan-
      gerous only to severely ill patients [56] and overall may be less virulent
      especially to "normal hosts." This does not appear to be the case. Both
      methicillin-resistant and methicillin-susceptible *S. aureus* are capable of
      producing toxins, and the frequency and spectrum of staphylococcal dis-
      eases caused by susceptible and resistant strains appear to be the same [56].
D. **Urgency of situation with multidrug-resistant bacteria.** In the recent report of the
   Rockefeller University Workshop on multidrug-resistant bacteria, the participants
   concluded that the epidemiologic data in the United States suggest that we have
   already "reached the point that health agencies should be able to (and need to)
   take steps to avert a potential crisis. In particular, the acquisition of resistance
   to vancomycin, either by MRSA or resistant *S. pneumoniae,* would create highly
   invasive clones that could not be controlled by any currently available chemotherapeutic agent. Indeed, the transfer and expression of vancomycin resistance to
   staphylococci have already been demonstrated in the laboratory, and their emergence in clinical strains may only be a matter of time" [56].
   Kunin [55] writes, "We have now reached an unacceptable situation. Some
   hospital strains of invasive gram-negative enteric bacteria and enterococci are
   not susceptible to any available drug. Multiply-resistant tubercle bacilli have
   appeared and spread rapidly . . . [Furthermore] the situation has now reached a
   crisis stage worldwide and is predicted to worsen with the introduction of new
   quinolones, macrolides, and oral cephalosporins."
E. **Proposed solutions to the problem**
   1. **Awareness of the problem.** Special efforts should be made to bring the issue
      of antibiotic resistance to the attention of microbiologists, government health

authorities, physicians [56], and especially the lay public, in an appropriate manner.

2. **More prudent use of antibiotics in humans and animals is critical** in developing and developed countries [52, 55, 56, 62, 63]. These are **global issues,** not just applicable to the United States.

   a. Provider education, antibiotic control programs, shorter courses of antibiotics when feasible (e.g., 3-day therapy for uncomplicated UTI; see Chap. 12), and narrow-spectrum agents when feasible (see prior discussion in sec. **X.B.2** under Antibiotic Checklist) are all appropriate approaches. The unrealistic demand for and, at times, poor compliance with antibiotic regimens by patients must also be dealt with.

   b. **Antibiotic control programs,** particularly involving third-generation cephalosporins [57, 64], help reduce the incidence of bacterial resistance associated with excess use. See Chap. 28F.

   c. Appropriate pharmaceutical advertising and promotion is essential [65, 66].

   d. Antimicrobial use in animals must be reviewed and improved [52].

3. **Improved surveillance.** Funding for, and interest in, surveillance systems at the state and national level has declined in recent years in the United States [56, 58, 61]. This needs to be rectified. Multidrug-resistant *S. pneumoniae,* drug-resistant group A streptococci, and vancomycin-resistant enterococci should be reportable to the Centers for Disease Control [56]. Better global surveillance has been suggested also [52, 56, 67].

4. **Increasing funding for basic research** in mechanisms of resistance, vaccine development, and development of novel interventions is needed. Unfortunately, in recent years, the funding for research of bacterial disease has been reduced substantially by the National Institutes of Health [56].

5. **New antibacterial agents** [56, 62]. With initial success of the many antibiotic agents released in the late 1980s and early 1990s, many pharmaceutical companies reduced their antibacterial research efforts in recent years. As a result, fewer antibiotics are expected to be released in the immediate future. New research in this area is needed [67a]. It is hoped that development can be expedited, possibly even with a "fast track" for new antibiotics for multidrug-resistant bacteria.

6. **Prevention of transmission with infection control** practices, improved sanitation conditions in developing countries, and improved care of the homeless, those in crowded conditions, and so on is needed. Rapid diagnostic tests and rapid treatment with effective antimicrobials also will help reduce transmission.

7. **Hospital administrations** are encouraged to support and pursue a **multidisciplinary** systems-oriented **approach** to these problems as recently emphasized in a 1996 report [67b]. Each hospital should establish its own strategies (1) to optimize the prophylactic, empiric, and therapeutic use of antimicrobials in the hospital, and (2) to detect, report, and prevent transmission of antimicrobial-resistant microorganisms [67b].

F. **Summary.** To deal with this increasing problem of multidrug-resistant bacteria and reverse this trend, we agree with Dr. Levy [62] who emphasizes, "The answer lies in efforts from all of us—physician, patient, microbiologist, public health official (and governmental policy officials), and manufacturer. No one can sit back and expect someone else to solve the problem. In the past, we have relied on the pharmaceutical companies to develop new drugs to deal with resistance—and they have largely succeeded. But, the ability to stay one step ahead of the bacteria has led to a complacency about the resistance problem. We can no longer maintain this attitude. No new family of antibiotics can be anticipated in the present decade."

III. **Excess antibiotic use is a worldwide problem** [68]. In the United States, antimicrobial agents are the second most commonly used class of drugs [63] (second to agents used for cardiovascular disorders). In hospitals, approximately 25–40% of patients receive antibiotics, accounting for nearly 25% of total drug acquisition, whereas about 15% of office-based private practice prescriptions are for antibiotics [69].

A. Several **studies suggest that approximately 50% of antibiotic use in the United States is inappropriate** (i.e., not indicated, wrong drug, wrong dose or duration). Kunin [69] has reviewed this problem and potential approaches to it in detail elsewhere. Guidelines are available to help hospitals improve their use of antibiotics.

B. **Should oral antibiotics be made available over the counter** (OTC)? In recent years, several agents previously available only by prescription are now OTC preparations. In 1993, nine of the ten top-selling OTC agents were available only by prescription in 1975 including ibuprofen (e.g., Advil, Nuprin, Motrin), miconazole (Monistat, Gyne-Lotrimin), pseudoephedrine (Sudafed, Afrin), brompheniramine and phenylpropanolamine (Dimetapp), and diphenhydramine (Benadryl) [70]. Whether some oral antibiotics should become available OTC is being considered [70]. We concur with Drs. Wenzel and Kunin [70] that **given the existing problems of antibiotic prescription drug abuse and emerging problems with bacterial resistance, overall society will not be well served if any antibiotics become OTC agents.** In particular, if a patient has a side effect from the currently available OTC agents (e.g., ibuprofen), the side effect will affect that one individual, whereas if OTC antibiotics were available and a person abused them and acquired a resistant pathogen, he or she might spread this resistant pathogen to multiple members of society.

IV. **Evaluating new agents** is difficult, if not impossible, for the practicing physician to do on his or her own. Much of the busy physician's information about antibiotics may come from biased advertising or from pharmaceutical company representatives. The hospital formulary or pharmacy and therapeutics committee is a useful resource for new drug evaluation. **Multiple factors** are involved in **evaluating new antibiotics** (see also discussions on individual agents later):
   A. **In vitro susceptibility.**
   B. **Pharmacokinetic studies.**
   C. **Toxicity or side effects.**
   D. **Results of clinical trials.**
   E. **Cost (not only on a grams-per-day basis but also in terms of the number of doses per day requiring preparation and administration).**
   F. **Local bias in terms of whether a specific agent is undergoing clinical trials at the institution, anecdotal experience with a new agent, and so on.**

References

1. Toshikawa, T.T. Unique Aspects of Infection in Older Adults. In T.T. Toshikawa and D.C. Norman (eds.), *Antimicrobial Therapy in the Elderly Patient.* New York: Marcel Dekker, 1994. Pp. 1–7.
   Useful textbook devoted to infections and antibiotic use in the elderly. See related papers by T.T. Yoshikawa and D.C. Norman, Treatment of infections in elderly patients. Med. Clin. North Am. *79:651, 1995; and K.B. Crossley and P.K. Peterson, Infections in the elderly.* Clin. Infect. Dis. *22:209, 1996.*
2. Norman, D.C. Clinical Approach to Diagnosis of Infection in Older Patients. In T.T. Toshikawa and D.C. Norman (eds.), *Antimicrobial Therapy in the Elderly Patient.* New York: Marcel Dekker, 1994. Pp. 23–31.
   Emphasizes the atypical presentation of infections in the elderly.
2a. Gleckman, R.A. Antibiotic concerns in the elderly: A clinician's perspective. *Infect. Dis. Clin. North Am.* 9:575, 1995.
3. Medical Letter. The choice of antibacterial drugs. *Med. Lett. Drugs Ther.* 38:25, 1996.
   Lists drugs of choice and alternative agents for most pathogens. Excellent reference. Revised approximately every 2 years.
4. Moellering, R., Jr. Principles of Anti-Infective Therapy. In G.L. Mandell, J.E. Bennett, and R. Dolin (eds.), *Principles and Practice of Infectious Diseases* (4th ed.). New York: Churchill Livingstone, 1995. Pp. 199–212.
5. Foran, R.M., Brett, J.L., and Wulf, P.H. Evaluating the cost impact of intravenous antibiotic dosing frequencies. *D.I.C.P. Ann. Pharmacother.* 25:546, 1991.
   Interesting study from the Robert Wood Johnson University Hospital (a private, 416-bed, not-for-profit, teaching hospital providing tertiary care) and the accounting firm of Price Waterhouse. Although cost estimates will vary from institution to institution, this study also estimated nursing time for administering each intravenous dose was about 4.6 minutes. For cost considerations in pediatrics, see J.M. Kaplan et al., Cost of antimicrobial therapy for infants and children. Pediatr. Infect. Dis. J. *9:722, 1990.*
6. Alan, J.D., and Moellering, R.C., Jr. Antimicrobial combinations in the therapy of infections due to gram-negative bacilli. *Am. J. Med.* 78(Suppl. 2A):65, 1985.
   Also see J.D. Alan, Antibiotic combinations. Med. Clin. North Am. *71:1079, 1987; and G.M. Eliopolous, Synergism and antagonism.* Infect. Dis. North Am. *3:399, 1989.*

7. Hughes, W.T., et al. Guidelines for the use of antimicrobial agents in neuropenic patients with unexplained fever. *J. Infect. Dis.* 161:381, 1990.
   This report from the Infectious Disease Society of America reviews this controversial area. For a related paper, see J.C. Wade, Antibiotic therapy for the febrile granulocytopenic cancer patient: Combination therapy vs. monotherapy. Rev. Infect. Dis. 11:S1572, 1989.

7a. Korzeniowski, O.M. Antibacterial agents in pregnancy. *Infect. Dis. Clin. North Am.* 9:639, 1995.
   Includes a discussion of the fetal risk stratification system shown in Table 28A-7.

8. Chow, A.W., and Jewesson, P.J. Pharmacokinetics and safety of antimicrobial agents during pregnancy. *Rev. Infect. Dis.* 7:287, 1985.

9. Safety of antimicrobial drugs in pregnancy. *Med. Lett. Drugs Ther.* 29:61, 1987.

10. Bennett, W.M., et al. *Drug Prescribing in Renal Failure: Dosing Guidelines for Adults.* (3rd ed.) Philadelphia: American College of Physicians, 1994.
   Contains good summary tables of antibiotic dose reduction recommendations in renal failure. Also has tables of dose reduction of cardiovascular, psychotropic, and other agents. Useful handbook.

10a. Livornese, L.L., Jr., et al. Antibacterial agents in renal failure. *Infect. Dis. Clin. North Am.* 9:591, 1995.
   Also contains a series of tables for dose reductions in renal failure.

11. Cockcroft, D.W., and Gault, M.H. Prediction of creatinine clearance from serum creatinine. *Nephron* 16:31, 1976.

12. Tschida, S.J., et al. Anti-infective agents and hepatic disease. *Med. Clin. North Am.* 79:895, 1995.

13. Singh, N., et al. B-lactam antibiotic-induced leukopenia in severe hepatic dysfunction: Risk factors and implications for dosing in patients with liver disease. *Am. J. Med.* 94:251, 1993.

14. Westphal, J.F., Jehl, F., and Vetter, D. Pharmacological, toxicologic, and microbiological considerations in the choice of initial antibiotic therapy for serious infections in patients with cirrhosis of the liver. *Clin. Infect. Dis.* 18:324, 1994.
   Report from France.

15. Bisno, A.L., and Waldvogel, F.A. (eds.). *Infections Associated with Indwelling Devices* (2nd ed.). Washington, DC: American Society for Microbiology, 1994.
   Entire text devoted to this topic.

16. Nightingale, C.H., Quintiliani, R., and Nicolau, D.P. Intelligent dosing of antimicrobials. *Curr. Clin. Top. Infect. Dis.* 14:252, 1994.
   Detailed discussion of concentration-dependent killing and concentration-independent killing of bacteria and possible clinical implications. For a related review by these same authors, see D.P. Nicalau et al., Antibiotic kinetics and dynamics for the clinician. Med. Clin. North Am 79:477, 1995.

16a. Levison, M.E. Pharmacodynamics of antimicrobial agents: Bactericidal and postantibiotic effects. *Infect. Dis. Clin. North Am.* 9:483, 1995.

17. Poretz, D.M., et al. Intravenous antibiotic therapy in an outpatient setting. *J.A.M.A.* 248:336, 1982.
   Study of more than 150 patients. See editorial comment in same issue. For an update on this topic, including reimbursement issues, emergency follow-up care, and other issues, see A.D. Tice, Growing pains in outpatient intravenous antibiotic therapy. Infect. Dis. Clin. Pract. 1:74, 1992.

18. Rehm, S.J., and Weinstein, A.J. Home intravenous antibiotic therapy: A team approach. *Ann. Intern. Med.* 99:383, 1983.

19. Eron, L.J., et al. Intravenous antibiotic therapy in ambulatory pediatric patients. *Pediatr. Infect. Dis.* 3:514, 1984.

20. Ingram, C., et al. Antibiotic therapy of osteomyelitis in outpatients. *Med. Clin. North Am.* 72:723, 1988.
   Reviews experience in 481 episodes.

21. Poretz, D.M. Home management of antibiotic therapy. *Curr. Clin. Top. Infect. Dis.* 10:27–42, 1989.
   For a special symposium on outpatient and home intravenous antibiotic therapy, see R.V. McCloskey et al., Home care symposium. Rev. Infect. Dis. 13(Suppl. 2) S141–195, 1991. Review by a clinician with extensive experience in this area, including a summary by S.L. Green, Practical guidelines for developing an office-based program for outpatient intravenous therapy, in this same issue, pp. S189–S192.

22. Tice, A.D. Outpatient parenteral antibiotic therapy: Management of serious infections. *Hosp. Pract.* 28(Suppl. 1 and 2):1–64, 1993.

A two-part symposium. The first part discusses medical (patient selection, antibiotic choice, delivery system), quality assurance, costs, and legal issues, among others. The second part addresses amenable infections (bacterial endocarditis, cellulitis, meningitis, pneumonia, pelvic inflammatory disease, pyelonephritis, osteomyelitis) and models for delivery (infusion centers and options in a variety of settings).

23. Kravitz, G.A. Advances in IV delivery. *Hosp. Pract.* 28(Suppl. 1):21, 1993.
    Good discussion of intravenous access devices and infusion devices.

24. New, P.B., et al. Ambulatory antibiotic infusion devices: Extending the spectrum of outpatient therapies. *Am. J. Med.* 91:455, 1991.
    Retrospective study of 98 patients who received antibiotics via ambulatory infusion pumps for mean duration of 18 days. Safe and effective approach in patients not eligible for minibag gravity infusions. Outpatient therapy will be cost-effective compared with hospitalization. See editorial comment, reference 25.

25. Poretz, D.M. High tech comes home. *Am. J. Med.* 91:453, 1991.
    Editorial comment on reference 24.

26. Jacoby, G.A., and Archer, G.L. New mechanisms of bacterial resistance to antimicrobial agents. *N. Engl. J. Med.* 324:601, 1991.
    Good review of this topic by knowledgeable experts. Authors emphasize the importance of rational and controlled antibiotic use in both humans and animals to prevent widespread resistance.

27. Mayer, K.H., Opal, S.M., and Medeioros, A.A. Mechanisms of Antibiotic Resistance. In G.L. Mandell, J.E. Bennett, and R. Dolin (eds.), *Principles and Practice of Infectious Diseases* (4th ed.). New York: Churchill Livingstone, 1995. P. 212.

27a. Fralmow, H.S., and Abrutyn, E. Pathogens resistant to antimicrobial agents: Epidemiology, molecular mechanisms, and clinical management. *Infect. Dis. Clin. North Am.* 9:497, 1995.

28. Dever, L.A., and Dermody, T.S. Mechanisms of bacterial resistance to antibiotics. *Arch. Intern. Med.* 151:886, 1991.

29. Chow, J.W., et al. Enterobacter bacteremia: Clinical features and emergence of antibiotic resistance during therapy. *Ann. Intern. Med.* 115:585, 1991.
    Authors conclude that more judicious use of third-generation cephalosporins may decrease the incidence of nosocomial multiresistant Enterobacter spp., *which in turn may result in lower mortality to* Enterobacter *bacteremia. See additional discussion in Chaps. 28F and 28H.*

30. Sanders, C. New B-lactams: New problems for the internist. *Ann. Intern. Med.* 115:651, 1991.
    Thoughtful editorial comment on reference 29, again emphasizing that microbial drug resistance must be controlled through the more judicious use of newer agents—for example, third-generation cephalosporins. See additional discussion in Chaps. 28F and 28H. See also C.C. Sanders, β-lactamases of gram-negative bacteria: New challenges for new drugs. Clin. Infect. Dis. *14:1089, 1992.*

31. Gustaferro, C.A., and Steckelburg, J.M. Cephalosporin antimicrobial agents and related compounds. *Mayo Clin. Proc.* 66:1064, 1991.
    Urges the use of first- and second-generation cephalosporins, rather than the broader third-generation cephalosporins, to help prevent resistance. For further discussion, see Chaps. 28F and 28H.

32. Garibaldi, R., and Burke, J. Surveillance and control of antibiotic use in the hospital. *Am. J. Infect. Control* 19:164, 1991.

33. DiNuble, M.J. Antibiotics: The antipyretics of choice? *Am. J. Med.* 89:787, 1990.
    Thoughtful editorial comment urging a more conservative approach to using antibiotics in the febrile patient.

34. Wilkowske, C.J. General principles of antimicrobial therapy. *Mayo Clin. Proc.* 66:931, 1991.

35. Bartlett, J.G. *Clostridium difficile:* Clinical considerations. *Rev. Infect. Dis.* 12(Suppl. 2):S243, 1990.
    A concise clinical review by an expert in the field. For an interesting editorial comment emphasizing the potential advantage of oral vancomycin over oral metronidazole for severe C. difficile infection, see S.L. Gorbach, Drugs for your mother-in-law: Metronidazole for Clostridium difficile. Infect. Dis. Clin. Pract. *1:46, 1992. See also discussion in Chap. 28P and reference 38.*

36. Fekety, R. Antibiotic-Associated Colitis. In G.L. Mandell, J.E. Bennett, and R. Dolin (eds.), *Principles and Practice of Infectious Diseases* (4th ed.). New York: Churchill Livingstone, 1995. Pp. 978–987.
    Also see R. Fekety et al., Treatment of C. difficile colitis. Am. J. Med. 86:15, 1989. Low-dose vancomycin (125 mg qid) was as effective as the high-dose drug (500 mg qid).

37. Fekety, R., and Shah, A.B. Diagnosis and treatment of *Clostridium difficile* colitis. *J.A.M.A.* 269:71, 1993.
    Still favors vancomycin for severe disease.
38. Bartlett, J.G. Antibiotic-associated diarrhea. *Clin. Infect. Dis.* 15:573, 1992.
    Good review published in October 1992. See related article by J.G. Bartlett, The 10 most common questions about Clostridium difficile–*associated diarrhea and colitis.* Infect. Dis. Clin. Pract. *1:254, 1992.*
39. Siegel, D.L., Edelstein, P.H., and Nachamkin, I. Inappropriate testing for diarrheal disease in the hospital. *J.A.M.A.* 263:979, 1990.
    Routine ordering of stool cultures and ova and parasite examination in patients hospitalized for more than 3 days was not cost-effective.
40. Peterson, L.R., and Kelly, P.J. The role of the clinical microbiology laboratory in the management of *Clostridium difficile*–associated diarrhea. *Infect. Dis. Clin. North Am.* 7:277, 1993.
41. Anand, A., and Glatt, A.E. *Clostridium difficile* infection associated with antineoplastic chemotherapy: A review. *Clin. Infect. Dis.* 17:109, 1993.
    C. difficile *can cause problems in these patients even without prior antibiotic use.*
42. Boland, G.W., et al. Antibiotic-induced diarrhea: Specificity of abdominal CT for the diagnosis of *Clostridium difficile* disease. *Radiology* 191:103, 1994.
    Retrospective review of 64 patients with C. difficile *diarrhea: Thirty-nine percent had normal CT scans; 17% had CT-specific diagnostic features of* C. difficile *disease such as nodular haustral thickening or the "accordion" pattern.*
43. Oliva, S.L., et al. Failure of intravenous vancomycin and intravenous metronidazole to prevent or treat antibiotic-associated pseudomembranous colitis. *J. Infect. Dis.* 159:1154, 1989.
44. Committee on Infectious Diseases. *1994 Red Book: Report of the Committee on Infectious Diseases* (23rd ed.). Elk Grove Village, IL: American Academy of Pediatrics, 1994. P. 163.
45. McFarland, L.V., et al. Nosocomial acquisition of *Clostridium difficile* infection. *N. Engl. J. Med.* 320:204, 1989.
    Also see L.V. McFarland et al., Risk factors for Clostridium difficile *carriage and* C. difficile–*associated diarrhea in a cohort of hospitalized patients.* J. Infect. Dis. *162:678, 1990; and M.S. Drapkin, Nosocomial infection with* C. difficile. Infect. Dis. Clin. Pract. *1:138, 1992.*
46. Gerding, D. Disease associated with *Clostridium difficile* isolation. *Ann. Intern. Med.* 110:255, 1989.
47. Johnson, S., et al. Prospective, controlled study of vinyl glove use to interrupt *Clostridium difficile* nosocomial transmission. *Am. J. Med.* 88:137, 1990.
48. Struelens, M.J., et al. Control of nosocomial transmission of *Clostridium difficile* based on sporadic case surveillance. *Am. J. Med.* 91(Suppl. 3B):138S, 1991.
    C. difficile *spores commonly contaminate areas such as bedpan storage sites, bedpan flushing devices, doorknobs, toilet seats, and tables and chairs in the rooms of* C. difficile–*infected patients.*
49. Snavely, S.R., and Hodges, G.R. The neurotoxicity of antibacterial agents. *Ann. Intern. Med.* 101:92, 1984.
    For a related update, see R.J. Thomas, Neurotoxicity of antibacterial therapy. South Med. J. *87:869, 1994.*
50. Medical Letter. Drug interactions update. *Med. Lett. Drugs Ther.* 26:11, 1984.
    For an update of these tables, see J.P. Sanford, Drug interactions to watch for during antibiotic therapy. J. Crit. Ill. *7:450, 1992, and Drug interactions with anti-fungals, antivirals, and other anti-infections.* J. Crit. Ill. *7:605, 1992.*
51. Gibaldi, M. Drug interactions (parts I and II). *Ann. Pharmacother.* 26:709, 1992.
52. Cohen, M.L. Epidemiology of drug resistance: Implications for a postantimicrobial era. *Science* 257:1050, 1992.
    Good review of extent of problem, risk factors, and potential solutions.
53. Neu, H.C. The crises in antibiotic resistance. *Science* 257:1065, 1992.
    Reviews specific pathogens involved.
54. Hooper, D., and Thornsberry, C. The epidemiology of emerging antimicrobial resistance. *Proceedings of the Thirty-Fourth Interscience Conference on Antimicrobial Agents and Chemotherapy,* Orlando, FL, American Society for Microbiology, Oct. 7, 1994.
    One of several symposia at this national meeting aimed at resistance problems.

55. Kunin, C.M. Resistance to antimicrobial drugs: A worldwide calamity. *Ann. Intern. Med.* 118:557, 1993.
    Emphasizes the global nature of this problem, including developing countries.
56. Tomasz, A. Multiple-antibiotic-resistant pathogenic bacteria: A report of the Rockefeller University Workshop. *N. Engl. J. Med.* 330:1247, 1994.
57. Meyer, K.S., et al. Nosocomial outbreak of *Klebsiella* infection resistant to the late-generation cephalosporins. *Ann. Intern. Med.* 119:353, 1993.
    See editorial comment in same issue and related discussions in Chap. 28F.
58. Berkelmen, R.L., and Hughes, J.M. The conquest of infectious diseases: Who are we kidding? *Ann. Intern. Med.* 119:426, 1993.
59. McCaig, L.F., and Hughes, J.M. Trends in antimicrobial drug prescribing among office-based physicians in the United States. *J.A.M.A.* 273:214, 1995.
    Study concluded that survey showed increased use of broader-spectrum and more expensive antimicrobial drugs, which has implications for all patients because of the impact on health care costs and the potential for the emergence of antimicrobial resistance.
60. DuPont, H.L., and Steele, J.H. Use of antimicrobial agents in animal feeds: Implications for human health. *Rev. Infect. Dis.* 9:447, 1987.
61. Berkelmen, R.L., et al. Infectious disease surveillance: A crumbling foundation. *Science* 264:368, 1994.
    Discusses impact of reduced financial support for surveillance studies.
62. Levy, S.B. Confronting multidrug resistance: A role for each of us. *J.A.M.A.* 269:1840, 1993.
    Commentary by a physician with a long-term interest in this topic.
63. Winker, M.A., et al. Emerging and reemerging global microbial threats: Call for papers. *J.A.M.A.* 273:241, 1995.
    Editorial comment, in part, on reference [59]. Also encourages reports on ideas about and research into this growing problem of resistance, to be studied and reported in a special series of J.A.M.A.-related publications for January 1996.
64. McGowan, J.E., Jr. Do intensive antibiotic control programs prevent the spread of antibiotic resistance? *Infect. Control Hosp. Epidemiol.* 15:478, 1994.
    Preliminary data suggest these efforts are worthwhile. Multicenter studies are needed.
65. Waud, D.R. Pharmaceutical promotions: A free lunch? *N. Engl. J. Med.* 327:351, 1992.
    A "sounding board" article.
66. Orlowski, J.P., et al. The efforts of pharmaceutical firm enticements on physician prescribing habits. *Chest* 102:270, 1992.
67. O'Brien, T.F. Global surveillance of antibiotic resistance. *N. Engl. J. Med.* 326:339, 1992.
    See related editorial comment update by M.A. Winkler and A. Flanagin, Infectious diseases: A global approach to a global problem. J.A.M.A. 275:245, 1996.
67a. Chopra, I., et al. New approaches to the control of infections caused by antibiotic-resistant bacteria: An industry perspective. *J.A.M.A.* 275:401, 1996.
67b. Goldmann, D., et al. Consensus statement: Strategies to prevent and control the emergence and spread of antimicrobial-resistant microorganisms in hospitals—a challenge to hospital leadership. *J.A.M.A.* 275:234, 1996.
    A multidisciplinary group of experts convened to provide hospital leaders with strategic goals and/or actions to help approach this problem at the hospital level.
68. Kunin, C.M., et al. Report of a symposium on use and abuse of antibiotics worldwide. *Rev. Infect. Dis.* 12:12, 1990.
69. Kunin, C.M. Problems in Antibiotic Usage. In G.L. Mandell, R.G. Douglas, Jr., and J.E. Bennett (eds.), *Principles and Practice of Infectious Diseases* (3rd ed.). New York: Churchill Livingstone, 1990. Pp. 427–434.
70. Wenzel, R.P., and Kunin, C.M. Should oral antimicrobial drugs be available over the counter? *J. Infect. Dis.* 170:1256, 1994.
    This discussion tries to look at the pros and cons of this issue.

B. Prophylactic Antibiotics

Prophylactic antibiotics are defined as **antibiotics used to prevent infection.** Approximately one-third of hospitalized patients receive antibiotics and, of these, one-half receive prophylactic antibiotics, primarily for surgical procedures. Although early studies in the 1950s and 1960s concluded that prophylaxis was not helpful, many of these studies were poorly done, and the basic principles of appropriate prophylactic antibiotic use were not understood. In reality, patients often were given therapeutic antibiotics; that is, the infection had already occurred. Since these early studies, **data have shown clearly that prophylactic antibiotics are useful in certain circumstances.**

Wound infections are the second or third most common nosocomial infections among all hospitalized patients. In many settings, appropriate prophylactic use of antimicrobial agents often can reduce the incidence of postoperative wound infections [1]. For some procedures, prophylaxis is not suggested and, in several situations, further studies will be needed to determine their usefulness clearly [1–8].

I. **Basic principles of surgical prophylaxis.** Animal model studies as well as clinical studies have established some basic guidelines for surgical antibiotic prophylaxis.

  A. **Timing of antibiotic administration**

    1. **Theory and animal studies.** Animal studies by Burke [9] and others [5] in the late 1950s and early 1960s showed that administration of antibiotics just before, during, and up to 3 hours after surgery effectively prevented infections in wounds experimentally inoculated with bacteria. This was called the **effective period of preventive antibiotic action or the "decisive period"** [5, 9]. The use of antibiotics for a brief period after this effective time period did not prevent wound infection [9].

      These experimental studies provided the data on which the timing of prophylactic antibiotics is based. Many clinical studies have been performed that support this principle [1–8]. A large, recent clinical study of patients receiving prophylactic antibiotics confirms that prophylactic antibiotics are most effective when given 0–2 hours before surgery. Beginning an antibiotic regimen 2–24 hours before surgery is not required or useful. In addition, if antibiotic administration begins more than 3 hours after the surgical incision, the prophylactic regimen is not effective [10].

    2. **Clinical application.** For surgical antibiotic prophylaxis to be successful, the **antibiotic must be given so that good tissue levels are present at the time of the procedure and for the first 3–4 hours after the surgical incision** [1, 2, 5, 9–12]. There is neither need nor reason to start prophylactic antibiotics days in advance.

    3. **Recommended timing.** Recent reviews [1, 4, 6a] suggest administering the parenteral antibiotic **30–60 minutes before the surgical incision is made** (i.e., with the induction of anesthesia).

      For cesarean section, antimicrobial prophylaxis should be delayed until the umbilical cord is clamped and then should be initiated immediately [1].

  B. **Duration of prophylaxis.** This **remains a controversial** issue and an important one in terms of the cost of prophylaxis [1–5, 6a]. **The optimal duration of perioperative antimicrobial prophylaxis is not known** [1]. Burke [11] has emphasized that since "the effective period lasts no longer than three hours after bacterial contamination of tissue and since bacterial contamination in most surgical procedures ends when the wound is closed, **there is little evidence to support prophylactic administration of antibiotics past the period of operation and recovery of normal physiology following anesthesia.**" Clinical studies by Stone and colleagues [12] and others [4, 6a, 12, 13] also support this approach.

    1. **Practical approach.** For many surgical procedures, a single dose of antibiotic given just before the procedure provides adequate tissue levels [4, 13], especially in **biliary tract** surgery, **hysterectomies,** and **gastric** operations. Some authors suggest that, in addition, two postoperative doses are reasonable [2]. Most experts recommend that antimicrobial prophylaxis should certainly be discontinued within 24 hours of the operative procedure [1].

      In prophylaxis for nonperforated appendectomy and colorectal surgery, up to 24 hours of prophylaxis often is recommended [2, 13]. In addition, when a prosthetic device is inserted, prophylaxis often is continued beyond one dose [14]. The optimal duration of prophylaxis in open heart surgery [1] and neurosurgery awaits further study [2, 3]. Many experts believe the continuation of prophylaxis until all catheters and drains have been removed is not appropriate [1]. Data are not available to resolve this issue clearly, and large-scale studies are needed [2].

    2. **Prolonged procedures.** If a procedure lasts for several hours, repeat doses of the antibiotic may be necessary intraoperatively to maintain adequate and

constant blood and tissue levels [1]. This is particularly important as the period of highest risk for bacterial contamination is most likely the close, not the beginning, of surgery [2]. In prolonged procedures, cefoxitin (with a short half-life) should be readministered every 2 hours until the wound is closed. Whether a similar cephalosporin, cefotetan, which has a longer half-life, is a better agent to use in colorectal surgery awaits further clinical experience with this agent (see Chap. 28F). When an agent with a longer half-life is used (e.g., **cefazolin), readministration is suggested every 4 hours** [1]. Common regimens are described in sec. **V.B. See Table 28B-1.**

3. **Prosthetic devices.** When a prosthetic device is inserted, prophylaxis often is given for 24–48 hours [3], although whether these patients need prolonged therapy is unclear. Some sources suggest single doses for prosthetic device surgery or an additional dose when patients are removed from bypass during open heart surgery [4]. Norden and coworkers [14] do not favor single-dose prophylaxis in prosthetic joint surgery, but short courses—regimens spanning 24 hours or less—are favored. Others also favor a three-dose regimen [2, 6], which is generally what we prefer.

II. **Which procedures benefit from prophylaxis?** In general, when a prosthesis is not involved, prophylaxis is not indicated for low-risk "clean" procedures.

A. **Agents are used when the inoculum of bacteria is high,** as in colonic surgery, surgery of the vagina, or infected biliary procedures **or** where the **insertion of an artificial device** (e.g., heart valve, total hip) reduces the inoculum required to cause infection, and when an infection may be catastrophic or may require repeat surgery.

B. **Clinical studies now support the use of prophylactic agents** in many settings and are reviewed in detail elsewhere [1–8, 13, 15]. Some examples include the following:

1. **Biliary tract surgery.** Clinical studies suggest that **surgical antibiotic prophylaxis is indicated for the high-risk group** but not for uncomplicated cholecystectomies in patients younger than 60 years. The biliary tract is normally sterile, with only a low rate of colonization when elective operations for stone-related disease are undertaken in young patients [1]. **High-risk** patients include those (1) older than 60 years of age [1], (2) with obstructive jaundice, (3) with acute cholecystitis or cholangitis, (4) with common duct stones [1, 4], (5) a nonfunctioning gallbladder [4], and (6) those who have undergone previous biliary surgery [1]. Prophylactic antibiotics decreased the infection rate from approximately 25% in controls to 5%. The role of prophylactic antibiotics in patients undergoing endoscopic retrograde cholangiopancreatography (ERCP) is discussed in sec. **VI.P.**

2. **Gynecologic surgery.** Local antibiotic irrigation has been used in some settings (e.g., prophylaxis of cesarean section [2]) but is not recommended [1, 3, 4, 16]. The role of prophylactic antibiotics in gynecologic and obstetric surgery has been summarized [16].

   a. **Hysterectomy.** Prophylaxis is beneficial in vaginal and possibly in abdominal hysterectomies [3, 4, 8, 16]. Antibiotics selected do not have to be

Table 28B-1. Recommended dose intervals for repeat doses in prolonged procedures

Agent	Half-life with normal renal function (hr)	Intraoperative dose interval (hr)*
Cefazolin	1.8	4
Cefoxitin	1	2
Cefotetan	3–4.5	6–8
Clindamycin	2.4–3	5–6
Metronidazole	8	
Vancomycin	3–9	

*The intraoperative dose can be given at 2 times the half-life of the agent to maintain adequate tissue levels.
Source: From E.P. Dellinger et al., Quality standard for antimicrobial prophylaxis in surgical procedures. *Clin. Infect. Dis.* 18:422, 1994.

active against all pelvic or vaginal organisms. First-generation cephalosporins (e.g., cefazolin) appear to be as effective as second- and third-generation cephalosporins [3]. In the cephalosporin-allergic patients, doxycycline, 200 mg IV (one dose) preoperatively, has been suggested [2]. Some authors favor oral doxycycline use in the cephalosporin-allergic patient: doxycycline, 100 mg PO at bedtime, and another identical dose orally 3–4 hours before the scheduled procedure. Clindamycin, 900 mg IV preoperatively, has also been proposed [16].

  b. Cesarean sections. Sections carried out in high-risk patients (e.g., those with premature rupture of membranes or emergency surgery) are associated with a lower rate of postoperative infection when prophylactic antibiotics are used. In this setting, an early infection may already have been established. A first-generation cephalosporin (cefazolin) can be given after the cord is clamped to avoid exposing the infant to the drug [3, 4, 16]. Alternative regimens in the patient truly allergic to cephalosporins have not been studied [16]. One source suggests that metronidazole, 500 mg IV, after clamping the cord is effective [2].

  c. Therapeutic abortion. Preoperative antibiotics can prevent infections after first-trimester abortion in women with previous pelvic inflammatory disease and after mid-trimester abortion [4, 16].

3. Orthopedics [4, 6, 15, 17, 18]

  a. Open fractures

   (1) For **simple open fractures,** a first-generation cephalosporin (e.g., cefazolin) is recommended for 18–24 hours [2, 17, 18].

   (2) For **more complex open fractures** requiring extensive debridement of environmental contaminants or insertion of a prosthetic device, therapeutic courses of antibiotics are recommended (e.g., for 10 days) [2]. (Although cefazolin is suggested in this setting [2], we have sometimes used ceftriaxone to ensure adequate activity against community-acquired gram-negative bacilli, which can be contaminants of the wound.)

  b. Closed fracture. The role of antibiotics in this setting is unclear and awaits further clinical study. Norden and colleagues [17] recommended that prophylaxis started immediately before surgery and lasting 12–18 hours should be offered to all patients with closed fractures undergoing operative fixation [17] while awaiting definitive studies.

  c. Total joint replacement. Antibiotic prophylaxis reduces the frequency of deep wound infection following total joint replacement [18]. Systemic antibiotic **prophylaxis is recommended** because the consequences of infection are so serious and prophylaxis is beneficial (e.g., short courses of cefazolin). In his review, Norden concluded that antibiotic-impregnated cement alone is effective in the prophylaxis of deep infection after joint replacement. In a recent report of a 10-year follow-up of more than 1,500 consecutive total hip arthroplasties, the incidence of deep infections in those patients who received systemic antibiotics versus gentamicin bone cement was not significantly different (1.6% versus 1.1%). The authors conclude that it would be beneficial to combine the use of systemic antibiotics and antibiotic-containing bone cement to decrease further the rate of deep infections, especially in those departments without an ultraclean-air environment [19]. However, the value of using both techniques over either alone has not been established.

  The role of ultraclean-air systems is controversial and has been reviewed by Norden and associates [14]. In summary, he emphasizes that ultraclean-air systems do offer protection against infection in total joint replacement, but that the benefit probably is small when antibiotic prophylaxis also is used [15].

  Operating rooms with ultraclean air help reduce wound infections, but these systems are expensive.

  d. Other orthopedic procedures

   (1) Antibiotic prophylaxis decreases postoperative wound infection when hip and other fractures are treated with **internal fixation by nails, plates, screws, or wires** [4, 20].

   (2) Whether antibiotic prophylaxis should be used for other orthopedic procedures (i.e., with no prosthetic device insertion) is unclear. However, there are data suggesting prophylaxis significantly reduced the frequency of infections in those **operations lasting longer than 2 hours** [20].

e. **Prophylaxis against hematogenous infection after total joint replacement.** Whether patients with indwelling prosthetic joints need antibiotic prophylaxis when undergoing dental, gastrointestinal, or genitourinary procedures is controversial [6, 14]. However, recent reviews of the data suggest antibiotics usually add little except expense [4, 6a, 20a, 20b].

Some experimental evidence indicates a high risk of infection of joint implants during bacteremia in a rabbit model, especially in the postoperative period [20]. We emphasize the following:

(1) Proper antibiotic therapy of focal infections is important (to prevent bacteremia), especially urinary tract and skin infections [15, 20].

(2) Prosthetic joint infections can occur after systemic bacteremias with gram-negative bacilli (e.g., *E. coli*) or staphylococci (e.g., *S. aureus*) especially early in the postoperative period [14], but there are few data to support joint seeding and subsequent prosthetic joint infection after dental procedures [20a, 20b]. See sec. **(3).** If a surgical procedure with a significant risk of bacteremia (see sec. **VI.C.2**) is indicated, in general, we do not use prophylactic antibiotics unless the prosthesis has only recently been inserted (e.g., within the preceding 8–12 weeks) or dental work has been performed as described in sec. **(3).**

(3) Dental work. Some orthopedic surgeons will use prophylaxis for dental procedures in patients with major joint arthroplasties even though there is no proof that antibiotics are needed in this setting [14, 21]. However, prosthetic joint infection with the type of organism (e.g., viridans streptococci) that commonly causes subacute bacterial endocarditis is a rare event, implying the absence of risk [20a, 20b].

Norden and colleagues [14] argue, as have others, that using available data and reasonable assumptions, routine dental prophylaxis may be unnecessary and may be associated with an unacceptable level of antibiotic-induced adverse effects if penicillins are used. Modeling indicates cost-effectiveness of administration of erythromycin or cephalexin for higher-risk patients, but there is a paucity of data to confirm these predictions. In the presence of overt or imminent dental sepsis or in immunocompromised patients, prophylaxis is strongly recommended by some against the probable or proven oral pathogen [14] until more data become available.

In their review, Hass and Kaiser [6] agree with the Working Party of the British Society for Antimicrobial Chemotherapy that more information is needed before the routine use of prophylactic antibiotics can be recommended for all patients with prosthetic joints who undergo procedures known to produce transient bacteremia [22]. Providing antibiotic prophylaxis for selected patients with prosthetic joints and particularly severe periodontal disease, however, may be reasonable, pending more data [6].

(4) Therefore, recent reviewers emphasize that most patients with indwelling prosthetic joints generally do not require antimicrobial prophylaxis when undergoing dental, gastrointestinal, or genitourinary procedures [4, 6a, 20a, 20b]. For long procedures, surgery in an infected area (including periodontal disease), or other procedures with a high risk of bacteremia, prophylaxis may be advisable [4].

4. **Gastrointestinal surgery**

a. **Elective colorectal surgery.** Preoperative antibiotics have been shown to reduce the incidence of postoperative infections [1, 2, 4, 6a, 23]. **Oral antibiotics,** which are poorly absorbed, have been given to reduce colony counts of resident colonic flora. **Parenteral antibiotics** have also been used perioperatively with success. In emergent bowel surgery, parenteral antibiotics are used alone, as time does not allow the use of the oral regimen. Whether oral and parenteral regimens together are better than oral alone remains to be determined [1, 4]. The most common practice in the United States is oral antibiotic administration along with mechanical bowel cleansing the evening before the operation and parenteral antibiotic administration in the operating room just before incision [1].

(1) **Oral.** A common oral regimen consists of an initial mechanical bowel preparation *and* neomycin sulfate (1 g) and erythromycin base (1 g) orally at 1 PM, 2 PM, and 11 PM, on the day prior to abdominal surgery [4]. The details of this oral regimen and the mechanical bowel preparation used with it are reviewed by Nichols [23].

(2) **Parenteral.** Data support the use of antimicrobial agents that are effective against both anaerobic and aerobic bowel organisms [4, 24]. **Cefoxitin** is an **appealing** agent in this setting, compared with the first-generation cephalosporins, because cefoxitin has greater activity against bowel anaerobes, including *Bacteroides fragilis* [2, 4]. A limited study suggested that cefoxitin (2 g q6h for 24 hours) was superior to cefazolin (1 g q8h for 24 hours) [15], although prior data had not shown any clear advantages of cefoxitin in this setting [25]. It is hoped that further studies will clarify this issue. Cefotetan, which has similar activity to cefoxitin but a longer half-life than cefoxitin or cefmetazole, has been used effectively in colorectal surgery and is another option [4]. See sec. **V.B.4.** Cefmetazole is another possible agent. (See Chap. 28F.) For other abdominal and pelvic procedures, including obstetric and gynecologic operations, cefazolin has been equally effective [4] and is less expensive compared to cefoxitin or cefotetan.

A combination of metronidazole and ceftriaxone has been shown to be effective in colorectal surgery [26]. Although metronidazole has been used extensively in the United Kingdom for prophylaxis, because of its potential carcinogenic risk (see Chap. 28P), it is not commonly recommended for prophylaxis in the United States [4] except as an alternate agent—for example, in a patient allergic to cephalosporins [2]. Furthermore, **the third-generation cephalosporins are not recommended for prophylaxis**: They are expensive, their activity against staphylococci often is less than cefazolin, their spectrum of activity against facultative gram-negative bacilli includes organisms rarely encountered in elective surgery, and their widespread use for prophylaxis promotes emergence of resistance to these potentially valuable drugs [4].

b. **Nonelective colorectal surgery.** In emergency surgery (e.g., for intestinal obstruction), there is no time to use the oral antibiotics plus mechanical bowel preparations. Therefore, a parenteral cephalosporin is advised. Cefoxitin and cefotetan have been commonly used (see sec. **4.a.(2)** and Chap. 28F). Cefmetazole is another option (see Chap. 28F), but it has a relatively short half-life, as does cefoxitin.

The third-generation cephalosporins are not recommended in this setting, as discussed in sec. **a**. If the operation reveals a bowel perforation, a full therapeutic course of antibiotics will be necessary.

c. **Gastroduodenal surgery.** Compared with lower GI surgery, upper GI surgery has a lower rate of infection because of the lower titer of bacterial flora in the upper GI tract. Ordinarily, patients undergoing surgery for uncomplicated duodenal ulcer require no prophylaxis [8]; in this situation, the highly acidic environment results in a very low endogenous bacterial density and, thus, rates of postoperative infection are low [1]. However **patients at high risk for infection may benefit from prophylaxis** [1, 3, 4, 8]. Included in this group are patients with diminished gastric motility or acidity (secondary to bleeding or obstructing duodenal ulcer, gastric ulcer, or gastric malignancy), or patients who have received effective acid-reducing therapy, whether medical (H_2-blockers such as ranitidine, or proton-pump inhibitors such as omeprazole [Prilosec]) or surgical. The risk of infection is also high in patients with morbid obesity [4]. In general, cefazolin is used in this setting [4]. Prophylactic cefazolin can also decrease infectious complications after gastric bypass surgery for obesity or percutaneous endoscopic gastrostomy [4].

d. **Appendectomy.** Preoperative antibiotics can decrease the incidence of infection following appendectomy [4]. Cefoxitin for one [4] to three doses [2] is commonly used. Cefotetan is another possibility. A perforated or gangrenous appendix requires full therapeutic regimens (see Chap. 11).

5. **Urologic procedures**
a. **If the urine is infected,** it is preferable to sterilize it before beginning an

elective procedure on the genitourinary tract. If that is not possible, then antimicrobial therapy targeting the responsible pathogens should be initiated before the procedure and continued until the urinary tract infection has resolved [1, 4].

b. If the urine is sterile, the role of antibiotics remains controversial.

   (1) Infectious disease experts do not recommend antimicrobials before urologic operations in patients with sterile urine [2, 4]. If the urine is sterile and the urologic procedure does not involve entry into the intestine, this is considered a clean procedure [1].

   (2) A wide majority of urologists in the United States believe that there is a role for prophylactic antibiotics in transurethral surgery even if the preoperative urine culture is sterile [27]. This belief is based on data indicating that postsurgical bacteriuria develops in many patients who had sterile urines preoperatively. Perhaps the prostate tissue itself may harbor urinary pathogens [28, 29]. See additional related discussion in Chap. 28S.

   (3) In general, we discourage the use of prophylactic antibiotics if the urine is sterile. At most, a single preoperative dose is suggested. Because of the lack of agreement about the value of prophylactic antibiotics for transurethral procedures, adhering to local practice may be reasonable in this setting [1].

6. Head and neck operations

   a. Prophylaxis decreases the incidence of wound infection after head and neck operations that involve an incision through the oral or pharyngeal mucosa [2–4, 30], **especially for cancer of the head and neck** [30]. Various regimens have been used typically for 24 hours: cefazolin, clindamycin, and gentamicin or ampicillin-sulbactam [2]. Even with antibiotic prophylaxis, when cancer patients undergo major head and neck surgery, significant postoperative wound infections may occur, in part due to the extensive excision and reconstruction in these debilitated patients [31].

   b. Infection rates in uncontaminated head and neck surgery (i.e., surgery in which there is no contamination with saliva—parotidectomy, thyroidectomy, rhinoplasty, myringoplasty, or tonsillectomy) are too low to justify prophylaxis [2, 3]. The role of antibiotic prophylaxis in surgery of the chronically draining ear and tonsillectomy awaits further study [30]. Gentamicin eardrops may decrease the incidence of purulent otorrhea after placement of a tympanostomy tube [4]. Prophylaxis for cochlear implant surgery has not been studied in controlled trials. Because of the devastating effect of cochlear implant infection, workers in the field recommend the use of strict aseptic techniques and prophylaxis with antibiotics active against staphylococci [3].

7. Neurosurgery. The **role** of prophylactic antibiotics in neurosurgery remains **unsettled.** In a recent review, Brown [32] emphasized that based on clinical studies, there are no unequivocal indications for the use of prophylactic antibiotics in neurosurgery.

   a. The effectiveness of prophylaxis in decreasing the incidence of infection has not been clearly established in cerebrospinal fluid **(CSF) shunt implantation,** with studies showing conflicting results [4, 30, 32]. This is in part because large enough studies have not been conducted [30]. While awaiting these data, it is reasonable to use prophylaxis in shunt surgery when the endemic rate of infection is higher than 3% [30]. Other reviews suggest prophylaxis if endemic rates of infection exceed 5% [33]. Some authors [3] suggest that no antibiotic prophylaxis is needed in institutions with low shunt infection rates ($< 10\%$). Consideration should be given to intravenous trimethoprim-sulfamethoxazole (TMP-SMX) perioperatively in institutions with high shunt infection rates ($> 20\%$) [2].

   b. The role of antibiotic prophylaxis in other types of neurosurgery is likewise unclear [30].

   (1) Antistaphylococcal antibiotics may decrease the incidence of wound infections after craniotomies [4] and are reasonable in this setting [33a].

   (2) Some reviewers believe the data may favor use of prophylaxis in clean and clean-contaminated neurosurgery and favor antibiotic prophylaxis [30].

(3) The literature does not support the use of antibiotic prophylaxis in patients with a closed skull fracture, with or without CSF leakage [3]. There are no controlled trials of antibiotic use in patients with open skull fractures. Because these types of injuries are culture-positive at the time of presentation, antibiotic use should be considered to be therapeutic rather than prophylactic. The optimal antibiotic regimen for these patients is undefined [3].

(4) In conventional lumbar diskectomy, the infection rate is so low that antibiotics are not justified. However, infection rates are higher after spinal procedures involving fusion, prolonged spinal surgery, or insertion of foreign material, and the use of prophylactic antibiotics is common, but controlled trials of such use are lacking [4].

8. Cardiovascular surgery. Prophylactic antibiotics can decrease the incidence of infection after cardiac surgery, including valvular procedures and coronary artery bypass grafting [4]. Single doses appear to be as effective as multiple doses, provided that high concentrations are maintained in the blood throughout the procedure [4]. In contrast, they are not indicated for cardiac catheterization [4].

9. Peripheral vascular surgery. Data support the use of prophylactic antibiotics for arterial reconstructive surgery of the abdominal aorta, vascular operations on the leg that include a groin incision, and amputation of the lower extremity for ischemia [4]. The *Medical Letter* indicates that many clinicians also recommend prophylaxis for implantation of any vascular prosthetic material, including grafts for vascular access in hemodialysis [4]. The utility of antibiotic prophylaxis in carotid artery surgery has not been established but, when infection rates are high, cefazolin for 24 hours has been used [2]. Routine use of prophylaxis is not recommended for carotid endarterectomy or brachial artery repair without prosthetic material [4].

10. Thoracic surgery
   a. Pulmonary resection. In patients undergoing this procedure a single preoperative dose of cefazolin caused a decrease in wound infection but no decrease in pneumonia or empyema [4]. Cefuroxime continued for 48 hours after pulmonary resection was more effective in preventing infection, particularly empyema, than one dose at induction and a second dose 2 hours later [33b].
   b. Other trials have found that multiple doses of a cephalosporin can prevent empyema after closed-tube thoracostomy for chest trauma [4].

11. Ocular surgery. The role of antibiotic prophylaxis for ocular surgery is unclear, but postoperative endophthalmitis can be devastating. Most ophthalmologists use antimicrobial eye drops for prophylaxis; many also give a subconjunctival injection at the end of the procedure, but controlled studies supporting a particular choice, route, or duration of antimicrobial prophylaxis are lacking [4].

12. Trauma
   a. Abdominal. The use of perioperative antibiotics as prophylaxis against infection in the patient with abdominal trauma and suspected ruptured hollow viscus is widely accepted [18]. If at surgery there is no injury to a hollow viscus, reducing the duration (e.g., with cefoxitin) to 12 hours is indicated [7]. For patients found to have intestinal perforation, then a short course of antibiotics (very early therapy for bacterial spillage) for 2–5 days with cefoxitin or a similar agent is advised [2].
   b. Chest. In penetrating thoracic trauma and in the placement of chest tubes in trauma management, prophylactic antibiotics have not been effective according to some reviews [2], but this is an unsettled area. See related discussion in sec. **10.b.**

13. Low-risk or "clean" procedures. Whether the benefits outweigh the risks of antibiotic prophylaxis for these procedures (e.g., hernia repair, breast operations, skin surgery) has been questioned. Some experts suggest prophylaxis [1] may be useful if the patient was at increased risk for infection (e.g., debilitated, diabetic, poor hygiene). Other experts emphasize that routine prophylaxis for these patients is not indicated [2].
   a. Breast surgery. Preliminary studies suggest perioperative cephalosporin therapy in excision of a breast mass, mastectomy, reduction mammoplasty, and axillary node dissection reduced the incidence of postoperative

infections [34], especially in patients at higher risk for infection. In a recent review, although controversial, the authors conclude prophylactic antibiotics are useful in this setting [35]. However, most *Medical Letter* consultants do not recommend prophylaxis routinely for breast procedures [4].

   b. **Herniorrhaphy.** Similarly, preliminary data suggest patients undergoing herniorrhaphy benefited from perioperative cephalosporin prophylaxis [34]. In a patient with additional risk factors for infection, single-dose prophylaxis is reasonable.

   14. **Other procedures.** Antibiotic **prophylaxis is not routinely recommended for** cardiac catheterization, GI endoscopy, repair of simple lacerations, outpatient treatment of burns, arterial puncture, paracentesis, or thoracentesis [1–4].

C. **"Dirty" surgery.** In such cases (e.g., bowel perforation, complex fracture), **antibiotics are used therapeutically for full courses.** These antibiotics are therapeutic, not prophylactic, because an early infection already is present. **Animal or human bites also deserve therapeutic courses** [4] **and are discussed in detail in Chap. 4.**

D. **Laparoscopic surgery.** Few data are available on the role of prophylactic antibiotics in this setting. The *Medical Letter* recently suggested that "until more data become available, the same standards should be applied to laparoscopic surgery as for operations through a traditional incision" [4]. For example, if a patient is in the high-risk group for an open (traditional) cholecystectomy (see sec. **B.1**), he or she should also receive prophylactic antibiotics for a laparoscopic cholecystectomy.

III. **Organisms involved.** An effective prophylactic regimen should be directed against the most likely infecting organisms but need not include drugs active against every potential pathogen. Regimens that only decrease the total number of pathogens permit host defenses to resist clinical infection [4]. Most surgical wound infections are acquired in the operating room from the patients' own microbial flora. The remainder are acquired mainly from the staff in the operating room during surgery. The inanimate environment (e.g., walls, floors, and surgical equipment) has little relevance to the spread of infection [36].

A. *Staphylococcus aureus.* **In wound infections after clean surgery, the major pathogen of concern is** *S. aureus,* which commonly colonizes the nose and the skin. The majority of these are penicillin-resistant. Therefore, any prophylactic agent would need to be effective against these organisms.

B. **Gram-negative bacteria** cause wound infections especially when surgery of the colon, genitourinary tract, or gynecologic organs is undertaken.

C. **Potential for resistant organisms.** In a given hospital, the prevalence of a specific organism may affect antibiotic selection. For example, if methicillin-resistant *S. epidermidis* is a problem in prosthetic device surgery, antibiotic choice is influenced by this fact (see Ayliffe [36]). If a patient has been on protracted antibiotic therapy, his or her flora may be different and a different, broader agent may be indicated.

D. It is unnecessary to use antibiotics active against all the organisms potentially involved in wound infections.

IV. **Potential disadvantages of prophylaxis**

A. **Superinfection with a resistant organism** is a concern. However, this risk is minimal if antibiotics are not initiated until just prior to the start of an operation, if their use postoperatively is for less than 24 hours, and if cephalosporins are used (see **V.B.4**). If antibiotics are used for less than 48 hours, normal flora usually will persist in sites such as the oropharynx.

B. **Toxic or allergic** reactions can occur whenever antibiotics are used. These can be minimized by using safe agents for short periods of time.

C. **Cost.** Antibiotics are expensive and should not be used unnecessarily. However, in patients clearly at risk of wound infections that have been shown to be decreased by antibiotic prophylaxis, the cost of the antibiotics is negligible compared with the hospitalization cost of a prolonged stay caused by a wound infection [2, 12]. When antibiotic prophylaxis is used, the least expensive effective agent for a brief period is chosen.

D. **A false sense of security** may be created by the use of antibiotics. **Meticulous surgery and careful preoperative and postoperative care are essential** in minimizing wound infections.

V. **Antibiotic agents used in surgical prophylaxis.** These agents must cover *S. aureus.* For distal ileum, appendix, or colon procedures, agents with activity against aerobic and anaerobic bacteria are preferred.

A. **Semisynthetic penicillin** (nafcillin or oxacillin) is, in clean surgery, active against *S. aureus* and is a potential agent. However, although the rationale could be debated, the cephalosporins are used more frequently for surgical prophylaxis.

B. **Cephalosporins are widely favored** in surgical prophylaxis. The cited reasons for preference of the cephalosporins include the following:

1. **Broad spectrum of activity.** These agents are active against most penicillin-susceptible and penicillin-resistant *S. aureus* as well as many *S. epidermidis* and many gram-negative strains, such as *Escherichia coli* and *Klebsiella* spp., which may cause wound infections (see sec. **6**). Cefoxitin and cefotetan are also active against most bowel-related anaerobes.

2. **Few side effects.** Side effects seen with these agents are few, and this is a crucial point for prophylactic antibiotics.

3. **Low incidence of allergic reactions.** With short duration of use, these agents rarely cause rashes or other allergic problems. They can be used in patients with delayed penicillin reactions.

4. **Which cephalosporin?** With the availability of first-, second-, and third-generation agents, the question arises as to which agent is preferable in routine surgical prophylaxis. **Because the first-generation agents are more active against *S. aureus,* are less expensive than the newer agents, and have a narrower spectrum of in vitro activity** (and therefore are less likely to select out resistant bacteria), **these agents are preferred for most surgical procedures.** Furthermore, of the first-generation agents, **cefazolin** has the added advantage of a moderately long serum half-life, making it a **preferred agent for prophylaxis** [1, 4]. In reviews [1, 4], **for colorectal surgery and appendectomy, cefoxitin or cefotetan is preferred** because these agents are more active against bowel anaerobes, including *B. fragilis* (see sec. **II.B.4**). For the other abdominal and pelvic procedures, including obstetric and gynecologic operations, cefazolin has been equally effective and is less expensive [4]. Single-dose cefotetan may be a more cost-effective agent than multiple doses of cefoxitin in colorectal surgery lasting for more than 2–3 hours. (See sec. **I.B.2** and Chap. 28F, sec. **II.F** under Individual Agents, for a discussion of cefotetan.)

   The *Medical Letter* emphasizes that the **third-generation cephalosporins should not be used** because they are more expensive, have less antistaphylococcal activity than cefazolin, and their spectrum of activity against gram-negative bacilli includes organisms rarely encountered in elective surgery. Their unnecessary and potential widespread use for prophylaxis may promote emergence of resistance to these potentially valuable therapeutic agents [4]. The optimal cephalosporin to use in cardiovascular surgery has been debated, with second-generation cephalosporins (e.g., cefamandole, cefuroxime) purported to have a broader spectrum of activity than the first-generation cephalosporins (e.g., cefazolin) and therefore presumed to be more effective [37]. However, recent studies do not reveal significant differences between the first- and second-generation agents in this setting [37, 38]. Therefore, the more cost-effective agent (cefazolin) seems rational.

5. **Prophylactic dosage.** Few reports have focused on the appropriate dose for prophylaxis [1].

   a. **Initial dose.** As discussed in sec. **I.A.3**, it is important to have good (i.e., therapeutic) antibiotic levels at the time of surgery. Ideally, perioperative antibiotics are given in the operating room just at the time of anesthesia (i.e., 30–60 minutes before the incision).

      (1) **Cefazolin,** a first-generation cephalosporin, is used commonly for many procedures, typically at a dose of 1–2 g. Although many regimes use 1 g of cefazolin per dose [4], others at times suggest 2 g per dose [1, 2], as in knee replacement when a tourniquet is used and in cholecystectomy [2].

      (2) **Cefoxitin or cefotetan.** Both 1-g [1, 4] or 2-g [1, 2] doses have been suggested. For colon surgery, we tend to use the 2-g dose. If cephalosporins are contraindicated, an aminoglycoside (1.7 mg/kg per dose of gentamicin or tobramycin) can be combined with clindamycin (600 mg per dose in adults) or metronidazole or aztreonam and clindamycin [1].

      (3) **In children,** 30–40 mg/kg per dose of the cephalosporin has been suggested [1].

      (4) **Vancomycin** can be given instead of cefazolin to patients who are allergic to cephalosporins or in institutions where methicillin-resistant

S. aureus (or coagulase-negative staphylococci) have become important pathogens; routine use of vancomycin for prophylaxis should be discouraged because it promotes emergence of vancomycin-resistant enterococci [4]. See Chap. 28O.

Because vancomycin provides no activity against facultative gram-negative bacilli, which may be involved in settings such as GI surgery, lower-extremity vascular surgery, or hysterectomy, another agent with gram-negative activity should be added to the regimen under these circumstances. If allergy to cephalosporins is the concern, aztreonam or an aminoglycoside can be used [1] (see sec. **d** for doses, and Chap. 28O).

   (5) **Cefuroxime** has also been studied in noncardiac thoracic surgery. See sec. **II.B.10.**

   b. **Intraoperative dosage for prolonged procedures.** It is desirable to maintain high tissue levels of the prophylactic agent throughout the surgical procedure. Therefore, repeat doses may be necessary intraoperatively in procedures lasting longer than 2 hours. When agents with a long biologic half-life are used (e.g., cefazolin), the dose can be repeated every 4 hours intraoperatively. When agents with a shorter half-life are used (e.g., cefoxitin), it is necessary to repeat doses every 2–3 hours intraoperatively. Usually, only one dose of cefotetan (1–2 g) is given preoperatively for a procedure lasting up to 5–6 hours. See sec. **I.B.** and **Table 28B-1.**

   c. **Postoperative dosage.** Postoperative administration of prophylactic antibiotics usually is unnecessary and, because of the frequent use of such agents, is expensive to the patient and hospital. Exceptions to this rule are discussed in sec. I.B.

   d. **For hospitals in which methicillin-resistant *S. aureus* or *S. epidermidis* frequently cause wound infections or for patients with cephalosporin allergies, vancomycin is an alternative agent** for patients undergoing prosthetic device surgery—for example, heart valve replacement, vascular procedures, and total hip replacement. Often 1 g of vancomycin is infused slowly intravenously over 120 minutes [4]. Vancomycin, 15 mg/kg, has also been used [2]. See detailed discussion of vancomycin dosing in Chap. 28O.

6. **Failures** of surgical prophylaxis with postoperative methicillin-susceptible *S. aureus* have been described despite the use of cefazolin [2, 39, 40]. The biologic explanation is very interesting, but the exact clinical application awaits further study.

   Presumably, failures occur because cefazolin is more susceptible to inactivation by some beta-lactamase-producing strains of *S. aureus* than other cephalosporins (e.g., cephalothin, cefuroxime, cefamandole) [39]. This in vitro observation has been known for years, but its clinical relevance in the past has been debated and is unclear. **While awaiting additional studies in this area, cefazolin still remains the agent of choice for most clinical situations** [1, 4].

   However, if methicillin-susceptible *S. aureus* infections continue to occur despite cefazolin (e.g., in cardiovascular or orthopedic procedures), infectious disease consultation is advised to help determine the optimal prophylactic agent to use in an institution if failures are seen with standard regimens.

C. **Ampicillin-sulbactam** (Unasyn) has been used for prophylaxis in head and neck cancer surgery because this agent will cover *S. aureus* and many gram-negative bacilli [41].

D. **Vancomycin** is indicated when prosthetic device infections due to methicillin-resistant staphylococci are a special problem and at times in the allergic patient.

E. **Topical antibiotic prophylaxis.** Early studies suggest that topical use of antibiotics may be effective in the prevention of surgical wound infections. However, the precise clinical implications of the use of topical agents await further well-controlled, comparative clinical studies. Therefore, unless topical agents are being used as part of a carefully designed clinical study, we do not advocate their use at this time.

VI. **Nonsurgical antibiotic prophylaxis.** There are a few indications for prophylactic antibiotics in the nonsurgical setting.

A. **Prevention of rheumatic fever.** The recommendations that follow are for most of the United States, where the incidence of rheumatic fever remains low. This has been reviewed elsewhere [42].

   1. **Prevention of initial attacks (i.e., "primary" prevention)** of rheumatic fever

involves the proper therapy of group A beta-hemolytic streptococcal infections of the upper respiratory tract. Studies have indicated that during epidemics, approximately 3% of acute streptococcal group A sore throats are followed by rheumatic fever; in endemic infections, attacks of rheumatic fever may be fewer [42].

  a. **Penicillin is the drug of choice** except in patients who are allergic to this drug. (See Chap. 7 for a detailed discussion of streptococcal pharyngitis and the role of cephalosporins in therapy.) It effectively prevents rheumatic fever even when therapy is started several days after the onset of the acute illness. A single dose of intramuscular benzathine penicillin G (600,000 units for patients weighing 60 lb [27 kg] or less, and 1.2 million units for patients weighing more than 60 lb) ensures treatment for an adequate time because this agent provides adequate blood levels for more than 10 days. **When oral therapy is used, a full 10-day course is necessary.** Penicillin V (in children, 250 mg bid or tid, and adults, 500 mg bid or tid) for 10 days often is advised [42]; 250 mg bid in children and 500 mg bid in adults is adequate [43].

  b. **In the penicillin-allergic patient,** erythromycin estolate (20–40 mg/kg/day to a maximum of 1 g/day) in two to four divided doses or erythromycin ethylsuccinate (40 mg/kg/day up to a maximum of 1 g) in two to four divided doses for 10 days has been advised [42]. In adults, 250 mg bid–qid commonly is used. The new macrolide, azithromycin, can be administered once daily and produces high tonsillar tissue concentrations. A 5-day course of azithromycin is approved by the Food and Drug Administration as a second-line therapy for patients 2 years of age or older with streptococcal A pharyngitis [42]. (See Chaps. 7 and 28M.) This may be a useful alternative in the penicillin-allergic patient in whom compliance may be improved with this regimen (e.g., a college student).

  Oral cephalosporins (e.g., cephalexin or cephradine) for 10 days also are acceptable alternatives and usually are better tolerated [43, 44]. (**See Chap. 7.**) Tetracycline and sulfonamides should not be used.

2. **Prevention of recurrent attacks of rheumatic fever (i.e., "secondary" prevention).** Patients with a prior history of rheumatic fever generally are at high risk of a recurrence if they develop a group A streptococcal upper respiratory tract infection. Because asymptomatic as well as symptomatic infection can trigger a recurrence, **continuous prophylaxis is recommended for patients with a well-documented history of rheumatic fever or Sydenham's chorea or those with definite rheumatic heart disease.**

  a. **The duration** of this continuous prophylaxis **is uncertain** [6a, 42]. Data suggest that recurrences decline with the advancing age of the patient and as the time interval after the most recent attack increases. Some clinicians argue that, ideally, prophylaxis is lifelong. Others will treat patients at least until they reach their early twenties and 5 years have elapsed since the last rheumatic attack [42] and then continue prophylaxis only in those who are at increased risk of exposure to streptococcal infections—for example, parents of young children, schoolteachers, others exposed to young children, as well as medical personnel and those in military service. Those living in crowded conditions and economically disadvantaged populations may also be at increased risk. Even after prosthetic valve surgery for rheumatic heart disease, prophylaxis should be continued, as these patients are theoretically at risk [42]. See detailed discussion in references [6a] and [42], which emphasize that the decision to discontinue prophylaxis must be individualized.

  b. **Regimens**

    (1) **Intramuscular benzathine penicillin G,** 1,200,000 units every month, is the recommended method [42]. In countries where the incidence of acute rheumatic fever is particularly high, or in certain high-risk patients, use of benzathine penicillin G every 3 weeks may be warranted [42]. This regimen is preferred for high-risk patients (e.g., young patients who have experienced a recent episode of rheumatic fever). However, the advantages of benzathine penicillin G must be weighed against the inconvenience to the patient and pain of injection, which causes some individuals to discontinue prophylaxis [42].

(2) **Oral regimens assume the compliance of the patient;** therefore, careful and repeated patient education is essential. Even with optimal compliance, risk of recurrence is still higher in those on regular oral prophylaxis compared with those receiving intramuscular benzathine penicillin G [42]. **Penicillin V,** 250 mg bid, is recommended. **Sulfadiazine,** 1 g once daily for patients weighing more than 60 lb and 500 mg once daily for patients weighing less than 60 lb, also is suggested. These regimens are about equally effective, and one of these regimens is preferred. For the exceptional patient who may be allergic to both penicillin and sulfonamides, erythromycin may be used [42], and 250 mg bid is suggested [42].

B. **Prevention of serious infections after splenectomy.** Overwhelming infection due to encapsulated organisms such as *S. pneumoniae, Haemophilus influenzae* and, rarely, *Neisseria meningitidis* can occur after splenectomy. Methods of preventing these overwhelming infections, which can occur months or years after splenectomy, remain unclear and controversial [45–49]. Children may be at particularly high risk, but it can also occur in adults.

An adult, splenectomized after trauma but otherwise healthy, is at risk for overwhelming pneumococcal sepsis, although at a much lower incidence than young children [46, 48], probably because of the adult's immune status, which supports the rest of the mononuclear-phagocytic system [47]. Recognition that adults as well as children are at increased risk of infection years after splenectomy has led to consideration of spleen-sparing surgical approaches after trauma [46, 47].

1. **Vaccines.** The **pneumococcal vaccine** usually is given to these patients, but its efficacy in this setting is unclear [46–48]. If an elective splenectomy is performed, the pneumococcal vaccine should be administered at least 2 weeks before the elective splenectomy [46]. The polysaccharide *H. influenzae* vaccine is another useful agent, although efficacy data with this vaccine for this use are not available. The role of **meningococcal vaccine** in this setting has not been established, but it seems a reasonable consideration and has been suggested [48]. (A single-dose vial of the quadrivalent vaccine is available now in the United States.)

2. **Prophylactic antibiotics.** Some experts recommend the use of oral penicillin daily (e.g., penicillin V, 125 mg bid in children and 250 mg bid in adults) in recently splenectomized patients. This is a particularly common practice in children [45, 48]. Whether to use prophylactic penicillin routinely in adults who are not otherwise compromised is a controversial issue [46–48]. We use prophylactic antibiotics in adults with Hodgkin's disease who have undergone splenectomy, chemotherapy, or radiation therapy. Less frequently, ampicillin is used on a daily basis as it is active against *H. influenzae* as well as *S. pneumoniae,* but it is more likely to cause side effects. Neither the optimal agent nor optimal duration of antibiotics in this setting has been established.

3. **Early therapeutic antibiotics.** Early empiric antibiotic therapy in patients who have undergone a splenectomy is an important consideration. Patients can be given a supply of antibiotic for use if an acute illness develops and medical attention is not immediately available [48]. Oral penicillin and amoxicillin have been used. When these patients present with nonspecific febrile illnesses, often flulike, early antibiotic therapy is rational for unexplained fever or chills. Ideally, appropriate cultures should be obtained, but if facilities for culture analysis are not immediately available, starting antibiotics without cultures is reasonable [46]. In community-acquired bacteremia of unclear primary focus of infection, therapy aimed at the likely pathogens should be instituted early while awaiting cultures. Cefuroxime and ceftriaxone are useful options. See Chap. 2 for a more detailed discussion.

4. **Identification warning.** Because these patients are at risk of fulminant sepsis, we encourage each patient to have some form of personal identification (e.g., medical alert necklace or bracelet, or note in his or her wallet or purse) indicating that he or she has undergone splenectomy. The patients' families should be aware of this potential complication.

5. **Summary.** Because the splenectomized patient is at risk of severe bacterial infections, especially if a remnant is not left behind, it seems prudent that these patients should receive the pneumococcal, *H. influenzae* b, and meningo-

coccal vaccines; however, they provide only partial protection against future bacteremias. We routinely use penicillin prophylaxis in children, at least for 2–4 years. In general, we neither routinely treat adults with prophylactic antibiotics after splenectomy nor use ampicillin in this setting unless the patient has received therapy for Hodgkin's disease. The medical records of these patients should indicate clearly that they have undergone splenectomy and, as stated earlier, we encourage patients to have some form of personal identification indicating that they have undergone splenectomy so that physicians caring for them can be immediately alerted. Early empiric antibiotics are a rational approach.

C. **Prevention of bacterial endocarditis** has been reviewed [50]. Although antimicrobial prophylaxis commonly is used in patients with certain types of valvular heart disease or prosthetic valves, **no adequate, controlled clinical trials of the effectiveness of antibiotic regimens for the prevention of bacterial endocarditis in humans have been done.** Therefore, recommendations are based on in vitro studies, clinical experience, data from animal models, and assessment of both the bacteria most likely to produce bacteremia from a given site and those most likely to result in endocarditis [50, 51]. The American Heart Association (AHA) stresses that its published report "represents recommended guidelines to supplement practitioners in the exercise of their clinical judgment and is not intended as a standard of care for all cases" [50], as it is impossible to make recommendations for all clinical situations in which endocarditis may develop.

1. **Underlying cardiac disease.** Certain cardiac conditions are more often associated with endocarditis than others. **See Table 28B-2.** What is meant by "insufficiency" in mitral valve prolapse is not fully clarified in the 1990 recommendations. This is a practical consideration for the clinician because, in patients with mitral valve prolapse, the murmur may vary from one examination to another and because Doppler echocardiography can detect nonaudible (and probably non-endocarditis-predisposing) amounts of valvular insufficiency even in normal valves [52]. In their editorial response, Kaye and Abrutyn [52] suggest that "on the basis of current knowledge, we believe that **prophylaxis is indicated for patients with mitral valve prolapse with a holosystolic murmur;** should be optional in cases of late systolic murmur, either spontaneous or evoked (e.g., standing or the valsalva maneuver); and is not indicated in the absence of a murmur."

   In their 1995 review of this topic, Dickinson and Bisno [6a] emphasize that clinical studies indicate that nearly all cases of infective endocarditis occur in patients with audible systolic murmurs, so prophylaxis is not recommended for patients with isolated systolic clicks. Patients with thickened and redundant valves clearly are at higher risk. They conclude by noting, "more convenient clinical markers are needed, however, to define with precision the subgroup of MVP patients at highest risk [for endocarditis]" [6a].

2. **Surgical and dental procedures** and instrumentations involving mucosal surfaces or contaminated tissue commonly cause transient ($\leq$ 15 minutes) bacteremia. Certain procedures are much more likely to initiate the bacteremia that results in endocarditis than are other procedures [50].
   a. **See Table 28B-3.**
   b. Edentulous patients may develop bacteremia from ulcers caused by ill-fitting dentures [50].

3. **Antibiotic regimens.** To reduce the likelihood of microbial resistance, it is important that prophylactic antibiotics be used only during the perioperative period. They should be initiated shortly before the procedure (1–2 hours) and should not be continued for an extended period (no more than 6–8 hours). In the case of delayed healing or of a procedure that involves infected tissue, it may be necessary to provide additional doses of antibiotics [50] (i.e., therapeutic courses).
   a. **For dental, oral, and upper respiratory tract procedures.** Antibiotic prophylaxis is recommended for all dental procedures likely to cause gingival bleeding, including routine professional cleaning. If a series of dental procedures is required, it may be prudent to observe an interval of 7 days between procedures to reduce the potential for the emergence of resistant strains [50].
      (1) **See Table 28B-4.** Therapy is aimed at viridans streptococci.

Table 28B-2. Cardiac conditions[a]

Endocarditis prophylaxis recommended
Prosthetic cardiac valves, including bioprosthetic and homograft valves
Previous bacterial endocarditis, even in the absence of heart disease
Most congenital cardiac malformations
Rheumatic and other acquired valvular dysfunction, even after valvular surgery
Hypertrophic cardiomyopathy
Mitral valve prolapse with valvular regurgitation

Endocarditis prophylaxis not recommended
Isolated secundum atrial septal defect
Surgical repair without residua beyond 6 mo of secundum atrial septal defect,
    ventricular septal defect, or patent ductus arteriosus
Previous coronary artery bypass graft surgery
Mitral valve prolapse without valvular regurgitation[b]
Physiologic, functional, or innocent heart murmurs
Previous Kawasaki disease without valvular dysfunction
Previous rheumatic fever without valvular dysfunction
Cardiac pacemakers and implanted defibrillators

[a]This table lists selected conditions but is not meant to be all-inclusive.
[b]Individuals who have a mitral valve prolapse associated with thickening or redundancy of the
valve leaflets may be at increased risk for bacterial endocarditis, particularly men who are 45
years of age or older.
Source: From A.S. Dajani, et al., Prevention of bacterial endocarditis: Recommendations by the
American Heart Association. *J.A.M.A.* 264:2919, 1990. Copyright 1990, American Medical
Association.

    (2) Amoxicillin now is recommended rather than oral penicillin because
amoxicillin is better absorbed from the GI tract and provides higher
serum levels [50].

    (3) In penicillin- (or ampicillin- or amoxicillin-) allergic patients, if eryth-
romycin is used, the erythromycin preparations shown in Table 28B-
4 are recommended because of their more rapid and reliable absorption
than other erythromycin formulations, resulting in higher and more
sustained blood levels [50]. In patients who have GI side effects with
erythromycin (or amoxicillin), clindamycin is preferred.

    (4) When the oral regimen cannot be given to a patient, an **alternative
parenteral regimen** can be used and is shown in Table 28B-5.

    (5) High-risk patients (i.e., individuals with prosthetic heart valves, a
previous history of endocarditis, or surgically constructed systemic-
pulmonary shunts or conduits) were considered candidates for parenteral regimens in prior endocarditis prophylaxis recommendations.
However, the recommendations [50] recognize that in practice there
are substantial logistical and financial barriers to the use of parenteral
regimens. In addition, oral regimens used by individuals who have
prosthetic valves in other countries have not been associated with
prophylaxis failures [50].

    Therefore, the **committee** "**recommends the use of the standard
prophylactic regimen** [see Table 28B-4] **in patients who have prosthetic heart valves and in other high-risk groups**" [50] (i.e., the oral
regimen). If a practitioner prefers to use parenteral regimens in these
high-risk patients, the regimens in Table 28B-5 can be used.

  b. For genitourinary and gastrointestinal procedures, antibiotics are **aimed
at enterococci,** for gram-negative bacilli rarely cause endocarditis [50].
**Prophylaxis is no longer recommended for gastrointestinal endoscopic
procedures even with biopsy** [50]. These procedures have rarely, if ever,
been implicated as the cause of endocarditis [52].

    (1) See Table 28B-6 for regimens.

Table 28B-3. Dental or surgical procedures[a]

Endocarditis prophylaxis recommended
Dental procedures known to induce gingival or mucosal bleeding, including
  professional cleaning
Tonsillectomy or adenoidectomy
Surgical operations that involve intestinal or respiratory mucosa
Bronchoscopy with a rigid bronchoscope
Sclerotherapy for esophageal varices
Esophageal dilatation
Gallbladder surgery
Cystoscopy
Urethral dilatation
Urethral catheterization if urinary tract infection is present[b]
Urinary tract surgery if urinary tract infection is present[b]
Prostatic surgery
Incision and drainage of infected tissue[b]
Vaginal hysterectomy
Vaginal delivery in the presence of infection[b]

Endocarditis prophylaxis not recommended[c]
Dental procedures not likely to induce gingival bleeding, such as simple adjustment
  of orthodontic appliances or fillings above the gum line
Injection of local intraoral anesthetic (except intraligamentary injections)
Shedding of primary teeth
Tympanostomy tube insertion
Endotracheal intubation
Bronchoscopy with a flexible bronchoscope, with or without biopsy
Cardiac catheterization
Endoscopy with or without gastrointestinal biopsy
Cesarean section
In the absence of infection for urethral catheterization, dilatation and curettage,
  uncomplicated vaginal delivery, therapeutic abortion, sterilization procedures,
  or insertion or removal of intrauterine devices

[a]This table lists selected procedures but is not meant to be all-inclusive.
[b]In addition to prophylactic regimen for genitourinary procedures, antibiotic therapy should be
directed against the most likely bacterial pathogen.
[c]In patients who have prosthetic heart valves, a previous history of endocarditis, or surgically
constructed systemic-pulmonary shunts or conduits, physicians may choose to administer
prophylactic antibiotics even for low-risk procedures that involve the lower respiratory,
genitourinary, or gastrointestinal tracts.
Source: From A.S. Dajani et al., Prevention of bacterial endocarditis: Recommendations by the
American Heart Association. *J.A.M.A.* 264:2919, 1990. Copyright 1990, American Medical
Association.

  (2) **For high-risk** patients (e.g., those with prosthetic heart valves or a
      previous history of bacterial endocarditis), **the parenteral regimen is
      still advised** [50], as in prior endocarditis prophylaxis recommenda-
      tions (see Table 28B-6).
  (3) **For low-risk** patients, an alternative oral regimen is provided in Table
      28B-6.
4. **Miscellaneous**
   a. **Recipients of secondary prevention of rheumatic fever.** Patients who
      take oral penicillin to prevent recurrent rheumatic fever (see section **A.2**)
      may have viridans streptococci in their oral cavities that are relatively
      resistant to penicillin or amoxicillin. In such cases, erythromycin or an-
      other of the alternative regimens listed in Tables 28B-4 and 28B-5 should
      be used rather than amoxicillin (or another penicillin) [50].

Table 28B-4. Recommended standard prophylactic regimen for dental, oral, or upper respiratory tract procedures in patients who are at risk[a]

Drug	Dosing regimen[b]
Standard regimen	
Amoxicillin	3 g PO 1 hr before procedure; then 1.5 g 6 hr after initial dose
Amoxicillin- or penicillin-allergic patients	
Erythromycin	Erythromycin ethylsuccinate, 800 mg, or erythromycin stearate, 1 g PO 2 hr
or	before procedure; then half the dose 6 hr after initial dose
Clindamycin	300 mg PO 1 hr before procedure and 150 mg 6 hr after initial dose

[a]Includes those with prosthetic heart valves and other high-risk patients.
[b]Initial pediatric doses are as follows: amoxicillin, 50 mg/kg; erythromycin ethylsuccinate or erythromycin stearate, 20 mg/kg; and clindamycin, 10 mg/kg. Follow-up doses should be one-half the initial dose. **Total pediatric dose should not exceed total adult dose.** The following weight ranges may also be used for the initial pediatric dose of amoxicillin: <15 kg, 750 mg; 15–30 kg, 1,500 mg; and >30 kg, 3,000 mg (full adult dose).
Source: From A.S. Dajani et al., Prevention of bacterial endocarditis: Recommendations by the American Heart Association. *J.A.M.A.* 264:2919, 1990. Copyright 1990, American Medical Association.

b. **Renal dysfunction.** In patients who have markedly compromised renal function, it may be necessary to modify or omit the second dose of gentamicin (see Chap. 28H) or vancomycin (see Chap. 28O).
c. **Concomitant anticoagulation use.** Intramuscular injections should be avoided in patients who receive heparin; warfarin use is a relative contraindication to intramuscular injections. Therefore, intravenous or oral regimens should be used whenever possible [50].
d. **Cardiac transplantation.** In the 1990 AHA recommendations, it was felt there were insufficient data to support specific recommendations for prevention of bacterial endocarditis in recipients of cardiac transplants [50].
e. **Open heart surgery.** Patients who undergo surgery for placement of prosthetic heart valves or prosthetic intravascular or intracardiac materials are also at risk for the development of bacterial endocarditis, usually caused by *S. aureus,* coagulase-negative staphylococci, or diphtheroids [50]. A first-generation cephalosporin commonly is used, but other considerations affect the antibiotic choice (see sec. II.B.8). Prophylactic antibiotics ideally should be continued for no more than 24 hours postoperatively to minimize emergence of resistant microorganisms [50].
f. **Adjunctive dental care** [50]. **Individuals who are at risk for developing bacterial endocarditis should optimize oral health to reduce the potential of bacterial seeding. Routine dental care and efforts to reduce gingival inflammation** (brushing, flossing, fluoride rinse, and chlorhexidine gluconate mouth rinse) **are important but often not emphasized enough.** Chlorhexidine that is painted on isolated and dried gingiva 3–5 minutes prior to tooth extraction reduces postextraction bacteremia. Other agents such as povidone-iodine or iodine and glycerin may also be appropriate. Irrigation of the gingival sulcus with chlorhexidine prior to tooth extraction reduces postextraction bacteremia in adults [50].
g. **Manipulation of subcutaneous abscesses** can be associated with staphylococcal or streptococcal bacteremias, although if a perineal abscess is manipulated, gram-negative bacilli or enterococci may be a concern (see Table 28B-3). **No formal guidelines are available. Possible approaches include the following:**
   (1) **For nonperineal abscess drainage**
      (a) **Oral regimen.** In adults, dicloxacillin, 500 mg PO or 500–1,000 mg cephalexin (higher dose in high-risk patients) PO 1 hour prior to drainage followed by a similar dose q6h once or twice after the procedure.

Table 28B-5. Alternative prophylactic regimens for dental, oral, or upper respiratory tract procedures in patients who are at risk

Drug	Dosing regimen[a]
Patients unable to take oral medications	
Ampicillin	Intravenous or intramuscular administration of ampicillin, 2 g, 30 min before procedure; then intravenous or intramuscular administration of ampicillin, 1 g, or oral administration of amoxicillin, 1.5 g, 6 hr after initial dose
Ampicillin-, amoxicillin-, and penicillin-allergic patients unable to take oral medications	
Clindamycin	Intravenous administration of 300 mg 30 min before procedure and an intravenous or oral administration of 150 mg 6 hr after initial dose
Patients considered high risk and not candidates for standard regimen	
Ampicillin, gentamicin, and amoxicillin	Intravenous or intramuscular administration of ampicillin, 2 g, plus gentamicin, 1.5 mg/kg (not to exceed 80 mg), 30 min before procedure; followed by amoxicillin, 1.5 g, orally 6 hr after initial dose; alternatively, the parenteral regimen may be repeated 8 hr after initial dose
Ampicillin-, amoxicillin-, and penicillin-allergic patients considered high risk	
Vancomycin	Intravenous administration of 1 g over 1 hr[b], starting 1 hr before procedure; no repeated dose necessary

[a]Initial pediatric doses are as follows: ampicillin, 50 mg/kg; clindamycin, 10 mg/kg; gentamicin, 2 mg/kg; and vancomycin, 20 mg/kg. Follow-up doses should be one-half the initial dose. **Total pediatric dose should not exceed total adult dose.** No initial dose is recommended in this table for amoxicillin (25 mg/kg is the follow-up dose).
[b]*Authors' note:* Some experts infuse 1 g vancomycin over 2 hours (see Chap. 28O).
Source: From A.S. Dajani et al., Prevention of bacterial endocarditis: Recommendations by the American Heart Association. *J.A.M.A.* 264:2919, 1990. Copyright 1990, American Medical Association.

      (b) Parenteral regimen. In adults, a semisynthetic penicillin (oxacillin or nafcillin) 1–2 g IV or 1 g cefazolin can be given a half hour prior to drainage. An oral dose of dicloxacillin or cephalexin could also be given at 6 and 12 hours after drainage as discussed in sec. **(a).**
    (2) For perirectal or perivulvar abscess drainage (which might involve staphylococci, enterococci and, to a lesser extent, gram-negative bacilli), the optimal regimen is not established.
      (a) Oral regimen. In the adult, Augmentin (500 mg amoxicillin–125 mg clavulanic acid) 1 hour before the procedure is an appealing agent in the non-penicillin-allergic patient. This could be repeated at 6 and 12 hours after the drainage procedure. In the penicillin-allergic patient, a single dose of intravenous vancomycin with an aminoglycoside is an option (see Table 28B-6) to ensure enterococcal coverage.
      (b) Parenteral. Vancomycin with an aminoglycoside can be used as described in Table 28B-6. Another potential regimen may be ampicillin-sulbactam (Unasyn) or piperacillin-tazobactam (Zosyn) with a single dose before the procedure (see Chap. 28E).
  D. Oral antibiotics to prevent infections in the leukopenic patient have been reviewed elsewhere [47, 53]. In general, we do not advocate their routine use unless as part of a special clinical study. See further discussions on TMP-SMX (Chap. 28K) and the fluoroquinolones (Chap. 28S).

Table 28B-6. Prophylactic regimens for genitourinary and gastrointestinal procedures

Drug	Dosage regimen[a]
Standard regimen	
Ampicillin, gentamicin, and amoxicillin	Intravenous or intramuscular administration of ampicillin, 2 g, plus gentamicin, 1.5 mg/kg (not to exceed 80 mg), 30 min before procedure; followed by amoxicillin, 1.5 g, orally 6 hr after initial dose; alternatively, the parenteral regimen may be repeated once 8 hr after initial dose
Ampicillin-, amoxicillin-, and penicillin-allergic patient regimen	
Vancomycin and gentamicin	Intravenous administration of vancomycin, 1 g, over 1 hr plus intravenous or intramuscular administration of gentamicin, 1.5 mg/kg (not to exceed 80 mg), 1 hr before procedure; may be repeated once 8 hr after initial dose[b]
Alternate low-risk patient regimen	
Amoxicillin	3 g orally 1 hr before procedure; then 1.5 g 6 hr after initial dose

[a]Initial pediatric doses are as follows: ampicillin, 50 mg/kg; amoxicillin, 50 mg/kg, gentamicin, 2 mg/kg, and vancomycin, 20 mg/kg. Follow-up doses should be one-half the initial dose. **Total pediatric dose should not exceed total adult dose.**
[b]*Authors' note:* We would give the vancomycin intravenously over 2 hours. We would repeat the gentamicin dose only.
Source: From A.S. Dajani et al., Prevention of bacterial endocarditis: Recommendations by the American Heart Association. *J.A.M.A.* 264:2919, 1990. Copyright 1990, American Medical Association.

    E. **Travelers' diarrhea.** Although this can often be prevented by prophylactic doses of TMP-SMX, TMP, or doxycycline, widespread use of this approach will increase problems of bacterial resistance. Short therapeutic courses therefore are preferred and are discussed in Chap. 21.

    F. **Influenza A** can often be prevented with immunization or amantadine (see Chap. 8).

    G. **Meningitis.** The use of rifampin and other agents to prevent the spread of meningococcal or *H. influenzae* type b meningitis from an index case to close contacts is discussed in Chap. 5.

    H. **Recurrent urinary tract infection.** The use of antibiotics to prevent recurrent episodes of urinary tract infection is reviewed in the individual discussions of these agents in Chap. 28: TMP-SMX, fluoroquinolones, nitrofurantoin, and mandelamine-ascorbic acid. Also see Chap. 12.

    I. *Pneumocystis carinii.* Prevention of recurrent *P. carinii* pneumonia is discussed in Chap. 24.

    J. **Chemoprophylaxis of tuberculosis.** See discussion of isoniazid in Chap. 9.

    K. **Lyme disease.** The use of prophylactic antibiotic treatment of tick bites in endemic areas generally is not indicated. See discussion in Chap. 23.

    L. **Recurrent otitis media in young children.** Although prophylactic regimens are used in this setting, the best regimens are unclear; further clinical studies are needed. This topic is discussed briefly in Chap. 7 and is reviewed elsewhere [54–56].

    M. **Prevention of infection in renal transplantation recipients.** Prophylaxis with TMP-SMX significantly reduces the incidence of bacterial infection following renal transplantation (especially infection of the urinary tract and bloodstream), can provide protection against *P. carinii* pneumonia, and is cost-beneficial [57]. Patients appear to tolerate this regimen well in this setting [57].

    N. **Prevention of infection in patients with chronic granulomatous disease.** Prophylaxis with TMP-SMX is useful in the prevention of infectious complications and does not appear to be associated with an increase of fungal infections [58].

    O. **Prevention of recurrent cholangitis.** Selected patients with a compromised biliary system (e.g., on account of an endoprosthesis in situ, history of choledochojejunos-tomy or hepaticojejunostomy or sphincteroplasty) who are prone to develop recur-rent bouts of cholangitis may benefit from chronic daily prophylactic antibiotics. The aim of suppressive antibiotic therapy is to prevent flare-ups of clinically overt cholangitis. Both TMP-SMX and fluoroquinolones have been used. This topic has been reviewed elsewhere [59].

P. **Complicated diagnostic or therapeutic endoscopic retrograde cholangiopan-creatography.** Although antibiotics have often been given for this procedure be-cause this seems reasonable, data now are supporting prophylactic antibiotic use in this setting [60, 60a].

Q. For postoperative T-tube cholangiography, routine prophylaxis does not appear to be necessary [61].

References

1. Dellinger, E.P., et al. Quality standard for antimicrobial prophylaxis in surgical procedures. *Clin. Infect. Dis.* 18:422, 1994.
   In this recent summary sponsored by the Infectious Disease Society of America, more than 50 experts in infectious diseases and 10 experts in surgical infectious diseases and surgical subspecialties reviewed the recommendations or suggested standards that might be applied without controversy in most hospitals. This is an excellent resource.
   For a related report, see T.K. Waddell and O.D. Rotstein, Antimicrobial prophylaxis in surgery: Committee on antimicrobial agents, Canadian Infectious Disease Society. Can. Med. Assoc. J. 151:925, 1994.
2. Kernodle, D.S., and Kaiser, A.B. Postoperative Infection and Antimicrobial Prophy-laxis. In G.L. Mandell, J.E. Bennett, and R. Dolin (eds.), *Principles and Practice of Infectious Diseases* (4th ed.). New York: Churchill Livingstone, 1995. Pp. 2742–2756.
   Excellent discussion by experts with a long interest in prophylactic antibiotics.
3. Conte, J.E., Jr. Antibiotic prophylaxis: Non-abdominal surgery. *Curr. Clin. Top. Infect. Dis.* 10:254–305, 1989.
4. Medical Letter. Antimicrobial prophylaxis in surgery. *Med. Lett. Drugs Ther.* 37: 79, 1995.
5. Waldvogel, F.A., et al. Perioperative antibiotic prophylaxis of wound and foreign body infections: Microbial factors affecting efficacy. *Rev. Infect. Dis.* 13(Suppl. 10):S782, 1991.
   Review of physiologic factors involved in surgical wound infections. Reviews the timing of effective antibiotic surgical prophylaxis. Includes discussion of bacterial factors, influence of foreign bodies, and so on.
6. Haas, D.W., and Kaiser, A.B. Antimicrobial Prophylaxis of Infections Associated with Foreign Bodies. In A.L. Bisno and F.A. Waldvogel (eds.), *Infections Associated with Medical Devices* (2nd ed.). Washington, DC: American Society for Microbiology, 1994. Pp. 375–388.
   See Table 2 on pages 382–383 for suggested regimens for various prosthetic device implants.
6a. Dickinson, G.M., and Bisno, A.L. Antimicrobial prophylaxis of infection. *Infect. Dis. Clin. North Am.* 9:783, 1995.
7. Page, C.P., et al. Antimicrobial prophylaxis for surgical wounds: Guidelines for clinical care. *Arch. Surg.* 128:79, 1993.
   Article developed by the Antimicrobial Agents Committee and approved by the Execu-tive Committee of the Surgical Infection Society as a set of guidelines for selection and use of prophylactic antibiotics for surgical wounds.
8. Hirschman, J.V., and Inui, T.S. Antimicrobial prophylaxis: A critique of recent trials. *Rev. Infect. Dis.* 2:1, 1980.
   Extensive review of early studies on prophylactic antibiotic use. For a related article, see Veterans Administration Ad Hoc Interdisciplinary Advisory Committee on Antimi-crobial Drug Usage, Prophylaxis in surgery. J.A.M.A. 237:1003, 1977, which provides an extensive reference list of early surgical prophylaxis studies.
9. Burke, J.F. The effective period of preventive antibiotic action in experimental inci-sions and dermal lesions. *Surgery* 50:161, 1961.
   This experimental study helped determine the appropriate timing of prophylactic anti-biotic administration. A classic.
10. Classen, D.C., et al. The timing of prophylactic administration of antibiotics and the risk of surgical wound infection. *N. Engl. J. Med.* 326:281, 1992.
    Prospective study of 2,847 patients undergoing elective clean or clean-contaminated

surgery. When antibiotics were given 0–2 hours before surgery, wound infections were significantly reduced. See editorial comment by D.R. Wenzel in the same issue, emphasizing the importance of preoperative administration.

11. Burke, J.F. Preventing bacterial infection by coordinating antibiotic and host activity: A time-dependent relationship. *South. Med. J.* 70(Suppl. 1):24, 1977.
   Emphasizes the importance of high levels of antibiotics intraoperatively.

12. Stone, H.H., et al. Prophylactic and preventive antibiotic therapy: Timing, duration, and economics. *Ann. Surg.* 189:691, 1979.
   When prophylactic antibiotics are started preoperatively in an appropriate way, it is not necessary to continue prophylaxis beyond the time in the recovery room. Further infections are not prevented, but costs rise unnecessarily if prophylactic antibiotics are prolonged.

13. DiPiro, J.T., et al. Single dose systemic antibiotic prophylaxis of surgical wound infections. *Am. J. Surg.* 152:552, 1986.

14. Norden, C., Gillespie, W.J., and Nade, S. Infections in Total Joint Replacements. In *Infections in Bones and Joints.* Boston: Blackwell Scientific, 1994. Pp. 291–319.

15. Maki, D.G., and Mackey, J. Cefazolin, cefoxitin, and cefamandole for prophylaxis in colorectal surgery [abstract no. 466]. Twenty-sixth Interscience Conference of Antimicrobial Agents and Chemotherapy, New Orleans, Sept. 30, 1986.
   Concluded that cefoxitin appears to provide greater protection against postoperative surgical infection in colorectal surgery.

16. Hemsell, D.L. Prophylactic antibiotics: In gynecologic and obstetric surgery. *Rev. Infect. Dis.* 13(Suppl. 10):S821, 1991.
   Good review with specific guidelines.

17. Norden, C., Gillespie, W.J., and Nade, S. Post-Traumatic and Contiguous Osteomyelitis. In *Infections in Bones and Joints.* Boston: Blackwell Scientific, 1994. Pp. 166–180.

18. Fiore, A.F., Joshi, M., and Caplan, E.S. Approach to Infection in the Multiply Traumatized Patient. In G.L. Mandell, J.E. Bennett, and R. Dolin (eds.), *Principles and Practice of Infectious Diseases* (4th ed.). New York: Churchill Livingstone, 1995. Pp. 2756–2761.

19. Josefsson, G., and Kolmert, L. Prophylaxis with systemic antibiotics versus gentamicin bone cement in total hip arthroplasty: A 10 year survey of 1688 hips. *Clin. Orthoped. Res.* 292:210, 1993.
   Follow-up report from this Swedish group who had earlier reported a significant difference at 2 and 5 years in favor of gentamicin bone cement but no difference at 10 years in the infection rate.

20. Norden, C.W. Antibiotic prophylaxis in orthopedic surgery. *Rev. Infect. Dis.* 13(Suppl. 10):S842, 1991.
   Good summary by a nationally recognized expert. See related reference [17] and related discussion by J. Segreti and S. Levin, The role of prophylactic antibiotics in the prevention of prosthetic device infections. Infect. Dis. Clin. North Am. 3:357, 1989.

20a. Wahl, M.J. Myths of dental-induced prosthetic device infections. *Clin. Infect. Dis.* 20:1420, 1995.
   Strong argument and review of data to stop the common practice of antibiotic prophylaxis for dental procedures to prevent late prosthetic joint infections as this approach is not based on scientific evidence but rather on "myths."

20b. Steckelberg, J.M., and Osmon, D.R. Prosthetic Joint Infections. In A.L. Bisno and F.A. Waldvogel (eds.), *Infections Associated with Prosthetic Indwelling Medical Devices* (2nd ed.). Washington, D.C.: American Society for Microbiology, 1994. Pp. 259–290.
   Data from the Mayo Clinic: in 39,000 large-joint implants with approximately 275,000 joint-years of follow-up, the overall incidence of large-joint implant infections due to dental pathogens (viridans streptococci) was 0.06 per 1000 joint-years—a rate similar to that for endocarditis in the general population. Therefore, routine prophylaxis is not warranted.

21. Nelson, J.P., et al. Prophylactic antimicrobial coverage in arthroplasty patients. *J. Bone Joint Surg.* [*Am.*]. 72:1, 1990.
   See related article by J.W. Little, Managing dental patients with joint prosthesis. J. Am. Dent. Assoc. 125:1374, 1994. Review shows transient dental bacteremias had little or no role in causing late infections of prosthetic joint replacements.

22. Simmons, N.A., et al. Case against antibiotic prophylaxis for dental treatment of patients with joint prosthesis. *Lancet* 339:301, 1992.

23. Nichols, R.L. Use of prophylactic antibiotics in surgical practice. *Am. J. Med.* 70:686, 1981.

Contains a good discussion of antibiotic prophylaxis in gastrointestinal surgery. For an update of this topic, see S.L. Gorbach, Antimicrobial prophylaxis for appendectomy and colorectal surgery. Rev. Infect. Dis. 13(Suppl. 10):S815, 1991.

24. Norwegian Study Group for Colorectal Surgery. Should antimicrobial prophylaxis in colorectal surgery include agents effective against both anaerobic and aerobic microorganisms? A double-blind, multicenter study. *Surgery* 97:402, 1985.

25. DiPiro, J.T., et al. Prophylactic parenteral cephalosporins in surgery: Are the newer agents better? *J.A.M.A.* 252:3277, 1984.
    Review of 17 published studies. Concludes there is no evidence that administration of second- or third-generation cephalosporins results in lower postoperative infection rates compared with administration of first-generation cephalosporins.

26. Weaver, M., et al. Oral neomycin and erythromycin compared with single-dose systemic metronidazole and ceftriaxone prophylaxis in elective colorectal surgery. *Am. J. Surg.* 151:438, 1986.

27. Mebust, W.K. Prophylactic antibiotics in transurethral surgery. *J. Urol.* 150:1734, 1993.

28. Klimberg, I.W., et al. A multicenter comparison of oral lomefloxacin versus parenteral cefotaxime as prophylactic agents in transurethral surgery. *Am. J. Med.* 92(Suppl. 4A):121S, 1992.
    Patients were required to have negative pretreatment urine cultures. Lomefloxacin (400 mg PO once 2–6 hours prior to surgery) or cefotaxime (1 g IV or IM 30–90 minutes before surgery) was given. Lomefloxacin was successful in preventing postoperative infections in 204 of 207 evaluable patients (98%). Cefotaxime was successful in 196 of 206 (95.1%) evaluable patients.
    See the two companion, related articles preceding this article in this symposium devoted to lomefloxacin.

29. Vitanen, J., et al. Randomized controlled study of chemoprophylaxis in transurethral prostatectomy. *J. Urol.* 150:1715, 1993.
    Concluded that single-dose antibiotic prophylaxis was useful to reduce postoperative infectious complications in this study from Finland of 599 patients who received no antibiotic (22% infections), one double-strength TMP-SMX tablet (12.3% infections), or 2 g ceftriaxone (7.6% infections). Initial urine cultures were sterile.

30. Shapiro, M. Prophylaxis in otolaryngologic surgery and neurosurgery: A critical review. *Rev. Infect. Dis.* 13(Suppl. 10):S858, 1991.

31. Phan, M., et al. Antimicrobial prophylaxis for major head and neck surgery in cancer patients: Sulbactam-ampicillin versus clindamycin-amikacin. *Antimicrob. Agents Chemother.* 36:2014, 1992.
    Even with perioperative prophylaxis, wound infections occurred in 20–30% of patients! See reference [41].

32. Brown, E.M. Antimicrobial prophylaxis in neurosurgery. *J. Antimicrob. Chemother.* 31(Suppl. B):49, 1993.
    See related article, Infection in Neurosurgery Working Party of the British Society for Antimicrobial Chemotherapy, Antimicrobial prophylaxis in neurosurgery and after head trauma. Lancet 344:1547, 1994.

33. Haines, S.J., and Walters, B.C. Antibiotic prophylaxis for cerebrospinal fluid shunts: A meta-analysis. *Neurosurgery* 34:87, 1994.
    See the related article, J.M. Langley et al., Efficacy of antimicrobial prophylaxis in placement of cerebrospinal fluid shunts: Meta-analysis. Clin. Infect. Dis. 17:98, 1993.

33a. Barker, F.G., III. Efficacy of prophylactic antibiotics for craniotomy: A meta-analysis. *Neurosurgery* 35:484, 1994.
    Analysis showed an advantage of antibiotics over placebo.

33b. Bernard, A., et al. Antibiotic prophylaxis in pulmonary surgery: A prospective, randomized, double-blind trial of flash cefuroxime versus forty-eight-hour cefuroxime. *J. Thorac. Cardiovasc. Surg.* 107:896, 1994.
    The 48 hour-regimen (1.5 g preoperatively and 1.5 g q6h for 48 hours postoperatively) was associated with a 46% infection rate versus a 65% infection rate in the 1.5 g preoperative dose and a similar dose once 2 hours later. The reduction in infection was significant at the p = .005 level.

34. Platt, R., et al. Perioperative antibiotic prophylaxis for herniorrhaphy and breast surgery. *N. Engl. J. Med.* 322:153, 1990.
    Although cefonicid was used in this study, presumably similar results would be achieved with more standard regimens (e.g., cefazolin). See related article by R. Platt et al., Prophylaxis against wound infection following herniorrhaphy or breast surgery. J. Infect. Dis. 166:556, 1992. In absence of formal guidelines, surgeons preferentially

used prophylaxis in patients at highest risk, e.g., more prolonged procedures, mastectomies, etc.

35. Platt, R., et al. Perioperative antibiotic prophylaxis and wound infection following breast surgery. *J. Antimicrob. Chemother.* 31(Suppl. B):43, 1993.
    Meta-analysis of published data of more than 2,587 surgical procedures. Multiauthored and numerous centers involved. Conclusion: Antibiotic prophylaxis (with cephalosporins) reduces the risk of postoperative infections.

36. Ayliffe, G.A.J. Role of the environment of the operating suite in surgical wound infections. *Rev. Infect. Dis.* 13(Suppl. 10):S800, 1991.
    See companion article by G.L. Archer, Alteration of cutaneous staphylococcal flora as a consequence of antimicrobial prophylaxis. Rev. Infect. Dis. 13(Suppl. 10):S805, 1991, which discusses how surgical prophylaxis changes the microflora and susceptibility of skin flora and how colonized patients and hospital staff make up a nosocomial reservoir for resistant bacteria.

37. Curtis, J.J., et al. Randomized, prospective comparison of first- and second-generation cephalosporins as infection prophylaxis for cardiac surgery. *Am. J. Surg.* 166:734, 1993.
    Randomized prospective study of 702 patients comparing cefazolin (1 g q8h for 48 hours) with one intraoperative dose at 4 hours versus cefuroxime (1.5 g q12h for 48 hours). There was no difference in the wound infection rates.

38. Townsend, T.R., et al. Clinical trial of cefamandole, cefazolin, and cefuroxime for antibiotic prophylaxis in cardiac operations. *J. Thorac. Cardiovasc. Surg.* 106:664, 1993.
    Randomized, double-blind study of 1,641 patients receiving cefazolin, cefamandole or cefuroxime. No differences in effectiveness in preventing operative site infections were demonstrated.

39. Sabath, L. Reappraisal of antistaphylococcal activities of first-generation (narrow-spectrum) and second-generation (expanded-spectrum) cephalosporins. *Antimicrob. Agents Chemother.* 33:407, 1989.
    Minireview of this topic, in which there has been a resurgence of interest.

40. Kernodle, D.S., et al. Failure of cephalosporins to prevent *Staphylococcus aureus* surgical wound infections. *J.A.M.A.* 263:961, 1990.

41. Weber, R.S., et al. Ampicillin-sulbactam vs. clindamycin in head and neck oncologic surgery. The need for gram-negative coverage. *Arch. Otolaryngol. Head Neck Surg.* 118:1159, 1992.
    Both agents were given preoperatively and for 48 hours postoperatively. Infections occurred in 13% of ampicillin-sulbactam recipients and 27% of clindamycin recipients from whom gram-negative organisms were more commonly isolated. Of greater interest would be a comparison of ampicillin-sulbactam and cefazolin because the latter covers many community-acquired gram-negative organisms.

42. Dajani, A., et al. Treatment of acute streptococcal pharyngitis and prevention of rheumatic fever: A statement for health professionals. *Pediatrics* 96:758, 1995.
    This October 1995 publication from the Committee on Rheumatic Fever, Endocarditis, and Kawasaki Disease of the Council on Cardiovascular Disease in the Young, the American Heart Association replaces the prior recommendations of this committee published in 1988.
        See related articles by A.D. Heggie et al., J. Infect. Dis. 166:1006, 1992, demonstrating that benzathine penicillin prophylaxis still is effective against group A streptococcal carriage and infection; and H.C. Lue et al., Long-term outcome of patients with rheumatic fever receiving benzathine penicillin G every three weeks versus every four weeks. J. Pediatr. 125(pt. 1):812, 1994, which favors the every-3-week schedule.

43. Bass, J.W. Antibiotic management of Group A streptococcal pharyngotonsillitis. *Pediatr. Infect. Dis. J.* 10:S43, 1991.

44. Klein, J.O. Management of streptococcal pharyngitis. *Pediatr. Infect. Dis. J.* 13:572, 1994.
    Group A streptococci remain uniformly susceptible to all penicillins and cephalosporins. Penicillin remains the treatment of choice. Alternative regimens are discussed.

45. Medical Letter. Prevention of serious infections after splenectomy. *Med. Lett. Drugs Ther.* 19:2, 1977.
    As of mid-1995, this topic has not been updated in The Medical Letter. For a related paper, see E.L. Francke and H.C. Neu, Postsplenectomy infection. Surg. Clin. North Am. 61:135, 1981.

46. Styrt, B. Infection associated with asplenia: Risks, mechanisms, and prevention. *Am. J. Med.* 88(Suppl. 5N):33N, 1990.
    A good review.

47. Schimpff, S.C. Infections in the Cancer Patient: Diagnosis, Prevention, and Treatment. In G.L. Mandell, J.E. Bennett, and R. Dolin (eds.), *Principles and Practice of Infectious Diseases* (4th ed.). New York: Churchill Livingstone, 1995. P. 2666.

48. Buchanan, G.R. Chemoprophylaxis in asplenic adolescents and young adults. *Pediatr. Infect. Dis. J.* 12:892, 1993.
    Editorial-like comment. The author typically recommends daily prophylaxis with penicillin for 3 years after splenectomy. He encourages those willing to take prophylaxis beyond that time to do so, but his alternative approach is to give the patient a supply of oral penicillin and, in the event of fever, to take a dose q8h if seeing a physician is delayed. By this method, the author hopes to prevent a fulminant pneumococcal sepsis, though he admits that no scientific evidence supports this approach.

49. Reid, M.M. Splenectomy, sepsis, immunisation and guidelines. *Lancet* 344:970, 1994.
    In this October 1994 editorial, the author basically reminds the reader that the best approach for this problem is still unclear and should be studied.

50. Dajani, A.S., et al. Prevention of bacterial endocarditis: Recommendations by the American Heart Association. *J.A.M.A.* 264:2919, 1990.
    Most up-to-date summary of SBE prophylaxis. Simpler and less costly regimens are emphasized. Published December 12, 1990. This is a statement from the Committee on Rheumatic Fever, Endocarditis, and Kawasaki Disease of the Council on Cardiovascular Disease in the Young of the American Heart Association. These recommendations are being updated in 1996 and will be published in late 1996 or early 1997. For an editorial comment on the 1990 recommendations, see E.A. Petersen, Prevention of bacterial endocarditis. Arch. Intern. Med. 150:2447, 1990.
    For a current discussion of the rationale and limitations of SBE prophylaxis, see recent review by D.T. Durack, Prevention of infective endocarditis. N. Engl. J. Med. 332:38, 1995.

51. Wehrmacher, W.H. Myths: Endocarditis. *Arch. Intern. Med.* 154:129, 1994.
    Editorial comment on the 1990 American Heart Association (AHA) recommendations of reference [50], again dealing with the issue of the lack of "hard data" for such recommendations and in response to a related article by dentist M.J. Wahl, Myths of dental-induced endocarditis. Arch. Intern. Med. 154:137, 1994, which also discusses some of the controversial recommendations in reference [50].
    Editorial comment points out that in 1992 the Endocarditis Working Party of the British Society for Antimicrobial Chemotherapy updated their recommendations for antibiotic prophylaxis. They are similar to the 1990 AHA guidelines.

52. Kaye, D., and Abrutyn, E. Prevention of bacterial endocarditis: 1991. *Ann. Intern. Med.* 114:803, 1991.
    Thoughtful editorial response of AHA recommendations (see reference [50]) pointing out the differences with prior AHA recommendations. Also discusses a rational approach to patients with mitral valve prolapse.
    For yet another editorial comment on these guidelines, see P.I. Lerner, Endocarditis prophylaxis: The new guidelines. Cleve. Clin. J. Med. 59:216, 1992. Concludes by reminding physicians that plaintiff lawyers will "be all too eager to challenge even minor deviations from the guidelines," a conclusion also pointed out in a more recent editorial (reference [51]).

53. Bodey, G. Antimicrobial prophylaxis for infection in neutropenic patients. *Curr. Clin. Top. Infect. Dis.* 1–43, 1988.

54. Paradise, J.L. Antimicrobial prophylaxis for recurrent acute otitis media. *Ann. Otol. Rhinol. Laryngol.* (Suppl. Jan) 155:33, 1992.
    Although questions remain about the choice of drug, optimal dosage schedules and therapy duration, risk of side effects, and the risk of selecting out resistant bacteria, antibiotic prophylaxis is a logical first step in managing recurrent otitis media in a child.

55. Giebink, G.S. Preventing otitis media. *Ann. Otol. Rhinol. Laryngol.* (Suppl. May) 163:20, 1994.

56. Williams, R.L., et al. Use of antibiotics in preventing recurrent acute otitis media and in treating otitis media with effusion. A meta-analytic attempt to resolve the brouhaha. *J.A.M.A.* 270:1344, 1993.
    Antibiotics appear to have beneficial but limited effect on recurrent otitis media and short-term resolution of otitis media with effusion. Longer-term benefits for otitis media with effusion have not been shown. See related comments in J.A.M.A. 271:430 and 272:203, 1994.

57. Fox, B.C., et al. A prospective, randomized, double-blind study of trimethoprim-sulfamethoxazole for prophylaxis of infection in renal transplantation: Clinical effi-

cacy, absorption of trimethoprim-sulfamethoxazole, effects on microflora, and the cost-benefit of prophylaxis. *Am. J. Med.* 89:255, 1990.

During the hospitalization after the transplantation surgery, 160 mg TMP and 800 mg SMX bid was given if creatinine clearance was greater than 30 ml/min. After discharge, a single daily dose of 160 mg TMP and 800 mg SMX was used. (If creatinine clearance was < 30 ml/min, one-half the usual dose per day was used.)

For a related article emphasizing the lack of side effects with TMP-SMX prophylaxis and lack of nephrotoxicity in cyclosporine recipients, see D.G. Maki et al., A prospective, randomized, double-blind study of trimethoprim-sulfamethoxazole for prophylaxis of infection in renal transplantation: Side effects of trimethoprim-sulfamethoxazole interaction with cyclosporine. J. Lab. Clin. Med. *119:11, 1992.*

58. Margolis, D.M., et al. Trimethoprim-sulfamethoxazole prophylaxis in the management of chronic granulomatous disease. *J. Infect. Dis.* 162:723, 1990.

59. Van der Hazel, S.J., et al. Role of antibiotics in treatment and prevention of acute and recurrent cholangitis. *Clin. Infect. Dis.* 19:279, 1994.

Good clinical discussion of this topic. Optimal duration of maintenance preventive doses is unclear. Authors suggest treating the patient for 3–4 months and then evaluating whether the antibiotics can be stopped without recurrence of infection. If infection recurs, therapy can be restarted. Lower-than-therapeutic doses may be effective (e.g., one double-strength tablet of TMP-SMX daily rather than bid).

60. Niederau, C., et al. Prophylactic antibiotic treatment in therapeutic or complicated diagnostic ERCP: Results of a randomized controlled clinical study. *Gastrointest. Endosc.* 40:533, 1994.

Prophylactic cefotaxime reduced the incidence of bacteremia.

60a. Byl, B., et al. Antibiotic prophylaxis for infectious complications after therapeutic endoscopic retrograde cholangiopancreatography: A randomized, double-blind, placebo-controlled study. *Clin. Infect. Dis.* 20:1236, 1995.

In this study, uninfected patients were assigned to receive piperacillin (4 g) or placebo tid; prophylaxis was started just before initial ERCP and was continued until biliary drainage was completely unobstructed. Authors concluded that antimicrobial prophylaxis significantly reduces the incidence of septic complications after therapeutic ERCP among patients presenting with cholestasis. No bacteremia was documented in the 30 patients receiving piperacillin. Seven (22%) of 32 patients receiving placebo had bacteremia; pathogens included Pseudomonas (3), E. coli (3), Streptococcus sanguis, and S. salivarius (1). All isolates were susceptible to piperacillin.

Nevertheless, the Medical Letter's antibiotic of choice for prophylaxis for biliary tract manipulation/surgery is cefazolin, and we also would favor use of cefazolin in most cases of ERCP, unless the patient had a long hospitalization and/or had been treated with protracted antibiotics so that a broader spectrum agent, e.g., piperacillin, aimed at hospital-acquired gram-negatives may be reasonable; in this case we might also give a single dose of an aminoglycoside.

61. Sheen-Chen, S.M., et al. Postoperative T-tube cholangiography: Is routine antibiotic prophylaxis necessary? A prospective controlled study. *Arch. Surg.* 130:20, 1995.

Study concludes that routine antibiotic prophylaxis to prevent infection following postoperative T-tube cholangiography is not necessary under selected conditions.

C. Penicillin G and Penicillin-Resistant *Streptococcus pneumoniae*

The term **penicillin** is the generic term for a broad group of agents including, but not limited to, penicillin G, penicillin V, oxacillin, dicloxacillin, nafcillin, ampicillin, amoxicillin, ticarcillin, and piperacillin. These agents are **bactericidal**. The precise mechanism of action of penicillins is unclear, but they interfere with the synthesis and promote lysis of bacterial cell walls [1, 2]. It is the binding to and inhibition of the high-molecular-weight penicillin-binding proteins that probably explain the antibacterial activity of penicillin and other beta-lactam antibiotics [1]. These agents provide good antibiotic levels in serum or urine, or in synovial, pleural, and pericardial fluids. Penetration into the spinal fluid is limited to approximately 5–10% of serum levels.

Many, but not all, of the penicillins are excreted primarily by the kidney by both glomerular filtration and tubular secretion. Dose reductions in severe renal failure are discussed under the individual agents. Some, however, are excreted mainly by the liver.

I. **Structure.** The penicillin nucleus and breakdown products are shown in Fig. 28C-1.
   A. **Structural modifications.** Penicillins with differing antimicrobial activity can be made from 6-aminopenicillanic acid. Alteration of the side groups has resulted in compounds with a broader spectrum of activity, resistance to penicillinases, stability in acid pH (important in oral preparations), and other different pharmacokinetic characteristics.
   B. **Common nucleus.** The intact structural nucleus is necessary for biologic activity. In addition, as a result of the common nucleus in the structure of the penicillins, the **potential for allergic cross-sensitivity** among the penicillins presumably is high.
   C. **Penicillinase** is a beta-lactamase enzyme that splits the beta-lactam ring (see site 1, Fig. 28C-1). The resulting penicilloic acid is inactive against bacteria. Penicillinase production is a principal mechanism of penicillin resistance in penicillin-resistant, coagulase-positive *Staphylococcus aureus, Pseudomonas* spp., and *Bacteroides fragilis,* and one of the mechanisms in *Escherichia coli* and *Proteus* spp. When a penicillin is combined with a beta-lactamase inhibitor (clavulanic acid or sulbactam; see Chap. 28E), many bacterial beta-lactamases can be inhibited [2].

II. **Spectrum of activity of penicillin G.** The advantages of penicillin G are its low cost, easy administration, excellent tissue penetration, relatively narrow spectrum of activity (when compared with cephalosporins, for example), and favorable therapeutic index [2]. Penicillin G remains the drug of choice in many clinical situations [3]. These include infection by the following organisms (see Table 28A-3).
   A. **Gram-positive aerobic cocci.**
      1. Penicillin is very active against *S. pyogenes* (group A), viridans streptococci, *S. bovis,* and penicillin-susceptible *S. aureus.* As a single agent, penicillin G is not effective against serious enterococcal infections (e.g., endocarditis).
      2. **Resistance of *Streptococcus pneumoniae* to penicillin is being seen with increasing frequency** [4–8a]
         a. **Definitions in laboratory** [4–6]
            (1) **Susceptible strains** have minimal inhibitory concentrations (MIC; see Chap. 25) of 0.1 μg or less of penicillin per milliliter.
            (2) **Intermediate resistance** is defined as strains with a MIC of 0.1–2 μg/ml.
            (3) **Highly resistant (or fully resistant** strains) have a MIC of 2 μg/ml or more. These strains are more likely to be resistant to other antipneumo-

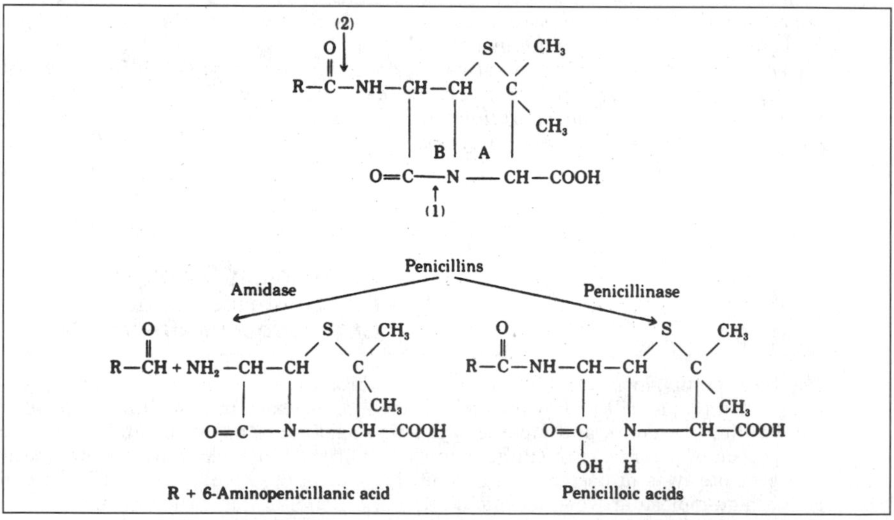

Fig. 28C-1. Penicillin: nucleus and breakdown products. *(1)* Site of beta-lactamase activity. *(2)* Site of amidase activity. (Amidase, an enzyme produced by microorganisms, cleaves penicillin at site 2.)

coccal agents. Strains resistant to three or more agents are defined as multidrug-resistant strains [4, 5].

(4) Laboratory testing. The National Committee for Clinical Laboratory Standards (NCCLS) recommends screening of at least blood and sterile fluid clinical isolates for penicillin resistance by disc diffusion, using a 1-μg oxacillin disc [8].

For those organisms that are not susceptible by screening, another test is necessary to determine the MIC. One useful technique for this is the E test (see Chap. 25). Other antibiotics (e.g., cephalosporins) can likewise be tested in vitro against *S. pneumoniae* using the E test.

b. Prevalence and frequency. Following early documentation of penicillin-resistant pneumococcal isolates in Australia and South Africa in the 1960s and 1970s, more widespread scattered resistance was reported in the 1980s. Penicillin resistance was uncommon in the United States at least through 1987 but, in recent years, the incidence has increased significantly.

(1) In a survey of *S. pneumoniae* isolates from normally sterile body fluids submitted to the Centers for Disease Control from October 1991 through September 1992 from 13 states, resistance (MIC ≥ 0.12 μg/ml) was seen in 6.6% of isolates, including 1.3% highly resistant isolates [4]. Rates of resistance varied among regions (range, 0–28%) [4, 6], so it is important for each hospital to ascertain its own frequency.

(2) Surveys of nasopharyngeal isolates from children revealed even higher rates of penicillin resistance: 29% in Tennessee and 33% in Kentucky, with rates as high as 60% in some daycare centers in the United States [6].

(3) In a 1994 symposium, it was estimated that in the United States up to 20–25% of *S. pneumoniae* isolates are, to some degree, penicillin resistant. Most of the resistance is intermediate, but approximately 20% is high level [7]. In a recent survey of invasive pneumococcal infections in Atlanta, Georgia, isolates from 25% of the patients were resistant to penicillin; 7% were highly resistant [4a]. In a 1996 report, for some areas in the United States, 25–30% of invasive pneumococcal isolates have either intermediate or high-level resistance [8a].

(4) In Europe, rates of penicillin-resistant *S. pneumoniae* vary from 1% or less in Belgium and Finland to 25% in Romania, 44% in Spain (with 15% high-level), and 59% in Hungary (36% high-level) [6].

c. Mechanisms and spread

(1) Pneumococcal resistance to penicillin results from **alterations in the generic structure** of the organism, **giving rise to changes in one** or **more of its penicillin-binding proteins** (PBPs), thereby reducing affinity for the drug. Several possible mechanisms have been proposed for such alterations including the selection of spontaneous mutants and the exchange of DNA from a resistant strain of pneumococci or from a streptococcal species of normal respiratory flora that is relatively insensitive to penicillin [4]. Because all beta-lactam antibiotics act by binding to PBPs, the PBP changes in penicillin-resistant strains also result in diminished susceptibility to other beta-lactam antibiotics [7a]. Penicillin-resistant strains are frequently, but not invariably, also resistant to other antimicrobial agents [7a].

(2) Selective pressure exerted by antibiotic use is often presumed to be a chief factor responsible for the development of resistance. However, resistant strains may be transported to geographically distant areas, where they may spread rapidly [6].

Clonal dissemination of resistant isolates has been demonstrated by use of molecular epidemiologic techniques. For example, resistant serotype 23F isolates from Cleveland, Ohio, appear to be identical to 23F strains previously isolated from Spain, and isolates from an outbreak in Iceland caused by serogroup 6B were found to be closely related to Spanish 6B strains [7a]. These observations support in vitro data that penicillin resistance is a stable characteristic and can persist and spread in the absence of antibiotic-selective pressure [7a].

In their 1995 review of this topic, Fraimow and Abrutyn suggest that low-level penicillin resistance probably has evolved independently under selective antibiotic pressure in a limited number of pneumococcal serotypes, and subsequent evolution to high-level resistance may have occurred by further recombination events. Particular high-level resistant strains then are capable of clonal spread through a wide geographic range [7a].

Local risk factors for the acquisition of penicillin-resistant strains include prior antibiotic exposure (e.g., for otitis media), prior hospitalization, exposure to childcare centers [7], and nursing homes [7a].

d. Effect on presentation and severity of illness

(1) Antibiotic-resistant pneumococci are neither more nor less virulent than susceptible strains [6]. In immunocompetent adults or children with community-acquired pneumococcal infections, the presentation and outcome of resistant pneumococcal infections have been similar to penicillin-susceptible infections. In the immunocompromised, disease outcome may be worse [6].

In a recent report from Spain, resistant *S. pneumoniae* were not associated with increased mortality in patients with pneumococcal pneumonia [5b].

The outcome of serious infections caused by resistant strains may be worse if there is a delay in initiating appropriate therapy [7a].

(2) **Factors associated with infection with resistant strains** include extremes of age, nosocomial acquisition, prior exposure to antibiotics [6], and immunocompromised status [7]. See related comments in sec. **c(2)**.

e. Susceptibility of penicillin-resistant *S. pneumoniae* to other antibiotics [5a, 6]

(1) Because all beta-lactam antibiotics interact with penicillin-binding proteins, changes in these proteins result in decreased susceptibility to all antibiotics of this type. See sec. **c**. Therefore, pneumococci resistant to penicillin usually are resistant to ampicillin, ticarcillin, and piperacillin. Because resistance is not dependent on the production of beta-lactamase, these organisms are resistant to amoxicillin-clavulanate and related beta-lactamase inhibitor combinations.

(2) For the cephalosporins (e.g., cefotaxime, ceftriaxone, and other cephalosporins), NCCLS defines susceptible strains as those with a MIC of less than 0.25 μg/ml, intermediate strains with a MIC of 0.5–1.0 μg/ml, and resistant strains with a MIC greater than 2.0 μg/ml [6]. Currently, these definitions apply strictly to cerebrospinal fluid (CSF) isolates, but probably apply to other isolates as well [6].

Because some isolates may be resistant to third-generation cephalosporins, susceptibility testing (e.g., E test) is suggested for clinical isolates from normally sterile body fluids. **For intermediate-resistant strains of *S. pneumoniae,*** the second- and third-generation cephalosporins usually are active [6, 7].

(3) **Highly resistant strains of *S. pneumoniae*** often are resistant also to erythromycin and clarithromycin, trimethoprim-sulfamethoxazole (TMP-SMX), and tetracycline. If these drugs are to be used, **it is imperative that susceptibility testing be performed** (e.g., with the E test).

The currently available fluoroquinolones are only modestly active against penicillin-susceptible *S. pneumoniae* (see Chap. 28S) and therefore do not solve the problem of therapy for resistant strains. **Vancomycin has been uniformly active against penicillin-resistant isolates;** imipenem is active against 90–100% [6].

(4) See Table 28C-1.

f. Serotypes involved and clinical implications

(1) Commonly involved serotypes of resistant isolates in the United States and elsewhere include 6B, 23F, 14, 9V, 19A, and 19F, with the highest rates seen in 6B and 23F isolates [4, 7, 7a]. The majority of isolates are serotypes present in the 23-valent pneumococcal capsular polysaccharide vaccine [4, 7]. See Chap. 9.

(2) Therefore, **the pneumococcal vaccine should be aggressively promoted** and **routinely administered to appropriate candidates** [4, 5, 7, 8]. (See Chap. 9.) Protection of the highly vulnerable pediatric population against pneumococcal infection will have to await the further devel-

Table 28C-1. Activity of cephalosporins against pneumococci susceptible, intermediate, and resistant to penicillin

Agent	MIC$_{90}$ (μg/ml)		
	Penicillin-susceptible	Penicillin-intermediate	Penicillin-resistant
Parenteral			
Cephalothin	0.125–0.25	1.0–8.0	8.0–32.0
Cefoxitin	1.0–2.0	4.0–8.0	≥32.0
Cefuroxime	0.03–0.12	1.0–4.0	4.0–8.0
Cefoperazone	0.12	1.0–2.0	2.0–8.0
Ceftizoxime	0.5–1.0	8.0–16.0	≥32.0
Ceftazidime	0.25–0.5	16.0–32.0	>32.0
Ceftriaxone	0.01–0.06	0.5–1.0	1.0–2.0
Cefotaxime	0.01–0.12	0.25–0.5	1.0–4.0
Oral			
Cefpirome	0.03–0.06	0.5	1.0
Cefepime	0.12	0.5	1.0–2.0
Cefpodoxime	0.06–0.25	1.0–4.0	4.0
Cefuroxime axetil	0.03–0.125	1.0–4.0	4.0–8.0
Cefaclor	0.5–2.0	8.0–16.0	16.0–≥32.0
Cefixime	0.25–1.0	8.0–32.0	≥32.0
Cefprozil	0.25–1.0	32.0	>32.0
Loracarbef	1.5–2.0	3.0–6.0, ⪯32.0	≥12.5, ≥32.0

MIC = minimal inhibitory concentration.
Source: From J.R. Schreiber and M.R. Jacobs, Antibiotic-resistant pneumococci. *Pediatr. Clin. North Am.* 42:519, 1995.

opment of a polyvalent polysaccharide-protein conjugate vaccine [4]. (See Chap. 22.)

g. **Clinical implications of penicillin-resistant** *S. pneumoniae* are discussed in the individual related chapters and in recent reviews [4b, 5a, 6a, 7a], but a few points deserve emphasis.

(1) **Pneumococcal meningitis.** Chloramphenicol is not an acceptable agent as the bactericidal activity against many penicillin-resistant strains is poor and sufficient bactericidal activity in the CNS to effect a cure may not be achieved [6]. Cefotaxime and ceftriaxone are reasonable initial empiric therapies for known or possible pneumococcal meningitis, but for known or highly suspected high-level resistance, combination therapy with vancomycin and ceftriaxone has been suggested [6]. Careful monitoring of CSF culture after 24–36 hours of therapy also is suggested to assess clearing of penicillin-resistant pneumococcal meningitis. (See related discussions in Chap. 5.)

The role of rifampin with vancomycin and/or a third-generation cephalosporin is undergoing evaluation [7a]. Imipenem has excellent in vitro activity against most resistant isolates but has a relatively high incidence of inducing seizures, particularly in association with other brain abnormalities [7a].

Recently, high doses of third-generation cephalosporins have been suggested for therapy of adults with meningitis due to resistant isolates [6b].

(2) **Sepsis and pneumonia.** The serum concentrations of penicillin and other beta-lactam antibiotics that can be achieved with intravenous penicillin (150,000–250,000 units of penicillin G per kilogram of body weight per day) or equivalent doses of other beta-lactam antibiotics are many times greater than the MIC for *S. pneumoniae* with intermediate penicillin resistance and even for many high-level penicillin-resistant strains. Therefore, most patients should respond to these regimens [4b, 5a, 6, 7a].

In a recent editorial, the author emphasizes that for now, high-dose penicillin (150,000 to 200,000 units per kg per day) remains effective therapy against resistant strains, at least those at the intermediate level [4b].

For patients in whom high-level penicillin resistance is expected (e.g., nosocomial pneumonia in debilitated patients), vancomycin or imipenem can be used; third-generation cephalosporins are likely to be effective in most cases [6]. See related discussion in Chaps. 2 and 9.

   (3) **Otitis media.** Because this is less serious than those infections in secs. **(1)** and **(2)**, a stepwise approach can be considered. As of mid-1994, Friedland and McCracken [6] suggested, and as of mid-1995 Schreiber and Jacobs [5a] again suggested, no change in the initial empiric therapy, which is still amoxicillin, even in areas with a high prevalence, of penicillin-resistant pneumococci.

   Ideally, for those patients who do not respond, myringotomy or tympanocentesis can be carried out so that the causative pathogen can be cultured and susceptibility tests performed. If antibiotic-resistant pneumococci are isolated, therapy should be guided by the antibiotic susceptibility results that are obtained [5a]. There is a paucity of information about the clinical efficacy of orally administered beta-lactam antibiotics for otitis media caused by penicillin-resistant *S. pneumoniae,* especially since the overall spontaneous clinical recovery rate for otitis media is high (50–60% from all causes) [6].

   See Chap. 7 for further discussion and alternative antibiotic options.

   h. **Methods to control** the rising incidence of penicillin-resistant *S. pneumoniae* still are being evaluated. However, the principles parallel those for control of increasing resistant bacteria discussed in Chap. 28A. These include more careful use of antibiotics, especially in the community; shorter courses of antibiotics; narrower-spectrum antibiotics; and so forth [7]. In early 1996, a special report was published on strategies to help minimize and control the impact of drug-resistant *S. pneumoniae* [8a].

   3. Resistance of group A streptococci to penicillin has not been observed. See sec. **IV.B.**

B. **Gram-negative aerobes.** Penicillin remains the antibiotic of choice for *Neisseria meningitidis* and *Pasteurella multocida* [3]. Penicillin is no longer a drug of choice for *Neisseria gonorrhoeae* (see Chap. 13).

C. **Anaerobes.** Penicillin is very effective against anaerobic species, including *Clostridium* spp., *Fusobacterium* spp., and *Actinomyces israelii* (actinomycosis). Although penicillin is active against many *Bacteroides* spp. (particularly oropharyngeal strains), it is not active against *B. fragilis.* If *B. fragilis* infections are suspected (e.g., intraabdominal or pelvic infections), another agent should be selected.

D. **Spirochetes.** Penicillin is the drug of choice for *Treponema pallidum* infection (see Chap. 13) and is active against *Borrelia burgdorferi.*

III. **Parenteral preparations of penicillin G (benzylpenicillin).** There are three main forms of parenteral penicillin G. The pharmacokinetics differ rather markedly.

A. **Aqueous penicillin G** is available in potassium and sodium salt forms (to provide stability in storage) for intravenous and intramuscular use. Ordinarily, the potassium salt form (1.7 mEq K^+/1 million units) is used. There is a sodium salt preparation available for special circumstances (e.g., renal failure) to avoid any additional potassium load. Aqueous penicillin **will produce high blood levels rapidly,** but excretion is rapid, yielding no detectable penicillin in the blood 4 hours after a dose. Therefore, for serious infections, the aqueous form should be given at least every 4 hours.

   1. **High-dose therapy. In adults with normal renal function,** 18–24 million units/day or 3–4 million units q4h is **used in serious infections** such as meningitis due to susceptible organisms, in some forms of endocarditis due to mildly penicillin-resistant organisms, and in severe clostridial infections. There is no indication for massive doses of penicillin (greater than 30 million units per day), because neurotoxicity of penicillin at that level is increased and alternate antibiotics are available. We favor giving aqueous penicillin G intravenously over 20–30 minutes rather than by constant infusion.

   2. **Intermediate doses** of aqueous penicillin (8–12 million units daily) are used

in aspiration pneumonias or lung abscess and in moderate to severe soft-tissue infections due to group A streptococci. This dose is used in conjunction with an aminoglycoside to provide a synergistic effect. Penicillin and gentamicin are used for synergy against enterococci and other resistant streptococci in endocarditis. Although the majority of enterococci are susceptible to the combination of penicillin and gentamicin, an increasing percentage of isolates have high-level resistance to gentamicin or penicillin [9]. In one study, the *Enterococcus (Streptococcus) faecium* strains had high-level resistance to penicillin, resulting in the loss of in vitro synergistic bactericidal activity of gentamicin combined with penicillin [9]. Therefore, **enterococci may no longer be assumed to be susceptible to a combination of penicillin and an aminoglycoside** (e.g., gentamicin) [10]. Special microbiologic screening tests for enterococci and special therapeutic implications are discussed in Chaps. 28H and 28O.

    3. Low doses. When lower blood levels are adequate, procaine penicillin may be used rather than the aqueous form. If the aqueous intravenous form of penicillin is used in known penicillin-susceptible pneumococcal pneumonia, the dose can be kept below 2.4 million units per day. High doses of penicillin are not necessary for known penicillin-susceptible pneumococcal pneumonia and may only increase the chances of superinfection [11]. In settings of known or suspected intermediate-resistant *S. pneumoniae,* higher doses of intravenous penicillin (e.g., 8–12 million units per day) may be effective. (For suspected or known high-level penicillin resistance, an alternative agent is indicated. See prior discussion in sec. **II.A.2** and related discussions in Chap. 9.)

    4. Pediatric dose. For children, 25,000–300,000 units/kg per day is recommended, depending on the severity of the infection.

B. Procaine penicillin G. Repository forms of penicillin have been developed to prolong the duration of penicillin in the blood. Procaine penicillin G (an equimolar ratio of penicillin G and procaine, which results in an insoluble crystalline salt) delays absorption. Peak levels (1–2 µg/ml) are reached in 2–4 hours, and detectable levels are present for 12–24 hours. Procaine penicillin is more likely to be allergenic than is aqueous crystalline penicillin G and is contraindicated in patients allergic to procaine [2].

    1. Doses usually are given **every 12 hours intramuscularly.** This preparation should not be given intravenously because of the risk of procaine toxicity. There is no direct correlation between increasing the dose at a single intramuscular site and peak serum level; that is, doubling the dose will not double the serum level. To increase the peak serum levels, two separate intramuscular injections must be used.

    2. Uses. Some authorities may still recommend procaine penicillin G, 300,000–600,000 units IM q12h, as a preferred regimen in uncomplicated known penicillin-susceptible pneumococcal pneumonia. Procaine penicillin is used in some of the alternative regimens for syphilis (see Chap. 13).

    3. Procaine reactions [12]. Immediately after the intramuscular injection of procaine penicillin, patients may complain of unusual tastes, dizziness, palpitations, auditory or visual disturbances, or fear of imminent death. Patients can be combative, have neuromuscular twitching, or experience grand mal seizures. These symptoms and signs usually clear spontaneously within 5–10 minutes. This type of reaction was seen in the therapy of gonorrhea, when 4.8 million units were used, but in fewer than 1% of patients. The syndrome probably results from the liberation of toxic quantities of procaine from the procaine penicillin G [12].

C. Benzathine penicillin G (long-acting) is an insoluble salt obtained by combining an ammonium base with penicillin G. **Very low blood levels** are achieved (approximately 0.10–0.15 units/ml), which can be detected for prolonged periods of time (i.e., 3–4 weeks). **Benzathine penicillin is used most commonly in the following conditions:**

    1. Syphilis (primary, secondary, and latent), in which a prolonged blood level is necessary to kill the slowly dividing treponemal organisms, which are very sensitive to penicillin (MIC = 0.03 unit/ml). However, insufficient levels are present in CSF or eye to eradicate these organisms at these sites. See Chap. 13.

    2. Rheumatic fever prophylaxis. A monthly injection (see Chap. 28B) will provide a serum level above that necessary to inhibit group A beta-hemolytic streptococci. This is the most effective regimen in adult patients with underlying rheumatic heart disease and avoids the problem of compliance with oral medications. In highly edemic areas, an every-3-week benzathine penicillin G (Bicillin) regimen has eliminated recurrent rheumatic fever.

3. **Streptococcal pharyngitis.** Many patients with group A beta-hemolytic streptococcal pharyngitis do not complete their oral antibiotic courses. In the high-risk patient (e.g., prior rheumatic fever) or the poorly compliant patient, use of benzathine penicillin will ensure maintenance of adequate levels (see sec. **VI.A.1.a** in Chap. 28B). A recent review [13] emphasizes that the highest cure rates for group A streptococcal pharyngitis are with benzathine penicillin at a dose of 600,000–1.2 million units. The major factor limiting use of this regimen is pain at the injection site. A combination of benzathine penicillin (900,000 units) and procaine penicillin (300,000 units) in a 2-ml injection was introduced in 1976, as Bicillin C-R 900/300, and was found to be effective in reducing the incidence and severity of local reactions while maintaining efficacy [13]. Although this combination is satisfactory therapy for most children, the efficacy of this combination for heavier patients (e.g., teenagers or adults) requires further study [13a].

IV. **Oral penicillin.** Oral penicillin G is partially inactivated by gastric acid. With a minor modification of the side chain, **penicillin V** (phenoxymethyl penicillin) is formed, and this congener **resists gastric acid breakdown and therefore provides higher serum levels** from the GI tract. On an equivalent-weight basis, oral penicillin V will provide blood levels 2–5 times greater than those attained with oral penicillin G. The potassium salt form of penicillin, penicillin VK, is well absorbed and provides good blood levels.

A. **Dosage.** For dose equivalents, 250 mg is equivalent to 400,000 units of penicillin G. The usual adult dosage is 1.6–3.2 million units/day divided into doses every 6 hours—that is, 400,000 units (250 mg)–800,000 units (500 mg) q6h. In children, the usual dosage is 25,000–100,000 units/kg/day divided into doses every 6 hours. A 500-mg dose results in a peak level of 3–5 μg/ml [2]. Penicillin VK is well absorbed even when ingested with meals. If necessary, higher blood levels can be achieved by adding probenecid as discussed in sec. **VI.C.**

B. **Uses.** Oral therapy has been shown to be useful in pharyngitis, minor oral or dental infections, and minor soft-tissue infections due to susceptible organisms, as well as completion of courses of treatment after initial intravenous therapy. **Group A streptococci remain uniformly susceptible to all penicillins** and cephalosporins. No evidence of resistance has been identified. The American Heart Association [13a] and the American Academy of Pediatrics continue to recommend a single dose of intramuscular benzathine penicillin or a 10-day course of oral **penicillin** V (500 mg bid or tid in adults and children older than 12 years and 250 mg bid or tid for children younger than 12 years) as the **standard for therapy** for group A streptococcal pharyngitis [13, 13a]. See Chap. 7 for related discussions.

C. **The spectrum of activity** of penicillin V is similar to that of penicillin G; however, **penicillin V is less active against gonorrhea.** If an oral regimen using a penicillin-related antibiotic is used in selected cases of gonorrhea, ampicillin or amoxicillin should be used as summarized in Chap. 13.

D. **Taste of suspensions.** In a study of taste acceptance, oral penicillin VK suspension (Vee Tids) was poor in taste, texture, and aftertaste in contrast to the majority of the other oral antimicrobial agents tested [14]. Because taste perception is considered to be the single most important factor in achieving compliance in children, especially children of preschool age, taste should be considered when selecting an antimicrobial suspension or liquid formulation for this age group [14].

V. **Untoward and toxic reactions**

A. **Penicillin allergy and hypersensitivity reactions** are discussed in Chap. 27. As many as 10% of recipients of penicillin G may develop an allergic reaction [2].

B. **Drug fever** may be the only manifestation of a penicillin side effect (see Chap. 28A).

C. **Eosinophilia** alone can occur with penicillin use. If the level exceeds 15% of the peripheral WBC count, it probably is reasonable to discontinue the drug. When eosinophilia occurs, rash may follow, and the presence of interstitial nephritis should be investigated.

D. **Interstitial nephritis** can occur with high doses but is relatively uncommon with oral penicillin G. This is discussed in Chap. 28D.

E. **Central nervous system toxicity.** An early clue to CNS toxicity owing to penicillin is **myoclonic twitching.** With very high blood levels and excessively high spinal fluid levels of penicillin, the patient may develop **seizures.** The seizure threshold of patients with meningitis may be lowered by their CNS infection. If they have renal failure and the usual meningeal doses of penicillin are used (i.e., 18–24 million units daily), these patients are at risk for CNS toxicity with seizures. This complication can be avoided by not using excessive doses in patients with normal renal function and by reducing high-dose intravenous therapy in renal failure patients (as discussed later), including the elderly, whose renal function is reduced by virtue of aging (see Chap. 28A).

VI. **Special considerations**

   A. **Dosage modification in renal failure**

      1. **High doses of intravenous aqueous penicillin.** Normally, penicillin G is eliminated rapidly, primarily by the kidney. In moderate to severe renal failure, **especially when high-dose** aqueous penicillin G **therapy** is used, penicillin can reach very high blood levels. **To avoid CNS toxicity, penicillin G doses must be reduced in renal failure and in the elderly.** A useful nomogram [15] is shown in Table 28C-2. Of the two doses suggested for each level of renal function, the lower dose is probably adequate for most patients. (The higher dose will provide an overestimate.) In severe renal failure, less than 10% of penicillin is inactivated by the liver. Consequently, in patients with severe renal failure (creatinine clearance < 10 ml/min) and liver disease, the lower of the two doses should always be used.

      2. When **moderate intravenous doses** (i.e., 8–12 million units/day) are to be used in patients with renal failure, we tend to reduce doses proportionately to the suggestions given in Table 28C-2 (i.e., approximately 50% of the high-dose recommendation).

      3. When a **low-dose intravenous penicillin** or oral penicillin [16] regimen is to be used, standard doses are employed.

   B. **Dialysis**

      1. **Hemodialysis** removes penicillin, but the amounts removed vary. When the equivalent of high-dose therapy is used (see Table 28C-2), Bryan and Stone [15] suggest an additional 500,000 units after each 6-hour dialysis. (A proportion of this supplemental dose could be given in a moderate- or low-dose regimen.)

Table 28C-2. Equivalent doses of aqueous penicillin G for high-dose therapy in renal failure[a]

Endogenous creatinine clearance (ml/min)	Penicillin G dose[b] and dose interval[c] (units)
125	1.7–2.0 million q2h or 2.6–3.0 million q3h
60	1.8–2.0 million q4h
40	1.3–1.5 million q4h
20	800,000–1 million q4h
10	800,000–1 million q6h
0	500,000–800,000 q6h or 700,000–1.1 million q8h
<10[d]	500,000 q8h

[a]**To achieve mean blood levels equivalent to 20 million units per day in the adult** with normal renal function, the above doses and dose intervals can be used in patients with renal failure.
   A **loading dose** of 750,000–1,200,000 units is suggested in patients with a creatinine clearance of less than 20 ml/min, and then the above doses and intervals can be followed. In patients with a creatinine clearance exceeding 20 ml/min, no loading dose is suggested.
[b]The lower dose is calculated to provide a mean serum level of 20 μg/ml for the "average" patient. The higher dose is an overestimate.
[c]After hemodialysis, an additional 500,000 units should be given to replace expected losses for an average full 6-hour dialysis.
[d]Because the extrarenal clearance of penicillin is impaired by liver disease, in patients with hepatic and renal failure (creatinine clearance <10 ml/min), even lower doses of penicillin G are suggested.
Source: Adapted from C.S. Bryan and W.J. Stone, "Comparable massive" penicillin G therapy in renal failure. *Ann. Intern. Med.* 82:189, 1975.

    2. Peritoneal dialysis likewise removes a variable amount of penicillin. Usually, doses are not specifically supplemented after peritoneal dialysis.

  C. Probenecid use. Penicillin G is eliminated primarily by the kidney, approximately 90% by tubular secretion and 10% by glomerular filtration. Probenecid blocks the renal tubular secretory transport of penicillin, and this, in turn, results in higher (usually approximately twofold) and more prolonged blood (plasma) levels of penicillin.

    1. Dosage. Probenecid, 500 mg PO qid, is recommended (in adults). Some patients may experience minor GI symptoms with probenecid use.

    2. Uses. Because the addition of probenecid increases the frequency of side effects, **we seldom use probenecid with oral therapy.** In moderate to severe infections requiring high blood levels, parenteral agents should be used. For mild infections routinely responding to oral penicillin therapy, probenecid addition is not necessary. Probenecid is used in some special circumstances.

      a. In the treatment of gonorrhea, probenecid has been used in some of the alternative regimens with amoxicillin (see Chap. 13).

      b. Prolonged oral penicillin therapy sometimes is indicated, as in the completion of therapy for actinomycosis. Probenecid in this setting may help to provide the higher blood levels necessary for adequate therapy. See Chap. 18.

  D. Cost. See Tables 28A-5 and 28A-6.

References

1. Chambers, H.F., and Neu, H.C. Penicillins. In G.L. Mandell, J.E. Bennett, and R. Dolin (eds.), *Principles and Practice of Infectious Diseases* (4th ed.). New York: Churchill Livingstone, 1995. Pp. 213–246.
2. Wright, A.J., and Wilkowske, C.J. The penicillins. *Mayo Clin. Proc.* 66:1047, 1991.
3. Medical Letter. The choice of antibacterial drugs. *Med. Lett. Drugs Ther.* 38:25, 1996.
   Lists drugs of choice and alternative agents for most pathogens. Excellent reference. Revised approximately every 2 years. Penicillin still is listed as the drug of choice for more than 15 organisms!
4. Breiman, R.F., et al. Emergence of drug-resistant pneumococcal infections in the United States. *J.A.M.A.* 271:1831, 1994.
   Isolates were from children and adults; 93% were blood culture isolates, 5% from the cerebrospinal fluid and the rest from pleural fluid, peritoneal fluid, and so on. See reference [8] also.
4a. Hofman, J., et al. The prevalence of drug-resistant *Streptococcus pneumoniae* in Atlanta. *N. Engl. J. Med.* 333:481, 1995.
   This August 1995 article from the CDC and Emory University looks at 431 isolates from patients with invasive disease in 1994. Multidrug resistance was common: isolates from 26% were resistant to TMP-SMX (7% highly resistant); 15% were resistant to erythromycin; and 9% were resistant to cefotaxime (4% highly resistant). Whites were more likely than blacks to have invasive infections caused by drug-resistant organisms. Among white children younger than 6 years, 41% of the S. pneumoniae *isolates were resistant to penicillin.*
4b. Tomasz, A. The pneumococcus at the gates. *N. Engl. J. Med.* 333:514, 1995.
   Editorial comment on references [4a] and [5a].
5. Austrian, R. Confronting drug-resistant pneumococci. *Ann. Intern. Med.* 121:807, 1994.
   Editorial comment.
5a. Schreiber, J.R., and Jacobs, M.R. Antibiotic-resistant pneumococci. *Pediatr. Clin. North Am.* 42:519, 1995.
   This June 1995 review article has an excellent summary, including detailed information of MIC data with alternative agents. See related summary by J.R. Lonks and A.A. Medeiros, The growing threat of antibiotic-resistant Streptococcus pneumoniae. *Med. Clin. North Am. 79:523, 1995.*
5b. Pallares, R., et al. Resistance to penicillin and cephalosporin and mortality from severe pneumococcal pneumonia in Barcelona, Spain. *N. Engl. J. Med.* 333:474, 1995.
6. Friedland, L.R., and McCracken, G.H., Jr. Management of infections caused by antibiotic-resistant *Streptococcus pneumoniae. N. Engl. J. Med.* 331:377, 1994.

6a. Bradley, J.S., et al. Consensus: Management of infections in children caused by *Streptococcus pneumoniae* with decreased susceptibility to penicillin. *Pediatr. Infect. Dis. J.* 14:1037, 1995.
   In this December 1995 publication, four infectious disease specialists with a particular interest in the problem of antibiotic-resistant pneumococci discuss their approach to meningitis, otitis media, pneumonia, and occult bacteremia.

6b. Viladrich, P.F., et al. High doses of cefotaxime in treatment of adult meningitis due to *Streptococcus pneumoniae* with decreased susceptibilities to broad-spectrum cephalosporins. *Antimicrob. Agents Chemother.* 40:218, 1996.
   In this small study, nine patients were treated with cefotaxime (300 mg/kg/day to a maximum of 24 g/day).

7. Doern, G. Emergence of antimicrobial resistance with *S. pneumoniae, H. influenzae,* and *Neisseria species.* Symposium: The Epidemiology of Emerging Antimicrobial Resistance. 34th Interscience Conference on Antimicrobial Agents and Chemotherapy, American Society for Microbiology, Orlando, FL, October 7, 1994.

7a. Fraimow, H.S., and Abrutyn, E. Pathogens resistant to antimicrobial agents: Epidemiology, molecular mechanisms, and clinical management. *Infect. Dis. Clin. North Am.* 9:497, 1995.
   An excellent summary published in September 1995.

8. Simberkoff, M.S. Drug-resistant pneumococcal infections in the United States: A problem for clinicians, laboratories, and public health. *J.A.M.A.* 271:1875, 1994.
   An editorial comment on reference [4].

8a. Jernigan, D.B., et al. Minimizing the impact of drug-resistant *Streptococcus pneumoniae* (DRSP): A strategy from the DRSP Working Group. *J.A.M.A.* 275:206, 1996.
   Strategy focuses on better surveillance systems, identifying risk factors and outcomes of DRSP infections, increasing the use of pneumococcal vaccine, and promoting judicious antimicrobial drug use. See related report from the CDC, Defining the public health impact of drug-resistant Streptococcus pneumoniae: *Report of a working group* M.M.W.R. 45(RR):1, 1996.

9. Bush, L.M., et al. High-level penicillin resistance among isolates of enterococci: Implications for treatment of enterococcal infections. *Ann. Intern. Med.* 110:515, 1989.
   Vancomycin and gentamicin therapy is indicated for these patients.

10. Herman, D.J., and Gerding, D.N. Antimicrobial resistance among enterococci. *Antimicrob. Agents Chemother.* 35:1, 1991.
   Nice review emphasizing that this problem is increasing and that in tertiary-care hospitals in the United States, up to 24.5% of enterococcal isolates in 1989 demonstrated high-level gentamicin resistance. See related article by D.J. Herman and D.N. Gerding, Screening and treatment of infections caused by resistant enterococci. Antimicrob. Agents Chemother. *35:215, 1991. See Chap. 28O also.*

11. Brewin, A., et al. High-dose penicillin therapy and pneumococcal pneumonia. *J.A.M.A.* 230:409, 1974.
   There is no advantage to treating patients with uncomplicated penicillin-susceptible pneumococcal pneumonia with more than 1,200,000 units daily of procaine penicillin G. The treatment of pneumococcal pneumonia has become more complex in cases where penicillin-resistant forms are known or highly likely to be causing the patient's infection. See text.

12. Green, R.L., et al. Elevated plasma procaine concentrations after administration of procaine penicillin G. *N. Engl. J. Med.* 291:223, 1974.
   Discusses setting, signs, and symptoms of procaine reactions.

13. Klein, J.O. Management of streptococcal pharyngitis. *Pediatr. Infect. Dis. J.* 13:572, 1994.
   Excellent summary by a recognized expert. Discusses current controversy of the role of cephalosporins as primary therapy in the nonallergic patient.

13a. Dajani, A., et al. Treatment of acute streptococcal pharyngitis and prevention of rheumatic fever: A statement for health professionals. *Pediatrics* 96:758, 1995.
   From the Committee on Rheumatic Fever, Endocarditis, and Kawasaki Disease of the Council on Cardiovascular Disease in the Young, the American Heart Association. This updates the 1988 statement. See related discussion in Chap. 28B.

14. Ruff, M.E., et al. Antimicrobial drug suspensions: A blind comparison of taste of fourteen common pediatric drugs. *Pediatr. Infect. Dis. J.* 10:30, 1991.
   Compared the smell, taste, and other characteristics of 14 commonly prescribed antimicrobial suspensions in a blind test in 30 adult volunteers to determine whether there was a difference in acceptability. Prior data have been anecdotal. See Chap. 28F for additional discussion. The oral cephalosporins ranked the best in terms of taste, texture,

and aftertaste compared with erythromycin, penicillin, and dicloxacillin. Children younger than 6 years of age may be more sensitive to taste than older children and adults.

15. Bryan, C.S., and Stone, W.J. "Comparable massive" penicillin G therapy in renal failure. *Ann. Intern. Med.* 82:189, 1975.
    Provides a convenient nomogram to use in this setting. See Table 28C-2. Still a useful reference.

16. Bennett, W.M., et al. Drug Prescribing in Renal Failure: Dosing Guidelines for Adults (3rd ed.). Philadelphia: American College of Physicians, 1994. P. 29.

D. Penicillinase-Resistant Penicillins

Penicillinase-resistant penicillins were developed by modifying the side chain of the common penicillin nucleus structure (see Fig. 28C-1), primarily to treat penicillinase-producing *Staphylococcus aureus*. They are bactericidal agents.

I. **Spectrum of activity**

A. *S. aureus*

1. **Initial therapy.** If infection in the nonallergic patient is known or highly likely to be due to *S. aureus,* these agents are preferred initially, because the majority of both community-acquired and hospital-acquired *S. aureus* pathogens are penicillin-resistant [1]. Although there are minor variations of the minimal inhibitory concentrations (MICs) against *S. aureus* and variations in protein-binding characteristics of oxacillin, nafcillin, and methicillin, these are not clinically relevant at the parenteral doses usually recommended.

2. **Penicillin-susceptible *S. aureus.* If susceptibility studies show that the *S. aureus* is susceptible to penicillin G,** penicillin G is the **preferred agent** (in the nonallergic patient) because it has a narrower spectrum of activity, has better in vitro activity than the penicillinase-resistant penicillins against susceptible *S. aureus,* and is less expensive.

3. **Methicillin-resistant *S. aureus*** (MRSA), or oxacillin-resistant *S. aureus* (ORSA), has emerged as an important nosocomial pathogen and has recently been reviewed elsewhere [2–3a]. Serious nosocomial outbreaks have occurred with MRSA. For example, in 1991, approximately 40% of isolates of *S. aureus* from large teaching hospitals were reported as methicillin resistant [2a]. The incidence of MRSA shows wide geographic variation and variation from hospital to hospital, demonstrating the importance of nosocomial or institutional environment in maintaining the isolates' transmission [2a]. MRSA and *S. epidermidis* strains can be resistant not only to the semisynthetic penicillins but also to the cephalosporins, to aminoglycosides, and to clindamycin.

   a. **Mechanisms of resistance** are reviewed elsewhere [2–3].

   b. **Pathogenesis and transmission.** Colonization with MRSA often precedes infection. The most common mechanism by which MRSA is introduced into an institution is the admission of an infected or colonized patient. A colonized or infected health care worker may disseminate the organism directly. Patients from a chronic-care facility may be a reservoir from which MRSA is introduced into an acute-care facility [2]. The principal mode of MRSA transmission within an institution is from patient to patient via the **transiently colonized hands of hospital personnel.** Transmission via the inanimate environment may be important for special populations such as in burn or intensive care units. Airborne transmission may be important for patients with tracheostomies who are unable to handle their secretions. Patients with severe dermatitis are at high risk not only for acquiring but also for disseminating nosocomial strains, probably via exfoliation of desquamated epidermal cells [2].

   Once established in a geographic area, "community-acquired" MRSA infections can occur among patients with increased risk of staphylococcal colonization and some direct or even indirect exposure to a hospital environment, but true community-acquired infections in otherwise healthy individuals without risk factors are still exceptional [2a].

   c. **Eradication** of the carrier state of MRSA is attempted to stop an outbreak in a health care setting or to prevent recurrent infection in an individual [2].

(1) **Topical treatment.** Bacitracin ointment has been used, but mupirocin, applied to the anterior nares for 5 days, is favored for eradication of nasal carriage [2]. (See Chap. 28U.) Unfortunately, some strains of MRSA are resistant to mupirocin [2a].

(2) **Oral systemic therapy** is necessary, especially in a colonized wound or an extranasal site. Rifampin and trimethoprim-sulfamethoxazole (TMP-SMX) have commonly been used [2, 3]. Minocycline and ciprofloxacin have been used if strains are susceptible [2a].

(3) **Combination therapy** with topical therapy of the nares and oral antibiotics is often employed. Nasal colonization can be eradicated from a significant proportion of carriers [2a]. Eradication of MRSA from respiratory tract secretions and colonized wounds (e.g., decubitus ulcer) is more difficult than elimination of nasal carriage and probably should not be attempted routinely [2a].

d. **Treatment of MRSA infections** and methicillin-resistant coagulase-negative staphylococci usually is with intravenous vancomycin. See Chap. 28O.

Gentamicin is synergistic with vancomycin in vitro against many MRSA strains and can be combined for bacteremic and endovascular staphylococci. Rifampin plus vancomycin may be either synergistic or antagonistic in vitro, but ample clinical data demonstrate the usefulness of this combination, particularly where tissue penetration of vancomycin may be suboptimal (e.g., CSF). Rifampin should not be used alone as resistance develops quickly [2a].

TMP-SMX and quinolones have been used for susceptible strains; quinolones should be used with caution because resistance may emerge on therapy [2a]. Minocycline has been used in selected infections, especially in Japan [2a].

e. **Infection control** practices are reviewed elsewhere [2, 3, 3a]. In response to the increase in prevalence of MRSA, some have recommended that isolation procedures be abandoned, arguing that the expenditure of time and money for these measures cannot be justified [3a].

A recent report favors isolation procedures for those patients colonized or infected with MRSA, emphasizing that MRSA is a virulent pathogen (30% of colonized patients become infected) and many MRSA infections are preventable [3a]. Furthermore, the report emphasizes that routine screening of patients transferred from nursing homes and hospitals to rapidly identify patients who are colonized and/or infected with MRSA (so they can be appropriately isolated) appears to be a cost-effective measure.

Contact isolation is commonly recommended [3a]. For patients with colonization and/or infection with burns, a major draining wound, extensive skin involvement, or a lower respiratory tract infection, strict isolation (i.e., a private room; gowns, gloves, and masks for all entering the patient's room) may be reasonable in an attempt to limit nosocomial spread, especially in hospitals with low endemic rates of MRSA (e.g., < 10% of *S. aureus* isolates are MRSA).

Very careful hand washing is mandatory after caring for patients colonized or infected with MRSA.

4. **"Tolerant"** *S. aureus.* The definition and the initial clinical significance of this phenomenon have been reviewed [4]. By definition, **tolerant** *S. aureus* consists of organisms whose minimal bactericidal concentration is 8–100 times higher than the MIC. **Whether this is an important laboratory finding or an artifact of technique remains unclear.** Some experts believe that a second antibiotic (e.g., an aminoglycoside) should be added to the semisynthetic penicillin when infections are due to documented tolerant *S. aureus*. Despite the initial enthusiasm for these observations, further studies have not clarified the importance of tolerance. A recent reviewer suggested that tolerance may, at times, be important in chronic infections associated with a foreign body [5].

B. **Other gram-positive aerobes.** These agents are active against *Streptococcus pneumoniae* and *S. pyogenes,* but the MICs for these organisms are higher for the penicillinase-resistant penicillins than for penicillin. Therefore, if final culture reports show the pathogen to be either *S. pneumoniae* or *S. pyogenes,* penicillin is preferred. If mixed infections with penicillin-resistant staphylococci and *S. pyogenes* (group A streptococci) or pneumococci occur, the penicillinase-resistant penicillin may be used alone, in the doses routinely recommended. Viridans streptococci are susceptible to the penicillinase-resistant penicillins but, in infections known to be caused by these and similar streptococci, penicillin is preferred. Alone, these agents are not effective against enterococci (see sec. **II.B.3**). The penicillinase-resistant penicillins are drugs of first choice only for penicillinase-producing *S. aureus* [1] when MRSA is not present.

C. **Gram-negative aerobes.** These agents are not effective against the Enterobacteriaceae (*Escherichia coli* and *Klebsiella* and *Enterobacter* spp.) or *Pseudomonas* spp. The penicillinase-resistant penicillins **are not recommended in the treatment of gonorrhea** [1]. For patients with infections due to *Pasteurella multocida,* penicillin is the preferred agent, and tetracycline (or cefuroxime) is recommended in the patient allergic to penicillin [1].

D. **Anaerobes.** Compared with penicillin, the penicillinase-resistant penicillins are less active against penicillin-susceptible anaerobes. These antistaphylococcal agents are not active against *Bacteroides fragilis.*

II. **Parenteral preparations.** There are no adequate studies to determine which antistaphylococcal agent is the best. Overall, oxacillin and nafcillin are very similar and, except as noted later, are probably interchangeable. Methicillin is more commonly associated with interstitial nephritis, especially in adults.

A. **Oxacillin**
   1. **Dose.** In adults, 6 g/day IV is recommended for moderate infections. For severe infections, 9–12 g/day IV is suggested, and the dose interval should be q4h. In children, the usual dose is 100–200 mg/kg/day in divided doses q4–6h. Because serum levels become very low 2.5–3.0 hours after intravenous doses administered over 20–30 minutes, in severe infections, a 4-hour dose interval is preferred.
   2. **In renal failure.** Oxacillin is excreted both renally and hepatically. In renal failure, doses do not have to be modified. **Hemodialysis and peritoneal dialysis** do not remove oxacillin. Therefore, no additional dose adjustments are necessary [6].
   3. **Side effects.** Allergic reactions can occur as with other penicillins (see Chap. 27). Rarely, neutropenia has been observed. Interstitial nephritis appears to occur less frequently than with methicillin [7–9]. Oxacillin-related **hepatitis** in prolonged intravenous use has been described. Therefore, **weekly liver function tests are advisable for patients receiving prolonged therapy** [10]. *Clostridium difficile* diarrhea can occur (see Chap. 28A).

B. **Nafcillin**
   1. **Dosage** is similar to that for oxacillin in adults and older children. **Nafcillin should not be used in premature or young infants with jaundice** as it is excreted primarily by hepatic mechanisms, which may be deficient in these neonates or infants (see Chap. 3).
   2. **In renal failure and dialysis,** dosage modification is not necessary. Therefore, nafcillin is an excellent choice in patients with renal impairment who require an antistaphylococcal semisynthetic penicillin [6].
   3. **Synergism with aminoglycosides.** Studies have demonstrated a synergistic effect of nafcillin and gentamicin against *S. aureus* and, to a lesser extent, enterococci. The value of adding an aminoglycoside to nafcillin in staphylococcal sepsis or endocarditis is not known [11]. Some clinicians, however, will add an aminoglycoside (low-dose regimens) in the first 4–7 days of therapy for severe staphylococcal sepsis. See related discussions in Chaps. 2 and 10.
   4. **Central nervous system penetration.** Studies have shown adequate penetration of nafcillin into the spinal fluid, particularly when pleocytosis is present. Some authors suggest that it **may be the drug of choice in staphylococcal meningitis** requiring penicillinase-resistant penicillins [12]. Adequate doses must be used—that is, 100–200 mg/kg/day. See related discussions in Chap. 5.
   5. **Side effects** are similar to those described previously for oxacillin. Interstitial nephritis can occur after nafcillin use, but it is less frequent than after methicillin use [13]. Neutropenia can occur. Phlebitis seems to occur more commonly with nafcillin than with oxacillin.

C. **Methicillin.** Many experts believe that this agent **should be avoided in adults** because of the increased risk of interstitial nephritis associated with its use. Consequently, the use of methicillin has decreased considerably in recent years [14]. In neonates, methicillin still is used (interstitial nephritis is unusual in this age group).

1. **Dosage**
   a. **Neonates.** See Chap. 3.
   b. **Children and adults.** Dosages as outlined in sec. **A.1** are used in patients with normal renal function.
2. **In renal failure,** doses must be reduced [6]. Nafcillin usually is preferred in renal failure patients, as discussed previously.
3. **Dialysis.** Methicillin is not removed by hemodialysis or peritoneal dialysis. Although intermittent doses of intravenous vancomycin are easy to use for susceptible staphylococcal infections, in an attempt to reduce the consumption of vancomycin (see Chaps. 28A and 28O), methicillin could be used in adult dialysis patients with susceptible *S. aureus* infection, as 3.0 g q24h gives adequate levels with minimal phlebitis.
4. **Interstitial nephritis** [7, 8, 15] occurs with the use of penicillin and other penicillin derivatives, but it is more common with methicillin use. This complication has been observed in all age groups. It does not appear to be dose-related and may represent a hypersensitivity reaction.
   a. **Signs and symptoms.** The major signs and symptoms usually appear after several days of antibiotic therapy and include hematuria, proteinuria, fever, a peripheral eosinophilia, morbilliform rash, and renal failure (in approximately 50% of cases). The renal failure may be severe and require dialysis. A nonoliguric renal failure can occur.
   b. **Diagnosis.** A minority of patients may have eosinophils in their urine sediments, which is a helpful diagnostic clue. Otherwise, the diagnosis depends on the clinical setting. A characteristic renal biopsy, which reveals an interstitial nephritis with eosinophilic aggregations, occurs.
   c. **Therapeutic approach.** The offending antibiotic should be discontinued. If additional staphylococcal therapy is necessary, a cephalosporin can often be used safely. However, cross-sensitization with the penicillins has been observed and, in some patients placed on cephalosporins, the renal failure may be aggravated. For these patients, if additional antistaphylococcal therapy is necessary, vancomycin is preferred. In patients with progressive azotemia, prednisone (40–60 mg daily in adults) has been used; however, its precise role in this setting is uncertain. In patients who are doing well clinically, steroids are neither routinely used nor recommended. In these difficult cases, a nephrology or immunology consultation (or both) seems prudent.
III. **Oral preparations** (cloxacillin, dicloxacillin)
   A. **Indications for use.** Penicillinase-resistant penicillins in oral form often are considered the oral drugs of choice for known or highly suspected penicillin-resistant mild staphylococcal infections. They are useful in treating soft-tissue infections due to susceptible *S. aureus* or mixed *S. aureus* and *S. pyogenes* (group A streptococci). In the nonallergic patient, as an ideal principle of antibiotic use, these narrow-spectrum agents are preferred over the oral cephalosporins [16]. If cultures reveal the pathogens to be penicillin-susceptible, then penicillin is less expensive and is an effective agent to use. However, if patients are prone to develop minor GI side effects (e.g., nausea) frequently while receiving oral antibiotics or when the taste of the liquid suspension may affect compliance, the oral cephalosporins may be better tolerated and therefore preferred over cloxacillin or dicloxacillin.

   In one study, oral dicloxacillin (Dynapen) suspension had the worst taste of the 14 antimicrobial agents tested, whereas cephalexin (Keflex) had one of the best taste scores [17]. Because taste perception is considered to be the single most important factor in achieving compliance in children, especially children of preschool age, we conclude that taste should be considered when selecting an antimicrobial suspension or liquid formulation for this age group [17]. Oral penicillinase-resistant penicillin agents and oral cephalosporins are both relatively expensive (see Table 28A-5). Overall, the decision about whether to use an oral penicillinase-resistant penicillin (e.g., dicloxacillin) versus an oral cephalosporin (see Chap. 28F) must be individualized. However, because appropriate doses of oral cephalexin appear to yield serum levels of drug that are sufficient to inhibit *S. aureus* and oral cephalexin causes fewer GI symptoms, an oral cephalosporin such as cephalexin is a reasonable choice.
   B. **Agents available**
      1. Oral nafcillin and oxacillin provide lower blood levels than do other available agents; therefore, these agents are not recommended.

    2. Cloxacillin and dicloxacillin provide acceptable blood levels. Higher blood levels can be achieved with dicloxacillin.

  C. Dosage. These drugs are better absorbed in the fasting states (i.e., 1 hour before or 2 hours after meals).

    1. Cloxacillin is available in an oral solution (125 mg/5 ml) and in 250-mg and 500-mg capsules. The usual dosage in children is 50–100 mg/kg/day and, in adults, 1–2 g per day divided into four equal doses.

    2. Dicloxacillin is available as a suspension (62.5 mg/5 ml) and in 125-mg and 250-mg capsules. The usual dosage in children is 25–50 mg/kg/day and, in adults, 1–2 g per day divided into four equal doses. The higher dose range may be preferable for adequate antistaphylococcal activity.

  D. Side effects. These agents commonly cause mild GI symptoms, and often the standard oral dosages (e.g., 500 mg q6h in adults) cannot be tolerated. In these patients, a first-generation oral cephalosporin may be better tolerated. If severe or persistent diarrhea occurs, antibiotic-related diarrhea must be considered (see Chap. 28A). The penicillin-allergic manifestations described in Chap. 27 and the side effects of parenteral agents (see sec. **II**) may occur.

IV. Cost. See Tables 28A-5 and 28A-6.

References

1. Medical Letter. The choice of antibacterial drugs. *Med. Lett. Drugs Ther.* 38:25, 1996.
   Excellent reference. Reviewed approximately every 2 years.
2. Mulligan, M.E., et al. Methicillin-resistant *Staphylococcus aureus:* A consensus review of the microbiology, pathogenesis, and epidemiology with implications for prevention and management. *Am. J. Med.* 94:313, 1993.
   Good review article.
2a. Fraimow, H.S., and Abrutyn, E. Pathogens resistant to antimicrobial agents: Epidemiology, molecular mechanisms, and clinical management. *Infect. Dis. Clin. North Am.* 9:497, 1995.
3. Martin, M.A. Methicillin-resistant *Staphylococcus aureus:* The persistent resistant nosocomial pathogen. *Curr. Clin. Top. Infect. Dis.* 14:170, 1994.
   Excellent review. Risk factors for nosocomial acquisition of MRSA colonization and infection include advanced age, length of hospital stay, previous hospitalization, stay in burn unit or intensive care unit, chronic underlying disease, prior antibiotic therapy, exposure to colonized or infected patient or colonized caregiver, surgical wound, and invasive devices.
   See related review by S.F. Bradley, MRSA in long term care: Fact, fiction, and controversy. Infect. Dis. Clin. Pract. *3:321, 1994.*
3a. Jernigan, J.A., et al. Control of methicillin-resistant *Staphylococcus aureus* at a university hospital: One decade later. *Infect. Control Hosp. Epidemiol.* 16:686, 1995.
   This December 1995 report concludes that screening cultures of transfer patients from facilities with a high prevalence of MRSA may offer significant benefit by preventing nosocomial infections and reducing patient days spent in isolation, thereby being cost effective.
   This report is from the University of Virginia Health Sciences Center at which all patients colonized or infected with MRSA are placed on **contact isolation;** *i.e., all contacts with patient wear a mask when within 5 feet of the patient, wear a gown for direct contact with the patient, and wear gloves for manual contact with the patient or other potentially contaminated surfaces.* **Again, true community-acquired MRSA colonization and/or infection was not noted in previously healthy people** *admitted for an isolated acute illness; MRSA was at times isolated from those who were chronically ill and frequently seen in outpatient facilities and/or patients tended by multiple hospital personnel at home.*
4. Kaye, D. The clinical significance of tolerance of *Staphylococcus aureus. Ann. Intern. Med.* 93:925, 1980.
   Concise discussion of the definition, potential clinical significance, and approach to patients with "tolerant" organisms.
5. Waldvogel, F.A. *Staphylococcus aureus* (Including Toxic Shock Syndrome). In G.L. Mandell, J.E. Bennett, and R. Dolin (eds.), *Principles and Practice of Infectious Diseases* (4th ed.). New York: Churchill Livingstone, 1995. P. 1757.
6. Bennett, W.M., et al. *Drug Prescribing in Renal Failure: Dosing Guidelines for Adults* (3rd ed.). Philadelphia: American College of Physicians, 1994.
   This is a useful handbook. Similar tables for dosing in renal failure appear in L.L.

Livornese, Jr., et al., Antibacterial agents in renal failure. Infect. Dis. Clin. North Am. *9:591, 1995; and S.K. Swan and W.M. Bennett, Drug dosing guidelines in patients with renal failure.* West. J. Med. *156:633, 1992.*

7. Linton, A.L., et al. Acute interstitial nephritis due to drugs: Review of the literature with a report of nine cases. Ann. Intern. Med. 93:735, 1980.
   See related discussion by R.M. Ten et al., Acute interstitial nephritis: Immunologic and clinical aspects. Mayo Clin. Proc. *63:921, 1988.*

8. Murray, K.M., and Keane, W.R. Review of drug-induced acute interstitial nephritis. *Pharmacotherapy* 12:462, 1992.

9. Tillman, D.B., Oill, P.A., and Guze, L.B. Oxacillin nephritis. *Arch. Intern. Med.* 140: 1552, 1980.

10. Bruckstein, A.H., and Attia, A.A. Oxacillin hepatitis. *Am. J. Med.* 64:519, 1978.
    The authors suggest weekly monitoring of serum transaminase levels in patients on prolonged therapy.

11. Sande, M.A., and Scheld, W.M. Combination therapy or bacterial endocarditis. *Ann. Intern. Med.* 92:390, 1980.

12. Kane, J.G., et al. Nafcillin concentration in cerebrospinal fluid during treatment of staphylococcal infections. *Ann. Intern. Med.* 87:309, 1977.

13. Barriere, S.L., and Conte, J.E. Absence of nafcillin-associated nephritis—a prospective analysis of 210 patients. *West. J. Med.* 133:472, 1980.

14. Wright, A.J., and Wilkowske, C.J. The penicillins. *Mayo Clin. Proc.* 66:1047, 1991.

15. Ditlove, J., et al. Methicillin nephritis. *Medicine* (Baltimore) 56:483, 1977.
    Still a useful review of this topic. Eosinophils in the urine may be a diagnostic clue. See references [7, 8].

16. Veterans Administration Ad Hoc Interdisciplinary Advisory Committee on Antimicrobial Drug Usage. Oral cephalosporins. *J.A.M.A.* 237:1241, 1977.

17. Ruff, M.E., et al. Antimicrobial drug suspensions: A blind comparison of taste of fourteen common pediatric drugs. *Pediatr. Infect. Dis. J.* 10:30, 1991.
    Compared the smell, taste, and other characteristics of 14 commonly prescribed antimicrobial suspensions in a blind test in 30 adult volunteers to determine whether there was a difference in acceptability. Prior data have been anecdotal. See Chap. 28F for additional discussion. The oral cephalosporins ranked the best in terms of taste, texture, and after taste compared with erythromycin, penicillin, and dicloxacillin. Children younger than 6 years may be more sensitive to taste than older children and adults.

E. Broad-Spectrum Penicillins and Beta-Lactam–Beta-Lactamase Combinations

Broad-spectrum penicillins possess variable activity against gram-negative bacilli. They sometimes are referred to as **second-generation penicillins** (e.g., ampicillin, amoxicillin), **third-generation** penicillins (e.g., carbenicillin and ticarcillin), and **fourth-generation** penicillins (e.g., azlocillin, mezlocillin, and piperacillin). In addition, some of these agents (e.g., amoxicillin, ampicillin, ticarcillin, and piperacillin) have been combined with a beta-lactamase inhibitor to increase the spectrum of the combination.

I. **Second-generation** broad-spectrum penicillins

  A. **Ampicillin and amoxicillin** [1] are semisynthetic compounds that have greater activity against some gram-negative bacteria than does penicillin G.

   1. **Spectrum of activity of ampicillin.** Ampicillin is active against pathogens listed under the spectrum of activity of penicillin G (see Chap. 28C and Table 28A-3). However, when one is dealing with an infection due to one of these pathogens, the narrower-spectrum and less expensive agent, penicillin, is preferred. The **expanded spectrum of ampicillin includes the following:**

    a. **Ampicillin is more active than penicillin against** enterococci, *Listeria monocytogenes,* and beta-lactamase-negative *Haemophilus influenzae.* At least 10–25% of *H. influenzae* strains are beta-lactamase-positive and ampicillin-resistant. Ampicillin should not be used for beta-lactamase-producing strains of *Staphylococcus* spp., *Haemophilus* spp., or *Moraxella (Branhamella) catarrhalis.* (See Table 28A-3.)

     b. Ampicillin is active against many but not all strains of *Escherichia coli* and *Proteus mirabilis,* particularly in community-acquired infections. It is also active against *Salmonella typhi* and many other *Salmonella* spp. as well as many *Shigella* spp.

     c. Ampicillin is not active against *Pseudomonas* spp. nor usually against hospital-acquired Enterobacteriaceae.

  2. Comparisons of ampicillin and amoxicillin (see Table 28E-1). **Amoxicillin** is currently available only as an oral preparation. Because, with similar doses, 95% of amoxicillin is absorbed from the GI tract, compared to 40% of ampicillin, one can achieve twice the blood levels with amoxicillin. Oral amoxicillin produces blood levels similar to those produced by intramuscular ampicillin [2]. Because of amoxicillin's improved absorption and good tissue penetration, it has essentially replaced ampicillin as an oral preparation except for *Shigella* infections.

     a. Spectrum of activity. Ampicillin and amoxicillin are susceptible to beta-lactamase. Their activity is **similar, but ampicillin is more effective against shigellae, and amoxicillin is more active against salmonellae.** In fact, **amoxicillin is not believed to be useful in the treatment of shigellosis,** even if the organism is susceptible in vitro [1, 2], perhaps because of its near-complete absorption.

     b. Toxicity. The frequency of rashes with amoxicillin is the same as that with ampicillin [1]. Amoxicillin seems to cause diarrhea less often [1, 2]. Allergic reactions are discussed in Chap. 27.

  3. Ampicillin and amoxicillin are **drugs of choice** [3] **for**

     a. Enterococci, *Streptococcus agalactiae* (group B streptococci), *L. monocytogenes* (often with an aminoglycoside).

     b. Susceptible *P. mirabilis* and *Eikenella corrodens.*

  4. Uses

     a. Amoxicillin is still considered the usual empiric agent of choice for acute otitis media (in areas with low prevalence of beta-lactamase-positive *H. influenzae*) [4, 5] and an excellent oral agent for bacterial sinusitis, bacterial exacerbations of bronchitis, susceptible bacteria in urinary tract infections (UTIs), and some *Salmonella* infections. It is not useful in the treatment of *Shigella* infections [2]. Amoxicillin is now the preferred agent for the prevention of endocarditis after dental procedures (see Chap. 28B). It has been used to eradicate *Helicobacter pylori* [6] associated with recurrent duodenal ulcer. See Chap. 11.

     b. Ampicillin can be used in the same situations as amoxicillin [3, 7, 8]. Because of resistant plasmids, strains of *Shigella* frequently are resistant to ampicillin; a fluoroquinolone is the empiric drug of choice [3]. If the *Shigella* spp. is ampicillin-susceptible, ampicillin (not amoxicillin) can be

Table 28E-1. Comparisons of amoxicillin and ampicillin

Characteristics	Amoxicillin	Ampicillin
Form available	Oral only	Oral and parenteral
Percentage absorbed from gastrointestinal tract	95%	40%
Effect of food	None	Decreased absorption
Concentration in urine	Very high	High
Concentration in sputum	High and persists	Lower and decreases
Activity against:		
Penicillin-resistant staphylococci	None	None
Salmonella	Good	Fair–good
Shigella	Poor	Good
Toxicity	Less diarrhea	Diarrhea, rash
Cost	Slightly more per tablet*	

*However, because a lower dose of amoxicillin often can be used, an equivalent course of amoxicillin may cost less than ampicillin.

used; an advantage of ampicillin is that a parenteral preparation is available for the hospitalized patient.

5. **Dosage**
   a. **Ampicillin**
      (1) **Intravenous.** In adults, 4–12 g daily is given depending on the organism involved and the severity and site of the infection. In adults with moderately severe infections, 1 g q4–6h often is given; for more severe infections, 1.5 g q4h may be necessary and, in meningitis in the adult, 2 g q4h is used. **In children,** the usual dosage range is 100–200 mg/kg/day in divided doses q6h. Higher doses (up to 400 mg/kg/day) are used in meningitis caused by known susceptible *H. influenzae.* Neonatal doses are outlined in Chap. 3.
      (2) **Oral.** The usual adult dose is 250–500 mg q6h **on an empty stomach.** If higher blood levels are desired, probenecid can be added, or amoxicillin is preferred (except in cases of *Shigella*). In children, 50–100 mg/kg/day in divided doses q6h is suggested.
      (3) **Intramuscular.** Ampicillin can be given intramuscularly, but the intravenous route generally is preferred.
      (4) **Renal failure.** Because ampicillin is excreted by the kidney, dosage is modified in patients with significant renal impairment, particularly when high-dose regimens are used. If the creatinine clearance is 10–50 ml/min, the standard dose can be given q6–12h. If the creatinine clearance is less than 10 ml/min, the standard dose can be given every 12–24 hours [9].
      (5) **Dialysis.** Ampicillin is partially removed by hemodialysis. After dialysis, a supplemental dose is required [9]. Peritoneal dialysis does not significantly lower ampicillin serum levels. For oral therapy, 250 mg q12h has been used [9].
      (6) **Pregnancy.** Ampicillin does cross the placenta. As with other penicillins, it should be used conservatively in pregnant women. See Chaps. 3 and 28A.
      (7) **Nursing mothers.** Ampicillin is excreted in human milk (see Chap. 3). In theory, the neonate could be sensitized by ampicillin in the mother's milk, so this agent should be used conservatively in nursing mothers as neonates commonly are treated with ampicillin.
   b. **Amoxicillin**
      (1) **Oral.** The usual adult dose is 250–500 mg q8h, and the fasting state is not essential. In children, 20–40 mg/kg/day is given in divided doses q8h. An oral suspension is available with 250 mg/5 ml and 125 mg/5 ml. For otitis media in children, 40 mg/kg/day in divided doses q8h typically is given. The usual adult dose (250 mg q8h) is given to children weighing more than 20 kg. Guidelines for the limited use of amoxicillin in alternative treatment regimens for gonorrhea are summarized in Chap. 13.
      (2) **Intravenous.** Currently, there is no parenteral preparation of amoxicillin.
      (3) **Renal failure.** If the creatinine clearance is 10–50 ml/min, the standard dose can be given q8–12h. If the clearance is less than 10 ml/min, the standard dose can be given q24h [9].
      (4) **Dialysis.** Dosage is as described for ampicillin; see sec. **a.(5).** In chronic ambulatory peritoneal dialysis (CAPD) patients, 250 mg q12h has been suggested [9].
      (5) **Pregnancy.** The package insert notes that safety for use in pregnancy has not been established. See **a.(6).**
      (6) **Is amoxicillin a superior oral agent?** A review of amoxicillin [1] concludes that, except in *Salmonella* or *Shigella* infections, there are few data to suggest that one agent is superior to the other if equivalent doses are taken (500 mg of ampicillin or 250 mg of amoxicillin). However, **many clinicians and formulary committees prefer to use amoxicillin,** because a lower dose can often be used, food does not interfere with its absorption, serum levels are 2–2.5 times as high as those achieved with a similar dose of ampicillin, and it can be given on an every-8-hour schedule. These factors improve patient compliance.
      (7) **Allergic reactions** are discussed in Chap. 27, with special emphasis on the morbilliform eruptions seen with ampicillin or amoxicillin.

B. Amoxicillin-clavulanate (Augmentin) is an **oral** agent that was released in the United States in 1984 [10–11b].

   1. Unique combination. This is an interesting combination agent of amoxicillin and clavulanic acid (potassium salt form). The clavulanic acid is a weak antibacterial, natural compound produced by *Streptomyces clavuligerus* and is a potent inhibitor of many beta-lactamases.

   Clavulanate has a ring structure similar to that of penicillin and, by a complex interaction, it functions as a suicide inhibitor, blocking the enzymatic breakdown of amoxicillin by beta-lactamases. This leaves the amoxicillin intact and able to inhibit the bacteria. See related discussion in sec. **III.A.**

   2. Spectrum of activity. Clavulanic acid inhibits the beta-lactamases of *S. aureus* (found in 80% of these organisms), *H. influenzae* (found in 10–25% or more of these organisms), and *Neisseria gonorrhoeae, Haemophilus ducreyi,* and *M. catarrhalis.* In addition, clavulanic acid inhibits beta-lactamases produced by many gram-negative bacilli, including *E. coli* and *Klebsiella* and *Proteus* spp. Therefore, the combination of amoxicillin-clavulanate is active against amoxicillin-susceptible as well as many previously amoxicillin-resistant organisms, including 97–100% of *S. aureus.* Most streptococci (including most enterococci), *N. gonorrhoeae, H. influenzae, E. coli,* and *Klebsiella* spp. are susceptible. It is not active against the beta-lactamases produced by *Enterobacter* or *Pseudomonas* spp. *Serratia* spp. also are resistant. *Streptococcus pneumoniae* with high-level resistance to penicillin will be resistant to amoxicillin-clavulanate. See Chap. 28C.

   Separate disc or broth testing with the combination must be performed.

   3. Pharmacokinetics

   a. Both components are **well absorbed orally,** with peak levels at 1 hour, independent of meals, antacids, or milk.

   b. The drugs penetrate peritoneal and pleural fluids well. **Very high urine levels** are achieved compared with modest serum levels. There is only fair penetration into pulmonary secretions; therefore, higher doses are necessary in pulmonary infections. The combination does not provide adequate CNS penetration, but it does cross the placenta.

   c. Both agents are excreted primarily by the kidney, although probenecid has no effect on the pharmacokinetics of clavulanic acid.

   4. Clinical application. Clinical trials have shown that this combination is effective in UTI, otitis media, sinusitis, skin and soft-tissue infections (including bite wounds), and some mild lower respiratory infections. The combination has been used successfully for oral treatment of the following [11–11b]:

   a. Otitis media or **sinusitis,** especially when patients are failing the initial amoxicillin trial or initially where there is a very high incidence of ampicillin resistance with *H. influenzae* or *M. catarrhalis.*

   b. Human and animal bite wounds. Because it has excellent activity against *S. aureus,* beta-lactamase-producing oral anaerobes, and *Pasteurella multocida,* **amoxicillin-clavulanate is the preferred oral agent in this setting** [12]. For a detailed discussion, see Chap. 4.

   c. Urinary tract infection. Although the fluoroquinolones and trimethoprim-sulfamethoxazole (TMP-SMX) are commonly used in UTI, for susceptible pathogens, amoxicillin-clavulanate provides another possible oral agent; it is not for uncomplicated UTI caused by amoxicillin-susceptible organisms.

   d. Other considerations include mild cases of diverticulitis meriting a trial of oral therapy (this combination is active against many *Bacteroides fragilis* as well as other bowel pathogens). A semisynthetic antistaphylococcal penicillin or first-generation cephalosporin still is the drug of choice for common soft-tissue infections. Because of its limited penetration into pulmonary secretions, we believe amoxicillin-clavulanate should be used cautiously in mild pulmonary infections caused by susceptible organisms and, if patients do not respond fairly rapidly, parenteral antibiotic therapy may be needed. This combination has been used in exacerbations of bacterial bronchitis in patients with chronic pulmonary disease. It has also been used for early, mild cases of community-acquired pneumonia (see Chap. 9).

   5. Side effects. Overall these are minor, but **GI side effects,** including nausea, vomiting, diarrhea, and abdominal cramps, are reported to occur in 10% of patients [11a]. These are related in part to the dose of clavulanate (i.e., more symptoms at higher doses) and **can sometimes be minimized if the combina-**

tion is taken with meals, without affecting bioavailability [11, 11a]. Anecdotally, we wonder if the percentage of GI side effects may be even higher than 10%, especially in adults. Gastrointestinal side effects are more common when this combination is used than when amoxicillin is used alone. Some patients cannot tolerate amoxicillin-clavulanate because of such side effects.

6. **Dosages.** The drug should be administered with food to decrease the incidence of GI side effects [11a].

   a. **Availability.** An injectable form is not available in the United States.

      (1) Oral **chewable tablets** in a **250-mg size** (250 mg amoxicillin and 62.5 mg clavulanate) and a **125-mg size** (125 mg amoxicillin and 31.25 mg clavulanate) for pediatric use.

      (2) An **oral suspension** with **125 mg/5 ml** (containing 125 mg amoxicillin and 31.25 mg clavulanate per 5 ml) and one with **250 mg/5 ml** (containing 250 mg amoxicillin and 62.5 mg clavulanate per 5 ml) for pediatric use.

      (3) **Adult-sized tablets: 500 mg** (500 mg amoxicillin and 125 mg clavulanate) and **250 mg** (250 mg amoxicillin and 125 mg clavulanate).

      (4) **Note: Two of the 250-mg amoxicillin/125-mg clavulanate tablets should not be taken at one time as the double dose of clavulanate is more likely to cause GI toxicity.** A cost-effective method of giving the higher dose is to give one 250-mg amoxicillin/125-mg clavulanate tablet along with one 250-mg generic tablet of amoxicillin.
      The chewable tablets and adult tablets have different amoxicillin-clavulanate ratios, as just listed, and should not be interchanged.

   b. **Adult dose.** The usual adult dose is one 250-mg amoxicillin/125-mg clavulanate tablet 3 times daily. If a higher dose is desirable, as in respiratory infections, the 500-mg amoxicillin/125-mg clavulanate tablet, or equivalent, can be used 3 times daily.

   c. **Children**

      (1) **Suspension for children:** 20–40 mg/kg/day (based on amoxicillin content) divided into 3 doses daily is advised. The higher dose range is suggested for sinusitis, otitis, and respiratory infections.

      (2) Children weighing 40 kg or more can follow adult dose regimens. The adult-size 250-mg tablet should not be used unless the child weighs more than 40 kg.

   d. **Renal failure.** Dosage guidelines in renal failure are not readily available [9]. Therefore, we would prolong the dose interval as described under amoxicillin. See sec. **A.5.b.(3).**

   e. **Pregnancy.** This is a category B agent. (See Chap. 28A). The package insert indicates that because there are no adequate and well-controlled studies in pregnant women, this agent should be used during pregnancy only if clearly needed. The combination has been used safely in studies of pregnant women with bacteriuria or UTIs [11a].

   f. **Nursing mothers.** Because amoxicillin is excreted into milk, the package insert suggests caution should be exercised if this agent is administered to a nursing woman.

C. **Ampicillin-sulbactam** (Unasyn) is discussed separately in sec. **III.B.**

D. **Bacampicillin hydrochloride (Spectrobid)** is an ampicillinlike oral antibiotic with a spectrum of activity similar to ampicillin [13]. The *Medical Letter* [13] concluded that there is **no evidence that bacampicillin offers any significant advantages over amoxicillin, which is much less expensive. Furthermore, there is no evidence that the twice-daily schedule (pulse dosing) is more effective than 3- (amoxicillin) or 4-times-daily regimens (ampicillin). We see no special advantages of this agent** and so it will not be further reviewed.

II. **Extended-spectrum penicillins.** To facilitate a clinical discussion of carbenicillin, ticarcillin, piperacillin, and so forth, these agents will be considered together as extended-spectrum penicillins.

   The so-called fourth-generation broad-spectrum penicillins (ureidopenicillins), which include mezlocillin, piperacillin, and azlocillin, are all derivatives of ampicillin. They have broader spectrums of activity than carbenicillin or ticarcillin and are more active in vitro on a weight basis. Although in vitro they often are more active against *Klebsiella* spp., *Serratia marcescens,* and *Pseudomonas aeruginosa* than the third-generation penicillins, this probably is not clinically important, as prospective, comparative studies have failed to demonstrate significant clinical superiority of these newer agents [7, 14, 14a]. They are active against *N. gonorrhoeae* and *H. influenzae,* which do not produce beta-lactamase [7].

None of these agents is the drug of choice for specific pathogens except for *P. aeruginosa* infections (usually not involving a localized UTI). For severe *P. aeruginosa* infections (e.g., pneumonia, wound, bacteremia), one of these agents combined with an aminoglycoside is the therapy of choice [3].

Generally, the pharmacy and therapeutic committee of each hospital selects one of these intravenous preparations for routine use. We favor piperacillin, as discussed later.

A. Carbenicillin (Geocillin)
  1. **Intravenous form.** Carbenicillin was the first of these intravenous agents that had increased activity against gram-negative bacteria. **In most hospitals in the United States by the mid-1980s, intravenous carbenicillin has been replaced by intravenous ticarcillin or piperacillin.** Since late 1991, intravenous carbenicillin has not been marketed in the United States.
  2. **Oral carbenicillin** (Geocillin) is still available and is the only oral preparation in this group of agents. Oral carbenicillin **provides very low blood levels** (6–10 μg/ml), which are inadequate to treat bloodstream or nonrenal tissue infections effectively. Consequently, oral carbenicillin **cannot and should not be used as an oral preparation for systemic infections.**
      a. **Uses. The oral form,** which is supplied as an indyl ester, breaks down in the liver to form free carbenicillin. It **provides excellent urine concentrations** (more than 1,000 μg/ml) and therefore can be used in UTIs with susceptible pathogens. For example, it may be potentially useful in treating infections by susceptible *Pseudomonas, Serratia,* or other gram-negative organisms that might otherwise require a parenteral drug. (Oral fluoroquinolones are an alternative. See Chap. 28S.) **In renal failure, insufficient urine levels are achieved and it therefore is not useful.**
      b. **Dosage.** One to two tablets (382-mg tablets) in adults qid is recommended for 10–14 days. For *Pseudomonas* infections, the two-tablet dose is recommended. This drug is not recommended for patients with a creatinine clearance of less than 10 ml/min [14a]. **This is an expensive oral agent,** an important fact if the susceptibility data allow the use of other less expensive oral agents (see Table 28A-5).
      c. A follow-up urine culture is suggested to ensure that the infection has been adequately treated when *P. aeruginosa* is the pathogen.
B. Ticarcillin (Ticar) [15]
  1. **Ticarcillin's spectrum of activity** is very similar to that of carbenicillin, but ticarcillin is more active on a weight basis, so that a lower dose of ticarcillin can be used. Ticarcillin is active against most strains of *P. aeruginosa,* especially when it is combined with an aminoglycoside for synergy. It also is active against many indole-positive *Proteus* spp. and other gram-negative organisms that are resistant to ampicillin. However, most strains of *Klebsiella* are resistant to ticarcillin. It is not active against penicillinase-producing staphylococci, and it is not acid-resistant. **Ticarcillin is not very active against enterococci** because of poor binding to their penicillin-binding proteins [7]. (Piperacillin is more active against enterococci.) Ticarcillin is effective against penicillin-sensitive anaerobes and most *B. fragilis.*
  2. **Uses.** Ticarcillin **seldom is used as a single agent because of the concern that resistance will develop rapidly.**
      a. **Pseudomonad infections.** The major clinical use of ticarcillin has been in combination therapy with gentamicin or another aminoglycoside to provide synergism against gram-negative agents, particularly pseudomonads. This combination has also been used commonly in the febrile leukopenic patient who has no obvious source of infection (see Chap. 2). In addition, because it is difficult to achieve adequate aminoglycoside levels in lung tissue and sputum, ticarcillin is used in susceptible gram-negative pneumonias together with an aminoglycoside for synergistic effect. One study [16] suggested that ticarcillin and tobramycin seemed superior to carbenicillin and gentamicin against susceptible *P. aeruginosa* pulmonary infections.
      b. **Second-line agent for *B. fragilis.*** Ticarcillin is effective against the penicillin-susceptible anaerobes, and, in vitro, 75–85% of *B. fragilis* strains are susceptible to ticarcillin. However, in vivo, *B. fragilis* organisms produce a beta-lactamase enzyme, which may inactivate the ticarcillin. For these

reasons, ticarcillin generally is a second-line agent against *B. fragilis*. (Cefoxitin and cefotetan are other second-line agents that are as effective as ticarcillin against *B. fragilis*.)

  c. **Urinary tract infections** with susceptible organisms sometimes are treated with ticarcillin alone. With the availability of third-generation cephalosporins and the fluoroquinolones, the need for ticarcillin in this setting is limited.

3. **Sodium load.** The sodium content of ticarcillin is approximately 5.2 mEq/g. This may be important in the patient with severe congestive heart failure or renal failure. Piperacillin and mezlocillin have even lower sodium loads per day.

4. **Dosage** (intravenous). See Table 28E-2.

  a. The usual dosage in **children and adults** is 200–300 mg/kg/day divided into q4h doses. (In adults with severe infections, the dose is usually 3 g q4h.) See Chap. 3 for doses in neonates.

  b. **In renal failure**, the dose interval can be prolonged, as shown in Table 28E-2.

  c. **Pregnancy.** There are no well-controlled studies in pregnant women; the package insert suggests ticarcillin should be used in pregnant women only when clearly indicated. See Chap. 28A (p. 1078).

5. **Allergies and side effects** are similar to those described for ampicillin. **Acquired platelet dysfunction with the potential for bleeding may occur**, especially in patients with renal failure or in those undergoing surgery. (See sec. **F.4** for further recommendations.)

C. **Mezlocillin (Mezlin)** is available only as a parenteral agent [14a, 17]. It is very similar to ticarcillin, although in vitro it may be more active against some strains of gram-negative bacilli (e.g., *Klebsiella pneumoniae*). Its activity against *P. aeruginosa* is comparable to that of ticarcillin. Mezlocillin contains 1.85 mEq of sodium per gram (less sodium than ticarcillin). Data suggest that mezlocillin is associated with less prolongation of bleeding time and fewer bleeding episodes than is ticarcillin [18]. The precise clinical implications of this await further clinical study and observation with the use of these agents. See further discussion in sec. **F.4.**

1. **Dosages**

  a. **Adults.** In adults, for life-threatening infections, 4 g q4h is suggested. For serious infections, 200–300 mg/kg/day given in four to six divided doses is suggested. The usual dose is 3 g q4h or 4 g q6h. Doses are reduced in renal failure [17], as summarized in Table 28E-2. This agent should not be mixed in solution with aminoglycosides, because in vitro it inactivates aminoglycosides.

  b. **Children.** The package insert indicates that there are only limited data on the safety and efficacy of this agent in infants and children with documented serious infection. In infants older than 1 month and children up to 12 years, 50 mg/kg of mezlocillin may be administered q4h (i.e., 300 mg/kg/day total), per the package insert. See Chap. 3 for dosages of mezlocillin and related agents (e.g., ticarcillin) in neonates.

  c. **In renal failure,** dosages are modified as in Table 28E-2.

  d. **Pregnancy.** This is a category B agent (see Chap. 28A). There are no adequate, well-controlled studies in pregnant women. The package insert suggests this agent should be used during pregnancy only if clearly needed. Mezlocillin crosses the placenta.

  e. **Nursing mothers.** Because mezlocillin is detected in low concentrations in milk, the package insert suggests caution should be exercised when mezlocillin is administered to a nursing woman.

2. **Cost.** See Table 28A-6.

D. **Piperacillin (Pipracil)** [19] has a broader spectrum of activity than ticarcillin. In vitro it is more active against *K. pneumoniae* and *P. aeruginosa*. Piperacillin contains 1.98 mEq of sodium per gram and therefore contains less sodium per gram than ticarcillin. Further clinical experience may determine whether use of this agent results in a lower incidence of hypokalemia or platelet-induced abnormalities when compared to ticarcillin, although early studies suggest that bleeding problems may be less frequent [19, 20].

1. **Dosages**

  a. **Adults.** The usual dose for serious infection is 3–4 g q4–6h in adults with normal renal function. For ease of administration, we commonly use 4 g q6h in adults. For serious infections, up to 18 g/day can be used.

  b. **Children.** In children 12 years of age or older, 200–300 mg/kg/day IV (not

Table 28E-2. Dosages of expended penicillins for serious infections based on renal function in adults

	Normal renal function			Mild–moderate renal failure			End-stage renal failure			Dosages (IV) if undergoing dialysis		
	Creatinine clearance (ml/min)	Suggested dose (g)	Interval[a] (hr)	Creatinine clearance (ml/min)	Suggested dose (g)	Interval (hr)	Creatinine clearance (ml/min)	Suggested dose (g)	Interval (hr)	Supplemental dose after hemodialysis (g)	Usual dose on hemodialysis	Dosages on peritoneal dialysis
Ticarcillin	>50	3–4	4	10–50	2–3	8	<10	2–3	12	3	2 g q12h	3 g q12h
Ticarcillin-clavulanate	>50	3	4	10–50	2	6–8	<10	2	12	3	2 g q12h	3 g q12h
Mezlocillin	>30	3–4	4	10–30	3	8	<10	2	8	3–4	3–4 g q12h	3 g q12h[b]
Piperacillin	>40	3–4	4	20–40	3–4	8	<20	3–4	12	1	2 g q8h	
Ampicillin-sulbactam[c]												
Piperacillin-tazobactam[d]												

[a] For normal renal function, interval can be lengthened to 6 hr and the dose increased by half to compensate. Also, 4 g q6h has been used with ticarcillin, mezlocillin, and piperacillin in adults with mild to moderate infections.

[b] Preliminary data suggest 2 g q12h during peritoneal dialysis and 3 g q24h in the interval based on H. Lange et al., Pharmacokinetics of piperacillin in patients undergoing peritoneal dialysis (abstract 398). In *Proceedings of the 21st Interscience Conference on Antimicrobial Agents and Chemotherapy.* American Society of Microbiology, Chicago, November 1981.

[c] See Table 28E-5.

[d] See Table 28E-6.

to exceed the adult daily dose) in divided doses q4–6h is suggested. Dosages for children younger than 12 years have not been established, and the safety of this agent in neonates is not known.

c. **Renal failure.** If the creatinine clearance is more than 40 ml/min, no dose reduction is necessary. For dosages in patients with renal failure, see Table 28E-2. Ideally, if patients have both hepatic failure and renal insufficiency, serum levels should be monitored.

d. **Pregnancy.** This is a category B agent (see Chap. 28A). Because there are no well-controlled studies in pregnant women, the package insert suggests this drug should be used during pregnancy only if clearly needed.

e. **Nursing mothers.** Piperacillin is excreted in low concentrations in milk; therefore, the package insert suggests that caution should be exercised if this agent is administered to nursing mothers.

2. **Cost** data are shown in Table 28A-6.

3. Because of its low sodium content, piperacillin is a useful agent in patients who should avoid an additional sodium load (e.g., in renal failure and congestive heart failure). Because of its additional in vitro activity against *P. aeruginosa,* it may be useful in severe infections due to this pathogen, when combined with an aminoglycoside to achieve synergy. At present, we would not use it as a single agent in serious systemic infections, in part because resistant organisms may develop. Approximately 20–40% of Enterobacteriaceae may be resistant to this single agent [7].

E. **Azlocillin** (Azlin) had no special advantages and, by mid-1991, was no longer marketed in the United States.

F. **Summary of these agents**

1. Despite minor in vitro susceptibility variations, the fourth-generation penicillins (piperacillin, mezlocillin) have shown **no clear clinical advantage** over the preceding third-generation agents—that is, ticarcillin [14, 14a]—except possibly less bleeding. (See sec. **4.**)

2. **Monotherapy** (except in localized UTI) with any of these agents (e.g., ticarcillin, piperacillin) **in serious infection is not advised,** because these agents are not bactericidal except at high serum concentrations, and resistance may emerge during therapy.

3. The fourth-generation penicillins (e.g., piperacillin or mezlocillin) have a **lower daily sodium load** compared to ticarcillin and therefore are an excellent choice for the patient with heart failure or renal failure.

4. **Platelet abnormalities and clinical bleeding.** Penicillin antibiotics, especially the carboxypenicillins (e.g., carbenicillin and ticarcillin), affect platelet membrane receptors and, in vivo, produce a prolongation of the bleeding time. This topic has been reviewed elsewhere [11, 21]. **Bleeding can occur with normal platelet counts** but usually there must be additional contributing factors such as surgery. Prior studies revealed that carbenicillin or ticarcillin causes prolongation of the bleeding time in patients who had received standard dosages for 7 days or more. The frequency and severity of the effect appeared to depend on dosage and duration of therapy [21]. By comparison, mezlocillin, piperacillin, and azlocillin caused less frequent and less profound prolongation of the bleeding time [21]. **Furthermore, clinical bleeding due to acquired platelet dysfunction was reported more often with carbenicillin and ticarcillin, especially in patients with renal failure or those undergoing surgery** [21].

5. **Recommendation. None of these agents appears to be superior.** Therefore, the formulary committee may want to select for availability one agent from this group based on cost and other factors (see secs. **3** and **4**). Although clinical efficacy for susceptible pathogens may be similar for these agents, **if one of these agents is used in a patient with renal failure or after surgery, it seems logical to reduce the risk of bleeding and sodium load by using a ureidopenicillin (i.e., piperacillin or mezlocillin) rather than ticarcillin.**

III. **Intravenous beta-lactam and beta-lactamase-inhibitor combinations.** Oral amoxicillin-clavulanate is discussed in sec. **I.B.**

A. **Background.** Many beta-lactam antibiotics, including the extended-spectrum penicillins, are subject to inactivation by a broad variety of beta-lactamases (enzymes) produced by pathogenic bacteria. The production of beta-lactamases is a common mechanism by which bacteria become resistant to antibiotics. See Chap. 28A.

A number of strategies have been developed to improve the effectiveness of beta-lactam antibiotics against beta-lactamase-producing organisms, including the combination of an enzymatic (beta-lactamase) inhibitor with beta-lactamase-susceptible penicillins (Table 28E-3). This topic is reviewed in detail elsewhere [22]; however, several points deserve emphasis.

1. The three beta-lactamase inhibitors have little intrinsic antimicrobial activity on their own.
2. Clavulanate itself is a strong inducer of chromosomal beta-lactamase production in organisms such as *Enterobacter cloacae* and *P. aeruginosa;* therefore, ticarcillin-clavulanate is less effective than ticarcillin alone against some strains of *E. cloacae.*

   Clavulanate is the most, and tazobactam the least, active inducer of type I chromosomal beta-lactamases. Sulbactam may induce production of beta-lactamase in *S. aureus;* the clinical significance of this is unclear.
3. The beta-lactamase inhibitors are irreversible ("suicide") inhibitors of a broad variety of beta-lactamases.
   a. All three beta-lactamases inhibit penicillinases found in *S. aureus* as well as chromosomal beta-lactamases in *Bacteroides* spp., *Proteus vulgaris,* and *Klebsiella* spp.
   b. Clavulanate is a potent inhibitor of staphylococcal and plasmid-mediated beta-lactamase, but it is not a particularly good inhibitor of the class I chromosomally mediated enzymes found in *Enterobacter* spp. or *Morganella morganii.* Sulbactam has little activity against class 1 beta-lactamases.
   c. Tazobactam has moderate activity against some class 1 chromosomal beta-lactamases (e.g., *M. morganii*) but not others (e.g., *E. cloacae*). See related discussion of tazobactam in sec. **D.**
4. The amount of beta-lactamase produced by a given organism is an important determinant of the clinical effectiveness of beta-lactamase-inhibitor combinations. Organisms that produce relatively small amounts of beta-lactamase are more easily inhibited by these combinations than those producing large amounts [22].
5. Mutations that alter the permeability of the outer cell envelope in gram-negative bacilli may lead to in vitro resistance and, at times, clinical failure of some combinations regardless of the beta-lactamase production.
6. **An important determinant of the effectiveness of these combinations is the in vitro activity of the active antibiotic. The overall intrinsic activity of piperacillin against gram-negatives is greater than that of ticarcillin or ampicillin** [22].

B. **Ampicillin-sulbactam (Unasyn)** [11–11b, 23, 24]
1. **In vitro activity.** Sulbactam inhibits many bacterial beta-lactamases, thereby extending the activity of ampicillin (discussed earlier). The combination in vitro is active against beta-lactamase-producing strains [24] of *H. influenzae, M. catarrhalis, N. gonorrhoeae,* many anaerobes (including *B. fragilis*) [25], *E. coli, Proteus* spp., *Klebsiella* spp., *Enterobacter aerogenes, Acinetobacter calcoaceticus, S. aureus,* and *S. epidermidis.*
   a. **Ampicillin-sulbactam is not active against *P. aeruginosa* and Enterobacteriaceae strains that have inducible beta-lactamases (*Serratia, Enterobacter,* and *Citrobacter* spp.)** [11] or methicillin-resistant staphylococcal species.
   b. **In addition, approximately 20–25% or more of *E. coli*** (including community-acquired) **are resistant** to this combination [11a, 26, 27]. Most of these

Table 28E-3. Available beta-lactamase inhibitor and beta-lactam antibiotic combinations

Active antibiotic	Beta-lactamase inhibitor	Trade name	Comment
Amoxicillin	Clavulanate	Augmentin	Only as oral agent
Ticarcillin	Clavulanate	Timentin	Only parenteral
Ampicillin	Sulbactam	Unasyn	Only parenteral
Piperacillin	Tazobactam	Zosyn	Only parenteral; most active antibiotic in vitro

E. coli strains have minimal inhibitory concentrations (MICs) that are very close to the breakpoint concentration for determining susceptibility (≤ 8 μg/ml). Although the clinical significance of this laboratory observation is unknown, a study in an animal model of infection caused by an ampicillin-sulbactam–resistant isolate of *E. coli* found the agent to be ineffective [11a, 27a].

  c. Overall, not as many gram-negative bacilli are inactivated by ampicillin-sulbactam in vitro as by other intravenous beta-lactam–beta-lactamase combinations or with many cephalosporins. **See Table 28E-4.**

 2. Pharmacokinetics. The pharmacokinetics of ampicillin are not altered by the coadministration of sulbactam [24]. Peak concentrations are attained immediately after an intravenous 15-minute infusion and in 1 hour after intramuscular administration. The serum half-life is approximately 1 hour, although it is prolonged in neonates, the elderly, and patients with renal insufficiency.

  a. **Excretion,** of both components, is primarily in the urine.

  b. **Tissue levels** are achieved in extravascular fluids, bile, and peritoneal and cerebrospinal fluid [24].

 3. Clinical trials. In controlled studies, ampicillin-sulbactam has been effective in treating intraabdominal and gynecologic infections and infections of the urinary tract, skin, soft tissue, bones, joints, ears, nose, and throat [23, 24].

Table 28E-4. Comparison of in vitro susceptibility data

Organism	Number tested	Antimicrobial	% Susceptible
Escherichia coli	10,942	Piperacillin-tazobactam	91.5
		Ticarcillin-clavulanate	88.8
		Ampicillin-sulbactam	65.4
		Cefoxitin	96.1
		Cefotetan	99.3
		Ceftriaxone	99.2
		Imipenem	99.7
		Aztreonam	98.1
		Ciprofloxacin	99.0
Klebsiella pneumoniae	4,405	Piperacillin-tazobactam	90.9
		Ticarcillin-clavulanate	91.3
		Ampicillin-sulbactam	75.2
		Cefoxitin	90.3
		Cefotetan	97.4
		Ceftriaxone	95.2
		Imipenem	99.6
		Aztreonam	94.1
		Ciprofloxacin	94.5
Proteus mirabilis	3,822	Piperacillin-tazobactam	96.2
		Ticarcillin-clavulanate	95.0
		Ampicillin-sulbactam	90.4
		Cefoxitin	94.7
		Cefotetan	97.7
		Ceftriaxone	98.5
		Imipenem	82.9
		Aztreonam	91.7
		Ciprofloxacin	96.6

Table 28E-4 (continued)

Organism	Number tested	Antimicrobial	% Susceptible
Serratia marcescens	1,392	Piperacillin-tazobactam	86.9
		Ticarcillin-clavulanate	84.3
		Ampicillin-sulbactam	9.1
		Cefoxitin	16.7
		Cefotetan	94.3
		Ceftriaxone	85.8
		Imipenem	90.5
		Aztreonam	86.0
		Ciprofloxacin	86.0
Pseudomonas aeruginosa	2,941	Piperacillin	88.6
		Piperacillin-tazobactam	91.5
		Ticarcillin-clavulanate	86.3
		Ampicillin-sulbactam	2.1
		Cefoxitin	1.5
		Cefotetan	3.2
		Ceftriaxone	17.5
		Imipenem	88.0
		Ciprofloxacin	79.4
Staphylococcus aureus	4,454	Piperacillin-tazobactam	96.6
		Ticarcillin-clavulanate	98.1
		Ampicillin-sulbactam	98.0
		Cefoxitin	98.1
		Ceftriaxone	98.4
		Imipenem	98.7
		Ciprofloxacin	91.7
Streptococcus agalactiae (group B)	701	Piperacillin-tazobactam	98.2
		Ticarcillin-clavulanate	97.0
		Ampicillin-sulbactam	99.6
		Cefoxitin	96.6
		Ceftriaxone	97.0
		Imipenem	99.4
		Ciprofloxacin	92.9
Streptococcus faecalis	2,624	Piperacillin-tazobactam	94.7
		Ticarcillin-clavulanate	23.2
		Ampicillin-sulbactam	97.0
		Cefoxitin	2.1
		Ceftriaxone	7.0
		Imipenem	95.5
		Ciprofloxacin	62.5

Source: Adapted from P.R. Murray et al. and the In Vitro Susceptibility Surveillance Group, Multicenter evaluation of the in vitro activity of piperacillin-tazobactam compared with eleven selected β-lactam antibiotics and ciprofloxacin against more than 42,000 aerobic gram-positive and gram-negative bacteria. *Diagn. Microbiol. Infect. Dis.* 19:111, 1994.

4. **Dosages. The efficacy and safety of this new agent has not been established in infants and children younger than 12 years.**
   a. The **usual dosage** in adults is 1.5–3 g (1 g ampicillin plus 0.5 g sulbactam to 2 g ampicillin plus 1 g sulbactam) given q6h if renal function is normal.
   b. **In renal failure,** the elimination of ampicillin and sulbactam is similarly affected and dose modification is necessary (**see Table 28E-5**).
   c. **Contraindicated in ampicillin-allergic patients.** Because this agent contains ampicillin, it is contraindicated in patients allergic to ampicillin or other penicillins (unless skin testing is performed). (See Chap. 27.) This seems obvious but is a concern if physicians order antibiotics by a trade name (Unasyn) rather than a generic name. This concern also applies to the combinations of ticarcillin-clavulanate (Timentin) and piperacillin-tazobactam (Zosyn), discussed later.
   d. **Pregnancy.** This is a category B agent. (See Chap. 28A.) Because there are no adequate studies in pregnant women, the package insert suggests this drug should be used during pregnancy only if clearly indicated.
   e. **Nursing mothers.** Low concentrations of this combination are excreted into milk. Therefore, the package insert suggests caution should be exercised when ampicillin-sulbactam is administered to a nursing woman.
5. **Side effects.** These are the same as those known to occur with ampicillin [11a].
   a. Ampicillin **allergic reactions,** commonly rashes, can occur (see Chap. 27).
   b. **Minor enzyme elevations** (serum aspartate aminotransferase and alanine aminotransferase) occur in approximately 6% of recipients [23, 24].
   c. Ampicillin-sulbactam can have a marked **effect on oral flora,** leading to colonization with gram-negative rods or fungi [24].
6. **Cost.** See Table 28A-6.
7. **Conclusion.** The role of this combination continues to evolve. Since its introduction in 1987, it has been a very popular agent for polymicrobial infections, diabetic foot ulcer infections, mild to moderate community-acquired intraabdominal and pelvic infections, mixed aerobic-anaerobic soft-tissue infections, selected cases of aspiration pneumonia, and severe UTI.
   In a survey of this book's contributors in early 1995, many infectious disease specialists believed this agent was often overused at his or her institution; many were also changing to piperacillin-tazobactam.
   a. **See sec. E for how we feel this agent fits in compared to similar** beta-lactam–beta-lactamase **combinations:** piperacillin-tazobactam may be preferred.
   b. We **would not use** ampicillin-sulbactam as monotherapy in patients with severe or life-threatening intraabdominal infection or mixed aerobic-anaerobic soft-tissue infections but prefer a combination of antibiotics in this setting (e.g., a third-generation cephalosporin and metronidazole). In addition, we would not use this agent alone for severe nosocomial infections, as many hospital-acquired gram-negative bacteria, including *E. coli* and *Klebsiella* spp., may be resistant; *Pseudomonas* spp. are also resistant. An aminoglycoside could be combined with it. It should not be used to treat methicillin-resistant staphylococcal infections.
   c. Ampicillin-sulbactam has not been studied extensively for treatment of infections in immunocompromised patients [11a].

Table 28E-5. Ampicillin-sulbactam dosages in patients with renal impairment*

Creatinine clearance (ml/min)	Recommended dosage
>50	1.5–3.0 g q6h
30–50	1.5–3.0 g q6–8h
15–29	1.5–3.0 g q12h
5–14	1.5–3.0 g q24h

*In patients undergoing hemodialysis, preliminary data suggest the ampicillin will be partially removed (approximately 60%) but not the sulbactam. One could therefore give a supplemental dose of ampicillin after dialysis or time the daily dose of ampicillin-sulbactam so that it is given after dialysis.

C. **Ticarcillin-clavulanate (Timentin)** is available for parenteral use [11a, 11b, 28–31].

1. **Spectrum of activity.** Ticarcillin-clavulanate is active against beta-lactamase-producing strains of *S. aureus, E. coli, Klebsiella* spp., *Proteus* and *Shigella* spp., *H. influenzae,* and some strains of *P. aeruginosa.*

   a. However, because bacteria with class 1 Richmond-Sykes beta-lactamases are not inhibited by clavulanic acid, strains of *Pseudomonas, Serratia, Citrobacter,* and *Enterobacter* that are resistant to ticarcillin and produce this inducible cephalosporinase are not susceptible to the combination [7, 11, 28, 29]. Many hospital-acquired *E. coli* are resistant to ticarcillin-clavulanate independent of beta-lactamase.

   b. **See Table 28E-4** for a comparison of in vitro activities of this agent.

   c. Enterococci are moderately resistant to this combination. (Ampicillin-sulbactam is more active against enterococci.) Methicillin-resistant staphylococci also are resistant to ticarcillin-clavulanate [7, 11].

   d. This agent is very active against anaerobes, including *B. fragilis* [30].

2. **Pharmacokinetics.** Ticarcillin is excreted primarily by the kidney, with very high urine levels achieved. The half-life of both agents is approximately 1 hour, necessitating a 4- to 6-hour dose interval. Dosage adjustments are necessary in significant renal failure. The combination penetrates tissues well.

3. **Clinical trials** indicate that this combination is effective for a variety of polymicrobial infections with susceptible pathogens, including intraabdominal infections, pelvic infections, osteomyelitis, pneumonia, bacteremias, UTI, and skin and soft-tissue infections [11, 28, 29].

4. **Dosages**

   a. **Adults.** Ticarcillin-clavulanate is available in 3.1-g vials containing 3 g ticarcillin and 0.1 g clavulanic acid as the potassium salt. The usual dosage in the average adult (60 kg) for systemic infection is one 3.1-g vial q4–6h if the creatinine clearance is more than 60 ml/min. For gynecologic infections, in moderate infection 200 mg/kg/day in divided doses q6h and for severe infection 300 mg/kg/day (based on the ticarcillin content) in divided doses q4h is suggested by the package insert. For patients weighing less than 60 kg, the recommended dosage is 200–300 mg/kg/day (based on the ticarcillin content) divided q4–6h.

      A vial containing 3 g ticarcillin and 0.2 g clavulanic acid is also available. This has been used in UTI, with a dosage of 3.2 g given q8h, per the package insert, when renal function is normal.

   b. **Children.** Dosages for children younger than 12 years and infants have not been established; nor has the efficacy and safety been established in this age group.

   c. **In renal failure,** dosing adjustments are necessary and are summarized in Table 28E-2.

   d. **Prior penicillin allergy precludes the use of this agent** unless skin testing is done. (See Chap. 27.)

   e. **Pregnancy.** This is a category B agent (see Chap. 28A). Because there are no adequate and well-controlled studies in pregnant women, the package insert suggests this agent should be used during pregnancy only if clearly indicated.

   f. **Nursing mothers.** The package insert suggests caution should be exercised when this agent is administered to a nursing woman.

5. **Side effects.** Although hypersensitivity reactions can occur, this drug appears to be well tolerated. A variety of problems, including oral candidiasis, hypokalemia, diarrhea, nausea, eosinophilia, and mild liver function test abnormalities have been noted [28]. Because this agent contains ticarcillin, the potential for platelet abnormalities or bleeding exists. (See sec. **II.F.4.**)

6. **Cost.** See Table 28A-6.

7. **Conclusion.** As with ampicillin-sulbactam, the role of this agent continues to evolve.

   a. After ticarcillin-clavulanate had been available for several years, reviewers concluded that "although the combination of ticarcillin and clavulanic acid is clinically efficacious in a variety of settings, it offers no advantage over more traditional antibiotics in uncomplicated infections due to susceptible organisms. **Its main indication for use is in the treatment of polymicrobial infections, particularly those involving susceptible beta-lactamase-producing organisms**" [7, 11, 11a]. Some experts believe that it is a useful agent in nosocomial pneumonias but that an aminoglycoside should be given in addition to ticarcillin-clavulanate when *P. aeruginosa* is a possible (or known) pathogen [32]. No evidence indicates that ticarcillin-clavulanate is more efficacious than other antibiotic regimens [7].

b. In a survey of this book's contributors in early 1995, many infectious disease subspecialists had replaced this agent with one of the new beta-lactam combinations and saw no special niche for this agent.

c. It is a useful agent in **mild to moderate community-acquired intraabdominal and pelvic infections** and mixed aerobic-anaerobic soft-tissue infections. However, piperacillin-tazobactam is more active.

d. We **would not use it** as monotherapy in severe or life-threatening infections in these settings but prefer a combination of antibiotics. We would also not use it as monotherapy for severe nosocomial infections, because many hospital-acquired gram-negative bacteria may be resistant to it. Finally, it should not be used to treat methicillin-resistant staphylococcal infections [11].

In febrile, granulocytopenic cancer patients, ticarcillin-clavulanate has been evaluated primarily in combination with an aminoglycoside [11a], and other options are available in this setting (see Chap. 2).

e. **See sec. E for** a comparison of beta-lactam–beta-lactamase combinations: **piperacillin-tazobactam may be preferred.**

D. **Piperacillin-tazobactam** (Zosyn) became available in the United States in late 1993 and has recently been reviewed [33–36a]. The tazobactam, a penicillanic acid sulfone, is a beta-lactamase inhibitor that extends the spectrum of activity of piperacillin. See sec. **A.**

Tazobactam has good inhibitory activity against Richman and Sykes types II, III, IV, and V beta-lactamases, staphylococcal penicillinase, extended-spectrum beta-lactamases, and class 1c chromosomal beta-lactamases, but limited activity against the remaining class 1 enzymes. Of chromosomally mediated enzymes, the class 1 enzymes are the most important clinically, particularly those in gram-negative bacteria with inducible class 1 enzymes (e.g., *Enterobacter, Citrobacter,* and *Providencia* spp. and *P. aeruginosa*) (see sec. **1**).

1. **Spectrum of activity.** This is **summarized in Table 28E-4** and is remarkably broad [14]. This agent has an in vitro spectrum of activity comparable to that of imipenem-cilastatin and superior to that of ceftazidime, ticarcillin-clavulanate, and ampicillin-sulbactam [11a].

a. **Gram-positive aerobes.** This combination is active against methicillin-susceptible *S. aureus, S. pyogenes, S. agalactiae,* and *S. pneumoniae* (but not highly penicillin-resistant strains; see Chap. 28C). Although active against *Enterococcus faecalis,* piperacillin-tazobactam is not active against *Enterococcus faecium* and methicillin-resistant *S. aureus* [33].

b. **Enterobacteriaceae.** Most community-acquired Enterobacteriaceae (e.g., *E. coli, Klebsiella* spp.) are susceptible but, because of poor activity of piperacillin-tazobactam against many of the class 1 beta-lactamases, *E. aerogenes, E. cloacae, Citrobacter* spp., *Serratia* spp., and *P. aeruginosa* may be resistant. See Table 28E-4.

c. Piperacillin-tazobactam has excellent activity against *H. influenzae, M. catarrhalis, Yersinia enterocolitica,* and *Plesiomonas shigelloides* but **not** *Salmonella* spp. or *Xanthomonas maltophilia.*

d. **Anaerobes.** Piperacillin-tazobactam has good activity against *B. fragilis* (but less than that of imipenem), *Bacteroides* spp. and *Clostridium perfringens* [33, 37]. Mouth anaerobes are typically susceptible to penicillin and piperacillin. Although some reviewers conclude there are no significant differences between the activity against anaerobes of piperacillin-tazobactam and other beta-lactamase inhibitor combination agents [11a], other reviewers have concluded that piperacillin-tazobactam inhibits a broader spectrum of anaerobes than does ampicillin-sulbactam or ticarcillin-clavulanate [36a] after review of the literature.

2. **Inoculum effect.** There is an inoculum effect with piperacillin alone with inocula in excess of 10^6 colony-forming units (cfu) per milliliter and with piperacillin-tazobactam with an inoculum of 10^7–10^8 cfu/ml in the presence of Enterobacteriaceae, *B. fragilis* group strains, enterococci, and *H. influenzae* [33]. The exact clinical implications of this are unclear currently.

3. **Pharmacokinetics** [33, 35, 38]. Piperacillin and tazobactam have similar half-

lives (approximately 1 hour), and tazobactam does not affect the pharmacokinetics of piperacillin. Preparations include an 8:1 ratio of piperacillin to tazobactam.

    a. Peak plasma concentrations of a 3.375-g dose provides peak piperacillin plasma concentration of approximately 240 μg/ml; a 4.5-g dose, 290–300 μg/ml [38]. See sec. **5.**

    b. Distribution is rapid as these hydrophilic agents distribute in most body fluids and tissue.

    c. Elimination. Renal excretion accounts for 50–60% of the administered dose. Probenecid can reduce excretion by 20–25%, indicating both components are also eliminated by renal tubular secretion. Doses must be reduced in patients with a creatinine clearance of less than 40 ml/min [33]. Although biliary excretion of both piperacillin and tazobactam is low, drug concentrations in the gallbladder may be high [33].

4. Clinical use. Piperacillin-tazobactam has been used in **polymicrobial infections.** Early clinical studies have recently been summarized [33, 36a]. The combination has been approved for use for moderate to severe infections with susceptible pathogens and appears effective in the following situations:

    a. Intraabdominal infections (especially appendicitis, including cases complicated by rupture or abscess). In one report, the combination appeared even more effective than imipenem, but the dose of imipenem used was only 500 mg q8h [39] and many of these patients appeared to have only mild to moderate infections, primarily appendicitis [33]. This topic has recently been reviewed [40].

    b. Pelvic infections in women [41, 42].

    c. Mixed aerobic **skin and soft-tissue** infections, including diabetic foot infections [35, 42].

    d. Community-acquired pneumonia, including beta-lactamase-producing *H. influenzae.* However, this agent is not active against *Mycoplasma* or *Legionella* [33, 43]. In addition, although it is an appealing agent for nosocomial pneumonia, it should not be used as monotherapy for suspected or known *P. aeruginosa* nosocomial pneumonia, for failures in this setting have been reported if piperacillin-tazobactam is used. Piperacillin-tazobactam has been combined with an aminoglycoside for nosocomial pneumonia therapy [33, 44].

    e. Clinical investigation. Piperacillin-tazobactam with an aminoglycoside has been used for empiric therapy of the febrile, leukopenic patient without a focal infection [33].

5. Dosages [38]

    a. Adults and children older than 12 years. The usual dose of piperacillin-tazobactam is 3 g/0.375 g q6h if the creatinine clearance is higher than 40 ml/min (i.e., 12 g piperacillin per day). A 4.5-g vial (piperacillin-tazobactam, 4 g/0.5 g) is also available as piperacillin is used in a higher dose in some settings. The higher doses should be used (4 g/0.5 g q6h or 3 g/0.75 g q4h) in combination with an aminoglycoside for empirical therapy when a *Pseudomonas* spp. may be present [36a]. (In documented pseudomonas infection, the addition of tazobactam will seldom add to the activity of piperacillin alone [36a]).

    b. In renal failure, doses need to be modified, as **shown in Table 28E-6.**

        (1) For patients receiving **hemodialysis,** the maximum dose of piperacillin-tazobactam is 2 g/0.25 g q8h. Because hemodialysis will remove 30–40% of the dose in a 4-hour dialysis, an additional 30% dose can be given after dialysis.

        (2) In chronic ambulatory peritoneal dialysis (CAPD), approximately 10% of the piperacillin dose is recovered [33]. Until further guidelines are available, in CAPD patients select the dose as if the creatinine clearance is less than 10 ml/min. See Table 28E-6.

    c. In **cirrhosis** or other hepatic disease, no dosage modifications are required [36a].

    d. In **children** younger than 12 years, the safety and efficacy of this agent have not been established.

    e. Pregnancy. This is a category B agent (see Chap. 28A). There are no adequate and well-controlled studies with piperacillin-tazobactam in preg-

Table 28E-6. Piperacillin-tazobactam dosages in renal failure

Creatinine clearance (ml/min)	Recommended dosage regimen
>40	12 g/1.5 g/day in divided doses of 3.375 g q6h
20–40	8 g/1.0 g/day in divided doses of 2.25 g q6h
<20	6 g/0.75 g/day in divided doses of 2.25 g q8h

Source: From *Physicians' Desk Reference* (50th ed.). Montvale, NJ: Medical Economics, 1996. P. 1422.

nant women. Therefore, the drug should be used during pregnancy only if clearly indicated [11a, 38].

f. **Nursing mothers.** Piperacillin is excreted in low concentrations in human milk; whether tazobactam is in human milk has not been studied. Therefore, the package insert suggests that caution be used if this agent is administered to a nursing woman [38].

6. **Side effects.** The toxicity of piperacillin-tazobactam is similar to that of other beta-lactam antibiotics [11a, 33, 36a]. The most common side effects include the following:

   a. **Gastrointestinal** disorders, primarily diarrhea and nausea, occur in 4.6% of recipients.

   b. Skin reactions occur in 2.2% of recipients, with fewer than 1% having a rash.

   c. No significant hepatic or renal dysfunction has been noted in early reports.

   d. Mild hypokalemia can occur, presumably due to the nonresorbable anion presented to the distal tubules, which cause an increase in the pH and a secondary loss of potassium ions.

E. **Ticarcillin-clavulanate versus ampicillin-sulbactam versus piperacillin-tazobactam.** The optimal agent for selected polymicrobial infections has not been clearly delineated in the medical literature. None of these beta-lactam–beta-lactamase combinations are listed as the antibiotic of first choice for any specific pathogen [3]. They are useful in polymicrobial infections.

In a recent review [11a], the authors concluded that "because of its broad spectrum of antibacterial activity, it [piperacillin-tazobactam] appears to be the best suited for treatment of mixed infections." In a 1996 summary of piperacillin-tazobactam, after an extensive review of the literature, the authors conclude, "The proven and theoretical advantages of piperacillin-tazobactam in comparison with those of ticarcillin-clavulanate appear to more than offset the modest difference in cost between the two compounds" [36a]. Furthermore, these reviewers conclude that clinical and microbiological outcomes "both indicated that piperacillin-tazobactam was superior to ceftazidime for the treatment of lower respiratory tract infections" [36a].

In a survey of this text's contributing authors in early 1995, there were obvious regional differences and anecdotal reasons for clinicians favoring one agent over another. When one of these drugs is indicated, we would offer the following considerations:

1. For situations in which *E. coli* is a likely pathogen, because 20–25% of *E. coli* strains are resistant to ampicillin-sulbactam, piperacillin-tazobactam is advised, although ticarcillin-clavulanate may be a reasonable alternative if one of these agents is to be used.

2. Because cefazolin is effective against most community-acquired *E. coli* strains, the more expensive beta-lactam–beta-lactamase inhibitor combinations should be used selectively. For community-acquired intraabdominal or pelvic infections, we favor the more cost-effective cefazolin-metronidazole combination (see Chap. 11).

   Piperacillin-tazobactam can be used selectively in the following situations:

   a. Severe (limb-threatening) diabetic foot ulcer infections, as discussed in Chap. 16.

   b. Selected patients with severe head and neck infections, complex sinusitis.

   c. Some non–intensive care unit–acquired early nosocomial pneumonia in patients at low risk for *P. aeruginosa* infection and in whom it is desirable to avoid an aminoglycoside.

    d. Selected intensive care unit (ICU) nosocomial pneumonias. If this drug is chosen, at least while awaiting cultures we would combine it with an aminoglycoside. Usually, we would use piperacillin and an aminoglycoside combination as a more cost-effective regimen in this setting.

3. None of these agents should be used as monotherapy for known or highly suspected severe *P. aeruginosa* infection (e.g., pneumonia, sepsis) or as monotherapy in febrile episodes in neutropenic patients. This would preclude monotherapy with one of these agents for serious nosocomial infections, especially acquired in an ICU setting [35].

4. For the situation in which monotherapy is indicated and we are deciding between one of these beta-lactam–beta lactamase combinations and imipenem, we tend to "save" imipenem for those patients who may have or develop resistant pathogens. See Chap. 28G.

5. Whether these agents are associated with less *Clostridium difficile* diarrhea compared with the second- and third-generation cephalosporins (see Chaps. 28A and 28F) is still unsettled, but this issue may be a consideration in some patients.

References

1. Neu, H.C. Amoxicillin. *Ann. Intern. Med.* 90:356, 1979.
2. Chambers, H.F., and Neu, H.C. Penicillins. In G.L. Mandell, J.E. Bennett, and R. Dolin (eds.), *Principles and Practice of Infectious Diseases* (4th ed.). New York: Churchill Livingstone, 1995. P. 233.
3. Medical Letter. The choice of antibacterial drugs. *Med. Lett. Drugs Ther.* 38:25, 1996.
4. Medical Letter. Drugs for the treatment of acute otitis media in children. *Med. Lett. Drugs Ther.* 36:19, 1994.
   Concludes that despite the increasing prevalence of resistant pathogens, Medical Letter consultants still consider amoxicillin to be the drug of choice for initial treatment of acute otitis media in most children.
5. Friedland, I.R., and McCracken, G.H. Management of infections caused by antibiotic-resistant *Streptococcus pneumoniae*. *N. Engl. J. Med.* 331:377, 1994.
   Authors still favor amoxicillin for initial empiric therapy of acute otitis media, even in areas with a high prevalence of penicillin-resistant pneumococci.
6. Hentschel, E., et al. Effect of ranitidine and amoxicillin plus metronidazole on the eradication of *Helicobacter pylori* and the recurrence of duodenal ulcer. *N. Engl. J. Med.* 328:308, 1993.
   For related discussion, see Medical Letter, Drugs for treatment of peptic ulcers, Med. Lett. Drugs Ther. 36:65, 1994, for a summary of antibacterial regimens, and see Chap. 11.
7. Wright, A.J., and Wilkowske, C.J. The penicillins. *Mayo Clin. Proc.* 66:1047, 1991.
8. Nathwani, D., and Wood, M.J. Penicillins: A current review of their clinical pharmacology and therapeutic use. *Drugs* 45:866, 1993.
9. Bennett, W.M., et al. *Drug Prescribing in Renal Failure: Dosing Guidelines for Adults* (3rd ed.). Philadelphia: American College of Physicians, 1994.
   Useful handbook. Also see dose reduction tables in L.L. Livornese, Jr., et al., Antibacterial agents in renal failure. Infect. Dis. Clin. North Am. 9:591, 1995.
10. Medical Letter. Amoxicillin-clavulanic acid (Augmentin). *Med. Lett. Drugs Ther.* 26:99, 1984.
11. Bush, L.M., Calmon, J., and Johnson, C.C. Newer penicillins and beta-lactamase inhibitors. *Infect. Dis. Clin. North Am.* 3:571, 1989.
11a. Bush, L.M., Calmon, J., and Johnson, C.C. Newer penicillins and beta-lactamase inhibitors. *Infect. Dis. Clin. North Am.* 9:653, 1995.
11b. Sensakovic, J.W., and Smith, L.G. Beta-lactamase inhibitor combinations. *Med. Clin. North Am.* 79:695, 1995.
12. Goldstein, E.J.C. Bite wounds and infection. *Clin. Infect. Dis.* 14:633, 1992.
    This is an outstanding state-of-the-art clinical review. See update in Mandell's textbook (see reference [2]).
13. Medical Letter. Bacampicillin hydrochloride (Spectrobid). *Med. Lett. Drugs Ther.* 23:49, 1981.
14. Drusano, G.L., et al. The acylampicillins: Mezlocillin, piperacillin, and azlocillin. *J. Infect. Dis.* 6:13, 1984.
14a. Tan, J.S., and File, T.M., Jr. Antipseudomonal penicillins. *Med. Clin. North Am.* 79:679, 1995.

15. Medical Letter. Ticarcillin. *Med. Lett. Drugs Ther.* 19:17, 1977.
16. Parry, M.F., and Neu, H.C. A comparative study of ticarcillin plus tobramycin versus carbenicillin plus gentamicin for the treatment of serious infections due to gram-negative bacilli. *Am. J. Med.* 64:961, 1978.
17. Medical Letter. Mezlocillin sodium (Mezlin). *Med. Lett. Drugs Ther.* 23:109, 1981.
18. Fass, A.J., et al. Platelet-mediated bleeding caused by broad-spectrum penicillins. *J. Infect. Dis.* 155:1242, 1987.
19. Medical Letter. Piperacillin sodium (Pipracil). *Med. Lett. Drugs Ther.* 24:47, 1982.
20. Gentry, L.O., Jamsek, J.G., and Natelson, E.A. Effects of sodium piperacillin on platelet function in normal volunteers. *Antimicrob. Agents Chemother.* 19:532, 1981. *Data suggest that piperacillin caused less platelet dysfunction than did ticarcillin or carbenicillin.*
21. Sattler, F.R., et al. Impaired hemostatis caused by beta-lactam antibiotics. *Am. J. Surg.* 155(5A):30, 1988.
22. Moellering, R.C., Jr. Importance of beta-lactamase inhibitors in overcoming bacterial resistance. *Infect. Dis. Clin. Pract.* 4(Suppl. 1):S1, 1995. *Concise clinical discussion. See also R.C. Moellering, Meeting the challenges of β-lactamases. J. Antimicrob. Chemother. 31(Suppl. A):1, 1993, for a related discussion.*
23. Lees, L., et al. Sulbactam plus ampicillin: interim review of efficacy and safety for therapeutic and prophylactic use. *Rev. Infect. Dis.* 8(Suppl. 5):S644, 1986. *Summary article at the end of a special symposium devoted to this agent.*
24. Medical Letter. Ampicillin/sulbactam (Unasyn). *Med. Lett. Drugs Ther.* 29:79, 1987.
25. Wexler, H.M., et al. In vitro efficacy of sulbactam combined with ampicillin against anaerobic bacteria. *Antimicrob. Agents Chemother.* 27:876, 1985.
26. Murray, P.R., Cantrell, H.F., Lankford, R.B., et al. and the In Vitro Susceptibility Study Group. Multicenter evaluation of the in vitro activity of piperacillin-tazobactam compared with eleven selected β-lactam antibiotics and ciprofloxacin against more than 42,000 aerobic gram-positive and gram-negative bacteria. *Diagn. Microbiol. Infect. Dis.* 19:111, 1994. *In vitro susceptibility data using Baxter Micro-scan susceptibility data from 79 medical centers for more than 42,000 clinical isolates. In one of our laboratories (R.E.R.), the incidence of* E. coli *resistant to ampicillin-sulbactam in 1994 was 24%.*
27. Pankey, G.A., Chambers, R.B., and the In Vitro Study Group. Activity of piperacillin-tazobactam, ampicillin-sulbactam, ticarcillin-clavulanate, cefoxitin, ceftazidime, ceftriaxone, cefotaxime, ciprofloxacin, and imipenem against 38,468 aerobic and facultative gram-negative and gram-positive clinical isolates. 34th Interscience Conference on Antimicrobial Agents and Chemotherapy. American Study of Microbiology, Orlando, FL: October 1994. Abstract #E42. *In this study, 35% of non–intensive care unit and 35% of intensive care unit isolates of* E. coli *were resistant to ampicillin-sulbactam, whereas only 9% of such isolates were resistant to piperacillin-tazobactam.*
27a. Rice, L., Carias, L., and Shlaes, D. Efficacy of ampicillin-sulbactam versus that of cefoxitin on treatment of *Escherichia coli* infections in a rat intra-abdominal model. *Antimicrob. Agents Chemother.* 37:610, 1993.
28. Roselle, G.A., et al. Clinical trials of the efficacy and safety of ticarcillin and clavulanic acid. *Antimicrob. Agents Chemother.* 27:291, 1985. *See related article by P.C. Appelbaum et al., β-lactamase production and susceptibilities to amoxicillin, amoxicillin-clavulanate, ticarcillin, ticarcillin-clavulanate, cefoxitin, imipenem, and metronidazole of 320 non-*Bacteroides fragilis Bacteroides *isolates and 129 Fusobacteria from 28 U.S. Centers. Antimicrob. Agents Chemother. 34:1546, 1990. These agents seem effective. The addition of clavulanate does not appreciably improve the efficacy of ticarcillin against these organisms.*
29. Moellering, R.C., Jr. β-lactamase inhibition: Therapeutic implications in infectious diseases—an overview. *Rev. Infect. Dis.* 13(Suppl. 9):S723-S777, 1991. *This is a multiauthored symposium with special emphasis on ticarcillin-clavulanate with clinical articles on skin and soft-tissue infections, aspiration pneumonia, nosocomial pneumonia, endometritis, and so on.*
30. Cuchural, G.J., Jr., et al. Susceptibility of the *Bacteroides fragilis* group in the United States: Analysis by site of isolation. *Antimicrob. Agents Chemother.* 32:717, 1988.
31. Medical Letter. Ticarcillin-clavulanic acid (Timentin). *Med. Lett. Drugs Ther.* 27:69, 1985.
32. Scheld, W.M., and Mandell, G.L. Nosocomial pneumonia: Pathogenesis and recent advances in diagnosis and therapy. *Rev. Infect. Dis.* 13(Suppl.) 9:S743, 1991.
33. Bryson, H.M., and Brogden, R.N. Piperacillin/tazobactam: A review of its antibacterial

activity, pharmacokinetic properties, and therapeutic potential. *Drugs* 47:506, 1994. *Extensive review with excellent summary for early clinical trial results. For a related review, see S.A. Marshall et al., Comparative antimicrobial activity of piperacillin-tazobactam tested against more than 5000 clinical isolates from five medical centers.* Diagn. Microbiol. Infect. Dis. *21:153, 1995.*

34. Greenwood, D., and Finch, R.G. Piperacillin/tazobactam: A new β-lactam/β-lactamase inhibitor combination. *J. Antimicrob. Chemother.* 31(Suppl. A):1–124, 1993.
    An entire symposium on this new agent.

35. Medical Letter. Piperacillin/tazobactam. *Med. Lett. Drugs Ther.* 36:7, 1994.
    See also Medical Letter, A reminder: Piperacillin/tazobactam is not for pseudomonas. Med. Lett. Drugs Ther. *36:110, 1994, in which the clinician is reminded that in an unpublished multicenter trial of 3 g/0.375 g of piperacillin-tazobactam q6h for nosocomial pneumonia due to P. aeruginosa, there were many failures. Therefore, monotherapy with this agent should not be used for serious P. aeruginosa infection.*

36. Moellering, R.C., Jr., et al. Piperacillin/tazobactam: A new dimension in antibiotic therapy. *Infect. Dis. Clin. Pract.* 4(Suppl. 1):S1–S36, 1995.
    A special supplement devoted to this agent.

36a. Sanders, W.E., Jr., and Sanders, C.C. Piperacillin/tazobactam: A critical review of evolving clinical literature. *Clin. Infect. Dis.* 22:107, 1996.

37. Appelbaum, P.C. Comparative susceptibility profile of piperacillin/tazobactam against anaerobic bacteria. *J. Antimicrob. Chemother.* 31(Suppl. A):29, 1993.

38. *Physicians' Desk Reference* (50th ed.). Montvale, NJ: Medical Economics, 1996. Pp. 1419–1422.

39. Brismar, B., et al. Piperacillin-tazobactam versus imipenem-cilastatin for treatment of intraabdominal infections. *Antimicrob. Agents Chemother.* 36:2706, 1992.
    In this open, randomized, comparative multicenter trial from Sweden, 69 patients received piperacillin-tazobactam (4 g/0.5 g q8h) and 65 received imipenem (500 mg q8h, which is a relatively low dose by US conventional dosing of 500 mg q6h). There were 4 failures or relapses in the piperacillin-tazobactam recipients versus 18 failures or relapses in the imipenem recipients . . . a significant difference. The majority of patients had appendicitis, and mortality was low compared with other studies of intraabdominal sepses (see reference [40]). We believe further studies using these two agents at comparable dosages and in very ill patients are needed before one can conclude piperacillin-tazobactam is superior to imipenem for serious intraabdominal sepsis.

40. Nord, C.E. Treatment of intra-abdominal infections: Worldwide clinical trials. *Infect. Dis. Clin. Pract.* 4(Suppl. 1):S17, 1995.
    Summary of four trials (from Sweden, Finland, United States and Canada, and Europe) demonstrating clinical efficacy of piperacillin-tazobactam. Data suggest this combination is at least as effective as either imipenem or clindamycin and gentamicin therapy.
    See related paper by H.C. Polk et al., Prospective randomized study of piperacillin/tazobactam therapy of surgically treated intra-abdominal infection. Am. Surg. *59: 598, 1993.*

41. Sweet, R., et al. Piperacillin and tazobactam versus clindamycin and gentamicin in the treatment of hospitalized women with pelvic infection. *Obstet. Gynecol.* 83:280, 1994.
    In this randomized, open-label trial at 12 hospitals, piperacillin-tazobactam (3 g/ 0.375 g) in 196 patients was compared with clindamycin (900 mg q8h) and gentamicin (2.5–5.0 mg/kg/day) in 103 patients. A favorable clinical outcome occurred with both regimens in approximately 85% of recipients. The most common diagnoses were endometritis (146 patients) and pelvic inflammatory disease (115 patients).

42. Sanders, C.V. Treatment of polymicrobial gynecologic and skin and skin-structure infections: Worldwide clinical trials. *Infect. Dis. Clin. Pract.* 4(Suppl. 1):S26, 1995.
    See related paper by J.S. Tan et al., Treatment of hospitalized patients with complicated skin and skin structure infections: Double-blind, randomized, multicenter study of piperacillin-tazobactam versus ticarcillin-clavulanate. Antimicrob. Agents Chemother. *37:1580, 1993. Study showed comparable response rates.*

43. Mouton, Y. Treatment of lower respiratory tract infections: Worldwide clinical trials. *Infect. Dis. Clin. Pract.* 4(Suppl. 1):S9, 1995.
    Summary of studies from Europe, Mexico, and the United States.

44. Smith, D.L. Parenteral piperacillin/tazobactam combined with amikacin for the treatment of severe pulmonary infections in intensive care units. *Infect. Dis. Clin. Pract.* 4(Suppl. 1):S33, 1995.
    When P. aeruginosa is a known or highly likely pathogen, an aminoglycoside should be used in combination rather than monotherapy with piperacillin-tazobactam.

F. Cephalosporins

The cephalosporins are the most commonly prescribed antibiotics in hospitals. Surveys show that they make up 30–50% of antibiotics prescribed for hospitalized patients. However, cephalosporins are listed infrequently as the drug of choice for known specific infections [1] (see Table 28A-3), but they are attractive because of their broad antimicrobial coverage and relative lack of toxicity. They are often overused. Cephalosporins often are characterized as first-, second-, and third-generation agents (Table 28F-1). The basic structure of cephalosporins is shown in Fig. 28F-1. Modification of the side chains will affect antibacterial or pharmacokinetic properties of the new compound. The structure-function relationships are reviewed elsewhere [2].

Although cefoxitin, cefotetan, and cefmetazole are technically cephamycins with a modification of the cephalosporin structure, clinically they are discussed with the cephalosporins [2].

General Concepts

I. **Advantages and disadvantages of the cephalosporins**
  A. **Advantages**
    1. **Bactericidal agents.** Like the penicillins, these agents inhibit bacterial cell wall synthesis.
    2. **Effective against penicillinase-producing *Staphylococcus aureus.*** These agents are all relatively resistant to the beta-lactamases produced by *S. aureus.* Some are more resistant than others, and **the first-generation agents** remain the most active against *S. aureus.*
    3. **Broad spectrum of activity.** These agents are effective against many gram-positive and gram-negative bacteria. However, they are not active against enterococci and, except for some third-generation agents and cefepime, are not active against *Pseudomonas* spp.
    4. **High therapeutic-toxic ratio.** The cephalosporins are well tolerated and produce fewer allergic reactions than do the penicillins. They have limited side effects even at high serum levels. Because of the high therapeutic-toxic ratio, **cephalosporins are often preferable to aminoglycosides** when susceptibility studies allow a choice [1, 2a]. The third-generation agents are extremely active against susceptible gram-negative enteric bacteria. In particular, cefotaxime and ceftriaxone are active against routine pathogens that cause meningitis; they have been shown to provide excellent cerebrospinal fluid (CSF) bactericidal levels in patients [1, 2].
  B. **Disadvantages**
    1. **Variable CSF penetration.** Neither the first-generation nor the second-generation agents provide adequate CSF bactericidal levels and are not recommended

Table 28F-1. The major cephalosporins

First-generation	Second-generation	Third-generation
Parenteral	Parenteral	Parenteral
Cephalothin (Keflin)	Cefamandole (Mandol)	Cefotaxime (Claforan)
Cefazolin (Ancef, Kefzol)	Cefoxitin (Mefoxin)[a]	Cefoperazone (Cefobid)
Cephapirin (Cefadyl)	Cefuroxime (Zinacef)	Ceftizoxime (Cefizox)
Cephradine (Velosef)	Cefonicid (Monocid)	Ceftriaxone (Rocephin)
	Cefotetan (Cefotan)[a]	Ceftazidime (Fortaz,
	Cefmetazole (Zefazone)[a]	Tazidime, or Tazicef)
		Cefepime (Maxipime)[b]
Oral	Oral	Oral
Cephalexin (Keflex)	Cefaclor (Ceclor)	Cefixime (Suprax)
Cephradine (Velosef,	Cefuroxime axetil (Ceftin)	Cefpodoxime (Vantin)
Anspor)	Cefprozil (Cefzil)	Ceftibuten (Cedax)
Cefadroxil (Duricef)	Loracarbef (Lorabid)[a]	

[a]A cephalosporinlike antibiotic. See text.
[b]Some authors have referred to this agent as a fourth-generation cephalosporin; see text.

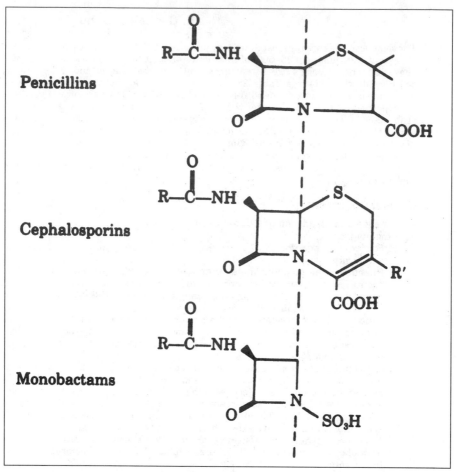

Fig. 28F-1. Structures of beta-lactam antibiotics. (From R.B. Sykes and D.P. Bonner, Aztreonam: The first monobactam. *Am. J. Med.* 78(2A):2, 1985.)

for meningitis. Although initially believed adequate for therapy in meningitis, cefuroxime (a second-generation agent) has been associated with treatment failures and relapses and is no longer recommended for meningitis [1]. (The third-generation cephalosporins do penetrate the CSF.)

2. **Limited activity or no activity against enterococci and pseudomonads.** See sec. **III.B** under Individual Agents later in this chapter.

Enterococci usually have "intrinsic resistance" against the cephalosporins. See Chap. 28A.

3. **Use may predispose patients to *Clostridium difficile* diarrhea.** Studies suggest that exposure to second- or third-generation cephalosporins may be independent risk factors for the development of *C. difficile* diarrhea [3]. Whether this preliminary observation is confirmed by other studies awaits further clinical experience and study.

II. **Sorting through the (parenteral) cephalosporin maze.** The prescriber has more than 15 parenteral agents from which to choose (see Table 28F-1). **Discussion of the parenteral cephalosporins under strict categories** (first- versus second- versus third-generation) **is often arbitrary** and probably is not as important to the clinician as understanding the role or niche for these agents. Therefore, **before reviewing the individual agents, we will first try to put these agents in perspective,** basing our discussion on the type of infection the clinician commonly encounters. We then will summarize the specific agents themselves. The final antibiotic decision becomes even more complex when one realizes that the other beta-lactam antibiotics (e.g., aztreonam, imipenem-cilastatin, and piperacillin-tazobactam combination) and the new fluoroquinolones (e.g., ciprofloxacin) have potential competing roles with the cephalosporins.

These topics are discussed in further detail in the individual sections of this chapter. This summary is provided as an overview only.

A. **Surgical prophylaxis.** The first-generation agents, particularly cefazolin, remain the mainstay agents. Some clinicians use cefoxitin or cefotetan for colon procedures. Surgical prophylaxis is reviewed in Chap. 28B. **The more expensive third-generation cephalosporins are not indicated for surgical prophylaxis.**

B. **Bacteremias**
 1. **Sepsis of unclear etiology.** Because staphylococci and gram-negative bacteria are important pathogens, a first-generation cephalosporin-aminoglycoside combination often is used. A third-generation agent alone (e.g., ceftriaxone or cefotaxime) may be reasonable, especially in community-acquired infection. (See Chap. 2.)
 2. A third-generation agent alone (e.g., ceftazidime) may not be sufficient in the bacteremic leukopenic patient with no focus of infection or for a nosocomial bacteremia. Double drugs, to achieve synergy, are favored in this setting.
 3. If susceptibility data on the blood isolate, in the nonleukopenic patient, reveal that a second- or third-generation agent is active and resistance (see sec. **III.C** under Individual Agents) is not a special concern, a third-generation agent should be used.
 4. None of the cephalosporins is effective against enterococcal infections.
 5. For known or highly suspected serious *Pseudomonas aeruginosa* infections (e.g., bacteremia or pneumonia), monotherapy with a cephalosporin is not advised. In susceptible *P. aeruginosa* meningitis, therapy with ceftazidime is the agent of choice (with or without an aminoglycoside), as aminoglycosides penetrate the CSF so poorly. In the patient with a delayed penicillin-allergic reaction history, an agent with activity against *Pseudomonas* (e.g., ceftazidime) may be combined with an aminoglycoside to achieve synergy.
 6. Endocarditis. See sec. **H.**

C. **Skin and soft-tissue infections**
 1. For **staphylococcal** or **streptococcal** infections, a **first-generation** agent (e.g., cefazolin) is the most active and usually the preferred cephalosporin when an antistaphylococcal penicillin cannot be used.
 2. For a mild to moderate, mixed aerobic-anaerobic infection (e.g., decubitus ulcer), cefoxitin is a reasonable agent because of its anaerobic, staphylococcal, and gram-negative activity. (Cefotetan or cefmetazole are other options.) For more severe or well-established infections, combinations of antibiotics directed at anaerobes and Enterobacteriaceae may be preferred. See Chap. 4.
 3. For mixed or susceptible gram-negative wound infections, a third-generation agent may allow one to avoid an aminoglycoside if beta-lactamase induction is not a major concern (see sec. **III.C** under Individual Agents).

D. **Central nervous system infections**
 1. **The first- and second-generation cephalosporins,** including cefuroxime, are **not recommended** for CNS infections.
 2. **Third-generation agents are the drugs of choice for gram-negative enteric meningitis,** which usually occurs in neonates or as a complication of neurosurgical procedures.
 3. **Meningitis. Increased interest has arisen in using the third-generation cephalosporins as empiric therapy in neonatal meningitis** (combining cefotaxime with ampicillin) and in **meningitis in children [4, 5] and adults [1, 2]** in whom most experts now favor ceftriaxone or cefotaxime as the drug of choice [1]. (In areas where highly resistant *S. pneumoniae* is a concern, vancomycin may be added while awaiting cultures.) See Chap. 5.
 4. **Brain abscess.** Although potentially useful in the treatment of brain abscesses, **combination therapy,** including an agent active against anaerobes, usually is **indicated** (e.g., the combination of penicillin, metronidazole, and ceftriaxone) unless reliable culture and susceptibility data clearly indicate that a third-generation cephalosporin alone is preferred.

E. **Eye infections**
 1. **Orbital cellulitis** may be a complication of sinus infections. A cephalosporin active against common sinus pathogens (e.g., *Streptococcus pneumoniae, S.*

aureus, Haemophilus influenzae) is appealing, and cefuroxime is a good choice. Ceftriaxone and cefotaxime are other options.

2. **Endophthalmitis** is difficult to treat, but cephalosporins, especially third-generation agents, often are used because of their potential penetration into the eye.

F. **Oral-dental infections.** Penicillin remains the drug of choice for most oral-dental infections. In patients either not responding to penicillin or allergic to penicillin, clindamycin is the usual alternative. Cefoxitin (or possibly cefotetan or cefmetazole) is another alternative, since it is active against anaerobes.

G. **Pulmonary infections**
   1. For *S. aureus* or *S. pneumoniae* therapy in the patient with a delayed penicillin allergy, a first-generation agent (e.g., cefazolin) is preferred if penicillin-resistant *S. pneumoniae* is not a concern. See Chap. 28C.
   2. For a mixed infection (e.g., postinfluenza bacterial infection with *S. aureus, S. pneumoniae,* or *H. influenzae*), cefuroxime is a useful agent. In the patient with chronic lung disease who is allergic to ampicillin or who may harbor ampicillin-resistant *H. influenzae,* cefuroxime has the advantage of not being as broad-spectrum as the third-generation agents, and superinfection with multiresistant bacteria may, therefore, occur less frequently. (See sec. **III.C** under Individual Agents.)
   3. Third-generation agents are especially useful when susceptibility data indicate activity (e.g., *Klebsiella* spp., *Escherichia coli,* or any *H. influenzae*). For *Enterobacter* spp. and other nosocomial gram-negative organisms, selection of organisms with chromosomally mediated beta-lactamase may preclude the use of a third-generation agent. (See sec. **III.C** under Individual Agents.)
   4. Severe *Pseudomonas* infections (e.g., pneumonia or bacteremia) should not be treated with one of the currently available agents alone; piperacillin and an aminoglycoside are preferred. In the patient with a delayed penicillin allergy in whom one wants to use combination therapy, a third-generation cephalosporin (e.g., ceftazidime) or cefepime combined with an aminoglycoside is an alternative to an expanded-spectrum penicillin such as a piperacillin-aminoglycoside combination.

H. **Cardiac infections (endocarditis)**
   1. For **staphylococcal** or **streptococcal** infections, when a cephalosporin is to be used, a first-generation agent is preferred. Some experts still favor cephalothin over cefazolin for susceptible *S. aureus* endocarditis and other severe nonmeningeal staphylococcal infections [2]. **No cephalosporin currently available is effective for enterococci.** Ceftriaxone has a role in the treatment of susceptible viridans streptococcal infections for which once-daily dosing regimens are important. (See sec. **III.B** under Individual Agents.)
   2. For the rare circumstance when a gram-negative organism causes endocarditis (e.g., *E. coli, Klebsiella* spp.), a third-generation agent is able to provide very favorable bactericidal levels. Caution must be exercised before using these agents for bacteria that rapidly develop resistance (see sec. **III.C** under Individual Agents).
   3. For **methicillin-resistant staphylococcal species** (e.g., methicillin-resistant *S. aureus* [MRSA]) even if there is in vitro activity of the agent, **cephalosporins are ineffective** in vivo [6, 7]. For methicillin-susceptible staphylococcal species, in vitro activity also implies in vivo activity.

I. **Intraabdominal or pelvic infections**
   1. For mild to moderate community-acquired infections, cefoxitin is a useful agent; cefotetan has also been used in this setting.
   2. Because of bleeding problems, moxalactam is no longer recommended. The other third-generation cephalosporins have no greater anaerobic activity than cefoxitin or cefotetan and therefore have little additional to offer.
   3. For a broad-spectrum yet relatively cost-effective agent (when compared with other antibiotics), a cephalosporin (e.g., cefazolin or ceftriaxone) combined with an antibiotic aimed at anaerobes (e.g., metronidazole) is a useful combination. See Chap. 11.
   4. Cefoxitin and cefotetan still play a role in the treatment of pelvic inflammatory disease (PID). See Chap. 13.

J. **Urinary tract infections (UTIs)**
   1. For community-acquired pyelonephritis in a patient who has had little previous therapy, a first-generation agent is useful.

2. For more complicated recurrent UTI, a second- or third-generation cephalosporin, based on susceptibility data, may allow one to avoid an aminoglycoside. An oral fluoroquinolone or parenteral aztreonam may be another option.
3. In nonbacteremic *Pseudomonas* UTI, monotherapy with ceftazidime or cefepime may be useful for susceptible pathogens.

K. **Sexually transmitted diseases.** Cefoxitin, cefotetan, and some of the third-generation agents, especially ceftriaxone, are used in gonorrhea and PID protocols. (See Chap. 13.)

L. **Septic joints**
1. For known or suspected **staphylococcal or nonenterococcal streptococcal** infection when a semisynthetic penicillin cannot be used, a first-generation agent (e.g., cefazolin or cephalothin) is preferred because of its enhanced *S. aureus* and gram-positive activity.
2. In a child younger than 5 years, when *H. influenzae* is also a concern, cefuroxime is an appealing single agent, although some clinicians would favor either ceftriaxone or cefotaxime.
3. In a young sexually active adult with monoarticular arthritis of unclear etiology in whom staphylococcal infection versus gonorrhea are the main concerns, cefoxitin, cefotaxime, or ceftriaxone is a useful agent while awaiting cultures because these agents are active against both pathogens.
4. The third-generation agents are used primarily for known or highly suspect gram-negative infections. They are also active against *Neisseria gonorrhoeae* (e.g., ceftriaxone).

M. **Osteomyelitis**
1. **For staphylococcal and nonenterococcal streptococcal** infections, a first-generation agent is preferred, as discussed in sec. **L.**
    Once-daily ceftriaxone is a consideration for the treatment of susceptible *S. aureus* infections, although the long-term cure rates after ceftriaxone therapy in this setting still are undergoing clinical evaluation. Because this is an evolving area, infectious disease consultation may be useful in this setting.
2. Cefuroxime (or cefotaxime or ceftriaxone) may be used for community-acquired osteomyelitis in a child younger than 5 years, as discussed in sec. **L,** as these agents will cover *S. aureus,* most streptococci, and *H. influenzae.*
3. The **third-generation** agents are useful for specific gram-negative infections when susceptibility data support their use and when resistance is not a major concern with prolonged use (see sec. **III.C** under Individual Agents). We would not use a third-generation agent alone for a *Pseudomonas* infection because adequate bone concentrations probably would not be achieved.

N. **Home intravenous therapy.** The cephalosporins with prolonged half-lives allow for once- or twice-daily home intravenous therapy. For example, ceftriaxone can be given once daily for non-CNS infections. However, its broad spectrum of activity or potential nonuniform activity against *S. aureus* must also be considered. Infectious disease consultation is advised to help choose the optimal home agent if a variety of agents are available. (See discussion of individual agents.)

III. **Overview of in vitro activity** of the (parenteral) cephalosporins
A. The **gram-positive** activity is summarized in **Table 28F-2.**
1. The first-generation agents remain the agents of choice for methicillin-susceptible *S. aureus* infections.
2. None of the cephalosporins are viewed as effective agents against enterococci or MRSA.
B. **Gram-negative and anaerobic** activity are summarized briefly in **Table 28F-3.**
1. The newer agents often are active against nosocomial pathogens.
2. Although the drug advertisements may list *P. aeruginosa* as being susceptible to the third-generation agents, especially cefoperazone, ceftazidime and cefepime, the minimum inhibitory concentrations (MICs) for *P. aeruginosa* usually are much higher than those for susceptible Enterobacteriaceae. Therefore, in life-threatening infections in which *P. aeruginosa* is a possible cause (e.g., bacteremia, pneumonia), these third-generation agents should not be used as monotherapy. An exception is meningitis due to a susceptible *Pseudomonas* spp., and in this setting ceftazidime alone has been effective.
3. Cefoxitin and cefotetan (and cefmetazole) are the most active agents against anaerobes, especially *Bacteroides fragilis.* (Moxalactam is no longer recommended.)

Table 28F-2. Cephalosporin gram-positive susceptibilities (MIC in μg/ml of most strains)

Organism	Cepha-lothin	Cefa-zolin	Cefu-roxime	Cefox-itin	Cefo-tetan	Cefmeta-zole	Cefo-taxime[a]	Cefopera-zone	Ceftri-axone	Ceftazi-dime	Cefe-pime
Staphylococcus aureus (penicillin-sensitive)	0.25	0.25	—	3.1	8–16	—	—	—	—	—	—
S. aureus (penicillin-resistant)	0.5	0.5	1.4	3.1	8–16	2.0	2–4	4.0	4.0	8–16	2.8–8.0
Streptococcus pneumoniae[b]	0.12	0.12	0.03–0.12	0.5	8	8.0	0.12	0.25	0.25	0.25	0.25
Streptococcus, group A	0.06	0.12	0.1	0.25	1.0–2.0	0.5	0.10	0.12	0.03	0.25	0.25
Viridans streptococci	0.5	1.0	—	4.0	4.0	—	0.25	1.0	0.25	4.0	—
Enterococci	R	R	R	R	R	R	R	R	R	R	R
Clostridium perfringens	0.5	0.12	1.3	1.0–2.0	1.0	—	2.0	—	—	—	2

R = resistant.

[a]Ceftizoxime has similar activity.

[b]Data for penicillin-susceptible strains. For data on penicillin-resistant strains, see detailed discussion in Chap. 28C and Table 28C-1.

Sources: Data adapted from A. Ward and D.M. Richards, Cefotetan: A review of its antibacterial activity, pharmacokinetic properties and therapeutic use. *Drugs* 30:382, 1985; W.E. Owens and S.M. Finegold, Comparative in vitro susceptibilities of anaerobic bacteria to cefmenoxime, cefotetan, and n-formimidoyl thienamycin. *Antimicrob. Agents Chemother.* 23:626, 1983; R.N. Jones and C. Thornsberry, In Vitro Antimicrobial Activity. Physical Characteristics and Other Microbiology Features of Cefuroxime: A New Study and Review. In R.C. Moellering, Jr. (ed.), *The Clinical Significance of the Newer β-Lactam Antibiotics: Focus on Cefuroxime* (Vol. 3 in *Therapeutics Today Series*). New York: ADIS Press, 1983. Pp. 30–45; H.C. Neu, The new beta-lactamase-stable cephalosporins. *Ann. Intern. Med.* 97:408, 1982; L.W. Ayers et al., Cefotetan: A new cephamycin, comparison of in vitro antimicrobial activity with other cephems. *Antimicrob. Agents Chemother.* 22:859, 1982; R.N. Jones, Cefotetan: A review of the microbiologic properties and antimicrobial spectrum. *Am. J. Surg.* 155(5A):16, 1988; and R.N. Jones, Review of the in vitro spectrum and characteristics of cefmetazole. *J. Antimicrob. Chemother.* 23(Suppl. D):1, 1989; J. Duval et al., In vitro antibacterial activity of cefepime: A multicentre study. *J. Antimicrob. Chemother.* 32(Suppl. B):55, 1993; B.A. Cunha and M.V. Gill, Cefepime. *Med. Clin. North Am.* 79:721, 1995.

Table 28F-3. In vitro activity of the parenteral cephalosporins

	Community-acquired E. coli, Klebsiella spp, P. mirabilis	H. influenzae[a] Beta-lactamase (+)	Enterobacter[b]		Other nosocomial gram-negatives	P. aeruginosa	B. fragilis[c]	Other Bacteroides spp.[c]
			E. cloacae	Other spp.				
Cephalothin	3+	0	0	0	0	0	0	0
Cefazolin	3+	0	0	0	0	0	0	0
Cefamandole[d]	3+	1+	0	0	0	0	0	0
Cefuroxime	3+	3+	0	0	1+	0	0	0
Cefoxitin	3+	1+	0	0	1+	0	3+	2+
Cefotetan	3+	2+	1+	0	2+	0	3+	1+
Cefmetazole	3+	1+	0	0	1+	0	2+	1+
Cefotaxime	3+	3+	1+	0	3+	1+	1+ to 2+	1+
Ceftriaxone	3+	3+	2+	1+	3+	1+	0	1+
Ceftizoxime	3+	3+	1+	0	3+	1+	1+	1+
Ceftazidime	3+	3+	2+	2+	3+	2+ to 3+	0	0
Cefoperazone	3+	2+	1+	1+	3+	2+	0	0
Cefepime	3+	3+	2+	2+	3+	2+ to 3+	0	0

3+ = most active; 2+ = moderately active; 1+ = modestly active; 0 = no clinically useful activity against.

[a]Agents active against beta-lactamase-positive H. influenzae are also active against ampicillin-susceptible, beta-lactamase-negative strains.

[b]Enterobacter species susceptible in vitro may develop resistance during therapy. See text.

[c]See text.

[d]Although in vitro H. influenzae may be susceptible to cefamandole, in vivo there may be a significant inoculum effect limiting its clinical effectiveness in severe H. influenzae infections. See text.

IV. **Special pharmacokinetic aspects** or properties
   A. **Table 28F-4 summarizes some of the pharmacokinetic properties of the cephalosporins.**
      1. **Dose interval.** Agents with a longer half-life allow for fewer doses per day and therefore may be cost-effective (see Chap. 28A).
      2. Dose modification in renal failure is variable and is discussed under the individual agent.
   B. **Cerebrospinal fluid penetration** with clinical efficacy in bacterial meningitis has been demonstrated with cefotaxime, ceftriaxone, and ceftazidime (against gram-negative bacilli).
   C. **Biliary penetration** has especially been demonstrated with cefazolin, cefamandole, cefoperazone, ceftriaxone, and ceftazidime.
   D. **Side effects** are discussed in detail in sec. **V** under Individual Agents. However, some special aspects of cephalosporin use are emphasized here.
      1. Hypoprothrombinemia and **bleeding** have been seen with moxalactam, cefamandole, cefoperazone and, less frequently, cefotetan, presumably because of the role the methylthiotetrazole ring plays in prothrombin synthesis. In severe renal failure, cefazolin has been associated with bleeding. (See discussion in sec. **V.D** under Individual Agents.) In addition, moxalactam has an antiplatelet effect that predisposes to bleeding; **it is no longer recommended for use** [6].
      2. **Ethanol intolerance** has been described especially with moxalactam and cefoperazone.
      3. **Phlebitis** is a potential problem, especially with cephalothin use.
V. **Cost.** Cost comparisons of the cephalosporins are shown in Table 28F-5. To compare the cost per day of cephalosporins with other antibiotics, see Tables 28A-5 and 28A-6.

Individual Agents

I. **First-generation agents.** These agents include the cephalosporins available before 1978. The prototype is cephalothin. These agents have **similar spectrums of antimicrobial activity.** Although there are minor differences, the similarities initially led to the use of the cephalothin disc for all first-generation agents except cefazolin. A separate disc is available for cefazolin, which is somewhat more active against gram-negative organisms [7], and should be used in the microbiology laboratory if disc susceptibility studies are done (if a hospital uses this agent), or separate MIC testing should be done. **These agents are active against** many gram-positive bacteria (except enterococci and methicillin-resistant staphylococci) (see Table 28F-2) and most community-acquired Enterobacteriaceae (see Table 28F-3). *P. aeruginosa* and other *Pseudomonas* spp. are routinely resistant to these agents. These first-generation agents

Table 28F-4. Pharmacokinetic properties of parenteral cephalosporins (in adults)

	Half-life (hr)	Standard dose (g)	Usual dose interval (hr)	Half-life (hr) in end-stage renal disease
Cephalothin	0.6	1.0–2.0	4	10
Cefoxitin	0.9	1.0–2.0	4–6–8	10–22
Cefotaxime	1.0*	1.0–2.0	6–8	3
Cefuroxime	1.0	0.75–1.5	6–8	15–20
Cefmetazole	1.2	2.0	6–12	
Cefazolin	1.8	1.0	6–8	18–36
Cefoperazone	1.8	2.0	6–8	2
Ceftizoxime	1.8	2.0	8	25–35
Ceftazidime	1.8	1.0–2.0	8	16–25
Cefonicid	4.6	1.0	24	65
Cefotetan	4.5	1.0–2.0	12	12–35
Ceftriaxone	7.0	1.0–2.0	24	12–15
Cefepime	2.0	1.0–2.0	12	14

*See text discussion.

Table 28F-5. Cost comparison of the cephalosporins

Antibiotic	Dose (g)	Dose interval	Cost of antibiotic[a]	Administration cost[b]	Total daily cost
Cefazolin (Ancef, Kefzol)	1	q6h	$12.00	14.00	$26.00
	1	q8h	9.00	10.50	19.50
Cefuroxime (Zinacef)	1.5	q8h	48.47	10.50	58.97
	750 mg	q8h	28.39	10.50	38.89
Cefoxitin (Mefoxin)	2	q6h	80.34	14.00	94.34
	2	q8h	60.26	10.50	70.76
Cefotetan (Cefotan)	2	q12h	46.04	7.00	53.04
Cefmetazole (Zefazone)	2	q8h	51.41	10.50	61.91
Cefotaxime (Claforan)	2	q8h	63.52	10.50	74.02
Ceftizoxime (Cefizox)	2	q8h	69.41	10.50	79.91
Ceftriaxone (Rocephin)	2	q24h	66.04	3.50	69.54
Ceftazidime (Fortaz)	2	q8h	86.44	10.50	96.94
Cefepime (Maxipime)	2	q12h	N/A	7.00	N/A

N/A = Drug approved but not marketed as of May 1996.
[a]Wholesale prices to pharmacist in the *American Druggist Blue Book* 1994–1995. Courtesy of Joseph S. Bertino, Jr., Pharm. D., Mary Imogene Bassett Hospital, Cooperstown, NY. **Note: Bidding practices affect actual hospital costs.**
[b]Based on a cost estimate of approximately $3.50 per intravenous dose. See study by R.M. Foran, et al., Evaluating the cost impact of intravenous antibiotic dosing frequencies. *DICP. Ann. Pharmacother.* 25:546, 1991, a report of a study at Robert Wood Johnson University Hospital showing that administration of an intravenous antibiotic dose IV costs approximately $3.35 for labor and material costs associated with admixture and administration (rounded off to $3.50 for this table).

have only limited activity against *H. influenzae*. For activity against *H. influenzae*, a second- or third-generation cephalosporin should be used. Penicillin-susceptible anaerobes are susceptible to these cephalosporins, but these agents are not active against *B. fragilis* [2]. Therefore, first-generation cephalosporins are appropriate treatment for methicillin-susceptible *S. aureus* and nonenterococcal streptococcal infections when it is desirable to avoid penicillins [2]. They are active against many community-acquired gram-negative bacilli but not *H. influenzae, Moraxella (Branhamella) catarrhalis* or *Pasteurella multocida.*

- **A. Cephalosporin (Keflin)** was the initial first-generation cephalosporin. It has, for the most part, been replaced by cefazolin, which requires less frequent administration and therefore is easier and more cost-effective to administer. See Tables 28F-4 and 28F-6 for a summary of the pharmacokinetic properties and dosages of cephalothin. Because of the pain associated with intramuscular use, the intravenous route is suggested [2].

    Among the cephalosporins, cephalothin is the least hydrolyzed by staphylococcal beta-lactamase and is considered still by some experts the optimal cephalosporin for treatment of methicillin-susceptible *S. aureus* endocarditis and other severe nonmeningeal susceptible *S. aureus* infections [2].

    1. Dose modification **in renal failure** is summarized in Table 28F-6 [8]. Although adequate blood levels can be achieved in renal failure, if moderately severe to severe renal failure exists in a patient with a UTI, cefazolin is preferred because it achieves good renal concentration even in severe renal failure [9].

    2. **Dialysis.** Because cephalothin is removed by hemodialysis and peritoneal dialysis, it is reasonable to give a dose after completion of hemodialysis and to continue an every-12-hour regimen (e.g., 1 g q12h) while the patient is on peritoneal dialysis [8].

    3. **Side effects.** See sec. **V.**

- **B. Cefazolin (Ancef, Kefzol)** [9] **has replaced cephalothin in most institutions.**

    1. **Pharmacokinetics.** Excellent blood levels can be achieved with either intravenous or intramuscular injection. Its half-life is 1.8 hours, compared with 30 minutes for cephalothin. (See Table 28F-4.) **In most moderate to severe infections, cefazolin can be given every 8 hours.** The dosage must be modified in renal failure, as indicated below. It achieves high therapeutic levels in bile

Table 28F-6. Typical dosages and summary of parenteral cephalosporins

Agent	Common adult single IV dose[a]	Usual dose interval in normal renal function[b] (hr)	Typical total adult daily dose (g)	Pediatric dose (d = day)	Dose interval (hr) with decreased creatinine clearance[c]				CSF penetration	Potential for bleeding side effects
					>50	30-49	10-29	<10		
First-generation										
Cephalothin (Keflin)	1-2 g	4-6	6-12	60-100 mg/kg/d; divided into q4-6h equal doses	4	6-8	6-8	12	Poor	No
Cefazolin (Ancef, Kefzol)	0.5-1 g	8	1.5-3.0	25-100 mg/kg/d; divided into q6-8h equal doses	8	12	12	24-48	Poor	In renal failure
Cephapirin (Cefadyl)	1-2 g	4	6-12	50-100 mg/kg/d; divided into q6h equal doses	As for cephalothin				Poor	No
Cephradine (Velosef)	1-2 g	6	2-8	50-100 mg/kg/d; divided into q6h equal doses	6	6-8	6-8	12	Poor	No
Second-generation										
Cefoxitin (Mefoxin)	2 g	6-8	6-8	80-160 mg/kg/d; divided into q4-6h doses	6-8	8-12	12-24	24[d]	Poor	No
Cefonicid (Monocid)	1 g	24[e]	1	Not advised	Reduce dose[f]				Poor	No
Cefuroxime (Zinacef)	750 mg-1.5 g	8	2.25-4.5	75-100 mg/kg/d; divided into q8h	8	8	12	24	Modest	No
Cefotetan (Cefotan)	1-2 g	12	2-4	Not advised	12	12	24	48	Poor	Yes
Cefmetazole (Zefazone)	2 g	8	6	Not advised	8-12[g]	16	24	48	?	Yes

Drug	Dose									
Third-generation										
Cefotaxime (Claforan)	1–2 g	8	3–6	50–180 mg/kg/d; divided into q6h[h]	8[i]	8–12	12	24	Excellent	No
Ceftizoxime (Cefizox)	2 g	8–12	4–6	150–200 mg/kg/d; divided q6–8h (if 6 months of age or older)	8–12	24–48	36–48	48–72	Excellent	No
Ceftriaxone (Rocephin)	1–2 g[j]	24	2	In meningitis, loading dose of 75 mg/kg and then 100 mg/kg/d (not to exceed 4 g/d) divided q12h. In other infections, 50–75 mg/kg/d (not to exceed 2 g) divided q12h or once-daily doses	24[k]	24[k]	24[k]	See text	Excellent	No
Ceftazidime (Fortaz, Tazidime, Tazicef)	1–2 g	8	3–6	90–150 mg/kg/d; divided q8h (to maximum 6 g/1)	8	12–24[a]	24–48[a]	48–72[a]	Excellent	No
Expanded-spectrum or fourth-generation										
Cefepime (Maxipime)	1–2 g	12	4	Not advised	12	See text			Modest	

[a] See text for details. Doses suggested for moderately severe infections.

[b] Or in patients with creatinine clearance >50 ml/min.

[c] See page 1079 (Chap. 28A) for the method of estimating creatinine clearance. Normal doses are used when the dose interval is prolonged.

[d] Dose is also reduced 50%. See text.

[e] Limited data on role in severe infections (see text).

[f] Doses are reduced per package insert.

[g] For creatinine clearance of >90 ml/min, the standard dose interval is used. Between 50 and 90 ml/min, a q12h interval can be used (see text). Neonatal dosages shown in Chap. 3.

[h] Higher dose range of cefotaxime used in meningitis. Use adult dosages in children weighing >50 kg.

[i] Dose interval for cefotaxime in children is usually q6h.

[j] In meningitis, 2 g q12h is advised (see text). In less severe infections, 1 g daily may be considered.

[k] In CNS infections, a q12h regimen is preferred. See text.

(unless there is biliary obstruction), bone, and pleural and joint fluid, and provides high urine levels. It does not penetrate into the CSF.

2. **Dosage** usually depends on the severity of the infection (see also Table 28F-6).
   a. In **adults,** the usual intramuscular or intravenous dose is as follows [9]. Intramuscular cefazolin is relatively pain-free.
      (1) In uncomplicated pneumococcal pneumonia in the patient with a delayed (late) penicillin allergy, 500 mg q12h.
      (2) In acute uncomplicated UTI, 1 g q12h.
      (3) In mild infections with susceptible gram-positive cocci, 500 mg q8h.
      (4) In moderate to severe infections, 1 g q8h. An every-6-hour schedule is used in the severely ill (e.g., bacteremic) patient.
   b. In **children,** the total daily dose is 25–100 mg/kg divided into three to four equal doses.
   c. For **surgical prophylaxis,** see Chap. 28B.
3. **In renal failure.** Cefazolin is eliminated primarily by renal excretion. If the creatinine clearance is greater than 50 ml/min, no dosage adjustments are necessary. If renal function deteriorates, there is an increase in the half-life and peak levels so that doses must be modified [8]. **(See Table 28F-6.)** Even in severe renal failure, cefazolin produces adequate urine concentrations [9].

   Peritoneal dialysis does not remove drug. In patients undergoing chronic ambulatory peritoneal dialysis (CAPD), doses of 500 mg q12h have been suggested [8]. **Hemodialysis** removes 40–60% of serum concentrations; a partial dose can be given to supplement serum levels.
4. **Side effects.** See sec. **V.**
5. Cefazolin is more readily hydrolyzed by staphylococcal beta-lactamase than is cephalothin. Although this relatively increased beta-lactamase vulnerability has not been clearly demonstrated to be of clinical significance, some experts prefer cephalothin for treatment of life-threatening methicillin-susceptible *S. aureus* infections [2].

C. **Cephapirin (Cefadyl) is very similar to cephalothin** in pharmacokinetics and spectrum of activity. If is available only as a parenteral agent. Although it can be given intramuscularly, the injections are painful [10] and the intravenous route is preferred [2]. (See Table 28F-6 for dosages.)
   1. **Side effects.** See sec. **V.**
   2. **Summary.** This agent has no special advantages when compared with cephalothin unless there are local pharmacy cost advantages based on local bidding. Rather than use this agent, most institutions appear to be using a first-generation agent that can be administered less frequently (e.g., cefazolin).

D. **Cephradine (Velosef)** is available in both an oral and a parenteral form.
   1. **Spectrum of activity** is similar to cephalothin, with only limited activity against *H. influenzae* [10].
   2. **Forms**
      a. **Oral (Velosef, Anspor)** forms are discussed later in this chapter. (See sec. **IV.A.**)
      b. **Parenteral (Velosef).** This form can be administered intravenously or intramuscularly. The intramuscular injections probably are more painful than intramuscular cefazolin. See Table 28F-6 for dosages.
   3. **Side effects.** See sec. **V.**
   4. **Summary.** Neither the oral form nor the parenteral form of cephradine offers any special advantages unless there are local cost factor advantages.

E. **Cephaloridine (Loridine) is no longer used** nor available because of its significant nephrotoxicity.

II. **Second-generation agents.** Since the introduction of the initial parenteral agents, cefamandole and cefoxitin, other agents have been released: ceforanide, cefonicid, cefuroxime, cefotetan, and cefmetazole (see Table 28F-1). These agents are expensive (see Tables 28A-6 and 28F-5). In terms of their clinical uses, those agents (e.g., cefuroxime) that are more active than the first-generation cephalosporins against common respiratory pathogens (*H. influenzae, M. catarrhalis, S. pneumoniae*) have become useful agents in treating infections of the respiratory tract and related appendages [2].

A second area of important use for those agents active against *B. fragilis,* community-acquired gram-negative bacilli, and *N. gonorrhoeae* (i.e., cefoxitin, cefotetan, and cefmetazole) is in intraabdominal, pelvic, and gynecologic infections, infected decubitus ulcers, diabetic foot ulcers, and mixed aerobic-anaerobic soft-tissue infections. Although the experience is most extensive with cefoxitin, available comparative trials suggest similar efficacy of cefoxitin, cefotetan, and cefmetazole [2]. Because up to 15% of *B. fragilis* may be resistant to these agents, they are not preferred in life-threatening infections. These agents often are inactive in the setting of induced (or derepressed) chromosomal beta-lactamases in Enterobacteriaceae (see sec. **III.C**) and are not highly active against *S. aureus,* so they are not optimal monotherapeutic agents for nosocomial infections [2]. See Table 28F-7.

A. **Cefamandole (Mandol).** After its introduction in the late 1970s and its initial popularity, several limitations of this drug have become obvious. **It has largely been replaced by another similar agent** (i.e., cefuroxime) or, in some institutions, by the third-generation agents. Because **an understanding of the limitations or problems associated with cefamandole help us to evaluate and understand the actual or potential problems with newer cephalosporins,** these issues will be summarized briefly.

1. **Disadvantages noted over time**
   a. **Inadequate CNS penetration** precludes its use in bacterial meningitis.
   b. **Inoculum effect.** It was soon recognized that cefamandole had variable activity against *H. influenzae* in vitro. Additional studies have clearly documented that cefamandole has an inoculum effect; that is, at low concentrations of bacteria, inhibition occurs, but at high concentrations of bacteria, the MIC of the organism dramatically increases. Cefamandole therefore is **not advised in life-threatening *H. influenzae* infections** (e.g., bacteremia, epiglottitis), and failures were described in severe pneumonias (i.e., settings with high bacterial inocula).
   c. **Hypoprothrombinemia and bleeding** were observed. Studies have shown that hypoprothrombinemia is relatively common and was seen in 13% of patients treated with cefamandole alone [11]. The possible mechanisms for this are discussed in sec. **F.4** and in sec. **V.**
   d. **Development of resistance during therapy** can occur, especially with *Enterobacter* spp. This is in part due to inducible beta-lactamases. See sec. **III.C.**
   e. **Relatively short half-life.** In severe infections, cefamandole is given every 4 hours. Similar agents (e.g., cefuroxime), which can be given less frequently, are easier and less expensive to administer.
   f. **Summary. Because of the aforementioned disadvantages and the availability of second-generation agents without these limitations (e.g., cefuroxime), most infectious disease experts and formulary committees no longer recommend cefamandole and have usually replaced this drug with cefuroxime or, at times, a third-generation cephalosporin.** Cefamandole is still an option in certain special settings for antibiotic surgical prophylaxis (see Chap. 28B). **We do not recommend cefamandole for therapeutic regimens.**

2. **Side effects.** See sec. **V.**

B. **Cefoxitin (Mefoxin)** [12, 13]. This cephamycin antibiotic (cephalosporinlike) has expanded activity against gram-negative bacteria. Against the common gram-negatives such as *E. coli* and *Klebsiella pneumoniae,* it is less active than cefazolin or cefamandole. After several years of experience, cefoxitin is **still a useful agent.**

1. **Spectrum of activity**
   a. **Gram-positive organisms.** Cefoxitin is slightly less active than first-generation agents. See Table 28F-2.
   b. **Gram-negative bacteria.** Cefoxitin has extended activity, but separate susceptibility testing (i.e., with a cefoxitin disc or dilutions) must be performed. It is active against *N. gonorrhoeae.* It is not active against *Enterobacter cloacae* or *P. aeruginosa* and is less active against *H. influenzae* than the true second-generation cephalosporins [2].
   c. **Anaerobes. Cefoxitin is active in vitro against 80–95% of strains of *B. fragilis* at clinically achievable concentrations** [13, 14], although in well-established infections, cefoxitin may not be as effective in vivo. It is active also against penicillin-susceptible anaerobes. The anaerobic activity of cefoxitin is better than that of most of the newer third-generation cephalosporins, and cefoxitin is viewed as the most potent of the cephalosporins against the *B. fragilis* group [2]. Moxalactam has similar anaerobic activity but, because of bleeding problems, generally is not recommended for use. Cefotaxime and its desacetyl metabolite have activity against anaerobes

Table 28F-7. Summary of major uses of cephalosporins

Class of agent	Clinical niche	Preferred agent
First-generation	1. Most active against methicillin-susceptible *S. aureus* and active against nonenterococcal streptococcal species; useful when desirable to avoid penicillins 2. Main agent for routine surgical prophylaxis not involving colon surgery. See Chap. 28B 3. Still active against many community-acquired gram-negative bacilli	Cefazolin[a]
Second-generation	Two major settings 1. Useful for respiratory-related infections (bronchitis, pneumonia, complicated sinusitis, complicated otitis media), taking advantage of enhanced activity against *H. influenzae* and *M. catarrhalis* as well as *S. pneumoniae* and activity for *S. aureus* 2. For mild to moderate mixed aerobic-anaerobic infections, as these agents are active against approximately 85% of *B. fragilis* strains, many community-acquired gram-negative bacilli, and *N. gonorrhoeae*. Therefore, useful in intraabdominal, pelvic, and gynecologic infections, decubitus ulcer, and diabetic foot ulcers	Cefuroxime Cefoxitin or cefotetan[b]

Third-generation	Two major settings
	1. Enhanced in vitro activity against *P. aeruginosa*
	  a. When a delayed penicillin allergy precludes the use of piperacillin or similar agents, usually combined with an aminoglycoside
	  b. For the febrile leukopenic patient without an obvious source of infection
	2. Enhanced activity against common meningeal pathogens[d] and community-acquired[e] and many nosocomially acquired Enterobacteriaceae
	  a. Therapy for meningitis
	  b. Gram-negative infections
		Ceftazidime[c]
		
		Ceftriaxone or cefotaxime[f]

[a]Some experts prefer cephalothin (Keflin) for methicillin-susceptible *S. aureus* bacteremia or endocarditis. See text. For streptococcal viridans endocarditis, ceftriaxone may be preferred. See text.

[b]Cefmetazole is another option. Both cefmetazole and cefotetan have the *N*-methylthiotetrazole (NMTT) side chain associated with hypoprothrombinemia. Therefore, for prolonged use, especially in a debilitated patient, we prefer cefoxitin. See text.

[c]Ceftazidime is preferred over cefoperazone. See text. Cefepime is also an option, but less experience with this agent. See text.

[d]Meningeal pathogens including *S. pneumoniae*, *H. influenzae* (beta-lactamase-positive and -negative) and *N. meningitidis*, but not *L. monocytogenes*. Ceftriaxone has also been effective therapy for meningitis caused by *S. pneumoniae* including species relatively resistant to penicillin but not those with high-level penicillin resistance. See text and Chap. 28C.

[e]For most community-acquired infections, the broad spectrum of a third-generation cephalosporin is not needed. Severe community-acquired infections with less susceptible organisms (e.g., in patients on prior antibiotics) may merit a third-generation agent.

[f]In neonates, cefotaxime is preferred over ceftriaxone (see Chap. 3). The role of cefepime is evolving (see text).

including *B. fragilis.* **Cefoxitin** (as well as cefotetan, which is discussed in sec. **II.F), has the best activity in vitro against oral and bowel anaerobes.** (See sec. **3.b.**) This activity against the anaerobes makes cefoxitin a useful agent in community-acquired mixed aerobic-anaerobic abdominal infections when therapy is initiated early after the insult and in other mild to moderate anaerobic infections.

2. **Pharmacokinetics.** Cefoxitin has properties similar to those of cephalothin (see Table 28F-4). The half-life is short (40–60 minutes) after intravenous administration. It is excreted unchanged in the urine, and doses must be reduced in renal failure (see sec. **7**). Cefoxitin can be administered intramuscularly or intravenously. The latter route is preferred in serious infections to help ensure adequate serum levels.

3. **Useful single agent.** Situations in which this drug may have an advantage over the other cephalosporins include the following:

   a. When susceptibility studies show that this cephalosporin is more effective than a first-generation cephalosporin agent.

   b. **Community-acquired mild to moderate intraabdominal infections** with mixed GI flora when treatment is begun before an established abscess develops. Cefoxitin appears to be a useful agent in diverticulitis, in cases of very early appendix rupture, and in bowel perforation before *B. fragilis* has become established in high titers.

      (1) **Advantages.** Cefoxitin will be less toxic than, for example, a combination of clindamycin and an aminoglycoside or other aminoglycoside-containing regimens. See Chap. 11.

      (2) **Disadvantages.** Cefoxitin is a potent beta-lactamase inducer (see sec. **III.C**). Some gram-negative bacteria may be resistant to cefoxitin, especially if the patient was recently hospitalized or was on broad-spectrum antibiotics. Some *B. fragilis* strains (approximately 5–15% typically) are not susceptible to cefoxitin. Enterococci are not susceptible but, in mild to moderately severe intraabdominal infection, it is not necessary to treat for enterococci (see Chap. 11). If a serum creatinine is drawn shortly after a dose of intravenous cefoxitin, the creatinine may be falsely elevated, as cefoxitin may interfere in some assays with the measurement of the serum creatinine in the laboratory [13].

   c. **Pelvic infections.** In mild to moderately ill patients, cefoxitin will cover *N. gonorrhoeae,* many gram-negative bacilli, and most anaerobes. Cefoxitin remains a reasonable drug for therapy of PID [15]. (See Chap. 13.)

   d. **Mild to moderate mixed aerobic-anaerobic soft-tissue infections.** These may respond well to cefoxitin, allowing one to use a single agent. The best results occur when the duration of illness, prior to the initiation of therapy, is short. Cefoxitin has often been used in mixed superficial foot ulcers in diabetic patients. Although cefoxitin is not active against enterococci, the significance of enterococci in mixed infections has recently been questioned; it probably is not necessary to treat routinely for enterococci. See Chap. 16, under Diabetic Foot Infections.

4. **Avoid cefoxitin, especially as a single agent in:**

   a. Known or suspected **bacteremia due to *B. fragilis.*** Because cefoxitin may not cover 5–15% of these organisms, metronidazole (routinely bactericidal against *B. fragilis*) is preferred. Until studies show otherwise, cefoxitin should be considered a second-line drug for *B. fragilis* infections.

   b. **Hospital-acquired intraabdominal sepsis.** As these patients may be colonized and subsequently infected with gram-negative organisms resistant to cefoxitin, an aminoglycoside may be necessary. In these seriously ill patients, rather than the use of cefoxitin with an aminoglycoside, other antibiotics often are preferable—for example, clindamycin or metronidazole and an aminoglycoside or ceftriaxone, or imipenem monotherapy.

   c. **Critically ill patients with intraabdominal sepsis or peritonitis.** In these patients, antibiotic coverage must be optimal while awaiting cultures. Coverage must be aimed primarily at *B. fragilis* and gram-negative bacteria. (See Chap. 11.) A third-generation cephalosporin (e.g., ceftriaxone) and metronidazole or possibly monotherapy with imipenem are options; the role of piperacillin-tazobactam in this setting awaits further clinical experience.

5. **Surgical prophylaxis.** The potential role of this cephalosporin in surgical prophylaxis (e.g., colonic surgery) is discussed in Chap. 28B.

6. **Dosage.** The following dosages are suggested (see also Table 28F-6):
   a. **Adults**
      (1) For uncomplicated UTIs and minor cutaneous infections (i.e., without bacteremia), 1 g IM or IV q6–8h.
      (2) For **moderately severe or severe infections,** 1 g q4h or 2 g q6–8h IV.
      (3) **For very serious infections** requiring maximal dosage, 3 g q6h IV can be used. (Often, alternative agents are used. See sec. **4.**)
   b. **Children.** Dosages of 80–160 mg/kg/day divided into four or six equal doses have been recommended for children older than 3 months.
7. **In renal failure,** the standard initial dose is given. Maintenance dosage depends on the severity of infection and degree of renal failure. No dosage modification is required if the creatinine clearance is more than 50 ml/min. (See Table 28F-6.)

   In adults, for a creatinine clearance of 30–50 ml/min, 1–2 g is given q8–12h; for a clearance of 10–29 ml/min, 1–2 g is given q12–24h; and, for a clearance of 5–9 ml/min, 500 mg–1 g is given q12–24h. If there is no renal function (i.e., clearance < 5 ml/min), 500 mg–1 g is given q24–48h.
8. **Dialysis.** Cefoxitin is removed significantly by **hemodialysis** so that a supplemental loading dose (e.g., 1–2 g) should be administered at the end of dialysis and usually should be repeated at 24–48 hours [16]. The effect of peritoneal dialysis on serum levels is being investigated. A preliminary study [17] suggests that peritoneal dialysis does not lower serum levels appreciably. In patients undergoing CAPD, 1 g daily has been suggested [8].
9. **Side effects.** See sec. **V.**

C. **Ceforanide (Precef).** Shortly after its release in 1984, the *Medical Letter* concluded that this agent is less active than previously available cephalosporins against *S. aureus, H. influenzae,* and enteric gram-negative bacilli, and there was "**no reason to use it**" [18]. This agent has not been available in the United States since 1991.

D. **Cefonicid (Monocid)** is a second-generation cephalosporin with a chemical structure similar to that of cefamandole.
   1. **Spectrum of activity** is similar to that of cefamandole and cefuroxime.
      a. **Gram-positive cocci.** This agent is less active against methicillin-susceptible *S. aureus, S. pyogenes,* and *S. pneumoniae* than are cefamandole and cefuroxime. Cefonicid is not active against enterococci or MRSA and may commonly show in vitro tolerance to *S. aureus* and group B streptococci [19, 20].
      b. **Gram-negative organisms.** Cefonicid is active against ampicillin-susceptible and ampicillin-resistant strains of *H. influenzae.* It is slightly more active against *N. gonorrhoeae,* including penicillinase-producing strains, than is cefamandole or cefoxitin, but it does not have the exquisite activity seen with the third-generation agents against *N. gonorrhoeae.* Like cefuroxime, cefonicid has an expanded gram-negative spectrum with good activity against *E. coli, K. pneumoniae,* and *Proteus mirabilis. Enterobacter* spp. usually are moderately susceptible. However, *Proteus vulgaris* and *Pseudomonas, Serratia,* and *Acinetobacter* spp. usually are resistant [19].
      c. **Anaerobes.** Many *Bacteroides* spp. are resistant to this agent, which offers no special anaerobic activity when compared with cefoxitin.
   2. **Pharmacokinetics**
      a. **Prolonged half-life.** The potential **special feature** of this second-generation cephalosporin is its **relatively long half-life** of approximately 4.5 hours in adults with normal renal function. (See Table 28F-4.) Serum concentrations of this antibiotic are in the therapeutic range 12 hours after a 1-g dose and are detectable after 24 hours, allowing for the possibility of once-daily doses [21]. However, serum levels at 12 hours after the usual 1-g dose IM or IV are only 15–20 μg/ml. The usual cutoff for susceptible pathogens is 16.0 μg/ml or less [19]. This has clinical implications in once-daily regimens for serious infections (see sec. **3**) because adequate serum bactericidal levels may not be achievable.
      b. **Elimination.** Cefonicid is eliminated by both glomerular filtration and tubular secretion, and 90–99% of a dose can be recovered in the urine within 24 hours [21]. Doses must be modified in renal failure. Routine doses provide urinary concentrations that remain in excess of the MIC for most susceptible bacteria for at least 24 hours [22].

    c. **Central nervous system penetration is inadequate;** therefore, cefonicid is not recommended for treatment in meningitis [21].

3. **Clinical studies** suggest that once-daily cefonicid therapy is efficacious in mild to moderately severe infection [21, 23, 24]. **Experience in serious infections is limited.** Cefonicid is effective in the treatment of bronchitis and pneumonia due to S. pneumoniae, H. influenzae, and E. coli [23], but many penicillin-susceptible pneumococci have relatively high MICs (1.6 μg/ml). Cefonicid is effective in the therapy of UTIs, soft-tissue and skin infections, and bone and joint infections due to susceptible pathogens. Because of the relatively low serum bactericidal levels 12–24 hours after a single daily dose and the relatively high MIC for S. aureus (6.3 μg/ml), we would not use this agent once daily for susceptible staphylococcal joint and bone infections.

    First-generation cephalosporins (e.g., cefazolin) are preferred for routine surgical prophylaxis. Efficacy data of cefonicid in the bacteremic patient are limited. Alternate agents should be used in bacteremic or very ill patients.

4. **Side effects.** Cefonicid has been **well tolerated,** with fewer than 1% of patients experiencing hypersensitivity reactions. A reversible influenzalike syndrome has been described in patients receiving long-term treatment for osteomyelitis [23]. **Because cefonicid is structurally similar to cefamandole, the potential for prolongation of the prothrombin time or overt bleeding exists.** (See sec. **V.**)

5. **Dosages.** See Table 28F-6.

    a. **Adults with normal renal function:** The usual dose is 1 g q24h IV, but doses up to 2 g (q24h) can be used for more severe infections [21].

    b. **Children.** Cefonicid is **not approved** for use in children, per the package insert.

6. **Renal failure.** Because the renal clearance of cefonicid declines linearly with decreasing renal function, dosages should be reduced in patients with renal insufficiency. Guidelines are provided in the package insert.

7. **Dialysis.** As 10% or less of a dose of cefonicid is removed by 4 hours of dialysis [22], supplemental doses are not necessary following hemodialysis. Dosage adjustment is not required for peritoneal dialysis [8].

8. **Cost.** If once-daily dosing with cefonicid is shown to be effective therapy for a problem, cefonicid may be a cost-effective agent [21]; however, if twice-daily treatment is given, the cost advantage may be lost. (See Table 28A-6).

9. **Summary. We do not use this cephalosporin.** In serious infections, other agents are preferred. In mild infections, oral agents may be available. Cefonicid does not seem to fill any unique niche.

E. **Cefuroxime** sodium (**Zinacef, Kefurox**) became available in the United States in 1984. Although it is similar to cefamandole in its antibacterial activity, cefuroxime's structure is different. In particular, **cefuroxime does not have the methylthiotetrazole group** at position 3 of the cephalosporin nucleus, which has been associated with prothrombin prolongation and bleeding in patients using cefamandole or other cephalosporins (see sec. **V**).

1. **Spectrum of activity** is similar to that of cefamandole [25, 26].

    a. **Gram-positive organisms.** (See Table 28F-2.) It is nearly as active in vitro as penicillin G against group A and B streptococci, penicillin-susceptible S. pneumoniae, and viridans streptococci. Generally, it is not as active against methicillin-susceptible S. aureus as are the first-generation cephalosporins, but still it has good activity against these organisms, with a MIC_{90} (i.e., level at which 90% of the organisms tested are susceptible) of 1.6 μg/ml or less.

    Methicillin-resistant S. aureus, enterococci, and Listeria monocytogenes are resistant to cefuroxime.

    Cefuroxime is active against most S. pneumoniae strains with intermediate resistance to penicillin but not highly resistant isolates [24a]. See related discussion in Chap. 28C.

    b. **Gram-negative organisms.** The activity of cefuroxime against these organisms can be categorized as follows [25]:

        (1) **Very active against ampicillin-susceptible or ampicillin-resistant** H. influenzae and M. catarrhalis as well as Neisseria meningitidis. In addition, there is no "inoculum effect" with cefuroxime.

        (2) Active against most N. gonorrhoeae, including penicillinase-producing strains.

   (3) Active against *P. multocida.*
   (4) Active against a wide variety of other gram-negative bacilli (*E. coli, P. mirabilis, Klebsiella, Citrobacter, Salmonella, Shigella,* and *Yersinia* spp., some *Enterobacter* spp., etc.) but is less active than the third-generation cephalosporins. Several studies have shown remarkable resistance of cefuroxime to most beta-lactamases produced by Enterobacteriaceae.
   (5) Not very active against *Providencia* spp., *P. vulgaris,* and *Serratia* and *Pseudomonas* spp.
   c. Anaerobes. Although cefuroxime appears to be active against most strains of *Clostridium* spp., *Fusobacterium* spp., and anaerobic gram-positive cocci, it is less active than cefoxitin (and cefotetan) against *B. fragilis* and other *Bacteroides* spp. Therefore, cefuroxime offers no special advantage in terms of a cephalosporin for anaerobic infections.
   d. *Borrelia burgdorferi* are susceptible.
 2. Pharmacokinetics. The half-life of cefuroxime is longer than that of cefamandole (see Table 28A-4), allowing less frequent dosing of cefuroxime. The major route of excretion is renal, and its half-life is prolonged in renal failure. Cefuroxime penetrates inflamed meninges, but CSF levels are borderline for treatment of bacterial meningitis due to susceptible pathogens. **Experts believe that cefuroxime does not provide adequate CSF bactericidal activity routinely [5], and it is no longer recommended in the therapy of meningitis** [1, 4, 5].
 3. Clinical studies. In addition to extensive clinical trials in the United States, cefuroxime has been used extensively in the United Kingdom and other countries. There have been excellent clinical results for susceptible pathogens [25–27]. Infections treated include UTI, sinus infections, lower respiratory tract infections, bone and joint infections, skin and soft-tissue infections, and bacteremias.
   Although effective in surgical prophylaxis, there is no reason to use this more expensive agent for routine surgical prophylaxis (see Chap. 28B).
   Oral cefuroxime is effective in streptococcal pharyngitis, but it is not the agent of choice. See related discussion in Chap. 7.
 4. Side effects. This agent has been very well tolerated. Occasionally, thrombophlebitis after intravenous use, pain after intramuscular use, and hypersensitivity reactions have been reported. Bleeding tendencies, which have been seen with cefamandole and other cephalosporin use, have not been reported [26]. Disulfiram-type reactions have not been described. (See sec. **V.**)
 5. Dosages. See Table 28F-6.
   a. Adults (with normal renal function). The usual dose range is 750 mg–1.5 g q8h depending on the severity of the infection.
     (1) In an uncomplicated community-acquired pneumonia, we typically give 750 mg q8h.
     (2) In a patient who is very ill with pneumonia or who has bone or joint infection, 1.5 g q8h is suggested. For less susceptible pathogens or very ill patients (e.g., postsplenectomy bacteremia), 1.5 g q6h is recommended at least initially.
   b. Children older than 3 months. For most infections, 75–100 mg/kg/day in divided doses q6–8h is recommended.
   c. The oral preparation is discussed in sec. **IV.B.2.**
 6. Renal failure. In the anuric patient, the normal half-life is prolonged to approximately 15–20.0 hours. If the creatinine clearance rate is greater than 20 ml/min/1.73 m^2, the usual doses can be given. See dose reductions in Table 28F-6. In significant renal failure, the manufacturer suggests the following: In adults, if the creatinine clearance is between 10 and 20 ml/min, 750 mg can be given q12h; if the creatinine clearance is less than 10 ml/min, 750 mg is suggested q24h.
 7. Dialysis. Cefuroxime is not removed by peritoneal dialysis and only modestly by hemodialysis; so a supplemental dose after hemodialysis is reasonable [8].
 8. Cost. See Tables 28A-5, 28A-6, and 28F-5.
 9. Summary and conclusions. Cefuroxime is an appealing agent. Infectious disease subspecialists and formulary committees in many hospitals have replaced cefamandole with cefuroxime.

a. **Advantages of cefuroxime**
   (1) Has a longer half-life than cefamandole and is therefore less expensive to administer than cefamandole.
   (2) Lacks the structural formula incriminated in the bleeding problems seen with moxalactam, cefamandole, and related antibiotics.
   (3) Has no inoculum effect.
   (4) Maintains excellent *H. influenzae* activity as well as good *S. aureus* and group B streptococcal activity; very active against *S. pneumoniae* strains, including those with intermediate resistance to penicillin.
   (5) Is well tolerated.
b. **Common clinical indications** for the use of cefuroxime include:
   (1) **Severe acute bacterial bronchitis** in patients with underlying chronic lung disease who are not responding to outpatient antibiotics or in a hospitalized patient allergic to ampicillin in whom intravenous antibiotics are desirable.
   (2) **Community-acquired pneumonia** in a patient allergic to penicillin or ampicillin or a patient not responding to amoxicillin or other oral antibiotics.
   (3) **Postinfluenza pneumonia** in which it is desirable to treat empirically for *S. pneumoniae, S. aureus,* and *H. influenzae.*
   (4) **Orbital cellulitis** in which it is desirable to treat empirically.
   (5) **Complicated sinusitis and epiglottitis** [2].
   (6) *P. multocida* wound infection in a patient with a delayed penicillin-allergic history.
   (7) **Lyme disease,** as an alternative agent [1] (see Chap. 23).
c. **Disadvantages of cefuroxime**
   (1) Not active against *B. fragilis,* enterococci, *L. monocytogenes, Pseudomonas* spp., high-level penicillin-resistant *S. pneumoniae,* and many nosocomial gram-negative bacilli. Therefore, unless susceptibility data are known, it should not be used alone for nosocomial infections potentially caused by resistant bacteria.
   (2) **Relatively expensive** agent. (See Table 28F-5.)
10. **Oral cefuroxime.** See discussion in sec. **IV.B.2.**
F. **Cefotetan (Cefotan)** was released in the United States in late 1986. It has characteristics of both second- and third-generation cephalosporins; it has enhanced gram-negative coverage similar to that of the third-generation agents but also has activity against anaerobes comparable to that of the second-generation cefoxitin. Because cefotetan often is promoted as "the cost-effective replacement for cefoxitin," it will be reviewed in some detail [28–31] here and considered clinically as a second-generation cephalosporin.
   1. **Spectrum of activity** [29, 31]
      a. **Gram-positive aerobes.** Cefotetan is active against pneumococci, group A and group B streptococci, and staphylococci, although it is less active against these organisms than many other cephalosporins and the penicillins. (See Table 28F-2.) Of interest, in the review by Jones [31], the MIC_{90} for *S. aureus* was 16 µg/ml, which is fairly high compared with other cephalosporins and in the range of ceftazidime, which has been considered a poor antistaphylococcal agent. Overall, **cefotetan is 2 to 4 times less active than cefoxitin against gram-positive cocci** [30]. It is inactive against enterococci.
      b. **Gram-negative aerobes.** The drug is active against gonococci, meningococci, and *H. influenzae.* In vitro, it is more active than cefoxitin against enteric gram-negative bacilli but less active than the third-generation cephalosporins (cefotaxime, ceftizoxime, ceftazidime, and ceftriaxone). Cefotetan is inactive against many strains of *Enterobacter* spp. and most strains of *P. aeruginosa* and *Acinetobacter* spp.
      c. **Anaerobes.** Cefotetan usually is considered comparable to cefoxitin in vitro against *B. fragilis* spp. but is less active against other *Bacteroides* spp. within the *B. fragilis* group, including many clinical isolates [16, 28, 31]. The clinical significance of this is uncertain [28, 30].
         In one report of the susceptibility data of all isolates of *B. fragilis* spp. from six hospitals in Chicago, 9% were resistant to cefoxitin, whereas 22% were resistant to cefotetan [31a]. Of the non-*fragilis* isolates of the

B. fragilis group, 5–33% were resistant to cefoxitin, compared with 43–100% that were resistant to cefotetan, depending on the institution [31a].

2. **Pharmacokinetics** [28]
   a. The **elimination half-life** of cefotetan is 3–4.5 hours compared to 1.0 hour or less for cefoxitin, **thus allowing twice daily dosing,** which would be more cost-effective dosing than cefoxitin.
   b. **Excretion is primarily by the kidney.** High concentrations of the drug are found in the urine 24 hours after a dose. A small amount is excreted in bile. **Dose adjustments are necessary in renal failure.**
   c. Data on **concentrations in bodily fluids,** especially CSF, are limited. Cefotetan is excreted in human milk in very low concentrations.

3. **Clinical studies.** In uncontrolled studies, cefotetan has been shown to be effective in the treatment of urinary tract, skin, soft-tissue, obstetric, gynecologic, intraabdominal, and head and neck infections and bacteremias [28, 29]. Early studies suggest that cefoxitin and cefotetan are equally effective in prophylaxis (typically, studies have compared single doses of cefotetan to multiple doses of cefoxitin) and in the treatment of acute PID, postoperative endometritis, and mild to moderate community-acquired intraabdominal infections [30].

4. **Side effects**
   a. **Risk of hypoprothrombinemia or bleeding. Cefotetan contains the *N*-methylthiotetrazole (NMTT) side chain** as in some other cephalosporins (cefamandole, moxalactam, cefoperazone), **which may cause hypoprothrombinemia (see sec. V.D.3).** Whether cefotetan is associated with more or less hypoprothrombinemia or clinical bleeding than other cephalosporins with the NMTT side chain or similar cephalosporin agents (e.g., cefoxitin, which does not have the NMTT side chain) is debated. However, cefotetan has been associated with hypoprothrombinemia and bleeding [2].
      (1) Although some reports suggest that there is no clear extra risk of bleeding in NMTT agents [32–34], other reviews suggest that the true risks have not yet been clearly defined [35, 36] except for moxalactam, or that indeed there is a risk with NMTT-containing agents [37, 38].
      (2) Of interest, the package insert of cefotetan (but not cefoxitin) indicates: "in common with many other broad-spectrum antibiotics, Cefotan [cefotetan] may be associated with a fall in prothrombin time activity [i.e., a prolongation of Pro Time] and, possibly, subsequent bleeding. Those at increased risk include patients with renal or hepatobiliary impairment, or poor nutritional state, the elderly, and patients with cancer. **Prothrombin time should be monitored and exogenous vitamin K administered as indicated**" [39].
         See Table 28F-8, which summarizes high-risk patients. (Also see Shevchuk and Conly [36].)

Table 28F-8. Nonantibiotic factors contributing to beta-lactam-associated hypoprothrombinemia

---

Impaired intestinal absorption of vitamin K
  Insufficient bile acids
    Gastric suctioning
  Impaired intestinal transport
    Ileus, peritonitis
    Bowel obstruction
  Damage to intestinal microvillae
    Cytotoxic chemotherapy
Nonintestinal factors
  Malnutrition with vitamin K depletion
  Renal failure
    Excessive NMTT concentrations

NMTT = *N*-methylthiotetrazole
Source: F.R. Sattler et al., Impaired hemostasis caused by beta-lactam antibiotics. *Am. J. Surg.* 155(5A):32, 1988.

(3) Obviously, researchers have not resolved all the issues of cefotetan's side effects. In the cefotetan symposium summary, Barza [30] said: "In my opinion, although antibiotic-related coagulopathies are clearly multifactorial, there is strong evidence for the role of the NMTT side chain in this adverse effect." He concludes his paper saying [30]: "In my opinion, there is a higher risk of hypoprothrombinemia with cefotetan than with cefoxitin in patients who are vitamin K–deficient. However, if physicians are aware of this liability and provide vitamin K supplementation (or avoid cefotetan altogether in patients who are nutritionally depleted), the benefits of cefotetan, especially the cost savings, make it an attractive substitute for cefoxitin."

We concur with Dr. Barza's conclusions but **suspect that many physicians who are using cefotetan in high-risk patients** (see sec. **V.D**) **are not monitoring their patients as the literature and package insert advise.**

b. **Other side effects** have been infrequent and not severe. Shared side effects of cephalosporins are **reviewed in sec. V.** Local pain after intramuscular injection and phlebitis after intravenous infusion have been reported. Rash, pruritus, fever and chills, nausea, vomiting, diarrhea, and superficial *Candida* infections have occurred. Agents with the NMTT side chain also are associated with a disulfiram reaction with alcohol (see sec. **V.E**).

5. **Dosage (intramuscular or intravenous)**
   a. **Adults.** The usual dose for moderately severe infections is 1–2 g IV or IM q12h. For life-threatening infections, the maximum dose, 3 g q12h, has been used [28]. For surgical prophylaxis, 1–2 g IV preoperatively is suggested (see Chap. 28B).
   b. **Children.** Effectiveness and safety have not been established in children.
   c. **Renal dysfunction** requires modification of the dosing regimen (see Table 28F-6). The manufacturer recommends the usual dosage for creatinine clearance that exceeds 30 ml/min; for a clearance of 10–30 ml/min, the usual dose can be given at 24-hour intervals. If the creatinine clearance is less than 10 ml/min, the dose appropriate to the severity of infection should be given every 48 hours. Cefotetan is dialyzable. After hemodialysis, one-fourth of the usual recommended dose is given every 24 hours on days between dialysis and one-half the usual recommended dose on the day of dialysis per the package insert. Another recommendation is 1 g after hemodialysis [8]. In patients undergoing CAPD, 1 g/day has been suggested [8].

6. **Summary and conclusions.** Cefotetan has an in vitro spectrum of activity similar to that of cefoxitin, although the gram-negative spectrum of cefotetan is comparable to that of many third-generation cephalosporins, but cefotetan is less active than cefoxitin against *S. aureus*. The cost of cefotetan per day is less than that of cefoxitin, especially considering the twice-daily dosing that the longer half-life of cefotetan allows. (See Table 28F-5.) The data currently available are not adequate to determine the precise risk of bleeding with protracted use.
   a. **For prophylaxis.** Cefotetan is not a primary agent. As discussed in Chap. 28B, a first-generation cephalosporin (e.g., cefazolin) is preferred for routine surgical prophylaxis. This is especially important when one considers the relatively poor activity of cefotetan against *S. aureus*.

   For colorectal surgery, if the procedure takes less than 2 hours, it is more cost-effective to use a single dose of cefoxitin than a single dose of cefotetan. If a colorectal surgical procedure is anticipated to be more than 2 hours, a single dose of cefotetan is more cost-effective and makes more sense than multiple doses of cefoxitin (see Chap. 28B). The risk of bleeding problems after one to three doses seems remote [36] (see sec. **V.D**).
   b. **For therapy**
      (1) **For patients with underlying risk factors for hypoprothrombinemia** (e.g., in patients who are malnourished or are allowed nothing by mouth for a significant length of time; **see Table 28F-8), we do not recommend using cefotetan or other NMTT-containing cephalosporins** such as cefmetazole (see sec. **G**) and, if a second-generation cephalosporin is indicated, we prefer cefoxitin.

(2) **If cefotetan is used in patients at risk for vitamin K deficiency, serial prothrombin times and vitamin K administration as indicated is advised (per the package insert).** Unfortunately, many hospitalized patients are at risk for vitamin K deficiency (see Table 28F-8), and whether the inconvenience of monitoring the patients or administering vitamin K is worth the cost savings is an individual institutional decision (see sec. **V.D**).

(3) For young women with pelvic infections or endometritis or mild to moderate community-acquired intraabdominal infections in healthy patients, cefotetan for short courses is reasonable and cost-effective.

c. In a recent publication of clinical practice guidelines, the Committee on Antimicrobial Agents of the Canadian Infectious Disease Society recommended that cefotetan could be considered an alternative single agent for prophylaxis of infection in patients undergoing elective bowel surgery, and it may be used to treat patients with acute PID and endometritis [39a], but hypoprothombinemia in debilitated patients is a concern.

G. **Cefmetazole (Zefazone)** was approved for release by the US Food and Drug Administration (FDA) in December 1989. This is a new cephamycin to European and North American clinicians, but it has been used widely in Japan since 1980. Its spectrum of activity is that of a second-generation cephalosporin and, therefore, is similar to cefoxitin and cefotetan [40, 41].

1. **Spectrum of activity.** The in vitro activity of cefmetazole closely resembles that of cefoxitin [42].

a. **Gram-positive cocci.** Methicillin-susceptible *S. aureus* strains have a MIC_{90} range of 1.0–4.0 μg/ml [42], similar to cefoxitin and more active than cefotetan against *S. aureus*. Methicillin-resistant *S. aureus* is not susceptible to cefmetazole, with a MIC_{90} of 25 μg/ml [42].

Cefmetazole is active against group A streptococci (see Table 28F-2). It has limited activity against *S. pneumoniae* and is active against *S. agalactiae* with a MIC_{90} of 2 μg/ml. It is not active against *L. monocytogenes* or enterococci.

b. **Gram-negative aerobes** [42]. Cefmetazole is two- to fourfold more active than cefoxitin against *E. coli, Klebsiella* spp., and *P. mirabilis* but has nearly equal activity against the indole-positive *Proteus* and *Providencia* species. Cefotetan is more active than either cefmetazole or cefoxitin [42] against most susceptible Enterobacteriaceae. Cefmetazole is active against *Salmonella* and *Shigella* spp., as well as *H. influenzae* (including beta-lactamase producers) and *M. catarrhalis*. Cefmetazole appears equally as effective as cefoxitin, or slightly less so (two- to fourfold), against *N. gonorrhoeae*. It is not active against *Citrobacter freundii, Pseudomonas* and *Enterobacter* spp., or *Serratia marcescens*.

c. **Anaerobes** [42]. Cefmetazole is active against gram-positive anaerobic cocci with a MIC_{90} of 0.12–8.0 μg/ml. Summary data show that against *B. fragilis,* cefmetazole may be equal to or up to twofold less active compared with cefoxitin. Against the *B. fragilis* group and other *Bacteroides* spp., cefmetazole was about as active as, or slightly less active than, cefoxitin.

2. **Pharmacokinetics.** According to the package insert, after a 2-g intravenous infusion, peak serum concentration in normal volunteers is approximately 140 μg/ml. More than 85% of the dose is excreted in the urine over a 12-hour period. Therefore, **in renal failure, dosages must be modified.** Cefmetazole provides excellent drug levels in urine, peritoneal fluid, skin tissue, bile, and ear exudate, but relatively low levels in sputum and prostatic tissue. Cefmetazole crosses the placenta, and trace amounts are in the milk of nursing mothers. The half-life after an intravenous dose is 1.2 hours. No data are available on CSF concentrations.

3. **Clinical studies.** In more than 4,000 patients studied by more than 75 investigators, cefmetazole was as effective as cefoxitin in the treatment of UTIs, skin and soft-tissue infections, lower respiratory infections, and intraabdominal infections, and in surgical prophylaxis [43].

4. **Dosages** are suggested in the package insert.

a. **For therapy.** The usual **adult dose,** depending on the severity of the infection, is 2 g IV q6–12h. For adults with normal renal function, the following guidelines are suggested:

      (1) For UTI, 2 g q12h IV.

      (2) For mild to moderate infections, 2 g q8h IV.

      (3) For severe or life-threatening infections, 2 g q6h.

  b. For prophylaxis. In colorectal surgery, 2 g given as a single dose 30–90 minutes before surgery or 2 g given 30–90 minutes before surgery and repeated at 8 and 16 hours later is recommended. If the operation lasts for more than 4 hours, the preoperative dose should be repeated per the package insert. See Chap. 28B for further discussion of surgical prophylaxis.

  c. Pediatric use. The safety and effectiveness in children has not been established.

  d. In renal failure. Doses are modified as shown in Table 28F-6. In the patient who has no renal function, 1–2 g q48h is advised, and the dose ideally is given after hemodialysis.

5. Side effects

  a. Overall, cefmetazole appears to be a safe agent, similar to other cephalosporins [40]. In a Japanese survey of more than 118,000 patients, there was a 2% incidence of adverse side effects, with rashes and minor GI symptoms the most common side effects [44].

  b. *N*-methylthiotetrazole and the risk of bleeding. In the Japanese surveillance study, there were no reports of hemorrhage due to hypoprothrombinemia, but there were cases of hypoprothrombinemia and prolonged bleeding time [44].

      Cefmetazole does contain the NMTT side chain, as does cefotetan; therefore, there is the potential to cause hypoprothrombinemia and, possibly, bleeding, as is discussed under cefotetan (see sec. **F.4** and **V.D**). The actual risk with this agent is unknown at this point and awaits further clinical experience with and study of this agent [2].

      Patients at risk for bleeding with other NMTT-containing agents (see Table 28F-8) would presumably be the same patients as are at risk with the use of this agent. (See sec. **F.4.a.**)

      The package insert indicates, "As with some other cephalosporins, cefmetazole may be associated with a fall in prothrombin activity [i.e., prolonged prothrombin times]. Those at risk include patients with renal or hepatic impairment, or poor nutritional state, as well as patients receiving a protracted course of antimicrobial therapy. Prothrombin time should be monitored for patients at risk and exogenous vitamin K administered as indicated" [39].

  c. A disulfiramlike reaction has been reported after ingestion of alcohol. See related discussion in sec. **V.E.**

6. Conclusions. At this point, we believe it is premature to determine how cefmetazole will fit in. It has not been shown to offer any clear clinical advantage over cefoxitin or cefotetan (see sec. **II.F.6**).

  a. Prophylaxis. For routine surgical prophylaxis, the first-generation cephalosporins are preferred (see Chap. 28B). Although approved for use in patients undergoing cesarean section or abdominal or vaginal hysterectomy and high-risk patients undergoing cholecystectomy, the first-generation cephalosporin agents usually are cost-effective in these situations (see Chap. 28B).

      For colorectal surgery, cefmetazole is a rational agent for prophylaxis, as are cefoxitin and cefotetan, although cefmetazole is not an agent of choice. (See Chap. 28B.) For colorectal surgery, the package insert of cefmetazole indicates that the usual preoperative mechanical preparation and oral neomycin or kanamycin and oral erythromycin, as described in Chap. 28B, had been given in prior studies of cefmetazole and colorectal surgical prophylaxis.

      Because of the relatively short half-life and, therefore, the need for a supplemental intraoperative dose at 4 hours in protracted procedures, **cefmetazole lacks the advantage of single-dose cefotetan in this setting** (see sec. **F.6.a**) (see Chap. 28B).

      Cefmetazole can be administered rapidly, with a 5-minute infusion for standard doses. This may be an appealing aspect for prophylactic antibiotic use.

  b. Therapy. Many of the same comments and concerns about cefotetan (see sec. **F.6** and **V.D**) apply to cefmetazole, which also is associated with the NMTT side effects.

c. **Cefoxitin versus cefotetan versus cefmetazole.** In patients requiring protracted therapy with one of these agents, we tend to favor cefoxitin unless serial prothrombin times are monitored.

III. **Third-generation agents.** Several agents are now available (see Table 28F-1) since the introduction of cefotaxime in 1981. These third-generation agents have even **broader gram-negative activity** than the first- and second-generation agents because they are more resistant to the beta-lactamases produced by gram-negative bacteria. Some of them have enhanced activity against *P. aeruginosa*. See summary Table 28F-7. In January 1996, yet another expanded-spectrum cephalosporin became available, cefepime. Although this has at times been referred to as a "fourth-generation cephalosporin," we have discussed this agent in sec. **F**. (The clinical implications of the term "fourth-generation" cephalosporin are not established at this point.)

A. **The dilemma.** Which agents to use remains a problem, even though we have now had more than a decade of experience with many of them [45–48]. **Most experts emphasize that these agents should be saved for situations in which their unique capabilities are required, in order to make them cost-effective and to avoid the development of widespread resistance.** This is not easy to accomplish, however. As Moellering [48] and others emphasized several years ago, the third-generation agents present "a situation where a large number of drug companies have spent millions of dollars developing these (agents) and all—reasonably—want to recoup their investment. There is going to be just tremendous competition to market the drugs both here in the United States and worldwide. The **clinician is going to be bewildered**." This concern, emphasized shortly after these agents were introduced in 1981, still remains.

B. **Special advantages of the third-generation agents.** Some general comments will be summarized here. **Individual agents are discussed in sec. III.E.**

1. **Spectrum of activity** [6, 46, 49]. The third-generation cephalosporins are drugs of choice only for a limited number of organisms. See Table 28F-9.

   a. **Gram-positive aerobes.** When these agents were released, they were considered less active against gram-positive aerobes [6, 49]. In his review, Neu [46] indicates, after further in vitro studies, that this may not always be the case.

   (1) *S. aureus.* First- and some second-generation cephalosporins are at least two- to fourfold more active than cefotaxime, ceftizoxime, and ceftriaxone against penicillin-susceptible *S. aureus* and against some, but not all, beta-lactamase-producing strains [46]. When considering cefotaxime, ceftizoxime, or ceftriaxone in suspected sepsis in which staphylococci cannot be excluded, one of these three cephalosporins provides adequate initial activity against staphylococci [46]. In patients with documented severe staphylococcal infections (e.g., *S. aureus* bacteremia), we would not use a third-generation cephalosporin as an agent of choice but would prefer an antistaphylococcal penicillin (e.g., oxacillin or nafcillin) or a first-generation cephalosporin.

   (2) **Coagulase-negative staphylococci.** If the organisms are methicillin-resistant, a cephalosporin is not recommended, even if the in vitro data suggest that a cephalosporin may be active. If methicillin-susceptible, cephalosporins are potential agents, although vancomycin often is used.

   (3) **Group A streptococci.** The third-generation cephalosporins (cefotaxime, ceftizoxime, and ceftriaxone) are very active against these pathogens, with MICs typically less than 0.03 µg/ml, comparable to benzylpenicillin and, in fact, more active than cefazolin or cefoxitin.

   (4) **Group B streptococci (*S. agalactiae*)** are also extremely susceptible to cefotaxime, ceftizoxime, and ceftriaxone, again with a MIC comparable to penicillin G and better than cefazolin.

   (5) **Groups C and G streptococci** are also very susceptible to the aforementioned third-generation agents.

   (6) **Most viridans streptococci and *Streptococcus bovis*** have lower MICs for these third-generation agents than the first- or second-generation cephalosporins. This has implications in alternate endocarditis therapeutic regimens (e.g., ceftriaxone once daily).

Table 28F-9. Bacteria for which third-generation cephalosporins are the antibiotic of choice

Organism	Cephalosporin of choice
Haemophilus influenzae (serious infections)	Cefotaxime or ceftriaxone[a]
Neisseria gonorrhoeae	Ceftriaxone[a] (or cefixime)
Salmonella typhi	Ceftriaxone[b]
Salmonella spp.	Ceftriaxone or cefotaxime (or a fluoroquinolone)
Escherichia coli *Klebsiella pneumoniae* Indole-positive *Proteus* spp. (*P. vulgaris*) *Providencia rettgeri* *Morganella morganii* *Providencia stuartii* *Serratia* spp.	Cefotaxime, ceftriaxone, ceftazidime, or ceftizoxime[c]
Pseudomonas pseudomallei	Ceftazidime
Haemophilus ducreyi (chancroid)	Ceftriaxone (or erythromycin or azithromycin)

[a]For both beta-lactamase-positive and beta-lactamase-negative strains.
[b]Ceftriaxone also provides high biliary concentrations.
[c]Some medical consultants would add an aminoglycoside in very serious infections.
Source. Adapted from *Medical Letter:* The choice of antibacterial drugs. *Med. Lett. Drugs Ther.* 38:25, 1996.

(7) *S. pneumoniae.* Cefotaxime, ceftizoxime, and ceftriaxone are very active against the usual highly susceptible organisms and relatively resistant strains but not against the highly penicillin-resistant strains [24a]. See related discussion in Chap. 28C.

(8) These agents are **not active** against the following:

(a) *L. monocytogenes.* **None** of the third-generation cephalosporins is **active** against these organisms. Thus, if these organisms are suspected (e.g., meningitis in the newborn or elderly, or meningitis or sepsis in the immunocompromised dialysis–renal transplant patient), different coverage is needed (e.g., with ampicillin or trimethoprim-sulfamethoxazole [TMP-SMX] in a penicillin- or ampicillin-allergic patient).

(b) Enterococci. **None** of the **cephalosporins inhibits enterococci** (*Enterococcus faecalis* or *Enterococcus faecium*) at concentrations that can readily be achieved.

(c) **Methicillin-resistant *S. aureus* and highly penicillin-resistant *S. pneumoniae.*** See sec. (7).

b. **Gram-negative aerobes**

(1) *H. influenzae* (and other *Haemophilus* spp.) and *N. gonorrhoeae* are extremely susceptible to the third-generation cephalosporins, including strains that produce beta-lactamases.

(2) *N. meningitidis* and *M. catarrhalis* are also very susceptible to the third-generation cephalosporins.

(3) **Enterobacteriaceae.** In the past decade, resistance to cephalosporins has increased in some, but not all, species. In fact, the excellent in vitro activity of the third-generation cephalosporins is a major advantage of these agents over the first- and second-generation cephalosporins. Bacteria resistant to the older cephalosporins and, at times, even the aminoglycosides are often susceptible to the third-generation cephalosporins.

(a) *E. coli,* both community-acquired and hospital-acquired, are usually very susceptible to the third-generation agents (i.e., cefotaxime, ceftizoxime, ceftriaxone, cefepime, and ceftazidime).

(b) Most *Klebsiella* spp. remain susceptible, but resistant strains are appearing in France and South America [46]; occasionally nosocomial strains isolated in the US are resistant (and these usually are susceptible to imipenem).

(c) *P. mirabilis, Providencia* and *Citrobacter* spp., and *P. vulgaris* generally are inhibited by very low concentrations.

(d) *S. marcescens'* susceptibility patterns can vary.

(e) *Enterobacter* spp., especially *E. cloacae,* have been a major weakness of the third-generation cephalosporins [46], and these organisms are important nosocomial pathogens. Approximately 10–30% of *E. cloacae* may initially be resistant to the third-generation cephalosporins, but even the isolates of *E. cloacae* with MICs of 1 μg/ml or less contain subpopulations of organisms that are easily selected for resistance to the third-generation cephalosporins. Presumably, the general use of cephalosporins, including the first- and second-generation cephalosporins, has caused the increase in isolation of this species over the last two decades. Also, *C. freundii* similarly develops resistance, although it has not become as prominent a nosocomial pathogen as *E. cloacae.* (See additional discussion of the clinical implications of this resistance in sec. C.2).

(f) Because of the variability in in vitro susceptibility data, individual susceptibility testing must be performed for each third-generation cephalosporin that may be used by the clinician.

(4) For *P. aeruginosa,* ceftazidime and cefoperazone can be considered potential agents [46]. Because cefoperazone is less active (and has the NMTT side chain), we believe that ceftazidime is the better third-generation cephalosporin for *P. aeruginosa* activity. Ceftazidime's MIC_{90} for *P. aeruginosa* is 8 μg/ml, signifying only modest activity. Some *Pseudomonas cepacia* strains are inhibited by ceftazidime.

Cefepime, released in January 1996, has similar in vitro activity against *P. aeruginosa* as does ceftazidime. See sec. F.

c. **Anaerobes.** Neu [46] noted that there is considerable controversy over the activity of third-generation agents against anaerobic species. A few summary comments are important [46].

(1) The anaerobic activity of cefotaxime, ceftizoxime, and ceftriaxone is suitable for respiratory pathogens (i.e., oral anaerobes).

(2) Neu [46] suggests that none of the third-generation agents currently used in the United States is very effective against pathogens that one would find in a postoperative abscess, after trauma to the abdomen in which the colonic flora has been released into the peritoneum, or if there is leakage of bowel contents after intraabdominal surgery, because none of the agents (except moxalactam) is truly stable to *Bacteroides* beta-lactamase [46].

(3) The second-generation cephalosporins (cefoxitin, cefotetan, and cefmetazole) are more active in vitro against anaerobes than any of the third-generation cephalosporins, but the meaning of this clinically with regard to cefotaxime interacting in vivo with its metabolite is uncertain [see sec. (4)].

(4) Cefotaxime and ceftizoxime have some anaerobic activity that may allow their use in early gynecologic infections [46]. Studies have shown synergy of cefotaxime and its desacetyl metabolite against *B. fragilis* group organisms, with up to 80–85% synergy of cefotaxime-desacetyl-cefotaxime [46]. Neu suggests that the clinical relevance of this synergy is that the presence of desacetylcefotaxime in abscess tissue at the same time as the parent compound increases the range of activity against many anaerobes when compared with either agent alone. Cefotaxime was as effective as cefoxitin at preventing abscesses in an animal model of *B. fragilis* abscess formation [46]. The exact role of cefotaxime in bowel anaerobic infections is still being evaluated. This agent has been shown to be an effective prophylactic agent after penetrating abdominal trauma [46a]. Of interest, cefotaxime is not listed as one of the alternative agents for *B. fragilis* therapy [1].

d. See Tables 28F-2 and 28F-3 for spectrum of activity.

2. **Pharmacokinetics.** Except for the long-acting agents, most of these agents display pharmacokinetics similar to that of cephalothin or cefazolin. Special aspects are discussed under the individual agent. (Also see Table 28F-4.)

3. **Toxicity** (see sec. **V**). **The cephalosporins are usually** very well tolerated.

C. **Potential disadvantages**

1. **Cost.** These are often relatively **expensive agents** in terms of the cost of the antibiotic per gram. However, the cost to use these agents per day, especially those agents with a long half-life, may be quite competitive compared with other agents. See Table 28F-5.

2. **Resistance**

   a. **Mechanisms** of resistance are reviewed elsewhere [2, 46, 50], but a few points warrant emphasis. Microbial resistance to cephalosporins can be mediated by three mechanisms [2] or a combination of these.

      (1) **Alteration of a penicillin-binding protein (PBP) target** that is essential for cell survival. Reduced affinity of PBP for beta-lactam antibiotics is a mechanism by which some *N. gonorrhoeae* and *S. pneumoniae* have become relatively resistant to penicillin and by which MRSA have become resistant to cephalosporins [2].

      (2) **Decreased ability of the antibiotic to reach its PBP target.** Gram-negative bacteria have a complex outer membrane composed of lipids, polysaccharides, and proteins, and this membrane constitutes a barrier to the cephalosporins. Cephalosporins penetrate the outer cell membrane primarily through water-filled channels called *porins* that are formed by various outer membrane proteins. Changes in porins as a consequence of exposure to an antibiotic may reduce penetration further and enhance resistance [2].

      (3) **Production of beta-lactamases that inactivate the cephalosporin.** This is the mechanism by which clinically relevant gram-negative bacteria are **most frequently** resistant to cephalosporins. These inactivating enzymes are encoded chromosomally or extrachromosomally through plasmids or transposons and may be produced constitutionally or may be induced.

         (a) High-level production of TEM-1 or SHV-1 beta-lactamases (common plasmid-mediated beta-lactamases among Enterobacteriaceae) has been associated with resistance to cephalothin, cefamandole, and cefperazone and penicillin–beta-lactamase inhibitor combinations.

         (b) *Enterobacter* spp., *C. freundii, Morganella, Serratia,* and *Providencia* spp., and *P. aeruginosa* **have an inducible chromosomally encoded cephalosporinase** (a Bush group 1-beta-lactamase), which can inactivate all the currently available cephalosporins. The induction or stable de-repression of this chromosomal beta-lactamase during prior exposure to the cephamycins or third-generation cephalosporins results in resistance to all the currently available cephalosporins. Emergence of this form of resistance is especially frequent when infection due to these organisms, especially *E. cloacae* and *P. aeruginosa,* are treated with broad-spectrum cephalosporins [2]. Therefore, it is essential to use these third-generation agents very conservatively, if at all, in infections caused by these pathogens and to avoid any unnecessary use of broad-spectrum cephalosporins that may help select out these organisms.

         (c) New plasmid-mediated extended-spectrum beta-lactamases (ESBLs) have been discovered and have been associated with decreased cephalosporin activity (e.g., especially to ceftazidime) and other beta-lactam agents (aztreonam), especially in *K. pneumoniae.* These strains usually remain susceptible to imipenem [2].

   b. The development of resistance of the original isolate during therapy with one of these agents (i.e., an initially susceptible organism, after days of therapy, is shown by repeat MIC testing to have become resistant), or the selection of resistant bacteria in patients who have received prior cephalosporins, is a growing clinical concern. This phenomenon is **important because it may affect one's decision about whether to use a third-generation agent.**

c. Organisms that may develop resistance during therapy with a third-generation cephalosporin include those listed in sec. **a.(3)(b).** In one report, 29% of *Enterobacter* spp. isolates, especially from patients who had received prior third-generation cephalosporin therapy, were resistant to third-generation cephalosporins. Emergence of resistance during cephalosporin antibiotic therapy occurred in 6% of patients with *Enterobacter* bacteremia [47]. In therapy for *P. aeruginosa* infections, emergence of resistance may occur in 20–30% of patients receiving these agents.

In contrast, the development of resistance during therapy is not a problem with susceptible *E. coli,* most *Klebsiella* spp., and with *Neisseria* spp. or *H. influenzae.*

d. **Clinical implications**

(1) **Therapeutic failures and relapses** can occur if resistance develops while the patient is receiving therapy. For example, a patient may have pneumonia due to *E. cloacae* with a susceptible pretreatment MIC to a third-generation cephalosporin (e.g., 4 µg/ml) but, after 12 days of therapy, *E. cloacae* isolated from sputum has a resistant MIC (e.g., > 64 µg/ml). The patient may deteriorate clinically. Furthermore, cross-resistance to multiple beta-lactam antibiotics is common. In one study, blood cultures revealed multidrug-resistant *Enterobacter* spp. (i.e., resistant to third-generation cephalosporins and extended-spectrum penicillins such as piperacillin). These usually were isolated in patients who had been treated in the preceding 14 days with third-generation cephalosporins. There were higher death rates than were seen in patients with the isolation of more sensitive *Enterobacter* spp. [47].

(2) **Nosocomial spread of these multidrug-resistant pathogens can occur.**

(3) **Intensive care units** (ICUs) may be particularly vulnerable to problems with increased cephalosporin resistance. Because of the heavy use of these cephalosporins in the ICU setting, serious nosocomial infections can occur. (See sec. **E.6.e.**)

(4) **The initial choice of a third-generation cephalosporin must be tempered by this very real potential problem.** Although the clinician may want to avoid using an aminoglycoside in an infection caused by one of the pathogens listed previously [see sec. **2.a(3)(b)**], especially if prolonged therapy is necessary, as in an infection that is difficult to eradicate (e.g., osteomyelitis) or occurring in association with a foreign body (e.g., endotracheal tube, urinary catheter, biliary drainage tube)—in these difficult-to-eradicate infections, the potential to develop resistance must be considered.

In particular, in one article [47], the **authors conclude that in *Enterobacter* bacteremia** "it may be prudent to avoid third-generation cephalosporin therapy regardless of in vitro susceptibility data." They suggested combination therapy (e.g., piperacillin and an aminoglycoside). The editorial response to this paper supports this recommendation and stresses that the **third-generation cephalosporins** "should not be viewed merely as newer cephalosporins with only an expanded spectrum and higher price tag than previous generations. They should be viewed as newer agents that can cause significantly greater problems in the area of multiply resistant pathogens. Because of these negative aspects, newer generation cephalosporins should never be used in settings where older cephalosporins or penicillins are efficacious.** This caution includes both therapeutic and prophylactic use" [51]. Other reviews concur [2a]. Therefore, the third-generation cephalosporins should be reserved for those very special circumstances in which they have a distinct advantage over other antibiotics.

e. **Combination antibiotic** therapy (e.g., an aminoglycoside plus a third-generation cephalosporin or a second beta-lactam antibiotic) does not prevent the development of this form of resistant bacteria. Beta-lactamase inhibitors (e.g., clavulanic acid) also do not solve this problem.

f. **Prevention. The judicious use of the newer antibiotics may help minimize this problem** [2, 46, 47, 51, 52]. Therefore, this resistance problem is another very important reason why formulary committees may want to encourage and monitor the proper use of these cephalosporins.

g. **Therapy** for these resistant prone organisms (e.g., *Enterobacter* spp.) ideally consists of an aminoglycoside and extended penicillin (e.g., piperacillin). Imipenem is another option if organisms are susceptible and is preferred by some [1].

If patients give a history of penicillin allergy, penicillin skin testing may allow use of an extended penicillin (e.g., piperacillin) and an aminoglycoside combination, which is preferable to a third-generation cephalosporin with or without an aminoglycoside.

h. See related discussion under **ceftazidime,** sec. **E.6.e.**

3. **Superinfection** can occur with enterococci or resistant gram-negative bacilli.

4. **Hypoprothrombinemia and bleeding,** at times, may occur (see sec. **V.D**).

D. **Indications for use.** The precise role of these agents continues to evolve. However, their exceptional activity against gram-negative bacilli and clinical experience with these agents provide useful guidelines [1, 2, 5–7, 46, 52–58].

1. **For enteric gram-negative bacillary meningitis** (e.g., due to susceptible *E. coli, Proteus* spp., and *K. pneumoniae*). These infections have been treated successfully with these agents. **In fact, these cephalosporins are probably the agents of choice in such difficult infections,** because high CSF bactericidal levels can be achieved [1, 2, 5, 45]. Except for ceftazidime, these agents are not active enough to treat a *P. aeruginosa* meningitis [59]. (Infectious disease consultation is advised for these difficult infections.)

2. **For empiric therapy for meningitis.** Third-generation cephalosporins are now believed to be the drugs of choice in empiric therapy for meningitis in children and adults [1, 2, 4, 5]. These agents are active against intermediately penicillin-resistant *S. pneumoniae* but, in areas where highly penicillin-resistant *S. pneumoniae* strains have been encountered, vancomycin should be added while awaiting cultures. See Chaps. 5 and 28C.

   a. **Neonates.** Although ampicillin and an aminoglycoside have been used, ampicillin and cefotaxime may be preferable, especially if gram-negative rods are seen on stained smears of the CSF, if cultures demonstrate a susceptible gram-negative pathogen, or if the meningitis occurs in the neonatal ICU (see Chap. 3). **Cefotaxime is preferred to other third-generation cephalosporins for use in neonates** both because it has been used more extensively and because it does not affect bilirubin-albumin binding as does ceftriaxone [4, 45].

   b. **Children.** Although ampicillin and chloramphenicol were used commonly in the past, either **cefotaxime or ceftriaxone** now is favored [1, 4, 5] as the initial drug of choice. See Chap. 5.

   c. **Adults.** Ceftriaxone and cefotaxime are common initial empiric agents. If *L. monocytogenes* is a concern (e.g., in those patients older than 55–60 years, immunocompromised patients), ampicillin (or TMP-SMX in a penicillin-allergic patient) often is added while awaiting cultures [1]. See Chap. 5.

3. **For susceptible gram-negative infections due to bacteria resistant to the first- and second-generation cephalosporins** (such as bacteremia, pneumonia, osteomyelitis, and intraabdominal infections). In this setting, the use of a third-generation agent alone is reasonable. However, the potential development of resistant pathogens must be considered (see sec. **C.2**).

4. **For certain multidrug-resistant bacteria** (e.g., resistant to aminoglycosides) in which separate susceptibility tests indicate the third-generation agent is active.

5. **Serious** bacteremias, pneumonias, empyemas, or other life-threatening **infections in which the enhanced bactericidal activity of the third-generation agents may be extremely desirable.** For example, in a patient with a serious *K. pneumoniae* pneumonia or bacteremia, the enhanced bactericidal activity of these agents may be very beneficial.

6. **For the allergic patient who cannot receive piperacillin or a similar agent along with an aminoglcoside for synergy against *P. aeruginosa.*** Data suggest that double-drug therapy, selected third-generation cephalosporins (e.g., ceftazidime), and an aminoglycoside may be synergistic and so may be useful in this setting [45]. The new agent cefepime may also be combined with an aminoglycoside for possible synergy (see sec. **F**). Penicillin skin testing

may be useful in some patients, especially those with vague allergic histories, for negative skin tests would allow expanded penicillins (e.g., piperacillin) to be used along with an aminoglycoside in an attempt to minimize resistance problems. (See Chap. 27.) Infectious disease consultation is advised in this setting.

7. **For life-threatening *H. influenzae* infections,** while awaiting cultures, a third-generation agent is the agent of choice [1].

8. **For infections due to multiple bacteria in which the third-generation cephalosporin allows the use of a single drug** rather than multiple drugs (e.g., wound infections due to susceptible bacteria).

9. **To be considered as monotherapy in certain settings**
   a. **Serious community-acquired infections** (e.g., pneumonia, UTI, wound infections) in which *Pseudomonas* is not a major concern may be reasonable settings for single-drug therapy. Smith [60] reported that cefotaxime alone was as effective, or more so, and less toxic than nafcillin plus tobramycin for nonneutropenic, noncancer patients with serious infections. Neu [46] has emphasized that cefotaxime and ceftriaxone have adequate antistaphylococcal activity while awaiting culture data in this setting.
   b. **Febrile leukopenic patients who are not bacteremic and are clinically stable** without an obvious focus are reasonable candidates for therapy with third-generation cephalosporins, although the **data are available only for ceftazidime** [61]. (See sec. **E.6.c.**)

10. **For infections due to bacteria for which** a third-generation cephalosporin is the drug of choice. **See Table 28F-9.**

11. Ceftriaxone has been used in the treatment of Lyme disease (see Chap. 23).

E. **Specific third-generation agents.** In addition to the generalizations made in secs. **B** and **D,** some specific points deserve emphasis because they may be useful in choosing a specific agent for a patient or hospital formulary [52–86].

1. **Cefotaxime (Claforan)** became available in the spring of 1981 [52]. Clinical studies have supported its effectiveness in serious infections, including those due to organisms resistant to other cephalosporins [2, 45, 46, 52, 60, 63].
   a. Cefotaxime has a **half-life** of 1 hour in persons with normal renal function but is metabolized to a desacetyl derivative, which has a half-life of 1.6 hours and possesses significant antimicrobial activity and may interact synergistically with its parent compound [3, 45, 46]. Approximately 50–60% of the drug is cleared by the kidney [49]. Cefotaxime given intravenously provides good CSF bactericidal levels against susceptible pathogens [2]. Serum levels of 200 µg/ml are achieved after a 2-g IV infusion. Cefotaxime can be given intramuscularly but, in the seriously ill patient, the intravenous route is preferred.
   b. **Dosage**
      (1) **Adults.** In his review, Neu [46] suggested that based on its pharmacologic properties and in vitro activity against susceptible pathogens, cefotaxime can be used at a dose of 1 or 2 g q8h depending on the severity of the infection (although the package insert allows up to 2 g q4h for life-threatening infections and 2 g q6–8h for severe infection). Of interest, because the half-life of cefotaxime increases as renal function declines, when the creatinine clearance is 30–50 ml/min (e.g., in many elderly patients with even normal serum creatinines), a dose every 12 hours may often be adequate.
         See Chap. 13 for dosages in gonorrhea regimens.
      (2) **Children.** For body weights of less than 50 kg, 50–180 mg/kg body weight per day IV is divided into four to six equal doses. The higher dosages are for the more serious infections, including meningitis. Based on the data presented in section (1), a dosage regimen of every 6 hours (rather than every 4 hours) seems reasonable in children. In children weighing more than 50 kg, the usual adult dosages can be used.
      (3) **Neonates.** See Chap. 3.
   c. **Renal failure.** Although the half-life of cefotaxime is not significantly increased with renal failure, its desacetyl and other metabolites accumulate appreciably so reduced cefotaxime dosing is warranted with severe azotemia [2]. Dosages are shown in Table 28F-6. The regular dose can be given at prolonged intervals (every 8–12 hours) when the creatinine

clearance is 10–50 ml/min, or a regular dose can be administered every 24 hours if the creatinine clearance is less than 10 ml/min [8]. After a 4- to 6-hour hemodialysis, approximately 50% of the drug is removed. Therefore, a supplemental dose of one-half of the loading dose can be given after hemodialysis. In patients undergoing CAPD, 1 g daily has been suggested [8].

   d. **Neonatal infections.** Cefotaxime combined with ampicillin is a combination of choice for empiric therapy of neonatal and infant meningitis (see sec. **D.2**). It is also an important agent in empiric therapy for meningitis of children [1]. In neonates, cefotaxime does not interfere with the metabolism of bilirubin, as ceftriaxone may.

   e. **Summary.** Cefotaxime remains a useful and important agent in children and adults.

   (1) **For neonatal infections, it is often the preferred third-generation cephalosporin,** as there is a great deal of experience with this agent in this population and it does not interfere with bilirubin metabolism.

   (2) **In children and adults,** although it is a useful agent, it has often been replaced by ceftriaxone, which can be given once a day in most infections (every 12 hours in meningitis) and is therefore often more cost-effective and more convenient to administer.

2. **Moxalactam (Moxam)** became available in the fall of 1981. **Bleeding disorders were reported subsequently as a complication.** Because of this well-recognized complication, **most experts now avoid this agent,** as there are many other third-generation cephalosporins from which to choose [1, 2, 45]. The proposed mechanisms and bleeding problems are discussed in sec. **V.** This agent has not been available in the United States since 1991.

3. **Cefoperazone (Cefobid)** was released in early 1983. See Andriole and Kirby [64] for an update of this agent.

   a. **Spectrum of activity.** In vitro, it is less active than cefotaxime against many Enterobacteriaceae but is more active against *P. aeruginosa*. Its activity against *Pseudomonas* is similar to that of piperacillin. Although active against many anaerobes, it is less active than cefoxitin against *B. fragilis* [53]. Studies vary, but 60% [45] to 85% of strains [65] of *P. aeruginosa* are considered susceptible to cefoperazone; the MIC_{90} is high at 32–64 µg/ml [45, 46, 65]. **Ceftazidime is more active in vitro, with a MIC_{90} (against *P. aeruginosa*) of 4–8 µg/ml** [45, 46]. Furthermore, over time, staphylococci (both coagulase-positive and coagulase-negative) resistance to cefoperazone is increasing [65].

   b. **Pharmacokinetics.** The drug is eliminated by biliary excretion so that **dosages do not require adjustment in renal failure.** The half-life of 1.8 hours may be prolonged in hepatic failure [53]. The half-life of cefoperazone is slightly reduced by hemodialysis, and dosing should be scheduled to follow a dialysis period, per the package insert.

   c. **Dosages.** For serious infections, 6–12 g daily (1.5–4.0 g q6–12h) is suggested [53]. In hepatic disease, dose adjustments may be necessary (i.e., increasing the dose interval to every 12 hours) [56]. Safety and efficacy in children have not been established. In patients with both hepatic and renal dysfunction, the package insert advises that the dosage should not exceed 1–2 g/day without close monitoring of serum levels.

   d. **Side effects. Hypoprothrombinemia with bleeding can occur** and can be reversed with vitamin K. (See sec. **V** for detailed discussion.)

   e. **Summary. We have little enthusiasm for this third-generation cephalosporin agent for several reasons.**

   (1) Other third-generation cephalosporins are more active against Enterobacteriaceae, and the MIC_{90} to *P. aeruginosa* is high compared with ceftazidime or cefepime. One reviewer concludes that cefoperazone does not have an important role in the treatment of serious infections caused by *P. aeruginosa* [2].

   (2) This agent has the NMTT side chain potentially associated with hypoprothrombinemia and bleeding (see sec. **V.D**). If used, prothrombin times would need to be monitored or vitamin K administered as indicated per the package insert, especially in high-risk patients. See Table 28F-8.

   (3) Although double beta-lactam agents have been and are being studied

in the treatment of febrile leukopenic patients [64], so has monotherapy with a third-generation cephalosporin (e.g., ceftazidime; see sec. **6**). In a commentary on this double-lactam antibiotic (e.g., cefoperazone and piperacillin) approach [66], it was noted that the major disadvantages are the occasional selection of resistant organisms, high cost, possibility of antagonism of some combinations with certain bacterial infections, and possible inadequate antistaphylococcal activity. Therefore, although a consideration, we see no major advantage of this approach.

(4) Cefoperazone's penetration into the CSF is relatively low, so its use in meningitis is not recommended.

4. Ceftizoxime (Cefizox) became available in 1983.

a. Spectrum of activity. In vitro, its activity against Enterobacteriaceae is very similar to that of cefotaxime [46, 54]. Many anaerobes are susceptible to ceftizoxime, but it is less active than cefoxitin against *B. fragilis* [54].

b. Pharmacokinetics. Although cefotaxime and ceftizoxime reach similar serum peaks, the latter is not metabolized in the liver and has a longer half-life (1.5 hours), allowing for less frequent dosing. Ceftizoxime is excreted primarily by the kidney. It penetrates tissues well, including the CSF.

c. Dosages

(1) Adults with severe infections: 2 g q8–12h is suggested. In life-threatening infections, 3–4 g q8h is suggested [54].

(2) Children. See Table 28F-6.

(3) Renal failure necessitates dosage reductions [8]. A standard dose can be given at prolonged intervals, as shown in Table 28F-6. In patients undergoing hemodialysis, no additional supplemental dosing is required following hemodialysis; however, dosing should be timed so that the patient is given the dose at the end of dialysis (per package insert).

d. Side effects (see sec. **V**). A disulfiramlike reaction and bleeding problems have not occurred with this agent.

e. Summary. This agent is very similar to cefotaxime but has a longer half-life, which permits dosing every 8–12 hours. However, ceftriaxone has an even longer half-life, allowing once- or twice-daily dosing, as discussed in sec. **5.e.** Many clinicians, ourselves included, prefer ceftriaxone because of its cost-effective and easier dosing schedules.

5. Ceftriaxone (Rocephin) has the longest half-life of the currently available third-generation cephalosporins, making once- or twice-daily dosing legitimate [55, 57]. In addition, it maintains the enhanced spectrum of activity of the newer agents. Rather than just a "me too" drug, in a symposium Moellering [57] argued that this agent represented a "major milestone" in antibiotic therapy; we agree. Therefore, this agent is discussed in some detail.

a. Spectrum of activity. See detailed discussion in sec. **III.B.1.** See Tables 28F-2 and 28F-3 for details on when ceftriaxone is the drug of choice for certain pathogens.

(1) Gram-positive aerobes. Ceftriaxone is very active against *S. pneumoniae*, including strains with intermediate resistance to penicillin but not those with high-level penicillin resistance (see Chap. 28C), and streptococci groups A and B. Although it is not as active as the first- or second-generation cephalosporins against methicillin-susceptible *S. aureus*, it has reasonable MICs for *S. aureus* (usually 4.0 µg/ml) (see Table 28F-2) but may not have uniform MICs for methicillin-susceptible *S. aureus* as would nafcillin or oxacillin. **It is not a useful agent against** enterococci, *L. monocytogenes,* or coagulase-negative or methicillin-resistant staphylococci [46, 67].

(2) Gram-negative aerobes. As with other third-generation cephalosporins, ceftriaxone is very active against *H. influenzae* and *N. gonorrhoeae* (including beta-lactamase producers), *N. meningitidis,* and most Enterobacteriaceae (i.e., *E. coli* and *Klebsiella, Serratia,* and *Proteus* spp.) [46, 67]. It is not very active against *Acinetobacter* and *Pseudomonas* spp.

(3) Anaerobes. Ceftriaxone is not as active as cefoxitin, cefotetan, or cefmetazole against anaerobes (especially *B. fragilis*).

(4) Spirochetes. Ceftriaxone (and cefotaxime) is active against *B. burgdorferi* (Lyme disease pathogen) [1, 68]. See Chap. 23.

b. **Pharmacokinetics**
  (1) **Prolonged half-life. The unique feature of ceftriaxone is its long elimination half-life** (6–8 hours in normal volunteers), which is by far the longest half-life of any available cephalosporin [69]. **This allows for safe once- or twice-daily dosing regimens.** Ceftriaxone can be given intramuscularly or intravenously. In the seriously ill patient, the intravenous route is preferred. For example, a single 2-g dose IV in volunteers produces plasma levels over a 24-hour period that exceed the inhibitory levels of *S. pneumoniae, S. pyogenes,* methicillin-susceptible *S. aureus, H. influenzae, Neisseria* spp., and 90% of Enterobacteriaceae [67]. Peaks exceed 200–250 μg/ml, with troughs in the 10- to 15-μg/ml range [69]. Using 2 g q24h results in average steady-state plasma concentrations comparable to those observed with 1 g q12h [69]. With a 1-g IV dose, peaks of up to 150 μg/ml and 24-hour troughs of 9 μg/ml can be achieved [39]. Doses do not have to be altered for the elderly or in patients with liver disease and moderate renal dysfunction.
  (2) **Excretion.** Ceftriaxone is **excreted primarily by the kidney.** High concentrations of the drug are achieved in the urine even 24–48 hours after a single dose. However, **dose adjustments are necessary only in very severe renal failure.** Children appear to eliminate the drug more rapidly than adults. Because nonrenal elimination of ceftriaxone occurs through biliary secretion of unchanged drug, **very high** and sustained **levels** are obtained in **unobstructed biliary tract.**
  (3) **Concentration in bodily fluids.** Ceftriaxone penetrates bodily fluids well. Excellent CSF bactericidal levels are achieved against susceptible pathogens [1, 4, 5, 45]. Transfer to placenta and breast milk occurs.
c. **Clinical studies**
  (1) Data suggest that ceftriaxone is a **drug of choice** for **empiric therapy of meningitis in children** [1, 4, 5]. For meningitis, an every-12-hour regimen is preferred. See Chaps. 3 and 5. (In geographic areas where high-level penicillin-resistant *S. pneumoniae* strains are a concern, vancomycin often is added until susceptibility data are available. See Chap. 28C.)
  (2) As a single agent given intravenously or intramuscularly once daily, ceftriaxone has been shown to be very effective for serious infections, including hospitalized patients, pneumonia, bacteremias, bone and joint infections, and skin and soft-tissue infections [45, 55, 70–74].
  (3) Once-daily therapy has also been used to allow home-outpatient therapy [73]. Because of its excellent in vitro activity against viridans streptococci, ceftriaxone once daily is a useful home intravenous agent in clinically stable patients with endocarditis due to this pathogen [75]. See Chap. 10.
  (4) Single low-dose intramuscular therapy is an excellent regimen in the treatment of uncomplicated gonorrhea in women [15]. See Chap. 13. Ceftriaxone therapy has also been shown to be effective for gonococcal ophthalmia neonatorum [15]; see Chap. 6.
  (5) Ceftriaxone has been used successfully in the therapy of **Lyme disease** (see Chap. 23) [1, 68].
  (6) Intramuscular ceftriaxone as a single dose has been suggested for treatment of acute otitis media in children, but this is controversial [75a]. Until further data clarify its use in this setting, we do not favor single-dose therapy in acute otitis media. In a setting where compliance with a usual 10-day oral regimen is extremely unlikely, a single dose of ceftriaxone may be a rational compromise but a second-line approach.
d. **Side effects.** Ceftriaxone appears to be a well-tolerated and safe agent [76, 77].
  (1) **Typical side effects** seen with any cephalosporin can occur with ceftriaxone (see sec. **V**). There is one report of a disulfiramlike reaction in a recipient of ceftriaxone [77]. **Ceftriaxone does not contain the NMTT side chain.**
  (2) **Cholecystitislike symptoms.** Ceftriaxone has the **unique ability to** cause sludge (also referred to as **"biliary pseudolithiasis"**) to form in

the gallbladder, particularly in children [77]. Associated symptoms may include nausea, epigastric distress, vomiting, and right upper quadrant tenderness. Biliary ultrasound studies show shadows suggesting sludge. Actual gallstones composed primarily of ceftriaxone have been described [78]. Symptoms subside with discontinuation of ceftriaxone, and conservative therapy is advised. The exact mechanism by which ceftriaxone induces sludge is unclear but is presumably related to the very high levels of ceftriaxone that can occur in bile (up to 100–200 times that found in serum) so that the solubility of the salt in bile is exceeded and precipitation occurs [78]. Persons with impaired gallbladder emptying (e.g., those with poor oral intake or on total parenteral nutrition) and those on maximal doses may be at a higher risk of developing biliary deposition that otherwise seems to be uncommon [78], especially in adults.

(3) **In neonates,** because ceftriaxone binds to serum proteins and may displace bilirubin, **ceftriaxone is not advised; cefotaxime is preferred** [77, 79].

e. **Dosages (intramuscular or intravenous)**

(1) **Adults.** The usual dose is 1–2 g once daily depending on the severity of infection. Because of the high peak serum levels achieved with a 1-g dose (i.e., 150 μg/ml), in all but life-threatening illness and meningitis we have commonly been using a 1-g/day dose, which is more cost-effective. The total daily dose should not exceed 4 g/day in life-threatening infections (e.g., 2 g q12h in meningitis in adults). In meningitis, an every-12-hour regimen is recommended.

(2) **Children.** For meningitis, a daily dose of 100 mg/kg/day (not to exceed 4 g), given in divided doses q12h, should be administered, usually with a loading dose of 75 mg/kg. In other serious infections, 50–75 mg/kg/day (not to exceed 2 g) in divided doses q12h is suggested.

(3) **Neonates.** Cefotaxime is preferred.

f. **Renal or hepatic dysfunction.** Because of the nonrenal (biliary) pathway of elimination, doses of ceftriaxone do not need reduction as long as the creatinine clearance is 5 ml/min or greater. In anephric patients, plasma concentrations should be monitored [8, 69].

Dose adjustments are not necessary in patients with liver disease and normal renal function. **If both hepatic and renal failure are present, the half-life of ceftriaxone is prolonged** significantly and accumulation can occur. In this setting, serum levels should ideally be monitored if alternate drugs are not available. If serum levels are not available and ceftriaxone is clearly the agent of choice, we have used a reduced dose (e.g., 500 mg/day) in non-CNS infections.

g. **Dialysis.** Hemodialysis does not significantly reduce serum levels [8, 69]. Ideally, serum levels should be monitored [8]; a dose of 500 mg/day may be a prudent regimen for non-CNS infections (while awaiting serum levels). In patients undergoing CAPD, a dose of 750 mg q12h has been suggested [8].

h. **Summary and conclusions. This is a very useful agent because** it:

(1) Maintains an expanded spectrum (similar to that of the third-generation agents already discussed).

(2) Has the longest half-life, allowing legitimate once-daily dosing or at least every-12-hour dosing, even in life-threatening infections (e.g., meningitis).

(3) Has the potential of cost-effective therapy when compared with more frequently administered agents (see Table 28F-5).

(4) Lacks the NMTT side chain associated with bleeding tendencies.

(5) Penetrates the CNS well.

(6) Has the potential for cost-effective outpatient use (e.g., patients who are clinically stable and have infections involving protracted courses such as gram-negative bone infections or selected cases of viridans streptococcal endocarditis) [75].

(7) Is a useful agent in gonococcal infection (Chap. 13), meningitis (Chap. 5), and Lyme disease (Chap. 23), as empiric therapy for intraabdominal infections (Chap. 11), and is the drug of choice for certain bacteria. See Table 28F-9.

6. **Ceftazidime (Fortaz, Tazidime, or Tazicef)** was released in the United States in July 1985 [80].
   a. **Spectrum of activity.** This has been reviewed in part in sec. **B.1.** Overall, the activity of ceftazidime against gram-positive cocci and anaerobes is inferior to that of most other third-generation agents [45] (see Table 28F-2). **Ceftazidime is the most active available cephalosporin against** *P. aeruginosa,* because it will inhibit 90% of strains at concentrations less than 8 μg/ml, especially in community and smaller hospitals [46]. However, this is a fairly high MIC, and resistance may develop during therapy. See sec. **C.2. Cefepime is also active against** *P. aeruginosa.* See sec. **F.**

      It is active against Enterobacteriaceae, similar to cefotaxime (see sec. **B.1**). Ceftazidime is more active against *P. aeruginosa* than are the antipseudomonal penicillins (e.g., piperacillin) [81].
   b. It is **excreted by the kidney,** and the half-life of 1.8 hours allows for dosing every 8–12 hours. A single 2-g dose IV will provide peak serum levels of approximately 180–190 μg/ml. It penetrates tissues well and has been used successfully in the treatment of meningitis [82], including *P. aeruginosa* meningitis [83].
   c. **Clinical role**
      (1) **Combination therapy for** *P. aeruginosa* **in penicilin-allergic patients.** For enhanced *P. aeruginosa* activity in the patient in whom ticarcillin or piperacillin cannot be used because of a delayed (late) penicillin allergy, ceftazidime can be combined with an aminoglycoside for possible synergy [45].
      (2) **Consideration for monotherapy**
         (a) *Pseudomonas* **UTI,** if susceptible, generally will respond well.
         (b) **Nonbacteremic, febrile leukopenic patients without an obvious focus** often are given antibiotic combinations (e.g., piperacillin and an aminoglycoside) (see Chap. 2). Ceftazidime alone has been found effective [61, 62, 66]. We would treat leukopenic patients with known or highly suspected gram-negative bacteremia with double-drug therapy to provide synergy. See Chap. 2.
         (c) **Selected cases of nosocomial pneumonia. If a Gram stain of sputum or culture can rule out** *S. aureus,* **ceftazidime may be a reasonable agent for very early gram-negative nosocomial pneumonias,** especially if an aminoglycoside is contraindicated [84]. For serious, well-established *P. aeruginosa* pneumonia, combination therapy (e.g., with an aminoglycoside) is necessary. (See Chap. 9.) Because the **development of resistance while on therapy with ceftazidime alone is also a concern** (see sec. **e**), we are very conservative and selective about the use of monotherapy with ceftazidime in this setting.
         (d) **Cystic fibrosis pulmonary infections.** Because of its enhanced activity against *P. aeruginosa* and, to a lesser extent, *P. cepacia,* ceftazidime has been useful in cystic fibrosis patients with pulmonary exacerbations. Early results were encouraging, and ceftazidime alone seemed as effective as, if not more so than, ticarcillin and tobramycin in this setting [81]. However, this is a difficult and special clinical problem. As with almost any antibiotic regimen in difficult-to-eradicate *P. aeruginosa* infections, resistance commonly occurs with prolonged therapy. (See sec. **e.**)
         (e) *Pseudomonas aeruginosa* **meningitis** has been treated successfully with intravenous ceftazidime [1, 2, 59, 82]. Infectious disease consultation is advised for this difficult problem.
         (f) **Malignant external otitis** has been treated successfully with ceftazidime [85].
   d. **Dosages** are summarized in Table 28F-6.
      (1) The **usual dose** of ceftazidime **in adults** for moderately severe infections is 1–2 g IV q8–12h. For serious or life-threatening infections, the maximum dose of 2 g q8h should be used [80]. **For children,** 30–50 mg/kg per dose IV q8h (to a maximum of 6 g/day) is customary. The higher dosage is used in immunocompromised children or in children with cystic fibrosis or meningitis. For dosages in neonates, see Chap. 3.

(2) **In renal failure,** doses must be modified. The manufacturer recommends that in adults, for creatinine clearances of 31–50 ml/min, 1 g q12h should be used. For a creatinine clearance of 16–30 ml/min, 1 g q24h is recommended. A dose of 500 mg is given once daily if the creatinine clearance is 6–15 ml/min, and once every 48 hours in the anephric patient.

(3) **In adult patients undergoing hemodialysis,** a loading dose of 1 g followed by 1 g after each dialysis session can be used. Ceftazidime, 500 mg q24h, is recommended for patients undergoing CAPD after a 1-g loading dose [8].

e. **Development of resistance.** As with any third-generation cephalosporin, resistance may develop over time, not only for a given patient but for isolates from a given hospital or part of a hospital (e.g., ICU). For example, after the introduction and use of ceftazidime in July 1986, the percentage of ceftazidime-susceptible hospital isolates of *P. aeruginosa, Citrobacter* spp., and *Enterobacter* spp. declined by mid-1988 from approximately 95% of strains susceptible to 50–70% of strains susceptible. After restrictions of ceftazidime use were instituted, susceptibility to ceftazidime improved [86]. In another study, multidrug-resistant *Enterobacter* bacteremia was correlated with ceftazidime use [47]. These data and related **data emphasize the need to use these third-generation cephalosporins wisely. Otherwise, their in vitro activity appears to decrease and therefore their clinical usefulness decreases if they are used excessively.** To help minimize this problem, many hospitals have antibiotic approval programs to try to curb excess use of the third-generation cephalosporins. See related discussion of resistance in sec. **III.C.2.**

f. **Side effects.** See sec. **V.** Ceftazidime has not been associated with bleeding problems and **does not have the NMTT side chain** [80].

F. **New expanded-spectrum cephalosporin. Cefepime (Maxipime)** was approved for use in mid-January 1996. It has recently been reviewed [86a–86c]. It is resistant to hydrolysis by Bush 1 beta-lactamases and many plasma-mediated extended-spectrum beta-lactamases [2, 86a], so it maintains activity against many gram-negative organisms resistant to third-generation agents and other beta-lactam antibiotics.

1. **Spectrum of activity.** Cefepime has a broader spectrum of activity than the third-generation cephalosporins and has been referred to as a prototypical **fourth-generation cephalosporin** by some [86c]. It has activity against gram-positive organisms comparable to cefotaxime and activity against gram-negative aerobic organisms comparable or superior to ceftazidime [86c]. It exerts its antibacterial effects by binding to PBPs. See Tables 28F-2 and 28F-3.

a. Regarding **gram-positive organisms,** cefepime is active (MIC_{90} data) against *S. pneumoniae* (≤ 0.25 µg/ml), including many strains resistant to penicillin, *S. pyogenes* (0.10–0.25 µg/ml), *S. agalactiae* (< 0.25 µg/ml), and methicillin-susceptible *S. aureus* (2.8–8.0 µg/ml). Methicillin-resistant *S. epidermidis,* MRSA, and enterococci are resistant. Cefepime is less active than the first- and second-generation cephalosporins against methicillin susceptible *S. aureus.*

b. **Against Enterobacteriaceae,** cefepime is very active. Among the organisms affected are *E. coli* (≤ 0.2 µg/ml), *K. pneumoniae* (2.0 µg/ml), and *Salmonella* spp. (0.12 µg/ml), as well as typically more resistant species such as *Enterobacter aerogenes* (1 µg/ml), *E. cloacae* (1 µg/ml), *C. freundii* (0.5 µg/ml), and *S. marcescens* (0.5 µg/ml).

c. Cefepime is active against *H. influenzae* (0.06 µg/ml), including beta-lactamase producers.

d. It is active against many strains of *P. aeruginosa* (6.4–13.8 µg/ml), similar to the in vitro activity of ceftazidime [86a, 86c].

e. It is not active against *B. fragilis.*

2. **Pharmacokinetics** [86a, 86c].

a. **Serum levels.** In healthy volunteers, a 2-g IM dose of cefepime provides a peak serum level of approximately 60 µg/ml, whereas 2 g IV reaches a peak of 130–140 µg/ml.

b. The elimination **half-life** is approximately 2 hours. Cefepime distributes widely into body tissues and fluids. Cefepime penetrates the CSF as do other third-generation cephalosporins, but experience in treating gram-negative bacillary meningitis is limited [86c].

   c. **Excretion** is primarily by **renal** mechanisms as unchanged drug. In renal failure, dosage reduction is necessary when the creatinine clearance is less than 60 ml/min. Hemodialysis and hemofiltration remove cefepime; continuous peritoneal dialysis removes cefepime to a lesser extent. Dose adjustment is not required in patients with hepatic dysfunction [86c].

3. **Clinical studies** suggest efficacy for bacteremia, upper and lower respiratory tract infections, UTI, and skin, bone, and gynecologic infections [86a]. When combined with an active anaerobic agent, cefepime has been used for intraabdominal infections. Many of the initial studies show similar efficacy of cefepime to that for ceftazidime. In addition, cefepime, in preliminary studies, has been effective as monotherapy in the febrile leukopenic patient without an obvious focus of infection [86a].

4. **Approved indications** for cefepime include:
   a. **Uncomplicated and complicated UTIs** caused by susceptible *E. coli* or *K. pneumoniae* when infection is severe, or *E. coli, K. pneumoniae*, or *P. mirabilis* when infection is mild to moderate.
   b. **Uncomplicated skin and skin structure** infections caused by methicillin-susceptible *S. aureus* or *S. pyogenes*.
   c. **Moderate to severe pneumonia** caused by *S. pneumoniae, K. pneumoniae, P. aeruginosa* (cefepime is usually combined with an aminoglycoside), or *Enterobacter* spp. (although resistance may occur; see related sec. **C.2**). See package insert also.

5. **Dosages**
   a. **For adults** usually 1–2 g IV or IM q12h is used depending on the severity of infection. In clinical trials, 2 g q8h has been used in the therapy of febrile leukopenic patients and *P. aeruginosa* pneumonias [86c]. Also, 500 mg q12h has been used in mild to moderately severe UTI.
   b. **In renal failure,** the package insert suggests normal doses can be used when the creatinine clearance is ≥ 60 ml/min. When the usual dose of 1–2 g given q12h is indicated: (1) for a creatinine clearance of 30–60 ml/min, the usual dose is given q24h; (2) for a creatinine clearance of 11–29 ml/min, 50% of the usual dose is given q24h; and (3) if the creatinine clearance is < 10 ml/min, 25% of the usual dose is given q24h. In patients undergoing hemodialysis, about 50% of cefepime is removed with the usual 3-hour dialysis and a repeat dose, equal to the initial dose, is suggested after each dialysis (per package insert). In patients undergoing continuous ambulatory peritoneal dialysis (CAPD), cefepime may be given at normal doses q48h (per package insert).
   c. **Pediatric use.** Cefepime is not recommended in children under 12 years although it has been studied in patients with cystic fibrosis [86a, 86c].

6. **Side effects.** In preliminary studies, cefepime has been **well tolerated,** with a safety profile similar to other cephalosporins (e.g., ceftazidime). **Gastrointestinal** side effects are the **most common,** including nausea (1.8%), diarrhea (1.7%), vomiting (1.5%), and constipation (1.2%). Headache (3.2%) and rash (1.8%) have been noted [86a]. Clinically relevant laboratory abnormalities were observed infrequently. The package insert notes that about 1.5% of patients discontinued cefepime due to adverse reactions in clinical trials.

7. **Summary.** The exact role for cefepime awaits further clinical study and experience. When susceptibility data allow, cefepime may permit the clinician to use a cephalosporin to treat infections resistant to other cephalosporin agents or other beta-lactam antibiotics.

   Cefepime is a broad-spectrum antibiotic. As with other broad-spectrum agents (e.g., imipenem, piperacillin-tazobactam), if these agents are used excessively, bacterial resistance presumably will develop. (See related discussions in sec. **III.C.2** and Chap. 28A).

   In difficult-to-treat infections (e.g., those associated with a foreign body), the development of resistance is a particular concern. In one review, the authors emphasize that although cefepime may help treat some infections resistant to currently available beta-lactam antibiotics, if cefepime is used "as injudiciously as the [current] third-generation cephalosporins," the usefulness of this new agent will be temporary: resistance will probably soon develop. They emphasize that "the rational and limited use of all antimicrobial agents may be the best long-term approach since resistance and drug use are directly and inevitably associated" [86b].

G. The **third-generation cephalosporins** are **not** indicated for:

1. **Empiric single-agent therapy in hospital-acquired sepsis of unknown etiology.** In this setting, *P. aeruginosa* or resistant gram-negative bacteria are potential pathogens. An aminoglycoside should be part of the antibiotic combination until culture data become available in these septic-appearing patients.

   Even in the elderly, an aminoglycoside can be used safely for 48 hours while awaiting culture results. Short-term aminoglycosides are not toxic. Also, ceftazidime has relatively poor *S. aureus* activity (and is not active against MRSA). (See Chap. 2.) In a patient with moderate to severe underlying hepatic disease in whom one would like to avoid an aminoglycoside (see Chap. 28H), aztreonam is an option for activity against gram-negatives. Imipenem is used in some settings if hospital-acquired bacteria have multidrug-resistant problems.

2. **Single-agent therapy in severe *P. aeruginosa* infections.** Although some of these third-generation agents have modest activity against *P. aeruginosa* and may provide adequate therapy in UTI, ceftazidime or cefepime should not be used as single agents for life-threatening pneumonia, bacteremias, or wound infections due to this pathogen. Ceftazidime is reasonable monotherapy in *P. aeruginosa* meningitis [5, 59, 82], but infectious disease consultation is advised for this unusual and difficult problem.

3. **Enterococcal infections.** The third-generation agents are not effective for enterococcal infections.

4. **Severe infections due to *E. cloacae* and *Acinetobacter calcoaceticus*.** Resistance may develop during therapy (see sec. **C.2**). Therefore, MIC and serum bactericidal levels ideally should be tested before one relies on these agents for infections due to these pathogens.

5. **Routine surgical prophylaxis.** The third-generation agents are not recommended for routine surgical prophylaxis (see Chap. 28B). These agents are more expensive, usually have less activity against *S. aureus* than older agents, and have not been shown to be superior in this setting.

6. **Severe intraabdominal sepsis** usually requires combination antibiotics or monotherapy with a drug such as imipenem.

IV. **Oral cephalosporins.** Even though these agents are among the most expensive, they are among the most commonly used oral antibiotics. Several years ago, the Veterans Administration Ad Hoc Interdisciplinary Advisory Committee on Antimicrobial Usage [87] stressed that there are "very few instances in which [older first-generation oral cephalosporins] are the primary drugs of choice for any infection. Less expensive and equally effective drugs should be used unless the organism is resistant to, or the patient exhibits an untoward reaction to, the agent of first choice." Although this concept is still valid, some of the initially preferred agents (e.g., dicloxacillin) have sufficient side effects (e.g., nausea, midepigastric discomfort) that oral cephalosporin agents (with fewer GI side effects) may be preferred to improve compliance. For example, in one report, Ruff and colleagues [88] studied the taste and aftertaste of 14 commonly prescribed antimicrobial suspensions, as taste perception is considered to be the single most important factor in achieving compliance in children. The three cephalosporin suspensions—cefixime (Suprax), cephalexin (Keflex), and cefaclor (Ceclor)—were superior in overall acceptability when compared with the other agents. The authors believed that taste should be considered when selecting an antimicrobial suspension or liquid formulation for use in children. They are also useful in penicillin-allergic patients. **These agents are useful in certain soft-tissue infections, UTIs, and in the special settings discussed.** See Table 28F-10, which summarizes their clinical role.

A. **First-generation agents [10]**

1. **Cephalexin (Keflex)**

   a. **Spectrum of activity.** This agent is active against methicillin-susceptible *S. aureus*, penicillin-susceptible *S. pneumoniae*, and *S. pyogenes*. It is not active against enterococci. The majority of urinary isolates of community-acquired *E. coli, Klebsiella* spp., and *P. mirabilis* are susceptible. Cephalexin is not active against *P. aeruginosa, S. marcescens,* or *Enterobacter* spp. It is not very active against *H. influenzae*.

   b. **Pharmacokinetics.** Cephalexin is very well absorbed, even in the presence of food. After a 500-mg oral dose, peak serum levels of 13–18 µg/ml are achieved. This provides blood levels adequate for susceptible gram-positive bacteria that cause soft-tissue infections (e.g., minor wounds or pharyngitis). The drug is excreted in the urine unchanged, so high urinary concentrations are achieved.

Table 28F-10. Common clinical uses of oral cephalosporins

Setting	Useful agent[a]	Comment[b]
Soft-tissue infections, cellulitis	First-generation agent preferred (e.g., cephalexin, cephradine)	When *S. aureus* and streptococci activity is desired. Provides poor gram-negative tissue levels. (Cefixime and ceftibuten have poor *S. aureus* activity; good gram-negative activity)
Otitis media, sinusitis	Cefaclor, cefuroxime, cefprozil[c]; cefixime,[c] ceftibuten[c]	Useful in delayed penicillin-allergic patients and when ampicillin-resistant *H. influenzae* are known or highly suspected. Cefixime and ceftibuten are less active against *S. pneumoniae*
Bronchitis	Cefaclor, cefuroxime, cefprozil,[c] loracarbef[c]	Alternative agents for delayed penicillin-allergic patients or patients on rotating antibiotic regimens. Cefixime and ceftibuten are not as active against *S. pneumoniae*
Streptococcal pharyngitis	First-generation agent; cefuroxime[d]	Alternative in the penicillin-allergic patient
Urinary tract infection	Cephalexin, cephradine Cefaclor, cefuroxime, loracarbef[c] Cefixime	When susceptibility data support use
Community-acquired pneumonia	Cefuroxime	For completion of therapy when intravenous cefuroxime has been required (see text); selected cases for oral therapy (see Chap. 9)

[a]Agent is usually not the drug of choice; often useful in the patient with a delayed penicillin allergy.
[b]See text discussion for details.
[c]See text for discussion of potential limitations of use in this setting.
[d]See Chap. 7.

c. **Uses.** Cephalexin is therefore **a useful agent in the treatment of UTI due to susceptible gram-negative organisms and minor *S. aureus* and streptococcal soft-tissue infections.** Because of the relatively high MICs of the susceptible gram-negative organisms and relatively low serum levels, this agent is not useful in soft-tissue infections due to gram-negative bacteria. Other oral agents are available. The role of cephalexin as oral therapy in osteomyelitis is undergoing study, but acceptable bactericidal levels against *S. aureus* are potentially achievable, and further studies are needed to determine the role of cephalexin in this setting [89].

d. **Dosage.** The usual adult dosage is 250–500 mg q6h. Based on one report, when maximal activity of cephalexin is desired in adults, 1 g q6h is a potentially useful dose [89]. In children, 25–50 mg/kg/day is divided into four equal doses.

e. **Renal failure.** In severe renal failure with a creatinine clearance of less than 10 ml/min, the dose interval is prolonged to every 12 hours.

2. **Cephradine (Anspor, Velosef)** is considered **an equivalent of cephalexin** with similar spectrum of activity, pharmacokinetics, and dosages.

a. **Renal failure.** In renal failure, dosages must be reduced. If the creatinine clearance exceeds 30 ml/min, no change is necessary. If the creatinine clearance is 15–30 ml/min, a dose is given q8–12h. If the clearance is 5–15 ml/min, the dose interval is 24–48 hours. With a creatinine clearance of less than 5 ml/min, a dose is given every 48–60 hours.

b. **Cost.** This agent may be available at a lower price than cephalexin to hospital pharmacies and therefore may be preferred. (See Table 28A-5.)

3. **Cefadroxil (Duricef)** is another analogue of cephalexin. It is promoted for UTIs and skin and soft-tissue infections [90]. A potential advantage is that doses can be given less frequently than most oral cephalosporins.

a. **Spectrum of activity.** This is similar to cephalexin and cephradine. It is not as active against *H. influenzae* as is cefaclor.

b. **Pharmacokinetics.** Cefadroxil will achieve peak serum and urine levels similar to those of cephalexin and cephradine. It is well absorbed orally, even in the presence of food. The drug is excreted more slowly, and the levels are sustained longer. Consequently, this agent can be administered 1–3 times rather than 3–4 times daily.

c. **Dosage.** In adults with normal renal function, 1 g bid or 2 g once daily is suggested for UTIs due to susceptible pathogens. For skin and soft-tissue infections, 1 g/day or divided doses bid is suggested. In children, for UTIs and skin and soft-tissue infections, 30 mg/kg/day in divided doses q12h is suggested. Dosages should be reduced in renal failure [8].

d. **Cost.** This agent is **very expensive,** even on a once-daily or twice-daily schedule (see Table 28A-5). Even if this agent is given once daily, it still is expensive for routine UTIs. Clearly, the cost of this agent will, and should, affect its use. **We do not advocate its use** (not even for group A streptococcal pharyngitis, as some have suggested). See Chap. 7.

B. **Second-generation oral agents.** These agents are particularly useful as alternative agents for otitis media not responding to amoxicillin (or when amoxicillin is contraindicated), sinusitis, bronchitis, and other respiratory infections. Trials comparing these agents among themselves, to amoxicillin-clavulanate, and to amoxicillin have not demonstrated a superior agent in a given infection. However, the studies examining the efficacy of these agents for respiratory tract infections have not contained large numbers of beta-lactamase-producing pathogens, a situation that might obscure differences in efficacy between the agents [2].

1. **Cefaclor (Ceclor)** has a structure similar to cephalexin except for a substitution of a chlorine atom for a methyl group. It is commonly promoted because of its enhanced in vitro activity against *H. influenzae* and, in particular, its potential usefulness in acute otitis media [90].

a. **Spectrum of activity.** This agent in vitro is active against *S. aureus, S. pneumoniae,* and *S. pyogenes.* It initially appeared to be more active than cephalexin and cephradine against *E. coli, Klebsiella* spp., and *P. mirabilis* but is susceptible to hydrolysis by beta-lactamases against some Enterobacteriaceae [91]. Cefaclor is not active against enterococci, *B. fragilis,* and many gram-negative bacteria, such as *Pseudomonas, Serratia,* and *Enterobacter* spp. In vitro, cefaclor is more active against *H. influenzae* than either cephalexin or cephradine, including ampicillin-sensitive and ampicillin-resistant *H. influenzae*. However, **variable susceptibility results are reported, the inoculum size affects results, and not all ampicillin-resistant strains of *H. influenzae* are susceptible to cefaclor. Studies have shown that 10–15% [90] or more of ampicillin-resistant *H. influenzae* strains also are resistant to cefaclor.** (Cefaclor is significantly destroyed by the TEM-1 and Bro-1 beta-lactamases of some *H. influenzae* and *M. catarrhalis* strains, respectively [2].) Cefaclor is not as active against ampicillin-resistant *H. influenzae* as is cefuroxime or parenteral third-generation cephalosporins or oral cefixime.

  b. **Pharmacokinetics.** Food intake will reduce absorption of cefaclor, and serum concentrations tend to be lower than levels achieved after comparable doses of cephalexin.

  c. **Dosage.** The usual adult dosage is 250–500 mg q8h. In children, the usual dosage is 20–40 mg/kg/day in divided doses q8h (with a maximum dose of 1 g/day), with the higher dose used in otitis media [90].

  d. **Clinical use.** It has been used primarily as an alternate agent in otitis media [92, 93], sinusitis [94], and upper respiratory tract infections. It is a possible alternate agent for UTI with susceptible pathogens.

  e. **Cost.** This oral cephalosporin is expensive. For a 10-day course of therapy, this agent will cost 3–4 times as much as a similar course of ampicillin, amoxicillin, or TMP-SMX. (See Table 28A-5.)

2. **Cefuroxime axetil (Ceftin)** is the acetoxyethyl ester of cefuroxime. After oral administration, it is deesterified in the intestinal mucosa and absorbed into the bloodstream as cefuroxime [95, 96].

  a. **Spectrum of activity.** Cefuroxime axetil owes its in vivo antibacterial activity to the parent compound, cefuroxime. This includes activity against many gram-negative aerobes (including *E. coli* and *K. pneumoniae*) and other gram-negative species, including beta-lactamase-positive and beta-lactamase-negative *H. influenzae* and *N. gonorrhoeae* as well as *M. catarrhalis,* and gram-positive aerobes (*S. aureus,* group A and B streptococci, and viridans streptococci, but not enterococci or methicillin-resistant staphylococci). (See sec. II.E.) Cefuroxime is more resistant to hydrolysis by beta-lactamases than is cephalexin or cefaclor but probably less so than cefixime [91]. Oral cefuroxime is active against *P. multocida* isolated from bite wounds, although cephalexin and cefaclor are not [97]. Oral cefuroxime is not active against *P. aeruginosa, Serratia* spp., *Acinetobacter* spp., and many hospital-acquired gram-negative bacilli.

  b. **Pharmacokinetics.** Of interest, there is **enhanced absorption of the oral tablets when cefuroxime axetil is administered with food,** compared with administration in the fasting state [3, 95, 96], but absorption is diminished by antacids and H_2-receptor agonists [2]. Peak serum levels are achieved 90–120 minutes after oral administration with peaks of approximately 4.5–5.0 μg/ml in children and adults receiving a 500-mg dose [95]. Infants and children may achieve slightly higher peak serum levels after receiving 15- to 20-mg/kg doses [95]. The serum elimination half-life is 1.2 hours [96]. The major route of excretion is renal.

  c. **Clinical uses.** Cefuroxime axetil was approved for use by the FDA in 1987. It has been effective in treating pharyngitis and tonsillitis, otitis media, bronchitis, UTI, and skin and soft-tissue infections due to susceptible pathogens [96]. It is considered an alternate agent for otitis media [93] and has been used in sinusitis [94]. Its effectiveness in lower respiratory tract infections in children has been somewhat variable [96].

  d. **Dosages.** Tablets are available in 125-, 250-, and 500-mg sizes. A recently introduced oral suspension is available and provides 125 mg/5 ml of suspension [39].

    (1) **For infants and children (3 months–12 years), the oral suspension** should be administered with food.

      (a) **For acute otitis media** (and impetigo), the package insert advises 30 mg/kg/day divided into a bid dose for 10 days (maximum daily dose is 1,000 mg).

      (b) **For pharyngitis or tonsillitis,** 20 mg/kg/day for 10 days is suggested (maximum dose of 500 mg/day).

    (2) For children (up to 13 years) who can swallow tablets whole:
       (a) For acute otitis media, 250 mg bid for 10 days.
       (b) For pharyngitis or tonsillitis, 125 mg bid for 10 days.
    (3) For children older than 13 years and adults:
       (a) For pharyngitis or tonsillitis, 250 mg bid.
       (b) For other infections, 250–500 mg bid depending on severity of infection. See Chap. 13 for doses in uncomplicated gonorrhea.

  e. Pregnancy. Regarding cefuroxime axetil's teratogenic effects, this is a category B drug (see Chap. 28A). There are no adequate and well-controlled studies in women. The drug should be used in pregnancy only if clearly needed [39].

  f. Nursing mothers. Because cefuroxime is excreted in human milk, consideration should be given to discontinuing nursing temporarily during treatment [39].

  g. Side effects. Gastrointestinal complaints are the most common.
    (1) With the oral suspension, diarrhea or loose stools (8.6%), dislike of the taste (5.0%), diaper rash (3.4%), and nausea and vomiting (2.6%) are the most frequently reported side effects [39].
    (2) With the tablets, nausea and vomiting and diarrhea are seen.
    (3) See sec. V for the general side effects potentially seen with the cephalosporins.

  h. Summary. The **indications** for cefuroxime axetil include the following [96]:
    (1) As an **alternate agent for otitis media** in children [93].
    (2) As a **possible agent in sinusitis and bronchitis,** especially in an allergic patient.
    (3) Possibly in UTI with more resistant bacteria, although for uncomplicated UTI, less expensive agents are available (e.g., TMP-SMX) [96].
    (4) For completion of therapy after intravenous cefuroxime, as in a patient with bronchitis or pneumonia, periorbital cellulitis, postinfluenza pneumonia, or a community-acquired pneumonia.

  i. Cost. This is an **expensive oral agent** (see Table 28A-5).

3. Cefprozil (Cefzil) is an oral second-generation cephalosporin released in the United States in early 1992 for treatment of pharyngitis, bronchitis, otitis media, and skin and soft-tissue infections [98, 99].

  a. Spectrum of activity. Cefprozil is similar in activity to cefaclor and cefuroxime axetil [98, 100]. Organisms with MICs of 8 μg/ml or less are viewed as susceptible [100]. Separate disc testing is advised [98].
    (1) Gram-positive aerobes. Cefprozil is active against beta-hemolytic streptococci, including groups A and B streptococci, penicillin-susceptible *S. pneumoniae,* methicillin-susceptible *S. aureus* (MIC_{90} = 1 μg/ml), and *L. monocytogenes* (MIC_{90} = 4 μg/ml). Cefprozil has only marginal activity against some enterococci [100]. Methicillin-resistant *S. aureus* are resistant to cefprozil.
    (2) Gram-negative aerobes. Cefprozil is active against *H. influenzae* (including beta-lactamase-producing strains) and *M. catarrhalis.* However, there may be an inoculum effect of cefprozil against *H. influenzae* [100]. Its activity against *H. influenzae* is only modestly increased beyond that of cephalexin and cefadroxil (first-generation agents) but comparable to that noted with cefaclor and less than that of cefuroxime [2].
      Its activity against Enterobacteriaceae is variable (and more active than the first-generation agents), but community-acquired *E. coli, Klebsiella* spp., and *P. mirabilis* are likely to be susceptible, whereas most strains of *Enterobacter* and *Serratia* spp., *Proteus vulgaris,* and *Pseudomonas* spp. are resistant. *Salmonella* and *Shigella* spp. have variable susceptibilities.
    (3) Anaerobes. Cefprozil is not active against *B. fragilis* or other *Bacteroides* spp. [98, 100]. Cefprozil is not viewed as an active agent against most common anaerobes.

  b. Pharmacokinetics. These data have been reviewed elsewhere [98, 101].
    (1) Absorption. Approximately 95% of an oral dose is absorbed from the GI tract, and absorption is **unaffected by food** or antacids. A 500-mg oral dose typically produces peak serum levels of approximately 9–10 μg/ml at 1 hour.

(2) **Metabolism and excretion.** Nearly 60–70% of cefprozil is excreted in the urine unchanged. With a creatinine clearance of less than 30 ml/min, dosage should be reduced by 50%. In patients with hepatic disease, the metabolism of cefprozil is minimally altered. The typical half-life of cefprozil is at least 1.3 hours. This relatively long half-life allows for the once-daily or twice-daily dosing schedules.

(3) **Excretion into breast milk.** In one study, less than 0.3% of the maternal dose was excreted in the breast milk. The authors concluded that the low excretion of cefprozil in breast milk and the excellent safety profile of cefprozil (see sec. **e**) suggest this cephalosporin may be administered to nursing mothers [102].

c. **Clinical use.** In randomized, controlled trials, cefprozil has been **effective** in treating children and adults with **pharyngitis** due to S. pyogenes; **bronchitis** due to penicillin-susceptible S. pneumoniae, H. influenzae, and M. catarrhalis; **otitis media; impetigo; and cellulitis** [98, 99]. It has been about as effective in these infections as erythromycin, cefaclor, cefuroxime axetil, and amoxicillin-clavulanate [98, 99].

Clinical studies are evaluating the role of cefprozil in UTI [99].

d. **Dosages.** Cefprozil is available as a 250-mg and 500-mg tablet as well as a liquid bubble-gum flavor oral suspension with 125 mg/5 ml and 250 mg/5 ml.

(1) **Adult** dosages per package insert are:
  (a) **For bronchitis,** 500 mg q12h.
  (b) **For skin and soft-tissue infections,** 250–500 mg q12h or 500 mg q24h, depending on the severity of infection.
  (c) For streptococcal pharyngitis, 500 mg q24h for 10 days.

(2) **Children** (6 months–12 years): 15 mg/kg bid, per the package insert.

(3) **In renal failure.** The dose should be halved in patients with a creatinine clearance of less than 30 ml/min [98, 101]. Cefprozil is removed by hemodialysis, and a supplemental dose of 50% of the maintenance dose is recommended following the dialysis procedure [101].

(4) In hepatic dysfunction, no dose adjustment appears necessary.

e. **Side effects.** Typical of the cephalosporins, cefprozil is generally well tolerated [98, 103]. Minor GI side effects (diarrhea, nausea, vomiting, abdominal discomfort) are the most common but appear to occur less frequently than with the use of amoxicillin-clavulanate or erythromycin [98, 103] and possibly cefixime [103]. Rashes can occur.

f. **Cost.** Cefprozil is an expensive oral agent compared with penicillin, generic TMP-SMX, and erythromycin, but is cost-competitive with amoxicillin-clavulanate, cefaclor, and cefuroxime axetil. (See Table 28A-6.) The wholesale cost for a 10-day course of cefprozil, 250 mg q12h, is approximately $55 [98].

g. **Summary.** Cefprozil is a new oral second-generation cephalosporin that has activity and clinical uses similar to those of cefaclor and cefuroxime axetil. The exact role of this agent awaits further study and clinical experience, but it does not appear to offer any unique advantages over existing agents and it is expensive.

(1) The *Medical Letter* concluded that cefprozil offers an alternative to cefaclor and cefuroxime axetil for the treatment of otitis media or bronchitis but emphasized that TMP-SMX can also be given twice daily and costs much less [98].

For routine empiric therapy of uncomplicated otitis media, amoxicillin remains the drug of choice. For patients who have otitis media with effusion for which treatment is indicated, amoxicillin is preferred also as initial therapy [104]. Failures to eradicate H. influenzae infection in otitis media have been seen in cefprozil therapy [99]; how frequently this occurs, especially in comparison with other alternative agents for otitis media, awaits further clinical experience. Even the package insert notes that "in treatment of otitis media, due to beta-lactamase producing organisms, cefprozil had bacteriologic eradication rates somewhat lower than those observed with a product containing specific beta-lactamase inhibitor." The twice-daily regimen for otitis media may improve compliance.

(2) Patients with recurrent episodes of acute exacerbations of chronic bronchitis can use cefprozil as another antibiotic in rotation with others.

(3) For streptococcal pharyngitis, penicillin remains the drug of choice [98], and studies support the use of twice-daily regimens of oral penicillin (250 mg bid for children younger than 12 years and 500 mg bid for children older than 12) rather than previously recommended three- or four-times-daily dosage regimens of penicillin [105]. In the penicillin-allergic patient, twice-daily regimens of erythromycin or a first-generation cephalosporin would be more cost-effective [105] than cefprozil.

(4) For skin and soft-tissue infections, the *Medical Letter* [98] concluded "there is no reason to use cefprozil rather than a penicillinase-resistant oral penicillin, such as dicloxacillin, or an oral first-generation cephalosporin such as cephalexin or cephradine."

(5) Cefprozil has not been approved for use in the therapy of pneumonia. Because cefprozil is not active against *Mycoplasma pneumoniae* or *Chlamydia pneumoniae* (TWAR strain) and is no more effective against *S. pneumoniae* than penicillin, it is not anticipated that cefprozil would play any special role in community-acquired pneumonia especially of young or middle-aged patients.

(6) **Because of these constraints, we see a limited role for this new agent, except as an alternative agent in otitis media,** where the twice-daily dosing schedule may help compliance. Further data are pending on its role in the treatment of UTI.

4. **Loracarbef** (Lorabid), released for use in the United States in 1992, is a new oral beta-lactam antibiotic of the **carbacephem class.** The carbacephems are similar in structure to the cephalosporins except that a methylene group in the tetrahydropyridine ring of the carbacephem nucleus has replaced the sulfur atom in the dihydrothiazine ring of the cephalosporin nucleus. This change renders the carbacephem nucleus more chemically stable than the corresponding cephalosporin nucleus [106], although the clinical significance of this is unclear. Because this structural modification of the cephalosporin molecule is minor, this agent is reviewed here with the cephalosporins. From a practical standpoint, loracarbef is clinically very similar to cefaclor.

   a. **Spectrum of activity.** Loracarbef inhibits cell wall synthesis. The in vitro activity of loracarbef is similar to that of other oral antibiotics currently available (e.g., cefaclor, amoxicillin-clavulanate, cefuroxime axetil, and TMP-SMX) [107]. A literature review summarizes the MIC_{90} of loracarbef in Table 28F-11. A range of MICs can be seen and is somewhat dependent on the specific test method used in a particular laboratory [107].

Table 28F-11. Susceptibility data for loracarbef

Organism	MIC_{90} (μg/ml)
Staphylococcus aureus (methicillin-susceptible)	
Penicillin-resistant	8.0
Penicillin-susceptible	1.0–2.0
Streptococcus pyogenes (group A streptococci)	≤0.06–1.0
S. pneumoniae (penicillin-susceptible strains)*	0.25–2.0
Haemophilus influenzae	
Beta-lactamase-negative	0.25–8.0
Beta-lactamase-positive	0.5–16.0
Moraxella (*Branhamella*) *catarrhalis*	
Beta-lactamase-negative	0.12–0.25
Beta-lactamase-positive	0.5–8.0
Klebsiella pneumoniae	0.25–8.0
Proteus mirabilis	1.0–8.0

*For penicillin-resistant strains, see Table 28C-1 (p. 1125).
Source: Based on summary data from G. Doern, In vitro activity of loracarbef and effects of susceptibility test methods. *Am. J. Med.* 92(Suppl. 6A):7S, 1992.

b. **Pharmacokinetics**
   (1) **Absorption.** Loracarbef is well absorbed from the GI tract, although **the ingestion of food will decrease and delay the peak serum concentrations** [108] (i.e., approximately 90% absorption after administration to fasting subjects versus 50–60% absorption with food.) After 400-mg doses (capsule), peak serum levels are approximately 12 μg/ml [108]. Following 15-mg/kg doses, peak serum levels achieved in middle-ear fluid are approximately 4 μg/ml. These levels are approximately 40–50% of the levels reached in plasma [108]. **The suspension is more rapidly absorbed than the capsules, resulting in higher peak concentrations** when administered in the same dose. **The suspension is recommended for otitis media per the package insert.**
   (2) **Metabolism and excretion.** Virtually all of an orally administered dose is excreted in the urine unchanged. Dosages must be reduced in patients with renal insufficiency [108].
   (3) The half-life of loracarbef in plasma is approximately 1 hour [108].
   (4) The pharmacokinetic profile of loracarbef in adults is comparable to that in children and the elderly [108].
c. **Clinical use.** Clinical trials have indicated that the efficacy of loracarbef is comparable to that of the comparison agents (e.g., amoxicillin, amoxicillin-clavulanate, cefaclor) in studies involving more than 9,000 patients. Of these patients, more than 4,500 received loracarbef [106, 109]. **Loracarbef has been approved for the following mild to moderately severe infections:**
   (1) Acute **bronchitis** and acute bacterial exacerbations of chronic bronchitis due to penicillin-susceptible *S. pneumoniae, H. influenzae* (including beta-lactamase-producing strains), and *M. catarrhalis* (including beta-lactamase-producing strains).
   (2) **Pneumonia caused by penicillin-susceptible *S. pneumoniae*** or non-beta-lactamase-producing strains of *H. influenzae.* The package insert notes that data are insufficient to establish efficacy in patients with pneumonia due to beta-lactamase-producing strains of *H. influenzae.*
   (3) **Otitis media** caused by penicillin-susceptible *S. pneumoniae, M. catarrhalis* (including beta-lactamase-producing strains), *S. pyogenes,* and *H. influenzae* (including beta-lactamase-producing strains). However, even the package insert notes that in patient populations with significant numbers of beta-lactamase-producing organisms, loracarbef's clinical cure and bacteriologic eradication rates were somewhat less than those observed with a product containing a beta-lactamase inhibitor. The exact role of loracarbef in this setting awaits further clinical study [110]. (See sec. **h.(3).**)
   (4) **Acute maxillary sinusitis** caused by penicillin-susceptible *S. pneumoniae, M. catarrhalis* (including beta-lactamase-producing strains), and *H. influenzae* (non-beta-lactamase strains only). The package insert again notes that data are insufficient to establish efficacy in patients with acute maxillary sinusitis caused by beta-lactamase-producing strains.
   (5) **Pharyngitis** or **tonsillitis** caused by *S. pyogenes.* However, the package insert indicates that data establishing the efficacy of loracarbef in the subsequent prevention of rheumatic fever are not yet available [see sec. **h.(2)**] and the first-generation cephalosporins are more cost-effective.
   (6) **Uncomplicated skin and soft-tissue infections** caused by *S. aureus* or *S. pyogenes.*
   (7) **Uncomplicated UTI** (cystitis and pyelonephritis) caused by susceptible *E. coli.*
d. **Dosages.** Loracarbef should be **administered at least 1 hour before meals or 2 hours after eating** to ensure maximal absorption. Loracarbef is available in 200-mg pulvules and as an oral suspension (100 mg/5 ml and 200 mg/5 ml). The package insert suggests:
   (1) **In adults** (≥ 13 years of age)
       (a) For pharyngitis or tonsillitis and uncomplicated skin and soft-tissue infections, 200 mg q12h. Pharyngitis or tonsillitis should be treated for 10 full days.
       (b) For acute bacterial bronchitis, 200–400 mg q12h.

(c) For acute exacerbations of chronic bronchitis, pneumonia, sinusitis, and uncomplicated pyelonephritis, 400 mg q12h.

(d) For uncomplicated cystitis, 200 mg q24h.

(2) **In children** (6 months–12 years of age)

(a) For otitis media, the **suspension** preparation at 30 mg/kg/day in divided doses q12h.

(b) For pharyngitis or tonsillitis, 15 mg/kg/day in divided doses q12h for 10 days.

(3) **In renal failure,** the usual dosage can be given to patients with a creatinine clearance of 50 ml/min or more. Patients with a creatinine clearance of 10–49 ml/min may be given half the recommended dose at the usual dosage interval or the normal recommended dose at twice the usual dosage interval [108]. In patients with severe renal insufficiency (creatinine clearance < 10 ml/min) who are not undergoing dialysis, the recommended dose can be given every 3–5 days per package insert. Patients on hemodialysis should receive a supplemental dose following hemodialysis.

e. **Contraindications.** Because it is similar in structure to the cephalosporins, **loracarbef is contraindicated in patients allergic to the cephalosporins.** In patients allergic to penicillin, there is a risk of a cross-hypersensitivity reaction and, until further data are available to clarify the incidence of this cross-hypersensitivity, **we avoid using loracarbef in patients with a history of allergy to the cephalosporins or an allergic reaction to penicillins.**

f. **Side effects.** In assessing the safety profile of 22 clinical trials involving more than 9,000 patients, of whom 4,500 patients received loracarbef, one review emphasizes that loracarbef was **well tolerated** by most patients, including children and elderly patients. Most adverse effects were mild and transient in nature; only 1.5% of recipients discontinued loracarbef therapy because of drug-related adverse effects [111].

(1) **Diarrhea** was the most common side effect but occurred less frequently than in patients receiving comparative agents (e.g., amoxicillin-clavulanate). Nausea and vomiting occurred infrequently.

(2) **Headache** occurred in fewer than 3% of recipients but was the second most common side effect and occurred at a slightly higher frequency in the loracarbef-treated group than in patients receiving comparable agents [111].

(3) **Rashes** can be seen in approximately 1.2% of recipients [111].

g. **Cost.** The wholesale cost for a 10-day course of 200 mg q12h loracarbef is $63. (See Table 28A-6.)

h. **Summary.** The exact role of this oral antibiotic awaits further study and clinical experience. Loracarbef, cefaclorlike in its clinical usefulness, provides a cephalosporin alternative for selected cases of otitis media and other respiratory infections such as sinusitis and bronchitis.

(1) In a symposium devoted to this agent [106], Drs. Moellering and Jacobs summarize loracarbef by concluding, "[A]nalysis of the data from clinical trials in terms of favorable post therapy clinical response by predominant pathogens suggests that loracarbef is an appropriate agent for the treatment of various respiratory, skin, and urinary tract infections" [109]. Of interest, Drs. Moellering and Jacobs do not emphasize any unique or special role for loracarbef and imply that it is a **reasonable alternative** for the approved clinical indications.

(2) For streptococcal pharyngitis, penicillin remains the drug of choice and can be given twice-daily. In the penicillin-allergic patient, a twice-daily regimen of erythromycin or a first-generation cephalosporin would be more cost-effective [105]. See related discussion in sec. **3.g(3)** and Chap. 7.

(3) For otitis media [105, 112] and acute maxillary sinusitis, amoxicillin is still the drug of choice in the nonallergic patient. For those patients not responding to amoxicillin therapy or those highly likely to have infection due to *H. influenzae* with beta-lactamase-positive organisms, drugs with a specific beta-lactamase inhibitor appear to be more effective than loracarbef. The package insert of loracarbef indicates that this agent is not ideal for these beta-lactamase-positive *H. influenzae*

infections. Although the precise relationship of MIC data and clinical efficacy is not clear, middle-ear fluid levels of loracarbef are approximately 4 μg/ml [108] and, as shown in Table 28F-11, the MIC_{90} of beta-lactamase-positive *H. influenzae* is variable, ranging between 0.5–16.0 μg/ml. In this setting, therefore, we believe TMP-SMX or amoxicillin-clavulanate often is preferred.

Similar limitations apply to an early pneumonia due to beta-lactamase-positive *H. influenzae*. In addition, for community-acquired pneumonia in young to middle-aged patients, loracarbef is not indicated as it is ineffective against *M. pneumoniae* and *C. pneumoniae* (TWAR strain) and is no more effective against *S. pneumoniae* than is penicillin or amoxicillin.

(4) For uncomplicated skin and soft-tissue infections caused by *S. aureus* or *S. pyogenes,* a penicillinase-resistant penicillin (e.g., dicloxacillin) or an oral first-generation cephalosporin (e.g., cephalexin or cephradine) is preferred.

(5) For acute bronchitis or exacerbations of chronic bronchitis, loracarbef may be a reasonable agent to rotate in these patients if beta-lactamase *H. influenzae* infections are not highly suspected or demonstrated. However, because *H. influenzae* organisms are common pathogens in this setting, the role of loracarbef needs to be determined by further clinical experience.

(6) For uncomplicated community-acquired UTI, loracarbef may be a useful agent, but many alternative agents already exist for UTIs.

(7) Therefore, **overall we believe this agent fills no unique niche.**

C. **Third-generation oral agents**

1. **Cefixime** (Suprax) became available in 1989 as a once- or twice-daily therapy for otitis media, pharyngitis, bronchitis, and UTI [113–115].

   a. **Spectrum of activity** [113]

      (1) **Gram-positive aerobes.** Cefixime is at least as active in vitro as other oral cephalosporins against group A streptococci but is slightly less active against *S. pneumoniae.* **S. aureus and other staphylococci are resistant to cefixime** because the drug has low affinity for a critical beta-lactam-binding protein. Enterococci and *L. monocytogenes* are resistant.

      (2) **Gram-negative aerobes**

         (a) Cefixime is highly active against *N. gonorrhoeae, H. influenzae,* and *M. catarrhalis,* including beta-lactamase producers. In one report, cefixime was very active against adult isolates of *H. influenzae* ($MIC_{90} = 0.125$ μg/ml) and *M. catarrhalis* ($MIC_{90} = 0.25$ μg/ml), including beta-lactamase-producing strains, and was more active in vitro than cefuroxime, cephalexin, or cefaclor against these pathogens [116].

         (b) Cefixime is a so-called third-generation oral cephalosporin because of its resistance to plasmid-mediated beta-lactamases produced by many gram-negative bacteria [91, 113]. However, cefixime is not resistant to some chromosomal beta-lactamases found in certain gram-negative strains [113]. **Cefixime is more active than other oral cephalosporins** against *E. coli, Klebsiella* spp., *P. mirabilis,* and *S. marcescens.* It has **no useful activity against** *Pseudomonas* spp. and many strains of *Enterobacter* and *Acinetobacter* spp. Cefixime is less active against gram-negative bacteria than the parenteral third-generation cephalosporins [113].

      (3) **Anaerobes.** Cefixime has **no useful activity** against anaerobes [113].

   b. **Pharmacokinetics.** Gastrointestinal absorption is slow and incomplete; whether taken with meals or not, approximately 40–50% of an oral dose is absorbed [113]. **The oral suspension is absorbed more rapidly and completely than the tablets and is preferred in the treatment of otitis media.** (See sec. **IV** for discussion of taste.) Cefixime apparently is not metabolized, and 50% of the absorbed dose is excreted in the urine within 24 hours; therefore, **dosages must be reduced in renal failure.** The average elimination half-life is 3 hours, and it becomes 2–4 times as long in patients with renal failure [113].

c. **Clinical trials.** In the treatment of otitis media, initial studies revealed cefixime to be about as effective as amoxicillin in eradicating beta-lactamase-negative *H. influenzae* and *Moraxella* spp. and more effective against beta-lactamase-positive *H. influenzae* but **less effective against** *S. pneumoniae* [113]. In other studies, cefixime was as effective as cefaclor for otitis media [113] [see sec. **f.(1)**]. Cefixime has also been as effective as amoxicillin in treating pharyngitis, tonsillitis, acute bronchitis, and UTI [113].

d. **Dosage.** Tablets are available in 200- and 400-mg sizes. The oral suspension contains 100 mg cefixime per 5 ml.

   (1) **Adults.** The recommended dose is 400 mg once daily or 200 mg bid.

   (2) **Children.** The dosage is 8 mg/kg/day of the suspension, once daily or in two divided doses. For children weighing more than 50 kg or older than 12 years, adult doses are recommended.

   The package insert suggests that the suspension be used in otitis media because the suspension may provide higher blood levels than the tablets. Efficacy and safety in infants younger than 6 months has not been established.

   (3) **In renal failure.** According to the package insert, normal dosages can be used if the patient's creatinine clearance exceeds 60 ml/min. For patients with a clearance of 21–60 ml/min or patients who are on hemodialysis, 75% of the standard dosage at the standard interval (e.g., in an adult, 300 mg daily) is used. Patients whose clearance is less than 20 ml/min or patients on CAPD may be given half the standard dosage at the standard interval (e.g., in an adult, 200 mg daily). Neither hemodialysis nor peritoneal dialysis removes significant amounts of the drug.

   (4) **In pregnancy.** The package insert indicates that this is a category B agent (see Chap. 28A). Cefprozil should not be used during pregnancy unless it is clearly indicated.

   (5) **Nursing mothers.** The package insert indicates it is not known whether cefixime is excreted in human milk; consideration should be given to discontinuing nursing during treatment with this drug.

e. **Side effects.** Gastrointestinal toxicity, mainly diarrhea, appears to be more frequent with cefixime than with cefaclor or amoxicillin. Severe diarrhea with antibiotic-related colitis (see Chap. 28A) has been reported [113]. For other side effects seen with cephalosporins in general, see sec. **V.**

f. **Clinical uses.** The exact role of this new oral agent still is evolving with clinical experience.

   (1) For otitis media and sinusitis, initial clinical trials have shown no advantage of cefixime over amoxicillin or cefaclor [117–119], but cefixime may be more efficacious than amoxicillin in treating *H. influenzae* otitis media [117]. Cefixime **may not routinely eradicate** *S. pneumoniae* **from middle-ear aspirates** [2a, 118]. In a recent review, Dr. Bluestone [119a] concluded that "in children, cefixime is similar in effectiveness to amoxicillin and cefaclor, but diarrhea and stool changes are more common with cefixime. Amoxicillin is still preferred for initial empiric treatment of uncomplicated acute otitis media." Cefixime is a viable alternative to amoxicillin when (1) a beta-lactamase-producing *H. influenzae* or *M. catarrhalis* is isolated from otorrhea or tympanocentesis; (2) the patient has delayed hypersensitivity to penicillins but not cephalosporins; (3) there is a high incidence of resistant bacteria in the community, or there is no improvement on amoxicillin; or (4) once-daily administration is more convenient [119a].

   In a recent review of the therapy for acute otitis media, amoxicillin remains the drug of choice for initial therapy in most patients. Cefixime was believed to have the disadvantage of relatively poor activity against *S. pneumoniae* [112].

   (2) For pharyngitis or tonsillitis, cefixime offers no advantage over penicillin.

   (3) For bronchitis, it has no advantage over TMP-SMX, which is less expensive.

   (4) For UTI, other less expensive agents are available for uncomplicated UTI. Cefixime will be potentially useful in the treatment of more

resistant bacteria as would the flouroquinolones, TMP-SMX, or amoxicillin-clavulanate.

(5) Studies have shown that oral cefixime was as effective as a single intramuscular dose of ceftriaxone for uncomplicated gonorrhea [120, 121]. (See Chap. 13.)

(6) The *Medical Letter* [113] stated that cefixime had no demonstrated advantage over previously available antibiotics that may cost much less. Unlike other cephalosporins, cefixime has no activity against staphylococci. This conclusion still appears valid.

(7) Summary. We see a potential role for this agent in selected patients with recurrent UTI and drug allergies when susceptibility data show that cefixime will be effective and possibly allow one to avoid a parenteral agent. It is an alternative agent in the patient not responding to conventional therapy for otitis media. Otherwise, at this time, it seems to have few advantages.

g. Cost. This is an expensive oral agent. (See Table 28A-5.)

2. Cefpodoxime proxetil (Vantin) was approved for use in late 1992 [122, 123].

a. Spectrum of activity (MIC_{90} in µg/ml). Cefpodoxime is active against *S. pyogenes* (MIC_{90}, 0.06 µg/ml), *S. agalactiae* (0.12 µg/ml), penicillin-susceptible *S. pneumoniae* (0.06–0.12 µg/ml), beta-lactamase-positive and -negative *H. influenzae* (0.12–0.25 µg/ml), *M. catarrhalis* (0.50–1.0 µg/ml), and *N. gonorrhoeae*. It is modestly active against *S. aureus* (MIC_{90}, 2.0 µg/ml) but not enterococci or MRSA. Cefpodoxime is active against many Enterobacteriaceae but not *Enterobacter, Serratia,* or *Morganella* spp.

b. Pharmacokinetics. Cefpodoxime is an ester prodrug; the ester enhances absorption from the small intestine but then is hydrolyzed during passage through the intestinal wall, and only free drug appears in the blood [122]. A 200-mg dose provides serum levels of approximately 2.2 µg/ml, whereas 400 mg provides a peak level of 3.8 µg/ml, per package insert. **Food increases bioavailability,** but concomitant use of antacids or H_2-blockers reduces plasma levels.

c. Clinical trials. Cefpodoxime has been studied in acute community-acquired pneumonia, acute otitis media, pharyngitis, UTI, skin and soft-tissue infections, acute and chronic bronchitis, and single-dose uncomplicated gonorrhea therapy (see Chap. 13) [122]. Penicillin still is considered the drug of choice in group A streptococcal pharyngitis. In the patient with a delayed (late) penicillin allergy, a first-generation cephalosporin is more cost-effective. See Chaps. 7 and 28C for detailed discussions.

d. Dosages. Both 100-mg and 200-mg tablets and an oral suspension (50 mg/5 ml and 100 mg/5 ml) are available. Per package insert:

(1) For adults (≥ 13 years old): 100 mg q12h for 7 days for uncomplicated UTI; 200 mg q12h for mild community-acquired pneumonia for 14 days and a similar dose for bacterial bronchitis for 10 days; 100 mg q12h for pharyngitis or tonsillitis for 10 days; 400 mg q12h for skin and soft-tissue infections for 7–14 days; and a 200-mg single dose for uncomplicated gonococcal infection (see Chap. 13).

(2) For children (6 months–12 years): 10 mg/kg/day divided q12h (maximum 400 mg/day) for 10 days for otitis media and 10 mg/kg/day divided q12h (maximum 200 mg/day) for 10 days for pharyngitis or tonsillitis.

(3) Pregnancy. Cefpodoxime should be used during pregnancy only if clearly indicated.

(4) Nursing mothers. Cefpodoxime is excreted into human milk. Because of the potential for a reaction in the nursing infant, a decision should be made whether to continue nursing or discontinue the drug, taking into consideration the importance of the drug to the mother. (These precautions are per the package insert.)

(5) Renal failure. Standard every-12-hour doses can be used for a creatinine clearance in excess of 50 ml/min. If the clearance is 10–50 ml/min, a standard dose can be given q16h; if less than 10 ml/min, a standard dose can be given q24–48h [8]. In patients undergoing hemodialysis, 200 mg after dialysis only is suggested. For patients undergoing CAPD, dose as if the creatinine clearance is less than 10 ml/min [8].

e. Cost. See Table 28A-5.

f. **Summary.** The *Medical Letter* [122] concluded in 1992: **"Cefpodoxime is a broad-spectrum oral cephalosporin that offers no clear advantage over previously available drugs for the treatment of any infection."** We still concur and see no unique role for this agent. When treatment with TMP-SMX or a fluoroquinolone is not feasible, selected cases of UTI, especially in women, may be treated with this agent, depending on susceptibility data.

3. **Ceftibuten** (Cedax) was approved for clinical use December 20, 1995. This agent was recently reviewed [123–123e].

   a. **Spectrum of activity.** Ceftibuten has structural characteristics of the third-generation cephalosporins, producing increased activity against gram-negative pathogens; like cefixime, ceftibuten has minimal activity against some gram-positive pathogens including staphylococci, some types of beta-hemolytic streptococci, and enterococci [123a].

   (1) Because this is a very new agent, detailed **MIC data** are **summarized in Table 28F-12.** The breakpoint concentration for susceptible pathogens is ≤ 8 μg/ml [123a]. An inoculum effect can be seen in vitro as with other new beta-lactams [123a]. For a detailed discussion of susceptibility data see reference [123a].

   (a) Among 2,930 Enterobacteriaceae, 92% of strains were susceptible.

   (b) Strains of *S. pneumoniae* resistant to penicillin (see Chap. 28C) are also resistant to ceftibuten.

   (2) Organisms resistant to ceftibuten include [123a] *S. aureus, Streptococcus agalactiae* (group B streptococci) and other streptococcal species (e.g., viridans streptococci, *S. bovis*), enterococci, **anaerobes** including *Clostridial* spp. and *Bacteroides* spp. Also, *Bordetella pertussis, Listeria monocytogenes, Pseudomonas* spp., *Acinetobacter* spp., and *Xanthomonas maltophilia* are resistant.

   b. **Pharmacokinetics.** Ceftibuten is rapidly and nearly completely absorbed from the upper portions of the gastrointestinal tract. Mean peak plasma concentrations of 15 μg/ml occur 2–3 hours after the administration of a single 400-mg oral dose to healthy young volunteers or after 9 mg/kg doses in children [123b]. The elimination half-life of ceftibuten is approximately 2.5 hours. Although administration of a ceftibuten capsule with a meal slightly delays the absorption, there is no major effect on the extent of absorption or half-life [123b]. The package insert emphasizes the suspension must be administered at least 2 hours before or 1 hour after a meal. Elderly patients absorb ceftibuten well, with a half-life of 3.2 hours related to a lower renal clearance in the elderly. After pediatric doses, middle-ear fluid concentrations are 13 μg/ml at 4 hours after a dose [123b].

   Ceftibuten has a postantibiotic effect (PAE) on common respiratory pathogens including *S. pneumoniae, H. influenzae, M. catarrhalis,* and *S. pyogenes* [123b]. The PAE may help explain the clinical responses seen in patients treated for respiratory pathogens.

   Based on these studies, Neu [123b] concludes that otitis media, pharyngitis, tonsillitis, and acute bacterial exacerbation of bronchitis due to susceptible pathogens can be treated with a single daily dose. See sec. **e.**

   c. **Clinical trials.** Ceftibuten has been successfully used in a variety of infections including acute uncomplicated and complicated UTIs, respiratory tract infections, acute otitis media, and streptococcal pharyngitis [123c].

   d. **Clinical indications.** Ceftibuten has recently been **approved for** mild to moderate infections caused by susceptible strains in the following settings. (Both beta-lactamase–positive and –negative strains of *H. influenzae* and *M. catarrhalis* are susceptible.)

   (1) **Acute bacterial exacerbation of chronic bronchitis** due to *H. influenzae, M. catarrhalis,* and penicillin-susceptible *S. pneumoniae.* The package insert notes that when *M. catarrhalis* was isolated from sputum, ceftibuten clinical efficacy was 22% less than controls.

   (2) **Acute bacterial otitis media** due to *H. influenzae, M. catarrhalis,* or *S. pyogenes.* The package insert notes that "although ceftibuten used empirically was equivalent to comparisons in the treatment of clinically and/or microbiologically documented acute otitis media, the efficacy against *S. pneumoniae* was 23% less than controls. Therefore,

Table 28F-12. In vitro susceptibility data for ceftibuten

Organism	No. tested	MIC$_{90}$
Streptococcus pneumoniae		
Penicillin-susceptible	127	4–8
Penicillin-resistant[a]	46[b]	>8–>32
Streptococcus		
Serogroup A	132	0.5–2
Serogroup C	28	1
Serogroup F	7	
Serogroup G	26	1–2
Enterobacteriaceae		
Citrobacter amalonaticus	16	1
Citrobacter diversus	58	≤0.06–0.25
Citrobacter freundii	202	1–>32
Enterobacter aerogenes	180	>32–64
Enterobacter agglomerans	36	8–>32
Enterobacter cloacae	358	32–>64
Escherichia coli	1367	0.25–0.5
Hafnia alvei	16	1–>32
Klebsiella oxytoca	110	0.03–0.13
Klebsiella pneumoniae	658	0.03–0.5
Morganella morganii	156	1–32
Proteus mirabilis	515	0.015–0.12
Proteus vulgaris	153	0.03–0.12
Providencia rettgeri	59	0.03–0.13
Providencia stuartii	72	≤0.06–1
Salmonella spp.	54	0.12–0.5
Serratia spp.	375[b]	2–32
Shigella spp.	51	0.25–1
Yersinia enterocolitica	45	0.25–4
Haemophilus influenzae		
Ampicillin-susceptible	357	0.03–0.5
Ampicillin-resistant		
Beta-lactamase-positive	196	0.06–2
Beta-lactamase-negative	18	4–7.68
Chloramphenicol-resistant	24	≤0.25
Haemophilus parainfluenzae	6	
Moraxella catarrhalis		
Beta-lactamase-positive	299	0.25–4
Beta-lactamase-negative	65	0.25–2
Neisseria gonorrhoeae	120[c]	0.015–0.5
Neisseria meningitidis	44	≤0.06–≤0.25

[a]See Chap. 28C for discussion of penicillin-resistant *S. pneumoniae.*
[b]Includes three species of *Serratia.*
[c]Beta-lactamase–positive and –negative strains have identical ceftibuten MICs.
Source: Modified from R.N. Jones, Ceftibuten: A review of antimicrobial activity, spectrum and other microbiologic features. *Pediatr. Infect. Dis. J.* 14:S77, 1995.

ceftibuten should be given empirically only when adequate anti-microbial coverage against *S. pneumoniae* has been previously administered" [emphasis added].
(3) **Pharyngitis and tonsillitis** due to *S. pyogenes*. The package insert indicates that data establishing the efficacy of ceftibuten for the prevention of subsequent rheumatic fever are not available.
e. **Dosage.** Ceftibuten is available in 400-mg capsules and a suspension (either 90 mg/5 ml or 180 mg/5 ml).

(1) **Adults and children over 12 years of age.** The recommended dose is 400 mg once daily for 10 days.

(2) **Children over 6 months of age.** The recommended dose is 9 mg/kg/day as a single dose (up to a maximum of 400 mg/day) for 10 days. The package insert emphasizes that the **suspension must be administered at least 2 hours before or 1 hour after a meal.**

Children weighing more than 45 kg should receive the maximum 400-mg dose daily.

(3) **In renal failure,** doses must be reduced when the creatinine clearance is less than 50 ml/min. According to the package insert, when the creatinine clearance is between 30–49 ml/min, 50% of the usual dose can be given q24h. When the creatinine clearance is 5–29 ml/min, 25% of the usual dose can be given q24h.

In patients undergoing hemodialysis 2–3 times weekly, the package insert suggests a single 400-mg dose or 9 mg/kg (maximum of 400 mg) administered at the end of each hemodialysis session.

(4) **Pregnancy.** This is a category B agent (see Chap. 28A). Because there are no well-controlled studies in pregnant women, the package insert suggests ceftibuten should be used in pregnancy only if clearly indicated. Ceftibuten did not have teratogenic effects or alter fertility in rats or rabbits [123d].

(5) **Nursing mothers.** The package insert indicates that, as of early 1996, it is not known if ceftibuten at recommended dosages is excreted in human milk and that caution should be exercised when ceftibuten is administered to a nursing woman. See related discussions in Chap. 28A.

f. **Side effects.** Typical of a cephalosporin, ceftibuten appears to be well tolerated [123d]. Less than 1% of children treated with ceftibuten had to withdraw from clinical studies because of clinical adverse effects. Diarrhea (approximately 3%), vomiting (2%), abdominal cramps (1%), and loose stools (1%) are the most common side effects reported in children [123d]. No cases of Stevens-Johnson syndrome, toxic epidermal necrolysis, or serum sickness–like reactions have been reported with use of the suspension in preclinical studies [123d].

In adults, the package insert suggests nausea [4%], headache [3%], diarrhea [3%], and dyspepsia [1%] are the most common side effects.

g. **Cost.** See Table 28A-5.

h. **Summary.** The exact niche for this new antibiotic will await further clinical experience with this agent. We would prefer other twice-daily treatment options for streptococcal pharyngitis as discussed in Chap. 7. Ceftibuten is not recommended for initial empiric therapy of acute bacterial otitis media, but it provides a once-daily regimen for patients who have not responded to initial therapy aimed at *S. pneumoniae.* See related discussions in sec. **d(2)** and Chap. 7. Ceftibuten also is another agent that can be used for acute exacerbations of chronic bronchitis, especially when a once-daily regimen is highly desirable or as an agent to rotate with other antibiotics in this setting, as described in Chap. 7.

D. **Uses and dosages of oral cephalosporins.** (See Table 28F-10.)

1. **Urinary tract infections.** These agents are useful in UTIs when organisms are not susceptible to less expensive agents (e.g., TMP-SMX or ampicillin) or as alternate agents in the ampicillin- or sulfa-allergic patient.

2. **Acute otitis media.** Ampicillin or amoxicillin still appears to be the drug of choice for uncomplicated infections. If *H. influenzae* resistant to ampicillin is known or highly suspected (e.g., the patient is not responding to ampicillin or amoxicillin) and TMP-SMX is contraindicated, the added expense of alternative agents such as cefprozil, cefaclor, oral cefuroxime, loracarbef, or cefixime is reasonable. In addition, these agents may be useful in the allergic patient.

3. **Soft-tissue infections.** For minor soft-tissue infections due to susceptible gram-positive bacteria, a first-generation cephalosporin (cephalexin or cephradine, 500–1,000 mg qid in adults) can be used. Because streptococci and *S. aureus* are the usual pathogens, there is no reason to use the second-generation oral agents, and cefixime and ceftibuten are not active against *S. aureus.*

4. **Acute sinusitis.** Because *H. influenzae* is an important pathogen in acute sinusitis of adults as well as children, cefaclor, oral cefuroxime, cefprozil, loracarbef and, possibly, cefixime are reasonable agents for the patient who cannot receive amoxicillin, ampicillin, or TMP-SMX.

V. **Side effects of cephalosporins.** These agents are very well tolerated, which is one reason they are so popular [3].

A. **Phlebitis.** With intravenous use, phlebitis is not uncommon. There are no clear data indicating significant differences among the cephalosporins in terms of their ability to cause phlebitis, although, anecdotally, cephalothin is more likely to cause phlebitis.

B. **Primary allergic reactions.** There is approximately a 1–5% incidence of primary allergic reactions to the cephalosporins: urticarial and morbilliform rashes, fevers, eosinophilia, serum sickness, and anaphylaxis [2a, 124]. In penicillin-allergic patients, the risk of allergic reactions to cephalosporins formerly was believed to be in the range of 5–15% [124], but this may be an overestimate; more recent estimates are as low as 1% [45]. **In the patient with a history of an immediate reaction to penicillin (i.e., anaphylaxis, bronchospasm, hypotension, etc.), cephalosporins should be avoided** [77] unless careful skin testing can be performed. In the patient with a late or delayed mild reaction to penicillin, cephalosporins commonly are used (with caution). See further discussions in Chap. 27.

Data suggest that **cefaclor may be more frequently associated with a mild, reversible serum sickness–like reaction** than other oral antibiotics [2a, 125]. The incidence of serum sickness–like reactions with the use of loracarbef is unclear but has been described. This is a potential concern because of the similar structure of cefaclor and loracarbef [125a]. Otherwise, there are no data to indicate that hypersensitivity reactions are more common with any individual cephalosporin [2].

C. **Nephrotoxicity**
   1. **Cephaloridine** is no longer available because of its nephrotoxicity.
   2. **When used alone, the cephalosporins have infrequently caused significant nephrotoxicity** [2, 2a]. Prior conflicting data suggest that, in patients treated with an aminoglycoside and cephalothin, there is increased nephrotoxicity compared to treatment with an aminoglycoside and penicillin derivative used in combination. Therefore, it may be prudent to avoid prolonged or unnecessary use of cephalothin and an aminoglycoside. Recent data do not suggest enhanced nephrotoxicity with the third-generation agents and aminoglycosides [77] and, in one review, cephalosporins were not believed to potentiate the toxicity of aminoglycosides [2a]. Whenever an aminoglycoside is used with a cephalosporin, renal function and aminoglycoside levels should be monitored, as nephrotoxicity of the aminoglycoside alone is a legitimate concern. (See Chap. 28H.) Interstitial nephritis can occur as a hypersensitivity response [2].

D. **Hematologic effects**
   1. **Positive Coombs' reactions** are relatively common (> 3%) in patients on high-dose parenteral cephalosporin therapy. Hemolytic anemia is rare [2, 126].
   2. Granulocytopenia and thrombocytopenia generally are believed to be rare complications [10, 127]. However, in patients with severe underlying hepatic dysfunction, various beta-lactam antibiotics, including the cephalosporins, have recently been associated with leukopenia [127a]. Such patients perhaps should receive lower doses of beta-lactam antibiotics [127a].
   3. **Hypoprothrombinemia and bleeding** (e.g., gastrointestinal) have been described with moxalactam, cefamandole, and cefoperazone especially [36]. (See secs. **II.F.4** and **II.G.5.**) Moxalactam and, to a lesser extent, cefoperazone have also been associated with platelet dysfunction [35].
      a. **Incidence.** The exact incidence of this problem is unclear and controversial. See secs. **II.F.4** and **II.G.5.** Cefamandole may be associated with hypoprothrombinemia in more than 10% of recipients [11]. Hypoprothrombinemia and bleeding have been noted even more frequently with moxalactam (up to 45%), with associated bleeding in fewer than 5% of patients [56]. One reviewer noted the frequency of hypoprothrombinemia in recipients of NMTT agents has varied from 4 to 68% [2].
      b. **Mechanism.** The most frequently proposed mechanisms are (1) destruction of menaquinone (vitamin K), producing GI flora (especially with agents providing high biliary-stool concentrations), or (2) interference

with prothrombin synthesis by agents with the NMTT side chain of cefamandole, moxalactam, cefoperazone, cefotetan, and cefmetazole. A detailed discussion of the mechanism is beyond the scope of this text but has been reviewed elsewhere [36, 128, 129].

   c. **Clinical implications.** Because of the bleeding problems associated with cefamandole and moxalactam use, most clinicians have stopped using these agents. The role of NMTT-containing new agents, especially cefotetan and cefmetazole, remains controversial. (See secs. II.F and II.G.)

   If an agent with the NMTT side chain is used, especially in a patient at risk for hypoprothrombinemia (see Table 28F-8), serial prothrombin times and careful clinical follow-up seem prudent [36]. Because of the many other cephalosporin agents from which to choose, many clinicians and formulary committees may elect to avoid the cephalosporins associated with bleeding problems despite the potential cost savings that these agents may offer. (See secs. II.F and II.G.)

E. **Ethanol intolerance. Disulfiramlike reactions** (flushing, tachycardia, nausea, vomiting, headache, hypotension) have been described in patients receiving moxalactam, cefoperazone, and cefotetan [130]. The reaction has been attributed to the methylthiotetrazole ring structure [56], which is similar to the structural configuration of disulfiram. **As a precaution, patients receiving these agents should be warned *not to consume alcohol or alcohol-containing medications,*** as small amounts of alcohol can trigger the reaction [56].

F. *Clostridium difficile* **diarrhea. See Chap. 28A.** As discussed earlier, preliminary studies suggest that use of the second- and third-generation cephalosporins put recipients at an increased risk for developing *C. difficile* diarrhea compared with other classes of antibiotic agents [3], although further clinical data are needed to confirm this *impression.*

References

1. Medical Letter. Choice of antimicrobial drugs. *Med. Lett. Drugs Ther.* 38:25, 1996.
   See related summary: article, Choice of cephalosporins. Med. Lett. Drugs Ther. *32:107, 1990.*
2. Karchmer, A.W. Cephalosporins. In G.L. Mandell, J.E. Bennett, and R. Dolin (eds.), *Principles and Practice of Infectious Diseases* (4th ed.). New York: Churchill Livingstone, 1995. Pp. 247–264.
   Useful text discussion by an experienced clinician. Good review of structure-function relationships.
   For additional discussion as to why cephalothin sometimes is preferred over cefazolin for therapy of life-threatening methicillin-susceptible S. aureus infections, see an in vitro animal model study conducted by S.W. Chapman and R.T. Steigbigel, Staphylococcal β-lactamase and efficacy of β-lactam antibiotics: In vitro and in vivo evaluation. J. Infect. Dis. *147:1078, 1983.*
2a. Gastaferro, C.A., and Steckelberg, J.M. Cephalosporin antimicrobial agents and related compounds. *Mayo Clin. Proc.* 66:1064, 1991.
3. Nelson, D.E., et al. Epidemic *Clostridium difficile*–associated diarrhea: Role of second- and third-generation cephalosporins. *Infect. Control Hosp. Epidemiol.* 15:88, 1994.
   Report from the Centers for Disease Control and a Veterans Administration medical center in which multivariate analyses revealed prior cephalosporin exposure was important in 32 patients. See related report by A. Anand et al., Epidemiology, clinical manifestations, and outcome of Clostridium difficile–associated diarrhea. Am. J. Gastroenterol. *89:519, 1994, in which prior ceftriaxone or ceftazidime use was associated with* C. difficile *diarrhea.*
4. Feigin, R.D., McCracken, G.H., Jr., and Klein, J.O. Diagnosis and management of meningitis. *Pediatr. Infect. Dis. J.* 11:785, 1992.
   For a related report, see A.R. Tunkel et al., Bacterial meningitis: Recent advances in physiology and treatment. Ann. Intern. Med. *112:610, 1990.*
5. McCracken, G.H., Jr., et al. Consensus report: Antimicrobial therapy for bacterial meningitis in infants and children. *Pediatr. Infect. Dis. J.* 6:501, 1987.
   See related article by U.B. Schaad et al., A comparison of ceftriaxone and cefuroxime for the treatment of bacterial meningitis in children. N. Engl. J. Med. *322:141, 1990. Concludes that ceftriaxone is superior.*
6. Donowitz, G.R., and Mandell, G.L. Beta-lactam antibiotics. *N. Engl. J. Med.* 318: 490, 1988.

7. Goldberg, D.M. The cephalosporins. *Med. Clin. North Am.* 71:1113, 1987.
8. Bennett, W.M., et al. *Drug Prescribing in Renal Failure: Dosing Guidelines for Adults* (3rd ed.). Philadelphia: American College of Physicians, 1994.
   A useful handbook. Similar tables for dosing in renal failure appear in L.L. Livingstone et al., Antibacterial agents in renal failure. Infect. Dis. Clin. North Am. 9:591, 1995.
9. Quintiliani, R., and Nightingale, C.H. Cefazolin. *Ann. Intern. Med.* 89(Part I):650, 1978.
10. Moellering, R.C., Jr., and Swartz, M.N. The newer cephalosporins. *N. Engl. J. Med.* 294:24, 1976.
    Reviews first-generation cephalosporins.
11. Kozak, A.J., et al. Hypoprothrombinemia associated with concurrent use of cefamandole in a rural teaching hospital. *Arch. Intern. Med.* 146:1125, 1986.
12. Neu, H.C. Cefoxitin: An overview of clinical studies in the United States. *Rev. Infect. Dis.* 1:233, 1979.
13. Sanders, C.V., Greenburg, R.N., and Marier, R.L. Cefamandole and cefoxitin. *Ann. Intern. Med.* 103:70, 1985.
14. Cuchural, G.J., et al. Susceptibility of the *Bacteroides fragilis* group in the United States: Analysis by site of isolation. *Antimicrob. Agents Chemother.* 32:717, 1988.
15. Centers for Disease Control. Sexually transmitted diseases treatment guidelines. *M.M.W.R.* 42(RR-14):1–102, 1993.
16. Humbert, G., et al. Pharmacokinetics of cefoxitin in normal subjects and in patients with renal insufficiency. *Rev. Infect. Dis.* 1:118, 1979.
17. Greaves, W.L., et al. Cefoxitin disposition during peritoneal dialysis. *Antimicrob. Agents Chemother.* 19:253, 1981.
18. Medical Letter. Ceforanide (Precef). *Med. Lett. Drugs Ther.* 26:91, 1984.
19. Actor, P. In vitro experience with cefonicid. *Rev. Infect. Dis.* 6(Suppl. 4):S783, 1984.
20. Conte, J.E., Jr. Clinical and economic impact of cefonicid: Overview and summary of the symposium. *Rev. Infect. Dis.* 6(Suppl. 4):S777, 1984.
21. Medical Letter. Cefonicid sodium (Monocid). *Med. Lett. Drugs Ther.* 26:71, 1984.
22. Barriere, S.L., et al. Pharmacokinetic disposition of cefonicid in patients with renal failure and receiving hemodialysis. *Rev. Infect. Dis.* 6(Suppl. 4):S809, 1984.
23. Jacob, L.S., and Layne, P. Cefonicid: An overview of clinical studies in the United States. *Rev. Infect. Dis.* 6(Suppl. 4):S791, 1984.
24. Kaye, D. An overview: Evaluation of cefonicid in infections of the urinary tract, lower respiratory tract, and skin and soft tissue. *Rev. Infect. Dis.* 6(Suppl. 4):S835, 1984.
24a. Friedland, I.R., and McCracken, G.H., Jr. Management of infections caused by antibiotic-resistant *Streptococcus pneumoniae*. *N. Engl. J. Med.* 331:377, 1994.
    See discussion of this important topic in Chap. 28C.
25. Jones, R.N., and Thornsberry, C. In Vitro Antimicrobial Activity, Physical Characteristics and Other Microbiology Features of Cefuroxime: A New Study and Review. In R.C. Moellering, Jr. (ed.), *The Clinical Significance of the Newer β-Lactam Antibiotics: Focus on Cefuroxime* (vol. 3 in *Therapeutics Today Series*). New York: ADIS Press, 1983. Pp. 30–45.
26. Medical Letter. Cefuroxime sodium (Zinacef). *Med. Lett. Drugs Ther.* 26:15, 1984.
27. Nelson, J.D. Cefuroxime: A cephalosporin with unique applicability to pediatric practice. *Pediatr. Infect. Dis.* 2:394, 1983.
28. Medical Letter. Cefotetan. *Med. Lett. Drugs Ther.* 28:70, 1986.
29. Ward, A., and Richards, D.M. Cefotetan: A review. *Drugs* 30:382, 1985.
30. Barza, M. Cefotetan: Summary of the symposium from an internist's viewpoint. *Am. J. Surg.* 155(5A):103, 1988.
    This excellent summary is from a published symposium. A related series of papers was also published in H.C. Neu and M. Barza. Am. J. Obstet. Gynecol. 158(3, Part II):687–746, 1988.
31. Jones, R.N. Cefotetan: A review of the microbiologic properties and antimicrobial spectrum. *Am. J. Surg.* 155(5A):16, 1988.
31a. Hecht, D.W., Osmolski, J.R., and O'Keefe, J.P. Variation in the susceptibility of *Bacteroides fragilis* group isolates from six Chicago hospitals. *Clin. Infect. Dis.* 16(Suppl. 4):S357, 1993.
    Data from two private medical centers and four university medical centers indicating variation in susceptibility data from hospital to hospital. See related discussions in Chap. 28I.
32. Jones, R.N. Hemorrhagic complications of cephalosporin therapy: A perspective for 1989. *The Antimicrobial Newsletter* 5:85, 1987.
33. Goldstein, N.H. Analysis of prothrombin time prolongation in North American cefotetan clinical trials: Questions and answers. *Am. J. Surg.* 155[5A]:64, 1988.

The incidence of hypoprothrombinemia was similar for cefotetan-treated patients [2.5%] and cefoxitin-treated patients [1.6%].

34. Grasela, T., et al. Prospective surveillance of antibiotic-associated coagulopathy in 970 patients. *Pharmacotherapy* 9:158, 1989.
    Nationwide surveillance program where study suggests that the frequency of antibiotic-associated coagulopathy is low, regardless of the antibiotic used, in patients who are not critically ill and not malnourished.

35. Sattler, F.R., et al. Impaired hemostasis caused by beta-lactam antibiotics. *Am. J. Surg.* 155(5A):30, 1988.
    Good discussion. Also contains useful discussion of therapy of patients who bleed while on antibiotics and discusses use of prophylactic vitamin K.

36. Shevchuk, Y.M., and Conly, J.M. Antibiotic-associated hypoprothrombinemia: A review of prospective studies 1966–1988. *Rev. Infect. Dis.* 12:1109, 1990.
    Extensive literature review in adult patients revealed that the incidence of hypoprothrombinemia varied from 3.7 to 64% with regimen containing N-methylthiotetrazole (NMTT) and from 0 to 24% with non-NMTT-containing regimens. Whether the NMTT side chain clearly is related to hypoprothrombinemia still is unclear, and more data are needed. Prophylactic use of antibiotics with or without the NMTT moiety is associated infrequently with significant hypoprothrombinemia. Certain high-risk factors (malnutrition, hepatic and renal dysfunction, older age, and severity of illness) may be important determinants of hypoprothrombinemia. Such high-risk patients need serial prothrombin monitoring.

37. McCloskey, R.V. Spontaneous reports of bleeding: Comparison of N-methylthiotetrazole side chain (MTT) and non-MTT cephalosporins. *J. Infect. Dis.* 158:1405, 1988.
    Review of adverse drug reports. Revealed use of MTT-containing cephalosporins, rather than non-MTT-containing compounds, is associated with more reports of hypoprothrombinemia, both with and without major bleeding. In conclusion, the author questions why MTT-containing cephalosporins continue to be used and why newer ones should be considered for clinical investigation.

38. Conjura, A., Bell, W., and Lipsky, J.J. Cefotetan and hypoprothrombinemia. *Ann. Intern. Med.* 108:643, 1988.
    Report of a 30-year-old woman with poor oral intake, azotemia, and cefotetan therapy for pneumonia. Patient developed hypoprothrombinemia and clinical bleeding, requiring transfusion after approximately 18 days of cefotetan therapy.

39. *Physicians' Desk Reference* (50th ed.). Montvale, NJ: Medical Economics, 1996.

39a. Committee on Antimicrobial Agents, Canadian Infectious Disease Society. Cefotetan: A second-generation cephalosporin active against anaerobic bacteria. *Can. Med. Assoc. J.* 151:537, 1994.
    Includes in the discussion of side effects that there have been several case reports of hypoprothrombinemia and bleeding associated with the use of cefotetan. The hypoprothrombinemia was viewed as a real risk when compared to the risk with cefoxitin use. Concluded that although use of cefotetan has cost advantages (e.g., over cefoxitin), these should not override safety and efficacy considerations. (Cefotetan is less active than cefoxitin against other species of the Bacteroides fragilis *group).*

40. Finch, R., Moellering, R.C., Jr., and Speller, D. Cefmetazole: A clinical appraisal. *J. Antimicrob. Chemother.* 23(Suppl. D):1, 1989.
    Issue devoted to a symposium on this new agent. For a related review, see the series of articles in Hosp. Ther. *15:(Suppl.):3, 1990.*

41. Medical Letter. Cefmetazole sodium (Zefazone). *Med. Lett. Drugs Ther.* 32:65, 1990.

42. Jones, R.N. Review of the in vitro spectrum and characteristics of cefmetazole. *J. Antimicrob. Chemother.* 23(Suppl. D):1, 1989.

43. Griffith, D.L., et al. Clinical experience with cefmetazole sodium in the United States: An overview. *J. Antimicrob. Chemother.* 23(Suppl. D):21, 1989.

44. Saito, A. Cefmetazole postmarketing surveillance in Japan. *J. Antimicrob. Chemother.* 23(Suppl. D):31, 1989.

45. Donowitz, G.R. Third-generation cephalosporins. *Infect. Dis. Clin. North Am.* 3:595, 1989.
    For a recent update see related review by N.C. Klein and B.A. Cunha, Third-generation cephalosporins. Med. Clin. North Am. *79:705, 1995.*

46. Neu, H. Pathophysiologic basis for the use of third-generation cephalosporins. *Am. J. Med.* 88(Suppl. 4A):3S, 1990.
    Updates these agents after a decade of use. Excellent review of susceptibility data; special emphasis on cefotaxime.

46a. Feliciano, D.V., et al. Single agent cephalosporin prophylaxis for penetrating abdominal trauma. *Am. J. Surg.* 152:674, 1986.
In this study, cefotaxime, 2 g q6h, was more effective than cefoxitin, 2 g q6h, in preventing infections. Both agents were given for 48 hours. However, the cefoxitin recipients may have been sicker patients, with more associated vascular injuries and intraoperative hypotension, and therefore may have been more prone to postoperative infections.
47. Chow, J.W., et al. *Enterobacter* bacteremia: Clinical features and emergence of antibiotic resistance during therapy. *Ann. Intern. Med.* 115:585, 1991.
Emphasizes that more judicious use of third-generation cephalosporins may decrease the incidence of nosocomial multiresistant Enterobacter *species, which in turn may result in a lower mortality for* Enterobacter *bacteremia.*
48. Maugh, T.H. A new wave of antibiotics builds. *Science* 214:1225, 1981.
49. Neu, H.C. The new beta-lactamase-stable cephalosporins. *Ann. Intern. Med.* 97:408, 1982.
50. Sanders, C.C., and Sanders, W.E., Jr. Microbial resistance to newer generation β-lactam antibiotics: Clinical and laboratory implications. *J. Infect. Dis.* 151:399, 1985.
51. Sanders, C. New β-lactams: New problems for the internist. *Ann. Intern. Med.* 115:651, 1991.
This editorial comment on reference 47 emphasizes the importance of using the third-generation cephalosporins prudently to avoid resistance.
52. Medical Letter. Cefotaxime sodium (Claforan). *Med. Lett. Drugs Ther.* 23:61, 1981.
53. Medical Letter. Cefoperazone sodium (Cefobid). *Med. Lett. Drugs Ther.* 25:29, 1983.
54. Medical Letter. Ceftizoxime sodium (Cefizox). *Med. Lett. Drugs Ther.* 25:109, 1983.
55. Medical Letter. Ceftriaxone sodium. *Med. Lett. Drugs Ther.* 27:37, 1985.
For an update symposium on ceftriaxone, see J. Remington et al. Update 1991: Ceftriax one in treatment of serious infections. Hosp. Pract. 262(Suppl. 5):5–64, 1991.
56. Barriere, S.L., and Flaherty, J.F. Third-generation cephalosporins: A critical evaluation. *Clin. Pharmacol.* 3:351, 1984.
57. Moellering, R.C., Jr. Introduction: Ceftriaxone—a long-acting cephalosporin. *Am. J. Med.* 77(4C):1, 1984.
58. Cherubin, C.E., et al. Penetration of the newer cephalosporins into cerebrospinal fluid. *Rev. Infect. Dis.* 11:526, 1989.
59. Rodriguez, W.J., et al. Treatment of *Pseudomonas* meningitis with ceftazidime with or without concurrent therapy. *Pediatr. Infect. Dis. J.* 9:83, 1990.
Ceftazidime is useful in this setting. Good bibliography.
60. Smith, C.R. Cefotaxime compared with nafcillin plus tobramycin for serious bacterial infection: A randomized, double-blind trial. *Ann. Intern. Med.* 101:469, 1984.
See editorial response in same issue.
61. Pizzo, P.A., et al. A randomized trail comparing ceftazidime alone with combination antibiotic therapy in cancer patients with fever and neutropenia. *N. Engl. J. Med.* 315:552, 1986.
See editorial response in same issue emphasizing the importance of not using monotherapy in the bacteremic patient. Additional support for using ceftazidime in combination with an aminoglycoside for bacteremias in cancer patients with granulocytopenia is shown in the study by EORTC International Antimicrobial Therapy Cooperative Group where ceftazidime is combined with a short or long course of amikacin for empiric therapy of gram-negative bacteremia in cancer patients with granulocytopenia. N. Engl. J. Med. *317:1692, 1987. See references 62 and 66.*
62. DePauw, B.E., et al. Ceftazidime compared with piperacillin and tobramycin for the empiric treatment of fever in neutropenic patients with cancer: A multicenter randomized trial. *Ann. Intern. Med.* 120:834, 1994.
In this large study (multicenter, randomized, controlled trial involving 876 patients including 83% acute leukemics and bone marrow transplant recipients), ceftazidime alone (2 g q8h) was as effective but safer than piperacillin (12–18 g/d) plus tobramycin (1.7–2.0 mg/kg per dose q8h if renal function was normal).
63. Young, J.P.W., et al. The evaluation of efficacy and safety of cefotaxime: A review of 2,500 cases. *J. Antimicrob. Chemother.* 6(Suppl. A):293, 1980.
64. Andriole, V.T., and Kirby, W.M.M. Overview/introduction: Cefoperazone. *Am. J. Med.* 85(Suppl. 1A):1, 1988.
Symposium emphasizes recent studies using double beta-lactam antibiotics (e.g., cefoperazone and mezlocillin or piperacillin) in neutropenic cancer patients.
65. Jenkins, S.G. Comparative susceptibility patterns of common clinical isolates to cefoperazone: 1981 to 1987. *Am. J. Med.* 85(Suppl. 1A):52, 1988.

66. Hughes, W.T., et al. Guidelines for the use of antimicrobial agents in neutropenic patients with unexplained fever. *J. Infect. Dis.* 161:381, 1990.
   Prepared by the Working Committee, Infectious Disease Society of America.
67. Cleeland, R., and Squires, E. Antimicrobial activity of ceftriaxone: A review. *Am. J. Med.* 77(4C):3, 1984.
68. Dattwyler, R.J., et al. Ceftriaxone as effective therapy in refractory Lyme disease. *J. Infect. Dis.* 155:1322, 1987.
   For a related article, see H.W. Pfister et al., Randomized comparison of ceftriaxone and cefotaxime in Lyme neuroborreliosis. J. Infect. Dis. 163:311, 1991.
69. Patel, I.H., and Kaplan, S.A. Pharmacokinetic profile of ceftriaxone in man. *Am. J. Med.* 77(4C):17, 1984.
70. Higham, M., Cunningham, F.M., and Teele, D.W. Ceftriaxone administered once or twice a day for treatment of bacterial infections of childhood. *Pediatr. Infect. Dis.* 4:22, 1985.
   Once-daily dosage in adequate in non-CNS infections.
71. Mandell, L.A., et al. Once-daily therapy with ceftriaxone compared with daily multiple-dose therapy with cefotaxime for serious bacterial infections: A randomized, double-blind study. *J. Infect. Dis.* 160:433, 1989.
   Daily single-dose therapy with ceftriaxone was comparable.
72. Smith, C.R., et al. Ceftriaxone compared with cefotaxime for serious bacterial infections. *J. Infect. Dis.* 160:442, 1989.
   Ceftriaxone, 2 g/d, was as safe and effective as cefotaxime, 2 g q4h.
73. Dagan, R., et al. Outpatient treatment of serious community-acquired pediatric infections using once-daily intramuscular ceftriaxone. *Pediatr. Infect. Dis. J.* 6:1080, 1987.
74. Frenkel, L.D., and the Multicenter Ceftriaxone Pediatric Study Group. Once-daily administration of ceftriaxone for the treatment of selected serious bacterial infections in children. *Pediatrics* 82:486, 1988.
75. Francioli, P., et al. Treatment of streptococcal endocarditis with a single daily dose of ceftriaxone sodium for 4 weeks. Efficacy and outpatient treatment feasibility. *J.A.M.A.* 257:264, 1992.
   A 2-g dose once daily was used. See favorable editorial response. See W.R. Wilson et al., Antibiotic treatment of adults with infective endocarditis due to streptococci, enterococci, staphylococci, and HACEK microorganisms. J.A.M.A. 274:1706, 1995. This December 1995 article summarizes the American Heart Association treatment guidelines in which ceftriaxone use is favored. See Chap. 10.
75a. Green, S.M., and Rothrock, S.G. Single-dose intramuscular ceftriaxone for acute otitis media in children. *Pediatrics* 91:23, 1993.
   A single intramuscular dose of ceftriaxone (50 mg/kg) was believed to be as effective as 10 days of oral amoxicillin for uncomplicated otitis media. Letters to the editor from A. Hoberman, J. Paradise, and P.H. Kaleida (Children's Hospital of Pittsburgh), Pediatrics 92:507, 1993, suggest that more data are necessary before adopting this approach.
   The Medical Letter concluded that a singe dose of intramuscular ceftriaxone could prove to be effective (therapy), but more data are needed; see Med. Lett. Drugs Ther. 36:21, 1994.
76. Moskovitz, B.L. Clinical adverse effects during ceftriaxone therapy. *Am. J. Med.* 77(4C):84, 1984.
   See companion article in same issue, pp. 89–97.
77. Fekety, F.R. Safety of parenteral third-generation cephalosporins. *Am. J. Med.* 88 (Suppl. 4A):38S, 1990.
78. Lopez, A.J., et al. Ceftriaxone-induced cholelithiasis. *Ann. Intern. Med.* 115:712, 1991.
79. Jacobs, R.F. Ceftriaxone-associated cholecystitis. *Pediatr. Infect. Dis. J.* 7:434, 1988.
80. Medical Letter. Ceftazidime. *Med. Lett. Drugs Ther.* 27:85, 1985.
81. Gold, R., et al. Controlled trial of ceftazidime vs. ticarcillin and tobramycin in the treatment of acute respiratory exacerbations in patients with cystic fibrosis. *Pediatr. Infect. Dis.* 4:172, 1985.
82. Norrby, S.R. Role of cephalosporins in the treatment of bacterial meningitis in adults. Overview with special emphasis on ceftazidime. *Am. J. Med.* 79(Suppl. 2A):56, 1985.
   See preceding article in same issue.
83. Korvick, J., and Yu, V.L. Antimicrobial agent therapy for *Pseudomonas aeruginosa*. *Antimicrob. Agents Chemother.* 35:2167, 1991.
   For severe pneumonia or bacteremia infections, an antipseudomonal penicillin and aminoglycoside still are preferred. In meningitis, ceftazidime as monotherapy is preferred.

84. Trenholme, G.M., et al. Use of ceftazidime in the treatment of nosocomial lower respiratory infections. *Am. J. Med.* 79(Suppl. 2A):32, 1985.
85. Johnson, M.P., and Ramphal, R. Malignant external otitis: Report on therapy with ceftazidime and review of therapy and prognosis. *Rev. Infect. Dis.* 13:173, 1990.
86. Koontz, F.B., et al. Antibiotic resistance: Experience at the University of Iowa hospitals and clinics. Presented at *Emerging Trends in Gram Negative Resistance: A new concern for critical care medicine* (symposium), Atlanta, Oct. 21, 1990.
    For a similar report, see R.L. Correlli et al., Thirty-first Interscience Conference on Antimicrobial Agents and Chemotherapy (Abstract 1006), Chicago, 1991.
86a. Barradell, L.B., and Bryson, H.M. Cefepime: A review of its antimicrobial activity, pharmacokinetic properties, and therapeutic use. *Drugs* 47:471, 1994.
    A comprehensive review. For a related symposium, see E.M. Brown, R.G. Finch, and L.O. White, Cefepime: A β-lactamase-stable extended-spectrum cephalosporin. J. Antimicrob. Chemother. 32(Suppl. B):1–214, 1994. See also C.C. Sanders, Cefepime: The next generation. Clin. Infect. Dis. 17:369, 1993.
86b. Ehrhardt, A.F., and Sanders, C.C. β-lactam resistance among *Enterobacter* species. *J. Antimicrob. Chemother.* 32(Suppl. B):1, 1993.
    Surveys in the United States and elsewhere have shown that there is an increased prevalence of multi-β-lactam-resistant strains of Enterobacter *spp., which is due to the increased use of available cephalosporins. Attempts to prevent these problems include the more judicious use of newer β-lactam antibiotics and the development of enhanced-potency cephalosporins (e.g., cefepime), which are able to avoid resistance because they have lower enzyme affinity and permeate more rapidly in the cell.*
    This article is the first in a series of articles in this special symposium devoted to cefepime. See E.M. Brown et al., Cefepime: A β-lactamase-stable extended-spectrum cephalosporin. J. Antimicrob. Chemother. 32(Suppl. B):1–214, 1993.
86c. Cunha, B.A., and Gill, M.A. Cefepime. *Med. Clin. North Am.* 79:721, 1995.
    See related paper by J.H. Schrank et al., Randomized comparison of cefepime and ceftazidime for treatment of hospitalized patients with gram-negative bacteremia. Clin. Infect. Dis. 20:56, 1995. Data suggested cefepime is as efficacious and well-tolerated as ceftazidime in this setting.
87. Veterans Administration Ad Hoc Interdisciplinary Advisory Committee on Antimicrobial Drug Usage. Oral cephalosporins. *J.A.M.A.* 237:1241, 1977.
88. Ruff, M.E., et al. Antimicrobial drug suspensions: A blind comparison of taste of fourteen common pediatric drugs. *Pediatr. Infect. Dis. J.* 10:30, 1991.
    Compared the smell, taste, and other characteristics of 14 commonly prescribed antimicrobial suspensions in a blind test in 30 adult volunteers. The oral cephalosporins ranked the best. Children younger than 6 years may be more sensitive to taste than older children and adults.
89. Baxter, R., Chapman, J., and Drew, W.L. Comparison of bactericidal activity of five antibiotics against *Staphylococcus aureus*. *J. Infect. Dis.* 161:1023, 1990.
    A bactericidal level of 1:8 or more has been associated with cure of osteomyelitis. See L.B. Reller, The serum bactericidal test. Rev. Infect. Dis. 8:803, 1986. The study by Baxter and colleagues demonstrated that in a small number of patients, cephalexin, 1 g PO q6h, provided peak bactericidal levels of 1:8, higher than those achieved with oral ciprofloxacin, dicloxacillin, and trimethoprim-sulfamethoxazole. These preliminary data further support the concept that at least with high doses, cephalexin can provide reasonably good bactericidal levels.
90. Medical Letter. Two new oral cephalosporins. *Med. Lett. Drugs Ther.* 21:85, 1979.
    Concise review of cefadroxil and cefaclor.
91. Sanders, C. Beta-lactamase stability and in vivo activity of oral cephalosporins against strains possessing well-characterized mechanisms of resistance. *Antimicrob. Agents Chemother.* 33:1313, 1989.
92. Blumer, J.L., Bertino, J.S., Jr., and Husak, M.P. Comparison of cefaclor and trimethoprim-sulfamethoxazole in the treatment of acute otitis media. *Pediatr. Infect. Dis. J.* 3:25, 1984.
93. Bluestone, C.D. Management of otitis media in infants and children: Current role of old and new microbial agents. *Pediatr. Infect. Dis. J.* 7:S129, 1988.
94. Sydnor, A.J., Jr., et al. Comparative evaluation of cefuroxime axetil and cefaclor for treatment of acute bacterial maxillary sinusitis. *Arch. Otolaryngol. Head Neck Surg.* 115:1430, 1989.
95. Ginsburg, C.M., et al. Pharmacokinetics and bactericidal activity of cefuroxime axetil. *Antimicrob. Agents Chemother.* 28:504, 1985.

96. Medical Letter. Cefuroxime axetil. *Med. Lett. Drugs Ther.* 30:57, 1988.
97. Goldstein, E.J., Citron, D.M., and Richwald, G.A. Lack of in vitro efficacy of oral forms of certain cephalosporins, erythromycin, and oxacillin against *Pasteurella multocida*. *Antimicrob. Agents Chemother.* 32:213, 1988.
98. Medical Letter. Cefprozil. *Med. Lett. Drugs. Ther.* 34:63, 1992.
99. Klein, J.O. Evaluation of a new oral antimicrobial agents and the experience with cefprozil—a broad-spectrum oral cephalosporin. *Clin. Infect. Dis.* 14(Suppl. 2):S183, 1992.
    Special supplement that reviews in vitro, pharmacokinetic, clinical efficacy, and safety profile of cefprozil. Supplement also has a good series of articles on how to evaluate new agents in the therapy of otitis media, sinusitis, pharyngitis, lower respiratory tract infections, and urinary tract infections.
100. Thornsberry, C. Review of the in vitro activity of cefprozil, a new oral cephalosporin. *Clin. Infect. Dis.* 14(Suppl. 2):S189, 1992.
    See related paper by J.C. Fung-Tome et al., Antibacterial activity of cefprozil with those of 13 oral cephems and 3 macrolides. Antimicrob. Agents Chemother. 39:533, 1995.
101. Barriere, S. Pharmacology and pharmacokinetics of cefprozil. *Clin. Infect. Dis.* 14 (Suppl. 2):S184, 1992.
102. Shyu, W.C., et al. Excretion of cefprozil into human breast milk. *Antimicrob. Agents Chemother.* 36:938, 1992.
103. Wiler, R.B., et al. Safety profile of cefprozil. *Clin. Infect. Dis.* 4(Suppl. 2):S264, 1992.
    Data on use in more than 4,000 children and adults, confirming the safety of this cephalosporin.
104. Bluestone, C.D. Current therapy for otitis media and criteria for evaluation of new antimicrobial agents. *Clin. Infect. Dis.* 14(Suppl. 2):S197, 1992.
    See associated discussions at the end of this article.
105. Bass, J.W. Antibiotic management of group A streptococcal pharyngotonsillitis. *Pediatr. Infect. Dis.* S43, 1991.
    Good discussion of antibiotic options and dosages. See related paper by J.O. Klein, Management of streptococcal pharyngitis. Pediatr. Infect. Dis. 13:572, 1994.
106. Moellering, R.C., and Jacobs, N.F., Jr. Advances in outpatient antimicrobial therapy: Loracarbef. *Am. J. Med.* 92(Suppl. 6A):1S, 1992.
107. Doern, G. In vitro activity of loracarbef and effects of susceptibility test methods. *Am. J. Med.* 92(Suppl. 6A):7S, 1992.
    Minimum inhibitory concentration data vary; loracarbef susceptibility tests may not predict therapeutic outcome.
108. DeSante, K.A., and Zeckel, M.L. Pharmacokinetic profile of loracarbef. *Am. J. Med.* 92(Suppl. 6A):16S, 1992.
109. Moellering, R.C., Jr., and Jacobs, N.F. Preclinical data and clinical experience with loracarbef: A summary. *Am. J. Med.* 92(Suppl 6A):1015, 1992.
    See related symposium: H.F. Eichenwald et al., New directions in antimicrobial therapy: Loracarbef. Pediatr. Infect. Dis. J. 11(Suppl. 8):S5, 1992.
110. Gan, V.N., et al. Comparative efficacy of loracarbef and amoxicillin-clavulanate for acute otitis media. *Antimicrob. Agents Chemother.* 35:967, 1991.
    See study by W.S. Foshee, J. Pediatr. 120:980, 1992. Loracarbef had similar efficacy but produced less diarrhea and vomiting.
111. Therasse, D.G. The safety profile of loracarbef: Clinical trials in respiratory, skin, and urinary tract infections. *Am. J. Med.* 92(Suppl. 6A):20S, 1992.
112. Medical Letter. Drugs for treatment of acute otitis media. *Med. Lett. Drugs Ther.* 36:19, 1994.
    Consultants conclude that despite the increasing prevalence of resistant pathogens, including penicillin-resistant Streptococcus pneumoniae, amoxicillin is still the initial treatment of choice for most children. The cephalosporins (second- and third-generation) offer expensive alternatives.
113. Medical Letter. Cefixime: A new oral cephalosporin. *Med. Lett. Drugs Ther.* 31:73, 1989.
114. McCracken, G.H., Jr. Introduction: Cefixime, clinical overview of a new oral third-generation cephalosporin. *Am. J. Med.* 85(3A):1, 1989.
115. Neu, H.C., and McCracken, G.H., Jr. Proceedings of a conference: Clinical pharmacology and efficacy of cefixime. *Pediatr. Infect. Dis. J.* 6:951, 1987.
116. Nash, D.A. Comparison of the activity of cefixime and activities of other oral antibiotics against adult clinical isolates of *Moraxella (Branhamella) catarrhalis* containing

BRO-1 and BRO-2 and *Haemophilus influenzae. Antimicrob. Agents Chemother.* 35:192, 1991.

117. Johnson, C.E., et al. Cefixime compared with amoxicillin for treatment of acute otitis media. *J. Pediatr.* 119:117, 1991.

Because Streptococcus pneumoniae *remains the most common cause of otitis media and amoxicillin is less expensive than the cephalosporins, amoxicillin still is the preferred agent for initial therapy when the pathogen is unknown. Cefixime is useful in the otitis-conjunctivitis syndrome, which is almost always caused by* H. influenzae, *and for children not responding to amoxicillin.*

118. Ottolini, M.G. Pneumococcal bacteremia during oral treatment with cefixime for otitis media. *Pediatr. J. Infect. Dis.* 10:467, 1991.

Discusses an 11-month-old patient who had positive blood cultures for Streptococcus pneumoniae *while on cefixime. Discusses other studies suggesting a trend toward cefixime failure to eradicate pneumococcus from middle-ear aspirates.*

119. Pippo, T., et al. Double-blind comparison of cefixime and cefaclor in the treatment of acute otitis media. *Scand. J. Infect. Dis.* 23:459, 1991.

119a. Bluestone, C.D. Review of cefixime in the treatment of otitis media in infants and children. *Pediatr. Infect. Dis. J.* 12:75, 1993.

120. Hansfield, H.H., et al. A comparison of single-dose cefixime with ceftriaxone as treatment for uncomplicated gonorrhea. *N. Engl. J. Med.* 325:1337, 1991.

A single dose of cefixime (400 mg or 800 mg) orally was as effective as 250 mg IM ceftriaxone. See Chap. 13; the 400-mg dose of cefixime is enough.

121. Plourde, P.J., et al. Single-dose cefixime versus single-dose ceftriaxone in the treatment of antimicrobial-resistant *Neisseria gonorrhoeae* infection. *J. Infect. Dis.* 166: 919, 1992.

A single oral dose of cefixime is effective.

122. Medical Letter. Cefpodoxime proxetil—a new oral cephalosporin. *Med. Lett. Drugs Ther.* 34:107, 1992.

See also H.S. Sader et al., In vitro activity of cefpodoxime compared with other oral cephalosporins tested against 5,556 recent clinical isolates from five medical centers. Diag. Microbiol. Infect. Dis. *17:143, 1993.*

123. Dabernat, H., et al. In vitro activity of cefpodoxime against pathogens responsible for community-acquired respiratory tract infections. *J. Antimicrob. Chemother.* 26(Suppl. E):1, 1990.

Special supplement devoted to cefpodoxime. See related symposium by D. Adam et al., Cefpodoxime proxetil: A new third generation oral cephalosporin. Drugs 42(Suppl. 3):1, 1991. Also see J.E. Frampton et al., Cefpodoxime proxetil. Drugs 44:889, 1992.

123a. Jones, R. Ceftibuten: A review of antimicrobial activity, spectrum and other microbiologic features. *Pediatr. Infect. Dis. J.* 14:S77, 1995.

Part of a special July 1995 supplement issue devoted to this new agent. Includes clinical study data on therapy of streptococcal pharyngitis and acute otitis media.

123b. Neu, H.C. Ceftibuten: Minimal inhibitory concentrations, post antibiotic effect and beta-lactamase stability—A rationale for dosing programs. *Pediatr. Infect. Dis. J.* 14:S88, 1995.

Discusses the pharmacokinetics and in vitro activity as basis for recommended once-daily dosing regimen.

123c. Wiseman, L.R., and Baljour, J.A. Ceftibuten: A review of its antibacterial activity, pharmacokinetic properties and clinical efficacy. *Drugs* 47:784, 1994.

123d. Reidenberg, B.E. Worldwide safety experience with ceftibuten pediatric suspension. *Pediatr. Infect. Dis. J.* 14:S130, 1995.

123e. Medical Letter. Ceftibuten: A new oral cephalosporin. *Med. Lett. Drugs Ther.* 38:23, 1996.

Concludes that this is an expensive new oral cephalosporin that seems like a poor choice for the indications for which it is being marketed!

124. Moellering, R.C., Jr. Penicillin allergy and cross-reaction to cephalosporins. *J.A.M.A.* 244:2562, 1980.

125. Heckbert, S.R., et al. Serum sickness in children after antibiotic exposure: Estimates of occurrence and morbidity in a health maintenance organization population. *Am. J. Epidemiol.* 132:336, 1990.

In this review, five cases of serum sickness due to cefaclor (in 3,553 courses); one case with amoxicillin (in 13,487 courses); and four cases with trimethoprim-sulfamethoxazole (in 5,597 courses) were noted. Risk of serum sickness was significantly elevated after cefaclor compared with amoxicillin. Cases of serum sickness were mild and did not require hospitalization. See also R. Platt et al., Infect. Dis. 158:474, 1988.

125a. Bravo, H.F., et al. Loracarbef, causing serum sickness–like reaction. *Infect. Dis. Clin. Pract.* 3:363, 1994.
Describes a case in an 18-year-old man. Loracarbef has a chemical structure identical to cefaclor except the sulfur atom in the dihydrothiazine ring of the cephalosporin has been replaced by a methylene group. A serum sickness–like reaction has been seen in 0.024 to 0.5% of cefaclor recipients; the incidence of serum sickness in loracarbef still is unclear.

126. Kauffman, C.A., et al. Cefotetan-induced immune hemolytic anemia. *Clin. Infect. Dis.* 15:863, 1992.

127. Kirkwood, C.F., et al. Neutropenia associated with β-lactam antibiotics. *Clin. Pharmacol.* 2:569, 1983.

127a. Singh, N., et al. β-lactam antibiotic–induced leukopenia in severe hepatic dysfunction: Risk factors and implications for dosing in patients with liver disease. *Am. J. Med.* 94:251, 1993.
*In patients with severe hepatic dysfunction (liver transplant recipients as well as patients with end-stage liver disease awaiting liver transplantation), leukopenia developed in 23% of recipients of β-lactam antibiotics. Usual dosages were given based on creatinine clearances. **The authors propose a reduction in dosages of beta-lactam antibiotics when used in patients with hepatic dysfunction.***

128. Lipsky, J. Review: Antibiotic-associated hypoprothrombinemia. *J. Antimicrob. Chemother.* 21:281, 1988.
Suggests that the hypothesis that the destruction of intestinal bacteria ultimately results in hypoprothrombinemia may not be justified. Antibiotics that contain the N-methylthiotetrazole side chain may inhibit the vitamin K–dependent step in clotting factor synthesis.

129. Sheradzan, R.R., et al. Comparative effects of cefoxitin and cefotetan on vitamin K metabolism. *Antimicrob. Agents Chemother.* 32:1446, 1988.

130. Kline, S.S., et al. Cefotetan-induced disulfiram-type reactions and hypoprothrombinemia. *Antimicrob. Agents Chemother.* 31:1328, 1987.

G. Unique Beta-Lactam Antibiotics: Aztreonam and Imipenem

I. **Aztreonam (Azactam).** In 1978–1979, after careful screening of naturally occurring beta-lactam products of microorganisms, a novel antibiotic was found and was given the family name *monobactam*. **Aztreonam is the first clinically useful monobactam** [1–7] and is not nephrotoxic, is weakly immunogenic, and has not been associated with abnormalities in coagulation [7]. It is promoted for the treatment of gram-negative aerobic infections as a safer agent than the aminoglycosides.

A. **Structure and activity**
1. **Basic structure.** Aztreonam is a beta-lactam antibiotic. The structural relationship of the monobactams compared with other beta-lactam antibiotics is shown in Fig. 28F-1.
2. **Molecular modification.** This naturally occurring parent compound has undergone multiple molecular modifications to achieve a clinically useful and active synthetic compound, **aztreonam.**
    a. Aztreonam **interferes** with the biosynthesis of **bacterial cell walls** by binding to penicillin-binding proteins [2].
    b. **Bactericidal** concentrations are similar to inhibitory concentrations; therefore, tolerance usually is not seen.
    c. Aztreonam is highly **resistant to** enzymatic inactivation by **beta-lactamases** produced by gram-negative bacteria (both plasmid- and chromosome-mediated). In addition, aztreonam is a poor inducer of chromosomal beta-lactamase production [2].

B. **In vitro activity.** The antibacterial spectrum of aztreonam **is unique among the beta-lactam antibiotics because it is active only against gram-negative aerobes.** The structure of aztreonam allows high-affinity binding of the drug to the penicillin-binding proteins of many aerobic gram-negative bacilli. Furthermore, aztreonam's structure provides a poor substrate for most beta-lactamases [6b].

1. **Gram-positive aerobes** (e.g., staphylococci, streptococci): little or no activity.
2. **Anaerobes:** little or no activity.
3. **Gram-negative aerobes**
   a. Highly active against many Enterobacteriaceae (e.g., *Escherichia coli, Klebsiella pneumoniae*), *Neisseria meningitidis, N. gonorrhoeae* (penicillin-susceptible and -resistant), and *Haemophilus influenzae* (ampicillin-susceptible and -resistant) with a minimum inhibitory concentration$_{90}$ (MIC$_{90}$) of 1.0 μg/ml or less (i.e., 90% of strains are susceptible to < 1.0 μg/ml). The activity of aztreonam is excellent and comparable to that of the aminoglycosides and third-generation cephalosporins [2–4, 6]. **See Table 28G-1.**
   b. Aztreonam is active against *Pasteurella multocida* and *Aeromonas* spp.
   c. Aztreonam inhibits 50% of *Pseudomonas aeruginosa* isolates at 4 μg/ml and 90% at 16–32 μg/ml; concentrations of aztreonam required to inhibit *P. aeruginosa* usually are twofold greater than those for ceftazidime [6]. Aztreonam is slightly less active in vitro than imipenem against *P. aeruginosa* but is more active than piperacillin, mezlocillin, or ticarcillin. Whether these in vitro differences are clinically important is unknown [2]. A recent review points out that about 12% of *P. aeruginosa* may be resistant to aztreonam [6b]. Some strains of *Pseudomonas* and *Enterobacter* spp. may be tolerant [7]. The combination of aztreonam and piperacillin (or mezlocillin) is synergistic against some strains of *P. aeruginosa* and *Enterobacter* spp. but not as frequently synergistic as is the combination of piperacillin-aminoglycoside [7a]. Aztreonam acts synergistically with aminoglycosides against *P. aeruginosa* and some Enterobacteriaceae [2].
   d. Strains of *Citrobacter freundii, Enterobacter aerogenes,* and *E. cloacae* usually are **resistant** to aztreonam, cefotaxime, and ceftazidime. Aztreonam is not active against *Legionella pneumophila,* most strains of *Acinetobacter* spp., and many strains of *Pseudomonas* spp. (e.g., *P. maltophilia* and *P. cepacia*) [3, 6].
   e. A 5-year (1983–1988) study of patterns of susceptibility revealed no change in susceptibility to aztreonam for Enterobacteriaceae, but an increase in resistance was seen with *P. aeruginosa* and *Acinetobacter* spp.; similar increases were seen with other beta-lactams and gentamicin [8].
   f. **See summary in Table 28G-1.**
4. **Susceptibility testing.** For dilution studies, susceptible organisms have MICs of 8.0 μg/ml or less, and resistant organisms have MICs of 32 μg/ml or more. Intermediately susceptible strains are those with a MIC equal to 16 μg/ml. Aztreonam generally does not show a significant inoculum effect. Based on these criteria, although aztreonam is active against *P. aeruginosa,* it often is only modestly so (i.e., intermediately susceptible), and *Acinetobacter* is resistant. See Table 28G-1.
C. **Pharmacokinetics** have been reviewed in detail elsewhere [6, 9].
   1. **Absorption**
      a. **Oral.** Aztreonam is poorly absorbed.
      b. **Parenteral. One hour after administration of an intravenous or intramuscular dose, serum levels are similar.** After 1 g, serum levels are 45–50 μg/ml at 1 hour; after a 2-g dose, levels are 90 μg/ml at 1 hour. After intravenous single doses of 500 mg, 1 g, and 2 g, peak serum levels are 55–65, 90–160, or 200–255 μg/ml, respectively [2].
      c. There is no apparent accumulation of the drug after multiple dosing [9].
   2. **Excretion and elimination**
      a. Aztreonam is excreted **primarily by the kidneys,** with two-thirds of an administered dose eliminated unchanged in the urine. Renal secretion, glomerular filtration, and nonrenal mechanisms are involved. Although probenecid can increase serum concentrations slightly, this is not clinically significant. No active metabolites have been found in the serum or urine [2].
      In adults with normal renal function, urinary concentrations are high. After 500-mg or 1-g doses intravenously, urinary concentrations at 4–6 hours are 250–330 and 710–720 μg/ml, respectively [2].
      b. Serum **half-life** for elimination is 1.6 hours, supporting the feasibility of 6- to 8-hour dosing regimens. Renal failure prolongs the half-life. (See sec. **F.**) The half-life is prolonged in neonates (see Chap. 3).
   3. **Penetration into body fluids and tissue**

Table 28G-1. Antibacterial spectrum of aztreonam compared with new cephalosporins

Organism	MIC$_{90}$ (μg/ml)*					
	Aztreonam	Cefuroxime	Cefotaxime	Ceftazidime	Cefoxitin	Cefoperazone
E. coli	0.25	1	0.25	0.5	8	4
K. pneumoniae	0.25	1	0.5	1	4	4
Klebsiella cloacae	8	>32	32	64	>32	32
E. aerogenes	4	>32	8	16	>32	8
Serratia marcescens	2	>32	16	8	16	16
Proteus mirabilis	<0.12	0.5	<0.12	0.12	4	4
Proteus vulgaris	<0.12	16	2	<0.12	8	4
Proteus rettgeri	<0.12	>32	0.25	4	8	4
Moraxella morganii	0.5	>32	2	1	8	4
Providencia stuartii	<0.12	>32	1	1	8	4
Salmonella spp.	0.25	0.5	0.5	1	4	8
C. freundii	8	>32	0.5	2	>32	16
A. calcoaceticus	64	>32	>64	32	>32	64
P. aeruginosa	8–16	>32	>64	4–8	>32	16
H. influenzae, ampicillin-sensitive	0.25	0.5	<0.12	0.25	4	0.12
H. influenzae, ampicillin-resistant	0.25	0.5	<0.12	<0.12	4	0.5
N. gonorrhoeae	0.25	0.5	<0.12	<0.12	2	0.25
S. aureus	>32	2	4	16	4	4
S. pyogenes	16	0.5	<0.12	0.25	2	0.12
S. pneumoniae†	>32	0.25	<0.12	0.5	2	<0.12
E. faecalis	>32	>32	>32	>32	>32	>32
B. fragilis	>32	>32	>32	>32	32	>32

*Concentration of antibiotic necessary to inhibit 90% of strains tested at inoculum of 5 × 10^6 colony-forming units.
†Editors' note: penicillin-susceptible strains.
Source: Adapted from H.C. Neu, Aztreonam activity, pharmacology, and clinical uses. *Am. J. Med.* 88(Suppl. 3C):3S, 1990.

a. Aztreonam penetrates pericardial fluid, peritoneal fluid, synovial fluid, pleural fluid, and blister fluid well. Aztreonam achieves concentrations in tissues of bone, liver, lungs, kidney, and prostate to inhibit most Enterobacteriaceae and many *P. aeruginosa* [2, 6].

b. Peak biliary concentrations at 2.5 hours of more than 40 μg/ml in the unobstructed biliary tree occur. Lower concentrations are achieved with partial or total obstruction.

c. Aztreonam penetrates inflamed meninges in a limited fashion [6]. In patients with uninflamed meninges, a 2-g dose of aztreonam produces concentrations of 0.5 μg/ml and 1 μg/ml in the cerebrospinal fluid (CSF) at 1 and 4 hours, respectively. Mean levels increased to 2 μg/ml and 3.2 μg/ml, respectively, when the meninges were inflamed [7]. Higher CSF concentrations have been noted in neonates and children [2]. The third-generation cephalosporins are preferred for meningitis due to gram-negative bacteria. (See Chaps. 5 and 28F.)

d. **Effect on fecal flora.** After either oral or parenteral administration, aztreonam markedly decreases the fecal aerobic gram-negative bacteria. These results suggest that aztreonam may be useful for oral prophylaxis of infection in immunocompromised patients because the drug may selectively decontaminate the intestinal tract without significantly altering the GI anaerobes or impairing their colonization-resistance function [9]. Preliminary data suggest that it may be effective in patients with bacterial gastroenteritis. However, it is not recommended for these purposes.

D. **Clinical trials and potential uses**

1. **Clinical trials.** Aztreonam has maintained an excellent efficacy and safety profile [5].

    a. **Efficacy** has been demonstrated in bacteremias and urinary tract, lower respiratory tract, skin and soft-tissue, intraabdominal, bone and joint, and pelvic infections, as well as infections in leukopenic patients [1–3, 6, 9].

    b. **Adverse reactions** are similar to those reported for other beta-lactam antibiotics (see sec. **E**), and nephrotoxicity does not seem to be a problem with aztreonam use.

2. **Clinical role in adults.** The clinical use of aztreonam has been reviewed [5–6b, 10–15]. **Aztreonam is active against gram-negative aerobes only. Combination therapy is required if mixed pathogens** (i.e., gram-positive aerobes or anaerobes) **are involved.**

    a. **Urinary tract infections (UTIs).** Multiple studies have shown the efficacy of aztreonam as a single agent in the treatment of upper and lower UTI caused by susceptible Enterobacteriaceae, *P. aeruginosa,* and *Providencia* spp., including organisms resistant to the aminopenicillins, first- and second-generation cephalosporins, and aminoglycosides [6, 10]. Pyelonephritis and urinary sepsis with resistant organisms constitute useful applications for aztreonam therapy as an alternative to the conventional use of aminoglycosides, especially in the elderly or in patients with renal or hepatic failure [5, 6, 10].

    b. **Intraabdominal infections.** Aztreonam can be used in combination therapy (with an antianaerobic agent such as clindamycin or metronidazole) [1, 5, 6, 10–12]. Aztreonam has been shown to be a safe and effective agent for the treatment of peritonitis caused by gram-negative organisms in patients undergoing continuous ambulatory peritoneal dialysis (CAPD) [16].

    c. **Obstetric and gynecologic infections.** A combination of aztreonam and clindamycin (or metronidazole in the nonpregnant patient) has been successful in postoperative gynecologic infections [1, 5, 6, 10].

    d. **Lower respiratory infections.** Aztreonam is an effective agent in the treatment of gram-negative pneumonia in nosocomial infection [6, 10, 13, 14].

        (1) **Hospital-acquired.** In nosocomial gram-negative pneumonias, aztreonam may be a useful alternative to an aminoglycoside [1, 6, 10, 13, 14, 17]. Clinical trials suggest aztreonam is as effective as the aminoglycosides in this setting [6a, 6b]. A reasonable alternative strategy to initial therapy with aztreonam is to begin with an aminoglycoside and then to switch to aztreonam after susceptibility data are available. Aztreonam has been useful for infections due to Enterobacteriaceae and susceptible *Pseudomonas* spp. It has been effective in treating exacerbations of pulmonary infections due to *P. aeruginosa* in patients with cystic fibrosis [10].

If aspiration pneumonia occurs in the hospital, clindamycin has often been added to ensure activity against gram-positive or anaerobic bacteria. However, this approach does not take advantage of the unique features of this antibiotic, and if *Pseudomonas* is not present, other single antibiotic treatment is less expensive and probably safer or as safe (e.g., second- or third-generation cephalosporins).

There are limited data on the in vitro synergy of aztreonam with beta-lactam antibiotics and aminoglycosides [13]. When aztreonam is combined with an aminoglycoside, approximately 30–60% of strains of gram-negative organisms reveal synergism [7]. When aztreonam is combined with beta-lactam antibiotics (e.g., piperacillin), a minority of strains (e.g., *P. aeruginosa*) are synergistic [7a]. Further studies are needed in this area to clarify the role of combinations of aztreonam and other antibiotics to provide synergy against gram-negative bacilli.

(2) **Community-acquired.** Because *S. pneumoniae* is the most common pathogen in this setting, an agent active against this pathogen is required, and less expensive options are available. (See Chap. 9).

(3) **Cystic fibrosis.** Symptoms in these patients appear to respond to aztreonam, which may allow it to be rotated with other agents (e.g., aminoglycosides, ceftazidime) or to be used as an alternative agent in the allergic patient. (See sec. **F.6.**)

(4) **Exacerbations** of chronic bronchitis are **not an indication** for aztreonam monotherapy, probably because gram-positive organisms are important pathogens in these patients [13].

e. **Bacteremias.** For bacteremia of unclear etiology, aztreonam can be used in combination therapy (e.g., with antistaphylococcal or antianaerobic agents, depending on the clinical setting). However, many other antibiotic options are possible in this setting. (See Chap. 2.) If a gram-negative bacteremia is demonstrated and the organism is susceptible only to an advanced-generation cephalosporin, yet susceptible to aztreonam, this may be the ideal setting for aztreonam. Aztreonam may avoid suppression of gram-positive and anaerobic flora and avoid overgrowth of colonized sites.

Currently, aztreonam is not recommended for use routinely in the leukopenic febrile patient, although aztreonam and vancomycin have been effective in this setting and are an alternative combination [6, 6b, 18].

f. **Skin and soft tissue.** In hospitalized patients or chronically institutionalized patients, mixed infections involving aerobic gram-negative bacilli may occur. If an aminoglycoside is indicated, aztreonam could be used in its place as part of combination therapy.

g. **Bone and joint infections.** Aztreonam is a useful agent in treating gram-negative osteomyelitis or septic arthritis as it has no deleterious impact on normal gram-positive and anaerobic bacterial flora and no significant nephrotoxicity [6a]. However, if susceptibility data allow, the oral fluoroquinolones are more appealing in this setting. (See Chaps. 16 and 28S.)

3. **Clinical role in pediatrics.** Aztreonam has been studied in children in the United States and elsewhere and has been shown to be effective in pyelonephritis, bacteremias, meningitis, skeletal infection, pneumonia (including patients with cystic fibrosis), and peritonitis [19–22]. It may not be an effective agent in infections caused by *Salmonella* spp. Further comparative clinical trials will delineate more specific indications [19].

E. **Toxicity.** Overall, aztreonam appears to be a safe agent, with side effects similar to other beta-lactams [6, 10]. Side effects have occurred in fewer than 7% of patients; only 2% have had to discontinue therapy because of adverse effects in one report [6]. A recent reviewer emphasizes that no major adverse reactions to aztreonam have been reported [2].

1. **Adverse reactions** include pain and phlebitis at the intravenous site, rash in 1%, and nausea, diarrhea, or other minor GI side effects. **No ototoxicity** has been seen. A mild, transient taste sensation during intravenous infusion has been reported (6% in one series) [9]. **Serious nephrotoxicity has not been reported** [9].

2. **Laboratory tests.** Eosinophilia and mild hepatic transaminase elevations (2–3 times normal) are commonly seen (similar to other beta-lactam antibiotics).

3. **Superinfections** can occur, and enterococcal infections have occurred [10].

F. Dosing. Aztreonam may be administered *intravenously or intramuscularly.* The intravenous route is recommended for patients requiring more than 1 g per dose and in those patients with bacteremias, abscesses, peritonitis, or other severe or life-threatening infections.

1. **Adult dosages are summarized in Table 28G-2.**
2. **Infants and children. The safety and efficacy of aztreonam have not been established in infants or children** (per package insert). Preliminary studies suggest that a dose of 30 mg/kg can be used, with the dose interval dependent on the age of the infant (i.e., if < 1 week of age, a dose is given q12h; for infants 1–4 weeks of age, a dose is given q8h; and for infants > 4 weeks of age, a dose q6–8h has been suggested). In children with meningitis or cystic fibrosis (and *P. aeruginosa* pulmonary infections), a higher dose of 50 mg/kg per dose q6h has been used in preliminary studies [19–22].
3. **Renal failure.** Because aztreonam is excreted by the kidneys, **dosage adjustment** is necessary in renal failure. The package insert and other sources [22a] suggest the following in adults:
   a. **For creatinine clearances between 10 and 30 ml/min/1.73 m²,** after an initial loading dose of 1–2 g, the dosages should be halved and standard dose intervals used.
   b. **For severe renal failure** (creatinine clearances < 10 ml/min/1.73 m²), the usual loading dose (500 mg–2 g) is followed by one-fourth of the usual dose given at the usual fixed interval of 6, 8, or 12 hours.

      In serious or life-threatening infections, in addition to the maintenance dose, **one-eighth of the initial dose should be given after each hemodialysis session** because after a standard 4-hour dialysis, approximately 50% of aztreonam is removed [6, 9]. Some sources suggest a 500-mg supplemental dose after hemodialysis [22a].

      Continuous ambulatory peritoneal dialysis clears only approximately 10% of an intravenous dose [6, 9]. Therefore, in patients on CAPD, dosing guidelines for a creatinine clearance of less than 10 ml/min can be followed [22a].
4. **Pregnancy.** Aztreonam crosses the placenta and is a category B agent (see Chap. 28A). There are no adequate and well-controlled studies of aztreonam use in pregnant women. The package insert suggests that aztreonam should be used during pregnancy only if clearly needed.
5. **Nursing mothers.** Aztreonam is excreted in breast milk at concentrations of approximately 1% of levels in the maternal serum. The package insert suggests that consideration should be given to temporary discontinuation of nursing and use of formula feedings while the mother receives aztreonam.
6. **Use in penicillin-allergic or cephalosporin-allergic patients.** Based on initial clinical experience and in vitro and animal model studies, it appears that **patients with immunologically mediated reactions to penicillins, and probably cephalosporins, are able to receive monobactams (e.g., aztreonam)** with little risk of cross-sensitivity [2]. This topic has been reviewed elsewhere [6, 10, 23] and has been carefully studied in patients with cystic fibrosis who are allergic to penicillin or cephalosporin antibiotics. Because these patients are chronically infected with *P. aeruginosa* and need serial antibiotic therapy, aztreonam is a potentially useful agent either as monotherapy or combination

Table 28G-2. Aztreonam dosages in adults with normal renal function

Type of infection	Dose[a]	Frequency (hr)
Urinary tract	500 mg–1 g	8 or 12
Moderately severe systemic infection	1–2 g	8 or 12
Severe systemic or life-threatening infections	2 g	6[b] or 8

[a]Higher doses used in more severe infection. Maximum recommended dose is 8 g/day in adults.
[b]In systemic or severe *P. aeruginosa* infections, 2 g q6–8h is advised.
Source: Copyright *Physicians' Desk Reference 1996,* 50th edition, published by Medical Economics Data, Montvale, New Jersey 07645. Reprinted by permission. All rights reserved.

therapy with an aminoglycoside. Moss and colleagues [24] concluded that "aztreonam appears to be safe and effective for the treatment of exacerbations of *P. aeruginosa*–associated endobronchitis in patients with cystic fibrosis who are allergic to antipseudomonal penicillins and/or cephalosporins. Cross-reactivity of pre-existing reaginic antibodies with aztreonam appears to be a rare but real occurrence, necessitating caution in the administration of aztreonam to a patient with cystic fibrosis who is known to be allergic to any beta-lactam antibiotic . . . [C]eftazidime may present a higher risk than other drugs because of the similarities of its side chain to that of aztreonam, but further investigation of this possibility is required." Furthermore, this report concludes that despite its low immunogenicity, aztreonam rarely can provoke immediate hypersensitivity reactions in patients with cystic fibrosis who receive multiple courses of aztreonam [24].

G. **Cost.** See Table 28A-6. The monotherapy costs of aztreonam compared with third-generation cephalosporin costs per day are competitive. If another antibiotic must be used with aztreonam (i.e., combination therapy), the daily antibiotic costs will be higher.

H. **Summary. The optimal way to use aztreonam still is debated.**

1. Aztreonam is a **rational alternative for gram-negative bacillary infections in the penicillin- and cephalosporin-allergic patient,** in whom one might ordinarily use an extended penicillin or third-generation cephalosporin. It is also an efficacious and safe alternative to aminoglycosides, especially in the elderly, in patients with hepatic insufficiency, and in patients with renal insufficiency [10, 11, 25, 26].

2. Despite the higher initial costs of aztreonam versus the aminoglycosides (see Table 28A-6), if one considers the potential costs of nephrotoxicity due to aminoglycosides [27] and the cost of monitoring aminoglycosides, aztreonam becomes potentially cost-effective or at least competitive. This was emphasized when Dr. Appel [25] wrote, "Although alternative treatments may seem to be more expensive than aminoglycosides at first look, consideration of this cost of nephrotoxicity, added to the expense of measuring serum aminoglycoside levels and renal function to monitor for nephrotoxicity, results in competitive cost-effectiveness for the two. Clearly, if non-nephrotoxic antibiotics, such as the third-generation cephalosporins or aztreonam, are equally efficacious and equally cost-effective in treating a given infection in a patient at high risk for renal damage, use of the alternative agent would be preferable to aminoglycoside." In the elderly person with reduced renal function or the patient with renal failure, the reduced dosage of aztreonam (see sec. **F.3**) will also help lower daily drug costs.

3. A contrasting opinion suggests that some of the assessments of nephrotoxicity of aminoglycosides have not adequately considered the use of **"individualized dosing" with pharmacokinetics,** which may help minimize nephrotoxicity (see Chap. 28H). **Further studies using this approach with cost assessments are needed.** Other potentially useful agents include the quinolones (see Chap. 28S).

4. In the *Medical Letter*'s listing of "The choice of antibacterial drugs" [28], **for specific pathogens, aztreonam is not listed as the "drug of first choice."**

5. We offer the following guidelines for consideration:

   a. In moderate to severe nosocomial infections, aminoglycoside therapy for gram-negative organisms for the initial 48–72 hours while awaiting cultures is prudent unless an aminoglycoside is contraindicated. Once susceptibility data are back, if the organism is susceptible to aztreonam, it often may be reasonable to switch to this agent. The development of resistance while on therapy is usually not a concern with aminoglycosides. The frequency with which bacteria develop resistance to aztreonam is not fully delineated. If the approach just outlined is used, the risk of resistance may be minimized.

   b. There is a recognized potential of increasing bacterial resistance and possible increased incidence of *C. difficile* diarrhea associated with the common use of advanced cephalosporins (see Chap. 28F). Aztreonam appears to be associated less often with these problems and therefore may be an appealing alternative. Aztreonam probably is underutilized currently.

   c. Because aztreonam is active only against gram-negative bacilli, when it is used empirically for mixed infections, combination therapy will be necessary, thereby increasing costs.

d. At times, an aminoglycoside may still be the preferred agent (see Chap. 28H) as, for example, in combination therapy against enterococcus and *Listeria monocytogenes* and in combination with antipseudomonal penicillin in severe *P. aeruginosa* infections [28].

e. Aztreonam has not been approved for use in infants and children by the US Food and Drug Administration (FDA). A New Drug Application (NDA) supplement has been submitted to the FDA, and approval is anticipated.

II. Imipenem (Tienam, Primaxin) is the **first carbapenem** antibiotic to be used in humans. Imipenem-cilastatin has undergone extensive clinical evaluation and has been reviewed in detail in an international symposium [29] and elsewhere [2, 10, 11, 30–31a]. **Imipenem is the widest-spectrum beta-lactam antibiotic introduced into clinical use** thus far [10, 11, 29, 30].

Imipenem binds with high affinity to penicillin-binding proteins, causing lysis of gram-positive and gram-negative bacteria. It is not hydrolyzed by most beta-lactamases, penicillinases, cephalosporinases, and plasmid- or chromosome-mediated *S. aureus* (methicillin-susceptible), many Enterobacteriaceae, *P. aeruginosa*, and most *P. cepaciae* [2].

A. Structure. Imipenem differs from other beta-lactam agents because of the lack of sulfur or oxygen in the bicyclic nucleus and the "trans" configuration [29]. This stereoscopic "trans" position of the hydroxyethyl side chain provides resistance to beta-lactamases.

B. Development of the imipenem-cilastatin combination. Imipenem is available only in combination with cilastatin.

    1. Imipenem. Thienamycin is the **parent compound.** In vitro this is an extremely active agent. It is unstable in concentrated solutions and in the solid state. The crystalline amidine **derivative *N*-formimidoyl thienamycin,** which was given the **generic name *imipenem,*** is stable.

    2. Cilastatin is not an antibiotic, and it does not interfere with the activity of imipenem in vitro. Cilastatin is a potent **selective enzyme inhibitor** that has two features.

        a. Ensures urinary antibiotic concentrations. The beta-lactam ring of imipenem is opened, converting the drug to an inactive metabolite by dehydropeptidase-I, an enzyme in the brush border of the kidney. Cilastatin coadministered with imipenem in a 1·1 concentration ratio [29, 31] selectively inhibits this enzyme, preventing inactivation and producing urinary concentrations. See sec. **D.2.b.**

        b. Has a "nephroprotective effect." Cilastatin appears to have a nephroprotective effect, first documented in animal studies in which prolonged administration of high doses of imipenem alone (over months) induced nephrotoxicity. The coadministration of imipenem-cilastatin prevents excessive intracellular antibiotic accumulation (at the tubular level) and consequent nephrotoxicity [31].

C. In vitro activity. In worldwide studies, imipenem inhibits 90% or more of clinically important bacteria [29, 32, 33]. The impressive activity of imipenem is due to three factors: (1) no permeability barrier in gram-negative bacteria, (2) stability against beta-lactamases, and (3) high affinity for penicillin-binding proteins [29].

    1. Gram-positive aerobes. Imipenem is very active against these organisms, similar to the first-generation cephalosporins and penicillins [10]. See Table 28G-3.

        a. Very susceptible, with a MIC_{90} of 0.1 µg/ml or less: penicillin-susceptible *Streptococcus pneumoniae,* group A and B streptococci, *Streptococcus bovis,* methicillin-susceptible *Staphylococcus aureus,* and *Staphylococcus saprophyticus.* Penicillin-resistant *S. pneumoniae* are susceptible to imipenem. See Chap. 28C for a detailed discussion of penicillin-resistant *S. pneumoniae.* Intermediately resistant strains of *S. pneumoniae* are routinely susceptible to imipenem; highly resistant strains are susceptible to imipenem 90–100% of the time [33a].

        b. Moderately susceptible. Enterococci usually are susceptible, with the MIC_{90} of *Enterococcus faecalis* approximately 1–3 µg/ml. Imipenem is bacteriostatic against susceptible enterococci [2]. Imipenem-aminoglycoside combinations may be synergistic against *E. faecalis* [32]. However, many strains of *E. faecium* are resistant to imipenem.

        c. Resistant. Methicillin-resistant *S. aureus* or coagulase-negative species are routinely **resistant.** Corynebacterium JK organisms are resistant, as are *E. faecium* strains [32].

Table 28G-3. Activity of imipenem and other antibiotics against aerobic gram-positive bacteria[a]

Bacteria	Imipenem	Cefazolin	Cefoxitin	Cefotaxime	Ceftriaxone	Ceftazidime	Piperacillin	Penicillin	Oxacillin	Vancomycin	Ciprofloxacin
S. aureus	<1	1	8–32	1–4	1–4	8–32	>32	>32	0.5	2	0.4–1[b]
Methicillin-resistant S. aureus	>8	>32	>32	>32	>32	>32	>32	>32	>32	2	0.25–1[b]
Coagulase-negative staphylococci	0.25	1	8–32	8–32	8–32	8–32	>32	6	0.5	2	0.25–1[b]
S. pneumoniae[c]	0.01	0.12	1–4	<1	<1	<1	0.02	0.01	0.04	1	1
S. pyogenes	0.1	0.1	<1	<1	<1	<1	0.02	0.01	0.04	0.5	2
E. faecalis (enterococcus)	0.8	>32	>32	>32	>32	>32	1.5	1	>32	1	0.5–2
E. faecium	>32	>32	>32	>32	>32	>32	—	2	>32	2	—
L. monocytogenes	1	>32	>32	>32	>32	>32	—	2	8	1	0.5–3

[a]Boldface titers are considered antibiotic-sensitive (susceptible).
[b]Editors' note: Recent data suggest many strains may be resistant or may develop resistance to ciprofloxacin (see Chap. 28S).
[c]Penicillin-susceptible strains. See Chap. 28C and text for discussion of penicillin-resistant strains.
Source: W.C. Hellinger and N.S. Brewer, Imipenem. *Mayo Clin. Proc.* 66:1074, 1991.

d. **Tolerant.** Minimum inhibitory concentrations of *L. monocytogenes* are low but tolerance occurs—that is, high minimum bactericidal concentrations (MBCs) are seen in vitro. This may also be seen with some strains of enterococci (e.g., *E. faecalis*), and its clinical significance remains uncertain.

2. **Gram-negative aerobic bacteria. See Table 28G-4.**

   a. **Nonenteric pathogens.** *N. meningitidis* and *N. gonorrhoeae* have a MIC$_{90}$ of less than 0.20 µg/ml, and *H. influenzae* with a MIC$_{90}$ of 0.6 µg/ml are very susceptible. The MICs for beta-lactamase–positive and –negative *N. gonorrhoeae* and *H. influenzae* are identical.

   b. **Enterobacteriaceae.** In a review of more than 8,000 isolates, three levels of imipenem activity were recognized [33].

      (1) A MIC$_{90}$ of 1.0 µg or less (very susceptible) was seen with *E. coli, Klebsiella* spp., *Salmonella* and *Shigella* spp., *Citrobacter diversus, Hafniae alvei,* and *Yersinia enterocolitica.*

      (2) A MIC$_{90}$ of approximately 1–2 µg/ml (susceptible) was seen with *Enterobacter* spp., *C. freundii,* and *Serratia* spp.

      (3) A MIC$_{90}$ of 2–4 µg/ml (less susceptible) was seen, especially with the *Proteus* spp.

   c. **Pseudomonas**

      (1) *P. aeruginosa* strains (more than 1,600 tested) have a MIC$_{90}$ of 5 µg/ml [33]. Similar MICs were noted for *Pseudomonas fluorescens.* Imipenem may show synergism with tobramycin or other aminoglycosides against *P. aeruginosa* [32].

      (2) *Pseudomonas cepacia* and *Pseudomonas maltophilia* strains are resistant. *P. maltophilia* (*Xanthomonas maltophilia*) produces a beta-lactamase that easily hydrolyzes imipenem [10].

      (3) *Pseudomonas stutzeri* was very susceptible.

   d. *Acinetobacter calcoaceticus* spp. are usually quite susceptible, but nosocomial infections due to resistant species can occur [33b].

   e. *Legionella pneumophila.* Although imipenem is active in vitro, it is not considered appropriate treatment for *Legionella* pneumonia because of the intracellular location of the organism [10, 32]. (See sec. G.)

3. **Anaerobes.** Imipenem has **excellent activity** against strict anaerobes, with the MIC$_{90}$ below 1 µg/ml for *Bacteroides fragilis* and other *fragilis* group spp., *B. melaninogenicus, Fusobacterium* spp., and anaerobic gram-positive cocci. The MIC$_{90}$ to *Clostridium perfringens* is higher (4 µg/ml), and some strains of *C. difficile* are relatively resistant, with a MIC$_{90}$ of 10 µg/ml.

   Based on in vitro susceptibility data, **imipenem is comparable in spectrum of activity to clindamycin, chloramphenicol, and metronidazole** [33]. In another study [34], imipenem and ticarcillin-clavulanate were the most active beta-lactam drugs studied, with imipenem demonstrating excellent activity against *B. fragilis* group anaerobes.

4. **Miscellaneous.** Other, less frequently isolated organisms have been shown to be susceptible to imipenem, including [33] *Campylobacter* spp., *Eikenella corrodens, Erysipelothrix rhusiopathiae, P. multocida, Actinomyces* spp., *Brucella melitensis, Moraxella* spp. [10], and *Nocardia* [32].

   Resistant organisms include *Flavobacterium* spp., *Corynebacterium* spp., *Mycobacterium fortuitum, Chlamydia trachomatis,* and **mycoplasma.**

5. **Imipenem is a potent inducer of beta-lactamases** that can cleave other beta-lactam antibiotics. The clinical significance of this phenomenon remains largely unknown [10]. Imipenem may show antagonism when combined with other beta-lactam antibiotics, particularly in the treatment of *P. aeruginosa* infections; this may be related to beta-lactamase induction by subinhibitory concentrations of imipenem [10]. Synergy with aminoglycosides against *P. aeruginosa* is uncommon [6b].

6. Imipenem does not penetrate into mammalian cells and therefore may be unsuitable for treatment of intracellular pathogens [10]. (See sec. **2.e.**)

7. **Imipenem** is considered the **antibiotic of choice for** hospital-acquired *Enterobacter* or *Acinetobacter* spp. [28]. See secs. **2.d.** and **E.2.j.**

D. **The pharmacokinetics of imipenem-cilastatin** have been reviewed [10, 35].

   1. **Route of administration and serum levels.** Imipenem and cilastatin are **not appreciably absorbed after oral administration.**

1228 Ch 28. Antibiotic Use

Table 28G-4. Activity of imipenem and other antibiotics against aerobic gram-negative bacteria*

Bacteria	Imipenem	Cefazolin	Cefoxitin	Cefotaxime	Ceftriaxone	Ceftazidime	Piperacillin	Amikacin	Ciprofloxacin
Escherichia coli	<1	64–128	8–32	<1	<1	<1	**8–32**	**1–4**	<1
Klebsiella	<1	>128	8–32	<1	<1	<1	64–128	–	<1
Enterobacter spp.	1–4	>128	>128	8–32	8–32	1–4	**8–32**	**1–4**	<1
Proteus mirabilis	1–4	8–32	1–4	<1	<1	<1	<1	**8–32**	<1
Indole-positive *Proteus*	1–4	>128	8–32	1–4	1–4	<1	**1–4**	**8–32**	<1
Serratia marcescens	1–4	>128	64–128	8–32	1–4	1–4	**8–32**	**8–32**	**0.125–1**
Pseudomonas aeruginosa	4	>128	>128	64–128	64–128	8	32	**8–32**	**0.25–2**
Pseudomonas (S.) maltophilia	>128	>128	>128	>128	–	25–32	>128	>128	**1–16**
Citrobacter	1–4	>128	>128	1–4	1–4	1–4	**8–32**	1–4	<1
Providencia	1–4	–	8–32	1–4	1–4	1–4	**8–32**	1–4	0.06–8
Acinetobacter	1–4	>128	>128	64–128	64–128	8–32	**8–32**	–	**0.06–1**
Salmonella	<1	8–32	–	<1	<1	<1	4	–	<1
Shigella	<1	8–32	–	<1	<1	<1	8	–	<1
Haemophilus influenzae	1–4	8–32	8–32	<1	<1	<1	–	8–32	<1
Neisseria gonorrhoeae	<1	1–32	**1–4**	<1	<1	<1	–	–	<1
Neisseria meningitidis	<1	<1	<1	<1	<1	<1	<1	–	<1

*Boldface titers are considered antibiotic-sensitive (susceptible).
Source: W.C. Hellinger and N.S. Brewer, Imipenem. *Mayo Clin. Proc.* 66:1074, 1991.

   a. After a 30-minute 1-g IV infusion, peak serum levels are 50–60 µg/ml; after 2 hours, 20 µg/ml; and after 6 hours, 0.8 µg/ml (the usual dosing interval). Plasma accumulation does not appear to occur after multiple doses [35].
   b. The serum half-lives of both imipenem and cilastatin are approximately 1 hour.
   c. The intramuscular preparation provides lower serum levels. At 1 hour, after 500 mg IM, plasma imipenem concentrations are 9–10 µg/ml (versus 21–22 µg/ml after 500-mg IV dosing) and, after 750 mg IM, plasma concentrations are typically 10 µg/ml (versus 28 µg/ml after 750-mg IV dosing) per the package insert.
 2. Elimination
   a. Renal excretion, primarily by glomerular filtration, is the major mechanism. In renal failure, doses must be modified as discussed in sec. **F.3.** Tubular secretion of imipenem blocked by probenecid is not clinically significant [35].
   b. Urinary levels. When cilastatin is coadministered with imipenem, approximately 70% of the imipenem is recovered in the urine. If imipenem is given alone, only 20% or so is recovered in the urine [35]. Urinary concentrations of 70 µg/ml, which exceeds the MICs of all common pathogens in UTI [35], occur after a 1-g infusion of imipenem-cilastatin.
   c. Biliary and GI levels. Although 99% of imipenem-cilastatin is recovered in the urine (over a period of 5 days), biliary levels of imipenem exceed the MICs of important biliary pathogens [29]. Because very little drug is found in the feces, there is little impact on normal bowel flora [2, 32]. Imipenem use is seldom followed by *C. difficile* diarrhea.
 3. Distribution. Imipenem is widely distributed in saliva, sputum, pleural fluid, synovial fluid, and bone. Early studies suggest that it penetrates the inflamed meninges, but levels are variable, ranging from 0.5 to 11 µg/ml [10] and 1–5 µg/ml in recent reviews [2]. After a 1-g IV dose, the mean peak aqueous humor level was 2.99 µg/ml at 2 hours after administration, and the mean vitreous level was 2.53 µg/ml at 2–3 hours after administration [36].
E. Clinical experience. Imipenem has been effective in a wide variety of infections [2, 6b, 10, 11, 30, 37].
 1. Clinical efficacy has been shown in patients with severe infections and serious underlying diseases [10, 11, 30, 37].
   a. Bacteremias. Against susceptible gram-positive, gram-negative, and anaerobic pathogens, patients had an excellent response. Limited experience in endocarditis shows efficacy for *S. aureus* [11].
   b. Pneumonia. An excellent response of pneumonia due to susceptible pathogens in severe community- and hospital-acquired infection was seen. However, whether this agent clearly improves mortality in bacteremic pneumonias or common nosocomial infections (e.g., *Enterobacter, Serratia*) awaits further clinical experience [38]. *Pseudomonas* infections remain difficult to eradicate, and monotherapy with imipenem alone is not advised [10, 11, 37a].
   c. Complicated UTIs, including *Pseudomonas* infections, have responded well. This is not surprising in light of the broad spectrum of activity and excellent urinary concentrations of imipenem-cilastatin.
   d. Pelvic and **intraabdominal** infections in conjunction with appropriate surgery, including infections in seriously ill patients, have responded very well [10, 11, 30, 38]. Imipenem-cilastatin is an active agent in treating severe intraabdominal infections [12, 38]. See Chap. 11.
   e. Skin and soft-tissue infections due to *S. aureus,* group A streptococci, enterococci, gram-negative bacilli, anaerobic, and polymicrobial infections respond well.
   f. Osteomyelitis. Imipenem-cilastatin has been used as monotherapy and is effective against *S. aureus,* gram-negative, and polymicrobial infections. In difficult gram-negative infections, it produced a response rate comparable to that of the new third-generation cephalosporins. Only 10% of gram-positive infections failed therapy in early studies [38].
 2. Considerations for use. Imipenem-cilastatin is an extremely potent antibiotic that appears to be well tolerated. It may be **especially useful in infections caused by pathogens resistant to other agents or for infections that would**

otherwise require multiple antibiotics [39]. It is too broad-spectrum to use when another single agent could be used (e.g., cefoxitin for mild to moderate community-acquired infections). **One might consider using imipenem-cilastatin as a single agent in the following** situations [10–12, 29, 38]:

a. **Bacteremias**
 (1) **Polymicrobial.** In patients with proven polymicrobial bacteremias, imipenem-cilastatin is appealing because it allows one to avoid the problems, expense, and toxicity of multiple agents.
 (2) **Initial treatment of patients with suspected bacteremias.**
  (a) **In community-acquired very severe illness** with presumed sepsis of unclear etiology, imipenem is a reasonable consideration. When susceptibility data of blood culture isolates are available, appropriate modifications of therapy (e.g., a narrower-spectrum agent) should be made.
  (b) **In hospital-acquired** bacteremia, imipenem is a very reasonable choice. In those instances in which *P. aeruginosa* was unsuspected and yet proved to be causative, imipenem is adequate for the first 48 hours of therapy. If *P. aeruginosa* is cultured from the bloodstream, imipenem should not be continued as monotherapy because resistance can develop.
   For known *P. aeruginosa* bacteremia (and pneumonia), standard combination therapy—that is, antipseudomonal penicillin such as piperacillin and an aminoglycoside or ceftazidime and an aminoglycoside in the patient with a delayed penicillin allergy—is advised [10, 11, 37]. **For *Acinetobacter* and *Enterobacter* spp., fairly common nosocomial pathogens, imipenem is viewed as the antibiotic of choice [28].**

b. **Febrile leukopenic patients without an obvious focal infection.** Monotherapy with a third-generation cephalosporin (e.g., ceftazidime) is often considered in febrile neutropenic patients without a focal infection. See Chaps. 2 and 28F. Studies suggest that imipenem can be used as monotherapy for the febrile leukopenic patient [40–43], including children [44]. Although imipenem has a broader in vitro spectrum of activity than ceftazidime, in a 1995 report, modification of therapy was appropriate in as many recipients of monotherapy with imipenem as with ceftazidime in this setting [44a].

c. **Hospital-acquired pneumonias.** For gram-negative hospital-acquired pneumonias, imipenem is adequate for 48 hours while awaiting cultures. However, for known established *P. aeruginosa* pneumonia, the development of resistance with imipenem monotherapy is common [11, 37, 37a], and conventional double-drug therapy is preferred. (See sec. **(2).(b)** above.) Imipenem has been combined with an aminoglycoside for some multiresistant strains of *Pseudomonas* (based on susceptibility data); this approach sometimes is used in patients with cystic fibrosis. However, some data suggest combination therapy may not be any more effective than imipenem monotherapy [44b].

d. **Complicated UTI.** Patients with recurrent UTI due to known or likely broadly resistant organisms may be candidates for imipenem. If the bacteria are susceptible to both aztreonam and imipenem, the narrower-spectrum aztreonam is preferred. If the bacteria also are susceptible to fluoroquinolones, these would be preferred because of the availability of oral therapy.

e. **Intraabdominal and pelvic infections.** Because of its activity against *B. fragilis,* gram-negative enteric bacilli, and gram-positive bacteria, imipenem-cilastatin is a very appealing agent for intraabdominal infections. (See Chap. 11.) For mild to moderate intraabdominal or pelvic infection, less expensive and narrower-spectrum agents (e.g., cefoxitin) are preferred [12]. In intraabdominal infection involving hospital-acquired bacteria that may be resistant to more standard combination regimens, imipenem may be preferred. Piperacillin-tazobactam may be another consideration. See Chap. 28E.

f. **Acute necrotizing pancreatitis.** The role of antibiotics for this difficult problem is reviewed in Chap. 11. Whether imipenem may play a special role in this setting is still undergoing clinical evaluation. (See discussion in Chap. 11, sec. **IV,** under Acute Necrotizing Pancreatitis, p. 445.)

    g. Serious soft-tissue infections (e.g., perirectal and perivulvar). In certain serious mixed aerobic-anaerobic infections, monotherapy is appealing, **especially when resistant bacteria are known to be involved or highly suspected.** These include **(1) mixed aerobic-anaerobic soft-tissue infections** and **(2) decubitus ulcers** with severe soft-tissue infection or sepsis.

    h. Special forms of osteomyelitis. Imipenem may be particularly useful in the following:

      (1) Polymicrobial osteomyelitis with all organisms susceptible to this single agent.

      (2) Initial empiric therapy, especially for an infection contiguous to a mixed wound infection.

      (3) Gram-negative infections when organisms are not susceptible to narrower-spectrum agents.

    i. Eye infections. Imipenem's role in this setting is still undergoing evaluation [36]. See Chap. 6.

    j. For serious hospital-acquired infections caused by susceptible strains of _Enterobacter_ or _Acinetobacter_ spp., imipenem is considered the agent of choice [28].

    k. It is an alternate agent for _Nocardia_ infections and for highly resistant _S. pneumoniae_ infections.

  3. Imipenem is not indicated for the following settings in which narrower or less expensive agents are preferred.

    a. Routine community-acquired pneumonia.

    b. Uncomplicated UTI.

    c. Routine streptococcal or staphylococcal skin and soft-tissue infections.

    d. _S. aureus_ or streptococcal bacteremias.

    e. Biliary tract infection. Because only 1% or so of the drug is excreted by the biliary tract, it may be appropriate to use other, more standard regimens for biliary infection, although adequate levels may be achieved. (See sec. **D.2.C.**)

    f. Endocarditis. The drug's precise role in endocarditis awaits further clinical study, but it appears effective in _S. aureus_ and streptococcal infections.

    g. Routine surgical prophylaxis. (See Chap. 28B.)

    h. Monotherapy of serious _P. aeruginosa_ infections. (See discussions in sec. **2.**)

F. Dosages. For a given patient, the dose of imipenem depends on (1) the severity of infection, (2) renal function (i.e., estimated creatinine clearance), **and (3) weight of the patient** (with dose reductions if the patient weighs < 70 kg).

  1. See Table 28G-5 for adult dosage regimens for adult patients weighing at least 70 kg. See Table 28G-6 for adult patients weighing less than 70 kg.

  2. Safety and effectiveness in infants and children younger than 12 years have not yet been established. Imipenem has been used for monotherapy in children older than 4 years who have fever and leukopenia due to chemotherapy [44a] and in other special settings.

  3. In renal failure, the serum half-life of imipenem-cilastatin increases; therefore, doses **must be reduced.** The package insert provides specific **guidelines,** which are **summarized in Table 28G-6.**

  4. Hemodialysis removes 40–70% of the imipenem and a variable amount of cilastatin, depending on the type and duration of dialysis. A supplemental dose can be given after hemodialysis.

    For dosages, see the footnotes of Table 28G-6.

    There is inadequate information to recommend usage of imipenem for patients undergoing peritoneal dialysis.

  5. Combination therapy

    a. Aminoglycosides and imipenem-cilastatin appear to be synergistic against many strains of _Pseudomonas_ spp. [40] and enterococci [10].

    b. Imipenem-cilastatin should not be combined with cephalosporins (e.g., a third-generation agent) **or expanded penicillins because antagonism has been described** [10, 40].

  6. Pregnancy. Imipenem is a category C agent (see Chap. 28A). The package insert indicates there are no adequate and well-controlled studies in pregnant women. Therefore, this agent should be used during pregnancy only if the potential benefit justifies the potential risk to the mother and fetus.

Table 28G-5. Intravenous[a] dosing schedule of imipenem-cilastatin for adults with normal renal function and body weight of at least 70 kg[b]

Type or severity of infection	Fully susceptible organisms, including gram-positive and gram-negative aerobes and anaerobes	Moderately susceptible organisms, primarily some strains of *P. aeruginosa*
Mild	250 mg q6h	500 mg q6h
Moderate	500 mg q6h–q8h	500 mg q6h–1 g q8h
Severe, life-threatening	500 mg q6h	1 g q6–8h[c]
Uncomplicated urinary tract infection	250 mg q6h	250 mg q6h
Complicated urinary tract infection	500 mg q6h	500 mg q6h

[a]An IM preparation of imipenem is available, but serum levels achieved after IM doses are lower than those achieved after IV doses. (See text.) **Therefore, in severe or life-threatening infections, the IV preparation is preferred** and, because imipenem usually is used in severe infection, the IV route is recommended. In adults with creatinine clearances in excess of 20 ml/min/1.73 m², the package insert suggests for mild to moderate skin and soft-tissue infection, lower respiratory tract infection, and gynecologic infection 500 or 750 mg IM q12h. In mild to moderate intraabdominal infection, 750 mg q12h is suggested.

Primaxin IM should be prepared with 1% lidocaine HCl solution (without epinephrine): The 500-mg dose is prepared with 2 ml, and the 750-mg dose is prepared with 3 ml of lidocaine HCl. **The IM formulation is not for IV use.** The IM preparation is contraindicated for use in patients allergic to imipenem or lidocaine. The IM dose should be administered by deep intramuscular injection into a large muscle such as the gluteal or lateral thigh. Total daily dosages greater than 1,500 mg are not recommended. See package insert.

[b]**Doses cited in table are based on a body weight of at least 70 kg. A further proportionate reduction in dose administered must be made for patients with a body weight of less than 70 kg as shown in Table 28G-6.**

[c]For *Pseudomonas aeruginosa* infections, maximum doses of 1 g q6h may be necessary; ideally double-drug therapy usually is indicated (see text).

Source: Adapted from Product Information on Primaxin. *Physicians' Desk Reference* (50th ed.) Montvale, NJ: Medical Economics Data, 1996.

Note: It is recommended that the maximum total daily IV dosage not exceed 50 mg/kg/day or 4 g/day, whichever is lower. However, patients older than 12 years with cystic fibrosis and normal renal function have been treated with IV imipenem at doses up to 90 mg/kg/day in divided doses, not exceeding 4 g/day (per package insert).

Table 28G-6. Reduced intravenous dosage of imipenem IV in adult patients with impaired renal function and/or body weight less than 70 kg

and body weight (kg) is	If TOTAL DAILY DOSE from Table 28G-5 is																			
	1.0 g/day				1.5 g/day				2.0 g/day				3.0 g/day				4.0 g/day			
	and creatinine clearance (ml/min/1.73 m²) is				and creatinine clearance (ml/min/1.73 m²) is				and creatinine clearance (ml/min/1.73 m²) is				and creatinine clearance (ml/min/1.73 m²) is				and creatinine clearance (ml/min/1.73 m²) is			
	≥71	41–70	21–40	6–20	≥71	41–70	21–40	6–20	≥71	41–70	21–40	6–20	≥71	41–70	21–40	6–20	≥71	41–70	21–40	6–20
	then the reduced dosage regimen (mg) is				then the reduced dosage regimen (mg) is				then the reduced dosage regimen (mg) is				then the reduced dosage regimen (mg) is				then the reduced dosage regimen (mg) is			
≥70	250 q6h	250 q8h	250 q12h	250 q12h	500 q8h	250 q6h	250 q8h	250 q12h	500 q6h	500 q8h	250 q8h	250 q12h	1000 q8h	500 q6h	250 q8h	500 q12h	1000 q6h	750 q8h	500 q8h	500 q12h
60	250 q8h	125 q6h	250 q12h	125 q12h	250 q6h	250 q8h	250 q8h	250 q12h	500 q8h	250 q6h	250 q8h	250 q12h	750 q8h	500 q8h	250 q8h	500 q12h	1000 q8h	750 q8h	500 q8h	500 q12h
50	125 q6h	125 q6h	125 q8h	125 q12h	250 q8h	250 q8h	250 q12h	250 q12h	250 q6h	250 q8h	250 q8h	250 q12h	500 q6h	500 q8h	250 q8h	250 q12h	750 q8h	500 q6h	500 q8h	500 q12h
40	125 q6h	125 q8h	125 q12h	125 q12h	250 q8h	125 q6h	125 q8h	125 q12h	250 q6h	250 q8h	250 q12h	250 q12h	500 q8h	250 q6h	250 q8h	250 q12h	500 q6h	500 q8h	250 q8h	250 q12h
30	125 q8h	125 q8h	125 q12h	125 q12h	125 q6h	125 q8h	125 q8h	125 q12h	250 q8h	125 q6h	125 q8h	125 q12h	250 q6h	250 q8h	250 q8h	250 q12h	500 q8h	250 q6h	250 q8h	250 q12h

Patients with creatinine clearances of 6–20 ml/min/1.73 m² should be treated with 125 mg or 250 mg IV q12h. There may be an increased risk of seizures when doses of 500 mg q12h are administered to these patients.

Patients with a creatinine clearance of <5 ml/min/1.73 m² should not receive imipenem IV unless hemodialysis is instituted within 48 hours.

For patients undergoing hemodialysis and with a creatinine clearance of <5 ml/min/1.73 m², dosage recommendations for patients with creatinine clearances of 6–20 ml/min/1.73 m² as shown in the table are advised. Both imipenem and cilastin are removed by dialysis; the patient should receive IV imipenem after hemodialysis and then q12h as indicated in the table.

Source: Copyright *Physicians' Desk Reference 1996*, 50th edition, published by Medical Economics Data, Montvale, New Jersey. Reprinted by permission. All rights reserved.

7. **Nursing mothers.** The package insert indicates it is not known whether imipenem is excreted in human milk. Because many drugs are excreted in human milk, caution should be exercised when this agent is administered to a nursing woman.

G. **Side effects and toxicity.** Data from the first 2,500 patients receiving imipenem indicate that imipenem-cilastatin has a safety profile similar to that of other beta-lactam antibiotics [45]; overall, imipenem has been reported in recent reviews to be well tolerated [2].

   1. **Adverse reactions**
      a. Minor **intravenous site irritation** occurs in 5% of patients or fewer.
      b. **Gastrointestinal symptoms** occur in nearly 5% [45] of patients receiving standard doses but in up to 20% [37] of patients when high-dose therapy is used. **Nausea and vomiting are the most common symptoms and may be decreased by decreasing the infusion rate or the dose.** Diarrhea occurs in 1.7–3.0% of patients. Pseudomembranous colitis can occur but seems to be rare.
      c. **Allergic reactions** such as drug fever, pruritus, rash, and urticaria are seen in fewer than 3% of patients [45]. **Patients allergic to penicillin should be considered allergic to imipenem** [46] unless skin tests can be done. In addition, imipenem should be avoided or administered under close monitoring to patients with a history of IgE-mediated hypersensitivity to other beta-lactam antibiotics [10]. See related discussion in Chap. 27.
      d. **Seizures** of unclear etiology occurred in early studies in approximately 1.5% of patients receiving imipenem-cilastatin, a percentage similar to that of other antibiotics [10, 45, 47]. In another study, of 1,700 patients treated with imipenem, it was concluded that imipenem-related seizures (possible, probable, or definite) occurred in 0.9% of recipients. Higher drug doses and decreased renal function, prior history of a seizure disorder, or prior CNS lesions were the main predisposing factors [47]. In this study, a similar incidence of seizures was seen in patients treated with other antibiotics. Focal or generalized tremor or myoclonus often indicates cortical irritability [10]. If a seizure, tremor, or myoclonus occurs during imipenem therapy, antibiotic dosages or continued need of the antibiotic should be reassessed, and anticonvulsant therapy and neurologic evaluation should be considered [45, 47].

      Because of the potential epileptogenic properties of imipenem, imipenem use in meningitis is not generally advised [32]. In clinical trials, an increased incidence of drug-related seizures was seen in children with meningitis [48]. An exception may be in a case of *S. pneumoniae* meningitis with high-level penicillin resistance and a contraindication to vancomycin use [48a]. See Chaps. 5 and 28C. **To help minimize the risk of seizures, dosages of imipenem should be appropriately reduced in the elderly and in patients with renal insufficiency.**
      e. **Hematologic effects.** Eosinophilia (4%) and direct Coombs' test positivity (2%) occur. Leukopenia and thrombocytopenia have been described. Prothrombin time prolongation rarely occurs, but bleeding has not been reported [10].
      f. **Nephrotoxicity and hepatotoxicity do not** seem to be associated with imipenem use [2].
      g. **No drug interactions** have been reported [2].
   2. **Bacterial colonization or superinfection**
      a. Colonization occurs more frequently than superinfection and does not appear to occur more frequently than with other broad-spectrum antibiotics [10, 37, 45].
      b. Resistant *Pseudomonas* spp. are recovered during therapy either because resistance develops or new colonization occurs with *P. aeruginosa* strains that are resistant to imipenem-cilastatin. This point was emphasized in a review of imipenem which summarized that in 17–60% of cases of *P. aeruginosa* pneumonia, 21% of *P. aeruginosa* bacteremia, 20% of cases of *P. aeruginosa* infection in patients with neutropenia, and 16% of *P. aeruginosa* osteomyelitis, the organism acquired resistance to imipenem during treatment—a situation that frequently led to clinical failure [32]. A recent review emphasizes the development of resistance mainly to *P. aeruginosa* also [31a].

Usually there is no cross-resistance with aminoglycosides, ceftazidime, or piperacillin.

c. Fungal overgrowth can occur.

d. The determination of the precise and comparative frequency of superinfection awaits further clinical use and study.

3. **Interaction with other antibiotics.** Antagonism may be seen between imipenem-cilastatin and either a third-generation cephalosporin or expanded penicillin (e.g., piperacillin). **Imipenem induces beta-lactamases, which can decrease the effectiveness of the cephalosporin or expanded penicillin [40].** See sec. C.5.

4. **Cost.** See discussion in Chap. 28A and Table 28A-6. Although imipenem is an expensive agent, its cost is approximately the same as that of most double-antibiotic regimens and less than that of most conventional triple-antibiotic regimens [32].

H. **Summary.** Imipenem is an extremely potent antibiotic. Its spectrum of activity is too broad for most community-acquired infections, and it should not be used for monotherapy of severe nosocomial *P. aeruginosa* infections. The indications for imipenem continue to evolve; the following are some guidelines:

1. In the *Medical Letter*'s 1996 "The choice of antibacterial drugs" [28], imipenem is listed as the drug of choice only for *Acinetobacter* and *Enterobacter* spp. (organisms typically acquired in the hospital) and for *Campylobacter fetus*.

2. Imipenem is used primarily in the treatment of seriously ill patients with nosocomial pathogens, especially when more than one pathogen is suspected [10] or known.

   a. See Table 28G-7.

   b. Imipenem is also a possible agent in critically ill patients with community-acquired intraabdominal sepsis, sepsis of unclear etiology, and severe aerobic-anaerobic soft-tissue infections while awaiting culture data, if monotherapy is highly desirable.

3. **Imipenem's broad spectrum of activity creates great temptation for indiscriminate use,** which may put the patient (and the hospital environment) at risk for colonization (or for infection) with very resistant organisms. (See related discussion in Chap. 28A.) **Imipenem's spectrum of activity is unnecessarily broad for most community-acquired infections.** To avoid abuse of this agent, Sobel [10] emphasizes the need for continual scrutiny of imipenem use and

Table 28G-7. Clinical use of imipenem

1. For serious nosocomial infections, especially those involving resistant organisms, polymicrobial infections (mixed anaerobes, aerobic, gram-positive and -negative, especially for diabetics)[a]
2. Used alone as an alternative to combination therapy for serious intraabdominal infections, thus avoiding ototoxic and nephrotoxic effects of aminoglycosides[b]
3. For *Pseudomonas* infections caused by organisms resistant to other antipseudomonal beta-lactam agents but, where possible, use in combination with an aminoglycoside
4. Possibly as monotherapy in febrile granulocytopenic patients

When *not* to use imipenem
1. **Not** alone in treatment of serious *Pseudomonas* infections,[c] especially pneumonia
2. **Not** for most community-acquired infections
3. **Not** for surgical prophylaxis
4. **Not** for methicillin-resistant staphylococcal infections
5. **Not** alone in therapy for serious enterococcal infections (*E. faecalis*)
6. **Not** in therapy for non-*aeruginosa* pseudomonal infections

[a]Editors' note: This agent is "saved for use" when cultures reveal or are likely to reveal resistant pathogens in someone usually already on antibiotics or who has recently received antibiotics. *Citrobacter freundii, Acinetobacter,* and *Enterobacter* spp. may be resistant to other antibiotics.
[b]Editors' note: Not for mild to moderate community-acquired infections where less broad agents are effective (e.g., cefoxitin, cefotetan, ampicillin-sulbactam, ticarcillin-clavulanate). Particularly useful in hospital-acquired intraabdominal infections in which resistant organisms may be involved.
[c]Editors' note: In general, for susceptible *P. aeruginosa* infections, an antipseudomonal penicillin and an aminoglycoside are preferred. (See Chap. 28H.)

prescribing patterns. Another reviewer has emphasized that "its broad spectrum and potency must be tempered with its judicious use so that its clinical life can be lengthened and maximized" [49]. A 1991 review of imipenem concluded that "indiscriminate use of imipenem should be avoided. In addition to the aforementioned toxic effects, emergence of resistance would limit the opportunities for its use in the future" [32]. This conclusion still holds. In a 1995 review, the authors conclude: "**Imipenem should be reserved for** [emphasis added] treating patients with serious disorders caused by bacteria suspected or proved resistant to less expensive and safer agents or for patients who are infected with multiple bacteria in whom imipenem alone could replace several antibiotic agents, such as patients with abdominal sepsis or diabetic foot infections" [6b]. To achieve these important goals, **many institutions have developed antibiotic control or approval programs** to help ensure the proper use of imipenem and other broad-spectrum agents (see Chap. 28A).

4. Imipenem has not been approved for use in infants and children by the FDA. Studies reviewing the use of imipenem in children have been published [50, 51].

III. **Meropenem** is a parenteral carbapenem with broad-spectrum in vitro activity similar to imipenem-cilastatin. As of May 1996, it is still an **investigational agent.** Meropenem is stable to human dehydropeptidase-I and, therefore, meropenem alone is administered (see related discussion under sec. **II.B.2.a**).

A. This agent has recently been **reviewed in detail** elsewhere [31a, 52–55].

B. **In clinical trials,** meropenem was effective in bacteremias, UTIs, lower-respiratory infections, intraabdominal infections, and meningitis [53].

C. **The safety profile** of this agent from trials in over 3000 patients is good. Adverse effects are similar in number and nature to those occurring with other beta-lactams [53]. Recipients appear to have fewer GI side effects compared with those receiving imipenem [31a]. There is a low incidence of seizures (lower than that seen with imipenem) and good tolerability at doses of up to 6 g/day in adults and 120 mg/kg/day in children [53]. Clinical trials suggest meropenem may be useful in the therapy of bacterial meningitis. Meropenem does not seem to precipitate seizures in this setting, as does imipenem, nor does it in patients with underlying CNS problems [53]. Therefore, meropenem may be useful for therapy of meningitis due to strains of *S. pneumoniae* resistant to penicillin but susceptible to meropenem, *H. influenzae,* and meningococci [31a].

D. **In clinical trials, intravenous dosing** in adults with normal renal function has been 500 mg to 1 g q8h in adults and 10–20 mg/kg q8h in children; in meningitis, adults have been given 2 g q8h and children 40 mg/kg q8h. **Doses are decreased in renal failure** [54]. Meropenem may be administered by IV bolus injection over approximately 5 minutes or by IV infusion over 15–30 minutes [53, 54].

References

1. Neu, H.C. Current state of infectious disease. Potential areas of directed therapy with aztreonam. *Am. J. Med.* 78(Suppl. 2A):77, 1985.
   An excellent editorial comment on initial potential use of this new agent. For an early summary see Medical Letter, *Aztreonam (Azactam).* Med. Lett. Drugs Ther. *29:45, 1987.*
2. Chambers, H.F., and Neu, H.C. Other β-Lactam Antibiotics. In G.L. Mandell, J.E. Bennett, and R. Dolin (eds.), *Principles and Practice of Infectious Diseases* (4th ed.). New York: Churchill Livingstone, 1995. P. 264.
3. Neu, H.C. Concluding statement. From a symposium entitled "Gram-negative aerobic bacterial infections: A focus on directed therapy, with special reference to aztreonam." *Rev. Infect. Dis.* 7(Suppl. 4):S840, 1985.
   Entire journal issue (Nov.–Dec. 1985) devoted to an extensive review of aztreonam.
4. Sykes, R.B., and Bonner, D.P. Aztreonam: The first monobactam. *Am. J. Med.* 78 (Suppl. 2A):2, 1985.
5. Neu, H.C. (ed.). Aztreonam's role in the treatment of gram-negative infections. *Am. J. Med.* 88(3C):1S–43S, 1990.
   Short symposium updating the efficacy and safety of this agent, which was well tolerated by more than 4,500 patients.
6. Neu, H.C. Aztreonam activity, pharmacology, and clinical uses. *Am. J. Med.* 88(Suppl. 3C):2S, 1990.
6a. Johnson, D.H., and Cunha, B. Aztreonam. *Med. Clin. North Am.* 79:733, 1995.

6b. Ennis, D.M., and Cobbs, C.G. The newer cephalosporins, aztreonam, and imipenem. *Infect. Dis. Clin. North Am.* 9:687, 1995.
7. Brewer, N.S., and Hellinger, W.C. The monobactams. *Mayo Clin. Proc.* 66:1152, 1991. *For a related article, see E. Westley-Horton and J.A. Koestner, Aztreonam: A review of the first monobactam. Am. J. Med. Sci. 302:46, 1991.*
7a. Greenberg, R.N., Meade, D.W., and Danko, L.S. Comparison of the synergistic activity of aztreonam or tobramycin plus piperacillin or mezlocillin. *J. Antimicrob. Chemother.* 32:342, 1993. *Using a checkerboard in vitro technique, 90% of isolates (50 species of P. aeruginosa, 10 species of Enterobacter) were synergistic or additive when tested against piperacillin-tobramycin, versus 66% when tested against piperacillin-aztreonam. There are limited in vitro data on this topic.*
8. Parry, M.F. Aztreonam susceptibility testing. *Am. J. Med.* 88(Suppl. 3C):7S, 1990. *Studied more than 5,800 clinical isolates in a 300-bed community hospital. Organisms susceptible to aztreonam with a MIC of 16 μg/ml or less.*
9. Swabb, E.A. Review of the clinical pharmacology of the monobactam antibiotic aztreonam. *Am. J. Med.* 78(Suppl. 2A):11, 1985. *For a related update, see H. Mattie, Clinical pharmacokinetics of aztreonam: An update. Clin. Pharmacokinet. 26:99, 1994.*
10. Sobel, J.D. Imipenem and aztreonam. *Infect. Dis. Clin. North Am.* 3:613, 1989. *Concise clinical summary. Also see B. Lipman and H.C. Neu, Imipenem: A new carbapenem antibiotic. Med. Clin. North Am. 72:567, 1988.*
11. Rice, L.B., and Eliopoulos, G.M. Imipenem and aztreonam: Current role in antimicrobial therapy. *Curr. Clin. Top. Infect. Dis.* 10:109, 1989.
12. Bohnen, J.M.A. Guidelines for clinical care: Anti-infective agents for intra-abdominal infection. *Arch. Surg.* 127:83, 1992. *This report from the Antimicrobial Agents Committee of the Surgical Infection Society suggests, for mild to moderate community-acquired infections, that single-agent therapy with cefoxitin, cefotetan, cefmatazole, or ticarcillin-clavulanate is recommended. For severe infections, monotherapy with imipenem or combination therapy with either a third-generation cephalosporin, aztreonam, or an aminoglycoside (with serum monitoring) plus clindamycin or metronidazole is recommended. For community-acquired infections, enterococci do not require specific therapy unless gram-positive cocci are seen on Gram stains of surgical specimens. In recurrent intraabdominal infection or hospital-acquired infections, enterococci may play a more important role. (See Chap. 11.) In the patient believed to be at risk for nephrotoxicity, we tend to favor a third-generation cephalosporin and metronidazole or clindamycin; imipenem; or aztreonam and clindamycin.*
For a related discussion, see E. Barboza et al., Clindamycin plus amikacin versus clindamycin plus aztreonam in established intraabdominal infections. Surgery 116:28, 1994. In this prospective, randomized, single-blind study from Peru, 31 patients received clindamycin (900 mg q8h) plus amikacin (5 mg/kg q8h) and 31 patients clindamycin (same dose) plus aztreonam (2 g q8h). Both regimens were highly effective.
13. Cook, J.L. Gram-negative bacillary pneumonia in the nosocomial setting. *Am. J. Med.* 88(Suppl. 3C):34S, 1990.
14. Colardyn, F., et al. Infections in patients in intensive care units: Can the combination of a monobactam and a penicillin replace the classic combination of a beta-lactam agent and an aminoglycoside? *Rev. Infect. Dis.* 13(Suppl. 7):S640, 1991. *This open, comparative, randomized study from Belgium of 76 patients in the intensive care unit, mostly with pulmonary infections, demonstrated that oxacillin (or cloxacillin) with aztreonam is as effective as the combination of a cephalosporin and tobramycin, if not more so. There was 11% nephrotoxicity in the aminoglycoside recipients. Larger clinical studies are pending. See related topics in this symposium on aztreonam.*
15. Conrad, D.A. Efficacy of aztreonam in the treatment of skeletal infections due to *Pseudomonas aeruginosa. Rev. Infect. Dis.* 13(Suppl. 7):S634, 1991. *Small, preliminary study of 10 patients with septic arthritis and 18 patients with osteomyelitis. Notes prior data indicating that more than 60% of serum levels of aztreonam are achieved in synovial fluid and approximately 13% of serum levels are achieved in cancellous bone.*
16. Dratwa, M., et al. Treatment of gram-negative peritonitis with aztreonam in patients undergoing continuous ambulatory peritoneal dialysis. *Rev. Infect. Dis.* 13(Suppl. 7):S645, 1991. *Intraperitoneal aztreonam (500 mg/liter was given in the first dialysate bag and 250*

mg/liter in subsequent bags). Pending cultures, a single dose of vancomycin also was used. No adverse reactions to aztreonam were seen.

17. Schentag, J.J., et al. Treatment with aztreonam or tobramycin in critical care patients with nosocomial gram-negative pneumonia. *Am. J. Med.* 78(Suppl. 2A):34, 1985.
   Aztreonam was superior in seriously ill patients.

18. Jones, P.G., et al. Aztreonam therapy in neutropenic patients with cancer. *Am. J. Med.* 81:243, 1986.
   Also see K.V. Rolston et al., Aztreonam in the prevention and treatment of infection in neutropenic cancer patients. Am. J. Med. *88(3C):24S, 1990.*

19. Stutman, H.R. Clinical experience with aztreonam for treatment of infections in children. *Rev. Infect. Dis.* 13(Suppl. 7):S582, 1991.
   Also see S.C. Aronoff, Aztreonam: New developments in the treatment of gram-negative infections in children. Pediatr. Infect. Dis. J. *8(Suppl. 9):S99–S132, 1989. According to* Physicians' Desk Reference *(50th ed.), Montvale, NJ: Medical Economics, 1996, P. 736, the safety and efficacy of aztreonam has not been established in children and infants.*

20. Lentnek, A.L., and Williams, R.R. Aztreonam in the treatment of gram-negative bacterial meningitis. *Rev. Infect. Dis.* 13(Suppl. 7):S586, 1991.
   Aztreonam can provide cerebrospinal fluid bactericidal levels against susceptible N. meningitidis, H. influenzae, and Enterobacteriaceae. It may provide an alternative agent in P. aeruginosa infections resistant to ceftazidime. It probably should not be used for Salmonella meningitis.

21. Sklavunu-Tsurutsoglu, S., et al. Efficacy of aztreonam in the treatment of neonatal sepsis. *Rev. Infect. Dis.* 13(Suppl. 7):S591, 1991.
   Aztreonam is a potentially useful agent in this setting, especially as it does not cause ototoxicity or renal toxicity and does not interfere with the binding of bilirubin and albumin.

22. Bosso, J.A., and Black, P.G. The use of aztreonam in pediatric patients: A review. *Pharmacotherapy* 11:20, 1991.

22a. Bennett, W.M., et al. *Drug Prescribing in Renal Failure: Dosing Guidelines for Adults* (3rd ed.). Philadelphia: American College of Physicians, 1994. P. 25.

23. Saxon, A., Swabb, E.A., and Adkinson, N.F., Jr. Investigation into the immunologic cross-reactivity of aztreonam with other beta-lactam antibiotics. *Am. J. Med.* 78 (Suppl. 2A):19, 1985.
   Also see N.F. Adkinson, Jr., Immunogenicity and cross-allergenicity of aztreonam. Am. J. Med. *88(Suppl. 3C):12S, 1990.*

24. Moss, R.B., et al. Evaluation of the immunologic cross-reactivity of aztreonam in patients with cystic fibrosis who are allergic to penicillin and/or cephalosporin antibiotics. *Rev. Infect. Dis.* 13(Suppl. 7):S598, 1991.
   Report from Johns Hopkins University that warns: aztreonam should be administered cautiously to patients with cystic fibrosis who are allergic to other beta-lactam antibiotics because it is potentially allergenic with repeated use. See accompanying related articles in this same symposium issue.

25. Appel, G.B. Aminoglycoside nephrotoxicity. *Am. J. Med.* 88(Suppl. 3C):16S, 1990.
   Also see discussion of symposium participants, pages 38S–42S in the same journal.

26. DeMaria, A., Jr. Randomized clinical trial of aztreonam and aminoglycoside antibiotics in the treatment of serious infections caused by gram-negative bacilli. *Antimicrob. Agents Chemother.* 33:1137, 1989.
   Aztreonam is compared with aminoglycosides in a randomized, prospective, non-blinded study of patients with serious gram-negative infections. Aztreonam was equally efficacious with fewer complications.

27. Eisenberg, J.M., et al. What is the cost of nephrotoxicity associated with aminoglycosides? *Ann. Intern. Med.* 107:900, 1987.

28. Medical Letter. The choice of antibacterial drugs. *Med. Lett. Drugs Ther.* 38:25, 1996.

29. Remington, J.S. Introduction: Carbapenems, a new class of antibiotics. *Am. J. Med.* 78(6A):1, 1985.
   This issue has a symposium on imipenem.

30. Medical Letter. Imipenem-cilastatin sodium (Primaxin). *Med. Lett. Drugs Ther.* 28:29, 1986.
   Also see M.M. Buckley et al., Imipenem-cilastatin: A reappraisal of its antibacterial activity, pharmacokinetics and therapeutic efficacy. Drugs *44:408, 1992.*

31. Birnbaum, J., et al. Carbapenems: A new class of beta-lactam antibiotics. *Am. J. Med.* 78(6A):3, 1985.

31a. Norrby, S.R. Carbapenems. *Med. Clin. North Am.* 79:745, 1995.

32. Hellinger, W.C., and Brewer, N.S. Imipenem. *Mayo Clin. Proc.* 66:1074, 1991.
    Concise clinical review.
33. Jones, R.N. Review of the in vitro spectrum of activity of imipenem. *Am. J. Med.*
    78(6A):22, 1985.
    See J.C. Pechere, Why are carbapenems active against Enterobacter cloacae *resistant
    to third generation cephalosporins?* Scand. Infect. Dis. *78(Suppl.):17, 1991.*
33a. Friedland, I.R., and McCracken, G.H., Jr. Management of infections caused by antibi-
    otic resistant *Streptococcus pneumoniae. N. Engl. J. Med.* 331:377, 1994.
    In vitro susceptibilities to imipenem for S. pneumoniae *include the following MIC$_{90}$
    data: for penicillin-susceptible strains, 0.01–0.03 µg/ml or less; for intermediately
    resistant strains, 0.03–0.12 µg/ml; and for highly resistant strains, 0.25–1.0 µg/ml.*
33b. Wood, C.A., and Reboli, A.C. Infections caused by imipenem-resistant *Acinetobacter
    calcoaceticus* biotype anitratus. *J. Infect. Dis.* 168:1602, 1993.
    Although Acinetobacter spp. *are almost universally susceptible to imipenem, imi-
    penem-resistant isolates have been reported and can cause nosocomial infections. Some
    isolates are susceptible to ampicillin-sulbactam. The polymyxins (e.g., colistimethate)
    appear active in vitro and may provide a therapeutic alternative. Infectious disease
    consultation is advised in the setting of an* Acinetobacter spp. *infection that is resistant
    to imipenem.*
34. Cuchural, G.J., Jr., et al. Susceptibility of the *Bacteroides fragilis* group in the United
    States: Analysis by site of isolation. *Antimicrob. Agents Chemother.* 32:717, 1988.
35. Drusano, G.L., and Standiford, H.C. Pharmacokinetic profile of imipenem/cilastatin
    in normal volunteers. *Am. J. Med.* 78(6A):47, 1985.
36. Axelrod, J.L., et al. Penetration of imipenem in human aqueous and vitreous humor.
    Am. J. Ophthalmol. 104:649, 1987.
    After a 1-g IV dose, levels were well above the MIC$_{90}$ of S. epidermidis, S. aureus, *and
    the* Enterobacteriaceae *commonly involved in bacterial endophthalmitis.*
37. Winston, D.J., McGrattan, M.A., and Busuttil, R.W. Imipenem therapy of *Pseudomo-
    nas aeruginosa* and other serious bacterial infections. *Antimicrob. Agents Chemother.*
    26:673, 1985.
37a. Fink, M.P. Treatment of severe pneumonia in hospitalized patients: Results of a
    multicenter, randomized, double-blind trial comparing intravenous ciprofloxacin with
    imipenem-cilastatin. *Antimicrob. Agents Chemother.* 38:547, 1994.
    *Ciprofloxacin (IV 400 mg q8h) or imipenem (1 g q8h) was used. Neither regimen was
    good for* P. aeruginosa, *but both regimens were effective for other susceptible pathogens.*
38. Neu, H.C. Summary of imipenem/cilastatin symposium. *Am. J. Med.* 78(6A):165, 1985.
39. Neu, H.C. New antibiotics: Areas of appropriate use. *J. Infect. Dis.* 155:403, 1987.
    *Clinically oriented summary of new agents, including third-generation cephalosporins,
    imipenem, aztreonam, and the fluoroquinolones.*
40. Wade, J.C., et al. Potential of imipenem as single-agent empiric antibiotic therapy
    of febrile neutropenic patients with cancer. *Am. J. Med.* 78(6A):62, 1985.
    *Also see J.C. Wade et al. Monotherapy for empiric treatment of fever in granulocytic
    cancer patients.* Am. J. Med. *80(Suppl. 5C):85, 1986.*
41. Bodey, G.P., et al. Imipenem-cilastin therapy of infections in cancer patients. *Cancer*
    60:255, 1987.
42. Hughes, W.T., et al. Guidelines for the use of antimicrobial agents in neutropenic
    patients with unexplained fever. *J. Infect. Dis.* 161:381, 1990.
43. Liang, R., et al. Ceftazidime versus imipenem-cilastin as initial monotherapy for
    febrile neutropenic patients. *Antimicrob. Agents Chemother.* 34:1336, 1990.
    *Study from Hong Kong in which 89 neutropenic patients were randomized to be treated
    with either agent as monotherapy. The in vitro susceptibilities and the clinical response
    suggested that with the exception of* P. aeruginosa, *imipenem was more effective than
    ceftazidime. The majority of failures, relapses, and superinfections were related to
    resistant organisms such as methicillin-resistant staphylococci,* Pseudomonas spp.,
    or fungi.
44. Riikonen, P. Imipenem compared with ceftazidime plus vancomycin as initial therapy
    for fever in neutropenic children with cancer. *Pediatr. J. Infect. Dis.* 10:918, 1991.
    *In this open, prospective randomized trial from Finland, in 89 patients, imipenem
    was well tolerated and effective as initial therapy for fever in neutropenic children.
    Imipenem will not be active against methicillin-resistant* S. epidermidis *infections.*
44a. Freifeld, A.G., et al. Monotherapy for fever and neutropenia in cancer patients. A
    randomized comparison of ceftazidime versus imipenem. *J. Clin. Oncol.* 13:165, 1995.
    *Report from the National Cancer Institute, National Institutes of Health, in which
    204 adult and pediatric patients received ceftazidime and 195 received imipenem.*

Both monotherapy regimens were effective (98% survival for both regimens) when modifications were made in response to clinical and microbiologic data. Imipenem appeared to have more GI side effects.

For a related discussion see A. Kojima et al., A randomized prospective study of imipenem-cilastatin with or without amikacin as an empirical antibiotic treatment for febrile neutropenic patients. Am. J. Clin. Oncol. 17:400, 1994. In this small study from Japan, 34 patients received combination therapy and 36 patients received imipenem alone. Data showed 91% of recipients of combination therapy responded versus 71% of those who received imipenem alone, suggesting combination therapy may be superior in this setting. Side effects were similar in each group in this report.

44b. Cometta, A., et al. Prospective randomized comparison of imipenem monotherapy with imipenem plus netilmicin for treatment of severe infections in nonneutropenic patients. *Antimicrob. Agents Chemother.* 38:1209, 1994.

Although combination therapy may achieve enhanced bacterial killing by synergism in vitro and in theory help prevent emergence of resistance, this may not be seen in vivo. In this study from Switzerland, 142 patients received monotherapy and 138 patients received combination therapy for nosocomial pneumonia, nosocomial sepsis, and severe peritonitis. Clinical outcomes were similar; the addition of netilmicin increased nephrotoxicity and did not prevent the emergence of P. aeruginosa resistant to imipenem. Therefore, for susceptible strains of P. aeruginosa causing established pneumonia, a piperacillin-aminoglycoside combination is preferred when not contraindicated.

45. Calandra, G.B. Review of adverse experiences and tolerability in the first 2,516 patients treated with imipenem/cilastatin. *Am. J. Med.* 78(6A):73, 1985.

46. Saxon, A., et al. Immediate hypersensitivity reactions to beta-lactam antibiotics. *Ann. Intern. Med.* 127:204, 1987.

47. Calandra, G., et al. Factors predisposing to seizures in seriously ill infected patients receiving antibiotics: Experience with imipenem/cilastatin. *Am. J. Med.* 84:911, 1988.

Offers some practical guidelines of assessment and treatment in this setting.

48. Wong, V.K., et al. Imipenem/cilastatin treatment of bacterial meningitis in children. *Pediatr. Infect. Dis. J.* 10:122, 1991.

Study terminated when 7 of 21 children developed seizure activity after imipenem therapy. Study concluded that the usefulness of imipenem for the treatment of bacterial meningitis in children may be limited by a possible increased incidence of drug-related seizures.

48a. Asensi, F., et al. Risk-benefit ratio in the treatment of children with imipenem-cilastatin for meningitis caused by penicillin-resistant pneumococcus. *J. Chemother.* 5:133, 1993.

49. Galpin, J.E., et al. Imipenem: A new beta-lactam antibiotic. *Infect. Dis. Alert* 4:21, 1984.

50. Ahonkhai, V.I., et al. Imipenem-cilastatin in pediatric patients: An overview of safety and efficacy studies conducted in the United States. *Pediatr. Infect. Dis. J.* 8:740, 1989.

Data suggest that imipenem should be safe and effective in selected pediatric patients.

51. Overturf, G.D. Use of imipenem-cilastatin in pediatrics. *Pediatr. Infect. Dis. J.* 8:792, 1989.

52. Davey, P., et al. Meropenem (SM7338): A new carbapenem. *J. Antimicrob. Chemother.* 24(Suppl. A):1–320, 1989.

Symposium on this agent emphasizing preclinical data: in vitro activity, pharmacokinetics, and activity in experimental animal models. Clinical data is provided in reference [53].

53. Finch, R.G., et al. Meropenem: Focus on clinical performance. *J. Antimicrob. Chemother.* 36(Suppl. A):1–223, 1995.

Symposium covering in vitro activity update, pharmacokinetics, and emphasizing clinical trial data.

54. Wiseman, L.R., et al. Meropenem: A review of its antibacterial activity, pharmacokinetics and clinical efficacy. *Drugs* 50:73–101, 1995.

55. Norrby, S.R. Carbapenems: Efficacy and safety profiles—focus on meropenem. *Scand. J. Infect. Dis.* (Suppl. 96):5–48, 1995.

H. Aminoglycosides

Since the introduction of streptomycin in 1944 and kanamycin in 1957, other more useful parenteral aminoglycosides, including gentamicin, tobramycin, netilmicin, and amikacin, have become available. These agents and their toxicity have been reviewed [1–8]. **The role aminoglycosides play in clinical medicine continues to evolve and to be modified as other classes of less toxic agents with expanded spectrum of activity** (e.g., third-generation cephalosporins, aztreonam, fluoroquinolones) **have become available.** Research and development of new aminoglycosides are at a standstill [1], reflecting the conservative approach of the pharmaceutical industry. In fact, the newest agent, netilmicin, failed to find a clear niche [1], again reflecting the reassessment of the role of aminoglycosides. Future efforts will likely be directed toward a better understanding and prevention, if possible, of resistance and toxicity [2]. Nevertheless, because of cost considerations, the only rare development of bacterial resistance while the patient is on therapy, reduced incidence of *Clostridium difficile* diarrhea, low risk of allergic reactions, and the better understanding of toxicity associated with these agents, the aminoglycosides remain very useful in selected settings [5].

These agents are, in most instances, bactericidal. They penetrate the cell wall and membrane and bind irreversibly to the 30 S bacterial ribosomes. The synthesized proteins are abnormal and nonfunctional, and bacterial death ensues. The precise mechanism through which the aminoglycosides cause bacterial cell death remains elusive [2] and is discussed elsewhere [5].

Paromomycin is discussed briefly at the end of this chapter.

I. **Important principles of aminoglycoside use**
   A. **Aminoglycosides versus other classes of antibiotics. Aminoglycosides have excellent activity against almost all aerobic gram-negative organisms.** If susceptibility data permit, most experts favor **the use of ampicillin or a cephalosporin** or, in certain settings, aztreonam (see Chap. 28C, sec. **I.H.**) or the fluoroquinolones (see Chap. 28S), as these agents are less toxic, and equal or higher therapeutic ratios can be achieved. However, **because of the potential for emergence of resistant organisms to these alternative agents, aminoglycosides retain their usefulness and, in some settings, may be preferred.** When to use the aminoglycosides rather than other agents (such as the third-generation cephalosporins or the fluoroquinolones or aztreonam) needs continued evaluation [1, 3, 4]. Despite these newer agents, the aminoglycosides are expected to remain important agents.
      1. **Community versus nosocomial infections.** Although aminoglycosides are active against gram-negative bacteria that cause community-acquired infection, cephalosporins too are usually active against these bacteria and are preferred. By contrast, bacteria that cause nosocomial infections are much more likely to be resistant to ampicillin or the cephalosporins. Therefore, **aminoglycosides are particularly useful in nosocomial infections,** especially when and if *Pseudomonas* spp. are a concern.
      2. **Modifying initial therapy.** In a nosocomial infection or, at times, in life-threatening community-acquired infections of unclear etiology, aminoglycosides are indicated as part of the initial treatment. If the causative pathogen is isolated and is demonstrated to be susceptible to ampicillin or a cephalosporin or other narrow-spectrum agents, appropriate modifications can be made.
   B. **Special problems with aminoglycoside use.** Before any of the individual agents are discussed, some special problems of aminoglycoside use need to be emphasized.
      1. **Toxicity.** Unlike the beta-lactam, monobactam, and fluoroquinolone antimicrobial agents, **the aminoglycosides have considerable intrinsic toxicity** [2]. Estimates suggest that 5–10% or more of patients receiving aminoglycosides may develop some degree of ototoxicity or nephrotoxicity [1, 2, 3, 5]. This risk of toxicity must be considered before and while using the aminoglycosides, especially for any extended period of time. **The toxicity of aminoglycosides is reviewed in detail in sec. II.D.**
      2. **Narrow toxic-therapeutic ratio. A related problem with the use of aminoglycosides is the narrow margin between effective and toxic concentrations.**
         a. **Therapeutic ratio.** An important principle in drug efficacy is the therapeutic ratio achieved after the administration of a standard dose. This is **defined** as the serum level of the bactericidal antibiotic divided by the minimal inhibitory concentration (MIC) of the organism being treated. This ratio can be estimated by knowing the pharmacology of the drug and the predicted MIC of the bacteria to that drug. It also is possible to measure, after a dose of antibiotic, the dilution of the patient's serum that will inhibit or kill the infecting organism. For bloodstream or soft-tissue infections, a therapeutic ratio of 4:1 to 8:1 usually is sufficient, whereas for pulmonary

infection, a ratio of 16:1 may be required to provide adequate tissue levels, as there is poor penetration of antibiotics into sputum. See related discussions in Chap. 25. The aminoglycosides demonstrate concentration-dependent bactericidal activity. See related discussion in sec. **III.E.1.a** and Chap. 28A (p. 1081).

b. **Low therapeutic ratios are achieved with aminoglycoside therapy.** The problem of achieving adequate therapeutic ratios with aminoglycoside therapy is emphasized in the following example comparing treatment of *Klebsiella pneumoniae* infections with gentamicin to treatment of *Streptococcus pneumoniae* with penicillin.

(1) If *K. pneumoniae*'s MIC for gentamicin is approximately 1.56 μg/ml,

$$\text{the therapeutic ratio with average serum levels} = \frac{\text{serum level of antibiotic}}{\text{MIC}}$$

$$= \frac{6 \ \mu g/ml}{1.56 \ \mu g/ml}$$

or approximately a fourfold ratio. This therapeutic ratio of 4:1 is adequate, in theory, for bloodstream infections. However, this peak is maintained for less than 1–2 hours, and suboptimal dosing is not uncommon with aminoglycosides. Even lower concentrations of the antibiotic are found at tissue levels. (See sec. **c.**).

(2) In contrast, for penicillin, this ratio is much higher and easier to achieve. For example, the average MIC for penicillin against group A streptococcus or penicillin-susceptible *S. pneumoniae* is 0.015–0.020 μg/ml.

(a) With low-dose penicillin,

$$\text{the approximate therapeutic ratio} = \frac{6.0 \ \mu g/ml}{0.02 \ \mu g/ml} = 300:1.$$

(b) With high-dose penicillin, one achieves a very high therapeutic ratio:

$$\frac{20 \ \mu g/ml}{0.02 \ \mu g/ml} = 1,000:1$$

c. **The site of infection and conditions at the site also affect potential activity.** Antibacterial activity is enhanced in media with an alkaline pH and reduced in media with an acid pH.

(1) In gram-negative bacterial pneumonias, less than half of the serum levels of gentamicin is measured in bronchial secretions. Furthermore, because the pH is less than 7.4 in inflammatory fluids such as sputum, activity of the drug is reduced.

(2) By contrast, in urinary tract infections (UTIs), gentamicin and other aminoglycosides are concentrated in the urine. Hence, even moderately resistant organisms can often be inhibited even when renal function is mildly to moderately impaired.

(3) Aminoglycoside activity is limited in an abscess, where the environment is hypoxic or the pH may be low, and in the presence of tissue necrosis containing divalent cations (which can inhibit aminoglycosides) [1, 9, 10]. See related discussion in Chap. 11, sec. **II.B.1** under Intraabdominal Infection (p. 418).

d. The currently accepted therapeutic range for aminoglycosides is discussed in detail in section **IV.** The clinician is unable to increase the dose of aminoglycosides significantly, to produce higher peak levels (and therefore higher therapeutic ratios), because of the risk of excess toxicity, which may be related to high serum levels. In contrast, beta-lactam agents can often be given in higher doses, achieving higher therapeutic ratios but without excess toxicity. See example in sec. **b.(2).**

3. **Monitoring of serum levels (concentrations). To ensure that serum levels are sufficient to be efficacious yet not so high as to be toxic, it is prudent to measure serum levels** of the aminoglycosides [11–13]. Many factors affect the levels of aminoglycoside achievable, such as the age of the patient, state of hydration, renal function, obesity, and certain settings (e.g., pancreatitis, cystic fibrosis). **This topic is discussed in detail in sec. IV.**

4. **Other limitations of use of aminoglycosides**
   a. **Poor oral absorption.** The aminoglycosides are not orally absorbed from the GI tract.
   b. **Central nervous system infection.** Aminoglycosides poorly penetrate the cerebrospinal fluid (CSF). Because their therapeutic ratio is marginal, CSF concentrations are usually insufficient.

      In gram-negative meningitis in adults, if aminoglycosides must be used, as in some cases of *P. aeruginosa* infections, intraventricular administration has sometimes been advised by infectious disease consultants, although this remains a controversial area and consultation is advised. Intravenous ceftazidime may allow monotherapy (see Chaps. 5 and 28F).
   c. Systemic therapy results in unreliable or inadequate therapeutic levels in vitreous fluid, prostate, and bile [2]. Parenteral administration results in low concentrations of active drug in bronchial secretions [5].

II. **Specific aminoglycosides: Gentamicin versus tobramycin versus netilmicin versus amikacin**
   A. **Clinical effectiveness. Against susceptible pathogens, these agents have been shown to be equally effective** [1, 4]. With some exceptions, after a standard dose, gentamicin, tobramycin, and netilmicin produce similar serum levels, whereas amikacin serum levels are approximately 4 times higher. However, the MICs of common community-acquired bacteria are 4 times as high for amikacin as for gentamicin, tobramycin, or netilmicin, so similar therapeutic (bactericidal) ratios are achieved.
   B. **Spectrum of activity.** There is usually no inoculum effect in vitro [5].
      1. **Gram-negative aerobes. The aminoglycosides are particularly active against**

Table 28H-1. Percentage of gram-negative bacilli susceptible to gentamicin and amikacin at specified concentrations—Mayo Clinic, 1989

Organism	No. of strains	Gentamicin (≤ 2 μg/ml)	Amikacin (≤ 8 μg/ml)
Acinetobacter calcoaceticus			
Var. *anitratus*	111	92	95
Var. *lwoffi*	78	97	100
Alcaligenes spp.	20	50	75
Citrobacter diversus	80	100	100
C. fruendii	248	96	100
Enterobacter aerogenes	340	99	99
E. agglomerans	35	100	100
E. cloacae	521	99	100
Escherichia coli	4,018	98	99
Klebsiella oxytoca	322	100	100
K. pneumoniae	1,045	97	100
Morganella morganii	163	91	98
Proteus mirabilis	533	97	100
P. vulgaris	47	96	100
Providencia rettgeri	16	94	100
P. stuartii	14	71	100
Pseudomonas aeruginosa	1,321	85	96
P. cepacia	17	6	6
P. fluorescens	45	93	100
Salmonella spp.	39	100	100
Serratia marcescens	246	97	98
Xanthomonas maltophilia*	242	11	12
Yersinia enterocolitica	10	100	100

*Formerly *Pseudomonas maltophilia* (recently renamed *Stenotrophomonas maltophilia*).
Source: From R.S. Edson and C.L. Terrell, The aminoglycosides. *Mayo Clin. Proc.* 66:1158, 1991.

the Enterobacteriaceae (*Escherichia coli* and *Klebsiella* and *Proteus* spp., etc.) and *Pseudomonas, Acinetobacter,* and *Providencia* spp. **See Table 28H-1.** Because these same gram-negative pathogens commonly cause hospital-acquired infections, the **aminoglycosides are especially useful as initial therapy in nosocomial infections,** usually in combination with an extended-spectrum penicillin (e.g., piperacillin) or a cephalosporin.

   a. **Against broadly susceptible community-acquired** gram-negative organisms, all four aminoglycosides have equal bactericidal levels.

   b. **Nosocomial gram-negative organisms.** In general, tobramycin in vitro is 2–4 times more active than gentamicin against *P. aeruginosa,* but the clinical implications of this are unclear. Netilmicin is less active than either tobramycin or gentamicin against susceptible *P. aeruginosa.* Against *Serratia* spp., gentamicin has 2–4 times the bactericidal activity of tobramycin. For other nosocomial organisms, there is less predictability, but generally, for susceptible pathogens, therapeutic or bactericidal ratios are equal for each of the three aminoglycosides.

   Amikacin usually will be the most active aminoglycoside against gentamicin-resistant strains, although some organisms resistant to gentamicin are susceptible to tobramycin.

   c. Aminoglycosides are minimally active against *Haemophilus* and *Legionella* spp. but are not used clinically for infections due to these pathogens [5].

2. **Gram-positive aerobes.** The aminoglycosides have some activity against these organisms but alone are never the preferred agents.

   a. **Staphylococci.** Against susceptible staphylococci, gentamicin and amikacin have equal bactericidal ratios, but there are some staphylococci that are resistant to gentamicin but susceptible to amikacin. The typical MIC_{90} for *S. aureus* (methicillin-susceptible) for gentamicin is 0.8 μg/ml [4]. An antistaphylococcal penicillin (e.g., nafcillin) and gentamicin are synergistic against *S. aureus.*

   b. **Viridans streptococci.** An aminoglycoside, usually gentamicin, sometimes is combined with penicillin to achieve synergy. See Chap. 10.

   c. **Enterococcus.* Gentamicin, together with ampicillin or penicillin, usually has the greatest activity against enterococci.** (Of the extended-spectrum penicillins, piperacillin is more active, in combination with gentamicin, against enterococci). The combination of a cell wall–active antibiotic (e.g., penicillin or ampicillin) to which the organism is susceptible and an aminoglycoside to which the enterococcus does not possess high-level resistance is preferred when such a combination is available [14].

   However, in recent years, at major medical centers there has been an increasing incidence of enterococci resistant to the combination of gentamicin-penicillin (so-called "high-level" gentamicin resistance, with a MIC to gentamicin > 2,000 μg/ml). Among 139 enterococcal isolates collected from eight US tertiary care hospitals in six geographic regions between July 1988 and March 1989, 24.5% demonstrated high-level resistance [14]. The details of this problem and alternative therapeutic approaches are reviewed elsewhere [14–18], and discussed further in sec. **F.2.**

   d. Nonenterococcal streptococci are not susceptible to aminoglycosides.

3. **Anaerobes.** The aminoglycosides are not active against anaerobes.

4. **Norcardia** is susceptible to amikacin [4].

5. **Mycobacterium.** Most *Mycobacterium tuberculosis* and *M. avium-intracellulare* isolates are susceptible to amikacin. (See Chaps. 9 and 19.)

C. **Pharmacokinetics**

1. **Gentamicin, tobramycin, and netilmicin have similar pharmacokinetics;** therefore, standard doses, peak levels achieved, and serum half-lives are essentially the same (see Table 28H-2). Their toxicity may differ, as noted later. The average half-life is 2–4 hours, and measurable levels may persist for 6

---

*There are now 12 enterococcus spp., and all but two have been isolated from human infections. These species can be identified in the microbiology laboratory. The majority of clinical isolates of enterococci will be *E. faecalis* (80–90%) and *E. faecium* (5–10%). Infrequently, *E. avium, E. raffinosus,* and *E. gallinarium* will be found. Clusters of infections with *E. raffinosus* have been reported. Other strains are isolated only rarely from human infections. (From A. Ballows et al. [eds.], *Manual of Clinical Microbiology* [5th ed.]. Washington, DC: American Society for Microbiology, 1991. Pp. 251–252.)

Table 28H-2. Expected peak and trough levels of respective aminoglycosides (in μg/ml)

	Peak[a,b]	Trough[c]	Toxic[b]
Gentamicin	6–8	≤0.8–1.2	>10
Tobramycin	6–8	≤0.8–1.2	>10
Amikacin	22–28	<4–6	>35
Netilmicin	6–8	≤0.8–1.2	>10

[a]One-half hour after a half-hour infusion.
[b]These peak toxic levels are with conventional dosage regimens. With once-a-day dosages, higher acceptable peak levels will routinely be achieved. See text.
[c]Level just before next dose.
Note: These ranges for peak and trough concentrations are used commonly, but their exact implications remain controversial, as reviewed in reference [19].

hours. The recommended dose interval is typically every 8 hours in adults (<60 years) with normal renal function and serious disease. However, individualized dosing may alter the interval. Once-daily dosing is also undergoing clinical evaluation. See sec. **III.E.**

2. **Amikacin is a semisynthetic kanamycin** derivative with pharmacokinetics nearly identical to those of kanamycin. The serum half-life is approximately 2–3 hours, and measurable serum levels may persist for 6–8 hours. The usual dose interval in adults is every 8 hours when renal function is normal, although the interval could be adjusted in individualized dosing.

3. **Excretion** of the aminoglycosides is 99% **renal** [5]. **In renal failure,** the drugs accumulate, and **dose reductions are therefore necessary.**

4. **Variation in pharmacokinetics.** There is **striking variation in the volume of distribution and rate of excretion of aminoglycosides** in patients with normal (as well as patients with abnormal) renal function [1, 3, 5]. **Thus, it appears to be important to monitor serum levels in the critically ill patient. Furthermore, monitoring of levels in the patient with renal failure** and in other populations listed in sec. **IV.B** is believed to be important not only to avoid toxic levels but to ensure adequate therapeutic levels.

5. **Tissue penetration.** Aminoglycosides achieve reasonable concentrations in bone, synovial fluid, and peritoneal fluid. Urinary concentrations are high and may exceed serum concentration by 100 times in patients with normal renal function [2]. Due to renal tubular cell absorption and subsequent release, the urine concentrations remain above therapeutic levels for several days after a single dose [5].

   As previously discussed, there is limited penetration into bronchial secretions and the CNS.

D. **Toxicity** [1, 3–7]. Hypersensitivity reactions are uncommon, phlebitis at the intravenous site is rare, and aminoglycosides do not induce hepatotoxicity or photosensitivity [5]. Important side effects include the following:

1. **Neuromuscular paralysis** rarely occurs but has occurred after intraperitoneal lavage (no longer used or recommended) or rapid intravenous bolus therapy, particularly in the setting of myasthenia gravis or concurrent use of succinylcholine or curare. This is usually reversible.

   Clinical manifestations of blockade may include weakness of respiratory muscles, flaccid paralysis, and dilated pupils. The risk of blockade is amplified in patients also administered D-tubocurare, succinylcholine, and similar agents. Neuromuscular blockade is reversed by rapidly infusing intravenous calcium gluconate; it can be prevented by infusing conventional doses of intravenous aminoglycosides over 20–30 minutes and once-daily regimens over 60 minutes [5]. There is no current indication for instillation of high concentrations of aminoglycoside into the peritoneal cavity or pleural space [5].

2. **Ototoxicity frequently is irreversible** and can appear after completion of therapy; repeated exposures engender cumulative risk. A given patient may suffer cochlear damage, vestibular damage or, rarely, both [5].

   a. **Cochlear (auditory) toxicity.** If audiometric studies are performed, 2–14% of recipients may demonstrate hearing loss. Clinically detectable hearing loss is uncommon [5]. The mechanism of auditory toxicity involves selective destruction of the outer hair cells of the organ of Corti [5]. Though this destruction originally was considered irreversible, clinical reports document at least some potential for regeneration of hair cells [5]. Patients particularly at risk for the development of ototoxicity are those who have received a high cumulative dose or a protracted course of aminoglycosides [19]. Other risk factors may include concomitant use of ethacrynic acid, toxic peak levels of aminoglycosides, and old age. **In general, routine audiograms are not possible and are not recommended** if renal function is normal. In a cooperative patient who needs protracted aminoglycoside therapy (e.g., > 2 weeks), audiograms carried out serially are a consideration. **Serum levels should be monitored carefully and adjusted in patients with renal failure. Protracted courses of aminoglycosides should be avoided whenever possible** [16]. Cochlear injury may be independent of nephrotoxicity, although the risk of either cochlear or vestibular toxicity is greater in patients with renal impairment [5]. Concomitant use of ethacrynic acid should be avoided. Netilmicin may be associated with less ototoxicity than the other aminoglycosides [6], but this is uncertain.

   b. **Vestibular** dysfunction manifested by nausea, vomiting, vertigo, dizziness, and unsteady gait with nystagmus is more difficult to evaluate in ill patients but presumably is related to the same predisposing factors that cause auditory toxicity [5]. This appears to occur in 1–3% of patients and has not been studied as thoroughly as auditory toxicity [6].

   Because vestibular injury can be compensated by visual and proprioceptive cues, patients can suffer considerable injury prior to the appearance of symptoms or clinical findings. Suspicion is raised at the bedside by complaints of nausea, vomiting, and vertigo. Symptoms are exacerbated in the dark, when the eyes are closed, or in other situations that block compensatory pathways [5].

   c. **If a patient is receiving an aminoglycoside and develops symptoms of hearing loss, tinnitus, vertigo, or nystagmus, the aminoglycoside should, if possible, be discontinued.** Some patients may complain of a sensation of fullness in the ears, which may represent early ototoxicity [5]. If alternative therapy is not available, very careful monitoring of peak levels and a slightly longer time of infusion should be considered.

3. **Nephrotoxicity** due to aminoglycoside use is a complicated topic. A review of the potential mechanisms is summarized elsewhere [1, 3, 5]. Toxicity appears to occur at the level of the proximal tubule. There is no agreement as to how injury or death of proximal tubule cells results in a decrease in the glomerular filtration rate. In some series, up to 7% of cases of acute renal failure in hospitalized patients were due to aminoglycosides [3]. In more recent studies, the overall incidence of aminoglycoside nephrotoxicity was 5–10% of recipients [3].

   a. Nephrotoxicity with aminoglycosides can manifest as rising BUN and creatinine, or proteinuria, or oliguria, or nonoliguric renal failure. The changes are **usually reversible when the drug is discontinued.** Progression to dialysis-dependent oliguric-anuric renal failure is rare [5].

   b. **Definition of** nephrotoxicity is usually an increase in serum creatinine above 1.5 or an increase of 0.4 mg/dl if the initial creatinine was normal. If the initial serum creatinine is elevated, nephrotoxicity is defined by a serum creatinine increase of at least 0.5 mg/dl if the initial creatinine was elevated but was less than 3.0 mg/dl, or a serum creatinine increase of more than 1.0 mg/dl if the initial creatinine exceeded 3.0. The serum creatinine is a convenient parameter to follow when monitoring for aminoglycoside nephrotoxicity [5]. Therefore, **serum creatinine levels should be obtained every 2–4 days in patients receiving aminoglycosides** [1].

   c. **Comparative nephrotoxicity of the aminoglycosides.** Prior studies have suggested that netilmicin and, to a lesser extent, tobramycin may be less nephrotoxic than gentamicin [3, 6]. However, these studies are very difficult to interpret, often involve relatively small numbers of patients, have many unexplained inconsistencies [6], and do not compare toxicity rates of empiric or nomogram regimens to individualized dosing. Other studies have been unable to confirm significant differences in nephrotoxicity among the aminoglycosides [3].

d. Risk factors associated with nephrotoxicity have not been fully defined nor universally accepted [5].

  (1) Concomitant liver disease appears to be important. In particular, we would avoid aminoglycoside use in patients with known early hepatorenal syndrome or at risk for this problem. Likewise, we would try to avoid aminoglycoside use in patients with prothrombin time prolongation due to underlying liver disease.

  (2) Hypotension, especially septic shock or sepsis syndrome, presents an increased risk for renal insufficiency. The role aminoglycosides play in this is unclear but, for community-acquired infections, it probably is prudent to avoid aminoglycosides in this setting. Prolonged hypovolemia with hypotension is also a potential risk factor.

  (3) Concomitant drug use may, at times, be important. Cephalothin use, along with an aminoglycoside, does not seem to enhance nephrotoxicity [3, 20], but even this is debated [5].

   (a) Aminoglycoside use along with vancomycin appears to increase toxicity in adults. (See Chap. 28O.)

   (b) Amphotericin B and cyclosporine increase toxicity when used with aminoglycosides. Concomitant use of furosemide or nonsteroidal antiinflammatory agents may also increase nephrotoxicity.

   (c) Intravenous furosemide, with the potential for relative hypovolemia, may be a risk factor.

   (d) Foscarnet may be a risk factor. (See Chap. 26.)

  (4) Other risk factors. Advanced age, previous courses of aminoglycosides (within 1 year), greater total dose of aminoglycoside, and prior renal disease have also been associated with toxicity [3], but their exact role is debated [5].

e. Course of nephrotoxicity

  (1) Typical. True nephrotoxicity seldom occurs in the first week of therapy [19]. The initial toxic manifestation generally is nonoliguric renal failure that usually is reversible if the drug is discontinued. Such reversal may take weeks or months to occur. Continued administration of the aminoglycoside (or failure to decrease the dose) may lead eventually to oliguric renal shutdown [1].

  (2) Rapid onset. Uncommonly, rapid onset of nephrotoxicity with aminoglycoside use occurs after only a few doses, for unclear reasons. The hallmark is a rise in creatinine from normal (or baseline) to renal failure in 1–2 days. Hypersensitivity or perhaps unrecognized major preexisting disease may be a mechanism. Unless there is no alternative, the aminoglycoside should be discontinued [1].

f. Prevention of nephrotoxicity is controversial [3, 8, 19].

  (1) Correction of hypovolemia, diminished renal perfusion, and congestive heart failure are indicated.

  (2) Careful monitoring of aminoglycoside serum levels in high-risk patients (see sec. **IV.B**) may help, but this has not been clearly established [19].

   (a) Individualized dosing of aminoglycosides has been advocated by Zaske [12] and Sawchuk [21] and their coworkers. This consists of obtaining levels at 0.5, 1, 3, and 8 hours; then, doses and intervals are adjusted for each patient (see sec. **III.C.1**). These same steps are repeated after the acute symptoms subside, usually after 72–96 hours of therapy. (Trough levels are kept at less than 2 μg/ml.) Sawchuk and colleagues [21] report an incidence of nephrotoxicity of 1% with gentamicin. In a large series of more than 1,400 patients who received individualized dosing, aminoglycoside nephrotoxicity was reported in 7.9% of carefully monitored patients [22]. Additional studies need to confirm the risk of nephrotoxicity with this dose method. This approach is discussed in detail in sec. **III.C**. The **authors believe that this approach may be the most prudent method to provide appropriate drug doses and possibly help minimize nephrotoxicity** when an aminoglycoside is clearly indicated. It is hoped that a prospective, controlled clinical study eventually will be done to clarify whether individualized dosing truly decreases the risk of nephrotoxicity (and ototoxicity).

      (b) Once-daily dosing of aminoglycosides may be associated with less nephrotoxicity [5]. This is discussed in sec. **III.E.**

     (3) Use the shortest appropriate course of aminoglycosides and use only when clearly indicated.

     (4) Consider alternative agents—for example, third-generation cephalosporins or aztreonam, especially in patients at high risk for nephrotoxicity and especially if aminoglycoside levels cannot be carefully monitored.

   4. Macular toxicity. Intravitreous injections for treatment or prophylaxis of endophthalmitis can be associated with macular toxicity. See Chap. 6.

E. Cost. The generic formulation of gentamicin is less expensive than all other aminoglycosides and cephalosporins. Amikacin is the most expensive aminoglycoside (see Table 28A-6). For a typical low-dose regimen, mean wholesale acquisition costs of the aminoglycosides are approximately $1.00 for gentamicin (80 mg), $4.00–5.00 for tobramycin (80 mg), and $50.00–55.00 for amikacin (500 mg) [2].

F. Resistance.

   1. Resistance to aminoglycosides, with the exception of streptomycin, **evolves very slowly.** Nonetheless, excess use of an antibiotic may be followed eventually by the development of resistance, though emergence of bacterial resistance during therapy is rare [5]. Based on this concept, many have reserved amikacin, the most active aminoglycoside, for patients with infections with a known or high likelihood of having resistant organisms, although this approach is controversial [1, 2, 4]. When gentamicin resistance is common, it is reasonable to use amikacin, especially if resistant blood isolates have been detected. In most instances, amikacin use will not lead to rapid emergence of amikacin resistance [23] and, while amikacin is used, gentamicin resistance may decline, allowing that institution to return safely to the use of gentamicin [24].

   2. High-level gentamicin-resistant enterococci [14–18].

     a. See laboratory definition in sec. **B.2.c.**

     b. Clinical significance. These enterococci are potentially very important nosocomial pathogens. The epidemiology of nosocomial enterococcal infections is very similar to that of nosocomial infections caused by methicillin-resistant staphylococci and by multidrug-resistant gram-negative bacilli. Probably these resistant bacteria spread among hospital patients via transient carriage on the hands of hospital personnel [16]. **Therefore, all enterococci isolated from normally sterile body fluids (e.g., blood) or serious wound infections should be tested in the microbiology laboratory for susceptibility to cell wall–active antibiotics (e.g., penicillin, ampicillin, piperacillin) and for high-level aminoglycoside resistance.**

     c. Therapy. If an organism is identified with high-level gentamicin resistance, optimal therapy is unclear [15]; **infectious disease consultation is advised.** Fluoroquinolones alone are not advised; nor is trimethoprim-sulfamethoxazole (TMP-SMX). If the isolate is susceptible to ampicillin, high-dose intravenous ampicillin is a possible approach [15]. Bacteremias associated with high-level gentamicin-resistant enterococci may result in higher mortality than those seen in patients with enterococcal bacteremia without high-level resistance [17]. Strains of *E. faecalis* with high-level gentamicin resistance can also produce beta-lactamase [18].

   3. Vancomycin-resistant enterococci are discussed in Chap. 28O.

G. Use of the aminoglycosides (gentamicin, tobramycin, netilmicin, amikacin)

   1. Aminoglycosides are seldom listed as drugs of choice [25] for specific pathogens **except** as follows:

     a. Gentamicin is used for synergy against certain pathogens [2, 5, 20]. In this setting, **lower doses** often are used for synergy (e.g., peaks of 4–5 μg/ml and troughs of <1.5 μg/ml), but whether this is the optimal approach is unclear.

       (1) Enterococci. In endocarditis or bacteremia, gentamicin typically is combined with penicillin G or ampicillin if there is no evidence of high-level gentamicin resistance in vitro.

       (2) Viridans streptococci may be treated with penicillin G and gentamicin, especially in endocarditis. See Chap. 10.

       (3) *S. aureus* **endocarditis.** Gentamicin sometimes is added to nafcillin for 72–96 hours. See Chaps. 2 and 10.

(4) **Methicillin-resistant *S. aureus* or *S. epidermidis*.** Prosthetic valve endocarditis usually is treated with vancomycin and gentamicin (and rifampin for *S. epidermidis*) (see Chap. 10).

(5) ***Listeria monocytogenes*** often is treated with ampicillin and gentamicin.

(6) Serious infections due to ***Pseudomonas aeruginosa,*** other *Pseudomonas* spp., and some Enterobacteriaceae (e.g., *Enterobacter* spp.) often are treated with full doses of an aminoglycoside in combination with an extended-spectrum penicillin (e.g., piperacillin) to achieve synergy (see Chap. 28A) [26].

(7) Empiric therapy for prosthetic valve endocarditis. (See Chap. 28O.)

   b. **Amikacin** has been used in some atypical mycobacterial infections [27].

   c. **Streptomycin or gentamicin** is an agent of choice [25] in brucellosis and tularemia. Streptomycin is the agent of choice for plague [20]; it remains a useful agent for *M. tuberculosis* therapy (see Chap. 9) and for *Mycobacterium kansasii* infections.

     Amikacin is the drug of choice for *M. fortuitum complex* infections [25].

   d. **Otherwise, the aminoglycosides are not listed as drugs of first choice** [25].

2. **However, there are several situations in which the aminoglycosides are used** [2]. Although netilmicin still is available, most institutions use gentamicin, tobramycin, or amikacin; netilmicin is no longer listed as an aminoglycoside of choice [25].

   a. **As empiric therapy in life-threatening community-acquired** infections potentially caused by resistant gram-negative bacteria (e.g., in a patient who has already received broad-spectrum oral antibiotics or who has recently been hospitalized and treated with antibiotics), an aminoglycoside may be used in combination initially. (The third-generation cephalosporins are also alternative agents in this setting.) Therapy can and should be modified when culture data become available. Gentamicin usually is preferred.

   b. **In hospital-acquired severe infections,** especially if *Pseudomonas* spp. or other cephalosporin-resistant gram-negative bacilli are suspected, the use of an aminoglycoside is indicated while awaiting culture data. Risk of toxicity often is small compared to the consequence of using an antibiotic that is ineffective.

     (1) **Amikacin versus gentamicin. In large medical centers or specialized areas** (e.g., intensive care units, burn units) where the frequency of resistance to gentamicin, tobramycin, or netilmicin may be high, amikacin is preferred at least until susceptibility data are available. If gentamicin resistance is low (e.g., 1–5%), gentamicin remains the most rational cost-effective choice unless the patient has recently received gentamicin. Under these circumstances, amikacin often still is reasonable while awaiting culture results in life-threatening infections.

     (2) **In most community hospitals** where resistance to gentamicin, tobramycin, or netilmicin is uncommon, we favor gentamicin because it is less expensive. An exception to this is the patient who has already received broad-spectrum antibiotics and therefore may have been colonized and possibly infected with a relatively resistant gram-negative bacteria. Until susceptibility data are available, amikacin is the preferred agent.

     (3) If a patient is potentially at high risk for aminoglycoside use (e.g., a patient with hepatic failure), an alternate agent can be used (e.g., aztreonam; see Chap. 28G).

     (4) If the gram-negative organism isolated is susceptible to all aminoglycosides, it is reasonable to use gentamicin, the most cost-effective agent.

   c. In **leukopenic, febrile patients** with no obvious focus of infection, an aminoglycoside and an extended-spectrum penicillin (e.g., piperacillin) have commonly been used [1, 28]. (See Chap. 2.) The choice of the particular aminoglycoside is guided by local susceptibility data.

   d. **For susceptible pathogens in which a less toxic agent is not available,** aminoglycosides have been used effectively in UTI, peritonitis, bone and joint infections, and in some cases of gram-negative bacillary endocarditis [1, 4]. Aminoglycosides along with an extended-spectrum penicillin (e.g., ticarcillin, piperacillin) have been used in malignant external otitis, but now other therapeutic options also are available (e.g., ceftazidime, ciprofloxacin).

e. **Intraabdominal infections**

(1) **Aminoglycosides are not ideal agents for intraabdominal infections,** in part because high tissue levels in an acid environment are difficult to achieve. Furthermore, it usually is not necessary to use agents active against enterococci (e.g., a common rationale for using ampicillin plus gentamicin in this setting).

See detailed discussion in Chap. 11, sec. **II.B.1,** under Intraabdominal Infection (p. 418).

(2) In the review by Ho and Barza [9], patients most likely to benefit from the inclusion of an aminoglycoside in the treatment regimen for intraabdominal infections presumably are the subset from whom *P. aeruginosa* or an *Enterobacter* spp. was isolated from the initial culture (peritoneal fluid or abscess cavity). This is not common except in nosocomially related infections; for hospital-acquired intraabdominal infections, aminoglycosides may still be necessary pending susceptibility data. See Chap. 11.

f. **For therapy for organisms that may develop resistance to monotherapy with a third-generation cephalosporin** (e.g., *E. cloacae, Citrobacter freundii,* and some *Acinetobacter* spp.), an aminoglycoside sometimes is combined with a cephalosporin with the hope of decreasing the likelihood that a resistant pathogen will emerge. Whether this is effective is unclear. A more attractive alternative is an aminoglycoside combined with an extended-spectrum penicillin (e.g., piperacillin if the organism is susceptible) for synergy. For *Enterobacter* spp., the latter combination is preferred. (See Chap. 28F.)

Imipenem often is preferred for treatment of nosocomially acquired *Acinetobacter* spp. and some *Enterobacter* spp. See Chap. 28G.

g. In special circumstances, the broadest-spectrum aminoglycoside, amikacin, may be the aminoglycoside suggested for routine use to help lower an unacceptably high level of gentamicin or tobramycin resistance at that institution or special care area [23, 24].

3. **Potential limitations**

a. **In lower respiratory tract infections,** the low pH of bronchial secretions may decrease the activity of aminoglycosides. We agree with other sources who **do not rely on aminoglycosides alone** in major lower respiratory tract infections [1] (e.g., *Pseudomonas* pneumonia).

b. **Sterilization of abscesses** may be difficult with aminoglycosides because of poor activity in the chemical presence of bivalent cations and anaerobic conditions [1].

c. **Prostatitis.** Aminoglycosides do not achieve useful levels in prostate tissue and are not considered effective therapy for infections of this organ [1].

d. **Intraabdominal infections.** See sec. **2.e** and Chap. 11.

III. **Aminoglycoside dosing.** Numerous dosage regimens have been proposed [5, 29–34], but studies comparing one regimen with another with respect to both effectiveness and safety are not available. Part of the dilemma is that any dosage regimen represents a compromise between several worthy objectives [29]: (1) the desire to achieve a high peak serum concentration that correlates with improved antibacterial efficacy in animals and patients [11], (2) the desire to have a low trough serum level, in part to reduce the potential of nephrotoxicity and possibly ototoxicity, and (3) the desire to have a reasonable dose interval for the nursing staff.

A. **General considerations**

1. Because aminoglycosides are highly water-soluble, their small solution volume makes **intramuscular injection** more feasible than with other antibiotics. Serum levels after intramuscular doses are somewhat lower than with intravenous dosing [1], with peak levels achieved in 30–90 minutes in normal subjects [5].

2. **Intravenous administration.** Standard doses of aminoglycosides can be administered intravenously over 30 minutes; if a large single daily dose is used, a 30- to 60-minute infusion is advised [5]. The **intravenous route is preferable, especially if** there is associated sepsis, hypotension, thrombocytopenia, or diabetes. The effects of more rapid intravenous infusion are being investigated.

3. **Dose adjustment in renal failure. Of all the available antibiotics, careful dose reduction in renal failure when using aminoglycosides is essential to try to avoid toxicity.** The options are reviewed in sec. **C.** An **estimation of creatinine clearance** is useful in dosing aminoglycosides and other antibiotics excreted by the kidney (see Chap. 28A).

B. **Loading dose** [5]. The purpose of this dose is to rapidly achieve therapeutic plasma levels.
  1. The loading dose is independent of renal function so a routine loading dose is given even if the serum creatinine is elevated.
  2. For most patients, it is **calculated based on ideal body weight** (IBW) in kilograms [5]:
    a. Women = 45 kg + 2.3 kg per inch of height over 5 ft.
    b. Men = 50 kg + 2.3 kg per inch of height over 5 ft.
    c. For example, for a male patient 5 ft. 10 in. tall, an estimated IBW would be 50 + 2.3(10) or 50 + 23 = 73 kg.
  3. **For very obese patients** whose actual body weight is more than 30% above IBW, another modification is suggested to calculate a loading dose [5, 31]. These patients can be more appropriately treated with aminoglycosides by using a revised body weight figure rather than the patient's actual weight [31].
    a. The ideal weight (lean body weight [LBW]) for the patient is determined from the formula in sec. **2.** Next, weight above LBW is determined (i.e., excess weight).
    b. **For dosage calculations,** revised weight equals LBW plus 40% excess weight (fat). This revised weight then is used in the routine dose calculations.
    c. For example, an obese woman has a wound infection requiring gentamicin or tobramycin. Her actual weight is 100 kg; her ideal weight is 60 kg; therefore, her excess weight is 40 kg.

$$\text{Weight for dosing} = \text{LBW} + 40\% \text{ excess}$$
$$= 60 \text{ kg} + 40\% \,(40 \text{ kg})$$
$$= 60 + 16$$
$$\text{Weight for dosing} = 76 \text{ kg}$$

This weight can be used in the aforementioned dose schedules.
  4. **Loading doses**
    a. For gentamicin, tobramycin, and netilmicin, 2 mg/kg typically is used [1, 5].
    b. For amikacin, a loading dose of 7.5 mg/kg has been suggested [1, 5].

C. **Maintenance dosing if renal function is normal (i.e., creatinine clearance ≥90 ml/min).** The calculation of an estimated creatinine clearance is shown in Chap. 28A, sec. **VI.C,** under Antibiotic Checklist (p. 1079).
  1. **Pharmacokinetics model.** Zaske [12] and Sawchuk [21] and their colleagues have devised a formula to help determine the pharmacokinetics of aminoglycosides in individual patients [30]. Timed serum samples are obtained to determine the volume of distribution and the half-life of the aminoglycoside for an individual patient. Using a kinetic model, they determined the appropriate doses needed for a given patient to achieve a desired peak and trough. Acceptable peak and trough levels can be maintained by adjusting doses and dose intervals. **This approach can be used in patients with either normal or impaired renal function.**
    a. Because of the **variations in the volume of drug distribution** and the patient's ability to excrete aminoglycosides, there is marked variation in levels achieved with conventional dosing techniques. The patient's age, renal function, state of hydration, presence or absence of fever, and degree of obesity all seem to affect eventual serum peak and trough levels and half-lives. **Individualized dosing allows adjustment for each patient** by measuring serum levels and calculating the aminoglycoside's half-life.
    b. Patients in whom pharmacokinetic studies reveal shorter half-lives than average need larger and more frequent doses to maintain adequate aminoglycoside peaks and to avoid prolonged periods of subtherapeutic levels. Patients in whom pharmacokinetic studies reveal longer half-lives require less drug and less frequent dosing to avoid toxic levels [12].
    c. **We believe that this may be the ideal way to manage the dosage of aminoglycosides.** However, it is labor-intensive and results in added costs.

2. **Standard dosage guidelines.** Listed here are commonly accepted **"rule-of-thumb" dosages** on a milligram-per-kilogram dose regimen. However, because of varying volumes of drug distribution and the effects of age, fever, and subtle renal dysfunction, **serum levels achieved often are highly variable,** particularly with gentamicin, tobramycin, and netilmicin. Therefore, monitoring of levels is an important part of continued use of these agents.

a. **For gentamicin, tobramycin, and netilmicin**

(1) **In neonates.** See Chap. 3.

(2) **In adults with normal renal function,** three dosage ranges are commonly used. The normal dose interval is every 8 hours. In elderly patients with a normal creatinine, the creatinine clearance should be estimated (see sec. **D.2**) as most will have some degree of renal dysfunction and therefore will require dose modification.

(a) **Low doses** of 0.5–1.0 mg/kg per dose (equivalent to 1.5–3.0 mg/kg/day) are used primarily **for UTIs.** Because aminoglycosides are primarily excreted by the kidneys, high urine levels are achieved even with low doses. In addition, the urine may be alkalinized to enhance the activity of aminoglycosides.

(b) **The standard dose** is 1.5–1.7 mg/kg per dose (4.5–5.1 mg/kg/day) for **tissue infections** (e.g., wounds and pneumonia).

(c) A **high dose** is 2 mg/kg per dose (6 mg/kg/day). This often is used **initially when the patient is clinically septic** and the risk of toxicity is outweighed by the seriousness of the infection. It **is a common initial, or loading, dose.** Once the patient has stabilized, the dose can be decreased to the 1.5–1.7 mg/kg range or, preferably, adjusted by the availability of drug levels.

(3) **In children,** the aminoglycosides are eliminated more rapidly. Therefore, higher doses often are used in children—for example, 1.0–2.5 mg/kg per dose (of gentamicin, tobramycin, or netilmicin), depending on the severity of the infection. The usual dose interval is every 8 hours, although shorter intervals commonly are required when individualized dosing is performed.

b. **For amikacin**

(1) The usual dose in adults, children, and older infants is 15 mg/kg/day divided into q8h doses.

(2) For neonates, see Chap. 3.

D. **Maintenance dosing in renal failure and in the elderly**

1. **Individualized dosing** with pharmacokinetics **is preferred** (see sec. **C.1**).

2. **Dose reduction, based on creatinine clearance, with normal dose interval.** The creatinine clearance or estimated creatinine clearance is used. The **serum creatinine may not accurately reflect the patient's renal function, especially in the elderly,** who may have decreased creatinine production [5]. The creatinine clearance is a better measure. By modifying the equation of Cockcroft and Gault [32], it is **possible to estimate the patient's creatinine clearance** from the patient's age, sex, body weight (in kilograms), and serum creatinine [1, 29] as discussed in sec. **VI.C.,** under Antibiotic Checklist (p. 1079) in Chap. 28A and summarized here:

a. **Male estimated creatinine clearance =**

$$\frac{(140 - \text{age}) \times (\text{weight})}{72 \times \text{serum creatinine}}$$

(1) **Female** estimated creatinine clearance = 85% of male value

(2) Some prefer to use IBW, especially in the obese patient, which can be calculated as:

(a) Male = 50 kg + 2.3 kg per each inch over 5 ft (in height).

(b) Female = 45.5 kg + 2.3 kg per each inch over 5 ft.

b. **If the patient is oliguric,** the creatinine clearance is estimated at less than 10 ml/min [29].

c. The ratio of the "estimated" creatinine clearance to normal creatinine clearance (100 ml/min) will approximate the ratio of aminoglycoside clearance [5]. This ratio (expressed as a percentage) is multiplied by the normal daily dose as though renal function were normal; this revised dose can be given at routine intervals. See the example that follows.

d. **Example:** A 70-year-old man has a weight of 70 kg and a serum creatinine of 2.2. His estimated creatinine clearance (C_{cr}) is [1]:

$$C_{cr} \, (\text{ml/min}) = \frac{(140 - 70) \times 70}{72 \times 2.2}$$

$$= \frac{4,900}{158.4} = 31 \text{ ml/min}$$

Therefore, 31/100 (see sec. **c**) = 31% of normal. If the normal dose of gentamicin per day were 70 kg × 5.0 mg/kg = 350 kg/day, then 31% of 350 mg = 108.5 kg/day. This can be divided up so that 36 mg can be given q8h. In practice, this is rounded off to the nearest 5 or 10 mg so that 35 mg is given q8h.

3. **Dose interval prolongation using a standard dose.** This method can lead to long periods of low levels of aminoglycoside, at trough times [1].
   a. **For gentamicin, tobramycin, and netilmicin.** To obtain an approximation of the **new** (corrected) **dose interval,** the serum creatinine is multiplied by 8. Hence, if the serum creatinine is 2.0, the routine dose can be given every 16 hours (serum creatinine of 2 × 8).
   b. **For amikacin,** the serum creatinine is multiplied by 9, and the routine dose is given at this interval. (If the creatinine level were 2.0, the adjusted interval would be 18 hours.)
4. **Dose reduction versus dose interval prolongation.** In general, in the acutely infected patient, some experts suggest that initially a dose-reduction approach and maintenance of frequent dosing is the best approach until the bloodstream is sterilized. This dose-reduction method may help to avoid any prolonged periods of inadequate antibiotic levels. Once the patient has begun to respond, one can use the dose interval–prolongation approach and measure levels to ensure adequate peaks and troughs in the hope of reducing nephrotoxicity associated with prolonged aminoglycoside use. See related discussions under once-daily-dosing regimens (sec. **E.2**).
5. **Whether the dose-reduction (sec. 2) or dose interval–prolongation method (sec. 3) is used, these are only guidelines. When renal failure exists, serum levels should be serially monitored.**
6. See discussion of serum monitoring in sec. **IV**.
E. **Once-daily aminoglycoside dosing.** In his recent 1995 review of this topic, Gilbert [5] introduces this approach noting: "It should be emphasized that data are currently not adequate to support an unqualified endorsement for once-daily dosing. Careful comparison of efficacy in a variety of infections will be required before one can conclude that efficacy is not reduced by extending dosing intervals."
   1. **The concept** of once-daily dosing **is based on three observations** [5, 33–35].
      a. Aminoglycosides are bactericidal agents, and their rate of bacterial killing increases as the antibiotic concentration is increased, regardless of the inoculum [5]. In theory, the higher serum levels with once-daily dosing will provide higher serum bactericidal levels and equivalent, or even enhanced, efficacy compared to conventional dosing (i.e., concentration-dependent killing [see p. 1081]). Transient high serum concentrations seem to be well tolerated.
      b. Aminoglycosides demonstrate a postantibiotic effect (PAE) [5] against aerobic gram-negative bacilli both in vitro and in vivo. The duration of the PAE is greater the higher the peak aminoglycoside concentration. The PAE is the persistent suppression of bacterial growth after short antibiotic exposure; therefore, the serum level of aminoglycoside can fall below the MIC of the pathogenic bacteria, without loss of efficacy.
      c. **Experimentally induced nephrotoxicity and ototoxicity were less severe in animals** administered a daily dose of drug as a single injection in contrast to the same daily dosage administered in two or three divided doses. Animals given a single daily dose accumulated less drug in the renal cortex; similar results were seen in patients who agreed to receive aminoglycoside prior to elective nephrectomy [5].
      d. Therefore, once-daily therapy provides the potential of reducing toxicity while not sacrificing efficacy, and yet it is easy to administer. Clinical studies are ongoing.
   2. **Clinical experience** has been reviewed [5, 34] and includes the following:
      a. In a prospective, randomized trial comparing a conventional multiple dos-

ing regimen of netilmicin with once-daily netilmicin and ceftriaxone once daily, both regimens had equal efficacy in adults, with similar overall rates of nephrotoxicity (16%), although the occurrence of nephrotoxicity in the once-daily regimens was more likely after prolonged use (i.e., >9 days) [33].

    b. Preliminary clinical data in more than 100 patients who received a single daily infusion over 60 minutes revealed no problems in terms of clinical response or toxicity.

    c. A recent report suggests the efficacy and safety of this approach in more than 2,000 patients. However, these patients had creatinine clearances in excess of 60 ml/min, the majority of patients were younger than 50 years, the duration of therapy was relatively short (3–5 days), and clinical efficacy was measured only in part [35].

  3. Additional clinical studies are needed to clarify the role of once-daily aminoglycoside dosing [5, 36]. This approach requires study in patients with various degrees of renal dysfunction before any guidelines for its routine use can be proposed [34]. Further studies also are needed to establish the safety and efficacy of large single-dose aminoglycoside therapy [2]. Serial monitoring of serum creatinine levels still is necessary in single- and multiple-dose regimens [33]. The dosage regimens used for single daily dosing are reviewed in detail elsewhere [5].

F. Miscellaneous

  1. Nomograms. Dosing by nomograms entirely, no matter how sophisticated, can lead to inadequate or excessive levels and consequently risk therapeutic failures or toxicity [1].

  2. In dialysis patients, approximately 50% of the predialysis levels are removed with a complete hemodialysis. Therefore, as an estimate after dialysis, one-half of the usual single dose usually is given to restore adequate serum levels. Because the type of dialysis machine used, the duration of dialysis, and the adequacy of the dialysis affect the amount of drug removed, **monitoring serum aminoglycoside levels is advised.** After a complete peritoneal dialysis, one-third to one-half of a usual single dose for a 24-hour period often is administered. Serum aminoglycoside levels are advised.

  3. Lumbar intrathecal instillation (or intraventricular instillation). In special circumstances and with infectious disease consultation, 4–8 mg gentamicin or tobramycin (without preservative) can be given intrathecally to adults once daily by barbotage. (*Barbotage* is the process whereby a portion of the agent is injected into the spinal fluid, after which the fluid is withdrawn and the maneuver is subsequently repeated until the entire amount is administered.) If direct intraventricular instillation of aminoglycoside is necessary, a reservoir (Richman, Ommaya) must be used.

  4. Gentamicin bone cement has been discussed in Chap. 28B.

  5. Gentamicin-impregnated polymethylmethacrylate beads have been used in orthopedic-related infections (e.g., osteomyelitis). A detailed discussion of their use is beyond the scope of this chapter, but their use has been reviewed in detail elsewhere [37].

  6. Aminoglycosides in peritoneal dialysis fluid have been used to treat susceptible peritoneal dialysis–associated infections. This topic is discussed in Chap. 11 and reviewed elsewhere [38]. This approach is not recommended for patients with systemic infection [5] because therapeutic serum levels are not achieved.

  7. Aerosolized aminoglycosides have been used primarily in two settings.

    a. Cystic fibrosis. Endobronchial infections with *P. aeruginosa*, which contribute to progressive airway disease, are a major cause of morbidity and mortality among patients with cystic fibrosis. The direct delivery of aminoglycosides to the lower airway by aerosol administration is attractive as it produces high concentrations of antibiotic at the site of infection. Prior studies have yielded conflicting data in this setting [39].

    In a recent multicenter, double-blind, placebo-controlled, crossover trial, compared with placebo, 600 mg tobramycin in saline, delivered tid by ultrasonic nebulizer, improved pulmonary function and reduced the sputum density of *P. aeruginosa* over the 28-day study period [39]. This approach was used when patients were not suffering pneumonia or a severe exacerbation of symptoms or a significant decline in pulmonary function tests, which would merit intravenous therapy.

    b. Purulent *P. aeruginosa* tracheobronchitis can sometimes occur in patients with underlying chronic obstructive lung disease. Typically, these patients raise large amounts of sputum, have *P. aeruginosa* isolated from sputum cultures, and have no evidence of pneumonia on the chest roentgenogram. We have used aerosolized aminoglycosides in carefully selected patients in this setting.

IV. **Monitoring of serum** levels or concentrations appears to be important to ensure maximum efficacy and minimal toxicity [1, 2, 5, 11, 12, 19].
   A. **See Table 28H-2** for ideal serum levels.
      1. **Peak levels** are the serum levels achieved 30 minutes after completion of an intravenous infusion. When the drug is given by the intramuscular route, peak levels occur at 45–60 minutes. In renal failure, the peak sample is usually drawn 120–150 minutes after the intramuscular dose, because drug continues to be absorbed and not excreted. **Peak serum levels** are obtained to ensure that enough drug was administered for therapeutic efficacy. Data from infected animals and analysis of clinical trial data support the correlation between high peak levels and antibacterial efficacy, although the clinical trial data are subject to some criticism [5]. (See related discussions in secs. **I.B** and **III.E.2.**) A peak level commonly is obtained after the first or second maintenance dose or after dosage adjustments (see sec. **C.2**).
      2. **Trough levels** represent concentrations persisting before the next dose. Trough levels are a measure of renal function, as is the serum creatinine, and generally are not believed to predict nephrotoxicity per se.
   B. **Indications for measuring aminoglycoside levels**
      1. **Renal failure** (see sec. **II.D.3**).
      2. **Seriously ill patients.** A peak level should be drawn early in therapy (e.g., after the second or third dose). This will help ensure adequate levels at the time of acute illness. Levels should be repeated after initial physiologic abnormalities that are part of the acute illness have been corrected. This will provide ideal levels later in therapy. Data have been presented that suggest the importance of a high peak concentration relative to the MIC, for an infecting organism is an important determinant of the clinical response to aminoglycoside therapy [11].

      Some experts believe that when drug doses are monitored and adjusted by serum levels (so-called individualized dosing with pharmacokinetics), less nephrotoxicity may occur, even when the doses are much greater than those routinely recommended [12] (see sec. **III.C**). However, some reviewers conclude there is no convincing evidence that individualized dosing has reduced the incidence of nephrotoxicity [5].

      If individualized dosing is not followed, some experts recommend that a trough level be measured on approximately the fifth day of therapy and intermittently thereafter as an indicator of drug accumulation. It is uncertain whether high trough levels lead to or merely reflect nephrotoxicity.
      3. **Patients with altered distribution or excretion. Obese** patients, **elderly** patients, patients with pancreatitis, patients with **ascites** or edema, and **dehydrated** patients belong in this category.
      4. **Children**
         a. **Younger than 3 months.** Monitoring of serum levels is routinely advised.
         b. **Older than 3 months.** Routine monitoring of serum levels is not indicated. Monitoring is advised if therapy extends beyond 10 days, renal function is impaired, higher-than-usual doses are needed (as in patients with cystic fibrosis, burns, or leukemia) or a potential nephrotoxin was administered in the preceding 3 months [13].
      5. **Protracted therapy.** Adult patients receiving therapy beyond 72 hours (e.g., after cultures are available) should have serum levels monitored [1].
   C. **Frequency of monitoring**
      1. **If individualized dosing** is carried out, serial aminoglycoside levels are measured per the pharmacokinetics protocol. (See sec. **III.C.1.**)
      2. **Otherwise,** the optimal frequency with which to measure serum levels is poorly defined. Measurement of peak level obtained in the first 48 hours of therapy is useful to ensure adequate levels, as discussed earlier. Similarly, a trough level measured in the same time period helps to rule out the possibility that this is elevated, which may necessitate prolonging the dose interval to achieve an acceptable trough level to help minimize toxicity.

      Peak and trough level measures can be repeated every 3–4 days if the patient is stable. In a patient who has major changes in hydration status or renal function, levels have to be repeated more frequently.

Infectious disease consultation or pharmacokinetic consultation is advised to help assist with aminoglycoside dosage adjustments.

D. **Inactivation of aminoglycosides in vitro.** Ideally, the serum levels should be measured immediately. If this is not possible, the serum should be frozen until the sample can be assayed. Gentamicin, tobramycin, and netilmicin can be inactivated in vitro or in vivo if the half-life is prolonged by renal failure by the antipseudomonal penicillins (e.g., ticarcillin or piperacillin).

E. **Summary. Therapy with the aminoglycosides must be carried out with care, providing adequate therapeutic blood levels, yet avoiding toxicity.** Even in normal patients, levels achieved with standard doses are highly variable. **Serum levels should be monitored in patients with** renal failure, in seriously ill or poorly responding patients and, ideally, in most patients on aminoglycosides for more than 3 days.

V. Other **aminoglycosides** are used less frequently and will be discussed only briefly.

A. **Streptomycin** was introduced in 1944 and was effective against many gram-negative bacteria and *M. tuberculosis.* However, resistance to streptomycin is now prevalent among gram-negative bacteria, so for these organisms, use is now limited.

The availability of streptomycin in the United States was limited in late 1991 [40]. However, by mid-1993, streptomycin became available from Roerig, a division of Pfizer Incorporated. As of mid-1996, physicians and hospital pharmacies can order streptomycin by calling 1-800-254-4445 (Monday through Friday 9 AM–5 PM E.S.T.).

1. **Current uses**

   a. **Tularemia.** Streptomycin (or gentamicin) is the drug of choice for susceptible strains of *Francisella tularensis* [25, 41].

   b. **Antituberculous therapy.** Streptomycin in combination with other agents still is used [25]. It requires parenteral administration and, with the availability of new oral antituberculous agents, streptomycin has assumed a lesser role in tuberculosis therapy (see Chap. 9). Nonetheless, it is still considered a drug of first choice [25].

   c. **Synergistic combinations.** Penicillin and streptomycin have been used to treat endocarditis due to viridans streptococci (e.g., *S. mutans*). Enterococcal endocarditis has been treated successfully with a combination of penicillin and streptomycin. However, in more recent years, in vitro studies have shown that streptomycin is not synergistic against at least 40% of enterococci. Therefore, unless susceptibility data are available, most clinicians believe that gentamicin is preferable as the aminoglycoside to be combined with penicillin, because this combination is synergistic against the majority of enterococci [25]. (See discussion of high-level gentamicin resistance in sec. **II.B.2.c.**)

   d. **Uncommon diseases** in which streptomycin is still a drug of choice [25] are brucellosis (with tetracycline), glanders (*Pseudomonas mallei*), and bubonic plague (due to *Yersinia pestis*). Although streptomycin can be used in listeriosis, many clinicians use gentamicin and ampicillin in this disease.

   e. **Alternate agent.** Streptomycin can be used in granuloma inguinale, and rat bite fever due to *Streptobacillus moniliformis* or *Spirillum minus* [25].

2. **Dosage.** In adults, for the unusual case of tularemia or plague, if renal function is normal a dose of 500–1,000 mg IM q12h can be used. In children, 20–30 mg/kg/day is given and divided into q12h doses.

   If renal failure is present, the dosage must be reduced. One approach [42] is to give a 1-g loading dose and then to prolong the interval. If the creatinine clearance is 10–50 ml/min, a dose interval of 24–72 hours is used. If the creatinine clearance is less than 10 ml/min, a dose interval of 72–96 hours is used. Streptomycin is removed by hemodialysis and peritoneal dialysis. If streptomycin must be used in dialysis patients, monitoring of serum levels is advisable.

   In tuberculosis therapy, intermittent dosage schedules are used. The average adult dose is 15 mg/kg up to 1 g (500–750 mg/day for patients older than 60 years) IM once daily for the first 2–8 weeks of therapy; thereafter, 25–30 mg/kg (to a maximum of a 1.5-g dose) twice weekly is used. Dosages are reduced in renal failure. For children with tuberculosis, 20–40 mg/kg/day initially (up to a maximum of 1.0 g) and 25–30 mg/kg 2 or 3 times weekly (maximum of 1.5 g) has been advised, per the package insert (see Chap. 9).

3. Toxicity. We tend to avoid using streptomycin in patients older than 55 years if an alternate agent is available.

    a. Ototoxicity. When given 2 g daily for more than 60 days, the majority of patients develop vestibular toxicity. The incidence is reduced by half if the dosage is reduced to 1 g daily. Deafness can occur. Patients particularly at risk are those with impaired renal function, elderly patients, and those receiving prolonged courses of therapy.

    b. Nephrotoxicity occurs much less commonly with streptomycin than with the other aminoglycosides.

    c. Hypersensitivity reactions include rash and drug fever.

B. Kanamycin is no longer indicated for use [1].

C. Sisomycin is an aminoglycoside whose structure and pharmacokinetics resemble those of gentamicin. Sisomycin may be active against gram-negative bacteria resistant to other aminoglycosides. Although sisomycin has been shown to be effective in the treatment of severe infections due to susceptible organisms and has been approved by the FDA, the manufacturer has decided not to market this agent in the United States.

D. Paromomycin (Humatin). Paromomycin sulfate is structurally related to streptomycin and is an amorphous powder with a saline taste [43]. It is too toxic for parenteral administration. Because it is not absorbed from the intestinal tract, it can be used safely as alternative therapy for infections due to *Entamoeba histolytica* (see Chap. 11) and, more recently, in AIDS patients infected with the protozoa *Cryptosporidium parvum* [5].

    1. Pharmacokinetics. Paromomycin is poorly absorbed from the GI tract, and most of an oral dose is excreted unchanged in feces. Impaired GI motility or ulcerations of the intestine may facilitate absorption of the drug, and that portion of a dose that is absorbed is slowly excreted in urine. Accumulation can occur in patients with impaired renal function.

    2. Uses

        a. Parasitic infections. Paromomycin is a drug of choice for asymptomatic carriers of *E. histolytica* and *Dientamoeba fragilis* infections. It is also an alternative agent for infections due to *Giardia lamblia* [44]. See Chap. 11.

        b. Cryptosporidiosis in patients with AIDS. Several recent reports suggest that paromomycin is useful in reducing symptoms due to cryptosporidiosis [45–47]. Common dose regimens have been 1 g PO bid initially (e.g., for 2–4 weeks) and then 500 mg bid as a maintenance dose. Symptoms of diarrhea may recur when the dose is reduced. Inhalation therapy has been reported for the treatment of rare cases of pulmonary cryptosporidiosis [47].

    3. Adverse side effects [43]

        a. Gastrointestinal effects are the most frequently seen side effects and include anorexia, nausea, vomiting, epigastric burning, cramps, and diarrhea.

        b. Other adverse effects include rash, eosinophilia, and headache.

        c. The use of paromomycin may result in overgrowth of nonsusceptible organisms (e.g., *Candida*).

    4. Precautions [43]. Like other aminoglycosides, paromomycin has potential nephrotoxic and ototoxic effects. It must be administered with caution to patients with ulcerative intestinal lesions, to avoid inadvertent absorption of the drug. Paromomycin is contraindicated in patients with impaired renal function or intestinal obstruction. In patients with cryptosporidiosis with AIDS, the potential benefit from this agent may outweigh these risks; this decision must be individualized.

VI. Summary. Because of the narrow toxic-therapeutic ratio of aminoglycosides and our current limited understanding of and limited ability to prevent their toxic side effects, **the aminoglycosides should be carefully used with goals in mind.**

A. Indications for use in initial therapy include:

    1. When aminoglycosides are clearly the drug of choice. (See sec. **II.G.1.**)

    2. For nosocomial infections and in life-threatening community-acquired infections in patients who may be infected with resistant gram-negative bacteria. (See sec. **II.G.2.**)

    3. In combination with another agent in the febrile leukopenic patient without an obvious focus of infection.

    4. In selected cases of intraabdominal infection, in combination therapy (usually with piperacillin), when *P. aeruginosa* or an *Enterobacter* spp. has been isolated from peritoneal fluid or surgically drained intraabdominal abscess cultures.

Furthermore, aminoglycosides and an antianaerobic agent (e.g., metronidazole or clindamycin) have often been used in combination therapy for severe intra-abdominal infection. (For community-acquired intraabdominal infections, an aminoglycoside usually is not indicated.)

5. In infections due to organisms that may rapidly develop resistance to monotherapy with the cephalosporins (or imipenem or aztreonam)—for example, especially *P. aeruginosa* and *E. cloacae* but also *C. freundii* and *Acinetobacter* spp.

   A compromise approach is to use an aminoglycoside combination in the setting in which resistance is likely to emerge if cephalosporins alone are used (see sec. **A.5**) for 1 week, and then, in a very high-risk patient for aminoglycoside toxicity, complete therapy with an alternative active cephalosporin agent, hoping that the bacterial inoculum will be decreased enough after 1 week of aminoglycoside therapy that the risk of emergence of resistance will be minimal.

B. **Use aminoglycosides for a limited time period whenever possible** (<3–5 days). If culture data allow a safer antibiotic to be used, switch to the safer agent if resistance is not anticipated to be a problem.

C. **Carefully assess the need for protracted aminoglycoside therapy** (i.e., >3–5 days), as prolonged use seems to be related to excess toxicity even with careful serum monitoring.
   1. Is the aminoglycoside the drug of choice? If so, it should be continued.
   2. Is the patient at potentially greater risk for aminoglycoside-associated ototoxicity or nephrotoxicity (e.g., underlying significant hepatic dysfunction, possibly the elderly patient or patient with underlying renal dysfunction), or does the patient have preexisting hearing or balance impairment such that any additional aminoglycoside ototoxicity may be very debilitating? If so, consider an alternate agent or at least consider limiting the duration of aminoglycoside therapy to approximately 7 days and then complete therapy with an alternate agent.

D. **Monitoring** patients on aminoglycosides [19]
   1. **Serum creatinines** should be measured before therapy and every 2–3 days during therapy.
   2. **Serum aminoglycoside concentrations should be monitored** in special settings and with prolonged therapy. (See sec. **IV.**)
   3. **Hearing and balance function should be assessed daily** by questioning the patient about the following symptoms: tinnitus, loss of hearing, a sense of fullness in the ears, headache, giddiness, lightheadedness, vertigo, nystagmus, ataxia, and unexplained nausea and vomiting. If these signs or symptoms occur, ideally the aminoglycoside should be stopped. Aminoglycoside-related ototoxicity, especially auditory, usually is irreversible and can have a significant impact on the future lifestyle of the patient [19]. Serial audiograms are a consideration in patients needing protracted courses (e.g., >14 days).

References

1. Pancoast, S.J. Aminoglycoside antibiotics in clinical use. *Med. Clin. North Am.* 72:581, 1988.
   Useful and concise review.
2. Edson, R.S., and Terrell, C.L. The aminoglycosides. *Mayo Clin. Proc.* 66:1158, 1991.
   Concise review.
3. Appel, G.B. Aminoglycoside nephrotoxicity. *Am. J. Med.* 88(Suppl. 3C):16S, 1990.
   Review of incidence, pathology, risk factors, and potential prevention of aminoglycoside nephrotoxicity.
4. Siegenthaler, W.E., et al. Aminoglycoside antibiotics in infectious diseases: An overview. *Am. J. Med.* 80(Suppl. 6B):2, 1986.
5. Gilbert, D. Aminoglycosides. In G.L. Mandell, J.E. Bennett, and R. Dolin (eds.), *Principles and Practice of Infectious Diseases* (4th ed.). New York: Churchill Livingstone, 1995. Pp. 279–306.
6. Kahlmeter, G., and Dahlager, J.I. Aminoglycoside toxicity: A review of clinical studies published between 1975 and 1982. *J. Antimicrob. Chemother.* 13(Suppl. A):9, 1984.
   Review covers 10,000 aminoglycoside-treated patients studied in 144 trials.
7. Brummett, R.E., and Fox, K.E. Aminoglycoside-induced hearing loss in humans. *Antimicrob. Agents Chemother.* 33:797, 1989.
8. John, J.J., Jr. What price success? The continuing saga of the toxic-therapeutic ratio in the use of aminoglycoside antibiotics. *J. Infect. Dis.* 158:1, 1988.

9. Ho, J.L., and Barza, M. Role of aminoglycoside antibiotics in the treatment of intraabdominal infection. *Antimicrob. Agents Chemother.* 31:485, 1987.
   *Literature review shows no evidence of a difference in efficacy for treatment of intraabdominal infection between regimens that contain and do not contain aminoglycosides. Likewise, there was no evidence of a difference in the incidence of superinfections between regimens with and without aminoglycosides. See Chap. 11, sec. **II.B.1,** under Intraabdominal Infections, for a more detailed discussion of this topic.*

10. Bohnen, J.M.A. Guidelines for clinical care: Anti-infective agents for intraabdominal infection. *Arch. Surg.* 127:83, 1992.
    This report from the Antimicrobial Agents Committee of the Surgical Infection Society suggests for mild to moderate community-acquired infections that single-agent therapy with cefoxitin, cefotetan, cefmetazole, or ticarcillin-clavulanate is recommended. For severe infections, monotherapy with imipenem or combination therapy with either a third-generation cephalosporin, aztreonam, or an aminoglycoside (with serum monitoring) plus clindamycin or metronidazole is recommended. In uncomplicated community-acquired infection, therapy aimed at enterococci probably is not necessary unless gram-positive cocci are noted on Gram stains of material obtained at surgery. See detailed discussion in Chap. 11.

11. Moore, R.D., Leitman, P.S., and Smith, C.R. Clinical response to aminoglycoside therapy: Importance of peak concentration to minimal inhibitory concentration. *J. Infect. Dis.* 155:93, 1987.

12. Zaske, D.E., Cipolle, R.J., and Strate, R.J. Gentamicin dosage requirements: Wide interpatient variations in 242 surgery patients with normal renal function. *Surgery* 87:164, 1980.
    Compared with routinely recommended regimens (3–5 mg/kg/d), 47% of the surgery patients required higher doses, and 14% required lower doses.

13. Massey, K.L., Hendeles, L., and Neims, A. Identification of children for whom routine monitoring of aminoglycoside serum concentrations is not cost effective. *J. Pediatr.* 109:897, 1986.

14. Herman, D.H., and Gerding, D.N. Antimicrobial resistance among enterococci. *Antimicrob. Agents Chemother.* 35:1, 1991.
    Part 1 of two-part minireview (see reference [15] also). Reviews incidence and mechanisms.

15. Herman, D.H., and Gerding, D.N. Screening and treatment of infections caused by resistant enterococci. *Antimicrob. Agents Chemother.* 35:215, 1991.
    See related article by M. Huyche et al., Bacteremia caused by hemolytic, high-level gentamicin-resistant Enterococcus faecalis. Antimicrob. Agents Chemother. *35:1626, 1991. Blood isolates with hemolytic colonies had higher death rates.*

16. Patterson, J.E., and Zervus, M.J. High level gentamicin resistance in *Enterococcus:* Microbiology, genetic basis, and epidemiology. *Rev. Infect. Dis.* 12:644, 1990.

17. Noskin, G.A., et al. High-level gentamicin resistance in *Enterococcus faecalis* bacteremia. *J. Infect. Dis.* 164:212, 1991.
    Prior cephalosporin therapy, prolonged hospitalization, and nosocomial acquisition were associated with these bacteremias. Patients commonly had natural protective barriers breached by catheters or ulcers. Urinary tract infection was a common portal of entry.

18. Wells, V.D., et al. Infections due to beta-lactamase-producing, high-level gentamicin-resistant *Enterococcus faecalis.* *Ann. Intern. Med.* 116:285, 1992.
    The risk for colonization with these recently described strains was strongly associated with severe underlying disease and previous antibiotic treatment. Hand carriage may spread this nosocomial pathogen. Ampicillin-sulbactam may be a potential therapeutic agent. See related article by M.L. Grayson et al., Increasing resistance to beta-lactam antibiotics among clinical isolates of Enterococcus faecium: A 22-year review at one institution. Antimicrob. Agents Chemother. *35:2180, 1991.*

19. McCormack, J.P., and Jevesson, P.J. A critical re-evaluation of the "therapeutic range" of aminoglycosides. *Clin. Infect. Dis.* 14:320, 1992.
    Review of literature on this topic from 1966 through 1989. A provocative paper which emphasizes that data really do not establish that clinical outcome is significantly related to peak, trough, or therapeutic levels. Furthermore, serum aminoglycoside levels do not correlate well with the development or prevention of ototoxicity or nephrotoxicity.

20. Moore, R.D., et al. Risk factors for nephrotoxicity in patients treated with aminoglycosides. *Ann. Intern. Med.* 100:352, 1984.

21. Sawchuk, R.J., et al. Kinetic model for gentamicin dosing with the use of individual patient parameters. *Clin. Pharmacol. Ther.* 21:365, 1977.
    Discusses individualized dosing model.

22. Bertino, J.S., Jr., et al. Incidence of and significant risk factors for aminoglycoside-associated nephrotoxicity in patients dosed by using individualized pharmacokinetic monitoring. *J. Infect. Dis.* 167:173, 1993.
Authors conclude that the prediction of aminoglycoside-associated nephrotoxicity based on currently identified risk factors is exceptionally difficult; individualized dosing may help lower the incidence of nephrotoxicity. Even preexisting renal failure was not a significant factor in predicting the development of nephrotoxicity with aminoglycoside use.

For a related paper, see J.B. Bertino et al., Cost considerations in therapeutic drug monitoring of aminoglycosides. Clin. Pharmacokinet. *26:71, 1994.*

23. Betts, R.F., et al. Five-year surveillance of aminoglycoside usage in a university hospital. *Ann. Intern. Med.* 100:219, 1984.

24. Gerding, D.A., et al. Aminoglycoside resistance and aminoglycoside usage: Ten years of experience in one hospital. *Antimicrob. Agents Chemother.* 38:25, 1996.

25. Medical Letter. The choice of antibacterial drugs. *Med. Lett. Drugs Ther.* 38:25, 1996.

26. Korvick, J., and Yu, V.L. Antimicrobial agent therapy for *Pseudomonas aeruginosa*. *Antimicrob. Agents Chemother.* 35:2167, 1991.
Minireview. For severe infections, an antipseudomonal penicillin (e.g., piperacillin) and aminoglycoside still are usually preferred. In meningitis, ceftazidime as monotherapy has evolved as the therapy of choice if the organism is susceptible.

27. Chin, J., et al. Treatment of disseminated *Mycobacterium avium* complex infection in AIDS with amikacin, ethambutol, rifampin, and ciprofloxacin. *Ann. Intern. Med.* 113:358, 1990.

28. Hughes, W.T., et al. Guidelines for the use of antimicrobial agents in neutropenic patients with unexplained fever. *J. Infect. Dis.* 161:381, 1990.

29. Gilbert, D.N., and Bennett, W.M. Use of antimicrobial agents in renal failure. *Infect. Dis. Clin. North Am.* 3:517, 1989.
See also reference [42].

30. Cipolle, R.J., et al. Systemically individualized tobramycin dosage regimens. *J. Clin. Pharmacol.* 20(10):570, 1980.

31. Schwartz, S.N., et al. A controlled investigation of the pharmacokinetics of gentamicin and tobramycin in obese subjects. *J. Infect. Dis.* 138:499, 1978.
Provides guidelines for initial dosing of aminoglycosides in the obese patient. For a related article, see A.M. Traynor, A.N. Nafziger, and J.S. Bertino, Jr., Aminoglycoside dosing weight correction factors for patients of various body sizes. Antimicrob. Agents Chemother. *39:545, 1995. Confirms that in obese patients, ideal body weight plus approximately 40% of their excess weight provides a good adjusted weight for use in dose calculations.*

32. Cockcroft, D.W., and Gault, M.H. Prediction of creatinine clearance from serum creatinine. *Nephron* 16:31, 1976.

33. Ter Braak, E.W., et al. Once-daily dosing regimen for aminoglycosides plus beta-lactam combination therapy of serious bacterial infections: Comparative trial with netilmicin plus ceftriaxone. *Am. J. Med.* 89:58, 1990.
Efficacy of both dosing regimens in adults was equal, but all patients received 2 g ceftriaxone daily. Multiple (bid or tid dosing based on a nomogram with peaks of 10–12 μg/ml and troughs <2 μg/ml) versus once-daily dose (total daily dose based on nomogram with troughs <2 μg/ml) versus once-daily dose . Nephrotoxicity and ototoxicity did not differ significantly in this small study. For related articles see P.J. deVries et al., Prospective randomized study of once-daily versus thrice-daily netilmicin regimens in patients with intraabdominal infections. Eur. J. Clin. Microbiol. Infect. Dis. *9:161, 1990, which showed efficacy and safety of both regimens, and L. Nordstrom et al., Does administration of an aminoglycoside in a single daily dose affect its efficacy and toxicity?* J. Antimicrob. Chemother. *25:159, 1990, demonstrating similar toxicity of daily versus three-times daily regimens.*

34. Gilbert, D.N. Once daily aminoglycoside therapy. *Antimicrob. Agents Chemother.* 35:399, 1991.
Good minireview of this topic. Data thus far is only in animals and patients with normal renal function. Further studies are indicated for this interesting approach. See related editorial on this topic by M.E. Levison, New dosing regimens for aminoglycoside antibiotics. Ann. Intern. Med. *117:693, 1992.*

35. Nicolau, D.P., et al. Experience with a once-daily aminoglycoside program administered to 2184 adult patients. *Antimicrob. Agents Chemother.* 39:650, 1995.
The authors concluded that this approach appears to be clinically effective, reduces the incidence of nephrotoxicity, and provides a cost-effective method for administration

of aminoglycosides by reducing ancillary service time and serum aminoglycoside determinations. See text comments on some of the limitations of this study.

36. Barclay, M.L., Begg, E.J., and Hickling, K.C. What is the evidence for once-daily aminoglycoside therapy? *Clin. Pharmacokinet.* 27:32, 1994.
   Extensive review concludes there is a need for clinical studies comparing individualized once-daily administration with conventional aminoglycoside therapy. See related reviews by R.D. Bates and M.C. Nahata, Once-daily administration of aminoglycosides. Ann. Pharmacother. *28:757, 1994, and editorial comment in the same issue; R.B. Dew and G.M. Sulsa, Once-daily aminoglycoside treatment.* Infect. Dis. Clin. Pract. *5:12, 1996; and R. Hatala et al., Once-daily aminoglycoside dosing in immunocompetent adults: A meta-analysis.* Ann. Intern. Med. *124:717, 1996.*

37. Seligson, D., and Henry, S.L. Newest knowledge of treatment for bone infection: Antibiotic-impregnated beads. *Clin. Orthop.* 295:2–118, 1993.
   An extensive symposium devoted to this important topic.

38. The Ad Hoc Advisory Committee on Peritonitis Management. Peritoneal dialysis-related peritonitis treatment recommendations, 1993 update. *Periton. Dialysis Int.* 13:14, 1993.
   Excellent summary, with dosage regimens.

39. Ramsey, B.W., Dorkin, H.L., Eisenberg, J.D., et al. Efficacy of aerosolized tobramycin in patients with cystic fibrosis. *N. Engl. J. Med.* 328:1740, 1993.
   *Authors conclude that the short-term (e.g., 4 weeks) aerosol administration of a high dose of tobramycin in patients with **clinically stable** cystic fibrosis is efficacious and safe for treating endobronchial infection with P. aeruginosa. By prolonging optimal pulmonary status in these patients, this approach may help decrease the frequency of courses of intravenous antibiotics for pulmonary exacerbations. Whether longer term administration of aerosolized tobramycin would increase the frequency of colonization by tobramycin-resistant bacteria is not known.*
      See related article by S.B. Fiel, Aerosol delivery of antibiotics to the lower airways of patients with cystic fibrosis. Chest *107(Suppl. 2):61S, 1995, for a review of this topic.*

40. Centers for Disease Control. Availability of streptomycin and para-aminosalicylic acid—United States. *M.M.W.R.* 41:243, 482, 1992.
   See same report reprinted in J.A.M.A. *267:2587, 1992.*

41. Enderlin, G., et al. Streptomycin and alternative agents for treatment of tularemia: Review of the literature. *Clin. Infect. Dis.* 19:42, 1994.
   Streptomycin remains the drug of choice, with higher cure rates than gentamicin.

42. Bennett, W.M., et al. *Drug Prescribing in Renal Failure: Dosing Guidelines for Adults* (3rd ed.). Philadelphia: American College of Physicians, 1994.
   A useful handbook. Similar tables for dosing in renal failure appear in S.K. Swan and W.M. Bennett, Drug dosing guidelines in patients with renal failure. West J. Med. *156:633, 1992, and L.L. Livornese et al., Antibacterial agents in renal failure.* Infect. Dis. Clin. North Am. *9:591, 1995.*

43. McEvoy, G.K., et al. *Drug Information.* American Society of Hospital Pharmacists. Bethesda, MD: American Hospital Formulary Service, 1994. P. 38.

44. Medical Letter. Drugs for parasitic infections. *Med. Lett. Drugs Ther.* 37:99, 1995.

45. White, A.C., Jr., et al. Paromomycin for cryptosporidiosis in AIDS: A prospective, double-blind trial. *J. Infect. Dis.* 170:419, 1994.
   In this small study of 10 patients, therapy resulted in improvement in both clinical and parasitologic parameters. A dose of 25–35 mg/kg/day (two 250-mg tablets tid or qid) of paromomycin was used.
      See related report by M.R. Wallace et al., Use of paromomycin for the treatment of cryptosporidiosis in patients with AIDS. Clin. Infect. Dis. *17:1070, 1993.*

46. Bissuel, F., et al. Paromomycin: An effective treatment for cryptosporidial diarrhea in patients with AIDS. *Clin. Infect. Dis.* 18:447, 1994.
   In this study from France, 22 of 24 patients responded clinically with 18 complete remissions. Clearance of cryptosporidia from stools occurred within 2–4 weeks of treatment. An initial dose of 1 g bid for 1 month, followed by a maintenance dose of 500 mg bid for 2 months, typically was given. On the maintenance dose, diarrhea may worsen and may respond again to full doses.
      See related report by M. Scaglia et al., Effectiveness of aminosidine (paromomycin) sulfate in chronic Cryptosporidium diarrhea in AIDS patients: An open, uncontrolled, prospective trial. J. Infect. Dis. *170:1349, 1994.*

47. Mohri, H., et al. Case report: Inhalation therapy of paromomycin is effective for respiratory infection and hypoxia by cryptosporidium with AIDS. *Am. J. Med. Sci.* 309:60, 1995.

I. Clindamycin

In 1962, lincomycin was isolated and later shown to have a unique antibiotic structure. This different structure helps to explain why this antibiotic class can be used in cephalosporin- and penicillin-allergic patients. Minor chemical modifications of the side chain of lincomycin produced clindamycin, which has an increased rate of absorption from the GI tract and an increased antibacterial activity compared to that of lincomycin. Consequently, in recent years, **clindamycin has virtually replaced lincomycin,** which is not discussed further in this text.

Clindamycin is an important antibiotic for intraabdominal or pelvic infections involving anaerobes [1–4]. In addition, it is a second-line alternative agent in penicillin-allergic patients. Clindamycin is bactericidal for some organisms but generally is bacteriostatic, depending on the bacterial species, inoculum of bacteria, and concentration of antibiotic available [2a, 3]. Clindamycin inhibits protein synthesis at the ribosomal level.

I. **Spectrum of activity**
  A. **Gram-positive aerobes.** Clindamycin is effective against group A streptococci and most *Staphylococcus aureus* strains. Of hospital isolates, 5–20% of strains of *S. aureus* may be resistant to clindamycin [2, 3]. The emergence of clindamycin-resistant *S. aureus* has been noted in clindamycin-treated patients, especially when the organisms initially had erythromycin resistance at the onset of treatment [2a, 3]. Methicillin-resistant strains of *S. aureus* usually are not susceptible to clindamycin. Clindamycin is not active against enterococci but is active against penicillin-susceptible *Streptococcus pneumoniae*. Penicillin-resistant strains of *S. pneumoniae* are typically resistant to macrolides and clindamycin [4a]. (See Chap. 28C.)
  B. **Gram-negative aerobes.** Clindamycin has **no useful activity** against gram-negative aerobes.
  C. **Anaerobes.** Clindamycin is active against gram-positive and gram-negative anaerobes, including most *Bacteroides fragilis* and *Clostridium perfringens* strains. Although clindamycin is active against *B. fragilis,* it is not always bactericidal. In the past decade, susceptibility data have shown increasing resistance of *Bacteroides* spp. to clindamycin at many but not all institutions [5, 6]. Approximately 5–10% of isolates of *B. fragilis* may be resistant to clindamycin. However, in one report from six hospitals in Chicago, rates of resistance against *B. fragilis* within this one city varied from 0 to 20% [7]. Non-*fragilis* members of the *B. fragilis* group (e.g., *B. distasonis, B. ovatus, B. thetaiotaomicron*) typically have even higher rates of resistance to clindamycin (15–40%) [3, 7].
  Approximately 10–20% of clostridial species, other than *C. perfringens,* are resistant to clindamycin [3]. *Clostridium perfringens* strains are very susceptible to clindamycin. Nearly 10–20% of peptococci strains are resistant to clindamycin [3].
  D. **Miscellaneous.** Clindamycin is not effective against *Mycoplasma pneumoniae,* but certain strains of *Toxoplasma gondii* are susceptible [2]. Clindamycin is also active against *Pneumocystis carinii, Babesia* spp. and *Plasmodium* spp. [2a].
  E. **Resistance.** The mechanism of resistance of *Bacteroides* spp. to clindamycin is reviewed in detail elsewhere and is mediated by ribosomal modification [7a]. As with resistance to aerobic pathogens (see Chap. 28A), resistance to anaerobes, including *Bacteroides* spp., reflects antibiotic use, at least in part [7, 7a].
II. **Pharmacokinetics**
  A. **Route and levels. Clindamycin is well absorbed from the GI tract** (i.e., 90% [2a]), and food does not decrease its absorption. Adequate blood levels can be achieved by the oral, intramuscular, or intravenous route. With oral therapy, approximately 90% bioavailability has been noted, and the resultant peak serum concentration is 3.6 µg/ml after a 300-mg dose [4]. In adult healthy volunteers, 600-mg and 900-mg IV doses provide peak serum levels of 10 and 11 µg/ml, respectively [3].
  B. **Penetration.** Clindamycin penetrates most body tissues well, including sputum, bile, bone, prostate, and pleural fluid, but does not penetrate the cerebrospinal fluid well [4]. It will cross the placenta. The antibacterial activity persists in feces for 5 or more days after parenteral therapy is discontinued, and growth of sensitive microorganisms in the colon remains suppressed for up to 2 weeks [2]. This antibacterial effect in the colon may explain, in part, why clindamycin use may be

a risk factor for the development of *Clostridium difficile* diarrhea. See Chap. 28A. High bioactivity is found in bile, when there is no obstruction, and in urine [3].

C. **Metabolism and excretion.** Clindamycin is metabolized primarily by the liver. **In severe hepatic insufficiency, the half-life of clindamycin is prolonged** to 8–12 hours [2a]; **therefore, doses of clindamycin should be reduced** in patients with severe liver failure or combined liver and renal failure [2a].

Clindamycin is actively transported into polymorphonuclear leukocytes and macrophages, significantly increasing the concentration of the drug within these cells. Animal studies have shown enterohepatic circulation of clindamycin and its metabolites, leading to prolonged presence of clindamycin in the stool, with gut flora changes up to 2 weeks after stopping clindamycin [2a]. This may play a role in predisposing patients to *C. difficile* diarrhea. See sec. **V.A** and Chap. 28A. The half-life of clindamycin is increased from 2.4 to approximately 6 hours in patients with severe renal failure,and peak blood levels after parenteral administration are nearly twice those in healthy people. If modified at all, parenteral doses should be halved in such patients [3]. (See secs. **IV.D.** and **IV.E.**)

III. **Indications for use. Clindamycin is not the agent of choice for any specific pathogen** [8]. It is a very useful alternative agent [2, 2a].

A. *Bacteroides fragilis* **infections.** In the 1988 *Medical Letter,* clindamycin and metronidazole were drugs of first choice for GI strains of *Bacteroides* spp. (e.g., *B. fragilis*) [9]. Since 1990, in the *Medical Letter*'s "Choice of antimicrobial agents," clindamycin is listed as the first **alternative drug** for GI strains of *Bacteroides* spp. [8, 9]; metronidazole is the drug of first choice. Because of the cost of clindamycin (see Tables 28A-5 and 28A-6), higher risk of *C. difficile* diarrhea when compared with metronidazole (see Chap. 28A and sec. **V.A**), and low incidence of *B. fragilis* resistant to clindamycin (see sec. **I.C**), **many experts favor metronidazole over clindamycin for GI infections.** Clindamycin has been effective for **intraabdominal and pelvic infections,** including peritonitis, abscess, and septic abortions [2a, 10]. Although many empiric regimens have been used for intraabdominal and pelvic infections due to anaerobes (e.g., combinations of clindamycin or metronidazole with an agent active against Enterobacteriaceae [usually gentamicin], cefoxitin or cefotetan, ampicillin with sulbactam, ticarcillin with clavulanate, impipenem), no consistent differences in clinical efficacy have been shown [3, 10, 11]. (See Chap. 11.) In endocarditis or other intravascular infections due to *B. fragilis,* metronidazole is the preferred agent, as it is more consistently bactericidal against *B. fragilis.*

B. **Alternative drug in allergic patients**
   1. In the penicillin-allergic patient, cephalosporins are often the alternative drugs initially used, especially in gram-positive infections. **In patients allergic to both penicillin and cephalosporins,** clindamycin is an effective alternative for susceptible aerobic gram-positive cocci (e.g., *S. aureus, Streptococcus pyogenes).* Clindamycin is considered a second-line alternate agent for penicilin-susceptible *S. pneumoniae* [8]. Clindamycin is an effective alternative to penicillin for *C. perfringens* therapy [3, 8]. In the animal model, clindamycin may be better for gram-positive infections [11a]. (See sec. **F.2.**)
   2. Because clindamycin may not be bactericidal against some *S. aureus* strains, it is not a reliable agent in patients with known *S. aureus* endocarditis or a staphylococcal bacteremia. Therapeutic failures with clindamycin in the treatment of staphylococcal endocarditis have occurred, and most experts think that in the allergic patient with staphylococcal bacteremia, a bactericidal agent such as a cephalosporin or vancomycin is preferable. In other staphylococcal infections (e.g., soft-tissue infections and bone infections), clindamycin is a useful alternative.

C. **Osteomyelitis.** Clindamycin penetrates bone very well, so it is a useful alternative for susceptible organisms in the allergic patient and has been used in carefully monitored oral programs [12]. It may have a special role in chronic recurrent osteomyelitis. (This is a difficult problem, and infectious disease consultation is, ideally, advised. See Chap. 16.) Although high concentrations of clindamycin are achieved in bone, an advantage of clindamycin in the treatment of osteomyelitis in patients has not been demonstrated [3]. Some investigators favor the use of clindamycin in diabetic foot osteomyelitis [2], especially when gram-negative aerobes and enterococci are not involved.

D. **Severe aspiration pneumonia or lung abscess.** When these infections are believed to be related to poor oral or dental hygiene and aspiration of oral anaerobes, penicillin has been the usual drug of choice, although clindamycin is also favored [8]. In the penicillin-allergic patient or the patient not responding to penicillin, clindamycin is a preferred agent [2a, 8]. Some experts favor the initial use of clindamycin in patients who are seriously ill with this problem, to ensure coverage for anaerobes that may be resistant to penicillin [13, 14].

E. **Diabetic foot infections.** Clindamycin, combined with an agent with good activity against aerobic gram-negative rods, is commonly used. See Chap. 16, under Diabetic Foot Infections.

F. **Miscellaneous uses**

1. **Invasive group A streptococcal infections** such as severe necrotizing fasciitis, streptococcal myositis, streptococcal toxic shock syndrome, and bacteremias have been reviewed [15]. **In these severe infections, penicillin may not be as effective** due to the slower growth rate of streptococci at large inoculum sizes, **and clindamycin may be more effective** in the mouse model [11a, 16] and clinically [15]. Why clindamycin may be more effective in this setting is not clear. **See** more detailed discussion in **Chap. 4.**

2. **Severe streptococcal or staphylococcal cellulitis.** For this problem, clindamycin is favored by some clinicians. See Chap. 4, sec. **I.**, under Cellulitis and Related Skin Infections, and reference [11a].

3. **Streptococcal group A pharyngitis.** Clindamycin has sometimes been considered an alternative agent in this setting [17], especially in the allergic patient and in patients with recurrent streptococcal pharyngitis [17a]. However, some reviewers point out that most recurrences of streptococcal pharyngitis are reinfections rather than relapses, and widespread use of clindamycin for this common problem will likely lead to the selection of clindamycin-resistant strains [3]. See related discussion in Chap. 7.

4. **Alternative agent for endocarditis prophylaxis for oral-dental procedures.** See Chap. 28B.

5. **Bacterial vaginosis** usually is treated with oral metronidazole, but oral clindamycin (300 mg PO bid for 7 days) or the 2% topical cream is an alternative [18]. (See sec. **IV.C** and Chap. 13.)

6. **Acne vulgaris.** A 1% **topical** clindamycin **gel** and lotion has been used in this setting.

7. **Central nervous system toxoplasmosis.** Clindamycin in combination with pyrimethamine has been used in patients with toxoplasmosis encephalitis lesions [19, 20] (see Chaps. 19 and 28U). Infectious disease consultation is advised for its use in this setting.

8. *Pneumocystis carinii* **pneumonia (PCP) in AIDS.** Clindamycin with primaquine is an effective alternative for patients in whom standard therapy for PCP has failed or could not be tolerated [21], but more recently it has been used in primary therapy for PCP [22]. Infectious disease consultation is advised (see Chap. 24).

9. **Babesiosis and malaria.** Clindamycin with quinine has been used in the treatment of babesiosis [2a, 3] and uncomplicated *Plasmodium falciparum* malaria [22a].

10. **Posttraumatic endophthalmitis** due to *Bacillus cereus* can be a fulminant infection. Clindamycin seems to be especially useful in this setting, because it is active against *B. cereus* and has fairly good penetration into the eye when given systemically and intraocularly. *B. cereus* is a known producer of beta-lactamases and is highly resistant to penicillins and cephalosporins, including the third-generation cephalosporins [2a, 23]. Also see Chap. 6.

11. **Odontogenic infections.** Orofacial infections may have a dental source and may lead to Ludwig's angina, maxillary sinusitis, and retropharyngeal and parapharyngeal abscess. (See Chap. 4 under Infections of Deep Spaces of the Neck). Although penicillin has been traditionally used, clindamycin in some trials has been more effective [2a]. The most likely cause of penicillin failure in these cases is infection with beta-lactamase–producing strains of *Prevotella melaninogenica* (formerly *Bacteroides melaninogenicus*) [2a].

12. **Chronic sinusitis or chronic otitis.** When specific bacteriologic data point to anaerobes as the contributing or sole etiologic agents, clindamycin has been used [2a].

IV. **Route and dosage.** Because of the possibility of *C. difficile* diarrhea, clindamycin should be prescribed with caution, if ever, in patients with inflammatory bowel disease [2a].

A. **Oral.** Tablets are available in 75- and 150-mg sizes. Flavored pediatric granules can be reconstituted into an oral solution with the equivalent of 75 mg/5 ml. In children, the recommended oral dosage is 10–25 mg/kg/day divided into q6h doses or for mild to moderately severe infections, 20–30 mg/kg/day in four divided doses has been used [23a]. In severe infections in children, such as osteomyelitis, 30–40 mg/kg/day (up to 50 kg of body weight) divided into q6h doses has been used. In adults, 300–450 mg q6–8h hours can be given, depending on the severity of the illness.

B. **Parenteral**
1. **In adults.** In the past, 600 mg IV q6h or 900 mg q8h in adults with severe infections was frequently recommended [24]. Even for severe infections, doses of 600 mg q8h are being used effectively; such a dosage is more cost-effective and appropriate [2a, 25, 26].
2. **In children** older than 1 month, 20–40 mg/kg/day is suggested, depending on the severity of the infection. The daily dose is divided into q6–8h doses.
3. **In neonates,** the dosages used are shown in Chap. 3.

C. **Clindamycin 2% vaginal cream** is an alternative agent for bacterial vaginosis and is given at a dose of 5 g intravaginally once daily for 7 days [18].

D. **In renal failure,** no change in the dosage is recommended [27]. Clindamycin is **not removed by either peritoneal dialysis or hemodialysis** [2a].

E. **In hepatic insufficiency,** the half-life is prolonged. Doses should be reduced or the dosage interval prolonged or, if possible, an alternative agent should be used. (See discussion in sec. **II.C.**)

F. **Pregnancy.** The package insert indicates that safety for use in pregnancy has not been established. See Chap. 28A.

G. **Nursing mothers.** Clindamycin has been reported in breast milk. Because of the potential for adverse reactions to clindamycin in neonates, the package insert suggests that the decision to discontinue the drug should be made, taking into account the importance of the drug to the mother.

H. **Potential for antagonism** with erythromycin. The attachment site of clindamycin at the ribosome is the same or overlapping with that of chloramphenicol and the macrolides. This explains the antagonism in vitro between **clindamycin and erythromycin;** these drugs **should not be used in combination.**

I. **Cost.** Clindamycin is a relatively expensive agent. See Tables 28A-5 and 28A-6.

V. **Side effects**
A. *C. difficile* **diarrhea.** Although clindamycin has received a great deal of attention as a cause of this condition, *C. difficile* diarrhea has been reported as a complication of almost all antibiotics. However, large series summarizing this problem emphasize that the most common agents associated with *C. difficile* diarrhea are clindamycin, ampicillin, and the cephalosporins [28, 29] (see Chap. 28A). In addition, one report points out that an outbreak of nosocomial *C. difficile* diarrhea, believed to be associated with clindamycin use, was controlled by subsequent restriction of clindamycin use [30].

B. **Allergic reactions** such as fever and rashes can occur. The reported incidence of rashes varies but may occur in 10% or more of recipients [1, 2, 2a].

C. **Hepatotoxicity.** Minor, reversible elevations of hepatocellular enzymes are frequent, especially with the parenteral route [3]. Overt jaundice and severe hepatitis are rare.

D. **Nephrotoxicity.** Clindamycin does not cause significant renal toxicity [1].

E. **Bone marrow suppression.** Occasionally, cases of neutropenia and thrombocytopenia have been reported [1, 3].

F. **A metallic taste** in the mouth when clindamycin is given parenterally occurs in up to 4% of recipients [2].

G. **In premature** infants, the benzyl alcohol that is used as a preservative in clindamycin phosphate has been rarely associated with a fatal *gasping syndrome* [2a].

References

1. Dhawan, V.K., and Thadepalli, H. Clindamycin: A review of fifteen years of experience. *Rev. Infect. Dis.* 4:1133, 1982.
2. Klainer, A.S. Clindamycin. *Med. Clin. North Am.* 71:1169, 1987.
2a. Falagas, M.E., and Gorbach, S.L. Clindamycin and metronidazole. *Med. Clin. North Am.* 79:845, 1995.
3. Steigbigel, N.H. Macrolides and Clindamycin. In G.L. Mandell, J.E. Bennett, and

R. Dolin (eds.), *Principles and Practice of Infectious Diseases* (4th ed.). New York: Churchill Livingstone, 1995. Pp. 341–346.
For another review, see F.M. Calia, Clindamycin. In S.L. Gorbach, J.G. Bartlett, and N.R. Blacklow (eds.), Infectious Diseases. Philadelphia: Saunders, 1992. Pp. 214–223.

4. Smilack, J.D., Wilson, W.R., and Cockerill, F.R. Tetracyclines, chloramphenicol, erythromycin, clindamycin, and metronidazole. *Mayo Clin. Proc.* 66:1270, 1991.

4a. Schreiber, J.R., and Jacobs, M.R. Antibiotic-resistant pneumococci. *Pediatr. Clin. North Am.* 42:519, 1995.

5. Chuhural, G.J., Jr., et al. Susceptibility of the *Bacteroides fragilis* group in the United States: Analysis by site of infection. *Antimicrob. Agents Chemother.* 32:717, 1988.
Data on susceptibility of more than 1,000 strains. For the clinically important B. fragilis and other B. fragilis group species, approximately 6.4% were resistant to clindamycin.

6. Scher, K.S. Emergence of antibiotic-resistant strains of *Bacteroides fragilis*. *Surg. Gynecol. Obstet.* 167:175, 1988.

7. Hecht, D.W., Osmolski, J.R., and O'keefe, J.P. Variation in the susceptibility of *Bacteroides fragilis* group isolates from six Chicago hospitals. *Clin. Infect. Dis.* 16 (Suppl. 4):S367, 1993.
Authors conclude that variation in the antimicrobial susceptibility of these bacteria is hospital-based and not attributable to the geographic region and therefore, for certain agents (e.g., clindamycin), in vitro susceptibility data cannot be assumed or predicted by large-scale surveys done elsewhere. Other agents are more predictably active against B. fragilis (e.g., metronidazole, imipenem, piperacillin-tazobactam).

7a. Rasmussen, B.A., Bush, K., and Tally, F.P. Antimicrobial resistance to *Bacteroides*. *Clin. Infect. Dis.* 16(Suppl. 4):S390, 1993.

8. Medical Letter. The choice of antimicrobial drugs. *Med. Lett. Drugs Ther.* 38:25, 1996.

9. Medical Letter. The choice of antimicrobial drugs. *Med. Lett. Drugs Ther. 30:37, 1988; 32:45, 1990; and 34:49, 1992; 36:53, 1994.*

10. Bohnen, J.M.A., et al. Guidelines for clinical care: Anti-infective agents for intraabdominal infection. *Arch. Surg.* 127:83, 1992.
This report from the Antimicrobial Agents Committee of the Surgical Infection Society suggests that for mild-to-moderate community-acquired infections, single-agent therapy with cefoxitin, cefotetan, cefmetazole, or ticarcillin-clavulanate is recommended. For severe infections, monotherapy with imipenem or combination therapy with a third-generation cephalosporin, aztreonam, or an aminoglycoside (with serum monitoring) plus clindamycin or metronidazole is recommended. For community-acquired infections, enterococci are not specifically treated unless identified presumptively on Gram stains of peritoneal fluid or abscess drainage or culture. For a detailed discussion of this topic, see Chap. 11.

11. Gorbach, S.L. Antibiotic treatment of anaerobic infections. *Clin. Infect. Dis.* 18(Suppl. 4):S305, 1994.
Discusses a variety of antibiotics used to treat intraabdominal infection. See Gorbach's related article, Treatment of intra-abdominal infections. J. Antimicrob. Chemother. 31:(Suppl. A):67, 1993, which emphasizes that it usually is not necessary to cover for enterococci. See Chap. 11.

11a. Stevens, D.L., Bryant, A.E., and Hackett, S.P. Antibiotic effects on bacterial viability, toxin production, and host response. *Clin. Infect. Dis.* 30(Suppl. 2):S154, 1995.
Study demonstrates that in addition to antibacterial properties, clindamycin is a potent suppressor of bacterial toxin synthesis and also has important immunomodulatory effects. These latter effects, the authors conclude, may explain, at least in part, why the efficacy of clindamycin in the treatment of infections due to certain gram-positive organisms is superior to, for example, penicillins.

12. Prober, C.G. Oral therapy for bone and joint infections. *Pediatr. Infect. Dis.* 1:8, 1982.

13. Bartlett, J.G., and Gorbach, S.L. Penicillin or clindamycin in primary lung abscess? *Ann. Intern. Med.* 98:546, 1983.
Excellent editorial. Not only is clindamycin useful in patients not responding to penicillin, but it also may be the preferred agent in seriously ill patients with anaerobic lung infections.

14. Gudiol, F., et al. Clindamycin vs. penicillin for anaerobic lung infection: High rate of penicillin failures associated with penicillin-resistant *Bacteroides melaninogenicus*. *Arch. Intern. Med.* 150:2525, 1990.
Almost 20% of anaerobes, usually B. melaninogenicus, initially isolated from transthoracic needle aspiration or bronchoscopic specimen brush cultures were penicillin-resistant, whereas none were resistant to clindamycin. Study reported from Spain.
Steigbigel points out in reference [3] that 15–25% of anaerobic pulmonary infections

involve beta-lactamase-producing strains of B. fragilis, B. melaninogenicus, P. rumini-cola, *and* B. ureolyticus, *which are resistant to penicillin.*

15. Stevens, D.L. Invasive group A streptococcus infections. *Clin. Infect. Dis.* 14:2, 1992.
    Excellent up-to-date review of this important topic.

16. Stevens, D.L., et al. The Eagle effect revisited: Efficacy of clindamycin, erythromycin and penicillin in the treatment of streptococcal myositis. *J. Infect. Dis.* 158:23, 1988.
    Clindamycin was superior in the mouse model.

17. Bass, J.W. Antibiotic management of group A streptococcal pharyngotonsillitis. *Pediatr. Infect. Dis. J.* 10:S43, 1991.
    This article is part of a special symposium, "Group A Streptococcal Infections: An Era of Growing Concern," published in October 1991. For a related update, see J.O. Klein, Management of streptococcal pharyngitis. Pediatr. Infect. Dis. J. *13:572, 1994, from a 1994 symposium devoted to streptococcal infections.*

17a. Orrling, A., et al. Clindamycin in persisting streptococcal pharyngotonsillitis after penicillin treatment. *Scand. J. Infect. Dis.* 26:535, 1994.
    After a routine 10-day course of oral penicillin, patients with persisting group A streptococci of the same T-type were retreated with either another course of oral penicillin or oral clindamycin. After retreatment, 14 of 22 patients receiving penicillin still had the same T-type streptococci, whereas none of 26 recipients of clindamycin still had streptococci on culture.

18. Medical Letter. Topical treatment for bacterial vaginosis. *Med. Lett. Drugs Ther.* 34:109, 1992.
    Vaginal clindamycin and vaginal metronidazole appear to be about as effective as oral metronidazole and better tolerated. The most frequent adverse effect of intravaginal clindamycin is vaginal candidiasis. The cream contains mineral oil, which may weaken latex or rubber condoms and diaphragms. The average wholesale cost for a 7-day course of vaginal clindamycin is $26.70. Approximately 5% of each vaginal dose is absorbed into the blood. See related article by J.D. Sobel et al., Long-term follow-up of patients with bacterial vaginosis treated with oral metronidazole and topical clindamycin. J. Infect. Dis. *167:783, 1993, which emphasizes high recurrence rates irrespective of initial treatment method. See related discussions in Chap. 13.*

19. Dannemann, B., et al. Treatment of toxoplasmic encephalitis in patients with AIDS: A randomized trial comparing pyrimethamine plus clindamycin to pyrimethamine plus sulfadiazine. *Ann. Intern. Med.* 116:33, 1992.
    This randomized, unblinded phase II multicenter trial of 59 patients suggests similar efficacy of these two regimens. All patients received at least 10 mg/day of folinic acid and pyrimethamine (200-mg loading dose, sometimes in divided doses over 24 hours), followed by 75 mg once daily) and either sulfadiazine (100 mg/kg, rounded to nearest gram, up to 8 g/day divided up into a qid schedule) or IV clindamycin (1,200 mg q6h for 3 weeks) and then PO clindamycin 300 mg/q6h or 450 mg q8h. Study period was 6 weeks. See Chap. 28U under Pyrimethamine.

20. Luft, B.J., et al. Toxoplasmic encephalitis in patients with the acquired immunodeficiency syndrome. *N. Engl. J. Med.* 329:995, 1993.
    Oral clindamycin (600 mg q6h) and pyrimethamine (200-mg loading dose, then 75 mg daily plus 10 mg/day of leucovorin) were effective treatment for toxoplasmic encephalitis. See related article by J. Blais et al., Effect of clindamycin on intracellular replication, protein synthesis and infectivity of Toxoplasma gondii. Antimicrob. Agents Chemother. *37:2571, 1993.*

21. Noskin, G.A., et al. Salvage therapy with clindamycin/primaquine for *Pneumocystis carinii* pneumonia. *Clin. Infect. Dis.* 14:183, 1992.
    Retrospective review of 26 patients. Clindamycin (usually 900 mg IV q8h initially and then PO) and primaquine (30 mg/day usually) were used. See Chap. 24.

22. Black, J.R., Feinberg, J., Murphy, R.L., et al. Clindamycin and primaquine therapy for mild-to-moderate episodes of *Pneumocystis carinii* pneumonia in patients with AIDS: AIDS clinical trials group 044. *Clin. Infect. Dis.* 18:905, 1994.
    Clindamycin (PO 600 mg q8h) and primaquine base (30 mg once daily), was an effective and well-tolerated regimen. See Chap. 24.

22a. Kremsner, P.G., et al. Clindamycin in combination with chloroquine or quinine is an effective therapy for uncomplicated *Plasmodium falciparum* malaria in children from Gabon. *J. Infect. Dis.* 169:467, 1994.

23. Davey, R.T., Jr., and Tauber, W.S. Post-traumatic endophthalmitis: The emerging role of *Bacillus cereus* infection. *Rev. Infect. Dis.* 9:110, 1987.

23a. Peter, G., et al. *1994 Red Book: Report on the Committee on Infectious Diseases* (23rd ed.). Elk Grove Village, IL: American Academy of Pediatrics, 1994. P. 550.

24. Flaherty, J.F., et al. Comparative pharmacokinetics and serum inhibitory activity of clindamycin in different dosing regimens. *Antimicrob. Agents Chemother.* 32:1825, 1988.
25. James, C.L. Treating intra-abdominal infections with clindamycin. *Clin. Pharm.* 5:955, 1986.
    Brief review of studies using 600 mg q8h.
26. Buchwald, D., et al. Effect of hospital wide change in clindamycin dosing schedule on clinical outcome. *Rev. Infect. Dis.* 11:619, 1989.
    A 600-mg q8h regimen of clindamycin was as effective as 600 mg q6h.
27. Bennett, W.M., et al. *Drug Prescribing in Renal Failure: Dosing Guidelines for Adults* (3rd ed.). Philadelphia: American College of Physicians, 1994.
    A useful handbook. Similar tables for dosing in renal failure appear in L.L. Livornese, Jr., et al., Antibacterial agents in renal failure. Infect. Dis. Clin. North Am. 9:591, 1995; and in S.K. Swan and W.M. Bennett, Drug dosing guidelines in patients with renal failure. West. J. Med. 156:633, 1992.
28. Bartlett, J.G. Antibiotic-associated diarrhea. *Clin. Infect. Dis.* 15:573, 1992.
    Excellent state-of-the-art clinical review by a national expert. Drugs that have a great impact on anaerobic fecal flora (e.g., clindamycin) will be associated with higher incidence rates of C. difficile diarrhea. Because metronidazole is well absorbed in the small intestine, there are far fewer changes in the fecal flora, with less C. difficile diarrhea. See Chap. 28A.
29. Fekety, R., and Shah, A.B. Diagnosis and treatment of *Clostridium difficile* colitis. *J.A.M.A.* 269:71, 1993.
30. Pear, S.M., et al. Decrease in nosocomial *Clostridium difficile*–associated diarrhea by restricting clindamycin use. *Ann. Intern. Med.* 120:272, 1994.

J. Chloramphenicol

Because of the irreversible fatal aplastic anemia that, on rare occasions, is associated with its use, chloramphenicol should be used only when clearly indicated. Although in the early 1980s there was renewed interest in chloramphenicol because it was active against *Bacteroides fragilis* (and therefore useful in anaerobic infections) **and** active against ampicillin-resistant *Haemophilus influenzae* (and therefore useful in meningitis and epiglottitis), in the mid-1990s, other agents usually are available for these problems. In addition to clindamycin, metronidazole, imipenem, ampicillin-sulbactam, ticarcillin-clavulanate, piperacillin-tazobactam and cefoxitin (or cefotetan or cefmetazole) are possible agents for anaerobic infections. The third-generation cephalosporins are exquisitely active against ampicillin-susceptible and ampicillin-resistant *H. influenzae*. Nevertheless, chloramphenicol remains a potentially useful agent in certain very well-defined settings [1–3].

I. **Mechanism of action.** Against *Staphylococcus aureus* and Enterobacteriaceae [4], chloramphenicol is a bacteriostatic antibiotic that inhibits protein synthesis at the ribosomal level. However, against common meningeal pathogens (*H. influenzae,* penicillin-susceptible *Streptococcus pneumoniae,* and *Neisseria meningitidis,* but not group B streptococci) data have shown that chloramphenicol is bactericidal [4]. Against penicillin-resistant strains (intermediate and high-level), tolerance may occur (i.e., the minimum bactericidal concentration [MBC] is much higher than the minimum inhibitory concentration [MIC] [see Chap. 25]) and cerebrospinal fluid [CSF] bactericidal levels may not be achievable for penicillin-resistant pneumococci [4a].

II. **Spectrum of activity.** Chloramphenicol is a broad-spectrum antibiotic active against many gram-positive and gram-negative bacteria, rickettsiae, chlamydiae, and mycoplasmas. However, it is not listed as the drug of first choice for any common pathogen [5], and alternative agents are available.

A. **Gram-positive bacteria.** Most gram-positive cocci, both aerobic and anaerobic, are susceptible to chloramphenicol, although the MICs are relatively high [1, 2]. Chloramphenicol is not considered a drug of choice against enterococci or staphylococci. Methicillin-resistant *S. aureus* usually is resistant to chloramphenicol [3]. Penicillin-resistant *S. pneumoniae* may be susceptible in vitro to chloramphenicol, but this agent may not be effective in vivo against this pathogen [4a]. See related discussion in Chap. 28C.

B. **Gram-negative bacteria.** *N. meinigitidis* and almost all ampicillin-resistant and ampicillin-susceptible *H. influenzae* strains are susceptible to chloramphenicol. Approximately 0.6% of strains of *H. influenzae* in the United States are resistant to chloramphenicol [2]. Some countries (e.g., Spain) have reported *H. influenzae* resistant to chloramphenicol and ampicillin [2]. Chloramphenicol has variable activity against other gram-negative bacilli; therefore, susceptibility studies are necessary. *Pseudomonas* spp. are resistant.

C. **Anaerobes.** Chloramphenicol has **excellent activity against gram-positive and gram-negative anaerobes,** including *B. fragilis*.

D. **Rickettsiae.** Chloramphenicol is active against the rickettsiae that cause Rocky Mountain spotted fever, Q fever, and typhus.

III. **Pharmacokinetics**

A. **Absorption.** Chloramphenicol is rapidly absorbed orally, although variable absorption may be seen in children. It penetrates body tissues well, including the spinal fluid and the unobstructed biliary tree. **Approximately 50% of serum levels appear in the CSF** in both the inflamed and uninflamed meninges. Formerly, the intramuscular route of administration was not recommended because of the inadequate serum levels achieved. However, one study suggests that adequate serum levels can be achieved in children with intramuscular administration [6], but intramuscular levels achieved in adults may be lower than those achieved intravenously; therefore, the intramuscular route should be used cautiously [2] and probably is best avoided [3]. The intravenous route provides good serum levels. Chloramphenicol readily passes the placental barrier and is present in breast milk.

B. **Inactivation.** Chloramphenicol is metabolized and inactivated primarily in the **liver** by glucuronyl transferase. This particular step is potentially important in neonates and adults with liver disease, in whom free chloramphenicol concentrations rise. These abnormally high levels of free chloramphenicol produce dose-related bone marrow suppression. There is wide variation in the metabolism and excretion of chloramphenicol in neonates and children; therefore, serum concentration monitoring is important in these age groups [2].

C. **Excretion. In renal failure,** the plasma half-life of the biologically active free chloramphenicol is not prolonged. Consequently, chloramphenicol is given in normal doses. However, partially metabolized inactive products do accumulate in renal failure; the significance of these is unclear, although they are believed to be nontoxic.

D. **Antagonism.** There has been some concern that antagonism may occur when a bacteriostatic drug such as chloramphenicol is used in combination therapy with bactericidal drugs such as penicillin. It is not clear whether this is clinically significant. This is discussed in more detail in Chap. 28A.

IV. **Toxicity.** Before the clinical usefulness of chloramphenicol is reviewed, it is important to review the major toxicity problems that have influenced chloramphenicol's clinical use. Although chloramphenicol can occasionally cause a hypersensitivity reaction (rash and fever) and, rarely, optic neuritis, its most important side effect is **bone marrow toxicity.**

A. **Dose-related bone marrow suppression. This may occur in any patient** on chloramphenicol, but it is especially likely in patients (1) who are on high doses (4 g or more daily), (2) who are on prolonged courses of therapy, and (3) who have blood levels of the free form of chloramphenicol in excess of 20–25 μg/ml. Consequently, neonates and patients with severe liver disease are at increased risk, as they are less able to inactivate the drug [7]. Anemia, reticulocytopenia, and neutropenia can occur. Occasionally, only thrombocytopenia is seen. Iron uptake by red blood cell normoblasts is inhibited by chloramphenicol, and serum iron levels may be elevated as a result. This reversible bone marrow depression is due to a direct pharmacologic effect of the antibiotic as a result of inhibition of mitochondrial protein synthesis [2].

1. **Monitoring patients**

a. **Serial blood counts.** Because this direct bone marrow toxicity can occur in any patient on chloramphenicol, it is important to perform **a complete blood cell count and platelet count or estimate every 2–3 days** while a patient is on chloramphenicol.

(1) If there is evidence of bone marrow suppression, the dose should be reduced and reassessment made of the need for this agent.

(2) If the bone marrow suppression worsens, usually the drug is discontinued.

   b. **Serum levels.** Direct bone marrow toxicity is related to levels of free chloramphenicol. **Therapeutic levels are between 10 and 20 μg/ml. The risk of direct bone marrow suppression increases when unconjugated (free drug) levels exceed 25 μg/ml** [2]. **Serum levels should be monitored, especially in neonates and with prolonged use.** Data indicate that when standard doses are administered intravenously to infants and children, the half-lives and levels achieved vary considerably from patient to patient [7]. High-pressure liquid chromatography and radioenzymatic methods are available to measure the unconjugated biologically active chloramphenicol.

   2. **Recovery.** Complete recovery occurs approximately 2 weeks after stopping the chloramphenicol **in this reversible form.**

B. **Unexplained aplastic anemia** is rare, occurring in only 1 in 25,000–40,000 courses of chloramphenicol.

   1. This rare complication usually is fatal. The precise mechanism in unknown, but there is a genetic risk. The aplasia is not dose-related and can become manifest weeks to months after the use of chloramphenicol. Aplasia has been observed after administration of eye ointment or ear drops containing chloramphenicol.

   2. **Oral versus intravenous therapy.** Anecdotal data have suggested that there may be a decreased risk of aplasia if the intravenous form of chloramphenicol rather than the oral preparation is used. This remains a controversial issue, but there are no detailed or controlled studies indicating that the intravenous route is associated with a lower frequency of aplasia. (However, the oral form of chloramphenicol is seldom used in the United States. See sec. **VII.B.2.**)

C. **Gray-baby syndrome.** Premature infants and newborns younger than 2 weeks have immature hepatic and renal function. Chloramphenicol can accumulate in the blood of these infants, especially when higher doses of the drug are used (i.e., 50–100 mg/kg/day for more than 3 days), causing the so-called gray-baby syndrome. Initial symptoms of this syndrome of chloramphenicol toxicity include vomiting, abnormal respiration, cyanosis, and abdominal distention. Over the next 24 hours, vasomotor collapse, hypothermia, and an ashen-gray skin color often develop. Approximately 40% of these infants die, although survivors appear to have no sequelae. The severity of this syndrome is related to the high level of **free** (unconjugated) chloramphenicol, which appears to result from (1) inadequate activity of the liver's glucuronyl transferase in conjugating the drug and (2) inadequate renal excretion of the unconjugated drug, which then continues to accumulate. **Therefore, chloramphenicol should be avoided in the premature infant and in the first 2 weeks of newborn life except in extreme life-threatening situations, in which decreased doses should be used and serum levels monitored.** Similar syndromes have been described in infants as old as 24 months [7]. (For dosages in neonates and related discussion, see Chap. 3.)

D. **Glucose-6-phosphate dehydrogenase deficiency.** Chloramphenicol may precipitate hemolysis in patients with a severe deficit of glucose-6-phosphate dehydrogenase.

E. **Childhood leukemia.** In a population-based case-control interview study of 309 childhood leukemia patients and 618 age- and sex-matched control subjects [8], a significant dose-response correlation was shown between chloramphenicol and the risk of acute lymphocytic and nonlymphocytic leukemia, especially in children treated for more than 10 days. Although additional studies may help clarify this risk, if chloramphenicol is believed to be initially indicated, whenever possible it seems prudent to change from chloramphenicol to a less toxic agent if clinical and susceptibility data allow [2].

V. **Clinical indications.** The *Physicians' Desk Reference* (PDR) [9] clearly notes the pharmaceutical manufacturer's warning that chloramphenicol **"must not be used when less potentially dangerous agents will be effective. . . It must not be used in the treatment of trivial infections or where it is not indicated, as in colds, influenza, infections of the throat, or as a prophylactic agent to prevent bacterial infections."** Because of the availability of less toxic antibiotics (e.g., third-generation cephalosporins, metronidazole), **chloramphenicol now is rarely the drug of choice** [1, 2] and seldom is used except in special settings or in the allergic patient. Chloramphenicol is not listed as the drug of first choice for any common pathogen [5].

A. **Potential indications for chloramphenicol use include the following** [1, 2, 3, 5]:

   1. **Alternative for life-threatening *H. influenzae* infections. The third-generation**

cephalosporins now are believed to be the drugs of choice in the empiric therapy of meningitis and acute epiglottitis in children [5, 10]. In the patient with an allergy history that precludes the use of cephalosporins, chloramphenicol alone remains an acceptable alternative [5].

2. **Alternative for bacterial meningitis due to a susceptible organism in a penicillin-allergic patient.** Although a third-generation cephalosporin (e.g., ceftriaxone) is often an appealing agent in the patient with a history of delayed penicillin allergy and not at high risk for *Listeria monocytogenes* infection or *S. pneumoniae* with high-level penicillin resistance, chloramphenicol is used also in meningitis of unclear etiology. **Chloramphenicol is an important alternate agent in the patient with bacterial meningitis and severe allergy to both penicillins and cephalosporins.** However, this agent is not indicated in meningitis due to Enterobacteriaceae. (See Chap. 5).

3. **Brain abscess.** Chloramphenicol may be used in this setting while awaiting culture results or if no culture data are available.

4. **Alternative agent in severe anaerobic infection.** With the availability of metronidazole, clindamycin, imipenem, cefoxitin, ticarcillin-clavulanate, ampicillin-sulbactam, and piperacillin-tazobactam, there seldom is the need to use chloramphenicol for anaerobic infections except possibly in the patient with multiple drug allergies that preclude the use of the more standard regimens. Chloramphenicol remains an alternative.

5. **Alternative drug in** *Salmonella typhi* infections, brucellosis, glanders, plague, rickettsial disease, *Chlamydia psittaci* infections (psittacosis), tularemia, and intraocular infections due to susceptible pathogens. (The latter can sometimes be treated with parenteral chloramphenicol, as it provides good aqueous and vitreous humor levels. The newer cephalosporins are preferred alternatives in these clinical situations, and the newer fluoroquinolones are other options.)

6. **Rickettsial infections** (Rocky Mountain spotted fever, typhus [murine], scrub typhus, tick-bite fever, Q fever). **Chloramphenicol may be the preferred agent when patients require parenteral therapy, in young children, and in pregnancy** [2]. Occasionally, chloramphenicol is useful when the differential diagnosis includes both meningococcemia and Rocky Mountain spotted fever [2].

7. **In susceptible** infections due to **vancomycin-resistant enterococci,** chloramphenicol may provide a possible alternative [11]. See related discussion in Chap. 28O.

B. **Severity of infections.** Most of the infections just outlined are unusual and serious or life-threatening. Patients are hospitalized for the initial therapy and may remain hospitalized for the duration of therapy. The oral preparation is seldom used or indicated in the United States (see sec. **VI.B**).

VI. **Contraindications to chloramphenicol use**
   A. In general, we avoid the use of chloramphenicol in **patients with leukopenia, severe anemias, or thrombocytopenia** because of the possibility of additional bone marrow suppression from chloramphenicol use. Occasionally, the initial leukopenia or thrombocytopenia may be due to the acute uncontrolled infection. In this setting, if chloramphenicol is still the drug of choice, it should be administered cautiously. Ideally, serum levels should be monitored.
   B. Because chloramphenicol readily crosses the placenta and is excreted in breast milk, **chloramphenicol should be avoided in pregnancy** (except in rickettsial infections; see sec. **V.A.6**) **and while breast-feeding.**

VII. **Route and dosage**
   A. **Neonatal doses** are reviewed by Meissner and Smith [7] and are listed in Chap. 3. **Serum levels should be monitored in neonates.**
   B. **Children and adults**
      1. **Intravenous.** The usual dosage is 50–100 mg/kg/day in divided 6-hour doses; although in adults we may limit the dose to 1 g q6h. Ideally, serum levels should be monitored periodically; if this is not possible, consideration should be given to reducing the dosage to 50–75 mg/kg/day after 48–72 hours if maximal doses are used initially. Serial blood cell counts or serum levels should be monitored. (See sec. **IV.A.1.**)
         a. **In renal failure,** routine doses and dose intervals can be used [12].
         b. **In hemodialysis or peritoneal dialysis,** no dosage adjustments are required [2, 12].
         c. **In hepatic failure,** patients may not be able to conjugate chloramphenicol and, consequently, free chloramphenicol levels may rise to toxic levels; this

is similar to the situation in neonates. Clear guidelines in this setting are not available. If chloramphenicol must be used, serum levels should be monitored. In adults, an initial loading dose of 1 g followed by 500 mg q6h sometimes is suggested; the course should be limited to 10–14 days [2].

2. **Oral chloramphenicol** is seldom indicated or used in the United States. In patients with known or highly suspected Rocky Mountain spotted fever, chloramphenicol at 50 mg/kg/day (divided into q6h doses) may be considered if tetracycline is contraindicated. Infrequently, a patient with multiple, severe allergies may be a candidate; infectious disease consultation is advised. A 250-mg capsule is available.

3. **Intramuscular.** There has been some interest in the intramuscular route as reported by Shann and colleagues [6]. In this study, performed in Papua, New Guinea, children older than 1 month and younger than 6 years were treated with 25 mg/kg of intramuscular chloramphenicol (buttock injections) q6h for severe infections (e.g., meningitis, pneumonia). Serum levels were monitored, and therapeutic levels were achieved routinely or even exceeded, although peak levels were highly variable. However, usually the intramuscular route is not recommended [2, 3]. Adults may not absorb intramuscular chloramphenicol as well as do children, especially if adipose tissue is injected [6].

4. **Drug interactions.** Chloramphenicol can prolong the half-life of chlorpropamide, phenytoin, tolbutamide, and warfarin derivatives. Toxic levels of these agents can be seen if the patient also is receiving chloramphenicol.

References

1. Francke, E.L., and Neu, H.C. Chloramphenicol and tetracyclines, *Med. Clin. North Am.* 71:1155, 1987.
2. Standiford, H.C. Tetracyclines and Chloramphenicol. In G.L. Mandell, J.E. Bennett, and R. Dolin (eds.), *Principles and Practice of Infectious Diseases* (4th ed.). New York: Churchill Livingstone, 1995. Pp. 310–317.
3. Smilack, J.D., Wilson, W.R., and Cockerill, F.R. Tetracyclines, chloramphenicol, erythromycin, clindamycin, and metronidazole. *Mayo Clin. Proc.* 66:1270, 1991.
4. Rahal, J.J., Jr., and Simberkoff, M.S. Bactericidal and bacteriostatic action of chloramphenicol against meningeal pathogens. *Antimicrob. Agents Chemother.* 16:13, 1979.
   Chloramphenicol is bactericidal at clinically achievable concentrations against H. influenzae, penicillin-susceptible S. pneumoniae, *and* N. meningitidis.
4a. Friedland, I.R., and McCracken, G.H., Jr. Management of infections caused by antibiotic resistant *Streptococcus pneumoniae*. *N. Engl. J. Med.* 331:377, 1994.
   Chloramphenicol is active in vitro against strains of S. pneumoniae *that are penicillin-susceptible, intermediately resistant, and highly resistant to penicillin, strains of* S. pneumoniae *with a minimum inhibitory concentration$_{90}$ of 2–4* μg/ml. *Nonetheless, cerebrospinal fluid bactericidal levels may be inadequate, or minimum bactericidal levels may be significantly higher than MIC levels.*
   Anecdotal evidence suggests chloramphenicol has poor clinical efficacy for penicillin-resistant pneumococcal meningitis in the United States. See discussions in Chap. 5. See related paper by J. Hofmann et al., The prevalence of drug-resistant Streptococcus pneumoniae *in Atlanta.* N. Engl. J. Med. *333:481, 1995, and related discussion in Chap. 28C.*
5. Medical Letter. The choice of antibacterial drugs. *Med. Lett. Drugs Ther.* 38:25, 1996.
6. Shann, F.S., et al. Absorption of chloramphenicol sodium succinate after intramuscular administration in children. *N. Engl. J. Med.* 313:410, 1985.
7. Meissner, H.C., and Smith, A.L. The current status of chloramphenicol. *Pediatrics* 64:348, 1979.
8. Shu, X.O., et al. Chloramphenicol use and childhood leukemia in Shanghai. *Lancet* 2:934, 1987.
9. Product information on Chloromycetin. *Physicians' Desk Reference* (50th ed.). Montvale, NJ: Medical Economics Data, 1996. Pp. 1900–1901.
10. McCracken, G.H., Jr., et al. Consensus report: Antimicrobial therapy for bacterial meningitis in infants and children. *Pediatr. Infect. Dis. J.* 6:501, 1987.
    See updated discussion of this topic by R.D. Feigin et al., Diagnosis and management of meningitis. Pediatr. Infect. Dis. J. *11:785, 1992. Also see further discussion in Chap. 5.*
11. Norris, A.H., et al. Chloramphenicol for the treatment of vancomycin-resistant enterococcal infections. *Clin. Infect. Dis.* 20:1137, 1995.

The authors suggest that chloramphenicol may be useful in selected patients, in this report from the University of Pennsylvania. However, at times, vancomycin-resistant enterococci were involved in mixed infection and therefore their precise role as pathogens in a single patient may be hard to assess. See related discussion in Chap. 28O.

12. Bennett, W.M., et al. *Drug Prescribing in Renal Failure: Dosing Guidelines for Adults.* (3rd ed.). Philadelphia: American College of Physicians, 1994.
A useful handbook. Similar tables for dosing in renal failure appear in S.K. Swan and W.M. Bennett, Drug dosing guidelines in patients with renal failure. West. J. Med. 156:633, 1992, and L.L. Livornese et al., Antibacterial agents in renal failure. Infect. Dis. Clin. North Am. 9:591, 1995.

K. Sulfonamides and Trimethoprim-Sulfamethoxazole

I. **Sulfonamides.** Sulfonamides were the first effective systemic antibacterial drugs used in humans. The sulfonamides are primarily **bacteriostatic** and act by interfering with bacterial synthesis of folic acid.

A. **Pharmacokinetics.** Sulfonamides generally are used in the oral form providing bacteriostatic blood levels. The sulfonamides are metabolized in the liver by acetylation and glucuronidation. Free drug and its metabolites are excreted by the kidney. Preparations less apt to become crystallized in urine have attained more widespread use. Sulfonamides compete for binding sites on plasma albumin and may increase blood levels of unconjugated bilirubin. (See sec. **I.C.**)

B. **Spectrum of activity.** Because **routine disc antibiotic sensitivity testing generally is unreliable, it is not used.** A minimum inhibitory concentration (MIC) can be performed if necessary. Community-acquired *Escherichia coli* often are susceptible, particularly at levels achieved in the urine. The sulfonamides also are active against many strains of *Neisseria meningitidis, Chlamydia, Toxoplasma,* and some *Nocardia* spp. A sulfonamide alone is not the drug of first choice for any bacterial pathogen [1]. Sulfonamides have in vitro activity against *Streptococcus pyogenes* and have been used in regimens to prevent recurrent attacks of rheumatic fever (see Chap. 28B), but they are not advised for treatment of streptococcal pharyngitis.

C. **Current clinical uses**
   1. **Situations in which sulfonamides are useful** include:
      a. ***Toxoplasma gondii*** infections (e.g., sulfadiazine or trisulfapyrimidine, with the drug pyrimethamine). (See Chap. 28U.)
      b. ***Nocardia asteroides*** infections, which respond well to sulfonamides. Trimethoprim-sulfamethoxazole (TMP-SMX) often is listed as the agent of choice [1].
   2. **Miscellaneous indications** for sulfonamide use are the following:
      a. Rheumatic fever prophylaxis (e.g., sulfadiazine, although this agent is not useful in established streptococcal pharyngitis infections). (See Chap. 28B.)
      b. Alternate agent in *Chlamydia* pneumonia.
   3. For initial uncomplicated urinary tract infection (UTI) due to *E. coli,* sulfonamides in the past were the empiric agents of choice. However, data suggest 25–35% of strains of *E. coli* causing outpatient cystitis are resistant to sulfonamides [2]. Therefore, **alone sulfonamides are no longer the agents of choice for empiric therapy of initial uncomplicated UTI.** However, in combination with trimethoprim, sulfonamides (i.e., TMP-SMX) are useful empiric agents in UTI.

D. **Preparations available and dosage regimen**
   1. **Short-acting** preparations usually are given 4 (and sometimes 6) times daily.
      a. **Sulfisoxazole** (e.g., Gantrisin, Azo Gantrisin) is excreted rapidly, is soluble in urine, and still is used sometimes in **UTIs.** Conventional therapy involved a 2- to 4-g loading dose and then 1 g q6h. (In children, the initial dose is half the 24-hour dose, and the maintenance dose is 150 mg/kg/24 hr divided into q6h doses.) Sulfisoxazole has also been used in single-dose therapy, at a dose of 1 or 2 g [3], in the carefully selected patient, as

discussed in sec. **II.D.** However, usually other single-dose regimens (e.g., TMP-SMX) or 3-day regimens are preferred (see sec. **II.F.1** and Chap. 12).

b. **Sulfadiazine** is less soluble in urine and therefore is less suitable for use in UTIs. It appears to be less protein-bound than sulfisoxazole, and one can achieve good blood and cerebrospinal fluid (CSF) levels with sulfadiazine. Therefore, it often is used when a sulfonamide is indicated, **as in nocardial infection, toxoplasmosis, and rheumatic fever prophylaxis** in the penicillin-allergic patient. Although it has a longer half-life than sulfisoxazole, sulfadiazine is given 4 times daily. The usual therapeutic dose in adults is a 2-g loading dose with a maintenance dose of 1 g 4 times per day.

Various dose regimens for the treatment of toxoplasmosis have been suggested, and infectious disease consultation is advisable. (See Chaps. 19 and 28U for a discussion of pyrimethamine and sulfadiazine therapy, including dosages.)

Sulfadiazine, 8–12 g daily, is the initial dose regimen for nocardiosis. Dosages should be adjusted to achieve peak concentrations of 10–20 mg/dl [4]. Duration of therapy is ill-defined but is usually 6–12 months.

c. **Triple sulfa drug** (trisulfapyrimidines; e.g., triple sulfa tablets #2) usually is made up of sulfadiazine and two other sulfa preparations. Theoretically, each drug maintains its solubility in the urine to decrease the chances for crystalluria. In adults, the usual dose is 1 g 4 times daily.

d. Other preparations appear to offer no major advantages (e.g., sulfamethizole [Thiosulfil]).

2. **Intermediate-acting** sulfonamides can be given 2 or 3 times daily. **Sulfamethoxazole** (Gantanol, Azo Gantanol) is less soluble than sulfisoxazole, is excreted more slowly, and therefore provides higher blood levels than sulfisoxazole. It can be given twice daily and has been used in UTIs, in which such a dose schedule helped with compliance. Because it has a greater tendency than short-acting sulfonamides to cause crystalluria, it is important to ensure a high urine output when it is used. The dose regimen in adults is a 2-g initial dose followed by 1 g bid. In children older than 2 months, the initial dose is 50 mg/kg; then, 25–30 mg/kg per dose is given bid. **Sulfamethoxazole has been combined with trimethoprim and is available as cotrimoxazole (Bactrim, Septra),** which is discussed in sec. **II** and is used more than any sulfonamides alone.

3. **Long-acting sulfonamides.** These are **no longer recommended,** because these preparations have the capacity to produce hypersensitivity reactions, which then become a prolonged problem.

4. **Common topical sulfonamides** [5]. Mafenide acetate (Sulfamylon) has been used topically on burns to help prevent bacterial colonization, particularly colonization with pseudomonads. Its use has been limited by the side effect of metabolic acidosis. Silver sulfadiazine has fewer side effects and is used extensively for burns. Outbreaks of silver-resistant infections in burn units may ultimately limit its usefulness [5]. Sulfonamides are used also in ophthalmic ointments.

5. **Sulfasalazine** (Azulfidine) is used in the treatment of ulcerative colitis.

E. **Toxicity.** Modern sulfonamides are more soluble, and crystalluria is much less of a problem, than in the past.

1. **Pregnancy and neonates. Sulfonamides should not be used in the last trimester of pregnancy** (especially the last month) because they are transplacentally transmitted and compete for bilirubin-binding sites on plasma albumin, increasing the risk of kernicterus [5]. Sulfonamides are **not recommended for therapy in neonatal infections or in nursing mothers** because the neonate's hepatic enzyme system may be immature.

2. **Hematologic considerations.** Sulfonamides should be avoided in patients with glucose-6-phosphate dehydrogenase (G-6-PD) deficiency, because hemolysis can be precipitated. However, one study showed that G-6-PD-deficient patients who received TMP-SMX did not have hemolytic reactions during therapy [6]. Bone marrow depression with anemia, leukopenia, or thrombocytopenia can occur with sulfonamide use, especially in those with folate deficiency.

3. **Hypersensitivity reactions** with rashes, vasculitis, erythema nodosum, erythema multiforme, and Stevens-Johnson syndrome can occur. These were

particularly common with the long-acting compounds, which are no longer recommended.

   F. Important drug interactions. Sulfonamides may displace drugs from albumin-binding sites, increasing the clinical effect of the displaced drug [5].

      1. Oral anticoagulants. The doses of oral anticoagulants (e.g., warfarin sodium) should be reduced while patients receive sulfonamides, which compete for albumin-binding sites and, in effect, increase the activity of a given anticoagulant dose.

      2. Methotrexate. Because sulfonamides displace methotrexate from its bound protein, the risk of methotrexate toxicity increases if sulfonamides are used concurrently.

      3. Oral hypoglycemic agents. The hypoglycemic effect of tolbutamide and chlorpropamide may be exaggerated by sulfonamides, although the precise mechanisms for this are unclear.

      4. Methenamine compounds should not be given concomitantly with sulfonamides because there is an increased risk of insoluble urinary precipitate formation.

   G. Sulfonamide use in renal failure. Because sulfonamides are excreted by way of the kidney, in renal failure doses must be reduced or dose intervals prolonged [7].

II. Trimethoprim-sulfamethoxazole (TMP-SMX) [5, 8–10], formerly called *cotrimoxazole,* is available commercially as Bactrim or Septra as well as generic preparations. This unique preparation was specifically formulated to include a combination of agents that would inhibit activity in two sequential steps of bacterial metabolism. The combination has two theoretic advantages: (1) It decreases the chances of bacterial resistance, and (2) the combination may act synergistically. The combination is available in oral and intravenous forms. The regular tablets contain 80 mg TMP and 400 mg SMX to provide an ideal blood ratio of 1:20 for optimal synergy. However, it is noteworthy that in different body fluids, the ratios of TMP to SMX are virtually never 1:20, so the value of the ideal ratio in the blood is uncertain. Alone, each agent is bacteriostatic, but together they are bactericidal and synergistic in vitro. Currently, sulfonamides are used most frequently in this combination [5].

   A. Mechanism of action. TMP-SMX sequentially blocks two steps in the synthesis of folic acid by bacteria (Fig. 28K-1).

   B. Pharmacokinetics. Oral TMP-SMX is well absorbed from the upper GI tract, even in the presence of acute gastroenteritis. Peak serum levels occur 1–4 hours after ingestion. The intravenous preparation provides excellent blood levels. TMP-SMX is excreted primarily by the kidneys, so doses must be reduced in renal failure. Excretion occurs over several hours, and this permits twice-daily dosing. This agent penetrates the CSF well (20–40% of serum levels). Concentrations of TMP in prostatic fluid usually are at least 3 times those of the serum concentrations [10].

   C. Spectrum of activity. Trimethoprim by itself has a wide spectrum of activity against gram-positive and gram-negative bacteria. Sulfamethoxazole is less active alone, but it enhances the activity of TMP when combined with it.

      1. Gram-positive cocci. TMP-SMX is active against the majority of *Staphylococcus aureus, S. epidermidis,* penicillin-susceptible *S. pneumoniae* strains, and viridans streptococci. In a recent survey of penicillin-resistant strains of *S. pneumoniae* in Atlanta, Georgia, 75% of the isolates resistant to penicillin were resistant to TMP-SMX [10a]. It is not useful clinically against enterococci. This agent is active against many methicillin-resistant *S. aureus* (MRSA) species. Despite the apparent in vitro sensitivity of MRSA, some reviews emphasize that clinical success with TMP-SMX therapy for MRSA is extremely variable and unpredictable [9a].

      2. Most Enterobacteriaceae, *Salmonella* **and** *Shigella* **spp.,** *Haemophilus influenzae* (ampillin-susceptible and ampicillin-resistant), **and** *Moraxella (Branhamella) catarrhalis* are susceptible. Although TMP-SMX is active against *N. gonorrhoeae,* the 1:20 blood ratio achieved does not appear to be optimal for synergism against gonococci; it is not an ideal agent in gonococcal infection [11]. TMP-SMX has activity against *Pasteurella multocida* [11a].

      3. TMP-SMX is **not active against** *Pseudomonas aeruginosa* or enterococci. However, *Burkholderia cepacia* (formerly *P. cepacia*) are susceptible, but *S. maltophilia* (formerly *P. maltophilia*) often are resistant [10].

      4. Anaerobes. TMP-SMX is not particularly active against anaerobes [10, 12].

      5. Miscellaneous [1]

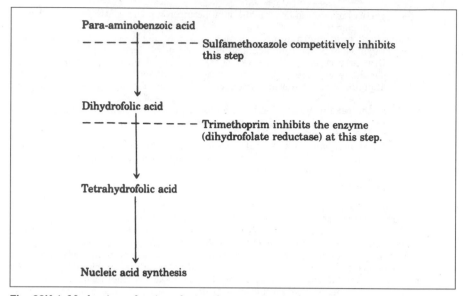

Fig. 28K-1. Mechanism of action of trimethoprim-sulfamethoxazole. Most bacteria cannot use exogenous folate but must make their own folate for nucleic acid synthesis. Trimethoprim-sulfamethoxazole can sequentially block the formation of tetrahydrofolic acid and thereby interfere with cell replication.

  a. TMP-SMX is active against *Listeria monocytogenes, Yersinia enterocolitica, Aeromonas* species, *Legionella micdadei,* and *Legionella pneumophila.*
  b. *Pneumocystis carinii* (a parasite) is susceptible.
  c. Many *Nocardia* spp. are susceptible.
  d. *Treponema pallidum* is resistant.
 6. Resistance to TMP-SMX has increased in recent years and is governed primarily by resistance to TMP. This is discussed in Chap. 28L and has recently been reviewed [12a]. Much of the resistance to TMP has been reported in developing countries where TMP has been used extensively as monotherapy and where antibiotics are available without prescription [9a]. Increasing resistance of TMP-SMX against *Salmonella typhi, Shigella* spp., MRSA, and *S. pneumoniae* is noted. Approximately 30–35% of nosocomial uropathogens are resistant to TMP-SMX [9a].
D. Current indications for use of TMP-SMX [5, 9, 10]. **For certain pathogens, TMP-SMX is considered the drug of first choice** [1]. These include *M. catarrhalis, H. influenzae* causing upper respiratory infections and bronchitis, *Y. enterocolitica, Aeromonas* spp., *Burkholderia cepacia* (formerly *P. cepacia, X. (S.) maltophilia,* Nocardia spp., and *P. carinii* (see Chap. 24).
 1. Urinary tract infections
  a. Acute initial uncomplicated UTI. The response and cure rates with TMP-SMX are as high as, or higher than, those obtained with ampicillin, cephalexin, or the sulfonamides. Although ampicillin (amoxicillin) or a sulfonamide alone has been effective and less expensive for the treatment of initial uncomplicated UTI, in many geographic areas in the United States, community-acquired *E. coli* causing these infections frequently are resistant (20–30%) to ampicillin or amoxicillin [2]. Therefore, TMP-SMX is indicated for an initial UTI, especially if there is concern about early upper urinary tract involvement [13]; TMP-SMX is a drug of choice in this setting [9a].
   TMP-SMX is commonly used for UTIs with organisms resistant to the less expensive antibiotics, in the penicillin- or ampicillin-allergic patient, or in special settings discussed next.

Virtually all strains of *Staphylococcus saprophyticus* are sensitive to TMP and therefore TMP-SMX [9a].

b. **Pyelonephritis.** Because TMP-SMX penetrates tissue well, it is a useful agent in this setting, especially as it can be given both intravenously and orally. In a study comparing ampicillin plus gentamicin to TMP-SMX plus gentamicin for women hospitalized with acute pyelonephritis, the TMP-SMX regimen was less costly and less likely to require modification due to antimicrobial resistance [14]. **If the Gram stain of unspun urine reveals gram-positive cocci suggesting enterococci, TMP-SMX is not a preferred empiric agent.**

c. **Recurrent UTI in adult women.** In women prone to recurrent UTI, TMP-SMX has helped decrease the rate of recurrence [15], presumably in part by decreasing colonization at the periurethral area. However, enterococcal colonization may result. An alternative regimen is a short course of antibiotic with a twice-daily dose of TMP-SMX for 3 days at the onset of symptoms. See detailed discussion in Chap. 12.

d. **Recurrent UTI in men.** In the absence of other genitourinary pathology, men with recurrent UTI often have chronic **bacterial prostatitis** that seeds the genitourinary tract [16]. Organisms in the prostate are extremely difficult to eradicate, because most antibiotics do not penetrate the prostate well. TMP-SMX penetrates the prostatic fluid and is very useful in these patients. (The fluoroquinolones also are useful in this setting.) See Chap. 12 also.

e. **Postcoital antibiotic prophylaxis for recurrent UTI** with TMP-SMX has been shown to be a safe, effective, and inexpensive approach to management in carefully selected young women with recurrent UTI [17]. See Chap. 12 also.

2. **Respiratory infections**
   a. *Pneumocystis carinii* **infections. TMP-SMX is considered the drug of choice in children and adults** for the treatment and prevention of *P. carinii* **pneumonia** (PCP) [18]. This topic is discussed in detail in Chap. 24.
   A high incidence of adverse effects occurs in patients with AIDS who are treated with TMP-SMX, especially when maximal doses are used [19]. See related discussion in sec. G and Chap. 24.

   b. **Acute exacerbations of chronic bronchitis.** Because TMP-SMX is active against penicillin-susceptible *S. pneumoniae, H. influenzae,* and *M. catarrhalis,* it is a useful agent in this setting [5, 19] or as part of a rotating antibiotic regimen or in the penicillin- and ampicillin-allergic patient.

   c. **Pneumonia.** For susceptible gram-negative pathogens, intravenous TMP-SMX has been used for lower respiratory tract infections [5]. TMP-SMX is an alternative agent for *L. micdadei* and *L. pneumophila* infections when erythromycin cannot be used [1].

   d. **Acute otitis media** in children is often due to *S. pneumoniae,* beta-lactamase-negative or beta-lactamase-positive strains of *H. influenzae,* and *M. (Branhamella) catarrhalis.* Most authorities believe that amoxicillin should be the initial agent of choice for uncomplicated otitis media [20]. TMP-SMX is an alternate agent in this setting, as is the combination of erythromycin and sulfisoxazole, and either combination can be used in the penicillin-allergic patient or in patients not responding to ampicillin or amoxicillin (implying that an ampicillin-resistant organism may be involved) or as initial therapy in some geographic areas where there is a known high incidence of ampicillin-resistant *H. influenzae.* (See Chap. 7.)

   e. **Sinusitis** has been treated effectively with TMP-SMX. See related discussion in Chap. 7.

3. **Gastrointestinal infections**
   a. **Shigellosis.** TMP-SMX is considered a useful alternative agent for enteritis caused by susceptible *Shigella* strains [1]. The fluoroquinolones are considered the drug of choice [1]. See Chap. 11 for further discussion.

   b. **Salmonella.** Although ceftriaxone usually is considered the drug of choice for *S. typhi* infections, and cefotaxime or ceftriaxone the treatment of choice for other *Salmonella* spp. infections requiring treatment, TMP-SMX is an excellent alternative agent [1]. See Chap. 11 for further discussion.

   c. **Travelers' diarrhea.** A few years ago, TMP-SMX was the most common agent used to treat travelers' diarrhea [21]. Now, the fluoroquinolones often are preferred since TMP resistance has become more common [21, 22]. See Chap. 21.

   d. **Prevention of spontaneous bacterial peritonitis** in patients with underlying cirrhosis. The use of TMP-SMX in this setting is discussed in Chap. 11.

4. **Some forms of meningitis. Gram-negative bacillary meningitis** caused by organisms only **moderately susceptible** to **third-generation cephalosporins** (e.g., *Enterobacter cloacae, Serratia marcescens*) or resistant to these antibiotics (*P. cepacia, Acinetobacter* spp.) may be candidates for TMP-SMX treatment if the organisms are susceptible [23]. TMP-SMX is an alternate agent in meningitis due to *L. monocytogenes* [1, 24], when ampicillin cannot be used. See Chap. 5.

5. **Prevention of infection in neutropenic patients.** The role of TMP-SMX in this setting remains controversial. It is an appealing agent to consider because it is an oral and well-tolerated antibiotic. It suppresses gram-negative enteric flora of the GI tract but without significant suppression of bowel anaerobes. Although initial studies suggested a potential role for use of TMP-SMX to prevent bacterial infections in the leukopenic patient [25], follow-up studies generally do not support these observations [26]. This is largely because, despite the use of TMP-SMX, the number of patients surviving or patients requiring other antibiotics is not appreciably changed. In addition, both the length of time before circulating WBCs can be detected and the numbers of patients with oral colonization with yeast are increased. The emergence of resistant Enterobacteriaceae in patients treated with prophylactic TMP-SMX is also an increasing concern [10].

   In a recent randomized, double-blind, placebo-controlled, cooperative study in granulocytopenic patients with acute leukemia, no significant differences in survival, frequency of bacteremia, overall infections, use of systemic antimicrobial therapy, or adverse effects, including myelosuppression, were observed between patients receiving TMP-SMX and those receiving placebo. The authors conclude that empiric administration of TMP-SMX for antibacterial chemoprophylaxis is not effective in adults undergoing remission-induction therapy for acute leukemia [27].

   In general, we believe the use of TMP-SMX in this setting should be restricted to patients monitored in clinical research protocols. We do not favor its use. See related discussion in Chap. 28S.

6. **Miscellaneous**
   a. **Endocarditis.** TMP-SMX has been used for susceptible pathogens causing bacteremias or endocarditis as an alternative agent [5, 28, 29].
   b. **Nosocomial infections.** Gram-negative nosocomial infections due to bacteria resistant to many antibiotics may be susceptible to TMP-SMX (e.g., *Enterobacter, Klebsiella*, and *Proteus* spp.), and patients will respond to this therapy. *Burkholderia cepacia* (formerly *P. cepacia*) infections that have relapsed or failed other agents often have responded well to TMP-SMX. **Prior to using TMP-SMX for these types of infections, in vitro data should show that the organism to be treated is susceptible to TMP-SMX.**
   c. *Nocardia.* TMP-SMX is an important agent for *Nocardia* infections and sometimes is viewed as the agent of choice [1].
   d. *Y. enterocolitica* and *Aeromonas* spp. infections can be treated with TMP-SMX.
   e. **Brucellosis.** TMP-SMX is an alternative agent for brucellosis.
   f. **Prevention of infection in renal transplantation recipients.** Prophylaxis with TMP-SMX significantly reduces the incidence of bacterial infection following renal transplantation (especially infection of the urinary tract and bloodstream), can provide protection against PCP, and is cost-beneficial [30]. Patients appear to tolerate this regimen well in this setting [30].
   g. **Prevention of infection in patients with chronic granulomatous disease.** TMP-SMX prophylaxis is useful in the prevention of infectious complications and does not appear to be associated with an increase of fungal infections [31].
   h. *Mycobacterium marinum.* TMP-SMX is an alternative agent [1].
   i. *Isospora belli* enteritis in patients infected with the human immunodeficiency virus (HIV) may have a clinical response to TMP-SMX [5].
   j. **Prevention of spontaneous bacterial peritonitis** in patients with underlying cirrhosis [32]: In this setting, TMP-SMX appears useful. See Chap. 11.

E. Forms available
   1. **Oral. Regular-strength** tablets contain 80 mg TMP and 400 mg SMX. The **double-strength** (DS) tablets contain 160 mg of TMP and 800 mg SMX. There are unflavored and cherry-flavored **suspensions** containing 40 mg TMP and 200 mg SMX per 5 ml.
   2. **Parenteral.** An intravenous form of TMP-SMX is supplied in 5-ml ampules* that contain 80 mg TMP and 400 mg SMX. The intravenous preparation is recommended for the following: (1) **severe UTIs** in patients who are vomiting or otherwise too ill to take an oral medication, (2) patients with severe **PCP,** (3) **severe *Shigella* infections,** and (4) certain serious multiresistant enteric gram-negative bacillary infections in which TMP-SMX is active in vitro. (Infectious disease consultation is advisable in this setting.) The intravenous form has also been used in the treatment of pneumonia, bacteremia, meningitis, and other serious infections [33].
F. Dosage. TMP-SMX is **not recommended for infants younger than 2 months** because of the **risk of kernicterus. In addition, its use in the pregnant woman, especially at term or in lactating women, is not recommended,** as sulfonamides cross the placenta and are excreted in breast milk and may cause kernicterus. The indications for oral versus intravenous therapy are discussed in sec. **E.** If the intravenous route is used initially, one often can switch to oral therapy as the patient improves. Adequate fluid intake should be encouraged to prevent sulfonamide crystalluria. **In renal failure, dosages must be adjusted.** In severe renal failure, because both TMP and SMX are excreted at different rates, in part depending on urinary pH, alternate drugs should be used when possible.
   1. **Urinary tract infections**
      a. **Cystitis.** For short-course **therapy of young female patients with uncomplicated acute cystitis,** single-dose therapy with two DS or one DS tablet bid for 3 days is very effective [10]. **We favor the 3-day regimen.** Conventional therapy for adult female or male patients with cystitis is one DS tablet bid for 7–10 days. For patients with known or suspected pyelonephritis, at least 14 days of therapy are suggested. For children, the same dosage used in otitis media is suggested (see sec. **2.d**) for 10 days (see Table 28K-1). See Chap. 12 also.
      b. **Prophylaxis for recurrent UTI** in adult women. After the urine has been sterilized with antibiotics, chronic suppressive therapy with one-half to one single-strength (SS) tablet TMP-SMX every other night at bedtime or one-half SS tablet nightly has usually been used for a variable number of months.
      c. **Intravenous therapy. For severe or complicated UTI,** 8–10 mg/kg/day (based on the TMP component) is recommended. The dose is divided into a q6h or q12h schedule until the patient improves enough to allow oral therapy.
      d. **Pediatric dose.** This is the same as for otitis media (see sec. **2.d**).
      e. **Prostatitis.** The recommended dose is usually two regular-strength tablets or one DS tablet bid. If the pathogen isolated on urine culture is susceptible to TMP-SMX and the initial clinical response is favorable, therapy can be continued at the preceding dosage for at least 2 weeks, but some experts suggest 30 days, if tolerated, to attempt to prevent the development of chronic prostatitis [34]. Chronic prostatitis is difficult to eradicate. It may respond to protracted courses of TMP-SMX, and 12 weeks of the dose regimens just cited have been used [16]. The oral fluoroquinolones also are used in this setting and are preferred by some clinicians. (See Chaps. 12 and 28S.)
      f. **Catheter-acquired UTI in women.** In women who undergo short-term Foley catheterization complicated by bacteriuria, for susceptible pathogens, a single dose of two DS TMP-SMX tablets was as effective as 10 days of therapy (one DS tablet bid) for asymptomatic bacteriuria in patients younger than 65 years [35]. In men and older women, a more conventional course of therapy is advised. See Chap. 12.

---

*Each 5-ml ampule usually is added to 125 ml of 5% dextrose in water by the pharmacy for intravenous administration. In some patients, this may represent a significant fluid load. The package insert suggests for patients on fluid restriction, each ampule may be added to 75 ml of 5% dextrose in water. (Also, the daily dose can be divided up into a q6h regimen rather than the q12h regimen. Supplemental diuretics may be needed in some patients.)

Table 28K-1. Pediatric dosages of TMP-SMX for UTI, otitis media, shigellosis, and the like[a] (pediatric suspension)

Weight		Dose—q12h	
lb	kg	Teaspoonsful	Tablets
22	10	1 tsp. (5 ml)	—
44	20	2 tsp. (10 ml)	1 tablet[b]
66	30	3 tsp. (15 ml)	1½ tablets
88	40	4 tsp. (20 ml)	2 tablets or 1 DS tablet

DS = double-strength
[a]For children 2 months of age or older.
[b]*Authors' note:* tablet = single-strength.
Source: Copyright *Physicians' Desk Reference* 1996 (50th ed.), published by Medical Economics Data, Montvale, NJ 07645. Reprinted by permission. All rights reserved.

2. **Respiratory tract infections**
   a. *P. carinii* **pneumonia.** Dosages are discussed in detail in Chap. 24.
   b. **Acute exacerbation of chronic bronchitis.** The equivalent of two regular tablets q12h for 7–10 days is suggested in adults.
   c. **Pneumonia.** For pneumonia infections, initially intravenous therapy can be used at 8–10 mg/kg/day (based on the TMP component) in divided doses q6h. After the patient improves, oral therapy can be used, often using the dosage for bronchitis.
   d. **Acute otitis media.** In children older than 2 months, the usual dose for otitis media is TMP, 8 mg/kg/day, and SMX, 40 mg/kg/day. The dose is given in two divided doses q12h for 10 days. A cherry-flavored oral suspension containing the equivalent of 40 mg TMP and 200 mg SMX in each 5 ml (teaspoonful) is available (Table 28K-1).
   e. **Sinusitis.** In adults, two regular tablets or one DS tablet of TMP-SMX bid for 10–14 days has commonly been used. In children, the dose for otitis media can be used. In a recent report, in adult patients with acute maxillary sinusitis, a 3-day course of TMP-SMX appeared as effective as a 10-day course [36]. See related discussion in Chap. 7.
3. **Gastrointestinal infections**
   a. **For** known susceptible *Salmonella* **and** *Shigella* **infections.** Oral or intravenous dosages recommended for acute UTI (see sec. **1.**) are used for 5 days.
   b. **For travelers' diarrhea,** various regimens have been used. One DS tablet bid for 3 days is effective in adults. A single dose of TMP-SMX (two DS tablets) and loperamide HCl (4-mg loading dose and 2-mg dose after each stool, up to 8 doses per day for a maximum of 2 days) is also effective, as is the combination of one DS tablet of TMP-SMX bid for 3 days and loperamide [21, 22].
4. **Meningitis.** If indicated, 10 mg/kg/day (based on the TMP component) IV divided q6h has been suggested in adults [23].
5. For **bacteremias** and **nosocomial infections** requiring intravenous therapy, 8–10 mg/kg/day (based on the TMP component) can be used. The dose can be divided into q6h or q12h schedule until the patient improves enough to allow oral therapy. For dosages in other unusual infections or when TMP-SMX represents alternative therapy, infectious disease consultation is advised. Also see the discussion by Remington [33].
6. **In renal failure,** a reduced dosage should be used, as shown in Table 28K-2.
7. **Pregnancy.** TMP-SMX is a category C drug. See Chap. 28A. It is generally **not recommended** for use in pregnancy unless the benefits justify the risk to the fetus [5]. See sec. **G.4.**
8. **Nursing mothers.** Because sulfonamides are excreted in human milk and may cause kernicterus, the package insert does not advise the use of TMP-SMX for nursing mothers. See sec. **G.4.**
9. **Dialysis.** Hemodialysis effectively removes TMP-SMX. Ideally, serum levels should be monitored in this setting. (See Table 28K-2.) Adult patients needing chronic peritoneal dialysis can receive the equivalent of one DS tablet of TMP-SMX q48h [5].

Table 28K-2. Dosages of TMP-SMX in renal failure

Creatinine clearance (ml/min)	Recommended dosage regimen
>30	Usual standard regimen
15–30	Half the usual regimen
<15	Use not recommended*

*If TMP-SMX is the agent of choice and no antibiotic alternatives are available and the creatinine clearance is 15 ml/min or less, *serum levels ideally should be monitored if this agent is used.* After an initial normal loading dose has been administered, subsequent total doses per 24 hours can be administered as a percent of the loading dose that equals the percent of renal function [10]. This dose can be given once daily or divided and given q12h. Patients who undergo hemodialysis should receive a normal loading dose after each dialysis procedure and a repeated fractional dose as necessary q24h between dialysis on the basis of peak and trough drug concentrations [10]. Infectious disease consultation is advised for use of this agent in patients with creatinine clearances of less than 15 ml/min.
Source: Copyright *Physicians' Desk Reference* 1996 (50th ed.), published by Medical Economics Data, Montvale, NJ. Reprinted by permission. All rights reserved.

   10. In significant **hepatic failure,** TMP-SMX should be avoided.
   11. **Serum monitoring** usually is not available or needed. In patients receiving high-dose therapy for PCP, pharmacokinetic monitoring of TMP concentrations may help reduce side effects, including myelosuppression. However, it may be difficult to obtain serum levels of TMP. See detailed discussion in Chap. 24.
G. **Toxicity and side effects.** This combination usually is well tolerated, even for prolonged periods. Reactions can occur either to the TMP (see Chap. 28L) or, more commonly, to the sulfonamide component (see sec. **I.E**). Adverse reactions have been reviewed [37]. **In patients with AIDS, drug toxicity** (rash, fever, neutropenia, thrombocytopenia, and transaminase elevation) **occurs more frequently,** but dose reduction and the use of corticosteroids, commonly used in PCP, may help reduce these reactions. See detailed discussion in Chap. 24. **In non-AIDS patients:**
   1. **Mild GI symptoms,** including nausea, vomiting, diarrhea, cramps, and similar symptoms, occur in 3–3.5% of patients [37] and are the most frequent adverse effects [9a].
   2. **Skin rashes** are relatively common, occurring in 3.5% (or more) of patients [8]. They are usually typical drug eruptions with a diffuse maculopapular rash or mild toxic erythema. Most rashes are benign and resolve with discontinuation of therapy. However, exfoliative dermatitis, Stevens-Johnson syndrome, or toxic epidermal necrolysis occur rarely. See Chap. 24 for a discussion of the increased frequency of rashes in AIDS patients receiving TMP-SMX.
   3. **Bone marrow.** Except for bone marrow transplant recipients in whom engraftment may be delayed, occasionally in pediatric patients, and in AIDS patients, severe hematologic reactions to TMP-SMX are rare [37].
      Thrombocytopenia can occur as with sulfonamide use. Although neutropenia has been attributed to TMP-SMX, the precise relationship to drug therapy is difficult to determine, as neutropenia (1) is common in randomly sampled young children (controls); (2) is seen with viral illnesses for which the patient, especially children, may receive antibiotics; and (3) in reviews has been seen with similar frequency in patients receiving amoxicillin therapy. Further studies are necessary to clarify this question. If neutropenia occurs in a patient receiving TMP-SMX, it is prudent to discontinue the TMP-SMX and use an alternative agent.
      Megalobastic bone marrow changes are uncommon except in those patients with preexisting depleted folate stores (e.g., alcoholics, the elderly, pregnant women, malnourished patients, and patients receiving phenytoin). It has been suggested that concomitant administration of folinic acid will reverse the antifolate effects of TMP-SMX, especially in patients not infected with HIV [10], without interfering with its antimicrobial effect [8]. (See sec. **VI.B.3** in Chap. 28L.) In a recent report, adjunctive folinic acid with TMP-SMX for PCP in AIDS patients was associated with an increased risk of therapeutic failure and death [38]. Therefore, empiric addition of folinic acid in this setting is not advised [38]. See Chap. 24.

Rarely, in patients with G-6-PD deficiency, hemolysis may be precipitated with TMP-SMX use (see sec. **I.E.2**). However, in one study, G-6-PD-deficient patients who received TMP-SMX did not have hemolytic reactions during therapy [6]. In patients with AIDS who receive TMP-SMX for PCP, dose reduction may help reduce bone marrow suppression (see Chap. 24).

4. **Potential for teratogenesis and kernicterus.** Because of the teratogenic effect seen in animal studies, **TMP-SMX is generally contraindicated in pregnant [5] or lactating women.** Furthermore, because the sulfonamide component displaces bilirubin from albumin-binding sites and may therefore increase the risk of kernicterus, **TMP-SMX is contraindicated in infants younger than 2 months and during lactation and pregnancy, especially at term.**

5. **Drug-drug interactions.** The sulfonamide-related interactions are reviewed in sec. **I.F.** and include interactions with oral anticoagulants and oral hypoglycemic agents. We try to avoid using sulfonamides, including TMP-SMX, in patients receiving warfarin. If TMP-SMX is used, serial prothrombin times should be monitored and, typically, the dose of warfarin should be reduced. TMP-SMX may prolong the half-life of phenytoin.

   One article emphasizes that coadministration of TMP-SMX and methotrexate (MTX) in children with leukemia may be associated with decreased renal clearance of free MTX and, therefore, a significant increase in systemic exposure to MTX and excess myelotoxicity [39]. (See related discussion in sec. **I.F.2.**)

6. **Nephrotoxicity** does not appear to be a significant side effect, particularly in patients with initially normal renal function [8].

7. Intrahepatic cholestasis rarely occurs [40]. Hepatitis can occur [41].

8. **Local thrombophlebitis** uncommonly occurs with IV administration.

9. **Acquisition of resistance** is discussed in Chap. 28L.

10. **Fever** can be seen as an adverse reaction [42] (see Chap. 1).

11. **Hyperkalemia** can occur in patients with AIDS during treatment for PCP with TMP-SMX. This is discussed in Chap. 28L, sec. **VI.B.2.**

H. Cost. See Tables 28A-5 and 28A-6.

III. Fansidar is a combination of pyrimethamine, a folate antagonist, and sulfadoxine, a long-acting sulfonamide. It has been used for malarial prophylaxis. See Chap. 21.

References

1. Medical Letter. The choice of antibacterial drugs. *Med. Lett. Drugs Ther.* 38:25, 1996.
2. Gruenberg, R.N. Antibiotic sensitivities of urinary pathogens, 1971–1982. *J. Antimicrob. Chemother.* 14:17, 1984.
   For updates, see W.E. Stamm et al., Urinary tract infections: From pathogenesis to treatment. J. Infect. Dis. 159:400, 1989; and W.E. Stamm and T.M. Hooton, Management of urinary tract infections in adults. N. Engl. J. Med. 329:1328, 1993.
3. Buckwold, F.J., et al. Therapy for acute cystitis in adult women. *J.A.M.A.* 247:1839, 1982.
4. Sarosi, G.A., et al. Treatment of fungal diseases. *Am. Rev. Respir. Dis.* 120:1393, 1979. *See also Chap. 18.*
5. Zinner, S.H., and Mayer, K.H. Sulfonamides and Trimethoprim. In G.L. Mandell, J.E. Bennett, and R. Dolin (eds.), *Principles and Practice of Infectious Diseases* (4th ed.). New York: Churchill Livingstone, 1994. Pp. 354–364.
   For a similar textbook discussion, see R.A. Gleckman and J.S. Czachor, Trimethoprim-Sulfamethoxazole. In S.L. Gorbach, J.G. Bartlett, and N.R. Blacklow (eds.), Infectious Diseases. Philadelphia: Saunders, 1992. Pp. 239–244.
6. Markowitz, N., and Saravolatz, L.D. Use of trimethoprim-sulfamethoxazole in a glucose-6-phosphate dehydrogenase-deficient population. *Rev. Infect. Dis.* 9:S218, 1987.
7. Bennett, W.M., et al. *Drug Prescribing in Renal Failure: Dosing Guidelines for Adults* (3rd ed.). Philadelphia: American College of Physicians, 1994.
   A useful handbook. Similar tables for dosing in renal failure appear in S.K. Swan and W.M. Bennett, Drug dosing guidelines in patients with renal failure. West. J. Med. 156:633, 1992.
8. Rubin, R.H., and Swartz, M.N. Trimethoprim-sulfamethoxazole. *N. Engl. J. Med.* 303:426, 1980.
9. Foltzer, M.A., and Reese, R.E. Trimethoprim-sulfamethoxazole and other sulfonamides. *Med. Clin. North Am.* 71(6):1177, 1987.

9a. Lundstrom, T.S., and Sobel, J.D. Vancomycin, trimethoprim-sulfamethoxazole, and rifampin. *Infect. Dis. Clin. North Am.* 9:747, 1995.

10. Cockerill, F.R., and Edson, R.S. Trimethoprim-sulfamethoxazole. *Mayo Clin. Proc.* 66:1260, 1991.

10a. Hofman, J., et al. The prevalence of drug-resistant *Streptococcus pneumoniae* in Atlanta. *N. Engl. J. Med.* 333:481, 1995.
    See related discussion in Chap 28C.

11. Rein, M.F., et al. Sulfamethoxazole-trimethoprim synergism for *Neisseria gonorrhoeae. Antimicrob. Agents Chemother.* 17:247, 1980.
    The 1:20 ratio achieved in the serum after oral TMP-SMX is minimally synergistic and sometimes antagonistic for gonococci.

11a. Sands, M., et al. Trimethoprim-sulfamethoxazole therapy of *Pasteurella multocida* infection. *J. Infect. Dis.* 160:354, 1989.
    In vitro activity suggests TMP-SMX may be a reasonable alternative agent for those who cannot take penicillin, cefuroxime, or tetracycline.

12. Wust, J., and Wilkins, T.D. Susceptibility of anaerobic bacteria to sulfamethoxazole-trimethoprim and routine susceptibility testing. *Antimicrob. Agents Chemother.* 14:384, 1978.

12a. Huovinen, P., et al. Trimethoprim and sulfonamide resistance. *Antimicrob. Agents Chemother.* 39:279, 1995.

13. Stamm, W.E., et al. Acute renal infection in women. Treatment with trimethoprim-sulfamethoxazole or ampicillin for two or six weeks. *Ann. Intern. Med.* 106:341, 1987.
    See editorial comment in same issue. See related articles by W.E. Stamm and T.M. Hooton, Management of urinary tract infections in adults. N. Engl. J. Med. 329:1328, 1993; and C.M. Kunin, Urinary tract infections in females. Clin. Infect. Dis. 18:1, 1994, as well as discussions in Chap. 12.

14. Johnson, J., et al. Therapy for women hospitalized with acute pyelonephritis. A randomized trial of ampicillin versus trimethoprim-sulfamethoxazole for 14 days. *J. Infect. Dis.* 163:325, 1991.
    All patients initially received gentamicin.

15. Stamm, W.E., et al. Antimicrobial prophylaxis of recurrent urinary tract infections. *Ann. Intern. Med.* 92:770, 1980.
    Still a classic reference on this topic. For updates, see L.E. Nicolle and A.R. Arkey, Recurrent urinary tract infections in adult women: Diagnosis and treatment. Infect. Dis. Clin. North Am. 1:793, 1987; and articles cited in the annotation for reference [13].

16. Smith, J.W., et al. Recurrent urinary tract infections in men: Characteristics and response to therapy. *Ann. Intern. Med.* 91:544, 1980.
    Emphasizes the importance of the prostate as the source of relapsing urinary tract infections in men. In prostatitis, prolonged courses of therapy (12 weeks) with trimethoprim-sulfamethoxazole result in higher cure rates than conventional 10-day courses.
        For an update, see B.A. Lipsky et al., Urinary tract infections in men. Epidemiology, diagnosis, and treatment. Ann. Intern. Med. 110:138, 1989.

17. Stapleton, A., et al. Postcoital antimicrobial prophylaxis for recurrent urinary tract infection. A randomized, double-blind, placebo-controlled trial. *J.A.M.A.* 264:703, 1990.
    The dose of postcoital TMP-SMX used was half a regular-strength tablet (i.e., 40 mg TMP–200 mg SMX).

18. Medical Letter. Drugs for parasitic infection. *Med. Lett. Drugs Ther.* 37:99, 1995.

19. Pines, A. Trimethoprim-sulfamethoxazole in the treatment and prevention of purulent exacerbations of chronic bronchitis. *J. Infect. Dis.* 128(Suppl.):S-706, 1973.
    For a related review, see D.T. Hughes and N.J. Russell, the use of trimethoprim-sulfamethoxazole in the treatment of chest infections. Rev. Infect. Dis. 4:528, 1982. Reviews some of the studies showing TMP-SMX is effective treatment for exacerbations of chronic bronchitis. For related discussion, see Chap. 7.

20. Medical Letter. Drugs for the treatment of acute otitis media in children. *Med. Lett. Drugs Ther.* 36:19, 1994.
    Although amoxicillin still is viewed as the drug of choice for initial empiric therapy, TMP-SMX is a useful alternative agent. See related discussions in Chap. 7.

21. Ericsson, C.D., et al. Treatment of traveler's diarrhea with sulfamethoxazole and trimethoprim and loperamide. *J.A.M.A.* 263:257, 1990.

22. Dupont, H.L. The 10 most common questions about travelers' diarrhea. *Infect. Dis. Clin. Pract.* 1:396, 1992.
    Practical summary. TMP-SMX still useful in areas where TMP resistance in bacterial enteropathogens is uncommon (such as the noncoastal interior of Mexico during the

rainy summer). Where TMP resistance is more common (e.g., South America, southern Asia, and northern Africa, and during the drier winter in virtually all areas), the fluoroquinolones are preferred in adults. A 3-day course of therapy is adequate.

23. Levitz, A.E., and Quintiliani, R. Trimethoprim-sulfamethoxazole for bacterial meningitis. *Ann. Intern. Med.* 100:881, 1984.

24. Spitzer, P.G., et al. Treatment of *Listeria monocytogenes* infection with trimethoprim-sulfamethoxazole: Case report and review of the literature. *Rev. Infect. Dis.* 8:427, 1986.

25. Gurwith, M.J., et al. A prospective controlled investigation of prophylactic trimethoprim-sulfamethoxazole in hospitalized granulocytopenic patients. *Am. J. Med.* 66:248, 1979.

26. Bow, E.J., et al. Randomized controlled trial comparing trimethoprim/sulfamethoxazole and trimethoprim for infection prophylaxis in hospitalized granulocytopenic patients. *Am. J. Med.* 76:223, 1984.
TMP-SMX itself may predispose toward an increased risk of infection by prolonging myelosuppression.

27. Ward, T.T., et al. Trimethoprim-sulfamethoxazole prophylaxis in granulocytopenic patients with acute leukemia: Evaluation of serum antibiotic levels in a randomized, double-blind, placebo-controlled Department of Veterans Affairs cooperative study. *Clin. Infect. Dis.* 17:323, 1993.
One of the few well-designed studies examining this problem. See thoughtful editorial response in this same issue by E.J. Bow and A.R. Ronald, who concur that TMP-SMX prophylaxis probably is not beneficial and further studies are needed with the fluoroquinolones.

28. Street, A.C., and Durack, D.T. Experience with trimethoprim-sulfamethoxazole in the treatment of infective endocarditis. *Rev. Infect. Dis.* 10:915, 1988.

29. Markowitz, N., et al. Trimethoprim-sulfamethoxazole compared with vancomycin for the treatment of *Staphylococcus aureus* infection. *Ann. Intern. Med.* 117:390, 1992.
Vancomycin was superior to TMP-SMX in efficacy in intravenous drug users with staphylococcal infections, but TMP-SMX is an alternative agent, especially for susceptible methicillin-resistant S. aureus.

30. Fox, B.C., et al. A prospective, randomized, double-blind study of trimethoprim-sulfamethoxazole for prophylaxis of infection in renal transplantation: Clinical efficacy, absorption of trimethoprim-sulfamethoxazole, effects on microflora, and the cost-benefit of prophylaxis. *Am. J. Med.* 89:225, 1990.
During the hospitalization after the transplantation surgery, 160 mg TMP and 800 mg SMX bid was given if creatinine clearance exceeded 30 ml/min. After discharge, a single daily dose of 160 mg TMP and 800 mg SMX was used. (If creatinine clearance was <30 ml/min, one-half the usual dose per day was used.)
For a related article emphasizing the lack of side effects with TMP-SMX prophylaxis and lack of nephrotoxicity in cyclosporine recipients, see D.G. Maki et al., J. Lab. Clin. Med. 119:11, 1992. Also see M.A. Lew et al., Ciprofloxacin versus TMP-SMX for prophylaxis of bacterial infections in bone marrow transplants. J. Clin. Oncol. 13: 239, 1995.

31. Margolis, D.M., et al. Trimethoprim-sulfamethoxazole prophylaxis in the management of chronic granulomatous disease. *J. Infect. Dis.* 162:723, 1990.

32. Singh, N., et al. Trimethoprim-sulfamethoxazole for the prevention of spontaneous bacterial peritonitis in cirrhosis: A randomized trial. *Ann. Intern. Med.* 122:595, 1995.

33. Remington, J.S. Update and advances in intravenous therapy with trimethoprim-sulfamethoxazole: Summary of a symposium. *Rev. Infect. Dis.* 9(Suppl. 2):S153, 1987.
Summary of this symposium on intravenous use of TMP-SMX.

34. Meares, E.M., Jr. Prostatitis. *Med. Clin. North. Am.* 75:405, 1991.
See detailed discussion of prostatitis in Chap. 12.

35. Harding, G.K., et al. How long should catheter-acquired urinary tract infection be treated? A randomized controlled study. *Ann. Intern. Med.* 114:713, 1991.

36. Williams, J.W., et al. Randomized controlled trial of 3 versus 10 days of trimethoprim-sulfamethoxazole for acute maxillary sinusitis. *J.A.M.A.* 273:1015, 1994.
The daily dose of TMP-SMX was one double-strength tablet bid. Eighty patients, median age of 48, were involved and clinically assessed 2 weeks after completion of antibiotics.

37. Gutman, L.T. The use of trimethoprim-sulfamethoxazole in children. A review of adverse reactions and indications. *Pediatr. Infect. Dis. J.* 3:349, 1984.

38. Safrin, S., Lee, B.L., and Sande, M.A. Adjunctive folinic acid with trimethoprim-

sulfamethoxazole for *Pneumocystis carinii* in AIDS patients is associated with an increased risk of therapeutic failure and death. *J. Infect. Dis.* 170:912, 1994.
39. Ferrazzini, G., et al. Interaction between trimethoprim-sulfamethoxazole and methotrexate in children with leukemia. *J. Pediatr.* 117:823, 1990.
40. Nair, S.S., et al. Trimethoprim-sulfamethoxazole-induced intrahepatic cholestasis. *Ann. Intern. Med.* 92:511, 1980.
    See related paper by I. Altraif et al., Cholestatic liver disease with ductopenia after administration of clindamycin and trimethoprim-sulfamethoxazole. Am. J. Gastroenterol. 89:1230, 1994.
41. Carson, J. L., et al. Acute liver disease associated with erythromycins, sulfonamides, and tetracyclines. *Ann. Intern. Med.* 119:576, 1993.
    Hepatitis associated with sulfonamides may be associated with fever, rash, and eosinophilia, suggesting hypersensitivity.
42. Boyce, T.G., et al. Fever as an adverse reaction to oral trimethoprim-sulfamethoxazole. *Pediatr. Infect. Dis. J.* 11:772, 1992.

L. Trimethoprim

Trimethoprim (TMP, Proloprim, Trimpex) not in combination with sulfamethoxazole (SMX) is available and is approved for use in uncomplicated urinary tract infections (UTIs) [1, 2].

I. **Mechanism of action.** By inhibiting dihydrofolate reductase, TMP interferes with the production of tetrahydrofolic acid in bacterial cells (see Fig. 28K-1).

II. **Spectrum of activity.** TMP is active and bactericidal against many gram-positive aerobic cocci and most gram-negative bacteria, except *Pseudomonas aeruginosa* and other *Pseudomonas* spp. [2a]. Enterococci usually are resistant. It is active against common urinary tract pathogens such as *Escherichia coli, Proteus mirabilis, Klebsiella pneumoniae*, and *Enterobacter* spp. Therefore, its spectrum of activity is very similar to that of the TMP-SMX combination. Most anaerobes are resistant [2].

III. **Pharmacokinetics.** TMP is well absorbed from the GI tract. The drug is excreted primarily unchanged by the kidneys, and urine concentrations are considerably higher than those in the blood. TMP penetrates prostatic and vaginal secretions well [2a]. TMP achieves high tissue levels in the kidney [2a]. Dosage must be altered in renal failure. TMP is excreted in breast milk. This drug increases the half-life of phenytoin.

IV. **Current clinical uses**
   A. **Acute, uncomplicated UTI.** The drug is approved for use in this setting. However, there are no data to indicate that this agent alone is any more effective in UTI than is TMP-SMX [1].
   B. **Recurrent UTI suppression.** TMP has been used in suppressive regimens for recurrent UTI in women [3]. The urine should be initially sterilized before chronic suppressive therapy is started.
   C. **Prostatitis.** Because TMP penetrates the prostate and is active against common urinary pathogens, it has been used successfully in regimens for both acute and chronic prostatitis [4], especially in the sulfa-allergic patient. TMP-SMX and the oral fluoroquinolones are alternative agents in this setting.
   D. TMP has been effective in the treatment of **travelers' diarrhea** [5]. See Chap. 21.
   E. TMP alone cannot be substituted for the combination of TMP-SMX in the therapy for *Pneumocystis carinii* infections. For this purpose, a combination of **dapsone and TMP** is required, and this **combination is effective for mild to moderate *P. carinii* pneumonia** in patients with AIDS [6–8]. This therapeutic combination is reviewed in detail in Chap. 24.

V. **Dosage**
   A. **Oral.** TMP is available only as an oral agent, in the form of scored 100-mg and 200-mg tablets. The effectiveness of TMP as a single agent in children younger than 12 years has not been established. The safety of TMP in infants younger than 2 months has not been demonstrated.
      1. **For acute, uncomplicated UTI.** The usual adult dose is 100 mg q12h or 200 mg q24h for 10 days. Also, 100 mg q12h for 3 days has been used.
      2. **For recurrent UTI suppression** therapy in women, 100 mg at bedtime has been used.

3. For single-dose therapy in uncomplicated UTI in women, 400 mg has been used. However, in one report, a significant number (29%) of women failed this regimen so that retreatment was common [9]. Consequently, the anticipated advantages of single-dose therapy (i.e., lower costs, convenience of administration, fewer adverse effects) were offset by the costs and inconvenience of retreatment. The authors suggest that a 3-day dose regimen is preferred over a single-dose regimen [9].

4. **For prostatitis,** 100 mg q12h or 200 mg q24h has been given for 4–12 weeks in patients allergic to sulfa in whom TMP-SMX could not be given. The oral fluoroquinolones are other alternatives.

5. **For travelers' diarrhea,** 100 mg bid for 3–5 days has been used. A 3-day course usually is adequate.

6. **For *P. carinii* pneumonia,** TMP and dapsone dosages are discussed in Chap. 24. See also Medina and colleagues [7] and the *Medical Letter* [8].

B. **In renal failure,** if the creatinine clearance is 15–30 ml/min, the dose should be reduced to 50 mg q12h. In the package insert, TMP is not recommended if the creatinine clearance is less than 15 ml/min.

C. **Pregnancy.** TMP is a category C agent (see Chap. 28A) and should be used during pregnancy only if the potential benefit justifies the potential risk to the fetus. See sec. **VI.B.4.**

D. **Nursing mothers.** TMP is excreted in human milk. Because TMP may interfere with folic acid metabolism, the package insert suggests caution should be exercised when TMP is administered to a nursing woman. See sec. **VI.B.4.**

VI. **Potential problems and adverse effects**

A. **Resistance to TMP.** There is concern that if TMP is used alone and, particularly, if use is prolonged, resistance may develop. Resistance to TMP in individual patients is not reported when TMP has been used for short periods. However, the global prevalence of TMP-resistant bacteria has increased in recent years [2a]. This is important, as resistance to TMP governs resistance to TMP-SMX. For example, from 1978 to 1981, *E. coli* resistance to TMP rose from 2 to 6% in Boston, from 8 to 30% in Paris, and to even higher rates (40%) in developing countries [10]. The liberal use of TMP-SMX for both veterinary and human disorders has been implicated.

In one report, children in daycare centers frequently were colonized with trimethoprim-resistant *E. coli,* and transmission of these *E. coli* among children within daycare centers and from children to household members is common [11].

In countries in which TMP-resistant bacterial enteric pathogens are common, an agent other than TMP-SMX will be necessary for effective therapy of travelers' diarrhea [12]. Resistance rates of gram-negative pathogens in developing countries have been reported to be clearly higher than those in the developed world. TMP resistance has been reported at high levels of 25–68% in South America, Asia, and Africa [12a]. In some developing countries, antibiotics may be more available without prescription and TMP may be used more often as monotherapy. Resistance to *Salmonella typhi* is worldwide. Also, resistance to TMP has become more common with *Shigella* spp., MRSA, and recently *S. pneumoniae* [2a].

B. **Adverse effects.** TMP is well tolerated.

1. **Skin rashes** have been noted in approximately 3% of patients, compared to 6% of patients receiving TMP-SMX [1]. Anaphylaxis has been described after TMP use [13]. In someone with a delayed diffuse rash from TMP-SMX, it may be reasonable to use TMP alone in the future as sulfonamides cause rashes more commonly. If someone had an immediate allergic reaction to TMP-SMX, we would avoid both TMP and sulfonamides in the future.

2. **Hyperkalemia** is seen commonly in patients with AIDS who are treated with high doses of TMP-SMX or TMP and dapsone for *P. carinii* pneumonia. TMP is a sodium-channel inhibitor and functions as a potassium-sparing diuretic agent [14, 15]. Hyperkalemia can be seen in hospitalized patients without AIDS [15a].

3. **Bone marrow effects.** The drug may interfere with folic acid metabolism, particularly in the folate-deficient patient [1]. Megaloblastic anemia, neutropenia, and thrombocytopenia have been described with prolonged use. The administration of folinic acid (e.g., 10 mg PO daily in adults) prevents or treats this effectively, but folinic acid is expensive. Prior reviews suggest that antibacterial activity is not impaired by folinic acid, except possibly against enterococci. However, because one report suggests adjunctive folinic acid with

TMP-SMX for *P. carinii* pneumonia in AIDS patients is associated with an increased risk of therapeutic failure and death [16], we do not add folinic acid in other regimens (e.g., TMP and dapsone for *P. carinii* pneumonia). See related discussion in Chap. 28K, sec. **II.G.3.** See Chap. 24.

4. Teratogenicity of TMP in humans has not been clearly established. **It seems prudent to use an alternate agent in pregnancy and nursing women** [2].

5. Abnormal liver function tests can occur [17].

C. Cost. See Table 28A-5.

VII. Summary. In the treatment of acute uncomplicated UTI, TMP alone offers no significant advantage over other agents. In the penicillin-, ampicillin-, or sulfa-allergic patient, TMP is a reasonable alternative. The role TMP will play in the treatment of prostatitis has yet to be defined as its protracted use in this setting may be associated with the acquisition of resistant organisms. TMP and dapsone have been used as alternative therapy in *P. carinii* pneumonia.

References

1. Medical Letter. Trimethoprim. *Med. Lett. Drugs Ther.* 22:69, 1980.
2. Zinner, S.H., and Mayer, K.H. Sulfonamides and Trimethoprim. In G.L. Mandell, J.E. Bennett and R. Dolin (eds.), *Principles and Practice of Infectious Diseases* (4th ed.). New York: Churchill Livingstone, 1995. Pp. 354–364.
2a. Lundstrom, T.S., and Sobel, J.D. Vancomycin, trimethoprim-sulfamethoxazole, and rifampin. *Infect. Dis. Clin. North Am.* 9:747, 1995.
3. Nicolle, L.E., and Ronald, A.R. Recurrent urinary tract infection in adult women: Diagnosis and treatment. *Infect. Dis. Clin. North Am.* 1:793, 1987.
4. Lipsky, B.A. Urinary tract infections in man. Epidemiology, pathophysiology, diagnosis and treatment. *Ann. Intern. Med.* 110:138, 1989.
5. Dupont, H.L., et al. Treatment of traveler's diarrhea with trimethoprim/sulfamethoxazole and with trimethoprim alone. *N. Engl. J. Med.* 30:841, 1982.
6. Leoung, G.S., et al. Dapsone-trimethoprim for *Pneumocystis carinii* pneumonia in the acquired immunodeficiency syndrome. *Ann. Intern. Med.* 105:45, 1986.
7. Medina, I., et al. Oral therapy for *Pneumocystis carinii* pneumonia in the acquired immunodeficiency syndrome. A controlled trial of trimethoprim-sulfamethoxazole versus trimethoprim-dapsone. *N. Engl. J. Med.* 323:776, 1990.
   This study showed that in patients with AIDS, oral therapy with TMP-SMX or TMP (20 mg/kg/day) and dapsone (100 mg/day) are equally effective for mild to moderate first episodes, but there are fewer serious side effects with the TMP-dapsone. See detailed discussion in Chap. 24.
8. Medical Letter. Drugs for parasite infection. *Med. Lett. Drugs Ther.* 37:99, 1995.
   TMP (5 mg/kg PO tid × 21 days) and dapsone (100 mg PO daily × 21 days) is listed as an alternative regimen for Pneumocystis carinii pneumonia therapy. See Chap. 24 for details.
9. Österberg, E., et al. Efficacy of single-dose versus seven-day trimethoprim treatment of cystitis in women: A randomized double-blind study. *J. Infect. Dis.* 161:942, 1990.
   In this study from Sweden, accumulated efficacy was 71% for single-dose and 87% for 7-day therapy in more than 300 patients. In a related study in children 2–16 years of age, single-dose TMP versus 7 days of TMP-SMX revealed that the single-dose TMP cleared the bacteria, but the risk of asymptomatic bacteria soon after treatment was high. See T. Nolan et al., Single-dose trimethoprim for urinary tract infection. Arch. Dis. Child. 64:581, 1989.
10. Goldstein, F.W., et al. The changing pattern of trimethoprim resistance in Paris, with a review of worldwide experience. *Rev. Infect. Dis.* 8:725, 1986.
    See C. Jansson et al., Trimethoprim resistance arising in animal bacteria and transferring into human pathogens. J. Infect. Dis. 167:785, 1993.
11. Fornasini, M., et al. Trimethoprim-resistant *Escherichia coli* in households of children attending day care centers. *J. Infect. Dis.* 166:326, 1992.
12. Dupont, H.L. The 10 most common questions about travelers' diarrhea. *Infect. Dis. Clin. Pract.* 1:396, 1992.
    Practical summary by a national expert. Emphasizes that for areas of the world where TMP-resistant enteric pathogens are uncommon (e.g., the noncoastal interior of Mexico during the rainy summer), TMP-SMX is effective. Where TMP resistance is more common (e.g., South America, southern Asia, and northern Africa, and during the drier winter in virtually all areas), the fluoroquinolones are preferred in adults. A 3-day course of therapy is adequate).
12a. Huovinen, P., et al. Trimethoprim and sulfonamide resistance. *Antimicrob. Agents*

Chemother. 39:279, 1995.

13. Alonso, M.D., et al. Hypersensitivity to trimethoprim. *Allergy* 47:340, 1992.
14. Choi, M.J., et al. Brief report: Trimethoprim-induced hyperkalemia in a patient with AIDS. *N. Engl. J. Med.* 328:703, 1993.
15. Velazquez, H., et al. Renal mechanism of trimethoprim-induced hyperkalemia. *Ann. Intern. Med.* 119:296, 1993.
15a. Alappan, R., et al. Hyperkalemia in hospitalized patients treated with trimethoprim-sulfamethoxazole. *Ann. Intern. Med.* 124:316, 1996.
16. Safrin, S., Lee, B.L., and Sande, M.A. Adjunctive folinic acid with trimethoprim-sulfamethoxazole for *Pneumocystis carinii* in AIDS patients is associated with an increased risk of therapeutic failure and death. *J. Infect. Dis.* 170:912, 1994.
17. Lindgren, A., and Olsson, R. Liver reactions from trimethoprim. *J. Intern. Med.* 236:281, 1994.

M. Erythromycin, Azithromycin, Clarithromycin, and Dirithromycin

Erythromycin

Erythromycin, a macrolide, has a chemical structure different from that of the cephalosporin or penicillin derivatives. Oral erythromycin is believed to be **one of the safest antibiotics in clinical use** [1, 2]. Erythromycin and the new macrolides inhibit protein synthesis by reversible binding to the 50 S ribosomal subunits of susceptible organisms [2]. Although it usually is considered a bacteriostatic agent, in high concentrations and against a low inoculum of bacteria it may be bactericidal. The *Medical Letter* lists erythromycin as a drug of first choice for several organisms and an alternative agent for several other pathogens [3, 4].

I. **Spectrum of activity.** Erythromycin is a broad-spectrum agent in that it is active against gram-positive and gram-negative bacteria, mycoplasmas, chlamydiae, treponemas, and rickettsiae (Table 28M-1).

A. **Bacteria**
1. **Aerobes**
   a. **Gram-positive organisms.** Erythromycin is active against and is an alternative agent for groups A, B, C, and G streptococci as well as *Streptococcus pneumoniae*. *S. pneumoniae* resistant to penicillin are often also resistant to erythromycin and other macrolide antibiotics; strains resistant to one macrolide are typically resistant to all macrolides [4a, 4b]. See related discussion in Chap. 28C. It is active against most group A streptococci isolated in the United States. Resistance in the United States is not as common as it is in some countries (e.g., Finland, where 5–45% or more of group A streptococci may be resistant [5]). However, in recent years the incidence of group A streptococci resistant to erythromycin in Japan has dramatically declined [6].

   Staphylococcus aureus usually is susceptible, but resistance emerges during treatment in an individual patient [1]. Interestingly, the *Medical Letter* does not list erythromycin as an alternative agent for *S. aureus* [3].

   Erythromycin is the drug of choice for *Corynebacterium diphtheriae* and is an alternative agent for *Bacillus anthracis* (anthrax) [3]. It is active against *Corynebacterium haemolyticum,* which can cause pharyngitis. High-level penicillin-resistant strains of *S. pneumoniae* are resistant to erythromycin and clarithromycin. See Chap. 28C.

   b. **Gram-negative organisms.** Erythromycin is an alternative agent for *Moraxella (Branhamella) catarrhalis*. It is an agent of first choice for *Campylobacter jejuni, Bordetella pertussis, Haemophilus ducreyi, Legionella micdadei,* and *Legionella pneumophila*. It is an alternative agent for *Eikenella corrodens*.

   Approximately 40% of H. influenzae strains are resistant to erythromycin [4]. Enterobacteriaceae (e.g., *Escherichia coli, Klebsiella* spp., *Enterobacter* spp.) are resistant.

2. **Anaerobes.** Erythromycin has activity against some species of gram-negative anaerobes, but *Bacteroides fragilis* strains and *Fusobacterium* spp. usually are resistant [1].

Table 28M-1. In vitro activity of selected macrolide antibiotics

Organism	Azithromycin, MIC_{90}	Clarithromycin, MIC_{90}	Erythromycin, MIC_{90}
Gram-positive aerobes			
Staphylococcus aureus			
Methicillin-susceptible	1.0[a]	0.12–0.25[a]	0.25–0.50
Methicillin-resistant	>128.0	>128.0	>128.0
Streptococcus pyogenes (group A)	0.12[a]	0.015[a]	0.03[a]
Streptococcus pneumoniae			
Erythromycin-susceptible			
(Penicillin-susceptible)	0.12[a]	0.015[a]	0.03–1.0[a]
Streptococcus agalactiae (group B)	0.5[a]	0.03–0.25[a]	0.03–0.25[a]
Streptococcus bovis	0.25		
Enterococci (group D)			
E. faecalis			
(Erythromycin-susceptible)	8.0		
(Erythromycin-resistant)	>64.0		
Viridans streptococci	16.0	0.03	0.06
Coagulase-negative staphylococci			
Methicillin-resistant	>128.0		
Methicillin-susceptible			
Listeria monocytogenes	4.0	0.12–2.0	0.5–2.0
Gram-negative aerobes[b]			
Haemophilus influenzae	1.0	2.0–16.0[b]	4.0–8.0
Moraxella catarrhalis	0.5	0.25–1.0	0.25–2.0
Neisseria gonorrhoeae	0.15	0.25–2.0	0.25–2.0
N. meningitidis	0.12	—	0.4–1.6
Pasteurella multocida	0.5	—	—
Bordetella pertussis	0.06	0.03	0.03
Legionella pneumophila	0.25–2.0	0.25	1.0–2.0
Campylobacter jejuni	0.12–0.5	1.0–2.0	1.0–2.0
Helicobacter pylori	0.25	0.03	0.25

Table 28M-1 (continued)

Organism	Azithromycin, MIC$_{90}$	Clarithromycin, MIC$_{90}$	Erythromycin, MIC$_{90}$
Anaerobes			
Gram-positive cocci (*Peptococcus*, *Peptostreptococcus*)	2.0	4.0->32.0	2.0->32.0
Bacteroides fragilis	8.0	2.0–8.0	4.0–32.0
Clostridium perfringens	1.0	0.5–2.0	1.0
Miscellaneous			
Chlamydia pneumoniae (formerly TWAR)	0.12–0.25–1.0	0.007	0.065–1.0
Chlamydia trachomatis	0.12–0.25	0.06–0.125	0.12–0.25
Mycoplasma pneumoniae	0.001	0.008–0.03	0.004
Borrelia burgdorferi[c]	0.015–0.04[c]	0.015	0.06–0.16[c]
Mycobacterium avium complex	32.0	4.0	64.0
M. cheloneae	—	0.25–0.5	—
M. fortuitum	0.5–2.0	0.5–2.0	8.0

[a]Erythromycin-resistant organisms will be resistant.

[b]See text.

[c]Minimum bactericidal concentration data.

Sources: Table summarized from data from H.C. Neu, Clinical microbiology of azithromycin. *Am. J. Med.* 91(Suppl. 3A):12S, 1991; A.P. Ball, Therapeutic considerations for the management of respiratory tract infections. *Infect. Med.* 8(Suppl. A):7, 1991; S.C. Piscitelli et al., Clarithromycin and azithromycin: New macrolide antibiotics. *Clin. Pharm.* 11:137, 1992; L.E. Welsh, In vitro evaluation of activities of azithromycin, erythromycin, and tetracycline against *Chlamydia trachomatis* and *Chlamydia pneumoniae. Antimicrob. Agents Chemother.* 36:291, 1992; B. Olsson-Liljequist and B.M. Hoffman, In vitro activity of clarithromycin combined with its 14-hydroxy metabolite against *Haemophilus influenzae. J. Antimicrob. Chemother.* 27(Suppl. A):11, 1991; and E. Eisenberg and M. Barza, Azithromycin and clarithromycin. *Curr. Clin. Top. Infect. Dis.* 14:52, 1994.

B. **Nonbacterial pathogens**
   1. **Mycoplasmas.** Erythromycin is very active against *Mycoplasma pneumoniae* and is a drug of choice for this pathogen as well as the drug of choice for *Ureaplasma urealyticum* [3].
   2. **Chlamydiae.** Erythromycin is active against *Chlamydia trachomatis* and *C. pneumoniae.*
   3. **Spirochetes.** Erythromycin is active against *Borrelia burgdorferi,* the causative agent in Lyme disease, and is an alternative agent for this pathogen. It also is active against *Treponema pallidum* but seldom is used for infections due to this pathogen.
II. **Pharmacokinetics** [1, 4, 7–9]
   A. **Oral absorption.** Erythromycin is acid-labile. In the stomach, it rapidly decomposes to two inactive metabolites, one of which may contribute to GI side effects. As a result of this instability and depending on the salt form, the rate of absorption may be unpredictable (35% ± 25%) [8]. Pharmaceutical preparations for oral use have been made with an aim toward diminishing destruction by gastric acid and promoting better absorption [1].
      1. Food in the stomach may decrease absorption of the drug, except in the estolate form [2] and possibly the stearate form [1].
      2. Average serum levels achieved by the different oral preparations (see sec. **IV.A**) are similar; therefore, no single oral formulation offers a clear advantage in adults [1, 4, 7]. In his review, Steigbigel [1] notes that "it would seem that in the treatment of infections of only moderate severity by organisms highly sensitive to erythromycin (*S. pneumoniae, S. pyogenes, M. pneumoniae*) differences in therapeutic results using various oral preparations will be insignificant. Limited clinical comparisons confirm that suspicion." In children, studies have suggested that erythromycin estolate has superior bioavailability over erythromycin ethylsuccinate [1, 9]. (See sec. **IV.A.1.**)
      3. Four hours after oral administration of a dose of 500 mg, peak serum concentrations are 1–2 µg/ml.
   B. **Intravenous.** Serum concentrations 1 hour after 500 mg to 1 g IV are approximately 10–15 µg/ml [2]. **Erythromycin should not be administered intramuscularly.**
      Intravenous preparations achieve appreciably higher serum levels and should be used to treat serious infections requiring erythromycin.
   C. **Half-life and excretion.** The serum half-life of erythromycin is approximately 1–2 hours, and levels persist for approximately 6 hours. Because erythromycin is excreted primarily by the liver, it must be **avoided or used carefully in patients with liver disease. Dose reduction is not necessary in mild to moderate renal failure.**
   D. **Miscellaneous**
      1. As a single agent, erythromycin provides adequate middle-ear levels against *S. pneumoniae* and *S. pyogenes* but probably not adequate to eradicate *H. influenzae* consistently [1].
      2. Erythromycin crosses the placenta, but it is not known to be teratogenic [4]. It also is excreted into breast milk [1].
      3. Limited data from patients with septic arthritis suggest that erythromycin penetrates the synovial fluid poorly [1].
      4. The very limited data available on concentrations of erythromycin achieved in the cerebrospinal fluid (CSF) of patients with meningitis suggest that large parenteral doses may be effective against highly susceptible pathogens such as *S. pneumoniae* [1].
III. **Indications for use**
   A. **Erythromycin** is considered a **drug of choice** [2, 3] in the following infections:
      1. *Mycoplasma pneumoniae* pneumonia. Tetracycline can also be used, but erythromycin is nearly 50 times more potent than tetracycline against *M. pneumoniae* in vitro [1, 10].
      2. *Legionella pneumophila* infections (i.e., Legionnaires' disease) as well as pneumonias due to *L. micdadei* and other *Legionella* spp. (often combined with rifampin).
      3. *Corynebacterium haemolyticum,* which appears to cause nonstreptococcal pharyngitis among young adults [11].
      4. *Chlamydia trachomatis* pneumonia, which is more common in children than adults. Erythromycin is used also for *C. trachomatis* conjunctivitis (see Chap. 6) and chlamydial pelvic infections, especially during pregnancy [12] (see Chap. 13).

5. *Bordetella pertussis* (whooping cough), for both therapy and prophylaxis.
6. *Campylobacter jejuni* infections.
7. *Corynebacterium diphtheriae* infections or carrier states.
8. *Haemophilus ducreyi* (chancroid) genital lesions [12].
9. *Bartonella (Rochalimaea) henselae,* the agent of bacillary angiomatosis [13].
10. *Ureaplasma urealyticum* infections (e.g., urethritis).
B. Erythromycin has also been used as an **alternative in the penicillin-allergic patient** for the following conditions:
   1. Group A streptococcal upper respiratory infections [5, 13a, 13b].
   2. *Streptococcus pneumoniae* pneumonia (penicillin-susceptible strains).
   3. Prevention of bacterial endocarditis following dental procedures (see Chap. 28B).
   4. Superficial minor staphylococcal skin infections. (Resistance to erythromycin may develop with its use over time, and erythromycin alone is not advised for deep-seated staphylococcal infections [1].)
   5. Rheumatic fever prophylaxis (see Chap. 28B).
   6. Rarely, in alternative regimens for early syphilis [12] (see Chap. 13).
   7. *Lymphogranuloma venereum.* Erythromycin is an alternative agent [12].
   8. Urethritis due to *C. trachomatis.* Erythromycin is an alternative agent [12, 14].
C. **Empiric therapy of (early) outpatient pneumonia, especially in the younger individual.** Erythromycin is used commonly in this setting, when an exact diagnosis often is not made [4] and the patient does not have severe underlying disease (e.g., alcoholism, chronic obstructive pulmonary disease [COPD]) and is not debilitated or immunocompromised. Erythromycin is an appealing agent because it is active against most important bacteria causing community-acquired pneumonia, including *S. pneumoniae, M. pneumoniae,* and even *Legionella* spp. [4].
D. Erythromycin base is used in combination with oral neomycin or kanamycin as preoperative GI prophylaxis (see Chap. 28B).
E. Erythromycin is not recommended for meningitis or endocarditis.

IV. **Preparations available**
   A. **Oral forms.** Several oral preparations are available: erythromycin base, stearate salt, ethylsuccinate ester, and the estolate form. Although the blood levels achieved with these forms vary somewhat, when the agents are used against very sensitive organisms, these minor differences are not believed to be clinically significant [1, 4, 7]. Also, no one formulation seems to cause substantially less GI upset than others [4].
      1. Although current advertisements for various formulations of oral erythromycin stress differences in serum concentrations, any of the preparations are absorbed well enough to attain serum concentrations higher than those needed to inhibit growth of susceptible pathogens. No data are available revealing clinical failure in adults of any oral erythromycin formulation (generic or brand name, taken while fasting or with food) due to inadequate bioavailability. However, **in children, erythromycin estolate appears to be more bioavailable than erythromycin ethylsuccinate** [7, 9], and absorption of the estolate is not affected by food [1].
      2. **Erythromycin estolate is no longer recommended for use in adults** [7] because of the associated incidence of cholestatic hepatitis. In children, however, erythromycin estolate rarely causes hepatitis, and it appears to be better absorbed, better tolerated, and more effective than ethylsuccinate [7, 9].
      3. In **bacterial endocarditis prevention,** erythromycin ethylsuccinate and erythromycin stearate are recommended because of (possibly) more rapid and reliable absorption, resulting in higher and more sustained serum levels than with other erythromycin formulations [15]. Although in the report by Dajani and colleagues [15] these preparations were favored, no references were cited to substantiate the recommendation.
      4. **Taste.** One study suggested erythromycin estolate (Ilosone) suspension had a superior taste and aftertaste when compared with erythromycin ethylsuccinate (erythromycin ES) [16]. Because taste perception is considered to be the single most important factor in achieving compliance in children, especially children of preschool age, the authors conclude that taste should be considered when selecting an antimicrobial suspension or liquid formulation [16].
   B. **Parenteral forms** of erythromycin are available for more serious infections requiring higher blood levels or for use when the patient cannot take oral medications. Erythromycin lactobionate and erythromycin gluceptate are available for parenteral (intravenous) administration [4].

V. Dosage
  A. Oral (preferably taken in the fasting state)
    1. Adults. The usual dosage recommended is 250–500 mg q6h. Patients may not tolerate the higher doses because of GI symptoms. **The estolate preparation is not recommended for use** [1]. (See sec. **IV.A.2.**)
    2. Children. The usual amount is 30–50 mg/kg/day divided into every-6-hour doses. In infants younger than 4 months, 20–40 mg/kg/day divided into every-6-hour doses has been suggested [4]. Erythromycin estolate and erythromycin ethylsuccinate are the most widely used preparations as they are both tasteless and available in suspensions.
  B. Parenteral. Erythromycin lactobionate or gluceptate use may be associated with thrombophlebitis. This may be avoided in part by dilution of the dose in at least 250 ml of intravenous fluid [1] and careful infusion over 40–60 minutes into a large peripheral vein or, if necessary, through a central venous line. The usual adult dosage is 1–4 g/day, divided into every-6-hour doses. A slow intravenous infusion may allow safe use (see sec. **VII.A**). For children, 50 mg/kg/day is recommended, divided into every-6-hour doses. The high doses are used commonly in *Legionella*-caused pneumonias. Intramuscular use should be avoided.
  C. Topical. There is a 1.5% and 2% erythromycin gel or solution that can be applied twice daily for treatment of acne skin lesions.
    There is also an ophthalmic ointment, which is discussed in Chap. 6.
  D. Renal failure. In mild to moderate renal failure, dose modification is not necessary [1]. **In severe renal failure,** with a creatinine clearance of 10 ml/min or less, **the drug may accumulate, and toxic side effects have been seen** in this setting [4]. Therefore, in severe renal failure the dose interval can be prolonged to 8 or 12 hours [4], or 50–75% of the usual dose can be given at the standard dose interval [17].
  E. Dialysis. Erythromycin is not removed by peritoneal dialysis or hemodialysis [17].
  F. Hepatic insufficiency. Because erythromycin is metabolized primarily by the liver, this agent should be avoided in patients with severe liver disease. If it is the agent of choice, dosages should be reduced and, ideally, serum levels should be monitored.
  G. Cost. See Tables 28A-5 and 28A-6.
VI. Drug interactions. Erythromycin may produce interactions with other drugs by interfering with their hepatic metabolism through the cytochrome P450 enzyme system [1].
  A. Theophylline. Concurrent use of high doses of oral theophylline and oral erythromycin salts may be associated with increased or toxic blood levels of theophylline [7]. This is an important potential interaction as many patients with underlying lung disease (and theophylline use) receive erythromycin. Reduction of the theophylline dose by 15–40% to compensate for an erythromycin-related decrease in theophylline clearance [4] or monitoring theophylline serum levels carefully is necessary.
  B. Warfarin. Erythromycin can increase the hypoprothrombinemic action of warfarin by an unknown mechanism, with a resultant need to reduce the dose of warfarin [4].
  C. Carbamazepine (Tegretol). The hepatic metabolism of this agent appears to be inhibited by erythromycin, and carbamazepine doses may require a 50% reduction [4].
  D. Digoxin. Erythromycin has the effect of improving digoxin absorption in some patients for it apparently inhibits one or more bacteria in the bowel that break down some of the administered digoxin before it is absorbed [4].
  E. Cyclosporine. Concurrent use of erythromycin and cyclosporine has led to elevated serum levels of cyclosporine and acute cyclosporine toxicity (e.g., abdominal pain and nausea) [18].
  F. Type 1 antiarrhythmic drugs (disopyramide, quinidine, procainamide). One report suggested that in two patients who had been stable on chronic disopyramide, antiarrhythmic therapy incited QT prolongation, ventricular tachycardia, and elevated disopyramide serum levels after erythromycin therapy [19]. The authors suggest that until this finding is confirmed, it may be prudent for clinicians to avoid erythromycin in patients receiving disopyramide. If erythromycin is clearly the drug of choice, disopyramide drug levels and QT electrocardiographic (ECG) intervals should be monitored [19].
    In a related report, a patient with a history of torsades de pointes arrhythmia

as an apparent complication of quinidine therapy had a similar adverse effect after intravenous erythromycin. **Erythromycin can produce a long QT syndrome** as a result of its direct physiologic actions. **The authors of this report believe that erythromycin should be avoided in patients with a history of the long QT syndrome** [20]. If it is the drug of choice, it should be used cautiously, with serial ECG monitoring in patients with a prior history of prolonged QT syndrome, especially if drug-induced [20]. Intravenous erythromycin has caused cardiac rhythm disturbances in premature infants [21].

G. **Terfenadine (Seldane) and astemizole (Hismanal) are contraindicated in patients taking erythromycin,** which may be associated with increased terfenadine or astemizole levels. Rare cases of serious cardiovascular adverse events, including death, cardiac arrest, torsades de pointes, and other ventricular arrhythmias, have been observed when these agents have been given concomitantly with erythromycin. The increased terfenadine or astemizole levels lead to electrocardiographic QT prolongation [22]. Similarly, erythromycin should not be taken with **cisapride (Propulsid).**

VII. **Toxicity and side effects.** Aside from the interactions already listed or when used intravenously in neonates, erythromycin is considered one of the least toxic commonly used antibiotics [1, 4, 7].

A. **Gastrointestinal symptoms.** With oral use, **epigastric distress is common,** as is diarrhea, but both can be diminished by taking the drug with meals. No adequate data are available in adults to indicate clearly that any type of erythromycin, or any one brand, causes less GI toxicity than any other.

Symptoms often improve if the dose is reduced. Gastrointestinal symptoms can occur with oral as well as intravenous therapy [1, 4]; a slow intravenous infusion (e.g., over 60 minutes) may help to decrease the associated nausea and vomiting, which may be seen more frequently in patients younger than 40 years [23, 24]. In one report, pretreatment with intravenous glycopyrrolate, a peripheral anticholinergic agent, and a 60-minute intravenous infusion of erythromycin helped to reduce the incidence of GI side effects in adults [24]. This recognized side effect has been put to good use in some situations. Of interest, erythromycin mimics the effect of the GI polypeptide motilin on GI motility, probably by binding to motilin receptors and acting as a motilin agonist.

Data suggest erythromycin may have therapeutic value in patients with severe diabetic gastroparesis [25]. The cramps, nausea, vomiting, and diarrhea appear to be due to the GI motility-stimulating effect of the macrolides.

B. **Allergic reactions** (rash, fever, eosinophilia) are uncommon. Erythromycin-induced allergic reactions are uncommon and generally mild and dermatologic. Cutaneous reactions occur in approximately 0.5–2.0% of treated patients; rashes are usually maculopapular and sometimes urticarial. Fixed drug eruptions, contact dermatitis, and anaphylaxis occur rarely. The risk of erythromycin hypersensitivity appears to be higher in patients allergic to other antibiotics [26].

C. **Cholestatic hepatitis** is rare and, although formerly associated with the estolate preparation in adults, usually after approximately 10 days of therapy [1], can occur with other erythromycin preparations [27].

D. **Deafness** may occur with high-dose use but usually reverses in 6–14 days after decreasing or discontinuing erythromycin [28]. This may occur more in elderly patients with renal failure [1]. In one report, hearing loss was dose- and serum concentration–dependent and was more likely to be seen in patients receiving 4 g/day IV. Other reviewers emphasize that higher dosages and depressed ability to eliminate erythromycin are more likely to result in ototoxicity. The hearing loss due to erythromycin appears to occur at those frequencies used for every day voice communication while simultaneously occurring at high frequencies. Therefore, the patient can recognize a change in hearing. This is different from the hearing loss associated with aminoglycosides, which begins at the very high frequencies and goes unnoticed by the patient until the damage progresses to the lower frequencies used in speech [29].

E. *Clostridium difficile* **diarrhea** occurs rarely with the use of erythromycin [1] (see Chap. 28A).

F. **Terfenadine and astemizole** interactions. See sec. **VI.G.**

Azithromycin (Zithromax)

Because erythromycin has certain characteristics that are less than ideal—relatively low bioavailability, propensity to produce GI side effects, and a proclivity to select resistant organisms in certain clinical settings [30]—new and improved agents have been sought.

In late 1991, the first new azalide antibiotic approved for clinical use was azithromycin. This is a novel 15-membered azalide antibiotic. Its nuclear structure differs from that of erythromycin in that the lactone ring contains a nitrogen atom. This molecular rearrangement has resulted in a compound with **remarkable and unique properties** [30], including an expanded in vitro spectrum of activity, high and **sustained tissue antibiotic levels,** which are much greater than the serum antibiotic levels, and a **prolonged tissue half-life, decreasing the doses per course of therapy.** Azithromycin inhibits protein synthesis, similar to erythromycin.

I. **Spectrum of activity.** Like erythromycin, azithromycin is a broad-spectrum agent that is active against gram-positive and some gram-negative bacteria, mycoplasmas, chlamydiae, and some spirochetes [31]. In an acid environment, the activity of macrolides decreases [32]. The in vitro activity of azithromycin is **summarized in Table 28M-1.** Most gram-negative bacteria are intrinsically resistant to the macrolides because of the inability of the macrolide to penetrate the outer cell membrane effectively. Azithromycin appears to be able to penetrate the outer membrane better than erythromycin and therefore has activity against some gram-negative organisms normally resistant to erythromycin [31a].

A. **Gram-positive aerobes.** Azithromycin is active against erythromycin-susceptible *S. aureus* (approximately 80% of strains), *S. pyogenes, S. pneumoniae, S. agalactiae,* and coagulase-negative staphylococci, but erythromycin and clarithromycin are more active against these gram-positive cocci. Enterococci usually are resistant [32]. **Strains of these organisms resistant to erythromycin will be resistant to azithromyoin.** Most methicillin-resistant *S. aureus* strains are resistant to erythromycin and azithromycin.

In addition, **azithromycin is two- to eightfold less active than erythromycin against staphylococci** and streptococci but is more active against *H. influenzae* [31].

B. **Gram-negative bacteria**
1. Azithromycin is severalfold more active against *H. influenzae* than is erythromycin or clarithromycin. It is more active than erythromycin against *M. catarrhalis* and *Neisseria* spp. It is very active against *L. pneumophila.*
2. However, **azithromycin's activity against many gram-negative bacilli is limited.**
   a. *Salmonella, Shigella,* and *Aeromonas* spp. and *E. coli* typically have MIC_{90} ranging from 4 to 16 mg/ml.
   b. Enterobacteriaceae such as *Klebsiella, Enterobacter, Citrobacter, Proteus, Providencia, Morganella,* and *Serratia* spp. are resistant [33].
   c. *Pseudomonas aeruginosa, P. cepaciae,* and *Xanthomonas maltophila* are resistant.
3. Azithromycin, as well as erythromycin and clarithromycin, are active against *B. pertussis* (whooping cough).
4. Azithromycin is active against *C. jejuni* and *Helicobacter pylori.* See Table 28M-1.

C. **Anaerobes.** Azithromycin inhibits many anaerobes at concentrations similar to or slightly lower than those for erythromycin [32, 33].

D. **Miscellaneous**
1. Most *B. burgdorferi* strains are inhibited by 0.015 μg/ml, suggesting azithromycin is more active in vitro than erythromycin or clarithromycin [32].
2. Preliminary data suggest that azithromycin inhibits *Toxoplasma gondii* and *T. pallidum* in animal models. However, clarithromycin and azithromycin may not eradicate infection in the animal model [32].
3. *Mycoplasma pneumoniae* usually is very susceptible at 0.25 μg/ml, but clarithromycin is more active against *Legionella* spp. and *C. pneumoniae* [32].
4. Against *Mycobacterium chelonae,* clarithromycin is 4- to 8-fold more potent than azithromycin and 10- to 50-fold more active than erythromycin. See Table 28M-1.

E. **Resistance** to erythromycin implies cross-resistance with azithromycin [32, 33].

II. **Pharmacokinetics.** Compared with other available antimicrobial agents, azithromycin has unique pharmacokinetic properties. **It yields high and sustained tissue levels** in excess of serum levels. This involves active movement from the serum into the intracellular sites.

A. **Background.** For concentration-dependent killing antibiotics, a serum bactericidal ratio of two- to eightfold is desirable to achieve adequate tissue levels. See Chap. 28A for further discussion of this principle.

Azithromycin provides tissue levels at the site of infection in excess of serum levels. In 1948, Eagle [34] wrote: "The concentration at the site of infection is the most important therapeutic consideration. Plasma levels are of importance only insofar as they are a measure of tissue concentration."

B. **Absorption.** Azithromycin is more stable than erythromycin at various pH ranges seen in the stomach, and approximately 37% of a single dose is absorbed, compared with 25% absorption of erythromycin [35].

   Food or concomitant use of antacids **decreases the bioavailability** of azithromycin by as much as 50% [31a]. **Azithromycin should be taken in the fasting state (i.e., at least 1 hour before or 2 hours after a meal)** [31]. This is especially important because this medication is taken once daily typically, and so its absorption should be maximized.

C. **Tissue kinetics** [35, 36]

   1. The concentration of azithromycin in most tissues exceeds the serum levels by 10- to 100-fold. Azithromycin appears to be concentrated intracellularly in lysosomes.

   2. The average tissue half-life is between 2 and 4 days.

   3. With recommended dosages daily for 5 days, therapeutic concentrations of azithromycin persist at the tissue level for 5 days or more after the completion of therapy.

   4. Azithromycin is rapidly and highly concentrated in a number of cell types, including polymorphonuclear leukocytes (PMNLs), monocytes, alveolar macrophages, and fibroblasts [35] (Fig. 28M-1).

      a. Cell uptake occurs to an extent beyond the levels of conventional antimicrobial agents. The function of PMNLs is not affected by antibiotic uptake [35]. **By migrating to sites of infection, these PMNLs may play a role in the transport of azithromycin to the actual site of infection.**

      b. Azithromycin is released spontaneously and slowly from phagocytes (and fibroblasts).

      c. Tissue concentrations do not peak until 48 hours after administration and persist for several days afterward [31a].

      d. Although it would seem an attractive hypothesis that high and persisting tissue concentrations of azithromycin should produce an enhanced effect against microbes in tissues, this effect has not been proved, especially with regard to intracellular pathogens [32].

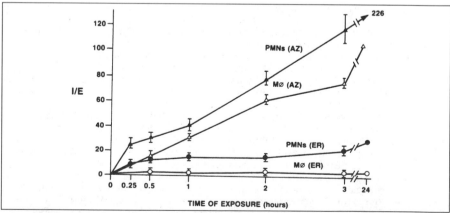

Fig. 28M-1. Uptake of azithromycin (*AZ*) and erythromycin (*ER*) by human polymorphonuclear leukocytes (*PMNs*) and murine peritoneal macrophages (*MΦ*). The differential between azithromycin and erythromycin was 10 to 1 for human PMNs and 26 to 1 for murine peritoneal macrophages after 24 hours of incubation. (From R.P. Gladue et al., In vitro and in vivo uptake of azithromycin (CP-62, 993) by phagocytic cells: Possible mechanisms of delivery and release at sites of infection. *Antimicrob. Agents Chemother.* 33:277, 1989).

   5. In animals, the concentrations of azithromycin in brain tissue are much higher than in the CSF. Concentrations in the CSF of humans without meningeal irritation are 0.01 µg/ml or less [32].
 D. **Metabolism and elimination** [35]
   1. The majority of azithromycin remains unmetabolized in the body.
   2. Preliminary data suggest that there is no evidence of hepatic cytochrome P450 induction or inactivation; therefore, azithromycin does not appear to interfere with the metabolism of theophylline.
   3. Approximately 20% of the drug is excreted unchanged in the urine, but no data are available for the effects of renal impairment on the pharmacokinetics of azithromycin [32]. One reviewer emphasizes that the intestinal tract is the major route of elimination for azithromycin; only 6–20% is eliminated renally. Therefore, in patients with mild renal failure, dose adjustment is not warranted. In patients with severe renal dysfunction, a decrease in the dose or dosing intervals may be indicated [8] but is not routinely recommended [17].
 E. **Clinical implications**
   1. The long half-life and prolonged tissue uptake of azithromycin allow for single-dose therapy of some problems (e.g., chlamydial urethritis) and constitute the rationale for a 5-day, once-daily regimen providing adequate tissue levels for at least 10 days.
   2. **Serum levels are low** and are not a measure of anticipated clinical efficacy. Furthermore, the low serum levels achieved with azithromycin should not be used in comparative evaluations of azithromycin with other more conventional antibiotics (e.g., erythromycin).
   3. Because serum levels are very low, azithromycin may not be useful in bacteremic patients.
   4. Because uptake in PMNLs may be an important factor in tissue distribution and effectiveness of azithromycin, the role of azithromycin in the leukopenic patient awaits further study.
III. **Indications for use**
 A. **Uses for adults only** (>16 years of age) **and for community-acquired infections approved by the US Food and Drug Administration** (FDA)
   1. **Upper respiratory tract.** Azithromycin is an **alternative to first-line therapy** (i.e., penicillin) of acute pharyngitis or tonsillitis due to *S. pyogenes* occurring in individuals who cannot take first-line therapy [3]. This is clearly emphasized in the package insert.
     a. **The package insert further emphasizes** the following:
       (1) Penicillin is the drug of choice in this setting.
       (2) Some strains of *S. pyogenes* may be resistant to azithromycin (e.g., erythromycin-resistant strains, see sec. **I.A.1** under Erythromycin). In one study, 2.2% of *S. pyogenes* strains were resistant to azithromycin. Susceptibility tests should be performed when patients are treated with azithromycin.
       (3) Data establishing efficacy of azithromycin in subsequent prevention of rheumatic fever are not available [30].
     b. Because penicillin can be given twice daily [37] and is significantly less expensive, penicillin is still the agent of choice for streptococcal pharyngitis or tonsillitis in the nonallergic patient.
     c. For susceptible strains in the penicillin-allergic patient, azithromycin provides an alternative that is easy to administer—that is, once daily for 5 days [13b]. See related discussions in Chap. 7.
     d. **Summary.** We believe that **azithromycin** plays a definite but **limited role in this setting.** It may be useful in selected allergic patients who have GI intolerance to erythromycin or in whom compliance is a major concern and antibiotic administration must be carefully supervised. See reference [37] and Chap. 7 for a detailed discussion of antibiotic alternatives in streptococcal pharyngitis (e.g., first-generation cephalosporins, clindamycin). Strains of *S. pyogenes* resistant to erythromycin are likely to be resistant to azithromycin.
       See related comments on pediatric use, sec. **B** and sec. **IV.B.**
   2. **Skin and soft-tissue infections.** Azithromycin has been effective in the treatment of **uncomplicated** skin and soft-tissue infections (e.g., early cellulitis, localized furuncle requiring antibiotics) due to *S. pyogenes, S. aureus,* or *S. agalactiae* [38]. Similar efficacy is achieved with 5 days of azithromycin or

10 days of cephalexin [32].

3. **Lower respiratory tract infections**
    a. **Bronchitis.** Acute exacerbations of bronchitis due to *H. influenzae, M. catarrhalis,* or *S. pneumoniae* in patients with COPD have been treated with azithromycin [32, 39]. Azithromycin would be another agent that may be rotated in patients with recurrent bronchitis. Its additional activity against *H. influenzae* and *M. catarrhalis* [3], in contrast to erythromycin, may be useful in this setting.
    b. **Pneumonia.** Azithromycin is approved for use in "**community-acquired pneumonias of mild severity** due to *S. pneumoniae* or *H. influenzae* in patients appropriate for outpatient oral therapy," per the package insert. The optimal role of azithromycin in this setting awaits further clinical experience with this agent.
        (1) **These patients must be selected very carefully** as many patients with pneumonia require hospitalization and intravenous therapy. Elderly, debilitated, or immunocompromised patients or those with a nosocomial pneumonia are not candidates for azithromycin outpatient therapy. Furthermore, if the patient's history suggests the possibility of bacteremia or this is documented, we would not rely on azithromycin because this agent provides low serum concentrations of antibiotics.
        (2) An interesting and appealing potential use of azithromycin may be in the completion of oral therapy in a patient hospitalized with a mild to moderate pneumonia due to susceptible pathogens and a clinical response to intravenous therapy. In this circumstance, a 5-day azithromycin regimen may be an effective way to complete the patient's antibiotic therapy.
        (3) At this time, although azithromycin is active in vitro against common pathogens in atypical pneumonia, it is not FDA-approved for use in this setting. Preliminary data suggest it is effective [40], but further clinical studies are needed. Because compliance with a 10- to 14-day course of conventional macrolide therapy for *M. pneumoniae* pneumonia often is difficult to achieve and preliminary studies are promising, we will use azithromycin for 5 days in selected patients, with careful serial follow-up evaluation.
4. **Nongonococcal urethritis and cervicitis due to *C. trachomatis*** has been effectively treated with a single dose of azithromycin, which ensures compliance and is extremely convenient when compared with other regimens requiring 7 days of therapy (see Chap. 13) [12].
B. **Pediatric use.** An oral suspension for pediatric use was approved by the FDA in 1995. Preliminary studies of its use in children for acute otitis media and group A streptococcal pharyngitis therapy have recently been reviewed. A once-daily regimen, for only 5 days, with an agent having a pleasant taste and requiring no food restrictions and no refrigeration is anticipated to enhance compliance, which will add to its appeal [41].
    Azithromycin has been approved, per package insert, for:
    1. **Acute otitis media** caused by *H. influenzae, M. catarrhalis,* and *S. pneumoniae* in children 6 months of age or older.
    2. As an alternative to first-line therapy (see Chaps. 7 and 28A) for pharyngitis/ tonsillitis caused by *S. pyogenes* in individuals who cannot use first-line therapy. See related discussion in sec. **A.1.**
C. **Investigational and non-FDA-approved uses** [32, 42]
    1. **Acute maxillary sinusitis** has been effectively treated with the 5-day dose regimen. Prior studies are reviewed elsewhere [32], with clinical results similar to those with amoxicillin.
    2. ***Mycobacterium avium* complex** infection in AIDS patients has been treated with clarithromycin and, to a lesser extent, with azithromycin [1, 32, 43]. The *Medical Letter* lists clarithromycin or azithromycin as one of the important drugs of choice used to treat AIDS patients [3]. See related discussion under clarithromycin.
    3. **Lyme disease.** Azithromycin is listed as an alternative agent [3]. See Chap. 23.
    4. **Other mycobacteria.** Azithromycin inhibits other atypical mycobacteria such as *M. chelonei, M. chelonei abscessus,* and *M. fortuitum.* Its potential role for treatment of these infections is being studied.
    5. **Miscellaneous.** Other potential uses, including treatment of toxoplasmosis in

AIDS patients, are discussed elsewhere [42]. Azithromycin also is being studied for eradication of *H. pylori* [42a].

IV. **Dosage**
   A. **For adults. Azithromycin** (Zithromax) is available as oral 250-mg capsules and a 1-g oral suspension dose packet, which **should be taken in the fasting state**—that is, 1 hour before or 2 hours after a meal. It is **approved for use in individuals 16 years of age or older.**
      1. **Single-dose therapy** for nongonococcal urethritis or cervicitis due to *C. trachomatis* is a single 1,000-mg dose.
      2. **The usual 5-day regimen** recommended for pharyngitis or tonsillitis (second-line therapy), susceptible skin and soft-tissue infections, and lower respiratory tract infections is 500 mg as a single dose on the first day, followed by 250 mg once daily on days 2–5 for a 1.5-g total dose. A "Z-pak" contains a 5-day supply (i.e., six tablets).
   B. **For children.** An oral suspension with either 100 mg/5 ml or 200 mg/5 ml was approved in 1995. According to the package insert, it has been approved for:
      1. **Acute otitis media.** In children 6 months of age or older, a 10-mg/kg dose is given once on day 1, followed by 5 mg/kg (given once daily) on days 2 to 5.
      2. **Pharyngitis/tonsillitis.** For patients 2 years and older, 12 mg/kg/day is given in a single dose daily on days 1 to 5.
   C. **Pregnancy.** Presumably azithromycin can cross the placenta. Azithromycin does not produce abnormalities in pregnant animals and is in pregnancy category B (i.e., should be used only if clearly needed; see Chap. 28A) [32].
   D. **Nursing mothers.** The package insert indicates that it is not known whether azithromycin is excreted in human breast milk and that caution should be exercised when azithromycin is administered to a nursing woman. However, it should be presumed that azithromycin is in human milk because it is present in the milk of lactating animals and because other macrolides are excreted into human milk [32].
   E. **In renal failure.** As with oral erythromycin, preliminary data suggest that no dosage modifications are necessary. Recommendations for end-stage renal disease are based on extrapolation as no data are yet available. Normal doses have been suggested [17].
   F. In **patients allergic to erythromycin.** In the rare patient who has a history of a severe allergic reaction to erythromycin, until further data are available, **azithromycin should be avoided.**
   G. **Potential interactions. Azithromycin does not appear to form complexes with the cytochrome P450 system.** Therefore, azithromycin does not seem to interact with theophylline, warfarin, and so forth, as does erythromycin (see sec. **V.A.5**). A potentially life-threatening interaction between terfenadine (Seldane) or astemizole (Hismanal) and erythromycin has been described [22]. (See sec. **VI.G** under Erythromycin.) Whether azithromycin will have a similar interaction with these agents is undergoing clinical study. Preliminary studies suggest that azithromycin and terfenadine do not interact [43a], and, in 1996, the package insert of azithromycin does not emphasize any contraindication of using these two agents [43b].
   H. **Hearing loss.** Reversible dose-related hearing loss has been reported with the use of high doses of azithromycin in the treatment of *M. avium* infections [31].
V. **Toxicity and side effects**
   A. **Adults.** Azithromycin, based on data from 3,995 adult patients who have received this agent [44], is well tolerated. The most common side effect is minor GI upset, and only 0.7% of recipients withdrew from therapy because they could not tolerate azithromycin. Elderly patients may tolerate azithromycin even better than younger patients. Ototoxicity or severe liver toxicity have not been reported [45].
      1. **Gastrointestinal.** Diarrhea (3.6%), nausea (2.6%), and abdominal pain (2.5%) can occur. Vomiting occurs in fewer than 1%. Gastrointestinal side effects are seen more commonly after the 1-g dose. Azithromycin seems to have fewer GI side effects than erythromycin.
      2. **Central and peripheral nervous system.** Approximately 1.3% of recipients had mild headache or dizziness.
      3. **Other side effects** (e.g., rash, vaginitis) are uncommon.
      4. **Liver function tests** may occasionally be minimally elevated.
      5. **Pharmacokinetic interactions.** Azithromycin does not seem to interact with theophylline, warfarin, cimetidine, carbamazepine, or methylprednisolone. Apparently, azithromycin does not inactivate cytochrome P450 enzymes [1].

Coadministration with antacids decreases the peak concentration of azithromycin but does not affect its overall absorption [36]. (See sec. **II.B.**)

B. Pediatric use. Preliminary data in 1,928 children aged 6 months to 15 years suggest azithromycin was well tolerated [46]. Treatment-related side effects occurred in 9.9% of azithromycin recipients versus 18.4% of recipients of a comparable drug in the study.

1. Only 0.9% of multidose azithromycin recipients discontinued therapy because of side effects.

2. **Common side effects** were diarrhea (3.1%), vomiting (2.5%), loose stools (1%), and abdominal pain (1.9%).

VI. Cost. This is an expensive agent [31]. See Table 28A-5.

A. The 1.0-g, single-dose actual wholesale price is approximately $24.15. The Food and Drug Administration has approved a single dose, 1-g oral suspension of azithromycin that will be available to wholesalers for approximately $15.00 and for $9.50 to public sexually transmitted disease clinics that are recipients of a grant from the Centers for Disease Control and Prevention [46a].

B. The 5-day 1.5-g total dose actual wholesale cost is approximately $36.33.

C. Patient costs will be higher still as these are wholesale costs to the pharmacy. However, because only a few tablets are necessary for a typical course of therapy, the cost of azithromycin may be very competitive compared with other agents requiring a 10-day course. (**See Table 28A-5.**)

VII. Summary. The pharmacokinetics of azithromycin are unique and fascinating. Tissue levels are significantly in excess of serum levels and are sustained. The once-daily dosage regimen is convenient but expensive. Because less expensive alternative agents are available, the exact role of azithromycin awaits further clinical experience. Unless there are major problems with compliance or allergies, we do not suggest this agent for pharyngitis or tonsillitis or soft-tissue infections. It may be useful as one of several agents to alternate in the treatment of acute exacerbations of chronic bronchitis. We would not use it in patients with pneumonia who may be bacteremic or need hospitalization, as discussed in sec. **III.A.3.** The *Medical Letter* concluded that azithromycin (and clarithromycin) is a well-tolerated, expensive alternative to erythromycin, and its most promising use may be in the treatment of *M. avium* and other difficult-to-treat infections associated with AIDS [31].

For **known** chlamydial urethritis or cervicitis, a single-dose regimen is appealing but expensive.

As suggested earlier, this agent may find its greatest use in areas currently undergoing clinical investigation—for example, in the treatment of AIDS patients with *M. avium* or toxoplasmosis and in patients with Lyme disease.

Clarithromycin (Biaxin)

Clarithromycin differs chemically from erythromycin by having an O-methyl substitution at position 6 of the macrolide ring. Its spectrum of activity is similar to that of erythromycin, except for enhanced *H. influenzae* activity, but it has better pharmacokinetic properties, including a twice-daily dose regimen [47, 48].

I. Spectrum of activity. Like erythromycin and azithromycin, clarithromycin is a broad-spectrum agent that is active against gram-positive and some gram-negative bacteria, mycoplasmas, chlamydiae, and some mycobacteria. The in vitro activity of clarithromycin is summarized in Table 28M-1.

A. Gram-positive aerobes. Clarithromycin is active against erythromycin-susceptible strains of *S. aureus, S. pyogenes, S. pneumoniae,* and *S. agalactiae.* **Strains resistant to erythromycin will be resistant to clarithromycin.** Most methicillin-resistant *S. aureus* strains are resistant to erythromycin (and, therefore, clarithromycin and azithromycin). High-level penicillin-resistant *S. pneumoniae* is resistant to clarithromycin.

B. Gram-negative bacteria.

1. **H. influenzae.** Against beta-lactamase-positive and beta-lactamase-negative organisms, clarithromycin alone has only modest activity, similar to that of erythromycin. However, a two- to fourfold decrease in the MIC has been reported when clarithromycin was combined with its active metabolite, 14-OH clarithromycin [36, 47].

2. **Enterobacteriaceae.** Clarithromycin is not considered an active agent against these pathogens.

C. **Anaerobes.** Clarithromycin's activity is similar to that of erythromycin [36] and, therefore, is only modest.
D. **Miscellaneous**
   1. Clarithromycin has activity similar to that of erythromycin against *M. pneumoniae* and *M. hominis* [36].
   2. Clarithromycin is also active against *H. pylori* and *T. gondii*.
   3. *Mycobacteria.* Preliminary data [42, 43] suggest that clarithromycin is active against *M. avium* complex, *M. chelonei*, *M. fortuitum*, and *M. chelonei abscessus*.
   4. Clarithromycin is active against *U. urealyticum* [3].
   5. **Clarithromycin is considered a drug of choice for *M. avium* complex and an alternative agent** [3] for *S. pyogenes*, *M. catarrhalis*, *H. pylori*, *H. influenzae* (upper respiratory infections), *Legionella* spp., *M. marinum*, *M. leprae*, *M. pneumoniae*, *U. urealyticum*, *B. burgdorferi*, and *C. pneumoniae* (TWAR).
II. **Pharmacokinetics**
   A. **Absorption. With or without food,** clarithromycin is **well absorbed orally** with an absolute bioavailability of 55% in healthy volunteers [31, 36]. This oral bioavailability of clarithromycin is more than twice that of erythromycin [32]. When taken with meals, bioavailability increases [31a]. An intravenous preparation is undergoing clinical evaluation.
   1. After a 250-mg oral dose, peak serum concentrations are 0.6–1.0 µg/ml, whereas after a 500-mg dose q12h, peak serum levels are 2–3 µg/ml [36].
   2. Similar serum levels can be achieved with the pediatric suspension in children: A dose of 7.5 mg/kg q12h in children attains serum levels similar to a dose of 250–500 mg q12h in adults [49].
   3. Concomitant **ingestion of food does not decrease bioavailability** and may actually enhance absorption [32].
   4. **Middle ear effusion (MEE) penetration** in chronic secretory otitis media [49].
      a. After the oral suspension of clarithromycin, clarithromycin and its OH metabolite penetrate adequately, with antibiotic concentrations exceeding the MICs of most otitis pathogens.
      b. The ratio of MEE to serum concentration was approximately 2.5 for clarithromycin and 1.7 for the OH metabolite [49].
      c. The penetration of clarithromycin into MEE was believed to be similar or superior to amoxicillin, trimethoprim-sulfamethoxazole (TMP-SMX), cefaclor, cefuroxime, and ceftriaxone [49].
   B. **Half-life.** The half-life of oral clarithromycin is approximately 4 hours (compared with 1.5–2.0 hours for erythromycin). This longer half-life of clarithromycin **allows for a twice-daily dose schedule.** The half-life of the 14-OH clarithromycin metabolite is nearly 3 hours.
   C. **Distribution.** Clarithromycin penetrates tissue well, including lung, kidney, liver, nasal mucosa, and tonsils [36]. Peak concentrations of clarithromycin in the CSF of dogs were less than 1% of peak serum concentrations. No data are available on the penetration of clarithromycin into the CSF of humans [32].
   D. **Metabolism and elimination.** Clarithromycin is metabolized extensively in the liver by both oxidative and hydrolytic mechanisms. The 14-OH metabolic breakdown product accounts for approximately 20% of the metabolites, with six other metabolites accounting for another 60%. Nearly 18% of clarithromycin is recovered unchanged in the urine, and 2–4% is recovered in the feces [36].
   When the creatinine clearance is less than 30 ml/min, marked increases in the half-life and peak levels can occur; dosing intervals should be prolonged.
III. **Indications for use**
   A. **FDA-approved uses in adults**
   1. **Pharyngitis or tonsillitis due to *S. pyogenes.*** Clarithromycin (250 mg bid) has been shown to be as safe and as effective as penicillin VK (250 mg qid) for streptococcal pharyngitis [50].
   However, as discussed in sec. III.A.1 under Azithromycin, penicillin remains the drug of choice and the most cost-effective agent. In the penicillin-allergic patient, other alternatives (e.g., erythromycin, cephalexin, clindamycin) are effective and usually well tolerated in twice-daily regimens [37], so that an expensive agent such as clarithromycin should play a limited role in streptococcal pharyngitis. Furthermore, erythromycin-resistant *S. pyogenes*, common in some countries (e.g., Japan), will be resistant to clarithromycin. See related discussions in Chaps. 7 and 28B.
   2. **Acute maxillary sinusitis** has been treated successfully with clarithromycin,

which works as well as amoxicillin in this setting [32, 51]. Clarithromycin is approved for use in sinusitis **due to** H. influenzae, M. catarrhalis, and susceptible S. pneumoniae.

Because clarithromycin in vivo appears to be more active against H. influenzae than erythromycin and is active against common sinus pathogens, including S. pneumoniae and M. catarrhalis, clarithromycin may be a particularly useful agent in this setting, especially in the allergic patient who cannot receive more conventional and less expensive therapy (e.g., amoxicillin or TMP-SMX).

3. **Bronchitis.** Clarithromycin has been used effectively in the treatment of **acute bacterial exacerbations of chronic bronchitis** [32, 36, 52]. Clarithromycin is approved for use for acute exacerbations of chronic bronchitis due to susceptible S. pneumoniae, M. catarrhalis, and H. influenzae.

Because this is a common clinical problem and because, in contrast to erythromycin, clarithromycin (1) has improved activity against H. influenzae, (2) can be given 2 rather than 4 times daily, and (3) has fewer GI side effects, clarithromycin is a useful but expensive alternative agent in this setting. Clarithromycin is another agent that can be alternated or "rotated" in some patients who serially receive antibiotics (e.g., 1-week therapy each month).

4. **Community-acquired pneumonia.** Clarithromycin is **approved for use in pneumonia due to** M. pneumoniae or S. pneumoniae [53]. However, often the etiologic agent is unknown, and erythromycin has become a commonly used agent in this setting in recent years. See Chap. 9.

Because of its enhanced activity against common respiratory pathogens, including H. influenzae, S. pneumoniae, M. pneumoniae, L. pneumophila, and C. pneumoniae (TWAR), convenient twice-daily dosing, and safety profile equivalent to erythromycin, as well as less GI intolerance when compared to erythromycin, clarithromycin is a useful agent for mild infection that can be managed on an outpatient basis. (See limitations for outpatient pneumonia therapy under Azithromycin, sec. **III.A.3.**) The Medical Letter lists clarithromycin as an alternative agent for M. pneumoniae and C. pneumoniae (TWAR) [3].

5. **Uncomplicated skin and skin structure infections** due to susceptible S. pyogenes or S. aureus [32]. More conventional therapy (e.g., erythromycin, dicloxacillin, or oral first-generation cephalosporins) may be more cost-effective therapy. (See Table 28A-5.) In the allergic patient or the patient who has GI side effects from erythromycin, clarithromycin provides a useful alternative.

6. *Mycobacterium avium* **complex** (MAC). **Clarithromycin** has been approved for treatment of disseminated MAC and is now viewed, along with azithromycin, as **one of the agents of choice** [3] for this pathogen, which commonly infects patients with AIDS [42, 43, 54, 55]. Because resistance to monotherapy commonly occurs, single-agent therapy is not advised [1].

7. *H. pylori.* In mid-April 1996, the Food and Drug Administration approved clarithromycin in combination with omeprazole for treatment to eradicate H. pylori. This combination [59] is an expensive therapeutic regimen [60]. This topic is reviewed in detail in Chap. 11.

B. **Approved uses in children** [43b, 56]
1. Clarithromycin has been approved for use in pharyngitis, tonsillitis, acute maxillary sinusitis, and skin and soft-tissue infections, with the same type of limitations as discussed under sec. **A.**
2. It is approved for otitis media in children. Clinical trials in the treatment of otitis media have shown similar efficacy for clarithromycin, amoxicillin, amoxicillin-clavulanate, and cefaclor [56, 57].
3. Clarithromycin has not been approved for lower respiratory infections in children [43b].

C. **Investigational uses** [42]
1. **Mycobacterial infections.** Clarithromycin is active against M. chelonei infections [58] as well as M. chelonei abscessus and M. fortuitum.
2. **Lyme disease.** Clarithromycin is listed as an alternate agent [3]. See Chap. 23.
3. **Toxoplasmosis.** Clarithromycin therapy is being studied in this setting [61].

IV. **Dosages.** Clarithromycin has been approved for use in adults and, currently, only oral tablets and an oral suspension are available.

A. **Specific adult dosages.** See Table 28M-2.

B. **Pediatric use.** For children 6 months of age or older, 15 mg/kg/day divided q12h for 10 days is recommended in the package insert. Suspensions are available with 125 mg/5 ml and 250 mg/5 ml.

C. Clarithromycin may be given with or without meals.

D. Renal failure. The package insert suggests that in the presence of severe renal failure, with or without coexisting hepatic impairment, decreased doses or prolongation of dosing intervals may be appropriate. Precise guidelines are not available but, based on the pharmacokinetics of clarithromycin, we would reduce the dose or prolong the interval if the creatinine clearance is less than 30 ml/min. (See sec. **II.D.**)

   1. Steigbigel [1] suggests, in severe renal failure, a 500-mg loading dose followed by 250 mg once or twice daily depending on the type of infection being treated.

   2. Another recommendation suggests 75% of normal doses if the creatinine clearance is 10–50 ml/min and 50–75% of normal doses if the creatinine clearance is less than 10 ml/min [17].

   3. A dose may be reasonable after hemodialysis [1], but no supplemental doses are suggested during continuous ambulatory peritoneal dialysis [1].

E. Hepatic failure. Dosage adjustments are not necessary; there is an increase in renal clearance [1].

F. Pregnancy. Clarithromycin has demonstrated adverse effects on pregnancy, outcome, and embryofetal development in animals. High doses of clarithromycin during pregnancy have caused cardiovascular anomalies in rats, cleft palates in mice, and fetal growth retardation in monkeys [31]. The package insert indicates there are no adequate and well-controlled studies in pregnant women. **Clarithromycin should be used in pregnancy only if the potential benefit justifies the potential risk to the fetus; it is a category C drug** (i.e., used only **if there is no alternative**) [32, 43b]. See Chap. 28A. If pregnancy occurs while taking this drug, the patient should be apprised of the potential hazard to the fetus.

G. Nursing mothers. The package insert notes that it is not known whether clarithromycin is excreted in human breast milk, and caution should be exercised when administering clarithromycin to a nursing mother as clarithromycin is excreted in the milk of lactating animals and other drugs of this class are excreted in human milk.

H. Contraindications. Clarithromycin should not be used in patients with severe allergies to erythromycin or other macrolide antibiotics **or in patients receiving terfenadine, astemizole, or cisapride.** See secs. **V.D** (p. 1304) and **VI.G** under Erythromycin (p. 1294).

I. For investigational use dosage. Dosages are available from the manufacturer. Further clinical trials are pending. Infectious disease consultation is advised.

V. Toxicity and side effects. The preclinical studies and early clinical experience suggest that clarithromycin is well tolerated and has a safety profile similar to that of erythromycin and other beta-lactam antibiotics. In phase II and phase III studies of 3,437 patients, only 1% of clarithromycin recipients had severe side effects, and most of these were gastrointestinal-related. There was no significant relationship between the

Table 28M-2. Clarithromycin dosage guidelines

Infection*	Dosage (q12h)	Normal duration (days)
Pharyngitis or tonsillitis	250 mg	10
Acute maxillary sinusitis	500 mg	14
Acute exacerbation of chronic bronchitis due to:		
S. pneumoniae	250 mg	7–14
M. catarrhalis	250 mg	7–14
H. influenzae	500 mg	7–14
Pneumonia due to:		
S. pneumoniae	250 mg	7–14
M. pneumoniae	250 mg	7–14
Uncomplicated skin and skin structure	250 mg	7–14

*For *M. avium* complex infections in adults, 500 mg bid is suggested. See text.

Source: Copyright *Physicians' Desk Reference* 1996, 50th edition, published by Medical Economics Data, Montvale, NJ 07645. Reprinted by permission. All rights reserved.

dosage of clarithromycin and the incidence of side effects. No significant hematologic, hepatic, or renal toxicity was reported [62]. Ototoxicity or severe hepatotoxicity have not been reported [45].

A. **Gastrointestinal** symptoms occur most commonly (approximately 9% of recipients) but are seen less frequently than with erythromycin use (approximately 20% of recipients) [62]. Other studies have shown 17% GI side effects in clarithromycin recipients versus 53% incidence in erythromycin recipients [36]. Diarrhea (3%), nausea (3%), abnormal taste (3%), dyspepsia (2%), and abdominal pain are noted in the package insert. These usually are mild.

B. **Headache** may occur in up to 2% of recipients [62].

C. **No significant hepatic, renal, or hematologic toxicity** appears to occur with clarithromycin use. Minor hepatic enzyme elevations can occur. In fewer than 1% of recipients, leukopenia and prothrombin time prolongation have been noted. Recently, a presumed case of clarithromycin-induced reversible thrombocytopenia was reported in an AIDS patient with a history of disseminated MAC infection [63].

D. **Drug interactions.** Only preliminary data are available. Clarithromycin appears to increase serum levels of theophylline and carbamazepine [36]. A potentially life-threatening interaction between terfenadine (Seldane), astemizole (Hismanal), or cisapride and erythromycin has been described [22]. (See sec. **VI.G** under Erythromycin.) Whether clarithromycin will have a similar interaction with these agents is undergoing clinical study. For now, **we think it prudent to avoid using clarithromycin and terfenadine, astemizole, or cisapride concomitantly.**

Preliminary studies of the effects of coadministration of zidovudine and clarithromycin do not indicate any alteration in the pharmacokinetics of either agent [42]. Clarithromycin can be given to patients on didanosine (ddI) [63a].

E. **Hearing loss.** Reversible dose-related hearing loss has been reported with the use of high doses of clarithromycin used to treat *M. avium* infections [31].

VI. **Cost.** Compared with erythromycin, clarithromycin is an expensive agent. (See Table 28A-5.) For a 10-day course of 250 mg PO bid or 500 mg PO bid, the average wholesale price is approximately $60.

VII. **Summary.** Clarithromycin is an interesting new erythromycinlike oral agent. It is expensive compared with erythromycin and other more conventional agents. (See Table 28A-5.) Whether the enhanced in vitro spectrum, especially against *H. influenzae*, convenient twice-daily dosing regimen, and decreased GI side effects are worth the added expense when compared with erythromycin must be considered for the individual patient. The exact role of this agent awaits further clinical trials and experience with clarithromycin. The *Medical Letter* concluded that clarithromycin (and azithromycin) is a well-tolerated, expensive alternative to erythromycin, and its most promising use may be in the treatment of *M. avium* or other difficult-to-treat infections associated with AIDS [31, 42, 43, 54, 55, 61]. (See sec. **F.**) In the meantime, we suggest the following:

A. **For pharyngitis or tonsillitis,** penicillin remains the drug of choice, and other more conventional and less expensive options are available for twice-daily therapy [37].

B. **For acute maxillary sinusitis,** clarithromycin is a potentially useful alternative agent in the allergic patient in whom less expensive agents may not be options.

C. **For bronchitis exacerbations,** other more conventional agents (e.g., amoxicillin, TMP-SMX, tetracycline) are more cost-effective, but clarithromycin is a potentially useful alternative in the allergic patient or in the patient in whom different antibiotics are used on a rotational schedule. (See sec. **III.A.3.**)

D. **For community-acquired pneumonia** in which erythromycin might be a preferred agent, clarithromycin offers enhanced *H. influenzae* activity, less GI intolerance, and a more convenient dosing regimen. However, relatively speaking, the clinical experience with clarithromycin therapy in patients with pneumonia is limited, and candidates for outpatient therapy with any oral agent must be carefully selected and closely followed.

In a patient with an atypical pneumonia who cannot tolerate high doses of oral erythromycin, clarithromycin may be a very useful alternative agent because of the decreased incidence of GI intolerance.

E. **For skin and soft-tissue infections,** we tend to use more conventional agents (e.g., an oral first-generation cephalosporin), but clarithromycin is an option, especially in the allergic patient.

F. **Investigational uses.** Because of its activity against unusual pathogens, clarithromycin is undergoing careful study in patients with MAC disease in AIDS [42, 43, 54, 55], other atypical mycobacterial infections, and *H. pylori*–related processes, and in therapy for Lyme disease. The *Medical Letter* listed clarithromycin as an alternative agent for *M. marinum* and *B. burgdorferi* [3]. Data from controlled clinical trials will be necessary to determine the role of clarithromycin in these settings. Clarithromycin was recently approved for use in eradicating *H. pylori*; see sec. **III.A.7.**

Dirithromycin (Dynabac)

Dirithromycin is an oral macrolide antibiotic that is similar to erythromycin, clarithromycin, and azithromycin. Dirithromycin was approved for marketing by the FDA in 1995; it has recently been summarized [64, 65].

I. **Spectrum of activity.** Dirithromycin in vitro is generally similar to erythromycin in its antibacterial activity; bacterial strains resistant to erythromycin are also resistant to dirithromycin. Many strains of *H. influenzae* are resistant to dirithromycin [64].

II. **Pharmacokinetics**
   A. **Absorption.** Absorption is slightly enhanced by the presence of food. After absorption from the GI tract, dirithromycin is rapidly converted by nonenzymatic hydrolysis to erythromycylamine, an active compound that reaches peak serum concentration in 4 to 5 hours [64]. Although serum concentrations are low, high concentrations are achieved in tissues [64].
   B. **Half-life and elimination.** Both dirithromycin and erythromycylamine are eliminated slowly, mainly in the bile and feces, with a half-life of 30 to 44 hours. Consequently, a once-daily dose can be used [65].

III. **Clinical trials** have been summarized elsewhere [64, 65] and indicate in relatively small studies that dirithromycin and erythromycin or other macrolides are similarly effective for community-acquired pneumonias, acute exacerbations of chronic bronchitis, skin and soft-tissue infections, and streptococcal pharyngitis.

IV. **Approved indications include** [64]
   A. Group A streptococcal pharyngitis.
   B. Community-acquired pneumonia due to susceptible *S. pneumoniae, Mycoplasma pneumoniae* and *Legionella pneumophila.*
   C. Acute exacerbations of chronic bronchitis due to susceptible *S. pneumoniae* or *M. catarrhalis* but not *H. influenzae,* which is a common pathogen in bronchitis [64].
   D. Skin and soft-tissue infections caused by susceptible *S. aureus* [64]. Most strains of MRSA will be resistant to dirithromycin.

V. **Dosages**
   A. The usual dose for adults is 500 mg once daily. For tonsillitis/pharyngitis caused by group A streptococci, a 10-day course is indicated.
   B. Dosage adjustments do not appear necessary in patients with mild or moderate hepatic, biliary, or renal impairment [65].
   C. **Cost.** The actual wholesale cost for a 7-day course is approximately $26.25 [64]. See Table 28A-5 for costs of other oral agents.

VI. **Adverse effects**
   A. The most common side effects are gastrointestinal (e.g., abdominal cramps, diarrhea) and the frequency at which these occur await further clinical experience with this agent, but presumably GI side effects will be similar to those with erythromycin.
   B. Because neither dirithromycin nor erythromycylamine binds to cytochrome P450 isozymes in vitro, significant adverse drug interactions are not anticipated nor have they been reported [64] in early studies.

VII. **Summary.** The role of this new agent awaits further clinical experience to assess its clinical efficacy and true incidence of adverse effects. In its November 1995 review of this agent, the *Medical Letter* concluded: "[D]irithromycin is a new macrolide antibiotic similar to erythromycin. The new drug offers the advantage of once-daily dosage, but **until more evidence of its effectiveness becomes available, older drugs are preferred**" [64]. We agree with this conclusion as of mid-1996.

References

1. Steigbigel, N.H. Macrolides and Clindamycin. In G.L. Mandell, J.E. Bennett, and R. Dolin (eds.), *Principles and Practice of Infectious Diseases* (4th ed.). New York: Churchill Livingstone, 1994. Pp. 334–341.
2. Smilack, J.D., et al. Tetracyclines, chloramphenicol, erythromycin, clindamycin, and metronidazole. *Mayo Clin. Proc.* 66:1270, 1991.

3. Medical Letter. The choice of antibacterial drugs. *Med. Lett. Drugs Ther.* 38:25, 1996.
4. Brittain, D.C. Erythromycin. *Med. Clin. North Am.* 71:1147, 1987.
   Concise clinical summary of this agent.
4a. Hofman, J., et al. The prevalence of drug-resistant *Streptococcus pneumoniae* in Atlanta. *N. Engl. J. Med.* 333:481, 1995.
   Isolates from 25% of patients were resistant to penicillin; 15% of isolates were resistant to erythromycin.
4b. Schreiber, J., and Jacobs, M.R. Antibiotic-resistant pneumococci. *Pediatr. Clin. North Am.* 42:519, 1995.
5. Seppala, H., et al. Resistance to erythromycin in group A streptococci. *N. Engl. J. Med.* 326:292, 1992.
   In Finland since 1988, there has been an increase in resistance of group A streptococci to erythromycin. The exact percentage depends on the specific geographic location, and rates vary from 5 to 45% resistance. See editorial in the same issue. See related paper by H. Seppala et al., Outpatient use of erythromycin: Link to increased erythromycin resistance in group A streptococci. Clin. Infect. Dis. 21:1378, 1995.
6. Fujita, K., et al. Decline of erythromycin resistance of group A streptococci in Japan. *Pediatr. Infect. Dis. J.* 13:1075, 1994.
   Although high levels of resistance were reported in the past (see S. Maruyama et al., Sensitivity of group A streptococci to antibiotics. Am. J. Dis. Child. 133:1143, 1979), this has declined dramatically. In the report by Fujita and colleagues, resistance rates of group A streptococci were 22% in 1981, with a marked decrease noted after 1983 and only one resistant isolate after 1986. The authors believe the rise in resistance was associated with the excessive use of erythromycin and the decline was associated with the reduced use of erythromycin.
7. Medical Letter. Oral erythromycins. *Med. Lett. Drugs Ther.* 27:1, 1985.
8. Kanatani, M.S., and Gugliclmo, B.J. The new macrolides: Azithromycin and clarithromycin. *West. J. Med.* 160:31, 1994.
   Review written by two doctors of pharmacy.
9. Hoppe, J.E., and the Erythromycin Study Group. Comparison of erythromycin estolate and erythromycin ethylsuccinate for treatment of pertussis. *Pediatr. Infect. Dis. J.* 11:189, 1992.
   Erythromycin estolate in a lower dose administered twice daily was equivalent to erythromycin ethylsuccinate given 3 times daily.
10. Jao, R.L., and Finland, M. Susceptibility of *Mycoplasma pneumoniae* to 21 antibiotics in vitro. *Am. J. Med. Sci.* 253:639, 1967.
11. Banck, G., and Nyman, M. Tonsillitis and rash associated with *Corynebacterium haemolyticum*. *J. Infect. Dis.* 154:1037, 1986.
   Reviews clinical aspects of 81 patients with this form of tonsillitis. Erythromycin is more effective than penicillin. Scarlatiniform, urticarialike, and erythema multiforme–like rashes are common. See companion article in same journal.
12. Centers for Disease Control. 1993 Sexually transmitted diseases treatment guidelines. *M.M.W.R.* 42(RR-14):1, 1993.
   For the background articles for these recommendations, see the recently published symposium by W.C. Levine et al., 1993 Sexually transmitted treatment guidelines. Clin. Infect. Dis. 20(Suppl. 1):S1, 1995, which includes a separate discussion of new treatments for Chlamydia trachomatis genital infections, with a review of the data on azithromycin.
   Contains good summary tables of dose regimens. Also see Chap. 13.
13. Tappero, J.W., et al. The epidemiology of bacillary angiomatosis and bacillary peliosis. *J.A.M.A.* 269:770, 1993.
   Appears to be a new zoonosis associated with both traumatic exposure to cats and infection with Rochalimaea spp. or a closely related organism. This article has a current bibliography. See related reports by J.W. Tappero et al., Bacillary angiomatosis and bacillary splenitis in immunocompetent adults. Ann. Intern. Med. 118:363, 1993; K.A. Adal et al., Cat scratch disease, bacillary angiomatosis, and other infections due to Rochalimaea. N. Engl. J. Med. 330:1509, 1994; and D.A. Relman, Bacillary angiomatosis and Rochalimaea species. Curr. Clin. Top. Infect. Dis. 14:205, 1994.
13a. Gerber, M.A. Antibiotic resistance in group A streptococci. *Pediatr. Clin. North Am.* 42:539, 1995.
   In the United States, based on susceptibility data, penicillin remains the drug of first choice, and erythromycin is a good alternative for the penicillin-allergic patient.

13b. Dajani, A., et al. Treatment of acute streptococcal pharyngitis and prevention of rheumatic fever: A statement for health professionals. *Pediatrics* 96:758, 1995.
Oral erythromycin remains an acceptable alternative for penicillin-allergic patients. See related discussion in Chaps. 7 and 28B. From the Committee on rheumatic fever, endocarditis, and Kawasaki Disease of the Council on Cardiovascular Disease in the Young, the American Heart Association.

14. Hooton, T.M., et al. Erythromycin for persistent or recurrent nongonococcal urethritis. A randomized placebo-controlled trial. *Ann. Intern. Med.* 113:21, 1990.
A 3-week regimen (500 mg qid) of erythromycin was more effective than placebo, especially in men with prostate inflammation.

15. Dajani, A.S., et al. Prevention of bacterial endocarditis: Recommendations by the American Heart Association. *J.A.M.A.* 264:2919, 1990.
See discussion of this reference in Chap. 28B.

16. Ruff, M.E., et al. Antimicrobial drug suspensions: A blind comparison of taste of fourteen common pediatric drugs. *Pediatr. Infect. Dis. J.* 10:30, 1991.

17. Bennett, W.M., et al. *Drug Prescribing in Renal Failure: Dosing Guidelines for Adults* (3rd ed.). Philadelphia: American College of Physicians, 1994.
A useful handbook. Similar tables for dosing in renal failure appear in L.L. Livornese, Jr., et al., Antibacterial agents in renal failure. Infect. Dis. Clin. North Am. 9:591, 1995; and S.K. Swan and W.M. Bennett, Drug dosing guidelines in patients with renal failure. West. J. Med. 156:633, 1992.

18. Martell, R., et al. The effects of erythromycin in patients treated with cyclosporine. *Ann. Intern. Med.* 104:660, 1986.

19. Ragosta, M., Weihl, A.C., and Rosenfield, L.E. Potentially fatal interaction between erythromycin and disopyramide. *Am. J. Med.* 86:465, 1989.
Concomitant use was associated with elevated levels of disopyramide, prolonged QT interval, and ventricular tachycardia in this preliminary report of two cases only.

20. Nattel, S., et al. Erythromycin-induced long QT syndrome: Concordance with quinidine and underlying cellular electrophysiologic mechanism. *Am. J. Med.* 89:235, 1990.
Authors conclude that erythromycin, especially intravenous use, should probably be avoided in patients with a history of drug-induced long QT syndrome.

21. Farrar, H.C., et al. Cardiac toxicity associated with intravenous erythromycin lactobionate: Two case reports and a review of the literature. *Pediatr. Infect. Dis. J.* 12. 688, 1993.
Intravenous erythromycin may be associated with cardiac conduction abnormalities, typically presenting as QT prolongation and torsade de pointes. This may be related to a quinidinelike effect.

22. *Marion Merrell Dow Pharmaceutical Drug Information Alert on Seldane* (Terfenadine), July 1992.
See also related warning: Reports of Dangerous Cardiac Arrhythmias Prompt New Contraindications for Hismanal. FDA Med. Bull. 23(1):2, 1993.

23. Seiffert, C.F., Swaney, J.R., and Bellanger-McCleery, R.A. Intravenous erythromycin lactobionate-induced severe nausea and vomiting. *DICP Ann. Pharmacother.* 23: 40, 1989.

24. Bowler, W.A. Gastrointestinal side effects of intravenous erythromycin. Incidence and reduction with prolonged infusion time and glycopyrrolate pretreatment. *Am. J. Med.* 92:249, 1992.
A 1-hour infusion of intravenous erythromycin combined with pretreatment with glycopyrrolate [Robinul injectable], 0.1 mg IV, infused over 15 minutes immediately prior to the scheduled erythromycin dose, reduced the incidence of nausea and vomiting in adult patients. There were no significant side effects from glycopyrrolate, which appeared to reduce the abnormal gastrointestinal motility caused by the intravenous erythromycin lactobionate preparation.

25. Janssens, J., et al. Improvement of gastric emptying in diabetic gastroparesis by erythromycin. *N. Engl. J. Med.* 322:1028, 1990.
See editorial comment on this interesting use of erythromycin in the same issue.

26. Boguniewicz, M., and Leung, D.Y.M. Hypersensitivity reactions to antibiotics commonly used in children. *Pediatr. Infect. Dis. J.* 14:221, 1995.

27. Carson, J.L., et al. Acute liver disease associated with erythromycin, sulfonamides, and tetracycline. *Ann. Intern. Med.* 110:576, 1993.
Data suggest that 2.8 cases of acute symptomatic hepatitis requiring hospitalization occur per million patients exposed to erythromycin. Incidence in the United States is estimated to be approximately 66 cases per year, as in the United States nearly 29

million prescriptions for erythromycin are written. In this study, no cases or controls were exposed to erythromycin estolate; other preparations do cause hepatotoxicity, however, as this study shows.

28. Swanson, D.J., et al. Erythromycin ototoxicity: Prospective assessment with serum concentrations and audiograms in a study of patients with pneumonia. *Am. J. Med.* 92:61, 1992.
    Patients receiving 4 g IV erythromycin daily should be monitored regularly for subjective evidence of sensorineural hearing dysfunction.

29. Brummett, R.E. Ototoxic liability of erythromycin and analogues. *Otolaryngol. Clin. North Am.* 26:811, 1993.
    No data in this review substantiate that clarithromycin or azithromycin are ototoxic, but these agents had been out for only a while.

30. Moellering, R.C., Jr. Introduction: Revolutionary changes in the macrolide and azalide antibiotics. *Am. J. Med.* 91(Suppl. 3A):1S, 1991.
    Overview of a special supplement discussing azithromycin.

31. Medical Letter. Clarithromycin and azithromycin. *Med. Lett. Drugs Ther.* 34:45, 1992.
    Note that occasional strains of group A streptococci may be resistant to erythromycin and clindamycin. See H. Seppala et al., N. Engl. J. Med. *326:292, 1992, and reference [5].*

31a. Zuckerman, J.M., and Kaye, K.M. The newer macrolides: Azithromycin and clarithromycin. *Infect. Dis. Clin. North Am.* 9:731, 1995.
    Both agents are bactericidal against susceptible S. pyogenes, S. pneumoniae, *and* H. influenzae. *Review of clinical uses. See related review by D. Schlossberg, Azithromycin and clarithromycin.* Med. Clin. North Am. *79:803, 1995.*

32. Eisenberg, E., and Barza, M. Azithromycin and clarithromycin. *Curr. Clin. Top. Infect. Dis.* 14:52, 1994.
    A good review.

33. Neu, H.C. Clinical microbiology of azithromycin. *Am. J. Med.* 91(Suppl. 3A):12S, 1991.
    Contains good tables with MIC data.

34. Eagle, H. Speculation as to the therapeutic significance of penicillin blood levels. *Ann. Intern. Med.* 28:250, 1948.

35. Schentag, J.J., and Ballow, C.H. Tissue directed pharmacokinetics. *Am. J. Med.* 91(Suppl. 3A):5S, 1991.

36. Piscitelli, S.C., Danziger, L.H., and Rodvold, K.A. Clarithromycin and azithromycin: New macrolide antibiotics. *Clin. Pharm.* 11:137, 1992.
    Extensive review.

37. Bass, J.W. Antibiotic management of group A streptococcal pharyngotonsillitis. *Pediatr. Infect. Dis. J.* 10:S43, 1991.
    Optimal treatment for children is with oral penicillin is 250–500 mg bid for 10 days. Twice-daily treatment regimens can be recommended for all antibiotics approved—for example, penicillin, erythromycin, first-generation oral cephalosporins, and clindamycin. For a related discussion, see J.O. Klein, Management of streptococcal pharyngitis. Pediatr. Infect. Dis. J. *13:572, 1994.*

38. Mallory, S.B. Azithromycin compared with cephalexin in the treatment of skin and skin structure infections. *Am. J. Med.* 91(Suppl. 3A):36S, 1991.
    A 5-day course of once-daily azithromycin is as effective as a 10-day course of twice-daily cephalexin in the management of minor infections.

39. Dark, D. Multicenter evaluation of azithromycin and cefaclor in acute lower respiratory tract infections. *Am. J. Med.* 91(Suppl. 3A):31S, 1991.

40. Schonwald, S., et al. Comparison of azithromycin and erythromycin in the treatment of atypical pneumonias. *J. Antimicrob. Chemother.* 25(Suppl. A):123, 1990.
    In this unblinded study conducted in Yugoslavia, 5 days of standard doses of azithromycin were as effective as 10 days of erythromycin (500 mg qid). Of 57 recipients of azithromycin, 31 had Mycoplasma pneumoniae *and 8* Chlamydia psittaci; *of 44 recipients of erythromycin, 24 had* M. pneumoniae *and 8 had* C. psittaci. *Adverse effects occurred in 1.8% of azithromycin recipients versus 13.6% erythromycin recipients.*
    See related article by S. Schonwald et al., Comparison of three-day and five-day courses of azithromycin in the treatment of atypical pneumonia. Eur. J. Clin. Microbiol. Infect. Dis. *10:877, 1991, which is also from Yugoslavia and involved fewer than 100 patients.*

41. Chartrand, S.A., et al. New approaches to the treatment of pediatric respiratory tract infections: Focus on azithromycin. *Pediatr. J. Infect. Dis.* 14(Suppl. 4):S29, 1995.
    Symposium on the rationale and early clinical data for otitis media and streptococcal pharyngitis.

42. Neu, H. New macrolide antibiotics: Azithromycin and clarithromycin. *Ann. Intern. Med.* 116:517, 1992.
    Editorial comment emphasizing the potential role of these agents in special settings.
42a. al-Assi, M.T., et al. Azithromycin triple therapy for *Helicobacter pylori* infection: Azithromycin, tetracycline, and bismuth. *Am. J. Gastroenterol.* 90:403, 1995.
    More studies are needed. A high dose of azithromycin was used (250 mg tid).
43. Cynamon, M.H., and Klemens, S.P. Activity of azithromycin against *Mycobacterium avium* infection in beige mice. *Antimicrob. Agents Chemother.* 36:1611, 1992.
    Study looks at clarithromycin also. See the related article by L. Heifets et al., Bacteriostatic and bactericidal activities of gentamicin alone and in combination with clarithromycin against M. avium. Antimicrob. Agents Chemother. 36:1695, 1992.
43a. Harris, S., et al. Azithromycin and terfenadine: Lack of drug interaction. *Clin. Pharmacol. Ther.* 58:310, 1995.
    However, this was a small study of only 24 healthy males between the ages of 18 and 45.
43b. *Physicians' Desk Reference* (50th ed.). Montvale, NJ: Medical Economics, 1996.
44. Hopkins, S. Clinical toleration and safety of azithromycin. *Am. J. Med.* 91(Suppl. 3A):40S, 1991.
45. Norrby, S.R. New macrolides and azalides: Any better than erythromycin? *Infect. Dis. Clin. Pract.* 3:405, 1994.
46. Hopkins, S.J., and Williams, D. Clinical tolerability and safety of azithromycin in children. *Pediatr. Infect. Dis. J.* 14:S67, 1995.
46a. Stamm, W.E., et al. Azithromycin for empirical treatment of nongonococcal urethritis syndrome in men: A randomized double-blind study. *J.A.M.A.* 274:545, 1995.
    See related discussions in Chap. 13.
47. Olsson-Liljequist, B., and Hoffman, B.M. In vitro activity of clarithromycin combined with its 14-hydroxy metabolite A-62671 against *Haemophilus influenzae. J. Antimicrob. Chemother.* 27(Suppl. A):11, 1991.
    The interaction of clarithromycin and its metabolite were additive in vitro. For a related article, see D.J. Hardy et al., Enhancement of the in vitro and in vivo activities of clarithromycin against Haemophilus influenzae by 14-hydroxy clarithromycin, its major metabolite in humans. Antimicrob. Agents Chemother. 34:1407, 1990. This is another study emphasizing that the in vivo activity of the parent compound and 14-OH derivative are synergistic or additive. Therefore, routine susceptibility tests may underestimate clarithromycin's potential efficacy against H. influenzae.
48. Neu, H.C. The development of macrolides: Clarithromycin in perspective. *J. Antimicrob. Chemother.* 27(Suppl. A):1, 1991.
49. Guay, D.R.P., and Craft, J.C. Overview of the pharmacology of clarithromycin suspension in children and comparison with that in adults. *Pediatr. J. Infect. Dis.* 12: S106, 1993.
50. Levenstein, J.H. Clarithromycin versus penicillin in the treatment of streptococcal pharyngitis. *J. Antimicrob. Chemother.* 27(Suppl. A):67, 1991.
51. Karma, P. The comparative efficacy and safety of clarithromycin and amoxicillin in the treatment of outpatients with acute maxillary sinusitis. *J. Antimicrob. Chemother.* 27(Suppl. A):83, 1991.
    Clarithromycin was as effective as amoxicillin and well tolerated.
52. Bachand, R.J. Comparative study of clarithromycin and ampicillin in the treatment of patients with acute bacterial exacerbations of chronic bronchitis. *J. Antimicrob. Chemother.* 27(Suppl. A):91, 1991.
    Both agents were effective and safe. See companion article in same supplement. Similar equivalent efficacy data are available for comparison with cefaclor.
53. Anderson, G., et al. A comparative safety and efficacy study of clarithromycin and erythromycin stearate in community-acquired pneumonia. *J. Antimicrob. Chemother.* 27(Suppl. A):117, 1991.
    Clarithromycin twice daily is at least as effective as 4-times-daily erythromycin and is better tolerated.
    For a more recent study, see S.M. Chien et al., Treatment of community-acquired pneumonia: A multicenter, double-blind, randomized study comparing clarithromycin with erythromycin. Chest 103:697, 1993. In 173 patients, both agents were effective. Patients had fewer GI side effects with clarithromycin (250 mg bid) than with erythromycin (500 mg qid).
54. Dautzenberg, B., et al. Activity of clarithromycin against *Mycobacterium avium* infection in patients with the acquired immunodeficiency syndrome. *Am. Rev. Respir. Dis.* 144:564, 1991.

See related article by N. Rastogi et al., Extracellular and intracellular activity of clarithromycin against MAL. Antimicrob. Agents Chemother. 35:462, 1991; and N. Mor and L. Heifets, MICs and MBCs of clarithromycin against Mycobacterium avium *within human macrophages. Antimicrob. Agents Chemother. 37:111, 1993.*

55. Chaisson, R.E., et al. Clarithromycin therapy for bacteremic *Mycobacterium avium* complex disease: A randomized, double-blind, dose-ranging study in patients with AIDS. *Ann. Intern. Med.* 121:905, 1994.
    Clarithromycin monotherapy acutely decreased M. avium *complex (MAC) bacteremia by 99% or more. Clarithromycin, 500 mg bid, was well tolerated and associated with better survival than other dosage regimens. Emergence of clarithromycin-resistant organisms was an important problem.*
    See editorial comment in same issue by M. Goldberger and H. Masur, which addresses some of the issues of multidrug therapy of MAC infection.
    For therapy for MAC in children, see R.N. Husson et al., Orally administered clarithromycin for the treatment of systemic Mycobacterium avium *complex infection in children with AIDS. J. Pediatr. 124:807, 1994. Also see L.L. Pelletier, Jr., et al. Clarithromycin therapy for* Mycobacterium avium–*complex infections in HIV-infected patients. Infect. Dis. Clin. Pract. 3:434, 1994.*

56. Nelson, J.D., and McCracken, G.H., Jr. (eds.). Clinical perspectives on clarithromycin in pediatric infections. *Pediatr. J. Infect. Dis.* 12(Suppl. 3):S98–S151, 1993.
    Symposium devoted to this topic, with several articles on otitis media and streptococcal pharyngitis and safety issues. See editorial comment at end by Dr. J.O. Klem.

57. Aspin, M., et al. Comparative study of the safety and efficacy of clarithromycin and amoxicillin-clavulanate in the treatment of acute otitis media in children. *J. Pediatr.* 125:136, 1994.
    A randomized, multicenter, investigator-blinded study of 180 patients 6 months–12 years of age. Compared clarithromycin (15 mg/kg in two divided doses) versus amoxicillin-clavulanate (40 mg/kg in three divided doses). Middle ear samples were obtained by tympanocentesis in 175 patients. Clinical response was similar, and recipients of clarithromycin had fewer GI side effects.

58. Wallace, R.J., Jr., et al. Clinical trial of clarithromycin for cutaneous (disseminated) infection due to *Mycobacterium chelonae. Ann. Intern. Med.* 119:482, 1993.
    Authors conclude clarithromycin may be the drug of choice for cutaneous (disseminated) disease due to M. chelonae, *although more data and longer follow-up studies are needed.*

59. Logan, R.P.H., et al. Eradication of *Helicobacter pylori* with clarithromycin and omeprazole. *Gut* 35:323, 1994.
    The MIC$_{90}$ of clarithromycin for H. pylori *is 0.03 µg/ml. A regimen of clarithromycin, 500 mg tid, and omeprazole, 40 mg/d, for 2 weeks was used. Therapy was associated with a 78% eradication rate. The majority of patients experienced a metallic taste, but only 5% of recipients could not complete the course due to side effects. This is an expensive regimen.*
    The therapy of H. pylori *continues to evolve. See related discussion in Chap. 11. See related paper by M. Forne et al., Impact of colloidal bismuth subnitrate in the eradication rates of* Helicobacter pylori *infection associated duodenal ulcer using a short treatment regimen with omeprazole and clarithromycin: A randomized study. Am. J. Gastroenterol. 90:718, 1995, in which the addition of bismuth was beneficial. Also see M.T. al-Assi et al., Clarithromycin, tetracycline, and bismuth: A new non-metronidazole therapy for* Helicobacter pylori. *Am. J. Gastroenterol. 89:1203, 1994.*

60. Medical Letter. Drugs for treatment of peptic ulcers. *Med. Lett. Drugs Ther.* 36:65, 1994.

61. Araujo, F.C., Prokocimer, P., and Remington, J.S. Clarithromycin-minocycline is synergistic in a murine model of toxoplasmosis. *J. Infect. Dis.* 165:788, 1992.

62. Wood, M.J. The tolerance and toxicity of clarithromycin. *J. Hosp. Infect.* 19(Suppl. A.):39, 1991.

63. Price, T.A., and Tuazon, C.U. Clarithromycin-induced thrombocytopenia. *Clin. Infect. Dis.* 15:563, 1992.

63a. Gillum, J.G., et al., Effect of clarithromycin on the pharmacokinetics of 2′-3′-dideoxyinosine in patients who are seropositive for HIV. *Clin. Infect. Dis.* 22:716, 1996.

64. Medical Letter. Dirithromycin. *Med. Lett. Drugs Ther.* 37:109, 1995.

65. Brogden, R.N., and Peters, D.H. Dirithromycin: A review of its antimicrobial activity, pharmacokinetic properties, and therapeutic efficacy. *Drugs* 48:599, 1994.
    Concludes by noting that studies comparing dirithromycin with the other newer macrolides are required to clearly define the place of dirithromycin among the many new members of this class of drugs.

N. Tetracyclines

The tetracyclines are active against many gram-positive and gram-negative bacteria, mycoplasmas, chlamydiae, and spirochetes. They are **bacteriostatic** and act by interfering with protein synthesis at the ribosomal level.

I. **Spectrum of activity.** Despite pharmacologic differences of the various preparations listed in Table 28N-1, there are no important clinical differences in terms of their antimicrobial activity. In vitro, minocycline and doxycycline are the most active.

   A. **Gram-positive aerobes.** Many gram-positive aerobic cocci are susceptible, but many strains of staphylococci, streptococci, and even some pneumococci are resistant to the tetracyclines. Group A streptococcal pharyngitis should not be treated with tetracycline because streptococci may persist in the pharynx and so may increase the risk of acute rheumatic fever [1]. Therefore, **the tetracyclines are not drugs of choice in infections due to gram-positive aerobes** [1, 2].

   B. **Gram-negative aerobes.** Urinary concentrations are adequate for some community-acquired *Escherichia coli* and, consequently, tetracyclines still are used in uncomplicated initial urinary tract infections (UTIs) [3] but less so than in the past [1]. **Tetracycline** also is active against, and **is the drug of choice for,** *Brucella* spp. (with gentamicin), *Calymmatobacterium granulomatis* (granuloma inguinale), *Vibrio cholerae* (cholera), and *Vibrio vulnificus* [2]. It is a drug of choice for *Helicobacter pylori* [1]. See Chap. 11. *Neisseria gonorrhoeae* strains resistant to penicillin G also tend to be resistant to tetracycline. **Tetracyclines are no longer a drug of choice or even an alternative agent for gonococcal infections** [2, 4]. (Tetracycline, especially doxycycline, is used in regimens to treat for simultaneous *Chlamydia trachomatis* infections. See Chap. 13.) Pseudomonads and many Enterobacteriaceae are resistant.

   C. **Anaerobes.** In recent years, there has been an increasing incidence of *Bacteroides fragilis* resistance to the tetracyclines (50% or more). Thus, these are not the drugs of choice for known or highly suspected *B. fragilis* infections. Doxycycline appears to have greater activity against *B. fragilis* than do other tetracyclines. Nevertheless, metronidazole, clindamycin, imipenem-cilastatin, ticarcillin-clavulanate, ampicillin-sulbactam, cefoxitin, or cefotetan is a preferred agent against *B. fragilis* [2, 3].

Table 28N-1. Preparations and administration of tetracyclines in adults

Generic name[a]	Half-life (hr)	Usual capsule dose (mg)	Usual interval between doses (hr)	Usual total daily dose
Short-acting				
Tetracycline hydrochloride[b]	8.5	250	6	1–2 g
Oxytetracycline[c]	9.6	250	6	1–2 g
Long-acting				
Doxycycline hyclate[d]	15–17	50–100	12–24	200 mg first day; then 100–200 mg daily
Minocycline[e]	17–19	50–100	12	200 mg initially; then 100 mg q12h

[a]Trade names given by footnotes.
[b]Achromycin; Panmycin; Sumycin; Tetracyn.
[c]Terramycin.
[d]Vibramycin Hyclate.
[e]Minocin.
Source: Adapted from E.M. Ory, The Tetracyclines. In B.M. Kagan (ed.), *Antimicrobial Therapy* (3rd ed.). Philadelphia: Saunders, 1980, p. 119; and H.C. Standiford, Tetracyclines and Chloramphenicol. In G.L. Mandell, J.E. Bennett, and R. Dolin (eds.), *Principles and Practice of Infectious Diseases* (4th ed.). New York: Churchill Livingstone, 1995, p. 307.

D. Miscellaneous [2]

1. **Spirochetes.** Tetracyclines are a drug of choice for *Borrelia burgdorferi* (Lyme disease; see Chap. 23); and *Borrelia recurrentis* (relapsing fever). Tetracyclines are alternative agents for *Treponema pallidum* and *Leptospira* spp.

2. **Rickettsiae.** Tetracyclines are the agent of choice for Rocky Mountain spotted fever, Q fever, endemic typhus (murine), typhus, scrub typhus, and human ehrlichiosis (see Appendix A).

3. **Mycoplasmas.** Tetracycline or erythromycin is a drug of choice for *Mycoplasma pneumoniae.* (Erythromycin is more active in vitro.) Tetracycline is an alternative agent for *Ureaplasma urealyticum.*

4. **Chlamydiae.** Tetracycline is the drug of choice for *Chlamydia psittaci* (psittacosis), *C. trachomatis* (e.g., urethritis, pelvic inflammatory disease [PID], and lymphogranuloma venereum), and *Chlamydia pneumoniae* (TWAR strain).

5. **Mycobacteria.** Minocycline is the drug of choice for *Mycobacterium marinum,* and doxycycline (and amikacin) is the drug of choice in *Mycobacterium fortuitum* complex infections.

6. ***Nocardia.*** Some strains of *Nocardia* are susceptible to this family of drugs, especially minocycline.

7. **Actinomycetes.** A tetracycline is an alternative agent for *Actinomyces israelii* (actinomycosis).

II. **Pharmacokinetics.** Although intravenous preparations are available, **usually the oral route is used** when tetracyclines are administered. The intravenous preparations are used in the protocols for treatment of PID and, infrequently, in Lyme disease, and doxycycline is recommended [4, 5]. Intramuscular preparations are available for the short-acting compounds but are not recommended because of the severe pain produced on injection [3].

A. **Gastrointestinal absorption.** These agents are incompletely absorbed from the GI tract primarily in the proximal small intestine. **Absorption is improved if the antibiotic is taken in the fasting state,** 1 hour before or 2 hours after meals; however, absorption of doxycycline is less affected by food [1]. **Absorption is impaired by milk, aluminum hydroxide, calcium, magnesium (e.g., in antacids), or iron preparations** [1]. The tetracyclines combine with the metallic ion calcium or magnesium, forming inactive chelates.

B. **Blood levels.** Although blood levels and serum half-lives vary with the preparation (see Table 28N-1), therapeutic blood levels for susceptible organisms generally are achieved if recommended doses are administered on an empty stomach. Therefore, there seems to be no major advantage in using one preparation rather than another [6], except in renal failure when doxycycline is the preferred agent for extrarenal infections (see sec. **E**). However, because the twice-daily dosing schedule of doxycycline improves compliance, doxycycline is used commonly to treat nongonococcal urethritis (see Chap. 13) and Lyme disease (see Chap. 23 and sec. **C**).

1. **Short-acting agents.** Of the agents available (e.g., oxytetracycline and tetracycline), **tetracycline** frequently is used and is a cost-effective agent.

2. **Long-acting agents**
   a. **Doxycycline** has the longest half-life (15–18 hours), which permits a dose interval of 12–24 hours, possibly improving compliance [4].
      Carbamazepine (Tegretol), phenytoin, and barbiturates decrease the normal half-life of doxycycline to almost one-half by increasing the hepatic metabolism of the antibiotic. Chronic ethanol ingestion has also shortened the half-life of doxycycline [3].
   b. **Minocycline** is used at times for nocardial infections [2]. (See also **sec. III.C.**)

3. **Intermediate-acting agents** are available (e.g., demeclocycline), but these seldom are used for infections. Demeclocycline has been used to treat inappropriate antidiuretic hormone syndrome [7].

C. **Distribution.** The tetracyclines diffuse reasonably well into sputum, urine, and peritoneal and pleural fluids. Good levels are achieved in synovial fluid and sinuses, with levels approaching serum concentrations [3]. Approximately 10–25% of tetracycline serum levels are found in the cerebrospinal fluid (CSF) [3].

Because of its increased lipophilic properties, doxycycline gives higher concentrations in the brain, and CSF than other tetracyclines. This may be particularly important in options for oral therapy for Lyme disease in which data suggest *B. burgdorferi* can invade the CNS early in the course of infection; therefore, oral antibiotic agents that penetrate the CNS seem prudent [8–10]. In a preliminary report, oral doxycycline, 100 mg bid, produced CSF levels of 0.6 µg/ml, whereas 200 mg bid produced levels of 1.1 µg/ml, which was more consistently above the estimated minimum inhibitory concentration (MIC) of *B. burgdorferi* (0.6–0.7 µg/ml) [8]. See Chap. 23.

All of the tetracyclines are concentrated in the liver. They are excreted via the bile into the intestine, from which they are partially reabsorbed. Antibiotic levels achieved in the bile and liver may be 5–20 times higher than simultaneous plasma levels [3].

D. Excretion. These antibiotics are excreted in the urine except for doxycycline, which is excreted primarily (90%) in the feces, largely as an inactive conjugate or chelate [1]. Renal failure prolongs the half-life of most of the tetracyclines except doxycycline. Unlike the other tetracyclines, doxycycline is excreted primarily in the GI tract. Therefore, **doxycycline is considered the tetracycline of choice for extrarenal infections when the patient has underlying renal failure** [3, 11].

E. Renal and hepatic insufficiency

1. **Renal failure. The tetracyclines, except doxycycline, should not be used in renal failure.** Neither the half-life nor the therapeutic dose of doxycycline varies with alterations in renal function [3, 11] for it is excreted in the GI tract in renal failure [3]. The tetracyclines are slowly removed by hemodialysis but are not effectively removed by peritoneal dialysis [3].

2. **Hepatic failure** is not known to cause elevated serum levels of the tetracyclines. However, these drugs should be used very cautiously in such situations because they have been noted to cause hepatotoxicity [3]. Some sources suggest that in patients with abnormal hepatic function, the dosage of tetracyclines should be reduced [1]. Because the half-life of minocycline in serum is not prolonged in patients with reduced hepatic function, some authors suggest that minocycline may be a safer tetracycline to administer to patients with hepatic failure [1].

F. Pregnancy and lactation. Tetracycline is transferred across the placenta and has caused dental deformities and dental discoloration in children whose mothers received tetracycline while pregnant. Tetracycline is excreted in breast milk. Therefore, the **tetracyclines should be avoided** by pregnant or lactating women.

III. Indications for use. These bacteriostatic agents should not be used in severe infections requiring bactericidal drugs (e.g., endocarditis, bacteremia, and meningitis).

A. Tetracycline is the drug of choice in the following infections [2–4, 7]:

1. **Rickettsial infections** (Rocky Mountain spotted fever, endemic and scrub typhus, Q fever, and human ehrlichiosis.).

2. *Mycoplasma pneumoniae* infections in adults. (Erythromycin is the other drug of choice here and is the drug of choice in children and pregnant women. For *C. pneumoniae* [TWAR strain] pulmonary infections, tetracycline is preferred [2].)

3. **Chlamydial infections.** Tetracyclines are used in psittacosis, trachoma, PID, urethritis, and lymphogranuloma venereum. Erythromycin is preferable for chlamydial pneumonia and in inclusion conjunctivitis therapy in infants (see Chap. 28M). Tetracycline (i.e., doxycycline) is the drug of choice in chlamydial infections coexisting with gonococcal infection or PID [11a]. (See Chaps. 13 and 14.)

4. **Nongonococcal or nonspecific urethritis.** Doxycycline twice daily usually is recommended over tetracycline hydrochloride 4 times daily as compliance is improved with the twice-daily regimen. (See Chap. 13.)

5. **Lyme disease.** Tetracycline is often a drug of choice for Lyme disease. See Chap. 23. Doxycycline is preferred because of its twice-daily schedule and because its GI absorption, tolerability, and penetration into the CNS are better than those of other tetracyclines [5].

6. **Brucellosis.** In this setting, streptomycin or gentamicin also is sometimes recommended.

7. *Helicobacter pylori.* Tetracycline is sometimes viewed as an agent of choice [2] in regimens designed to eradicate *H. pylori* infection associated with peptic ulcer disease. The optimal regimen to eradicate *H. pylori* continues to undergo clinical study, even when involving tetracycline [11b]. See Chap. 11.

8. **Ehrlichiosis.** This emerging disease is discussed in detail in the appendix. The therapy of choice is tetracycline, usually in the form of doxycycline.

9. **Miscellaneous** infections, including granuloma inguinale, cholera, glanders *(Pseudomonas pseudomallei;* usually jointly with streptomycin), relapsing

fever due to the spirochete *B. recurrentis,* and *V. vulnificus* infections [12, 12a]. Minocycline is used in *M. marinum* infections [1]. Minocycline is uniquely active against some strains of methicillin-resistant *Staphylococcus aureus* (MRSA).

B. **Other common uses** for tetracyclines include the following:

1. **Urinary tract infections** with susceptible organisms (including the **acute urethral syndrome** in women).
2. **Bronchitis** in patients with known underlying chronic lung disease.
3. **Pelvic inflammatory disease** and other sexually transmitted diseases (STDs) regimens [4]. (See Chap. 14.)
4. **Travelers' diarrhea.** Doxycycline has proved useful in prophylaxis [13], which usually consists of a single 100-mg/day (adult) dose. **Routine prophylaxis of travelers is not recommended.** Prophylaxis may be useful for persons visiting high-risk areas on critical (e.g., business or political) missions for a limited time; for persons with underlying health problems that might increase susceptibility to diarrhea (e.g., achlorhydria); or for persons who may be at special risk if severe diarrhea caused dehydration (e.g., cardiac patients) [13]; but it is not encouraged [13a]. See detailed discussion of travelers' diarrhea in Chap. 21.
5. **Acne.** See sec. **V.B.1.e.**
6. **Prostatitis.** Although tetracyclines sometimes are used in this setting, trimethoprim-sulfamethoxazole (TMP-SMX) and the fluoroquinolones penetrate the prostate tissue better, and these latter agents are more active against organisms that cause prostatitis.
7. **As an alternative agent in the penicillin-allergic patient** with syphilis (see Chap. 13). **Tetracycline is also an alternative agent in** *Pasteurella multocida, Campylobacter jejuni, Francisella tularensis* (tularemia), *Clostridium tetani, Moraxella catarrhalis, Bacillus anthracis* (anthrax), *Yersinia pestis* (plague), and *Bartonella (Rochalimaea) henselae* (agent of bacillary angiomatosis) infections [2].
8. **Anaerobic infections** with susceptible organisms.
9. As an alternative agent in travelers for short-term prophylaxis for chloroquine-resistant *Plasmodium falciparum* malaria in Africa when mefloquine cannot be used [14]. (See Chap. 21.)
10. **Sexually acquired epididymitis** usually is caused by *C. trachomatis* or *N. gonorrhoeae.* (When the causative organism is not known, epididymitis can be treated with a single dose of ceftriaxone followed by doxycycline for 10 days [4].)

C. **Minocycline** was formerly recommended as the drug of choice for meningococcal prophylaxis but, because of the very high incidence of vestibular side effects with this preparation, rifampin now is recommended. (See Chap. 5.) Minocycline is an alternative agent for susceptible *Nocardia* infections.

    Preliminary studies suggest that minocycline may be useful in selected patients with MRSA infections [2, 15, 16]. Further studies are needed to define the role of minocycline in this setting; infectious disease consultation is advised (see related discussions in Chap. 28D). Minocycline has also been used in the treatment of mild rheumatoid arthritis [16a].

IV. **Contraindications to use**
A. **Pregnancy and lactation**
B. **Children younger than 8 years.** See discussion of side effects in sec. **VI.A.** Alternate agents usually are available. Experts believe that, except in patients suspected of having Rocky Mountain spotted fever [3], there are **no indications for the use of tetracycline in children younger than 8 years [17].**

V. **Preparations available.** No one preparation has superior antibacterial activity. No clear-cut clinical advantages among the different preparations have been established. **Tetracycline hydrochloride is still the most cost-effective oral agent, but** compared with generic doxycycline, **the added cost of doxycycline is no longer a major factor** (see Table 28A-5) **and compliance may be better with doxycycline** because it can be taken twice-daily without regard to meals [3]. **Doxycycline also is recommended for uremic patients with infections outside the urinary tract for which a tetracycline is indicated.** The standard protocols for treatment of STDs often use doxycycline because compliance usually is improved with a twice-daily regimen (for doxycycline) versus a 4-times-daily regimen (for tetracycline) [4]. As discussed in sec. **III.A.5, doxycycline is preferred** in Lyme disease therapy.

A. **Route.** Tetracycline **usually** is given **orally** as capsules, although most of the preparations are available also in the liquid form. Absorption is improved if the oral preparations are taken **while fasting.** (See sec. **II.A.**) Intramuscular injection is not indicated due to local pain. **Intravenous therapy** occasionally is used in patients who cannot tolerate oral regimens because of nausea and vomiting or because adequate levels must be ensured (e.g., doxycycline in PID).

B. **Dosage regimens**

1. **Oral.** The common oral preparations available are shown in Table 28N-1.

   a. **Generic tetracycline.** For patients without renal failure, the generic form of tetracycline hydrochloride is clinically as effective as other agents (except possibly for Lyme disease) and is least expensive (see Table 28A-5).

      (1) **In adults,** 250–500 mg of tetracycline hydrochloride q6h, or qid, is used.

      (2) **In children > 8 years,** 20–40 mg/kg/day is divided into q6h doses.

   b. **Doxycycline.** If a generic preparation of tetracycline is used, generic doxycycline is now only slightly more expensive than tetracycline hydrochloride; doxycycline can be given q12–24h, which will improve compliance.

      (1) **In adults,** the usual first-day dosage is 200 mg administered as 100 mg q12h, and then 100 mg is given q12–24h, depending on the severity of the infection. For dose regimens in Lyme disease, see Chap. 23 and reference 8; for regimens in urethritis and PID, see Chaps. 13 and 14.

      (2) **In children older than 8 years** who weigh less than 45 kg, 4.4 mg/kg is given on the first day, divided into two doses given at 12-hour intervals, followed by 2.2 mg/kg/day as a single dose or divided into every-12-hour doses. Adult regimens can be used in patients weighing more than 45 kg.

      (3) **Drug interactions.** See sec. **VII.**

      (4) **In very unusual circumstances, it may be reasonable to administer a single course of tetracycline to children under 8 years old** for specifically defined indications where the alternative regimen may produce more severe toxicity [3]. For example, Standiford points out that the tetracyclines may be indicated for children suspected of having Rocky Mountain spotted fever who can tolerate oral medications [3]. Doxycycline is suggested in this setting since it binds less with calcium than do other tetracyclines and may cause dental changes less frequently in children [3]. Doxycycline [2] is a rational agent in the child with ehrlichiosis. See Appendix A (p. 1404).

   c. **Minocycline** may be useful in **special settings** as in alternative therapy of *Nocardia* or MRSA infections. Infectious disease consultation is advised in these special settings. (See sec. **III.C.**) If renal function is normal, 100 mg bid has been used [15] in adults. (See Table 28N-1.) In the patient with renal failure, including the elderly, the dose should be reduced as per the package insert and used only if this agent is clearly indicated. Vestibular side effects can occur. (See sec. **III.C.**)

   d. **In renal failure, tetracyclines should not be used. The exception is doxycycline** (and possibly minocycline [17a], although the use of this agent in renal failure and dosages are controversial), which can be used for nonrenal infections in the patient with renal failure. In this setting, the extra cost is justifiable, because routine doses can be used (see sec. **II.E**).

   Neither **peritoneal dialysis** nor **hemodialysis** alters the half-life of doxycycline. Therefore, postdialysis dose adjustments for patients receiving doxycycline are not necessary [17a].

   e. **Specific regimens** (in adults with normal renal function).

      (1) **In acne.** If systemic antibiotics are indicated (e.g., severe cystic acne, patients not responding to topical antibiotics, extensive lesions), 250 mg PO qid can be used initially, for up to 6 months, and then the dose can be tapered to 250 mg bid [18, 19].

      (2) **In nongonococcal urethritis** in adults, doxycycline, 100 mg PO bid for 7 days, typically is suggested. Tetracycline hydrochloride, 500 mg PO qid for 7 days, can be used [4]. (See Chap. 13.)

      (3) **In STD** regimens. See Chap. 13.

      (4) **In syphilis.** See Chap. 13.

      (5) **In bronchitis or mycoplasma infections,** 250–500 mg qid of tetracycline hydrochloride commonly is used for 10–14 days; doxycycline 100

mg qd or bid is an option. **In UTIs,** 500 mg tetracycline hydrochloride qid may be commonly used for either a 3-day or a 10- to 14-day course. As an alternative, doxycycline 100 mg qd or bid can be used.

(6) In Lyme disease. See Chap. 23.

2. **Parenteral**

a. **Tetracycline hydrochloride** is no longer commercially available.

b. **Doxycycline is used intravenously in PID regimens,** as an alternative in patients with Lyme disease [5], and at times in patients with renal failure who have extrarenal infections that require intravenous tetracycline. The infusion should be given slowly, usually over 1–4 hours, with 1 hour being the minimal infusion time. Intravenous solutions should not be given intramuscularly, and extravasation should be avoided. The usual intravenous dose for adults and children older than 8 years and weighing more than 45 kg is 200 mg on the first day of therapy, given in one or two divided infusions, followed by 100–200 mg daily depending on the severity of infection, with 200 mg given in one infusion or two divided infusions at 12-hour intervals.

In children older than 8 years who weigh less than 45 kg, 4.4 mg/kg is given on day 1 in two divided doses at 12-hour intervals, and 2.2 mg/kg/day typically is given once daily subsequently.

Doxycycline is not affected by dialysis [17a].

Intravenous doxycycline is commonly used in PID regimens. In this setting, for adults, doxycycline, 100 mg IV bid, and cefoxitin, 2.0 g IV q6h, is recommended for at least 48 hours after the patient improves [4]. Then oral doxycycline, 100 mg bid, is used to complete a 14-day course. (See Chap. 14.)

c. **Minocycline** rarely is given IV. Infectious disease consultation is advised.

VI. **Toxicity and side effects**

A. **Teeth and bone.** Tetracycline can cause depression of bone growth, permanent gray-brown discoloration of the teeth, and enamel hypoplasia when given during tooth development (i.e., during the latter half of pregnancy, during infancy, and in childhood [children younger than 8 years]). Tetracycline use should be avoided in children younger than 8 years and in pregnant and lactating women [3, 17].

B. **Hypersensitivity** reactions such as anaphylaxis, urticaria, and rashes are uncommon. Minocycline pneumonitis has been described [19a]. **Photosensitivity reactions consisting of a red rash on areas exposed to intense sunlight can occur with all tetracyclines;** these may be toxic rather than allergic reactions [3]. **Patients receiving doxycycline, especially high-dose regimens, should either avoid intense sun exposure or use sunscreens with a reasonably high protection factor.** In a recent report, the authors conclude doxycycline should be avoided during intense sun exposures and that alternative tetracyclines be used [19b].

C. **Gastrointestinal effects. Epigastric distress and nausea are seen commonly after oral administration,** and these symptoms are somewhat dose-related. The tetracyclines are irritative substances to the GI tract [3]. Vomiting can occur. The administration of food with doxycycline or minocycline may decrease some of these GI side effects [3]. (Food decreases the absorption of the other tetracyclines.)

D. **Accentuated prerenal azotemia.** Tetracyclines appear to aggravate preexisting renal failure by inhibiting protein synthesis, which increases the azotemia from amino acid metabolism [3].

E. **Benign intracranial hypertension.** This entity rarely may be seen in adults, especially women, on tetracycline. In adult patients who present with headache, have papilledema, and are taking tetracycline, it should be considered [20].

F. **Esophageal ulcerations** associated with various tetracyclines and doxycycline have been reported [21]. In most cases, the patients were taking the capsules with little or no fluid before going to bed [3]. **To help minimize this, oral doses should be given with adequate amounts of fluid.**

G. **Hepatitis** has been described usually after high doses of intravenous therapy or usual doses in patients with renal dysfunction [22].

H. **Skin pigmentation** changes can occur with prolonged minocycline use [23].

I. **Thrombophlebitis** can occur with intravenous use.

J. **Vestibular** side effects can occur, especially with minocycline. (See sec. **III.C.**)

K. **Superinfections with** oral and anogenital **candidiasis** are relatively common in patients taking tetracyclines.

VII. Drug interactions. (See secs. **II.A.** and **II.B.2.**) **It has been reported that women receiving oral contraceptives have become pregnant while receiving tetracyclines.** This may be caused by the reduction in bacterial hydrolysis of conjugated estrogen in the intestine [3].

Teteracyclines may potentiate the effects of oral anticoagulants, making careful monitoring of prothrombin times essential.

References

1. Smilack, J.D., et al. Tetracyclines, chloramphenicol, erythromycin, clindamycin, and metronidazole. *Mayo Clin. Proc.* 66:1270, 1991.
2. Medical Letter. The choice of antibacterial drugs. *Med. Lett. Drugs Ther.* 38:25, 1996.
   Lists drugs of choice and alternative agents for most pathogens. Excellent reference. Revised approximately every 2 years. For a review of resistance problems with tetracycline, see B.S. Speer et al., Bacterial resistance to tetracycline: Mechanisms, transfer, and clinical significance. Clin. Microbiol. Rev. 5:387, 1992.
3. Standiford, H.C. Tetracyclines and Chloramphenicol. In G.L. Mandell, J.E. Bennett, and R. Dolin (eds.), *Principles and Practice of Infectious Diseases* (4th ed.). New York: Churchill Livingstone, 1995. Pp. 306–310.
   Chapter contains good tables of minimum inhibitory concentration (MIC) data for many organisms against various tetracycline preparations. Also see related summary by N.C. Klein and B.A. Cunha, Tetracyclines. Med. Clin. North Am. 79:789, 1995.
4. Centers for Disease Control. 1993 Sexually transmitted diseases treatment guidelines. *M.M.W.R.* 42 (RR-14):1–102, 1993.
   Latest recommendations for therapy. For a recent symposium on the background papers for this 1993 report, see W.C. Levine et al. (eds.), 1993 Sexually transmitted diseases treatment guidelines. Clin. Infect. Dis. (Suppl.1) S1, 1995.
5. Rahn, D.W., and Malawista, S.E. Lyme disease: Recommendations for diagnosis and treatment. *Ann. Intern. Med.* 114:472, 1991.
   For another update, see A.C. Steere et al., Treatment of Lyme arthritis. Arthritis Rheum. 37:878, 1994, and Chap. 23. *Also see E.M. Massarotti et al., Treatment of early Lyme disease.* Am. J. Med. 92:396, 1992, *emphasizing that doxycycline therapy had fewer side effects than did oral amoxicillin and probenecid (500 mg tid of each).*
6. Ory, E.M. The Tetracyclines. In B.M. Kagan (ed.), *Antimicrobial Therapy* (3rd ed.). Philadelphia: Saunders, 1980.
7. Francke, E.L., and Neu, H.C. Chloramphenicol and tetracyclines. *Med. Clin. North Am.* 71:1155, 1987.
8. Dotevall, L., and Hagberg, L. Penetration of doxycycline into cerebrospinal fluid in patients treated for suspected Lyme neuroborreliosis. *Antimicrob. Agents Chemother.* 33:1078, 1989.
   Small study from Sweden. Showed higher cerebrospinal fluid (CSF) levels of doxycycline in the 10 patients receiving 200 mg PO bid compared with 12 patients receiving 100 mg bid. Because early CNS infection with acute infection may be more common than previously considered (see reference [9]), the higher doses of oral doxycycline may be prudent.
9. Luft, B.J. Invasion of the central nervous system by *Borrelia burgdorferi* in acute disseminated infection. *J.A.M.A.* 267:1364, 1992.
   Interestingly, preliminary study from Stony Brook, NY, in which 8 of 12 patients with acute disseminated Lyme borreliosis with less than 2 weeks of active disease had B. burgdorferi–specific DNA in their CSF using the polymerase chain reaction (PCR). Some patients with positive PCR had no CNS signs or CSF abnormalities with routine studies, again emphasizing the potential of early CNS dissemination. Exact clinical implications await further studies.
10. Kaslow, R. Current perspective on Lyme borreliosis. *J.A.M.A.* 267:1361, 1992.
    Good overview of Lyme disease. Again emphasizes that optimal therapy of early disease, with possible CNS dissemination of infection, is unclear.
11. Whelton, A. Tetracyclines in renal insufficiency: Resolution of a therapeutic dilemma. *Bull. N.Y. Acad. Med.* 54:223, 1978.
    Discusses the use of doxycycline in renal failure.
11a. Weber, J.T., and Johnson, R.E. New treatments for *Chlamydia trachomatis* genital infection. *Clin. Infect. Dis.* 20(Suppl. 1):S68, 1995.
11b. Sung, J.J., et al. Triple therapy with sucral fate, tetracycline, and metronidazole for *Helicobacter pylori* associated duodenal ulcers. *Am. J. Gastroenterol.* 90:1424, 1995.
12. Abrutyn, E. New uses for old drugs. *Infect. Dis. Clin. North Am.* 3:653, 1989.

12a. Fang, F.C. Use of tetracycline for treatment of *Vibrio vulnificus* infections. *Clin. Infect. Dis.* 15:1071, 1992.
Emphasizes that tetracyclines seem to be agents of choice for V. vulnificus *infections.*

13. Dupont, H.L., and Ericsson, C.D. Chemotherapy and chemoprophylaxis of travelers' diarrhea. *Ann. Intern. Med.* 102:260, 1985.

13a. DuPont, H. The 10 most common questions about travelers' diarrhea. *Infect. Dis. Clin. Pract.* 1:396, 1992.
Very good practical review by an expert. Emphasizes that most travelers should not rely on antibiotic prophylaxis but therapeutic courses as needed. In recent years, trimethoprim-sulfamethoxazole or fluoroquinolones, rather than doxycycline, are used in 3-day bid regimens for therapeutic courses. (See discussion in Chap. 21.) Where trimethoprim resistance is common (e.g., South America, southern Asia, and northern Africa and during the drier winter months in virtually all areas), the fluoroquinolones are preferred in adults.

14. Centers for Disease Control. *Health Information for International Travel 1995.* Washington, DC: US Government Printing Office. HHS Publication No. (CDC) 95-8280.
Excellent source that is revised annually. See related article by M.J. Shmaklersky et al., Failure of doxycycline as a causal prophylaxis against P. falciparum *malaria in healthy nonimmune volunteers.* Ann. Intern. Med. *120:294, 1994.*

15. Lawlor, M.T., et al. Treatment of prosthetic valve endocarditis due to methicillin-resistant *Staphylococcus aureus* with minocycline. *J. Infect. Dis.* 161:812, 1990.
Case report of a patient who failed initial therapy with vancomycin plus gentamicin (and rifampin) and trimethoprim-sulfamethoxazole.

16. Yuk, J.H., et al. Minocycline as an alternative antistaphylococcal agent. *Rev. Infect. Dis.* 13:1023, 1991.
See related report by R. Darouiche et al., Eradication of colonization by methicillin-resistant Staphylococcus aureus *by using oral minocycline-rifampin and topical mupirocin.* Antimicrob. Agents Chemother. *35:1612, 1991. See related discussions in Chap. 28D.*

16a. Tilley, B.C., et al. Minocycline in rheumatoid arthritis: A 48 week, double-blind, placebo-controlled trial. *Ann. Intern. Med.* 122:81, 1995.
Minocycline was a safe and effective agent for patients with mild to moderate rheumatoid arthritis. Its mechanisms of action remain to be determined.
In same issue, see editorial comment by H.E. Paulus entitled "Minocycline treatment of rheumatoid arthritis."

17. Food and Drug Administration. Pediatric tetracycline use. *FDA Drug Bull.* 9(5):29, 1979.
Because of bone and dental problems, tetracyclines are not recommended during pregnancy or in patients younger than 8 years.

17a. Bennett, W.M., et al. *Drug Prescribing in Renal Failure: Dosing Guidelines for Adults* (3rd ed.). Philadelphia: American College of Physicians, 1994.

18. Cunliffe, W.J. Evolution of a strategy for the treatment of acne. *J. Am. Acad. Dermatol.* 16:591, 1987.
Also see P.E. Pochi et al., An update on acne management. Patient Care *23:85, 1989. This is a useful concise review.*

19. Maibach, H. Second-generation tetracyclines, a dermatologic overview: Clinical uses and pharmacology. *Cutis* 48:411, 1991.
Discusses role of doxycycline and minocycline in dermatology. For a related article, see J.K. Wilkin and S.D. Witt, Treatment of rosacea: Topical clindamycin versus oral tetracycline. Int. J. Dermatol. *32:65, 1993. Study showed topical clindamycin in a lotion base is as safe and effective as oral tetracycline.*

19a. Sitbon, O., et al. Minocycline pneumonitis and eosinophilia. A report on eight patients. *Arch. Intern. Med.* 154:1633, 1994.
Also see related article by J.M. Guillon et al., Minocycline-induced cell-mediated hypersensitivity pneumonitis. Ann. Intern. Med. *117:476, 1992.*

19b. Bjellerup, M., and Ljunggren, B. Differences in phototoxic potency should be considered when tetracyclines are prescribed in the summer-time. *Brit. J. Dermatol.* 130:356, 1994.

20. Walters, B.N.J., and Gubbay, S.S. Tetracycline and benign intracranial hypertension: Report of five cases. *Br. Med. J.* 282:19, 1981.
Benign intracranial hypertension should be suspected in patients complaining of headache while on tetracycline.

21. Amendola, M.A., and Spera, T.D. Doxycycline-induced esophagitis. *J.A.M.A.* 253:1009, 1985.

22. Carson, J.L. Acute liver disease associated with erythromycins, sulfonamides, and tetracyclines. *Ann. Intern. Med.* 119:576, 1993.

23. Dwyer, C.M., et al. Skin pigmentation due to minocycline treatment of facial dermatoses. *Brit. J. Dermatol.* 129:158, 1993.

O. Vancomycin

Vancomycin was introduced into widespread clinical use in 1958. In the 1960s and 1970s, vancomycin was relegated to a second-line antibiotic status because of the popularity of the antistaphylococcal penicillins and cephalosporins. In addition, early preparations of vancomycin contained substantial amounts of fermentation broth impurities that probably contributed significantly to the toxicity associated with its early use [1].

In recent years, there has been renewed interest in and use of vancomycin. This is in part because of improved production techniques that made vancomycin preparations very nontoxic. However, perhaps the most important factor is the advent of infections due to methicillin-resistant coagulase-positive and -negative staphylococci, including infections associated with intravascular catheters or prosthetic devices in the immunocompromised or debilitated host [2]. Furthermore, the etiology of antibiotic-related diarrhea has been ascribed to *Clostridium difficile* (see Chap. 28A), and oral vancomycin was the drug of choice for *C. difficile* diarrhea until recently. See sec. III.A.3.

Vancomycin is a **bactericidal** agent inhibiting bacterial cell wall synthesis. There is no competition between vancomycin and penicillin for binding sites, and cross-resistance between the two drugs does not occur.

I. **Spectrum of activity** [3–9]. Vancomycin is usefully **active only against gram-positive bacteria,** particularly aerobes.

A. **Gram-positive bacteria.** The activity of vancomycin is summarized in Table 28O-1. Vancomycin is bactericidal at achievable serum concentrations against these organisms. The exception is most strains of enterococci, against which it is only bacteriostatic [3]. There **are** vancomycin-resistant enterococci (VRE). The development of resistance to vancomycin occurred only rarely from the time it was introduced into clinical use more than 30 years ago [4]. Since 1991, however, the occurrence of VRE has increased dramatically.

  1. ***Staphylococci.*** Vancomycin is active against methicillin-susceptible and -resistant *Staphylococcus aureus* (MRSA) and almost all strains of methicillin-susceptible and -resistant coagulase-negative staphylococci. Rare isolates of methicillin-resistant coagulase-negative staphylococci are resistant to vancomycin [5]. A coagulase-negative staphylococcus, speciated as *S. haemolyticus,* may be relatively resistant to vancomycin [7, 9].

    Against *Staphylococcus epidermidis,* the combination of vancomycin and rifampin commonly is synergistic and rarely demonstrates antagonism. However, vancomycin-rifampin synergism has been demonstrated against only one-fifth to one-third of *S. aureus* isolates, and antagonism is noted frequently [4].

    Biofilms of slime produced particularly on plastic foreign bodies by *S. epidermidis* may be associated with treatment failures [1, 10].

  2. **Enterococci.** Although enterococci may not be major pathogens in mixed intraabdominal or pelvic infections (see Chap. 11) or diabetic foot infections (see Chap. 16), enterococci commonly cause urinary tract infections (UTIs) and, not infrequently, bacteremia. In addition to community-acquired infections, enterococci have become increasingly important nosocomial pathogens: They are now the second or third most common nosocomial pathogen [11]. This may be explained in part by selective pressure by frequent cephalosporin use (see Chap. 28F) and patient-to-patient or hospital personnel–to–patient spread.

    Enterococcus faecalis makes up the bulk of clinical isolates (85–90% in most laboratories), and *Enterococcus faecium* accounts for 5–10% of clinical isolates. Infrequently encountered strains are *E. durans, E. avium, E. raffinosus, E. gallinarium,* and *E. casseliflavus* [11].

    a. If resistance is not present (see **b** and **c**), vancomycin is bacteriostatic

Table 28O-1. Minimal inhibitory concentrations (MIC) of vancomycin for various organisms

Organism	MIC (µg/ml)
Staphylococcus aureus	
Methicillin-sensitive	0.8–5.0
Methicillin-resistant	0.06–2.0
S. epidermidis	0.39–3.12
Streptococcus pyogenes	0.25–0.5
S. pneumoniae	0.25–1.0
Viridans streptococci	0.06–8.0
Enterococcus faecalis	0.2–6.25*
Clostridium difficile	1.0–8.0
Listeria monocytogenes	0.625–5.0
Corynebacterium jeikeium	0.20–6.25

*Some strains of enterococcus may be resistant.
Source: A. Kucers and N.M. Bennett, *The Use of Antibiotics* (4th ed.). Philadelphia: Lippincott, 1987. Pp. 1045–1068.

against enterococci, and the combination of vancomycin and gentamicin is bactericidal [3, 6, 7].

   b. High-level gentamicin-resistant enterococci are discussed in Chap. 28H. Although resistant to penicillin-, ampicillin-, or vancomycin-gentamicin combinations, some of these strains are susceptible to penicillin-streptomycin combinations. If the organism is resistant to streptomycin, no aminoglycoside combination is bactericidal [11].

   c. Vancomycin-resistant enterococci are being isolated more frequently, especially in larger hospitals. Often these are strains of *E. faecium* [10]. In a 1993 survey, vancomycin resistance was in 3.6% of enterococci in hospitals with more than 500 beds, in 1.8% of enterococci in hospitals with 200–500 beds, and in no hospitals with fewer than 200 beds [12]. This represented a 20-fold increase in the percentage of VRE from January 1989 through March 1993 [12]. Vancomycin-resistant strains of *E. faecalis, E. faecium,* and *E. gallinarium* have been detected [8].

   (1) Patients infected with VRE often are very debilitated, have had prolonged hospitalizations and have often received multiple antibiotics, including vancomycin [7, 13].

   (2) There is concern that vancomycin resistance may spread to other organisms (e.g., MRSA or penicillin-resistant *Streptococcus pneumoniae*) [13a].

   (3) Control of VRE is reviewed elsewhere [13], but general principles include the following:

   (a) Testing all clinical isolates of enterococci for vancomycin resistance.

   (b) Careful isolation of infected or colonized patients with VRE in a private room and the **use of gowns and gloves** for all caregivers entering the room.

   (c) Prudent use of vancomycin (see sec. III). This may help reduce VRE [13–15].

   (4) Therapy for VRE. See sec. **IX.**

   (5) Colonization is often more common with VRE than actual infection [15a]. However, bacteremias can and do occur [15b].

   3. *Streptococci.* Vancomycin is bactericidal against *Streptococcus pyogenes,* group C and G streptococci, viridans streptococci, and *S. pneumoniae,* including multidrug-resistant strains [4, 7].

   4. Miscellaneous. Vancomycin is active against *Corynebacterium diphtheriae, Corynebacterium JK* group, and *Clostridium difficile.*

B. Gram-negative bacteria. Vancomycin has no clinically useful activity against these organisms.

C. Anaerobes. Although vancomycin has some activity against *Clostridium* spp., (see sec. **A**), it is not used as an agent for anaerobic infections.
II. **Pharmacokinetics.** Vancomycin is excreted by the kidneys by glomerular filtration, and **doses therefore must be reduced in renal failure.**
    A. **Oral preparation.** Vancomycin is poorly absorbed after oral administration; undetectable serum levels are achieved except in patients with both severe inflammatory bowel disease and impaired renal function [6]. Very high stool concentrations are achieved, making this agent useful in *C. difficile* diarrhea and staphylococcal enterocolitis.
    B. **Intravenous preparation.** After intravenous administration, therapeutic levels are achieved in the serum and in synovial, pericardial, and pleural fluids. Vancomycin penetrates the inflamed meninges [1, 6], but treatment failures in meningitis have occurred. Vancomycin penetration into brain abscess fluid is greater than penetration into the cerebrospinal fluid (CSF) [1].
        1. **Half-life.** The serum half-life in adults with normal renal function is 4–8 hours. In anuria, the half-life is prolonged to 7–12 days [1].
        2. Increased dosage requirements of vancomycin in pregnant women (with endocarditis) have been documented, which is presumably due to increased urinary clearance and vastly increased volume of distribution in this population [1]. Pharmacokinetics are variable in children [16].
        3. Bile levels are inadequate for treating biliary infections [1]. Vancomycin does not penetrate well into ocular tissue after IV administration [17]. See Chap. 6.
        4. **Penetration** of vancomycin from serum **into peritoneal dialysis fluid** is variable and unpredictable [3]. Therefore, in the setting of peritonitis due to gram-positive organisms (e.g., in patients receiving chronic intermittent peritoneal dialysis), the intraperitoneal route is recommended and convenient for the patient [4, 18].
        5. **Serum levels** achieved after intravenous dosages are discussed in sec. **V.A.**
    C. Intramuscular administration is not advised. Because of the pain on injection, no satisfactory preparation is available [7].
III. **Indications for use.** Vancomycin is used in serious infections in the allergic patient or in the patient with certain resistant organisms [1, 6, 7, 19–21]. **Because the administration of vancomycin is a frequently cited risk factor for subsequent colonization or infection with VRE, prudent use of vancomycin is emphasized** [13, 14]. It is anticipated that if only a few VRE are present, for example, per gram of feces, these will proliferate rapidly in the presence of vancomycin. Such an increase means there will be a much greater chance of spread of these organisms to other persons and that there will be many more potential donors to transfer vancomycin resistance to other species [13, 13a] of bacteria.
    Guidelines for proper use of vancomycin should be a part of a hospital's quality improvement program and should include the participation of the pharmacy and therapeutics committee, infection control, and infectious disease, medical, and surgical staffs [14].
    A. **Situations in which the use of vancomycin is appropriate or acceptable** [14]
        1. **Treatment of serious infections due to beta-lactam-resistant gram-positive microorganisms.** Clinicians should be aware that vancomycin may be less rapidly bactericidal than beta-lactam agents for beta-lactam-susceptible staphylococci (see sec. **2**).
            a. This includes **MRSA** (see Chaps. 28A and 28D), coagulase-negative staphylococci, *Corynebacterium jeikeium,* and highly resistant strains of *S. pneumoniae* (see Chap. 28C).
            b. **Coagulase-negative staphylococci (including *S. epidermidis*) infections.** Surveys indicate that 35–65% of clinically important coagulase-negative staphylococci isolates are resistant to methicillin [5]. Vancomycin, sometimes combined with gentamicin or rifampin for synergy, has become the treatment of choice for these infections [5, 6, 21, 22]. Rare strains may become resistant to vancomycin [5]. **Vancomycin appears to be effective in prosthetic device infections and CSF shunt infections [23], especially if combined with rifampin. It also is effective against staphylococci-associated nosocomial infections in intensive care nurseries.** (See additional discussion in Chap. 28D.)
            c. **Serious diphtheroid infections** (e.g., endocarditis of prosthetic valves, CSF shunt infections, and infections in the compromised host) that are

penicillin-resistant (or that occur in the severely allergic patient) can be treated with vancomycin.

2. **Treatment of infections due to gram-positive microorganisms in patients with a history of anaphylaxis to beta-lactam antimicrobials.** Patients with other types of allergic history should be skin-tested for verification.

In patients with delayed penicillin allergy, cephalosporins often are used (Chap. 28F). Because it is structurally unrelated to other antibiotics, vancomycin is useful in the penicillin- and cephalosporin-allergic patient (see Chap. 27).

a. **Serious *Staphylococcus aureus* (coagulase-positive) infections.** Intravenous vancomycin is an effective agent [21, 22, 24, 25]. However, vancomycin may be slow to sterilize the bloodstream of patients with *S. aureus* endocarditis [3, 26, 27]. (Therefore, for bacteremias due to methicillin-susceptible *S. aureus*, a semisynthetic penicillin [nafcillin, oxacillin] is preferred over the convenient dosing schedule of vancomycin [27] in the nonallergic patient.) Vancomycin is preferred over trimethoprim-sulfamethoxazole (TMP-SMX) [28].

b. **Endocarditis** due to viridans streptococci or susceptible streptococci, such as *Streptococcus bovis,* can be treated with vancomycin. Because vancomycin may be only bacteriostatic against some enterococci, most authorities recommend vancomycin plus an aminoglycoside as the treatment of choice for enterococcal endocarditis [4, 6, 21, 29, 29a].

c. **Central nervous system infections** [7, 23, 30, 31]. The penetration of vancomycin into the CSF may be variable when intravenous vancomycin is used [30, 31]. In the severely allergic patient with staphylococcal meningitis, infectious disease consultation is advisable to help adjust doses and monitor CSF drug levels if necessary.

3. **Antibiotic-associated colitis (AAC) that fails to respond to metronidazole therapy or AAC that is severe and potentially life-threatening** [6, 7, 21, 32]. Intravenous vancomycin produces low fecal concentrations, and so oral therapy is used [4]. Because of the concern for selecting out VRE, **vancomycin is no longer used for primary treatment of AAC** [13, 14, 21]. See related discussion in Chap. 28A.

4. **Prophylaxis** is recommended by the American Heart Association **for preventing endocarditis** in patients at risk. See detailed discussion in Chap. 28B.

Vancomycin is used in prophylactic regimens to prevent endocarditis in ampicillin- or amoxicillin-allergic patients who are undergoing GI or genitourinary manipulations, in patients with artificial heart valves, or in other high-risk patients undergoing dental procedures.

5. Prophylaxis for surgical procedures involving implantation of prosthetic materials or devices at institutions with a high rate of infections due to MRSA or methicillin-resistant *S. epidermidis.* A single dose administered immediately preoperatively is sufficient unless the procedure lasts more than 6 hours, in which case the dose should be repeated. Prophylaxis should be discontinued after a **maximum** of two doses. See detailed discussion in Chap. 28B.

B. **Situations in which the use of vancomycin should be discouraged** [13, 14]

1. Routine surgical prophylaxis (see Chap. 28B).

2. Empiric antimicrobial therapy for a febrile neutropenic patient, unless there is strong evidence at the outset that the patient has an infection due to gram-positive microorganisms (e.g., inflamed exit site of Hickman catheter), and the prevalence of infections due to beta-lactam-resistant gram-positive microorganisms (e.g., MRSA) in the hospital is substantial.

Gram-positive bacteremias in patients with leukopenia after chemotherapy are common [2]. This is due in part to an increase in the use of central lines (e.g., Hickman catheters), leading to catheter-related *S. aureus* and coagulase-negative staphylococcal infections. Contamination of platelet packs with coagulase-negative staphylococci as well as GI sources of coagulase-negative staphylococci may also contribute.

An early study favored the empiric use of vancomycin for fever of unclear etiology in treatment-induced granulocytopenic patients [33]. By contrast, conclusions from another early study did not favor empiric use of vancomycin in febrile leukopenic cancer patients and encouraged the addition of vancomycin only when clinical (e.g., exit site infections or critical illness) or microbiologic (e.g., blood cultures positive for gram-positive cocci) data support its use [34]. Mortality is similar if vancomycin is given empirically or started only when culture data support its use. **We do not use vancomycin empirically for an initial episode of fever in the leukopenic patient unless there is evidence of a line-related infection** (e.g., increasing tenderness, erythema, or exudate at the exit site or tunnel of the catheter) early in the course of chemotherapy. Other infectious disease consultants favor this approach [35] as do the recent CDC guidelines [14]. In recurrent episodes of undefined fever in patients with prolonged neutropenia and a central line in place, we would repeat blood cultures and add vancomycin if the blood cultures reveal gram-positive cocci. Data also favor adding vancomycin after identification of gram-positive infection in most institutions, although some have argued that empiric use of vancomycin (until culture data are back) can be justified in specific centers where bacteremias are caused almost exclusively by methicillin-resistant staphylococci [36].

   3. Treatment in response to a single blood culture positive for coagulase-negative staphylococcus, if other blood cultures drawn in the same time frame are negative (i.e., if contamination of the blood culture is likely). Because contamination of blood cultures with skin flora (e.g., *S. epidermidis*) may cause vancomycin to be inappropriately administered to patients, the phlebotomist and other personnel who obtain blood cultures should be properly trained to minimize microbial contamination of specimens. See Chap. 2 for related discussion.
   4. Continued empiric use for presumed infections in patients whose cultures are negative for beta-lactam-resistant gram-positive microorganisms.
   5. Systemic or local (e.g., intravenous catheter or lock) prophylaxis for infection or colonization of indwelling central or peripheral intravascular catheters or vascular grafts.
   6. Selective decontamination of the digestive tract.
   7. Eradication of MRSA colonization. See related discussions in Chap. 28D.
   8. Primary treatment of AAC. See sec. **A.3.**
   9. Routine prophylaxis for very low birth weight infants. See sec. **C.4.**
   10. Routine prophylaxis for patients on continuous ambulatory peritoneal dialysis.
   11. Treatment (chosen for dosing convenience) of infections caused by beta-lactam-sensitive gram-positive microorganisms in patients who have renal failure.
   12. Use of vancomycin solution for topical application or irrigation.

C. **Miscellaneous**
   1. **Methicillin-resistant staphylococcal hemodialysis shunt infections** in patients undergoing hemodialysis have been effectively treated with single, 1-g IV doses every 7–10 days or doses with pharmacokinetic monitoring (see sec. **V.C.4**).
   2. **Chronic ambulatory peritoneal dialysis** can be associated with gram-positive coccal **peritonitis.** Vancomycin is a useful agent in this setting. See Chap. 11.
   3. **Staphylococcal enterocolitis** rarely occurs but, if a case is documented, oral vancomycin is indicated.
   4. Although two recent studies suggest that continuous low-dose vancomycin intravenous infusion will reduce significantly the incidence of coagulase-negative staphylococcal bacteremia in neonates weighing less than 1,500 g, their routine use is not advised, in part because of the risk of selecting for VRE and potentially more difficult infections to eradicate [15].

IV. **Dosage**
A. **Oral.** An oral preparation is available but is expensive (see Table 28A-5). Anecdotally, some hospital pharmacies have made up an oral solution dose from the intravenous powder formulation to provide a more cost-effective oral preparation.
   1. **For *C. difficile* diarrhea** in adults, 125 mg q6h for 10 days is as effective a regimen as the previously used 500-mg PO qid regimen [37]. In children, the dose is 40 mg/kg/day in four divided doses. See Chap. 28A for further discussion of *C. difficile* diarrhea.
   2. **For staphylococcal enterocolitis,** 500 mg q6h in adults has been suggested. (It is unclear whether this entity really exists.)
B. **Intravenous**
   1. **Adults.** A common dosage in adults with normal renal function has been 500 mg (infused over 60 minutes) q6h. However, a more convenient and more cost-effective dosage regimen, and one providing higher peaks, is 1 g q12h (given over 2 hours to avoid the so-called red man syndrome). In seriously ill

patients, 1 g of vancomycin q8h for the first few days (if renal function is normal) has been suggested [3]. When vancomycin is given together with an aminoglycoside, many authorities recommend a reduced dose (e.g., 500 mg q8h [or, preferably, pharmacokinetic monitoring]). When used for prophylaxis in cardiac surgery, some authors favor a 15-mg/kg preoperative dose [38]. **In meningitis,** doses of 1 g q8h for 2–3 days (in adults with normal renal function) have been suggested [1]. **See sec. V.C for dosages in renal failure.**

2. **Children and neonates.** There is less experience with the use of vancomycin in children. For infants and children with non-CNS infections, 10-mg/kg doses IV over 60 minutes q6h (40 mg/kg/day) often are suggested. In CNS infections, 15-mg/kg doses IV over 60 minutes q6h are suggested.

In neonates, during the first week of life, 15-mg/kg doses IV q12h have been recommended and, in infants 8–30 days of age, 15-mg/kg doses IV q8h have been recommended [16]. However, one study suggests these dosages frequently produce serum levels greater than the desired therapeutic range, especially in low-birth-weight infants [25]. This may be due in part to the immaturity of the neonatal liver, which allows the drug to accumulate. Therefore, for premature infants of up to 9 weeks' postnatal age or 41 weeks' postconceptional age, an initial loading dose of 15 mg/kg can be given, followed by doses of 10 mg/kg q8h [1]. **In neonates, close monitoring of vancomycin serum levels is important to ensure therapeutic efficiency without toxicity** [25]. **See Chap. 3 for other dose regimens in neonates.**

3. **Pharmacokinetic monitoring can be performed** to ensure adequate serum levels. (See sec. **V.**) Often, a once-a-day dosage regimen is feasible, and this may be useful in home intravenous regimens especially.

C. **Intraperitoneal administration.** In patients on chronic ambulatory peritoneal dialysis, a vancomycin dose of 30 mg/kg per 2-liter intraperitoneal dose once weekly for 2 weeks was effective for susceptible gram-positive organism peritonitis [4, 39, 40]. Another dosing regimen of 2 g intraperitoneally (in one 6-hour exchange) every 7 days for two doses has been suggested [18]. See Chap. 11.

D. **Vancomycin administration into the CSF.** Because of the somewhat limited or variable penetration of intravenous vancomycin into the CSF, for inadequately responding staphylococcal meningitis or meningitis due to high-level penicillin-resistant *S. pneumoniae,* injection of vancomycin into the lumbar subarachnoid space or intraventricular injection may be a consideration. This topic has been reviewed in detail elsewhere [41]. **Infectious disease consultation is advised.**

V. **Monitoring serum vancomycin.** Although monitoring serum vancomycin levels has become a common practice in the last few years in the United States, in a recent excellent careful review of prior studies, the authors emphasize: **There are no data to support a cause-and-effect relationship between serum levels of the drug and either its efficacy or its presumed toxicities** [42].

A. Vancomycin pharmacokinetics are sufficiently predictable that adequate serum drug concentrations can be obtained by empiric dosing methods (e.g., see sec. **C**) that take into account the patient's age, weight, and renal function. This is especially true when renal function is normal. **Therefore, routine vancomycin serum monitoring is not advised.**

B. In a thoughtful editorial comment of the preceding review, **Moellering** [43] concurs that routine monitoring of serum vancomycin concentration is not necessary or useful. However, he **suggests a limited number of clinical settings in which following the vancomycin level in the serum or other body fluids may be prudent.** These include the following:

1. **Patients receiving vancomycin-aminoglycoside combinations.** Although it is not clear that monitoring serum vancomycin levels will prevent nephrotoxicity in this setting, increasing trough levels of vancomycin may be a sensitive indicator of nephrotoxicity and may provide an early warning to the clinician that the doses of both vancomycin and aminoglycosides should be adjusted.

2. **Anephric patients undergoing hemodialysis and receiving infrequent doses of vancomycin for serious systemic infection** (especially if the newer high-flux dialysis membranes are used). It may be reasonable to monitor serum trough levels occasionally to make certain that serum vancomycin concentrations are adequate.

3. **Patients receiving higher-than-usual doses of vancomycin** (e.g., patients being treated for high-level penicillin-resistant *S. pneumoniae* meningitis). It may be prudent to monitor serum or CSF levels to determine whether they

are adequate. Cerebrospinal fluid levels may also be useful when vancomycin is used to treat staphylococcal meningitis.

4. **Patients with rapidly changing renal function.** In these patients, it may be easier to monitor serum levels than to attempt repeatedly to adjust dosages based on nomograms or other formulas.

C. **In renal failure, maintenance doses must be reduced.** Often, dose adjustments are made from nomograms based on the apparent linear relationship between creatinine clearance and vancomycin clearance.

   1. **Moellering and coworkers [44] have devised a nomogram and table** for determining vancomycin dosage in patients with various degrees of renal failure (Table 28O-2). This approach is designed to achieve an average steady-state concentration of 15 μg/ml (rather than peak and trough levels), and it assumes a fixed volume of distribution of 0.9 liters/kg.

   2. **Matzke and colleagues [45] published a very useful nomogram** designed to achieve peak and trough concentrations of 30 μg/ml and 7.5 μg/ml, respectively [1]. After an initial loading dose of 25 mg/kg (infused at 500 mg/hr), the vancomycin maintenance dose remains constant at 19 mg/kg (infused at 500 mg/hr), but the dosage interval depends on the creatinine clearance (Fig. 28O-1) [1]. Doses are based on actual total weight, not ideal patient weight. (See Chap. 28A for instructions on how to estimate creatinine clearance, which is based on ideal body weight.)

   3. **Individualized dosing. Ideally, vancomycin dosage can be individualized based on serum concentrations** [1], usually with the help of pharmacokinetic consultation. Initial vancomycin dosage is calculated on a per-body-weight basis with the use of the nomogram (see sec. **2**) followed by adjustments to attain peak serum levels of 30–40 μg/ml and trough levels of 5–10 μg/ml [1].

      Individualized dosing of vancomycin is not as well developed as with aminoglycosides (see Chap. 28H) but would be ideal in patients described in sec. **V.B.**

   4. **Hemodialysis** or **peritoneal dialysis** does not remove significant amounts of vancomycin [1]. One dosing regimen in this setting suggests that dialysis patients receive an initial 1-g IV dose followed by 500 mg every 8 days [46]. Ideally, we prefer individualized dosing in this setting, with an initial loading dose of 25 mg/kg (infused at 500 mg/hr) and, typically, patients can be maintained on 19 mg/kg given every 5–7 days. (If on day 5 after the prior dose, the serum level is < 10 μg/ml, a maintenance dose is given. If on day 5 after the prior dose, the serum level is > 10 μg/ml, the maintenance dose can be given usually in 48 hours [i.e., on day 7].)

D. **Miscellaneous issues**

   1. **Serum concentrations.** In adults, at 1–2 hours after a 500-mg dose of IV vancomycin, peaks range from 8 to 12 μg/ml. When 1-g doses are given intrave-

Table 28O-2. Dosage table for vancomycin in patients with impaired renal function*

Creatinine clearance (ml/min)	Vancomycin dose (mg/24 hr)
100	1,545
90	1,390
80	1,235
70	1,080
60	925
50	770
40	620
30	465
20	310
10	155

*The initial dose should be no less than 15 mg/kg, even in patients with mild to moderate renal insufficiency.
Source: Modified from R.C. Moellering, Jr., D.J. Krogstad, and D.J. Greenblatt, Vancomycin therapy in patients with impaired renal function: A nomogram for dosage. *Ann. Intern. Med.* 94:343, 1981.

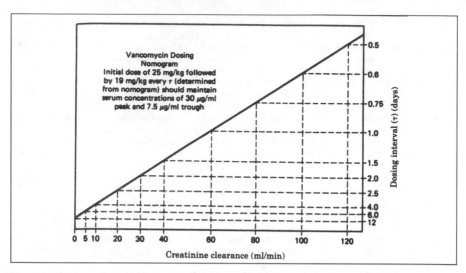

Fig. 28O-1. Nomogram for vancomycin dosage in patients with renal failure. (From G.R. Matzke et al., Pharmacokinetics of vancomycin in patients with varying degrees of renal function. *Antimicrob. Agents Chemother.* 25:433, 1984.)

nously, **peaks of 20–50 μg/ml and troughs of 5–12 μg/ml are achieved, and these are probably more desirable levels [7].**

2. The **peak level** should be drawn 1–2 hours after completion of the intravenous infusion. Moellering [43] suggests that peak levels be drawn 2 hours after completion of the intravenous infusion.

VI. **Toxicity.** Currently available purified parenteral preparations are very well tolerated. **Only when another drug with nephrotoxic or ototoxic potential** (e.g., an aminoglyco-side) **is used simultaneously is there significant risk** [1, 7, 47–50]. The major adverse effects of vancomycin are summarized in Table 28O-3.

A. **Ototoxicity** is a potential side effect but is relatively uncommon [4]; it appears to occur when very high serum levels (>80 μg/ml) are reached [7]. The greatest risk of hearing loss occurs when vancomycin doses are not adequately adjusted or monitored in renal failure.

B. **Nephrotoxicity** is very **uncommon** if standard doses are used in the patient with normal renal function or if doses are appropriately reduced in the patient with renal failure [1, 7]. **When vancomycin is used with an aminoglycoside, it is important to monitor serum levels of both antibiotics to decrease the risk of nephrotoxicity (and ototoxicity).**

C. **Red man syndrome (RMS).** If vancomycin is infused too rapidly, it may cause the so-called **red man (red neck) syndrome,** which includes **flushing of the face, neck, or torso, pruritus** [1, 6, 7, 51–54], **or hypotension.** This reaction is believed to result from nonimmunologically mediated histamine release secondary to hyperosmolarity associated with the rapid infusion of vancomycin [1, 7]. **Rapid bolus infusions also can cause pain and muscle spasms of the chest and back** [6]. It is vital to recognize these syndromes so that the patient is not mistakenly labeled allergic to vancomycin.

1. **Infusion rate. Most of these reactions can be avoided if vancomycin is infused slowly**—that is, each 500 mg over 1 hour (or 1.0 g over 2 hours, 1.5 g over 3 hours, etc.).

2. **Dose relationship.** These reactions are less likely to occur if infusions of 500 mg rather than 1,000 mg are given over 1 hour [51]. (If the 1-g dose is used, it should be infused over 2 hours. See sec. **1.**)

3. **Prevention.** Studies have shown that in normal adult volunteers, prior administration of a histamine antagonist (50 mg of oral or intravenous diphenhydramine 45–60 minutes before the first dose of intravenous vancomycin or hydroxyzine hydrochloride, 50 mg PO approximately 2 hours before the intravenous infusion of vancomycin) provided significant protection against vanco-

Table 28O-3. Adverse effects associated with the use of vancomycin

Ototoxicity
  Hearing loss: often irreversible; rare; associated with drug levels >30 μg/ml
  Enhanced risk with concomitant aminoglycoside therapy
Infusion-related side effects
  Red man syndrome
  Pain and spasm syndrome
  Hypotension
Thrombophlebitis–associated with peripheral venous cannulas
Hypersensitivity reactions
  Drug fever (rare)
  Allergic rash (rare)
Neutropenia
  Reversible
  Develops after prolonged use
Nephrotoxicity
  Rare
  Enhanced risk with concomitant aminoglycoside therapy
  Reversible

Source: M.P. Wilhelm, Vancomycin. *Mayo Clin. Proc.* 66:1165, 1991.

mycin-induced RMS compared with prior placebo administration [52, 55].

4. **Clinical implications.** Although the RMS resembles an allergic reaction, one should recognize that it is not immunologically mediated and that such reactions do not preclude continued administration of vancomycin [53]. **Broncho-spasm and angioedema are not part of the RMS and, if seen, suggest a true allergic reaction to vancomycin.** If the RMS occurs with the first dose of vancomycin, pretreatment with an H_1 blocker (e.g., 50 mg oral diphenhydramine 45–60 minutes before intravenous vancomycin) and a slower infusion is advised [52]. We do not routinely pretreat patients with an H_1-blocker but favor a slow infusion rate.

D. **Rashes** have been reported in approximately 5% of patients treated with vancomycin [1, 7]. Stevens-Johnson syndrome may occur rarely [56].

E. **Phlebitis** at the site of infusion **can be minimized if the vancomycin is diluted in 100–200 ml dextrose and water or saline solution and infused slowly** at a rate not exceeding 15 mg/min [4].

F. **Fever and chills** after intravenous administration occur much less frequently with the more recent preparations of vancomycin, which contain fewer impurities.

G. **Neutropenia** can occur, especially with prolonged use, and agranulocytosis has been described [57]. Therefore, **serial blood counts are indicated (at least weekly) for any patient on prolonged vancomycin therapy.**

H. **Intracranial pressure elevation.** A study suggests that intracranial pressure rises with intravenous vancomycin infusions [58].

I. **Anaphylaxis** has been described, and desensitization of patients with a history of anaphylaxis has been reported [59].

VII. **Cost.** Vancomycin is **expensive.** (See Tables 28A-5 and 28A-6.) Inappropriate use of this agent should be avoided (see sec. **III**).

VIII. **Teicoplanin** (Targocid) is an antibiotic chemically similar to vancomycin but with important differences responsible for the unique physical and chemical properties of the complex [7].

A. **Investigational agent.** Although widely used in Europe for the treatment of gram-positive infections [3], teicoplanin was an investigational agent in the United States until late 1995 when even **clinical investigations were suspended.** As of mid-1996, there is no "compassionate-use" availability of this agent either.

B. A brief summary of this agent would emphasize the following [7]:

1. Its long half-life allows for administration intramuscularly or intravenously once daily.

2. It has excellent bactericidal activity against gram-positive bacteria, similar to vancomycin [60, 61]. It is more active than vancomycin and ampicillin

against enterococci, although concomitant aminoglycoside therapy is necessary for bactericidal effect [3].

3. It has been used for clinical indications similar to those for vancomycin (see sec. **III**) with the advantage of less frequent dosing. It may be useful for patients who have had neutropenic or allergic reactions to vancomycin [7].
4. Whether teicoplanin will be less toxic than vancomycin awaits further clinical experience with this agent. Rare ototoxicity has been reported [3].
5. Teicoplanin does not penetrate into the CSF well after intravenous use but, in a preliminary report, has been given by using an external ventricular drainage device [62].
6. Wilhelm [3] concluded that concern about the occurrence of teicoplanin-resistant staphylococci and reports of clinical failures with use of teicoplanin in patients with bacteremic staphylococcal infections have prompted serious questions about the overall advantages of teicoplanin over vancomycin. Currently, it seems unlikely that teicoplanin will usurp the prominent and important role of vancomycin in clinical practice in the United States [3].

IX. **Therapy for VRE**
   A. The **optimal therapy for** documented infection with **VRE is not established. Infectious disease consultation is advised.**
   B. **Several approaches have been tried.**
      1. Chloramphenicol may be useful in some patients with susceptible VRE [63].
      2. A few strains of VRE have been susceptible to teicoplanin.
      3. Antibiotic combinations in vitro may at times reveal bactericidal combinations [64].
      4. Quinupristin/dalfopristin (RP59500: Synercid, Rhône, Poulene Rorer) is an investigational drug (from the streptogramin class of antibiotics) available on a compassionate-use basis (610-454-3071) [21]. Kirby-Bauer discs for in vitro susceptibility tests are also available (610-454-3071).
      5. Polymicrobial surgical infections that include VRE may respond to antibiotics aimed at other susceptible organisms [21]. See Chaps. 11 and 16 for the role of enterococci in these settings.
      6. In VRE endocarditis, surgical replacement of the infected valve may be required [21].
      7. Bacteremia associated with intravenous lines may respond to removal of the lines [21].
   C. **Infection control practices** are important to prevent the spread of this organism. At this point, we favor careful isolation of these patients [13].
      1. **Single room** (or cohorting of VRE-colonized or -infected patients).
      2. **Gowns and gloves for all** those entering the patient's room.

References

1. Ingerman, M.J., and Santoro, J. Vancomycin: A new old agent. *Infect. Dis. Clin. North Am.* 3:641, 1989.
   See related update by T.S. Lundstrom and J.D. Sobel, Vancomycin, trimethoprim-sulfamethoxazole, and rifampin. Infect. Dis. Clin. North Am. 9:747, 1995.
2. Ena, J., et al. The epidemiology of intravenous vancomycin usage in a university hospital. A 10-year study. *J.A.M.A.* 269:598, 1993.
3. Wilhelm, M.P. Vancomycin. *Mayo Clin. Proc.* 66:1165, 1991.
   See related clinical summary by B.A. Cunha, Vancomycin. Med. Clin. North Am. 79:817, 1995.
4. Glew, R. Vancomycin. In S.L. Gorbach, J.G. Bartlett, and N.R. Blacklow (eds.), *Infectious Diseases*. Philadelphia: Saunders, 1992.
5. Schwalbe, R., Stapleton, J.T., and Gilligan, P.H. Emergence of vancomycin resistance in coagulase-negative staphylococci. *N. Engl. J. Med.* 316:927, 1987.
6. Medical Letter. New preparations of vancomycin. *Med. Lett. Drugs Ther.* 28:121, 1986.
7. Fekety, R. Vancomycin and Teicoplanin. In G.L. Mandell, J.E. Bennett, and R. Dolin (eds.), *Principles and Practice of Infectious Diseases* (4th ed.). New York: Churchill Livingstone, 1995. Pp. 346–354.
   For a more detailed summary of teicoplanin, see D.M. Campoli-Richards, R.N. Brogden, and D. Faulds, Teicoplanin: A review of its antibacterial activity, pharmacokinetic properties and therapeutic potential. Drugs 40:449, 1990; and K.W. Shea and B.A. Cunha, Teicoplanin. Med. Clin. North Am. 79:833, 1995.
8. Handwerger, S., et al. Concomitant high-level vancomycin and penicillin resistance in clinical isolates of enterococci. *Clin. Infect. Dis.* 14:655, 1992.

Infectious disease consultation is advised for therapy of vancomycin-resistant entero-cocci. See related discussions in Chaps. 28A and 28H. Also see B.E. Murray, Antibiotic resistance among enterococci: Current problems and management strategies. Curr. Clin. Top. Infect. Dis. *11:94, 1991.*

9. Schwalbe, R.S., et al. Selection for vancomycin resistance in clinical isolates of *Staphylococcus haemolyticus. J. Infect. Dis.* 161:45, 1990.

10. Darouiche, R.D., et al. Vancomycin penetration into biofilm covering infected prostheses and effect on bacteria. *J. Infect. Dis.* 170:720, 1994.
    Failure to cure prosthesis–related infections is not due to poor penetration of vancomycin into the biofilm but likely due to diminished antimicrobial effect on bacteria in the biofilm environment. For a review of prosthesis–related infections, including pathogenesis and therapy, see A.L. Bisno and F.A. Waldvogel (eds.), Infections Associated with Indwelling Devices *(2nd ed.). Washington, DC: ASM Press, 1994.*

11. Moellering, R.C., Jr. Emergence of enterococcus as a significant pathogen. *Clin. Infect. Dis.* 14:1173, 1992.

12. Centers for Disease Control. Nosocomial enterococci resistant to vancomycin: United States, 1989–1993. *M.M.W.R.* 30:597, 1993.
    Emphasizes dramatic 20-fold increase in vancomycin-resistant enterococci during this time frame. The percentage of nosocomial enterococci resistant to vancomycin increased from 0.3% in 1989 to 7.9% in 1993 and, among patients in intensive care units with nosocomial infections, the increase was from 0.4% in 1989 to 13.6% in 1993.
    See reprint in J.A.M.A. 270:1796, 1993. Also see V. Sastry et al., Vancomycin-resistant enterococci: An emerging pathogen in immunosuppressed recipients. Transplant Proc. *27:954, 1995. Also see L.B. Rice and D.M. Shlaes, Vancomycin resistance in the enterococcus: Relevance in pediatrics.* Pediatr. Clin. North Am. *42:601, 1995.*

13. Murray, B.E. What can we do about vancomycin-resistant enterococci? *Clin. Infect. Dis.* 20:1134, 1995.
    Editorial discussion emphasizing risk factors for vancomycin-resistant enterococci (VRE) and potential methods of prevention. Discusses related reference in same issue and suggests that because of heavy environmental contamination of VRE, **gowns and gloves may be useful for caregivers entering the rooms of VRE-infected or -colonized patients.** *Discusses possible mechanisms of how VRE are introduced into humans (e.g., animal-derived food products or inadvertent contamination of bacterial preparations that are consumed orally). See A.D. Luber et al., Relative importance of oral versus intravenous vancomycin exposure in the development of vancomycin-resistant enterococci.* J. Infect. Dis. *173:1292, 1996 (oral may be more important); and R. Shekar et al., Household transmission of vancomycin-resistant* Enterococcus faecium. Clin. Infect. Dis. *21:1511, 1995 (discusses person-to-person spread and risks at home).*

13a. Edmond, M.B., Wenzel, R.P., and Pasculle, A.W. Vancomycin-resistant *Staphylococcus aureus:* Perspectives on measures needed for control. *Ann. Intern. Med.* 124: 329, 1996.

14. Centers for Disease Control. Preventing the spread of vancomycin resistance. Report from the Hospital Infection Control Practice Advisory Committee. *Fed. Reg.* 59:25758, (May 17) 1994.
    Preliminary recommendations of expert group emphasizing how to control the increasing problems with VRE. Prudent vancomycin use, careful infection control practices, screening for VRE, and hospital staff education all are emphasized.
    These recommendations also have been published in Infect. Control Hosp. Epidemiol. *16:105, 1995;* Am. J. Infect. Cont. *23:87, 1995; and more recently, in final form, in* M.M.W.R. *44(RR-12):1–13, 1995.*

15. Barefield, E.S., and Philips, J.B., III. Vancomycin prophylaxis for coagulase-negative staphylococcal bacteremia. *J. Pediatr.* 125:230, 1994.
    Good editorial review of this bacteremia in neonates. Reviews two articles published in same journal demonstrating that intravenous vancomycin will reduce coagulase-negative bacteremias, but routine use of vancomycin for this purpose is not advised.

15a. Montecalvo, M.M., et al. Natural history of colonization with vancomycin-resistant *Enterococcus faecium. Infect. Control Hosp. Epidemiol.* 16:680, 1995.

15b. Shay, D.K., et al. Epidemiology and mortality risk of vancomycin-resistant enterococcal bloodstream infections. *J. Infect. Dis.* 172:993, 1995.

16. Schaad, U.B., et al. Clinical pharmacology and efficacy of vancomycin in pediatric patients. *J. Pediatr.* 96:119, 1980.

17. Baum, J., and Barza, M. Infections of the Eye. In S.L. Gorbach, J.G. Bartlett, and N.R. Blacklow (eds.), *Infectious Diseases.* Philadelphia: Saunders, 1992.
    Includes data on pharmacokinetics of vancomycin in vitreous and aqueous humor.

18. The Ad Hoc Advisory Committee on Peritonitis Management. Peritoneal dialysis–related peritonitis treatment recommendations—1993 update. *Peritoneal Dialysis Int.* 13:14, 1993.
19. Banner, W., Jr., and Ray, C.G. Vancomycin in perspective. *Am. J. Dis. Child.* 138:14, 1984.
    Editorial comment on pediatric use.
20. Levine, J.F. Vancomycin: A review. *Med. Clin. North Am.* 71:1135, 1987.
21. Medical Letter. The choice of antibacterial drugs. *Med. Lett. Drugs Ther.* 38:25, 1996.
22. Grieble, H.G., et al. The prevalence of high-level methicillin resistance in multiply resistant hospital staphylococci. *Medicine* (Baltimore) 60:62, 1981.
    Both S. aureus and S. epidermidis can be resistant to multiple antibiotics and cause severe infections. Vancomycin is the drug of choice.
23. Gardner, P., et al. Infections of mechanical cerebrospinal fluid shunts. *Curr. Clin. Top. Infect. Dis.* 9:185, 1988.
    Also see reference [31].
24. Mulligan, M.E., et al. Methicillin-resistant *Staphylococcus aureus:* A consensus review of the microbiology, pathogenesis, and epidemiology with implications for prevention and management. *Am. J. Med.* 94:313, 1993.
    Extensive review of this topic.
25. Alpert, G., et al. Vancomycin dosages in pediatrics reconsidered. *Am. J. Dis. Child.* 138:20, 1984.
    Close monitoring of serum levels is important, especially in neonates and infants. See related article by R.V. Jarrett et al., Individualized pharmacokinetic profiles to compute vancomycin dosage and dosing interval in preterm infants. Pediatr. Infect. Dis. J. 12:156, 1993.
26. Levine, D.P., et al. Slow response to vancomycin or vancomycin plus rifampin in methicillin-resistant *Staphylococcus aureus* endocarditis. *Ann. Intern. Med.* 115:674, 1991.
    Slow clinical improvement is common. The median duration of bacteremia was 9 days. See reference [17] for an editorial comment on this article.
27. Karchmer, A.W. *Staphylococcus aureus* and vancomycin: The sequel. *Ann. Intern. Med.* 115:739, 1991.
    For methicillin-susceptible S. aureus severe infections, in the nonallergic patient, the semisynthetic penicillins (e.g., oxacillin, nafcillin) are preferred over vancomycin, which may take longer to sterilize the bloodstream. For a related discussion, see A.W. Karchmer, Ask the expert: Is vancomycin versus S. aureus optimal therapy? Infect. Dis. Clin. Pract. 1:143, 1992.
28. Markowitz, N., et al. Trimethoprim-sulfamethoxazole compared with vancomycin for the treatment of *Staphylococcus aureus* infection. *Ann. Intern. Med.* 117:390, 1992.
    Vancomycin was superior in efficacy and safety when treating intravenous drug users. Trimethoprim-sulfamethoxazole may be an alternative to vancomycin in some methicillin-resistant S. aureus infections.
29. Sande, M.A., and Scheld, W.M. Combination therapy of bacterial endocarditis. *Ann. Intern. Med.* 92:390, 1980.
29a. Wilson, W.R., et al. Antibiotic treatment of adults with infective endocarditis due to streptococci, enterococci, staphylococci, and HACEK microorganisms. *J.A.M.A.* 274:1706, 1995.
30. McLaurin, R.L., and Frame, P.T. Treatment of infections of cerebrospinal fluid shunts. *Rev. Infect. Dis.* 9:595, 1987.
    Discusses use of intrashunt injections of vancomycin and oral therapy with trimethoprim-sulfamethoxazole and rifampin. Also see Annotation of reference 31.
31. Yogev, R. Cerebrospinal fluid shunt infections: A personal view. *Pediatr. Infect. Dis.* 4:113, 1985.
    For a recent review, see A.L. Bisno and L. Sternau, Infections of central nervous system shunts. In A.L. Bisno and F. Waldvogel (eds.), Infections Associated with Prosthetic Devices (2nd ed.). Washington, DC: ASM Press, 1994. Chap. 5.
32. Bartlett, J.G. *Clostridium difficile:* Clinical considerations. *Rev. Infect. Dis.* 12(Suppl. 2):S243, 1990.
    Concise review. See updated references and detailed discussion in Chap. 28A.
33. Karp, J.E., et al. Empiric use of vancomycin during prolonged treatment-induced granulocytopenia. Randomized, double-blind, placebo-controlled clinical trial in patients with acute leukemia. *Am. J. Med.* 81:237, 1986.
34. Rubin, M., et al. Gram-positive infections and the use of vancomycin in 550 episodes of fever and neutropenia. *Ann. Intern. Med.* 108:30, 1988.
35. Hughes, W.T., et al. Guidelines for the use of antimicrobial agents in neutropenic

patients with unexplained fever. *J. Infect. Dis.* 161:381, 1990.
See related article by R. Ramphal et al., Vancomycin is not an essential component of the initial empiric regimen for febrile neutropenic patients receiving ceftazidime: A randomized prospective study. Antimicrob. Agents Chemother. *36:1062, 1992.*

36. European Organization for Research and Treatment of Cancer International Antimicrobial Therapy Cooperative Group and the National Cancer Institute of Canada—Clinical Trials Group. Empiric use of vancomycin in the febrile neutropenic patient. *J. Infect. Dis.* 165:591, 1992.
   Comment on prior EORTC data published on this topic in J. Infect. Dis. *163:951, 1991, which does not support the empirical addition of vancomycin to initial antibiotic therapy in cancer patients with fever and granulocytopenia.*

37. Fekety, R., et al. Treatment of antibiotic-associated *Clostridium difficile* colitis with oral vancomycin: Comparison of two dosage regimens. *Am. J. Med.* 86:15, 1989.
   The 125-mg PO qid dose was as effective as the 500-mg qid dose.

38. Farber, B.F., et al. Vancomycin prophylaxis in cardiac operations: Determination of an optimal dosage regimen. *J. Thorac. Cardiovasc. Surg.* 85:933, 1983.

39. Morse, G.D., Nairn, D.K., and Walshe, J.J. Once weekly intraperitoneal therapy for gram-positive peritonitis. *Am. J. Kidney Dis.* 4:300, 1987.

40. Boyce, N.W., et al. Intraperitoneal vancomycin therapy for CAPD dialysis. *Am. J. Kidney Dis.* 12:304, 1988.
   Two doses of intraperitoneal vancomycin, given once weekly, were effective.

41. Luer, M.S., and Hatton, J. Vancomycin administration into the cerebrospinal fluid: A review. *Ann. Pharmacother.* 27:912, 1993.

42. Cantú, T.G., Yamanaka-Yuen, N.A., and Leitman, P.S. Serum vancomycin concentrations: Reappraisal of their clinical value. *Clin. Infect. Dis.* 18:533, 1994.
   Review of literature emphasizing that there are no data clearly showing vancomycin serum level monitoring improves efficacy or reduces toxicity over careful conventional dosing regimens.

43. Moellering, R.C., Jr. Monitoring serum vancomycin levels: Climbing the mountain because it is there? [editorial]. *Clin. Infect. Dis.* 18:544, 1994.
   Routine monitoring of serum levels is not necessary. Editorial comment on reference [42].

44. Moellering, R.C., Jr., et al. Vancomycin therapy in patients with impaired renal function: A nomogram for dosage. *Ann. Intern. Med.* 94:343, 1981.

45. Matzke, G.R., et al. Pharmacokinetics of vancomycin in patients with various degrees of renal function. *Antimicrob. Agents Chemother.* 25:433, 1984.
   See also G.R. Matzke et al., Evaluation of the vancomycin clearance–creatinine clearance relationship for predicting vancomycin dosage. Clin. Pharmacol. *4:311, 1985. See related article by K. Vance-Bryan et al., Effect of obesity on vancomycin pharmacokinetic parameters as determined by using Bayesian forecasting technique.* Antimicrob. Agents Chemother. *37:436, 1993. Data shows that using actual body weight is superior to using lean body weight to calculate dose requirements in these patients with normal renal function.*

46. Cunha, B.A., et al. Pharmacokinetics of vancomycin in anuria. *Rev. Infect. Dis.* 3(Suppl.):269, 1981.

47. Brummett, R.E., and Fox, K.E. Vancomycin- and erythromycin-induced hearing loss in humans. *Antimicrob. Agents Chemother.* 33:791, 1989.

48. Farber, B.F., and Moellering, R.C., Jr. Retrospective study of the toxicity of preparations of vancomycin from 1974 to 1981. *Antimicrob. Agents Chemother.* 23:138, 1983.
   In a study by M.A. Cimino et al., Am. J. Med. *83:1091, 1987, in which vancomycin was used with gentamicin, nephrotoxicity occurred less frequently when vancomycin trough levels were less than 10 μg/ml.*

49. Downs, N.J., et al. Mild nephrotoxicity associated with vancomycin use. *Arch. Intern. Med.* 149:1777, 1989.

50. Appel, G.B. Aminoglycoside nephrotoxicity. *Am. J. Med.* 88(Suppl. 3C):16S, 1990.

51. Healy, D.P., et al. Comparison of steady-state pharmacokinetics of two dosage regimens of vancomycin in normal volunteers. *Antimicrob. Agents Chemother.* 31:393, 1987.
   When compared to 500 mg q6h, 1 g vancomycin IV q12h is associated with a greater incidence of the red man syndrome.

52. Wallace, M.R., Mascola, J.R., and Oldfield, E.C., III. Red man syndrome: Incidence, etiology, and prophylaxis. *J. Infect. Dis.* 164:1180, 1991.
   Good summary. Emphasizes that slow infusions (e.g., 1 g over 2 hours) reduces this side effect. If a patient has red man syndrome (RMS) after the first dose and vancomycin

is the ideal agent to continue, the second dose should be given slowly (over longer than 2 hours) after pretreatment with an H₁-blocker (50 mg oral diphenhydramine 45–60 minutes before vancomycin infusion). Although RMS presumably occurs less frequently with teicoplanin use, it has been reported. See S. Dubettier et al., Red man syndrome with teicoplanin. Rev. Infect. Dis. 13:770, 1991.

53. Deresinski, S.C. Vancomycin and the red man syndrome. *Infect. Dis. Alert* 11:34, 1992.
54. Southern, D.J., et al. Adverse effects of vancomycin administered in the perioperative period. *Mayo Clin. Proc.* 61:721, 1986.
55. Sahai, J., et al. Influence of antihistamine pretreatment on vancomycin-induced red man syndrome. *J. Infect. Dis.* 160:876, 1989.
56. Laurencin, C.T., et al. Stevens-Johnson type reaction with vancomycin treatment. *Ann. Pharmacother.* 26:1520, 1992.
57. Adrouny, A., et al. Agranulocytosis related to vancomycin therapy. *Am. J. Med.* 81:1059, 1986.
    A rare complication.
58. Gaskill, S.J., and Marlin, A.E. Vancomycin: Its effect on intracranial pressure. *Pediatr. Neurosurg.* 18:139, 1992.
59. Anne, S., et al. Vancomycin anaphylaxis and successful desensitization. *Ann. Allergy* 73:402, 1994.
    Describes a several-day desensitization protocol.
60. Greenberg, R.N. Treatment of bone, joint, and vascular access–associated gram-positive bacterial infections with teicoplanin. *Antimicrob. Agents Chemother.* 34: 2392, 1990.
    For related reference, see J.L. Schmit, Efficacy of teicoplanin for enterococcal infections: 63 cases and review. Clin. Infect. Dis. 15:302, 1992, in which teicoplanin showed good efficacy. Further studies are needed to determine optimal dosing and combination therapy.
61. Van der Auwera, P., et al. Randomized study of vancomycin versus teicoplanin for the treatment of gram-positive bacterial infections in immunocompromised hosts. *Antimicrob. Agents Chemother.* 35:451, 1991.
62. Cruciani, M., et al. Evaluation of intraventricular teicoplanin for the treatment of neurosurgical shunt infections. *Clin. Infect. Dis.* 15:285, 1992.
63. Norris, A.H., et al. Chloramphenicol for the treatment of vancomycin-resistant enterococcal infections. *Clin. Infect. Dis.* 20:1137, 1995.
    Chloramphenicol may be useful in selected patients in this report from the University of Pennsylvania. However, at times, VRE was involved in mixed infection and therefore its precise role as a pathogen in a single patient may be difficult to assess.
64. Hayden, M.K., et al. Bactericidal activities of antibiotics against vancomycin-resistant Enterococcus faecium blood isolates and synergistic activities of combinations. *Antimicrob. Agents Chemother.* 38:1225, 1994.
    Using time-kill studies, bactericidal activity was attainable against 7 of 13 VRE isolates at 24 hours.

P. Metronidazole

Metronidazole has been used for several years for *Trichomonas vaginalis* infections, for amebiasis, and for giardiasis. In recent years, it has become an extremely important agent in anaerobic infections [1–5].

I. **Spectrum of activity**

   A. **Aerobes. Metronidazole is not active against *Staphylococcus aureus* and other staphylococci, streptococci (including enterococci), and Enterobacteriaceae.** There are some animal model data suggesting that it may be active against *Escherichia coli* and some strains of *Klebsiella* and *Proteus* spp. [1, 3] but, from a practical standpoint, metronidazole is not viewed as an agent useful for Enterobacteriaceae.

   Gardnerella (Haemophilus) vaginalis is susceptible to metronidazole.

   B. **Anaerobes.** Metronidazole is **very active and bactericidal** against anaerobes [1–7], including *Bacteroides fragilis* and other *Bacteroides* spp., *Clostridium* spp. (including *C. perfringens* and *C. difficile*), and *Fusobacterium, Peptococcus,* and *Peptostreptococcus* spp., although some studies suggest somewhat less activity against anaerobic gram-positive cocci. *Propionibacterium acnes* is highly resistant

[1, 2, 6]. In addition, metronidazole is not active against microaerophilic strepto-cocci [2]. (See sec. **IV.C.3.**)

In the 1996 *Medical Letter,* **metronidazole is listed as the agent of choice for GI strains of *Bacteroides* spp.** (i.e., *B. fragilis*) [5]. (See Chap. 28I, sec. **I.C.**, (p. 1262) for additional discussion of *B. fragilis* susceptibility data.)

Metronidazole is active against *C. difficile.*

In their review, Finegold and Mathisen conclude that metronidazole has the best bactericidal activity of all the drugs active against anaerobic bacteria [1].

C. **Parasites.** Metronidazole is very active against *Entamoeba histolytica, Giardia lamblia,* and *T. vaginalis* [8], although some strains of *T. vaginalis* may be resistant [3]. (See discussions in Chaps. 11 and 13.)

D. **Resistance.** Initially susceptible bacteria rarely develop resistance to metronidazole; this is discussed elsewhere [1]. A combination of several mechanisms may be required for emergence of high-level resistance [1].

II. **Pharmacokinetics**

A. **Oral absorption.** Metronidazole is **very well absorbed** from the GI tract. **Serum levels are similar following equivalent oral and intravenous doses.** Although total absorption of the drug is not affected by administration with food, peak serum levels are delayed [2].

B. **Serum concentrations.** The intravenous preparation provides excellent serum levels against susceptible pathogens, with peak levels averaging 25 μg/ml and trough levels of 18 μg/ml with standard intravenous regimens [1].

C. **Half-life.** The serum half-life is approximately 8 hours, so dosage intervals of longer than 6 hours are feasible [2] (Table 28P-1).

D. **Tissue penetration.** Metronidazole has **excellent penetration** into almost all sites and has been shown to provide therapeutic levels in bone, unobstructed biliary tract, cerebrospinal fluid, brain abscess contents, empyema fluid, hepatic abscesses, middle ear, pelvic tissue, and vaginal secretions [1, 2]. Penetration into aqueous humor results in levels one-half to one-third of serum levels [2].

E. **Metabolism and excretion.** Metronidazole is metabolized primarily in the liver and excreted in the kidney.

F. **Placenta and breast milk.** Metronidazole readily crosses the placenta and penetrates breast milk (in therapeutic concentrations).

G. A 0.75% **vaginal gel formulation** (MetroGel-Vaginal, Curatek) was approved for treatment of bacterial vaginosis [8a]. Approximately 50% of an intravaginal 5-g dose (containing nearly 37.5 mg of metronidazole) is absorbed, but peak serum concentrations are only about 2% as high as those with a 500-mg oral dose [8a]. See Chap. 13.

III. **Carcinogenic potential.** The **package insert** contains a **warning** that metronidazole has been shown to be carcinogenic in mice and rats [9]. The precise risk for humans is unclear and remains controversial. Though data are incomplete, some experts believe that, because metronidazole is a carcinogen for animals, it is a potential carcinogen for humans [10]. Metronidazole has not been shown to be teratogenic, but many experts believe that it **should not be used in pregnancy** or should be used during pregnancy only if no alternative agent is available. It **should be avoided especially during the first trimester** [1–3, 8, 10]. In a recent metaanalysis, metronidazole does not appear to be associated with an increased teratogenic risk [10a]. **Because it is excreted into breast milk, nursing should be discontinued during and for 2 days after therapy with metronidazole** [1]. There is concern that with prolonged use or repeated courses of metronidazole, the potential carcinogenic effect may be increased [3, 11].

IV. **Clinical uses**

A. **Indications for oral or intravenous form**

1. **Anaerobic infections.** Metronidazole has been used extensively in the treatment of a variety of anaerobic infections, including soft-tissue infections, intraabdominal and pelvic infections, and brain abscess. See individual chapter discussions.

Metronidazole is not active against Enterobacteriaceae. Therefore, in mixed GI or pelvic aerobic and anaerobic infections, an additional agent is necessary [12].

Metronidazole has been shown to be consistently bactericidal against *B. fragilis;* it is the agent of choice in patients with *B. fragilis* bacteremia with known or suspected endocarditis or other vascular infections. It usually is active

Table 28P-1. Metronidazole dosage regimens

Indication	Route of administration	Adult dosage[a]
Susceptible anaerobic infections[b]	IV[c]	Loading dose of 15 mg/kg, then 7.5 mg/kg q6h[d]
	PO	1–2 g/day in 2–4 doses q6–12h[e]
C. difficile diarrhea	PO	250 mg qid for 10–14 days [14][f]
	IV[g]	500 mg q6–8h
Trichomonas vaginitis	PO	2 g in a single dose[h]
Bacterial vaginosis (nonspecific vaginitis, Gardnerella vaginalis vaginosis)	PO	500 mg bid for 7 days[i]
	Topical	See footnote[i]
Giardiasis	PO	250 mg tid for 5 days[j]
Amebiasis (intestinal or extraintestinal)	IV or PO	750 mg tid for 10 days[k]

[a]Dosages must be modified if creatinine clearance < 10 ml/min or if there is significant hepatic dysfunction. See text. Also see footnotes for pediatric regimens.

[b]For serious infection, duration of therapy may be 2–4 weeks, depending on clinical response and type of infection.

[c]Intravenous therapy is preferred initially in very ill patients or those unable to take oral medication. Once the patient improves, oral therapy can be used. See text.

[d]Intravenous dose usually infused over 60 minutes.

[e]Because of the relatively long half-life of metronidazole, oral doses have been administered at q6h, q8h, or q12h intervals [1, 2]. An oral regimen of 7.5 mg/kg q6h can also be used.

[f]Oral metronidazole is useful in mild to moderately severe cases [13, 14]. In seriously ill cases, oral vancomycin, 125 mg PO q6h, is preferred [5, 16]. See text.

[g]For patients unable to take oral therapy, intravenous metronidazole is preferred (not intravenous vancomycin). See text and related discussion in Chap. 28A.

[h]Experience has shown that single-dose therapy is as effective as the longer, multiple-dose regimens previously recommended (i.e., 250 mg tid or 500 mg bid for 7 days). The single-dose regimen of 2.0 g metronidazole given simultaneously to the index case and all sexual partners is suggested [17]. Metronidazole should not be given during pregnancy. See related discussions in Chap. 13.

[i]Single-dose therapy with metronidazole is less effective in this setting. If metronidazole is contraindicated, clindamycin, 300 mg PO bid for 7 days, can be used [17]. A 0.75% vaginal gel formulation of metronidazole (MetroGel-Vaginal) is available in a 70-g tube and packaged with a 5-g vaginal applicator. The dose is 5 g intravaginally bid for 5 days. Women using any formulation of metronidazole should not drink alcohol because the drug may interact with alcohol to cause disulfiramlike symptoms [8a]. (See text and sec. II.G.)

[j]In children, giardiasis has been treated with 5 mg/kg/dose tid for 5 days [8].

[k]In amebiasis therapy, after 10 days of metronidazole, iodoquinol, 650 mg tid for 20 days, is recommended [8] in adults. The pediatric dose of metronidazole is 35–50 mg/kg/day divided into three doses for 10 days; iodoquinol, 30–40 mg/kg/day in 3 divided doses, is given (after completion of metronidazole) for 20 days [8].

Source: Modified from G.E. Mathisen and S.M. Finegold, Metronidazole and Other Nitroimidazoles. In S.L. Gorbach, J.G. Bartlett, and N.R. Blacklow (eds.), *Infectious Diseases*. Philadelphia: Saunders, 1992. P. 262; and Medical Letter. Drugs for parasite diseases. *Med. Lett. Drugs. Ther.* 37:99, 1995.

against the 5–15% of isolates of *B. fragilis* that are resistant to clindamycin (see Chap. 28I). The cost per day of metronidazole is typically less than that for clindamycin (see Tables 28A-5 and 28A-6), and metronidazole may be associated with less *C. difficile* diarrhea than is clindamycin (see Chap. 28A). **For these reasons, metronidazole is viewed as the agent of choice for B. fragilis infections in adults** [5].

2. **Antibiotic-associated diarrhea due to C. difficile** responds to metronidazole (see further discussion in Chap. 28A [13–14a]). Oral therapy is most effective and less expensive than intravenous therapy, but intravenous administration of metronidazole may be effective in patients who cannot receive oral therapy [15]. For most cases of *C. difficile* diarrhea and initial empiric therapy, hospital formulary committees favor the use of oral metronidazole rather than oral vancomycin, because metronidazole is more cost-effective. Because of these advantages of metronidazole and as excessive use of oral vancomycin may contribute to the increasing problem of vancomycin-resistant enterococci (VRE),

metronidazole is usually viewed as the initial drug of choice for *C. difficile* diarrhea [5]. See related discussions in Chap. 28O. However, **for very severe or refractory cases of *C. difficile* diarrhea, oral vancomycin** is still used [14, 14a, 16]. (See Chaps. 28A and 28O.)

3. **Trichomoniasis.** Metronidazole is the preferred therapy unless contraindicated. See Chap. 13.
4. **Bacterial vaginosis** (nonspecific vaginitis, *G. vaginalis* vaginosis). Metronidazole is the drug of choice in this common vaginitis [17]. A new topical agent recently was approved for this use also [8a]. See Chap. 13.
5. **Giardiasis** has been treated effectively with metronidazole. Although it is not approved for the treatment of giardiasis in the United States, metronidazole frequently is prescribed [8] because quinacrine hydrochloride is no longer available. See Chap. 11.
6. **Amebiasis.** Intestinal and hepatic disease due to *E. histolytica* often are treated with metronidazole followed by iodoquinol [8]. See Chap. 11.
7. **Perineal** fistula associated with Crohn's disease has been treated with metronidazole (see sec. **C.5**).
8. **Eradication of *Helicobacter pylori* in peptic ulcer disease.** Metronidazole has been used in various regimens to eradicate *H. pylori* [18, 19]. This topic is reviewed in detail in Chap. 11 under *Helicobacter pylori* and Peptic Ulcer Disease (see pp. 403–406).
9. **Tetanus.** Although historically penicillin has been the usual recommended agent [5], a study from Indonesia suggests metronidazole is more efficacious and therefore may be the drug of choice for tetanus [20].

B. **Topical metronidazole gel** is an effective and safe therapeutic agent for rosacea [21]. A 0.75% vaginal gel formulation of metronidazole is available for treatment of bacterial vaginosis [8a]. (See sec. **II.G** and Chap. 13.)

C. **Contraindications or areas of limited use**
1. **Pregnancy. Metronidazole use is contraindicated during the first trimester** (see sec. **III**). Metronidazole is classified in pregnancy as category B agent (see Chap. 28A). The package insert emphasizes that use in the second and third trimesters of pregnancy should be restricted to those patients in whom alternative therapy has been inadequate [9]. In their review, Finegold and Mathison emphasize that the use of metronidazole during pregnancy should be reserved for situations in which it is clearly needed [1].
2. **Lactating women.** Metronidazole use is contraindicated as metronidazole is excreted into breast milk (see sec. **III**). Nursing should be discontinued during metronidazole use and for 2 days after therapy with metronidazole [1].
3. **Pulmonary anaerobic infections.** Metronidazole is less-than-optimal therapy [1, 2] for mixed aerobic and anaerobic pulmonary infections, at least in part because of the relative resistance of microaerophilic streptococci to metronidazole.
4. **Prophylaxis.** Although metronidazole has been shown to be an effective agent (in combination with another agent such as ceftriaxone) for GI surgical procedures [9], other agents are favored [22]. (See discussion in Chap. 28B.)
5. **Crohn's disease.** Although metronidazole has been used in Crohn's disease since 1975, its efficacy remains unproved [3]. With prolonged or repeated courses, there is concern regarding the development of peripheral neuropathy, carcinogenicity, and emergence of resistant microorganisms [1, 3]. Metronidazole is effective therapy for severe perineal disease associated with Crohn's disease elsewhere in the GI tract that has been unresponsive to previous medical and surgical therapy [23].

V. **Preparations and doses.** As stated previously, this agent **should be avoided in pregnancy, particularly in the first trimester.** Because metronidazole is so well absorbed orally and blood levels comparable to intravenous therapy can be achieved with oral therapy, once the patient's condition allows, oral therapy can be used instead of intravenous therapy [1]. Minor infections typically are treated with oral therapy. **The package insert indicates that safety and effectiveness in children have not been established except for the treatment of amebiasis** [9].

A. **Adult dosage regimens.** See Table 28P-1.
B. In **renal failure,** doses do not require modification, except in the case of severe renal failure (i.e., creatinine clearance <10 ml/min), where a 50% reduction in the usual dose is suggested to prevent the possible accumulation of toxic metabolites [24]. Hemodialysis rapidly removes metronidazole, and a dose after hemodial-

ysis is suggested [24]. The drug also is eliminated during peritoneal dialysis, and dose reduction generally is not recommended during chronic ambulatory peritoneal dialysis [2], although some sources suggest a 50% dose reduction in these patients [24].
   C. **In patients with significant hepatic impairment,** with or without renal impairment, **plasma clearance of metronidazole is delayed** and dose adjustments are advisable [1]. Although data are limited, pharmacokinetic studies in patients suggest that doses should be reduced by at least 50% in this patient population [1, 2].
VI. **Adverse effects.** In general, metronidazole is well tolerated.
   A. **Carcinogenic potential.** This controversial subject is discussed in sec. **III.**
   B. **Alcohol intolerance.** Alcoholic beverages should not be consumed by patients **taking any formulation of metronidazole,** because of a disulfiramlike effect (i.e., nausea, vomiting, abdominal cramps, strange taste sensations, and headaches).
   C. **Peripheral neuropathy,** manifested as numbness and tingling of the extremities, has rarely been seen with a short course of metronidazole therapy but is more commonly seen after therapy lasting a few months [23]. If the agent is discontinued when symptoms first begin, the symptoms usually will disappear. This problem is more likely to occur in patients on high doses. Generalized **seizures** have been reported. Metronidazole should be used with caution in patients with a history of seizures or other CNS disorders [1]. If seizures occur with metronidazole use, the drug should be discontinued (unless there is another obvious explanation for the seizure and an alternate agent is not available).
   D. **Anticoagulation interference.** Metronidazole can potentiate the effect of warfarin and thus produce prolongation of the prothrombin time.
   E. **Miscellaneous. Mild GI symptoms** of nausea, abdominal discomfort, diarrhea, and so on can occur. Nausea may be seen in up to 12% of recipients of oral metronidazole [4]. Patients not uncommonly complain of a **metallic, unpleasant taste** while on oral therapy. Furring of the tongue, glossitis, stomatitis, and dry mouth can occur [1]. Reversible neutropenia has been observed. Metronidazole may be a cause of **acute pancreatitis,** and its use should be discontinued if no other risk factor is found [25]. Rarely, metronidazole has caused pseudomembranous colitis [2].
   F. The recently released vaginal gel formulation appears to be well tolerated; nausea, abdominal cramps, and a metallic taste have occurred but to a much lesser degree than with the oral drug [8a].
VII. **Cost.** See Tables 28A-5 and 28A-6.
VIII. **Tinidazole is similar to metronidazole** in its mechanism of action, antimicrobial spectrum, and toxicity. **It is not clinically available in the United States,** nor are there plans by the pharmaceutical company to have it released in the United States in the near future. It has a prolonged serum half-life (12.5 hours), with the potential for simpler dosage regimens. There is far less clinical experience with this agent than with metronidazole [2].

References

1. Finegold, S.M., and Mathisen, G.E. Metronidazole. In G.L. Mandell, J.E. Bennett, and R. Dolin (eds.), *Principles and Practice of Infectious Diseases* (4th ed.). New York: Churchill Livingstone, 1995. Pp. 329–334.
2. Mathisen, G.E., and Finegold, S.M. Metronidazole and Other Nitroimidazoles. In S.L. Gorbach, J.G. Bartlett, and N.R. Blacklow (eds.), *Infectious Diseases.* Philadelphia: Saunders, 1992. Pp. 260–265.
   Good discussion by a couple of national authorities. An update of the discussion in reference 1.
3. Scully, B.E. Metronidazole. *Med. Clin. North Am.* 72:613, 1988.
   See related update by M.E. Falagas and S. Gorbach, Clindamycin and metronidazole. Med. Clin. North Am. *79:845, 1995.*
4. Smilack, J.D., et al. Tetracyclines, chloramphenicol, erythromycin, clindamycin, and metronidazole. *Mayo Clin. Proc.* 66:1270, 1991.
5. Medical Letter. The choice of antibacterial drugs. *Med. Lett. Drugs Ther.* 38:25, 1996.
6. Musial, C.E., and Rosenblatt, J.E. Antimicrobial susceptibilities of anaerobic bacteria isolated at the Mayo Clinic during 1982 through 1987: Comparison with results from 1977 through 1981. *Mayo Clin Proc.* 64:392, 1989.
   For B. fragilis *group, 0% of 677 isolates were resistant to metronidazole.*
7. Cuchural, G.J., Jr., et al. Susceptibility of the *Bacteroides fragilis* group in the United

States: Analysis by site of infection. *Antimicrob. Agents Chemother.* 32:717, 1988. *For B. fragilis group, 0% for 673 isolates were resistant to metronidazole. In a brief report from Spain, 2% of clinical isolates were resistant to metronidazole. See M.T. Pelaez et al., Resistance of anaerobic bacteria to antimicrobial agents. Rev. Infect. Dis. 13:183, 1991.*

8. Medical Letter. Drugs for parasitic infections. *Med. Lett. Drugs Ther.* 37:99, 1995.

8a. Medical Letter. Topical treatment for bacterial vaginosis. *Med. Lett. Drugs Ther.* 34:109, 1992.
Concludes that although published data are limited, vaginal metronidazole and 2% vaginal clindamycin both appear to be nearly as effective as oral metronidazole and are better tolerated. The dose of clindamycin vaginal cream is 5 g intravaginally once daily for 7 days. The average wholesale cost for the clindamycin vaginal cream is $26.70 and for the metronidazole vaginal gel, $20.40. In a related article by J.D. Sobel et al. (Long-term follow-up of patients with bacterial vaginosis treated with oral metronidazole and topical clindamycin. J. Infect. Dis. 167:783, 1993), the authors point out the long-term recurrence rates observed in bacterial vaginosis irrespective of treatment method.

9. *Physician's Desk Reference* (50th ed.). Montvale, NJ: Medical Economics Data, 1996.

10. Goldman, P. Metronidazole. *N. Engl. J. Med.* 303:1212, 1980.

10a. Burtin, P., et al. Safety of metronidazole in pregnancy: A meta-analysis. *Am. J. Obstet. Gynecol.* 172:525, 1995.
All published articles reporting on metronidazole use during pregnancy were screened.

11. Krause, J.R., Ayuyang, H.Q., and Ellis, L.D. Occurrence of three cases of carcinoma in individuals with Crohn's disease treated with metronidazole. *Am. J. Gastroenterol.* 80:978, 1985.

12. Bohnen, J.M.A., et al. Guidelines for clinical care: Anti-infective agents for intra-abdominal infection. A Surgical Infection Policy Statement. *Arch. Surg.* 127:83, 1992.
Metronidazole is a mainstay agent for antianaerobic activity, especially in severe infections. Useful clinical discussion.

13. Teasley, D.G., et al. Prospective randomized trial of metronidazole versus vancomycin for *Clostridium difficile*–associated diarrhea and colitis. *Lancet* 2:1043, 1983.

14. Bartlett, J.G. *Clostridium difficile:* Clinical considerations. *Rev. Infect. Dis.* 12(Suppl. 2):S243, 1990.
A good concise clinical review by an expert in the field. For an update of this topic, see J.G. Bartlett, Antibiotic-associated diarrhea. Clin. Infect. Dis. 15:573, 1992, which emphasizes the role of vancomycin for seriously ill patients and also discusses options for patients with multiple recurrences. See reference [16].

14a. Fekety, R., and Shah, A.B. Diagnosis and treatment of *Clostridium difficile* colitis. *J.A.M.A.* 269:71, 1993.
Also favors oral vancomycin for severe illness. See additional references in Chap. 28A.

15. Bolton, R.P., and Culshaw, M.A. Faecal metronidazole concentrations during oral and intravenous therapy for antibiotic associated colitis due to *Clostridium difficile*. *Gut* 27:1169, 1986.
Intravenous metronidazole was associated with therapeutic fecal concentrations and clinical response. Also see Chap. 28A.

16. Gorbach, S.L. Drugs for your mother-in-law: Metronidazole for *Clostridium difficile*. *Infect. Dis. Clin. Pract.* 1:46, 1992.
See related comment on viewing oral vancomycin as the "gold standard" of therapy for C. difficile diarrhea by M.S. Drapkin, Nosocomial infection with C. difficile. Infect. Dis. Clin. Pract. 1:138, 1992; and J.G. Bartlett, The 10 most common questions about Clostridium difficile–associated diarrhea/colitis. Infect. Dis. Clin. Pract. 1:254, 1992.

17. Centers for Disease Control. 1993 Sexually transmitted diseases treatment guidelines. *M.M.W.R.* 42(RR-14):1, 1993.

18. Walsh, J.H. *Helicobacter pylori:* Selection of patients for treatment. *Ann. Intern. Med.* 116:770, 1992.
Good editorial overview of this controversial topic and commentary on reference [19].

19. Graham, D.Y., et al. Effect of treatment of *Helicobacter pylori* infection on the long-term recurrence of gastric or duodenal ulcer: A randomized controlled study. *Ann. Intern. Med.* 116:705, 1992.
Triple therapy consisted of tetracycline HCL 500 mg PO qid, metronidazole 250 mg PO tid, and bismuth subsalicylate (5–8 Pepto-Bismol tablets daily) for 2 weeks. All patients received ranitidine 300 mg at bedtime until the ulcer was healed or 16 weeks had elapsed. See detailed discussions in Chap. 11.
The use of this regimen is suggested also in the Medical Letter *(see reference [5].)*

20. Ahmadsyah, I., and Salim, A. Treatment of tetanus: An open study to compare the efficacy of procaine penicillin and metronidazole. *Br. Med. J.* 291:648, 1985.
    In this trial, 76 patients received penicillin and 97 metronidazole. Patients in the metronidazole group had a significantly lower mortality, a shorter hospital stay, and improved response to treatment.
21. Medical Letter. Topical metronidazole for rosacea. *Med. Lett. Drugs Ther.* 31:75, 1989.
22. Medical Letter. Antimicrobial prophylaxis in surgery. *Med. Lett. Drugs Ther.* 37: 79, 1995.
    Metronidazole is not encouraged.
23. Babb, R.R. The use of metronidazole (Flagyl) in Crohn's disease. *J. Clin. Gastroenterol.* 10:479, 1988.
    Editorial comment. Good summary of this controversial area. Doses of 1.5–2.0 g daily have been used.

    Also see the editorial comment by D.H. Present, The prevention of Crohn's disease after surgery: Metronidazole is a small but continuous medical advancement. Gastroenterol *108:1935, 1995; and related paper by P. Rutgeerts et al., Controlled trial of metronidazole treatment for prevention of Crohn's recurrence after ileal resection.* Gastroenterol. *108:1617, 1995.*
24. Bennett, W.M., et al. *Drug Prescribing in Renal Failure: Dosing Guidelines for Adults* (3rd ed.). Philadelphia: American College of Physicians, 1994.
    Useful handbook.
25. Corey, W.A., et al. Metronidazole-induced acute pancreatitis. *Rev. Infect. Dis.* 13: 1213, 1991.
    Case report and review of the literature of this rare complication. See additional discussion of this report by Y. Romero et al., Metronidazole and pancreatitis. Clin. Infect. Dis. *15:750, 1992.*

Q. Rifampin and Rifabutin

Rifampin (Rifadin)

Rifampin was discovered in 1965. Its mechanism of action involves inhibiting DNA-dependent RNA polymerase by binding to the subunit of the enzyme in susceptible microorganisms, thus interfering with protein synthesis [1]. Rifampin is bactericidal. Resistant strains of bacteria have altered RNA polymerase that is not inhibited by rifampin [1].

Although rifampin **currently is approved for use only in patients with tuberculosis and in nasopharyngeal carriers of *Neisseria meningitidis*, its use in the treatment of patients with other infections is under active investigation [1a]. Clinically relevant aspects of its use are summarized in this chapter** [1–3].

I. **Spectrum of activity.** Rifampin is a **broad-spectrum** agent, active against bacteria, mycobacteria, and chlamydiae.
   A. **Bacteria.** The in vitro activity of rifampin as a single agent is summarized in Table 28Q-1.
   B. **Mycobacteria.** Most strains of *Mycobacterium tuberculosis* are susceptible to rifampin (minimum inhibitory concentration$_{90}$ [MIC$_{90}$] = 0.6 μg/ml) to a degree comparable to isoniazid (INH) [3], but **resistant strains are being isolated** with greater frequency in recent years [3a]. See Chap. 9. The susceptibility of other mycobacteria is variable: *M. kansasii* and *M. marinum* are susceptible with a MIC$_{90}$ of 2.5 μg/ml, whereas most strains of *M. intracellulare* have a MIC$_{90}$ of 20, and *M. fortuitum* and *M. chelonei* are resistant with a MIC$_{90}$ of more than 20 μg/ml [1].
   C. **Chlamydiae.** Many species of *Chlamydia*, particularly *C. trachomatis*, are susceptible to rifampin.
II. **Resistance**
   A. **Rapid emergence of resistant bacteria occurs with monotherapy.** Susceptible bacteria develop resistance to rifampin by one-step mutations that alter the subunit of the RNA-polymerase enzyme [1].
   B. **Except for short-term prophylaxis, rifampin should not be used alone** [1].
III. **Pharmacokinetics.** Rifampin is red-orange in color in the crystalline state. The **oral** form is well absorbed from the GI tract in the fasting state. In late 1989, an **intravenous preparation** of rifampin became available for use in patients for whom the oral route

Table 28Q-1. In vitro activity of rifampin

Organism	MIC$_{90}$ (μg/ml)[a]
Gram-positive	
Staphylococcus aureus[b]	0.015
S. epidermidis[b]	0.015
Streptococcus pyogenes	0.12
S. pneumoniae (penicillin susceptible)	4.0
Viridans streptococci	0.12
Enterococcus faecalis	16.0
J K diphtheroids	0.05
Listeria monocytogenes	0.25
Clostridium difficile	≤0.2
C. perfringens	≤0.1
Peptococcus, Peptostreptococcus spp.	1.6
Proprionibacterium acnes	≤0.1
Gram-negative	
Neisseria gonorrhoeae	0.5
N. meningitidis	0.12
Moraxella (Branhamella) catarrhalis	0.03
Haemophilus influenzae	0.5
H. ducreyi	0.03
Legionella pneumophila	0.03
Brucella spp.	1.25
Escherichia coli	16.0
Klebsiella pneumoniae	32.0
Enterobacter spp.	64.0
Pseudomonas aeruginosa	64.0
Bacteroides fragilis	0.8
B. melaninogenicus	0.2

[a]MIC$_{90}$ = concentration below which 90% of tested organisms are inhibited.
[b]In most cases, the MIC for methicillin-resistant strains is similar to those for methicillin-susceptible strains [1].
Source: Modified from W.A. Craig, Rifampin and Related Drugs. In S.L. Gorbach, J.G. Bartlett, and N.R. Blacklow (eds.), *Infectious Diseases*. Philadelphia: Saunders, 1992. Pp. 265–266.

is not an option. (This preparation should not be given intramuscularly.) The same dose per day is given either orally or intravenously. The usual dosage per day (as a single daily dose) for tuberculosis is 600 mg for adults and 10–20 mg/kg, not to exceed 600 mg, for children. See Chap. 9. For pediatric and adult patients in whom capsule swallowing is difficult or in whom lower doses are needed but the oral route is desirable, a liquid suspension can be made up according to the package insert.

A. **Distribution.** The drug is well distributed, with levels in body fluids and tissue similar to those observed in serum. Therapeutic concentrations are obtained in serum, urine, saliva, bone, pleura, pancreatic juice, and cerebrospinal fluid (CSF) [1, 2].

B. **Metabolism.** Rifampin is cleared from the circulation primarily by hepatic metabolism and biliary excretion. Its half-life is 2–5 hours and is prolonged in hepatic disease. **In renal failure,** when the creatinine clearance is 10–50 ml/min, a 50–100% dose is suggested. When the creatinine clearance is less than 10 ml/min, 50% of the usual dose now is suggested [4].

Hemodialysis and chronic ambulatory peritoneal dialysis do not remove rifampin [4].

C. **Peak serum concentrations** after an oral dose of 600 mg or 10 mg/kg are variable but usually are in the range of 7–15 μg/ml [1].

D. **Patients taking rifampin often develop a harmless red-orange coloring of the urine, saliva, sweat, and tears; they should be forewarned of this to prevent unnecessary anxiety.**

E. Concurrent use of *p*-aminosalicylate acid will decrease absorption of rifampin.

IV. **Clinical use.** Rifampin is approved officially for use only in the treatment of patients with tuberculosis and carriers of *N. meningitidis* [5].

A. **Tuberculosis.** Rifampin is an important agent in the treatment of *M. tuberculosis* and some of the atypical mycobacteria [6, 7]. (See also Chap. 9.) Rifampin also is used in multidrug regimens to treat *Mycobacterium avium-intracellulare* (MAI) complex infections in patients with AIDS [8] (see Chap. 19). Rifampin has been used for chemoprophylaxis of tuberculosis in the rare isoniazid-allergic patient and for prophylactic therapy of contacts exposed to isoniazid-resistant organisms [7].

B. **Bacterial meningitis contacts.** Rifampin has been used successfully in eradicating the carrier state of close contacts of meningococcal and *Haemophilus influenzae* meningitis [9]. See the rationale and specific recommendations in Chap. 5, sec. **VII.B** under Meningitis (pp. 165–166).

C. **Investigational studies.** When rifampin is used alone for specific infections, resistance rapidly develops. Thus, there has been increased interest in the **use of rifampin with other antibiotics to avoid this** [1a]. For a detailed discussion of rifampin use in a variety of conditions and for conditions for which use is not approved, see reference [3].

   1. **Therapy of methicillin-resistant *Staphylococcus aureus* (MRSA)**
      a. **Rifampin in combination with a second agent (e.g., trimethoprim-sulfamethoxazole) has been used to try to eradicate nasal carriage of MRSA** [10, 10a]. See related discussion in Chap. 28D.
      b. For **other MRSA infections,** vancomycin is the therapy of choice (see Chap. 28O). There are no data to support the routine addition of rifampin to vancomycin, but if there is an inadequate response to vancomycin alone, then the addition of rifampin, gentamicin, or both should be considered. In his review, Farr emphasizes that rifampin resistance has been reported during therapy for MRSA infections with rifampin plus vancomycin, and the addition of gentamicin to the regimen may help prevent the development of rifampin resistance [3].

   2. **Endocarditis and bacteremias.** Rifampin has been studied particularly in **endocarditis** due to *S. aureus* and *S. epidermidis.* For endocarditis due to *S. aureus,* there are conflicting in vitro data as antagonism may be seen with combination therapy [11, 12]. Infectious disease consultation is advised before using rifampin in this setting. Bactericidal levels should be compared before and after adding rifampin.

      In the animal model of endocarditis caused by MRSA, the combination of vancomycin with rifampin was significantly more effective than was vancomycin alone [10a, 11]. In the experimental model of endocarditis caused by *S. epidermidis,* the addition of gentamicin or rifampin to vancomycin was beneficial, even though in vitro synergistic studies may not predict a beneficial effect [11]. For *S. epidermidis* prosthetic valve endocarditis, vancomycin given in combination with rifampin (300 mg PO q8h) and gentamicin (1.0–1.3 mg/kg q8h if renal function is normal) often is advocated [13, 13a]. The vancomycin and rifampin typically are given for 6 weeks and the gentamicin for the initial 2 weeks. See detailed discussion in Chap. 10.

   3. **Severe *Legionella* infections.** In treating severe infections due to *Legionella pneumophila* and other *Legionella* spp., rifampin has often been combined with erythromycin [1a, 6], even though there are no clinical randomized trials that demonstrate improved response of such combined therapy [1, 3].

   4. **Cerebrospinal fluid shunt infections.** In combination with another agent (e.g., vancomycin), rifampin has been used to treat staphylococcal coagulase-negative infections [14, 14a].

   5. **Chronic osteomyelitis** due to *S. aureus* has been treated with a combination of nafcillin and rifampin [1, 15]. In the treatment of experimental osteomyelitis caused by MRSA, a ciprofloxacin-rifampin combination was more effective than rifampin alone or in combination with vancomycin [11].

   6. ***Brucella* infections.** Prolonged therapy with doxycycline plus rifampin has a clinical response similar to that of tetracycline plus streptomycin [1, 1a, 6].

   7. **Orthopedic implant infections.** In a preliminary report, prosthetic device infections were treated with rifampin-containing antibiotic combinations [15a].

   8. **High-level penicillin-resistant *S. pneumoniae* meningitis** merits therapy with vancomycin. Some experts have suggested rifampin may be added [6], but this is an unresolved area. See Chaps. 5 (p. 154) and 28C.

V. **Adverse reactions.** The **most common side effect** observed with rifampin **is an orange-red discoloration of the urine.** (See sec. **III.D.**) Permanent staining of soft contact lenses can occur during rifampin therapy [1]. The adverse reactions of rifampin often are classified into the following four types [2]:

A. **Immunosuppression.** In in vitro and animal studies, rifampin has been shown to suppress the secretion of migration inhibition factor by lymphocytes, the response of lymphocytes to stimulation by nonspecific mitogen, and the production of antibody by cultured lymph node cells [2]. The precise implications of these studies for humans are unclear [3]. In addition, tuberculin skin test reactivity may be diminished in patients receiving rifampin.

B. **Immunologic reactions**

 1. **Allergic or hypersensitivity reactions** such as drug fever, skin rashes, and eosinophilia are uncommon.

 2. **A flulike syndrome** with fever, malaise, and headache can occur, particularly with irregular administration. It is very infrequent with routine intermittent tuberculosis regimens (i.e., twice weekly on the same 2 days) and also infrequent with routine daily use. Renal failure, thrombocytopenia, hemolysis, and the hepatorenal syndrome can occur in this flulike syndrome [2, 3]. Interstitial nephritis is a rare complication. Most patients improve with supportive care and withdrawal of the agent. Presumably, the risk of these reactions can be reduced if the doses are given on a regular schedule.

C. **Toxic reactions**

 1. **Hepatotoxicity** has been seen in patients with overdose, prior hepatic disease, and concurrent use of hepatotoxic agents (e.g., halothane anesthesia). There is some concern about whether the combined use of isoniazid and rifampin increases hepatotoxicity. In patients with mild liver function test abnormalities, rifampin must be used with caution, and liver function tests ideally should be monitored carefully if the drug is employed. For other uses of rifampin (i.e., when not treating mycobacterial infections) in patients without underlying hepatic dysfunction, serial liver function tests are not routinely recommended. See further discussion in Chap. 9. In one review, Craig [1] emphasized that although elevated liver enzyme values are observed in approximately 5–10% of recipients of rifampin, "hepatitis occurs in only 0.15–0.43% of persons treated with rifampin alone. The incidence of hepatitis rises to 2.5% in patients receiving multiple drug therapy for tuberculosis; however, most studies suggest that rifampin does not enhance the hepatotoxicity of isoniazid" [1]. In marked rifampin overdoses with associated liver damage, bright red urine, saliva, and tears and red discoloration of the skin have occurred.

 2. **Renal injury** is uncommon [2, 3].

 3. **Exudative conjunctivitis,** which is reversible once the drug has been discontinued, has been reported.

D. **Drug interactions. By potentiating hepatic microsomal cytochrome P450– related enzymatic reactions, rifampin induces increased hepatic excretion of a number of drugs** and other compounds metabolized by the liver [1, 3, 16].

 1. Examples

 a. **Oral contraceptives and levonorgestrel implants (Norplant). Concurrent use of rifampin has been associated with an increased rate of pregnancy** and menstrual irregularity.

 b. **Oral anticoagulants** (e.g., warfarin). Rifampin can antagonize the anticoagulant activity of warfarin. Doses of warfarin must be adjusted upward after rifampin is started and doses reduced when rifampin is discontinued.

 2. **These interactions** have been reviewed in detail and **are summarized in Tables 28Q-2 and 28Q-3** and in references [16] and [17]. One report emphasizes rifampin's interactions with the azole antifungal agents [17].

VI. **Precautions**

A. **Pregnancy.** Rifampin crosses the placenta readily and is teratogenic in animals. There are no adequate and well-controlled studies in pregnant women in terms of the effects on the fetus. Rifampin is a category C agent (see Chap. 28A). The package insert emphasizes that rifampin should be used during pregnancy only if the potential benefits justify the potential risks to the fetus [5]. Rifampin has been used to treat severe cases of tuberculosis in pregnant women [1]. Rifampin is not recommended for pregnant women who are contacts of infected patients with *H. influenzae* meningitis. Pregnant women in close contact with an index case of *N. meningitidis* meningitis can be treated with ceftriaxone if the woman is not allergic to cephalosporins. See related discussion in Chap. 5, sec. **VII.B** under Meningitis (pp. 165–166).

B. **Nursing mothers.** The package insert suggests that because of the potential for tumorigenicity for rifampin in animal studies, a decision should be made whether

Table 28Q-2. Previously described rifampin drug interactions[a]

Drug	Comments
Anticoagulants, oral[b]	Increase anticoagulant dose based on monitoring of prothrombin time
Beta-blockers	May need to increase propranolol or metoprolol dose
Chloramphenicol	Monitor serum chloramphenicol concentrations; increase dose if needed
Contraceptives, oral[b]	Use other forms of birth control; document patient counseling in chart
Cyclosporine[b]	Monitor serum cyclosporine concentrations; increased dose will likely be needed
Digitoxin[b]	Monitor serum digitoxin concentrations; monitor for arrhythmia control and signs and symptoms of heart failure; increase dose if needed
Digoxin	Monitor serum digoxin concentrations; monitor for arrhythmia control and signs and symptoms of heart failure; clinically significant interaction most likely in patients with decreased renal function
Glucocorticoids[b]	Increase glucocorticoid dose twofold to threefold with concomitant rifampin therapy
Ketoconazole[b]	Avoid this combination if possible; monitor serum ketoconazole concentrations; increase dose if needed; space rifampin and ketoconazole doses by 12 hours
Methadone[b]	Increase methadone dose with concurrent rifampin therapy; control withdrawal symptoms
Phenytoin[b]	Monitor serum phenytoin concentrations; increase phenytoin dose if needed
Quinidine[b]	Monitor serum quinidine concentrations; monitor for arrhythmia control; increase dose if needed
Sulfonylureas	Increase sulfonylurea dose based on blood glucose control; monitor blood glucose with discontinuation of rifampin therapy
Theophylline[b]	Monitor serum theophylline concentrations; increased dose will likely be needed
Verapamil[b]	Use alternative agent to verapamil if possible, because even very large increase in oral verapamil may not be sufficient; monitor serum verapamil concentrations; monitor patient for clinical response

[a]Carefully adjust doses when rifampin is discontinued; enzyme induction effect is gradually reduced over 1–2 weeks. For details see reference [16].
[b]Major clinical significance is well established.
Source: S.M. Borcherding, A.M. Baciewicz, and T.H. Self. Update on rifampin drug interactions. *Arch. Intern. Med.* 152:711, 1992. Copyright 1992, American Medical Association.

to discontinue nursing or to discontinue the drug, taking into account the importance of the drug to the mother [5].
  C. Liver disease. The use of rifampin in patients with liver disease is not recommended except in case of necessity; in such patients, the drug's half-life usually is doubled [1].
  D. Drug interactions. See sec. **V.D.**

Rifabutin (Ansamycin)

Rifabutin (Mycobutin) [18–21] is a semisynthetic ansamycin that was approved for the prevention of disseminated *Mycobacterium avium* complex (MAC) in patients with advanced human immunodeficiency virus (HIV) infection [20, 21] by the US Food and Drug Administration in late December 1992. It also is used in regimens to treat disseminated MAC.
  Rifabutin is active against most strains of MAI (i.e., MAC) isolated from HIV-

Table 28Q-3. Updated rifampin drug interactions[a]

Drug	Comments
Antacids	May need to space rifampin and aluminum hydroxide doses apart by several hours; more study needed
Haloperidol	Monitor serum haloperidol concentrations; alter dosing regimen if needed; limited initial study indicates serum concentrations and half-life are reduced by about 50%
Tocainide	Monitor arrhythmia control; increase dose if needed; 1 trial in healthy subjects found nearly 30% decrease in tocainide serum half-life
Disopyramide	Monitor arrhythmia control; increase dose if needed; initial study indicates decrease in disopyramide serum half-life of about 50%
Propafenone	Monitor plasma propafenone concentrations; monitor arrhythmia control; increase dose if needed
Ciprofloxacin	No interaction noted in humans to date; more study needed
Dapsone	Decrease serum concentrations; studies needed in patients with *Pneumocystis carinii* pneumonia
Fluconazole	May need to increase fluconazole dose; monitor signs and symptoms of infection; one trial in healthy subjects found 22% decrease in fluconazole serum half-life
Nifedipine	Monitor clinical response; may need to increase dose; controlled study needed
Diltiazem[b]	Consider alternative agent to diltiazem if possible, because even very large increase in oral diltiazem may not be sufficient; may monitor serum diltiazem concentrations (see Table 28Q-2 regarding similar interaction with verapamil); monitor clinical response
Diazepam	Monitor clinical response; may need to increase diazepam dose; 300% increase in diazepam oral clearance has been reported

[a]Agents available in the United States; for each interaction, carefully adjust doses when rifampin is discontinued; enzyme induction effect is reduced gradually over 1 to 2 weeks.
[b]More study needed in patients; probably of major clinical significance.
Source: S.M. Borcherding, A.M. Baciewicz, and T.H. Self, Update on rifampin drug interactions. *Arch. Intern. Med.* 152:711, 1992. Copyright 1992, American Medical Association.

positive and HIV-negative people. The MIC_{90} of MAI is typically approximately 2 µg/ml [1]. Rifabutin is also active against all rifampin-sensitive *M. tuberculosis* strains and about one-third of rifampin-resistant strains [3].

I. Pharmacokinetics
   A. Bioavailability. Rifabutin is absorbed rapidly, and absolute bioavailability is in the range of approximately 20% [1].
   B. Metabolism is similar to that for rifampin. The elimination half-life is long (45 hours) and as a result of a very large volume of distribution, average plasma concentrations remain relatively low after repeated standard doses [18]. The drug is taken up by all tissues and is especially concentrated in the lungs where levels may be 10-fold higher than in the serum [3]. Animal models suggest rifabutin has less of an effect on hepatic microsomal enzyme activity than rifampin.
   C. Clinical studies
      1. Rifabutin has been used **in therapeutic regimens** for disseminated MAI infections in patients with AIDS [6, 19–22]. See Chap. 19.
      2. Rifabutin also has been used **to prevent MAC** in patients with HIV infection. This topic has recently been reviewed elsewhere [23], but prophylaxis with rifabutin should be considered for HIV-infected adults and adolescents who have $CD4^+$ lymphocyte counts of <75/mm³, although some experts would wait until the count is <50/mm³ [23]. Disseminated MAC should be ruled out before starting prophylaxis (i.e., with a negative blood culture for mycobacterium). See related discussion in Chap. 19.

II. Dosages
   A. Prevention of MAC. A 150-mg capsule is available. For the prevention of MAC in patients with advanced HIV infection, 300 mg PO daily is recommended in adults by the package insert. This can be administered as a once-daily dose or,

in patients with a propensity to nausea, vomiting, or other GI upset, 150 mg bid with meals.

B. **Pediatric use.** The safety and effectiveness of rifabutin for prophylaxis of MAC in children have not been established, per the package insert. However, recent recommendations suggest consideration for children infected with HIV and CD4+ cell counts $<75/mm^3$ as reviewed elsewhere in detail [23], and a dosage of 5m/kg has been used in pharmacokinetic studies [23].

C. **Pregnancy.** The package insert suggests that rifabutin should be used in pregnant women only if the potential benefit justifies the potential risk to the fetus. Data are still pending. Rifabutin is viewed as a category B agent (see Chap. 28A). Information is insufficient for recommendations concerning the use of rifabutin for prevention of MAC in pregnancy [23].

D. **Nursing mothers.** It is not known whether rifabutin is excreted in human milk. The package insert suggests a decision should be made whether to continue nursing or discontinue rifabutin, taking into account the importance of the drug to the mother. See related discussions in Chap. 19.

E. The current package insert does not contain any dose modifications for renal or hepatic dysfunction [24].

F. **For therapeutic regimens,** rifabutin, 300–450 mg PO daily, is often suggested along with clarithromycin or azithromycin, and ethambutol and/or clofazamine and/or ciprofloxacin [25]. See related discussions in Chap. 19.

Because of the potential for side effects at higher doses, see sec. **III**, 300 mg/day of rifabutin may be a rational compromise [26].

III. **Side effects.** Rifabutin is generally well-tolerated at the prophylaxis dose of 300 mg/day. Rash, GI intolerance, and neutropenia are seen in 2–4% of recipients [24]. In therapeutic regimens for MAC and at higher doses (e.g., ≥600 mg/day), adverse effects can be seen in the majority of patients, especially leukopenia, GI intolerance, diffuse polyarthralgia syndrome (19%), and anterior uveitis (6%) [26].

IV. **Investigational uses.** Rifabutin is undergoing ongoing clinical evaluation for therapy for MAC in patients with AIDS and in therapeutic regimens for *M. tuberculosis.* Rifabutin also is undergoing clinical investigation for the treatment of Crohn's disease.

References

1. Craig, W.A. Rifampin and Related Drugs. In S.L. Gorbach, J.G. Bartlett, and N.R. Blacklow (eds.), *Infectious Diseases*. Philadelphia: Saunders, 1992. Pp. 265–271.
1a. Morris, A.B., et al. Use of rifampin in nonstaphylococcal, nonmycobacterial disease. *Antimicrob. Agents Chemother.* 37:1, 1993.
2. Sanders, W.E., Jr. Rifampin: The Prototype Rifamycin. In B.M. Kagan (ed.), *Antimicrobial Therapy* (3rd ed.). Philadelphia: Saunders, 1980. Pp. 153–161.
3. Farr, B.M. Rifamycins. In G.L. Mandell, J.E. Bennett, and R. Dolin (eds.), *Principles and Practice of Infectious Diseases* (4th ed.). New York: Churchill Livingstone, 1995. Pp. 317–329.
   Contains a good discussion of some of the therapeutic, though unapproved, uses of rifampin.
3a. Freiden, T.R., et al. The emergence of drug-resistant tuberculosis in New York City. *N. Engl. J. Med.* 328:522, 1993.
   In April 1991, 19% of isolates were resistant to rifampin and INH! See companion article on therapy for these patients. See also Chap. 9.
4. Bennett, W.M., et al. *Drug Prescribing in Renal Failure: Dosing Guidelines for Adults* (3rd ed.). Philadelphia: American College of Physicians, 1994.
5. *Physicians' Desk Reference* (50th ed.). Montvale, NJ: Medical Economics Data, 1996. P. 1529.
6. Medical Letter. The choice of antibacterial drugs. *Med. Lett. Drugs Ther.* 38:25, 1996.
7. American Thoracic Society and Centers for Disease Control. Treatment of tuberculosis and tuberculosis infection in adults and children. *Am. J. Resp. Crit. Care Med.* 149:1359, 1994.
8. Abruntyn, E. New uses for old drugs. *Infect. Dis. Clin. North Am.* 3:653, 1989.
9. Committee on Infectious Diseases, American Academy of Pediatrics. In G. Peter et al. (eds.), *Report of the Committee on Infectious Diseases* (23rd ed.). Elk Grove Village, IL: American Academy of Pediatrics, 1994.
10. Fekety, R. The management of the carrier of methicillin-resistant *Staphylococcus aureus. Curr. Clin. Top. Infect. Dis.* 8:169, 1987.
10a. Mulligan, M.E., et al. Methicillin-resistant *Staphylococcus aureus:* A consensus re-

view of the microbiology, pathogenesis, and epidemiology with implications for prevention and management. *Am. J. Med.* 94:313, 1993.
A comprehensive review. See related discussions in Chap. 28D.

11. Fantin, B., and Carbon, C. In vivo antibiotic synergism: Contribution of animal models. *Antimicrob. Agents Chemother.* 36:907, 1992.

12. Kaatz, G.W., et al. Ciprofloxacin and rifampin, alone and in combination, for therapy of experimental *Staphylococcus aureus* endocarditis. *Antimicrob. Agents Chemother.* 33:1184, 1989.
Although the combination may decrease the risk of acquisition of ciprofloxacin resistance, with respect to improved efficacy in this rabbit model the combination of ciprofloxacin and rifampin is unpredictable and strain-dependent and cannot be assumed to result in better therapeutic outcome than is achieved with ciprofloxacin alone.

13. Karchmer, A.W. Staphylococcal endocarditis: Laboratory and clinical basis for antibiotic therapy. *Am. J. Med.* 78(Suppl. 6B):116, 1985.

13a. Wilson, W., et al. Antibiotic treatment of adults with infective endocarditis due to streptococci, enterococci, staphylococci, and HACEK microorganisms. *J.A.M.A.* 274:1706, 1995.

14. Gardner, P., Leipzig, T.J., and Sadigh, M. Infections of mechanical cerebrospinal fluid shunts. *Curr. Clin. Top. Infect. Dis.* 9:185, 1988.

14a. Bisno, A.L., and Sternau, L. Infections of Central Nervous System Shunts. In A.L. Bisno and F.A. Waldvogel (eds.), *Infections Associated with Indwelling Devices.* Washington, D.C.: ASM Press, 1994. Pp. 91–109.
This is an excellent review.

15. Norden, C.W., et al. Chronic osteomyelitis caused by *Staphylococcus aureus:* Controlled clinical trial of nafcillin therapy and nafcillin-rifampin therapy. *South. Med. J.* 79:947, 1986.
Authors concluded that combination therapy should be considered for patients with chronic staphylococcal osteomyelitis.

15a. Widner, A.F., et al. Antimicrobial treatment of orthopedic implant–related infections with rifampin combinations. *Clin. Infect. Dis.* 14:1251, 1992.
Preliminary report from Switzerland in which 9 of 11 patients with infected prosthetic implants (e.g., total knee, hip) that could not be removed were successfully treated with a protracted course of at least 2 months with oral rifampin in combination with a second agent (e.g., fluoroquinolones). Authors indicated a multicenter, double-blind controlled trial comparing regular antimicrobial treatment with and without rifampin for this type of patient was started in 1992, with results anticipated to be published in 1996–1997.

16. Borcherding, S.M., Baciewicz, A.M., and Self, T.H. Update on rifampin drug interactions. *Arch. Intern. Med.* 152:711, 1992.
See summary Tables 28Q-1 and 28Q-2. For related earlier summary of agents listed in Table 28Q-1, see A.M. Baciewic, T.H. Self, and W.B. Bekemeyer, Update on rifampin drug interactions. Arch. Intern. Med. 147:565, 1987.

17. Tucker, R.M., et al. Interactions of azoles with rifampin, phenytoin, and carbamazepine: In vitro and clinical observations. *Clin. Infect. Dis.* 14:165, 1992.
Patients receiving therapy with an azole agent (ketoconazole, itraconazole, or fluconazole) for systematic myoses may have drug interactions that decrease azole concentrations in serum and, in turn, decrease clinical efficacy.

18. Skinner, M.H., and Blaschke, T.F. Clinical pharmacokinetics of rifabutin. *Clin. Pharmacokinet.* 28:115, 1995.
For a related paper, see R.N. Brogden and A. Fitton, Rifabutin: A review of its antimicrobial activity, pharmacokinetic properties and therapeutic efficacy. Drugs 47:983, 1994.

19. Medical Letter. Rifabutin. *Med. Lett. Drugs Ther.* 35:36, 1993.

20. Agins, B.D., et al. Effect of combined therapy with ansamycin, clofazimine, ethambutol, and isoniazid for *Mycobacterium avium* infection in patients with AIDS. *J. Infect. Dis.* 159:784, 1989.

21. Hoy, J., et al. Quadruple-drug therapy for *Mycobacterium avium-intracellulare* bacteremia in AIDS patients. *J. Infect. Dis.* 161:801, 1990.
Patients received rifabutin, clofazimine, isoniazid, and ethambutol. Mycobacteremia was cleared in 22 of 25 patients who received this regimen, and 18 patients who received this regimen experienced complete resolution of symptoms associated with the infection. The regimen used appeared to be effective in clearing mycobacteremia and in ameliorating symptoms of infection.

22. Sullam, P.M., et al. Efficacy of rifabutin in the treatment of disseminated infection due to *Mycobacterium avium* complex. *Clin. Infect. Dis.* 19:84, 1994.

In combination with other antimicrobial agents (e.g., clofazimine and ethambutol), rifabutin (600 mg/d) may be effective in the treatment of disseminated MAC infection.

23. USPHS/IDSA Prevention of Opportunistic Infections Working Group. USPHS/IDSA guidelines for the prevention of opportunistic infections in persons infected with human immunodeficiency virus: Disease-specific recommendations. *Clin. Infect. Dis.* 21(Suppl. 1):S32, 1995.
    This is an excellent resource. Discusses pediatric considerations. See related discussions in Chap. 19.
24. *Physicians' Desk Reference* (50th ed.). Montvale, N.J.: Medical Economics, 1996.
25. Medical Letter. Drugs for AIDS and associated infections. *Med. Lett. Drugs Ther.* 37:87, 1995.
26. Griffith, D.E., et al. Adverse events associated with high-dose rifabutin in macrolide-containing regimens for the treatment of *Mycobacterium avium* complex lung disease. *Clin. Infect. Dis.* 21:594, 1995.
    Authors conclude that a rifabutin dose of 300 mg/day may be optimal in multidrug regimens for MAC that includes macrolides.

R. Spectinomycin

Spectinomycin (Trobicin) was approved by the US Food and Drug Administration (FDA) in 1971 for use in certain gonococcal infections. The structure of spectinomycin is similar, but not identical, to that of the aminoglycosides. Spectinomycin inhibits protein synthesis at the ribosomal level, and its activity against gonococci is bactericidal. **Spectinomycin is used only as an alternative agent for some infections caused by *Neisseria gonorrhoeae*** [1–4].

Spectinomycin is not effective against *Treponema pallidum* or *Chlamydia trachomatis* [3]. Resistant strains of *N. gonorrhoeae* have been reported in the United States [2].

I. **Indications for use**
   A. **Alternative regimens for gonococcal infections.** See Chap. 13.
      1. **Uncomplicated urethral, endocervical, or rectal infections.** When the drugs of choice (cephalosporin or quinolone) cannot be used, spectinomycin is an alternative [2, 4]. It is active against penicillin-resistant strains of gonococci.
      2. **Treatment of gonococcal infections in pregnancy.** Pregnant women who cannot tolerate cephalosporins can be treated with spectinomycin [2].
      3. **Disseminated gonococcal infections.** Patients who are allergic to beta-lactams can be treated with spectinomycin [2].
   B. **Actual or potential resistance.** Spectinomycin does not produce sustained, high bactericidal levels in blood, and resistant strains have been reported in the United States and elsewhere [4].
      Whether the drug should be used more often in initial infections has been reviewed in the past. Prior data suggest that extensive use of spectinomycin in initial gonococcal therapy might lead to the emergence of spectinomycin-resistant gonorrhea [5]. The need for careful use of spectinomycin has also been emphasized in a report by Boslego and coworkers [6]. After only 3 years of using spectinomycin as the primary treatment for uncomplicated gonococcal urethritis in US military men in the Republic of Korea, more than 8% of recipients were treatment failures [6].

II. **Contraindications and limitations to use**
   A. **Pharyngeal gonococcal infection.** Spectinomycin **is ineffective** against this infection, probably because the drug is not secreted in saliva in adequate concentrations.
   B. **Incubating syphilis.** Spectinomycin **will not abort incubating syphilis** and may actually prolong the incubation period. Thus, **patients treated with spectinomycin should have a syphilis serology test** at the time of treatment and again in 2–3 months to rule out this associated diagnosis.
   C. **Nonspecific urethritis** (nongonococcal urethritis [NGU]). At least 50% of cases are due to *C. trachomatis* that are not susceptible to spectinomycin. Although a minority of cases may be due to *Ureaplasma urealyticum* (T-mycoplasmas), against which spectinomycin is active, the drug is not a very useful agent in NGU.
      Tetracycline is the preferred agent for NGU because it is effective against both major etiologic organisms. See Chap. 13.

III. Route and dosage. Spectinomycin is given intramuscularly and is well absorbed by this route. In uncomplicated anogenital gonococcal infection, 2 g spectinomycin is given intramuscularly as a single dose in men or women and, in children, 40 mg/kg (maximum 2 g) IM is given once [2]. For alternative treatment of inpatients with disseminated gonococcal infections who are allergic to beta-lactam agents (i.e., cephalosporins), spectinomycin, 2 g IM q12h, can be used [2] and can be given every 12 hours for 3 days [3] in adults.

In renal failure, no dose adjustment of spectinomycin is required. Neither hemodialysis nor chronic ambulatory peritoneal dialysis removes spectinomycin [7]. Spectinomycin is relatively expensive [2]. See Table 28A-6.

IV. Toxicity appears very limited, perhaps because the total dose is low. There are no known serious adverse reactions.

V. Conclusions. Spectinomycin has a **limited but useful role in gonococcal infections.** The best use of this agent is in the treatment of gonorrhea in persons who cannot tolerate cephalosporins or quinolones [4].

References

1. Medical Letter. The choice of antibacterial drugs. *Med. Lett. Drugs Ther.* 38:25, 1996.
2. Centers for Disease Control. 1993 Sexually transmitted disease treatment guidelines. *M.M.W.R.* 42(RR-14):S57–S67, 1993.
3. Gilbert, D.N. Aminoglycosides. In G.L. Mandell, J.E. Bennett, and R. Dolin (eds.), *Principles and Practice of Infectious Diseases* (4th ed.). New York: Churchill Livingstone, 1995. P. 299.
4. Moran, J.S., and Levine, W.C. Drugs of choice for the treatment of uncomplicated gonococcal infection. *Clin. Infect. Dis.* 20(Suppl. 1):S47, 1995. *Background studies for recommendations in reference* [2].
5. Karney, W.W., et al. Spectinomycin versus tetracycline for the treatment of gonorrhea. *N. Engl. J. Med.* 296:889, 1987.
6. Boslego, J.W., et al. Effect of spectinomycin use on the prevalence of spectinomycin-resistant and of penicillinase-producing *Neisseria gonorrhoeae*. *N. Engl. J. Med.* 317:272, 1987.
7. Bennett, W.M., et al. *Drug Prescribing in Renal Failure* (3rd ed.). Philadelphia: American College of Physicians, 1994. P. 26.

S. Fluoroquinolones

Quinolone antibiotics have been available for decades. The prototype quinolone is **nalidixic acid,** which has been available since the mid-1960s. Because of the rapid development of bacterial resistance, even during therapy, this agent is not recommended. **Oxolinic acid** is a synthetic derivative related to nalidixic acid. Because of the emergence of bacterial resistance during treatment and frequent adverse CNS effects, it is a poor choice for treatment of urinary tract infection (UTI). **Cinoxacin** is related chemically to nalidixic acid. It offers no special advantages. **These older quinolone antibiotics will not be discussed further, because they have been replaced by the newer fluoroquinolones.**

In the **newer synthetic fluoroquinolones,** the original two-member ring of nalidixic acid has been modified. (See sec. **I.A.**) These new fluoroquinolones include **norfloxacin, ciprofloxacin, ofloxacin, enoxacin,** and **lomefloxacin,** as well as some investigational agents. Norfloxacin was released in 1986, ciprofloxacin in late 1987, ofloxacin in 1991, and, in 1992, temafloxacin (also removed in 1992), lomefloxacin, and enoxacin became available.

Their broad spectrum of antimicrobial activity, bioavailability, penetration into tissues, long serum half-lives, and general safety have made the new fluoroquinolones very attractive agents for treating numerous infections [1]. However, an alarming rate of resistance has developed. This plus the inappropriate use of these agents concerns many experts [1–4]. Because the basic structure can easily be modified synthetically, new fluoroquinolones are anticipated to be released in the next few years and, as with the numerous cephalosporin derivatives, this proliferation of agents will make appropriate clinical use even more difficult.

We first will review several shared properties of the fluoroquinolones (sec. **I**) and then review each available fluoroquinolone (secs. **II–VII**). This discussion will involve some repetition, since the reader may use only portions of this chapter. We will use the terms *fluoroquinolone* and *quinolone* interchangeably, as in the literature. Several general reviews are available [1–5].

I. **General properties**
   A. **Basic structure.** The basic structure of the fluoroquinolones is shown in Fig. 28S-1 [3].
      1. **In vitro activity.** Critical to this is the carboxy group at position C-3 and the keto group at C-4. **All the agents currently available contain a fluorine at C-6** (not present in nalidixic acid or oxolinic acid), which provides increased activity against staphylococci and Enterobacteriaceae [3].
      2. C-7 and C-8 substitutions significantly change the antimicrobial activity, the pharmacokinetics, and the metabolism of these compounds [3].
      3. Because these are synthetic compounds, the potential for many structural modifications exists.
   B. **Mechanism of action.** Quinolones interfere with DNA synthesis by inhibiting DNA gyrase, a bacterial enzyme essential for DNA replication. Fluoroquinolones inhibit DNA supercoiling that is produced by DNA gyrase in vitro, and they promote gyrase-mediated double-stranded DNA breakage at specific sites [4]. The details of the mechanism of action are reviewed elsewhere [1–4].
   C. **In vitro activity** has been reviewed [1–6] and is summarized in Table 28S-1.
      1. **Gram-positive cocci. Most quinolones are not as active against gram-positive bacteria as they are against gram-negative bacteria.**
         a. The currently available fluoroquinolones have relatively high minimum inhibitory concentrations (MICs) against *Streptococcus pneumoniae* and other streptococci. (See Table 28S-1.)
         b. The fluoroquinolones are active against streptococci and enterococci at levels achievable in the urine.
      2. **Gram-negative cocci**
         a. *Neisseria gonorrhoeae, Moraxella (Branhamella) catarrhalis,* and *Haemophilus influenzae,* including beta-lactamase-positive and beta-lactamase-negative strains, are very susceptible. Strains of *N. gonorrhoeae* resistant to the quinolones may be an emerging problem [6a, 6b]. See sec. **F.2.**
         b. **Enterobacteriaceae.** More than 90% of isolates are inhibited by less than 2 μg/ml [4] (see Table 28S-1). Ciprofloxacin is the most active of the available fluoroquinolones and inhibits 90% of Enterobacteriaceae at concentrations of less than 0.5 μg/ml [4].
            (1) *Escherichia coli, Klebsiella pneumoniae,* and *Enterobacter* spp. are all very susceptible, with most having a MIC_{90} of less than 1 μg/ml.
            (2) Gastrointestinal pathogens (e.g., *Salmonella* and *Shigella* spp. and *Campylobacter jejuni*) are very susceptible, with a MIC_{90} of less than 0.5 μg/ml.
            (3) *Serratia marcescens* and *Acinetobacter* spp. have intermediate susceptibility.
            (4) *Pseudomonas aeruginosa* has intermediate susceptibility, with a MIC_{90} ranging from 0.5 to 8.0 μg/ml. Ciprofloxacin is the most active agent, inhibiting most *P. aeruginosa* strains at concentrations of 1 μg/ml or less [4]. *Stenotrophomonas maltophilia* (formerly *P. maltophilia*) and *Burkholderia cepacia* (formerly *P. cepacia*) are relatively resistant, with MICs ranging from 1 to 8 μg/ml among the fluoroquinolones [4].

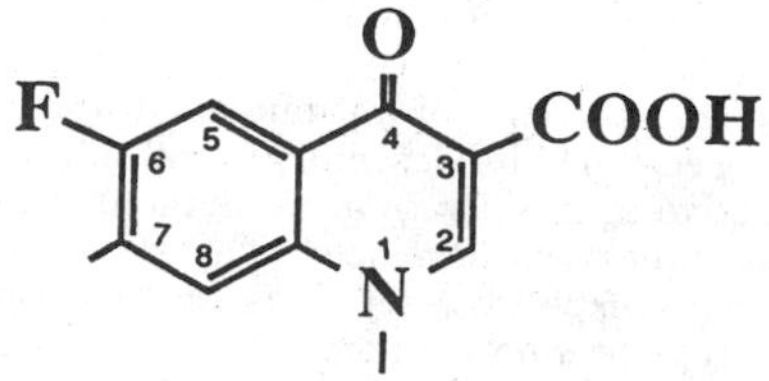

Fig. 28S-1. The nucleus of a four-quinolone antibacterial agent. (From H. Neu, Use of the fluoroquinolones: Mini-review. *Infect. Dis. Clin. Pract.* 1:1, 1992.)

Table 28S-1. The minimum inhibitory concentrations (MIC_{90}) in vitro of quinolone antibiotics (measured in µg/ml)[a]

Organism	Ciprofloxacin	Norfloxacin	Ofloxacin	Enoxacin	Lomefloxacin	Sparfloxacin[c]
Escherichia coli	0.12	0.25	0.25	0.25	0.25	0.12
Klebsiella pneumoniae	0.12	0.5	0.25	0.25	0.5	0.25
Enterobacter spp.	0.12	1	0.25	0.5	0.5	0.25
Citrobacter spp.	0.12	1	0.25	0.25	1	1.12
Serratia marcescens	0.25	2	2	2	2	1
Shigella spp.	0.12	0.25	0.25	0.25	0.25	0.12
Proteus mirabilis	0.12	0.25	0.25	0.25	0.25	0.12
Proteus, other	0.25	0.5	0.5	0.5	1	0.5
Morganella morganii	0.12	0.5	0.12	2	0.5	0.5
Providencia spp.	0.25	2	0.5	2	0.25	0.5
Yersinia enterocolitica	0.12	0.25	0.12	0.25	4	0.12
Pseudomonas aeruginosa	0.5	8	4	2	0.5[b]	2
Acinetobacter spp.	1	8	1	8	4	0.25
Staphylococcus aureus						
Methicillin-susceptible	0.5	1	0.5	2	4	0.25
Methicillin-resistant	0.5	4	0.5	4	2	0.25
Staphylococcus epidermidis	0.5	2	2	8	2	0.06
Enterococci	2	8	4	6	1	0.5
Streptococcus (group A)	1	4	2	8	16	0.5
Streptococcus (group B)	1	8	2	16	8	0.25
Streptococcus pneumoniae[d]	2	8	2	16	16	<0.06

Table 28S-1 (continued)

Organism	Ciprofloxacin	Norfloxacin	Ofloxacin	Enoxacin	Lomefloxacin	Sparfloxacin[c]
Haemophilus influenzae	<0.06	<0.12	<0.12	<0.12	8	<0.06
Neisseria gonorrhoeae	<0.06	<0.12	<0.12	<0.12	0.12	<0.06
Neisseria meningitidis	<0.06	<0.12	<0.12	<0.12	0.12	<0.06
Campylobacter spp.	0.05	0.05	1	1	0.12	0.12
Bacteroides fragilis	16	>32	8	>32	—	2
Bacteroides melaninogenicus	8	>32	8	>32	64	2
Peptostreptococcus	4	>32	2	>32	16	0.5
Mycobacterium tuberculosis	1	—	1	—	16	2
Branhamella catarrhalis	<0.12	<0.12	<0.12	<0.12	<0.12	<0.12
Brucella spp.	1	8	2	8	0.12	—
Listeria monocytogenes	2	4	2	8	8	0.25
Corynebacterium JK	1	4	1	8	8	0.25
Legionella spp.	<0.12	0.5	<0.25	0.5	0.25	0.25
Chlamydia trachomatis	2	8	1	8	0.25	0.25
Mycoplasma hominis	1	8	1	8	2	0.25
Ureaplasma	16	32	2	16	4	—
Mycoplasma pneumoniae	1	8	1	8	—	0.5

[a]Median MIC_{90} of the new quinolone antibiotics was 1 μg/ml. Based on published results from multiple studies.
[b]In another review, the MIC_{90} was 8.0 μg/ml for more than 4,000 strains. See K.H. Mayer and Judy A. Ellal, Lomefloxacin: Microbiologic assessment and unique properties. *Am. J. Med.* 92 (Suppl. 4A):58S, 1992.
[c]Investigational agent as of May 1996.
[d]Penicillin-susceptible strains.
Source: Modified from H.C. Neu, Quinolone antimicrobial agents. Reproduced, with permission, from the *Annual Review of Medicine* Vol. 43, © 1992 by Annual Reviews Inc.

3. **Anaerobes.** The currently available quinolones have limited anaerobic activity; other agents are preferred for anaerobic infections.
4. **Miscellaneous**
   a. *Legionella* spp. are susceptible, and clinical studies are under way to assess the role of quinolones in respiratory tract infections caused by *Legionella* spp.
   b. *Mycoplasma pneumoniae* strains are susceptible to some of the fluoroquinolones (see Table 28S-1), but erythromycin is much more active, with MICs in the range of 0.004–0.063 μg/ml [7, 8]; therefore **erythromycin still is preferred** for infections due to these pathogens.
   c. Several *Mycobacterium* spp., both atypical and typical, and rickettsiae are susceptible [6].
   d. *Bordetella pertussis* often is susceptible.
5. **Synergistic combinations.** The combination of ciprofloxacin and an antipseudomonal penicillin or imipenem is synergistic for approximately 20–50% of isolates of *P. aeruginosa*. In contrast, the combination of quinolones and aminoglycosides rarely showed synergy for *P. aeruginosa,* Enterobacteriaceae, or enterococci [9, 10].

   The combination of beta-lactams or aminoglycosides or imidazoles with a fluoroquinolone is usually indifferent against Enterobacteriaceae and gram-positive bacteria. Combinations of rifampin with quinolones tested against *Staphylococcus aureus* can show either synergy or antagonism in in vitro tests, but most animal experiments of staphylococcal infections suggest that the combination of rifampin and quinolones is synergistic [4]. In one report, the activity of ciprofloxacin against clindamycin-susceptible strains of *S. aureus* was antagonized by coadministration of clindamycin [11]. The clinical implications of this preliminary observation are unclear.

   In general, Neu [4] **suggests that the fluoroquinolones should be combined with other agents not to achieve synergy, which is extremely variable, but to provide activity against bacteria inadequately inhibited by the fluoroquinolones.**
6. **Other in vitro features.** There appears to be **no** significant **inoculum effect,** and fluoroquinolones generally are bactericidal. MICs are higher in an acidic environment (pH <5.5). The fluoroquinolones have a significant **postantimicrobial suppressive effect** for Enterobacteriaceae, staphylococci, and *P. aeruginosa* [4]. The clinical significance of this is unclear.
7. The fluoroquinolones have **concentration-dependent bactericidal activity.** The potential clinical significance of this is reviewed in Chap. 28A, under Antibiotic Checklist sec. **VII.A.3** (pp. 1080–1081).

D. **Pharmacokinetics** [1–4, 12–14]
   1. **Oral absorption.** All fluoroquinolones are **well absorbed after oral administration,** although the degree of absorption varies from 55% with norfloxacin to 95% or more with ofloxacin and lomefloxacin [4].
      a. Peak serum concentrations are reached in 1–2 hours after ingestion in the fasting state and in approximately 2 hours when ingested after a meal [4] (Table 28S-2).
      b. **Urinary concentrations** are high and may be 100-fold the serum concentrations.
      c. **Medications decreasing bioavailability**
         (1) **Antacids** containing aluminum, magnesium, and calcium substantially decrease fluoroquinolone absorption. This can be minimized by administering the antacid 2 hours after the fluoroquinolone is taken [4].
         (2) **Sucralfate,** when coadministered with the fluoroquinolones, **reduces bioavailability** of the fluoroquinolone by 85–90%. This effect can be minimized by administering sucralfate at least 6 hours before the fluoroquinolone [4]. The H₂-blockers (e.g., cimetidine, ranitidine) do not appear to affect absorption of the fluoroquinolones [4].
         (3) **Iron** tablets, **zinc** in vitamins, **calcium** supplements, and didanosine **(ddl)** tablets can decrease absorption.
   2. **Intravenous preparations** are available for ciprofloxacin and ofloxacin. Intravenous preparations are undergoing clinical study for lomefloxacin and enoxacin. The agents in general provide 1 μg/ml per 100 mg of drug infused intravenously [4, 12].

Table 28S-2. Pharmacokinetic parameters of quinolones

Parameter	Norfloxacin	Ciprofloxacin	Ofloxacin	Enoxacin	Lomefloxacin	Sparfloxacin*
Dose	400	500	400	600	400	400
C_{max} (μg/ml)	1.5	2.5	5.5	4	4	1
$T_{1/2}$ (hr)	4	4	7	6	8	18
$T_{1/2}$ (hr) $C_{cr} < 10$ ml	8	10	30	9.4	25	30
Urinary recovery (%)	25	30	90	60	76	30
Urine concentration (μg/ml)	>200	>200	>200	>200	>200	>100
Metabolism (%)	20	20	3	20	5	—

$T_{1/2}$ = serum half-life; C_{max} = maximum concentration; C_{cr} = creatinine clearance.
*Investigational agent as of May 1996.
Source: Modified from H.C. Neu, Quinolone antimicrobial agents. *Annu. Rev. Med.* 43:463, 1992.

3. **Tissue penetration.** Fluoroquinolones penetrate well into most tissues, including sputum, bile, saliva, blister fluid, bone, aqueous humor, and prostate [4, 13]. The fluoroquinolones enter polymorphonuclear leukocytes and alveolar macrophages where they produce concentrations of 3–8 μg/ml. In general, the concentrations of fluoroquinolones achieved in the cerebrospinal fluid (CSF) are low [4].
4. Serum **half-lives** of the available fluoroquinolones range from 3–4 hours to 8 hours, allowing for every-12- or every-24-hour dosing (see Table 28S-2).
5. **Excretion** is primarily by way of the kidney, and elimination half-lives are prolonged in the presence of renal failure; however, drugs achieve therapeutic concentrations within the urine even with markedly reduced renal function [4].
6. **Miscellaneous**
   a. **Some of these agents interfere with the excretion of theophylline** (e.g., ciprofloxacin and enoxacin, but not norfloxacin, lomefloxacin, or ofloxacin).
   b. **In elderly patients,** the peak concentrations of **ciprofloxacin and enoxacin** increase with age, without a concurrent increase in serum half-life. Presumably, there is a more efficient absorption of these drugs in the elderly [14]. Therefore, renal function in the elderly should be estimated and doses modified as needed.

E. **Resistance.** Although it initially appeared that bacterial resistance to the fluoroquinolones would not be a serious problem, this has not proved to be the case. Clinically important resistance has been an increasing problem, especially for *S. aureus, P. aeruginosa* and, to a lesser extent, *S. marcescens.* This topic is reviewed in detail elsewhere [1, 4, 15–20].
   1. **Mechanisms**
      a. **Alterations in DNA gyrase.** Bacterial DNA gyrase is composed of two subunit A proteins and two subunit B proteins. Quinolone resistance (e.g., to *P. aeruginosa*) has been associated with point mutations, which result in single amino acid substitution of the genes for either of these subunits. Such alterations in DNA gyrase confer resistance to quinolones beyond the one to which the bacteria were initially exposed [1].
      b. **Decreased permeability.** Exposure to gradually increasing levels of fluoroquinolones can result in high-level resistance (mutations in gram-negative bacteria), probably attributable to changes in the outer membrane protein and lipopolysaccharides [1, 4].
      c. Plasmid-mediated resistance to fluoroquinolones does not appear to occur or is rare [1, 4]. However, historically, a "plasmid-free" grace period of several decades of clinical use was observed with other antimicrobial agents before plasmid-mediated resistance developed [1].
   2. **Clinical relevance.** Resistance to the fluoroquinolones has been an increasingly important problem in the following settings [1, 2, 4, 15–20].
      a. *P. aeruginosa.* Resistance has been found in the treatment of UTI, especially when an indwelling catheter is left in place [17], with prolonged use in respiratory infections in patients with cystic fibrosis, and following therapy of skin and soft-tissue infections both with and without contiguous osteomyelitis or a foreign body.
      b. **Staphylococci**
         (1) **Methicillin-resistant *S. aureus* (MRSA)** now commonly is resistant to ciprofloxacin. In a report from the Centers for Disease Control (CDC), 79% of recently isolated MRSA strains were resistant to ciprofloxacin. Typically these are nosocomially acquired infections, although approximately half of the patients had a prior history of ciprofloxacin use [18]. Other investigators have reported similar rates of MRSA resistant to ciprofloxacin, and prior use of ciprofloxacin seemed to be an important factor for the selection of ciprofloxacin-resistant strains [19]. These investigators conclude that **ciprofloxacin has limited usefulness in treating MRSA infections [18–19a].**
         (2) **Methicillin-susceptible *S. aureus*** strains likewise are being reported as showing an increased resistance to ciprofloxacin to the level of 10–30% [1, 2, 4, 18].
         (3) **Coagulase-negative staphylococci** often are resistant to ciprofloxacin. Patients who have received fluoroquinolones prophylactically for chemotherapy-induced leukopenia have developed bacteremias with

fluoroquinolone-resistant coagulase-negative staphylococci. Nosocomial spread of these pathogens has been well described [1, 20].

   c. ***Serratia marcescens*** fluoroquinolone resistance is common now in some countries (e.g., Japan) and is anticipated to increase in the US [1, 4].

   d. *E. coli* ciprofloxacin-resistant bacteremias have recently been described in Spain in patients with chronic underlying diseases and prior fluoroquinolone use [20a].

   e. Cross-resistance among the various fluoroquinolones to the aforementioned pathogens and other resistant pathogens generally is complete [4, 20b].

  3. Approaches to decrease clinically relevant resistance are discussed later in sec. I (pp. 1359–1361).

F. Clinical uses. Fluoroquinolones are potent, broad-spectrum antibacterial agents that have changed therapeutic approaches to a variety of infections [1–5, 21–56]. The fluoroquinolones are only occasionally listed as drugs of choice (e.g., for *C. jejuni* infections, *Shigella* and *Salmonella* infections, UTI due to *P. aeruginosa, Bartonella henselae,* and in combination therapy for *Mycobacterium avium* complex) [21].

  1. Urinary tract infections [22–28]. All the fluoroquinolones are highly effective against the majority of bacteria causing UTI [1–4].

   a. **Complicated (e.g., pyelonephritis) or recurrent UTI. The fluoroquinolones should be saved for treatment of more resistant pathogens** (e.g., *P. aeruginosa,* hospital-acquired gram-negative bacteria) **and should not be used for uncomplicated initial UTI** (i.e., cystitis) for which many other agents are available. For complicated UTI, an oral quinolone can often be used instead of a parenteral agent, allowing one to avoid a hospitalization or shorten the hospital course. (If the fluoroquinolones are used in uncomplicated UTI, resistant organisms may be associated with future infections, precluding their use in a patient later on.)

   b. **Prostatitis.** The fluoroquinolones penetrate the prostate well and therefore are appealing in the treatment of prostatitis [1–4, 24]. After 4–6 weeks of therapy, the quinolones have cure rates of 65–90%; these results are comparable or superior to what has been seen with other agents (e.g., trimethoprim-sulfamethoxazole [TMP-SMX]) [1, 4]. *P. aeruginosa* infections are difficult to eradicate.

   c. **Uncomplicated UTI in patients with multiple antibiotic allergies.** There is no evidence that the fluoroquinolones are more effective than TMP-SMX if the organisms are susceptible to both agents [4]. However, in the sulfonamide-allergic patient who may be allergic to other antibiotics commonly used for cystitis (e.g., amoxicillin, oral cephalosporins), the fluoroquinolones are effective alternatives. Although single-dose regimens have been used for selected patients with uncomplicated UTI, 3-day regimens have proven more effective and are preferred by most experts [3, 4, 26–28]. See related discussions in Chap. 12.

   d. **Chronic suppressive therapy** in patients with recurrent UTI. Preliminary studies suggest the quinolones can be used in selected patients. (See sec. **II.C.1** and Chap. 12.)

   e. There are no conclusive data indicating that fluoroquinolones should be used as chronic prophylaxis in patients with chronic renal lesions such as renal calculi or in patients with indwelling urethral catheters. In these patients, the fluoroquinolones eventually will select out more resistant urinary pathogens. Lithotripsy may be useful in patients with calculi; urologic evaluation is advised.

  2. Sexually transmitted diseases (STDs)

   a. **Gonococcal infections.** The fluoroquinolones are very active against *N. gonorrhoeae* [1–4, 25]. (See Table 28S-1.) A single oral dose of ciprofloxacin (500 mg) or ofloxacin (400 mg) is a recommended regimen for **uncomplicated gonococcal urethritis, cervicitis, or rectal infections** [29]. Norfloxacin (800 mg) or enoxacin (400 mg) or lomefloxacin (400 mg) as single doses are effective also [29]. Failures of therapy for pharyngeal infection can occur after fluoroquinolone treatment. Ciprofloxacin, 500 mg PO bid, has been used to complete therapy for disseminated gonococcal infection after initial conventional therapy [30]. See Chap. 13.

Until 1992, virtually all strains of *N. gonorrhoeae* tested were suscepti-ble to fluoroquinolones. Recent reports from Southeast Asia, Australia, Ohio, Hawaii, Colorado, and Washington suggest the emergence of resis-tance in *N. gonorrhoeae* [6a, 6b]. Isolates with decreased susceptibilities to ciprofloxacin have decreased susceptibilities to other fluoroquinolones. (See sec. **e.**)

   b. ***Chlamydia trachomatis.*** None of the fluoroquinolones is effective as single-dose therapy. **Ofloxacin,** 300 mg PO bid for 7 days, has proven **effective** for chlamydial urethritis, cervicitis, or proctitis [4, 30]. Norfloxacin is not effective, and ciprofloxacin is less effective than doxycycline [4, 31].

   c. **Chancroid.** The fluoroquinolones are effective alternative regimens in the therapy of chancroid [25] due to *Haemophilus ducreyi;* ciprofloxacin, 500 mg PO bid for 3 days, has been suggested [30].

   d. There is **no** established **role** for the use of **fluoroquinolones in the treat-ment of pelvic inflammatory disease (PID)** [4, 29].

   e. **The fluoroquinolones are not effective against incubating syphilis; therefore, if they are used as treatment for STDs, patients should be monitored with serologic tests for syphilis** [29]. The fluoroquinolones have usually failed in the eradication of *Ureaplasma urealyticum* [3].

3. **Osteomyelitis and septic arthritis** [1–4, 32–37].

   a. **Gram-negative bacteria.** Fluoroquinolones are very effective for suscepti-ble gram-negative bacteria causing osteomyelitis. Oral ciprofloxacin has been evaluated extensively [32–36]. Whenever possible, the site of infec-tion should be surgically debrided, especially in chronic osteomyelitis, before initiating therapy. If possible, foreign metallic material should ideally be removed; otherwise, resistance may be acquired by the pathogen during therapy, especially when *P. aeruginosa* and *S. marcescens* are involved. If the prosthesis cannot be removed, infections tend to relapse as soon as the antibiotic has been stopped [4]. In malignant external otitis caused almost exclusively by *P. aeruginosa,* ciprofloxacin especially has been effective as monotherapy (see sec. **III**).

   b. ***S. aureus* and other gram-positive bacteria.** The role of fluoroquinolones for *S. aureus* infections still is unsettled. Because of the relatively higher MIC_{90} for *S. aureus* (compared to Enterobacteriaceae [see Table 28S-1]) and the concerns about the emergence of potential bacterial resistance (see sec. **E**), some experts believe that the treatment of *S. aureus* osteomy-elitis with a quinolone is still investigational [2]. Other experts believe that oral ciprofloxacin or ofloxacin is appropriate therapy for susceptible *S. aureus* infections after careful surgical debridement when indicated [34–37].

      At this point, we favor a conservative approach to the treatment of osteomyelitis caused by *S. aureus* alone and agree with one reviewer's conclusion that "despite many anecdotal reports of the efficacy of quino-lones for the treatment of staphylococcal infections, the pooled data are inconclusive" and further data are needed [32]. **We do not advocate use of a fluoroquinolone as first-line therapy for *S. aureus* osteomyelitis.**

      If a fluoroquinolone is used as alternative therapy in *S. aureus* osteomy-elitis, combination therapy with rifampin has been suggested [32]. Also, in mixed infections with susceptible *S. aureus* and gram-negative bacilli, after appropriate surgical debridement and initial intravenous antibiotic therapy, a protracted course of an oral fluoroquinolone may be a useful approach in certain patients.

      Because the role of fluoroquinolones for *S. aureus* osteomyelitis is an unsettled area, infectious disease consultation is suggested.

   c. **Septic arthritis.** The role of the fluoroquinolones in these infections has not been as well studied [4]. Some of the aforementioned principles can be extrapolated to this setting while awaiting further clinical data.

4. **Respiratory tract infections** [1–4, 38–41]

   a. **Fluoroquinolones are not drugs of choice for empiric therapy of common community-acquired pneumonias** because *S. pneumoniae* are the most common pathogens. Likewise, they are **not drugs of choice for acute exacerbations of acute bronchitis** unless a sputum Gram stain shows predominantly gram-negative pathogens, as *S. pneumoniae* also is a common pathogen in community-acquired bronchitis.

Treatment of pneumococcal infection in animal models has demonstrated that fluoroquinolones often are not effective in this setting [40, 41]. Furthermore, treatment of *S. pneumoniae* infections with currently available fluoroquinolones has resulted in clinical failures, and pneumococcal bacteremia and pneumococcal meningitis have developed in patients who received oral ciprofloxacin. Therefore, in particular, the fluoroquinolones should be avoided in patients who may have pneumococcal disease associated with a bacteremia [3].

b. Fluoroquinolones are **useful for pneumonia and bronchitis due to susceptible gram-negative pathogens.** After the patient has completed an initial course of intravenous antibiotics, an oral fluoroquinolone can often be used to substitute for intravenous therapy. The fluoroquinolones are highly effective when *H. influenzae* or *M. catarrhalis* are the primary pathogens. Ciprofloxacin has proven effective therapy for nosocomial pneumonia due to gram-negative bacteria, including *P. aeruginosa* and many Enterobacteriaceae [3].

c. **Cystic fibrosis exacerbations.** Monotherapy with fluoroquinolones (e.g., ciprofloxacin) for susceptible pathogens has been as effective as traditional therapy with intravenous beta-lactams and aminoglycosides [39]. The fluoroquinolones do not eliminate colonization with *P. aeruginosa,* and emergence of resistant strains during treatment, with cross-resistance to other fluoroquinolones, is common. (See sec. **E.**)

   Chronic, long-term prophylaxis is not recommended [39].

d. **Fluoroquinolones are not agents of choice for aspiration pneumonia** in patients with poor dental hygiene. Other agents with activity against anaerobes, such as penicillin or clindamycin, are indicated.

e. Although some fluoroquinolones inhibit *M. pneumoniae, Chlamydia pneumoniae,* and *Legionella* spp. (see Fig. 28S-1), it is difficult to determine the precise role of the fluoroquinolones in these infections, because the number of well-documented cases treated with fluoroquinolones is limited [3]. Further clinical studies are needed to define their role in this setting.

5. **Bacterial gastroenteritis.** All the fluoroquinolones are effective in the treatment of diarrhea by bacterial pathogens [1–4]. (See Table 28S-1.)

a. *Shigella.* Fluoroquinolones now are listed as the drug of choice for these infections [21], although the optimal duration of therapy (e.g., one dose versus 3 days versus 5 days) is unclear [3, 41a].

b. *Salmonella.* Initially, the fluoroquinolones were believed to be promising in attempts to eradicate *Salmonella* carrier states, as they had intracellular penetration, high concentrations in the stool, and increased concentrations in bile [1, 42]. Despite these favorable attributes, clinical relapses and prolonged fecal excretion have been reported [1].

   In one report, several patients who received oral ciprofloxacin for 14 days continued to excrete *Salmonella* in the stool for a period of time [43]. Therefore, the fluoroquinolones may not dramatically reduce the likelihood of a posttherapy carrier state. Because of these data, careful serial stool culture monitoring is necessary after such attempts to eradicate *Salmonella* [1, 43]. Infectious disease consultation is advisable.

   In one review, Neu [3] recommends treatment of salmonellosis in those who are toxic, hypotensive, or otherwise critically ill with the suggestion of a bacteremic illness. For a more detailed discussion of the therapy for *Salmonella* infections, see Chap. 11.

   The fluoroquinolones are effective in treating typhoid fever [3, 4].

c. **Travelers' diarrhea** has been effectively treated with 3 days of norfloxacin, ciprofloxacin, ofloxacin, and enoxacin [1–4, 44–47]. Three days of therapy often is suggested [44, 45, 47, 47a]. See Chap. 21.

d. *Campylobacter jejuni.* A fluoroquinolone or erythromycin is listed as the agent of choice for therapy for these infections [21]. However, treatment failures have been documented as has the development of resistance [46, 48].

e. **Empiric therapy of presumed bacterial gastroenteritis.** The fluoroquinolones have been used to treat patients with severe presumed bacterial gastroenteritis (e.g., associated fever, dehydration, positive fecal leukocyte smears) while awaiting cultures. However, if patients have *Salmonella* infections, the carrier state may persist (see sec. **b**) and, if patients have *C. jejuni* infections, therapeutic failures are common (see sec. **d**).

If the patient may have had an associated transient bacteremia, a fluoroquinolone providing adequate blood levels (e.g., ciprofloxacin) is preferred.

6. **Soft-tissue infections**
   a. **Fluoroquinolones are not intended for routine *S. aureus* or group A and group B streptococcal infections or anaerobic soft-tissue infections.** Because streptococci are common pathogens in cellulitis, in his review, Neu [3] emphasizes that it is important to be very cautious in using fluoroquinolones in cellulitis. We concur and prefer more conventional therapy with antistaphylococcal penicillinase-resistant penicillins (e.g., oxacillin) or a first-generation cephalosporin (e.g., cefazolin, cephalexin, or cephradine) for routine cellulitis or clindamycin in severe infection not complicated by an open wound and not in the perirectal or perineal area. (See Chap. 4.)
   b. The fluoroquinolones are effective agents in mixed aerobic, gram-negative, and gram-positive skin infections with cellulitis, wounds, and ischemic ulcers. In these settings, an oral fluoroquinolone often is combined with an anaerobic agent (e.g., clindamycin), for the fluoroquinolones are primarily active against the aerobic gram-negative pathogens. Resistance can occur with *P. aeruginosa* and *S. aureus,* especially if there is poor perfusion of the tissues or low concentrations of the drug at the site of infection [3].

7. **Miscellaneous**
   a. **Prevention of infection and outpatient treatment of infection in leukopenic patients**
      (1) The fluoroquinolones have been investigated for prophylaxis in leukopenic patients because they can eradicate pathogenic aerobic gram-negative bacilli, including *P. aeruginosa,* while sparing the anaerobic bacteria. However, this type of prophylaxis may just change the spectrum of infections and give rise to resistant *Staphylococcus epidermidis* or alpha-hemolytic streptococci that originate in the oropharynx [1]. The prophylactic use of fluoroquinolones in this setting is more common in Europe than in the United States [49].

      The use of fluoroquinolones to prevent infections in leukopenic patients remains unsettled. There is no consensus on their use in this setting [2]. Because of the potential for selecting resistant pathogens, occasional cases of gram-positive bacteremia despite prophylaxis [4], possible side effects, unchanged death rates in recipients of prophylaxis, and the potential usefulness of these agents in therapeutic regimens for these patients later, **we currently would not advise routine use of the fluoroquinolones or other oral agents** (e.g., TMP-SMX) **to prevent infectious complications in the leukopenic patient** unless the patient is part of a controlled clinical trial trying to assess the role of these regimens. This topic has recently been reviewed [49a].
      (2) A recent report discusses the potential **role of oral quinolones in the outpatient management of low-risk neutropenic febrile patients** who are not on quinolone prophylaxis [49b]. These patients need careful selection and follow-up; further experience with this approach is under clinical evaluation.
   b. **Meningococcal carrier state.** Fluoroquinolones (e.g., ciprofloxacin) have been used in this setting [50, 51] and may provide alternatives to rifampin. See Chap. 5, sec. **VII.B.2** under Meningitis.
   c. **CNS infections.** Some of the quinolones penetrate the CSF and brain tissue. However, their relatively low activity against *S. pneumoniae* and anaerobes and the presumed need for a 10–20:1 ratio of drug CSF level to MIC for clinical efficacy indicates that they will have a limited role in the treatment of CNS infections. This topic is reviewed elsewhere [50].
   d. **Malignant external otitis** is discussed in sec. **3.a.**
   e. Fluoroquinolones have been used as prophylaxis of postoperative UTI when administered prior to surgery. (See sec. **VI.C.2,** p. 1373, and Chap. 28B, pp. 1102–1103.)
   f. The role of the fluoroquinolones in peritonitis, spontaneous peritonitis, and peritonitis associated with continuous ambulatory peritoneal dialysis

(CAPD) is undergoing clinical evaluation [3]. These topics are discussed in Chap. 11 (see sec. **III.F** under Intraabdominal Infection, pp. 423–426).

g. *Mycobacterium* **infections.** The fluoroquinolones are being evaluated for treatment of these infections. Ciprofloxacin and ofloxacin are considered alternative agents for *M. tuberculosis,* and ciprofloxacin is one of the drugs of choice in *M. avium* complex [21]. This use is discussed elsewhere [3, 52, 53]. See Chaps. 9 and 19.

The exact role of the fluoroquinolones in this setting awaits further study. Infectious disease consultation or pulmonary consultation is advised for use of these agents in mycobacterial infections.

h. **Cat-scratch disease** (due to *Bartonella henselae)*. A few patients have been treated with ciprofloxacin [21, 54]. (See Chap. 17.)

i. **Malaria.** The fluoroquinolones are being evaluated for use in some forms of malaria [55, 56].

j. **Methicillin-resistant** *S. aureus* **infection.** See sec. **E.2.b.**

G. **Adverse reactions.** The fluoroquinolones are well tolerated, and the adverse effects are fairly similar among all the various agents. In general, the overall percentage of adverse reactions is 2–8% [1–4].

1. **Gastrointestinal symptoms** (e.g., primarily nausea, but also abdominal discomfort, vomiting, diarrhea, anorexia) **are the most common** (approximately 5%) but seldom are severe enough to necessitate discontinuing treatment. *Clostridium difficile* diarrhea is seen infrequently [1]. See Chap. 28A.

2. **CNS symptoms** can occur in 1–4% of patients. The most common symptoms have been headache (mild), slight dizziness, mild sleep disturbance, and alteration of mood with agitation, anxiety, or depression.

Seizures have rarely been reported and may be seen in patients receiving other medications simultaneously—for example, theophylline with ciprofloxacin or enoxacin, or nonsteroidal antiinflammatory agents (NSAIDs) with enoxacin. The possible mechanisms are unclear and are reviewed elsewhere [57, 58]. Some experts have suggested that fluoroquinolones should not be prescribed for patients with a history of convulsions or psychotic episodes and that the concomitant use of NSAIDs and fluoroquinolones should be avoided [57].

3. **Dermatologic reactions** occur in fewer than 1–2% of patients, and usually consist of a nonspecific rash or photosensitivity. Neu [3] has advised patients to be cautious about exposure to ultraviolet light when taking these drugs, particularly in high doses. Lomefloxacin in particular may have an increased incidence of phototoxicity. See sec. **VI.E.2.**

4. Mild laboratory abnormalities (e.g., leukopenia, abnormal liver function tests) occur infrequently.

H. **Precautions in use of fluoroquinolones**

1. **Do not use in patients allergic to older analogues** (e.g., nalidixic acid, oxolinic acid, or cinoxacin) or other fluoroquinolones.

2. **Do not use in children.**

a. **Cartilage development.** Nalidixic acid and other fluoroquinolones can produce cartilage erosions in young animals. Therefore, this possibility is a concern in pediatric populations, and **fluoroquinolones are not recommended for use in children** (see sec. **d**), **pregnant women, and nursing mothers.** The potential of this toxicity in children continues to be evaluated [1–4].

There have been no major arthralgias, myalgias, or joint damage noted in adult patients taking quinolones for long periods of time.

b. Children with **cystic fibrosis** have been treated with quinolones because the benefits are believed to outweigh the risks. Fulminant diarrhea due to a multiresistant *Shigella* strain for which other agents are not active is another potential use in children [3].

c. The age above which fluoroquinolones currently are safe is unclear (i.e., 14 versus 16 versus 18 years of age). One pharmaceutical company suggested avoiding them in teenagers (except those with cystic fibrosis) unless one obtains informed consent from a family member. The CDC guidelines for sexually transmitted disease therapy suggest that children should be 17 years of age or older before using ciprofloxacin for gonococcal infections [29]. Many package inserts suggest avoiding fluoroquinolones in those younger than 18 years.

    d. In special situations, fluoroquinolones may be justified in children when alternative safe therapy is not available. See a recent discussion of this [58a].

3. **Avoid in pregnancy and lactation** because of the potential effect on developing cartilage in the fetus or infant (see sec. **2**).

4. **Do not take with antacids containing magnesium or aluminum,** which markedly diminish the absorption of oral fluoroquinolones. **Sucralfate** should either be avoided because it can impair absorption [57, 58] or be taken 6 hours before the fluoroquinolone is taken. (See sec. **D.1.**)

5. **Monitor theophylline serum levels** in patients receiving theophylline with ciprofloxacin or enoxacin. See individual agent discussions.

    Norfloxacin and ofloxacin do not seem to elevate serum levels of theophylline.

6. **Caffeine interaction.** All the fluoroquinolones produce some change in caffeine metabolism, especially enoxacin and ciprofloxacin. This is reviewed in detail elsewhere [58]. Neu [3] suggests that patients should be warned to avoid taking these drugs late in the evening with a heavy caffeine load.

7. **Warfarin.** The question of whether a warfarin-fluoroquinolone interaction actually occurs in patients remains unanswered. While awaiting data on this issue, close monitoring of the prothrombin time of patients receiving warfarin and fluoroquinolones seems prudent [58]. See related discussion in sec. **III.F.5.**

8. **Cyclosporine.** Whether there is a drug interaction of cyclosporine with the fluoroquinolones is unclear. Until more data are available, careful monitoring of serum concentrations of cyclosporine and measures of renal function in patients receiving therapy has been suggested [58].

    A recent review concludes that controlled studies involving cyclosporine pharmacokinetic profiles do not support a pharmacokinetic or pharmacodynamic drug interaction between ciprofloxacin and cyclosporine [58b].

9. **Possible tendon rupture.** Postmarketing data suggests that quinolone use may be associated with a risk of tendon rupture. This usually involves the Achilles tendon (unilateral or bilateral) but has also been reported in the shoulder joint and hand. The pathogenesis of this potential complication is not understood. Some patients may have been on excessive doses or corticosteroids, but 9 of 25 patients had no obvious risk factor [58c].

    The US Food and Drug Administration (FDA) will be updating labeling for all fluoroquinolones to include a warning about the possibility of tendon rupture, **including the recommendation to discontinue treatment with quinolones at the first sign of tendon pain or inflammation and to refrain from exercise until the diagnosis of tendonitis can be confidently excluded** [58c].

10. **Remember that these agents are expensive** compared with alternatives. They should be used only when clearly indicated (e.g., to allow one to avoid an agent or avoid hospitalization) to make them cost-effective (see Table 28A-5).

I. **Inappropriate or excessive use of fluoroquinolones.** As discussed in Chap. 28A, prior studies have revealed that between 25 and 50% of antibiotics prescribed in the United States are unnecessary or inappropriately used. Therefore, it is not surprising to learn that the fluoroquinolones have been used inappropriately and excessively. This may have not only a negative impact on their future usefulness, but patients also are receiving a drug for some clinical conditions that is less effective or more expensive than conventional therapy.

1. **The problem of excessive use of the fluoroquinolones** has been specifically addressed. **In 1990, Drs. Frieden and Mangi (from Yale University** School of Medicine, New Haven, CT) reported on the inappropriate use of oral ciprofloxacin [59]. The authors emphasized that "sophisticated, expensive antibiotics are becoming first-line therapy, even where they may be unnecessary or insufficient treatment. Ciprofloxacin exemplifies this pattern . . . and inappropriate therapy may be common with other oral and intravenous antibiotics, but this problem seems particularly acute with ciprofloxacin" [59]. They emphasized the inappropriate use, especially in situations in which streptococcal species or *S. aureus* is likely—for example, outpatient, community-acquired pneumonias or cellulitis. The authors point out that ciprofloxacin has been heavily marketed and noted that in the first 6 months of 1988, ciprofloxacin was the second most advertised product in the pharmaceutical journals. The authors then reviewed the appropriate use of ciprofloxacin.

The authors' concluding paragraph reads: "Properly used, ciprofloxacin is effective and can save money by shortening or preventing hospitalization. However, indiscriminate use leads to unnecessary expense, treatment failures, increased resistance, and adverse reactions. We cannot quantitate the extent of misuse of ciprofloxacin; we suspect an epidemic. Each day, Americans spend $700,000 on ciprofloxacin. Our experience suggests that much of this expenditure is inappropriate" [59].

2. **Response of the infectious disease experts.** Reviewers of the fluoroquinolones have tried to respond to the known excessive use of these agents.

   a. **In 1991, Drs. Hooper and Wolfson (Massachusetts General Hospital,** Boston, MA) [2] concluded their review of the fluoroquinolones by emphasizing conditions in which these agents were preferred over previously available agents including complicated UTIs, especially those caused by *P. aeruginosa* or resistant pathogens; very ill patients with suspected bacterial gastroenteritis; pulmonary exacerbations in cystic fibrosis patients when due to susceptible *P. aeruginosa;* invasive, malignant, external otitis caused by *P. aeruginosa;* and therapy for susceptible gram-negative osteomyelitis, usually after initial intravenous conventional therapy. They went on to emphasize that "the use of the quinolones should, in our view, focus on infections in which there is a differential benefit over conventional agents in terms of efficacy, safety, or cost or in infections for which few alternative treatments exist" [2]. It is hoped that such focused application would help to minimize the development of resistance that will "compromise the usefulness of these drugs."

   b. **Also in 1991, Drs. Walker and Wright (Mayo Clinic,** Rochester, MN) [1] stressed in their review of the fluoroquinolones that "although the fluoroquinolones have proved effective in various types of infections, they should seldom be the drugs of choice . . . (their) misuse will inevitably result in increased bacterial resistance and eventual loss of clinical utility. When treatment with fluoroquinolones is considered for a specific infection, certain guidelines should be followed." After listing these guidelines and situations in which fluoroquinolones should not be used, they conclude: "The safety, broad spectrum of activity, clinical efficacy, and convenience of an antibiotic do not obviate the use of reason and careful clinical judgement by physicians . . . The rapidly increasing problem of resistance to the fluoroquinolones and their widespread, indiscriminate use are likely no coincidence. This resistance is spreading directly between patients . . . Physicians should reevaluate their prescribing behavior so that patients who truly need these excellent agents will be able to benefit from them now and in the future" [1].

   c. **In 1992, Dr. H. Neu (College of Physicians and Surgeons, Columbia University,** New York, NY) [4] concluded his review by emphasizing "inappropriate use of fluoroquinolones has the potential of rapidly destroying the efficacy of these agents . . . With the tremendous increase in resistance of MRSA and *P. aeruginosa,* it is difficult to predict how useful the agents will be in 5 years. Hence, **unless there is more rational use of the compounds in the community, they will become as ineffective for many bacteria as are penicillin G and the tetracyclines.**"

   d. **In 1994, Dr. Pickering and colleagues (Brigham and Women's Hospital,** Boston, MA) [59a] reviewed the appropriate use, or abuse, of fluoroquinolones in a large academically oriented **long-term care facility.** Only 25% of the orders were judged appropriate! The authors concluded that the study indicated less-than-optimal prescribing of oral fluoroquinolones in the long-term care setting, with the potential complications of the development of resistant bacterial strains and increased costs [59a].

   e. **In the *Medical Letter's* 1996 version of "The Choice of Antimicrobial Drugs,"** the fluoroquinolones are listed as the agents of first choice only a few times: (1) for UTI due to susceptible *P. aeruginosa,* (2) for *Shigella* infections, (3) for *S. typhi* or other *Salmonella* spp. (ceftriaxone is the other drug of choice), (4) for *C. jejuni* gastroenteritis for which erythromycin is the other drug of choice, (5) for *M. avium* complex infections (as a possible drug of first choice usually in a multidrug regimen), and (6) for *Bartonella henselae* (cat-scratch bacillus) [21].

3. **A rational response.** The fluoroquinolones, including ciprofloxacin, are extremely useful agents in the proper setting. They may be lifesaving, allow the patient to avoid or shorten hospitalization, or be very cost-effective. The bacterial resistance problems will only worsen if these drugs are used unnecessarily.

As emphasized in sec. **2,** to maintain the usefulness and longevity of these agents, they should be used only when clearly indicated. These indications have been reviewed in sec. **F** and in Table 28S-3. In addition, the fluoroquinolones are not indicated in several circumstances that have likewise been reviewed in sec. **F** and in Table 28S-4.

II. **Norfloxacin (Noroxin)** became available in 1986 and is the first antimicrobial in the fluoroquinolone class to be marketed in the United States. It is **approved for use in adults** with uncomplicated and complicated UTI.

A. **In vitro activity** [60]. See Table 28S-1.

1. **Gram-positive aerobes.** Norfloxacin is not active against most *Streptococcus* spp., although at concentrations achievable in the urine, it is active against enterococci (group D streptococci).

2. **Gram-negative aerobes.** Norfloxacin is active against most Enterobacteriaceae with MIC_{90} values of 2.0 μg/ml or less. (See Table 28S-1.) Norfloxacin is less active against strains of *P. aeruginosa* than is ciprofloxacin. **Urinary pathogens with a MIC of less than or equal to 16 μg/ml are considered susceptible** [60].

Norfloxacin is active against a variety of enteric pathogens, including *Salmonella* and *Shigella* spp., toxogenic *E. coli, Campylobacter* spp., *Vibrio cholerae, Yersinia enterocolitica,* and *Aeromonas* spp. Norfloxacin is active against penicillin-susceptible and penicillin-resistant *N. gonorrhoeae.*

3. **Anaerobes.** Norfloxacin is **not active** against anaerobes, including *Clostridium difficile* [60].

B. **Pharmacokinetics. See general discussion in sec. I.D.**

1. **Oral absorption.** If norfloxacin is ingested on an empty stomach, oral doses are well absorbed, producing peak serum levels of 1.5–2.0 μg/ml. Therapeutic urinary levels are maintained for 12–24 hours, with a level of more than 100 μg/ml in the urine for more than 8 hours after a 400-mg oral dose [61].

2. **Metabolism and excretion.** The liver is the primary site of metabolism, whereas the urine is the major route of excretion. Dose modifications are necessary when the glomerular filtration rate falls below 30 ml/min.

C. **Clinical indications. See also sec. I.F.**

1. **Urinary tract infections.** Norfloxacin is useful in the treatment of adults with uncomplicated and complicated UTI caused by susceptible strains. It is as effective as conventional therapy with no documented advantage over any prior agent (e.g., TMP-SMX and amoxicillin) for uncomplicated acute UTI, unless organisms such as *P. aeruginosa* are involved.

Although levels in renal tissue are excellent, **blood levels are not sufficiently high to treat bacteremic patients.** Norfloxacin has been used for the prophylaxis of recurrent UTI in adult women [62]. Because norfloxacin penetrates prostatic tissue well, it has been used in the therapy of bacterial prostatitis. See related discussions in Chap. 12.

2. **Alternative agent in uncomplicated gonococcal infections** [29]. See sec. **I.F.2.** Ciprofloxacin or ofloxacin usually is preferred [29]. Norfloxacin has limited activity against *C. trachomatis.*

3. **Prevention and treatment of diarrheal disease.** The quinolones are active against most bowel pathogens. Norfloxacin has been shown to be effective in the treatment of travelers' diarrhea [1–4]. (See sec. **I.F.5** and Chap. 21.)

4. **Prevention of infection in leukopenic patients** undergoing chemotherapy is an unsettled issue, which has been summarized in sec. **I.F.7.** (We do not favor its use in this setting.)

D. **Dosages.** Only an oral preparation is available as a 400-mg tablet. Norfloxacin should be given with water 1 hour before or 2 hours after meals. Adequate hydration is suggested by the manufacturer to prevent the crystalluria that has sometimes been observed with total doses of greater than 800 mg daily. Concomitant use of antacids should be avoided. (See routine precautions, sec. **I.H.**)

1. **In normal renal function** or creatinine clearance of more than 30 ml/min.

Table 28S-3. Summary of appropriate indications for fluoroquinolones

Indications	Comments	Preferred fluoroquinolone[a]
UTI	1. Reserve for complicated UTI in which resistance to usual oral antibiotics exists (e.g., *P. aeruginosa*) 2. Alternative regimen in patients with multiple allergies to other antibiotics	If susceptible, any will work
Chronic bacterial prostatitis	1. When organisms are resistant to TMP-SMX 2. When TMP-SMX cannot be used or has failed	If susceptible, any probably will work (ofloxacin is approved for prostatitis)
Uncomplicated gonococcal urethritis, cervicitis, or rectal infection	As an alternative to ceftriaxone As an alternative regimen	Ciprofloxacin[b] or ofloxacin[b] Norfloxacin,[b] enoxacin,[b] or lomefloxacin[b]
Chlamydial cervicitis, urethritis, or proctitis	Only as an alternative regimen	Ofloxacin for 7 days
Osteomyelitis due to susceptible gram-negative bacilli	1. May save the need for prolonged IV therapy 2. Initial debridement important 3. Role in *S. aureus* osteomyelitis is minimal (see text)	Ciprofloxacin
Invasive ("malignant") external otitis	1. When due to susceptible *P. aeruginosa,* will save protracted IV therapy 2. In severe cases, conventional double-drug antipseudomonal IV therapy advised initially	Ciprofloxacin
Gram-negative nosocomial pneumonia	1. Initially conventional IV antibiotics typically used[c] 2. Oral fluoroquinolones may help shorten hospitalization or need for IV therapy (see text)	Greatest experience with ciprofloxacin
Exacerbations of pulmonary infections in patients with cystic fibrosis	Avoid chronic, continuous use, which will facilitate resistance	Greatest experience with ciprofloxacin. Ofloxacin also useful
Shigella infections	Fluoroquinolones are the drugs of choice [21] in adults	
Travelers' diarrhea	Fluoroquinolones often are preferable to TMP-SMX[d]	Greatest experience with norfloxacin and ciprofloxacin[e]
Severe bacterial gastroenteritis	When patient is sufficiently ill that antibiotics need to be started empirically	If bacteremia is a concern, ciprofloxacin may be preferred. For gastroenteritis alone, any agent should be effective

Table 28S-3 (continued)

Indications	Comments	Preferred fluoroquinolone[a]
Gram-negative soft-tissue infections	1. In mixed aerobic-anaerobic infections and when gram-negatives not susceptible to other cheaper oral agents; an agent aimed at anaerobes will need to be addressed 2. Resistance can occur to *S. aureus*	Ciprofloxacin
For susceptible gram-negative infections in patients with multiple drug allergies (e.g., to cephalosporins, sulfa)		
For certain forms of mycobacterial infections	See text and Chaps. 9 and 19	See text and Chaps. 9 and 19

[a]See text for dosages.
[b]Fluoroquinolones are not active against incubating syphilis. See text and Chap. 13.
[c]Often combination IV antibiotic therapy is used initially (e.g., antipseudomonal penicillin and an aminoglycoside) for 7–10 days and then an additional 7–10 days of oral fluoroquinolone to complete a protracted course. See text.
[d]See reference [47a] and its annotation.
[e]Ciprofloxacin provides higher blood levels.

Table 28S-4. When fluoroquinolones are not indicated

1. Uncomplicated UTI that can be treated with cheaper or alternative agents.
2. Bacteriuria or UTI associated with foreign bodies (e.g., Foley catheter, renal calculi)[a] in which prolonged therapy will just select out resistant bacteria.
3. Pelvic inflammatory disease or syphilis, including incubating syphilis.
4. Primary agent for initial therapy of *S. aureus* osteomyelitis. See text.
5. Community-acquired pneumonia.[b]
6. Community-acquired bronchitis due to *S. pneumoniae*.[b]
7. Aspiration pneumonia secondary to poor oral or dental hygiene.
8. Group A or non–group A streptococcal skin infections or routine cellulitis possibly due to group A streptococci or *S. aureus*.
9. Otitis media or sinusitis.
10. Streptococcal pharyngitis.
11. Anaerobic infections.
12. Children, pregnant women, nursing mothers.

[a]Patients with renal calculi need urologic evaluation for possible lithotripsy therapy.
[b]Currently available fluoroquinolones are not very active against *S. pneumoniae*. See text.

a. **For uncomplicated UTI in adults,** 400 mg twice daily for 7–10 days is recommended by the package insert for conventional therapy. Although single-dose therapy has been tried in carefully selected young women with uncomplicated UTI, one study suggests that a 3-day course is preferable [28]. Most experts now favor 3-day regimens. See Chap. 12.

b. **For complicated UTI in adults,** 400 mg twice daily for 10–21 days.

2. **In renal failure,** in patients with a creatinine clearance of 30 ml/min or less, one 400-mg tablet daily for the above duration is suggested. For patients with severe renal insufficiency (i.e., creatinine clearance <10 ml/min) or in patients on hemodialysis or peritoneal dialysis, an alternative agent is advised [63].

3. In patients with hepatic dysfunction, doses do not require modification.

4. **Drug interactions.** Norfloxacin does not interfere with theophylline or caffeine metabolism.

E. **Side effects.** Overall, norfloxacin is tolerated well. The most frequent side effects have been nausea, dyspepsia, headache, and dizziness [1–4, 64]. (See sec. **I.G.**)

F. **Contraindications.** See the detailed discussion in sec. **I.H.**

G. **Cost.** Compared with other conventional oral agents (see Table 28A-5) used for UTI, norfloxacin is expensive.

H. **Summary.** After the approval and release of norfloxacin, the *Medical Letter* [61] concluded that norfloxacin should prove useful for oral therapy of complicated UTI caused by Enterobacteriaceae resistant to multiple antibiotics, *P. aeruginosa,* and enterococci. For more routine and uncomplicated UTI, older and less expensive drugs still are preferred.

Although many newer and even more active fluoroquinolones are available, norfloxacin remains a useful agent in the treatment of susceptible UTI and is effective in travelers' diarrhea.

Norfloxacin does not provide acceptable serum or nonrenal tissue concentrations. It does not interfere with theophylline metabolism. Like many other clinicians, **we have, for the most part, replaced norfloxacin with ciprofloxacin,** which provides higher serum levels and enhanced *P. aeruginosa* activity.

III. **Ciprofloxacin (Cipro)** was released in late 1987. This agent has been extensively reviewed [1–5, 65].

A. **In vitro activity.** Overall, ciprofloxacin remains as active in vitro as any of the available fluoroquinolones. (**See related discussion in sec.** I.C.)

1. **Gram-positive aerobes.** As with the other fluoroquinolones, ciprofloxacin is less active against gram-positive aerobes than gram-negative aerobes. In fact, MIC values are 10- to 100-fold greater for gram-positive aerobes than those for the enteric bacilli [66, 67]. (See Table 28S-1.)

a. **S. aureus** is only moderately susceptible with an MIC_{90} of approximately 0.5–1.0 μg/ml. (Resistance can develop during therapy; see sec. **I.E.**)

b. *S. epidermidis* is slightly more susceptible, with a MIC_{90} of 0.12–0.50 μg/ml for methicillin-susceptible and some methicillin-resistant strains.

c. Although *S. pyogenes* and enterococci (group D) are moderately susceptible, with a MIC_{90} of 1–2 μg/ml, **other streptococcal species** (*S. pneumoniae,* group B streptococci, viridans streptococci) are relatively resistant with a MIC_{90} of 2.0–8.0 μg/ml.

d. *Staphylococcus saprophyticus* strains are susceptible.

2. **Gram-negative aerobes.** Ciprofloxacin is very active against these organisms. Overall, the antimicrobial potency of ciprofloxacin in vitro against gram-negative aerobes is two- to fourfold greater than that of norfloxacin (see Table 28S-1). Based on the proposed breakpoint for susceptibility of 1 μg/ml or less [66, 67]:

a. **Highly susceptible** pathogens include Enterobacteriaceae; *N. meningitidis;* ampicillin-susceptible and ampicillin-resistant *N. gonorrhoeae; H. influenzae;* and *M. catarrhalis.* Also *Aeromonas* spp., *Pasteurella multocida, H. ducreyi,* and Vibrionaceae (including *Vibrio* spp.) are highly susceptible.

b. **Moderately susceptible** pathogens include *P. aeruginosa* (MIC_{90} = 0.5 μg/ml).

c. **Resistant** bacteria include *Burkholderia cepacia* (formerly *P. cepacia*) and *Stenotrophomonas maltophilia* (formerly *P. maltophilia*).

3. **Anaerobes** generally are **not susceptible** to ciprofloxacin at clinically achievable concentrations.

4. **Miscellaneous**

a. Ciprofloxacin is active against *Legionella* spp. and is marginally active against *M. pneumoniae* and *C. trachomatis,* although the clinical implications of this are still being studied. (See sec. **I.C.4.**)

b. Ciprofloxacin is active against *M. tuberculosis* (as an alternative agent) and *M. avium* complex (as an agent of first choice) [21]. See Chaps. 9 and 19.

c. Ciprofloxacin is not active against *Treponema pallidum.*

d. **Postantibiotic effect.** Ciprofloxacin appears to have a significant postantibiotic effect (i.e., persisting suppression of bacterial growth following exposure to the antibiotic) against Enterobacteriaceae, *S. aureus,* and *P. aeruginosa.* The clinical significance of this is unclear [68].

e. **Antibiotic combinations** to achieve possible synergy are discussed in sec. **I.C.5.**

B. Pharmacokinetics
1. **Oral absorption.** Ciprofloxacin is well absorbed. Antacids decrease absorption if they are used concomitantly. After a 500-mg oral dose, mean serum levels are 2.0–2.5 μg/ml. After 500 mg PO bid, urine concentrations are more than 200 μg/ml and are therefore far in excess of the MICs of susceptible pathogens. (See Table 28S-2.)

   With the high antibacterial activity of ciprofloxacin, serum levels of 0.25 μg/ml will inhibit approximately 95% of susceptible organisms (e.g., in bacteremias complicated by UTI or bacterial gastroenteritis). Serum levels are maintained above 0.25 μg/ml for at least 10 hours after oral doses of 500 mg.
2. **Half-life.** The half-life in patients with normal renal and hepatic function is 3.0–4.5 hours. Metabolism of the drug does occur. In marked renal failure, the half-life is prolonged two- to threefold. Although the drug is excreted in part by the kidney, elimination also occurs through the intestinal mucosa, providing high intestinal levels useful in intestinal infections.
3. **Intravenous ciprofloxacin.** The serum half-life of intravenous ciprofloxacin is approximately 5 hours. A 400-mg IV dose given over 1 hour produces plasma concentrations comparable to a 750-mg oral dose and an "area under the curve" comparable to a 500-mg oral dose. A 200-mg IV dose is equivalent to a 250-mg oral dose [69].

   This oral-intravenous pharmacoequivalence correlates with the bioavailability of oral ciprofloxacin, which is approximately 70–80% that of intravenous ciprofloxacin. Thus, a larger dose is needed when ciprofloxacin is given orally [70], or a proportionate intravenous dose is 80% of the oral dose [71].

   After a 60-minute infusion IV of 200 mg and 400 mg ciprofloxacin, mean peak serum concentrations of 2.1 and 4.6 μg/ml are achieved [70]. There may be slight pain and irritation at the intravenous site if the drug is administered over less than 60 minutes or if a small peripheral vein site is used [71].
4. **Distribution.** Ciprofloxacin penetrates tissues well, including prostate and bone. Biliary elimination is negligible. (See discussion in sec. **I.D.**)
5. **In renal failure,** dosages must be reduced.
6. **Drug Interactions. Theophylline blood levels are elevated** typically in patients receiving both ciprofloxacin and theophylline. The serum level elevations are variable, ranging from 17 to 87% in reported series [57, 58]. In one study, 30% of patients developed toxic theophylline levels when ciprofloxacin was given concomitantly [72]. **Therefore, theophylline doses should be reduced and serum theophylline levels should be monitored when patients receive theophylline and ciprofloxacin.** (See sec. **I.H.5.**)
7. **In liver disease.** No dosage adjustments are necessary in patients with chronic cirrhosis [70].
C. Clinical uses
1. **A review of the appropriate use of the fluoroquinolones is presented in sec. I.F and in Tables 28S-3 and 28S-4.**
2. The **approved uses** of ciprofloxacin include the following:
   a. **Urinary tract infections.** Ciprofloxacin is especially useful in patients with UTI due to susceptible pathogens resistant to other oral antibiotics or in patients with multiple antibiotic allergies. In patients with underlying structural abnormalities of the urogenital tract, renal calculi, or chronic indwelling catheters, a cure is unlikely with any antibiotic. (See sec. **I.F.1.**)
   b. **Osteomyelitis.** If compliance can be ensured and appropriate surgery is done to remove devitalized tissue, oral ciprofloxacin can be very effective for susceptible gram-negative pathogens, including *P. aeruginosa* [3, 43]. This includes malignant external otitis caused by *P. aeruginosa* [3, 73]. (See sec. **I.F.3.**) We do not believe that ciprofloxacin is a primary agent for gram-positive osteomyelitis (see sec. **I.F.3.b.**).
   c. **Respiratory infections.** The role of the quinolones in this setting is reviewed in sec. **I.F.4.**
      (1) **Gram-negative pneumonias.** Ciprofloxacin use is very appealing in this setting (see sec. **I.F.4**).
      (2) **Cystic fibrosis.** See sec. **I.F.4.**
      (3) Acute bacterial bronchitis appears to respond to ciprofloxacin if gram-negative bacteria are seen on Gram stains.
      (4) As discussed previously in sec. **I.F.4,** ciprofloxacin is not recommended in the following settings:

   (a) Because of the limited activity of quinolones against group A
   streptococci and *S. pneumoniae,* these agents are not useful in
   pharyngitis, nor are they drugs of choice in otitis media or
   sinusitis.
   (b) Community-acquired pneumonia is commonly due to *S. pneumoniae* in adults and mycoplasma in children and young adults, and
   other agents are preferred.
   (c) Orofacial or dental infections and aspiration pneumonias should
   not be treated with ciprofloxacin or other quinolones, which have
   little anaerobic activity.
 d. **Infectious diarrhea.** See prior general discussion in sec. **I.F.5.**
   (1) Travelers' diarrhea. Ciprofloxacin is very effective in treating **travelers' diarrhea** [47a] and often is viewed as a drug of choice. See Chap. 21.
   (2) Ciprofloxacin and other fluoroquinolones have excellent antibacterial
   activity against all the common diarrheal pathogens, including toxicogenic *E. coli; Shigella* and *Salmonella* spp. (including *S. typhi*); *Aeromonas* spp., *Vibrio parahemolyticus; Y. enterocolitica;* and *C. jejuni.*
   This includes strains from areas of the world where multiple drug
   resistance is common. Therefore, ciprofloxacin has been effectively
   used in the empiric therapy of severe presumed or known **bacterial
   gastroenteritis.** (See sec. **I.F.5.**)
 e. **Skin and soft-tissue infections.** Ciprofloxacin is very useful in patients
   with decubitus ulcers and chronic cutaneous infections due to susceptible
   pathogens, especially gram-negative bacteria. It has also been a useful
   agent in soft-tissue infections of the extremities in diabetes or associated
   with peripheral vascular disease [74]. (See sec. **I.F.6** and Chap. 16 under
   Diabetic Foot Infections.)
 3. **Other uses**
 a. **Initial recommended regimen** [31] for single-dose therapy for uncomplicated gonococcal urethritis, cervicitis, or rectal infection. (See sec. **I.F.2.a.**)
   This regimen is not effective in the treatment of nongonococcal urethritis
   due to *C. trachomatis* or *U. urealyticum* or incubating syphilis. See
   Chap. 13.
 b. **Prostatitis.** Because ciprofloxacin penetrates prostate tissue well and is
   active against most pathogens associated with bacterial prostatitis, clinicians have used ciprofloxacin in this setting even though it is not an
   official FDA-approved use.
 c. **Prophylaxis in neutropenic patients** is discussed in sec. **I.F.7.a.** We do
   not favor the routine use of empiric oral ciprofloxacin in this setting. Also
   as a single agent, intravenous ciprofloxacin is not advocated for empiric
   therapy in the granulocytopenic patient without an obvious source of fever
   [20a, 75]. See Chap. 2.
 4. **To compare, contrast, or emphasize special aspects of ciprofloxacin** versus
   other fluoroquinolones, we cite the following:
 a. **Advantages** (see also Table 28S-3).
   (1) This fluoroquinolone has as good if not better in vitro activity against
   P. aeruginosa compared with the other fluoroquinolones.
   (2) Ciprofloxacin is the only fluoroquinolone currently approved for bone
   and joint infections. It has been a very useful agent in malignant
   external otitis due to *P. aeruginosa.*
   (3) It provides blood levels often adequate to treat bacteremias associated
   with UTI, GI infections, and skin and soft-tissue infections.
 b. **Disadvantages**
   (1) Ciprofloxacin interferes to a variable degree with theophylline and
   caffeine metabolism.
   (2) Resistance to ciprofloxacin may develop, especially when it is used
   for *S. aureus* or difficult-to-eradicate *P. aeruginosa* infections. (See
   sec. **I.E.**) Many MRSA strains are now resistant to ciprofloxacin.
   (3) **This very useful agent often is overutilized.** (See sec. **I.I**, p. 1359.)
D. **Dosages. Ciprofloxacin should not be used in children** (see ref. [58a] and sec.
 I.H.2.) **or pregnant women. See the general precautions in sec.** I.H.
 1. **Oral dosage** guidelines are shown in **Table 28S-5.**
 a. **Availability.** Ciprofloxacin is available in 250-mg, 500-mg, and 750-mg
   tablet sizes.

Table 28S-5. Ciprofloxacin dosage guidelines*

Location of infection	Type of severity	Dosage
Urinary tract	Mild–moderate	250 mg q12h
	Severe–complicated	500 mg q12h
Lower respiratory, bone and joint, skin and skin structure	Mild–moderate	500 mg q12h
	Severe–complicated	750 mg q12h
Infectious diarrhea	Mild–moderate–severe	500 mg q12h

*Dosages when renal function is normal.
Source: Copyright *Physicians' Desk Reference* 1996 (50th ed.), published by Medical Economics Data, Montvale, NJ 07645. Reprinted by permission. All rights reserved.

    b. In renal failure. Dosage modification is required for patients with severe renal insufficiency. In severe infections, serum levels should be monitored. If the creatinine clearance is more than 50 ml/min, the usual dosages can be used (see Table 28S-5). If the creatinine clearance is 30–50 ml/min, 250–500 mg q12h can be used as ciprofloxacin is metabolized and partially excreted through the biliary system of the liver. If the creatinine clearance is 5–29 ml/min, 250–500 mg q18h is suggested.

    Another approach is to use the normal dose interval but reduce the dose by 50% for a creatinine clearance of 10–50 ml/min and to one-third of the normal dose if the creatinine clearance is less than 10 ml/min [63]. For patients on hemodialysis or peritoneal dialysis, 250 mg q12h has been recommended [63] or, after dialysis, 250–500 mg q24h.

  2. Intravenous ciprofloxacin was the first fluoroquinolone to become available in the United States in an intravenous formulation (1991).

    a. Dosage

      (1) For a mild to moderate UTI, 200 mg IV q12h infused over 60 minutes.

      (2) For severe or complicated UTI and other infections, 400 mg IV q12h infused over 60 minutes.

      (3) In significant renal failure, the dose interval can be adjusted to q18–24h as discussed in sec. **1.b.**

    b. Intravenous versus oral ciprofloxacin

      (1) Cost. Intravenous ciprofloxacin is much more expensive than oral therapy, approximately tenfold more so [69]. The average wholesale price (AWP) for 400 mg q12h of the intravenous formulation for 1 day is $60.02. The AWP for oral ciprofloxacin 500 mg bid is $6.26 per day. (See Tables 28A-5 and 28A-6.)

      (2) Achievable serum concentrations are similar to those achieved with oral therapy, so there is no advantage to using the intravenous form to obtain higher blood levels.

      (3) Indications for intravenous form. If ciprofloxacin is the preferred agent in a patient who is unable to take oral medications (i.e., because of nausea, vomiting, NPO status, perioperative, etc.), the more expensive intravenous preparation is indicated [20b].

    c. So-called streamlined intravenous and then oral therapy is discussed in sec. **E.**

  3. Ophthalmic formulation. An ophthalmic formulation of ciprofloxacin (Ciloxan-Alcon) was marketed in the United States in 1991 for treatment of bacterial keratitis and conjunctivitis. In its review, the *Medical Letter* concluded that ciprofloxacin is active in vitro against most ophthalmic pathogens, and the ophthalmic formulation may be able to sterilize corneal ulcers. (See related discussion in Chap. 6, sec. **IV** under Infectious Keratitis.) Widespread use of ophthalmic ciprofloxacin could add to the growing number of bacterial strains resistant to the drug, limiting its usefulness for systemic treatment of serious infections [76].

  4. Contraindications. As with other fluoroquinolones, ciprofloxacin is not approved for use in children and pregnant or nursing women. (See sec. **I.H.**)

5. **Drug interactions** of the fluoroquinolones were discussed earlier in secs. **I.D** and **I.H.**

Ciprofloxacin does interfere with theophylline metabolism. Some reviewers have suggested that patients with an initial serum concentration of theophylline at the upper end of the therapeutic range should have their daily dose of theophylline reduced by 30–50%. Patients with an initial serum concentration of theophylline at the low end of the therapeutic range can continue to take the same dose during treatment with ciprofloxacin but should be monitored closely because the changes in theophylline clearance may be greater than 50% [58]. Serial theophylline monitoring seems prudent.

Because **ciprofloxacin may reduce the clearance of caffeine,** it probably is prudent to advise patients to decrease their daily consumption of caffeine while taking ciprofloxacin. Ciprofloxacin should not be taken with **antacids** or **sucralfate.** (See sec. **I.D.**)

E. **"Sequential" or "streamlining" antibiotic therapy from intravenous to oral therapy.** In recent years, some of the fluoroquinolone pharmaceutical companies and some articles have emphasized the potential usefulness of certain agents (e.g., ciprofloxacin, ofloxacin) initially administered intravenously and then switched to a more cost-effective oral regimen [71, 77, 78]. We believe that this aspect may at times be overemphasized by the pharmaceutical industry, and we do not agree with some authors who suggest that hospitals "should look to the pharmaceutical manufacturers to help 'market' the fluoroquinolones for the Pharmacy and Therapeutics Committee and thus promote the concept of streamlining therapy from intravenous to oral antibiotics" [79]. In fact, in a review of intravenous ciprofloxacin, the authors concluded that "intravenous ciprofloxacin does not represent an important advance in the treatment of infectious diseases . . . Furthermore, intravenous ciprofloxacin should be reserved for patients who are unable to take oral fluoroquinolones" [20b].

In fact, this is not a novel approach. For decades clinicians have initially treated *S. pneumoniae* pneumonia with intravenous penicillin and then switched to oral penicillin after an initial clinical response. Similarly, clinicians have treated tracheobronchitis (with and without pneumonia) in patients with chronic obstructive pulmonary disease (COPD) with intravenous ampicillin first, followed by oral ampicillin or amoxicillin.

In 1975, Feigin and colleagues [80] reported on the use of oral clindamycin in the treatment of *S. aureus* osteomyelitis. In our first edition of *A Practical Approach to Infectious Diseases* (1983), while discussing the therapeutic options for osteomyelitis, Dr. S. Chapman [81] wrote: "[I]n attempt to circumvent the complication of long-term intravenous therapy, recent articles (from 1975–1979) have evaluated short-term parenteral therapy followed by oral antibiotics in children with hematogenous osteomyelitis. Oral therapy is appealing since it is more comfortable for the patient and may reduce the risk of intravenous-related phlebitis and/or bacteremia." Since the availability of an intravenous form of TMP-SMX in 1981, serious *Pneumocystis carinii* pulmonary infections have been treated with initial intravenous TMP-SMX and then oral therapy to allow cost-effective outpatient therapy.

Tuomanen and coworkers [82], **in 1981,** demonstrated that oral chloramphenicol achieved equivalent blood levels to that of intravenous therapy, and oral chloramphenicol could be used to complete the course of therapy for *H. influenzae* meningitis in children if compliance could be ensured and serial serum levels were monitored.

When the fluoroquinolones are indicated as discussed in secs. I.F and C, we advocate their use. At times, this may involve a specific fluoroquinolone initially intravenously and then oral or other antibiotics intravenously followed by oral fluoroquinolones, depending on the clinical circumstances. Streamlining is not unique to ciprofloxacin.

F. **Toxicity and side effects.** Prior studies and clinical experience suggest that ciprofloxacin appears to be well tolerated, with most reactions mild to moderate in severity. (**See sec.** I.G.)

1. **Gastrointestinal symptoms,** including abdominal cramps, nausea, and vomiting, can occur. In patients receiving theophylline therapy concomitantly, theophylline excess should be ruled out.

2. **CNS-related symptoms** can occur. Theophylline or caffeine serum excess may intensify these symptoms. (See sec. **I.G.**)

3. **Interstitial nephritis** can occur [20b].
4. **Tendon rupture** may occur. See discussion in sec. **I.H.9.**
5. **Interaction with warfarin.** Whether the quinolones can significantly increase the response to warfarin continues to be evaluated. (See related discussion in sec. **I.H.7.**) A review of case reports submitted to the Food and Drug Administration concluded that the quinolone-warfarin interaction is clinically important and that patients receiving therapy with the two drugs at the same time should be monitored closely [82a, 82b]. However, a recent study in early 1996 concludes that ciprofloxacin use has little effect on prothrombin time [82b]. Nevertheless, the authors conclude: "[A]s with any new drug that is added to therapy for a patient receiving warfarin treatment, it is still prudent to monitor the anticoagulation response" [82b].

G. **Cost.** Typical of the fluoroquinolones, ciprofloxacin is an expensive oral agent. For a 10-day course, the average wholesale price of the pharmacist for 250 mg bid is $54.10; for 500 mg bid, it is $62.61; and for 750 mg bid, it is $108.60. (See Table 28A-6.)

H. **Resistance and issues of excessive use have already been discussed** in detail. (See sec. **I.E.**)

I. **Summary.** Ciprofloxacin is an extremely useful and often cost-effective oral agent if used when indicated. Unfortunately, this agent often is overutilized, and resistance to this and other fluoroquinolones may eventually limit the usefulness of this agent.

IV. **Ofloxacin (Floxin)** was released in 1990 and has been reviewed [1–4, 83–86].
A. **In vitro activity.** Overall, the in vitro activity of ofloxacin is similar to that of ciprofloxacin; both are more active than norfloxacin [84, 87]. **See Table 28S-1.**
1. **Gram-positive aerobes.** Many streptococci are susceptible to ofloxacin but much less so than penicillin [84]. The MIC_{90} for *S. pneumoniae* is 2.0 μg/ml [4, 87], which is relatively high compared with the MIC_{90} data for gram-negative bacteria (see Table 28S-1) and achievable serum levels. (See Table 28S-2.) Ofloxacin and ciprofloxacin have similar activity against susceptible *S. aureus*. The MIC_{90} for enterococcus is likewise relatively high at 4 μg/ml [4, 87], but organisms are susceptible to concentrations achievable in the urine.
2. **Gram-negative aerobes**
   a. **Highly susceptible organisms** include Enterobacteriaceae, *N. gonorrhoeae* (including penicillin-resistant strains), *H. influenzae*, and *M. catarrhalis* (ampicillin-susceptible and ampicillin-resistant strains).
   b. **Moderately susceptible pathogens** include *P. aeruginosa* (MIC_{90} = 4 μg/ml) [4, 87]. Typically, **ofloxacin is approximately fourfold less active against *P. aeruginosa* than is ciprofloxacin.**
3. **Anaerobes** generally are not susceptible to ofloxacin at clinically achievable concentrations.
4. **Miscellaneous**
   a. *Chlamydia trachomatis.* **Ofloxacin is more active against this pathogen than are other quinolones.**
   b. See sec. **I.C** and Table 28S-1. Ofloxacin is active against *C. pneumoniae, M. pneumoniae, M. tuberculosis* [21], and *M. leprae* [21].
   c. Ofloxacin, like other fluoroquinolones, has poor activity against *T. pallidum* [84].

B. **Pharmacokinetics.** Both an oral and an intravenous preparation are available. (See sec. **I.D.**)
1. **Oral absorption.** Ofloxacin is well absorbed and is 98% bioavailable (higher than other fluoroquinolones), with peak serum concentrations achieved in 1–2 hours. The elimination half-life is approximately 5–8 hours [84]. (See Table 28S-2.)
2. **Intravenous preparation.** An intravenous preparation is available. Intravenous ofloxacin provides serum levels comparable to those achieved with oral doses [1–4, 88], as the oral form is so well absorbed. Even the package insert emphasizes that the intravenous formulation does not provide a higher degree of efficacy or more potent antimicrobial activity than an equivalent dose of the oral formulation. The intravenous form is used, therefore, when patients are not candidates for oral therapy. It is about tenfold more expensive than the oral preparation. See Tables 28A-5 and 28A-6.
3. **Metabolism and excretion.** More than 70% of the oral or intravenous dose is recovered in the urine as unchanged ofloxacin. Only minimal amounts

(less than 5% of the dose) are recovered as metabolites. The intravenous preparation demonstrates a similar pharmacokinetic profile to that seen after oral doses, supporting the interchangeability of both forms of therapy. Dosage adjustment seems necessary only in renal impairment [89].

4. **Distribution.** High concentrations are found in the lung, gallbladder, liver, muscle, tonsils, sinus mucosa, kidney, and prostate. CSF concentrations have not been studied adequately [84].

5. **In renal failure,** dosage adjustments are recommended when the creatinine clearance falls below 50 ml/min.

6. **Drug interactions.** (See secs. **I.D.** and **I.H.**) Several clinical studies indicate that **ofloxacin does not interfere with theophylline metabolism** [58, 84] **or caffeine metabolism** [58].

C. **Clinical uses**

1. **A review of the appropriate uses of the fluoroquinolones is provided in sec. I.F and is summarized in Tables 28S-3 and 28S-4.**

2. **Approved uses** of ofloxacin

   a. **UTI,** both uncomplicated and complicated, for which ofloxacin is comparable in efficacy to TMP-SMX [84]. A 3-day regimen is effective for uncomplicated UTI.

   b. **Prostatitis** (primarily due to *E. coli*) [86].

   c. **Sexually transmitted diseases,** as recommended agent for uncomplicated urethral and cervical gonorrhea and nongonococcal urethritis and cervicitis due to *C. trachomatis*. See Chap. 13.

   d. **Lower respiratory tract infections and acute exacerbations of bacterial bronchitis** due to *H. influenzae* and *S. pneumoniae*. Although small studies are available showing the efficacy of oral ofloxacin for community-acquired pneumonia [90], some pneumococcal infections have been resistant to ofloxacin [84] and the MIC_{90} of ofloxacin for *S. pneumoniae* is relatively high. (See Table 28S-1.) Consequently, we do not advocate the use of ofloxacin for community-acquired pneumonias. (See sec. **I.F.4** for further discussion.) Ofloxacin appears to be equivalent to ciprofloxacin for treating bronchopulmonary disease caused by *P. aeruginosa* in patients with cystic fibrosis [84].

   e. **Mild to moderate skin and soft-tissue infections.** However, fluoroquinolones are not agents of choice for *S. aureus* or group A streptococcal skin infections. (See sec. **I.F.6.**)

3. Unfortunately, there are no head-to-head comparisons of the quinolones [86]. **To compare, contrast, or emphasize special aspects of ofloxacin versus other fluoroquinolones,** we cite the following:

   a. **Advantages**

      (1) **Ofloxacin does not interfere with theophylline or caffeine metabolism.** This is an advantage in patients with underlying COPD who need fluoroquinolone therapy but are receiving concomitant theophylline therapy.

      (2) **Ofloxacin is an alternative to tetracyclines for the treatment of chlamydial urethritis** [21, 86] (and is approved for use as single-dose therapy for uncomplicated gonococcal urethritis).

   b. **Disadvantages**

      (1) **Ofloxacin is at least fourfold less active against *P. aeruginosa;* therefore, in infections due to this pathogen (e.g., complicated UTI, malignant external otitis), ciprofloxacin is preferred [86].**

      (2) **Only a limited number of cases of prostatitis were studied** in this drug's new drug application (NDA), and the majority of cases were due to *E. coli*. Therefore, the FDA limited its approval of ofloxacin for treatment of *E. coli* prostatitis [86, 90a]. However, in practice, this quinolone and others are used for treating patients with prostatitis, with quinolones aimed at susceptible pathogens that have been cultured from the patient's urine (see sec. **I.F.1** and Chap. 12).

      (3) **Ofloxacin currently is not approved for the treatment of osteomyelitis,** and the experience of its use in this setting is limited [86, 90a].

      (4) Although ofloxacin is active in vitro against *S. pneumoniae* and *S. aureus,* one review emphasizes that emergence of resistance, therapeutic failures, and superinfections have been observed with these organisms when they are exposed to fluoroquinolones; therefore, cau-

tion is prudent. For patients in whom pneumococcal or staphylococcal infection has been documented or is strongly suspected, the use of a beta-lactam agent, vancomycin, or a macrolide is preferable [86].

(5) Ofloxacin has not been approved for use in GI infections.

D. **Dosages for adults**
1. **Oral** tablets of ofloxacin are available in 200-mg, 300-mg, and 400-mg sizes. The dosage regimens for approved uses are shown in **Table 28S-6.**
2. **Intravenous** ofloxacin, 200–400 mg, is given by **slow infusion over 60 minutes.** Because the pharmacokinetics of oral and intravenous ofloxacin are similar, the same dosage regimen used in Table 28S-6 can be used for intravenous dosages. The intravenous preparation is more expensive than the oral tablets, so the **oral preparation is preferred if the patient can take oral medications.**
3. **In renal failure**
   a. For a creatinine clearance of 10–50 ml/min, the usual dose interval is prolonged, and the usual dose is given every 24 hours.
   b. When the creatinine clearance is less than 10 ml/min, one-half of the usual dose is given every 24 hours.
   c. **In patients undergoing dialysis.** In patients undergoing hemodialysis, 100 mg bid has been suggested [63]. In patients undergoing CAPD, dosages in sec. **b** have been suggested [63].
4. **Contraindications.** As with other fluoroquinolones, this agent is not recommended for use in children and in pregnant or nursing women [84]. (See sec. **I.H.**)
5. **Drug interactions** of the fluoroquinolones are reviewed in sec. **I.H.** Ofloxacin does not interfere with theophylline or caffeine metabolism. Antacids and sucralfate should not be used concomitantly.
E. **Toxicity and side effects** have been reviewed [86]. Most of these effects were mild and did not shorten the course of therapy. Approximately 1–3% of recipients discontinued ofloxacin therapy due to side effects. (**See related discussion in sec. I.G.**)
   1. **Gastrointestinal symptoms** were the most common side effect (5.4% recipients), especially nausea, diarrhea, dysgeusia, and vomiting [86].
   2. **CNS symptoms** were seen in 5.1%, with insomnia, headache, and dizziness reported most frequently.
   3. **Skin symptoms** were seen in 1% and included rash, pruritus, and diaphoresis.
   4. **Tendon rupture** may occur. See discussion in sec. **I.H.9.**
F. **Cost.** Typical of the fluoroquinolones, ofloxacin is an expensive oral agent. The AWP for a 10-day supply of 400 mg bid is approximately $73.16. (See Table 28A-6.) For a similar intravenous dose, the AWP is about ten times the cost of the oral agent. See Tables 28A-5 and 28A-6.
G. **Resistance and potential for excessive use.** The increasing problem with the development of resistance and the potential for the abuse of these agents is discussed in sec. **I.E.** Just as if ciprofloxacin were used excessively, the same issues and concerns apply if ofloxacin is excessively used. See sec. I.I, p. 1359.
H. **Summary.** In its review of ofloxacin, the *Medical Letter* concluded: "Ofloxacin, a new oral fluoroquinolone, appears to be equivalent to ciprofloxacin for treatment of urinary tract, lower respiratory tract, prostate, and skin or soft tissue infections . . . it can be used to treat chlamydial infections. A penicillin or a cephalosporin is preferred over either ofloxacin or ciprofloxacin for treatment of known or suspected streptococcal or pneumococcal infection. Overuse leading to the development of bacterial resistance presents a serious threat to the long-term usefulness of these drugs" [84]. We would add that ofloxacin does not interfere with theophylline or caffeine metabolism as does ciprofloxacin.

Ofloxacin has not been used as extensively for, nor has it been approved for, use in osteomyelitis.

V. **Temafloxacin (Omniflox) was voluntarily withdrawn from worldwide markets** in mid-1992 by the manufacturer as a result of an unexpected profile and incidence of reported serious adverse reactions after the introduction of this agent. These reports included symptoms of severe hypoglycemia in elderly patients, hemolytic anemia, hepatic dysfunction, renal failure requiring dialysis in some instances, anaphylaxis, and death [91].

VI. **Lomefloxacin (Maxaquin)** was released in 1992 as a once-daily oral fluoroquinolone for the treatment of UTI and bronchitis caused by *H. influenzae* and *M. catarrhalis.* The agent has been reviewed [92–96].

Table 28S-6. Adult oral (IV) dosages for ofloxacin with normal renal function*

Infection	Description	Unit dose	Frequency	Duration	Daily dose
Lower respiratory tract infections	Exacerbation of chronic bronchitis	400 mg	q12h	10 days	800 mg
	Community-acquired pneumonia	400 mg	q12h	10 days	800 mg
Sexually transmitted diseases	Acute, uncomplicated gonorrhea	400 mg	Single dose	1 day	400 mg
	Cervicitis or urethritis due to C. trachomatis	300 mg	q12h	7 days	600 mg
	Cervicitis or urethritis due to C. trachomatis and N. gonorrhoeae	300 mg	q12h	7 days	600 mg
Skin and skin structure infections	Uncomplicated infections	400 mg	q12h	10 days	800 mg
Urinary tract	Cystitis due to E. coli or K. pneumoniae	200 mg	q12h	3 days	400 mg
	Cystitis due to other susceptible organisms	200 mg	q12h	7 days	400 mg
	Complicated UTIs	200 mg	q12h	10 days	400 mg
Prostatitis	Prostatitis due to E. coli	300 mg	q12h	6 weeks	600 mg

*When creatinine clearance is greater than 50 ml/min. See text for dose reduction in renal failure.
Source: Copyright *Physicians' Desk Reference* 1996 (50th ed.), published by Medical Economics Data, Montvale, NJ 07645. Reprinted by permission. All rights reserved.

A. **In vitro activity.** Lomefloxacin has no unique in vitro activity [94]. (**See Table 28S-1.**)
   1. **Gram-positive aerobes.** Most pneumococci and streptococci have relatively high MICs to lomefloxacin [92, 93]. In one report, 45% of *Enterococcus faecalis* and 66% of *E. faecium* strains were resistant to lomefloxacin [94]. Methicillin-resistant *S. aureus* with acquired high-level resistance to ciprofloxacin are now common and probably will be resistant to lomefloxacin as well [93]. (See sec. I.E.)
   2. **Gram-negative aerobes.** Lomefloxacin is active against most Enterobacteriaceae, *H. influenzae,* and *M. catarrhalis* (including ampicillin-resistant strains). The MIC_{90} for *P. aeruginosa* ranges from 0.5 µg/ml (see Table 28S-1) to 8 µg/ml in other reviews [96].
   3. **Anaerobes** are not susceptible to lomefloxacin at clinically achievable concentrations.
   4. **Miscellaneous**
      a. Lomefloxacin is active against *C. trachomatis, Legionella* spp., and *M. pneumoniae* [8], but the clinical significance of this awaits further clinical study.
      b. Lomefloxacin does not inhibit *T. pallidum.*
B. **Pharmacokinetics**
   1. **Oral absorption** of lomefloxacin is excellent, as it is almost completely absorbed (95–98%) [93].
   2. A 400-mg oral daily single dose provides peak plasma concentrations of approximately 3–3.4 µg/ml, and urine concentrations are maintained at roughly 100 times concurrent plasma concentrations. Plasma trough concentrations are 0.3 µg/ml [95]. Urine concentrations of more than 80 µg/ml during the 12- to 24-hour period after a 400-mg dose are provided [95].
   3. The **elimination half-life** of lomefloxacin is 7–8 hours, **allowing a once-daily dosage regimen** [95].
   4. Lomefloxacin penetrates tissue well, including urine, stool, bile, bronchial fluid, prostate, and bone [92, 93]. Cerebrospinal fluid concentrations have not been well studied, but, based on data from other fluoroquinolones, penetration is inadequate to treat meningitis [93].
   5. **In renal failure.** More than half of the orally administered dose is normally excreted in the urine as unchanged drug. In renal failure, the elimination half-life is prolonged so that a **reduction of the dose is advised when the creatinine clearance is less than 30 ml/min** [92].
   6. **Liver failure** has no effect on the pharmacology of lomefloxacin; therefore, in hepatic dysfunction, no dosage adjustment is necessary.
   7. **Drug interactions.** Lomefloxacin affects hepatic microsomal enzyme function minimally; hence, it has **no effect on theophylline or caffeine clearance.** See sec. I.H.
C. **Clinical uses**
   1. **A review of the appropriate uses of the fluoroquinolones** is presented in sec. I.F and Tables 28S-3 and 28S-4.
   2. The **approved uses of lomefloxacin** include the following:
      a. **Urinary tract infection,** both complicated and uncomplicated, caused by susceptible pathogens. Because all the available fluoroquinolones are effective in the therapy of susceptible UTI, it is not surprising that lomefloxacin, 400 mg once daily, is as effective as twice-daily TMP-SMX and twice-daily norfloxacin or ciprofloxacin [92]. Although preliminary data suggest that lomefloxacin is as effective in acute pyelonephritis as is TMP-SMX, additional clinical studies are needed to assess the role of lomefloxacin in acute pyelonephritis [92].
      b. **Acute bacterial exacerbations of chronic bronchitis** caused by *M. catarrhalis* and *H. influenzae.* Note that the package insert indicates that lomefloxacin is not indicated for exacerbations due to *S. pneumoniae,* as in vitro resistance to lomefloxacin is relatively common. Therefore, before lomefloxacin is used, the diagnosis of bronchitis due to *H. influenzae* or *M. catarrhalis* should be supported by an evaluation of the sputum Gram stain (typically showing > 25 polymorphonuclear leukocytes, < 10 squamous epithelial cells per high-power field, and coccobacillary gram-negative forms with a paucity of gram-positive cocci) and culture of sputum to help rule out an exacerbation due to probable or known *S. pneumoniae.*

Neu [92] emphasizes this limitation by stating, "[I]t is important to note that these lomefloxacin studies of bacterial bronchitis focused on gram-negative pathogens and that there was a clear attempt to avoid gram-positive pathogens such as *S. pneumoniae* . . . clearly, based upon its activity in vitro, lomefloxacin cannot be considered appropriate therapy of pneumococcal infection."

    c. Prophylaxis of UTI prior to transurethral surgery. Patients with infected urine preoperatively have usually been treated with antibiotic prophylaxis to prevent postoperative UTI or bacteremia. (See Chap. 28B.) **Whether prophylaxis is needed if preoperative urine cultures are negative is a controversial issue.** Although some reliable sources suggest that antimicrobials are not recommended before urologic operations on patients with sterile urine [97], some authors have supported antibiotic prophylaxis in this setting, citing data that confirm that after transurethral surgery, postsurgical bacteriuria developed in most patients who had sterile urines preoperatively and the prostate tissue itself may harbor urinary pathogens [98]. See related discussion in Chap. 28B, sec. **II.B.5.**

    Because lomefloxacin is well absorbed, penetrates the prostate well, and has a long half-life, studies have shown that it is an effective prophylactic agent when given as a single 400-mg dose 2–6 hours before transurethral surgery [92, 98]. It is approved for use for antibiotic prophylaxis in patients undergoing transurethral surgery.

  3. To compare, contrast, or emphasize special aspects of lomefloxacin versus other fluoroquinolones, we cite the following:

    a. The **exact role of lomefloxacin** currently is unclear and **awaits further clinical experience** with this agent.

    b. As with other fluoroquinolones, it will be useful in the treatment of UTI. The once-daily dose regimens of lomefloxacin may be especially useful when supervision of oral medications is mandatory (e.g., when a family member must dispense the medication to another family member, or in an adult home setting, when a caregiver must administer doses to a resident). Otherwise, we are not sure a once-daily regimen is significantly more convenient and ensures better compliance than the twice-daily regimens of other agents.

    c. Because *S. pneumoniae* is a common pathogen in acute exacerbations of bacterial bronchitis and because these exacerbations often are treated empirically by the clinician, we do not view lomefloxacin or other fluoroquinolones as first-line agents in this setting. We prefer amoxicillin, TMP-SMX, or a second-generation oral cephalosporin.

    d. Lomefloxacin is not approved for use in osteomyelitis or GI infections.

    e. In transurethral surgery, antibiotic prophylaxis may be indicated and can be used preoperatively. We would advocate its use in those patients with a positive preoperative urine culture or history of bacterial prostatitis. (See sec. **2.a.**) See Chap. 28B, sec. **II.B.5.**

D. Dosages. Lomefloxacin is available only as an oral 400-mg scored tablet, which may be taken without regard to meals.

  1. Adult dosage regimens. As per the package insert, when the creatinine clearance is greater than 40 ml/min.

    a. For UTI. In uncomplicated cystitis, one 400-mg tablet daily for 10 days. For complicated UTI, the same dose is given for 14 days.

    b. For acute exacerbations of chronic bronchitis, one 400-mg tablet for 10 days.

    c. For preoperative prophylaxis for transurethral surgical procedures, a single 400-mg dose of lomefloxacin has been given 2–6 hours prior to surgery.

  2. In renal failure

    a. For a creatinine clearance of 10–39 ml/min, an initial loading dose of 400 mg once, followed the next day and thereafter by a daily dose of 200 mg (one-half tablet) for the duration of therapy.

    b. For a creatinine clearance of less than 10 ml/min or for patients undergoing hemodialysis. Hemodialysis removes only a negligible amount of lomefloxacin. Per package insert, hemodialysis patients should receive (as in sec. **a**) an initial loading dose of 400 mg followed by daily maintenance doses of 200 mg once daily for the duration of treatment.

    c. Peritoneal dialysis. The effect of peritoneal dialysis on lomefloxacin is undergoing clinical evaluation; preliminary recommendations for dosing in this setting are to use dosages for creatinine clearance of <10 ml/min.
  3. Contraindications. As with other fluoroquinolones, this agent is not approved for use in **children and pregnant or nursing women.** See sec. **I.H.**
  4. Drug interactions for fluoroquinolones are discussed in sec. **I.H.** Lomefloxacin does not interfere with theophylline dosages, but antacids and sucralfate should not be used concomitantly.
  5. In cirrhosis, the package insert indicates that the nonrenal clearance does not change. No special dose modification is needed for hepatic dysfunction.
E. Toxicity and side effects. Prior studies suggest that lomefloxacin appears to be well tolerated, with most adverse events of mild to moderate severity. In general, the incidence of adverse events for patients was similar to that for recipients of other fluoroquinolones [99]. (See sec. **I.G.**) The most common adverse events were as follows:
  1. Gastrointestinal symptoms with nausea in 3.7% and diarrhea in 1.4% of recipients.
  2. Photosensitivity in 2.4% or more of recipients. With postmarketing experience, it became apparent that phototoxicity was more common than was initially appreciated. These phototoxic reactions have occurred with and without the use of sunscreens or sunblocks and have occurred after a single dose. Therefore the manufacturer has advised: **"Exposure to direct or indirect sunlight (even when using sunscreens or sunblocks) should be avoided while taking lomefloxacin and for several days following therapy. Lomefloxacin therapy should be discontinued immediately at the first signs or symptoms of phototoxicity"** [99a].
  3. CNS-related symptoms of headache in 3.2% and dizziness in 2.3% of recipients.
  4. Miscellaneous
    a. Concurrent administrations of theophylline did not increase the incidence of adverse events [99].
    b. None of the observed laboratory abnormalities that were attributable to lomefloxacin were clinically significant or serious enough to interrupt therapy.
  5. Tendon rupture may occur. See sec. **I.H.9.**
F. Cost. Typical of the fluoroquinolones, lomefloxacin is an expensive oral agent. (See Table 28A-6.) For a 10-day course of 400 mg daily, the average wholesale price to the pharmacist is $61.07 (see Table 28A-5).
G. Resistance and excessive use of fluoroquinolones. The increasing problem of the development of resistance and abuse of fluoroquinolones is reviewed in sec. **I.E.**
    In a symposium devoted to lomefloxacin and an introductory article on the use of fluoroquinolones, Neu [100] concludes his comments by emphasizing: "It is important to understand that extensive use of the fluoroquinolones, use of inadequate doses, or inappropriate timing of doses will diminish efficacy and select resistance. Significant problems have already occurred with MRSA in many parts of the United States. Many pseudomonads have already become resistant to the drugs, and further resistance has recently been reported in organisms such as *E. coli* when the agents were used inappropriately in treatment of selected urinary tract infections."
H. Summary. Lomefloxacin is a new oral fluoroquinolone with a long half-life, allowing for once-daily dosing, which may be useful in some settings. Whether a once-daily regimen truly improves compliance versus a twice-daily regimen is unclear in the literature. Lomefloxacin is approved for use in UTI due to susceptible strains and acute exacerbations of chronic bronchitis when the Gram stain or culture shows *H. influenzae* or *M. catarrhalis*. Lomefloxacin is not indicated for therapy of bronchitis due to *S. pneumoniae* or community-acquired pneumonia. As with other fluoroquinolones, lomefloxacin is an expensive agent.
VII. Enoxacin (Penetrex) was approved for use in the treatment of UTI and for single-dose therapy for gonorrhea in late 1991 and was marketed in late 1992. This agent has been reviewed elsewhere [1–4, 101–105].
  A. In vitro activity. The in vitro activity of enoxacin is **summarized in Table 28S-1;** it has no unique activity when compared with other fluoroquinolones.
    1. Gram-positive aerobes. Penicillin-susceptible *S. pneumoniae,* streptococci group A and B, enterococci, and *S. epidermidis* have high MIC$_{90}$s, ranging from 8 to 16 µg/ml. Even **methicillin-susceptible *S. aureus*** has a relatively

high MIC$_{90}$ of 2 μg/ml. Therefore, this agent offers no enhanced activity against gram-positive aerobes compared with other fluoroquinolones.

In vitro, ofloxacin and ciprofloxacin are more potent inhibitors of gram-positive organisms than is enoxacin [102]. Enterococci are relatively resistant to enoxacin but might be susceptible to the high concentrations achievable in urine [105].

2. **Gram-negative aerobes.** Typically, Enterobacteriaceae are highly susceptible. *H. influenzae, B. catarrhalis,* and *N. gonorrhoeae* are very susceptible, including beta-lactamase-positive strains. Overall, enoxacin is less active against gram-negative aerobes than is ofloxacin or ciprofloxacin [102].

3. **Anaerobes** are not susceptible to enoxacin at clinically achievable concentrations.

4. **Miscellaneous.** In contrast with some of the other fluoroquinolones, enoxacin is not very active against *M. pneumoniae* or *C. trachomatis,* but it is active in vitro against *Legionella* spp. As with other fluoroquinolones, enoxacin is not active against *T. pallidum.* See Table 28S-1.

B. **Pharmacokinetics.** Enoxacin currently is available only as an oral tablet, although an intravenous preparation is undergoing clinical evaluation.

1. **Oral absorption** is excellent, with approximately 90% bioavailability after an oral dose [103]. However, **absorption is decreased in the presence of food or drugs that lower gastric acidity [105].** After a 400-mg dose, serum concentrations of 2.0 μg/ml are achieved [103]; after a 200-mg dose, serum concentration of approximately 1.0 μg/ml is achieved. The amount of enoxacin absorbed is not changed by the ingestion of food [103]. The rapid and extensive oral absorption of enoxacin results in plasma drug concentrations that are similar to those observed after intravenous administration. Thus, either route should give similar therapeutic effect [103].

2. The **elimination half-life** for enoxacin ranges from 4 to 6 hours, allowing for a twice-daily dosing schedule. Metabolic clearance accounts for approximately half of the clearance of enoxacin; high concentrations of active unchanged drug are achieved in the urine [103].

3. **In renal failure,** the half-life is prolonged and reduction of dosages is necessary. Hemodialysis is not an effective way to remove enoxacin [63, 103].

4. **Drug interactions. Enoxacin can inhibit some isozymes of the cytochrome P450 hepatic microsomal enzyme system.** Enoxacin is associated with a decrease in theophylline and caffeine clearance [1–4, 58, 103]. Therefore, **concurrent treatment with enoxacin should be accompanied by a 50% reduction in the dose of theophylline and serial monitoring of theophylline serum levels [58]. The package insert also suggests that patients avoid consumption of caffeine-containing products during enoxacin therapy.**

Other drug interactions are reviewed in sec. **I.H.** The coadministration of antacids and sulcralfate should be avoided.

C. **Clinical uses.** Although enoxacin has undergone clinical studies in a variety of settings, including respiratory tract infections, skin and soft-tissue infections, and GI infections [1–4, 101, 102], it has been **approved for use only in UTI and single-dose therapy of uncomplicated urethral or cervical gonorrhea.**

1. A review of the appropriate uses of the fluoroquinolones is presented in sec. **I.F.** and Tables 28S-3 and 28S-4.

2. A summary of the **approved uses of enoxacin** include the following:

   a. **Urinary tract infection.** For uncomplicated and complicated UTI, enoxacin has been shown to be clinically effective, as have all the other fluoroquinolones [1–4, 101, 102, 104], and similar in efficacy to TMP-SMX [101]. Prostatic concentrations after 200 mg bid orally were 4 μg/g [101].

   b. **Uncomplicated urethral or cervical gonorrhea.** All the fluoroquinolones are effective in single-dose therapy for this problem, including infections caused by beta-lactamase-producing strains. (See sec. **I.F.2.**) None of the quinolones are active against *T. pallidum* or *C. trachomatis* (as single-dose therapy).

3. **To compare, contrast, or emphasize special aspects of enoxacin versus the other fluoroquinolones,** we cite the following:

   a. Enoxacin appears to offer no unique role when compared with other fluoroquinolones, as all these agents are effective for treatment of susceptible UTI and as single-dose therapy for uncomplicated gonorrhea [105].

b. In patients who receive theophylline, the dose of oral theophylline should be reduced and serum theophylline levels monitored, ideally, as discussed in sec. **B.4.** Daily caffeine intake should be reduced when patients take enoxacin. Because this is not necessary when norfloxacin, ofloxacin, or lomefloxacin is used, these other fluoroquinolones may be preferred by some clinicians.

D. Dosages. Enoxacin is available as 200-mg and 400-mg oral tablets, which should be taken at least 1 hour before or 2 hours after meals [105].

    1. Adult dosage regimens per package insert

        a. Uncomplicated UTI: 200 mg q12h for 7 days.

        b. Complicated UTI: 400 mg q12h for 14 days.

        c. Uncomplicated urethral or cervical gonorrhea: 400 mg as a single dose, as an alternative regimen (see sec. **I.F.2**). See also Chap. 13.

    2. In renal failure

        a. Normal dosages can be used in patients with a creatinine clearance exceeding 30 ml/min.

        b. For a patient with a creatinine clearance of 30 ml/min or less, after a normal initial dose, one-half of the recommended dose q12h is given for the duration of therapy.

        c. For patients undergoing hemodialysis or peritoneal dialysis, the dose is reduced as in sec. **b,** with no supplemental dose after hemodialysis [63].

    3. Contraindications. As with other fluoroquinolones, enoxacin is not recommended for use in **children** younger than 18 years or in **pregnant** or **nursing** women. See sec. **I.H.**

    4. Drug interactions for fluoroquinolones are discussed in sec. **I.H.** Enoxacin **does** interfere with caffeine and theophylline metabolism. More than any other fluoroquinolone, enoxacin inhibits hepatic metabolism of methylxanthines; it may cause serious theophylline toxicity and possibly caffeine toxicity as well [105] (see sec. **B.4**). Antacids and sucralfate should not be used concomitantly. Ranitidine and dietary supplements containing iron or zinc may interfere with absorption of enoxacin [105].

E. Toxicity and side effects. Prior studies suggest that enoxacin appears to be well tolerated, with most adverse effects mild and similar to those of other fluoroquinolones [1–4, 101, 102] unless patients are receiving theophylline therapy also and the theophylline dose has not been properly reduced and serum levels monitored. A review of 2,407 patients treated with enoxacin in Japan [102] and data in the package insert report the following:

    1. Gastrointestinal symptoms, especially nausea, were the most common side effect (occurring in approximately 3–8% of recipients). Abdominal discomfort, anorexia, diarrhea, and vomiting can also occur.

    2. CNS-related symptoms. Dizziness (1–2%), headache (1%), and nervousness or anxiety (1%) have also been reported. **If theophylline dosages are not reduced and properly monitored** in patients receiving theophylline and enoxacin, nausea, vomiting, headache, tachycardia, and so on may be due to theophylline excess [58]. **Restlessness or insomnia may also be due to caffeine excess if caffeine intake is not reduced** while taking enoxacin. **Seizures** have been described, including patients receiving NSAIDs with enoxacin. (See sec. **I.G.2.**)

    3. Rashes (1%), unusual taste (1%), and pruritus (1%) have also been described.

    4. See general discussion of fluoroquinolone toxicity in sec. **I.G.**

    5. Tendon rupture may occur. See sec. **I.H.9.**

F. Cost. Typical of the fluoroquinolones, enoxacin is an expensive oral agent. The AWP of a single 400-mg dose is $2.60; therefore, for a 14-day, 400-mg bid course, the AWP would be approximately $72.80 [105]. See Table 28A-5 for cost comparison with other quinolones.

G. Resistance will occur if enoxacin is not used properly. See sec. **I.E.**

H. Summary. The precise role of this new oral fluoroquinolone awaits further clinical experience. At this point, we do not see a special niche for enoxacin, as other fluoroquinolones that do not interfere with theophylline or caffeine metabolism are equally effective for UTI and uncomplicated gonorrhea therapy. The *Medical Letter* concluded that enoxacin offers no advantage over ciprofloxacin, ofloxacin, or many other drugs that can be used to treat UTI or gonorrhea [105].

VIII. Investigational agents include [106]:

A. **Levofloxacin,** which is a variation of ofloxacin but has about twice the in vitro activity of ofloxacin.
B. **Sparfloxacin** has increased in vitro activity against gram-positive aerobes, including *S. pneumoniae,* but less activity against *P. aeruginosa* than ciprofloxacin.
C. **Grepafloxacin** has increased in vitro activity against gram-positive aerobes but less activity against gram-negative aerobes.
D. **Clinafloxacin** has increased in vitro activity against gram-positive aerobes and *B. fragilis,* with possible activity against vancomycin-resistant enterococci.
E. **Trovafloxacin** has increased activity against gram-positive aerobes and *B. fragilis.*
F. **DU6859a** is broad spectrum in its in vitro activity, with enhanced activity against gram-positive aerobes, anaerobes, and *P. aeruginosa.*

References

1. Walker, R.C., and Wright, A.J. The fluoroquinolones. *Mayo Clin. Proc.* 66:1249, 1991.
   See related summary by F.A. Kahn, Quinolones and macrolides: Roles in respiratory infection. Hosp. Pract. *28:149, 1993.*
2. Hooper, D.C., and Wolfson, J.S. Fluoroquinolone antimicrobial agents. *N. Engl. J. Med.* 324:384, 1991.
   Emphasizes the need for appropriate use of these agents to prolong their clinical usefulness as much as possible. For a related article emphasizing the appropriate use of quinolones, see the report of the Committee on Antimicrobial Agents: Canadian Infectious Disease Society by T.J. Louie, Can. Med. Assoc. J. *150:669, 1994.*
3. Neu, H.C. Use of the fluoroquinolones: Mini-review. *Infect. Dis. Clin. Pract.* 1:1, 1992.
   See related updates by E.F. Hendershot, Fluoroquinolones. Infect. Dis. Clin. North Am. *9:715, 1995; and B. Suh and B. Lorber, Quinolones.* Med. Clin. North Am. *79:869, 1995.*
4. Neu, H.C. Quinolone antimicrobial agents. *Annu. Rev. Med.* 43:463, 1992.
   Good overview of this topic.
4a. Moellering, R.C., Jr. Quinolone Antimicrobial Agents: Overview and Conclusions. In D.C. Hooper and J.S. Wolfson (eds.), *Quinolone Antimicrobial Agents* (2nd ed.). Washington, DC: American Society for Microbiology, 1993. Chap. 29, pp. 527–537.
   Summary chapter in an excellent text devoted to the quinolones.
5. Andriole, V.T. Quinolones. In G.L. Mandell, R.G. Douglas, Jr., and J.E. Bennett (eds.), *Principles and Practice of Infectious Diseases* (3rd ed.). New York: Churchill Livingstone, 1990. Pp. 334–345.
   For an updated version, see D.C. Hooper, Quinolones. In G.L. Mandell, J.E. Bennett, and R. Dolin (eds.), Principles and Practice of Infectious Diseases *(4th ed.). New York: Churchill Livingstone, 1995, pp. 364–376. Also see related discussions in reference [4a] edited by this same author.*
6. Bellido, F., and Pechère, J.C. Laboratory survey of fluoroquinolone activity. *Rev. Infect. Dis.* 11(Suppl. 5):S917, 1989.
6a. Centers for Disease Control. Decreased susceptibility of *Neisseria gonorrhoeae* to fluoroquinolones—Ohio and Hawaii, 1992–1994. *M.M.W.R.* 43:325, 1994.
   Thus far, the CDC does not recommend changes in the treatment of gonorrhea in the United States based on these reports. However, because infections with N. gonorrhoeae *strains with minimum inhibitory concentrations of 1.0–2.0 μg/ml of ciprofloxacin have been acquired in Southeast Asia and Australia, clinicians treating persons believed to have been infected in these areas should consider using other antimicrobials. This report is reprinted in* J.A.M.A. *271:1733, 1994.*
   See related reports in Antimicrob. Agents Chemother. *38:2196, 2200, 1994.*
6b. Centers for Disease Control. Fluoroquinolone resistance in *Neisseria gonorrhoeae*—Colorado and Washington, 1995. *M.M.W.R.* 44:761, 1995.
7. Cassell, G.H., et al. Comparative susceptibility of *Mycoplasma pneumoniae* to erythromycin, ciprofloxacin, and lomefloxacin. *Rev. Infect. Dis.* 11(Suppl. 5):S992, 1989.
8. Kenny, G.E., and Cartwright, F.D. Susceptibility of *Mycoplasma pneumoniae* to several new quinolones, tetracycline, and erythromycin. *Antimicrob. Agents Chemother.* 35:587, 1991.
   Most active fluoroquinolones were two investigational agents, sparfloxacin and WIN57273.
9. Neu, H.C. Synergy of fluoroquinolones with other antimicrobial agents. *Rev. Infect. Dis.* 11(Suppl. 5):S1025, 1990.
10. Neu, H.C. Synergy and antagonism of antimicrobial combinations with quinolones. *Eur. J. Clin. Microbiol. Infect. Dis.* 10:255, 1991.

11. Weinstein, M.P., et al. Crossover assessment of serum bactericidal activity and pharmacokinetics of ciprofloxacin alone and in combination in healthy elderly volunteers. *Antimicrob. Agents Chemother.* 35:2352, 1991.
12. Lode, H. Pharmacokinetics and clinical results of parenterally administered new quinolones in humans. *Rev. Infect. Dis.* 11(Suppl. 5):S996, 1989.
13. Gerding, D.N., and Hitt, J.A. Tissue penetration of the new quinolones in humans. *Rev. Infect. Dis.* 11(Suppl. 5):S1046, 1989.
    Contains a series of tables showing percentage penetration into various sites.
14. Norrby, S.R., and Ljungberg, B. Pharmacokinetics of fluorinated 4-quinolones in the aged. *Rev. Infect. Dis.* 11(Suppl. 5):S1102, 1989.
15. Wolfson, J.S., and Hooper, D.C. Bacterial resistance to quinolones: Mechanisms and clinical importance. *Rev. Infect. Dis.* 11(Suppl. 5):S960, 1989.
    Emergence of resistance occurs relatively often in infections caused by P. aeruginosa *and* S. aureus *and other bacteria for which the therapeutic ratio of the currently available quinolones is quite low.*
16. Kotilainen, P., et al. Emergence of ciprofloxacin-resistant coagulase-negative staphylococcal skin flora in immunocompromised patients receiving ciprofloxacin. *J. Infect. Dis.* 161:41, 1990.
    Septicemias in neutropenic leukemic patients were associated with cross-resistance.
17. Parry, M.F., et al. Quinolone resistance: Susceptibility data from a 300-bed community hospital. *Am. J. Med.* 87(Suppl. 5A):12, 1989.
18. Blumberg, H.M., et al. Rapid development of ciprofloxacin resistance in methicillin-susceptible and methicillin-resistant *Staphylococcus aureus. J. Infect. Dis.* 163:1279, 1991.
    High-level resistance to ciprofloxacin developed in from 0% to 79% of methicillin-resistant S. aureus *(MRSA) over a 1-year period. In a similar time period, 13.6% of methicillin-susceptible* S. aureus *developed* S. aureus *resistance. Study concluded that ciprofloxacin appears to have limited usefulness in treating staphylococcal infections and colonization, especially those due to MRSA.*
19. Raviglione, M.C., et al. Ciprofloxacin-resistant *Staphylococcus aureus* in an acute-care hospital. *Antimicrob. Agents Chemother.* 34:2050, 1990.
    Study revealed a progressive increase in the rate of resistance to ciprofloxacin during the first year of use, with initial rates being approximately 10% and recent rates being higher than 80%. Methicillin-susceptible strains remained susceptible in this study. Authors concluded that ciprofloxacin has limited usefulness against MRSA.
19a. Mulligan, M.E., et al. Methicillin-resistant *Staphylococcus aureus:* A consensus review of the microbiology, pathogenesis, and epidemiology with implications for prevention and management. *Am. J. Med.* 94:313, 1993.
20. Trucksis, M., Hooper, D.C., and Wolfson, J.S. Emerging resistance to fluoroquinolones in staphylococci: An alert. *Ann. Intern. Med.* 114:424, 1991.
20a. Pena, C., et al. Relationship between quinolone use and emergence of ciprofloxacin-resistant *E. coli* in bloodstream infections. *Antimicrob. Agents Chemother.* 39:520, 1995.
    Report of 27 cases of bacteremia (18 community-acquired) in nonneutropenic adults. Overall rates of E. coli *bacteremia with resistant strains increased from 0% in 1988 to 7.5% in 1992. Prior quinolone use seems to be the most important risk factor.*
20b. Maddix, D.S., and Warner, L. Do we need an intravenous fluoroquinolone? *West. J. Med.* 157:55, 1992.
    Major conclusions in this review include (1) intravenous ciprofloxacin does not represent an important advance in the treatment of infectious diseases; (2) intravenous ciprofloxacin should be reserved for patients unable to take oral fluoroquinolones; and (3) there is little evidence to support the use of fluoroquinolones as first-line agents for the treatment of common nosocomial or community-acquired bacterial infections.
21. Medical Letter. The choice of antibacterial drugs. *Med. Lett. Drugs Ther.* 38:25, 1996.
22. Lee, C., and Ronald, A.R. Norfloxacin: Its potential in clinical practice. *Am. J. Med.* 82(Suppl. 6B):27, 1987.
23. Neu, H.C. Ciprofloxacin: An overview and prospective appraisal. *Am. J. Med.* 82 (Suppl. 4A):395, 1987.
    Good clinical summary of the potential role of ciprofloxacin and other quinolones from a symposium devoted to this agent.
24. Nather, K.G. Use of the quinolones in urinary tract infections and prostatitis. *Rev. Infect. Dis.* 11(Suppl. 5):S1321, 1989.
25. Wolfson, J.S., and Hooper, D.C. Minireview: Treatment of genitourinary tract infections with fluoroquinolones. *Antimicrob. Agents Chemother.* 33:1655, 1662, 1989.

26. Neu, H. Urinary tract infections. *Am. J. Med.* 92(Suppl. 4A):635, 1992.
Good review of this topic.
27. Norby, R. Short-term treatment of uncomplicated lower urinary tract infections in women. *Rev. Infect. Dis.* 12:458, 1990.
28. Saginur, R., et al. Single dose compared with 3-day norfloxacin treatment of uncomplicated urinary tract infection in women. *Arch. Intern. Med.* 152:1233, 1992.
From the Canadian Infectious Diseases Society Clinical Trials Group. Three days is more effective for S. saprophyticus, whereas both regimens were equally effective for E. coli. The dose of norfloxacin used was two 400-mg tablets as a single dose. See related article by L.E. Nicolle et al., comparing 3-day therapy of lomefloxacin with 3-day norfloxacin in Antimicrob. Agents Chemother. *37:574, 1993. Both regimens effective for uncomplicated urinary tract infections.*
29. Centers for Disease Control. 1993 Sexually transmitted diseases treatment guidelines. *M.M.W.R.* 42(RR-14):1, 1993.
See complete discussion of sexually transmitted diseases in Chap. 13.
30. Levine, W.C., et al. 1993 Sexually transmitted treatment guidelines. *Clin. Infect. Dis.* 20(Suppl.):S1, 1995.
This April 1995 supplement contains the ten background papers drafted prior to the recommendations reviewed in reference [29].
31. Hooton, T.M., et al. Ciprofloxacin compared with doxycycline for nongonococcal urethritis: Ineffectiveness against *Chlamydia trachomatis* due to relapsing infection. *J.A.M.A.* 264:1418, 1990.
Ciprofloxacin is inadequate for treatment of chlamydial infections in men, often resulting in relapsing infections.
32. Waldvogel, F.A. Use of the quinolones for the treatment of osteomyelitis and septic arthritis. *Rev. Infect. Dis.* 11(Suppl. 5):S1259, 1989.
33. Dan, M., et al. Oral ciprofloxacin treatment of *P. aeruginosa* osteomyelitis. *Antimicrob. Agents Chemother.* 34:849, 1990.
Surgical debridement is essential before oral therapy. Protracted therapy is used—that is, 2–4 months—but prolonged therapy is feasible because the oral route is employed.
34. Mader, J.T., et al. Oral ciprofloxacin compared with standard parenteral antibiotics therapy for chronic osteomyelitis in adults. *J. Bone Joint Surg.* [Am.] 73:104, 1990.
Oral ciprofloxacin was as effective. Note that in their discussions, the authors advise careful evaluation of susceptibility data before using oral ciprofloxacin for gram-positive infections. For a related article, see L.O. Gentry and C.G. Rodriguez, Antimicrob. Agents Chemother. *34:40, 1990.*
35. Gentry, L.O. Antibiotic therapy for osteomyelitis. *Infect. Dis. Clin. North Am.* 4:485, 1990.
36. Gentry, L.O. Oral antimicrobial therapy for osteomyelitis. *Ann. Intern. Med.* 114:986, 1991.
Editorial comment that concludes: "Given a precise diagnosis and thorough debridement, oral therapies should be as successful as parenteral therapies, except in patients with diabetes mellitus or severe peripheral vascular disease, for whom an initial regimen of parenteral therapy may be necessary." Even this advocate of oral therapy goes on to emphasize that "although oral quinolones are currently effective for many staphylococcal infections, there are concerns that increasing or indiscriminate use of the oral quinolones may serve to diminish their future efficacy in staphylococcal osteomyelitis."
37. Gentry, L.O., and Rodriguez-Gomez, G. Oral ofloxacin versus parenteral therapy for chronic osteomyelitis. *Antimicrob. Agents Chemother.* 35:538, 1991.
38. Thys, J.P., Jacobs, F., and Motte, S. Quinolones in the treatment of lower respiratory tract infections. *Rev. Infect. Dis.* 11(Suppl. 5):S1212, 1989.
39. Grenier, B. Use of the new quinolones in cystic fibrosis. *Rev. Infect. Dis.* 11(Suppl. 5):S1245, 1989.
40. Gisby, J., Wrightman, B.J., and Beale, A.S. Comparative efficacies of ciprofloxacin, amoxicillin, amoxicillin-clavulanic acid, and cefaclor against experimental *Streptococcus pneumoniae* respiratory infections in mice. *Antimicrob. Agents Chemother.* 35:831, 1991.
The efficacy of ciprofloxacin against these experimental respiratory infections was poor, despite good penetration into lung tissue, and is a reflection of the low in vitro activity of this quinolone against S. pneumoniae, *one of the most common pathogens in community-acquired pneumonia.*
41. Azoulay-Dupuis, E., et al. Antipneumococcal activity of ciprofloxacin, ofloxacin, and

temafloxacin in an experimental mouse pneumonia model at various stages of the disease. *J. Infect. Dis.* 163:319, 1991.
Treatment in this model, with ofloxacin and ciprofloxacin, did not significantly improve survival rates compared with those of untreated animals. Temafloxacin was effective, but this fluoroquinolone has been withdrawn (see text).

41a. Bennish, M.L., et al. Treatment of shigellosis: III. Comparison of one- or two-dose ciprofloxacin with standard 5-day therapy. *Ann. Intern. Med.* 117:727, 1992.
A single 1-g dose of ciprofloxacin is effective therapy for patients infected with species of Shigella *other than* S. dysenteriae *type 1, which merits 5-day therapy.*

42. Rodriguez-Noriega, E., et al. Quinolones in the treatment of *Salmonella* carriers. *Rev. Infect. Dis.* 11(Suppl. 5):S1179, 1989.

43. Neill, M.A., et al. Failure of ciprofloxacin to eradicate convalescent fecal excretion after acute salmonellosis: Experience during an outbreak in health care workers. *Ann. Intern. Med.* 114:195, 1991.
In this small randomized, placebo-controlled, double-blind study, four of eight recipients of ciprofloxacin (at 750 mg PO bid for 14 days) had positive stool cultures 14–21 days after completing therapy. This high relapse rate could not be explained by noncompliance, presence of biliary disease, or development of resistance to ciprofloxacin. Therapy may have prolonged fecal excretion of salmonella.

44. Taylor, D.N., et al. Treatment of travelers' diarrhea: Ciprofloxacin plus loperamide compared with ciprofloxacin alone. A placebo-controlled randomized trial. *Ann. Intern. Med.* 114:731, 1991.
Concluded that in a region in Egypt where enterotoxigenic E. coli was the predominant cause of travelers' diarrhea, loperamide combined with ciprofloxacin was not better than treatment with ciprofloxacin alone. Both regimens were safe. Ciprofloxacin, 500 mg bid for 3 days, was used.

45. Petruccelli, B.P., et al. Treatment of travelers' diarrhea with ciprofloxacin and loperamide. *J. Infect. Dis.* 165:557, 1992.
Regimens compared were a single 750-mg dose of ciprofloxacin versus 750 mg of ciprofloxacin plus loperamide versus 500 mg oral ciprofloxacin bid for 3 days plus loperamide. Patients receiving 3 days of ciprofloxacin and loperamide reported a lower cumulative number of liquid bowel movements at 48–72 hours after therapy started. Loperamide use appeared safe.

46. Wistrom, J., et al. Empiric treatment of acute diarrheal disease with norfloxacin: A randomized, placebo-controlled study. *Ann. Intern. Med.* 117:202, 1992.
Norfloxacin, 400 mg PO bid for 5 days, was used versus placebo. Most patients had travelers' diarrhea. Empiric therapy was beneficial to culture-positive and severely ill patients. Data suggested that the limited beneficial effect of empiric norfloxacin may be outweighed by prolongation of the Salmonella *carrier state and by the development of resistance to* Campylobacter *(seen in six of nine recipients of norfloxacin).*

47. Dupont, H.L., et al. Five versus three days of ofloxacin therapy for traveler's diarrhea: A placebo controlled study. *Antimicrob. Agents Chemother.* 36:87, 1992.
Double-blind study of 232 visitors to Guadalajara, Mexico. Ofloxacin, 300 mg PO bid for 3 or 5 days, was used versus placebo. Authors concluded that ofloxacin was effective in shortening the illness and in eradicating the pathogen from patients with diarrhea caused by bacterial enteropathogens (e.g., E. coli, Shigella) and those with fecal leukocytes. Three-day courses were as effective as 5-day courses; therefore, a 3-day course is recommended.

47a. Dupont, H.L. The 10 most common questions about travelers' diarrhea. *Infect. Dis. Clin. Pract.* 1:396, 1992.
Practical summary by national expert. Emphasizes that for areas of the world where trimethoprim-resistant enteric pathogens are uncommon (e.g., noncoastal interior of Mexico during the rainy summer), trimethoprim-sulfamethoxazole is effective. Where trimethoprim resistance is more common (e.g., South America, southern Asia, and northern Africa and during the drier winter months in virtually all areas), the fluoroquinolones are preferred in adults. A 3-day course of therapy is adequate.

48. Goodman, L.J., et al. Empiric antimicrobial therapy of domestically acquired acute diarrhea in urban adults. *Arch. Intern. Med.* 150:541, 1990.

49. The GIMEMA Infection Program. Prevention of bacterial infection in neutropenic patients with hematologic malignancies: A randomized, multicenter trial comparing norfloxacin with ciprofloxacin. *Ann. Intern. Med.* 115:7, 1991.
Study from Italy comparing oral ciprofloxacin, 500 mg bid (300 patients), to oral norfloxacin, 400 mg bid (319 patients), in patients with neutrophil counts of fewer

than 1,000/mm³. Ciprofloxacin appeared to be more effective in preventing fever; norfloxacin recipients received more empiric antibiotics. However, overall mortality was the same in both study groups.

49a. Bow, E.J., and Ronald, A.R. Antibacterial chemotherapy in neutropenic patients: Where do we go from here? [editorial]. *Clin. Infect. Dis.* 17:333, 1993.
Reviews article suggesting empiric therapy with trimethoprim-sulfamethoxazole is not effective in adults undergoing remission-induction therapy for acute leukemia. Authors conclude that well-defined studies with the quinolones still need to be done to define the benefits and limits of chemoprophylaxis in this setting.

49b. Malik, I.A., et al. Feasibility of outpatient management of fever in cancer patients with low-risk neutropenia: Results of a prospective randomized trial. *Am. J. Med.* 98:224, 1995.
This report from Pakistan examined the results of 400 mg of oral ofloxacin bid in 182 low-risk patients. More than 75% of patients had resolution of fever without other antibiotic modification. Patients were split: 50% received outpatient therapy; 50% received inpatient therapy. Mortality was 4% in outpatients and 2% among inpatients.
See editorial comment in the same issue advising a conservative approach to this type of therapy in patients not on quinolone prophylaxis (which may select out resistant pathogens).
See also related article by I.A. Malik et al., Self-administered antibiotic therapy for chemotherapy-induced, low-risk febrile neutropenia in patients with nonhematologic neoplasms. Clin. Infect. Dis. *19:522, 1994.*

50. Scheld, W.M. Quinolone therapy for infections of the central nervous system. *Rev. Infect. Dis.* 11(Suppl. 5):S1194, 1989.

51. Darouiche, R., et al. Levels of rifampin and ciprofloxacin in nasal secretions: Correlations with MIC_{90} and eradication of nasopharyngeal carriage of bacteria. *J. Infect. Dis.* 162:1134, 1990.

52. Kemper, C.A., et al. Treatment of *Mycobacterium avium* complex bacteremia in AIDS with a four-drug oral regimen: Rifampin, ethambutol, clofazimine, and ciprofloxacin. *Ann. Intern. Med.* 116:466, 1992.
A reduction in symptoms and bacteremia can be achieved as early as 2 weeks after therapy is begun. Prolonged therapy is necessary to eradicate systemic infection.

53. Hussey, G., et al. Ciprofloxacin treatment of multiple drug–resistant extrapulmonary tuberculosis in a child. *Pediatr. Infect. Dis. J.* 11:408, 1992.
Brief report.

54. Holley, H.P., Jr. Successful treatment of cat-scratch disease with ciprofloxacin. *J.A.M.A.* 65:1563, 1991.
Five adult patients treated with 500 mg bid are briefly discussed.

55. Sarna, P.S. Norfloxacin: A new drug in the treatment of *Falciparum malaria. Ann. Intern. Med.* 111:336, 1989.
See editorial comment in the same issue.

56. Watt, G., et al. Ciprofloxacin treatment of drug-resistant *Falciparum malaria. J. Infect. Dis.* 164:602, 1991.

57. Davies, B.J., and Maesen, F.P.V. Drug interactions with quinolones. *Rev. Infect. Dis.* 11(Suppl. 5):S1083, 1989.

58. Radandt, J.M., Marchbanks, C.R., and Dudley, M.N. Interactions of fluoroquinolones with other drugs: Mechanisms, variability, clinical significance, and management. *Clin. Infect. Dis.* 14:272, 1992.
See related review by D.E. Nix, Drug-Drug Interactions with Fluoroquinolone Antimicrobial Agents. In D.C. Hooper and J.S. Wolfson (eds.), Quinolone Antimicrobial Agents. Washington, DC: American Society for Microbiology, 1993. Chap. 11.

58a. Schaad, U.B., et al. Use of the fluoroquinolones in pediatrics: Consensus report of an International Society of Chemotherapy commission. *Pediatr. Infect. Dis. J.* 14:1, 1995.
Potential indicators in pediatric patients include respiratory infections in cystic fibrosis patients, very complex urinary tract infections, chronic suppurative otitis media due to Pseudomonas aeruginosa, *and selected GI problems (e.g., resistant invasive* Salmonella *or* Shigella *infection).*

58b. Hoey, L.L., and Lake, K.D. Does ciprofloxacin interact with cyclosporine? *Ann. Pharmacother.* 28:93, 1994.
Cyclosporine and ciprofloxacin may be used together safely at the recommended dosages without increased cyclosporine monitoring.

58c. Szarfman, A., et al. More on the fluoroquinolone antibiotics and tendon rupture. *N. Engl. J. Med.* 332:193, 1995.

Brief review and recommendations from the US Food and Drug Administration. Ruptures occurred 2–42 days after initiation of quinolone therapy.
59. Frieden, T.R., and Mangi, R.J. Inappropriate use of oral ciprofloxacin. *J.A.M.A.* 264:1438, 1990.
Interesting and discouraging statistics. In 1989, more than 5 million prescriptions filled. It often is misused.
59a. Pickering, T.D., et al. The appropriateness of oral fluoroquinolone-prescribing in the long-term care setting. *J. Am. Geriatr. Soc.* 42:28, 1994.
60. Goldstein, E.J.C. Norfloxacin, a fluoroquinolone antimicrobial agent: Classification, mechanism of action, and in vitro activity. *Am. J. Med.* 82(Suppl. 6B):3, 1987.
61. Medical Letter. Norfloxacin (Noroxin). *Med. Lett. Drugs Ther.* 29:25, 1987.
62. Nicolle, L.E., et al. Prospective, randomized, placebo-controlled trial of norfloxacin for the prophylaxis of recurrent urinary tract infections in women. *Antimicrob. Agents Chemother.* 33:1032, 1989.
A dose of 200 mg at bedtime was effective and well tolerated for the 12 months of this study. See a related article by W. Brumfitt et al., Norfloxacin vs. macrodantin for the prophylaxis of recurrent urinary tract infection in women. Rev. Infect. Dis. 11(Suppl. 5):S1338, 1989.
63. Bennett, W.M., et al. *Drug Prescribing in Renal Failure: Dosing Guidelines for Adults* (3rd ed.). Philadelphia: American College of Physicians, 1994.
This is a useful handbook. Similar tables for dosing in renal failure appear in L.L. Livornese, Jr., et al. Antibacterial agents in renal failure. Infect. Dis. Clin. North Am. 5:591, 1995; and S.K. Swan and W.M. Bennett, Drug dosing guidelines in patients with renal failure. West. J. Med. 156:633, 1992.
64. Corrado, M.L., et al. Norfloxacin: Review of safety studies. *Am. J. Med.* 82(Suppl. 6B):22, 1987.
65. Medical Letter. Ciprofloxacin. *Med. Lett. Drugs Ther.* 30:11, 1988.
Also see H. Thadepalli et al., Ciprofloxacin: In vitro, experimental, and clinical evaluation. Rev. Infect. Dis. 10:505, 1988, and related articles in same issue.
66. Barry, A.L., and Jones, R.N. In vitro activity of ciprofloxacin against gram-positive cocci. *Am. J. Med.* 82(Suppl. 4A):27, 1987.
67. Sanders, C.C., et al. Overview of preclinical studies with ciprofloxacin. *Am. J. Med.* 82(Suppl. 4A):2, 1987.
68. Spivey, J.M. Postantibiotic effect. *Clin. Pharm.* 11:865, 1992.
Concludes noting that although data are limited, animal and human studies provide support for the clinical importance of this effect. Further research is necessary.
69. Medical Letter. Intravenous ciprofloxacin. *Med. Lett. Drugs Ther.* 33:75, 1991.
70. Rodvold, K.A. Pharmacokinetics of IV ciprofloxacin. *Infect. Med.* 8(Suppl. C):12, 1991.
71. Beam, T.R., Jr. The sequential advantage. *Infect. Med.* 8(Suppl. C):9, 1991.
Discusses how ciprofloxacin is the first fluoroquinolone that can be switched from intravenous to oral therapy.
72. Raoof, S., et al. Ciprofloxacin increases serum levels of theophylline. *Am. J. Med.* 82(Suppl. 4A):115, 1987.
73. Lang, R., et al. Successful treatment of malignant external otitis with oral ciprofloxacin: Report of experience with 23 patients. *J. Infect. Dis.* 161:537, 1990.
See related article by H. Giamarellou, Malignant external otitis and the newer quinolones. Rev. Infect. Dis. 11(Suppl. 5):S1109, 1989.
74. Peterson, L., et al. Therapy of lower extremity infections with ciprofloxacin in patients with diabetes mellitus, peripheral vascular disease, or both. *Am. J. Med.* 86:801, 1989.
75. Meunier, F., et al. Prospective randomized evaluation of ciprofloxacin versus piperacillin plus amikacin for empiric antibiotic therapy of febrile granulocytopenic cancer patients with lymphomas and solid tumors. *Antimicrob. Agents Chemother.* 35:873, 1991.
This study does not support the use of intravenous ciprofloxacin, which had inconsistent activity against gram-positive organisms. Study from the European Organization for Research on Treatment of Cancer International Antimicrobial Therapy Cooperative Group.
76. Medical Letter. Ophthalmic ciprofloxacin. *Med. Lett. Drugs Ther.* 33:51, 1991.
77. Kahn, F.A. Sequential intravenous-oral administration of ciprofloxacin vs. ceftazidime in serious bacterial respiratory tract infection. *Chest* 96:528, 1989.
78. Paladino, J.A., et al. Clinical and economic evaluation of oral ciprofloxacin after an abbreviated course of intravenous antibiotics. *Am. J. Med.* 91:462, 1991.

After 3 days of conventional intravenous antibiotics, patients were placed on oral ciprofloxacin, 750 mg PO bid.

For a related review on intravenous ofloxacin and its potential use intravenously and then orally, see L.O. Gentry, Intravenous ofloxacin: Clinical overview and literature evaluation. Infect. Dis. Clin. Pract. *1:363, 1992.*

79. Nightingale, C.H., et al. Determining the formulary status of quinolone antibiotics: One institution's approach. *Hosp. Formul.* 27:509, 1992.

Effective pharmacy bidding to control costs is important, but we would hope that the hospital prescriber will be educated about appropriate antibiotic use by the pharmacy and physician staff and not primarily by pharmaceutical company representatives!

80. Feigin, R.D., et al. Clindamycin therapy of osteomyelitis and septic arthritis in children. *Pediatrics* 55:213, 1975.

Patients received intravenous clindamycin until they were afebrile for 3 days, then oral therapy for weeks.

81. Chapman, S.W. Osteomyelitis. In R.E. Reese and R.G. Douglas, Jr. (eds.), *A Practical Approach to Infectious Diseases.* Boston: Little, Brown, 1983. P. 621.

82. Tuoman, E.I., et al. Oral chloramphenicol in the treatment of *Haemophilus influenzae* meningitis. *J. Pediatr.* 99:968, 1981.

82a. Jolson, H.M., et al. Adverse reaction reporting of interaction between warfarin and fluoroquinolones. *Arch. Intern. Med.* 151:1003, 1991.

82b. Isreal, D.S., et al. Effect of ciprofloxacin on the pharmacokinetics and pharmacodynamics of warfarin. *Clin. Infect. Dis.* 22:251, 1996.

Adult patients received 750 mg PO bid for 2 weeks. Authors conclude that warfarin therapy is not a contraindication to the use of ciprofloxacin.

83. Moellering, R.C., Jr., and Neu, H.C. Ofloxacin: A pharmacodynamic advance in quinolone antimicrobial therapy. *Am. J. Med.* 87(Suppl. 6C):1S–81S, 1989.

84. Medical Letter. Ofloxacin. *Med. Lett. Drugs Ther.* 33:71, 1991.

For a more detailed review of intravenous ofloxacin, see L.O. Gentry, Intravenous ofloxacin: Clinical overview and literature evaluation. Infect. Dis. Clin. Pract. *1: 363, 1992.*

85. Sanders, C.C. Review of preclinical studies with ofloxacin. *Clin. Infect. Dis.* 14:526, 1992.

86. Sanders, W.E., Jr. Oral ofloxacin: A critical review of the new drug application. *Clin. Infect. Dis.* 14:539, 1992.

87. Fuchs, P.C. In vitro antimicrobial activity and susceptibility testing of ofloxacin: Current status. *Am. J. Med.* 87(Suppl. 6C):10S, 1989.

88. Guay, D.R.P., et al. Safety and pharmacokinetics of multiple doses of intravenous ofloxacin in healthy volunteers. *Antimicrob. Agents Chemother.* 36:308, 1992.

89. Flor, S. Pharmacokinetics of ofloxacin: An overview. *Am. J. Med.* 67(Suppl. 6C): 24S, 1989.

90. Sanders, W.E., Jr., et al. Oral ofloxacin for the treatment of acute bacterial pneumonia: Use of a nontraditional protocol to compare experimental therapy with "usual care" in a multicenter clinical trial. *Am. J. Med.* 91:261, 1991.

In this study, 69 patients were treated with ofloxacin, 400 mg PO q12h, versus 64 patients treated at least initially with "usual" parenteral antibiotics. There were 22 patients with presumed S. pneumoniae *pneumonia in the ofloxacin group. Both groups did well with therapy. Very sick patients were excluded from the study, and ofloxacin-treated patients were clinically followed very carefully.*

Also see B. Lipsky et al., Ofloxacin treatment of Chlamydia pneumonia *(strain TWAR) lower respiratory tract infections.* Am. J. Med. *89:722, 1990, in which ofloxacin was effective in four patients.*

90a. *Physicians' Desk Reference* (50th ed.). Montvale, N.J.: Medical Economics, 1996.

91. Kroll, R.L. Drug recall information letter. Abbott Laboratories, Abbott Park, IL, June 6, 1992.

92. Neu, H.C. Lomefloxacin: Development of a once-a-day quinolone. *Am. J. Med.* 92 (Suppl. 4A):136S, 1992.

Summary of a special supplement devoted to the in vitro activity, pharmacokinetics, clinical efficacy, and safety profile of this new fluoroquinolone.

93. Medical Letter. Two new fluoroquinolones. *Med. Lett. Drugs Ther.* 34:58, 1992.

94. Jones, R. Fluoroquinolone (Lomefloxacin) international surveillance trial: A report of 30 months of monitoring in vitro activity. *Am. J. Med.* 92(Suppl. 4A):52S, 1992.

More than 500,000 facultative organisms tested by standardized disc diffusion methods in 36 countries.

95. Mant, T.G.K. Multiple-dose pharmacokinetics of lomefloxacin: Rationale for once-a-day dosing. *Am. J. Med.* 92(Suppl. 4A):26S, 1992.
96. Mayer, K.H., and Ellal, J.A. Lomefloxacin: Microbiologic assessment and unique properties. *Am. J. Med.* 92(Suppl. 4A):58S, 1992.
    Has good minimum inhibitory concentration data in summary tables.
97. Medical Letter. Antimicrobial prophylaxis in surgery. *Med. Lett. Drugs Ther.* 37:79, 1995.
98. Klimberg, I.W., et al. A multicenter comparison of oral lomefloxacin versus parenteral cefotaxime as prophylactic agents in transurethral surgery. *Am. J. Med.* 92(Suppl. 4A):121S, 1992.
    Patients were required to have negative pretreatment urine cultures. Lomefloxacin (400 mg PO once 2–6 hours prior to surgery) or cefotaxime (1 g IV or IM 30–90 minutes before surgery) was given. Lomefloxacin was successful in preventing postoperative infections in 204 of 207 evaluable patients (98%). Cefotaxime was successful in 196 of 206 (95.1%) evaluable patients.
    See the two companion-related articles preceding this article in this symposium devoted to lomefloxacin.
99. Rizk, E. The U.S. clinical experience with lomefloxacin, a new once-daily fluoroquinolone. *Am. J. Med.* 92(Suppl. 4A):130S, 1992.
    Overview of all clinical studies of lomefloxacin conducted in the United States prior to this publication. Data based on 2,869 patients who received lomefloxacin.
99a. Medical information letter: Important drug safety information for maxaquin. G.D. Searle and Co., Skokie, IL, July 19, 1993.
100. Neu, H.C. Pharmacokinetics, microbiology, cost: Interrelated problems for the 1990's that impact on the use of fluoroquinolone antimicrobial agents. *Am. J. Med.* 92(Suppl. 4A):2S, 1992.
    Lead article in this recent symposium on lomefloxacin.
101. Zinner, S.H. Clinical overview of enoxacin. *Clin. Pharmacokinet.* 16(Suppl. 1):59, 1989.
102. Henwood, J.M., and Monk, J.P. Enoxacin: A review of its antibacterial activity, pharmacokinetic properties, and therapeutic use. *Drugs* 36:32, 1988.
    For a similar review, see D. Speller and R. Wise, Enoxacin a laboratory and clinical assessment. J. Antimicrob. Chemother. 21(Suppl. B):1, 1986.
103. Toothaker, R.D. Enoxacin absorption and elimination characteristics. *Clin. Pharmacokinet.* 16(Suppl. 1):52, 1988.
104. Childs, S.J. Tissue penetration and clinical efficacy of enoxacin in urinary tract infections. *Clin. Pharmacokinet.* 16(Suppl. 1):32, 1989.
105. Medical Letter. Enoxacin—a new fluoroquinolone. *Med. Lett. Drugs Ther.* 34:103, 1992.
    Concludes that enoxacin offers no advantage over ciprofloxacin, ofloxacin, or many other drugs that can be used to treat urinary tract infection or gonorrhea.
106. Hooper, D.C. Symposium on Future Antibiotics: Quinolones. Infectious Disease Society of America Annual Meeting. San Francisco: September 17, 1995.

T. Urinary Antiseptics

Urinary antiseptics are agents that concentrate in the urine but do not produce adequate levels in the serum. Therefore, these agents are **useful** primarily in the prevention or therapy of lower **urinary tract infections** (UTIs) and not for severe pyelonephritis or associated systemic infection (i.e., urosepsis).

I. **Nitrofurantoin** presumably inhibits various enzymes within bacteria, although the precise mechanism of action is poorly understood [1].

   A. **Spectrum of activity.** Nitrofurantoin is active against most *Escherichia coli* and a minority of *Enterobacter* and *Klebsiella* spp. *Pseudomonas* spp. are resistant, as are most *Proteus* spp. Nitrofurantoin also is active against gram-positive bacteria that sometimes produce UTIs, such as enterococcus, *Staphylococcus aureus*, *S. epidermidis*, and *S. saprophyticus* [2].

   B. **Pharmacokinetics.** Nitrofurantoin is well absorbed from the GI tract, but inadequate therapeutic levels are achieved in the serum and body tissues. Nitrofurantoin penetrates the interstitial tissue of the renal medulla [2]. For susceptible pathogens, adequate urinary concentrations are achieved. **The drug is contraindicated in renal failure** (i.e., creatinine clearance <40 ml/min) because adequate urinary antibiotic levels may not be achieved in that condition. In addition, serum

levels increase in renal failure, presumably increasing the toxicity of this agent.
   In an alkaline urine, the antibacterial effect of nitrofurantoin is decreased; therefore, the urine should not be alkalinized [1].
C. **Preparations available**
   1. **Furadantin** is the microcrystalline form and has been available since 1953.
   2. **Macrodantin** is the macrocrystalline form, and it appears to be associated with a **lower incidence of GI side effects** and better patient tolerance than the microcrystalline form [1, 3]. Macrodantin has activity and pharmacokinetics similar to furadantin.
   3. An intravenous preparation of nitrofurantoin [4] is no longer available.
D. **Uses.** Nitrofurantoin is used in the treatment or prophylaxis of UTIs [1, 5].
   1. **Therapy for UTIs due to susceptible pathogens.** The macrocrystalline form is available in 25-, 50-, and 100-mg capsules. The usual adult dose is 50–100 mg qid. In elderly patients, lower dose ranges are advisable [4] (see sec. **E.2.b**). In children, 5–7 mg/kg/day is given in divided doses qid. Nitrofurantoin is used in the treatment of **lower** UTIs. In a recent review, the authors emphasize that patients with acute pyelonephritis respond inconsistently to nitrofurantoin. Thus, nitrofurantoin should not be used for treatment of pyelonephritis [1]. We would avoid it in a moderately to severely ill patient with pyelonephritis. **In lower UTI with susceptible enterococci, nitrofurantoin may provide an alternative agent for the ampicillin-allergic pateint** [5]. Nitrofurantoin should not be used in neonates.
   2. **Prophylaxis of UTIs.** Macrodantin has been given at bedtime as a single 50- or 100-mg dose to women with recurrent, uncomplicated UTI.
   3. **In renal failure, the drug is contraindicated,** as discussed in sec. **B.**
   4. **In hepatic failure,** the drug probably should be avoided because of its association with hepatotoxicity.
   5. **In pregnancy,** caution should be used; this is a category B agent (see Chap. 28A). Nitrofurantoin may be used to treat UTIs in pregnancy when clearly indicated, but it should not be used at term [1].
E. **Toxicity.** Nitrofurantoin is associated with a long list of adverse reactions, and **adverse reactions are very common,** varying from mild, reversible effects to severe reactions to nitrofurantoin, other than mild GI symptoms, were severe enough to necessitate hospitalization, and 1% of reactions were fatal [7].
   1. **Gastrointestinal irritation** is the most common side effect, with anorexia, nausea, and vomiting. This may be decreased by using the macrocrystalline preparation (Macrodantin) and may be dose-related [2].
   2. **Pulmonary reactions are the most common severe problem associated with nitrofurantoin use** [1, 7].
      a. **Acute pneumonitis** with fever, cough, and eosinophilia can occur after a few hours or days of therapy. On chest roentgenography, pulmonary infiltrates or pleural fluid is seen. This pneumonitis probably is hypersensitivity phenomenon and is rapidly reversible by discontinuing treatment. Acute reactions do not generally progress to chronic reactions [1].
      b. **Chronic pulmonary reactions** with interstitial pneumonitis may be more common in older patients on prolonged, and even low-dose, treatment. This may be related to a toxic reaction (i.e., nitrofurantoin generates toxic oxygen radicals that produce this lung injury) [2]. This syndrome has an insidious onset (malaise, cough, and dyspnea on exertion), and fever and eosinophilia are seen less frequently. In some cases, improvement occurs with discontinuing the nitrofurantoin. A beneficial effect of corticosteroid therapy has not been convincingly demonstrated in patients with chronic nitrofurantoin pulmonary reactions [1]. Permanent pulmonary fibrosis can occur. **In very elderly patients (>80 years of age) in whom renal function is declining as a part of the aging process, the dose should be limited to no more than 100 mg/day in conventional courses (e.g., 7–14 days) even when the serum creatinine is normal** (see sec. **B.**). We avoid prolonged use of this agent in the elderly.
      c. **Frequency of pulmonary reactions.** One report suggests that nitrofurantoin may cause acute severe pulmonary illness approximately once in every 5,000 first administrations and that chronic fibrosis serious enough to warrant hospitalization may occur in about 1 in 750 long-term users [8].

3. **Polyneuropathies** with demyelination and degeneration of sensory and motor nerves is a severe side effect that may occur more often in patients with renal failure as well as in protracted courses of therapy [1]. The mechanisms are unclear, but it is believed to be related to a direct toxic effect of the drug. **The drug should be stopped if early signs of a neuritis,** such as paresthesias, develop.

4. **Bone marrow** depression may occur. In patients with glucose-6-phosphate dehydrogenase deficiency, acute hemolysis may be precipitated by nitrofurantoin use. However, based on one report, clinically important hemolytic reactions appear to be rare [9]. Megaloblastic anemias, leukopenia, and thrombocytopenia can occur [2].

5. **Hepatotoxic reactions,** including cholestatic jaundice and hepatocellular damage, have been described. Nitrofurantoin has been associated with the development of **chronic active hepatitis** [10], although this is a rare reaction that is presumably immunologically based. Usually these patients have been on chronic therapy. Because of this association, some authors [10] have recommended monthly liver function tests in patients on chronic therapy. Deaths have been reported in patients who have continued to take nitrofurantoin after the onset of hepatitis. Discontinuation of nitrofurantoin often results in clinical and laboratory improvement [2, 11].

6. **Dermatologic** problems, including urticaria, maculopapular rashes, and angioneurotic edema, can occur; discontinue if these reactions are seen.

7. **In children.** There has been some concern that the side effects of nitrofurantoin in children may outweigh the benefits. This issue has been reviewed with the conclusion that serious adverse reactions to nitrofurantoin in children are rare and that the vast majority of patients recovered from their reactions once the drug was discontinued. Therefore, this agent remains **potentially useful** in pediatric patients [12].

II. **Methenamine** [1] is not an active antibacterial agent.

A. **Mechanism of action.** Under the proper pH conditions, methenamine can be hydrolyzed to form formaldehyde and ammonia. **Formaldehyde is the active agent,** and its formation depends on many factors.

1. **Acid environment.** For hydrolysis to occur, an acid pH is required. Ideally, the urine pH must be **6.0 or less [1]** so that hydrolysis can take place. (This is a very important clinical point. To be effective, the drug must be given to a patient with an acidic urine.) In addition, because the serum is not acidic, hydrolysis does not occur in the serum and formaldehyde is not generated there. In many patients, in the absence of diuresis, a sufficiently acid urine to liberate free formaldehyde exists.

2. **Time needed for hydrolysis.** In addition to the acid pH, adequate time must be allowed for hydrolysis to occur. Ideally, 2–3 hours are necessary to generate adequate concentrations of formaldehyde. Therefore, **in a patient with a chronic indwelling bladder catheter, it is not surprising that this is a useless agent,** as adequate contact time cannot be achieved in the catheterized patient [13]. However, this agent may be helpful in patients with partial outlet obstruction (e.g., prostatic hypertrophy), in which adequate contact time is available. Although methenamine will not work in the patient with a chronic indwelling Foley catheter, it may have a beneficial effect in preventing UTI in patients with neurogenic bladders who are in a program of intermittent catheterization and bladder retraining, because the urine may remain in the bladder long enough between catheterizations [14].

3. **Adequate concentrations.** To form adequate levels of formaldehyde (even if the aforementioned two conditions are met), adequate doses of methenamine must be used.

B. **Spectrum of activity.** An appealing property of methenamine is that if enough formaldehyde is generated, all gram-positive and gram-negative bacteria are susceptible. In addition, bacteria do not become resistant to formaldehyde.

C. **Pharmacokinetics.** Methenamine is well absorbed from the GI tract and is excreted into the urine. Even in the presence of the proper urine pH, only 2–20% of the drug is broken down into the active free formaldehyde. Because ammonia is generated with methenamine degradation, **the agent is contraindicated in hepatic insufficiency** [1].

D. **Preparations available.** Methenamine has been combined with acids, theoretically to help acidify the urine. For example, methenamine with mandelic acid is methenamine mandelate (Mandelamine), and methenamine is combined with hippuric acid as methenamine hippurate (Hiprex or Urex). However, when given in the usual recommended doses, the organic acids in these combinations generally are inadequate to acidify the urine [1]. Methenamine alone has been given with large doses of ascorbic acid (2–6 g daily) in an attempt to acidify the urine.

E. **Uses.** Methenamine with ascorbic acid has been used primarily in chronic suppressive therapy for UTIs in patients without an indwelling catheter. Methenamine hippurate has also been used [15]. The urine must have a pH of 5.5 or less for formaldehyde to be generated. In UTI due to *Proteus* spp. it may be impossible to achieve adequate pH levels because of the high urinary pH generated by *Proteus*. It is important to sterilize the urine initially with another agent before using chronic methenamine and ascorbic acid suppression therapy [16]. This regimen may be particularly useful in the patient with a partial obstruction that allows adequate contact time.

F. **Dosage**

1. In **adults,** 1 g of methenamine mandelate (Mandelamine) or methenamine hippurate (Hiprex or Urex) is given PO bid to qid. Ascorbic acid (e.g., 1 g PO qid) often is given in an attempt to acidify the urine adequately and keep the pH less than or equal to 6.0. The urinary pH should routinely be monitored (e.g., daily or every other day). Higher doses of ascorbic acid may be necessary to acidify the urine and, in some patients, adequate urinary acidification cannot be achieved with 4–6 g daily of ascorbic acid. For children between 6–12 years old, the dose is 500 mg to 1 g bid. An oral suspension (methenamine mandelate, 500 mg per 5 ml) is available for younger children; for children younger than 6 years old, the usual dose is 250 mg per 30 pounds of body weight PO qid [1].

2. In **renal failure,** limited guidelines are available. Methenamine mandelate is not advised if the creatinine clearance is less than 50 ml/min [17].

3. In **patients with gout or hyperuricemia, these agents should be avoided.** Acidification of the urine and the use of acid salts may promote uric acid crystals and calculi formation.

4. **Methenamine should not be administered in conjunction with sulfonamides,** which may precipitate when formaldehyde is released [2] (see Chap. 28K, sec. I.F.4).

5. In **hepatic insufficiency, methenamine should be avoided** because of the ammonia produced [1].

G. **Toxicity.** Methenamine generally is well tolerated. Minor GI side effects, such as gastric discomfort, nausea, and vomiting, can occur, especially at high doses. With prolonged high doses, some patients note urinary frequency, dysuria, and hematuria, which may be caused by formaldehyde irritating the mucosal lining of the genitourinary tract. The dysuria often diminishes with continued use as the mucosa becomes less sensitive.

H. **Summary.** Methenamine is not useful for acute UTIs. It is a **potential agent for chronic suppressive therapy** [15, 16]. For the drug to be effective, the urinary pH must be acidic (i.e., 5.5 or less) and there must be adequate time to form the active degradation product, formaldehyde. Consequently, this agent is **not effective in chronically catheterized patients.** In general, before initiating chronic suppressive therapy, we use another agent to decrease colony counts of the pathogenic bacteria. This is especially important in *Proteus* spp. infections because these urea-splitting organisms increase the pH of urine.

References

1. Hooper, D.C. Urinary Tract Agents: Nitrofurantoin and Methenamine. In G.L. Mandell, J.E. Bennett, and R. Dolin (eds.), *Principles and Practice of Infectious Diseases* (4th ed.). New York: Churchill Livingstone, 1995. Pp. 376–381.
2. Meyers, B.R., and Gurtman, A.C. Miscellaneous Drugs. In S.H. Gorbach, J.G. Bartlett, and N.R. Blacklow (eds.), *Infectious Diseases.* Philadelphia: Saunders, 1992. Pp. 271–280.
3. Kalowski, S., Radford, N., and Kincaid-Smith, P. Crystalline and macrocrystalline nitrofurantoin in the treatment of urinary tract infection. *N. Engl. J. Med.* 290: 385, 1974.
4. Medical Letter. Nitrofurantoin. *Med. Lett. Drugs Ther.* 22:36, 1980.

5. Medical Letter. The choice of antibacterial drugs. *Med. Lett. Drugs Ther.* 38:25, 1996.
   For uncomplicated urinary tract infection due to susceptible enterococci, nitrofurantoin is listed as the first alternative agent when ampicillin or amoxicillin cannot be used.
6. Medical Letter. Nitrofurantoin in pregnancy. *Med. Lett. Drugs Ther.* 28:32, 1986.
7. Holmberg, L., et al. Adverse reactions to nitrofurantoin. An analysis of 921 reports. *Am. J. Med.* 69:733, 1980.
8. Jick, S.S., et al. Hospitalizations for pulmonary reactions following nitrofurantoin use. *Chest* 96:512, 1989.
   Study from the Boston Collaborative Drug Surveillance Program and the Group Health Cooperative of Puget Sound. More than 16,000 first courses of therapy and 742 chronic users (i.e., recipients of 10 or more prescriptions). The frequency of less severe pulmonary reactions, not requiring hospitalizations, is not known and awaits further study.
9. Gait, J.E. Hemolytic reactions to nitrofurantoin in patients with glucose-6-phosphate dehydrogenase deficiency: Theory and practice. *D.I.C.P.* 24:1210, 1990.
   Since 1953, approximately 130 million courses of nitrofurantoin have been distributed in the United States alone. Retrospective analysis of Norwich Eaton adverse reaction data base contains 127 reports of hemolytic reactions; a "worst case" estimate of the incidence rate was 1 in 100,000 courses of therapy. For cases in which outcome was reported, complete recovery occurred in 87% of patients.
10. Sharp, J.R., et al. Chronic active hepatitis and severe hepatic necrosis associated with nitrofurantoin. *Ann. Intern. Med.* 92:14, 1980.
    All patients were women. Liver damage can be severe and even fatal if not recognized. See editorial comment in same journal issue. Also see recent related paper by M.F. Hebert and J.P. Roberts, Endstage liver disease associated with nitrofurantoin requiring liver transplantation. Ann. Pharmacother. *27:1193, 1993.*
11. Reinhart, H.H., et al. Combined nitrofurantoin toxicity to liver and lung. *Gastroenterology* 102:1396, 1992.
    Patient described with pulmonary fibrosis and chronic active hepatitis. Both resolve after nitrofurantoin is discontinued.
12. Coraggio, M.J., Gross, T.P., and Roscelli, J.D. Nitrofurantoin toxicity in children. *Pediatr. Infect. Dis. J.* 8:163, 1989.
13. Vainrub, B., and Musher, D.M. Lack of effect of methenamine in suppression of or prophylaxis against chronic urinary tract infection. *Antimicrob. Agents Chemother.* 12:625, 1977.
14. Kevorkian, C.G., Merritt, J.L., and Ilstrup, D.M. Methenamine mandelate with acidification: An effective urinary antiseptic in patients with neurogenic bladders. *Mayo Clin. Proc.* 59:523, 1984.
    See accompanying editorial comment in the same issue.
15. Cronberg, S., et al. Prevention of recurrent acute cystitis by methenamine hippurate: Double-blind cross-over long-term study. *Br. Med. J.* 294:1507, 1987.
16. Freeman, R.B., et al. Long-term therapy for chronic bacteriuria in men: U.S. Public Health Service cooperative study. *Ann. Intern. Med.* 83:133, 1975.
17. Bennett, W.M., et al. Drug Prescribing in Renal Failure (3rd ed.). Philadelphia: American College of Physicians, 1994.

U. Miscellaneous Agents

Pyrimethamine

I. **Introduction. Pyrimethamine (Daraprim), along with a sulfonamide, is the treatment of choice for *Toxoplasma gondii* infections [1–3].** Unfortunately, the pyrimethamine and sulfonamide combination is plagued with toxicity rates that may preclude its use in up to 40% of patients. Pyrimethamine plus clindamycin is considered an acceptable alternative combination [4, 5].

Because of the AIDS epidemic, approximately 10% of patients infected with the human immunodeficiency virus (HIV) in the United States and up to 25% of AIDS patients in some European countries (in which undercooked meat commonly is consumed) may develop toxoplasmic encephalitis [1, 2]. Pyrimethamine has been used more extensively in the last decade and therefore is summarized here with special emphasis on the treatment of toxoplasmic encephalitis.

Pyrimethamine is also in Fansidar (see Chap. 21).

II. **In vitro activity.** Pyrimethamine is active against susceptible *Plasmodium* spp. and *T. gondii*. It is also active against *Pneumocystis carinii* when used in combination with a sulfonamide (e.g., sulfadiazine).

III. **Mechanism of action.** Pyrimethamine is a folic acid antagonist and has a mechanism of action similar to that of trimethoprim [6]. (See Fig. 28K-1 and Chap. 28K.) Pyrimethamine inhibits the formation of tetrahydrofolic acid in *T. gondii* by interfering with dihydrofolate reductase. **When combined with a sulfonamide, the combination sequentially blocks folic acid metabolism** of the proliferative form **of *T. gondii* and is synergistic against this organism** in vitro and in vivo. The tissue cyst form of toxoplasma is resistant to presently available agents, including pyrimethamine and sulfonamides [1].

IV. **Pharmacokinetics.** The pharmacokinetics of pyrimethamine are poorly understood [2]. Pyrimethamine is available only in 25-mg tablets; there is no parenteral form [1].

   A. **Absorption.** Pyrimethamine usually is well absorbed, though slowly, from the GI tract, with peak serum concentrations achieved within 2 hours of administration [6, 7].

   B. **Distribution and metabolism.** Pyrimethamine is distributed mainly to the kidneys, lungs, liver, and spleen [6]. It is highly protein-bound (87%) and lipophilic and has a half-life of 2–5 days. It appears to be cleared by hepatic metabolism [8], and doses are not modified in renal failure [9].

   Because of its use in toxoplasmic encephalitis, Weiss and colleagues [8] studied serum and **cerebrospinal fluid (CSF) levels** of pyrimethamine and showed that achievable serum levels varied widely after standard dosages and were not predictable. The CSF concentrations were approximately 12–25% of simultaneous plasma levels [8].

   C. Pyrimethamine is **excreted in** the **milk** of nursing mothers [6, 7].

V. **Clinical uses**

   A. **Malaria prophylaxis.** Pyrimethamine (combined with sulfadoxine [Fansidar]) use in this setting is described elsewhere [10]. (Also see Chap. 21.)

   B. **Toxoplasmic encephalitis and *T. gondii* therapy in HIV-related infections.** The regimen of choice is the combination of pyrimethamine and a sulfonamide (e.g., sulfadiazine) [1, 3]. These agents are active against trophozoites (the proliferative form of *T. gondii*) and are synergistic in combination. Because the tissue cyst form of *T. gondii* is resistant to these and other presently available agents [1, 2], suppressive therapy becomes necessary in HIV-infected patients.

      1. **Primary therapy** (aimed at proliferative forms of *T. gondii*) **for** the initial **3–6 weeks** of therapy (adult regimens shown)

         a. **Pyrimethamine**

            (1) **A loading dose** for an adult is 200 mg/day given in two divided doses on day 1. Then 75–100 mg/day (or 50–75 mg/day) is given usually for 3–6 weeks. In children, 2 mg/kg/day for 3 days and then 1 mg/kg/day (maximum of 25 mg/day) for 4 weeks has been suggested [3]. (A different dosage regimen is advised for congenital toxoplasmosis; see reference 3.)

            (2) **Folinic acid** (leucovorin) is given orally each day in a starting dose of 10 mg/day. This can be increased incrementally to 50 mg/day if hematologic toxicity develops [2]. Folinic acid may help decrease the bone marrow toxicity of pyrimethamine. (See sec. **VI.A.1.**) The parenteral form of folinic acid is well absorbed orally when given with orange juice at the same time as the pyrimethamine [1]. Folinic acid does not inhibit the action of pyrimethamine on *T. gondii* trophozoites. Folinic acid can be given intravenously.

         b. **Plus a sulfonamide.** For example, sulfadiazine with an adult loading dose of 75 mg/kg up to 4 g is given; thereafter, 100 mg/kg/day rounded off to the nearest gram up to 8 g/day is given in two or four divided oral doses. Adequate hydration of oral fluid intake should be encouraged to avoid renal crystalluria, with possible renal failure, when sulfonamides are used. (See Chap. 28K.) The pediatric dose of sulfadiazine is 100–200 mg/kg/day for 3–4 weeks [3].

         c. **Plus clindamycin. If a patient cannot take sulfonamides,** clindamycin is an effective alternative agent [3–5]. Clindamycin is combined with pyrimethamine. (See Chap. 28I and references [3] and [5].)

         d. Pyrimethamine alone is not advised [1]. Trimethoprim-sulfamethoxazole (TMP-SMX) alone is not recommended [1, 2].

2. **Maintenance or chronic suppressive therapy** (adult regimens shown) of toxo-plasmic encephalitis is important in HIV-infected patients to prevent relapses that have been described when chemotherapy is stopped [1]. **Suppressive therapy is lifelong** in HIV-infected patients.
   a. **Pyrimethamine** is given at 25–50 mg daily.
   b. **Sulfadiazine** is given 500 mg PO q6h in AIDS patients [1]. Again, clinda-mycin may be an alternative in the sulfa-allergic patient. (See Chap. 28I.)
3. For therapy for *T. gondii* in the non-HIV-infected patient, dosages of pyrimeth-amine and sulfonamides are reviewed elsewhere [1].
4. **Pyrimethamine doses in renal failure.** Data suggest standard dosage regimens can be used [9]. Supplemental doses are not necessary in patients undergoing peritoneal dialysis or hemodialysis [9].
5. **Serum levels of pyrimethamine** achieved after oral therapy are variable and, if malabsorption is a concern or if the patient is responding poorly, monitoring serum levels may be reasonable [8].
C. **Alternative regimen for *Pneumocystis carinii* prophylaxis.** Although pyrimeth-amine and sulfadiazine combination therapy has been investigated in the treat-ment of *P. carinii* pneumonia (PCP), other regimens are preferred. (See Chap. 24.) However, for the patient already receiving pyrimethamine and sulfadiazine for toxoplasmosis therapy, separate PCP prophylaxis (e.g., with TMP-SMX, dapsone) does not appear to be necessary [11].

VI. **Toxicity of pyrimethamine**
   A. **Bone marrow suppression.** The most notable toxic effect of pyrimethamine is bone marrow suppression with megaloblastic anemia, granulocytopenia, and thrombocytopenia. The suppression is **dose-related** and, in primary therapy of toxoplasmic encephalitis in AIDS patients, hematologic side effects should be anticipated but may be difficult to differentiate from those associated with HIV infection per se or other drugs the patient may be receiving [1, 2]. High dosages of pyrimethamine may deplete folic acid stores and cause reversible bone marrow depression [6].
      1. **Folinic acid (leucovorin) may ameliorate the bone marrow toxicity** of pyri-methamine, and folinic acid does not interfere with the activity of pyrimeth-amine or sulfadiazine on *T. gondii* [2].
         a. See sec. **V.B.1.** for dosages.
         b. **Do not use folic acid** because it will prevent the action of pyrimethamine on *T. gondii* [2].
      2. **Serial CBCs** (e.g., twice per week initially and then once weekly) should be performed in patients receiving pyrimethamine, **to help monitor** for **hemato-logic toxicity.**
   B. **Other side effects** [6]
      1. **Gastrointestinal.** Anorexia, abdominal cramps, and vomiting can occur at high doses of pyrimethamine. Administering the drug with meals (or at a reduced dose) may help prevent vomiting.
      2. **Dermatologic. Skin rashes** can occur (but are more likely to be related to sulfonamide use). (See Chap. 28K.)
      3. **Central nervous system.** High doses may result in adverse reactions, including ataxia, tremors, and seizures. In patients with a history of a seizure disorder, starting therapy with a lower dose and building up to standard dosages may be reasonable.

VII. **Contraindications** or special limitations [6]
   A. **Known hypersensitivity** to pyrimethamine.
   B. **Documented folate-deficiency anemia.**
   C. **Children younger than 2 months.**
   D. **Pregnancy, especially near term.** Generally, sulfonamide use is avoided in preg-nancy at term because of the risk of kernicterus. (See Chap. 28K.) Otherwise pyrimethamine should be used with caution in pregnancy, as teratogenic effects have been shown in animals. There are no adequate or well-controlled studies on the use of pyrimethamine in pregnancy in humans (per package insert). Therefore, it should be used only if the potential benefits outweigh the risks to the fetus. Infectious disease consultation is advised in this setting.
   E. **Nursing. Pyrimethamine is excreted in milk.** Because of its potential bone marrow suppressive effects, it would seem prudent to avoid nursing, especially in mothers receiving high-dose therapy as in toxoplasmic encephalitis primary or suppressive therapeutic regimens.

References

1. Beaman, M.H., et al. *Toxoplasma gondii.* In G.L. Mandell, J.E. Bennett, and R. Dolin (eds.), *Principles and Practice of Infectious Diseases* (4th ed.). New York: Churchill Livingstone, 1995. Pp. 2455–2475.
Authoritative and excellent review. Good discussion of dosage regimens for toxoplasmic encephalitis. For a review of a related topic, see C. Renold et al., Toxoplasma encephalitis in patients with the acquired immunodeficiency syndrome. Medicine *71:224, 1992, which is a review of 86 cases.*
2. Israelski, D.M., and Remington, J.S. Toxoplasmic encephalitis in patients with AIDS. *Infect. Dis. Clin. North Am.* 2:429, 1988.
Useful concise article emphasizing therapy. Discusses potential role of clindamycin in patients who cannot receive sulfonamides.
3. Medical Letter. Drugs for parasitic infection. *Med. Lett. Drugs Ther.* 37:99, 1995.
Contains pediatric regimen for pyrimethamine doses.
4. Luft, B.J., and Remington, J.S. Toxoplasmic encephalitis in AIDS. *Clin. Infect. Dis.* 15:211, 1992.
One of the "AIDS Commentary" series. Written by national experts on toxoplasmosis. Good clinical summary.
5. Dannemann, B., et al. Treatment of toxoplasmic encephalitis in patients with AIDS: A randomized trial comparing pyrimethamine plus clindamycin to pyrimethamine plus sulfadiazine. *Ann. Intern. Med.* 116:33, 1992.
Randomized, unblinded phase II multicenter trial from the California Collaborative Treatment Group. All patients received pyrimethamine (200-mg loading dose divided up over 24 hours, followed by 75 mg/d with at least 10 mg folinic acid daily) and 26 patients received clindamycin (initially 1,200 mg IV q6h for 3 weeks and then 300 mg PO q6h or 450 mg PO q8h) versus 33 patients who received sulfadiazine (at 100 mg/kg/d, rounded off to nearest gram, up to 8 g/d, divided up into a qid schedule for 6 weeks). Patients were treated for 6 weeks, and the results suggested that clinical efficacy of pyrimethamine and clindamycin was equivalent to pyrimethamine and sulfadiazine. Therefore, the study concluded that pyrimethamine-clindamycin appears to be an acceptable alternative in patients unable to tolerate pyrimethamine and sulfadiazine. (d = day)
6. American Hospital Formulary Service. *Drug Information.* Pyrimethamine. Bethesda, MD: American Society of Hospital Pharmacists, 1990. Pp. 396–400.
7. Webster, L.T., Jr. Drugs Used in the Chemotherapy of Protozoal Infections: Malaria. In A.G. Goodman et al. (eds.), *The Pharmacological Basis of Therapeutics.* New York: Pergamon, 1990. Pp. 985–987.
8. Weiss, L.M., et al. Pyrimethamine concentrations in serum and cerebrospinal fluid during treatment of acute encephalitis in patients with AIDS. *J. Infect. Dis.* 157:580, 1988.
Achievable serum levels vary; 12–25% of serum levels penetrate CSF. Monitoring serum drug levels may be useful.
9. Bennett, W.M., et al. *Drug Prescribing in Renal Failure: Dosing Guidelines for Adults* (3rd ed.). Philadelphia: American College of Physicians, 1994.
This is a useful handbook. Similar tables for dosing in renal failure appear in S.K. Swan and W.M. Bennett, Drug dosing guidelines in patients with renal failure. West. J. Med. *156:633, 1992; and L.L. Livornese et al., Antibacterial agents in renal failure.* Infect. Dis. Clin. North Am. *9:591, 1995.*
10. Centers for Disease Control. Recommendations for the prevention of malaria among travelers. *Health Information for International Travel.* Atlanta: US Department of Health and Human Services (HHS publication no. (CDC) 95-8280), 1995. (For sale by the Superintendent of Documents, US Government Printing Office, Washington, DC 30402.)
11. Heald, A., et al. Treatment for cerebral toxoplasmosis protects against *Pneumocystis carinii* pneumonia in patients with AIDS. *Ann. Intern. Med.* 115:760, 1991.

Mupirocin

Mupirocin (Bactroban) is a topical antibiotic initially introduced for the treatment of impetigo [1–3]. It is also a useful agent for the eradication of nasal carriage of staphylococci. Mupirocin interferes with bacterial RNA and protein synthesis by binding to bacterial isoleucyl transfer-RNA synthetase and preventing incorporation of isoleucine into protein chains. Because of this unique mechanism of action, mupirocin has little cross-resistance with other antibiotics [1, 2].

I. **In vitro activity**

A. **Gram-positive aerobes.** Mupirocin is active against *Staphylococcus aureus, S. epidermidis,* and *S. saprophyticus,* including methicillin-resistant strains [1, 2]. It also is active against *Streptococcus pyogenes* (group A streptococci) but not enterococci (group D) [1].

B. **Gram-negative aerobes.** Mupirocin is not active against Enterobacteriaceae or *Pseudomonas aeruginosa* [1].

C. **Anaerobes.** Mupirocin is not active against anaerobes.

II. **Pharmacokinetics.** Mupirocin, formerly called *pseudomonic acid,* is a naturally occurring antibiotic derived from the fermentation of *P. fluorescens.* Trace amounts absorbed into the systemic circulation are hydrolyzed rapidly. The inactive metabolite has a plasma half-life of less than 30 minutes [1].

III. **Clinical use**

A. **Impetigo.** Impetigo is a superficial, usually self-limited infection of the skin characterized by macules or papules progressing rapidly to vesicles, pustules, and exudative crusts. It occurs most frequently in children and often is associated with insect bites or rhinorrhea. Impetigo generally is caused by group A streptococci, but staphylococci are frequent secondary invaders; both organisms can often be cultured from the lesions [1].

Before the availability of mupirocin, systemic antibiotics (e.g., erythromycin, a first-generation cephalosporin, a penicillinase-resistant penicillin, clindamycin) have been used effectively to treat impetigo. The use of previously available topical antimicrobial antibiotics for the treatment of impetigo had been discouraged after a series of well-designed studies showed systemic antibiotics to be superior to topical agents [4]. Streptococcal impetigo has been associated with acute glomerulonephritis; whether any antibiotic treatment prevents this complication is unknown [1]. Oral erythromycin has often been viewed as a favorite and cost-effective agent for impetigo. See related discussion in Chap. 4.

Topical mupirocin appears to be as effective as systemic antibiotics in the treatment of impetigo [5–8]. The 3-times-daily mupirocin regimen and fewer side effects associated with its use (as compared to oral erythromycin) make mupirocin an appealing agent to patients and their families [8].

B. **Use in eradication of nasal staphylococcal colonization.** Early studies have shown that mupirocin applied to the anterior nares twice daily for 5 days often is effective in eradicating staphylococci, **including methicillin-resistant strains** [9, 10]. Chronic regimens in hemodialysis patients have also been tried [11].

1. **The calcium-base ointment** (recently made available in the United States in spring 1996) **is preferred** in this setting, because it tends to irritate the mucosal lining less than the polyethylene glycol base formulation. However, the polyethylene glycol base formulation has also been used for this purpose [12].

2. Nasal colonization with *S. aureus,* including methicillin-resistant forms, has been associated with the eventual development of staphylococcal infections, particularly in patients in long-term facilities and patients undergoing hemodialysis [13, 14]. Using mupirocin to reduce nasal colonization and, therefore, future infections is a consideration [13, 14], but long-term use may select out resistant MRSA [14a].

IV. **Preparations and dosages**

A. The **2% mupirocin ointment in polyethylene glycol** currently is available in the United States in a 15-g tube. For impetigo, a small amount of the ointment should be applied to the affected area 3 times daily, typically for 10 days. The package insert suggests that the involved area may be covered with a gauze dressing if desired. Patients not showing a clinical response within 3–5 days should be reevaluated.

1. The ointment is not for ophthalmic use.

2. It should not be used in patients with extensive open wounds or burns because of the risk of nephrotoxic effects from systemic absorption of the polyethylene glycol [4].

3. The package insert suggests that the drug should be used in pregnancy only if clearly needed. It is not known whether mupirocin passes into breast milk; nursing should be temporarily discontinued while using mupirocin.

4. We would not use mupirocin topically for treatment of impetigo if there is a concomitant group A streptococcal pharyngitis that may be associated with impetigo of the face (e.g., impetigo contiguous to or below the nares); we favor oral systemic therapy in these patients.
    B. **Two percent mupirocin calcium ointment for intranasal use (Bactroban Nasal) is indicated for eradication of nasal colonization with MRSA in adult patients and healthcare workers as part of a comprehensive infection control program to reduce the risk of infection among high-risk patients during MRSA outbreaks [9, 10]. It was approved in early 1996 and is available in single-use applicator tubes (1 g): half the ointment is applied to each nostril bid for 5 days.**
V. **Side effects.**
    A. **Local adverse reactions can occur with the polyethylene glycol formulation.** Mupirocin appears to be well tolerated, with few side effects when compared with systemic erythromycin [5–8]. Burning, stinging, or pain occur in 1.5–3% of patients, and itching occurs in 1% [2, 4]. Contact dermatitis (rarely), nausea, tenderness, and rash can occur but in fewer than 1% of recipients [2]. Photosensitivity reactions have not occurred [1, 4]. The polyethylene glycol–containing formulation is irritating when used on broken skin or mucous membranes (see sec. **III.B.1**). Owing to the possibility of absorption and serious renal toxicity should this formulation be applied to open wounds or burns [1], such application should be avoided.
    B. **Nasal mupirocin** is generally well tolerated. The two most common adverse effects are rhinitis and headache. Avoid contact with the eyes.
VI. **Cost.** A 15-g tube of the currently available polyethylene glycol–containing formulation is $15.80 (average wholesale price). The 2% nasal calcium formulation may vary in price: for a single-course purchase, the cost is about $40; with bulk purchases, up to 50% of the cost can be saved.

References

1. Medical Letter. Mupirocin—a new topical antibiotic. *Med. Lett. Drugs Ther.* 30:55, 1988.
2. *Physicians' Desk Reference* (50th ed.). Montvale, NJ: Medical Economics Data, 1996. P. 2470.
3. Committee on Infectious Diseases, American Academy of Pediatrics. *Report of the Committee on Infectious Diseases* (23rd ed.). Elk Grove Village, IL: American Academy of Pediatrics, 1994. P. 425.
   The "Red Book" supports the use of mupirocin in impetigo.
4. Infectious Diseases and Immunization Committee, Canadian Paediatric Society. Mupirocin in the treatment of impetigo. *Can. Med. Assoc. J.* 142:543, 1990.
   Concluded that adequate randomized, controlled clinical trials were needed before mupirocin could be recommended over systemic antibiotics.
5. Goldfarb, J., et al. Randomized clinical trial of topical mupirocin versus oral erythromycin for impetigo. *Antimicrob. Agents Chemother.* 32:1780, 1988.
   Sixty-two children received either mupirocin (3 times daily) or erythromycin (4 times daily). Mupirocin was safe, and data showed a trend toward more rapid response with mupirocin than with erythromycin. See a similar early report by S. McLinn, Topical mupirocin vs. systemic erythromycin treatment for pyoderma. Pediatr. Infect. Dis. J. 7:785, 1988.
6. Britton, J.W., et al. Comparison of mupirocin and erythromycin in the treatment of impetigo. *J. Pediatr.* 117:827, 1990.
   Fifty-four children received either mupirocin (3 times daily) or oral erythromycin (4 times daily) in a double-blind placebo-controlled study. Both agents were equally effective. Compliance was better with the 3-times-daily mupirocin.
7. Dagan, R., and Bar-David, Y. Double-blind study comparing erythromycin and mupirocin for treatment of impetigo in children: Implications of a high prevalence of erythromycin-resistant *Staphylococcus aureus* strains. *Antimicrob. Agents Chemother.* 36:287, 1992.
   In this study from Israel, 28% of the S. aureus strains isolated were erythromycin resistant. All strains were susceptible to mupirocin, which was believed to be an appropriate and effective alternative to erythromycin.

8. Rice, T.D., Duggan, A.K., and DeAngelis, C. Cost-effectiveness of erythromycin versus mupirocin for the treatment of impetigo in children. *Pediatrics* 89:210, 1992.
   Erythromycin has commonly been a preferred agent for impetigo. Study from Johns Hopkins in which children were randomly assigned to receive oral erythromycin 4 times daily (46 patients) or topical mupirocin 3 times daily (47 patients) for 10 days. **Both regimens were equally effective.** *Although the overall costs (medication plus office visits) were more for the mupirocin recipients (because of a couple of extra clinic visits to assess slow resolution of lesions in this group), those receiving erythromycin were more likely to have side effects or interference with their usual daily schedule. Therefore, mupirocin may be preferred by parents. See related article by J.J. Leyden,* Clin. Pediatr. *31:549, 1992.*

9. Scully, B.E., et al. Mupirocin treatment of nasal staphylococcal colonization. *Arch. Intern. Med.* 152:353, 1992.
   Intranasal use twice daily for 5 days. This preparation of calcium in a paraffin base was effective in eliminating S. aureus *nasal carriage in medical staff at Columbia University College of Physicians and Surgeons. All 34 recipients of mupirocin tolerated this agent well.*

10. Reagan, D.R., et al. Elimination of coincident *Staphylococcus aureus* nasal and hand carriage with intranasal application of mupirocin calcium ointment. *Ann. Intern. Med.* 114:101, 1991.
    In this study of 68 health care workers with stable S. aureus *nasal carriage, either mupirocin or placebo intranasally twice daily for 5 days was given. Mupirocin was safe and effective in eliminating* S. aureus *nasal carriage in healthy persons for up to 3 months and appears to have a corresponding effect on hand carriage at 72 hours after therapy. Authors conclude that this agent may be useful in therapy for limiting autoinoculation and nosocomial spread of* S. aureus.
    In same issue, see thoughtful editorial comment by Dr. R. Haley, MRSA: Do we just have to live with it? *Also see reference 14.*

11. Boelaert, J.R., et al. Once weekly nasal mupirocin in hemodialysis patients [abstract 34]. Thirty-first Interscience Conference on Antimicrobial Agents and Chemotherapy, Chicago, Sept. 30, 1991.
    Nasal calcium mupirocin 2% was given once a week to 60 hemodialysis patients, with clearing of nasal colonization in 96% of recipients and reduction of staphylococcal bacteremias. Similar data had been shown with the use of mupirocin 3 times per week in patients undergoing hemodialysis. See related article on the use of nasal mupirocin to eradicate nasal carriage of S. aureus *in hemodialysis patients by C. Watanakunakorn et al.* Am. J. Infect. Control *20:138, 1992.*

12. Darouiche, R., et al. Eradication of colonization by methicillin-resistant *Staphylcoccus aureus* by using oral minocycline-rifampin and topical mupirocin. *Antimicrob. Agents Chemother.* 35:1612, 1991.
    Concludes that when the individual circumstances of a medical facility justify eradication of methicillin-resistant S. aureus *(MRSA) colonization, a multidisciplinary approach, which includes antibiotic therapy with oral minocycline and rifampin, along with 2% mupirocin intransally twice daily for 5 days, may be successful.*

13. Ena, J., et al. Epidemiology of infections in nasal carriers of *S. aureus* on hemodialysis [abstract 28]. Thirty-first Interscience Conference on Antimicrobial Agents and Chemotherapy, Chicago, Sept. 30, 1991.
    When colonized patients became infected, the infections were caused by strains persistently carried in their nares.

14. Muder, R.R., et al. Methicillin-resistant staphylococcal colonization and infection in a long-term facility. *Ann. Intern. Med.* 114:107, 1991.
    In this study, 197 patients were followed with regular surveillance cultures of the anterior nares; 25% of the MRSA carriers had an episode of staphylococcal infection. Colonization of the anterior nares by MRSA predicts the development of staphylococcal infection in long-term care patients. Most infections arise from endogenously carried strains. Also see reference 10.

14a. Kauffman, C.A., et al. Attempts to eradicate methicillin-resistant *Staphylococcus aureus* from a long-term care facility with the use of mupirocin ointment. *Am. J. Med.* 94:371, 1993.
    Mupirocin ointment (polyethylene glycol base) is effective at decreasing colonization with MRSA. Long-term use of mupirocin selected for mupirocin-resistant MRSA. Authors conclude that mupirocin should be saved for use in outbreak situations and not used over the long term in facilities with endemic MRSA colonization. See related report by M.E. Mulligan et al., Am. J. Med. *94:313, 1993.*

Appendixes

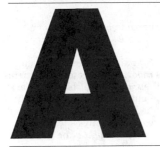

Ehrlichiosis: An Emerging Infectious Disease

Gerald A. Landry
and David H. Walker

The first description of human ehrlichial infection in the United States in 1987 was a catalyst for increased interest in ehrlichiae and their clinical manifestations. Although the clinical manifestations of ehrlichioses encompass a wide spectrum, the recognized febrile illness that follows these infections parallels other tickborne diseases in many respects. However, awareness of key differences between these disease entities should facilitate early diagnosis.

There are two species of *Ehrlichia* known to cause human disease in the United States. *E. chaffeensis* infects mainly mononuclear phagocytes and is the etiologic agent of human monocytic ehrlichiosis (HME). The second species, which is related to the veterinary *E. phagocytophila* and *E. equi,* infects granulocytes and is the etiologic agent of human granulocytic ehrlichiosis (HGE). Despite similar clinical presentations, comparison of these two human chrlichioses demonstrates significant differences.

Clinicians must maintain a high index of suspicion in order to diagnose human ehrlichiosis promptly. Ehrlichial infection should be considered in patients who present with constitutional symptoms of fever, headache, myalgias, and a history of tick bite or exposure in an endemic area during times of peak incidence. HME occurs from spring through autumn; HGE is seen year-round. The peak incidence of both diseases is from May through July. Typical clinical laboratory data include leukopenia, thrombocytopenia, anemia, and elevation of hepatocellular enzymes. Variable clinical expression is known to occur. **Rash is seen in a minority of patients.** Demographically, older males are likely to manifest the most severe disease and, consequently, seek medical attention.

I. Overview
A. The organism
1. Ehrlichioses are zoonotic infections caused by small obligate intracellular **gram-negative bacteria** of the family Rickettsiaceae and the genus *Ehrlichia*. Originally described as canine pathogens, ehrlichiae are bacteria capable of infecting human granulocytes and monocytes. Ehrlichiae are known to reside and proliferate intracellularly within cytoplasmic phagosomes. They can be visualized rarely after Romanowsky staining of a peripheral blood smear in HME but can be visualized in a substantial proportion of patients with HGE.
2. Three genogroups of ehrlichiae are currently known to exist. Human disease may result following infection with any genogroup [1, 2].
   a. *E. canis* group: *E. canis, E. chaffeensis, E. muris, E. ewingii,* and *Cowdria ruminantium.*
   b. *E. phagocytophila* genogroup: *E. equi, E. platys, E. phagocytophila,* and *Anaplasma marginale.*
   c. *E. sennetsu* genogroup: *E. sennetsu, E. risticii,* and *Neorickettsia helminthoeca.*
B. Historical background
1. *E. canis* infection was first described in Algerian dogs in 1935 and is the known etiologic agent of canine monocytic ehrlichiosis [3, 4]. *E. sennetsu,* the first ehrlichia known to be a human pathogen, is the cause of a self-limited infectious mononucleosis-like syndrome described in Japan in 1954 [5]. The first documented case of human ehrlichiosis in the United States occurred in Arkansas in 1986 in a 51-year-old man with a history of tick exposure. Morphologic analysis and indirect immunofluorescent antibody testing suggested *E. canis* as the infecting agent [6].
2. In 1991, *E. chaffeensis* was isolated using a canine histiocytoma cell line and was identified by a method based on amplification and sequencing of the 16S

rRNA gene (rDNA) [7]. This species was shown to be genetically and antigenically related to *E. canis* and was thought to be the sole etiologic agent of human ehrlichiosis in the United States [8].

3. In 1994, polymerase chain reaction (PCR) analysis of an organism in blood (using eubacterial universal primers) was reported for six febrile patients from northern Minnesota and Wisconsin. In their peripheral blood smears, these patients were found to have inclusions in neutrophils, a target cell that is not characteristic of *E. chaffeensis*. This was the first report of HGE caused by an *Ehrlichia* species demonstrated by DNA sequence analysis to have more than 99.8% homology of the 16S rDNA with *E. phagocytophila* and *E. equi* [9]. The agent of HGE has recently been successfully isolated in horses and propagated in cell culture [9a,9b].

C. **Two human ehrlichioses are known to exist in the United States**; both appear to be tickborne [1]. The clinical manifestations of these diseases are difficult to distinguish from other flulike illnesses and are characterized by the acute or subacute onset of fever, headache, and myalgias. Typical laboratory features include leukopenia, thrombocytopenia, and elevation of serum aminotransferases. The clinical presentation is discussed in detail in sec. **IV.A.**

   1. **HME** is an infection of mononuclear phagocytes in tissue and blood by *E. chaffeensis.*
   2. **HGE** is an infection of granulocytes due to a phylogenetically distinct organism.

II. Epidemiologic features

A. As of early 1995, more than 400 cases of HME had been identified by the Centers for Disease Control (CDC), and hundreds of other cases have been documented by other laboratories. Most cases occur in the Southeastern and South Central United States. Approximately 150 cases of HGE have been documented, and greater recognition of this disease is expected to reveal many more cases in the future.

   1. **HME** has been **documented most frequently** in Oklahoma, Missouri, Georgia, Virginia, Texas, and Arkansas.
   2. **HGE** has been **reported** in Wisconsin, Minnesota, Massachusetts, Connecticut, Pennsylvania, Rhode Island, and New York. Infections also have been acquired in California, Maryland, Arkansas, and Florida [1, 10].

B. **Both species of ehrlichia are believed to be tickborne.**

   1. **HME.** It is now well documented that the lone star tick, *Amblyomma americanum,* is a vector for the agent of HME.

      a. Epidemiologic surveys have demonstrated that *E. chaffeensis* infection tends to occur within the geographic distribution of the tick vector *A. americanum* [11].

      b. PCR has detected *E. chaffeensis* in *A. americanum* in four states [11a].

      c. In nature, the mammalian hosts of HME are deer [1]. Dogs are experimental hosts, but there have been no documented natural infections [12].

      d. Experimentally infected deer have transmitted *E. chaffeensis* to the feeding larvae and nymphs of *A. americanum,* which maintain the ehrlichiae transstadially to the adult stage. Adult and nymphal ticks have subsequently transmitted infection to other deer when feeding [13].

      e. The dog tick, *Dermacentor variabilis,* also has been implicated as a carrier of *E. chaffeensis*. Sporadic cases of ehrlichiosis have occurred in West Coast states within the known geographic range of *D. variabilis* [1].

      f. The majority of patients with HME report tick exposure in a tick-infested area or an actual tick bite (83% and 68%, respectively) [14].

   2. **HGE.** There is highly suggestive evidence that *Ixodes scapularis (dammini)* is the tick vector for the agent of HGE.

      a. HGE has been most closely linked to the bite of the deer tick *I. scapularis (dammini)* [15]. Ehrlichiae are found in the salivary glands of this vector [16].

      b. There is a suspected association between HGE and the tick *Ixodes pacificus* in California [1]. *I. pacificus* is a documented experimental vector of *E. equi* [17].

      c. The mammalian hosts of HGE are thought to be deer, horses, sheep, cattle, goats, dogs and, white-footed deer mice [1].

      d. HGE occurs year-round but **the peak incidence** of disease in **endemic rural areas** is from **May to July.** This appears to coincide with the peak exposure time between nymphal *I. scapularis* ticks and humans.

    e. The majority of patients with HGE report tick exposure in a tick-infested area or an actual tick bite (100% and 67%, respectively) [15].

III. **Pathogenesis**

  A. The pathogenesis of the human ehrlichioses **has not been fully elucidated.** Although monocytes or granulocytes appear to be the targeted cells of infection, host pathogenic inflammatory or immune events may be the final common pathway dictating disease severity [1].

  B. **In human infection, a working model for HME has been proposed.** However, given the similarities in clinical presentation between HME and HGE, a common pathophysiology is suggested.

    1. *E. chaffeensis* are inoculated by tick bite into the dermis.

    2. The organism spreads via lymphatics and blood vessels.

    3. The ehrlichiae are phagocytosed by monocytes, macrophages or their precursors in the bone marrow, liver, spleen, lymph nodes, and, occasionally, the lung and the meninges.

    4. Once a cell is infected, the ehrlichiae replicate by binary fission, becoming vacuole-contained microcolonies called *morulae.* (*Morula* is Latin for mulberry, which these cytoplasmic inclusions resemble on Giemsa smears of peripheral blood.)

    5. Proliferation of the organism takes place with injury to heavily infected cells, particularly in immunocompromised patients, and possibly by indirect injury of tissue by cytokines or other mediators [18–20].

    6. The morulae are released presumably via exocytosis or when the infected cell ruptures and the cycle begins again.

    7. Subsequently, there is stimulation of immunologic and inflammatory mechanisms, which leads to sequestration, destruction of infected cells, or granuloma formation.

    8. The severity of infection may be determined by the balance between induced protective immunity, ehrlichia-associated immunosuppression, and mediation of cytolysis by ehrlichiae or immunopathologic mechanisms [1].

IV. **Clinical manifestations.** The clinical manifestations of ehrlichiosis are **notoriously nonspecific.** The clinical presentations of HME and HGE are similar.

  A. **Clinical manifestations of HME** [14]

    1. **Fever, malaise,** and **headache** were the most common presenting symptoms found by Fishbein et al. [14], but no single symptom was present in more than 75% of patients on the first day.

    2. **Myalgia,** the next most frequent symptom, occurs at some point during the illness in 68% of people.

    3. **Other symptoms** include rigors, arthralgia, nausea, diaphoresis, vomiting, cough, and confusion.

    4. A **rash** appears **in 36% of patients** but in only 6% at disease onset and in 25% within the first week. The rash is usually macular or papular or both but may be petechial. It is located most often on the trunk, legs, arms, and face.

    5. In a laboratory-based study of human ehrlichiosis from 1985 to 1990 [14], the **median age** of case-patients was **44 years,** which is substantially older than that for Rocky Mountain Spotted fever (RMSF). The **majority** of these patients were **male** [74.5%]. Age-specific incidence rates increased steadily with increasing age; these rates were highest for persons 60–69 years of age.

    6. Occasionally, patients may present with signs, symptoms, and laboratory evidence suggesting predominant involvement of a single organ system. These presentations might include cough with infiltrates on chest x-ray, gastroenteritis, meningitis, or acute abdominal pain [1].

    7. When examined, cerebrospinal fluid may show a lymphocytic or neutrophilic pleocytosis [21].

    8. The **median duration** of illness **exceeds 3 weeks** [1].

    9. There is a complication rate of approximately 16%. **Complications include** renal dysfunction or failure, disseminated intravascular coagulation, cardiomegaly, opportunistic infection, seizure, and coma. The mean age of patients who die is older than those who are hospitalized without complications or do not require hospitalization [14].

    10. The mortality rate of HME is estimated to be approximately 2–3% [1, 11].

  B. **Clinical manifestations of HGE.** HGE like HME is a multisystem disorder. Most patients also demonstrate hepatocellular injury, mild azotemia, anemia, and nausea. To date, there have been no large geographically widespread surveillance studies characterizing HGE's epidemiologic, clinical, or laboratory features.

1. In a recent study of 41 patients by Bakken et al. [22], the typical presentation of patients with HGE was **fever** (100%), **chills** (98%), **myalgias** (98%), and **headache** (85%). Other symptoms during the course of illness included **malaise** (98%), **nausea** (39%), **vomiting** (34%), **cough** (29%), and **confusion** (17%). The histologic correlates of respiratory signs and elevated serum transaminases are interstitial pneumonia and focal hepatocellular necrosis, respectively [15].

2. Demographically, **78%** of patients were **male,** and the range of ages was 6 to 91 years (**median** age = **59 years**). Tick exposure was reported by 90% of patients, with actual tick bite reported by 73% a median of 8 days prior to the onset of disease.

3. Most patients demonstrated variable degrees of **thrombocytopenia, leuko-penia,** or **anemia.** The mean aspartate aminotransferase (AST) value was 148 units/liter. Intracytoplasmic morulae in peripheral neutrophils were seen in the majority of cases, although they may be less frequent in HGE in the Northeastern states.

4. Thrombocytopenia and coagulopathy in severe infection may predispose to hemorrhagic complications; neutropenia or other defects in host defenses may predispose to opportunistic infections [15].

5. Rash is very uncommon [21].

6. The mortality rate of HGE is estimated to be 5% [22]. This rate may be higher in untreated patients and substantially lower with early empiric therapy.

C. **Signs and symptoms of HGE and HME.** See Table A-1 [1, 14, 15, 22].

D. The **differential diagnosis of ehrlichiosis** includes RMSF, Colorado tick fever, Q fever, leptospirosis, Lyme disease, typhus, legionnaires' disease, tularemia, typhoid or paratyphoid fever, brucellosis, viral hepatitis, enteroviral infections, meningococcemia, and influenza [23].

E. **Miscellaneous issues**

1. Undoubtedly, there is a bias toward representation of more severely afflicted patients in laboratory-based surveillance studies. Indeed, the majority of HME patients identified serologically in a longitudinal study were asymptomatic with a ratio of asymptomatic to symptomatic patients of 2 to 1 [23a].

2. It is uncertain whether ehrlichiae are capable of producing a chronic, asymptomatic infection. Dumler et al. [1, 24] have demonstrated that persistent human infection can occur and might represent an ecological adaptation for ehrlichial survival in the natural host. A mammalian reservoir for maintenance in nature would be required for the ehrlichiae because transovarial transmission of ehrlichial species in ticks has not been shown to occur. Delayed sequelae, months after initial infection as in Lyme disease, have not been described in humans but are well documented in canine monocytic ehrlichiosis.

3. While elderly patients are likely to develop more severe manifestations of disease with higher mortality, the exact cause of mortality is unknown. It is clear, however, that secondary infections with either nosocomial or opportunis-

Table A-1. Signs and symptoms of HME and HGE (%)

Sign/symptom	HME	HGE
Fever	97	100
Malaise	84	98
Myalgia	68	98
Headache	81	85
Rigors	61	98
Nausea	48	39
Vomiting	37	34
Cough	26	29
Rash	36	2
Confusion	20	17

Source: Data from [1, 14, 15, 22].

tic pathogens occur frequently in severely ill patients. For example, in a case report documenting persistent infection with *E. chaffeensis,* postmortem examination revealed pulmonary aspergillosis and active cytomegalovirus infection in the lungs, stomach, and pancreas after 68 days of hospitalization, despite antibiotic therapy [24].

4. Evidence suggests that infection with some species of ehrlichiae imparts defects in host phagocytic defenses as well as T and B cell function [25, 26].

5. The duration of time a tick must be attached to the host to transmit infection is unknown but is presumed to be 12–24 hours or longer [21].

6. Serologic surveys for Lyme disease performed in endemic areas suggest that some patients probably have had concomitant tickborne infections, including ehrlichiosis, borreliosis, and babesiosis. The interaction of one tickborne illness with another may affect the clinical manifestations of both diseases; however, the clinical implications await further study [27, 28].

V. **Laboratory data.** A definitive diagnosis cannot be made on the basis of the nonspecific clinical presentation.

A. The **classic clinical laboratory findings** in HME and HGE are seen in the majority of patients and include the following [1, 14].

1. **Progressive leukopenia** (often with a left shift) and **thrombocytopenia.** The leukocyte count and the platelet count reach a nadir at the end of the first week of illness.

2. **Anemia.** The hematocrit tends to fall steadily during the first few weeks of infection.

3. **Hepatic enzymes.** Mild to moderate elevations of AST, alanine aminotransferase (ALT), alkaline phosphatase, and lactate dehydrogenase (LDH) occur, with a tendency toward a rapid increase in the first days of illness and subsequent slow resolution.

B. **Bone marrow examination.** In HME, bone marrow examination most often demonstrates **nonspecific** myeloid hyperplasia, megakaryocytosis, and granulomas. Occasionally, histiocytic infiltration, myeloid or pancellular hypoplasia, or normocellular marrow is seen. Widespread perivascular lymphohistiocytic infiltrates, focal hepatocellular necrosis, and evidence of mononuclear phagocyte activation in the liver, spleen, lymph node, and bone marrow also are present [29]. Activation of the mononuclear phagocyte system is hypothesized to result in peripheral white blood cell and platelet destruction. In severely immunocompromised patients, extensive ehrlichial growth is accompanied by necrosis of many infected macrophages.

C. **Detection of morulae in peripheral blood leukocytes** aids the early diagnosis of HGE but is extremely insensitive with respect to HME and time consuming with unknown sensitivity in HGE [1]. In HGE, neutrophil-containing morulae may be seen, if searched for carefully, in peripheral blood smears in more than half of patients in the upper Midwest [D.H. Walker, unpublished data, 1996].

D. **Serologic diagnosis.** Initially, all cases of HME were diagnosed by indirect fluorescent antibody assay (IFA) testing cross-reaction with *E. canis* [6, 11, 30].

1. The **current CDC recommendation for serologic diagnosis of HME** is a fourfold increase in antibody titer against *E. chaffeensis* antigens (minimum titer = 64) or a single high serum antibody titer (>128) for a patient with a clinically compatible history [1, 14].

2. The **current recommendation for** confirmation of infection with **HGE** is an IFA serologic reaction at a titer of 80 or greater or a fourfold increase in titer to *E. equi* antigen [1, 15]. The etiologic organism of HGE resembles *E. phagocytophila* and *E. equi.* Antigens prepared by isolation of *E. equi*–infected equine leukocytes or *E. phagocytophila*–infected bovine leukocytes have proved useful in the identification of IFA serologic responses of humans after infection with the agent of HGE [1, 15].

E. **Polymerase chain reaction.** Specific oligonucleotide PCR primers have been designed on the basis of the nucleotide sequences of the 16S rDNA for *E. chaffeensis* and for the HGE agent. **PCR has been used for clinical identification of patients with HME** [31] **and HGE** [15]. Although not currently widely available, **PCR facilitates early confirmation of acute infection.** The results of diagnostic testing, however, should not delay initiation of empiric treatment.

VI. **Therapy.** Delays in antibiotic therapy have been shown to be associated with an increased risk of complications or death [11, 14].

A. **HME**

1. Historically, tetracycline has been the antibiotic of choice for rickettsial infec-

tion. **The efficacy of tetracycline** in the treatment of **HME** is now **well established.** Tetracycline [31a], nearly always in the form of doxycycline, has been shown to cause prompt defervescence and to reduce both the rate of hospitalization and the duration of illness [11, 14].

  a. In adults and children, oral or intravenous **doxycycline** is recommended. Adults should receive doxycycline 100 mg, PO or IV, bid; children require 3 mg/kg/day (up to maximum of 200 mg/day), PO or IV, in two divided doses. If the diagnosis of ehrlichiosis is confirmed, tetracycline remains a rational agent in the child under 8 years of age because chloramphenicol may not be uniformly effective in this life-threatening illness [21]. In RMSF, therapy is continued for 2 or 3 days after defervescence, for a minimum total of 5–7 days [1]. Similar schedules, therefore, might be made for the duration of therapy for ehrlichiosis.

  b. Although in vitro data suggest that rifampin may be a practical alternative therapy for HME, the paucity of clinical experience precludes its use at this time.

  2. Retrospective analysis has shown that chloramphenicol may be used successfully to treat human ehrlichiosis; however, caution is advised.

  a. To date, the number of patients treated with chloramphenicol has been small, and in at least one study the patients were younger, and presumably less severely ill, than those treated with other antibiotics [14].

  b. In vitro susceptibility data have demonstrated that *E. chaffeensis* is resistant to chloramphenicol, ciprofloxacin, erythromycin, trimethoprim-sulfamethoxazole, penicillin, and gentamicin, which had minimum inhibition concentrations (MICs) of 16, 4, 8, 4, 40, and 32 µg/ml, respectively. Doxycycline and rifampin were found to be bactericidal with minimum bactericidal concentrations (MBCs) of 0.500 and 0.125 µg/ml, respectively [32].

  c. Cases have been reported wherein patients did not respond to courses of treatment with chloramphenicol [6].

 B. HGE. There have been no susceptibility data or therapeutic trials published to date for HGE; clinical experience indicates that doxycycline is efficacious [1].

 C. Prophylaxis. It is unclear at this point whether prophylactic antibiotics should be used after tick bites in endemic areas [21].

 VII. Conclusion. It is clear that clinicians must maintain a high index of suspicion in order to diagnose HME and HGE. Ehrlichiosis should be considered in the differential diagnosis of an acute or subacute febrile illness in patients exposed to tick bites in endemic areas. Suggestive laboratory data include leukopenia, thrombocytopenia, anemia, and elevation of ALT, AST, alkaline phosphatase, and LDH. Early recognition, presumptive diagnosis, and empiric treatment are of paramount importance in the successful outcome of this disease. For adults and children, doxycycline is the treatment of choice.

References

1. Dumler, J.S., and Bakken, J.S. Ehrlichial diseases of humans: Emerging tick-borne infections. *Clin Infect Dis.* 20:1102–1110, 1995.
2. Walker, D.H., and Dumler, J.S. The emergence of ehrlichioses as human health problems. *Emerg. Infect. Dis.* 2:18–29, 1996.
   See *D.H. Walker, Human ehrlichiosis: More trouble from ticks.* Hosp. Pract. *31:47, 1996.*
3. Donatien, A., and Lestoquard F. Existence en Algerie d'une Rickettsia du chien. *Bull. Soc. Pathol. Exot.* 28:418–419, 1935.
4. Nims, R.M., et al. Epizootiology of tropical canine pancytopenia and southeast Asia. *J. Am. Vet. Med Assoc.* 158:53–63, 1971.
5. Fukuda, T., et al. Studies on causative agent of 'Hyuga netsu' disease. *Med. Biol.* 23:200–205, 1954.
6. Maeda, K., et al. Human infection with *Ehrlichia canis,* a leukocytic rickettsia. *N. Engl. J. Med.* 316:853–856, 1987.
7. Dawson, J.E., et al. Isolation and characterization of an *Ehrlichia* sp. from a patient diagnosed with human ehrlichiosis *J. Clin. Microbiol.* 29:2741–2745, 1991.
8. Anderson, B.E., et al. *Ehrlichia chaffeensis,* a new species associated with human ehrlichiosis. *J. Clin. Microbiol.* 29:2838–2842, 1991.
9. Chen, S.M., et al. Identification of a granulocytotropic *Ehrlichia* species as the etiologic

agent of human disease. *J. Clin. Microbiol.* 32:589–595, 1994.
9a. Madigan, J.E., et al. Transmission and passage in horses of the agent of human granulocytic ehrlichiosis. *J. Infect. Dis.* 172:1141–1144, 1995.
9b. Goodman, J.L., et al. Direct cultivation of the causative agent of human granulocytic ehrlichiosis. *N. Engl. J. Med.* 334:209, 1996. *See editorial comment in same issue.*
10. Telford III, S.R., et al. Human granulocytic ehrlichiosis in Massachusetts. *Ann. Intern. Med.* 123:277–279, 1995.
11. Eng, T.R., et al. Epidemiologic, clinical, and laboratory findings of human ehrlichiosis in the United States, 1988. *J.A.M.A.* 264:2251–2258, 1990.
11a. Anderson, B.E., et al. *Amblyomma americanum:* A potential vector of human ehrlichiosis. *Am. J. Trop. Med. Hyg.* 49:239–244, 1993.
12. Dawson, J.E., et al. Susceptibility of dogs to infection with *Ehrlichia chaffeensis,* a causative agent of human ehrlichiosis *Am. J. Vet. Res.* 53:1322–1327, 1992.
13. Ewing, S.A., et al. Experimental transmission of *Ehrlichia chaffeensis* among white-tailed deer by *Amblyomma americanum J. Med. Entomol.* 32(3):368–374, 1995.
14. Fishbein, D.B., et al. Human ehrlichiosis in the United States, 1985 to 1990. *Ann. Intern. Med.* 120:736–743, 1994.
15. Bakkan, J.S., et al. Human granulocytic ehrlichiosis in the upper Midwest United States. *J.A.M.A.* 272:212–218, 1994.
16. Pancholi, P., et al. *Ixodes dammini* as a potential vector of human granulocytic ehrlichiosis. *J. Infect. Dis.* 172:1007–1012, 1995.
17. Richter, P.J., et al. *Ixodes pacificus* as a vector of *Ehrlichia equi. J. Med. Entomol.* 33:1–5, 1996.
18. Chen, S.M., et al. Cultivation of *Ehrlichia chaffeensis* in mouse embryo, vero, BGM, and L929 cells and study of *Ehrlichia*-induced cytopathic effect and plaque formation. *Infect. Immun.* 63:647–655, 1995.
19. Paddock, C.D., et al. Brief report: Fatal seronegative ehrlichiosis in a patient with HIV infection. *N. Engl. J. Med.* 329:1164–1167, 1993.
20. Marty, A.M., et al. Ehrlichiosis mimicking thrombotic thrombocytopenic purpura: Case report and pathological correlation. *Human Pathol.* 26:920–925, 1995.
21. Walker, D.H., and Dumler, J.S. Ehrlichiosis: Emerging Bacterial Pathogens Symposium. 35th Interscience Conference on Antimicrobial Agents and Chemotherapy. San Francisco, CA: September 18, 1995.
22. Bakken, J.S., et al. Human granulocytic ehrlichiosis: Clinical and laboratory characteristics of human granulocytic ehrlichiosis. *J.A.M.A.* 275:199–205, 1996.
23. Fine, D.P. Ehrlichiosis. In P.D. Hoeprich et al. (eds.), *Infectious Diseases* (5th ed.). Philadelphia: Lippincott, 1994. Pp. 1281–1283.
23a. Yevich, S.J., et al. Seroepidemiology of infections due to spotted fever group Rickettsiae and Ehrlichia species in military personnel exposed in areas of the United States where such infections are endemic. *J. Infect. Dis.* 171:1266–1273, 1995.
24. Dumler, J.S., et al. Persistent infection with *Ehrlichia chaffeensis. Clin. Infect. Dis.* 17:903–905, 1993.
25. Woldehiwet, Z. The effects of tick-borne fever on some functions of polymorphonuclear cells of sheep. *J. Comp. Path.* 97:481–485, 1987.
26. Larsen, HJS, et al. Immunosuppression in sheep experimentally infected with *Ehrlichia phagocytophila. Res. Vet. Sci.* 56:216–224, 1994.
27. Pancholi, P., et al. Serological evidence of human granulocytic ehrlichosis in Lyme disease patients from the upper midwest. Infectious Disease Society of America 33rd Annual meeting. San Francisco, CA: September 16, 1995. (Abstract #21)
28. Dumler, J.S., et al. Human granulocytic ehrlichiosis, Lyme disease and babesiosis in the upper midwest: Evidence for concurrent infection. 35th Interscience Conference on Antimicrobial Agents and Chemotherapy. San Francisco, CA: Sept 18, 1995. (Abs K29)
29. Dumler, J.S., et al. Human ehrlichiosis: Hematopathology and immunohistologic detection of Ehrlichia chaffeensis. *Human Pathol.* 24:391–396, 1993.
30. Dawson, J.E., et al. Diagnosis of human ehrlichiosis with the indirect fluorescent antibody test: Kinetics and specificity. *J. Infect. Dis.* 162:91–95, 1990.
31. Anderson, B.E., et al. Detection of the etiologic agent of human ehrlichiosis by polymerase chain reaction. *J. Clin. Microbiol.* 30:775–780, 1992.
31a. Medical Letter. The choice of antibacterial drugs. *Med. Lett. Drug Ther.* 38:25, 1996. *No alternative agent is listed for ehrlichiosis.*
32. Brouqui, P., and Raoult, D. In vitro antibiotic susceptibility of the newly recognized agent of ehrlichiosis in humans, Ehrlichia chaffeensis. *Antimicrob. Agents Chemother.* 36:2799–2803, 1992.

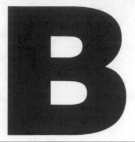

Infectious Disease Aspects of Employee (Occupational) Health: A Brief Overview

Sally H. Houston,
John T. Sinnott,
and JoAnn Palumbo Shea

Employee Health and Safety

Health care workers (HCWs) are an important link in the control of infection. Many states already regulate minimal health and immunization requirements for employment in health care facilities. A comprehensive employee health program should be developed utilizing guidelines and regulations from the Centers for Disease Control (CDC), Occupational Safety and Health Administration (OSHA), National Institute for Occupational Safety and Health (NIOSH), and state health departments. This discussion does not attempt to define such a comprehensive program, which has been addressed in other references [1–5]. **Rather, the intent of this discussion is to alert** the student, house officer, practicing physician, and other **health care providers about those employee health issues that overlap with infection control issues; that is, how to protect the HCWs from acquiring or spreading infections in the hospital, clinic, or office setting.**

I. Employee health program
   A. **Major objectives** of an employee health program should include the following:
      1. Screen periodically to identify occupational health risks, implement preventive measures [1], and comply with respiratory agency minimal standards.
      2. Provide management of occupationally related illness and communicable disease or bloodborne pathogen exposure among HCWs.
      3. Monitor and investigate exposures and disease outbreaks among personnel.
      4. Emphasize preventive health practices and health maintenance habits and promote individual responsibility for infection control.
   B. **Baseline and periodic health assessment.** At the time of employment, it is useful to establish a baseline health and immunization history. If documentation of immunization is not possible, **serologic testing for rubella, rubeola, varicella-zoster virus,** and **hepatitis B virus** (HBV) is warranted [6]. A comprehensive medical history and physical examination is not necessary for infection-control purposes but may be required by state regulations and serves as an important resource for determining preexisting medical problems. Many facilities have adopted "position-specific" screening that targets risks associated with specific tasks. Yearly, each worker's health status should be reassessed and immunizations updated [1].
   C. **Tuberculosis control.** OSHA regulations include the following. A baseline intermediate purified protein derivative (PPD) tuberculin skin test is required for all new employees whose tuberculosis status is unknown or whose reaction is negative by history. Two-step testing will eliminate potential false positive PPD conversions as a result of the booster effect [7, 8] (see Chap. 9 under Tuberculosis.) A current chest roentgenogram to rule out active disease is recommended for individuals exhibiting a positive reaction to PPD, with assessment for active pulmonary disease and consideration of isoniazid (INH) prophylaxis (see Chap. 9). The need for repeat PPD testing should be dictated by exposure or the prevalence of tuberculosis in the hospital population or geographic area. State regulations may also affect this interval [1]. Health care workers at increased risk for exposure to tuberculosis should be PPD-tested every 3–6 months depending on hospital risk assessment data. Potential high-risk employees include emergency department personnel, respiratory therapists, microbiology laboratory workers, pathologists, specialists in pulmonary medicine, and nurses in some settings [8–9a]. For further discussion, see Chap. 9 and related references [8, 9].

D. **Immunization program.** Immunization of hospital staff helps reduce the risk of transmissible diseases [1, 6, 10, 11] (see also Chap. 22).

1. **Rubella. All HCWs, regardless of age or gender, should be immune to rubella.** This is a vital strategy for preventing congenital rubella syndrome, and some states have made it mandatory. Many hospitals require immunity as a condition of employment. **New employees** without documentation of immunization after his or her first birthday **should be screened for rubella antibody and offered immunization if seronegative** [10] (see Chap. 22).

2. **Hepatitis B immunization.** OSHA requires that all employees whose job activities place them at risk for blood exposure be **offered** the hepatitis B vaccine at the employer's expense. Prescreening is not required unless specifically requested by the employee but may be helpful and cost-effective if risk factors for hepatitis B are present [12]. For the details of hepatitis B vaccination, see Chap. 22. Postvaccination testing for antibody to HBV surface antigen should be performed to document antibody response. This will assist in determining the need for further immunization or appropriate postexposure prophylaxis [13]. OSHA mandates that employers document vaccination history (including employee refusal of vaccine) as well as provide training in both the prevention of exposure to bloodborne pathogens and the correct use of personal protective equipment (PPE).

3. **Influenza.** Influenza can spread quickly through a health care facility, particularly one with a residential environment. Therefore, aggressive efforts should be made to immunize staff, particularly those with direct patient contact, in November of each year [11] (**see Chap. 8**). Nosocomial transmission of influenza has been demonstrated and may have dramatic effects on patient outcome [6].

4. **Rubeola.** Measles may present a significant risk to both HCWs and their patients. Persons born before 1956 are, in general, considered immune to measles. Among HCWs born after 1956, up to 14% are susceptible to measles [14, 15]. The Infectious Diseases Society of America recommends that hospitals require evidence from all HCWs of measles infection or receipt of two doses of live virus vaccine [16]. If this documentation is lacking, serologic testing should be done and live measles virus vaccine should be administered at employment and repeated 1 month later for all HCWs who are not immune. Live virus vaccines are contraindicated during pregnancy [16, 17].

5. **Tetanus-diphtheria.** It is important to update tetanus-diphtheria immunization at the time of employment (if need be) and every 10 years thereafter. See detailed discussion in Chap. 6.

6. **Mumps.** Susceptible adult HCWs, especially males, are candidates for vaccination [1]. See Chap. 22.

7. **Varicella.** Knowledge of the varicella-antibody status of employees who provide direct patient care has become more important as the immunosuppressed patient population increases. Consequently, most hospitals, particularly those with large pediatric or immunocompromised populations, have initiated varicella screening of all employees. Documentation of serology will prevent unnecessary work restrictions and disruption of patient services should exposure occur [1, 6].

   The live-attenuated varicella vaccine is discussed in detail in Chap. 22. Precise guidelines for the use of this vaccine in HCWs have not yet been published. Susceptible HCWs who have direct patient contact would seem to be potential candidates for this vaccine; this must be individualized until guidelines are available.

8. **Other immunizations.** Booster doses of poliomyelitis immunization generally are not indicated. Administration of oral poliovirus vaccine to an HCW is contraindicated due to the risk of transmitting the live virus. Some hospitals provide vaccine against pneumococcal pneumonia. Consideration should be given to offering hepatitis A vaccine to food handlers, hospital childcare workers, and selected research personnel (see Chap. 11).

E. **Screening for carriage of bacterial, viral, or parasitic pathogens.** Unless an HCW is or has been epidemiologically implicated in disease transmission, or has symptoms of infection, routine screening for pathogens (e.g., HBV, the human immunodeficiency virus [HIV], *Salmonella* spp., *Staphylococcus aureus*) is not indicated (see sec. II). However, some state or local regulations may require screening of food handlers for enteric pathogens.

F. **Work restrictions for acute, chronic, or recurrent infections.** In certain situations, HCWs will need to be placed on work restrictions, complete or partial, depending on the infection and risk of transmission [1]. Table B-1 summarizes these recommendations.
G. **Prophylaxis after exposure to various illnesses** has been reviewed elsewhere in this book.
   1. **Hepatitis A.** See Chap. 11.
   2. **Hepatitis B.** See Chaps. 11 and 22.
   3. **Hepatitis C.** Results have been equivocal in studies attempting to assess the value of prophylaxis with immunoglobulins against parenterally transmitted non-A, non-B hepatitis. For persons with percutaneous exposure to blood from a patient with parenterally transmitted non-A, non-B hepatitis, it may be reasonable to administer immunoglobulin (0.06 ml/kg) as soon as possible after exposure [1]. See related discussions in sec. **II.A.2** and Chap. 11.
   4. **Meningococcal disease.** See Chap. 5.
   5. **Rabies.** Health care workers who either have been bitten by a human with rabies or have scratches, abrasions, open wounds, or mucous membranes contaminated with saliva or other potentially infective material from a human or animal with rabies should receive a full course of antirabies treatment [1]. See Chap. 4.
II. **Occupational issues related to bloodborne disease transmission**
   A. **Risk of transmission to HCWs**
      1. **Hepatitis B virus.** As of November 1991, in the United States there were an estimated 1–1.25 million chronic carriers of HBV (HBsAg-positive). These persons represent a continuous risk to uninfected persons. In the United States, there are between 200,000 and 300,000 new cases reported annually. In part because of such figures, the CDC now recommends that all children in the United States receive hepatitis B vaccine [13]. (See Chaps. 11 and 22.) Still, approximately 300 HCWs annually die of HBV or its complications [18]. Individuals in occupations that involve the performance of invasive procedures or frequent contact with blood are at increased risk of exposure. Surveys of personnel in high-risk occupations have shown high rates of seropositivity: between 5 and 30% or more for hospital-based physicians and laboratory personnel [10, 11]. The risk for HBV infection following a single percutaneous exposure to blood contaminated with hepatitis B "e" antigen (HBeAg-positive) is estimated to be 27–43%, with a 6–24% risk for developing subsequent clinical hepatitis [19]. **These data underscore the importance of hepatitis B immunization as a preventive measure. See Chap. 22.**
      2. **Hepatitis C virus (HCV).** Second-generation immunoassays have improved the positive predictive value of the antibody test for HCV. However, the rate of HCV transmission and risk factors for transmission remain to be determined. OSHA guidelines regarding prevention of exposure to bloodborne pathogens were intended to prevent transmission of HCV and other yet-to-be-identified bloodborne pathogens. Contraction of HCV infection has been documented to occur via needlestick transmission [19]. The risk of transmission appears to be less than 4%, compared to up to 67% for HBeAg-positive serum [20]. Approximately 50% of those infected with HCV will go on to develop chronic liver disease with increased risk for cirrhosis and hepatocellular carcinoma [21]. See related discussions in Chap. 11.
      3. **Human immunodeficiency virus.** Health care workers are at low risk for acquiring HIV from their patients. However, studies and individual case reports have documented several cases of occupational transmission [22]. Currently, the risk from a single percutaneous exposure to HIV-infected blood is estimated to be approximately 0.3% (see Chap. 19). Projections of individual lifetime risk have been proposed based on the seroprevalence of HIV in the geographic area and the frequency with which an individual sustains accidental injuries that represent a risk for bloodborne disease transmission [23]. In a 1993 report, approximately 40 cases of occupationally acquired HIV had been reported [18]. Circumstances resulting in occupational **HIV transmission** have **involved blood or bloody fluids only** and transmission has occurred primarily through hollow-bore needlestick injury [18]. **Prolonged contact** with HIV-positive blood on nonintact skin or mucous membranes also may have transmitted the virus [22]. Several instances of HIV transmission in laboratory settings have been

Table B-1. Work restrictions for hospital workers exposed to or infected with selected infectious diseases

Disease or problem	Relieve from direct patient contact	Partial work restriction	Duration
Conjunctivitis, infectious	Yes		Until discharge ceases
Cytomegalovirus infections	No		
Diarrhea			
Acute stage (diarrhea with other symptoms)	Yes		Until symptoms resolve and infection with *Salmonella* is ruled out
Convalescent stage *Salmonella* (nontyphoidal)	No	Personnel should not care for high-risk patients	Until stool is free of the infecting organism on two consecutive cultures not less than 24 hours apart
Enteroviral infections	No	Personnel should not care for infants and newborns	Until symptoms resolve
Group A streptococcal disease	Yes		Until 24 hours after adequate treatment is started
Hepatitis, viral			
Hepatitis A	Yes		Until 7 days after onset of jaundice
Hepatitis B			
Acute	Possibly	Personnel should use barrier precautions for procedures that involve trauma to tissues or contact with mucous membranes on non-intact skin	Until antigenemia resolves
Chronic antigenemia	Possibly	HCWs who are HBeAg-positive may be restricted in certain situations	Until antigenemia resolves
Hepatitis C (parenterally transmitted non-A, non-B)	No	Personnel should use barrier precautions for procedures that involve trauma to tissues or contact with mucous membranes on non-intact skin	Period of infectivity has not been determined

Table B-1. (continued)

Disease or problem	Relieve from direct patient contact	Partial work restriction	Duration
Herpes simplex			
Genital	No		
Hands (herpetic whitlow)	Yes	(Note: It is not known whether gloves prevent transmission)	Until lesions heal
Orofacial	No	Personnel should not care for high-risk patients	Until lesions heal
Human immunodeficiency virus	Possibly	HCWs may be restricted in certain situations	
Measles			
Active	Yes		Until 7 days after the rash appears
Postexposure (susceptible personnel)	Yes		From the fifth through the twenty-first day after exposure or 7 days after the rash appears
Mumps			
Active	Yes		Until 9 days after onset of parotitis
Postexposure (susceptible personnel)	Yes		From the twelfth through the twenty-sixth day after exposure or until 9 days after onset of parotitis
Pertussis			
Active	Yes		From the beginning of the catarrhal stage through the third week after onset of paroxysms, or until 7 days after start of effective antimicrobial therapy
Postexposure (asymptomatic personnel)	No		
Postexposure (symptomatic personnel)	Yes		Same as active pertussis

	Restriction	Comments	Duration
Rubella			
Active	Yes		Until 5 days after rash appears
Postexposure (susceptible personnel)	Yes		From the seventh through the twenty-first day after exposure
Scabies	Yes		Until treated
Staphylococcus aureus (skin lesions)	Yes		Until lesions have resolved
Upper respiratory infections	No	Personnel with upper-respiratory infections should not care for high-risk patients	Until acute symptoms resolve
Varicella (chickenpox)			
Active	Yes		Until all lesions dry and crust
Postexposure (susceptible personnel)	Yes		From the tenth through the twenty-first day after exposure and, if varicella occurs, until all lesions dry and crust
Zoster (shingles)			
Active	No, if lesions localized and covered	Appropriate barrier desirable	Until lesions dry and crust, personnel should not care for high-risk patients (regardless if lesions are covered)
Postexposure (personnel susceptible to chickenpox)	Yes		From the tenth through the twenty-first day after exposure and, if varicella occurs, until all lesions dry and crust

HBeAg = hepatitis B e antigen.

Source: J.A. Polder, O.C. Tablan, and W.W. Williams. Personnel Health Services. In J.V. Bennett and P.S. Brachman (eds.), *Hospital Infections* (3rd ed.). Boston: Little, Brown, 1992. Pp. 36–37.

documented [24]. Recently, this topic has been extensively reviewed elsewhere [25].

B. **Screening employees for HBV, HCV, or HIV.** Routine preemployment or periodic screening of employees for HBV, HCV, or HIV **has been discouraged** [26]. Such testing should be linked to the provision of employee health services (i.e., screening after hepatitis B vaccine administration or as part of postexposure management). **Screening should not be used, and is prohibited in some states, to exclude or modify employment in health care settings.**

C. **Postexposure management.** Employees who have sustained percutaneous or mucous membrane or nonintact skin exposures to blood or body fluids (i.e., serous fluids) that may contain a bloodborne virus should be evaluated, counseled, and offered appropriate medical follow-up. **When possible, individuals who are the source of such exposures should be screened for HBV and HIV. Requirements for obtaining informed consent of the source patient vary from state to state.** Recommendations for testing source patients for HCV remain controversial, though most authorities would agree that testing of high-risk patients is reasonable [27]. Testing for HIV in exposed employees should be accompanied by appropriate pretest and posttest counseling; informed consent must be obtained [24].

1. Chapter 22 provides guidelines for **HBV postexposure prophylaxis,** which takes into consideration the HBV status of both the source individual and the employee.

2. Geberding and Henderson [28] recommend that HCWs exposed to HCV undergo testing for HCV antibody and liver function tests at the time of exposure. Follow-up testing should be repeated at 3 and 6 months, or sooner if the HCW becomes symptomatic [28]. Administration of serum immunoglobulin (ISG 0.06 ml/kg) to HCWs as soon as possible after parenteral exposure to a confirmed case of HCV has been suggested, but failures have been reported [27].

3. Health care workers who have been exposed to an HIV-positive source should be offered the following:

   a. Baseline HIV antibody testing to determine the employee's serostatus at the time of exposure and periodically thereafter (e.g., 6 weeks, 3 and 6 months) to rule out seroconversion.

   b. Pretest and posttest counseling is required in most states to manage postexposure anxiety and to provide risk-reduction education to prevent third-party transmission during the period when seroconversion may occur.

   c. Consideration may be given to zidovudine (ZDV; formerly azidothymidine [AZT]) postexposure prophylaxis. Although not proven effective, some clinicians believe it may be beneficial. ZDV can be offered to employees after accidental exposure to HIV-infected blood [29].

      In 1990, the CDC issued a statement about ZDV prophylaxis, indicating that there are insufficient data on which to base a recommendation for or against its use in the management of HIV exposures. However, the CDC did provide suggestions on the use of ZDV for clinicians who choose to prescribe it [30].

      In 1993, a report from the CDC described the results of an ongoing surveillance program. The CDC has been tracking persons exposed to HIV who have taken ZDV prophylaxis; eight exposed HCWs have seroconverted despite prophylaxis, whereas five other cases of ZDV prophylaxis failure have been reported in other settings [31]. However, in a recent preliminary report from the CDC, ZDV appeared to have a beneficial effect when used in this setting, but this was a retrospective study [32]. In 1996, the role of ZDV, with or without other antiretroviral agents, for postexposure prophylaxis remains an unsettled, evolving area. See related discussion in Chap. 26 (p. 1004).

      Emphasis must be placed on decreasing the risk of exposure to bloodborne pathogens via proper barrier techniques and appropriate handling of sharps as well as the implementation of needle safety devices [26].

4. For a more detailed discussion of this topic, see reference [25].

D. **Management of HCWs infected with HIV, HBV, or HCV.** This topic is reviewed in references [19, 33–35] as well as in a thoughtful editorial by Geberding [26].

1. **HIV-infected workers.** Every industry, including health care, has HIV-positive workers at all levels. A topic of some concern is whether infected HCWs pose a risk for HIV transmission to patients. Although a potential may exist in settings where invasive procedures are performed, as of March 1996, there was only one highly publicized reported case of suspected transmission [26,

36, 37]. Screening of more than 19,000 patients of HIV-infected HCWs has failed to reveal another case of HIV transmission from infected HCW to patient [38]. Currently, the CDC recommends that individual institutions establish a task force with a mandate to define exposure-prone procedures and to evaluate the competency of HIV-infected and HBeAg-positive HCWs who perform such procedures [19, 39, 40]. According to a CDC analysis, the risk of death from HIV or HBV infection acquired during an invasive procedure performed by an infected surgeon is similar to that of acquiring HIV infection from a transfused unit of screened blood [26].

2. **HBV-infected workers.** Hepatitis B has uncommonly been transmitted from an HCW to a patient, despite the fact that the CDC estimates that approximately 1900 U.S. surgeons are chronically infected with HBV [35]. An unusual outbreak of HBV was described recently in patients operated on by a surgeon who was positive for HBeAg [35]. Furthermore, HBV is known to have been transmitted during invasive procedures from 34 infected HCWs to at least 350 patients in the United States and elsewhere since the early 1970s [26].

It is suggested that HCWs who perform invasive procedures know their HBV status. However, if a worker is HBeAg-positive or epidemiologically linked to patient transmission, work practices need to be reviewed and, if modifications cannot be reasonably accommodated, work restrictions should be imposed [10, 19].

3. **HCV-infected workers.** Our current knowledge regarding transmission of HCV is limited. (See related discussions in Chap. 11.) A recent report identifies two patients who appeared to have contracted HCV from a cardiac surgeon infected with HCV [34]. Therefore, specific guidelines to reduce risk of transmission from infected HCW to patient remain unclear. Proper hand-washing, use of approved barriers, and appropriate surgical technique with regard to prevention of exposure to sharps should be emphasized [21].

III. **Education and training** of all HCWs is a vital component of the infection control and employee health program. All employees should receive initial job orientation and in-service education about disease transmission, their role and responsibility for disease prevention, the infection control aspects of employee health, and the use of employee health services [1]. Employees also should receive specific training on the use of barrier precautions and preventive practices as they relate to implementation of universal precautions. Such training has been mandated by OSHA.

IV. **OSHA regulations.** On December 6, 1991, OSHA published its standard, "Occupational Exposure to Bloodborne Pathogens" (*Federal Register* 29 CFR Part 1910.1030). By issuing this standard, OSHA indicates that HCWs face a significant health risk as a result of occupational exposure to bloodborne pathogens such as HBV and HIV.

A. **Purpose of the standard.** The purpose of this standard is to minimize or eliminate occupational risk to bloodborne diseases by the provision of engineering and work practice controls, personal protective equipment, training, vaccination, and postexposure evaluation and follow-up. This standard applies to employees in all health care facilities including hospitals, clinics, dentists' and physicians' offices, blood banks and plasma centers, long-term care homes, hospices, clinical laboratories, funeral homes, and institutions for the developmentally disabled.

B. **Components of the program**

1. **Exposure control plan.** This is a written plan that identifies employees with risk of occupational exposure. It contains a schedule and method for implementation of standard requirements and postexposure evaluation procedures. The plan should be reviewed and updated annually and be made available to all employees at risk.

2. **Methods of compliance.** The standard requires employers to implement methods and training to comply with provisions for worker protection to minimize or eliminate exposures. Areas addressed include:

   a. Administration of policies and procedures.

   b. Engineering and work practice controls.

   c. Personal protective equipment (PPE) must be provided, must be accessible, and must be utilized when indicated.

3. **Hepatitis B vaccination.** This standard requires that the hepatitis B vaccine be made available at no cost to all employees at risk of occupational exposure, within 10 days of initial job assignment, and after training on bloodborne pathogen exposure is completed. Employees declining vaccination must sign a declination form and may request vaccination at a later date.

4. **Postexposure evaluation and follow-up.** The employer must make a postexposure evaluation available immediately after the exposure incident. Requirements for HIV and HBV testing of the source individual and exposed employee, provision of postexposure prophylaxis, and counseling are included.
5. **Training program.** The OSHA standard requires that all employees at risk for occupational exposure attend a training program at the time of initial employment and annually thereafter. The components of the training program include an explanation of the epidemiology and transmission of bloodborne diseases, an explanation of methods to eliminate or minimize exposures (e.g., hand-washing, use of PPE), and postexposure follow-up, as well as labeling and record-keeping requirements.
6. **Record keeping.** Records of postexposure evaluations and hepatitis B vaccination must be kept for the length of employment plus 30 years.

References

1. Polder, J.A., Tablan, O.C., and Williams, W.W. Personnel Health Services. In J.V. Bennett and P.S. Brachman (eds.), *Hospital Infections* (3rd ed.). Boston: Little, Brown, 1992. Pp. 31–62.
2. Sherertz, R.J., Marosok, R.D., and Streed, S.A. Infection Control Aspects of Hospital Employee Health. In R.P. Wenzel (ed.), *Prevention and Control of Nosocomial Infections*. Baltimore: Williams & Wilkins, 1993. Pp. 295–332.
3. Rosenstock, L., and Cullen, M.R. *Textbook of Clinical Occupational and Environmental Medicine*. Philadelphia: Saunders, 1994.
4. Centers for Disease Control. *Guidelines for Protecting the Safety and Health of Health Care Workers*. Atlanta, GA: National Institute for Occupational Safety and Health (publication No. 88-119), 1988.
5. Mayhall, C.G. (ed.). *Hospital Epidemiology and Infection Control*. Baltimore: Williams & Wilkins, 1996.
    Contains an excellent series of chapters under the heading of "epidemiology and prevention of nosocomial infections in healthcare workers" (e.g., viral hepatitis, HIV, tuberculosis, etc.).
6. Williams, W.W., et al. Vaccines of importance in the hospital setting: Problems and developments. *Infect. Dis. Clin. North Am.* 3(4):701–719, 1989.
    See related discussion in reference [11].
7. McGowan, J.E., Jr. The booster effect—A problem for surveillance of tuberculosis in hospital employees. *Am. J. Infect. Control* 11:57, 1983.
    See discussion of this topic in Chap. 9 and reference [8].
8. Centers for Disease Control. *Core Curriculum on Tuberculosis: What the Clinician Should Know* (3rd ed.). 1994.
    This is an extremely useful monograph. It can be ordered by calling the CDC Voice Information Center (404-639-1819) or by faxing the CDC Fax Information Center (404-332-4565).
    Also see related discussions in Chap. 9 under Tuberculosis.
9. Centers for Disease Control. Essential components of a tuberculosis prevention and control program. *M.M.W.R.* 44(RR-11):1–34, 1995.
9a. Sepkowitz, K.A. AIDS, tuberculosis, and the health care worker. *Clin. Infect. Dis.* 20:232, 1995.
    Detailed discussion of TB as an occupational risk and review of guidelines to prevent transmission of TB in health care facilities.
10. Williams, W.W. CDC guidelines for infection control in hospital personnel. *Infect. Control* 4(Suppl.):326, 1983.
11. Fedson, D.S. Immunization for Health Care Workers and Patients in Hospitals. In R.P. Wenzel (ed.), *Prevention and Control of Nosocomial Infections* (2nd ed.). Baltimore: Williams & Wilkins, 1993. P. 214.
12. Centers for Disease Control. Protection against viral hepatitis. *M.M.W.R.* 39:(RR-2):1, 1990.
13. Centers for Disease Control. Hepatitis B virus: A comprehensive strategy for eliminating transmission in the United States through universal childhood vaccination. Recommendations of ACIP. *M.M.W.R.* 40(RR-13):1–25, 1991.
14. Kim, M., Lapointe, J., and Liu, F. Epidemiology of measles immunity in a population of healthcare workers. *Infect. Control Hosp. Epidemiol.* 13(7):399–402, 1992.

15. Houck, P., Scott-Johnson, G., and Krebs, L. Measles immunity among community hospital employees. *Infect. Control Hosp. Epidemiol.* 12(11):663–668, 1991.
16. Krause, P.J., et al. Quality standard for assurance of measles immunity among health care workers. *Clin. Infect. Dis.* 18:431–436, 1994.
17. Centers for Disease Control. Measles prevention: Recommendations of the Immunization Practices Advisory Committee (ACIP). *M.M.W.R.* 38(S-9):1–18, 1989.
18. Fry, D.E. Occupational risks of infection in the surgical management of trauma patients. *Am. J. Surg.* 165(Suppl. 2A):26S–33S, 1993.
    See related paper by M.E. Chamberhand et al., Human immunodeficiency infection among health care workers who donate blood. Ann. Intern. Med. 121:269, 1994, in which HIV infection due to occupational exposure was uncommon.
19. Doebbeling, B.N., and Wenzel, R.P. Nosocomial Viral Hepatitis and Infections Transmitted by Blood and Blood Products. In G.L. Mandell, J.E. Bennett, and R. Dolin (eds.), *Principles and Practice of Infectious Diseases* (4th ed.). New York: Churchill Livingstone, 1995. P. 2618.
20. Kiyosawa, K., et al. Hepatitis C in hospital employees with needlestick injuries. *Ann. Intern. Med.* 115:367–369, 1991.
21. Davis, J.M., et al. The Surgical Infection Society's policy of human immunodeficiency virus and hepatitis B and C infection. *Arch. Surg.* 127:218–221, 1992.
22. Centers for Disease Control. Update: Acquired immune deficiency syndrome and HIV infection in health-care workers. *M.M.W.R.* 37:229, 1989.
23. Centers for Disease Control. Guidelines for prevention and transmission of human immunodeficiency virus and hepatitis B virus to health care and public safety workers. *M.M.W.R.* 38(S-6):1–37, 1989.
24. Centers for Disease Control. 1988 Agent summary statement for HIV and report on laboratory-acquired infection with HIV. *M.M.W.R.* 37(S-4):1–17, 1988.
25. Beekman, S.E., and Henderson, D.K. Nosocomial Human Immunodeficiency Virus Infection in Health Care Workers. In C.G. Mayhall (ed.), *Hospital Epidemiology and Infection Control.* Baltimore: Williams & Wilkins, 1996. Chap. 63.
26. Geberding, J.L. The infected health care provider. *N. Engl. J. Med.* 334:594, 1996.
    Thoughtful editorial comment on bloodborne pathogens (HBV, HCV, and HIV); discussed in references [34, 35]. Routine screening of HCW is not the solution; better preventive methods need to be developed and implemented.
27. Lettau, L.A. The A, B, C, D, and E of viral hepatitis: Spelling out the risks for healthcare workers. *Infect. Control Hosp. Epidemiol.* 13(2):77–81, 1992.
28. Geberding, J.L., and Henderson, D.K. Management of occupational exposures to bloodborne pathogens: Hepatitis B virus, hepatitis C virus, and human immunodeficiency virus. *Clin. Infect. Dis.* 14:1179–1185, 1992.
29. Henderson, D.K., and Geberding, J.L. Prophylactic zidovudine after occupational exposure to the human immunodeficiency virus and interim analysis. *J. Infect. Dis.* 160:321, 1989.
30. Centers for Disease Control. Public Health Service statement on management of occupational exposure to human immunodeficiency virus, including considerations regarding zidovudine postexposure use. *M.M.W.R.* 39:RR-1, 1990.
31. Tokars, J.I., et al. Surveillance of HIV infection and zidovudine use among health care workers after occupational exposure to HIV infected blood. *Ann. Intern. Med.* 118(12):913–919, 1993.
32. Centers for Disease Control. CDC study: AZT reduces HIV risk from needle-sticks. *Am. Med. News* 39:40, 1996.
33. Henderson, D.K. Human Immunodeficiency Virus in Patients and Providers. In R.P. Wenzel (ed.), *Prevention and Control of Nosocomial Infections.* Baltimore: Williams & Wilkins, 1993. Pp. 42–57.
    See related review by D.K. Henderson, HIV-1 in the Health Care Setting. In G.L. Mandell, J.E. Bennett, and R. Dolin (eds.), Principles and Practice of Infectious Diseases (4th ed.). New York: Churchill Livingstone, 1995.
34. Esteban, J.I., et al. Transmission of hepatitis C virus by a cardiac surgeon. *N. Engl. J. Med.* 334:555, 1996.
    Study provides evidence that a cardiac surgeon with chronic HCV may have transmitted HCV to five patients during open-heart surgery. See thoughtful editorial comment in reference [26].
35. Harpaz, R., et al. Transmission of hepatitis B virus to multiple patients from a surgeon without evidence of inadequate infection control. *N. Engl. J. Med.* 334:549, 1996.
    A thoracic surgeon-to-patient HBV outbreak occurred despite apparent compliance with infection-control measures. See thoughtful editorial comment in reference [26].

36. Centers for Disease Control. Possible transmission of human immunodeficiency virus to a patient during an invasive dental procedure. *M.M.W.R.* 39:489, 1990.
See also CDC Update: Transmission of HIV infection during invasive dental procedures — Florida. M.M.W.R. *40:377, 1991.*
37. Ciesielski, C., et al. Transmission of human immunodeficiency virus in a dental practice. *Ann. Intern. Med.* 116:798–805, 1992.
38. Mishu, B., and Schaffner, W. HIV-infected surgeons and dentists. Looking back and looking forward. *J.A.M.A.* 269(14):1843–1844, 1993.
39. Centers for Disease Control. Recommendations for prevention of HIV transmission in health-care settings. *M.M.W.R.* 36(Suppl. 2S):1S–19S, 1987.
40. Centers for Disease Control. Recommendations for preventing transmission of human immunodeficiency virus and hepatitis B virus to patients during exposure-prone procedures. *M.M.W.R.* 40:1–9, 1991.

Index

Index